■ Vital Signs

BLOOD PRESSURE

Blood Pressures for Girls and Boys, Ages 1-17 Years*, for 95th Percentile in Height†

Age	Height Percentile	GIRLS: Systolic 5%	50%	95%	GIRLS: Diastolic 5%	50%	95%	BOYS: Systolic 5%	50%	95%	BOYS: Diastolic 5%	50%	95%
1	95th	100	104	107	56	58	60	98	103	106	54	56	58
2	95th	102	105	109	61	63	65	101	106	110	59	61	63
3	95th	104	107	110	65	67	69	104	109	113	63	65	67
4	95th	105	108	112	68	70	72	106	111	115	66	69	71
5	95th	107	110	113	70	72	74	108	112	116	69	72	74
6	95th	108	111	115	72	74	76	109	114	117	72	74	76
7	95th	110	113	116	73	75	77	110	115	119	74	76	78
8	95th	112	115	118	75	76	78	111	116	120	75	78	80
9	95th	114	117	120	76	77	79	113	118	121	76	79	81
10	95th	116	119	122	77	78	80	115	119	123	77	80	82
11	95th	118	121	124	78	79	81	117	121	125	78	80	82
12	95th	119	123	126	79	80	82	119	123	127	78	81	83
13	95th	121	124	128	80	81	83	121	126	130	79	81	83
14	95th	123	126	129	81	82	84	124	128	132	80	82	84
15	95th	124	127	131	82	83	85	126	131	135	81	83	85
16	95th	125	128	132	82	84	86	129	134	137	82	84	87
17	95th	125	129	132	82	84	86	131	136	140	84	87	89

*Blood pressure percentile determined by a single measurement.
†Height percentile determined by standard growth curves.
Complete tables found in Chapter 30 of this text.
From National High Blood Pressure Education Program Working Group on High Blood Pressure in Children and Adolescents: The Fourth Report on the Diagnosis, Evaluation, and Treatment of High Blood Pressure in Children and Adolescents, *Pediatrics*, 114(2):555-576, 2004. Available at www.nhlbi.gov or www.pediatrics.aappublications.org/cgi/reprint/114/2/S2/555. Accessed December 17, 2010.

RESPIRATIONS

Normal Respiratory Rates In Children

Age (years)	Respiratory Rate (breaths/minute)
0-1	24-38
1-3	22-30
4-6	20-24
7-9	18-24
10-14	16-22
15-18	14-20

Slightly higher respiratory rates in the neonatal period (i.e., 40-50 breaths/min) may be normal in the absence of other signs and symptoms.

PULSE

Normal Heart Rates (Beats per Minute) in Infants and Children

Age	Resting (Awake)	Resting (Asleep)	Exercise/Fever
Newborn	100-180	80-160	Up to 220
1 week-3 months	100-220	80-200	Up to 220
3 months-2 years	80-150	70-120	Up to 220
2-10 years	70-100	60-90	195-215
10-20 years	55-90	50-90	195-215

■ Nutrition

CALORIC NEEDS OF INFANTS AND TODDLERS

Daily Estimated Energy Requirements (EER) for Infants and Toddlers in Kilocalories

Age	Calculation of Daily Kilocalorie Needs	Estimate Based on 50th Percentile of Weight
0-3 months	EER = (89 × weight of infant [kg] − 100) + 175 (kcal for energy deposition)	100 kilocalories/kg/day
4-6 months	EER = (89 × weight of infant [kg] − 100) + 56 (kcal for energy deposition)	85 kilocalories/kg/day
7-12 months	EER = (89 × weight of infant [kg] − 100) + 22 (kcal for energy deposition)	80 kilocalories/kg/day
13-35 months	EER = (89 × weight of child [kg] − 100) + 20 (kcal for energy deposition)	83 kilocalories/kg/day

From Robertson J, Shilkofski N: *The Harriet Lane handbook: a manual for pediatric house officers*, ed 17, Philadelphia, 2005, Mosby.

Estimated Calorie Needs per Day by Age, Gender, and Physical Activity Level: Children Ages 2-18 Years*

Gender	Age in years	Sedentary	Moderately Active	Active
Males	2-3	1000-1200†	1000-1400†	1000-1400†
	4-8	1200-1400	1400-1600	1600-2000
	9-13	1600-2000	1800-2200	2000-2600
	14-18	2000-2400	2400-2800	2800-3200
Females	2-3	1000	1000-1200	1000-1400
	4-8	1200-1400	1400-1600	1400-1800
	9-13	1400-1600	1600-2000	1800-2200
	14-18	1800	2000	2400

*Estimated calories needed to maintain calorie balance for various gender and age groups at three different levels of physical activity. The estimates are rounded to the nearest 200 calories. An individual's calorie needs may be higher or lower than these average estimates.

†The calorie ranges shown are to accommodate needs of different ages within the group. For children and adolescents, more calories are needed at older ages. From U.S. Department of Agriculture (USDA) and U.S. Department of Health and Human Services (HHS): *Dietary guidelines for Americans, 2010*, ed 7, Washington, DC, 2010, U.S. Government Printing Office.

Fluid Replacement Calculations for Dehydration

Mild	ORS	40-50 mL/kg over 4 hours
Moderate	ORS	60-100 mL/kg over 4-6 hours
Severe	IV fluids	See Chapter 32 for protocol

ORS, Oral rehydration solution.

Number of Servings and Serving Sizes for Age and Calorie Intake

Food Groups	1-3 YEARS OLD* Servings	4-6 YEARS OLD* 1200	1600	2000	6-21 YEARS OLD 2600	3100	Serving Size: 1600-3100 Calorie Diets
Grains	6: ¼-½ slice bread; 4 tbsp cooked cereal, rice, pasta; ¼ cup dry cereal; 1 or 2 crackers	4-5	6	6-8	10-11	12-13	1 slice bread; 1 cup of ready to eat cereal; ½ cup rice, pasta, or cereal
Vegetables	2-3: 1 tbsp/year age cooked vegetable	3-4	3-4	4-5	5-6	6	1 cup raw leafy, ½ cup cooked or raw other vegetables; ½ cup vegetable juice
Fruits	2-3: ½ piece fresh fruit, ¼ cup fruit canned/cooked, ¼-½ cup juice	3-4	4	4-5	5-6	6	1 medium fruit; ¼ cup dried fruit; ½ cup fresh, frozen, canned fruit; ½ cup fruit juice
Fat-free or low-fat milk and milk products	2: 1-2 year olds should have whole milk, 500 mg calcium/day	2-3: 800 mg calcium/d	2-3: 1200-1500 mg calcium/d 9-18 years of age	2-3	3	3-4	1 cup milk, 1 cup yogurt, 1½ oz cheese
Lean meats, poultry, fish, eggs	2	3 or less	3-4 or less	6 or less	6 or less	6-9	1 oz cooked meats, poultry, fish; 1 egg
Nuts, seeds, legumes	2: (a) 2 tbsp cooked beans or peas; (b) only creamy peanut butter spread thinly on a cracker/bread; (c) omit seeds and nuts	3/week	3-4/week	4/week	1	1	⅓ cup or 1½ oz nuts, 2 tbsp peanut butter, 2 tbsp or ½ oz seeds, ½ cup cooked legumes (dried beans or peas)
Fat, oils	Moderate use until 2 years of age (about 30% of total calories)	1	2	2-3	3	4	1 tsp soft margarine; 1 tsp vegetable oil; 1 tbsp mayonnaise; 1 tbsp salad dressing
Sweets and added sugars		3 or less per week	3 or less/ week	5 or less/ week	Less than 2	Less than 2	1 tbsp sugar; 1 tbsp jelly or jam; ½ cup sorbet, gelatin dessert; 1 cup lemonade
Adequate sodium intake	1,000 mg/day	1,200 mg/ day	1,500 mg/ day	1,500 mg/ day	1,500 mg/ day	1,500 mg/ day	
Maximum sodium limit		2,300 mg/ day	2,300 mg/ day	2,300 mg/ day	2,300 mg/ day	2,300 mg/ day	

*Because of the inconsistency in recommendations for calorie intake in young children among expert sources, the table focuses on the areas of agreement in terms of serving sizes and number of servings.

Data from American Academy of Pediatrics: *Pediatric nutrition handbook*, ed 5, Elk Grove Village, IL, 2004, American Academy of Pediatrics; Dietz WH, Stern L, editors: *Guide to your child's nutrition*, New York, 1999, Villard; U.S. Department of Health and Human Services and US Department of Agriculture: *Dietary guidelines for Americans, 2010*, ed 7, Washington, DC, 2010, U.S. Government Printing Office.

Pediatric
Primary Care

Pediatric Primary Care

Fifth Edition

Catherine E. Burns, PhD, RN, CPNP-PC, FAAN
Professor Emeritus
Primary Health Care Nurse Practitioner Specialty
School of Nursing
Oregon Health & Science University
Portland, Oregon

Ardys M. Dunn, PhD, RN, PNP
Associate Professor Emeritus
University of Portland School of Nursing
Portland, Oregon;
Professor, Retired
School of Nursing
Samuel Merritt College
Oakland, California

Margaret A. Brady, PhD, RN, CPNP-PC
Professor
School of Nursing
California State University Long Beach
Long Beach, California;
Co-Director, PNP Program
School of Nursing
Azusa Pacific University
Azusa, California

Nancy Barber Starr, MS, APRN, BC (PNP), CPNP-PC
Pediatric Nurse Practitioner
Advanced Pediatric Associates
Aurora, Colorado

Catherine G. Blosser, MPA:HA, RN, APRN, BC (PNP)
Pediatric Nurse Practitioner
Albertina Kerr Health Services
Portland, Oregon

Associate Editor

Dawn Lee Garzon, PhD, PNP-BC, CPNP-PC, PMHS, FAANP
Teaching Professor
College of Nursing
University of Missouri–St. Louis
St. Louis, Missouri

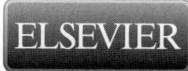

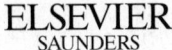
ELSEVIER
SAUNDERS

1600 John F. Kennedy Blvd.
Ste 1800
Philadelphia, PA 19103-2899

Pediatric Primary Care, ed 5   ISBN: 978-0-323-08024-8
Copyright © 2013 by Saunders, an imprint of Elsevier Inc.

Notice

Knowledge and best practice in this field are constantly changing. As new research and experience broaden our understanding, changes in research methods, professional practices, or medical treatment may become necessary.

Practitioners and researchers must always rely on their own experience and knowledge in evaluating and using any information, methods, compounds, or experiments described herein. In using such information or methods they should be mindful of their own safety and the safety of others, including parties for whom they have a professional responsibility.

With respect to any drug or pharmaceutical products identified, readers are advised to check the most current information provided (i) on procedures featured or (ii) by the manufacturer of each product to be administered, to verify the recommended dose or formula, the method and duration of administration, and contraindications. It is the responsibility of practitioners, relying on their own experience and knowledge of their patients, to make diagnoses, to determine dosages and the best treatment for each individual patient, and to take all appropriate safety precautions.

To the fullest extent of the law, neither the Publisher nor the authors, contributors, or editors, assume any liability for any injury and/or damage to persons or property as a matter of products liability, negligence or otherwise, or from any use or operation of any methods, products, instructions, or ideas contained in the material herein.

Previous editions copyrighted 2009, 2004, 2000, 1996

Library of Congress Cataloging-in-Publication Data

Pediatric primary care / Catherine E. Burns ... [et al.]. — 5th ed.
    p. ; cm.
    Includes bibliographical references and index.
    ISBN 978-0-323-08024-8 (hardcover : alk. paper)
    I. Burns, Catherine E.
    [DNLM: 1. Pediatrics—United States. 2. Primary Health Care—United States. WS 100]
    618.92—dc23

                                                                 2011052232

Executive Content Specialist: Lee Henderson
Content Development Specialist: Jacqueline Twomey
Publishing Services Manager: Jeff Patterson
Design Direction: Amy Buxton

Printed in the United States of America

Last digit is the print number: 9 8 7 6 5

Contributors

Denise C. Abdoo, RN, MSN, CPNP-AC/PC
Senior Instructor of Pediatrics, Nurse Practitioner
Kempe Child Protection Team & Pediatric Emergency
    Medicine
University of Colorado Denver, School of Medicine
Denver, Colorado
Role Relationships

Michele E. Acker, MN, ARNP
Pediatric Nurse Practitioner
Department of Anesthesiology
Seattle Children's Hospital;
Senior Lecturer
University of Washington, School of Nursing
Seattle, Washington
Dental and Oral Disorders

Anne C. Albers, MSN, RN, CPNP
Nurse Practitioner, Department of Pediatric Neurology
Washington University School of Medicine
St. Louis, Missouri
Neurologic Disorders

Nancy Barber Starr, MS, APRN, BC (PNP), CPNP-PC
Pediatric Nurse Practitioner
Advanced Pediatric Associates
Aurora, Colorado
*Cognitive-Perceptual Disorders: Attention-Deficit/Hyper-
    activity Disorder, Learning Problems, Sensory Process-
    ing Disorder, Autism Spectrum Disorder, Blindness, and
    Deafness*
Self-Perception Issues
Gynecologic Disorders
Dermatologic Disorders

Jan Bazner-Chandler, RN, MSN, CNS, CPNP
Assistant Professor, Nurse Practitioner
Azusa Pacific University
Azusa, California
Musculoskeletal Disorders

Shirley Becton McKenzie, MS, APRN, PNP-BC, AE-C
Pediatric Nurse Practitioner
Emergency Department
The Children's Hospital
Denver, Colorado;
Colorado Kids Pediatrics
Centennial, Colorado
Ear Disorders

Roberta Bentson Royal, RN, MSN, CPNP, CSPI
Oregon Poison Center
Oregon Health & Science University
Portland, Oregon
Infectious Diseases and Immunizations

Anita D. Berry, MSN, CNP, APN
Director, Healthy Steps for Young Children Program
Pediatric Integration
Advocate Health Care
Oak Brook, Illinois
Developmental Management in Pediatric Primary Care
Developmental Management of Infants
Developmental Management of Toddlers and Preschoolers

Catherine G. Blosser, MPA:HA, RN, APRN, BC (PNP)
Pediatric Nurse Practitioner
Albertina Kerr Health Services
Portland, Oregon
Physical Activity and Sports for Children and Adolescents
Sexuality
Infectious Diseases and Immunizations
Neurologic Disorders
Eye Disorders
Cardiovascular Disorders
Gastrointestinal Disorders
Complementary Medicine
Prescribing Medications in Pediatrics

Cris Ann Bowman-Harvey, RN, MSN, CPNP
Faculty, Emergency
University of Colorado
CPNP, Emergency
Children's Hospital Colorado
CPNP, Pediatrics
Advanced Pediatric Associates
Aurora, Colorado
*Cognitive-Perceptual Disorders: Attention-Deficit/Hyper-
    activity Disorder, Learning Problems, Sensory Process-
    ing Disorder, Autism Spectrum Disorder, Blindness, and
    Deafness*

Margaret A. Brady, PhD, RN, CPNP-PC
Professor
School of Nursing
California State University Long Beach
Long Beach, California
Co-Director, PNP Program
School of Nursing
Azusa Pacific University
Azusa, California
Role Relationships
Introduction to Disease Management
Pediatric Pain Management
Infectious Diseases and Immunizations
Atopic and Rheumatic Disorders
Respiratory Disorders
Gastrointestinal Disorders
Dermatologic Disorders
Musculoskeletal Disorders

Constance B. Brehm, PhD, MS, MPh, RNP, RN
Professor of Nursing
Azusa Pacific University
Azusa, California
Common Injuries

Catherine E. Burns, PhD, RN, CPNP-PC, FAAN
Professor Emeritus
Primary Health Care Nurse Practitioner Specialty
School of Nursing
Oregon Health & Science University
Portland, Oregon
Child and Family Health Assessment
Introduction to Functional Health Patterns and Health
*   Promotion*
Sleep and Rest
Cognitive-Perceptual Disorders: Attention-Deficit/Hyper-
*   activity Disorder, Learning Problems, Sensory Process-*
*   ing Disorder, Autism Spectrum Disorder, Blindness, and*
*   Deafness*
Gastrointestinal Disorders
Genetic Disorders
Environmental Health Issues
Growth Charts
Pediatric Laboratory Values

Donald L. Chi, DDS, PhD
Acting Assistant Professor of Dental/Public Health
   Sciences
University of Washington
Seattle, Washington
Dental and Oral Disorders

Sara D. DeGolier, RN, MS, CPNP
Pediatric Nurse Practitioner, Emergency Department
The Children's Hospital
Aurora, Colorado
Self-Perception Issues
Common Injuries

Joy S. Diamond, MS, RN, CPNP
Pediatric Nurse Practitioner
Advanced Pediatric Associates
Centennial, Colorado
Role Relationships

Mary Ann Draye, MPH, ARNP
Assistant Professor, Director of Family Nurse Practitioner
   Program
School of Nursing
University of Washington
Seattle, Washignton
Dental and Oral Disorders

Karen G. Duderstadt, PhD, RN, CPNP, PCNS
Clinical Professor, Department of Family Health Care
   Nursing
University of California San Francisco
Pediatric Nurse Practitioner, Children's Health Center
San Francisco General Hospital
San Francisco, California
Health Status of Children: Global and Local Perspectives

Ardys M. Dunn, PhD, RN, PNP
Associate Professor Emeritus
University of Portland School of Nursing
Portland, Oregon;
Professor, Retired
School of Nursing
Samuel Merritt College
Oakland, California
Cultural Perspectives for Pediatric Primary Care
Developmental Management of Adolescents
Introduction to Functional Health Patterns and Health
*   Promotion*
Nutrition
Elimination Patterns
Role Relationships
Sexuality
Values and Beliefs
Gastrointestinal Disorders
Environmental Health Issues

Maxine Fookson, RN, MN, PNP
Pediatric Nurse Practitioner, School Based Health Program
Multnomah County Health Department
Portland, Oregon
Physical Activity and Sports for Children and Adolescents
Cognitive-Perceptual Disorders: Attention-Deficit/Hyper-
*   activity Disorder, Learning Problems, Sensory Process-*
*   ing Disorder, Autism Spectrum Disorder, Blindness, and*
*   Deafness*

Lynne A. Frost, DNP, RN, CPNP-PC
Nurse Practitioner
University of Portland
Portland, Oregon
Sleep and Rest

Bonnie Gance-Cleveland, PhD, RNC, PNP, FAAN
Associate Professor, Nurse Practitioner
Arizona State University
Phoenix, Arizona
Developmental Management of School-Age Children

Dawn Lee Garzon, PhD, PNP-BC, CPNP-PC, PMHS, FAANP
Teaching Professor
College of Nursing
University of Missouri–St. Louis
St. Louis, Missouri
Developmental Management in Pediatric Primary Care
Developmental Management of Adolescents
Coping and Stress Tolerance: Mental Health and Illness
Common Injuries

Nan M. Gaylord, PhD, RN, CPNP
Associate Professor
College of Nursing
University of Tennessee
Knoxville, Tennessee
Genitourinary Disorders
Perinatal Disorders

Teral Gerlt, MS, RN, WHCNP-E
Instructor
Oregon Health & Science University
School of Nursing
Portland, Oregon
Sexuality
Gynecologic Disorders

Steven Goodstein, MS, MT (ASCP)
Assistant Professor
Department of Pathology
Oregon Health & Science University
Portland, Oregon
Pediatric Laboratory Values

Denise A. Hall, BS, CMPE
Administrator
Advanced Pediatric Associates
Centennial, Colorado
Strategies for Managing a Health Care Practice

Pamela J. Hellings, RN, PhD, CPNP-R
Professor Emeritus
Oregon Health & Science University
Portland, Oregon
Breastfeeding

Rita Marie John, DNP, EdD, CPNP
Associate Professor of Clinical Nursing
School of Nursing
Columbia University
New York, New York
Introduction to Disease Management
Atopic and Rheumatic Disorders
Respiratory Disorders

Barbara Jones Deloian, PhD, RN, CPNP
Pediatric Nurse Practitioner
Director, Health Services for Children with Special Needs
Colorado Department of Public Health and Environment
Denver, Colorado
Developmental Management in Pediatric Primary Care
Developmental Management of Infants

Veronica Kane, PhD, RN, MSN, CPNP
Clinical Assistant Professor, Coordinator - Pediatric Nursing
    Specialty
MGH Institute of Health Professions, School of Nursing
Boston, Massachusetts;
Pediatric Nurse Practitioner, Pediatrics, Urgent Care
Harvard Vanguard Medical Associates
Braintree, Massachusetts
Hematologic Disorders

Julie Martchenke, RN, MSN, CPNP
Pediatric Cardiology Nurse Practitioner
Oregon Health & Science University
Portland, Oregon
Cardiovascular Disorders

Peter M. Milgrom, DDS
Professor of Dental Public Health Sciences
Director of Northwest Center to Reduce Oral Health
    Disparities
University of Washington
Seattle, Washington
Dental and Oral Disorders

Teri Moser Woo, PhD, RN, CPNP
Associate Professor
School of Nursing, University of Portland;
Pediatric Nurse Practitioner, Ambulatory Pediatrics
Kaiser Permanente
Portland, Oregon
Eye Disorders

Mary A. Murphy, CPNP, PhD
Developmental Consultant
The Children's Hospital
University of Colorado at Denver and Health Sciences Center
Denver, Colorado
Developmental Management of Toddlers and Preschoolers

Jennifer Newcombe, RN, MSN, CNS, CPNP
Nurse Practitioner, Pediatric Cardiothoracic Surgery
Loma Linda Children's Hospital
Loma Linda, California
Pediatric Pain Management

Ann M. Petersen-Smith, PhD, RN, CPNP-AC
Assistant Professor, PNP Option Coordinator
Division of Women, Children, and Family Health
College of Nursing
University of Colorado Denver
Aurora, Colorado
Ear Disorders
Gastrointestinal Disorders
Genitourinary Disorders
Dermatologic Disorders

Melissa Reider-Demer, MSN, CPNP
Neurology Pediatric Nurse Practitioner
Children's Hospital of Los Angeles
Los Angeles, California
Neurologic Disorders

Arlene Smaldone, DNSc, CPNP, CDE
Assistant Professor of Nursing
School of Nursing
Columbia University
New York, New York
Endocrine and Metabolic Disorders

Robert D. Steiner, MD
Credit Unions for Kids Professor of Pediatric Research
Oregon Health & Science University
Portland, Oregon
Endocrine and Metabolic Disorders

Martha K. Swartz, PhD, RN, CPNP
Professor and Associate Dean
Office of Clinical and Community Affairs
School of Nursing
Yale University
New Haven, Connecticut
Hematologic Disorders

Ohnmar K. Tut, BDS, MPhil
Affiliate Faculty, Dental Public Health Sciences
School of Dentistry
University of Washington
Seattle, Washington;
Honorary Lecturer, Periodontology Department
Otago Unviersity, Otago Dental School
Dunedin, New Zealand
Dental and Oral Disorders

Peggy Vernon, RN, MA, C-PNP
Nurse Practitioner
Highlands Ranch, Colorado
Dermatologic Disorders

Becky J. Whittemore, MN, MPH, FNP
Nurse Practitioner
Child Development and Rehabilitation Center
Oregon Health & Science University
Portland, Oregon
Endocrine and Metabolic Disorders

Robert J. Yetman, MD
Professor of Pediatrics
Director, Division of Community and General Pediatrics
The University of Texas Medical School at Houston
Houston, Texas
Perinatal Disorders

Yvonne Yousey, RN, CPNP-PC, PhD
Associate Professor of Nursing
School of Nursing
University of Northern Colorado
Greeley, Colorado
Developmental Management of School-Age Children

We are delighted to introduce the fifth edition of *Pediatric Primary Care*. This book was first developed as a resource for advanced practice nurses serving the primary health care needs of infants, children, and adolescents. Pediatric nurse practitioners (PNPs) and family nurse practitioners (FNPs) were, and still are, our primary audience. However, our audience has grown so that physician assistants, pediatricians, family physicians, pediatric clinical nurse specialists, community health nurses, pediatric ambulatory care nurses, school nurses, and other primary care providers also find the book to be a valuable resource. The field of pediatric primary care has also grown and changed since the first edition of this book. Evidence-based practice is now acknowledged as essential and is the foundation for this book. The interdisciplinary Institute of Medicine (IOM) has now explicitly recognized the critical role of nurse practitioners and nurses in providing health care to the population in the United States (IOM Report, 2010).

Our goal has been to provide a textbook for health care students, as well as a resource for clinicians. Feedback from our readers over the past several years indicates that we have achieved that goal: both students and experienced clinicians find *Pediatric Primary Care* to be a key resource for their work and study. The first edition won an award from *Nurse Practitioner* journal, and the third edition received an *American Journal of Nursing* Book-of-the-Year Award for primary care—indicators of the quality of our work.

Each of the editors brings a special perspective to the subject of pediatric primary health care: nurse practitioner educators, practicing PNPs, and a PNP with years of experience working in and teaching community health. Each editor has unique areas of expertise—development, nursing theory, cultural competence, and extensive experience with a variety of health care problems. Additionally, we have drawn on contributors from a variety of specialties to address specific content of the book. For this edition, we have added an Associate Editor who has experience in psychosocial and mental health and is a nurse practitioner educator.

Organization of the Book

We recognize that children are a special population and that providing health care to them must be approached using four unique perspectives: their developmental changes over time, their dependency on their parents, the differential epidemiology of child health, and the different demographic patterns of children and their families (Rothman et al, 2009). These themes are carried throughout the text.

After three introductory chapters that discuss child health issues and assessment of children in the context of their families and cultures, the book is organized into three major sections—Management of Development, Approaches to Health Management in Pediatric Primary Care, and Approaches to Disease Management. Some features of the fifth edition about which we are particularly excited include the following:

- Introduction of health literacy as an important variable in primary care
- Discussion of the most current model for primary care relationships: the provider-child-family triad, with family-centered collaborative negotiations taking the place of top-down provider-to-family-and-child care
- Discussion of the concept of motivational interviewing in provider-client interaction
- Additional color photos of some important ear, skin, and dental pathologies to help with diagnosis
- A chapter devoted to pain management
- An updated chapter on genetics that discusses the new paradigm for genetic practice, including an introduction to epigenetics
- Discussion of health care for immigrants and refugees
- Expanded discussion of the management of childhood obesity
- In-depth discussion of management of mental health problems in primary care
- More in-depth discussion of cognition and emerging developmental neuroscience
- Updated tables to facilitate differential diagnoses of related conditions or conditions that have some common elements
- Updated tables to summarize management strategies for common conditions

Every chapter has been updated to bring the most current information available to the reader. We have maintained key features that have made previous editions so successful:

- An assessment chapter that emphasizes a holistic approach, including identification of development, disease, and functional health problems within the context of the family
- Attention to cultural factors
- Emphasis on prevention and management of problems from the primary care provider's point of view and scope of practice
- Explicit reference to *Healthy People* guidelines (U.S. Department of Health and Human Services, 2010), *Bright Futures* (Hagan et al, 2008), practice guidelines from the U.S. Preventive Services Task Force, the American Academy of Pediatrics, and others
- A chapter on practice management
- Introduction of key concepts and foundations for care in a narrative format followed by a discussion of the identification and management of diagnoses using an outline format
- Organization of information into tables and appendices for quick access and efficient use by clinicians
- Emphasis on best practice guidelines for well child care, development, and acute and chronic illness

- Additional resources for each chapter, located in Appendix D, include websites to access organizations and printed materials that may be useful for clinicians and their clients
- Discussion Questions for each chapter, located in Appendix E, written by nurse practitioner educators to assist students to think about the implications for practice of the material they have just read

PEDIATRIC PRIMARY CARE FOUNDATIONS SECTION

Chapter 1 begins with a review of the major morbidity and mortality statistics highlighting the health problems of children in the United States and worldwide. The chapter then identifies the important goals for health care of children and describes several sets of current guidelines and standards designed to safeguard primary care of children. Working with managed care organizations is discussed. Chapter 2 presents health assessment of the child and family, including both history and physical examination data. The chapter uses a model that supports identification and management of development, functional health patterns, and disease problems. Chapter 3 highlights important cultural components of care to be incorporated into the assessment and management plans for all clients.

MANAGEMENT OF DEVELOPMENT SECTION

The development section includes five chapters—an introduction to development for primary care and chapters on infants, toddlers and preschoolers, school-age children, and adolescents. Each chapter begins with a review of the major developmental theories used to understand children in a particular age group. The assessment of developmental needs of children in primary care is then reviewed. Topics for discussion with parents are outlined, including parenting and discipline. Several important developmental issues for each age group are discussed from a problem-oriented perspective. Application of principles of child development to primary care is the key feature for these chapters. Red flags are described to alert the clinician to key developmental problems.

APPROACHES TO HEALTH MANAGEMENT IN PRIMARY CARE SECTION

Functional health patterns (Gordon, 1987, 2010) serve as the organizational framework of this section. Eleven patterns are common to people of all cultures and ages. The first chapter introduces the section, using the concepts of health maintenance and health promotion. Chapters on nutrition, breastfeeding, elimination, sleep, and activity and sports participation follow, emphasizing healthy lifestyle choices as well as identifying common concerns seen by the primary health care provider. The remaining functional health pattern chapters are more psychosocial in nature:

- Self-perception
- Role relationships where issues of child abuse are addressed
- Coping and stress tolerance to explore mental health problems of children
- Cognitive/perceptual patterns to discuss attention-deficit/hyperactivity disorder, learning disabilities, sensory

perception, autism, and sensory problems of blindness and deafness
- Sexuality
- Values and beliefs

In all of these chapters, foundations of psychology and the basic sciences are first introduced and then applied to common problems of children. Normative behaviors are discussed, and the assessment process is reviewed. Current guidelines, standards for care, and management strategies with which the clinician should be familiar are identified. Common problems of each pattern are presented with the aid of a problem-oriented framework.

APPROACHES TO DISEASE MANAGEMENT SECTION

This section of the book is devoted to pediatric diseases or disorders and their management. It includes 23 chapters. An introductory chapter reviews essential components of illness diagnosis and is followed by a separate chapter on pain management. The infectious diseases chapter reviews key communicable diseases and includes a comprehensive subsection on immunizations. A major set of chapters focuses on principal body systems, with additional chapters devoted to neonatology, genetics, and uncomplicated trauma. An environmental health chapter discusses these important emerging issues. A chapter on complementary therapies promotes the primary care provider's knowledge about many of the less traditional health care strategies that families may be using.

Each chapter follows the same format throughout. Standards and guidelines for care are highlighted, the physiologic and assessment parameters are discussed, management strategies are identified, and management of common problems is presented in a problem-oriented format. Each disease or condition is explained as follows:

- Description
- Epidemiology
- Clinical findings (history, physical examination, laboratory and other studies)
- Differential diagnoses
- Management
- Complications
- Preventive and patient education measures

Tables highlight and summarize differential diagnoses, management, and other pertinent information. The scope of practice of the primary care provider is always kept in mind with appropriate referral and consultation points identified.

PRACTICE MANAGEMENT CHAPTER

In the current healthcare marketplace, it is increasingly important that the clinician be aware of issues of productivity, compliance with state and federal laws, quality-of-care indicators, and successful business practices that will ensure viability. The chapter on practice management provides information for developing practices.

APPENDICES

The appendices, located in the back of the book, include sections on the use of drugs in children and guidelines for increasing adherence to medication regimens in pediatric practice; growth parameters; laboratory data; useful resources, such as national organizations for various disorders; and discussion questions. The appendices are designed for easy access to reference data.

SUMMARY

This book is written by and for nurse practitioners and other clinicians devoted to primary health care of children. It provides a comprehensive resource for graduate students and serves as a reference for practicing clinicians. The editors assume that the reader has a baccalaureate degree in nursing or a related field and advanced coursework in physiology, child development, health assessment, pharmacology, and family systems. Thus, this book guides clinical application of concepts important to primary health care of children and their families. The book is conceptually organized around domains of interest to pediatric primary care providers—development; functional health patterns related to health maintenance and psychosocial well-being of children and their families; and diseases of children that require intervention, monitoring, and/or referral. The book uses a problem-oriented focus consistent with the education of nurse practitioners and other health care providers and has been written using the latest standards and guidelines available. Content is consistent with the major recommendations for primary care of children. We are delighted to bring forward a fifth edition of this much-needed resource.

Editors

Catherine E. Burns, PhD, RN, CPNP-PC, FAAN
Ardys M. Dunn, PhD, RN, PNP
Margaret A. Brady, PhD, RN, CPNP-PC
Nancy Barber Starr, MS, APRN, BC (PNP), CPNP-PC
Catherine G. Blosser, MPA:HA, RN, APRN, BC (PNP)

Associate Editor

Dawn Lee Garzon, PhD, PNP-BC, CPNP-PC, PMHS, FAANP

REFERENCES

Gordon M: *Nursing diagnosis: process and application*, New York, 1987, McGraw-Hill.
Gordon M: *Manual of nursing diagnosis*, ed 12, Sudbury, MA, 2010, Jones and Bartlett.
Hagan J, Shaw JS, Duncan PM: *Bright Futures: guidelines for health supervision of infants, children, and adolescents*, ed 2, Elk Grove, IL, 2008, American Academy of Pediatrics.
Institute of Medicine of the National Academies: *The future of nursing: leading change, advancing health*, 2011. Available at www.iom.edu/Reports/2010/The-Future-of-Nursing-Leading-Change-Advancing-Health (accessed November 4, 2011).
Rothman RL, Yin HS, Mulvaney S et al: Health literacy and quality: focus on chronic illness and patient safety, *Pediatrics* 124(suppl 3):S315–326, 2009.
U.S. Department of Health and Human Services: *Healthy People 2020*, Washington, DC, 2010, U.S. Government Printing Office.

Acknowledgments

A book of this size and complexity could never have been completed without considerable help—the work of the contributors who researched, wrote, and revised content; the consultation and review of experts in various specialties who critiqued drafts and provided important perspectives and guidance; and the essential technical support from those who managed the production of the manuscript and the final product. We appreciate the authorship and review work of Ann Petersen-Smith, and Lee Henderson, Executive Content Strategist; Jackie Twomey, Content Development Specialist; and Jeanne Genz, Project Manager, at Elsevier, who have provided essential support and expertise throughout the writing and production of this edition. We could not have done it without our family and friends who offered unending support and encouragement for the duration of the project. We are indebted to so many people and want to say thanks to them all. The following are some of the many people we want to acknowledge.

CONTRIBUTORS TO THE FOURTH EDITION

These people were instrumental in helping us develop the fourth edition of the book. Although they are not authors in this edition, their ideas and work have contributed greatly to our work, and we are deeply indebted to them:

Janet Williams, Kathleen Shelton, Bridget O'Boyle-Jordan, Barbara Jones Deloian, Catherine Goodhue, Melissa L. R. Burchett, Cheryl E. Hanna, William J. Muller, Sheila M. Kodadek, Mary Margaret Gottesman, and Gail M. Houck

OUR THANKS TO FAMILY AND FRIENDS

Thanks so very much for giving me the time and support to work on this text one more time! To my husband, Jerry Burns; my daughters Jennifer and Jill and their families; other family and friends; and to the many PNPs, FNPs, and NP faculty who have expressed their appreciation for this text and encouraged us to continue the project.

Catherine E. Burns

My thanks to Marvin Dunn; Malcolm and Megan Dunn; Philip Dunn and Liz Flynn, grandchildren Miles Christopher, and Claire Sylvia Dunn (from "the craziest Nana in the whole wide world!" Thanks for being my joy and inspiration); and other family and friends.

Ardys M. Dunn

With appreciation for your caring and support to Martha, Larry, Greg, Katie, and the rest of the Brady clan, my dear friends, and in memory of Grandma Mary.

Margaret A. Brady

Jon, Jonah and AnnaMei Starr—mahalo for your patience with me each and every time you had to delay something you wanted for me "to work on the book." Aloha! Thanks as well to my APA colleagues who give me room to practice and grow.

Nancy Barber Starr

To my husband, Terry, whose attention to keeping the home fire burning and food in my stomach, allowed me long hours at the computer; to other family; and, in honor of the 100th year of my mother (plan on taking that hot air balloon ride, Mom).

Catherine G. Blosser

My thanks to the students, parents, and families who make me a better person; to Alonso, Rachel, and Elizabeth Garzon who give my life meaning; and to Amy DiMaggio, friends, and family for loving me and giving me wings.

Dawn Lee Garzon

The Child's Name is Today

We are guilty of many errors and faults,
but our worst crime is abandoning the children,
neglecting the fountain of life.
Many of the things we need can wait.
The child cannot.
Right now is the time his bones are being formed,
his blood is being made,
and his senses are being developed.
To him we cannot answer, "Tomorrow."
His name is "Today."

Gabriela Mistral (1889-1957) 1945
Nobel Laureate in Literature, Chile

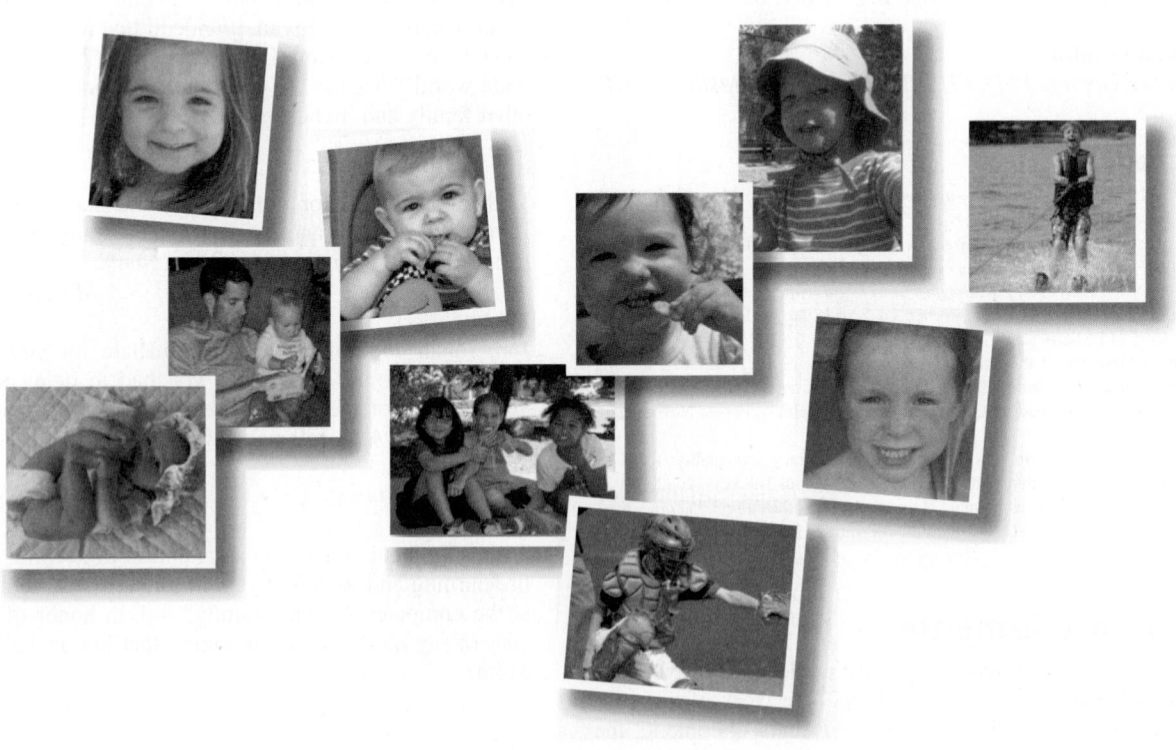

This book is dedicated to the infants, children, and adolescents and their families about whom this book was written, wishing them health, loving support, and happiness, the real goals of this book.

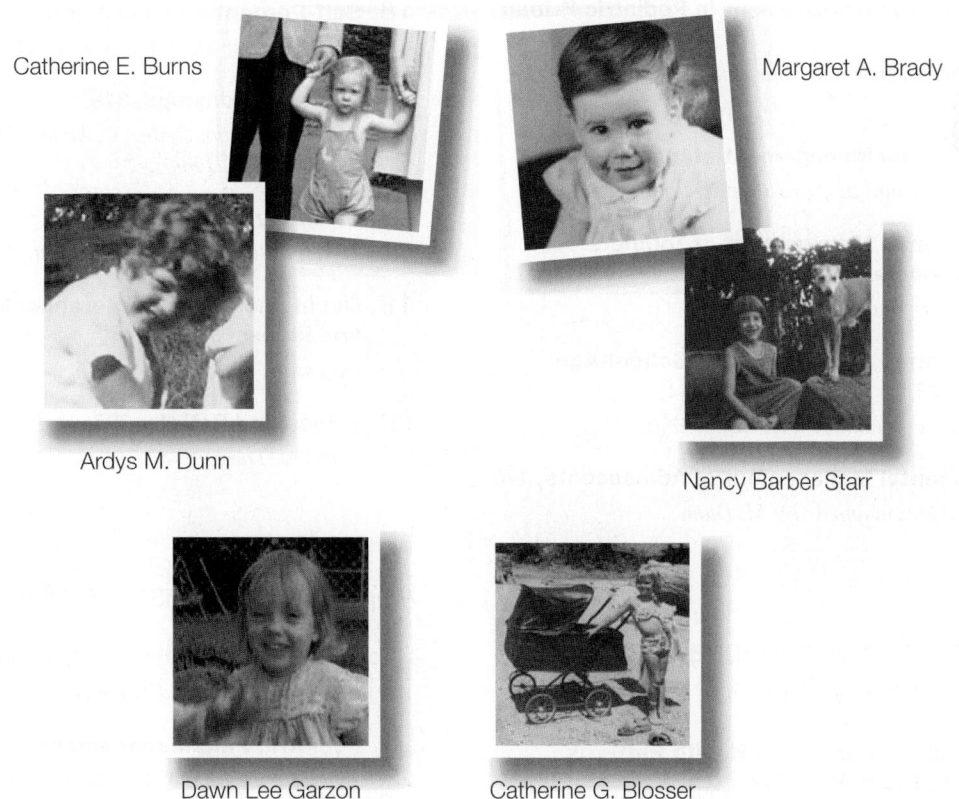

Catherine E. Burns

Margaret A. Brady

Ardys M. Dunn

Nancy Barber Starr

Dawn Lee Garzon

Catherine G. Blosser

Contents

Appendixes

APPENDIXES

Pediatric Primary Care Foundations

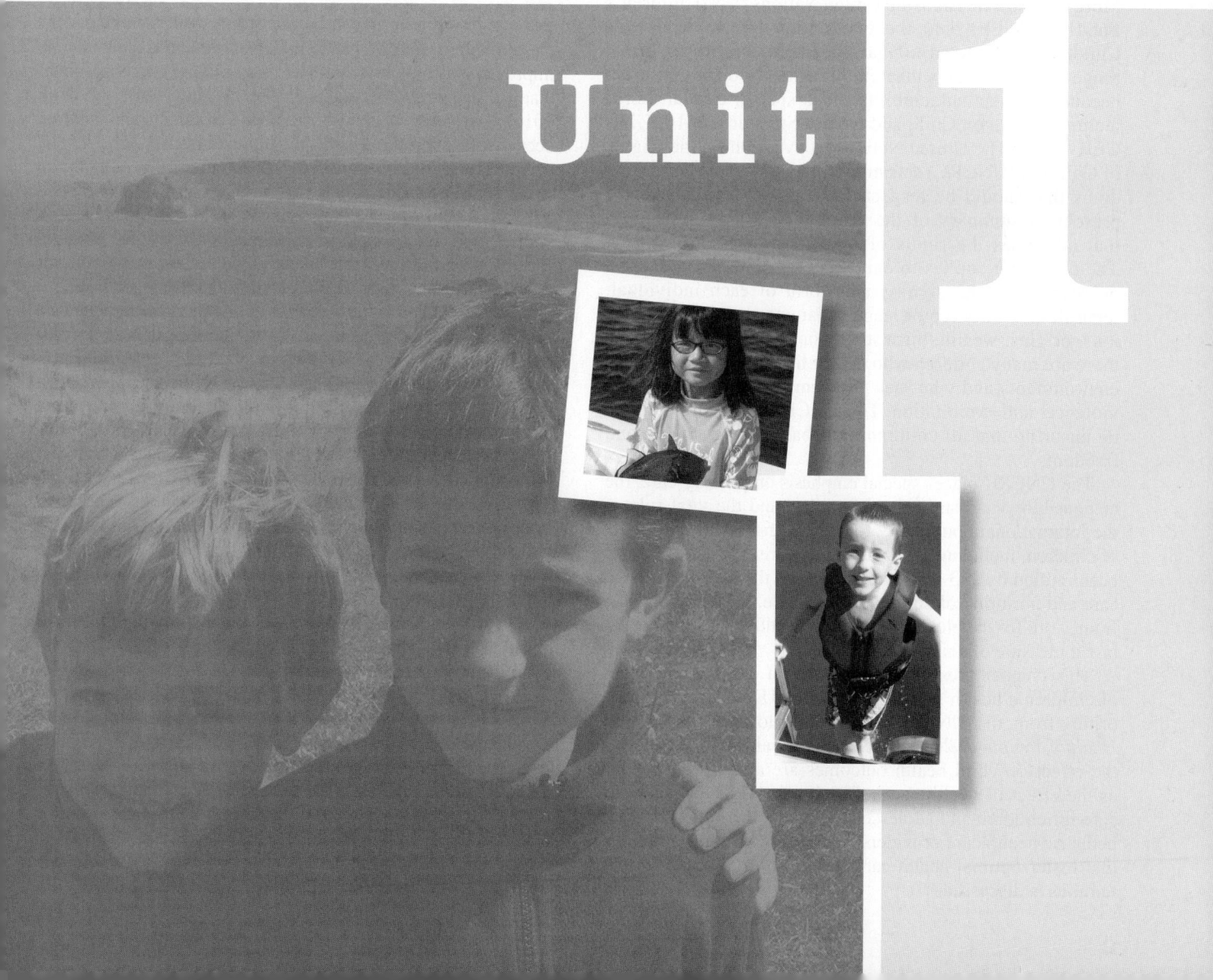

Unit

1

Health Status of Children:

Global and Local Perspectives

KAREN G. DUDERSTADT

More than 20 years ago, the United Nations (UN) Children's Fund (UNICEF) held the Convention on the Rights of Children and enacted a legal document asserting a broad range of human rights inherently due to children. Children, because of their vulnerability, need special care and protection (Forum on Child and Family Statistics, 2010; UNICEF, 2009). The United Nations Convention on the Rights of Children (UNCRC) sets minimum entitlements and freedoms that should be respected by governments. Box 1-1 presents a summary of the articles from the Convention that addresses the rights of protection (UNICEF, 2009). The document applies to children globally and is founded on respect for the dignity and worth of each individual, regardless of race, color, gender, language, religion, opinions, origins, wealth, birth status, or ability. Unfortunately there are many children who do not live in nurturing family environments and who lack freedom from armed conflict, violence, and exploitation. The UNCRC continues to work on ensuring that all children have basic human rights and freedoms.

The UNCRC places special emphasis on primary care, the responsibility and strength of families, and the vital role of the international community to protect and secure the rights of children, including access to health care. The UNCRC has been ratified by 193 nations and remains the standard for the care and nurturing of children everywhere. It also provides a framework for the global definition of health of children and a broad measure of child health status.

This chapter presents an overview of the current status of children's health globally and in the U.S. The health priorities from the UN Millennium Development Goals and *Healthy People 2020* are presented. Health disparities and the effect on child health outcomes are addressed, as well as the effect of health care reform in the U.S. on access to care for children and adolescents. Finally, the important role pediatric health care providers have in advocating for polices that foster optimal health care services for all children and families is discussed.

■ Global Health Status of Children

Despite improved child health interventions and socioeconomic improvements in many countries, 8.8 million children younger than the age of 5 years die each year worldwide (Black et al, 2010). Sixty-eight percent of the deaths in infants and children occur from often-preventable infectious diseases. The largest percentage of deaths is due to pneumonia; 18% of children younger than 5 years of age die from pneumonia worldwide, 15% from diarrheal diseases, and 8% from malaria. Although malnutrition is a primary contributory factor to neonatal and childhood deaths from infectious diseases, it is often not reflected in census data. Vitamin A and zinc deficiencies, suboptimal breastfeeding patterns, and overall nutritional deficiencies contribute as underlying causes in one third of deaths globally for children younger than 5 years of age (Black et al, 2008).

Forty-one percent of all deaths globally occur in neonates. Birth asphyxia and preterm birth complications comprise the largest proportion of these neonatal deaths. Half of the mortality worldwide occurs in children in five countries—India, Nigeria, Democratic Republic of Congo, Pakistan, and China. The high rate of mortality concentrated in these countries is due not only to economic and social conditions but also large concentrations of populations of children younger than 5 years; 43% of the pediatric population globally lives in these five countries (Black et al, 2010). Afghanistan and Ethiopia also have high rates of death due to pneumonia and diarrheal diseases. Fifty-one percent of all deaths due to acquired immunodeficiency syndrome (AIDS) occur in South Africa, Nigeria, Mozambique, Tanzania, and Uganda. Malaria accounts for 57% of the deaths in Nigeria, Democratic Republic of Congo, Uganda, Sudan, and Tanzania (Black et al, 2010).

Successful vaccination programs have markedly reduced the mortality caused by some infectious diseases, particularly measles and tetanus; however, tetanus is still responsible for 1% of deaths in children younger than 5 years of age. Figure 1-1 illustrates the global, regional, and national causes of child mortality (Black et al, 2010).

BOX 1-1 Convention on the Rights of the Child: Summary of Protection Rights

According to the Convention on the Rights of the Child, every child has the right to protection from:

	Articles
Illicit transfers and illegal adoption	11, 21
Violence, abuse, exploitation, and neglect	19
Armed conflict	22, 38-39
Child labor, trafficking, sexual and other forms of exploitation, and drug abuse	32-36, 39
Torture and deprivation of liberty, and capital punishment	37-39

In addition, the Convention ensures special protection, assistance and care for children who are:

Deprived of the family environment	20, 22
Disabled	23
In conflict with the law	37, 39-40

From United Nations International Children's Fund: *The state of the world's children*, ed 2, New York, 2009, UNICEF, p 25.

The Child Health Epidemiology Reference Group (CHERG) of the World Health Organization (WHO) and UNICEF have been charged with developing improved evidence on the causes and determinants of neonatal and childhood morbidity and mortality and evaluating the effectiveness of interventions to inform global priorities and programs (CHERG, 2009). Their goal is to provide timely estimates on the causes and determinants of child mortality, improve knowledge on the causes of maternal mortality, determine the relationship between disease burden and risk factors for maternal and childhood morbidity and mortality, and assist countries in planning and monitoring child health interventions. The CHERG estimates on mortality and determinants of death have assisted countries to target programs and interventions to reduce health disparities.

MILLENNIUM DEVELOPMENT GOALS

The UN Millennium Development Goals aim to reduce childhood mortality by two thirds in children younger than 5 years of age by 2015 and to provide benchmarks for tackling extreme poverty both globally and locally (United Nations, 2000). The eight goals consist of 21 quantifiable targets that are measured by 60 health indicators (Fig. 1-2). They provide a framework for

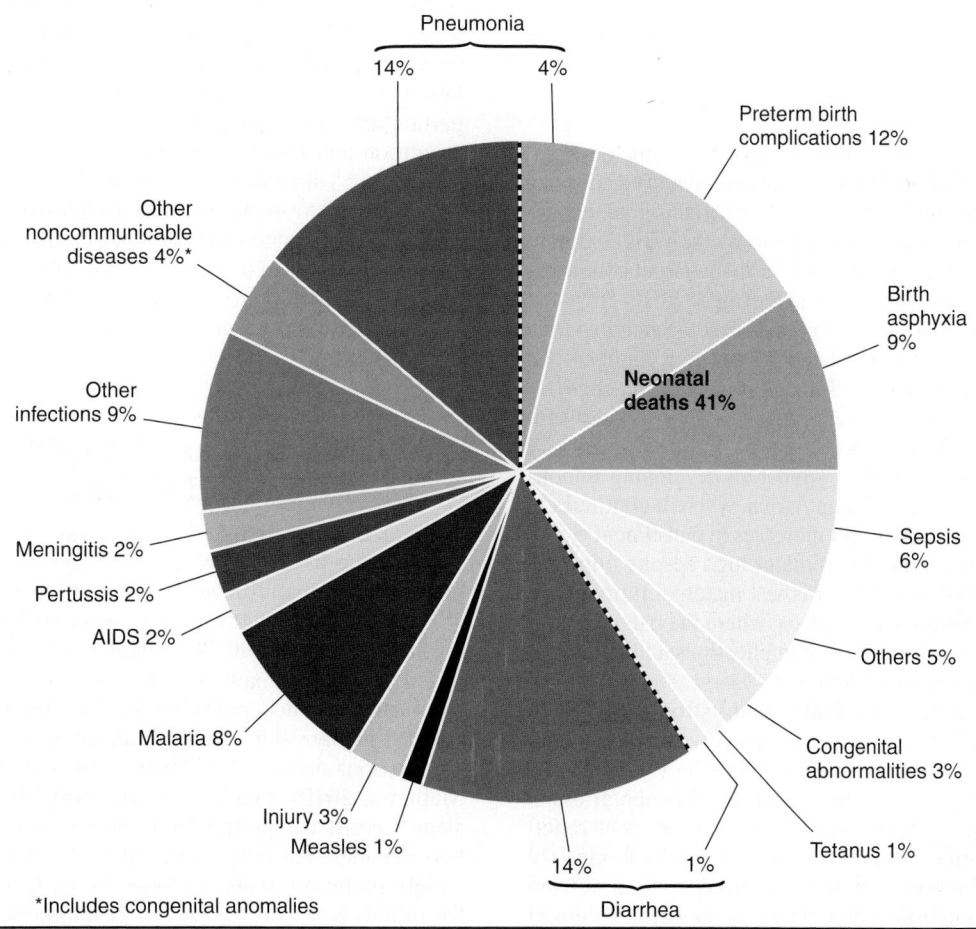

*Includes congenital anomalies

FIGURE 1-1 Global, regional, and national causes of child mortality. Data are separated into deaths of neonates 0-27 days and children aged 1-59 months. Causes that led to less than 1% of deaths are not presented. (From Black RE, et al: Global, regional, and national causes of child mortality in 2008: a systematic analysis, *Lancet* 375(9730):1973, 2010.)

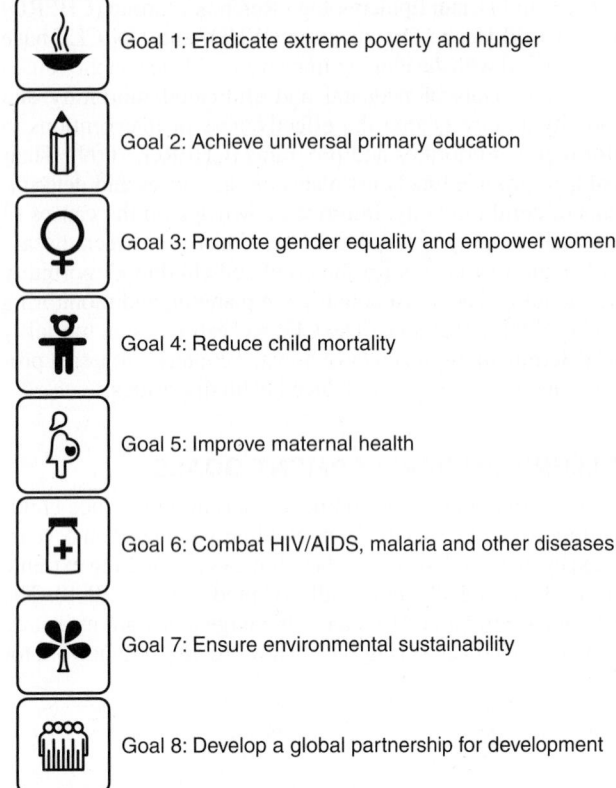

Goal 1: Eradicate extreme poverty and hunger

Goal 2: Achieve universal primary education

Goal 3: Promote gender equality and empower women

Goal 4: Reduce child mortality

Goal 5: Improve maternal health

Goal 6: Combat HIV/AIDS, malaria and other diseases

Goal 7: Ensure environmental sustainability

Goal 8: Develop a global partnership for development

FIGURE 1-2 United Nations Millennium Development Goals.

the international community to ensure socioeconomic development reaches all children. If these goals are achieved, poverty could be reduced by 50% worldwide. To reach this goal, expansion and acceleration of the interventions by the WHO to target the leading causes of death are required in the target countries.

The UN has made progress toward these goals in many regions. Malaria prevention has expanded to sub-Saharan Africa with the use of insect-treated bed nets for children younger than 5 years of age. Access to safe drinking water has reached 1.6 billion people over the past decade, but the safety of water supplies remains a challenge. Enrollment of children in primary school reached 90% in 2006 in almost all developing regions with the exception of sub-Saharan Africa, where it continues to hover around 70% despite recent increases in enrollment (UNICEF, 2009). Maternal mortality remains high despite improvements in some regions, with the highest maternal mortality in southern Asia and sub-Saharan Africa, where the risk of maternal death from pregnancy-related complications and childbirth is 1 in 22 births during the childbearing years.

The economic growth potential remains strong in many of the developing regions, and partnerships between developing countries and nongovernmental organizations (NGOs) continue to provide significant sources of developmental assistance. Developing countries will require further debt relief, reduced trade barriers, improved access to technologies for renewable energy production, and enhanced protection from and response to environmental disasters to sustain current advances. Further, global political efforts will be required to support achievement of the Millennium Development Goals by 2015 and a renewed commitment to the future health and well-being of children everywhere.

FOOD INSECURITY AND EFFECT ON CHILD HEALTH

Hunger and undernutrition are the largest contributing risk factors in the mortality of children less than 5 years of age in developing countries. Undernutrition refers to a form of malnutrition resulting in stunting and wasting caused by deficiencies of essential vitamins and minerals (Black et al, 2008). Globally, undernutrition is an important determinant of maternal and child health and is estimated to cause 3.5 million deaths annually. It is a known underlying cause of 35% of the global disease burden in children less than 5 years of age. Vitamin A and zinc deficiencies remain the largest disease burden among the nutritional deficiencies, with vitamin A deficiency causing 600,000 deaths annually in children less than 5 years of age (Black et al, 2008). Although rates of exclusive breastfeeding have increased for infants less than 6 months of age in all but one of the developing regions, suboptimal breastfeeding remains responsible for 1.4 million deaths annually (UNICEF, 2009). Preventable nutritional deficiencies are a compelling case for further implementation of the Millennium Development Goals and increased support for micronutrient supplementation for children in developing regions.

Hunger and undernutrition are often referred to as food insecurity, the condition that exists when people do not have "physical and economic access to sufficient, safe, nutritious, and culturally acceptable food to meet their dietary needs" (United Nations Millennium Project, 2006, p 20). Poverty and food insecurity are primary contributors to maternal and child undernutrition. Food insecurity occurs in impoverished populations in developing countries and in industrialized nations particularly among migrant populations. Children affected by migration and family separation are at risk for food insecurity and are vulnerable to further health consequences including exposure to exploitation and child trafficking. Growing evidence on climate change indicates the dramatic effect on food crops that lead to food distribution issues, one of the primary contributors to food insecurity. Figure 1-3 illustrates the relationship between climate change, food availability, and malnutrition.

■ Health Status of Children in the United States

Despite improvements in some areas of child health status over the past decade, the U.S. lags significantly behind other economically developed countries in some measures of child health. Infant mortality is an important indicator of the health of a nation. The infant mortality rate in the U.S. has remained stagnant over the past decade (6.9 per 1000 live births) and depending on the data source, the U.S. ranks approximately 30th when compared with other industrialized nations on this child health indicator (MacDorman and Mathews, 2010). The high infant mortality rate reflects the steady increase in preterm birth rates in the U.S. over the past two decades. Although mortality rates for very low-birth-weight preterm infants are lower in the U.S., mortality rates for infants born at 37 weeks of gestation or term infants are significantly higher in the U.S. than in most industrialized countries (MacDorman and Mathews, 2010). One in 8 babies in the U.S. is born preterm as compared to 1 in 18 babies in Ireland and Finland.

Health effects

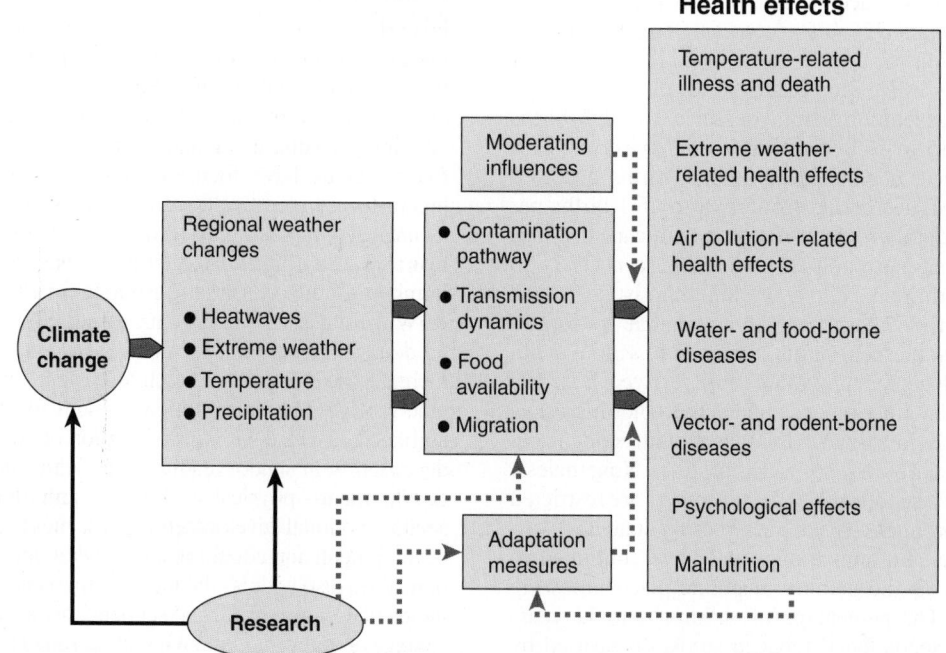

FIGURE 1-3 Pathways by which climate change affects health. (Used with permission from World Health Organization: *Children's health & environment: a review of the evidence,* p 29, 2002. [WHO adapted from Patz JA, McGeehin MA, Bernard SM et al: The potential health impacts of climate variability and change for the United States: executive summary of the report of the health sector of the US National Assessment, *Environ Health Perspectives,* 108:367-376, 2000]).

Child poverty rates in the U.S. remain significantly higher than in other economically developed nations. Twenty percent of U.S. children, including 1 in 3 Hispanic, 1 in 3 African American, and 1 in 10 white/non-Hispanic children, live in poverty (Forum on Child and Family Statistics, 2010). There are also 5.9 million children, or 8% of the pediatric population, living in extreme poverty in the U.S. with incomes less than half of the federal poverty threshold[1] (Forum on Child and Family Statistics, 2010).

Most concerning among the child health indicators in the U.S. is the percent of overweight children. Based on international standards for overweight, U.S. youth have the highest rate of obesity (25.1%) as compared to Australia (23.9%), Canada (19.5%), and the United Kingdom (15.8%) (Foundation for Child Development, 2007). In the U.S., 20 states have 1 in 3 children who have a body mass index (BMI) greater than the 97th percentile for age. The rate of obesity has tripled among adolescents in the past three decades. Obese and overweight youth are more at risk for associated adult health problems including heart disease, type 2 diabetes, stroke, and osteoarthritis (Ogden et al, 2010).

Poor eating patterns are a major factor in the high rate of obesity among children and adolescents. Over the past decade, children's diets have been out of balance, with too much added sugar and saturated fats and limited nutrient-rich foods, particularly fruits, vegetables, and whole grains. Children ages 2 to 5 years are the only age group to meet the standards for

total fruit and milk intake (Forum on Child and Family Statistics, 2010). Of all the child health indicators, overweight and obesity will significantly affect the cost of providing health care services in the U.S. and in the economically developed nations for the next generation.

HEALTH INDICATORS IN CHILDREN AND FAMILIES

Several health indicators of child health indicate significant progress in the U.S. Seventy-six percent of children ages 19 to 35 months received the recommended combined six-vaccine series[2] in 2008. Coverage rates for pneumococcal vaccine continue to improve and reached 80% in 2008 (Forum on Child and Family Statistics, 2010). These improvements remain below the *Healthy People 2010* goal of 80% vaccine coverage for the combined vaccines and 90% vaccine coverage for individual vaccines. Children living in low-income families had lower rates of vaccine coverage (72% as compared to 78% for children living in higher-income families). Among adolescents, vaccination rates reached more than 90% coverage for hepatitis B and the second dose of measles, mumps, and rubella (MMR) vaccine. Coverage for pertussis in adolescents 13 to 17 years of age remains low, but increased to 40.8% in 2008 with administration of Tdap (tetanus, diphtheria

---

[1]The average poverty threshold for a family of three in 2010 was $18,310, and for a family of four, the threshold was $22,050. Families in extreme poverty in 2010 were living on less than $11,000 annually.

[2]The combined series consists of four doses of diphtheria, tetanus toxoids, and acellular pertussis (DTaP) vaccines; three doses of poliovirus vaccines; one dose of any measles, mumps, and rubella vaccine; three doses of *Haemophilus influenzae* type B (HIB) vaccines; three doses (or more) of hepatitis B vaccines; and one dose of varicella vaccine.

and acellular pertussis) vaccine. For human papillomavirus (HPV4) vaccine, about 37% of adolescent females had initiated the vaccination series (≥1 dose) in 2008 (Centers for Disease Control and Prevention [CDC], 2009).

The 2008 adolescent birth rate declined to 21.7 births per 1000 females 15 to 17 years of age, the lowest rate ever recorded. The largest decline in adolescent births occurred in Hispanic females, decreasing from 47.8 to 46.1 births per 1000 in females 15 to 17 years of age. Significant declines also occurred among black, non-Hispanic adolescents (35.8 to 34.9 per 1000) (Forum on Child and Family Statistics, 2010). School-based health centers have the potential to further reduce the rate of adolescent births. Students in schools with school-based health centers providing reproductive health services have reported neither more sexual activity nor increased frequency of sexual intercourse compared with students in schools without school-based health centers. Nonetheless, more than one in five school-based health centers are restricted from providing reproductive health services by state law.

Rates of secondhand smoke exposure have continued to decline in the U.S. as the number of public places allowing smoking declines. The percentage of children 4 to 11 years of age exposed to secondhand tobacco smoke, measured by blood cotinine levels, decreased from 88% in 1994 to 53% in 2008. Teen smoking rates have also declined. The percentage of adolescents who smoke regularly has reached its lowest level since monitoring began in 1997. In 2009, daily cigarette smoking declined from 10% to 3% in eighth graders, 18% to 6% in tenth graders, and 25% to 11% in twelfth graders (Forum on Child and Family Statistics, 2010).

NEW MORBIDITIES: FAMILY VIOLENCE AND CHILDHOOD DEPRESSION

Depression can adversely affect the development and well-being of children and adolescents and the health and stability of families. In 2008, 8% of adolescents 12 to 17 years of age had at least one major depressive episode (MDE) during that year. The prevalence of MDEs was lowest in youth 12 to 13 years of age (5%) and highest among those 16 to 17 years of age (11%). The rate of MDEs is nearly three times higher among females (12%) compared with males (4%). The percentage of youth receiving mental health services for depression has not kept pace with the increase in episodes. In 2008, 40% of youth with at least one MDE received treatment for depression (Forum on Child and Family Statistics, 2010). There is also a large gap between mental health needs and the availability of mental health services for children and adolescents, and an increasing demand on pediatric primary care providers for early assessment and intervention for children and families with chronic mental health conditions.

Family violence can be a contributing factor to childhood depression. Exposure to domestic violence during childhood can be associated with increased aggressive behavior, emotional problems such as depression and anxiety, and poorer school performance (Fantuzzo and Mohr, 2003). Children who are exposed to domestic violence have exhibited similar effects to those children who are direct victims of abuse. As incidents of family violence and domestic violence continue to rise, increased awareness and data about the short- and long-term effects of exposure to violence care needed to ameliorate the effects on child development.

HEALTHY PEOPLE 2020

Over the past three decades, *Healthy People* has been measuring the effect of health promotion activities on the health status of children and families. Setting benchmarks for improved quality of health care services has spotlighted prevention activities in a disease-focused health care system. The *Healthy People* goals have focused on specific disparities in child health to improve health care services and health outcomes. *Health People 2020* emphasizes the need for continued progress toward optimal health and has proposed benchmarks for a number of new prevention activities for child health.

With increased proportions of children with developmental delays, *Healthy People 2020* focuses on new objectives to increase the percentage of children less than 2 years of age who receive early intervention services for developmental disabilities and to increase the proportion of children entering kindergarten with school readiness in all five domains of healthy development—physical well-being and motor development, social emotional development, approaches to learning, language development, and cognition and general development. The new objectives also address the increase in maladaptive behaviors in the pediatric population and set benchmarks to increase the percentage of young children who are screened for autism and other developmental delays at 18 and 24 months of age. To address the trend in the increase in major depressive disorders, *Healthy People 2020* includes an objective to decrease the prevalence of MDEs among children with depression and mood disorders, and to increase the proportion of primary care providers screening for depression in the primary care setting (USDHHS, 2010).

Healthy People 2020 sets new goals for reducing the proportion of overweight and obese children with an objective focusing on reducing consumption of calories from solid fats and added sugars in the pediatric population younger than 2 years of age. Also, *Healthy People 2010* objectives were modified to monitor the dietary intake of children beginning at 2 years of age with benchmarks to increase the variety and contribution of fruits and vegetables and whole grains in the diet and reduce the consumption of sodium beginning at 2 years of age (*Healthy People, 2010*). This recommendation is consistent with the recent trends in overweight beginning in the first 2 years of life and continuing into the school years. There is also a goal to increase the proportion of pediatric primary care providers who regularly measure the BMI of their patients (*Healthy People, 2010*) to improve early surveillance of trends in overweight and obesity in the early years.

Finally, in relation to access to health services, the *Healthy People 2020* objectives address the need for increasing the proportion of practicing primary care providers, including nurse practitioners, to improve access to quality health care services. The demand for primary care services will increase as more children, adolescents, and young adults qualify for health insurance plans and seek preventive health care. The health workforce needs to stand ready to offer appropriate evidence-based clinical preventive services to fulfill the objective of health care reform to reduce overall health care costs. Further, *Healthy People 2020* goals that address children's health and drive public policy are now spread throughout the topic areas and could be organized to more specifically provide a child health framework (Halfon et al, 2007). This would assist in designing an improved integrated system of care coupled with improved access for all children and a more integrated system of communication to facilitate continuity of care for children and families.

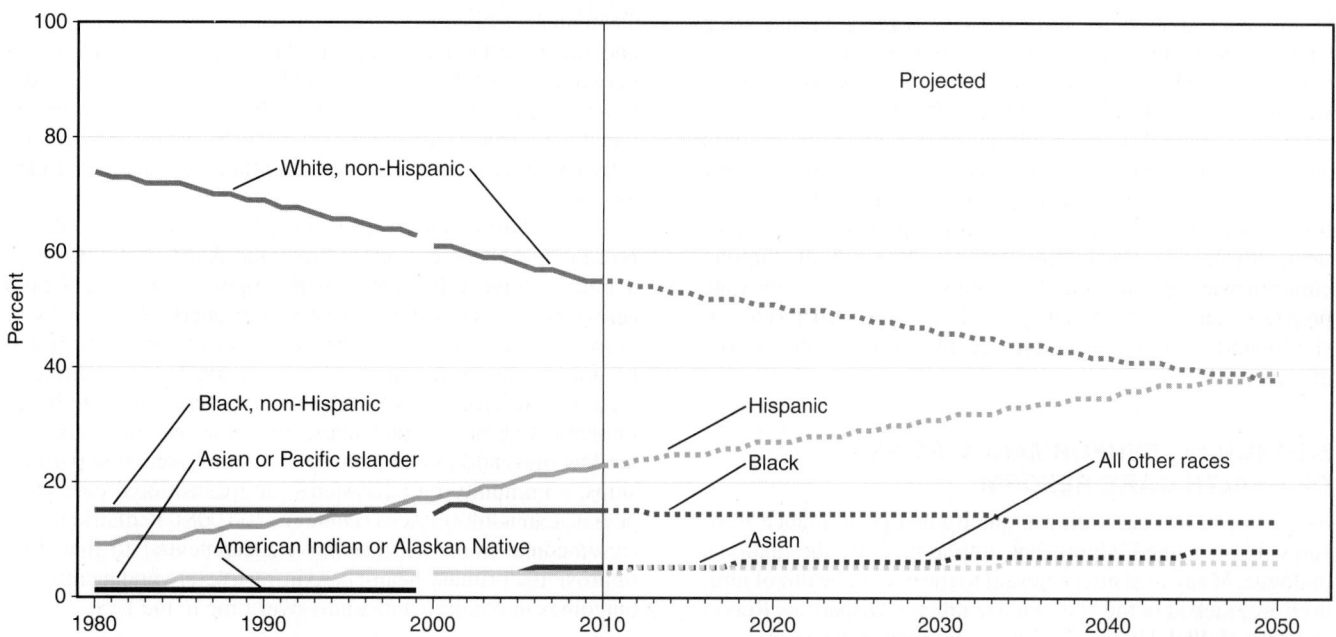

NOTE: Data from 2000 onward are not directly comparable with data from earlier years. Data on race and Hispanic origin are collected separately; Hispanics may be any race. In 1980 and 1990, following the 1977 Office of Management and Budget (OMB) standards for collecting and presenting data on race, the decennial census gave respondents the option to identify with one race from the following: White, Black, American Indian or Alaskan Native, or Asian or Pacific Islander. The Census Bureau also offered an "Other" category. Beginning in 2000, following the 1997 OMB standards for collecting and presenting data on race, the decennial census gave respondents the option to identify with one or more races from the following: White, Black, Asian, American Indian or Alaska Native, and Native Hawaiian or Other Pacific Islander. In addition, a "Some other race" category was included with OMB approval. Those who chose more than one race were classified as "Two or more races." Except for the "All other races" category, all race groups discussed from 2000 onward refer to people who indicated only one racial identity. (Those who were "Two or more races" were included in the "All other races" category, along with American Indians or Alaska Natives and Native Hawaiians or Other Pacific Islanders.)

FIGURE 1-4 Percentage of U.S. children ages 0 to 17 by race and Hispanic origin, 1980-2009 and projected 2010-2050. (From Forum on Child and Family Statistics: *America's children in brief: key health indicators for well-being,* 2010. Available at http://childstats.gov [accessed Aug 17, 2010].)

HEALTH EQUITY AND CHILD HEALTH IN THE UNITED STATES

The overall number of children in the U.S. has increased in the past decade by 2 million and the racial and ethnic distribution of those children has changed. In the most recent U.S. census, there were 74.5 million children, constituting 24% of the population (Forum on Child and Family Statistics, 2010). By 2023, fewer than 50% of U.S. children are projected to be white, non-Hispanic, whereas the number of Hispanic children has been steadily increasing over the past 2 decades and is projected to reach 39% of the pediatric population by 2050 (Forum on Child and Family Statistics, 2010) (Fig. 1-4). Understanding the changing demographics of the pediatric population is critical to shaping the health care workforce and health care services for future generations of children. Further, the debate on whether to expand health care to immigrant children would need to become part of the dialogue in order to further decrease health disparities.

Two measures of health disparities for children from the recent National Healthcare Disparities Report (NHDR) were particularly concerning—disparities in physical activity in children and disparities in pediatric asthma care (U.S. Department of Health and Human Services [USDHHS], 2009). Parents reporting that they did not receive advice about the recommendations for daily physical activity for children showed the largest gap; children living in higher-income families were almost twice as likely to report receiving advice as children living in poor families. Increasing physical activity has shown to be the most effective strategy for reducing childhood overweight.

The second major health care disparity is the management of asthma. More than 7 million children less than 18 years of age have asthma (USDHHS, 2009). The cost of asthma care totals more than $20 billion annually for children and families. Closing the gap in the quality of asthma care is key to reducing overall health care costs. The rate of emergency department visits and hospitalizations for African-American children remains twice the rate of white, non-Hispanic children. Black and Hispanic children also have more indicators of poorly controlled asthma, including more daily rescue medicine use and lower use of inhaled corticosteroids, compared with white, non-Hispanic children (Crocker et al, 2009). Access to specialized quality health care services for children with chronic health conditions is critical to attaining health equity among diverse populations and limiting the effect of health disparities.

■ Health Care Reform

The passage of the Children's Health Insurance Program Reauthorization Act of 2009 (CHIPRA) marked a tremendous step forward in providing quality affordable health care to children and their families. More than half the states took advantage of new options in CHIPRA and/or made other improvements in their children's coverage programs since CHIPRA was enacted. U.S. Census Bureau data released in September 2009 indicated the number of uninsured children was at the lowest level since 1987. With employer-based coverage becoming less available and affordable for children and adults alike, Medicaid and CHIP are chiefly responsible for the insurance gains among children, more than offsetting losses in private coverage. Still, significant disparities in health care insurance coverage exist, especially among children who are in racial and ethnic minorities. Coverage progress achieved in recent years has not helped reduce or significantly narrow the difference in coverage rates across groups of children.

MEASURING PERFORMANCE AS PART OF HEALTH CARE REFORM

As part of health care reform, quality and performance measures have gained significant importance in the national dialogue. Many measures relevant to the overall health of children are tracked in the National Healthcare Disparities Report (NHDR) (USDHHS, 2009). The section reporting on children specifically focuses on four components of health care: prevention, treatment, management, and access to care. Core report measures for both quality of health care and access to health care were developed based on selected criteria such as prevalence and clinical significance. These will continue to be refined over the next decade as provisions of the health care reform legislation are implemented.

Lack of health care insurance is the single strongest predictor of quality of care for U.S. children—greater than the effects of race, ethnicity, family income, or education (USDHHS, 2009). Quality of care is measured by the timeliness and effectiveness of care, as well as the safety of the care delivered. Measures of access to care include health insurance coverage, utilization of health care services, and barriers to care. Both access and quality are required to eliminate the impact of disparities in health. The true challenge for eliminating health disparities lies in our ability to shift the public focus to policies that favor health care for all children.

ADVANCED PRACTICE NURSES' ROLE AND HEALTH CARE REFORM

A growing body of evidence demonstrates that advanced practice nurses (APNs) deliver high-value primary care services (Naylor and Kurtzman, 2010). APNs provide continuity of care for underserved populations at greater risk for ambulatory care–sensitive conditions such as asthma, pneumonia, and vaccine-preventable conditions contributing to hospitalizations that increase the cost of health care delivery. Increasing access to APNs who deliver quality primary care services would reduce health care costs, improve health outcomes, and produce health care savings, all steps toward allowing the U.S. to lead rather than trail the other economically developed countries in child health indicators.

Health care reform places a greater emphasis on primary care infrastructure including medical home. *Medical home* is defined by Berwick as "a practice team that coordinates a person's care across episodes and specialties" (2009, p w555). The concept of a medical home is being promoted

as an answer to cost containment, quality clinical outcomes, and higher patient satisfaction. The American Academy of Pediatrics' (AAP) model of medical home has been redefined as a *patient-centered medical home* and is supported by the Institute of Medicine and the Patient Centered Primary Care Collaborative (PCPCC) and emphasizes quality of care outcomes.

The *pediatric health care/medical home* is a model of care promoting holistic care of children and their families through a collaborative relationship with qualified pediatric health care providers inclusive of nurse practitioners (National Association of Pediatric Nurse Practitioners [NAPNAP], 2009). Exemplary innovative models in pediatric health care/medical home services delivered by nurse practitioners are being implemented in several states. Interventions in successful models must address the concepts of family-centered partnerships, community-based systems, and transitional care from pediatric to adult services (Duderstadt, 2008). Pediatric health care/medical home services have the potential to markedly improve the primary health care infrastructure and health care outcomes in children and adults over time in the U.S.

■ Evidence-Based Clinical Preventive Services and Health Promotion

HEALTH SUPERVISION GUIDELINES

The quality of preventive health care services for children varies greatly, and many children are not receiving the recommended preventive services and developmental surveillance required for health promotion. There are many barriers to effective well-child care—time constraints, low level of reimbursement for preventive care and developmental screening services, and lack of community referral sources to assist children, adolescents, and families. Also, limited training of pediatric health care providers in development surveillance and in emotional and behavioral problems has contributed in some areas to inconsistent quality of preventive health care services affecting children and families.

Improving and strengthening primary care requires a strong evidence-based foundation. Lack of funding and infrastructure to support primary care research stands in sharp contrast to the organized commitment and emphasis on advancing knowledge in disease entities and treatment options. There remains a significant gap between the application of clinical research to strengthen primary care and the science of primary care management focused on single diseases entities. Much of the basis for primary care is not yet evidence based. This gap provides an area of research open to pediatric nurse researchers and other pediatric health care providers trained in clinical research. Increased evidence in the primary health care domain would help to move the public dialogue toward a greater focus on primary prevention and away from a disease-focused health care system.

AAP GUIDELINES

The AAP guides well-child care and published the *Recommendations for Preventive Pediatric Health Care* annually (AAP, 2000) for many years. However, it became clear that the number of recommended health directives for well-child care had far surpassed the time available to pediatric health care providers to meet the expectations of quality care. Recent recommendations from the AAP to improve the efficiency and effectiveness of health promotion and preventive pediatric care have placed a greater emphasis on behavioral and developmental issues. Their recommendations suggest uncoupling the periodicity of well-child visits with the required immunizations and providing greater emphasis on healthy growth and developmental surveillance (Schor, 2004; Tanner et al, 2009). Part of the revision includes basing well-child care on the evidence-based research available on child and family development rather than the periodicity of required immunizations. This will necessitate a revision of the current recommendations that guide practice, which can be found in the *Bright Futures* publication (Hagan et al, 2008).

BRIGHT FUTURES

Bright Futures is a national health promotion initiative dedicated to the principle that "every child deserves to be healthy and that optimal health involves a trusting relationship between the health professional, the child, the family, and the community as partners in health practice" (Hagan et al, 2008, p 1). *Bright Futures* not only helps providers deliver prevention-based, developmentally oriented care but it is also family-focused care and fosters relationships between families, pediatric health care providers, and communities. The parent tools accompanying the current edition of *Bright Futures* empower families with great skills and knowledge to be active partners in the child's healthy growth and development. The complete guide to *Bright Futures* is available to health care providers and to parents at www.brightfutures.org.

Child and Family Health Assessment

CATHERINE E. BURNS

Family-centered, community-based primary care for children is recognized as the best possible practice model for providing health care services to children and their families. The family is the most influential factor in a child's life (American Academy of Pediatrics [AAP], 2003) and its functioning is totally intertwined with the child's health and well-being. However, pediatric primary care providers face significant challenges in implementing family-centered care. At minimum, family-centered care is perceived as time consuming. In addition, families are still too often viewed from a pathology-based model borrowed from psychiatry and psychology, and primary care providers often report feeling inadequate to the task of working with the complex and often stressed families they meet in their practices.

Delivery of family-centered care for children requires the provider to shift focus from child-as-the-unit-of-analysis to family-as-the-unit-of-analysis depending on the problem at hand. Although the child's welfare is ultimately the goal, the family is so integral to a child's well-being that unless the family is healthy, the child cannot achieve true physical, developmental, and psychological health. Moving from child to family and back again during the assessment process is a complex task but an essential one for providing excellent care.

This chapter presents a child assessment model that integrates some family issues and a family assessment model that is useful when greater focus on the family is needed.

The outline for assessment of children in this chapter is consistent with the organization of the entire text in which development, functional health issues, and diseases are the three domains for pediatric practice and are the major units of this book. Each chapter provides comprehensive coverage of topics that are categorized within one of these domains. Throughout the book, family is considered integral to the child's life and care. This chapter provides foundations for an integrated assessment of the child, using a family-centered approach.

■ Foundations for Child and Family Assessment

CHILD HEALTH ASSESSMENT FOUNDATIONS

A careful, complete, and thoughtful assessment of the child's health status is absolutely essential to providing excellent primary health care. This assessment is based on knowledge of child development, family structure and functions, culture, anatomy and physiology, pathophysiology, pharmacology, health care delivery systems, communities, and standards of primary health care for children. The assessment must also be viewed through the lens of the provider's experience to allow the provider to modify perceptions and validate data on the basis of previous work. When providers analyze patient care situations, they are engaged in critical thinking. This chapter cannot teach critical thinking nor does it teach physical assessment. Rather, it provides frameworks for gathering data to facilitate expert decision-making in areas of pediatric practice. It is assumed that the reader knows how to do a complete physical examination and has some experience working with children and families in health care settings. It is also assumed that clinicians have the requisite knowledge in the foundation areas listed previously.

When analyzing patient problems most providers are comfortable with classification of diseases using categories found in the *International Classification of Diseases, edition 9 revised, Clinical Modification* (*ICD-9-CM*) (USDHHS, 2003), including infectious, endocrine, nutritional, metabolic, immunologic, respiratory, and cardiovascular. *ICD-10-CM* will be effective October 2013. Providers consistently record the disease diagnoses they make for problems in these body systems. One reason that providers use this classification system so easily is that the classic health history format drives diagnostic decisions into these categories. Box 2-1 shows this classic health history format.

The classic medical history is written to expand on the chief complaint, which is generally a physical problem. Issues such as nutrition, development, and activities of daily living

BOX 2-1　The Classic Health History

I. Patient-identifying information: name, birth date, sex, address, record number, and name of historian, along with relationship to the patient stated

II. Chief complaint (CC)

III. History of present illness (HPI)

IV. Past medical history (PMH)
   A. Prenatal, natal, postnatal
   B. Past illnesses
   C. Allergies
   D. Accidents
   E. Hospitalizations
   F. Immunization history
   G. Nutrition history
   H. Growth
   I. Development

V. Review of systems (ROS): as found in disease domain database described in Tables 2-3 and 2-4 with the following added:
   A. Psychological—colic, breath-holding, thumb sucking, head banging, fears, tics, behavior disorders, temper tantrums, nail biting, hair pulling, masturbation. Adjustment to home, school, neighborhood. Temperament—activity level, predictability, moods, intensity of reactions, adaptability, initial responses, distractibility. Sleep—amount, habits, problems.

VI. Family history (FH)

VII. Socioeconomic (SE)
   A. Occupations of father and mother
   B. Time spent with child by parents, activities together
   C. Finances—adequacy
   D. Persons in the home
   E. House or apartment living arrangements
   F. General relationship of family members
   G. Community support systems—friends, church, agencies involved with family
   H. Safety precautions

are included, primarily as they relate to various diseases. This classification system works well and has generally been taught to physicians, nurse practitioners (NPs), and other providers. The system fails, however, to provide a framework for integrating the daily living (also called functional health patterns) and developmental issues of children into the problem lists and management plans. Without that framework, primary care providers, especially NPs who emphasize developmental and functional health areas of practice, may fail to clearly identify and document many of the unique contributions they make to child health care. Without that identification, the special aspects of their work with patients remain invisible.

An alternate model is offered in this chapter that integrates the nursing and medical aspects of primary care work conceptually and clinically (see discussion of Box 2-3 later). This assessment model (Burns, 1991, 1992a,b) is based on the assumption that patient problems can be grouped into three distinct domains: developmental problems, functional health problems, and diseases (Box 2-2). Although it was originally developed for NPs, the framework is useful to all pediatric health care providers.

Developmental Problems

This domain includes the long-term issues of development and maturation over the life span. In pediatrics, developmental issues are prominent. The National Survey of Children's

Health estimates that 15.8% of children are at moderate risk for developmental, behavioral, or social delays and another 10.6% are at high risk for similar delays (Child and Adolescent Health Measurement Initiative, 2009). Failing to identify a developmental problem or to plan for its management is as serious as missing diabetes mellitus or a dislocated hip. Physical as well as developmental problems can affect a child's entire future if not remedied or managed to minimize their effects. Clinicians assess for developmental problems in the areas of gross motor, fine motor, speech and language, cognitive, social/emotional, and adaptive behaviors.

Developmental surveillance is considered integral to every pediatrics visit (AAP, 2006). However, Halfon and colleagues (2004) found that developmental assessments were completed for only 57% of children ages 10 to 35 months. Schonwald and colleagues, in a 2009 article, present a study that demonstrates that developmental screening does not change the length of visits and increases parental reports so that they discussed more developmental concerns and had their questions answered. Significant increases in developmental screening and parent reports of quality of care occurred in practices in which extra education related to development was given to providers and additional systems to promote childhood development were instituted (Margolis et al, 2008; McKay, 2006).

Zero to Three has developed a taxonomy of developmental diagnoses (Zero to Three, 2005), which may be a useful resource for developmental problem diagnoses.

Functional Health Problems

Functional health problems are derived from Gordon's functional health patterns (Gordon 1987, 2010) and are incorporated into the international taxonomy of nursing diagnoses (NANDA International, 2009). These patterns provide a way of thinking about the problems that nurses have always managed independently. Other primary care providers are also asked to manage functional health problems of children. These patterns represent the universal health behavior patterns of all humans, regardless of culture, sex, age, or economic status. Gordon's 11 patterns include health beliefs and behavior, nutrition, elimination, activity, sleep, role relationships, coping, self-perception, cognition and perception, sexuality, and values and beliefs. All functional health problems involve the family because the family really is the primary caregiver for infants and children. NPs and other providers become involved when the family's knowledge and experience are insufficient to meet the needs of the child or when the family directly contributes to the child's problems as with the role-relationship problem of child abuse.

Labels for many problems in the functional health domain are found in the NANDA taxonomy terms (NANDA International, 2009), which is expanded and updated every 2 years. Many terms are also found in the *ICD-9-CM* and other taxonomies such as the *International Classification of Sleep Disorders* (American Academy of Sleep Medicine, 1997).

Diseases

Diseases are conditions assessed and managed at the tissue or organ level of analysis. The diagnoses found in the disease domain generally come from the *ICD-9-CM*. Otitis media, streptococcal pharyngitis, and appendicitis are examples of

BOX 2-2   Suggested Integrated Classification System of Diagnoses for Use by Primary Care Providers

Domain I: Development Diagnoses
Cognitive Development
- Cognitive delay
- Learning disorder

Language Development
- Language delay
- Speech delay

Motor Development
- Gross motor delay
- Fine motor delay

Social Development
- Social developmental delay
- Attachment failure

Domain II: Functional Health Diagnoses
Health Perception and Health Management Pattern
- Adjustment impaired
- Decisional conflict
- Health maintenance alteration
- Health-seeking behavior
- Home-care resources inadequate
- Home-maintenance management impaired
- Knowledge deficits
- Noncompliance
- Risk of injury—suffocation, poisoning, trauma, aspiration
- Self-care deficits—dressing, toileting, hygiene
- Skill deficit
- Therapeutic regimen management ineffective—individual or family

Nutritional—Metabolic Pattern
- Anorexia
- Anorexia nervosa
- Breastfeeding ineffective, interrupted, or effective
- Bulimia
- Colic
- Infant-feeding pattern ineffective
- Nausea
- Nutrition alterations less than or more than body requirements
- Swallowing impaired

Elimination Pattern
- Constipation
- Encopresis
- Enuresis
- Incontinence, bowel or urinary

Activity and Exercise Pattern
- Activity intolerance
- Diversional activities deficit
- Fatigue
- Physical mobility impaired

Sleep Pattern
- Sleep pattern disturbance

Cognitive and Perceptual Pattern
- Attention-deficit disorder
- Disorganized infant behavior
- Memory impaired
- Potential for enhanced organized infant behavior
- Sensory-perceptual alteration
  - Blind
  - Deaf

Self-Perception and Self-Concept Pattern
- Body image disturbance
- Personal identity disturbance
- Self-esteem disturbance, chronic or situational

Role Relationships Pattern
- Abuse
- Caregiver role strain
- Communication impaired—verbal
- Family coping ineffective, disabling, compromised, potential for growth
- Family process alteration
- Family process alteration: alcoholism
- Loneliness, risk for
- Parenting alteration
- Parental role conflict
- Risk of alteration in parent-infant-child attachment
- Role performance alteration
- Social interaction impaired
- Social isolation

Sexuality Pattern
- Pregnancy
- Sexual dysfunction
- Sexual pattern alteration

Coping and Stress Tolerance Pattern
- Anxiety
- Comfort alteration
- Coping—individual, ineffective, defensive
- Depression
- Fear
- Grieving—anticipatory, dysfunctional
- Hopelessness
- Ineffective denial
- Pain, chronic
- Posttrauma response
- Powerlessness
- Rape-trauma response
- Self-mutilation risk
- Substance misuse
- Violence potential, self or others

Values and Beliefs Pattern
- Potential for enhanced spiritual well-being
- Spiritual distress

BOX 2-2 Suggested Integrated Classification System of Diagnoses for Use by Primary Care Providers—cont'd

Domain III: Pediatric Disease Diagnoses (Diagnoses included are examples, not an exhaustive list)

Infectious Diseases
- Candidiasis
- Chickenpox
- Chlamydia
- Diarrheal infection
- Giardiasis
- Gonorrhea (or other sexually transmitted disease [STD])

Endocrine, Nutritional, Metabolic, and Immune Diseases
- Diabetes mellitus
- Fluid volume excess or deficit
- Food allergy
- Immunodeficiency disease
- Thyroid disorders

Diseases of Blood and Blood-Forming Organs
- Anemias and red blood cell disorders
- Jaundice
- Leukemia and white blood cell disorders
- Platelet disorders

Neurologic and Sense Organ Diseases
- Central nervous system—epilepsy or seizures, cerebral palsy
- Ear—otitis externa, otitis media, serous otitis
- Eye—amblyopia, conjunctivitis, dacryocystitis, myopia, strabismus
- Macrocephaly, hydrocephaly, microcephaly

Circulatory System Diseases
- Cardiac output decreased
- Congenital heart disease
- Hypertension

Respiratory System Diseases
- Acute nasopharyngitis
- Allergic rhinitis
- Asthma
- Bronchiolitis
- Pharyngitis
- Pneumonia

Digestive System Diseases
- Acute abdomen
- Constipation (not encopresis)
- Diarrhea
- Gastroesophageal reflux disease
- Hernia
- Vomiting

Dental Disorders
- Caries
- Malocclusion
- Oral mucous membrane alteration

Genitourinary System Disorders
- Adhesions
- Cryptorchidism
- Hydrocele
- Hypospadias
- Incontinence
- Urinary tract infection

Gynecologic Disorders
- Menstrual disorder
- Vaginitis

Skin Diseases
- Acne
- Atopic dermatitis
- Cellulitis
- Congenital lesion
- Contact dermatitis
- Folliculitis
- Impetigo
- Nevus
- Seborrhea
- Urticaria

Musculoskeletal Diseases
- Developmental dislocated hip
- Genu varum or valgum
- Internal tibial torsion
- Lordosis
- Metatarsus adductus
- Osgood-Schlatter disease
- Scoliosis
- Strain or sprain

Symptoms, Signs, Ill-Defined Conditions
- Hypotonia
- Jaundice
- Temperature alteration—hypothermia, hyperthermia

Injury and Poisoning
- Abrasion
- Bee sting
- Burn
- Contusion
- Corneal abrasion
- Fracture
- Insect bite
- Sprain or strain
- Injury, high risk for

Environmental
- Exposure to toxin (specify)
- At risk for environmental exposure

Data from Burns C: Development and content validity testing of a comprehensive classification of diagnoses for use by pediatric nurse practitioners, *Nurs Diagn* 2:93-104, 1991; and Burns C: *Development and content validity testing of a comprehensive classification of diagnoses for use by pediatric nurse practitioners,* unpublished doctoral dissertation, University of Oregon, Eugene, 1989.

disease diagnoses. Providers should use the diagnosis that guides understanding of etiology and management.

The *International Classification of Diseases* (USDHHS, 2003) is designed to represent the phenomena of concern to physicians. It is broad and mature in scope. It represents physiologic problems of patients extremely well but includes few labels, or rubrics, for the behavioral, social, and developmental problems that NPs also manage. The *ICD-9-CM* listings are recognized by many insurance carriers for billing purposes and, as such, have become the "currency" for much health care delivery in the U.S., whereas the NANDA nursing diagnoses have not yet achieved that recognition. Fortunately, a variety of diagnoses similar to those in the NANDA classification can be found among the medical listings, thus facilitating reimbursement for management of functional health patterns.

Problem Interactions

The concept of interactions of problems across domains is important to understand. For instance, iron deficiency anemia can be considered a disease if looked at from the effects of lack of iron on heme production, red blood cells, oxygen transport, and cellular metabolism. The clinician can diagnose this disease and prescribe an iron supplement to manage the problem at this physiologic level. However, if the problem is found to be related to a lack of iron in the diet, the provider can choose to intervene at the functional health-nutrition level, call the problem "Nutrition: Less Than Body Requirements for Iron," and teach the family how to increase the selection of iron-rich foods for the table. Iron deficiency has also been shown to cause developmental delays (Glader, 2007). If a goal for the visit is to provide additional support in the school setting, a developmental problem would be diagnosed.

A particular domain can also serve as the context for the problem in another area. For instance, Down syndrome, a chromosomal disorder, can be the cause or context for a cognitive development problem. If the intervention is for cognition, a developmental problem of cognitive delay is listed. Content issues for which the clinician is planning interventions are the diagnoses. The contextual issues are not the diagnoses.

The most important point to remember is that interventions must be based on or derived from diagnoses. A situation should never arise in which the provider intervenes without explicit reasons for doing so. The reasons are stated as diagnoses, either actual or potential, and enumerated in the problem list. The preventive work (i.e., to avoid potential problems) done by clinicians also needs to be identified. Diagnoses, in addition to interventions, must be recorded. The *ICD-9-CM* provides the lists of reimbursable diagnoses and the CPT codes provide the therapeutic intervention codes. Some common CPT codes are listed inside the back cover of this book.

FAMILY ASSESSMENT FOUNDATIONS
The Family's Role in Health Care of Children

However daunting the perceived barriers to family-centered care seem to be, investing in family assessment and management is essential in contemporary pediatric primary care practice. Duffy (1988) wrote that understanding family health promotion begins with understanding family dynamics. Research has repeatedly demonstrated that a mother's level of education, her beliefs and attitudes about health, and her own health practices have significant influences on the health status of her children. Parental stress and mental health problems such as depression affect health care for children. Nationally, nearly 13% of children live in households with at least one parent experiencing high stress. Children in those families are more likely to seek emergency care for their children rather than using a medical home for care and experience more injuries (Brown and Wissow, 2008; Minkovitz et al, 2005; Phelan et al, 2007; Raphael et al, 2010). Maternal depression in the first year of her infant's life has been associated with poorer caregiving and resulting poorer language development at 3 years of age (Stein et al, 2008) and maternal depressive symptoms were predictive of asthma symptoms in inner-city African-American families (Otsuki et al, 2010). As fathers become increasingly involved in their children's health care, questions about relationships between characteristics of fathers and family health behavior are being raised. Fathers, too, need to be involved with the health care of their children. It is not surprising that parents who believe that they can improve their health status by practicing health promotion behaviors tend to raise children who share similar beliefs.

Research has provided definitive evidence that children, from birth through adolescence need nurturing and attention from the significant adults in their lives. These adults most often are the child's birth or adoptive parents, but they may also be grandparents, extended family members, or foster parents. Evidence is strong that when children are raised without this consistent, affectionate attention and without sensitive interactions with a caring adult, the results can be devastating for both child and society (Kazak et al, 2010). For example, family cohesion, beyond dyadic family relationships, is related to adolescent hostility; the functioning of the family as a whole affects adolescent behavior and emotional health (Richmond and Stocker, 2006). In contrast, when a parent or another significant adult responds consistently and sensitively to a child's needs, such as a need to play, to eat, to sleep, to be comforted, or to be left alone, the child is likely to grow up competent to initiate and build strong, nurturing relationships. Although inadequate or poor parenting is linked in the literature to factors such as poverty, substance abuse, and minimal education, research suggests that a poor "fit" between a child and a significant adult can occur in any family, including those in which the adults are well educated, socially competent, and economically successful. Issues of family relationships and family disruption are discussed in Chapter 17 more fully.

Family Assessment Basic Elements

Family assessment begins with the assumption that families are central to and inseparable from the health of children. It is based on a family health promotion framework that assumes that the vast majority of family members are competent, want to do what is best for their children, and desire to be active participants in their children's health care. Family assessment in primary care practice with children requires attention to family structure, family life cycle stage, family functioning, and social network. In other words, a basic family assessment addresses characteristics of the family, transitions that the family is experiencing, how family members interact and get things done, what they believe and value, and how they interact with the community.

It is important to recognize that providers' own definitions of family and healthy family functioning are culturally and temporally bound, determine who is and who is not family, and can profoundly affect assessment, treatment, and outcomes. Providers might find it useful to periodically examine their own assumptions and beliefs regarding families and use the knowledge gained to foster increased sensitivity and openness to the rich diversity that their clients present.

Legal definitions of family usually address bonds of blood, marriage, and adoption. A significant number of contemporary families do not fit such restrictive definitions. To address this reality, Whall (1986, p 240) defined family as "a self-identified group of two or more individuals whose association is characterized by special terms, who may or may not be related by bloodlines or law, but who function in such a way that they consider themselves to be a family." Wherever practitioners' personal definitions might fall on a continuum of inclusiveness, it is imperative that they know and understand the implications of that definition in practice.

Essential components of the assessment of the child's family are discussed later.

Family Structure and Roles. Assessment of a family's structure and roles includes the composition of the family or household, demographic data, intergenerational data, and information about family roles. Implicit in the data is the way the family defines itself and how the family gets its work done.

There are many types of families, including two-parent, single-parent, grandparent, or other family member–headed, blended or stepfamilies, foster, gay, extended families, and others. Specific issues for various family types are addressed in the section on targeted assessments later in this chapter with the genogram and ecomap and in Chapter 17 as well.

Family Life Cycle. Family life cycle assessment includes data on the present family life cycle stage (such as a family with young children), family life cycle transitions or developmental crises (such as serious illness of a frail, elderly grandparent), and family life cycle events that are untimely or "out of sync" (such as the terminal illness of a young wife and mother).

Family Functioning. Healthy family functioning should result in what Terkelsen, in his classic paper, called the "good-enough family" (Terkelsen, 1980). Families have both strengths and limitations, but the majority of families are able to meet most of their members' needs most of the time. This is a hopeful stance, one that allows for the less than perfect family to feel successful and empowered. Family resilience is a helpful concept referring to healthy family functioning (Benzies and Mychasiuk, 2009).

Characteristics of healthy family functioning have been identified by a number of researchers. Open communication, mutual respect and support, differentiation, shared problem-solving, shared decision-making, flexibility, enhancement of members' personal growth, sense of play and humor, and a shared value of service to others are some of these assets (Curran, 1983; deChesnay, 1986). The American Academy of Pediatrics (AAP) states that a child will thrive best when cared for by two mutually committed parents who respect and support each other, who have adequate social and financial resources, and who both are actively engaged in the child's upbringing. Characteristics of the successful family are described by the AAP as being cohesive, enduring, and mutually appreciative. Such families communicate effectively and often, adapt to changing circumstances, spend time together, are committed to the family, and embrace a common religious or spiritual orientation (AAP, 2003).

Protective factors for family resilience include individual, family, and community factors. Some individual factors include internal locus of control, emotional regulation, effective coping skills, and others. Some family factors include structure, stable partner relations, cohesion, social support, and adequate income, while some supportive community factors include community involvement, peer acceptance, supportive mentors, a safe neighborhood; and access to quality school, daycare, and health care (Benzies and Mychasiuk, 2009).

Family Social Network. Positive social support exists when the family feels emotional support, tangible help, and informed (Benzies and Mychasiuk, 2009). The family's social network includes those individuals, activities, agencies, and institutions that have the potential to support, harm, or drain energy from the family. Assessing the family's relationships with extended family, friends, and the community provides information on which to base recommendations and further assessment. The ecomap provides an efficient way to assess family social networks.

Parenting Issues for Different Family Structures

Family-related factors, such as the composition and structure of the family, socioeconomic status, and health status, have the potential to influence the health and well-being of children and adolescents in significant ways. Although much about family assessment remains constant across families, it is useful to pay attention to some of the unique potential family variations. Chapter 17 provides a broader discussion of family issues for different variations that must be considered in the assessment process. Some of these family structures and family issues include:

- Two-parent families
- Working parents and child care
- Poverty and families
- Single-parent families
- Displaced and homeless families
- Blended families
- Adolescent parents
- Gay and lesbian parent families
- Adoptive parent families
- Grandparents raising grandchildren
- Foster parent families
- Families raising children with special needs
  - Multiple births
  - Premature infants
  - Children with special needs

Some assessment questions that should be considered for these family situations are found in Table 2-1 later in the chapter.

◼ The Environment for Data Collection

SETTING UP THE ASSESSMENT ENVIRONMENT

Health care is a family event in pediatrics, and pediatric primary health care is delivered in many settings, not just examination rooms in outpatient clinics. Wherever the patient and the family are to be cared for, privacy must be ensured. People should have places to sit down, and the room in which the examination is conducted should be well lighted and allow the patient to lie down comfortably. The examiner must be able to work comfortably, too. The health care provider should sit down during the history to make data collection a conversation, to equalize the status of clients and examiner, and to help clients feel that they have time to talk. Sitting also helps the provider conserve energy for a busy day. The environment must be safe, given the developmental ages of the children to be cared for, and should present an atmosphere of warmth and welcome.

COMMUNICATION WITH CHILDREN AND FAMILIES

"Communication is the most common 'procedure' in medicine" (Levetown and AAP Committee on Bioethics, 2008, p 1441). In an excellent discussion by these authors, communication is identified as critical to the provision of health care. It must be responsive to the needs of the child and family within the context of their own dynamics. It is essential to diagnosis and successful treatment planning, and results in better patient outcomes including physical and psychosocial benefits, increased patient satisfaction, patient knowledge, adherence, functional status, and adaptation to challenging situations. "Poor communication, on the other hand, can prompt lifelong anger and regret, can result in compromised outcomes for the patient and family, and can have medicolegal consequences for the practitioner" (Levetown and AAP Committee on Bioethics, 2008, p 1441).

The three elements they identify as essential to excellent communication are as follows:
- Communication needs to provide information.
- Communication should be sensitive interpersonally, with affective behaviors indicating the provider's attention to and interest in the parents' and child's feelings and concerns.
- Communication should help to build a partnership among the three parties, allowing discussion of concerns, perspectives, and suggestions from all.

Health care communication is different from normal discourse because very personal issues are discussed—hopes and fears; sexuality; mental health issues; painful issues such as abuse, drug use, school and personal failure; and serious or terminal illness. Communication involves both cognitive and affective elements. When drug use, alcohol consumption, and smoking were addressed with mothers, parent-provider relationships were positively affected (Garg et al, 2010). Similarly, discussion of maternal stress also results in greater maternal satisfaction with care (Brown and Wissow, 2008).

The pediatric health history has several unique aspects. First, the participants in the conversation include the child, caregiver, and provider, more than just the patient and provider as in the adult care model. Second, the topics emphasized vary significantly depending on the child's developmental stage. Third, the process of communication with the child and the extent to which he or she is involved with health care decisions varies with his or her age. Those readers with an adult health care background need to especially heed these differences.

Families want to be addressed by their last names, shake hands with the provider, and have the provider introduce himself or herself (Amer and Fischer, 2009). For young children, the conversation time gives them the opportunity to become familiar with the examiner and setting, which is essential for cooperation when needed. Remember that young children are learning the "script" for health care visits. The visit should help them learn a script that is understandable and not too stressful. When the script is to be varied (e.g., no immunizations this visit), alert them to the change with cues and explanations for the new experiences of this visit and the likelihood that the new script will be repeated at future visits.

The provider is also observing parent-child interactions during the visit. For example, are the parents responding to their baby? Do the parents contribute to the school-age child's self-esteem? Cues to mental health problems in any family member or the child should be addressed.

For adolescents, the history can be started with the parents and teen together; however, they then need to separate, with the provider getting information from the parents and the teen independently. Interviewing teens requires patience as they are learning to take responsibility for their own health care. Interactions will change as teens mature developmentally or as the situation is modified.

Data can be collected verbally, through record review, via written forms completed by the family, or through a combination of these methods. It might not be practical for data to be fully collected on the first visit; rather, the collection can be staged according to the visit priorities. When time with patients is limited, it is common to ask new families to come early for their first appointment to complete a written history before meeting the clinician. Notation of any missing data should be made so that further baseline data can be collected at the next visit.

In 2008, more than 23% of children in the U.S. lived in immigrant families. In these families, 81% of children spoke English very well; however, only 37% of their parents spoke English very well (Mather, 2009). Thus, interpreter services must be available if the clinician and family are not fluent in each other's languages. These services are mandated by law. Use of family members as interpreters is not recommended. Family members may try to protect the patient by hiding important information. Legally, the provider may be at risk if information was not transmitted correctly or completely either to or from the clinician (Lehna, 2005).

▓ The Database

THE CHILD HEALTH HISTORY

It is said that 80% of diagnoses are made on the basis of the history. The physical examination only provides a partial view of the situation as it is at the moment. It is often a cloudy picture because the body frequently responds similarly to different assaults. It is the history of the problem—its onset, duration, progress, associated symptoms, meaning, and effects on daily living—that brings the health care provider to an understanding in sufficient depth to choose appropriate management. Functional health and developmental problems present the same issues for the provider. A thorough, thoughtful history is essential.

The database described in this chapter summarizes the child health history and physical examination and the family assessment. The model presented uses a basic problem-oriented format that begins with subjective data (the history), moves to objective data (the physical examination, laboratory, and test data), then lists the problems by domain (identified through

BOX 2-4 Problem-Oriented History for Adolescents

I. Database—Contextual and Family Information
  A. With Whom Do You Live?
  B. In the Past Year Have There Been Any Changes in Your Immediate Family, Such As:
  Marriage, separation, divorce
  Serious illness or injury
  Loss of job
  Move or change of address
  Change of school
  Births, deaths
  Other (explain):

  C. What Languages are Spoken in Your Home?

II. Disease Database
  A. Chief Complaint
  B. Past Medical History
    1. In the past year have you had any injury or illness that made you miss school or cut down on activities, or that required medical care?
    2. Have you been hospitalized or used Emergency Department Services in the past year?
    3. Do you have any illnesses or medical conditions?
    4. Are you taking any medications?
    5. Have you been exposed to tuberculosis in the past year?
    6. Have you stayed overnight in a homeless shelter, jail, or detention center in the past year?
    7. Girls only: Have you had a period? Date of last one. Do you do breast self-examinations?
    8. Boys only: Have you had wet dreams? Do you do testicular self-examinations?

  C. Review of Systems
    1. Do you have any questions or concerns about any of the following?
    Height or weight
    Blood pressure
    Headaches and migraines
    Eyes or vision
    Hearing, ears or earaches
    Nose
    Frequent colds
    Mouth and teeth (frequency of tooth brushing, flossing)
    Neck and back
    Chest pain
    Coughing and wheezing
    Breasts
    Heart
    Stomach
    Nausea and vomiting
    Diarrhea and constipation
    Skin (rash, acne, sore, use of sunscreen)
    Muscle or joint pain
    Frequent or painful urination
    Sexual organs or genitals
    Menstruation or periods
    Sexual activity
    Future plans or job
    Physical or sexual abuse
    Masturbation
    Cancer or dying
    Other (explain):

III. Functional Health Database
  A. Health Maintenance and Health Perception
    1. Do you usually wear a helmet for inline skating, bicycle, skateboard, motorcycle, or all-terrain vehicle use?
    2. Do you usually wear a seat belt when riding in a car, truck, or van?
    3. In the past year, have you been in a car when the driver has been drinking or using drugs?
    4. Do you use electric tools or heavy equipment at work or home?
    5. Do you have questions or concerns about preventing accidents or injuries?

  B. Nutrition
    1. Do you eat from the four food groups almost every day?
    2. Do you have any diet, food, or appetite concerns?
    3. Are you eating in secret?
    4. Are you satisfied with your eating patterns?
    5. Do you prefer a change in your current weight?
    6. Have you tried to lose weight or control weight by vomiting, taking diet pills or laxatives, or starving yourself?
    7. Do you have concerns about your weight?

  C. Activities
    1. Do you watch television or play video games more than 2 hours per day?
    2. Are you involved with exercises that make you sweat and breathe hard at least three times per week?
    3. What do you do after school?
    4. Do you have physical problems that limit your exercise?
    5. Do you have questions or concerns about exercise or physical activity?

  D. Sleep
    1. Do you have trouble sleeping?
    2. Do you have trouble with tiredness?

  E. Elimination Habits
    1. Do you sometimes wet the bed?

  F. Role Relationships
    1. Do you have at least one friend you really like and feel you can talk to?
    2. Do your parents or guardian usually listen to you and take your feelings seriously?
    3. Do you and your parents or guardian do things together on a regular basis, such as eating meals, attending religious activities, performing chores or errands, playing sports, or watching television?
    4. Is there a lot of tension or conflict in your home?
    5. Do you have questions or concerns about family or friends?

  G. Coping, Temperament, and Discipline
    1. Alcohol
    In the past year, did you or friends get drunk or very high on alcoholic beverages?
    Have you ever consumed alcohol and then done any of the following: driven a vehicle, gone swimming or boating, gotten in a fight, used tools or equipment, done something you later regretted?
    Have you been criticized or gotten in trouble because of drinking?
    Do you have any questions or concerns about alcohol?

Continued

BOX 2-4   Problem-Oriented History for Adolescents—cont'd

2. Drugs

Do you or your friends ever use marijuana or street drugs?

Do you ever use nonprescription drugs or drugs prescribed for someone else to get to sleep, stay awake, calm down, get high, or enhance your sports performance?

Have you ever used steroids without a physician telling you to do so?

Do you have any questions or concerns about drugs or drug use?

3. Tobacco

Do you or your friends ever smoke cigarettes or use smokeless tobacco?

Does anyone you live with smoke cigarettes or use smokeless tobacco?

Do you have any questions or concerns about cigarettes or other tobacco products?

4. Emotions

Have you had fun during the past 2 weeks?

In general are you happy with the way things are going for you these days?

During the past few weeks, have you often felt sad or down with nothing to look forward to?

Have you ever seriously thought about killing yourself, made a plan to kill yourself, or actually tried to kill yourself?

Do you think counseling would help you or someone in your family?

Do you have any questions or concerns about physical, sexual, or emotional abuse?

5. Weapons and violence

Do you or does anyone you live with have a gun, rifle, shotgun, or other firearm in your home?

In the past year, have you ever carried a gun, knife, razor blade, club, or other weapon?

Have you been in a physical fight during the past 3 months?

Are guns or violence a problem in your neighborhood?

Have you ever witnessed a violent act?

When you are angry, do you ever get violent?

Do you have any questions or concerns about violence or your safety?

Has anyone threatened to harm you in the last year?

H. Cognitive and Perceptual Problems

1. In general do you like school? Why?
2. Are your grades this year better or worse than the year before? What are your usual grades?
3. Have you ever had to repeat a grade in school?
4. Do you cut classes or skip school?
5. How many days of school have you missed this year?
6. Have you ever been suspended or dropped out of school?
7. Do you have any questions or concerns about school or your learning?

I. Self-Perception and Self-Concept

1. Do you have any concerns about the size or shape of your body or your physical appearance?
2. What do you like about yourself?
3. What do you do best?
4. If you could, what would you change about your life or yourself?

J. Sexual and Menstrual

1. Do you date?
2. Do you or your friends have sexual intercourse or oral or anal sex?
3. Do you think you might be gay, lesbian, or bisexual?
4. Have you ever been told that you have a sexually transmitted disease, such as gonorrhea, genital herpes, chlamydia, trichomonas, syphilis, hepatitis, genital warts, AIDS, or HIV infection?
5. Do you have any questions or concerns about sex or relationships?
6. Are you worried about getting pregnant (girls) or do you worry about getting someone pregnant (boys)?
7. Have you ever been forced to do something sexual that you did not want to do?
8. Do you practice abstinence?
9. Do you use a birth control method? If so, which one(s)?
10. Do you want information or supplies to prevent pregnancy or sexually transmitted diseases, including HIV?

K. Values and Beliefs and Religious Orientation

1. Are you involved with any religious groups or activities on a regular basis?
2. Do you have any strong ethical, moral, or religious beliefs?

IV. Development Database

Throughout the history, listen for data that allow you to assess the following areas (see Chapter 8).

A. Motor Development

1. All teens should be active and skilled in a variety of physical activities and sports.
2. Fine motor development should also be mature. Special arts or crafts or occupational activities may be learned.

B. Cognitive Development

1. Early adolescents are still concrete and generally present rather than future oriented. Questions can be answered quite literally.
2. Middle adolescents can use and understand if-then statements. They are able to understand long-term consequences and think of the future. They might challenge many ideas and rules with their newfound skills in logic and reasoning.
3. Late adolescents are able to consider options before making decisions, engage in sophisticated moral reasoning, and use principles to guide their decisions.

C. Social Development

1. Early adolescents are egocentric in thinking. They can vacillate between childish and mature behavior, especially around their parents. Their peers are usually of the same sex. Group activities are the norm.
2. Middle adolescents are concerned with their identity within society and less concerned with their sexual identity unless they are struggling with recognizing their homosexuality. They tend to distance themselves from parents, spend less time at home, and increasingly challenge parental control. Cliques or friends prevail, with only a few close friends. Physical intimacy can occur during this stage, and romantic partners are common.

BOX 2-4 Problem-Oriented History for Adolescents—cont'd

3. Late adolescents have distanced themselves from parents and then reestablished relationships with family on a new basis of independence. Romantic and emotional intimacy appears.

D. School and Vocational Development

1. Early adolescents are usually adjusting to the expectations of middle school. Setting priorities and completing homework independently can be a challenge. Future goals are often unrealistic and change frequently.

2. Middle adolescents are entering high school and beginning to develop an awareness that their performance in school will affect their future options for work or college. They do not usually have specific ideas about future vocations in mind.

3. Late adolescents are making decisions about vocations, college, working, or entering the military.

Adapted from American Medical Association, Department of Adolescent Health: *Guidelines for adolescent preventive services (GAPS) user's manual*, Chicago, 1994, American Medical Association.

reader a sense of the probability that the history is accurate, complete, and from a knowledgeable source.

The Database-Subjective Information
Chief Complaint and History of Present Problem

- *Concerns:* The health care visit should begin with open-ended questions to allow the child and family to voice their concerns. What brings the child to the clinic today? The chief complaint is a brief statement of the problem and its duration. Remember that new concerns can arise at any point during the visit. Agendas can be hidden or unconscious. The chief complaint or complaints can involve disease, the functional health pattern, or development, and the problem may lie primarily with either the child or family.

- *Present problem history:* For each concern, a chronologic description should be made that includes a symptom analysis (i.e., onset, duration, characteristics or symptoms, exposure to illnesses or other causative factors, similar problems in other family members or neighbors, previous episodes of similar illnesses or symptoms, previous diagnostic measures, pertinent negative data, things that have been tried in attempts to manage the concern and their success, and the meaning of the concern for the family and child). (See Box 2-5 for symptom analysis.)

Even though the patient comes in for a specific problem, always ask some screening questions that tap into the other domains of the history—disease, functional health, and developmental. At visits for minor illnesses, health promotion and disease prevention issues should be considered in addition to the problem at hand. An immunization history, if appropriate, should be completed at every visit.

Disease Domain Database
Past medical history:

- *Prenatal:* Planned pregnancy? When did prenatal care begin? What was the mother's health during pregnancy? Drug, alcohol, and tobacco use? Illnesses and medications? Weight gain? Accidents? (With age and history of a healthy baby, these sections may become less significant.)

- *Perinatal:* Where was the baby born and who delivered the infant? Duration and process of labor? Vaginal or cesarean delivery and process? Infant response to labor and delivery (breathing, crying)? Resuscitation needed? Apgar scores? Birthweight, length, and head circumference? Gestational age? Neonatal course: infections or other health problems, physiologic stabilization, feeding, responsiveness?

BOX 2-5 Symptom Analysis

1. Onset—initial and episodic; date and time, sudden or gradual, setting
2. Location of pain—local, radiation, generalized, superficial, or deep
3. Duration—how long, has it eased, gotten worse?
4. Characteristics and course:
   - Symptom quality: nature of symptoms
   - Symptom quantity: severity, frequency, volume, number, size or extent, degree of functional impairment
   - Course: continuous or intermittent, pattern of variation
5. Activating (precipitating) and aggravating factors
6. Relieving factors
7. Tests and treatment, including complementary therapies: what, when, where, who, and results, including complications and sequelae
8. The meaning of the symptoms to patient and family and patient's reactions to symptoms

Jaundice? Weight at discharge? Hospital duration? Neonatal follow-up over the first few weeks? (Again, with age and health, this section is given less attention.)

- *Past disease profile:* What health problems has the child experienced, and what have the outcomes been? Who has provided care? Infectious diseases?

- *Other current health problems (not related to the chief complaint):* What problems does the child have now? What was the date of onset? Who is the principal health care provider for each problem, and what is the current status (e.g., medications, awaiting surgery, problem in remission)?

- *Operations, hospitalizations, emergency department visits:* Has the child been hospitalized for any reason? Why, when, where, outcomes? Response to hospitalization? Problems resolved? Emergency department visits? Why, when, and outcomes?

- *Injuries:* What significant injuries has the child experienced? What care was needed, was care sought at emergency department(s), and does the child have any sequelae?

- *Allergies:* Allergies to foods, medications, or environmental factors? How are the allergies manifested? When did the allergies develop? What care is given?

- *Growth:* What has the child's growth pattern for height, weight, and head circumference been? (Always plot growth data and body mass index [BMI] on a growth grid to assess progress.) Is the child similar in size to peers? Are clothing sizes changing? Has growth been a worry for the child or family?
- *Immunizations and laboratory tests:* Obtain a record with dates for all immunizations received in the past. Reactions? Blood tests and screening tests?
- *Medications:* Is the child taking any medications (prescription drugs, over-the-counter agents, or folk remedies)? What? Why? How much? Responses to the medication?

Review of systems: Remember that this section documents the history of body systems, not the physical assessment findings. The goal is to seek information about all the body systems that may be related to the present problem or the patient's general health status.

- *General:* Is the child considered to be well, happy, and developing normally?
- *Skin:* History of birthmarks, lesions, or skin conditions including hair and nails?
- *Head:* Head trauma? Head growth—microcephaly, macrocephaly? Headaches?
- *Eyes, ears, nose, throat:* Vision and eye problems? Hearing and ear problems? Nose—discharge or bleeding episodes, breathing interference? Throat problems or infections?
- *Respiratory:* Breathing problems? Respiratory infections? Blue spells? Cough? Snoring at night or obstructive sleep apnea?
- *Cardiovascular:* Heart murmur history? Cyanosis? Blood pressure problems? Activity intolerance? Syncope?
- *Gastrointestinal:* Infections, diarrhea, constipation, vomiting, or reflux? Structural problems? Anal itching or fissures? Stomachaches? Weight loss?
- *Genitourinary:* Infections, discharges? Structural problems? Stream appearance? Frequency or burning?
- *Gynecologic:* Menarche and menstrual history including length of menses, frequency of cycle, cramps, and clots? Vaginal discharge or bleeding? Itching?
- *Musculoskeletal:* Movement or structural problems? Broken bones or joint sprains? Joint inflammation?
- *Neurologic:* Seizures? Movement disorders? Tremors? Tics? Loss-of-consciousness episodes? Headaches?
- *Endocrine:* Problems with growth or pubescence?
- *Hematologic:* Anemia history or symptoms? Blood transfusions? Bleeding disorders?
- *Dentition:* Number of teeth and eruption pattern? Dental trauma? Dental care? Use of fluoride? Teeth brushing? Toothaches? Use of appliances?

Family history of diseases: Classically the three-generation pedigree is used to map out risks for genetic diseases in families, but can be used more broadly to detect conditions with modifiable risk factors. In a broader form, the pedigree is also a genogram (Wattendorf and Hadley, 2005). The genogram is described in more detail later in this chapter. Families can use checklists to note conditions or construct a pedigree online (www.hhs.gov/familyhistory). Now that the human genome has been mapped out, genetic diseases are receiving more attention, making the three-generation genogram an important component of the health history (Maradiegue and Edwards, 2006).

- *Mother and father:* Ages and health history.
- *Mother's pregnancy history:* Number of pregnancies, births, status of offspring.
- *Familial diseases:* Age, sex, and health status of each family member. Familial and communicable diseases, such as diabetes, epilepsy, tuberculosis, hypertension or heart disease, cancer, sickle cell anemia, birth defects, known genetic disorders?
- *Genogram or pedigree:* Draw out a genogram of the family members, including sex, age, and health status of each member. (See Chapter 40 for pedigree notations.)

Environmental history: This section is used to consider toxic exposures. What foods does the child eat and how are they prepared? What is the quality of the child's living environment(s)—water and air quality? Pesticides used? Are chemicals or heavy metals stored in or near the home? Has the child been exposed to tobacco smoke or lead? Exposure? What are the noise levels in the child's environment?

Functional Health Domain Database. The questions in this section are organized by functional health patterns. This text devotes an entire chapter to each of the 11 patterns, including assessment and management of identified problems.

Health maintenance and health perceptions: All people take steps to influence and protect their health. These choices include selection of health care providers, use of safety devices, learning how to take care of oneself, and daily care of the body. Problems identified might include health-seeking behavior, altered health maintenance, or noncompliance with a preventive or adaptive health care regimen. Usual data include the following:

- Usual primary care provider: last visit?
- Dentist: last visit?
- Child's self-care or caregiver needs for more knowledge of caregiving?
- Health care recommendations that the family chooses not to or is unable to follow?
- Safety measures used: Car seats or seat belts? Smoke and carbon monoxide alarms? Window screens? Home safety measures? Pools? Firearms in the home? Helmet use?
- Routine health promotion regimens?
- Home and health management resource issues for the chronically ill or handicapped child? Home nursing? Equipment needs? Transportation needs?

Nutrition: Quality and quantity of the daily diet and the processes of feeding and swallowing, in addition to data to support diagnoses, such as nutrition, less than or greater than body requirements; anorexia; bulimia; impaired swallowing; and breastfeeding issues would be found in this section.

- Daily diet: Breakfast, lunch, snacks, and dinner? Aversions and preferences?
- Cultural patterns related to nutritional preferences and eating?
- Supplements and vitamins?
- Feeding patterns: Mealtimes and snack times? Feeding strategies? Self-feeding skills?
- Breastfeeding and bottle-feeding issues?
- Nutritional restrictions or special needs: calories, other?
- Satisfaction with weight?
- Difficulties chewing or swallowing? Reflux?

Activities: Physical mobility and the diversional and occupational activities of daily life should be described here.

- Amount, timing, and types of physical activities? Other play opportunities and activities?

- Television and computer or electronic games time?
- Reading time?
- Sports, organized activities, and hobbies of older children and adolescents?
- Activity limitations caused by health problems?
- Special equipment used or needed to support mobility?

Sleep: Sleep and rest patterns are described here. Hours? Disturbances for the child or family? Sleep aids? Sleep position for infants? Signs of sleepiness?

Elimination: Problems of elimination can be analyzed at the physiologic level of the genitourinary or gastrointestinal systems or in terms of daily living patterns. Enuresis and encopresis are daily living problems (bowel and bladder habits) that fall in this area. Physiologically, the child is well, but the elimination habits are problematic.

- Urinary patterns: Bed-wetting? Toilet training? Voiding schedule?
- Bowel patterns: Constipation or soiling? Stooling patterns? Toilet training?

Role relationships: Role relationships include family relationships and relationships with peers and friends in the community. Both family and individual diagnoses need to be considered here. Family coping, family process alteration, parenting alteration, abuse, and social interaction or isolation can be addressed. This section assesses family functioning in greater depth than the introductory family functioning section of the history.

- Family interactions: Between parents? Parents and children? With other family members?
- Parenting style and activities?
- Peers and social supports for the child and family? Special adults in the child's life?
- Communication with and by the child: Verbal? Nonverbal?
- School performance for school-age children and teens.
- Concerns that anyone has abused the child.

Coping and temperament, mental health, and discipline issues: People select and use a variety of coping strategies in their daily lives. Temperament is also important to understand child behavior and likely responses to the environment. Discipline strategies used in families are important to identify. Anxiety, fear, hopelessness, grief, powerlessness, substance abuse, pain, and potential for violence might be identified diagnoses.

- Stressors for the child and family? Losses?
- Coping strategies of the child and caregivers?
- Use of alcohol or drugs?
- Temperament characteristics of the child and the "fit" with other family members?
- Problem behavior, discipline strategies used and their outcomes?
- Indications of depression, suicide, violent behavior, anxiety?

Cognitive and perceptual: Cognitive or perceptual problems are identified here. Attention-deficit disorder is an example.

- Hearing or vision problems?
- Learning disorders or attention problems?
- Adaptations made at home and school to assist the child, especially for problems of comprehension?

Self-perception or self-concept: Personal role identity, body image, and self-esteem are issues identified in this functional health domain.

- Satisfaction with self?
- Feelings of depression?

Sexuality: All people have sexuality issues that affect their lives. Within their sexual preferences and habits, problems are identified when these patterns are interrupted or viewed as problematic by the client or family. Pregnancy, viewed from the psychosocial perspective, is also a sexual issue that should be explored.

- Sexual habits?
- Sexual relationships?
- Development of sexual identity?

Values and beliefs: This last section explores spiritual patterns and personal values and beliefs that affect the child's health.

- Involvement with church?
- Religious rituals?
- Sense of alienation?
- Sense of spiritual meaning in one's life?
- Values the family wants to impart to their children?

Development Domain Database. The levels of different aspects of development are assessed and documented in this area. Both past milestones and current functioning are important. Developmental surveillance is expected at all visits, and screening tests should be administered periodically to infants and young children (AAP, 2006).

- *Motor landmarks*–gross and fine motor: sitting, standing, walking, use of hands and arms, and so on
- *Language landmarks*—words, sentences, intelligibility, comprehension
- *Personal and social*—play, attachment, self-care, peer and family relationships
- *Scholastic grade and progress*

Family Database. The intent of this section is to identify basic family, daycare, school, work, or community agency factors that form the context of the child's life and need to be considered in planning care. The provider also needs to shift to the family-as-unit-of-care here to identify family problems—another level of issues. Family problems might include impaired communication among family members, social isolation, family violence, impaired parents, alterations in parenting, caregiver role strain, and others. This section of the history could be obtained using a genogram and/or ecomap format, both of which are discussed in greater detail later or, at least, provide preliminary data if those assessment strategies are used. In general, families appreciate concerns and inquiries related to the health of their family although, in one study, mothers preferred to answer domestic violence questions away from the children (Zink et al, 2006). Providers should not hesitate to ask questions about the family.

Family Composition and Structure. The provider needs to know who makes up the family as the family defines it. Who lives in the home—family and others? How are they related? What is the meaning of the family structure to the child? In other words, does the child feel like a member of the family—cared for and supported? Does the family feel whole or is it missing members from the child's or another's point of view?

Current Family Situation. An understanding of the current family situation is helpful, especially if a significant period has elapsed since the child and family were last seen. Understanding changes that the family is facing and where they are in the family life cycle is also important. Are there family problems that put the family at risk—"out of sync" issues, such as a seriously ill parent, young teen parent, or grandparenting by an ill elder?

Extended Family Context. Data about the extended family may not seem relevant to parents or children, but patterns that can have an effect on children's health often do not become evident until this kind of intergenerational mapping is done. This more extensive mapping of a family may be used when the clinical picture includes conflicting information or when the effectiveness of a prevention activity is a concern. For example, knowing that both the mother and grandmother of the young adolescent in your office became pregnant at 14 and dropped out of high school may be helpful in deciding how to best use a brief visit.

"It would help me to help your child if I knew more about your child's grandparents, aunts, uncles, and other relatives. Let's begin with your mother's family...."

Demographic Data. Demographic data include dates of birth, death, adoption, marriage, separation, divorce, significant illness, and major family events; culture and ethnicity; religion; education; and occupations. The provider can probe for more information about specific data as they appear to be significant in a given situation. For example, faith and strength of adherence to a specific religion may have an unexpected effect on care decisions for a child. Disagreement about adherence within a family may result in mixed messages and uneven follow-through with a treatment plan.

Historical Perspective. Knowledge of the timing and repetition of significant family events or behavior may be helpful. For example, adolescent pregnancy, alcohol abuse, dropping out of high school, and suicide may be patterns of behavior in a family's intergenerational history.

If gaps in data become evident, they need to be explored. It is also helpful to keep in mind events external to the family that may have influenced family choices. For example, the years of conflict in Iraq and Afghanistan have interrupted many life plans. Immigration, voluntary or forced, can have an effect on family health status. Natural disasters such as floods, hurricanes, and droughts have changed family histories and the health status of family members.

Family Relationships and Roles. In developing the database, providers can begin to probe for family relationships and roles. For example, understanding how parents make decisions and solve problems can be useful in helping parents improve health promotion practices or to recognize the positive actions they take with their families.

- Primary caregiver? Who helps? Stresses of caregiver: is the caregiver well both physically and emotionally?
- Does anyone require more attention from the primary caregiver than the patient?
- How much time do parents and child spend in the home together?
- How are family decisions made? How are arguments worked out?
- What is the relationship between caregiver and partner?
- Do the family members consider household relationships to provide a safe environment for all?

Family Social and Community Network. What community resources and family support systems are used? What agencies work with this child and family? Where does the child go for daycare, school, work (teens), and what is the quality of each setting?

Family Environment and Resources. What is the home environment: apartment, home, or farm? Fenced yard or perceived unsafe neighborhood? Family financial resources: health insurance, money for necessities? What are the sources of money for the family—jobs or government assistance? Family stresses over resources and home environment?

Genograms and Ecomaps. The construction of genograms and ecomaps, two approaches to developing a family database, are described in the following sections. Neither requires the purchase of standardized assessment tools, and both can be updated over time, a characteristic making them valuable to pediatric providers in understanding patterns in children and families. Together, the genogram and ecomap assist clinicians in assessing family structure and roles, life cycle transitions, family functioning, and social networks in a relatively quick and efficient manner. Both have the advantage of providing a means for interacting with children and their family members in a focused, nonthreatening way around potentially complex and difficult issues. Both also are inherently appealing to families. They help families see themselves in new ways and provide ways for families to be partners in their own diagnosis and management. Even if not explicitly constructed during a visit, conceptually, they assist the provider to organize family data for analysis and identification of problems (Olsen et al, 2004). Thus every pediatric provider should be familiar with these two models. Assessment of family issues and resources does not always occur in primary care, but families generally welcome the opportunity to discuss the family-as-the-unit-of-care with clinicians.

Providers who use genograms and ecomaps in their practice frequently come to the conclusion that the tools are as useful for intervention as they are for assessment. In addition, those working with children find that including the children in the construction and updating of genograms and ecomaps helps children be active in their own care and provides data on family interactions.

Genogram Construction. Genograms are sociometric paper-and-pencil tools used to depict a family's composition and history across generations (Fig. 2-1). Although not essential, computer programs to facilitate genogram data management have become available and can be easily included in computerized patient records. These programs have made updating genogram data easy and efficient. Genograms are appealing to providers because they provide graphic representations of complex family data; they allow the providers to map the family structure clearly and to update the picture as it emerges. Further, genograms are an efficient clinical summary making it easier for providers to keep in mind family members, patterns, and events that may have recurring significance in a family's ongoing care. Genograms also help providers think systematically about how events and relationships in their clients' lives are related to patterns of health and illness, and they are a subjective, interpretive tool to help generate tentative hypotheses for further systematic evaluation.

Priorities for organizing genogram data for clinical use rely less on formal blood and legal links and more on repetitive symptoms and relationships or patterns of functioning seen across the family or over generations. They are most effective when constructed during an initial visit with children and their families and then revised as new information becomes available.

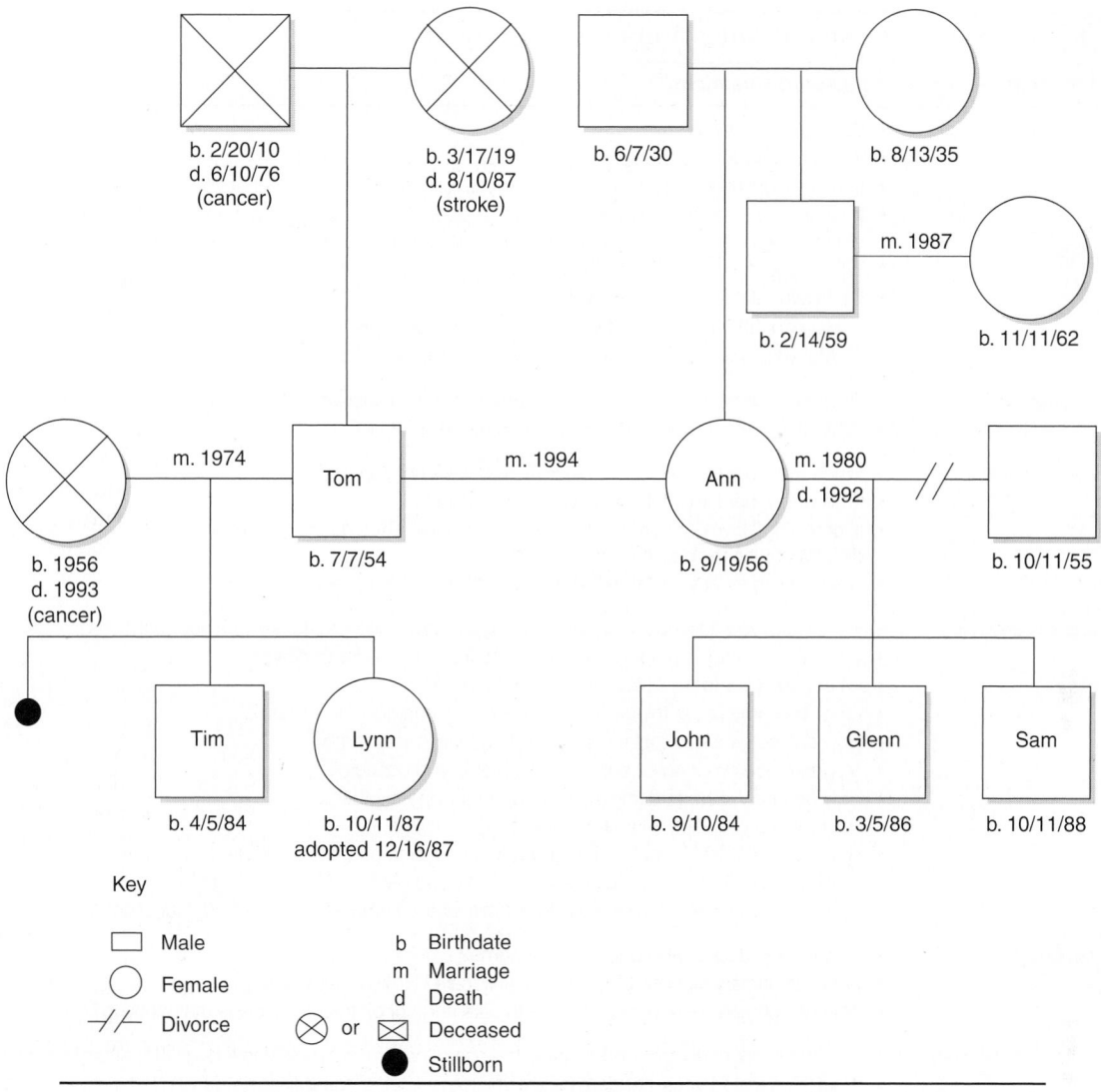

b. 2/20/10
d. 6/10/76
(cancer)

b. 3/17/19
d. 8/10/87
(stroke)

b. 6/7/30

b. 8/13/35

m. 1987

b. 2/14/59

b. 11/11/62

m. 1974

Tom

m. 1994

Ann

m. 1980

d. 1992

b. 1956
d. 1993
(cancer)

b. 7/7/54

b. 9/19/56

b. 10/11/55

Tim

Lynn

John

Glenn

Sam

b. 4/5/84

b. 10/11/87
adopted 12/16/87

b. 9/10/84

b. 3/5/86

b. 10/11/88

Key

☐ Male   b Birthdate

◯ Female   m Marriage
             d Death

–/ /– Divorce   ⊗ or ⊠ Deceased

              ● Stillborn

FIGURE 2-1 A three-generational genogram of a blended family.

The provider begins by drawing a basic family tree, with the present family members guiding identification of family members. It is clinically useful to identify members of the current household in which children live. In fact, it can be more informative and useful to learn who is living in a household than who is related by blood or birth. This objective can be met by drawing a circle around the members of the genogram who currently live together (e.g., the circle may include parents and three children, or it may include one of two parents, two of three children, and a grandparent). It is also useful to include at least three generations of the family. Standardized symbols can be found at www.genopro.com/genogram_components/default.htm.

Health history information, including serious medical, behavioral, and emotional problems, can be noted on the genogram (e.g., drug or alcohol problems, serious problems with the law, and causes of death). Likewise, family information that is significant to the health of the child can be included, such as ethnic background, language spoken in the home, education of parents, occupations, religious affiliation, major family moves, and current location of family members. Significant others who live with or are important to the family should be included, for example family friends, foster

children, and babysitters. In some cases, the significant other is a family pet.

Practical pointers include using pencil instead of pen, unless there are legal or institutional requirements to use a pen; leaving space at the bottom of the page for notes; and including a key to notations or unusual symbols. It also is useful to provide child patients with their own paper and pencils or crayons to use while conducting the interview; they might even draw a picture of their family for you.

The genogram interview can begin with an open question, such as, "Tell me about your family." It can be addressed to children, parents, or both. As the genogram is being constructed, questions can be used to elicit information about family functioning. Specific suggested questions are found in Table 2-1. They are examples only and should not be viewed as exhaustive. Therapeutic interviewing questions relate to all the issues of the genogram discussed later.

Ecomaps. Ecomaps are similar to genograms in their inherent and deceptive simplicity (Fig. 2-2). They depict the systems and relationships essential to the functioning of the family. A lack of family social support is related to feelings of isolation, hopelessness, depression, and other negative

TABLE 2-1	Family Assessment Questions for Genogram	
Family History Topic	**Suggested Questions**

Family composition and structure	• Who is in your family?
	• Who currently lives with you and your child?
	• If the relationships are not clear: How are you related to the members of your household?
	• If divorce or separation is involved: Where does the child's other parent live? What are the custody and visitation agreements? How often does the child see or hear from the other parent?
	• Who in your family was involved in the decision to come here today?
	• If a health-related problem is involved:
	  ○ How do other members of your family see this problem?
	  ○ With whom will you discuss today's visit when you go home?

Current family situation	• Have there been any changes in your family since your last visit? • What, if any, changes do you anticipate in the near future?
Extended family situation	• When was your mother born? Where? Who were her parents? • Who was in her family while she was growing up? • Is she living? If yes: Where does she live now? How often do you have contact with her? If no: When did she die? What was the cause of death? • How did she meet your father? When were they married (if applicable)?
Family relationships and roles	• How would you describe your parenting style? How does it compare with your partner's? • Who in your family is responsible for monitoring your children's health? • What does your family enjoy most about this child? • What are some of the things you do together as a family? How often? • How do you generally make important decisions in your family? • To whom does your child tend to tell problems and concerns? • How do family members show their support for one another? • How well do you think your family adapts to change? • How does your family nurture the interests and talents of each individual family member? • To whom do you go for advice about being a good parent? Why do you go to that person? • How do you deal with unwanted advice from family members about raising your child(ren)?
Two-parent families	• How do you decide who does what at home? • Who has primary responsibility for daily childcare? How is that working? • Who has primary responsibility for health care and appointments? How is that working?
Working parents and childcare	• How many hours do you work outside the home in a typical week? How does that affect your family life? • What tensions do you anticipate (or are you experiencing) to be associated with balancing work and home? • What child care arrangements have you made? How satisfactory are they? What would you change if you could? • How do you manage care for a child who is ill on a workday?
Multiple births	• Have things gone as you expected with the babies? • When you have questions about their care, whom do you ask? • Have you had help from your partner? Family members? Friends? • How are your babies similar? How do they differ from one another? • How have you managed those times that happen to all new parents when you feel overwhelmed? • How have the babies' sibling(s) responded to them?
Families with a child with a chronic illness	• How are things going on a day-to-day basis with your child's care? • How is the child's illness affecting your child's relationships with other children? • How is school going? • How is the child's illness affecting family life? • What are your hopes for the future? Your concerns? • What do you need most right now to better care for your whole family?
Blended families	• Have things gone as you expected they would in your new family? • How is each child coping with the new family? • How are the children responding to the situation? • How has their childcare or school situation changed, and how have they responded? • What do the parents identify as the most significant loss for each child in the blended family? The most significant benefit? • How are the relationships between parents (including stepparent) and children? • How are the relationships among the stepsiblings? • How are the parents handling discipline issues?

TABLE 2-1	Family Assessment Questions for Genogram—cont'd
Family History Topic	**Suggested Questions**
Single-parent families	• What is the best thing about being your child's only parent? • What is most challenging for you about being a single parent? • How do you get the support you need as a parent? • What would most help you raise your child at this point in time?
Foster parents	• What is the best thing about being a foster parent for this child? • What challenges do you have in taking care of this child? • What other information do you need to understand and care for this child? • How do you manage the loss when you must relinquish a child? • What support systems do you have to help you provide care to this foster child and still maintain your own mental health and sense of happiness?
Gay/lesbian families	• What support systems do you use as a gay family with a child/children? • Have your children had any difficulties at school or elsewhere when they explain that they have two dads or moms instead of a mom and dad at their house? How have you helped them cope? • Is one of you a biological parent and the other has adopted the child or is there some other arrangement that we should know about? Are there any legal issues that we should be aware of so that if the child needs emergency care or hospitalization that care can be authorized and both of you will have visitation rights as you want?

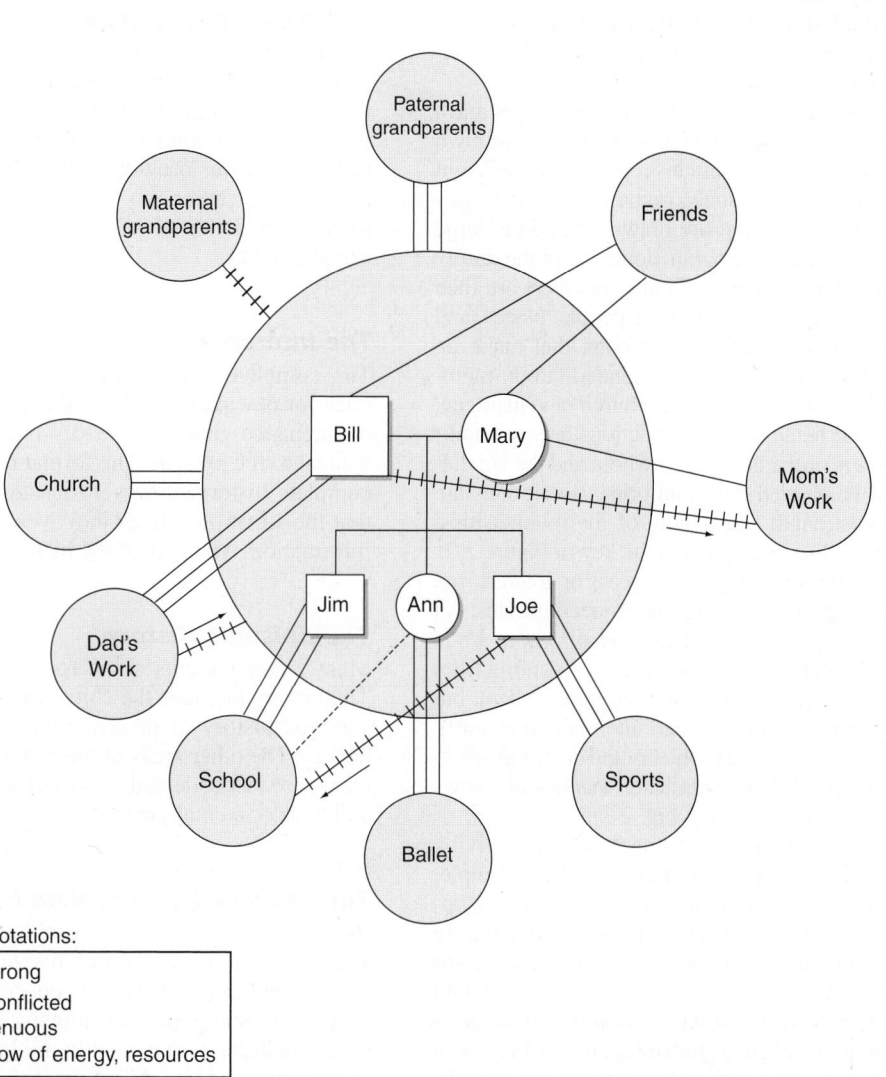

Key to notations:
≡ Strong
+++ Conflicted
--- Tenuous
⇄ Flow of energy, resources

FIGURE 2-2 Ecomap of family with three children. Ecomaps can provide additional data about the major systems in a family's life and the nature of the family's relationships with those systems.

BOX 2-6 Family Assessment Tools

Comprehensive Family Assessment Models

These models provide ways to organize family assessment material. They can provide a database characterized by both breadth and depth.

- Calgary Family Assessment Model (CFAM) (Wright and Leahey, 2005)
- Family Health Assessment Form (Friedman, 1986)

Family Assessment Screening Tool

This screening tool is quick to administer (5 minutes) and provides an overview assessment of family functioning.

- Family Apgar (Smilkstein, 1978)

Family Functioning Tools

These tools vary in length and complexity, but all are easy to score and provide in-depth data about family functioning.

- Family Adaptability and Cohesion Evaluation Scale (FACES IV) (Olson and Gorall, 2006)
- Family Environment Scale (FES) (Moos and Moos, 1994)
- Feetham Family Functioning Survey (FFFS) (Feetham and Humerick, 1982)

Family Stress and Coping Tools (McCubbin et al, 1996)

These tools provide clinicians with information about how families define and manage stress. They can be used to help families self-diagnose their strengths and identify areas needing modification.

- Assessing adolescent stress: Adolescent-Family Inventory of Life Events and Changes (A-FILE)
- Family Inventory of Life Events (FILE)
- Family Coping Strategies (F-COPES)

feelings, which will secondarily affect the child's well-being. Mapping of family relationships within and outside family boundaries highlights the nature of those relationships, their potential for support, conflicts in the relationships, and areas of current or potential strain and stress. The ecomap uses a genogram as a foundation, so the genogram should be constructed first (McGuiness et al, 2005).

As with genograms, all that is needed is a piece of paper and a pencil. A large circle representing the family boundary is drawn in the center of the paper; smaller circles representing different parts of the environment (individuals, organizations and institutions, hobbies, work, and so on) are drawn around the large circle. Inside the large circle, a genogram depiction of the family members in the household is drawn. Family members are then asked to label the smaller circles with those people, places, and activities, whether enjoyable, stressful, or both, that make up their world. Examples of labels include extended family members, friends, work, school, band practice, church or synagogue, camping, exercise, and health care. Connections between individual family members or the family as a whole and the smaller circles are then drawn. Coded lines and brief descriptions are used to indicate the strength and quality of the relationships. Common codes for the lines are found in the key in Figure 2-2.

Direction of the flow of energy, resources, or interest can be indicated by drawing arrows along the connecting lines. An example is a family with three children, one of whom loves school and does well (three solid lines with arrows pointing from school to the child); one of whom is an indifferent student, but likes the social aspect of school (a dotted line with no arrows); and one who has serious academic problems and dreads going to school each morning (a solid line with hatch marks and arrows pointing from the child to school) (see Fig. 2-2).

Sometimes the whole family is connected to an activity, and the energy flow is similar for all members. For example, a family might identify a particular family friend as supportive. In other cases, the experience differs across family members. For example, family vacations may be positive for all members of the family except adolescents, who would prefer to stay home near their friends. A scarcity of connections outside the household suggests isolation and may be a problem if the family needs significant support during a crisis. A sheet full of circles may indicate a family overcommitted and overwhelmed by activities and responsibilities.

In summary ecomaps provide both additional data about a family's social network and potential for social support. They also provide a way of validating information from the genogram interview, especially around family relationships and roles.

Selected Family Assessment Tools. The process of constructing a genogram and ecomap results in a fairly complete picture of the family's composition, social network, and family functioning. However, at times additional information is needed. Examples of assessment models and tools found in Box 2-6 offer providers other resources that are clinically relevant and reasonably efficient. In addition, the tools have research evidence of reliability and validity supporting their use in practice.

The Interval History

The complete history usually needs to be completed only once for new patients. After that for routine scheduled health maintenance visits, the history is updated only from the last contact to the present. The format remains the same as for the complete history; however, questions are modified to verify that the situations are as they were in the past or to add new information. All areas of the history should be assessed.

The Episodic History

Many times patients come for help with specific problems. The history includes the chief complaint with symptom analysis and history of present illness sections of the complete history. The other areas of the history should be updated since data were last collected. Always listen for emerging problems and developmental progress.

The Psychosocial Problem History

Psychosocial or behavioral problems also must be assessed. Some considerations are summarized in Box 2-7. Much of the data related to psychosocial concerns will be collected in the functional health pattern domain database. Additional suggested material is included in the Family Database section to be discussed later in this chapter.

For adolescents, the HEEADSSS (home, education and employment, eating, activities, drugs, depression, sexuality,

Adapted from Green M, Sullivan P, Eichberg C: Avoid a "Swiss cheese" history when psychosocial complaints are on the menu, *Contemp Pediatr* 19:115, 2002.

BOX 2-7 Suggestions for the Psychosocial Complaint History

1. Use good communication skills—listen. Nonjudgmental approach. Seek a balanced give and take of information.
2. Interview the child or adolescent alone and with parents. Time alone with the preschooler may be used for play or drawing.
3. Have questionnaires or checklists from parents, teachers, and childcare workers available. Use the information in the interview.
4. Be alert to emotional tone and interactions among family members.
5. Review the context for the concern:
   - Information about parents and family members: illnesses, mental health problems, poverty, employment, violence, social isolation
   - Information about the child: school, peer relationships, temperament, neglect or abuse history, foster home placements, losses
   - Information about child-parent relationships: attachment disorder, unrealistic expectations, poor family communication, lack of knowledge of child development and appropriate parenting
6. The history of present illness becomes an amalgam of information from the multiple sources—child, parents, others. Do not assume that both parents have the same views of the issues.
7. Remember that the interview itself may be therapeutic.

---

suicide, and safety) method is often recommended as a psychosocial review of systems (Goldenring and Rosen, 2004).

THE PHYSICAL EXAMINATION

The physical examination is conducted following the history, although younger children might do better with developmental testing preceding the physical examination. Height, weight, head circumference, BMI, and vital signs are recorded. Principal findings that the provider is expected to identify are presented Box 2-8. Screening tests for hearing and vision, in addition to laboratory data and data from other disciplines, are included as other types of objective information. More experienced providers collect some of the history while conducting the physical examination. Content of the examination will vary depending on the child's age and the various problems under consideration. Further discussion of physical examination techniques and findings are found in specific disease chapters.

OTHER DATA
Laboratory and Radiographic Data

Record hearing, vision, hematocrit or other blood tests, lead, urinalysis, newborn screening tests, and tuberculosis screening.

Developmental and Psychological Test Scores

Scores need to be recorded and considered when problems are being identified.

Data from Other Disciplines

Summarize social work, nutrition, physical therapy, occupational therapy, medical specialist, speech pathology, education, and other reports.

Creating the Problem List

The problem list is derived from analysis of the subjective and objective data collected. Differential diagnosis is the clinical decision-making process used to derive the problems listed (Fig. 2-3). To use this process the provider considers all the possible diagnoses for the problems presented by the patient. Then the factors that support or rule out each of the various options considered are analyzed. Identification of the best fit of the patient's subjective and objective data with the possible diagnoses is the goal. If further data are needed to confirm a diagnosis, collection of these data is incorporated into the plan. For example, the differential diagnoses for coryza (a runny nose) include, among others, allergic rhinitis, upper respiratory infection, and a foreign body in the nose. The clinician uses data about related symptoms (e.g., itchy eyes, a sore throat, systemic symptoms, or bilateral or unilateral drainage from the nostrils) to choose which diagnosis best fits the child's picture. That analysis for fit is the diagnostic reasoning process.

Functional health problems and developmental problems are also subject to the notion of differential diagnosis. For example, a child who is not sleeping well might be fearful, a trained night feeder, or might experience episodes of obstructive sleep apnea. The interventions for each problem are different. Thus the provider must use the differential diagnosis process to identify the problem or problems at hand. A problem should never be included on the problem list that is not supported by subjective and objective data found and recorded in the database. "Rule out" should not be listed as a diagnosis (it may be considered part of a plan). The diagnosis would be the unexplained symptom (e.g., "dysuria").

AVOIDING DIAGNOSTIC ERRORS

Data collection for clinical practice, just as for research, must be as reliable and valid as possible. To assist with reliability, consider the following techniques: test-retest, interrater reliability, and internal consistency.

- **Test-retest:** Ask the question again later. Take a blood pressure reading twice. Look for the physical finding a second time a bit later.
- **Interrater reliability:** Ask someone else to listen, palpate, and so on for the same finding. Does someone else get the same answer to the same question you asked?
- **Internal consistency:** Look for a logical consistency to the findings obtained. If something is "out of sync," question it. For example, do the height points on the graph line up, or is one significantly off the trajectory? If there is significant variation, consider a measuring error before looking for a health problem that has altered growth. Does the history support the physical findings? Does the story keep changing?

Algorithms, computer algorithms, protocols, and flowsheets can improve the consistency and reliability of the data

---

BOX 2-8 Essential Physical Examination Data to Collect

General appearance: Ill or well, distressed, alert, cooperative, body build; reaction to parents; characteristic position, movements, nutrition, developmental appearance as contrasted with the stated age

Skin: Color—pigmentation, cyanosis, jaundice, carotenemia, erythema, pallor; vascular—visible veins, arteries; eruptions, petechiae, ecchymosis, hives, rashes; lesions; texture, scaling, striae, scars; sweat, edema, turgor; subcutaneous tissue; distribution and color of hair; nail appearance

Lymph nodes: Occipital, postauricular, preauricular, cervical, parotid, submaxillary, sublingual, axillary, epitrochlear, inguinal; size, mobility, tenderness, heat

Head: Position, shape, sutures, fontanelles; size—circumference, microcephaly, macrocephaly, hydrocephaly; facial paralysis, twitching

Eyes: Vision, visual fields, cover test; blinking; position—exophthalmos, enophthalmos, hypertelorism, hypotelorism; movements—strabismus, extraocular movements, nystagmus; ptosis—eyelids, sclera, conjunctivae; lesions—styes, chalazion; corneas—corneal reflex; discharge; pupils—accommodation, iris; retina—red reflex, fundus

Ears: Anomalies; position; discharge; tenderness; canals; tympanic membranes—redness, light reflex, landmarks, bulging or retraction, perforation, mobility; mastoid; hearing; vestibular function

Nose: Shape; alae nasi, flaring; mucosa, secretions, bleeding, airway; septum; polyps, tumors

Mouth: Odor; teeth—number, edges, occlusion, caries, formation, color; gums—discoloration, bleeding; buccal mucosa; tongue—coating, protrusion, color, tremor, lesions; palate—cleft, arch; tonsils—size, color, exudate; pharynx—appearance, color, lesions

Neck: Size; anomalies—webbing, edema, nodes, masses; sternocleidomastoid; trachea; thyroid; vessels; motion—head drop, tilting, nodding, range of motion

Chest: Shape—circumference, symmetry, Harrison groove; movement—flaring, expansion, abdominal or thoracic breathing, intercostal retractions

Breasts: Tanner stage of development, symmetry, redness, heat, tenderness, lumps; gynecomastia

Lungs: Respiration—type, rate, dyspnea; exercise tolerance; cough, hemoptysis, sputum; palpation—masses, tenderness, fremitus; percussion—dullness, hyperresonance, diaphragm location; auscultation—breath sounds, crackles (rales), rubs, rhonchi, wheezes, vocal resonance

Cardiovascular and heart: Blood pressure and pulse rate; inspection—vascularity, bulging, impulse; distress, cyanosis, edema, clubbing, pulsations, venous distention; palpation—femoral pulses, point of maximal impulse, thrill; auscultation—first and second heart sounds, rhythm, split, third heart sound, gallop, friction rub, venous hum, murmurs

Abdomen: Inspection—shape, distention, transillumination; umbilicus, diastasis rectus, veins; peristaltic, gastric waves; auscultation—bowel sounds, bruits; palpation—superficial or deep tenderness, rebound; spleen, liver, masses, kidneys, bladder, uterus; percussion—masses, fluid, flatus

Genitalia: Discharge, foreign body; *male and female*—Tanner staging; *female*—tags; labia, adhesions, vagina, clitoris; vaginal, bimanual examination for teenage girls (pelvic examination observations are discussed further in Chapter 35); *male*—penis—hypospadias, epispadias, phimosis, meatus; scrotum, testes, hydrocele, hernia; cremasteric reflex

Anus and rectum: Buttocks, fistula, fissure, prolapse, polyps, hemorrhoids, rashes; rectal—rectum, fistula, megacolon, masses, prostate, tenderness; sensation

Musculoskeletal: Anomalies, length, clubbing, pain, tenderness, temperature, swelling, shape, symmetry; gait—stance, balance, limp; foot position; spine—tufts of hair, dimples, masses, spina bifida, tenderness, mobility, scoliosis; posture—lordosis, kyphosis; joints—heat, tenderness, mobility, swelling, effusion; muscles—development, pain, tone, spasm, paralysis, rigidity, contractures, atrophy

Nervous system: General impression, abilities, responsiveness, position, spontaneous movements, play activity; development—consistent with age or current level; state of consciousness, irritability, seizure activity; gait, stance, limp, ataxia; coordination, Romberg sign; tremors, twitching, choreiform movements, athetosis, spasticity, paralysis, flaccidity; reflexes—superficial, deep tendon, clonus, Chvostek sign; primitive reflexes for infants and children with neurologic impairments—Moro, tonic neck, Babinski, grasp, suck; thumb position; sensation—hyperesthesia, paresthesia, temperature, touch; stereognosis; cranial nerves I to XII; hearing and vision

---

collected, especially when several staff members are involved with the data for a given patient.

To assess the validity, or meaning, of data collected, the provider should consider sources of error:
- Do the cumulative data fit and support a given diagnosis? If not, perhaps the diagnosis was inadequate or an error in data collection, sequencing, or interpretation occurred. Providers constantly need to attend to age, sex, race, culture, and other issues when they consider data. Is it likely for a caucasian child to have sickle cell disease? What diagnoses should one consider when a teenage girl has abdominal pain, as opposed to the diagnoses possible for a boy of the same age?
- Was the diagnosis made on the basis of one isolated finding or a cluster? For instance, diagnosing pneumonia after hearing a cough and diagnosing failure to thrive with one growth measurement are mono-operation bias errors.
- Sometimes two problems occur with overlapping findings. One problem might be missed, whereas the other is pursued.

- The patient might change the data provided because of stress or worry about the outcomes of the assessment visit. Both findings and their meaning to patients need to be explored with the patient and family.
- Provider expectations can also threaten accurate diagnosing.
- Were cues missed or questions unasked?
- Data are often compared with specific criteria (e.g., heights and weights for age are known, developmental milestones are established, laboratory norms are set for children of different ages). Which test has been used? What is its specificity and sensitivity? Is the right criterion being used?
- Were all data such as laboratory studies reviewed promptly?

■ Creating the Management Plan

A plan must be developed for every identified problem. It is helpful to consider diagnostic, therapeutic, and educational interventions for every problem listed. Of course, not every problem requires work in all three areas, but they should be

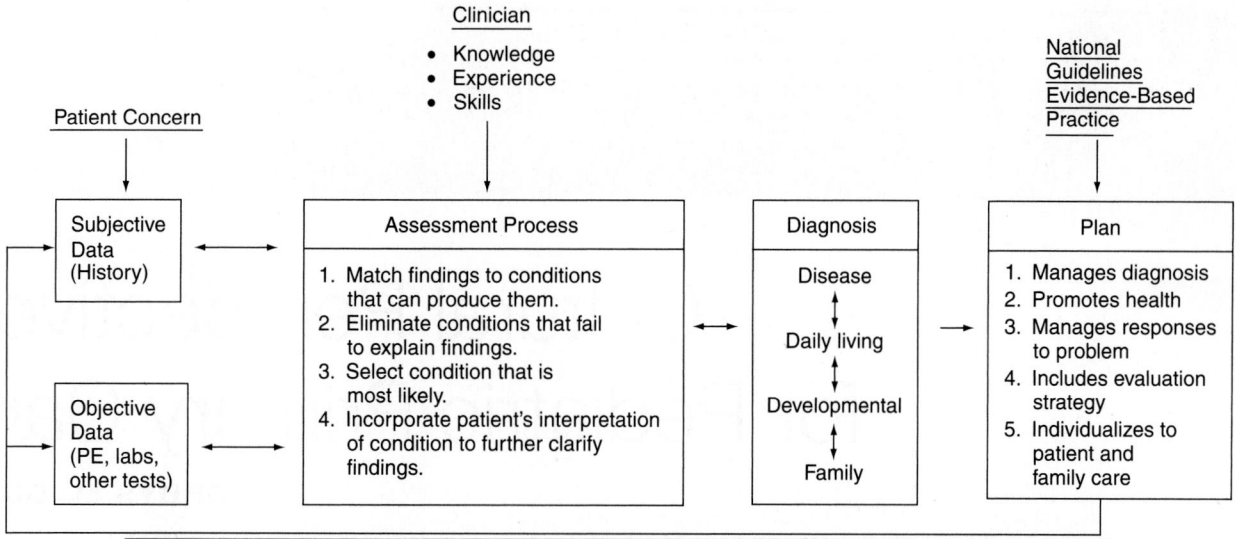

FIGURE 2-3 Model for clinical decision-making. The provider takes the patient's concern and clarifies it with subjective and objective data, using past experience and skills to facilitate the assessment process. The process, which happens both during and after data collection, involves decision-making to find the best match between standardized diagnoses and the patient's findings. Once the diagnosis is made, a plan is developed, using national evidence-based guidelines where appropriate, to achieve the five goals listed. Sometimes the development of the plan requires further data collection. (Data from Burns C: Development and content validity testing of a comprehensive classification of diagnoses for use by pediatric nurse practitioners, *Nurs Diagn* 2:93-104, 1991.)

considered. The management activities are listed in the record. The plan should always include a recommendation for the next visit and what is to be done at that visit in an attempt to move the patient into a health maintenance pattern rather than being seen only episodically. Just as the problem list must be consistent with the data at hand, plans must address diagnoses that are included in the problem list. In other words, the plan is internally consistent with the data and diagnoses.

Using newer models of family collaborative decision-making (see Chapter 9 for further information), plans for care should be communicated to the family with a discussion of alternatives for management of issues with risks and benefits for each option. Active parent-child involvement with creation of the plan of care is the most desirable. Studies have shown that this process is more likely to occur with college graduate parents and female, more experienced physicians. Parents may raise more concerns about the risks than the benefits about various options for care (Cox and Raaum, 2008). Deliberation time with families averaged about 3 minutes per visit with a mean of four plans proposed. Passive involvement with parents occurred in 68% of visits (Cox et al, 2007).

Thus more work needs to be done to develop these skills for clinicians.

■ Communicating Assessment Data

An important corollary to health assessment is the skill to communicate information obtained in both oral and written forms. A record of the care given must always be written to communicate the provider's logical thinking based on data obtained. This record is important because it provides information for later care, serves as a communication link with other providers, documents the quality of care provided, may be used for research purposes, and serves as a legal and billing document. Verbal communication of health care information is also essential. The words must paint a picture of the child and family for the reader or listener (e.g., a consultant). Knowledge of the classic format used by other health care providers is important. Using that same format or one that is closely related facilitates efficient communication about patient problems.

Cultural Perspectives for Pediatric Primary Care

ARDYS M. DUNN

The ethnic and cultural face of America has changed rapidly in the past decade, and the population continues to become more diverse. From 2000 to 2009, more than half a million refugees or asylum seekers entered the U.S. Each year between 500,000 and 1 million immigrants were naturalized as U.S. citizens, and more than a million immigrants were granted legal permanent residence or "green card" status (Department of Homeland Security, 2010).

Many immigrants to the U.S. are unauthorized; that is, they entered the U.S. without documents or, having entered with proper documents (e.g., student visa), have overstayed their time limit. A recent review of U.S. census data by the Pew Research Center concluded that nearly 12 million unauthorized immigrants live in the U.S. This group is more likely than U.S. citizens or documented immigrants to live in families with children, and about 73% of children in these families are born in the U.S., making them U.S. citizens (Passel and Cohn, 2009). The stress of immigration, especially if exacerbated by an unauthorized entry or a history of having come from an area of war, famine, or dislocation puts families and children at risk for physical and psychological health problems. Health care providers must consider these circumstances when assessing and managing care for immigrant and refugee clients.

In addition, significant health disparities continue among minority cultural groups in the U.S. For example, the 2005 infant mortality rate for non-Hispanic blacks was 13.3 per 1000 live births, in contrast to an overall rate of 6.8 per 1000 live births and 5.7 for non-Hispanic whites (Centers for Disease Control and Prevention [CDC], 2011a). These disparities have not changed since 1995 and have been attributed in part to a lack of communication between providers and patients that may be related to cultural differences (Fadiman, 1997; Pavlish et al, 2010).

In response to demographic changes and in an effort to mitigate health disparities, many health education institutions have created curricula to develop more culturally competent providers (Calvillo et al, 2009; Kripalani et al, 2006). Evaluation of these curricula is just beginning and data vary on the difference they make in provider attitudes and health outcomes as well as how to best evaluate the programs (Bhui et al, 2007; Lie et al, 2008; Mostow et al, 2010; Sequist et al, 2010).

Because of the complex circumstances of immigrant and ethnic communities, cultural competence needs to be expanded to incorporate a "critical awareness" of broad social, economic, and political dynamics. Educational programs must prepare clinicians to deal effectively with the complex interrelationship of variables that influence health behaviors, decisions, and outcomes, only one of which is culture per se (Airhihenbuwa and Liburd, 2006; Kumagai and Lypson, 2009; Underwood et al, 2005). Having this skill gives clinicians the ability to provide high-quality health care to all populations.

This chapter reviews some of the basic principles of cultural dynamics, emphasizing that environmental, economic, and social factors are integrally woven into the fabric of every client-provider encounter and that clinicians must consider the reality of individual history, experience, and meaning in every interaction. A new section has been added outlining care of recent immigrants and refugees. A more comprehensive discussion of the challenge of providing culturally competent care and eliminating health disparities for immigrants in the U.S. can be found in Walker and Barnett's *Immigrant Medicine* (2007).

■ Culture

Culture is defined as a set of "patterns, explicit and implicit, of and for behavior," "acquired and transmitted by symbols" and based on "traditional [i.e., historically derived and selected] ideas and … their attached values. Culture systems may, on the one hand, be considered as products of action, on the other as conditioning elements of further action" (Kroeber, 1952). In an anthropologic and sociologic sense, culture is a social construction of the relationships within and among groups of human beings, specifically created through the ongoing interactions of individuals with others and with their environment (Berger and Luckmann, 1966). It is based on ethnicity, race, religion, class, and geography. The term *ethnicity* is used to identify groups of people within society, each of which shares distinctive traits and customs. *Race*, in contrast, classifies humans according to specific physical characteristics (e.g., pigmentation, facial features). Humans also differ by religion, social class, and the physical place or environment in which they experience life. All of these qualities contribute to shaping the culture of the social group.

UNIVERSAL CHARACTERISTICS OF CULTURE

Although a cultural group may possess unique qualities, all cultures have certain common characteristics. These universal characteristics of culture represent the framework within which cultures exist. Understanding these characteristics gives health care providers a starting point from which to learn about the more specific culture of their client base. One must take care, however, not to assume that all members of a group share the same qualities; no one quality is definitive of a culture, and within cultural groups, individuals show great variation in behavior and beliefs.

Culture Is Dynamic and Shared

As both a product and function of human interaction, culture is constantly evolving; there is no absolute, reified quality that can be attributed to a group of humans. In most societies, a dominant group is clearly evident. The culture of this group largely shapes the lifestyle and collective consciousness of the community, functions as the guardian and sustainer of the controlling value system, and allocates rewards. Generally, individuals in a society learn to identify with the dominant cultural framework and incorporate its traditions and customs into their daily life and decision-making. The extent to which this adaptation of culture occurs is termed *cultural embeddedness.* Many factors influence the degree of cultural embeddedness, including level of education, socioeconomic status, social class, country of origin of individuals or their ancestors, exposure to other cultures, lifestyle, length of stay in the host country, and the exact region of the host country in which individuals grow up, reside, or both.

Individuals may also identify with a minority group (i.e., a group that shares racial or ethnic characteristics that differ from those of the majority group) or may have a number of subcultural affiliations based on gender, social class, religion, occupation, or socioeconomic status. In diverse societies, especially where minority groups are large or their members are vocal proponents of retaining their cultural integrity, assimilation into the dominant culture may not be easy or automatic, and cultural confusion or conflict may occur. Characteristics (e.g., skin color, religion) that set a minority group apart from the dominant group may result in collective discrimination within the society. Ethnocentrism and racism create and perpetuate the distinctions of dominant and minority groups. *Ethnocentrism* is the belief that one's own ethnic culture or subculture is superior to all others. *Racism* is the assumption of inherent racial superiority or inferiority with consequent discrimination.

An individual or group that straddles two or more cultures and embraces more than one set of values is termed *bicultural,* but efforts to achieve this status can be a source of considerable stress. Tremendous intraethnic diversity may exist in life perspective, values, problem-solving strategies, and customs among individual members of dominant and minority groups. Thus one can expect to see variations within and between cultures. In diverse societies, all cultural groups will change as a result of their interactions.

Culture Is Learned

The elements of culture are transmitted from one generation to another through a complicated process of social interaction. This socialization process shapes a child's reality; children learn how to perceive the world, the values, ideologies, and rules that motivate and define behavior. This learning is facilitated by the long period of dependency that humans have before reaching physical and social maturity and depends on the child's temperament and biologic capabilities. Social institutions such as the family, school, peer groups, and media influence and support cultural socialization.

Family. The family is the first socializing force an individual encounters. A powerful primary group, the family provides material and psychological support and exposes the child to a set of values in the context of intensely personal relationships. Children first learn patterns of socially appropriate (or inappropriate) behavior in the family. Each culture possesses its own values, attitudes, and practices with regard to families and child rearing, and care and guidance are provided in culturally prescribed ways. Family dynamics can facilitate conformity to the prevailing standards and codes of behavior. As active family members, children develop their own personalities and a sense of self; the family provides the opportunity to identify feelings and emotions, express ideas and thoughts, and practice interactional skills that children will use throughout their lives.

School. The school functions to expand the child's socialization beyond the boundaries of the family. Schools serve as models for much of the adult social world, teaching children strategies for negotiating one's way within the institutions of adult society (e.g., workplace, politics, or organized recreation). For many children, schools may provide stability, opportunities for creative expression, and learning. A sense of collective identity and responsibility to the group may grow as children engage in school activities. For others, school experiences can have a negative effect on the child's sense of self, leading to a feeling of rejection and isolation from the group.

Peer Group. Peer groups play a powerful role in socializing children to their culture, especially among older children. Peer groups can place children in a position of social equality unlike the socially inferior position that they may experience at home or in their school or community role. Through peer interactions, children explore their identities, give and receive validation of appropriate behavior, and further consolidate a sense of self.

Media. Television, radio, magazines, newspapers, films, and electronic media (e.g., phones, internet, texting, blogging) have an enormous influence on the cultural socialization of children, especially in the developed world. As an audience, contemporary Americans are conditioned to receive mass culture passively via these vehicles. Through the media, the child is exposed to a wide array of values, many of which conflict with those of the family and/or the school.

Culture Is Symbolic

Communication takes place between humans using cultural symbols such as language (verbal and nonverbal), dress, food, music, dance, sports, and other activities. The extent to which individuals understand and master these cultural symbols will shape their self-concept, how others perceive them, and their ability to function within and contribute to their culture.

Culture Is Integrated

Culture is reflected in and influences all aspects of an individual's life. The cultural values, beliefs, and behaviors one learns are embedded in the fabric of one's life and can be generalized from one social arena to another. Ideas about the appropriate behavior of children may extend from the family to the school to the community (e.g., "children should be respectful to adults"). On the other hand, a cultural group may have different expectations in different roles; for example, language used among peers in the street may be very different from that used in the school or at home.

Attitudes and behaviors regarding health, wellness, disease, and disability are an intricate part of this cultural framework.

CULTURES IN AMERICAN SOCIETY

The population of the U.S. consists of numerous ethnic groups, races, and subcultures and is becoming increasingly diverse. It is often broken down into the dominant white middle class and a number of minority groups, including African Americans, Hispanic Americans, Asian Americans, Native Americans, Russian Americans, and Arab Americans. Within each of these categories, there are many subgroups. For example, most providers would include families from Iran, Syria, and Iraq in the category of "Arab Americans," yet the cultural differences between each are immeasurable, and, though they may share some common characteristics, each is unique and constantly changing.

To present descriptions of each cultural group is beyond the scope of this text. Instead Table 3-1 lists some of the more common health issues found in some cultural groups. It must be remembered that these health issues are not exclusive to a particular culture; they may be, however, overrepresented in some groups (e.g., lead poisoning in African-American children) because of environmental, social, economic, and class factors, not intrinsic cultural characteristics. Thus, though cultural competence on the part of providers is essential, institutional, political, and social change will also have to occur before full equity in health care is realized. That, too, is a discussion beyond the scope of this text.

▪ Providing Culturally Competent Care

DEVELOPING CULTURAL COMPETENCE

Today's U.S. health care providers should be culturally competent in the care they provide. The effort to develop cultural competence is an excellent example of the dynamic nature of culture: U.S. health care providers are members of a particular personal and professional cultural group; their clients represent different cultures, and the intercultural exchange among clients and providers will change the nature of health care in America.

Cultural competence is the ability to communicate among cultures and demonstrate cultural skill outside one's culture of origin. It is based on empathy, respect, and knowledge and requires a fundamental recognition and valuing of culture as a distinctive way of life. The culturally competent provider's focus is not on how to interact with clients so that they will comply with a medical regimen. Instead, culturally competent providers work with clients to increase mutual

TABLE 3-1	Common Health Issues Found in Some Specific Cultural Groups
Cultural Group	**Health Issue**
African American	High infant mortality rate Sickle cell trait and disease Hypertension Obesity Type 2 diabetes mellitus Type 1 diabetes mellitus with beta-cell destruction Slipped capital femoral epiphysis Blount disease Lead poisoning caused by environmental exposure in urban areas Violence
Asian American	Lactose intolerance Tuberculosis Dental caries Cleft lip and palate
Caucasian	Rett syndrome (girls) Tay-Sachs disease (Ashkenazi Jew; French Canadian) Tyrosinemia (French Canadian; Scandinavian) Celiac disease Cystic fibrosis Phenylketonuria (Northern European) Pyloric stenosis (Northern European) Blount disease (Northern European) Lactose intolerance Type 1 diabetes mellitus Glutaric aciduria type 1 (Amish and Hutterites; Canadian) Lice
Latino	Dental caries Obesity Type 2 diabetes mellitus Blount disease Asthma
Native American (American Indian)	Otitis media Poor prenatal care, low-birthweight babies, high infant mortality rate Alcoholism Unintentional injury
Samoan or Polynesian	Dermatological conditions Obesity Slipped capital femoral epiphysis
Russian	Obesity
American	Alcoholism

understanding, share information and knowledge, strengthen clients' control of their health, and construct more healthful decisions.

To achieve cultural competence, providers must work to:
- Understand and, if necessary, change their *worldview*
- Become familiar with *core cultural issues*

- Increase their knowledge about *core cultural issues related to health and illness*
- Become knowledgeable about the particular *cultural groups to whom they deliver care and with whom they work*, in general, and in terms of health and illness
- Develop skills that provide a basis for *effective communication and negotiation* between client and provider

Worldview

A worldview is a conceptual framework that allows members of a social group or culture to answer fundamental questions such as "How does the world function?" "Why does it operate that way?" "Where is it going?" "What does it mean? "What values, ethics, and moral standards is it working from?" "How should we act?" and "What is true or false?" "What is knowledge?" In the U.S., for example, the dominant worldview tends to reflect an activist, rational-mastery, future-oriented approach to life. It is based on a perception of independence and autonomy, and it values acquisition and power. Diversity of ideas, race, ethnicity, and lifestyle may be given little value unless they are useful to those in power. Incidents of discrimination based on race, gender, age, or sexual orientation can be outcomes of this perception.

Various aspects of worldviews have been identified and are often presented as dichotomies for purposes of comparison: for example, individualism versus collectivism; masculinity versus femininity; linear thinking versus global thinking. An example related to health care would be the U.S. culture of "individualism," in which clients make their own decisions about treatment, as opposed to a Southeast Asian culture of "collectivism" (e.g., Hmong), in which the family is actively involved in deciding what treatment will be done. The dualistic thinking reflected in these taxonomies has come under criticism as being too simplistic, however, because it does not help explain the subtle nuances of cultures or the complexities of behaviors of members of social groups (Turiel, 2004). To understand human behavior, one must look at interaction within the larger socioecological context. Not all Hmong clients rely on family members to help them make decisions about health treatments, for example; nor do all Americans make their decisions independently. Though culture is a vital element in why people make the choices they do, those choices depend on many other factors as well.

For health care providers working with clients from a cultural group other than their own, this means two things: first, they need to examine their own worldview, look at what social and cultural dynamics affect their thinking and behavior, and determine how this influences their practice and interaction with clients. A relevant example might be clinicians who work with adolescents. Clinicians are part of an "adult culture." To effectively work with adolescents, they need to reflect on what their "adult" perceptions are regarding teenagers and how those perceptions structure their approach to the client. There are additional dynamics to consider: Providers have experienced their own adolescence and have had their worldview shaped by that experience. They bring those perceptions to the interaction with their adolescent client (some providers have said, "Two people walk into the exam room when I see an adolescent—me as an adult caregiver, and me when I was 16 years old"). How do health care providers' worldviews affect their thinking about this client? How, in turn, does this thinking influence the way they interact with adolescent clients? Additionally the current life situation of the provider may be important to consider; perhaps he or she is struggling with a rebellious teenager at home. This personal concern could change the provider's ability to provide high-quality care to adolescents.

Second, health care providers must be open to understanding the worldview of their clients and be willing to adapt their own in order to find the most effective way of providing health care. For example, problem-solving approaches vary among cultures. Not everyone solves problems in the linear, cause-and-effect way often attributed to the dominant culture in the U.S. If clinicians present a health problem and its solution in a linear fashion and insist that their patients and families use the same perspective, they should not be surprised if the patient is sometimes "noncompliant." An example might be a child who has a fever. Based on their worldview, clinicians begin a diagnostic process of examination and laboratory testing to rule out causes, with some idea of an infectious agent in the back of their mind that may need to be treated with an antibiotic. The family, however, may attribute the fever to a nonbiologic cause, and may have a more reflective, circuitous problem-solving style, part of which is a wait-and-see attitude. They may typically let the child's body do what it will in response to the fever or may provide support in traditional cultural ways that involve preparation and time (e.g., sweats, prayer, chicken soup). Of added concern, conflicts in cultural worldviews may contribute to psychological problems created by stress that go beyond simple culture shock (Caldwell-Harris and Ayçiçegi, 2006) or to the labeling of clients as having problems, primarily psychological, when their behavior is actually consistent with their own deep-seated cultural expectations (Chen et al, 2009).

Core Cultural Issues

Core cultural issues are those qualities that are "universal (i.e., every culture has them) but specific (i.e., every culture expresses them differently)" (Dunn, 2002, p 107). One cannot know all there is to know about all cultural groups, but clinicians can work with their clients from specific cultural groups to identify how that culture expresses these core issues. Table 3-2 outlines these issues and provides several examples of each.

Core Cultural Issues Related to Health and Illness

Cultural beliefs and values influence clients' understanding and management of health and illness in the following areas:

- Understanding how the body functions
- Definition, classification, or meaning of illness
- Causes of illness or disease
- Appropriate ways in which an individual should behave when ill
- Best treatments and appropriate individuals to seek out for treatment and healing

Assessment questions that allow clients and families to explain how they believe their body functions and how they understand their illness, what they think the illness means, what they believe about the causes of their illness, and what they think might be a way to treat it can give providers

TABLE 3-2   Core Cultural Issues

Cultural Issue	Example
Physical and biological characteristics	Bone structure, hair, skin
Self-orientation and worldview	Individualistic (centered on self and one's needs) versus collectivistic (person is part of larger whole, functions within context of community and history)
Concepts of time, space, and physical distance	What is the comfortable distance between individuals during conversation; when and how is it appropriate to touch a client?
Style and pattern of communication	Who speaks for the family, and when they do so, what language is used; are introductory comments or questions expected; is language formal?
Physical and social activities expected of group members	Muslim women may be expected to cover their faces when in public; young Latino women may be expected to have a male family member escort when they go out.
Relationships with others, often based on gender, age, or social class	Father in family may make decisions for other family members; grandmother may be first person consulted for health problems.
Systems of social organization	Older children in Southeast Asian family may live at home with parents, contribute to family income; attendance at religious services and participation in church activities may be focus of social life.
Relationships with nature	Belief in animism (inanimate natural objects [e.g., wind, earth, rocks] have spiritual quality); sense of responsibility and stewardship toward environment; view that environment is unsafe (e.g., "cleanliness is next to godliness")

BOX 3-1   Identifying Cultural Meaning of Illness for Families

- What is the problem or illness called?
- What does the family believe is happening?
- What do you think caused the problem or illness?
- Why do you think it started when it did?
- How has this illness affected you and the family?
- What are the chief problems this sickness has caused?
- How severe is the sickness?
- Will it have a short or long course?
- What kind of treatment should the patient receive?
- What are the most important results you hope to have happen from this treatment?
- What treatments have you already tried?
- What helped in the past?
- What do you fear most about this illness?
- Are you afraid to tell your relatives or friends? What are you fearful might happen?

Data from Kleinman A, Eisenberg L, Good B: Culture, illness and care: clinical lessons from anthropologic and cross-cultural research, *Ann Intern Med* 88(2):251-258, 1978.

harmful, however, and may comfort both parent (being able to do something) and child (because of the massage and attention). If the family wishes to use it, it should be encouraged. Another folk remedy for gastritis, however, is *greta*, a lead-based powder that is mixed with water and given to the child orally. *Greta* does not treat the cause of the gastritis and is a serious health risk to the child; it is the provider's responsibility to explain why it should not be given and explore with the family what alternatives are possible. Most families will not persist in treating their children with clearly harmful remedies.

Specific Cultural Groups

Interaction with and study about specific cultural groups, languages, and worldviews can greatly increase one's knowledge base and is essential to sensitive, relevant care. When doing cultural assessments, however, cultural characteristics must be viewed as being on a continuum; the provider must recognize that not all individuals from the same social group have the same characteristics. Intraethnic variations must be anticipated and incorporated into the plan of care for a truly individualized approach. Attempting to fit a family or individual into any preconceived cultural framework is not cultural sensitivity—it is stereotyping. Stereotyping and cross-cultural comparisons are to be avoided because they interfere with the development of basic trust and threaten the success of the therapeutic relationship and the plan of care.

Communication and Negotiation Strategies

Communication strategies used in interactions with clients can facilitate trust and convey the message that the clients' beliefs and approaches to health and illness are recognized and respected. This allows both clinicians and clients to actively negotiate for mutually acceptable interventions of care. A basic communication course discusses these strategies. Successfully using them in the clinical setting requires ongoing practice, evaluation of their effectiveness, and reflection on ways to change them to strengthen communication.

significant insight into how to best work with clients (Kleinman et al, 1978) (Box 3-1).

When developing the plan of care, incorporate culture-related practices whenever possible and appropriate. Delivering care in a respectful, accepting, nonjudgmental manner that is congruent with the individual's cultural beliefs and practices does not mean that providers must lower their standards. Rather they should think in terms of the context within which those standards exist. It is helpful to ask the following questions: Is the culture-related practice efficacious? Is it safe? If it is beneficial, the clinician should encourage it. A home remedy may be safe but have no therapeutic benefit; the client, however, may believe in it, and this belief can have a powerful placebo effect that should be encouraged. If the treatment is not safe, further negotiation must ensue with an explanation as to why the practice is harmful and what options would be better. An example might be treatments for gastrointestinal distress in children used by some Mexican families: one treatment involves rubbing the child's abdomen and body with an uncooked egg in the shell, a technique that is not likely to affect the biologic cause of the gastritis. The egg treatment is not

In the health care setting, effective communication requires listening in a way that allows clients to explain what the situation means to them (see Box 3-1). Providers must clearly explain their perspective and understanding of the situation, explore a common ground of understanding with clients, and discuss and adapt possible solutions to meet the client's needs (Box 3-2). As previously mentioned, generating a solution based on the client's cultural context does not mean that providers compromise quality of care; care should be enhanced because it is tailored to the unique needs of the client.

Although the style of each provider and the characteristics and needs of clients vary in each client-provider interaction, several considerations should be kept in mind when communicating with clients in a pediatric health care setting.

Respect. All communication should be respectful. Though this seems obvious, providers do not always convey a clear message of respect. Initially addressing parents, grandparents, and other adults by their formal name can be a good beginning. Acknowledging all individuals in the room is important. Taking notes should be deferred if it interferes with conversation and engagement with the child and family. Actively listening and speaking clearly, calmly, and responsively encourages the child and family members to express their ideas and concerns. Include the child in conversation as is age-appropriate, encourage questions, and check frequently for understanding. Be alert to the style of interaction of the family: a direct approach can be threatening to some; in these situations, indirect questions, hypothetical situations, and open-ended questions can be more helpful.

Context. In some cultural groups the context in which a message is presented may have more significance than the words that are used. Generally, cultures can be seen as high-context or low-context.

In high-context cultures, individuals tend to be less direct in their verbal statements and extremely sensitive to nonverbal and situational cues, such as body language. Communication is facilitated by use of nonverbal methods rather than direct verbal statements, and understanding is derived primarily from experience, observation, and interaction, not necessarily from words or explanations. Relationships and kinship are important and many family members in high-context cultures may be involved in decisions about a child's care. The opinion of a grandmother might be considered valuable and could be solicited and listened to carefully (e.g., if extended family members are present at a health care visit, ask about their concerns and ideas; if only the primary caregiver is present, ask what the family is thinking and concerned about [see Box 3-1 for a framework of questions to use in this approach]).

In low-context cultures, the emphasis is on the content of the verbal message. Verbal communication is direct, explicit, and concrete; nonverbal and situational cues are less significant than in high-context cultures. The provider should be very clear in verbal communication with clients from low-context cultures, recognizing that they may not pick up on situational and nonverbal cues.

Time and Space as Forms of Nonverbal Communication

Time. Some cultures view time as steady, predictable, and mobile. It is always moving forward, and the impressions of past, present, and future are distinct—it is "monochronic," one thing at a time. For example, individuals who make lists and schedules, planning when to do certain tasks and following an ordered timeline demonstrate a monochronic approach to life. For others, the reality of time exists only in relation to events occurring. "Polychronic" time is characterized by "the simultaneous occurrence of many things and by a great involvement with people" (Hall, 1990, p 14). For example, individuals who plan to finish a task by a set time but coincidentally meet an old friend they haven't seen for a while may stop to talk for hours, the planned task forgotten in the moment. From this perspective there is no such thing as early or late. The future is less important than the present, and problems of daily survival take priority over far-reaching goals. An understanding of these differences can aid providers in looking at their clients' actions, especially failed treatment plans, from a different and more accepting perspective.

Space. Human beings seek to maintain a certain spatial distance from others. An expression of boundaries, this desire for control over a certain amount of personal space is known as *territoriality*, and although it varies from one individual to another, based on gender, age, and situation, there is a correlation between personal space requirements and culture (Watson, 1980). Three dimensions or zones of spatial distancing are recognized: The *intimate zone* allows close proximity and is reserved for family members and those in the roles of caregiver, comforter, and protector; the *personal zone* provides more spatial distance between individuals and is reserved for friends and close acquaintances; and the *public zone* is the spatial distance expected between coworkers and individuals in business encounters. This sense of personal space can be perceived not only visually, as with the establishment of a comfortable distance or with direct or indirect eye contact, but also through sound, smell, and touch.

Most people are not consciously aware of their personal space requirements and unconsciously may give nonverbal cues, such as turning to avoid direct face-to-face contact or stepping back, to indicate that they need more personal space. A tendency to move closer, lean forward, and maintain direct eye contact for sustained periods indicates the need for less spatial distance.

Failure to recognize and respect an individual's personal space needs may be interpreted as a threatening invasion of personal space or a lack of caring and compassion, depending on the situation. An awareness of boundaries, territoriality, and appropriate responses to cues received with regard to the spatial needs of an individual client or family enhance the development of a satisfactory client-provider relationship.

Language and Use of Interpreters. Providers are encouraged to become "linguistically appropriate." As a part of this effort, federal standards relating to linguistic competence have been developed—Culturally and Linguistically Appropriate Services (CLAS). These guidelines encourage providers to recognize that there are linguistic variations within cultural groups and that individuals who speak the same language may not share the same cultural background. There also may be a wide range of literacy levels in all language groups (U.S. Department of Health and Human Services [USDHHS] Office of Minority Health, 2001).

It is helpful to speak the client's language, but that ability alone is not sufficient and may not always be possible or necessary to be linguistically appropriate. Interpreters can be used very effectively; the quality of care for clients with limited English proficiency is improved with professional interpreter services (Karliner et al, 2007). Federally-funded managed care networks and community health centers are required to have interpreters accessible for all non–English-speaking clients. The importance of using a qualified interpreter cannot be overemphasized. Interpreters who are familiar with the culture and the language are especially helpful because they are likely to be more sensitive to the nonverbal cues inherent in a patient's presentation of a complaint. The term *cultural broker* is used to describe an individual who bridges two or more cultures and can translate both linguistic and cultural meaning.

In some immigrant communities, especially those that are small, there may be few qualified interpreters. Also, as members of a small, closely knit community, both interpreter and client may find it awkward to discuss sensitive personal information in a clinical setting and then return to their culturally prescribed social roles in the community. In larger immigrant communities, several languages or dialects may be spoken; language barriers may arise even among people who speak the same language because communication patterns differ among classes, subcultures, and regions of the country of origin. Some health care facilities do not have adequate interpreter services and providers rely on family members or unqualified facility staff to translate. In all these cases, patient confidentiality, provider-family understanding, and quality of care can be jeopardized. Although not an ideal solution, contracting with a commercial telephone interpreter service may be a possibility in these instances.

Interpreters and providers may experience conflict related to control of the clinical situation: providers do not understand what is being said, and may not be clear as to whether the interpreter is accurately conveying their (the provider's) message or completely relaying the client's comments. Interpreters may perceive themselves as part of the medical team and take on a "co-diagnostician" role in which they make decisions affecting care. Something as "minor" as neglecting to fully disclose what the client has said because the interpreter did not think it important, or offering the client advice beyond that given by the provider can compromise care (Hsieh, 2007). A good working relationship between provider and interpreter and a clear understanding of the role of each is necessary and must be actively negotiated (Hsieh, 2010; Hsieh et al, 2010).

The qualified interpreter stands or sits behind the provider so as not to interfere with eye contact between the client, the parent, and the provider. If privacy is an issue, the interpreter can stand or sit behind a screen. If topics related to sexuality are to be discussed, interpreters should be of the same sex as the patient.

The interpreter should make an effort to translate the dialogue as closely and accurately as possible for both parties. When a provider's yes or no question results in a lengthy response, the interpreter must ensure that the provider is apprised of the whole statement, including any seemingly unrelated data. It is especially difficult to convey emotion through verbal translation, and this component of communication may be lost or diminished when interpreters are used. This should not be perceived as lack of concern on the part of the client or family, and the provider should be alert for nonverbal cues. Nonverbal cues may have their own cultural connotative meaning, however, so clarification may be necessary (e.g., "You seem very upset; I noticed your face changed when we talked about _____. Are you worried about _____?"). Regarding instructions for home management, it may be helpful if the interpreter can write instructions for the family in the family's language and review them again before the family leaves.

Interpreters should work toward the following goals:
- Make the clients' description and understanding of the problem clear to the provider.
- Communicate accurately the provider's interpretation and explanation of a health problem (e.g., pathophysiology) to the client.
- Facilitate the discussion to develop a management plan.
- Assess patient and parents' level of knowledge and understanding of what is being said.

Culturally Sensitive Patient Education. It is incorrect to assume that all clients and their families value and benefit from printed patient education material. Although members of low-context cultures may seek and appreciate written material, it may be overwhelming for members of high-context cultures who are trying to interpret myriad nonverbal and situational cues as well as the verbal message associated with the visit. The best approach is to make clients aware of the written material that is available and let them know they may take it if they wish.

Any instructions for home management should be written in simple terms in the client's native language or in the language in which parents or caregivers are literate (which may be different from the native language), and educational efforts should be directed toward all adult family members present. Abbreviations should be avoided, and all written material should be reviewed with the patient, parent, or both, with the help of an interpreter when necessary. Assessing literacy must be done with sensitivity because illiteracy is a source of shame for some people.

RECOGNIZING CULTURE SHOCK

The process of emigrating—leaving one's homeland to settle in a different country—presents the individual and the family with many challenges. Changes in diet, exposure to unfamiliar environmental hazards, and lack of appropriate immunity may threaten physical health. Familiar resources are absent, and unfamiliar behaviors, expectations, symbols, and language are barriers to meeting basic daily needs. Considerable energy is required to interpret and respond to this new environment. Feelings of helplessness and exhaustion that may ensue are part of the phenomenon known as culture shock, first identified by anthropologists in the 1950s (Oberg, 1960).

Culture shock affects the physical, emotional, and psychological well-being of every member of the family and may take many months to overcome. Generally, individuals progress through stages of culture shock. Initially they may be fascinated with the novelty of the new culture, then become hostile or highly critical before moving on to adjustment and acceptance. The degree of culture shock experienced depends on many variables, including social status, personality characteristics, age, occupation, available support systems, familiarity with the dominant language, general state of health, and the extent of cultural differences between the home and host countries. For immigrants who have experienced displacement, violence, trauma, abuse, and fear, culture shock is complicated by post-traumatic responses and difficulty coping with other stressors.

Clients and family members experiencing culture shock may appear noncompliant, inappropriately complacent, or overreactive to health care providers. Successful management of culture shock can be facilitated by clearly and patiently explaining what is happening with the client; providing clear, relevant information about how the health system works; acknowledging the client's sense of confusion as normal; and giving positive feedback for the client's efforts. The provider can be a source of stability in the client's bewildering world.

Health care providers working with clients and families from culturally diverse backgrounds frequently experience culture shock, too. Lack of knowledge of differences in diseases, cultural practices, beliefs, and values can result in feelings of helplessness, frustration, and inadequacy for everyone involved in the helping relationship. Clinicians can reduce their own culture shock and that of their clients by learning about the different cultural groups they work with and recognizing the signs of culture shock in their clients and themselves.

■ Health Care for Immigrant and Refugee Populations

Immigrants represent the large category of individuals from other countries (aliens) who apply for permanent resident status in the U.S. Refugees and asylum seekers are a subset of immigrants who have been displaced by trauma or war in their country of origin, or who seek asylum from their country of origin due to risk of life, safety, or well-being. All aliens, whatever their history or circumstance, have the same health requirements when requesting permanent immigration or resident status in the U.S. These requirements serve to identify health problems and necessary care for immigrants and to protect the U.S. population from diseases that may be introduced by new arrivals.

In order for immigration to be considered, applicants must complete a health assessment (Box 3-3). These assessments are conducted by physicians in the alien's country of origin who are appointed by the U.S. Department of State Consulates (panel physicians) or by physicians in the U.S. appointed by the U.S. Citizenship and Immigration Service (civil surgeons). If applicants are found to have an inadmissible health condition (Box 3-4) or are underimmunized, treatment may be given or vaccines administered to help them meet the requirement for admission. Because a vaccine series can take months to complete, applicants become eligible for immigration after the series is begun. The applicant may also request a waiver for an inadmissible condition. The decision to admit

---

BOX 3-3 Health Assessment Required for Immigrants and Refugees

History

- Current signs and symptoms
- Medications: prescribed, over the counter (OTC), traditional, or herbal
- Allergies
- Family medical history (e.g., diabetes, hypertension, severe illness)
- Social history
  - ○ Travel
  - ○ Family structure
  - ○ Current living situation, safety, support
  - ○ Occupational history
  - ○ Use of alcohol, tobacco, nonprescription drugs, other substances from country of origin (e.g., betel nuts in Thailand; khat in East Africa)
  - ○ Educational level, literacy
- Past medical history
  - ○ Hospitalization
  - ○ Severe illness
  - ○ Chronic conditions
  - ○ Mental health conditions
  - ○ Injuries
  - ○ Surgeries, including dental
  - ○ Blood transfusions
- Vaccinations
- Review of systems (ROS)

Physical

Thorough head-to-toe physical examination, including nutritional assessment, growth and development, and sexual maturity. Genital examination may be deferred to a later health visit if not deemed appropriate (e.g., different gender provider, obvious reluctance on part of client).

---

an applicant rests with the U.S. Citizenship and Immigration Service, but is based in part on the health findings. Aliens who present at a port of entry to the U.S. with an inadmissible condition or who have been exposed to such a condition (e.g., severe acute respiratory syndrome [SARS]) may be placed in isolation or quarantine at the discretion of the U.S. Surgeon General (CDC, 2011b).

Individuals who apply for a temporary visitor status are not required to have a health assessment (Yanni et al, 2009). Unauthorized immigrants would also not be examined but, as with temporary visitors, could require medical care and/or represent a health risk to the U.S. population.

Once in the country, ongoing settlement issues influence health needs and decisions. Currently, ten voluntary private agencies (VolAgs) and one state agency work with the U.S. Department of State to provide "initial reception and placement" of new refugees (Box 3-5). Refugees may be "anchored" (i.e., have a family member or friend who assumes some responsibility for their placement) or "free" (i.e., having no contact in the U.S.). In early 2008, all refugees from Burma and Bhutan were designated as "free" because this population is so new to the U.S. that there is no well-established community here to support new immigration. "Free" refugees have no role in deciding where they will be placed. However, if a Burmese/Karen or Bhutanese refugee does have a family member or friend in the U.S., the individual may request placement

Inadmissible Conditions for U.S.
Immigration Purposes*†

- Communicable diseases of public health significance
  - Infectious tuberculosis
  - Syphilis
  - Other sexually transmitted diseases (chancroid, gonorrhea, granuloma inguinale, lymphogranuloma venereum)
  - Hansen disease (leprosy)
- No documentation of vaccination against vaccine-preventable diseases‡
- Required vaccines include:
  - Mumps
  - Measles
  - Rubella
  - Polio
  - Tetanus
  - Diphtheria
  - Pertussis
  - *Haemophilus influenzae* type B (HIB)
  - Rotavirus
  - Hepatitis A
  - Hepatitis B
  - Meningococcal disease
  - Varicella
  - Pneumococcal pneumonia
  - Influenza
- Physical or mental disorders with associated harmful behaviors
- Substance-related disorders (drug abusers or addicts)

*The final health assessment may demonstrate successful treatment of these conditions, making the applicant eligible for admission based on current health status.
†Effective January 4, 2010, human immunodeficiency virus (HIV) testing is no longer required for immigration and HIV infection was removed from the list of inadmissible conditions.
‡As of December 14, 2009, human papillomavirus (HPV) and zoster vaccines are not required for immigrants.
From CDC: Medical examination of immigrants and refugees. Available at www.cdc.gov/immigrantrefugeehealth/exams/medical-examination.html (accessed January 27, 2011).

Voluntary and State Agencies
(VolAgs) Contracted with U.S.
Department of State to Provide
Refugee Resettlement Services,
2011

- Church World Service
- Ethiopian Community Development Council
- Episcopal Migration Ministries
- Hebrew Immigrant Aid Society
- International Rescue Committee
- Kurdish Human Rights Watch
- U.S. Committee for Refugees and Immigrants
- Lutheran Immigration and Refugee Service
- United States Conference of Catholic Bishops
- World Relief
- State of Iowa, Bureau of Refugee Services

and be designated "free with geographical preference" or "free-o," even though the family or friend (who also may be a recent immigrant) has limited responsibility for resettlement; the VolAg assumes primary responsibility. Not all states are able to accept "free" refugees.

VolAgs assist new arrivals to settle into the community. Each refugee family is assigned a VolAg caseworker who meets the refugees at the airport; arranges housing and basic household supplies; provides an orientation to the community; assists in application for Social Security cards, draft status (if applicable), public assistance (if necessary), school and English class (English as a second language [ESL]) enrollment, and employment; arranges for medical care and refugee screening; facilitates travel for family reunification; and gives special care to separated or unaccompanied minors.

Medical care and screening with a primary care provider are to be arranged for refugees within 90 days of entry into the community. If an applicant has a medical waiver for entry, health care should be arranged sooner than the 90 days. The CDC Division of Global Migration and Quarantine is responsible for notifying state and local health departments of new arrivals who need medical treatment and/or follow-up (Maloney et al, 2007).

In response to large immigrant populations, some states and municipalities work with VolAgs to develop coordinated, integrated programs of service, support and information for both clients (i.e., immigrants) and providers (e.g., the Minnesota Refugee Health Program can be accessed at www.health.state.mn.us/divs/idepc/refugee) and many volunteer groups provide services both in countries of origin and in the U.S. (e.g., American Refugee Committee International [www.arcrelief.org]).

In contrast, immigrants applying for resident status who are not refugees or are not seeking asylum are not assigned caseworkers or considered for service under refugee programs. Depending on their resources, immigrants may enter the health care system as any resident client would do; they may pay "out of pocket," have insurance through a job, or apply directly for public assistance and Medicaid. They may also access public health resources in their community.

Underutilization of health care services is characteristic of immigrant populations, contributes to health discrepancies seen between immigrants and native-born Americans, and presents a health risk because many conditions go untreated. A Harvard Medical School study found that health care expenditures for immigrants were about 55% less than for native-born Americans; for immigrant children, expenditures in 1998 were 74% less (Mohanty et al, 2005). Most immigrants are insured (44% of recent and 63% of established immigrants), yet still use health resources less than insured native-born, effectively subsidizing the care of native-born residents (Ku, 2009).

Many new immigrants, including those who are unauthorized, use public sector resources (e.g., county and state public health departments) for health care, but, though they represent 5% of the population, recent immigrants used only about 1% of public health resources (Ku, 2009). Unauthorized immigrants, in particular, may make efforts to avoid public scrutiny and remain isolated from services and agencies.

INITIAL HEALTH CARE VISIT

The goal of the immigrant's initial visit with the primary care provider is to begin to establish trust with the clients; such trust will foster communication and, it is hoped, health-seeking by clients.

Assessment

Care given at the initial visit should include a thorough history and physical examination (see Chapter 2; Box 3-3; Box 3-6) and assessment for both acute and chronic conditions (Dicker et al, 2010; Hulme, 2010). Although the evaluation is standard, rounding up all the usual suspects, there are some special considerations to keep in mind when working with new immigrants and refugees, including:

- The provider should emphasize that the examination is aimed at benefiting the client and has no effect on the client's immigrant status. Confidentiality should be explained to the client.
- The provider should explain that he or she is learning and interested in learning more about the client's culture; explanations from the client are welcome and the provider may need to ask questions related to culture.
- It may be extremely difficult or impossible to get a complete and accurate history.
- Include traditional, herbal, or other complementary medications when soliciting medication history.
- Include use of substances (e.g., betel nut in Thailand, khat in East Africa) when soliciting alcohol, tobacco, or drug use history.
- Ask about education level and literacy.
- Attend especially to mental health and nutrition concerns.
- Provide for same-gender examiners when conducting examinations of genitalia or asking questions related to personal or intimate matters.
- Get a thorough vaccination history; ask to see any documentation the client has from other providers (e.g., the panel physician who conducted the admission examination overseas; vaccine card given to parents in Mexico). Remember that immigrants may not have received all vaccinations prior to arrival. See Box 3-4 for a list of vaccination requirements for U.S. immigration.
- Anticipate the need for referral, and assist the client to make contact with referral sources as needed. Work closely with caseworkers and public health nurses assigned to clients.

Management

Primary care providers face heightened challenges when working with new immigrants and refugees. The same cultural barriers discussed earlier operate: differences in language, worldviews, and perceptions and interpretations of the meaning of health and illness. Added to these barriers are the dynamics of rapid transition, major shifts from rural to urban living, and, for refugees, experience with violence, dislocation, extreme poverty, and fear. In the dislocation process, families experience changes in gender roles, social expectations, and family responsibilities. All of the rules change: children may be lost, orphaned, or abandoned; women may take a more visible public role; and adolescents may be unsupervised, largely operating in peer groups. The ability to cope that derives from a strong social support network is jeopardized, and families are uprooted and disoriented. Seeking health care and adhering to health care recommendations may be low on the list of survival needs.

In addition to the skills of cultural competence discussed previously, providers of care to refugees need to develop a

---

BOX 3-6 Immigrant Health Needs: Considerations for Primary Care Providers

- Acute conditions: infectious diseases (tuberculosis [TB], hepatitis B), dental caries, diseases of malnutrition
- Chronic conditions: diabetes, malaria, parasites, others (e.g., thalassemia, sickle cell)
- Mental health conditions: both acute and chronic, and related to both circumstances of immigration and intrinsic variables (i.e., the condition would have manifested without immigration)
- Conditions related to the social circumstances of immigration:
  - Stress of transition, particularly a move from rural to urban environment (Steffen et al, 2006)
  - Posttraumatic stress disorders: although children suffer psychologic trauma of war, dislocation, and violence, there are many factors (e.g., family attachment, peer support, extended social networks) that serve to help the child cope and demonstrate resilience (Betancourt and Khan, 2008; Crowley, 2009)
  - Exposure to environmental and safety hazards in new location (e.g., traffic and population density; farmworkers' occupational health; see Chapter 41)
  - Malnutrition secondary to poverty and lack of access to high-quality nutrients

Adapted from Hulme P: Cultural considerations in evidence-based practice, *J Transcult Nurs* 21(3):271-280, 2010.

---

knowledge base related to the following (Suurmond et al, 2010):

- Political situation and experience of clients in the country of origin
- Transition time experienced by clients: were they in refugee camps? Where? What were conditions there?
- Diseases common in the country of origin and in transition sites
- Effects on health that result from being a refugee (e.g., stress, malnutrition, etc.)
- Legal context for refugees in the U.S.
- Effective management of trauma

Primary care providers must also be skilled at explaining the U.S. health care system to clients. Fortunately, the use of community-based participatory action to meet refugee health needs has been shown to be effective (Culhane-Pera et al, 2010). In some immigrant communities, clients are involved in planning systems, and primary care providers have support from a larger system, including public health nurses, interpreters, social workers, and voluntary community agencies. A community-based approach is essential to counter the low use of health services by members of the immigrant or refugee community and provide effective care (Birman et al, 2008).

Providing culturally competent care is a challenge that requires personal reflection as well as significant change in beliefs, attitudes, and practices. By working sensitively with clients of diversity, sharing ideas and information, learning from and about each other, and celebrating differences and similarities, clients and clinicians can become full participants in creating a new cultural context for the health and illness experience.

Management of Development

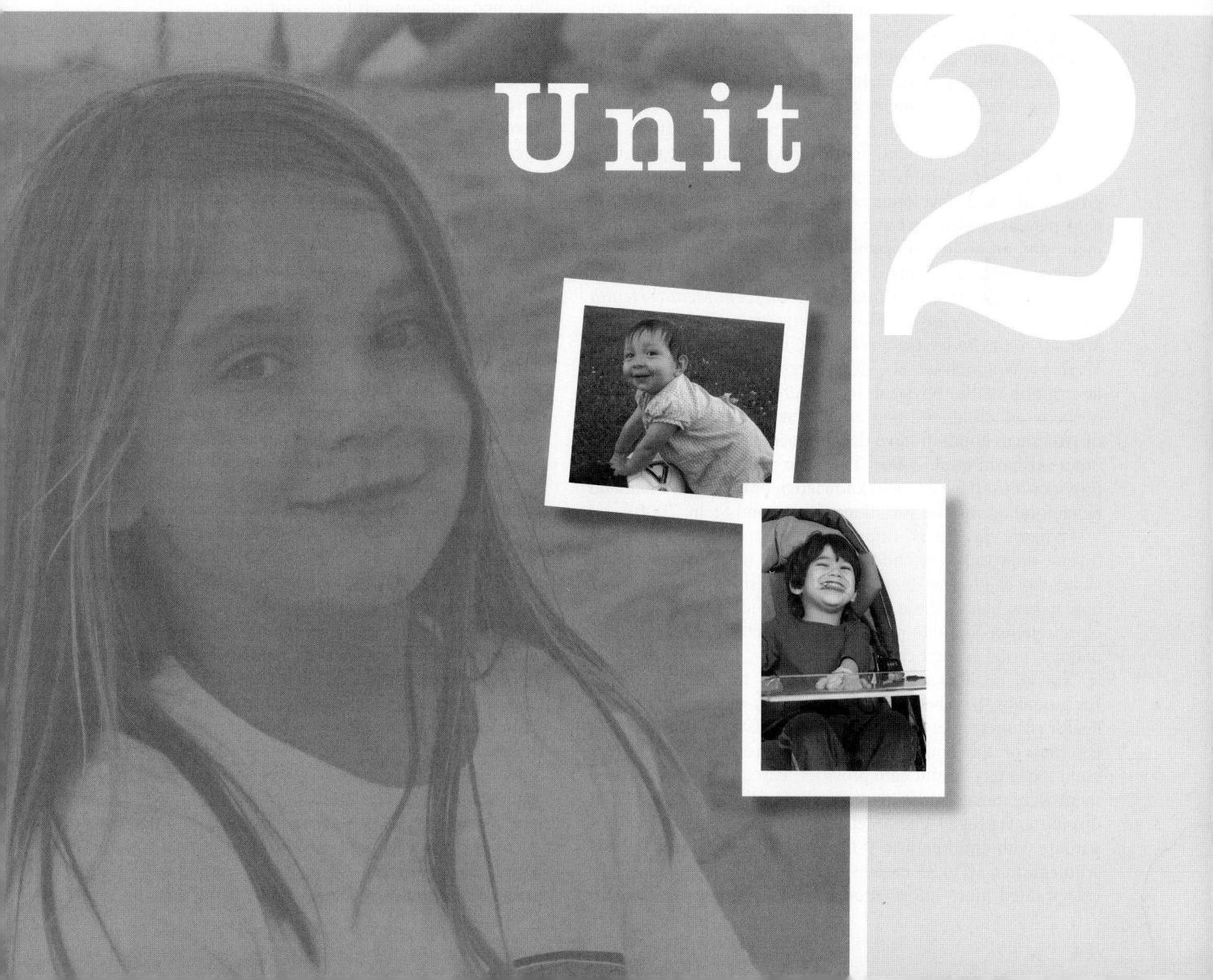

Unit

2

Developmental Management in Pediatric Primary Care

ANITA D. BERRY, DAWN LEE GARZON, AND BARBARA JONES DELOIAN

Modern approaches to managing children's well-being differ dramatically from those that prevailed at the turn of the last century, when health supervision often consisted of a brief examination to detect communicable or contagious diseases. In the twenty-first century significant social, economic, and demographic changes continue to influence the American family and affect children's health. Children's health supervision uses a broader approach than that necessary for disease detection. Pediatric primary care providers have a responsibility to monitor children's overall physical, cognitive, and psychosocial development, and to provide anticipatory guidance to families as children grow. This requires a strong background in child development, knowledge of strategies that help parents understand and adjust to their child's development, and an ability to establish effective relationships with children and their parents.

The Classification of Child and Adolescent Mental Health Diagnoses in Primary Care: Diagnostic and Statistical Manual for Primary Care (DSM-PC), Child and Adolescent Version (Wolraich et al, 1996) presents a comprehensive description of the physical and psychosocial developmental concerns of childhood and adolescence. An estimated 17% of American children have developmental or behavioral disorders (Bhasin et al, 2006). Thus, the pediatric primary care provider must have a sound knowledge of developmental and behavioral norms and variations (Dixon and Stein, 2006).

Pediatric providers offer parents support and suggest diverse approaches to childrearing. They help parents understand the challenges that new accomplishments create and how to best handle these challenges. Providers who develop a close relationship with parents and their children share in the parents' pride as their child grows.

Not all health care providers satisfy the parents' needs for guidance, however. A national survey of early childhood health (Blumberg et al, 2004) gathered data on parents' perceptions of the anticipatory guidance received from their child's primary health care provider. Parent reports indicated there were unmet needs, particularly for discussion related to discipline strategies and toilet training (expressed by 36% of parents with children 4 to 9 months old and 56% of parents with children 10 to 35 months old). Other areas in which parents wanted more information included reading, vocabulary

development, social development, childcare, and burn prevention (Olson et al, 2004). To meet the needs of parents and children, it is imperative for primary care providers to have a sound foundation regarding all aspects of evaluating, assessing, and managing child development.

This chapter presents an introduction to principles of development, developmental theories, methods of developmental assessment, and identification and management of developmental problems. Chapters 5 through 8 review developmental theories, describe normal patterns of development, identify "red flags" related to development, and recommend anticipatory guidance for families of infants, toddlers and preschoolers, school-age children, and adolescents.

■ Developmental Principles

Development is a lifelong, dynamic process. Achievement of milestones in one phase sets the stage for the next phase. Development is also a dynamic and reciprocal process that occurs between the child's internal and external environments. Key principles provide a context to understand concepts of development. Exactly how these principles manifest in a particular child depends on the child's genetic background, personality, and intrauterine and extrauterine environmental factors.

Principle 1. Growth and development are orderly and sequential. Although children differ in rates and timing of developmental changes, they generally follow certain predictable stages or phases. Specific examples include the rapid growth during the first year of life, progress toward independence throughout childhood, and the development of secondary sex characteristics during adolescence.

Principle 2. The pace of growth and development is specific for each child. Developmental changes vary considerably for each child. Some children demonstrate early skill in motor coordination, others in language acquisition. These changes represent the uniqueness of each child.

Principle 3. Development occurs in a cephalocaudal and proximodistal direction. An example of this principle is seen as infants develop increasing motor coordination, gaining head control before sitting and walking. Similarly, developmental progress is seen in controlled movements that occur first near the midline of the body, such as rolling over. Eventually distal coordination of the hands, such as mastery of the pincer grasp, occurs.

Principle 4. Growth and development become increasingly integrated. Behavior that is taken for granted, such as self-feeding, occurs as a result of numerous small changes and skills acquired by the child. Simple skills and behaviors are integrated into more complex behaviors as the child grows and develops.

Principle 5. Developmental abilities increasingly organize and differentiate. As a result of increasing maturation and experience, children's behaviors and responses to internal and external cues become more regulated, organized, and differentiated. The infant's crying and body movements in response to hunger cues are different from the toddler's walking to the refrigerator in response to the same cues.

Principle 6. The child's internal and external environments affect growth and development. Opportunities for play, societal norms, cultural values, family traditions, and family beliefs all influence the development of children. Similarly, children influence their environment to achieve desired experiences and opportunities.

Principle 7. Certain periods are critical during growth and development. Critical periods are points of time when developmental advances occur and are particularly susceptible to alterations due to internal and external influences. The development of congenital anomalies when the fetus is exposed to certain viruses during fetal growth is one example.

Principle 8. Growth and development are dynamic processes influenced by many factors. Development is a continual process, often without smooth transitions. Phases of development are marked by periods of change, growth, and stability plateaus. Developmental predictors must incorporate the individual nature of development and the numerous individual factors that influence developmental outcomes (Cech and Martin, 2002).

■ Developmental Theories

Developmental theories include an array of ideas about how children progress from infancy through adolescence and provide many perspectives on children's growth and development. Health care providers need to stay abreast of changing ideas regarding child development and appreciate new developmental theories relating to children. Developmental theories are based on various cultures, personalities, environmental issues, philosophical beliefs, and investigative methods. Thus, when using a developmental perspective in practice, the provider should understand how the theory was developed and how it may relate to a particular family and child. Developmental theories provide guidelines for understanding the unfolding of the child's behavior, personality, and physical abilities. It is usually necessary to combine several theories to understand the child as a whole person.

Criticism of the work of early child development theorists stated that they lacked an evidence base, failed to consider the child in different cultural and socioeconomic settings, and had a linear focus that missed the subtleties of the interaction of "nature" and "nurture." More research is being conducted to validate and test developmental theories,

incorporate new concepts, and gain a better understanding of children's learning mechanisms, especially children who have special needs.

ETHOLOGY: ANIMAL STUDIES

The study of animal behavior, looking at the concepts of bonding, altruism, social intelligence, and dominant and submissive behavior led to theoretic assumptions that frame the study of child development. Bowlby (1969) first generalized theories developed about animal behavior to bonding for humans, articulating the concept of attachment theory. Ainsworth and colleagues (1971) examined the elements of early attachment and separation in child development and personality. This was followed by Klaus and Kennel's work (1976), which emphasized the importance of early mother-infant contact. Their work later became the basis for changes in hospital rooming-in care.

MATURATIONAL THEORIES: DEVELOPMENTAL MILESTONES

Early theories about human behavior set the stage for studies of child development. Rousseau's descriptions in 1762 of the natural, innately good growth of the child, if not misled by a "corrupt social environment," provided the foundation for maturational theories. Gesell (1940) is credited with the term *maturation* in reference to the orderly, sequential developmental changes that occur over time. He described cycles of behavior that correspond to certain chronologic ages. His work resulted in the chronologic growth and development norms for motor, affective, linguistic, and social domains that are now used to assess developmental progress.

Lewin (1936) identified growth principles and the currently acknowledged stages of infancy, early childhood, and adolescence. He provided an understanding of the play and decision-making phases through which children progress.

Havighurst's work (1953), a summation of ideas from many theorists, popularized the concept of developmental tasks as "successful achievement which leads to happiness and to success with later tasks, while failure leads to unhappiness in the individual, disapproval by society, and difficulty with later tasks."

COGNITIVE-STRUCTURAL THEORIES: LANGUAGE AND THOUGHT

Cognitive-structural theories examine the ways in which children think, reason, and use language. They are based on assumptions about central nervous system maturation and children's interactions with their environment. Individual differences are ascribed to genetic endowment and environmental influences.

Jean Piaget's observations, many of which were of his own children, provide an understanding of children's cognitive development and their perception and interaction with the world around them. Piaget (1969) described how children actively use their life experiences, incorporating them into their own mental and physical being over time. He emphasized how children modify themselves depending on their environmental experiences and their stage-related competency level. Piaget described four stages of cognitive development (Table 4-1).

| TABLE 4-1 | Comparison of Early Developmental Theorists |

Age	Freud	KOHLBERG	
		Stages	
0-12 mo	Oral stage	Stage 1 "premoral" pre-conventional level	1: Punishment avoidance and obedience
12-18 mo			
18-36 mo	Anal stage	Stages 1-2 pre-conventional level	2: Instrumental realistic orientation—recognizes needs in others as long as own needs are met
3-6 yr	Oedipal stage	Stages 1-2 pre-conventional level	
6-11 yr	Latency stage	Pre-conventional (stage 2)—to 7 yrs Conventional (stages 3 and 4)— 7-10 yrs Post-conventional (stage 5)—10-11 yrs	3: Interpersonal acceptance of "nice" girl and "good" boy social concept—does not want relationships with others harmed 4: The "law and order" orientation—rules are not flexible or changeable 5: Social contract and utilitarian orientation—rules can change on social needs
12-17 yr	Adolescence (Oedipus complex)	Stages 5-6 post-conventional level	6: Universal ethical orientation principles are source of rules. Inner conscience present.
17-30 yr	Young adult	Stages 5-6	

Sensorimotor Stage (Birth to 2 Years)

At this stage children learn about the world through their actions and sensory and motor movements. Key concepts during this period include object permanence, spatial relationships, causality, use of instruments, and combination of objects. The child's framework for learning is the self, and there is little cognitive connection to objects outside the self.

Preoperational Stage (2 to 7 Years)

Children next attempt to make sense of the world and reality. However, this is based on an egocentric perspective and is accomplished through certain mental operations that are linked to concrete objects. Children at this stage are not able to understand cause and effect. Therefore, their reasoning is often flawed. Children begin to use semiotic functioning, or the use of one thing to represent another. Intuitive reasoning emerges toward the end of this stage, but reasoning continues to be connected to the concrete reality of the here and now.

Concrete Operational Stage (7 to 12 Years)

Children use symbols to represent concrete objects (here and now) and perform mental operations in their head. This requires cognitive skills to organize experiences and classify increasingly complex information. Most schoolwork requires functioning at this level with flexibility of thought, declining egocentrism, logical reasoning, and greater social cognition.

Formal Operational Stage (13 Years through Adulthood)

At this stage, children begin to think abstractly and imagine different solutions to problems and different outcomes. Adolescents begin to develop increased awareness of degrees of illness and personal control of one's health. Renewed egocentrism may be noted early in this stage as a result of a lack of differentiation between what others are thinking and one's own thoughts. This egocentric thinking eventually gives way to an appreciation of the differences in judgment between the adolescent and other individuals, societies, and cultures. It

PIAGET		ERIKSON	
Stages/Substages	Characteristics	Psychological Crisis	Themes
Sensorimotor stage			
Reflexive stage: 0-1 mo	Innate infant reflexes	Trust vs. mistrust	To get; to give in return
Primary circular stage: 1-4 mo	Repetitive responses		
Secondary circular stage: 4-8 mo	Outward-directed behaviors		
Coordination of secondary circular stage: 8-12 mo	Object permanence and goal-directed behaviors		
Tertiary circular reactions stage: 2-18 mo	Causality and object permanence through several steps	Autonomy vs. shame	To hold on; to let go
Mental combinations stage: 18-24 mo	Memory used for problem-solving		
Preoperational stage: Preconceptual stage: 2-4 yr Intuitive stage: 4-7 yr	Increased use of symbols, especially language; representational thought, egocentrism, assimilation, and symbolic play Increased symbolic functioning, language, decreasing egocentricity, imitation of reality	Initiative vs. guilt	To make things; to play
Concrete operational stage	*Flexible thought:* understands rules of reversibility and deconcentration, conservation, and identity *Declining egocentrism:* ability to understand another's perspective *Local reasoning:* understands concepts of relation, ordering, conservation; able to classify objects *Social cognition:* improved sense of equality and justice	Industry vs. inferiority	To make things; to complete
Formal operational stage	Development of logical thinking, able to work with abstract ideas; able to synthesize and integrate concepts into larger schemes	Identity vs. role confusion	To be oneself; to share being oneself or not being oneself
Formal operational stage		Intimacy vs. isolation	To lose and find oneself in another

becomes the basis of an adolescent's ability to think about politics, law, and society in terms of abstract principles and benefits rather than focusing only on the punitive aspects of societal laws.

Piaget's work was expanded by theorists such as Flavell (1977) and Siegler and colleagues (1973), who looked at specific intellectual capabilities via the information processing model. This model included concepts of attention, perception, memory, and making inferences and provided an initial understanding of how mental activity leads progressively to more sophisticated ways of handling information.

Kohlberg (1969) focused on theories of moral development and socialization, emphasizing the process by which children learn the expectations and norms of their society and culture (see Table 4-1). Kohlberg's work primarily involved male participants. Gilligan (1982) suggested that female thoughts and actions involve significantly different objectives and goals, specifically that girls tend to think more in terms of caring and relationships, basing their moral judgments on complexities they perceive in human interactions.

Fowler's theory (1981) described the spiritual dimension of human life, or the development of faith. This theory addressed the process by which humans develop meaning for daily life. Faith is described as the structure that people use to build their lives. Fowler emphasized that achieving the stages is not due to intelligence but rather occurs through valuing, thinking, and interacting with others.

The Role of Social Interaction in Cognitive Development

Vygotsky's theory of child learning states that as children interact with others, they develop as individuals within cultural contexts. They simultaneously develop memory, problem-solving skills, attention, and concept formation (1978). Core to Vygotsky's theory is the "zone of proximal development," which is the difference between what a child can do on his or her own and what he or she can do with help from others.

Vygotsky believes that children learn by watching adults and other children and that children learn best when their parents and caregivers provide them with opportunities in the child's zone of proximal development. This theory holds that cognitive development occurs in a social, historical, and cultural context, and that adults guide children to learn. Development depends on the use of language, play, and extensive social interaction. One of Vygotsky's examples is the process of the child learning to point his or her finger. Initially, the infant points his or her finger without meaning; however, as people, and especially caregivers, respond to the finger pointing, the infant learns there is meaning to the movement. What starts as a muscle movement becomes a means of interpersonal connection between two people (Vygotsky, 1978). This theory further holds that play and learning should be constructed to take into consideration the child's needs, inclination, and incentives. This theory supports the benefit of adult social learning opportunities via group interaction and observation.

PSYCHOANALYTIC THEORIES
Personality and Emotions

Psychodynamic theorists study factors that influence the emotional and psychological behavior of individuals. Personality includes the characteristics of temperament and motivation, in addition to concepts related to self-esteem and self-concept. Sigmund Freud (1938) was one of the most influential theorists in this area. Freud sought to find links between the conscious mind and the body through the unconscious mind (see Table 4-1). Some of his most significant contributions were his descriptions of the interactions of id, ego, and superego (Thomas, 1985).

Anna Freud continued the work of her father, focusing particularly on children. It was through her studies that the implications of psychoanalysis for raising normal children were developed. She believed that psychoanalytic theory could help parents gain "insight into the potential harm done to young children during the critical years of their development by the manner in which their needs, drives, wishes, and emotional dependencies are met" (Freud, 1974).

Erikson (1964) expanded Freud's theories, describing the stages of the individual throughout the life span (see Table 4-1). Each stage presents problems that the individual seeks to master. Erikson believed that if problems were not resolved, they would be revisited again at future stages.

Sullivan (1964) emphasized the importance of self-concept and the environmental influences that modulate it. He defined the most crucial cultural environment as the home and the parent. Sullivan posited that progression toward mature relationships is based on communication skills and the integration of social experiences inhibited or enhanced by the parents' relationship between themselves.

Mahler and colleagues (1975) analyzed the development of an infant's evolving independence through study of the mother-infant dyad. Three phases of development were proposed: autism, symbiosis, and separation-individuation. They posited that these phases account for the gradually increasing awareness of the infant's sense of self and others. In the autistic phase (3 to 5 weeks old), the infant has no concept of self but is working, physiologically, to achieve homeostasis in the extrauterine world. The second phase, symbiosis, refers to a period of undifferentiation or fusion with the mother in which infant and mother form a dual unity. Separation-individuation (from about 4 to 5 months old onward) is characterized by a steady increase in awareness of the separateness of the self and the other.

Infant attachment within the context of separation and connectedness has been explored by Stern (1985), Emde and Buchsbaum (1990), and Rogoff (1990). They propose that the quality and consistency of infant-caregiver relationships help the infant develop an affective, or emotional, sense of self. The early beginnings of the sense of self are based on three biologic principles: self-regulation, social fittedness, and affective monitoring (Emde, 1988). Infants with attachment security and a sense of connectedness are more likely to explore and be autonomous; they also have what is called an *internal working model* to guide them in later attachments.

The concept of *intersubjectivity,* or mutual understanding of meaning and mutual engagement in social interactions, underlies attachment theory. Observing that even very young infants demonstrate an ability to interact beyond an instinctive or reflexive manner with a sympathetic individual, Trevarthen and Aitken conducted an extensive review of the literature on the topic of infant intersubjectivity (2001). They concluded that the infant's capacity for self-regulation may be based in the operation of an intrinsic motive formation (IMF) developed in the parietotemporal region of the prenatal brain. Studies of the brain and infant behavior suggest that this IMF guides the newborn's ability to integrate sensory-motor coordination, orient to preferred stimuli (e.g., mother's voice), sustain mutual attention with an affectionate other, and anticipate what to expect in the environment. Successful development of the infant's "purposive consciousness" and the ability to cooperate with and learn from another depends on the neurologic functioning and the presence of a supportive environment. The parent guides the infant to connect with others and experience mutuality. Social interactions and infant engagement with their parents and objects in their world are major developmental influences.

These theories help the provider assist parents to understand why, for example, 9-month-old infants (who now understand object permanence) will look over the side of the highchair for food or a toy that has fallen to the floor and smile and laugh when they spot it because they knew it would be there. These same infants may call a parent to their room in the middle of the night; they now have "person permanence." They can picture their parent in their mind and, perhaps experiencing normal separation anxiety, they want the parent to come to them. The provider can use the concepts of attachment theory and intersubjectivity to explain that this behavior is that of a normal developing infant trying to have his or her needs met. The behavior reflects an infant who is attached and who uses the parent as a secure base from which to explore the world. It is not a problem, nor is the child being "bad."

BEHAVIORAL THEORIES: HUMAN
Actions and Interactions

Behaviorism, the study of the general laws of human behavior, focuses on the present and ways that the environment influences human behavior. Skinner's view of child development examined learning that was controlled through classic operant conditioning (1953). Behavior modification therapy is largely based on Skinner's work. Bandura's social learning theory looked at imitation and modeling as a means of learning, emphasizing the social variables involved (Mott, 1990; Thomas, 1985). Bijou and Baer (1965) responded to critics of behaviorism's view of the child as a passive object, arguing that children's responses to environmental stimuli are dependent on their genetic structure and personal history (Thomas, 1985).

HUMANISTIC THEORIES
Innermost Self
Maslow (1971), Buhler and Allen (1972), and Mahrer (1978) are among the most well-known humanistic theorists, examining development throughout the life span. Maslow's hierarchy of needs included physiologic, safety, belongingness and love, esteem, and self-actualization needs. He differentiated deficiency needs from growth or self-actualization needs. Rather than proposing stages through which children or adults mature, the humanists believe that individuals and those around them are responsible for any movement they make from one plateau of needs to another; intrinsic forces do not move them along.

ECOLOGIC THEORIES
The key concepts of human ecology theory (Bronfenbrenner, 1979) emphasize the interdependence between environmental settings (roles, interpersonal relations, and activities) and the developing child. Development is described as the growing capacity to discover, sustain, or alter the self or the environment. Children are viewed as dynamic entities who are increasingly able to restructure the settings in which they live. Environments are seen as influencing children, leading to mutual accommodation and reciprocity. Children's perceptions of the environment influence their behavior and development more than the objective reality does.

Children are influenced by the home and family, child care settings, schools, entertainment and recreational activities, their parents' work, and broad economic opportunities in society. Recognition is given to ecologic transitions or changes in an individual's role or setting, such as the birth of a sibling or changes in family structure. Routine and ritual within the family system can be powerful mediators of children's development (Fiese, 2002; Kubicek, 2002). The parent-child interaction also may be inhibited or enhanced by the parents' relationships. When parents experience positive mutual feelings, the parent-child relationship is strengthened. Alternatively, when parents experience mutual antagonism or interference, the parent-child relationship may be impaired (Kelly and Barnard, 2000). These theories are especially useful to better understand the impact of domestic violence on a child's development and future.

TEMPERAMENT
The work of Chess and Thomas (1995) explains the role that temperament plays in children's behavior. They identified characteristics or qualities of temperament and introduced the concept of "goodness of fit" to describe the degree to which the child's environment and parents' characteristics, including the parents' temperament, are congruous with the child's natural temperamental characteristics. Understanding the child's unique temperament prepares the health care provider

to help parents and other caregivers to better understand the child's behavior, especially when the behavioral reactions are confusing or problematic for the parents. The provider can discuss with parents their view of their child's temperament, how it "fits" with the parents' temperament or that of other family members, and what parent-child strategies can be used if conflicts emerge between the child's temperament and the caregivers' personal style. The intent is to alleviate guilt and frustration and to assist parents to develop skills that enhance positive behaviors rather than exaggerate difficult temperamental characteristics. Being able to support both the parent and child's needs can prevent significant problems later on. Table 4-2 further defines characteristics of temperamental differences.

SELF-REGULATION
Self-regulation involves a transition from mutual regulation between mother and newborn and emphasizes the importance of both "nature and nurture" in a child's development (Shonkoff and Phillips, 2000; Trevarthen and Aitken, 2001). Examples of self-regulation are early infant sleep patterns and the ability to self-soothe, the toddler's ability to manage emerging emotions, the preschooler's ability to transition from home to school, the school-age child's ability to focus attention on important tasks, and the adolescent's sense of

TABLE 4-2	Characteristics of Temperament
Temperament Characteristic	**Description**
Activity	What is the child's activity level? Is the child moving all the time he or she is awake, some of the time, or rarely?
Rhythmicity	How predictable is the child's sleep-wake pattern, feeding schedule, and elimination pattern?
Approach or withdrawal	What is the child's response when presented with something new such as a new toy, a new experience, or a new person? Does he or she immediately approach or turn away?
Adaptability	How quickly does the child get used to new things? Quickly or not at all?
Threshold of response	How much stimulation does the child require for calming? A quiet voice and touch or more intense, loud voice or firm grasp?
Intensity of reaction	Are the child's responses (crying or laughing) very subtle or extremely intense?
Quality of mood	Is the child's mood usually outgoing, happy, joyful, pleasant or unfriendly, withdrawn, or quiet?
Distractibility	How easily is the child distracted by outside disturbances such as a phone ringing, TV, siblings?
Attention span and persistence	How long will the child continue to play with a particular toy or engage in a certain activity? Does this continue even when there are distractions?

confidence and competence. Learning self-regulation is influenced by differences in temperament, genetics, child abilities, and characteristics of the child's environment (Kochanska et al, 2001). The ways in which the social environment interacts with the individuality of the child and the types of interventions that will contribute to successful self-regulation continue to be explored. One important variable influencing the child's development appears to be a need for a predictable and consistent environment and a caring, emotionally available caregiver (Bronson, 2000).

EARLY BRAIN DEVELOPMENT

On October 3, 2000, the National Research Council and the Institute of Medicine of the National Academies released *From Neurons to Neighborhoods: The Science of Early Childhood Development*, an update and synthesis of current scientific knowledge of child development from birth to age 5, including discussion of the latest research in early brain development (Shonkoff and Phillips, 2000). By 8 months of age, brain synapses have increased from 50 trillion to 1000 trillion and remain at this level throughout early childhood. During the rest of childhood and adolescence, the efficiency of the neuronal networks, especially the prefrontal cortex which is responsible for judgment and impulse control, is refined. Studies cited in this report confirm the fact that early experiences affect the development of the brain and lay the foundation for intelligence, emotional health, and moral development. Positive early experiences have a positive effect on formation of brain cells. The report emphasizes the following developmental concepts: healthy early development depends on nurturing and dependable relationships; how young children feel is as important as how they think, particularly with regard to school readiness; and, although society is changing, the needs of young children are not being met in the process. Ultimately, the report recommends that our society make a major reassessment of how we address the needs of young children. The health care provider plays an important role in helping parents understand how daily experiences such as feeding, playing, diapering, calming, and sleep influence infants' brain development. Specifically, providers can teach parents that providing predictable, consistent, and loving care helps the infant learn trust, the first stage of psychosocial development, according to Erikson.

Research on the developing brain confirms a number of key points, including:

- Some physical brain characteristics are genetically determined, and most neurons are present at birth.
- The capacity to build the brain structures that support social, emotional, and mental development is greatest in early childhood and decreases over time.
- Pruning of unused synapses hinders some learning in later life.
- Early stimulation is necessary for optimal brain development.
- The brain grows rapidly in early childhood; by 6 years old the brain is about 95% of its adult size.
- Ongoing stress, including child abuse, neglect, maternal depression, substance abuse, or family violence can damage the growing brain (McCrory et al, 2010).
- Normal brain development requires good nutrition.

Cultural Influences on Development

Cultural and ethnic traditions shape the development of infants, children, adolescents, parents, and families. Some cultural groups manifest childhood developmental milestones differently than others. Group differences, however, may be irrelevant when providing individualized care for a particular child and family. More accurate assessments of families and children come from understanding the specific culture of a family and community. To understand family culture, additional assessment is needed beyond the traditional health history and physical examination.

Tools such as the genogram, ecomap, and family functioning model (Minuchin, 1974) can help identify family structure, strengths, resources, and health responses, beliefs, and practices. The childhood health assessment questionnaire (CHAQ) and child health questionnaire (CHQ) have been adapted to a number of cultural groups (Ruperto et al, 2001), and cross-cultural tools to be used with specific illnesses (e.g., lupus erythematosus, rheumatoid arthritis) are being developed (Moorthy et al, 2010). The interview process clarifies families' unique qualities and resources, and serves as an avenue for communicating interest in, and understanding of, individual families and their ethnic or cultural values, differences, and commonalities (see Chapters 2 and 3).

Health care providers should understand that there are variations in normal for different cultures. Early milestones, such as eating solid food, weaning from the breast or bottle, sleeping through the night, and toilet training, may occur at different ages and be considered normal. Parental responses to their children's needs also vary by culture. Using a validated screening tool with high sensitivity, specificity, and reliability helps the provider to better determine which children need referrals. Once the child reaches kindergarten, children from all cultural backgrounds should have similar development (Hagan et al, 2008).

Providers need to recognize their own cultural biases and how their culture and ethnic traditions affect approaches to certain aspects of the well-child visit. By gaining this awareness and understanding, they more effectively work with others, especially those who are very different from themselves (see Chapter 3).

Developmental Assessment

SIGNIFICANCE FOR THE HEALTH CARE PROVIDER

Monitoring children's developmental progress brings the pleasure of watching them master expected developmental milestones. With time, many providers develop an intuitive sense about the general ages at which particular milestones should occur. Experience also brings an appreciation of individual differences in infants, families, and ethnic groups.

Many variables can make it difficult to appreciate intuitively all the various developmental skills of any particular child. For example, a premature infant at or below the fifth percentile for height and weight may physically appear much younger. The discrepancy between size and age can lead to an inaccurate estimate of the child's abilities. Consider an infant who is 15 months chronologically, 12 months adjusted age, but physically and developmentally at the 9-month level. If the provider evaluated this infant developmentally based on physical size, the development level might appear appropriate (size and development at 9 months). Adjusting for age because of the infant's prematurity (adjustment to 12 months), the infant might still appear normal, and the need for intervention and referral might be missed. When a valid and reliable standardized developmental screening tool is used, it is more readily apparent that the infant requires referral and intervention services. It is important to note that even the developmental assessment tools with the highest standards may not be predictive for extremely low-birth-weight infants (Hack et al, 2005).

As a result of the understandable inconsistency in a practitioner's intuitive knowledge of child development and the importance of early identification of developmental concerns, the American Academy of Pediatrics (AAP) Committee on Children with Disabilities recommends that developmental surveillance be incorporated into each well-child preventive visit. Further, a standardized screening test is recommended for children at 9 months, 18 months, and 24 to 30 months (AAP, 2006). Many developmental screening tools have psychometric qualities including sensitivity, specificity, validity, and reliability and have been standardized on diverse populations.

DEVELOPMENTAL SURVEILLANCE

The concept of developmental surveillance as described by Dworkin (1989; 1993) provides the framework for this discussion. Surveillance encompasses all primary care activities related to the monitoring of the development of children, including the following:
- Eliciting and attending to parental concerns
- Obtaining a relevant developmental history
- Making accurate and informative observations of children
- Sharing opinions and concerns with other relevant professionals

Developmental surveillance involves more than simply asking developmental questions, completing a developmental screening checklist, asking how a child is doing in school, or completing a school physical examination. Emphasis is placed on monitoring development over time within the context of the child's overall well-being rather than viewing development during an isolated testing session.

Several assumptions underlie developmental surveillance. These include the following:
- Development is a self-fueling, ongoing process that requires physical and emotional energy.
- Development occurs in stages and is dynamic and interactional.
- Development is influenced by the child and his or her environment.
- Development occurs in "spurts and lulls." Periods of disorganization, disharmony, and turbulence are usually followed by periods of harmony, balance, and organization as new skills are integrated.
- All areas of development are interrelated.

Providing supportive care for children through developmental surveillance also is based on certain assumptions. These include the following:
- Children are generally healthy and have adaptive capabilities. Therefore, the goal of the provider is to maximize health and development and a child's overall potential, rather than solely to resolve problems.
- Individual differences among children are reflected in developmental variations that reflect the unique characteristics of families, cultures, and social circumstances. Individual developmental variations and positive adaptations should be appreciated and facilitated.
- Children and families have the capacity to learn from and grow beyond their limitations when interventions are based on their abilities.
- Preventive health care for children includes developmentally supportive mental health care.

One focus of developmental surveillance is to build parental competence and confidence, which in turn enhances the child's overall well-being. When providers teach parents about the child's unique development strengths and skills, parents increase their knowledge of development and create their own parenting style. When parents feel success in their current parenting role, they do a better job meeting their child's future needs. Developmental surveillance is further supported by developmental screening and assessment as discussed in the following text (Rydz et al, 2005).

DEFINITIONS
Developmental Screening
Screening is considered a first-level contact with an individual to identify potential and actual developmental concerns. Developmental screening is a brief, inexpensive method to identify children who may need a more comprehensive assessment and diagnostic evaluation. It allows the practitioner to document a child's progress over time and objectively identify and reinforce a child's developmental strengths. It may also serve as a tool to stimulate parent questions about development and facilitate parent education (Perrin and Stancin, 2002).

Developmental screening strategies are appropriate for all children, although culture and life experiences may affect some outcomes and need to be taken into consideration. Screening is conducted with the assumption that some children's developmental skills will fall outside the normal limits identified by the screening tool, thus requiring a referral for a more in-depth developmental assessment. In addition, parent education to facilitate the "next steps" of development for the child may also be needed.

Developmental Assessment
A developmental assessment, more in-depth than a developmental screening, is conducted when a definitive diagnosis and a more individualized approach to guide the plan of care and manage the child's concerns are required. Assessment is a second level of analysis, focusing on a narrower, often complicated problem. Generally, assessments confirm a developmental problem, identify the type of problem, describe the level of functioning in one or more developmental domains, and provide parents with anticipatory guidance and referrals to appropriate therapy, early intervention services, or community resources.

AREAS OF DEVELOPMENTAL SCREENING AND ASSESSMENT

Typical areas of developmental screening and assessment include language, motor, social-emotional, and cognitive skills. Screening and assessment should also examine the

TABLE 4-3 Areas of Child Development

Developmental Area	Definition
Physical development	Physical stability, growth, sexuality
Regulatory skills	State control and modulation, ability to manage sensory (e.g., light, noise, touch, movement) input from the external and internal environment; self-regulation and control
Adaptive skills and fine motor skills	Self-care skills that are involved in daily routines (e.g., feeding, bathing, dressing, brushing teeth)
Motor skills	Skills that facilitate overall movement and locomotion
Communication and language	Verbal and nonverbal communication skills including behaviors, gestures, signs
Social-emotional development and parent-child interaction	Ability to interact with others and the environment and overall affect; the reciprocal relationship between the child and his or her caregivers
Cognitive and intellectual development	Cognitive and intellectual skills, including problem-solving, decision-making, and goal setting

regulatory and sensory systems as a part of the child's overall development and functioning. Regulation refers to infants' daily patterns of sleep-wake cycles that include sleeping, eating, moving, responding, and reacting to their internal and external environments. Sensory system evaluation includes assessment of the child's ability to receive, process, and respond to both internal and external stimuli. Finally, although it is conceptually a part of the child's social skill set, it is important to review parent-child interactions and the family and environmental context in which the child is living. A comprehensive approach to developmental screening and assessment that includes the areas of regulation and adaptive skills in daily routines will be presented for each age group in the following chapters. Table 4-3 provides examples of information to gather within each of these areas.

STRATEGIES FOR DEVELOPMENTAL SCREENING AND ASSESSMENT

Several key strategies are involved in developmental screening and assessment:
- Parent interview
- Child interview
- Observation of child's behavior
- Observation of child-parent interaction
- Parent questionnaire

Success using these strategies begins when the health care provider builds rapport and a trusting relationship with parent and child. Gaining the parents' and child's trust and engagement in the interview process is critical to obtaining accurate and reliable information. The parent interview requires the provider to encourage parents to share sensitive information, ask questions,

BOX 4-1 Interview Guide for Daily Routines

- Tell me about your child's typical day.
- What aspects of your child's day are easy? What aspects are more challenging?
- How does your child communicate what he or she wants?
- Does your child show an ability to understand the feelings of others?
- How does your child act around others?
- To what extent has your child developed independence in eating, dressing, and toileting? Responsibilities at home, school, and community?
- How does your child get from one place to another (e.g., running, walking, transportation)?
- What do you like best about your child?
- What nicknames does your child have?

BOX 4-2 Observations During a Feeding

- Positioning of the infant or child and the caregiver
  - Eye contact
  - Infant holding
  - Minimization of environmental distractions
- Suck, swallow, breathing coordination, and physiologic stability
- Infant or child comfort with eating
- Oral motor functioning
- Lip closure, tongue, jaw movements, swallowing
- Endurance for feeding
- Sustained attention to feeding
- Stability of head and trunk control
- Ability to reach, grasp, hold, transfer objects
- Self-feeding skills and utensil use
- Coordination and quality of movements during feeding
- Infant's or child's anticipation of feeding
- Clarity of behavioral cues (engagement and disengagement cues) and use of vocalizations
- Responsiveness to caregivers' actions and verbalizations

and express concerns about their child's development. The child interview requires an understanding of child development and ages. The provider must be skilled in the use of age-appropriate strategies to engage the child and be sensitive to the unique needs of each child. Providers need to have the ability to relate to the child verbally and nonverbally. One example is to sit at the same level as the child in order to establish eye contact. Targeted questions around daily routines often provide insight into a child's daily activities and parents' areas of concern. Examples of these questions are provided in Box 4-1.

A trusting relationship also enhances the health care provider's ability to accurately observe the child's behaviors. Observation of the child and the child's attention, activities, verbalization, connection with the parent, processing of information, quality of movements, cooperation, and ability to follow requests are all components of developmental screening and assessment. Box 4-2 lists specific observations that may be made during an infant feeding in a clinic or home visit, and Box 4-3 lists observations that can be made during a play or teaching activity with the parent.

Many standardized screening tools are available and recommended for developmental screening. Many of these tools

BOX 4-3	Observations During Spontaneous Play or a Teaching Activity

- Positioning of the infant or child and the caregiver
  - Eye contact
  - Placement of toys within reach
  - Minimization of environmental distractions
- Success of gaining child's attention and sustained attention to play or teaching activity
- Tracking or following both visually or with verbal instructions and modeling
- Initiation of play activity
- Anticipation of songs or games
- Ability to reach, grasp, hold, transfer objects
- Coordination and quality of movements
- Clarity of behavioral cues and use of vocalizations
- Responsiveness to caregivers' actions and verbalizations
- Use of a toy in the manner it was meant to be used
- Ability to use representational play

have been developed to meet the demands of a busy, efficient office practice. Each of the following chapters provides suggested developmental screening or assessment tools that are age-appropriate.

Strategies Specific to Developmental Screening

Aspects of the screening should be incorporated into the physical examination. By doing this the provider not only sees the child "in action," but also has an opportunity to demonstrate to parents the infant or child's current or emerging skills. After completion of developmental screening, the provider should review the findings with parents. A parent-report screening tool can be completed by the parent in the waiting room or examination room, scored by a nurse or medical assistant, and then reviewed by the provider with the parent. This discussion helps families focus on concerns they may have, provides opportunities to answer specific parent questions, addresses parenting issues, and is conducive to providing anticipatory guidance.

When developmental screening is omitted or delegated to medical assistants or volunteers and not reviewed by the primary provider, the significance of subtle variations of normal behavior or behavior that is very near the abnormal range may be overlooked. Nurse practitioners (NPs) should be leaders in the use of standardized developmental screening tools in their practices to enhance the efficiency and quality of the practice. Such tools provide a consistent, reliable, and efficient method of documentation of care provided and set standards for referral. Use of developmental screening tools involves engaging other providers and office staff with some minimal training and imparting knowledge of community resources. Implementing this standard of practice increases parent satisfaction and engagement as experts on their child and recognizes the provider-parent partnership in the care of the child (Earls and Hay, 2006).

Strategies Specific to Developmental Assessment

Developmental assessment tools are significantly different from screening tools and are appropriate when concerns require more in-depth developmental or diagnostic evaluation.

Assessment tools for developmental and behavioral diagnosis, home assessment, family assessment, parent-child interaction assessment, parent stress, and parental competency are most frequently used in research but may also be of value in the clinical setting. These tools can be used for a thorough assessment of the child within the family context, to look at the parent-child interaction, and to develop a substantiated diagnosis for the child. The information also improves the practitioner's ability to structure individualized interventions for both the child and the parents, and it can be used to evaluate the effectiveness of recommended interventions. Tools used for overall development include the Bayley Scales of Infant Development (Aylward, 1995), Ages and Stages (ASQ-3) (Squires et al, 2009), the Child Developmental Inventory (Ireton, 1992), and the Mullen Scales of Early Learning (Mullen, 1989). Tools used to evaluate specific behaviors or characteristics include the Autism Diagnostic Observation Scale—Generic (ADOS—G) (Lord et al, 1994), Childhood Autism Rating Scale (CARS) (Schopler et al, 1986), and the Nursing Child Assessment Satellite Training (NCAST) Feeding and Teaching Scales (Barnard, 1976, 1979).

Because of the complexity of issues that might need evaluation, developmental assessment tools require more knowledge, practice, and skill to perform reliably, interpret the findings, and plan appropriate interventions. These tools generally require special training or credentials to administer accurately.

■ Management Strategies in Child Development

PROMOTING PARENT DEVELOPMENT AND PARENT-CHILD INTERACTION: ANTICIPATORY GUIDANCE

Anticipatory guidance as defined in past years in which specific topics were scripted for discussion at specified well child visits is a relatively ineffective means of improving child and parent outcomes (see Chapter 9). However, parents need clear information about expectations for child development and providers must educate parents and families about normative development and best practices for managing development. The broadly defined goal of anticipatory guidance is to help parents plan for and cope with anticipated changes and to increase parenting skills, confidence, and competence in problem solving. The guidance is intended to assist parents to adapt parenting styles and strategies to their child's temperament, growth, and development. The following should be included:

- Assess the child's developmental status.
- Determine the parents' knowledge of child development.
- Determine the parents' knowledge of and experience with the parent role.
- Assess the parents' problem-solving and coping skills.
- Instruct parents about normal child development and variations of that development as indicated. Provide educational information and materials as appropriate. Most parents value written materials that are developmentally and age-appropriate.
- Assist parents to develop realistic expectations of their child's development.
- Instruct parents about parenting strategies and concepts.
- Guide parents to appropriate community resources and support networks.

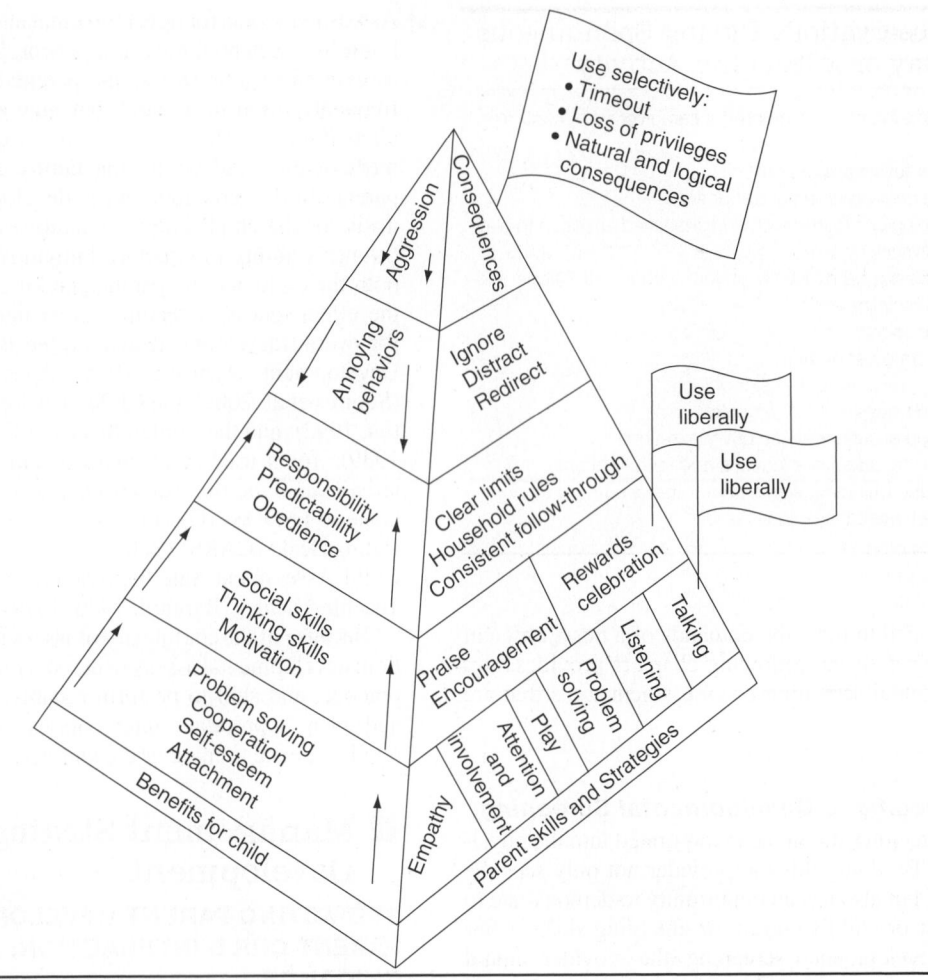

FIGURE 4-1 Parenting pyramid. (From Webster-Stratton C: *The incredible years: a trouble shooting guide for parents of children aged 2-8,* Seattle, WA, 2005, Incredible Years Press.)

- Reassess and obtain feedback; reinforce healthy parental role development.

The responsibility of promoting parent development through anticipatory guidance may be more challenging than providing physical care, especially in primary care practices in which time is limited. The standard of care in pediatric practices should include opportunities for providers to address parenting issues or concerns. Quick, pat answers to complex parenting issues do not facilitate parental growth. Creative strategies can be used to structure prenatal visits, hospital discharge rounds, early discharge newborn follow-up, breastfeeding consultations, well-child visits, and referrals to achieve this standard. An organized parent support program in practice settings, for example, can help providers listen, hear, and act on parents' concerns. Without an organized plan that connects the child's developmental needs, parents' concerns and educational needs, providers' abilities and resources, and community resources, it is easy to overlook, delay, or deny important parenting issues.

The interview and counseling conducted during anticipatory guidance should be based on a consistent framework. Programs such as *Touchpoints* (Brazelton and Sparrow, 2006), *Bright Futures* (Hagan et al, 2008), *Healthy Steps* (Minkovitz et al, 2001), and *The Incredible Years* (Webster-Stratton, 2005) (Fig. 4-1) can be used. Specific questions

are suggested to elicit responses from parents and guide the visit, and to provide anticipatory guidance and counseling. Stein (1998) emphasized the need for an organized framework when approaching developmental and behavioral issues. He suggested focusing on four basic areas: developmental themes, temperament, family support, and resiliency (the ability to withstand stressors). He emphasized the use of the teachable moment and role modeling during the office visit.

There is a wealth of popular literature available to guide parents as they raise their children. The primary pediatric health care provider can be an invaluable resource for parents in three major ways: by accurately assessing and competently caring for the child's needs; by supporting positive parent behaviors or actions; and by providing the information, suggestions, strategies, and guidance they need to be good parents. Giving parents positive feedback, being open to teaching, and listening to parents' concerns builds parent confidence, creates a trusting relationship, and establishes comfort for bringing forth more difficult concerns if such discussion is necessary. The provider-family relationship can be a powerful tool to guide family members' management of their child's temperament, behavior, and development. The benefit of establishing a long-term, continuous relationship with a child and family cannot be overestimated.

BOX 4-4	Parenting Red Flags

Moderate Concern

- Disinclination to separate from child or prematurely hastening separation
- Signs of despondency, apathy, or hostility
- Fearful, dependent, apprehensive
- Disinterested in or rejecting of infant or child
- Overly critical, mocking, and censuring of child; tendency to undermine child's confidence
- Inconsistent in discipline or control; erratic in behavior
- Highly restrictive and overly moralistic environment
- Turning away from eye-to-eye contact

Extreme Concern

- Extreme depression and withdrawal; rejection of child
- Intense hostility; aggression toward child
- Uncontrollable fears, anxieties, guilt
- Complete inability to function in family role
- Severe moralistic prohibition of child's independent strivings
- Domestic abuse or violence in the home
- Self-destructive behaviors: alcohol or drug abuse
- Untreated mental health issues (e.g., parent with diagnosis of bipolar disorder schizophrenia, delusional disorder)

Certain "red flags" related to parent-child interactions indicate that further assessment of the home environment, parent-child interaction, and child's development is indicated. Box 4-4 identifies some of these parental red flags.

DISCIPLINE

Children do not always behave the way their parents want them to. The question of how parents should deal with children's misbehavior has led to a wealth of parenting books, books on discipline, strategies for child development, and many frustrated parents. Parents tend to use a combination of strategies—spanking, yelling, timeout, taking away a favorite toy, or reasoning with the child (Regalado et al, 2004), and each family brings differing temperaments, styles, and beliefs to the process. There are, however, some basic principles and guidelines about discipline that providers can discuss with parents to help them handle discipline. The AAP, in its 1998 policy statement (reaffirmed in 2004), stated that "effective discipline requires three essential components: [1] a positive, supportive, loving relationship between the parent(s) and child; [2] use of positive reinforcement strategies to increase desired behaviors; and [3] removing reinforcement or applying punishment to reduce or eliminate undesired behaviors" (AAP, 1998, p 723). All three of these components guide the principles discussed below:

- Parents should talk with each other to come to agreement on how they will handle discipline and their child's misbehavior.
- A distinction must be made between discipline and punishment.
  - Discipline is training or education that molds the behavior, mental capacities, or moral character of an individual. Discipline is used by the parent to teach the child appropriate behavior and to keep the child safe.
  - Punishment, on the other hand, is loss, pain, or suffering that is administered in response to behavior; it is a form of retribution.

- Parents should focus their interactions with children on discipline, rather than punishment. As with the food pyramid in which wholesome grains, proteins, fruits, and vegetables form the base for good nutrition, a "parenting pyramid" describes teaching, play, guidance, role modeling, and thoughtful correction of a child's behavior as the broad base for parent-child interactions (see Fig. 4-1; Webster-Stratton, 2005). Like nutrient-empty foods, punishment should be used as little as possible.
- Misbehavior can often be prevented. When a child appears willful, bored, or out-of-sorts, distraction and active engagement with the parent (e.g., giving the child something to do; talking to, playing with, dancing with the child) can be used to stop misbehavior before it starts.
- Parents need to be alert to when children are reaching their limits (i.e., are nearing "meltdown" because they are tired, hungry, or overstimulated) and intervene to prevent problems from occurring.
- Children who are at a "meltdown" stage are not able to relate rationally to a parent's reasoned explanation or request; the underlying problem—hunger, lack of sleep, etc.—must be dealt with first. Conversely, parents are not always at their best and may need a "timeout" from the child to cool down and regain self-control. Parents should have a plan for help when they need respite.
- All children need rules, limits, and expectations that should be reasonable and appropriate to the age and developmental capabilities of the child. A 3-month-old, for example, cannot be expected to stop crying when her parents tell her to. As children grow they should negotiate with their parents to help set the rules. This parent-child interaction helps children learn how to be active, valued family members and builds their social skills.
- Parents should be sure that the rules are clear and specific and should strive for consistency in adhering to them. Even young children benefit when the parent explains what the rules are and why they are necessary.
- Be flexible when responding to a child's behavior. Parents should agree about what issues are important to stand firm on. A wise mother said she had learned to "not sweat the small stuff," and chose to ignore very minor infractions while rewarding positive behaviors.
- Parents should role model expected behaviors.
- Adhering to rules should be rewarded. Parents should be encouraged to catch their children "being good" and give praise, encouragement, or rewards. Praise and encouragement are powerful reinforcements for good behavior. Some parents find a 4:1 ratio to be a good rule of thumb: four positive reinforcements for every negative.
- Praise and rewards for following the rules are different from "bribes" for being good (e.g., "If you stop crying, I'll get you an ice cream cone"), which should be discouraged.
- Children should be treated with respect and empathy, even when being reprimanded for misbehavior.
- Breaking rules should lead to natural and logical consequences.
- Consequences should be given immediately, be fair, and should relate to the rule broken.
- Consequences should be appropriate to the age and developmental capabilities of the child. Timeout, being sent to

the child's room, restricting a favorite activity, and turning off the television or video games are all examples of consequences that have been successfully used. For example, if a 6-year-old child begins to play with his food, he can be sent to his room for "alone time," without his dinner. If a 4-year-old pushes or punches her sibling, she can be given a timeout or not be allowed to play with a friend. If a 10-year-old breaks the neighbor's window with her baseball, she can be expected to apologize, help clean up the mess, and work to pay for the new window. As children grow they should help determine the consequences for misbehavior.

- Parents should follow through on limits set. Frequent threats ("If you do that one more time, I'll send you to your room!") without follow-through teach the child that they can continue their misbehavior without consequence. Learning early that they are accountable for their behavior is an invaluable lesson for children.
- Punishment should never be a withdrawal of the parent's love or affection.
- Corporal punishment is unnecessary and has the potential to cause physical and/or psychic damage.

No parent is perfect, and parents bring their own upbringing to the role. Parental behavior may reflect efforts to "be like my parents were" or, as seems more often the case, "not do things wrong, like my parents did with me." Providers should acknowledge that parents are trying to do the best they can and encourage them to relax and discover how they and their child can best interact.

Concerns About Delayed Development

DEVELOPMENTAL RED FLAGS

Child development is exceptionally varied. A 2-year-old girl may use full complex sentences, whereas her 3-year-old neighbor relies on three-word directives (e.g., "want milk, peeze") to get what he desires. Both can be normal, but the differences may be striking, and parents may express concern that their child is "delayed." Prevalence estimates of developmental and behavioral disorders in the United States range from 15% to 18% (Glascoe, 2000). Health care providers should keep in mind certain red flags related to normal child development when seeing infants and children for well-child care or minor acute illnesses. These red flags are highlighted in each of the following chapters in this unit.

If a concern is noted during a routine visit, a standardized developmental screening is the next step, followed by a developmental assessment as appropriate. Subsequently, a decision must be made as to whether the child is progressing appropriately or whether intervention is indicated. Information from the history, physical examination, developmental screening and assessment, hearing and vision screening, and other tests that are indicated is essential in making this decision. It is also important to consider the cause of developmental delays when making a judgment to intervene directly or refer (Box 4-5).

Children with screening findings that are very near normal may be mildly delayed, but not eligible for early intervention services (criteria for early intervention vary from state to state, and a child may need to be between 25% and 50%

BOX 4-5 Etiologies of Developmental Delays

- Central nervous system dysfunction
- Mental health problem
- Chronic disease affecting either functional abilities or activity tolerance (e.g., cardiovascular, visual, auditory)
- Child abuse and neglect
- Maternal or paternal stress
- Developmentally inappropriate animate or inanimate environment, or both
- Lack of parental knowledge of development
- Genetic syndromes
- Depression
- Attention-deficit hyperactivity disorder
- Autism spectrum
- Regulatory or sensory dysfunctions
- Unknown causes

delayed to be eligible in some states). Children with a mild delay and/or those who are at risk may benefit from activities such as encouraging "tummy time" when awake (for an infant who is not yet rolling over). Providers can use a manual such as *The Hawaii Early Learning Program (HELP) at Home Manual* to assist them with suggestions to parents for mild delays in various domains. They can also make referrals to programs such as Early Head Start and YMCA classes. These suggestions can also allow parents to begin working on an area while waiting for early intervention services to begin.

Understanding the possible cause helps the provider plan appropriate developmental care, including parent counseling, educational programs, and referral choices (e.g., Which developmental specialist is most appropriate to further assess the child? Which treatment modality, such as speech or physical therapy, would be most effective?). The discussion in Chapter 27 of the management of cerebral palsy illustrates the decision-making process used in cases of developmental delay. One should not assume that waiting will remedy a problem when parents express a concern or when developmental delays are noted; even though developmental progress may occur, the rate and quality can be abnormal. In addition, parent's stress and anxiety about their child can cause further problems. Neither can one assume that all developmental problems can be fixed with home remedies (e.g., changing parenting or environmental factors). Sometimes developmental problems are indicators of serious systemic, particularly neurologic, dysfunctions.

Vulnerability and resilience are two characteristics under current discussion in the child health literature. *Vulnerability* refers to a person's sensitivity and inclination to decompensate in the face of life stressors. *Resilience* (sometimes called *hardiness*), in contrast, is a person's capacity to survive intact, both psychologically and physically, despite adversity. In children these characteristics affect outcomes as stressors come and go in the child's life experiences. Many children demonstrate remarkable resilience despite significant risks; others are less capable of coping. Any child who fails to move ahead as expected, or begins to deteriorate developmentally requires an immediate developmental assessment and diagnostic evaluation.

TALKING WITH PARENTS ABOUT DEVELOPMENTAL DELAYS

Talking with parents on a routine, ongoing basis about their child's development will usually make it easier should a specific developmental problem appear. It can be a challenging process. Typically, parents notice differences in the child first and seek reassurance or confirmation of problems from their health care provider. Should a problem be found, a "strength-based" approach can help soothe the experience of receiving "bad news." Each infant and child has areas in which development is progressing, even if the progress is not consistent with usual development. Discussing these areas, in addition to the parents' concerns, is important. Discussing these areas *first* provides parents with a framework for understanding their child's unique strengths along with any particular developmental challenges.

Parents may be overwhelmed with the news that their child has a developmental problem. To determine whether parents understand what they have been told, the provider can ask the parent how they are going to explain what has been discussed to others at home. To increase parents' follow-through, providers need to be very familiar with referral resources. They should walk the parent through the next steps in the process, and after allotting time for the family to complete the referral visit, follow up with a phone call or office or home visit with the family.

Above all, it is important to be honest, positive, and realistic. Most often, the long-term prognosis for developmental delays is unknown because of continuing brain development. Parents want to know what they can do and, specifically, how they can assist their child. They also need support and time to cope with their own feelings. Different families have different expectations for their children, so a child with mild delay may be more devastating to one family than a child with severe developmental delays may be to another. Parents may report that they have expressed their concerns to their health care provider only to be reassured or told let's "wait and see." Later on, as problems become more obvious and a referral is finally made, they are frustrated that they were not listened to initially and that services to their child have been delayed.

Implementing Individualized Interventions

Early Intervention Programs. Children with developmental delays should receive appropriate referral or more frequent visits, or both, particularly during the first year of life (see Chapter 21 for a discussion of issues related to children with chronic illnesses). Many difficulties with parent-child interaction, and/or learning, behavioral, and attachment problems can be avoided or more effectively managed by offering parental counseling or referral to appropriate community services (e.g., a social emotional consultant or someone with experience in infant mental health) during the first year of life. The longer the problem lasts, the more difficult it is to resolve. Most communities have early infant education programs for infants and young children (birth to 3 years old) provided for under Public Law 108-466. This law, the Individuals With Disabilities Education Improvement Act of 2004, a reauthorization of P.L. 99-457, was enacted at the federal level in 1986. This law requires developmental screening and early intervention programs for infants and young children at risk

for developmental delay. The individualized family service plan (IFSP) is a process that includes the family in planning services for children. Primary care providers may be asked to participate in the meetings in which the IFSP is developed with the family. These programs can be established through school systems, health departments, or developmental programs and vary significantly in quality and comprehensiveness from one community to another. The importance of structured programs that stimulate growth of all children cannot be overestimated (Emde et al, 2001). Providers need to be familiar with community resources and educate community leaders and legislators about the developmental and health needs of children and families.

There are a number of comorbidities associated with developmental disorders that occur because of the functional impairment or occur secondary to the medical management of these conditions. Common complications of developmental disorders include alterations in gastrointestinal motility, malnutrition, urinary tract infections, impaired airway clearance, frequent upper respiratory tract infections, and altered neuromuscular tone (Garzon et al, 2010). Children with developmental delays may require special attention in many areas, including assessment of medical and dental needs, feeding, sleep, elimination, activity, temperament, and behavior. Nursing interventions, such as education regarding medications, modifications of therapies as a result of the child's health status, referrals to parent groups, and assistance regarding organization of the child's health records, are greatly appreciated by the family.

School Intervention Resources. Public Law 94-142, enacted in 1975, addresses the needs of children older than 3 years. Under this legislation schools are mandated to provide appropriate education to all children with developmental delays, including opportunities for mainstreaming children with developmental delays or handicaps into regular classrooms. Special education services assist in this process through the development of an individualized education plan (IEP).

Planning sessions for IFSPs or IEPs determine the developmental or school services offered during a designated period of time for a particular child, usually each calendar year or each school year. If a child's or family's needs are not identified, services are not made available. Often health care needs are not considered in these planning sessions. Primary health care providers should advocate for families and children. In this role, they help clarify children's health needs and ensure that parental concerns, health care services, and educational services are appropriately coordinated (Jackson Allen et al, 2010).

Family-Centered Care. The National Association of Pediatric Nurse Practitioners (NAPNAP) pediatric health care home position statement (NAPNAP, 2009), Public Law 99-457, and the AAP (AAP, 2001) all emphasize the importance of the family within the child's life. The need to develop a partnership with the family is crucial so that families are comfortable and engaged in creating the plan of care for their own child. Each family's cultural values, learning styles, and health beliefs and practices must be respected. The shift from child-centered to family-centered care is represented in Table 4-4.

Care Coordination. The Maternal and Child Health Bureau (MCHB) and the AAP define children with special needs as "children with special health care needs beyond

TABLE 4-4	Comparison of Child-Centered and Family-Centered Care
Child-Centered Care	**Family-Centered Care**
Goal: To take care of the child for the short term.	*Goal:* Parental empowerment and child advocacy for the life of the child.
Child's needs are primary focus.	Family needs to assist the child are the focus.
Professionals decide on the plan of care.	Family and professionals decide on the plan of care.
Parents' opinions are not consistently requested.	Parents' ideas are requested and valued.
Families are considered part of a particular group.	Families are all considered to be unique.
Parents participate as observers.	Parents are considered to be equal members at whatever level they are comfortable.
Parental differences are judged as not being in the best interest of the child.	Family culture, language, ethnicity, and structure are respected.
Test results of the child are the most important factor used to plan care.	Focus is on addressing parental concerns, issues, questions, and their need for assistance in problem-solving.
One-way communication, professional to parent.	Two-way communication, with parents encouraged to have input into the child's care plan.

those who have or are at increased risk for chronic physical, developmental, behavioral, or emotional conditions and who require health and related services of a type or amount beyond that required by children generally" (McPherson et al, 1998). Care coordination is one of the key elements for children with special needs, and the primary care provider is ideally suited to direct the medical home (AAP, 1999; Antonelli and Antonelli, 2004). Nurse practitioners (NPs) have the unique skills to function in this role as a result of their nursing background and appreciation for the complex needs of families and children with special health care needs. NPs help families understand the importance of accessing parent and community resources to sustain their long-term care of the child. It is important for the NP to become "community wise" through professional networks, parent groups, and educational connections. It is essential to develop a system within the office of up-to-date referral agencies and contact information. Through public health agencies these resources may also be easily identifiable and invaluable in assisting parents. However, it is not enough simply to give a family a name and phone number of a referral source. All too often, parents' calls lead to busy signals, disconnected numbers, or the wrong agency for their needs. These deterrents can discourage even the most willing family from pursuing needed resources for their child. Parents may hesitate to seek resources because of apprehension about the outcome of the referral, costs, time constraints, or lack of understanding about the need for timely follow-up. When the provider intervenes to guide families through the referral process and coordinate services, parents have greater confidence in the new health care or educational resource and are more likely to achieve appropriate follow-up for their child.

Developmental Management of Infants

BARBARA JONES DELOIAN AND ANITA D. BERRY

Infancy is an exciting time for everyone involved—the infant, his or her immediate family, extended family members, and others in the infant's community. Pediatric health care providers are privileged to be able to work with families during this period of rapid, predictable (yet unique), and challenging change. When providing care to infants and their families, practitioners have a responsibility to assess and monitor growth and development; educate parents about child development; offer guidance about ways to foster healthy growth and development; identify and manage health problems; guide, counsel, and support parents when dealing with their infant's health or illness; and collaborate with other providers as necessary.

Learning, reading, and writing do not start in kindergarten or first grade. Language and literacy skills begin at birth through everyday loving interactions—sharing books, telling stories, singing songs, and talking to one another. Adults—parents, grandparents, and teachers—play a very important role in preparing young children for future school success and in becoming self-confident and motivated learners. Responsive relationships with consistent caregivers help build positive attachments, support healthy social-emotional development, and are the foundation of mental health for infants, toddlers, and preschoolers. During pregnancy and early life, internal physiologic and neurologic factors and external factors such as light, sound, touch, positioning, taste, and movement affect the infant. Physical growth, brain development, the surrounding environment, and, particularly, the actions of the infant's caregivers influence an infant's ability to develop consistent and predictable responses to internal and external stimuli during the first year of life. Nurturing relationships between infants and their adult caregivers strengthen all aspects of an infant's development (Dixon and Stein, 2006).

■ Birth Rates and Infant Mortality

National trends in birth rates and infant mortality are important measures of population-based infant health. Between 2007 and 2009, birth rates dropped from 14.3 per 1000 to 13.5 per 1000 (Tejada-Vera and Sutton, 2010). Between 2005 and 2007 the total birth rate among those ages 15 to 19 years

increased by 5%, but there was a slight drop in 2008. In all age groups the populations with the highest birth rates are Hispanics and non-Hispanic African Americans, whereas Asians and non-Hispanic whites have the lowest birth rates (Hamilton et al, 2010). The infant mortality rate in 2007 was 6.8 deaths per 1000 births, a slight but statistically insignificant increase over a mortality rate of 6.7 per 1000 in 2006 (Xu et al, 2010). The infant death rate in African-American infants (13.2 per 1000) and other racial groups (10.6/1000) is more than double that of white infants (5.63/1000) (Xu et al, 2010). The disparity of infant mortality rates between black, non-Hispanic, and white American infants is of grave concern. The leading causes of infant mortality are birth defects, low birthweight and prematurity, sudden infant death syndrome (SIDS), newborn complications of pregnancy, and unintentional injuries. According to the Centers for Disease Control and Prevention (CDC), of the 4.38 million babies born in the U.S. every year, approximately 4600 infants die for no obvious reason. Of these deaths, about one half are caused by SIDS, the third leading cause of infant death in the U.S. It is also the leading cause of death among infants between 1 and 12 months old (Xu et al, 2010). The SIDS rate declined significantly since 1992 when the American Academy of Pediatrics (AAP) began their "Back to Sleep" campaign (AAP, 2005).

■ Development During the First Year

BIRTH TO 1 MONTH
Physical Development

Newborn assessment begins with a determination of gestational age using the Dubowitz/Ballard exam or similar gestational age scale (see Chapter 38). It is important to document significant prematurity, intrauterine growth restriction (IUGR), and size for gestational age (i.e., either large for gestational age [LGA] or small for gestational age [SGA]). Comparisons are made between the reported gestational age, birthweight and length, and head circumference.

The infant may initially lose up to 5% to 8% of birthweight but should regain it within 10 to 14 days. Weight loss of 10% or more requires close monitoring and may require further evaluation. Weight gain after the initial loss averages 0.5 to 1 ounce (14 to 28 g) per day, or about 2 pounds (1 kg) per month. Nutritional needs to promote growth are about 110 kcal/kg/day (see Chapter 10).

The stability of the infant's autonomic nervous system can be evaluated through heart rate, respiratory rate, temperature control, and color changes. The infant should demonstrate some degree of regulation of state and ease of transitions from deep sleep through quiet alert to active alert and crying. A variety of techniques can be used to arouse the newborn for feedings. The newborn sleeps about 16 out of 24 hours and, if encouraged to breastfeed every 2 to 3 hours, may have one longer stretch of 4 hours at night. It is important to assess for a normal-pitched cry because problems such as hypothyroidism and genetic disorders (e.g., cri du chat syndrome) can cause voice alterations.

Motor Skills Development

The newborn's flexed posture provides the infant with the ability to self-console when positioned so that the hands reach the face and mouth. Primary reflexes, such as sucking, rooting, asymmetric tonic neck, Moro, and grasp, should be present and symmetric. Passive muscle tone is evaluated within gestational age scales through observation of shoulder (scarf sign) and knee flexibility (popliteal angle). Arm and leg recoil provide information about the infant's active movements, particularly symmetry and coordination. Jerkiness and tremors may be noted. The neonatal period begins a remarkable series of fine and gross motor skill milestones for the infant (Table 5-1).

Communication and Language Development

The newborn gives clear signals of distress, such as crying, arching, or gagging. These help the caregiver respond to the infant's needs. The newborn should be able to habituate to sound and light. Newborns use self-consoling or self-calming behaviors, such as sucking, moving hand to mouth, or grasping clothing.

Articulation, or the way that the structures of the nose and mouth mold the sounds emitted by the larynx, begins at birth with the infant's first cry. In the first few weeks of life, infants make sounds of comfort and discomfort.

Social and Emotional Development and Maternal Postpartum Depression

Social skills are evident as the newborn quiets readily, turns to the parent's voice, and demonstrates a brief smile. Using a soft voice, touching, and picking up the baby are ways the caregiver consoles the newborn.

Social and emotional development is closely linked to the mother's emotional state—60% to 80% of mothers experience "baby blues" in the first 2 weeks of life, 10% to 15% have postpartum depression during the first year of the infant's life, and 0.1% to 0.2% present with postpartum psychosis. Postpartum depression can occur anytime during the first year of the infant's life, whereas postpartum psychosis generally presents in the first weeks after delivery. The rate of postpartum psychosis is significantly higher if there is maternal schizophrenia or bipolar disease, or when the mother's history is positive for previous postpartum psychosis (Spinelli, 2009).

The pediatric health care provider sees mothers frequently during the infant's first year of life. Infants' well-child visits should be used as opportunities to screen mothers and families for factors that can affect the infant's growth and development including depression and intimate partner violence. A screening tool such as the 10-question Edinburgh Postnatal Depression Scale can be used to identify mothers needing further evaluation, referral, and close follow-up (Cox et al, 1987; Wisner et al, 2002) (see Chapter 38 for a copy of this scale).

Cognitive-Sensory Development

Vision is limited, but the newborn has the ability to focus briefly on a face or bright object when it is brought into visual range (about 8 to 12 inches from the infant's face). Newborns visually track objects to midline. Of all the senses, the sense of smell is most acute in newborns. Hearing is also fairly well developed.

1 THROUGH 3 MONTHS

Physical Development

During months 1 through 3 the infant experiences many physical and developmental changes. Length increases about 1.4 inches (3.5 cm) per month and head circumference about 0.8 inch (2 cm) per month, with more rapid growth for the younger infant. The infant typically gains 0.5 to 1 ounce (14 to 28 g) per day and has 8 to 10 feedings in 24 hours, each lasting 20 to 30 minutes. Feedings lasting longer than 30 minutes need to be evaluated. At about 6 to 8 weeks, the infant may experience a growth spurt and fuss to eat more frequently. Mothers who are breastfeeding need extra encouragement during this time because they may believe that they do not have enough milk for their baby. Provider reassurance can be backed up by an interval infant weight check if the mother is overly concerned. Providers should instruct mothers to follow their infant's cues for feeding; pointing out that the extra suckling will increase the milk supply sufficiently to meet their growing infant's needs. Elimination patterns become more regular. Infants go from defecating with each feeding to having one or two bowel movements daily or every other day if formula fed, and bowel movements that range from once or twice daily to once every 3 to 5 days if breastfed. Wet diapers occur after each feeding.

Sleep cycles become more regular, about 15 to 16 hours per day, with defined sleep-wake patterns. The infant may need more organized play periods as sleep periods consolidate with consistent naps. Many infants have fussy periods in the late evening that may last 1 to 3 hours. Infant crying tends to peak at this age, but fortunately this fussiness usually lasts only a few weeks. Regular nap or nighttime routines help keep infants calmer. The provider should discuss with parents plans to cope with crying before this time is upon them. This is a good time to explain "shaken baby syndrome" to parents and encourage them and others who care for the infant to have a repertoire of coping skills.

Motor Skills Development

Fine motor skills begin to emerge as primitive reflexes become integrated. Infants attempt to grasp rattles, fingers, and clothing. They are able to demonstrate visible head control, lifting

TABLE 5-1	Fine Motor and Gross Motor Development Milestones for Infants and Preschoolers		
Age	**Fine Motor Movement**	**Oral Movement**	**Motor Movement**
Birth	Flexion	Suckling tongue movements, extension-retraction of tongue, up-and-down jaw movements, low approximation of lips	Momentary head control when held sitting
1 mo	Extension, nondirected swipes	Rooting	Turns head when prone
4 mo	Directed swipes, corralling, reaching		Sits with support, begins to roll over, head steady in sitting
4-5 mo	Ulnar-palmar grasp		"Swims" in prone position, no head lag
6-7 mo	Radial-palmar grasp, raking	Sucking with negative oral cavity pressure, rhythmic jaw movements, firm approximation of lips	Sits independently, rolls over, rocks on hands and knees, free head lift in supine position
7-8 mo	Radial-digital grasp	Phasic bite reflex, rhythmic bite and release pattern	Supports weight standing, bounces when held
7-9 mo	Scissors grasp	Munching, early chewing	Sits alone well, may crawl
9-10 mo	Voluntary release		Cruises, pivots while seated, pulls to stand
12 mo	Picks up pellet with pincer grasp	Chewing with spreading and rolling tongue movements, tongue lateralization, rotary jaw movements, controlled sustained bite	Walks with one hand held, stands alone momentarily
18 mo	Makes tower of 4 cubes, imitates scribbling, dumps pellet, puts blocks in large holes, drinks from cup with little spilling, can take off socks		Directed throwing, walks well independently, climbs into adult chair
24 mo	Makes tower of 7 cubes, does circular scribbling, folds paper once imitatively, turns doorknobs, turns pages one at a time, unbuttons or unzips large fasteners, puts on coat with assistance		Throws overhand, runs well, kicks ball, walks up and down stairs placing both feet on each step
30 mo	Makes tower of 9 cubes, makes vertical and horizontal strokes, imitates circle, buttons large buttons, uses fork in fist, twists jar lids		Jumps off ground with both feet
36 mo	Makes tower of 10 cubes, imitates bridge of 3 cubes, copies circle, snips with scissors, can brush teeth but not well, puts shoes on feet		Broad jumps, walks up stairs alternating feet, may pedal tricycle, balances on one foot 2 to 3 seconds
48 mo	Copies bridge from model, copies cross and square, cuts curved line with scissors, dresses self, strings small beads		Pedals tricycle, runs smoothly, hops on one foot, catches large ball
60 mo	Some can print name; copies triangle, opens lock with key, bathes self, cuts out simple shapes, pours from small pitcher		Walks downstairs alternating feet, catches bounced ball, skips, stands on one foot 7 to 8 seconds

the head off the bed about 45 degrees when in the prone position and showing little head droop when held in suspension. All normal body movements are symmetric (see Table 5-1).

Communication and Language Development

Parents should be encouraged to notice how their infant looks at them when they are talking and how intently the infant looks at faces, especially during the quiet alert state, the time when the infant is most interactive. Infants "connect" with parents, even if only for a few moments. By talking to their infant during caregiving activities, parents encourage early language development. Infants start to make cooing and babbling sounds, much to the delight of their parents (Table 5-2 lists receptive and expressive language skills for children from birth to 5 years old). However, body movements (e.g., snuggling, turning the head, arching the body) continue to be the primary form of communication, and providers can help parents identify and become more skilled at interpreting their infant's cues.

TABLE 5-2	Speech and Language Milestones: Areas for Surveillance	
Age	**Receptive Language**	**Expressive Language**
0-3 mo	Attends to voice, turns head or eyes Startles to loud sounds Quiets in response to voice Smiles, coos, gurgles to voice	Undifferentiated but strong cry Coos and gurgles Single-syllable repetition *g, k, h,* and *ng* appear
3-6 mo	Actively seeks sound source May look in response to name Responses may vary to angry or happy voice	Increased babbling, vocal play Increased repetitive babbling (gaga) Laughs Vocalizes to toys Spontaneous smile to verbal play Increased intensity and nasal tone Vocalizes to removal of toy Experiments with own voice
6-9 mo	May look at family member when named Inhibits to "no" Begins interest in pictures when named Individual words begin to take on meaning	Babbles tunefully Increased sound combinations Uses *m, n, b, d, t* Initiates sounds such as click or kiss Uses nonspecific "mama" and "dada"
9-12 mo	Will give toy on request Understands simple commands Turns head to own name Understands "hot," "where's...?" Responds with gestures to "bye-bye"	Increased imitating efforts Has one word with specific reference Accompanies vocalizations with gestures Jargon increases Imitates animal sounds
12-18 mo	Follows simple one-step commands Understands new words weekly Increased interest in named pictures Differentiates environmental sounds Points to familiar objects and body parts when named Understands simple questions Begins to distinguish "you" from "me"	All vowels, many consonants present Increased use of true words Jargon is sentence-like Shows "no" behavior Names a few pictures, 10 words Can imitate non-speech sounds (cough, tongue click) Names some body parts
18-24 mo	Follows two-step commands Vocabulary increases rapidly Enjoys simple stories Recognizes pronouns	Imitates two-word combinations Dramatic increase in vocabulary Speech combines jargon and words Names self Answers some questions Begins to combine words
24-30 mo	Understands prepositions *in* and *on* Seems to understand most of what is said Understands more reasoning ("when you are finished, then...") Identifies object when given function (wear on feet, cook on)	Jargon reduced Two- to three-word sentences Repeats two numbers Increased use of pronouns Asks simple questions Joins in songs and nursery rhymes Can repeat simple phrases and sentences
30-36 mo	Listens to adult conversations Understands preposition *under* Can categorize items by function Begins to recognize colors Begins to take turns Understands "big" and "little," "boy" and "girl"	Child answers questions ("wear on feet," "to bed") Repeats three numbers Uses regular plurals Can help tell simple story
36-42 mo	Understands *fast* Understands prepositions *behind* and *in front* Responds to simple three-part commands Increasing understanding of adjectives and plurals Understands "just one"	Understands and answers ("cold," "tired," "hungry") Mostly three- to four-word sentences Gives full name Begins rote counting Begins to relate events Lots of questions, some beginning prepositions (*on, in*)

TABLE 5-2	Speech and Language Milestones: Areas for Surveillance—cont'd	
Age	**Receptive Language**	**Expressive Language**
42-48 mo	Recognizes coins Begins to understand future and past tenses Understands number concepts—more than one	Uses prepositions Tells stories Can give function of objects Repeats larger than six-word sentences Repeats four numbers Gives age Good intelligibility
48-60 mo	Responds to three-action commands	Asks "how" questions Answers verbally to questions such as "How are you?" Uses past and future tenses Can use conjunctions to string words and phrases together

Social and Emotional Development

The infant becomes highly social, imitating the parent's expressions and visually following the parent. Infants are more responsive to sounds in their environment, attending to sounds by quieting body movements or demonstrating visual responses. By three months, infants demonstrate a social smile and will usually smile in response to their parent's voice. As infants become more active, alert, and responsive, parents may mistakenly assume that the infant can handle more activity and irregular stimulation than capable of managing. It is important for caregivers to develop sensitivity to infant cues for the need to rest or to have decreased stimulation.

Cognitive Development

By 4 to 8 weeks infants readily begin to take in more of their environment. When a face or toy is brought into visual range, the infant visually tracks past midline, vertically, and horizontally. Even very young infants demonstrate various facial expressions, respond to sounds, and attempt to imitate mouthing movements. By 3 months infants begin to enjoy toys and may wave their arms when a toy is brought into sight.

4 THROUGH 5 MONTHS

Physical Development

Infants 4 through 5 months old usually begin to settle into regular patterns of eating, sleeping, and playing. They sleep 12 to 15 hours a day with five feedings during the day and one during the night. By this age infants begin to sleep through the night without feeding. Somewhere between 4 and 6 months, infants double their birthweight, and slow growth to gain about 5 ounces (140 g) a week. Their length increases about 0.8 inch (2 cm) per month, and head circumference increases about 0.4 inch (1 cm) per month. Growth may appear in spurts although the overall growth chart will show a steady upward curve. Weight gain can be influenced by the amount of play activity and the sleep schedule. Although the infant's primary source of nutrition comes from breast milk or formula, parents may ask about when to begin feeding solid foods. Many parents introduce some infant cereals by 4 months, but nutritionally, full-term babies need nothing other than breast milk or iron-fortified formula until 6 months old (see Chapter 10). As solid food is added, changes in stool consistency will be noted.

Motor Skills Development

Fine motor skills are demonstrated as infants play with their hands and begin to reach for and pull at clothing or other objects that are close. Eventually they grasp toys and begin to grab at other objects, such as the parent's hair, earrings, or eyeglasses. They also start to place their hands on the breast or the bottle in an attempt to hold or pat it.

Motor skills progress (see Table 5-1) as the Moro and asymmetric tonic neck reflexes are integrated, and there is no longer the obligation of arm extension with head turning. The Landau reflex emerges. Infants who are given sufficient tummy time generally begin to roll, first from front to back and then from back to front. Head control becomes stronger and more sustained, and there should be no head lag when the baby is pulled to sit. When in the prone position, infants hold their head up at 45 degrees, gradually progressing to 90 degrees for sustained periods of time. The infant learns to sit, first in the tripod stance, then unassisted with the head held erect. When lying supine, infants are able to lift their legs and bring their feet to their mouth. They bear full weight when standing and enjoy bouncing up and down in a parent's lap. All their body movements should be symmetric.

Communication and Language Development

Infants' social skills increase and verbal skills become more evident (see Table 5-2). They begin babbling, using vowel sounds, cooing, and laughing quietly and experiment with variations in tone and pitch, such as low-pitched chuckles and deeper laughs. Eventually they laugh out loud, much to the enjoyment of those around them. Infants' responses to sounds gradually become more localized, and they search for the sound of a bell or rattle.

Oral-motor development is a prerequisite for speech. Throughout infancy oral development progresses from sucking and rooting to rhythmic biting and chewing. Beginning at about 6 months and continuing through 2 years, the child learns to chew by moving the jaw up and down while flattening and spreading the tongue, and to control biting by using rotary jaw movements with lateralization of tongue placement. These motor skills, essential for the production of speech, are among the most complex movements that the young child must master.

Social and Emotional Development

During this time, infants' social skills become more evident. Usual behavior includes spontaneous smiling at parents and others while visually following the caregiver around the environment and turning the head a full 180 degrees. At this age they promptly look at an object when it is placed in front of them; they notice things. The infant's increasing awareness of the environment facilitates more complex social interactions. Infants begin to recognize that their parents are responding to their needs. They notice, for example, as the parent prepares to offer the breast or get a bottle ready for feeding. Because infants notice other things, parents can often distract them from demanding immediate gratification by talking, playing, or using other social interactions such as reciprocal vocalizations and eye contact. As a result, infants learn that their hunger needs will be met, but that there are other satisfying interactions they can have with their parents. Infants at this age begin to more actively reciprocate their parents' attention and enjoy playing with their parents. Crying may reflect tiredness or a need for social interaction, not just hunger. Parents are able to acknowledge their child's unique personality, and this reciprocal recognition is an important aspect of infant-parent attachment.

Cognitive Development

Visual exploration increases during this age, as infants seek out objects in the environment such as mobiles, mirrors, their hands, and the toys that they are holding. Their preference, however, is looking at their parents' or another person's face. Chewing and mouthing are other means of exploration used to differentiate textures, tastes, and shapes. As their muscle control improves, they are able to bring a toy to their mouth first when lying on their back and then when sitting.

6 THROUGH 8 MONTHS

Physical Development

As infants reduce their breast milk or formula intake and add solids to their diet, growth velocity changes. Weight gain slows to 3 to 4 ounces (85 to 110 g) a week, or about 1 pound (0.5 kg) a month; length gains are about 0.5 to 0.6 inch (1.2 to 1.5 cm) per month; and head circumference increases about 0.2 inch (0.5 cm) per month. If concerns about a large head circumference exist, note each parent's head circumference and graph them to determine percentile for comparison with their infants, and continue to monitor the infant carefully (see Chapter 27 for a discussion of macrocephaly). Teething symptoms can begin at about 6 months as the central incisors emerge and at 8 months when the lateral incisors emerge. The first childhood illness might occur at the same time as teething behaviors start and these events can disrupt the infant's previous sleep routine.

Motor Skills Development

Motor skills at this age need little encouragement for development because of the infants' desire to explore the environment. Infants sit erect for longer periods of time and may scoot while in a sitting position. Crawling begins with the infant pushing up to the hands and knees and rocking in place, then eventually mastering the rhythm of hands and knees working together. Many infants will pull themselves along on the floor with their arms, and use one foot or toe to push while their stomachs remain on the floor, prior to beginning to use hands and knees to crawl. Infants may stand, fully supporting their weight, when their hands are held at shoulder height.

Fine motor skills continue to be honed, and babies are more adept at using their palm and all of their fingers to pick up objects. Initially they rake at small objects and are able to hold a small cube, lifting it off the table. Gradually they use fingers and thumb to pick up objects. They reach for and grasp toys, can hold a toy in each hand at the same time, and can transfer objects from one hand to another.

Communication and Language Development

Vocalizations continue to show increasing variety in pitch and tone, and imitation of specific speech sounds begins. Infants articulate single-sound units that may be vowels, consonants, or blends such as "ah," "ba," "da," "ga," "ch," and "bl." Gradually, they progress to double-consonant sounds (e.g., "dada") and occasionally will vocalize using three or more different syllables. They use "mama" and "dada," but not specifically for their parents. Infants can delight their parents as they respond to verbal cues and play at making sounds and noises when alone. They enjoy imitating oral sounds such as "raspberries" and coughing.

Although infants' expressive language skills are limited, their receptive language is evident when they listen and respond to their parents' talking. Infants distinguish facial expressions and gestures, may stop or quiet when their parent uses "no" or a different tone of voice, and turn toward their parents' voices and other sounds, localizing directly to the sound.

It is important to encourage parents to begin reading to their child daily at a very young age, at least by 6 months, if not sooner. This can be introduced as part of the bedtime routine. Watching TV or videos should be discouraged because it is a passive medium, and infants learn language best when they interact with another person, by listening to parents' voices and looking at a face that responds to them.

Social and Emotional Development

Infants at this age greatly enjoy social play, and their individual personality and temperament continue to be expressed. At times, infants' increased ability to do things for themselves puts them at odds with their parents. Even if parents have learned to understand their infant's cues and engage with the infant responsively, giving and taking and control issues can arise. Infants use gestures such as pointing, reaching with outstretched arms, tugging, and throwing things to get their parent's attention and communicate their needs. As infants' abilities and desires become more complex, and they expand their repertoire of communication cues, parents need to learn new parenting skills (e.g., how to handle a determined child) to meet their infant's social development needs.

Stranger anxiety may appear at this time, depending on the variety of caregivers infants have had and their individual temperament.

Cognitive Development

From 6 through 8 months there is significant growth in infant cognitive development. The infant understands cause-and-effect relationships in activities such as ringing a bell; pulling on a string to retrieve a ring, train, or phone; and dropping a toy from the crib or highchair. They follow a toy if it falls and remains within their visual field. For some older infants, beginning object permanence is evident because they will look for partially hidden objects and play peek-a-boo. The infant is increasingly aware of surroundings and begins to express individual preferences more clearly. This is often a time when resistance to bedtime, feeding, and parental separation occurs.

9 THROUGH 12 MONTHS
Physical Development
At 9 to 10 months the infant's growth may follow a different growth curve than the one established early in infancy. Growth spurts become more apparent to parents as the infant seems to outgrow clothes "overnight." At the same time, illnesses, decreased solid food intake caused by teething, and the infant's increased activity level can slow the growth rate. It is important to estimate the infant's total caloric intake if there is a significant decrease in the infant's growth or if feeding problems are present. Early intervention for feeding problems at this time can result in a much easier resolution (see Chapter 10).

Infants show regular patterns in bowel and bladder elimination. Some parents interpret their ability to predict their infant's bowel movements as toilet training (see Chapter 12). Sleep problems, if managed with consistency, begin to resolve, although there might still be struggles with bedtime.

Between 11 and 12 months infants gain about 1 pound (0.5 kg) per month. Growth in length continues to occur in spurts. Eleven- to 12-month-olds usually eat solids well, want to feed themselves, and are able to recognize their own hunger or satiation needs. They usually do not eat the same amount at each meal and often demonstrate specific food preferences. Because infants do not have full dentition, food choices should be limited to soft or pureed foods or foods that turn soft when chewed (e.g., breadsticks). Feedings begin to follow a routine of breakfast, lunch, and dinner, with midmorning and afternoon snacks.

Motor Skills Development
Fine motor development allows older infants to entertain themselves for extended times. They hold objects of different sizes and pick up small objects using the sides of the fingers and eventually a fine pincer grasp, most often transferring the object directly to their mouth. Infants at this age enjoy putting objects into containers and taking them out again and, by 11 or 12 months, can stack blocks one on top of the other. They often begin to hold a cup with two hands, but may still have difficulty sealing their lips around the edge of the cup to take sips.

At 9 to 10 months most infants sit for long periods and crawl on hands and knees. They "cruise," walking around furniture holding on with both hands, and pull themselves off the floor to a standing position. They begin to let themselves down from furniture with fairly good control and take steps if someone holds two hands and then one hand. Eventually they take a few steps from one object or person to another. Some may momentarily stand alone, and others may walk independently.

Communication and Language Development
Receptive language skills improve, and infants participate in games such as pat-a-cake and peek-a-boo. Babies at this age momentarily stop activity when they hear "no," but they do not truly understand what "no" means. They are still very focused on observing activities in their environment and, when given names of things, attend well to the new information. They enjoy songs and rhymes and may participate by "singing" along.

By 12 months, infants' expressive language has expanded to a total of three or four words. Words such as "dada," "mama," or "ba-ba" (for bottle) can be recognized. They are able to name a picture in a book, visually look for an object when named, and follow simple one-step requests.

Social and Emotional Development
Infants at this age demonstrate stranger anxiety, and some demonstrate fear of new situations or experiences. As a result they will look to their parent for reassurance and attempt to engage the parent in eye contact while watching their parent's expression. Emotions, such as affection, anger, jealousy, and anxiety become more evident in late infancy. However, once familiar with new people, particularly if introduced by their parents, babies enjoy initiating interactive games and social interchanges. Overall, 11- to 12-month-olds appear to be in love with the world, love to explore, and have little understanding of those things that can cause them harm. They help with dressing by extending an arm or leg and retrieve the bottle if it is dropped. Most take great pride in mastering new skills or overcoming their fears, and they look to others around them to take notice as well.

Cognitive Development
Cognitively, older infants complete more complicated tasks, such as stacking and container play. They master object permanence and easily locate a toy placed out of sight or under a cloth. This skill allows them to take a more active role in playing hide-and-seek or peek-a-boo. They hold a crayon or pencil with their whole hand and make dots on a piece of paper imitating a drawn line.

Infants' curiosity blossoms as they begin to explore visually, and with mouthing and chewing, grasping, poking, shaking, pushing, pulling, and stacking. They develop their own games or explore different ways of playing with familiar toys or objects. Play and other activities become more spontaneous and self-directed, and the parent follows the lead of the child in play, imitating the child's interest and modeling newer activities related to the same toy or game (e.g., playing pat-a-cake and then adding a song).

■ Developmental Assessment of Infants
Monitoring the overall growth and development of the infant is critical because of the rapid changes during this time. If a delay or concern is detected early, prompt treatment improves the likelihood of positive outcomes. It is important to discuss the infant's development with parents so that they can anticipate changes and plan ways to support their infant's emerging

developmental skills. Effective assessment occurs with consistent visits with the same provider. Seeing the same provider on a regular basis strengthens the parent-child-provider relationship and makes it easier to pursue follow-up questions and concerns, validate the efforts of parents, and reinforce their successes. It is important to explain to parents what is being done during the examination so that they know the provider has completed a thorough and complete examination.

SCREENING STRATEGIES FOR INFANTS

As noted in Chapter 4, there is a distinction between screening and diagnostic assessment. Providers use both strategies when working with infants. One of the most informative questions that can be asked of the parent is, "Tell me about your infant's day." This elicits information about daily routines of feeding, bathing, naps and sleep, elimination, and play activities. It also gathers data about what areas may be most difficult for the parents and areas where suggestions may be most helpful. Listening carefully to parents' responses to this question from visit to visit helps providers truly understand the life of the infant and how best to assist an individual family.

Every well-child visit should include developmental surveillance in which the provider assesses parents' concerns, obtains a relevant developmental history, and completes a thorough and accurate examination, looking particularly at the child's development over time. Screening, using a standardized, valid, and reliable screening tool, should be conducted at the 9-, 18-, 24-, or 30-month well-child visit and whenever there is a parent or provider concern (AAP, 2006). The Ages & Stages Questionnaire (ASQ) or the Parents' Evaluation of Developmental Status (PEDS) is recommended for infants and young children and can be completed by parents while waiting to see the provider. Other tools may be used for specific areas of concern, such as speech and language, social and emotional behavior: ASQ: Social Emotional (ASQ: SE), the Infant-Toddler and Family Instrument (ITFI), the Temperament and Atypical Behavior Scale (TABS), and the Receptive-Expressive Emergent Language (REEL) Scale. Simply completing a checklist of developmental milestones or asking about specific milestones does not adequately screen an infant for developmental status, especially an infant who was born prematurely.

DIAGNOSTIC DEVELOPMENTAL ASSESSMENT STRATEGIES FOR INFANTS

Developmental assessment tools include the Brazelton Neonatal Behavioral Assessment Scale, the HOME Scale, the Bayley Scales of Infant Development, and the Nursing Child Assessment Satellite Training (NCAST) scales (feeding scale, teaching scale, sleep activity record, and personal environment assessments). These tools require special training to use and take longer to administer than screening tools. Use of developmental assessment tools can ensure timely, appropriate referrals and help establish individualized intervention strategies for clients.

It is beyond the scope of this chapter to provide a complete review of the screening and assessment tools available in the areas of infant development, parent-child interaction, and family assessment.

■ Anticipatory Guidance for Infants

Many of the issues of infancy can be addressed through education and anticipatory guidance of parents. New parents can be bombarded with more information and opinions than they can manage—from their own parents, neighbors, friends, the media, and others. When confronted with a question as common as, "When do I begin to feed my baby solid foods?" parents, especially first-time parents, can be confused by all their options. Health care providers help parents sort through the information, understand what it means, and decide what is best for their family. Providers have several goals in mind as they work with new parents of infants, specifically to help parents:

- Develop a set of skills that they can use as their child grows
- Understand how infants in general develop and what their capabilities are
- Understand and appreciate their own child's abilities during infancy
- Interact with their child in a way that strengthens the child-parent bond, nurtures and cherishes the child, and increases their self-confidence as parents

To achieve these goals, providers must listen carefully to parents. If parents express a concern, listening carefully to their perception of the problem is essential. Information can then be structured to more directly address specific concerns. New information or anticipatory guidance expands the parents' knowledge base, gives them more choices about how to handle a situation, and puts them in charge, making them feel more competent to succeed as parents. Education helps parents learn about infant development, what activities promote healthy development, and what the parent can do to provide secure, safe relationships in an environment that supports their child's development. Too much information, or information that the parent feels is irrelevant, however, can be overwhelming, so providers must be sensitive to the parents' learning needs. Frequently, time limitations in a clinic or office setting lead to use of a "laundry list" of topics for anticipatory guidance rather than information individualized to the infant and family being seen. Alternative approaches such as parent groups or classes that focus on commonly shared parenting issues can be used effectively.

Providers must also validate the parents' efforts to do their job as parents. Acknowledging specific positive aspects of the parents' skills before offering anticipatory guidance helps ensure that parents are more receptive to new ideas. Parents should always be asked what they have tried that has worked, and their successes should be reinforced. Providers should be alert for developmentally appropriate parent-child interactions in the office and reinforce the parents' behavior with immediate positive feedback.

Observing and commenting on aspects of the child's development during the office visit is a "teachable moment," allowing the provider to initiate discussions with parents about concerns or anticipatory guidance topics. Providers can also model developmentally appropriate activities during the well-child examination. They can show parents ways to interact with their infant that stimulate, comfort, or soothe the baby. During these demonstrations, parents can be asked to give examples of things they have done at home as they care for their infant. If a problem was discussed at a previous well-child care visit and a plan made to try certain activities (e.g., creating a nighttime ritual to manage a 10-month-old who refuses to go to sleep in her own bed), providers should review the outcome, and provide positive feedback and encouragement for the efforts made and successful results.

Health education and anticipatory guidance can help parents become knowledgeable about their child's needs and capabilities, better able to read their infant's cues, and provide timely and appropriate care. Parents gain the skill to become their child's advocates. In turn, support from providers and the infant's responsive behaviors strengthen the parents' confidence and aid their receptiveness to future anticipatory guidance. The following are specific topic areas in which practitioners' anticipatory guidance can help parents through the remarkable, fast-moving first year of their child's life.

THE PRENATAL VISIT

Prenatal visits provide an opportunity to assess parents' knowledge and receptiveness to anticipatory guidance. The prenatal visit includes a discussion of the partnership between the primary care provider and the parent, instruction about newborn care, assessment of feeding preferences (i.e., breast versus formula), injury prevention, and the management of possible sibling rivalry or toddler jealousy situations. The prenatal visit is a time to look for risk factors for perinatal depression (e.g., previous history of depression or previous postpartum depression; lack of social support). These meetings provide a foundation for later visits and establish the pediatric provider as a resource for the parents.

THE NEONATAL VISIT

The newborn visit in the hospital should focus on family readiness, infant behaviors, feeding, safety, and routine baby care. Practice guidelines for newborn care during the immediate postnatal period should be provided in writing; the hospital visit is the least opportune time to discuss infant care because of the mother's physiological state, which reduces her ability to absorb new information. Parents should leave the hospital knowing how to interpret their infant's hunger and discomfort signs, and what signs and symptoms related to feeding (breast milk or formula), jaundice, and infant care (e.g., umbilical cord) are of concern and warrant a call to the provider. Written information should include the phone numbers of the practice and specifics about how to reach the provider after hours and on weekends. A follow-up visit in the office should be within 48 hours of discharge.

BIRTH TO 1 MONTH
Regulation and Sleep-Wake Patterns
- Infants need assistance to develop day-night cycles because they do not distinguish between days and nights. Using a consistent daily routine helps the infant establish a good sleep-wake cycle.
- Placing the infant in a bassinet or crib for naps during the day allows an easier transition from the parent to bed at night.
- Infants need a variety of movement, voice, or touch to move them from sleep to wake states. Rhythmicity of voice, movement, or touch calms infants or lowers their

state, and a parent's slow, easy movements during caregiving will lessen the infant's startle or Moro reflex.
- Some infants benefit from external stimuli such as music, voice, or movement to help calm them and support their self-regulation. Gentle massage or swaddling helps some infants adjust to state changes.

Strength and Motor Coordination
Infants' gradual increase in strength makes it possible for them to lift their heads. Parents should place their infants in the supine position for sleep, but give their babies "tummy time" when awake and alert, as soon as the newborn comes home from the hospital. Tummy time consists of supervised time spent playing with the baby in a prone position. Initially 2 to 3 minutes, two or three times a day, is sufficient, but time intervals should gradually increase until the infant spends a total of 1 hour daily while prone (Ma, 2009). Time spent prone allows infants to develop strong neck muscles and decreases the likelihood of positional plagiocephaly.

Feeding and Self-Care
- A primary developmental activity of the newborn is organizing feeding responses. Bringing the infant slowly to an awake state for feeding is the first step. If the infant is overstimulated or disorganized, it may be necessary to reduce external stimuli (e.g., lights and noise), increase the infant's flexion of arms and legs, or bundle the infant to assist with central nervous system control and improve feeding responses.
- Infants need a regular suck-swallow and breathing rhythm for feeding. If milk flows through the breast or bottle too rapidly or too slowly, adjustments are needed to help the baby manage the feeding. Feedings that are longer than 40 minutes or shorter than 20 minutes should be evaluated further.
- The face-to-face feeding position is important because it encourages eye contact and parent-child communication and interaction.
- The infant's reach for breast or bottle represents beginning exploratory learning and should be encouraged. Parents also can encourage the grasp reflex while the baby is feeding through finger play or finger holding.
- Infants are good at regulating how much they need to eat. It may not always be consistent from one meal to the next. Understanding and respecting an infant's hunger and satiation cues help protect against later feeding and nutritional problems, such as obesity. Burping techniques may also be different for each infant and is an important time for a rest during feeding, in addition to social interaction.
- Urinary output is one indicator of adequate intake, but not the only one. Weight gain, feeding type (breast milk or formula), frequency and duration, frequency of spit-ups, and infant activity level must be evaluated to ensure the infant's adequate nutrition.
- Some infants need more opportunities for sucking. Evidence indicates that the use of a pacifier during sleep decreases the risk of SIDS (AAP, 2009; Hauck et al, 2005). The evidence for nipple confusion and breastfeeding difficulties with use of a pacifier is not clear. However, it is recommended that pacifier use begin in breastfed infants

after 1 month of age (Hauck et al, 2005). Parents should be encouraged to provide their infants with pacifiers when they place their infant to sleep, but not to reinsert them after the infant is asleep. If the infant refuses the pacifier, he or she should not be forced to take it, and the pacifier should not be coated with sweet solutions. Pacifiers should be cleaned frequently and replaced after a few weeks.

- Support and guidance for breastfeeding mothers may require additional counseling, observation of feedings, and referral to a lactation consultant, in addition to guidance on strategies for returning to work while breastfeeding (see Chapter 11).

Communication and Language

- Newborn's communication skills are seen during state changes, periods of alertness, feeding, and sleep routines. Parents must be alert to nonverbal infant communication (e.g., fussiness, turning the head away) to understand their infant's needs.
- Attending promptly to infant crying helps the infant to develop a sense of trust.
- Imitating infant sounds encourages an infant to vocalize and experiment with different types of sounds.

Social and Emotional Growth

- Newborns are able to tolerate brief periods of social interaction when they are in an alert state. Orienting to visual stimuli (e.g., a parent's smiling face) helps the infant keep a stable alert state. Parents need to learn how to help the infant achieve this alert state and how to avoid overstimulating a newborn. These are discussed more fully later.
- Being gently touched and held are very important for the newborn. Encourage parents to hold their infant and assure them that holding does not spoil a baby, but meets their need for emotional support and tactile contact and fosters infant-parent bonding.
- Facilitating overall family development and emotional growth is important, especially for siblings. Based on the age of the sibling, parents may need ideas of what would be appropriate involvement for them with the newborn.
- Parental development is fostered by pointing out concrete ways that parents are meeting the needs of their infant (more than just "You are doing a good job"). Parents' concerns should be followed up closely with support, guidance, and reassurance when appropriate. It is important for parents to have early success while caring for the new infant.

Cognitive and Environmental Stimulation

Parents should encourage opportunities for the infant to look at things in the environment. Placing mobiles at the side of the bassinet or crib helps prevent overstimulation. As infants develop, a variety of objects encourage them to visually explore their surroundings and move their heads from side to side. It is also helpful to place infants at different ends of the bed periodically. Including infants in family activities during their awake times exposes them to many sounds and visual images.

1 THROUGH 3 MONTHS

Regulation and Sleep-Wake Patterns

- Structuring an infant's day helps meet the infant's ongoing need for external routines and facilitates state organization.
- The use of repetitive stimulation (e.g., rocking or a soothing voice) for quieting and a variety of stimulation to help the infant achieve an alert state (e.g., undressing, stroking, or voice intonations) are important parenting strategies.
- Parents need to understand their infant's need for swaddling and sensitive movements because of the immature nervous system (e.g., continuation of Moro or asymmetric tonic neck reflex).
- Sleep location, safety, position ("back to sleep"), and the establishment of a naptime and nighttime ritual all influence later sleep habits for the infant. Helping infants learn to go to sleep on their own begins with becoming drowsy in their parent's arms and then being placed in the bassinet or crib while still awake.

Strength and Motor Coordination

- Placing the infant in different positions for playtime and when awake, especially the prone position, encourages upper body strength, and neck, arm, and head control. Other family members may be especially good at encouraging this as the infant lies prone on the chest and looks up into their face.
- The supine position stimulates movement of the fingers, hands, feet, and legs, and makes it easier to hold toys.

Feeding and Self-Care

- Feedings become more consistent, and the infant continues to have a strong need for sucking, especially for nonnutritive sucking, such as sucking on fingers and toys. A pacifier may be helpful.
- Feedings continue to be important to meet both nutritional and developmental needs. This is a time for close, affectionate communication between parent and baby.
- Each infant will demonstrate unique cues for readiness to eat and satiation. As the parents get ready for the feeding, they will recognize that their infant begins to anticipate that they will be fed. Reinforce the parents' responsiveness to the infant's cues that he or she has eaten enough and does not overfeed.
- Positive reinforcement for continued breastfeeding is still needed and problem-solving strategies for the mother who is returning to work are beneficial (see Chapter 11).

Communication and Language

- Talking and singing to infants during routine daily activities should be encouraged. The value of hearing the parent's voice is great, even if the infant does not understand the words.
- Helping parents understand and respond to their infant's cues and sleep-wake states supports communication between parent and infant.
- Reading as part of daily or evening routine should be encouraged.

Social and Emotional Growth

- Parents' observations and intuitions about their infant need to be reinforced. Recommendations associated with the parents' own observations are the most supportive and educational; parental competence will grow as their increasing skills are validated.
- An infant's hands are often described as an infant's "first toy." In addition, they are used for self-consoling and hand-to-mouth exploration.
- Continuing to respond to infants' cries as soon as possible reassures them that their needs will be met and decreases the chances of crying later on.
- The infant's emerging temperament and the parents' perceptions of the infant's behaviors will need to be resolved if there are conflicts.
- Infants have an increasing social need and desire to play with the caregiver. Often fussing or crying is misinterpreted for hunger. Parents may need assistance to set up "play stations" (different play activities) so the infant can be moved easily from one activity to another. As a result of the infant's short attention span, approximately 10 to 15 minutes at each station over an hour's time will usually lead to a tired, happy baby.
- Parents need to develop strategies to have time together as a couple. Providers can help them identify criteria for childcare resources and locate those resources.

Cognitive and Environmental Stimulation

- The infant's visual awareness is increasing and more visual diversity is needed, such as changes in position and location and changes in stimulating objects, such as a mobile or mirror.
- Toy selection and equipment should include criteria for safety and developmental appropriateness for the infant. Toys should be semirigid, unpainted, and have varying textures. Toys that rattle and make sounds are appropriate. These encourage waving arms and kicking legs.

4 THROUGH 5 MONTHS

Regulation and Sleep-Wake Patterns

- Infants need to resume sleep independently when they awaken at night. Help parents prepare for future changes in the infant's sleep-wake pattern by putting the infant to sleep in the crib while drowsy but not yet asleep. If the infant awakens at night, he or she is more likely to resume sleep without comforting from the parent.
- Nighttime rituals continue to be an important aspect of helping the infant anticipate what is going to happen next, which builds a sense of security.
- Parents' perception of their infant's temperament plays an important role in how they respond to their infant. They may describe their infant as easy, average, or challenging, and they may compare their infant with other babies. Parents may need encouragement to understand their infant's uniqueness and can be shown how individualizing their activities to their baby's style makes parenting much easier.
- Varied parenting approaches to infants of different temperaments, including patterns of eating and sleeping, can be discussed.
- Consistent, prompt responses to infant crying continue to be essential.

Strength and Motor Coordination

As the infant becomes more mobile, safety measures become more critical; parental supervision and childproofing the home, relatives' homes, and child care or daycare settings are essential for safety (e.g., locks on cabinets and gates for stairs).

Floor-time play encourages motor strength and coordination. Playpens can be limiting, but can be effectively used as a safety measure. Movable walkers have been found to be unsafe and should be discouraged (Hagan et al, 2008). If parents choose to use a walker, it should not have wheels and should only be used for brief periods (e.g., 10 to 15 minutes) as a safe place to set a child.

Feeding and Self-Care

- Drooling is less about teething and more about salivary gland maturation. The infant gradually develops the ability to swallow excessive saliva.
- Responding appropriately to the infant's hunger cues and satiation cues continues to be important.
- Infants are ready for solids as their gastrointestinal tract matures, and they mature developmentally. They should have good head control and be able to sit alone before solids are started. Listen closely to parents' questions and beliefs and the influence of others on the introduction of solids. Although the AAP recommends exclusive breastfeeding until 6 months old, they also note that it is appropriate to start solid foods between 4 and 6 months; not every infant is ready to start solids at the same age (AAP, 2005; American Heart Association et al, 2006).
- When solids are introduced, a spoon should be used. Cereal should not be given in a bottle. This helps the infant develop new oral-motor skills. Skills needed to suck and swallow milk from a bottle or breast differ from those needed to take cereal from a spoon.
- Interacting with the infant during feeding fosters the parent-child relationship and makes feeding time fun rather than just a routine.
- Allowing infants to pat the breast or bottle and place their hands on the bottle promotes self-feeding later as they learn to hold their bottle or cup. Bottles should not be propped because the infant can aspirate.

Communication and Language

- Parents' use of reciprocal or "back-and-forth talking" with their infant, especially using changes in voice inflection and intonation, is important in developing communication skills.
- Parents' talking to their infant during caregiving activities holds the infant's attention, especially when the infant is fussy. Talking to the infant makes it easier to change diapers, prepare meals, and attend to the infant's needs in other ways. It also stimulates the infant's language skills.
- Reading to an infant and looking at picture books, describing the pictures, colors, and actions, is beneficial even at this early age. The importance of developing habits of quiet time, reading time, and parent-child together time can also be stressed. Providers may want to participate in Reach Out and Read, the national early literacy program for children 6 months through 5 years old.

Social and Emotional Growth

- The infant continues to need nonnutritive sucking as a means of self-regulation. Sucking on fingers or toys requires different oral-motor movements from those needed to suck on a pacifier.
- Discipline can be discussed and differentiated from punishment. The important role of "parents as teachers" may be a new concept to some parents. Helping parents understand the importance of modeling desired behaviors and redirecting behavior should be discussed before it is needed (see Chapters 4 and 17).
- Information about age level child development and strategies to deal with difficult behaviors is important. Referral to parenting classes that provide information on developmental milestones and anticipated changes may be helpful. Although parents may have books on development, a one-page handout addressing a particular subject of immediate concern, given to the parents by the provider, is likely to be more useful. Such handouts are available through *Healthy Steps* and *Bright Futures*.
- Both parents need to be involved in ongoing communication about their roles, responsibilities, and expectations. Fathers may be more comfortable handling the infant at this age, as the infant becomes responsive. Differences between parental expectations need to be discussed (e.g., to allow an infant to cry at bedtime or not).
- Caregivers may need help finding time for themselves, managing life stresses, or when returning to work. Infant behaviors often mirror the emotional state of their caregivers.
- The parents' emotional well-being and availability is an important aspect of the infant's overall care. Helping parents value their time together may need to be reinforced.
- Also important is counseling about how to select safe and appropriate child care and toys.

Cognitive and Environmental Stimulation

- With the infant's increasing activity and awake time, parents will need strategies to provide more attention and play activities. The infant will make every effort to obtain the parents' attention by smiling, making sounds, or crying. Using a variety of activities and toys such as soft stuffed toys, rattles, a crib gym or busy box, and toys of different sizes, weights, shapes, materials, and colors can be suggested. Home objects that infants see every day can be used as "toys" for stacking, shaking, and rolling.
- Infants may also enjoy looking at themselves in a mirror, and placing a mirror next to the changing table is a good diversion.
- Activities such as walks to the park, visiting neighbors, or trips to the grocery store are all part of an infant's learning experiences.

6 THROUGH 8 MONTHS
Regulation and Sleep-Wake Patterns

- Infants may have settled into a good sleep routine through the night, only to have it interrupted with teething or illness. They may need assistance to resume their regular sleep-wake patterns. Parents may need to go to the infants to assure them they are safe, but should not feed infants for comfort or to help them return to sleep.
- An increased need for consistency of nighttime rituals to help the infant transition from playtime to sleep time (e.g., bath time and a story) may be evident.
- Teaching infants to sleep in their own crib can be a struggle for some parents. Begin by putting them to bed while they are drowsy but still awake. If the infant wakes in the night, parents can help them return to sleep with the least amount of intrusion (e.g., use face, voice, touch, and then holding).
- Infants are now more capable of waiting for gratification and parents can use talking and tone of voice to distract, calm, and reassure infants that their needs will be met.

Strength and Motor Coordination

- Floor time is essential for the infant to learn to crawl and walk. Parents must provide for infant safety. Movable walkers are unsafe and may actually hinder walking. Stationary walkers are also not recommended.
- Childproofing the home becomes increasingly important. Putting gates on stairs, padding sharp corners, covering electrical outlets, removing small objects and latex balloons from within the infant's reach, and keeping the cord on an iron safely out of the way needs to be stressed. Make sure that parents and other caregivers have the telephone number for a poison control center handy (1-800-222-1222). Some parents find it helpful to lie on the floor where the infant plays to find hazards visible to the infant.
- Bath-water temperature must be checked, and infants should never be left alone even for a few seconds in the tub.
- Active supervision is the best way to prevent injuries as an infant becomes more mobile, and requires parents to be within reach and free of distractions while watching their infant.

Feeding and Self-Care

- If not already started, solids should be introduced at 6 months. Breastfed infants need iron-fortified foods. Parents often need specific information about types of foods to start with, quantity, and feeding positions (see Chapter 10). Use an infant seat or a highchair (properly seated high enough that the infant's back and sides are supported and arms are at the level of the tray).
- Structured mealtimes are important to help the family maintain regular infant routines.
- Allowing the child to hold a spoon or cup encourages self-feeding and begins preparing the infant for later weaning from bottle or breast.
- Often parents are uncomfortable with the messiness of infant feeding. Discuss ways they can minimize the mess (e.g., sheet or plastic tablecloth on the floor, small portions of food) and still allow the infant to explore, look at, touch, smell, and taste the new foods. Assure the parents that there will always be some mess.
- Introducing solid foods and infant teething often occur simultaneously. Cleansing the teeth (use a soft cloth or soft toothbrush) and providing fluoride supplements, if the water supply is not fluoridated, are important at this time (see Chapter 33).

Communication and Language

- Using the names of objects, encouraging gestures, talking about everyday activities, and responding to the infant's increasing vocalizations are important.
- Early lessons in "reading to an infant" include showing the infant picture books and magazines and talking about the pictures.
- Naming body parts while changing diapers and during bath time is an enjoyable activity for parents. To demonstrate the infant's responsiveness, the provider can model this behavior during the physical examination.

Social and Emotional Growth

- Identifying and encouraging the child to have a "transitional object" (e.g., a favorite toy or blanket) can ease the coming developmental phase of separation anxiety.
- Discussing parents' feelings regarding limit setting, consistency of care, and parental consensus about discipline is important.
- Positive parental responsiveness and attention supports infant social and emotional growth.

Cognitive and Environmental Stimulation

- Toys that involve cause-and-effect reactions, stacking, and container play can be demonstrated and encouraged. Most often, favorite toys are common household objects such as wooden spoons, plastic bowls, pull toys, or a telephone. Especially popular is any object that the parents use.
- Interactive games are important, and infants should be encouraged to initiate actions and guide play.

9 THROUGH 12 MONTHS
Regulation and Sleep-Wake Patterns

- A "transitional object" can ease the infant's experience in new situations and provide a sense of comfort or familiarity.
- Predictability in the daily schedule allows the infant to gain mastery over new situations. Efforts to establish and maintain regular mealtimes, a nighttime routine, and consistent caregivers increase the infant's sense of security during transitions.
- The infant's temperament becomes more evident in activity level, curiosity level, and ease in adjusting to new situations. The infant's temperament may not always be compatible with that of other family members. This discrepancy can become an area of conflict and turmoil. Inquiring about such, and discussing positive parenting strategies, can generate creative solutions.

Strength and Motor Coordination

- The parents' natural tendency to "cheer" their infants on as they refine old and achieve new motor skills is an example of positive reinforcement for the child in other areas of development.
- Childproofing the environment is critical because the infant is increasingly mobile and curious. Parents need help to anticipate their infant's next major developmental achievement and prepare for the child's natural curiosity. Babies at this age are able to get into trouble but not get themselves out (e.g., falling in a slippery bathtub).

- Safe storage of medicines, cleaning agents, matches, and firearms (in locked cabinets, not just out of reach) are essential precautions for mobile older infants with increased fine motor skills and unbounded curiosity.
- Bath-water temperature must be checked, and infants should never be left alone even for a few seconds in the tub.
- Plastic bags, balloons, and small objects must be kept away from the curious, exploring infant.
- As fine motor skills improve, oral exploration is still one of an infant's primary learning methods, so most everything ends up in the mouth. Having the 24-hour poison control telephone number available and posted for caregivers is critical.
- Active supervision, with the parent within reach and without distractions, is the best way to prevent injuries as an infant becomes more mobile. Once the infant can pull to stand in the crib, the crib mattress should be lowered to the lowest rung. Outings for both parents and child help relieve stress and provide wonderful learning opportunities for the infant.

Feeding and Self-Care

- The division of responsibility in feeding becomes more obvious during this time. Parents are responsible for providing healthful foods in an environment that is pleasant and conducive to eating. Children are responsible for determining how much of the healthful foods they will eat. Nine- to 12-month-old infants begin to self-feed and demonstrate clear preferences and dislikes. Discussing the division of responsibilities and the control issues that may arise at this time can help families establish healthy eating patterns for a lifetime (see Chapter 10).
- Dental hygiene and caries prevention include use of a soft cloth or soft toothbrush to cleanse teeth and gums. Toothpaste is not necessary, but when used should not contain fluoride. Fluoride supplements should be given if the family's water supply is not fluoridated (see Chapter 33).
- Transitioning from purees to blended foods, finger foods, and soft solids involves major changes for infant and parents. Remind parents that it can take 10 to 20 exposures for infants to accept a new food into their diet.
- Practicing with spoons and cups in play and at mealtime helps develop the infant's skills in using them and promotes eventual self-feeding. Infants should be weaned from the bottle and pacifier by about 12 months of age.
- Establishing consistent mealtimes and snack times and avoiding the habit of "grazing" (i.e., having food constantly available) will encourage appropriate intake of foods. Because hunger is inconsistent for infants, three meals and two or three snacks will ensure adequate nutrition. Having the infant sit in a highchair to eat sets a pattern and expectation for eating at the table, rather than grazing.
- Eating together at least once a day as a family is important for infants. The likelihood that infants will try new foods increases as they observe others eat. Eating with others keeps the infant focused on meals. Distractions, such as toys and television, should be avoided. Mealtime conversation should be pleasant, helping all family members enjoy their time together.

Communication and Language

- Reinforcing the infant's effort to communicate through gestures, pointing, and ambiguous vocalizations should be encouraged. This "practice" with language provides the groundwork for future speech skills. Parents should not try to anticipate exactly what the child needs.
- Naming utensils and the color, smell, taste, and texture of foods builds language skills and keeps the infant engaged during mealtime.
- Naming body parts and pointing to them provides distraction during diaper changes and bath time.
- Reading is more interactive as the infant points to pictures in a book, imitates animal sounds, and assists in turning pages. Encourage parents to read to their infant often.

Social and Emotional Growth

- As infants reach 12 months, their emerging will, desire for autonomy, need for control, and sense of initiative become more evident. They begin to distinguish themselves from their parents.
- It is important to help parents understand discipline is a guidance process used to teach positive behaviors (as compared with punishment in which constraints are applied to negative behaviors).
- Distraction is very effective when guiding an infant's curiosity by redirecting behavior to desirable activities.
- The infant's stranger anxiety may be difficult for parents to handle. Parents may need help in establishing a separation ritual that helps the infant understand the parent is leaving but will return. They may need to express their feelings of concern or even disappointment when their infant enjoys the time away from the parent.
- Parents may have difficulty finding the energy needed to deal with busy, mobile infants and appreciate suggestions on how to cope when exhaustion occurs.
- Two-parent families may need the opportunity to discuss how to delegate and share parental roles and responsibilities.
- Parents need positive reinforcement for their continually developing skills, just as their children do.

Cognitive and Environmental Stimulation

- Playing with the child strengthens the parent-child bond and stimulates the infant's cognitive development.
- Allowing the child to take the lead in play activities is important, but parents can use play to model new activities and skills.
- Interactive games such as peek-a-boo, pat-a-cake, and rolling a ball back and forth encourage reciprocal social play. Interaction with the caregiver is still the most important activity for the infant.
- Books, music, blocks, stacking toys, container toys, and pull toys all allow self-initiated activities.
- Many 12-month-old children have a box of toys that they enjoy dumping out for play. An infant's curiosity and interest can be sustained if toys are "cycled" (some put away and brought out at a later date).
- Bath time and sandboxes provide safe opportunities to engage in messy play that most infants enjoy. Infants need this type of tactile stimulation.

- Parents need factual information regarding the physiologic and cognitive development that is necessary for toilet training. This prevents unrealistic expectations later on (see Chapter 12).

▪ Common Developmental Issues for Infants

Parents' concerns during the infant's first year of life are often related to inexperience or lack of knowledge about infant growth and development. Few infants have developmental delays. Having a "normal" baby does not make the parents' concern any less compelling, and the health care provider has a responsibility to answer parents' questions; provide essential information about development; make accurate assessments to rule out problems; treat or refer problems appropriately; and provide follow-up care and support. Some of the more common developmental issues that trouble parents are discussed in this section. When parents understand the complexity of infant growth and development, they are better able to make healthy decisions for their infants and family.

SLEEP

Should babies sleep in the same bed with their parents? How much sleep does an infant need? How can an 8-month-old be encouraged to sleep through the night? These are just a few of the questions parents may have about their infant's sleep. The answers to these and other questions will differ for each family and infant. A full discussion of children's sleep and rest patterns is found in Chapter 14. There are some general principles to help guide parents, including the following:

- The first month of life is one of transition from the warm, dark uterine environment in which the fetus lived with the rhythm of the mother's body, heartbeat, and respirations. Being in a similar environment, close to those rhythms, helps many infants relax and sleep.
- Parents must ensure a safe environment for their infant's sleep: a supine sleep position on a firm surface in a crib or bassinet, from which the infant cannot fall. Parents should consider using a sleeper or other sleep clothing as an alternative to blankets. If using a blanket, put the baby with feet at the foot of the crib. Tuck a thin blanket around the crib mattress that reaches only as far as the baby's chest. Waterbeds, pillows, bumper pads, and soft toys can suffocate and are not recommended. Co-sleeping is not recommended. Factors that increase the risk of suffocation while co-sleeping include parental obesity and parental use of alcohol, drugs, or medications that cause the parent to sleep more soundly than usual.
- Self-regulation of state is an important skill for infants to learn. Learning to put themselves to sleep and to sleep as long as they need is an important developmental task, but infants often need assistance transitioning from an awake state into sleep. As the infant matures neurologically, ease of state transition increases and self-regulation skills develop. Helping parents understand the natural consolidation of sleep states in the first year of life will help them appreciate this challenge. A consistent and predictable sleep routine, in a consistent and predictable location (for both naps and nighttime sleep), provides the infant with a foundation to establish self-regulation.

FEEDING

Exclusive breastfeeding for the first 6 months of life, and breast milk with solids from 6 to 12 months are recommended (see Chapters 10 and 11). Infant feeding concerns or problems (particularly a less than expected weight gain or decrease in weight) should be assessed through an observation of a feeding in the clinic (or at home, if resources allow). A detailed feeding history, a minimum 3-day diet history, and calorie analysis is needed. The infant's oral motor skills and general development should be assessed because early feeding issues may indicate other subtle developmental delays that can benefit from early intervention. A standardized feeding assessment, using a tool such as the NCAST Feeding Scale, provides information about the parent-child relationship and assists in the development of individualized recommendations for the parents.

CRYING

Infant crying and irritability can cause parents to worry that something is wrong. It can disrupt the family and create a strained parent-child relationship. Labeling the crying as "colic" when it occurs more than 3 hours a day, 3 times a week, and begins between 3 weeks and 3 months of age may or may not console stressed parents (see Chapter 32). It is advisable to evaluate the crying duration and intensity, what factors contribute to it, and what factors offer relief. Assessment of the infant's sleep-wake activity and amount of direct holding also provides insight into how to assist the family. Parents can use the NCAST sleep activity record to evaluate the infant's daily feeding, sleep routine, and fussiness.

Teaching parents to understand their infant's behavioral cues and communication is an important first step in resolving frequent crying. Most often, infant irritability is reduced as the infant establishes a consistent sleep-wake cycle, especially daily naps. The sleep-deprived infant is likely to become irritable and demonstrate poor feeding routines. Parents should be alert to the infant's cues of tiredness and assist their infant to transition from the wake to sleep state.

SPITTING UP

Providing appropriate care involves differentiating between normal infant "spit-up," regurgitation, reflux, and vomiting. In addition to describing the differences to parents, it helps to have them complete a 3-day diary with the frequency and events surrounding these episodes. Spitting up may be influenced by the infant's daily routine and schedule, including feeding and burping pattern and lack of a sleep routine. Incomplete feedings that result in grazing or overfeeding can contribute to spitting up. Reflux, crying and arching while feeding, and vomiting require more in-depth assessment and management and are discussed in Chapters 10 and 32.

DISCIPLINE AND BEHAVIORAL GUIDANCE

Parents may express concern that their infant does "not mind," misbehaves, or is "spoiled." The first year of life is one in which the infant needs to establish a sense of trust and attachment. Infants need to feel secure and safe, to trust that the parents and/or caregiver will meet their needs. From this base, the infant learns self-regulation and the ability to reciprocate in affectionate, mutually satisfying interactions with others. If parents struggle with behavioral or discipline concerns in the first year of life, the provider should intervene early with education about child development, what parents should expect of their infant, and how parents can most effectively respond. Time is well spent helping parents understand the needs of infants and developing an appropriate parenting style. Establishing a regular routine, especially for sleep and feeding, facilitates the infant's social and emotional growth. At times there is a mismatch in temperament between the parent and child. (See Chapter 18 for strategies to help parents of children with different temperaments.) The child's challenging behaviors or external demands on the parent can leave the parent little energy to provide the assistance the child needs.

■ Classification of Developmental Disorders in Infants

Developmental delay in infants involves disorders that manifest as motor problems (e.g., cerebral palsy), communication problems (e.g., receptive or expressive communication and behavior), or cognitive problems (e.g., problem solving, mental retardation, specific deficits in processing information). Processing disorders include peripheral problems such as deafness and blindness; central processing that results in motor, language, and perceptual dysfunction; and behavioral problems.

Although there are some limits to the history, it usually provides the best clues to the diagnosis of developmental delay. Some problems, such as fetal alcohol syndrome, uterine drug exposure, autism, and fragile X syndrome may not have clear symptoms in infancy. Early behaviors of autism, for example, are just beginning to be defined and there are beliefs that some signs of autism appear as early as 3 to 4 months (see Chapter 15) (Johnson et al, 2007). In some cases parents may not be able to recall exactly when their child achieved a particular milestone or how long the infant has demonstrated a particular behavior.

It is important to determine whether the problems are the result of neurodegeneration as opposed to a static encephalopathy. Developmental delays that appear during infancy are usually connected to dysfunctions of major organs, physiologic abnormalities, and physiologic imbalances. Thus early indications include alterations in feedings, sleep, or interactions. Later presentations include motor coordination problems, hearing and vision problems, or more severe interaction problems. Gross motor deficits are most often identified after 9 months, although parents may report concerns earlier. The *Bright Futures* Tool and Resource Kit includes resources for primary care providers, including parent/family education, and developmental, behavioral, and psychosocial assessment information.

■ Red Flags for Infants

Infant developmental problems may be difficult to identify, but the provider must be alert to "red flags" that place the infant at risk or indicate a potential problem. Providers should also listen carefully to parents' concerns about their child's development. Often it is the parent who first notices "something

TABLE 5-3   Developmental Red Flags: Newborns and Infants

Age	Physical Development (Autonomic Stability, Regulation, Sleep, Temperament)	Gross Motor (Strength, Coordination)	Fine Motor (Feeding, Self-Care)	Language and Hearing	Psychosocial and Emotional Skills	Cognitive and Visual Abilities
Newborn to 1 mo	Lack of return to birthweight by 2-wk examination; Poor coordination of suck-swallow; Tachypnea or bradycardia with feedings; Poor habituation to external stimuli	Asymmetrical movements; Hypertonia or hypotonia; Asymmetrical primitive reflexes	Hands held fisted; Absent or asymmetrical palmar grasp	No startle to sound or sudden noises; No quieting to voice; High-pitched cry	Diffuse nonverbal cues; Poor state transitions; Irritable	Doll's eyes; No red light reflex; Poor alert state
3 mo	Poor weight gain; less than 1 lb (0.5 kg) weight gain in 1 mo; Head circumference increasing greater than 2 standard deviations on growth curve or showing no increase in size; Continuing problems with poor suck-swallow; Difficulty with regulation of sleep-wake cycle; Fussy baby	Asymmetrical movements; Hypertonia or hypotonia; No attempt to raise head on stomach	Hands fisted with oppositional thumb; No hand-to-mouth activity; Feedings taking longer than 45 min; Consistently awakening hourly for feeding	Does not turn to voice, rattle, or bell; No sounds, coos, squeals	Lack of social smile; Withdrawn or depressed; Lack of consistent, safe childcare; Lack of eye-eye contact	No visual tracking; Not able to fix on face or object
6 mo	Less than double birthweight; Head circumference shows no increase; Continuation of poor feeding or sleep regulation; Difficulty with self-calming	Persistent primitive reflexes; Does not attempt to sit with support; Head lag with pull to sit; Scissoring	Does not reach for objects, hold rattle, hold hands together; Does not grasp at clothes	No babbling; Does not respond to voice, bell, rattle, or loud noises even with startle	No smiles; No response to play; Solemn appearance; Lack of eye-eye contact	Not visually alert; Does not reach for objects; Does not look at caregiver
9 mo	Parent control issues with feeding or sleep; Night awakening that persists; Offered bottle in bed for sleep; Difficulty with self-calming, self-regulation	Does not sit even in tripod position; No lateral prop reflex; Asymmetrical crawl, handedness, or other movements	No self-feeding; No high chair sitting; No solids; Does not pick up toy with one hand	Lack of single- or double-consonant sounds; Lack of response to name or voice; Does not respond to any words; Lack of reciprocal vocalizations	Intense stranger anxiety or absent stranger anxiety; Does not seek comfort from caregiver with stress; Poor eye-eye contact	Lack of visual awareness; Lack of reaching out for toys; Lack of toy exploration visually or orally
12 mo	Less than triple birthweight; Losing more than 2 standard deviations on growth curve for weight, length, or head circumference; Poor sleep-wake cycle; Extreme inability to separate from parent	Not pulling self to stand; Not moving around the environment to explore	Persistent mouthing; Not attempting to feed self or hold cup; Not able to hold toy in each hand or transfer objects	Inability to localize to sound; Not imitating speech sounds; Not using two or three words; Does not point, or uses only gestures or pointing	No response to game playing; No response to reading or interactive activities; Withdrawn or solemn; Poor eye-eye contact	Not visually following activities in the environment

Mo, month(s); *wk*, week(s); *min*, minute(s).

is not quite right," without knowing what the problem might be. Potential problems need closer developmental surveillance and more frequent developmental and social-emotional screening, and often require referral to developmental centers for more in-depth assessments. As the well-child history is taken, specific risk factors for development delays can be identified, including the following:

- Prenatal exposure to street drugs or alcohol
- Prematurity
- Low birthweight, SGA, intrauterine growth retardation
- Anoxia or birth trauma
- Neonatal intensive care and long-term hospitalization
- Cardiovascular illnesses
- Endocrine and metabolic problems
- Genetic syndromes
- Failure to thrive
- Cerebral palsy
- Sensory problems
- Parental or environmental deficit in meeting the infant's needs (e.g., alcohol or drug abuse by parent; parental depression)

Table 5-3 outlines developmental findings that are indications for referral to a child development center, a state's early child development identification program, or a child development specialist. When clear indicators are present, referral should be made rather than waiting some months to validate observations. If autism is suspected, referral to a behavioral/developmental specialist is most appropriate.

Some primary care practices have providers with expertise in minor developmental problems. These professionals, in consultation with a specialist, may take an initial "wait-and-see" approach. They can also provide more in-depth expertise in developmental, sleep, feeding, behavioral assessments, and parenting issues. They may also conduct ongoing assessments as the infant grows and help parents implement interventions to foster healthy development. If the infant needs referral, primary health care providers work with the parents to connect them to community resources, advocate for necessary services, and continue to provide the infant with long-term primary care.

Developmental Management of Toddlers and Preschoolers

MARY A. MURPHY AND ANITA D. BERRY

Developmental changes in the second through fifth years of life are subtler than those seen in the first year, yet they are highly significant. Children enter toddlerhood as babies, dependent on parents and caregivers for their survival and leave as accomplished children with elaborate and sophisticated skills. Ready to enter the social world of school and community, 5-year-olds have a sense of self that shapes the quality of their character as older children, adolescents, and adults. Children begin this change process by refining abilities acquired in the first year, learning, for example, to walk smoothly with control and speed, to run and climb, and to combine words into phrases and sentences. They add to their repertoire of skills, growing stronger, bigger, and more socially, emotionally, and intellectually capable. This chapter reviews some of the many changes that occur for toddlers (usually defined as a child 12 to 24 months old) and preschoolers (a child 2 to 5 years old), and describes the primary health care provider's role when working with these children and their families.

■ Development of Toddlers and Preschoolers

PHYSICAL DEVELOPMENT

Physical and physiologic changes in toddlers and preschoolers continue at a much slower pace than in the first year of life. Statistically, children gain weight faster and earlier than children in earlier decades (Trifiletti et al, 2006); however, growth charts continue to show the average 2-year-old weighs 26 to 28 pounds (12.5 to 13.5 kg), with boys being slightly heavier than girls, and is 34 to 35 inches (85 to 90 cm) tall. Head circumference in the average 2-year-old is 19 to 19.5 inches (48 to 50 cm). Although most toddlers have no palpable fontanelles by 12 months, the anterior fontanelle should completely close by 18 to 19 months. During the fourth and fifth years, skeletal growth continues as additional ossification centers appear in the wrist and ankle and additional epiphyses develop in some

of the long bones. For the 4- to 5-year-old, the legs grow faster than the head, trunk, or upper extremities. Changes related to body systems are highlighted in Table 6-1. More detailed discussion of development, systems, and disease processes can be found in Units 3 and 4 of this text.

MOTOR DEVELOPMENT

Motor development is divided into two components—gross and fine. Gross motor refers to the development and use of the large muscles. Fine motor includes hand and finger development and oral-motor development (see Table 5-1 for a review of gross and fine motor milestones by age).

Use of the dominant hand may appear as early as 8 to 12 months but generally emerges between 2 and 4 years. There are some children, however, who do not show a hand preference until 5 to 6 years old. The 4-year-old can thread small beads on a chain; grasp a pencil appropriately to copy some letters (v, h, t, o); draw a person with head and features, legs, trunk, and arms; use scissors to cut on a line; fasten buttons; and eat with a fork. By 5 years these movements expand to copying a square and additional letters (x, l, a, c, u, y), writing some letters spontaneously, producing identifiable pictures, counting fingers on one hand, and using all eating utensils appropriately.

Two-year-olds may still be "toddling," using their arms for balance and frequently falling as they try to run or move quickly. They begin to master climbing and by 3 to 4 years are walking smoothly. The following are gross motor behaviors that average toddlers and preschoolers demonstrate:

2-year-old
○ Tosses or rolls large ball
○ Walks up stairs with help (may or may not alternate feet)
○ Walks with control

3-year-old
○ Jumps with both feet
○ Climbs stairs with alternate feet both up and down to any height, up ladders

TABLE 6-1	Physical Development of Toddlers and Preschool-Age Children
Body System	**Developmental Changes**
Dental	By 12 mo, the child usually has 6 to 8 primary teeth. By 2 yr, the child has a complete set of 20 primary teeth. By 3 yr, the second molars usually erupt. During the second year, calcification begins for the first and second permanent bicuspids and second molars. Most growth and calcification of the permanent teeth occur within the gums; it is not visible.
Neurologic	Continued myelinization and cortical development occurs. Fine motor movements are more detailed and sustained: • 2-year-olds can easily manipulate fingers to stack 4 blocks. • 3-year-olds can create a tower of 8 or more blocks. • 4-year-olds can easily build a 12-block step design. • 5-year-olds can grasp a pencil appropriately to copy simple geometric designs accurately and write their name in block letters. Gross motor skills are smoother and more coordinated. Sensory function is more mature. Visual acuity is 20/70 for 2-year-olds; 20/30 for 5- to 6-year-olds.
Cardiovascular	Little change occurs in the second and third year. By the fifth year, the heart has quadrupled in size since birth. By 5 years, the heart rate is typically 70 to 110 bpm. Normal sinus arrhythmia may continue, and innocent murmurs are common. The hematologic system should produce only adult hemoglobin by the fifth year. The hemoglobin level stabilizes at 12 to 15 g/dL.
Pulmonary	Abdominal respiratory movements continue until the end of the fifth or sixth year. Respiratory rate slows to about 30 breaths per minute.
Gastrointestinal	By 2 years, the salivary glands reach adult size. The stomach becomes more bowed and increases its capacity to about 500 mL. Many children still require a nutritious snack between meals because of small stomach size. During the second year, the liver matures and becomes more efficient in vitamin storage, glycogenesis, amino acid changes, and ketone body formation. The lower edge of the liver may still be palpable. By 4 to 5 years, the gastrointestinal system is mature enough for the child to eat a full range of foods. Stools are more like those of adults.
Renal	Kidneys begin descending deeper into the pelvic area and grow in size. Ureters remain short and relatively straight. A 2-year-old may excrete as much as 500 to 600 mL of urine a day. A 4- to 5-year-old excretes between 600 and 750 mL daily.
Endocrine	Quiescent time for sexual growth, with few physical or hormonal changes. Growth hormone stimulates body growth.

bpm, Beats per minute.

   ○ Rides a tricycle using the pedals to move from place to place
   ○ Kicks ball forward
4-year-old
   ○ Tries to skip using alternate feet
   ○ Catches a bouncing ball
   ○ Runs around corners lightly on toes and stops voluntarily

COMMUNICATION AND LANGUAGE DEVELOPMENT

Language uses symbols for thoughts; thus it emerges with Piaget's preoperational stage of development. Beginning around 2 years old, toddlers use words to convey their thoughts and feelings. Once the process begins, it develops rapidly. Cognitive development is a basic requirement for language development because the child must decipher the rules of language independently, problem solve to understand the communication of others, and create symbols that reflect his or her ideas and emotions and can be understood by others. Language development requires mastery of the following:
• Oral-motor ability to articulate sounds
• Auditory perception to distinguish words and sentences
• Cognitive ability to understand syntax, semantics, and pragmatics
• Psychosocial-cultural environment to motivate the child to engage in language use

Language milestones are evident in two general categories—receptive and expressive language. These are presented for infants and children younger than 5 years old in Table 5-2.

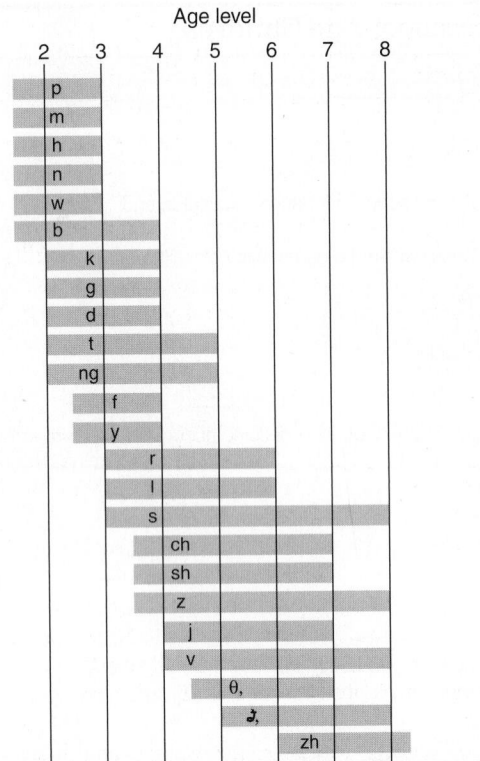

Age level

FIGURE 6-1 Norms for development of speech sounds. θ, *th* as in *thin*; ʒ, as in *this*. (From Van Riper C, Erickson RL: *Speech correction: an introduction to speech pathology and audiology,* ed 9, Needham Heights, MA, 1996, Allyn & Bacon, p 98. Reprinted by permission.)

Articulation

Young children practice articulation skills daily, and by 24 months speech sounds are 25% intelligible to a stranger. The intelligibility rate jumps to about 66% between 24 and 36 months, with 90% intelligibility by 3 years old. By 4 years, speech should be completely intelligible with the exception of particularly difficult consonants. By 5 years the tongue-contact sounds of "n," "t," "d," "k," "g," "y," and "ng" are more intelligible. Some sounds, such as the "zh" sound, are not added until the child is 6 to 8 years old. Figure 6-1 identifies sounds articulated by children at specific ages.

During the second year the child practices playful changes in pitch and loudness. Three- and 4-year-olds show normal hesitance in speech or stuttering. They "stutter" by repeating words, especially those at the start of a sentence, or when excited such as when they want to convey an important message (e.g., "Mommy, I…Mommy, I…Mommy, I want to tell you I hear the ice cream truck"). This normal speech variant does not include syllable repetition or cause undue stress for the child. These dysfluencies should pass if ignored; they can be considered abnormal if they occur in 5-year-olds or if they involve syllable repetition instead of word repetition.

Children usually progress through a regular sequence of mispronunciations as they learn new articulation skills. At first they simply omit the new sound, and then they try to substitute a more familiar sound for the new one (e.g., the "w" for "r" substitution, as in "wabbit" for "rabbit"). Distortion is followed by "addition" as the child adds an extra sound (e.g., "gulad" for "glad"). Knowing each of these steps allows the

examiner to assure the parent that the child is developing normally or needs monitoring.

Lexicon

Lexicon refers to vocabulary. Vocabulary size is influenced by many factors, including environment, stimulation, intelligence, multilingualism, culture, and personality. Children usually understand more words than they are able to express, and addition of words to their expressive vocabulary comes with continued practice. Girls typically say their first word between 8 and 11 months, boys about 14 months. Most 2-year-olds have more than 200 words in their vocabulary, and most 4- to 5-year-olds add approximately 50 words a month to their vocabulary. Five-year-olds should be able to define some words with other words (e.g., "cup" is "you drink with it," or "chair" is "to sit on").

Syntax

Syntax, or grammar, refers to the structure of words in sentences or phrases. The ability to construct sentences that convey meaning is a complex skill, proceeding through several stages in children: receptive, holophrastic, and telegraphic speech. Much of this skill is developed between 8 months and 3.5 years. By 8 months children develop receptive language (i.e., they understand others who use a new word or structure before they are able to use it themselves). When asked "Where is the ball?" an 8-month-old searches for the ball. Between 12 and 18 months, children begin to use holophrases or single words to express whole ideas. The child says "milk," perhaps to mean the whole sentence, "Give me a glass of milk." A complex idea is expressed in one succinct word. Holophrastic sentences are denominative (labeling) or imperative (commanding).

Around 18 months children begin using telegraphic speech, phrases that have many words omitted and sound like a telegram, to convey their message (e.g., "get milk," "go bye-bye"). At around 2 years of age, children begin to expand their vocabulary and to form short sentences like "my big ball" and "the yummy cookie." This is the age when toddlers begin to mimic phrases and gestures used by caregivers like "Oh, my goodness." Sentence structure becomes more complex as children move from active sentences, to questions, to passive and negative construction, and then add plurals (at 3 years old) and past tenses (at 4 years old) to their grammar. Three- or four-word sentences should be evident by 3 years, and by 5 years old, the child's syntax is close to adult style, including use of future tense and complete sentences of five or six words in length.

Semantics

Semantic development, the understanding that words have specific meaning and the child's use of words to convey specific meaning, is an ongoing process extending into adulthood. This development occurs in stages from global to more specific and requires interaction through conversation, listening, and reading. Words used in any language have both denotative (the specific, concrete referent of the word) and connotative (a broader range of feelings aroused by the word) meanings. Even though children may be quite adept at using words correctly, they may have only a vague, diffuse connotative understanding of these words. For example, the 3-year-old who drops a toy and uses an expletive she heard when her father dropped a dish does not understand the connotative meaning of what she has said. As language progresses from simple to more complex, meaning and cognitive understanding evolve.

Bilingualism

Raising children to be bilingual can help preserve the family culture and heritage, and studies suggest that fluent bilingual children have greater mental flexibility and enhanced employment and lifestyle opportunities. Initially, normal toddlers from bilingual homes show mild delays in initial spoken words and mixing of the words and phrases from the two languages. Children who associate a clear environmental context for each language (e.g., home is Spanish, and school is English) may progress faster in acquiring both languages (Feldman, 2005). Maintaining bilingualism should be encouraged, but it requires time and effort as the child learns to read and write to maintain fluency in both. For families anxious to integrate culturally in a society with a different language, emphasizing skill in the language of the new community may be viewed as a first priority.

Simultaneous bilingualism occurs when children hear and learn two languages from infancy. These bilingual children should be equally competent in both languages by 3 years old. Sequential bilingualism occurs when the child, usually 3 years or older, learns one language and then is immersed in another. Children learning sequentially may have more apparent differences in their skills from language to language until they have developed proficiency in both.

Bilingual preschoolers experience no delays in vocabulary development and are proficient in sorting one language from the other, although they may "code switch" to the other language for clarity as they talk. They switch languages depending on the person with whom they are speaking and the circumstances. Some even translate for others, seeming to understand that not everyone speaks or understands both languages. Ultimately, whether a second, third, or even more languages are learned simultaneously or sequentially, most children have one dominant language. Bilingual children with significant vocabulary delays require the same evaluation as delayed monolingual children.

SOCIAL AND EMOTIONAL DEVELOPMENT

Psychosocial changes in toddlers and preschoolers are remarkable. Emotions and cognition are interconnected so that assessment of any one area of development is somewhat arbitrary. Toddlers spend most of their time up, running about, verbalizing, and demanding to join in family activities. These are years of intense learning about and managing feelings such as love, happiness, anger, frustration, aggression, and jealousy, and social skills such as sharing, giving, and receiving affection. They learn the words that go with their feelings and, with guidance, the appropriate behaviors. A major developmental milestone for this age is the achievement of a sense of independence and autonomy. The road from depending on parents for everything to doing some things for themselves, however, can be rocky and uneven.

The toddler and preschooler's ability to achieve independence is influenced, in part, by the strengths in their social environment. In particular, maternal depression (chronic and postpartum) has a significantly negative effect on the development of normal infant engagement behaviors that can persist into the toddler and preschool years. Based on the child's emerging sense of identity, maternal depression can lead to social, emotional, and language concerns (Pascoe et al, 2006). Specifically, research indicates that young children whose mothers have depression are significantly more likely to have emotional dysregulation at age 4 years and altered perceived competence at age 5 (Maughan et al, 2007).

Toddlers need a great deal of love, warmth, and comfort, primarily from their parents and caregivers. Toddlers learn to give love and find satisfaction in pleasing their parents. They learn to respond to kisses, hugs, and cuddles they have received by giving kisses, hugs, and cuddles in return. Toddlers who make these early attempts at giving love and are rejected or ignored soon stop trying and begin to find pleasure elsewhere. Toddlers with sensory issues learn to avoid some gestures unless they are in control and decide they can handle the tactile or sensory feelings. Some toddlers find that thumb sucking, rhythmic body movements, and body manipulation are more pleasurable and reliable than person-to-person contacts.

Preschoolers develop more sophisticated ideas about feeling, giving, and sharing. The 4- to 5-year-old moves away from the extremely self-centered attitude of earlier toddlerhood. Parents are viewed as the epitome of wisdom, power, integrity, and goodness. If early stages of the love relationship are not satisfied, preschoolers show more fears, inhibitions, explosive behavior, and demands for attention.

Toddlers and preschool-age children gradually increase their ability to follow commands consistently as they work to gain and maintain approval of adults and to behave as "good" children are expected to do. By preschool years, children begin to show interest in table manners, being polite, saying "thank you" without a reminder, sharing, saying (and meaning) "I'm sorry," and taking turns. These social skills are learned through daily interactions at home, school, and church, from parents, peers, relatives, and neighbors. Children learn to read social cues of others' behavior (e.g., the voice tone, slight facial expression, posture) and correct their own behavior. Some children, frequently boys, find these cues vague and difficult to learn, and parents can help by modeling, explaining, and discussing them.

Children at this age vacillate between being a big boy or big girl and a mommy's baby. They take great pride in doing as many things as possible for themselves, yet they need to feel totally secure in their parents' care. On some days, toddlers cling to Mother's skirt, not letting her out of sight; on other days, the child can play for short periods in the next room, trotting back every so often to see, touch, and hear the mother and be reassured by her presence. The child who is securely attached uses the parent as a secure base from which to go out and safely explore the world. Gradually the periods of separation lengthen, and the child needs only to hear the mother's voice or to check occasionally for security. Separation anxiety is frequent during these years and can be traumatic for both parents and child.

Preschool children are much less dependent on their parents and frequently tolerate physical separation for several hours. As this sense of separateness increases, children are more aware that they are different from their surroundings, their families, and their friends. They begin to realize that other persons also have feelings, fears, and doubts. Peer dependence and learning about how to have and be friends begin to be important.

Toddlers like to have a choice in matters and quickly learn the power of the word "no." They can become extremely negative, practicing the power of "no" every day for months. As toddlers practice making choices, they are clumsy, awkward, and frequently wrong. This can be very frustrating for them, and their outraged responses can be equally annoying for their parents. Toddlers discover the delights of control over others and themselves. This increases their sense of power but can also lead to misunderstandings and hurt feelings if their parents do not read their moods properly. With time they become more skilled, make better choices, have more successes, and feel more powerful. They no longer have to work so hard to show others their power, and the negative stage passes.

Preschool-age children are more verbal than toddlers and are able to perform many more self-care tasks (e.g., feed themselves using appropriate utensils, blow their own noses, and go to the bathroom unassisted). Interactions become easier and more enjoyable as the child learns to verbally express needs and feelings.

Sibling Interaction

Interaction patterns between siblings vary and are affected by factors such as opposite gender, temperament, insecure attachment, family discord, corporal punishment, and perceptions of unequal treatment. Many toddlers or preschoolers regress when a new baby arrives, whereas older children may experience excitement, love, and enhanced self-esteem with a new sibling. Parents need to promptly limit any aggression expressed by the older child, provide love and attention, and talk about feelings. When older children fight, parents need to describe the situation and provide even-handed control. Blaming a child, except in a clear-cut instance of misbehavior, is usually unproductive. Promoting support, loyalty, and friendship is important for sibling interactions (see Chapter 17).

Morality

Morality, or the ability to know right from wrong, is based on external control during the toddler years and stems from children's love of their parents and a desire to please them. Parent teaching generally focuses more on helping the child to make safe decisions rather than moral ones. Toddlers cannot be expected to make correct choices if left alone in potentially dangerous situations because their internal sense of conscience is rudimentary and judgment is absent. Any room with electrical sockets, knobs for technical equipment, open windows, or hot food represents a risk. As toddlers gain language skills, they begin to echo the parent's firm "no," but they do not understand the full meaning of the term. By 24 months many toddlers show beginning internalization by saying "no" to themselves and stopping the act; they may continue with the act as they talk to themselves, still saying "no."

Preschoolers form a foundation for their moral development as they develop socioemotionally and cognitively. For the 4- to 5-year-old, morality is more internally controlled.

Instead of basing all decisions on the knowledge of the consequences of the act (e.g., "If I take a cookie, I will be sent to my room"), older children show an elementary understanding of what is right and wrong, fair or unfair. They recognize others' needs and may express a desire to help or comfort others. They begin to think ahead and are able to plan and control their urges, thus avoiding punishment. Four-year-olds can internalize some demands from their parents, and feelings of guilt can be elicited after some transgressions.

Peer Relationships

Toddlers may be fascinated by children their own age and demonstrate curiosity by physically examining the other child closely, poking and probing. However, they generally do not engage with their peers in an interactive way. Play is an essential component of cognitive, physical, emotional, and social development (Ginsburg and American Academy of Pediatrics [AAP], 2007). Parallel play is the norm. Preschoolers learn to interact with peers as their social world grows. Play is the major mechanism through which toddlers and preschoolers practice gender roles, such as housekeeping, caring for baby dolls, "fixing" household items, and caring for the garden and yard. As symbolic language develops, play becomes more interactive, cooperative, and shared. Imaginary play leads to "let's pretend," role-playing, and creation of imaginary friends. Fantasy and make-believe are very important during these years. Children need both structured and free play. Children today spend less time playing outside than previous generations and they are more likely to play in their yard than any other location. Research indicates that children have greater free play time when parents perceive their neighborhoods to be safe, when parents have social relationships within their neighborhoods, and when playgrounds are close (Veitch et al, 2010).

Shared or cooperative play makes simple games of hide-and-seek and tag possible. Games with complicated rules can be frustrating to the preschooler, who prefers simple games with the option of making up the rules as the game proceeds. Cheating is common because the boundaries of acceptable play are not yet clear, and the earliest stages of moral behavior are only beginning to emerge.

Body Image

Toddlers are often highly concerned about body image. They realize that they are separate persons and begin to take notice of their own bodies. They may become fascinated with the different parts of the body and how they work. Bodily injury becomes a concern, and cuts and bruises elicit much discussion. Toward the end of the second year, children may notice the inner feelings of their bodies (e.g., the urge and tension to move the bowels, the release and relaxation resulting from going to the bathroom, the discomfort of hunger, and the pleasure of eating). These are abstract feelings that toddlers cannot put into words but can show with actions.

Preschoolers are equally curious about their bodies but are more capable of understanding and expressing themselves. They reexamine themselves frequently, and worries over a lost tooth or a skinned knee are common. Curiosity about their bodies and those of others generates a wealth of innocent questions that generally require only a simple answer. They learn that genital manipulation brings pleasure, and masturbation peaks around 3 to 4 years.

COGNITIVE DEVELOPMENT

Cognitively, toddler thinking is highly concrete. According to Piaget (see Table 4-1), 18- to 24-month-old children use mental imagery and infer causality when they can see only the effect. By the end of the second year children enter the preoperational stage with preconceptual and intuitive thinking. Primitive conceptualization processes begin with the development of symbolic thinking. A block becomes a car; words become symbols for ideas. The 3-year-old continues to develop symbolic thinking, and this manifests through drawing and acting out elaborate play scenarios. However, children at this age generally are unable to take another's perspective but continue to view the world egocentrically. Attending to one characteristic at a time is another feature of preschool thinking. For example, the child will try to fit a jigsaw puzzle piece using either color or shape but not both.

Parents may have difficulty understanding the thoughts of preschool children. On the surface preoperational thinking has many characteristics that resemble adult thinking, and parents are often deceived into believing that children are able to think as adults do. Preschool children, for example, are developing the use of language and the ability to symbolize concepts mentally. Some of their verbalizations appear quite precocious, as evidenced by the 3-year-old who stares out the window and then states, "Look, mommy, the trees are saying yes and no." Preschool children continue to be concrete and egocentric in their thinking, and their logic is the source of many communication problems between parents and children. Table 6-2 identifies major characteristic of preschool thinking and gives examples of each.

Language development through the toddler and preschool years remains one of the most sensitive indicators of cognitive development, and assessment tools plot language ability as a way of measuring cognitive levels. Social development and adaptive skills are a major factor during this development. Differentiation of the self from others, with increasing

TABLE 6-2 Examples of Preschool Children's Thinking Using Piaget's Preoperational Stage	
Characteristic	**Example**
Egocentricism	"It's snowing so I can go play in it."
Unable see another's viewpoint	If John is holding a doll with its face toward Ann, Ann thinks John can also see the doll's face.
Mental symbolization of the environment	"The wind is crying." "The (flushing) toilet is an angry animal."
Incomplete understanding of sequence of time	Knows names of time components: today, tomorrow, yesterday, minutes, days, weeks, etc., but uses them inconsistently: "I'm not going to take a nap yesterday." Yesterday means any time before now; tomorrow means any time in the future. Historical events are conceptualized in terms of the present: "Mommy, do you know George Washington?"
Developing sense of space: from experiencing space as a part of their activity to moving through it to understanding space in terms of detail and direction	Frequently used words: *in, on, up, down, at, under.*
Evolving ability to categorize or order objects and phenomena	Early preschooler: no understanding of concept of class or groups; undisturbed to see new Santa Claus on every corner. Cluster phenomena: when asked to sort a series of blocks, the child may cluster a small, medium, and large block as a "baby," "mommy," and "daddy" block. By 4-5 years, child is able to consistently use 1 or 2 categories to arrange objects in some order (color, number, form, or size).
Developing ability to establish causality (realism, animism, artificialism)	*Realism:* Intellectual (dreams are actually real) and nominal (a horse can only be called a horse, not, for example, a stallion or filly). *Animism:* 2- to 3-year-olds think objects possess innate person-like qualities that cause results: "The chair made me fall down." *Artificialism:* 3- to 4-year-olds think things are caused by some controlling force that controls the world.
Transductive reasoning: from particular to particular	If the child does not like one particular vegetable, he or she will not like another particular fruit: "I can't eat my banana because my potatoes are burned."
Developing sense of conservation of quantity, weight, mass	Preschooler is usually unable to conceptualize that change in shape does not affect quantity, weight, or mass of an object. Generally, 50% of 5-year-olds have mastered conservation of quantity, and 50% of 6-year-olds have mastered conservation of weight or mass.
Rigidity	Generally, children in the preoperational stage are very rigid in their thinking.

TABLE 6-3	Screening Tools for Toddler and Preschoolers	
Screening Tool	**Appropriate Age; Screening Time**	**Characteristics**
ASQ-3: Ages & Stages Questionnaire 3: A parent completed child-monitoring system	2-60 mo; 10-20 min or less	32 individual questions FM, GM, communication, personal-social, and problem solving
ASQ: Ages & Stages Questionnaire: Social-Emotional (ASQ:SE)	3-60 mo; 10-20 min or less	32 individual questions social and emotional
BDI: Battelle Developmental Inventory screening test (BDI-2)	0-8 yr; 10-30 min; complete test 1-2 hr	100 standardized items, personal and social, adaptive, motor communication, cognitive
CDI: Child Development Inventory	15 mo-6 yr; 10-20 min	Questions: social, self-help, GM, FM, expressive language, language comprehension, letters, and numbers
DASE: Denver Articulation Screening Examination	2.5-7 yr; 5 min	30 repeated words
ESI-R: Early Screening Inventory Revised	3-6 yr; 15-20 min	Standardized items motor, language, and cognition; parent interview about self-help skills, social-emotional
HSQ: Home Screening Questionnaire	0-3 and 3-6 yr; 15-20 min	Parent questionnaire, 80 questions on environment
MAP: Miller Assessment for Preschoolers	2.9-5.8 yr; 20-30 min	Screens for preschool readiness for kindergarten: motor, language, sequencing, memory, visuospatial perception
PEDS: Parent's Evaluation of Developmental Status	Birth-8 yr; 2 min	Parent interview with open-ended questions
PDQ-II: Prescreening Developmental Questionnaire	0-9 mo, 9-24 mo, 2-4 yr, 4-6 yr; 5-10 min	Parent questionnaire, FM, GM, social, language
TABS: Temperament and Atypical Behavior Scale	Birth-6 yr; 15-20 min	Parent interview, 55 questions on detached, hypersensitive and hyperactive, underreactive, dysregulated behaviors
SSP: Short Sensory Profile	Birth-adult; 15-20 min	Parental questions in seven areas: tactile sensitive, taste-smell sensitivity, movement, underresponsive, auditory filtering, low energy and weakness, visual and auditory

FM, Fine motor; *GM,* gross motor.

sensitivity not only to the rules and norms for social interaction but also to the perception of the perspectives and feelings of others, requires ever increasing cognitive capability. Finally, play quality is an indicator of cognitive development. Through play, children manipulate and learn to control their environment in safe, yet stimulating ways.

■ Developmental Assessment of Toddlers and Preschoolers

Developmental assessment is an essential part of each health maintenance visit and includes both screening and diagnostic testing. Its goal is to monitor the child's growth and development and to determine at an early stage if problems exist. The process begins by building rapport with the parents, encouraging them to share developmental concerns, and listening to their comments with care and attention. Data are collected through parent interviews, screening tools, observation of the interactions between the child and parents, physical examination, and laboratory or other diagnostic measures. If there are questions about the child's development, a thorough diagnostic assessment is needed to determine the degree of developmental delay and to identify management priorities.

SCREENING STRATEGIES FOR TODDLERS AND PRESCHOOLERS

Toddlers and preschoolers need screening for physical and motor skills, communication and language, and social, emotional, and cognitive development. This can be done at well-child visits and at visits for episodic illnesses. Validated screening tools provide a quick, inexpensive method of identifying potential delays or concerns. These tools are generally appropriate for all children, although culture and experience can affect outcomes and must be taken into consideration. Parents can complete a screening tool in the waiting room or providers can directly ask the parent questions. Providers should make sure they understand the parents' responses and follow up with more probing questions to clarify any concerns. Table 6-3 lists a variety of developmental screening tools. Tables 6-4, 6-5, 6-6, and 6-7 list questions that can be used to assess behavior and include the purpose or rationale for these questions.

Physical Development

Annually, toddlers and preschool children need anthropometric measurement including, after 3 years old, blood pressure. Hearing and vision assessment is recommended at ages 4 and 5 years (Hagan et al, 2008). The AAP advocates for regular

TABLE 6-4	Assessment of Physical Development and Motor Skills: Questions and Rationales
Question	**Rationale for Question**
Tell me about your child's health.	Invites discussion of somatic issues and complaints.
Does your child appear to be developing in a way similar to other children of the same age?	Assesses parent perceptions of physical development; developmental milestones.
Describe your child's elimination patterns.	Provides parents' framework for systematically assessing child; can be especially helpful for children with a chronic illness.
Has any illness interfered with your child's daily activities?	Assesses possible chronic medical problem and effects on development.
Tell me about your child's daily habits: toilet training, sleeping, eating.	Assesses parent understanding of readiness, child's cues, changing behaviors, and current status.
How does your child get from place to place?	Assesses gross motor skills (e.g., walks, climbs, runs, pedals tricycle).
How does your child feed himself or herself (e.g., cup, bottle, utensils)?	Assesses fine motor skills.
Tell me about your child's play activities.	Assesses gross and fine motor skills.

TABLE 6-5	Assessment of Communication and Speech Development: Questions and Rationales
Question	**Rationale for Question**
How does your child communicate needs and desires?	Assesses verbal and nonverbal communication strategies, vocabulary, and expressive language.
What do you think your child understands?	Evaluates cognitive level and receptive language.
How does your child respond to simple commands? To two- or three-step commands?	Evaluates receptive language; evaluates short-term memory and auditory sequencing.
Does your child use plurals, pronouns, phrases, and sentences?	Indicates increased understanding of more complex structures.
How well can you understand your child's speech? How well can others?	Indicates increased articulation ability.

dental home visits after 1 year of age and routine primary care evaluation for dental caries (AAP, 2003 [reaffirmed 2009]).

Motor Skills Development

Toddlers and preschoolers continue to develop and refine their motor skills, driven by curiosity, desire for independence, and endless energy. Gross and fine motor skills are best assessed using standardized screening tools, such as the Ages & Stages Questionnaire (ASQ), or by asking parents about the child's development.

Fine motor development is evaluated by assessing finger, hand, and oral movements. Gross motor skills are evaluated by assessing the child's ability to crawl, sit, walk, run, hop, skip, and climb. The quality of the child's movements during these activities is important to note as well.

Communication and Language Development

Communication is a vital part of being a happy, functioning human being, and language assessment is important during early childhood. A careful history of the child's abilities and pattern of learning (e.g., when did the child first articulate words?) provides much of the essential information. Physical examination helps to determine if physical structures necessary for speech are intact (e.g., a cleft uvula may indicate an occult cleft palate that could interfere with the child's ability to shape words). Finally, diagnostic testing, using tools such as the Early Language Milestone (ELM) test or the Denver Articulation Screening Exam (DASE) may be necessary to refine the assessment (Table 6-8). Listening to children and talking with their parents is essential, but the provider should also remember that parents may not be fully sensitive to speech problems because they are accustomed to hearing the child's current speech.

Language screening is divided into expressive and receptive language skills (see Table 5-2). Because language and cognitive skills are intricately interwoven, most intelligence tests have language sections that can be useful in assessing the total child. Expressive language screening places emphasis on articulation and vocabulary. Receptive language looks at comprehension, repetition, and follow-up of language heard (e.g., child's ability to follow directions).

Social and Emotional Development

Assessment of psychosocial and emotional development addresses children's roles in the family, success in making friends and working with peers, self-esteem, and feelings of contentment and security. The social emotional section of the ASQ assesses these behaviors but a more complete screening can be done by using the specific ASQ: Social-Emotional (ASQ:SE).

Cognitive Development

After 2 years old, as thinking moves into the preconceptual stages, cognitive development is increasingly expressed through symbol systems and language. Toddlers begin to

TABLE 6-6 Assessment of Psychosocial and Emotional Development: Questions and Rationales

Question	Rationale for Question
Is your child able to feed, dress, and take care of his or her own toileting?	Assesses adaptive skills, comfort with own abilities.
How does your child behave within the family and with other family members?	Assesses child's development of roles within the family system; attachment should be evident.
How do you guide or discipline your child without always saying "no"?	Evaluates adaptability, creativity, repertoire of parent's skills in response to child's behaviors.
How does your child respond when you set limits?	Assesses child's understanding of limits of appropriate behavior, social rules, and self-control.
How does your child react to strangers or new situations?	Evaluates child's ability to deal with increasingly complex social situations.
Tell me about any tantrums your child has. What causes them? How does he or she behave? How do you respond?	Evaluates responses to stress, development of independence, and social control.
What does your child do for play?	Indicates social and emotional well-being.
How does your child behave around other children?	Considers social development with peers and development of appropriate play.
What is your child's best friend's name? Does he or she have shared activities with peers?	Indicates child is developing a social circle and increasing opportunities for practicing new social skills.
Does your child seem to understand the feelings of others?	Assesses empathy.
Is your child afraid of anything in particular? How do you handle that fear?	Evaluates parents' responses to child's emotional stresses and understanding of child's view and feelings.
Does your child have imaginary friends? Does she or he have a fantasy play time?	Allows child to explore emotions and developing roles in a safe way.

TABLE 6-7 Assessment of Cognitive Development: Questions and Rationales

Questions Asked of 1- to 3-Year-Olds	Rationale for Questions
Tell me about a typical day. What sorts of things does your child do? Who does she or he play with? (ask of parent)	Assesses complexity of manipulation of objects, parallel and cooperative play, role-playing.
What is your name? Are you a boy or girl? How old are you? (ask of child)	Three-year-olds should know beginning facts.
Can your child follow simple instructions? (ask of parent)	Assesses ability to retain and process instructions and respond to input.
Does your child speak clearly? How much do you understand when your child speaks to you? Can your child understand what you say to him or her?	Assesses progress in decoding, encoding, and using a language system effectively.
How does your child behave in the family and with other children?	Indicates understanding of social systems and norms.

Questions Asked of 4- to 5-Year-Olds	Rationale for Questions
Ask child general information questions (e.g., colors, numbering, objects).	Assesses general fund of knowledge.
Ask child what makes the sun come up.	Illustrates child's belief about causality.
Ask child about concepts of time.	Assesses understanding of a relatively sophisticated concept.
Ask child about spontaneous play (e.g., with puppets or dolls), imaginative use of play materials (e.g., clay, crayons, other toys).	Assesses imagination and magical thinking.
Ask child to draw a person.	50% of 4-year-olds draw a three-part person; by 5 years old, child can draw an eight-part person.
How does the child behave in preschool? (ask of parent)	Assesses language, social, and play development in relation to peers in a setting where expectations differ from those at home.

TABLE 6-8	Speech and Language Evaluation Tools	
Evaluation Tool	**Age Assessed and Test Characteristics**	**Source**
The Capute Scales: Cognitive Adaptive Test and Clinical Linguistic and Auditory Milestone Scale (CAT/CLAMS)	0-36 mo Interview. Tests language and problem-solving skills to help clearly identify between the two.	Paul H Brookes Publishing www.pbrookes.com
Clinical Evaluation of Language Fundamentals—Preschool (CELF-P)	3-6 yr Assesses receptive and expressive language.	Harcourt Assessment The Psychological Corporation (Publisher) www.psychcorp.com
Clinical Evaluation of Language Fundamentals— School Age (CELF-3)	6-21 yr Assesses receptive and expressive language.	Harcourt Assessment The Psychological Corporation (Publisher) www.psychcorp.com
Denver Articulation Screening Examination (DASE)	2.5-7 yr Screens articulation only (not a complete assessment).	Denver Developmental Materials www.denverii.com/DASE.html
Fluharty Preschool Speech and Language Screening test	3-6.11 yr Direct testing of vocabulary, articulation, comprehension, repetition (expressive).	Pearson Assessments www.ags.pearsonassessments.com
Early Language Milestone (ELM) Scale (ELM Scale-2)	0-36 mo Tests visual and auditory receptive, auditory expressive. History, testing, observation 3-5 min.	Pro-Ed www.proedinc.com
Goldman-Fristoe Test of Articulation	2-22 yr Assesses articulation skills.	Pearson Assessments www.ags.pearsonassessments.com
Peabody Picture Vocabulary test	2.5-90+ yr Screens for receptive vocabulary.	Pearson Assessments www.ags.pearsonassessments.com
REEL: Receptive and Expressive Emergent Language	0-36 mo Interview or direct observation of expressive and receptive language.	Pearson Assessments www.ags.pearsonassessments.com

enjoy make-believe, and preschoolers love stories and become masters at games of pretend and fantasy.

DIAGNOSTIC ASSESSMENT STRATEGIES FOR TODDLERS AND PRESCHOOLERS

Once a child is identified through screening as having a possible problem, more definitive diagnostic testing or referral to an appropriate specialist is necessary.

■ Anticipatory Guidance for Toddlers and Preschoolers

Anticipatory guidance for toddlers and preschoolers helps parents and children transition from a highly dependent relationship to one in which the child has an established sense of autonomy with an evolving understanding of the self as a separate, creative, and powerful being. During the process, parents learn new communication and interaction skills with their children. Although the toddler and preschool years can be frustrating at times, the ultimate outcome of good communication and relationships that support the potential of both child and parent is worth the effort. Providers should offer anticipatory guidance in all of the following areas of growth and development: family support, child development, mental health, healthy weight, healthy nutrition, physical activity, oral health, healthy sexual development and sexuality, safety and injury prevention,

and community relationships and resources (Hagan et al, 2008).

REGULATION AND SLEEP-WAKE PATTERNS

- Discuss the need to assist toddlers and preschoolers to transition from one state to another. Consistent sleep and naptime schedules are essential. Use of a comfort object (e.g., teddy bear) and bedtime rituals help.
- Explain how children at this age process information and control themselves. They can be overwhelmed if they have too much stimulation.
- Explain that some children may have sensory integration problems that require even more structuring and modulation of their environment.
- Discuss how to help children identify and name their feelings. This ability will help them to more successfully organize and integrate the sensations they experience and respond appropriately (Brazelton and Sparrow, 2006).
- Encourage parents to provide opportunities for children to have some control and choice in daily activities (e.g., can select the story to be read at bedtime), while maintaining important rituals.
- Discuss sleep problems that may appear at this time, including sleep resistance, bruxism, nightmares, and somnambulism (see Chapter 14).
- Encourage parents to offer naps and opportunities for rest but not to force them on children. It is the parents' job to make sure the child has ample time to rest.

- Encourage parents to form good sleep routines, to provide positive reinforcement of healthy sleep behavior, and to use firm, loving, and consistent discipline when dealing with sleep refusal and other behavioral sleep problems.

STRENGTH AND MOTOR COORDINATION

- Discuss the importance of play as a way for toddlers and preschoolers to practice their developing physical, social, and emotional skills and to maintain a healthy lifestyle and weight (Ginsburg and AAP, 2007).
- Encourage parents to provide their children with a variety of play activities that use both fine and gross motor skills and that expose children to nature, such as the following:
  - Take children to a park to run, throw balls, play on the swing set, and roll on the grass.
  - Provide children with pencils, crayons, paper, paints, utensils, blocks, and age-appropriate building toys.
  - Encourage children to play with natural materials, water, sand, grass, and leaves.
- Explain how parents can incorporate practice with motor skills as part of daily routines (e.g., have child help pour the milk, hold the cup, or squeeze the toothpaste; encourage child to do own buttons, snaps, and zippers).
- Emphasize the need for constant adult supervision of children's activities.
- Discuss how parents can make the environment safer for their child: securing doors and windows; removing toxic substances and dangerous objects; providing toys that are developmentally appropriate and safely constructed.
- Reinforce teaching about car seat use and explain the need for larger car seats and booster seats as the child grows.

FEEDING AND SELF-CARE

- Provide parents with information about healthy foods and nutritional needs of their child (see Chapter 10). Three meals and two nutritious snacks per day are encouraged, if possible.
- Discuss the parents' responsibility to provide children with healthy foods and to allow children to make choices from healthy food options. Many families find the "bite rule" helpful. This means that children need to have at least one bite of everything on their plate for each year of age. So, 2 year-olds would have two bites, 3 year-olds three bites, and so on. Discourage parents from making separate meals for their young children. Allowing children to restrict their foods often makes a picky palate worse.
- Young children may go on "food jags," refusing some foods or requesting the same food day after day. Parents need to make sure the food eaten is nutritious.
- Explain how changes in toddlers' eating habits are caused by developmental changes (e.g., child has a decrease in appetite, is easily distracted, demonstrates more curiosity about what is going on around him or her than in eating, is more interested in using gross motor skills than in sitting still).
- Explain nonnutritive value of food and eating (e.g., finger foods stimulate fine motor and cognitive development, in addition to child's sense of control and independence; eating together as a family can strengthen relationships and develop social skills).
- Encourage self-feeding to help child gain new skills.

- Encourage parents to structure family mealtimes that are pleasant and interactive; this may mean offering the toddler foods that can be eaten in short periods of sitting. Avoid making meals a power struggle.
- Discuss weaning (if not already done by 12 months).
- Explain the importance of the child gaining mastery of self-care (e.g., toileting, bathing, dressing, eating) and the valuable role the parent plays as teacher in the process. Assist parents to cope with the frustration or tensions generated by toddlers and preschoolers wanting to "do it myself."
- Ask if parents are concerned about child becoming overweight.

COMMUNICATION AND LANGUAGE

Children learn and refine communication and language skills best through their interactions with others. When parents and caregivers listen to them, talk interactively with them, and read to them, the child's language blossoms (Hammer et al, 2010). Encourage parents to stimulate their child's language skills by doing the following:

- Read to children daily, using short, simple stories or picture books.
- Model appropriate language.
- Talk to the child, explaining in clear, simple language what is happening around the child; this helps increase vocabulary and the child's understanding of the world.
- Listen with care and respond actively to the child's verbalizations.
- Provide the child with opportunities to interact verbally with other children and adults.

Providers can also suggest the following strategies to parents to enhance their child's language development:

- No television viewing for children younger than 2 years old and limit television viewing and videos to 1 to 2 hours or less of appropriate programs per day for older children. Remove televisions from children's bedrooms (Hagan et al, 2008; National Association of Pediatric Nurse Practitioners [NAPNAP], 2009).
- Explain that children need constant reinforcement of their speech and language efforts, but that nonverbal language, especially touch, continues to be crucial.
- Give parents an opportunity to explain their expectations for their child; discourage parental pressure on child to perform (e.g., use of flash cards, requirement that child articulate sounds correctly) but point out that daily activities provide a wealth of opportunities to practice language skills.
- Reassure parents that language errors of young children usually disappear as the child grows.
- Inform parents that children learn receptive language first, then expressive, and that they may not fully understand the meaning, especially connotative meaning, of what they hear or say (e.g., a 4-year-old may innocently ask a stranger about their private body parts). Parents should explain clearly, simply, and unemotionally which words are appropriate and in which settings.

SOCIAL AND EMOTIONAL GROWTH

The emotional development of toddlers is an area in which parents may need a great deal of anticipatory guidance and support. The balance between dependence and independence is constantly in flux for young children and their parents, and conflict can develop as a result of inconsistent or extreme behavior. Toddlers and preschoolers need to master multiple social tasks during these years. They need to learn how to identify, control, and manage their feelings and emotions around anger, joy, love, and frustration. They learn about making and keeping friends, sharing, cooperative play, and living socially within a family. They learn to handle separation from parents, home, and neighborhood (Hagan et al, 2008). To help families with this process, providers should do the following:

- Reemphasize the role of parents as guides of their child's social and emotional growth. Parents must actively engage with their children, showing interest in their activities and giving them guidance on appropriate behavior.
- Encourage parents to give their children opportunities to expand social skills and form important attachments outside the immediate family by doing the following:
  ○ Provide toys that children can use creatively.
  ○ Allow children to explore, guiding them to activities that are fun.
  ○ Structure time for children to play in natural settings. "Nature play" enhances physical, mental, and emotional health of children (McCurdy et al, 2010).
  ○ Allow children to make choices when possible; do not give children a "choice" when there really is none (e.g., "Do you want to go to bed?"). Instead, use "toddler's choices" that allow the child to have a say and yet still get toward the final objective (e.g., "Do you want to put your pants on or your shirt on? Do you want to take the bunny or the bear with you during your nap?").
  ○ Discuss differences among people openly and positively.
  ○ Help children identify, name, and express feelings, both positive and negative.
  ○ Teach children to manage anger and resolve conflicts without violence.
  ○ Discuss television programs and movies to help children distinguish fantasy from reality.
  ○ Take children on trips to places of interest in the community.
  ○ Arrange play times with other children; encourage cooperative play (e.g., tag, hide-and-seek).
  ○ Reinforce positive child behavior ("catch the child being good").
  ○ Make the limits of what is expected of children clear, consistent, and achievable.
- Differentiate discipline and teaching from punishment.
- Discuss parenting and discipline (see Chapters 4 and 17).
- Clarify each parent's expectations of child's behavior.
- Discuss how parents plan to resolve differences in expectations.
- Provide information to parents related to child development and what parents can expect their child to be able to do.
- Recommend parenting classes that provide information on developmental milestones, anticipated changes, and management strategies as children grow.
- Encourage parents to show affection in the family.
- Explain to parents that myths or fables can be important ways of teaching children abstract concepts, such as love, sharing, and giving.

- Inform parents of the need to provide children a feeling of safety and security. Parents can do the following:
  ○ Support use of comfort or transitional objects to allay fears (e.g., blanket).
  ○ Consider use of a nightlight.
  ○ Provide reassurance if nightmares or fears occur and respond to child's fears.
  ○ Explain about "good" and "bad" touches to private parts.
  ○ Reinforce that the child can always come to the parent for comfort.

COGNITIVE AND ENVIRONMENTAL STIMULATION

- Explain to parents that toddlers and preschoolers are concrete and preoperational in their thinking. As a result, parents need to be ready to explain things over and over patiently, without expecting the child to understand the adult's interpretation clearly. Also, children may use words to convey thoughts and feelings, but many responses are repetitive, and trial-and-error problem solving is usually crude. They frequently attend to only one aspect of a problem, giving partial answers.
- Emphasize that parents should avoid putting their own meaning on the child's behavior or statements. For example, the child's statement, "What if you just bought a new house, and I was allergic to something in the house? I guess you'd have to get rid of me," should not be interpreted to mean the parents have somehow failed to show the child how much they love him or her. Rather the child can be exploring the concepts of place, ownership, belonging, size, or importance. In the child's mind, a house is much bigger than he or she is and may be more important. An appropriate response from the parent might be, "No, we'd probably have to get a new house or take out whatever you are allergic to. Even if we just bought it, you are more important than any house, and we wouldn't want to lose you."
- Reassure parents that "Why?" will not continue to be the child's most frequent question. Toddlers and preschoolers are actively exploring meaning in their world and have learned that asking "Why?" brings them more information—and attention. As parents answer them, children begin to show threads of symbolic and more abstract thought.

■ Common Developmental Issues for Toddlers and Preschoolers

FEARS

As the 2- to 3-year-old's world expands and the ability to fantasize develops, fears appear about things that might happen. "Magical thinking," characteristic of preschoolers, can accentuate these fears. Early fears include fear of separation, strangers, water, loud noises, crowds, the dark, and animals. Four- to 5-year-olds add wild animals, masks, and aggressive actions to the list. Fears may be expressed in a variety of ways: flight, requests for help, sudden shyness, irritability, hyperactivity, frustration, or aggressive actions (Dixon and Stein, 2006). By 4 years old, children identify nightmares as "not real," although they may still be afraid. Adults should not dismiss the fears as trivial but offer reassurance with words and their presence; this helps children work through the anxiety and tension they feel. Preschool children may still express fear of the dark or of harm to their bodies, but if the fears do not decrease with time, the child and family need referral for counseling (see Chapter 19). TV should be limited to 1 to 2 hours a day and should be monitored by parents or caregivers so as not to include programs that show violence (AAP, 2009).

TEMPER TANTRUMS

Temper tantrums are episodes in which the child is frustrated and angry and loses control of his or her feelings. The tantrum may be as mild as whining and pouting, or it may be a full-blown display of crying, yelling, flinging oneself on the floor, kicking, and screaming. Some children can hold their breath until they turn cyanotic and/or lose consciousness (Dixon and Stein, 2006).

Temper tantrums are common, with as many as 50% to 80% of children experiencing them; they usually peak at about 18 to 28 months. Tantrums stem from the child's attempts for power and control and the sudden loss of both, or because of frustration that is compounded by differences between receptive and expressive language. There are so many activities that toddlers want and struggle to do but are not developmentally ready to perform. Being tired or hungry exacerbates the frustration children can feel when their wishes are thwarted.

Ultimately, children will learn how to self-regulate, to identify a feeling and manage the actions appropriate to that feeling, and will thus "outgrow" the temper tantrums of toddlers. Management involves helping children master self-regulation and learn that there are better ways to handle frustration; this is a process that requires parents to engage in many of the interactions discussed earlier in this chapter (see "Anticipatory Guidance for Toddlers and Preschoolers"). Management also requires that parents deal with the immediate event of the tantrum itself. Some parents are aghast that their child would show such a violent display of emotions; others may express being frightened. Parents' responses usually depend on their comfort level. Some parents go to the child and hold, comfort, and distract him or her; some remove the child from the stimulation of the moment, putting him or her in "timeout"; and some physically restrain the child in a "bear hug" until the crying and thrashing-about behavior subsides. Generally, the most effective measures are thought to be the following:
- Ignore the child's behavior (give no physical or eye contact).
- Ensure that the child is safe and will not be injured.
- Use positive reinforcement when the child self-regulates and avoids a tantrum.

Health care providers can prepare parents for the possibility of temper tantrums by discussing them at the 12-month visit. It is important to describe the developmental stages the child will progress through (autonomy, independence, and preoperational thinking) and to explain how those stages contribute to high levels of frustration for the child. When parents understand the dynamics of tantrums, they can minimize the likelihood that they will occur. Parents can do this by not putting children in positions that they cannot easily handle, providing support for the child or redirecting the child early in the emotional cycle if frustration appears to be building, and making sure that external factors (e.g., hunger, sleepiness) are

managed well. Providers should also give parents the opportunity to discuss how they would like to handle the tantrum should it come. Parents should be counseled to avoid hitting or spanking the child because it only teaches the child that hitting is permitted if you are an adult, and, when emotions are high, hitting can quickly escalate to abuse.

DISCIPLINE

Limit setting and discipline are methods of helping a child learn rules, regulations, guidelines, and goals that make the world a more predictable place and are best taught by someone who loves the child (see Chapter 4). Discipline should encompass love, self-esteem, guilt, praise, and discomfort. Parents teach the child how to live within their family, what activities are expected, limits, and consequences. The child is helped to learn respect for authority, even if they disagree. Discipline protects and keeps the child safe from environmental dangers.

Discipline as guidance begins at birth when babies begin learning what brings smiles, warmth, and food. By toddlerhood the parents must control the child's environment while offering limited challenges (e.g., a verbal "no" and physical removal). Reasonable consistency helps. Parents need to understand their limits and tolerances in how they guide their toddler. Methods include verbal "no," physical removal, isolation, withdrawal of privileges, and natural and logical consequences. Modeling good behavior, encouraging, and rewarding reinforce "appropriate" behavior. Cause and effect need to be short and timely because toddlers may not remember what they did after minutes or hours.

CHILD CARE AND PRESCHOOLS

Many parents return to work during the first year of their child's life and must make arrangements for childcare. In 2009, more than 59% of mothers with preschool-aged children (younger than 6 years) were employed and 76% of those worked full-time. During the same year, 72% of women with children between 6 and 17 years old were employed (Bureau of Labor Statistics, 2010). According to the U.S. Census Bureau (2006), 36% of children younger than age 5 years who live at home with an employed mother regularly received child care by a nonrelative, whereas another 34% had no regular arrangement, yet received out-of-home care. As a result, childcare issues affect millions of people and can be a source of significant parental concern. Parents need to be able to evaluate child care options for their children and feel secure that their children are in safe, appropriate situations.

It can be stressful for young children and their families to enter a setting outside the home that has a teacher, curriculum, and learning expectations. Suddenly, parents find their child compared with 20 other children. A child with developmental delays (e.g., speech, motor, physical) may be singled out as different, not fitting in, or a behavior problem. Preschool and kindergarten were originally intended to help children learn separation, sharing, listening, paying attention, and some simple social skills. Kindergarten children are often expected to show pre-academic skills such as writing, counting, and letter and word recognition in addition to the preschool social skills of paying attention and sitting still. In making their childcare selection, parents should select a play-based learning curriculum because this is the most comfortable way for young children to learn.

School readiness criteria are outlined in Table 7-5. By considering school readiness factors, parents can make more appropriate decisions about their child's ability to handle the demands of a structured preschool setting. It is also important to consider the following child characteristics:

- Social skills (e.g., ability to separate from parent for several hours)
- Language skills, both expressive and receptive
- Physical size
- Energy level (e.g., ability to actively participate)
- Neurologic maturation required for fine and gross motor activities (e.g., writing, cutting, coloring, climbing, running, walking)
- Neurologic maturation of sensory and cognitive function (e.g., visuospatial perception, tactile maturation, auditory processing, attending skills, memory)

TOILETING

Toileting skills and training are a major milestone for a child and the parents. It is a complex developmental skill that many children master effortlessly, but some children and families need guidance and support along the way (see Chapter 12).

SAFETY

As children grow and develop, their world expands and exposes them to ever-increasing dangers. Safety should be a topic of every well-child visit, and the discussion should focus on the developmental age of the child. The focus of injury prevention at this age is active supervision. This means that the caregiver must be able to physically reach the young child and not be distracted from supervision by other things like phone calls, alcohol, and so on. Toddlers and preschoolers are not old enough to learn and remember safety rules, so the best approach is to control their environment because it is generally restricted to the house, the yard, or the parent's side. For preschoolers the world is bigger and more dangerous and includes the house, the yard, the neighborhood, the preschool, and traveling (e.g., car, bike, scooters). See Chapter 39 for a discussion of causes and management of unintentional injuries.

◼ Red Flags for Toddlers and Preschoolers

Although a wide range of normal development may be seen when assessing children, the provider needs to be alert to developmental red flags, signs of delayed or abnormal development. In addition to obvious abnormalities, minor problems that are left untreated can develop into major concerns; minor signs and symptoms that persist can indicate a more serious underlying problem, or a major problem can occur as a one-time event (e.g., child who sets a fire). Some children and families are at high risk and need careful monitoring and guidance to detect problems at an early stage or to prevent their occurrence (e.g., very early premature infants, families with history of violence, families with chronic medical or mental health problems, some single-parent families). The warning signs, or red flags, can be found in Table 6-9. Children who

demonstrate these behaviors should be referred. Immediate referral is required for children who stop eating, demonstrate cruelty to animals or other people, are self-harmful, start fires, or talk of harming themselves, their peers, or others.

PHYSICAL DISORDERS

Children should be monitored for physical growth milestones. Further investigation, screening, and referral may be appropriate when children fall outside normal growth parameters or when children follow a normal growth pattern and begin to level off or fall below that range. If children have symptoms—stop eating, complain of tiredness, are not as active as usual, or the parents state that the child has regressed—it is time to investigate.

COGNITIVE DISORDERS

Mental and cognitive delays are more difficult to recognize and categorize without the help of a screening tool or more in-depth assessment. These tools rank children on the basis of a standardized score or against standardized criteria (e.g., word definition). Children with scores below 85 on intelligence scales, for example, predictably have more difficulty in school. Significant discrepancies between test scores taken over time also suggest problems. The causes of delay must be carefully assessed as well because some children may have a neurologic limitation, whereas others may be delayed as a result of material or environmental deprivation. Identifying the causes is necessary to plan effective interventions. In any case, when delays are suspected, prompt referral to developmental specialists or early childhood intervention programs for more detailed assessment is essential.

LANGUAGE DISORDERS

Language delays or disorders are problems in learning the communication systems and, when present, affect other areas of development, especially cognitive, social, and emotional development. Because language development is the best indicator of cognitive development, language delays may indicate serious issues that require developmental and educational intervention.

Children with language delays experience problems in either receptive or expressive language, or both. They may start talking late, talk very little as toddlers, or have prolonged stages of normal stuttering, distortion, and substitution.

Cognitive, familial, environmental, or cultural factors cause language delays. Language delays or disorders may occur if the child does not hear, is not immersed in a language-rich environment, or has a psychological disorder, such as severe deprivation or autism. Speech disorders (problems producing sounds) are associated with physical problems (e.g., cleft lip, cleft palate, cerebral palsy, hearing impairments), or they can be idiopathic.

Language evaluation involves assessment of the total child, including physical, cognitive, social, emotional, and perceptual characteristics. Expressive and receptive language must be evaluated. The inability to use the symbols of language may be characterized by the following:

- Improper use of words and their meanings
- Inappropriate grammatical patterns

- Improper use of speech sounds

Speech disorders involve problems producing correct speech sounds and may be characterized by difficulty in the following:
- Producing speech sounds (articulation)
- Maintaining speech rhythm (fluent speech)
- Controlling vocal production (voice)

Management of children with language disorders requires a clear understanding of the nature of the problem. Referral to a specialist (e.g., pediatric speech pathologist) to make that determination is often the first step. Deficits identified in Table 6-9 are cause for referral for additional testing. Other criteria that warrant referral include the following:
- There is excessive, indiscriminate, irrelevant verbalizing after 18 months old.
- The child is using only single words by 16 months, or two-word phrases by 2 years.
- There is consistent and frequent omission of initial consonants, which are generally mastered early in the second year; the child uses mostly vowel sounds after 1 year.
- There are unusual confusions, reversals, or telescoping in connected speech.
- There is a loss of previously acquired language skills.
- The child stops talking.
- The child reacts to his or her own speech with embarrassment or withdrawal.
- The child's voice is monotone, extremely loud, largely inaudible, or of poor quality.
- Pitch is not appropriate to the child's age and gender.
- Hypernasality or lack of nasal resonance occurs.

TABLE 6-9   Red Flags of Development: Toddlers and Preschoolers

Age	Growth, Rhythmicity, Sleep, and Temperament	Psychosocial and Emotional Skills	Cognitive and Visual Abilities	Gross Motor, Language, and Hearing	Fine Motor, Feeding, and Self-Care	Strength and Coordination
15 mo	No nighttime ritual Difficulty with transitions Parents express concern about temperament or control issues	Problems with attachment to caregiver	Lack of object permanence	Lack of consonant production Does not imitate words No gestures or pointing	No self-feeding	No attempts at walking
18 mo	Poor sleep schedule Problems with control and behavior	Does not pull person to show something	Primary play: mouthing of toys No finger exploration of objects Lack of imitation	Unable to follow simple directions (e.g., "no," "jump")	Does not try to scribble spontaneously Unable to use spoon	Not yet walking or frequently falls when walking
24 mo (2 yr)	Less than four times birth weight or falling off growth curve Poor sleep schedule Awakens at night; unable to put self back to sleep	Absent symbolic play No evidence of parallel play Displays destructive behaviors Always clings to mother		No two-word phrases Use of noncommunicative speech (echolalia, rote phrases) Unable to identify 5 pictures Unable to name body parts No jargon History of greater than 10 episodes of otitis media	Unable to stack 4 or 5 blocks Still eating pureed foods Unable to imitate scribbles on paper Unable to dump pellet from bottle	Unable to walk downstairs holding a rail Persistent waddle walk Persistent toe walking
30 mo	Resistance to regular bedtime Beginning behavior issues	Problems with biting, hitting playmates, parents	Does not try to get toy with stick	No two-word sentences Unable to name some body parts	Unable to feed self Unable to build a tower of 6 blocks Unable to imitate circle shape Unable to imitate vertical stroke	Unable to jump in place Unable to kick ball on request

TABLE 6-9 Red Flags of Development: Toddlers and Preschoolers—cont'd

Age	Growth, Rhythmicity, Sleep, and Temperament	Psychosocial and Emotional Skills	Cognitive and Visual Abilities	Gross Motor, Language, and Hearing	Fine Motor, Feeding, and Self-Care	Strength and Coordination
36 mo (3 yr)	Problems with toilet training Unable to calm self	Not able to dress self Does not understand taking turns No pretend play		Unable to give full name Unable to match two colors Does not use plurals Does not know two or three prepositions Unable to tell a story Unclear consonants Unintelligible speech Unable to construct a sentence	Unable to build a tower of 10 blocks Holds crayon with fist Unable to draw circle	Unable to balance on one foot for 1 sec Toeing-in causes tripping with running
48 mo (4 yr)	Lack of bedtime ritual Behavior concerns: withdrawn or acting out Stool holding Problems with toilet training	Unable to play games, follow rules Unable to follow limits or rules at home (e.g., put toys away) Cruelty to animals, friends Interest in fires, fire starting Persistent fears or severe shyness Inability to separate from mother	Unable to count 3 objects Unable to recall 4 numbers Unable to identify what to do in danger, fire, with a stranger Consistently poor judgment	Difficulty understanding language Problems understanding prepositions Limited vocabulary Unclear speech	Lack of self-care skills—dressing feeding, Unable to button clothes Unable to copy square	Unable to balance on one foot for 4 sec Unable to alternate steps when climbing stairs
60 mo (5 yr)	Continued sleep problems Concerns with night terrors Hair pulling— scalp or eyelashes	Difficulty making and keeping friends; no friends Difficulty understanding sharing, school rules, organization of daily activities Cruelty to animals, friends Interest in fires, fire starting Bullying or being bullied Prolonged fighting, hitting, hurting Withdrawal, sadness, extreme rituals	Unable to count to 10 Unable to identify colors Difficulty following three-step command	Speech pattern not 100% understandable Cannot identify a penny, nickel, or dime Abnormal rate or rhythm of speech	Unable to copy triangle Unable to draw a person with a body	Difficulty hopping, jumping

Developmental Management of School-Age Children

BONNIE GANCE-CLEVELAND AND YVONNE YOUSEY

School-age children are busy, active, curious, and creative. With guidance and encouragement they eagerly apply the skills they learned as toddlers and preschoolers as they move into more structured school environments, home schooling, or community settings. Their physical abilities advance, and they join organized sports activities and engage in casual play with friends or siblings. Cognitively and emotionally, school-age children face daunting challenges. They must master the intellectual skills of reading, writing, mathematics, science, and other academic work. They are expected to become skilled socially, separating from home and family, establishing friendships, negotiating with siblings and other family members, and developing a sound sense of who they are as unique members of the community.

School-age children pass through several phases on their way from preschool innocence to the complexity of adolescence. The school-age years are divided into early childhood (5 to 7 years), middle childhood (8 to 10 years), and late childhood (11 to 12 years). Children in each of these phases demonstrate different developmental goals and achievements. Each school-age child is unique, and patterns of "normal" development have broad parameters. The goals of school-age children's development include laying the groundwork for achievement, creating a sense of self-worth, developing the ability to contribute to the group, and, ultimately, gaining satisfaction with life.

Primary health care providers who care for school-age children must be familiar with psychosocial theoretical models of development in this age group as well as physical growth parameters. Parents often turn to their health care provider for understanding and guidance. Some authors characterize the school-age period as one of quiescence, but a remarkable amount of growth takes place, and the route is not always smooth. Providers support children and their families to successfully achieve during these important years.

■ School-Age Child Development

PHYSICAL DEVELOPMENT

School-age children gain strength and coordination and become more physically capable, setting the stage for participation in sports, dance, gymnastics, and other activities.

Success and enjoyment of physical activities establishes healthy patterns for a lifetime. Social status among children is often based on physical competence; therefore, the child's feelings about physical development can be as important as the physical growth itself.

The growth rate of school-age children increases significantly from that of the toddler and preschooler and occurs in "spurts." The child literally "grows out of his or her clothes" in a matter of weeks. Children from this age group need height, weight, and body mass index (BMI) evaluation. Head circumference increases slowly, although it is not routinely measured. By middle childhood the brain is about 90% of its adult size. Full adult brain size is reached by about 12 years old. Myelination of the brain, which is necessary for information processing, is not complete until early adulthood. The cerebral cortex (responsible for intelligence) and the frontal lobe (responsible for problem-solving, judgment, and decision-making) are the last to fully develop. The increasing maturation of the brain allows children to complete increasingly complex skills and have greater control over their bodies (see Chapter 2). Organ development is complete. Most school-age children sleep about 10 hours per night (range 8 to 14 hours) without naps, particularly during the school year. Night terrors or sleepwalking may emerge (see Chapter 14).

Traditionally, school-age children are lean; however, recent national data indicate a steady increase in overweight school-age children. National Health and Nutrition Examination Survey data indicate that in 2007 to 2008, 35.5% of children 6 to 11 years old were overweight or obese, up from 29.8% in 1999 to 2000; 19.6% of all children and adolescents were obese. The number of overweight girls, 6 to 11 years old, increased from 13.8% in 1999 to 2000 to 18% in 2007 to 2008. For boys the increase was from 14% overweight in 1999 to 2000 to 21.2% in 2007 to 2008. Although these data represent a significant increase, even more alarming is the fact that in 1980, only 5% to 6% of children were overweight (Ogden et al, 2010). In less than 25 years, the number of overweight children in the U.S. has more than tripled, and the trend continues.

Table 7-1 includes a description of the significant physical changes that occur in school-agers. Discussion of school-age

TABLE 7-1	Physical Development of School-Age Children
Body System	**Developmental Change**
Skin and lymph	• At about 6 yr, tonsils and adenoids are their largest. • Prepubescence is characterized by more active sebaceous glands and vasomotor instability that can lead to uncontrolled blushing.
Head, eyes, ears, nose, and mouth	• By early childhood, head size becomes smaller in proportion to body size. • Developing frontal sinus cavities contribute to increased susceptibility to upper respiratory infections, sinus irritation, and sinus headaches. • By 6 to 7 yr, the retinas are fully developed, and visual acuity is 20/20. • By middle childhood, the Eustachian tubes grow longer, narrower, and more slanted. • By 5 to 6 yr, first primary teeth are shed, and first permanent teeth erupt, usually the central incisors. • Each year after 6 yr, approximately four teeth are replaced, one set in the upper jaw, one set in the lower jaw.
Pulmonary	• Through childhood, the lungs gradually descend into the thoracic cavity. • By 8 yr, alveolar development is complete. • During middle childhood, tidal volume increases; normal adult respiratory rate is achieved, 18 to 30 breaths per minute. • Increased maturation of macrophagocytic activity of mucus and ciliary function in lungs make child more resistant to respiratory infections.
Cardiovascular	• By 5 yr, the heart is four times larger than at birth. • By 7 yr, the left ventricle thickens and is two to three times greater in size than the right; blood pressure increases to 90 to 108/60; cardiac volume increases; heart rate declines to 60 to 100 beats per minute. • Atherosclerosis begins in childhood.
Gastrointestinal	• By middle childhood, the gastrointestinal system is of adult size and function.
Genitourinary	• By 6 yr, elimination patterns are established; greater than 90% of children are toilet trained. • Bladder capacity continues to expand. • Between 10 and 14 yr, puberty begins but can be normal in any child after 8 yr. • Delayed puberty is diagnosed as no secondary sex changes (e.g., breast budding; penis or testicle growth) at 13 yr in girls and 14 yr in boys.
Musculoskeletal	• Long bones grow, leading to taller, thinner appearance. • Spine becomes straighter; legs become straighter. • Facial bones are actively changing, as nasal accessory sinuses grow.
Immune system	• Rapid maturation of immune system during middle childhood. • Allergic conditions may appear.

health issues and disease processes is found in Units 3 and 4 of this text.

MOTOR SKILLS DEVELOPMENT

In middle childhood gross motor skills continue to be refined, allowing children to hop, skip, tandem walk, alternate their foot patterns, and use an overhand motion. Activities that require balance and coordination such as riding a bicycle, swimming, roller skating, and skateboarding demonstrate children's expanding skills. In late childhood, gross motor skills become more controlled and purposeful. Skills are perfected with practice. A sense of competition is high as children try to outlast or outperform one another. Consequently, school-age children enjoy participating in competitive sports.

Mastery of fine motor skills includes finer dexterity and better control of scissors and writing tools such as crayons and pencils. In early childhood, children become adept at dressing themselves, including being able to tie knots and manage buttons and zippers. Their drawings become more recognizable, showing details of eyes, ears, and other body parts. Self-care skills (e.g., combing hair, brushing teeth) improve. In late childhood, hand-eye coordination improves, and the child uses each hand independently with speed and smoothness. During this time skill in playing musical instruments emerges.

COMMUNICATION AND LANGUAGE DEVELOPMENT

The child's language patterns provide insight into the neurologic system's status because the maturing brain is capable of increasingly complex language skills. Both receptive and expressive language skills improve. Six-year-olds have a well-developed vocabulary and retrieve words quickly. They have simple syntactic abilities and follow more complex directions than preschoolers. The language demands of school can be challenging for 6-year-olds. First, they may not be accustomed to attending to total auditory stimuli as in the classroom environment. Second, they are still mastering connotative and semantic skills such as understanding the concepts "before" and "after," relative clauses (e.g., "the cat was chased by the dog"), and the structures of sentences. These factors can make it difficult for some to follow complicated directions or to cope with the increased demand to recall information within a specific time frame. Narrative skills can be poor, and reading may be difficult. The expressive language of 6-year-olds should be fully intelligible. Stuttering usually resolves by school age but may be seen if young children are overly eager to express themselves. Stuttering should be ignored at this age as long as it does not involve repetition of syllables or cause distress for the child.

Seven-year-olds' receptive language is strong as they move from the ability to simply decode language to the more complex process of encoding information. They can organize previous knowledge and express it verbally or in writing. They solve word problems. Articulation mastery of the sounds of "l" and "th" may not be achieved until 7 or 8 years of age.

Eight- to 9-year-old children demonstrate significant syntactic growth with better use of pronouns, allowing them to understand convoluted sentences. Comparatives are learned, and the child distinguishes qualities such as more or less, near or far, and heavy or light. By 8 years old, children follow complex directions. They begin to tell jokes because they understand different meanings of words. In their expressive language, children have better narrative abilities and significantly improved storytelling and summarization skills needed for such activities as explaining a task to other children. Vocabulary grows, and there are gradual improvements in grammar (e.g., noted by the use of past and future tenses and plural forms of nouns, particularly irregular nouns and verbs).

At 10 years, children discuss ideas and understand inflections and metaphors. Their ability to understand ambiguities of sentence structure, word meaning, and language contributes to their increasing ability to enjoy jokes and riddles. Using concrete operational thinking, they analyze and interpret language and become more aware of the inconsistency in spoken languages. Children in late childhood understand that the literal meaning of words may not be the only meaning. By 12 years old, children should be able to answer questions involving sophisticated concepts. Expressively, their sentences should be grammatically correct, and they have more detail in their verbal skills. The ability to express emotions also develops. Language has become a means of socializing, and fewer gestures are used. Language can become a game as children make up words and participate in storytelling using proper sequence and pronouns.

Language impairment is linked with motor coordination disorders. Forty to 90% of children with specific language impairment meet criteria for developmental coordination delay. In addition, the overlap between language impairment and attention-deficit/hyperactivity disorder is estimated as high as 90%. Fifty-one percent of children with a language learning disability met the criteria for another developmental disorder (Campbell and Skarakis-Doyle, 2007).

The development of speech and auditory skills is crucial to long-term literacy skills in children. It is necessary to assess these skills throughout the school years to determine the need for remedial efforts with those children who demonstrate literacy difficulties (Shapiro et al, 2009).

SOCIAL AND EMOTIONAL DEVELOPMENT

The psychosocial development of school-age children puts to rest the notion that childhood is a "quiescent" period. Challenges that school-age children face are especially difficult because the child's skill and ultimate success are dependent on abilities that are only just evolving. Gaining social acceptance from one's peers, for example, depends on skills such as being socially responsive, understanding the group "rules," using the group jargon, being appropriately assertive, and being empathic. Children who do not yet have those skills can experience a sense of failure when they are compared with their peers who do. Erikson stated that school-age children are eager to learn and internally motivated to achieve mastery and recognition (see Chapter 4). They need to be given experiences in an environment that recognizes, adjusts for, and supports their maturing set of skills, where they can explore creatively, learn actively, and be recognized for their successes.

The stages through which children progress as they become more socially and emotionally mature are sequential and build on earlier skills (Table 7-2) (see Table 4-1 and discussion in Chapter 4 of the theoretical models of development). In particular, school-age children must develop social interactional skills including how to:

- Understand meaning in social situations and interpret the social cues of others
- Initiate interactions
- Terminate interactions positively
- Gain impulse control and manage emotions
- Resolve conflicts
  Mastering these skills enables children to:
- Refine their role within the family system
- Separate self from family
- Develop and maintain peer friendships
- Develop positive relationships with adults outside the family
- Achieve social acceptance
- Strengthen a sense of self

The earliest school-age milestone in the psychosocial area occurs when children learn to separate easily from family, allowing them to go to school. As they move into the community, children maintain their role and feelings of belonging to a family, but also develop secondary attachments with other adults outside the home. Having good relationships with adults outside the home and supports within the community are especially important when the family is not wholly functional—not responsive and supportive—to the child (Vanderbilt-Adriance and Shaw, 2008).

Peer Relationships

A major task of school-age children is to develop competence in social relationships. Friendships are an important part of the school-ager's life. They allow children to practice learned social skills, provide emotional support, and help children identify a healthy self-image. Social acceptance is especially important at this age. Friends are generally chosen because of shared skills, interests, personality, and loyalty. Children come to see themselves in the eyes of their friends. As early as 7 years old, some children are more concerned about a friend's opinion than about adults' opinions. They develop "best friends" and dress and talk like their peers. A special-friend phase should occur at around 10 years old. This is an intense attachment to a same-sex child. With that friend, the child expands the self, learns altruism, shares feelings, and learns how others manage problems. Talking on the telephone and sleepovers become more common. These early

TABLE 7-2	Developmental Characteristics of School-Age Children			
Approximate Stages and Ages	**Psychosexual Development**	**Social and Emotional Development**	**Cognitive and Problem-Solving Development**	**Moral Development**
Early childhood (5-7 yr; carried over from the toddler and preschool years to about 6 yr)	*Phallic stage (Freud):* Attachment to the parent of the opposite sex. Usually sexual identity occurs at the end of this phase, and sexual urges are submerged.	*Initiative vs. guilt (Erikson):* Moving into a larger social environment and thus able to initiate activities on their own. Begin to learn to modulate their own behaviors through development of a consciousness as to what is considered appropriate by parents and society.	*Preoperational period (Piaget):* Representative language and early reasoning. Problem-solving intuitive rather than logical. Thought process involves magical thinking, egocentrism, centration, syncretism, juxtaposition, animism, artificialism, participation, and irreversibility.	*Preconventional stage (Kohlberg):* Stage 1: Reasoning based on rewards and punishment or the consequences of behavior. Stage 2: Begin to base behaviors on own needs and at times the needs of others. Reciprocity is concrete. Others' feelings are secondary.
Middle childhood (7-10 yr)	*Latency stage (Freud):* The superego or conscious is internalized. Energy is put into acquiring cultural and social skills. Guidelines established by the family are followed.	*Industry vs. inferiority (Erikson):* Begin to appreciate individual interests and skills and seek to become successful members of a group. Internal motivation to achieve, compete, and obtain recognition. If unsuccessful, learning motivation can be lost.	*Early concrete operational (Piaget):* Begin to use logic and become more objective, using an external point of view. Thinking involves *decentration* (keeping track of both color and shape when working on a jigsaw puzzle), *conservation* (one cookie though broken in two is still one cookie), *transitivity* (if a first-grade rule is to sit still and all grades have that rule, one must sit still in second grade), *seriation* (ordering shapes from smallest to largest), *classification* (separating out objects on the basis of common features [i.e., circles from triangles]), *reversibility* (ability to reverse a process or action—water to ice to water). Develop the ability to understand size and shape when the physical properties can be manipulated.	*Conventional stage (Kohlberg):* Stage 3: Begin to act to please others. Stage 4: Begin to conform to rules.
Late childhood (10-12 yr; carried into adolescence)	*Genital stage (Freud):* Reemergence of sexual impulses.	*Industry vs. inferiority (Erikson):* Continuation of socialization with other children and groups. Development of hobbies and interests outside of school allows recognition of individual worth.	*Late concrete operational (Piaget):* Able to conceptualize size, shape, quantity, space, and thus able to problem-solve using abstract thought. Able to classify items into a hierarchical system.	*Postconventional stage (Kohlberg):* Stage 5: Begin to appreciate that their behaviors benefit society. Stage 6: Begin to form principles from conscience, even if they differ from what is generally acceptable in society. Look for rationale in rules. Respect for authority and maintaining social order.
			Formal operational (Piaget): Distinguished by the ability to use abstract thinking, complex reasoning, flexibility, and hypothesis formation. Become more aware of contradictions, falsehoods, and shortcomings in previous beliefs. Become aware of how others think of them.	

friendships are the basis for later relationships. Family conflicts can arise when peer activities and expectations conflict with family rules and values.

Children's temperaments affect the way they interact with peers, teachers, family, and others in their environment. Emotional problems during these years often follow frustrations, losses, and situations in which the child's self-esteem is threatened or the child is faced with adversity.

Morality

Although there is variability in moral development, moral reasoning in early childhood is usually determined by the consequences of behavior: to avoid punishment, receive rewards, or meet one's needs. There is some consideration of the feelings of others, but only as it serves one's needs. By 7 years old, most children name a site for their conscience (heart or brain), and, consistent with concrete thinking, school-age children tend to be rather rigid in their views of right and wrong. They can understand the relationships between responsibility and privileges and realize that choices between right and wrong behaviors are within their control. Some children at this age act appropriately to get a direct reward, whereas others view moral behavior as following the rules of higher authority (see Table 20-2). In late childhood children begin to move into Kohlberg's postconventional stage (Kohlberg, 1981), where respect for authority and social norms develops.

The ability to reason through difficult situations with a variety of factors operating depends on cognitive development; however, school-age children do not have the cognitive maturity to cope with all situations. The school environment, where rules and values differ from those of the immediate family, must be confronted and negotiated daily. This presents a challenge to the child's concepts of right and wrong. Social pressures may make it difficult to choose actions that the child believes are right. The pressures of gangs, drugs, and peers push many children to make decisions about their activities and behaviors before they are developmentally ready. Furthermore, family values are challenged as the child learns that other families make decisions and have beliefs that differ from their own.

Body Image

School-age children can appear to be totally unaware of their bodies (e.g., the 9-year-old who does not change his shirt for 3 days), perhaps because they are so busy with their daily lives. In fact, children at this age are extremely curious about changes happening to them as they grow, and they are sensitive to others around them. Highly literal in their thinking, they can be very frank with questions to people they trust (e.g., "Grandma, why are you growing a mustache?"). At the same time, they learn the importance of social politeness—what is appropriate in certain situations and how to behave themselves—so they may be uncomfortable or shy about new or unusual situations. Modesty is characteristic of school-age children.

Sexual exploration, including masturbation, is common. Children in early childhood, 5 to 7 years old, often play "doctor." In middle childhood, children compare their bodies with friends of the same sex.

Physical growth and neurologic maturation give children the ability to master many new physical skills. Young

swimmers, runners, skateboard enthusiasts, soccer players, musicians, and artists all emerge at this time. Their achievements—and failures—help them define who they are and are the basis for their evolving self-image. The images they have about their bodies come from the experiences they have and from the feedback from family, peers, teachers, and others in the community. This feedback clarifies their understandings and allows the child to gain in self-confidence and feelings of worth (see Chapter 16).

Coping Skills

As a part of the process of developing relationships with others, school-age children refine their ability to identify, label, and manage their feelings. However, their experiences are limited and their cognitive abilities are still expanding. They continue to need help labeling complex emotions such as sadness, depression, worry, and envy. They also need help to consciously manage feelings in acceptable ways.

Impulse control is an important coping skill learned by school-age children. Without impulse control, random behavior occurs; on the other hand, overly controlled children appear hostile, uncreative, or both. By 7 years old, children develop sufficiently to function in a variety of settings (e.g., home, school, playground) with increasing competence.

School-age children face a variety of stressors in society today, including violence, parental divorce, substance abuse in the family, early responsibilities, and lack of support in school. Violence is a constant problem for many, not only in neighborhoods where they live and play but also within their families and schools. Anxiety disorders are one of the most common mental disorders seen in children, with most cases being diagnosed before age 12 years (Beesdo et al, 2009).

Based on the Substance Abuse and Mental Health Services Administration's (SAMHSA) National Survey on Drug Use and Health in 2008, 8.3 million parents of children less than 18 years old reported drug abuse in the past year. More than 11.9% of all parents stated they abused drugs (USDHHS and SAMHSA, 2008). Substance abuse by parents has led to many children being placed in foster care. In some states, 60% to 70% of all foster care placements are drug related, and many directly connected to methamphetamine use (Smith et al, 2007).

Some children are given heavy responsibility at a young age. When parents work, many children must care for themselves after school. Latchkey children remain alone, housebound and unsupervised, until adults return at the end of the day. Some also have the responsibility of caring for younger siblings.

Many schools lack resources to maintain small class sizes or offer special programs for children with learning difficulties. As a result, children with learning problems are passed on from grade to grade without remediation and with the stigma of failure. Children with chronic illnesses or disabilities may have trouble adapting during the school-age years and may need special help to foster independence and a sense of self-esteem. The child's physical differences may lead to isolation and rejection by peers. Academic success may be difficult if the child is also cognitively impaired, or if the condition limits exposure to opportunities for cognitive development. Latchkey children with chronic illnesses are especially vulnerable because they may need to make decisions about a health care situation without adult advice. Such children need to understand their illness, medications, where to go for emergency care, how to write down instructions or messages, and how to follow important rules. Children mature at different rates in their ability to manage their self-care throughout the school-age years. A child's capacity for self-care of chronic illnesses depends on the illness, its stability, the child's age and cognitive skills, and the child's support network.

COGNITIVE DEVELOPMENT

In early childhood, children transition from preoperational thinking that uses intuitive problem-solving to early concrete operational thinking. One of the signs of school readiness at this age is the presence of logical thought processes (Box 7-1). Magical thinking and egocentric logic fade, and concepts of conservation, transformation, reversibility, decentration, seriation, and classification emerge. Children's ability to mentally manipulate the world, relationships, and viewpoints of others is facilitated when they have the opportunity to physically manipulate concrete materials (e.g., using paints, paper, and glue; building things; making dams and forts of mud, snow, or rocks).

By middle childhood, children need to understand relationships of mass and length and multiple variables relating to objects. School-age children normally classify or group materials in relation to other information they have. By late childhood, children have well-developed concrete operational thinking. They should be able to focus on more than one aspect of a problem and use logical thinking. For effective cognitive work, young people must process information, recognize salient cues in the environment, organize their thoughts, consider relationships with other information, use short- and long-term memory retrieval

---

BOX 7-1	Screening and Assessment

Screening Tests to Evaluate School Readiness

Test	Source	Content
Beery Visual-Motor Integration, Fifth Edition (VMI-5)	Pro-Ed Inc. www.proedinc.com	Test of visual motor integration
Denver Developmental Screening Test II	Denver Developmental Materials, Inc. www.denverii.com	Divided into four areas: Gross motor Language Fine motor Personal and social
Pediatric Examination of Educational Readiness (PEER-2) and Pediatric Examination of Educational Readiness at Middle Childhood (PEERAMID-2)	Educators Publishing Service, Inc. www.epsbooks.com	Combined neurodevelopmental, behavioral, and health assessment

Screening and Assessment Tools for the School-Age Child

Tools	Ages	Reference	Reporter	Item No.	Strengths	Weaknesses
Pediatric Symptoms Checklist (PSC)	6-12 yr	Jellinek et al, 1988; Jellinek et al, 1999	Parent report for 6-16 yr. List of behaviors followed by never, sometimes, often.	35	Measures psychosocial dysfunction. Normative data, reliable, valid. Specificity of 68% and sensitivity of 95%. Used extensively in pediatric populations.	Not for older adolescents. No depression-specific subscore; measures global dysfunction.
Child Behavior Checklist (CBCL)	6-18 yr	Jensen et al, 1996	Parent report for 4-18 yr. Checklist.	138	Multidimensional. Widely accepted and used; provides normative data for age and gender. Reliable and valid. Validated in many languages and countries. Often used to validate other screens.	Requires 20-25 min. Not easily scored. Computer scoring recommended. May not be feasible for mass screening. Subscales may have lower sensitivity than total scores.
Child Depression Inventory (CDI)	7-16 yr (used up to 18 yr)	Brooks and Kutcher, 2001; Myers and Winters, 2002	Child selects 1 of 3 statements.	27	Well studied, reliable, and internally consistent.	CDI scores vary with age and sample, making cutoff scores difficult for mass screening. Some studies failed to distinguish between depressed and non-depressed children. Does not ask if suicide was attempted.

Continued

BOX 7-1 Screening and Assessment—cont'd

Tools	Ages	Reference	Reporter	Item No.	Strengths	Weaknesses
Child Depression Inventory—Parent (CDI-P)	6-16 yr	Wierzbicki, 1987	Parent selects one choice from three statements.	27	Ability to ask a second informant. Studied in a nonclinical population.	Fewer validation studies than the instruments from which it was derived (CDI and BDI).
Psychosocial Screening (PSC–youth)	9-14 yr	Gall et al, 2000	Self-report. List of behaviors followed by never, sometimes, often.	35	Addresses psychosocial impairment. Used in nonclinical populations.	Fewer validation studies than the parent version.
Children's Depression Rating Scale (CDRS)–revised	6-12 yr	Brooks and Kutcher, 2001	Interviewer based; 14 items for parents, 3 items based on child observation.	17	Reliable. Valid. Combines multiple informants. Interviewer does not need to be qualified clinician. All depressive symptoms.	Takes more than 30 min to complete. Recommended method is for trained interviewer to speak separately with parent, child, and another adult, such as the teacher. Involves training.
Youth Outcome Questionnaire (YOQ-12)	4-17 yr	Tzoumas et al, 2007	Self-report of behaviors. Parent completed. Based on YOQ-2.01, a 64-item test.	12	Has potential for computer-based administration. Comparable to DSC and DISC-PS.	Newer test but has good reliability and sensitivity.

BDI, Beck Depression Inventory.

and storage skills, make decisions based on the analysis of information, take action, and use feedback to further their learning.

Concrete operational abilities allow children to read, write, and communicate thoughts effectively. It is now possible to learn about the world, its people, and the views and values of others. Logical thinking and new social skills appear with the ability to understand the viewpoints of others and the decline of egocentricity. Empathy, or the ability to share and understand another's feelings, emerges and with it the capacity for making deep friendships.

Developmental Assessment of School-Age Children

Health promotion ensures physical, cognitive, and social emotional health and protects children from infectious diseases and injuries (intentional and unintentional) (Hagan et al, 2008). The real value of preventive health visits may be in the monitoring, screening, and anticipatory guidance related to developmental, behavioral, and emotional issues. It is by reviewing the child's progress, offering suggestions, and validating parent's efforts that providers best assist families as they move through the school-age years.

Developmental surveillance (see Chapter 4) is an essential aspect of each contact with the school-age child because visits are less frequent during the school years. Most visits are for minor acute illnesses rather than health maintenance.

Data must be collected on the child's physical, nutritional, neurodevelopmental, psychosocial, behavioral, and emotional status during these visits. As with all children, assessment of the family system is crucial. For the school-age child, it is particularly important to evaluate how well the family nurtures the child while supporting the child's efforts to separate, become more independent, and create a unique self in the community.

The assessment process begins by building rapport with the parents and the child. Ask direct questions first to the child, encouraging him or her to share aspects of daily routines, family experiences, school activities, and sensitive developmental concerns. Parents can then be invited to expand on data collected, providing information not only about the child's abilities but also about interactions between child and parents.

SCREENING STRATEGIES FOR SCHOOL-AGE CHILDREN

Formal developmental screening tools and/or questionnaires should be used with all children (Hagan et al, 2008). These tools allow the child, parent, and teachers to provide specific information about a child's development, behaviors, and emotional status. They also document a baseline status, highlight potential need for referrals, and evaluate the effectiveness of intervention strategies. Differing parental, school, and child perceptions about specific issues may be noted. Parental reports of skills and concerns about language, fine motor, cognitive, and emotional-behavioral development are highly predictive of true problems. The information gives the provider insights into areas needing further investigation and those that may require counseling, therapy, or other intervention strategies. In addition, the *Bright Futures: Guidelines for Health Supervision of Infants, Children, and Adolescents* (3rd edition) recommends annual routine health visits for children from 5 through 12 years (Hagan et al, 2008).

Physical Development

Physical development is assessed through history taking, physical examination, and documentation of findings (Table 7-3). Growth measurements (weight, height, BMI) and blood pressure should be evaluated and compared with age-appropriate norms at each visit. Hearing and vision should be screened at routine health visits. Hemoglobin or hematocrit is done during early childhood (between 15 months and 5 years) and again during late childhood (about 13 years); girls should be screened again after beginning menstruation. Perform fasting glucose, insulin, lipid analysis; total cholesterol, and liver function tests to assess for diabetes mellitus, hyperlipidemia, and metabolic syndrome in children 4 years or older with a BMI equal to or greater than 95% or if BMI is greater than 85% and other risk factors are present such as family history of diabetes or cardiovascular disease. Lead screening should be conducted if no previous screen has been done, if a previous screen was positive, or if there is a change in risk factors (see Fig. 41-5 for lead screening criteria). Likewise, a tuberculin skin test should be performed if screening indicates risk factors (see Chapter 23). Review immunization status at all visits and update immunizations as appropriate. Tanner staging should be done at all visits because school-age children can begin pubertal changes as early as 8 years old, and some endocrine problems may emerge in the school years (see Chapters 8 and 25). If a child does not have a regular dentist, oral health screening and referral to a dental home are indicated.

Motor Skills Development

Strength and coordination can be evaluated using a systematic musculoskeletal and neurologic examination as identified in Table 7-4. Concerns about balance, coordination, strength, and mobility should be followed up depending on attention, school performance, and overall developmental function. Problems in this area may account for school performance or learning problems.

Communication and Language Development

Assessment of communication and language development is ongoing during the health care visit as the provider talks directly with the child; probes for the child's understanding (e.g., can child; follow directions? does the child understand explanations given by the provider?); listens to the child's articulation, vocabulary, sentence structure, and grammar; and notes the child's ability to interact socially with the examiner, the parent, and others. Ask the child to write something on a sheet of paper to assess writing skills. Assessment also includes reports from the parent and/or teachers.

Social and Emotional Development

Assessment of social and emotional development is an important aspect of the well-child examination because many children are affected by mental health, psychosocial problems, and risk-taking behaviors. Thirteen percent of parents with school-age children have concerns about their child even though their child functions well (Foy et al, 2010). Key components of emotional and developmental assessment include evaluation of the child's coping, mood, self-esteem, and interpersonal relationships (including parent-child, siblings, and friendships). It is also important to observe the interaction between parents and child during the examination and to examine children's roles in the family, discuss their success in making friends and working with peers, and explore their feelings of contentment and security (see Fig. 2-2 and Chapter 19).

Cognitive Development

Assessment of cognitive development is difficult in school-age children. Generally, standardized paper-and-pencil tests are more accurate than clinical judgments. Knowledge about the child's performance compared with that of peers in the classroom, the child's grades, and information from conferences with teachers provide some data. Often a psychologist performs psychological testing of the child if more definitive information is needed.

DIAGNOSTIC ASSESSMENT STRATEGIES FOR SCHOOL-AGE CHILDREN

If problems are suspected, additional testing can be performed (e.g., bone age can be determined by using x-rays of the wrist to determine epiphyseal fusion; intelligence testing establishes cognitive abilities). Further endocrine, nutrition, genetic, or other assessments may be necessary if the child does not meet the norms for physical growth.

▪ Anticipatory Guidance for School-Age Children

Anticipatory guidance involves individualized discussion with parents to help them understand, respond to, and guide their child's behavior and development. A family-centered approach that includes motivational interviewing is an effective way of eliciting the family's understanding of current risks, and negotiating a plan for behavior change (see Chapters 4 and 9). This section includes anticipatory guidance discussion points. Because children assume more responsibility for self-care as they grow, these topics should be discussed with them, as is age-appropriate. The information provided here is not intended to be used exhaustively at visits, but to illustrate how developmental concepts can be applied in everyday living. The management of problems that may be identified through this process follows in later chapters (e.g., sleep problems are discussed in Chapter 14).

PARENT DEVELOPMENT

The role of parents is central in preparing and supporting their child's transition during the school-age years. Often families have social and economic constraints as they raise their children, and parents need help to fulfill their responsibilities.

TABLE 7-3	Guidelines for the History and Physical Examination of the School-Age Child

Assessment Area	Findings
Chief Complaint	Main concern (e.g., school performance: inattention, fidgeting, difficulty completing tasks, stays on tasks forever, forgetful, angry, frustrated, poor academic performance, moody, irritable, talks excessively)
Subjective Data and History	
Birth history	Early development, including feeding, sleep-wake cycles, colicky or fussy baby, poor suck; Apgar scores; length of hospitalization; oxygen or phototherapy
Past medical history	Illnesses that may explain the child's problems (e.g., otitis media, chronic illness, vision problems, dental problems, food allergies, reflux, voiding and stooling issues, undiagnosed pain); chronic conditions such as asthma, congenital cardiac conditions, accidents, injuries, hospitalizations, or surgeries
Allergies	Type of allergies and reactions
Past development	Age attained early developmental milestones, especially language and social skills
Interim history	Onset of problem; description of when it occurs; note child's use of alcohol, drugs, and cigarettes; review of systems related to any chief complaint; any medications taken for acute or chronic conditions
Daily activities	Daily sleep-wake pattern, routines and schedule, amount of passive activities (TV and computer) vs. active play and recreational activities; note family routines, family activities, family expectations of the child, and child's ability to complete chores or jobs around the house
Temperament and personality	Identify difficulty with change and transitions, establishing routines, or finishing tasks; difficulty with mood, new situations, making or keeping friends
School history	School progress, subjects liked and disliked, peer relationships, match with teacher and school philosophy
Family history	Family and home routines and environment, family support systems, activities, involvement in social and school activities, parent's knowledge of child's friends and involvement with child's friends
Family review of systems	Family history of medical problems, congenital anomalies, ADHD, learning problems, mental retardation, autism, emotional or psychiatric problems, sleep problems, drug or alcohol abuse, diabetes, obesity, asthma or allergies, domestic violence, criminal activities
Objective Data and Physical Examination	
Measurements and vital signs	Child's growth percentiles, especially if below the 5th percentile or above the 85th percentile; note head circumference where appropriate; note BMI and blood pressure and compare with norms for age of child; hematocrit
General	Child's overall appearance, cooperation, parent-child interaction, parent's responsiveness to the child, and the child's responsiveness to the parent
Skin and lymph	Rashes, lesions, edema, and shape of the nails, hemangiomas, hirsutism, fat tissue, and skinfolds; note enlarged lymph nodes, or mottling of the skin
Head, eyes, ears, nose, mouth	*Head:* Unusual skull shape, hair swirls and unruly hair, and hairline; identify any problems with the temporomandibular joint *Face:* Flat midface, short mandible, asymmetrical facial movements, and unusual facies, fetal alcohol syndrome facies *Eyes:* Eye position (hypertelorism/hypotelorism), asymmetries, small epicanthal folds or palpebral fissures; lid: ptosis; conjunctiva: clarity; pupils: PERRLA and cover test, especially for strabismus; EOM: visual fields, nystagmus; fundus: light reflex, vessels, disc, and macula, visual acuity *Nose:* Size, shape, bridge, and anteverted nostrils *Mouth, lips, fulcrum, tongue:* Thin upper lip, micrognathia or retrognathia, long or flat philtrum, prognathism or malocclusion; tongue: fasciculations, symmetry, suck, swallow, and strength *Teeth:* Enamel, shape, dentition, and signs of bruxism *Palate:* Pharynx, palate shape, size of tonsils, movement of uvula, gag reflex *Neck:* Symmetry and strength of movement, swallow, trachea, lymph; thyroid: position, symmetry, movement
Chest	Shape, pectus excavatum, and short xiphoid
Breasts	Tanner stage; symmetry; presence of supernumerary nipples
Lungs	Inspiratory and expiratory wheezing or absence of breath sounds; peak flow if history of asthma
Cardiac	PMI, heart sounds, murmurs, and thrills; pulses: equality, symmetry, and strength

TABLE 7-3	Guidelines for the History and Physical Examination of the School-Age Child—cont'd

Assessment Area	Findings
Abdomen	Bowel sounds, abdominal shape and movements, umbilicus position, tenderness, masses, organ size, bladder or bowel distention
Musculoskeletal	Note size of muscles, symmetry, hypertonia or hypotonia, range of motion, posture, joints, dactyly *Back:* Evaluate spine for scoliosis, cysts, dimples, hair tufts, and CVA tenderness *Upper and lower extremities:* Evaluate active and passive strength (tone), symmetry, hyperextension of fingers and joints, and presence of tremors; movement: observe body while sitting, standing, running, walking, jumping, skipping, hopping, and kicking; note hip dysplasia, foot position, palmar creases, short fifth finger, incurved fifth finger, tapered phalanges, nail hypoplasia, flexion of elbow
Genitourinary, gynecologic	Evaluate anatomy and Tanner stage *Male:* Note testes size, placement; note if circumcised or not; evaluate for hydrocele, hernia, or hypospadias *Female:* Note hypoplastic labia; evaluate for hernia

ADHD, Attention-deficit/hyperactivity disorder; *BMI,* body mass index; *CVA,* costovertebral angle; *EOM,* extraocular movements; *PERRLA,* pupils equal, round, reactive to light and accommodation; *PMI,* point of maximal impulse.

TABLE 7-4	Guidelines for Neurodevelopmental Assessment of the School-Age Child

Assessment Area	Findings
Overall impression	Behavior, attention and distractibility, motor activity level, impulsivity, degree of cooperativeness, strategies for and persistence in task completion, problem-solving, organizational skills, ability to follow directions and ask for assistance.
Cerebral	Attention, behavior, orientation, cooperation, participation, and separation from parents. Are judgment, orientation, memory (short- and long-term ability to remember eight familiar objects in "memory box"), affect, and calculation age appropriate or immature?
Cranial nerves	Note any asymmetries or oral-motor dyspraxia.
Cerebellar functioning	Fine motor movements: Evaluate for dysfunctions, including problems with balance, fine motor control (rapid alternating movements), and pincer or pencil grasp. Coordination: Evaluate coordination, including balance (Romberg, balance on one foot), tandem walk (heel-toe walk), duck walk, and coordination while throwing and catching a ball (use a small ball with older children).
Sensory functioning	Evaluate problems recognizing body parts or body position, sensitivity to touch, asymmetrical or poor graphesthesia (letters or numbers) or stereognosis (objects).
Gross motor function	Evaluate overall gait, coordination for age while skipping, running, walking on balance beam. Appropriateness for age. Note posture, ability to sit straight in chair vs. leaning on desk. Ability to stand for periods of time without leaning on something.
Extraneous movement, tremors	Evaluate for synkinesis (motor overflow), dyskinesis (incomplete or fragmented movements), mild dyspraxic movements, dysdiadochokinesia (inability to perform rapid movements), motor impersistence.
Auditory perceptual abilities	Evaluate discrimination, processing, integration, memory, and comprehension of auditory information. Evaluate ability to detect changes in volume, discrimination of vowel or consonant sounds. Note directionality and consistent or inconsistent use of right or left eye, hand, foot. Note ability to remember series of spoken words and numbers forwards and backwards and ability to understand or comprehend a written paragraph. Note expressive language ability (word retrieval, formulation, and articulation). Evaluate conversation spoken spontaneously through story or history. Evaluate ability to define words appropriate for age.
Visual perceptual	Identify memory recall (short- and long-term), visual discrimination, visuospatial perception, visual memory for objects, visual discrimination of subtle differences in words (e.g., *ten* and *tin*), colors, shapes, and sizes, object assembly, and decoding.
Organization	Observe problem-solving of math problems.
Visual motor integration	Note ability to copy a design (+, 0, square, or triangle) and handwriting. Evaluate picture of a person and coordination drawn by the child for age appropriateness.
Learning style	Evaluate concrete and abstract thinking, sequential or stimulus processing, thought integration, perseveration, ritual and routine; control; adaptation to changes; modulation of behaviors; exaggeration (overdo or underdo) activities.

Parents welcome the support, suggestions, and connection to resources that providers can give them.

A child's entry into school can be emotionally stressful for parents because they must adjust to a new social situation, routine, and a changing relationship with their child. Some parents feel that they have "lost" their child, watching him or her move from dependence on the family to participation in a new world of which the parent is not a part. Other parents anticipate the new opportunities facing the child and family and are ready to help their child cope with challenges that emerge in the school environment. Parents need to support the school's standards, and research indicates that parents' education expectations for their children help determine the child's school success (Dubow et al, 2009). Parents also have a responsibility to provide an environment that reinforces their children's educational efforts; research indicates that frequent television viewing, little parental control of media content, and viewing of R-rated movies damage children's school performance (Sharif and Sargent, 2006).

The Internet and other forms of technology introduce new risks for school-age children. With the widespread availability of social networking websites and cell phones, Internet safety is becoming a growing concern for school-age youth. Although these technologies allow expanded opportunities to practice newly acquired social skills, they can also be used negatively (e.g., bullying and sexual exploitation). There is growing evidence that bullying and peer pressure outside of school now largely occur through electronic devices like computers and cell phones. Research suggests that the greatest risks for Internet-initiated victimization are family-conflict, depression, conversing with unknown people about sex, sending personal information to strangers, and being a victim of child abuse (Noll et al, 2008). Other risky child behaviors include visiting chat rooms, participating in activities with provocatively dressed avatars, and being solicited sexually online. Studies suggest that youth who experience higher rates of online sexual advances are more likely to agree to offline meetings. Many reported sex crimes stemming from online interactions involve youth who are aware that the other person is older, who engage in online discussion of sexual activity, and who know the meeting would involve sexual activity. Parents need to monitor Internet sites that their children access and discuss with their children the dangers of offline meetings with people met online (Noll et al, 2009). Software programs are available to assist parents to monitor their child's Internet and cell phone communication.

As children move through the years from 6 to 12, parents continue to extend freedoms and add new responsibilities. They need to provide opportunities that allow children to experience and master new challenges and adjust family patterns of nutrition, sleep, activities, health maintenance, safety, and communication to fit with the child's needs and emerging skills. Resiliency and coping are learned skills, and it is important that parents understand that learning occurs in both failure and success. Parents need to be available to children to ensure the child has both the social and emotional skills essential to move into and succeed in school and community environments.

REGULATION AND SLEEP-WAKE PATTERNS

Family routines provide a support to the daily life of the child and help the child self-regulate. If children have routines that they can rely on, they are more comfortable exploring new areas and trying new skills. Family routines strengthen the relationship between parent and child, provide family stability and continuity, and serve as a buffer during times of change and transition. Strong family relationships are protective against divorce, alcoholism, substance abuse, and violence. Suggestions the provider can make to parents include the following:

- Encourage the family to establish and recognize traditions or family activities that are special (e.g., birthday celebrations, Sunday afternoon walks, videos, and popcorn on Saturday night).
- Help parents explore ways to adapt the child's new schedule in an effort to maintain previous routines or readjust routines to meet the new schedule (e.g., if the child must meet a school bus at an early hour, making a school lunch the night before can become part of a new evening routine).

School-age children who do not receive adequate sleep often demonstrate irritability, fatigue, poor attention, and poor learning. Bedtime is still difficult, and delay tactics are not uncommon. Parents can be encouraged to do the following:

- Continue a regular nighttime routine to transition from active daytime play to evening quiet play. Consistency between workweek and weekend bedtimes is important.
- Encourage reading at bedtime. School-agers will transition from parents reading to them to the child independently reading.
- Set a regular time for morning awakening, giving the child extra time to come fully awake without being rushed.
- Minimize stimulation (e.g., no scary television programs) before bedtime.

STRENGTH AND MOTOR COORDINATION

Because of the maturity of the central nervous system and cognitive advances, most children are physically capable. Most enjoy playing hard so that they can develop physical skills, strength, and coordination. Parents can support this growth if they do the following:

- Encourage children's participation in daily exercise.
- Provide for activities that are fun, involve family or peers, and require cognitive or social skills, including rules, strategies, and skills.
- Include children's friends in family activities (e.g., hiking, skiing, swimming).
- Support children's interest in preferred physical activities that are healthful; personal achievement in an activity helps develop healthy self-image.
- Encourage hobbies and activities that foster fitness and increased motor skills.
- Encourage activities that require training, commitment, and effort, especially for older children.
- Help children prevent the stress of over scheduling.
- Limit activities that include TV, video games, or computer time to no more than 2 hours a day.
- Let the children "own" the activity (e.g., Little League baseball games should be fun for the children, not a contest among parents over whose child is the best).
- Explore ways children with physical limitations can participate in preferred activities and with their peers (see Chapter 13 on the health care for the young athlete regarding Special Olympics sports activities for families and children with physical challenges).

NUTRITION, SELF-CARE, AND SAFETY
Nutrition
School-age children have good appetites and many are overweight or obese, so careful assessment of nutrition is important. Diets can be deficient in iron, calcium, or vitamin C, and high-fat snack foods can become a habit. School-age children need to learn to choose nutritious foods while away from home and to try new foods. Because food is not readily available all day at school, eating well at breakfast and dinner becomes especially important. High-calorie snacks and other high-calorie foods have contributed to obesity in school-age children; nearly 35% are overweight (Ogden et al, 2010), and monitoring and weight control programs are needed at earlier ages (see Chapter 10). Parents should be advised to do the following:
- Ensure that the child has three nutritious meals and two nutritious snacks daily.
- Know that food jags are common.
- Establish an eating routine, with at least one daily meal together as a family. Maintain family meals as much as possible to preserve family time and share interests and experiences from the day's activities.
- Monitor food choices and opportunities to determine best foods.
- Teach children to understand the importance of eating healthy foods.
- Encourage participation in meal planning, food shopping and selection, and meal preparation.
- Discuss making nutritious choices at fast-food restaurants and when "on the go."

Self-Care
For school-age children, learning to take responsibility for their own health begins with simple goals and moves to more complex decision-making strategies. For example, children may begin by deciding to have a fruit or vegetable at each meal and then progress to helping plan some meals and participate in their preparation. Other areas in which children take increasing responsibility are dental health, hygiene and grooming, snacking, and exercise. Children at this age see health in positive terms and equate it with being able to participate in desired activities. Parents can do the following things to assist the child's achievement in self-care:
- Explain the relationship between good health and self-care.
- Supervise personal hygiene such as brushing teeth, combing hair, and doing nail care; for older school children, supervision is minimal, with an occasional reminder.
- Set clear limits on expectations for cleanliness, healthy exercise, hours of sleep, and other health-promotion behaviors.
- Recognize that children may be "noncompliant" as a means of exerting independence; a discussion about decision-making and healthy choices may be needed to resolve the issue.
- Be flexible.
- Provide children with opportunities to experiment with appropriate healthy behaviors that allow them to develop self-expression (e.g., school-age children can enjoy new hairstyles or having their hair dyed).
- Encourage shared decision-making and self-care during illnesses and for chronic disease management.
- Give children an opportunity to ask questions about sexuality, drugs, alcohol, and tobacco; encourage discussion about these topics as a family; teach about puberty changes.
- Model healthy behaviors.

Safety
Unintentional injuries are common among school-age children. Often their growing bodies allow them to get themselves into situations that they cannot get out of without help. They need guidance and direction to be safe and make safe choices. Although parents do not provide the constant supervision they did for toddlers and preschoolers, it is important that they work with their school-age child to ensure safety. The health care provider can give guidance to parents and encourage them to do the following:
- Help children learn "survival skills" (e.g., name, telephone number, address, use of 911, how to ask adults for help, what to do if lost).
- Require use of protective gear when riding bicycles, skateboards, or scooters.
- Require seatbelts and use booster seats.
- Encourage use of sunscreen (sun protection factor 15 or higher) before going outside to play.
- Teach children to swim, but always supervise their activities near water.
- Educate children about physical and social hazards (e.g., pedestrian traffic on busy streets; facts about pregnancy, intercourse, and sexually transmitted diseases; what to do if they find a weapon or syringe).
- Monitor children's use of website chat rooms; limit access with use of parental filters. Control children's access to TV programming with use of V-chip.
- Monitor TV, video, cell phone, instant messaging, and Internet use.
- Use security tools to protect children from instant messages and IP addresses of strangers on the Internet.
- Educate children on the use of the Internet as an opportunity, not a right.
- Get rid of firearms or ensure that they are unloaded and locked, with ammunition in a different location.
- Help children to think about safety aspects of activities; talk about safety.

COMMUNICATION AND LANGUAGE
Mastering the ability to read, comprehend, and write is essential for the school-age child's academic success. Parents can help children learn these skills by doing the following:
- Provide structured time and space for children to complete school writing and reading assignments.
- Read stories to children; even older children enjoy listening to stories that are exciting or relevant to them.
- Listen to the child read aloud.
- Role model by reading and writing often.
- Encourage the child to make notes, keep a journal, and write letters to friends and family members. Skill with writing supports reading and vice versa.
- Play word games with the child (e.g., finding all the things that "start with B" while on a road trip can entertain a

6-year-old; Junior Scrabble or Boggle is fun for older children). Let the child lead the play; the parent should not be "out to win," and the child should not be made to feel inadequate for not knowing everything.
- Talk with the child and actively listen as the child talks.
- Enroll the child in structured, voluntary afterschool programs that offer an opportunity to engage in active conversation with other children and adults (Mahoney et al, 2010).
- Never punish a child by removing books or writing materials.
- Limit TV, computer activities, and video games to 1 to 2 hours per day.

SOCIAL AND EMOTIONAL GROWTH

Finding support in the family system and peer group while establishing individuality and independence is the hallmark of successful social and emotional growth for the school-age child. Siblings and parents fulfill a crucial role in contributing to social and emotional growth of children through their roles, relationships, and activities in everyday life (Tucker and Updegraff, 2009). Providers can help foster that growth by encouraging parents to do the following:
- Negotiate goals and priorities with the child.
- Enhance goal setting with charts, calendars, and tally sheets. Care should be taken not to reward children too much because this can decrease motivation. Let children set goals while parents monitor activities and point out options.
- Appreciate the products of the child's work at home and at school; encourage successful activities.
- Provide positive expressions of love, concern, and pride to promote a sense of belonging to the family.
- Share family history and visits with relatives to help children be proud of their heritage.
- Help children feel that the home base is secure to increase their confidence as they move into other domains.
- Make home rules and expectations clear and use consistency in applying them.
- Discuss family values and rules and explain the differences that the child may face when away from home.
- Play and work together as a family to teach children how to work together with their classmates and to function as a team; children should maintain their responsibilities to the family (e.g., jobs or chores around the house).
- Provide opportunities for children to make and develop friendships with a variety of children, teaching them how to initiate, sustain, and terminate relationships with friends.
- Include the child's friends in some activities and outings.
- Teach children how to read social cues.
- Provide social skills training and supervise experiences in which children can practice new skills successfully.
- Help children learn to communicate well with other adults.
- Teach respect for authority and rules away from home.
- Help children identify and appropriately express their emotions.
- Provide fantasy play opportunities to allow children to deal safely with their emotions and concerns and to develop their creativity.
- Provide guidance about how to appropriately express feelings of aggression and emerging sexuality; discuss sexual values.

- Help children with decision-making and accepting consequences of actions.
- Model positive conflict resolution and good communication.
- Teach anger management and conflict-resolution skills.
- Help children learn delayed gratification and increase their frustration tolerance, while still remaining sympathetic.
- Provide children with opportunities for appropriate behavior when values are challenged (e.g., "You can say, 'No, my mom won't let me do that,' and then walk away").
- Recognize that parents are role models and that children internalize parental values as they begin to form a conscience.
- Recognize that children may identify with a special person, such as a movie star or athlete.
- Recognize that having a strong sense of self-esteem helps "inoculate" children against some of the negative peer pressures they may experience.
- Monitor activities on social networking sites.
- Set and adhere to rules for Internet use and social networking sites both inside and outside the home.
- Set aside time to listen to the child talk about how his or her day went. Talk about things that went well and those that went poorly.

COGNITIVE AND ENVIRONMENTAL STIMULATION

School is a major source of intellectual stimulation and an arena in which the child experiences cognitive growth. Expectations for performance increase over the school years with examinations, graded papers, and homework assignments. Reading becomes a tool to attain and master knowledge rather than being an end in itself. Thus poor readers begin to experience broader academic failure and can become increasingly frustrated. Unless these children are provided with social and remedial support, they may see school as an unpleasant burden, develop feelings of failure, and look for validation through nonacademic experiences. Social supports can help children cope with this stress, and interacting with healthy, interested, and caring adults is the strongest support children can have. The family also provides the child with stimulation for cognitive growth. Parents can be counseled to do the following:
- Read to the child and have the child read to the parent.
- Establish and build trust with children through joint use of computers and online activities.
- Stimulate the younger child's thinking about comparisons and differences (e.g., changes in shape and volume of objects; directions to and from school) to facilitate cognition at the concrete operations level.
- Discuss variables in objects or situations as experienced, seen on television, or read about to help move the child's thinking away from the earlier egocentric style.
- Provide opportunities to gain knowledge through books, outings, classes, and family discussions.
- Engage children in experiences with other languages, music, and cultural groups.
- Explore and explain the environment and community to the child to promote broader understanding of the world.
- Establish a regular homework time and place to help the child maximize time for cognitive practice.
- Establish an environment that encourages children to focus and complete tasks with limits clearly defined.

- Provide help early if children experience school problems to lessen secondary problems with emotions and conflict.
- Volunteer at the child's school or participate in school activities for parents.
- Recognize academic achievement because success motivates further work.
- Stay involved with school assignments and evaluate progress to support the child's work.
- Encourage problem-solving efforts.
- Provide more complex opportunities to plan and complete projects that use skills learned at school, such as planning and cooking meals, planning family outings, and managing money and a budget.

■ Common Developmental Issues for School-Age Children

SCHOOL READINESS

Description

School readiness is a complex concept that depends on a child's physical, cognitive, and emotional development, and how well the child's developmental abilities match with the school and family environment and expectations. School entrance is currently based on chronologic rather than developmental age. What children bring with them from other life experiences to their school years either enhances or inhibits their capacity to learn (McAllister et al, 2005). School entry is stressful for all children, but immature children have increased stress because the expectations for performance are beyond their abilities; they may not have adequate coping resources. Children who lack necessary skills to meet school demands and expectations may be unsuccessful, and early school failure can lead to significant negative consequences. Health care providers have a responsibility to work with parents and their communities to promote optimal development and school readiness for children.

School participation requires skills to perform self-care, interact with a variety of new people, act with a sense of responsibility, and emotionally separate from the family and home base. Children need to meet school standards, which may be different from those at home. There is a social expectation to gain an awareness of "the group"—an ability to go along with the group while meeting some personal needs through the group's achievements.

Studies conducted in the early 1990s indicated that teachers believed up to 35% of children were not ready for school due to deficiencies in language, emotional maturity, general knowledge, social confidence, and physical maturity (Boyer, 1993). More recent studies indicate that many parents have ambivalent attitudes toward the schools that their children attend and do not feel that the schools have the capacity to meet children's educational needs (McAllister et al, 2005). Socially and economically disadvantaged children are at greatest risk for difficulties. Head Start or comparable early childhood education experiences have been shown to improve school readiness in these high-risk populations (Bierman et al, 2008). Attention to social and emotional factors and to nurturing relationships in the life of a child facilitate healthy child development and foster school success (Currie, 2005).

Children who are not ready to begin school should not be kept out of school waiting for maturation. Rather, schools, health care providers, and parents need to help provide remedial activities to promote readiness, diagnose learning disabilities and developmental delays, and find alternative methodologies to assist the child to "catch up." Community education systems and developmental specialists can help support parents in this process.

Clinical Findings

History

- *Child experiences:* Evaluate opportunities for participating in activities away from home, following directions, playing with other children, habits, and interest in school.
- *Parents and family:* Assess the parents' feelings about their child entering school. What do they think their child will experience at school (e.g., racism, bullying, teachers who do not recognize or appreciate their child's unique strengths)? What do they think the school will expect of their child (e.g., to be appropriately sociable, to sit still, to learn quickly)? Do they think their child will be able to handle the demands of school? Do they think that the chosen school can meet the child's needs? Reluctance on the parents' part may be communicated to their child. Ask what parents have done to prepare their child for school. Ask about family activities, sibling school experiences, traumatic events, or separation on the part of the child or parents. Communicate that parent expectation is the strongest predictor of school success.
- *Home environment:* Inquire about daily routines, family activities together, and parent- versus child-initiated activities for learning.
- *Developmental progress:* Ask about the child's developmental opportunities and skills in communicating needs, fine motor and gross motor activities, behaviors, fears, separation from parents, and play with other children.
- *Other issues:* Ask about other concerns (e.g., chronic illness, economic issues, homelessness, family stressors) that might compromise regular school attendance or school success.

Physical Examination.
The child should have a complete physical examination with special focus on the following:

- Neurologic development, including sensory, cognitive, and language
- Height, weight, BMI, blood pressure
- Dental health
- Immunization status

Diagnostic Tests

- Hearing
- Vision
- Hematocrit
- Lead screening, if indicated

Other Testing or Evaluations

Developmental Evaluation. Normative skills are included in Table 7-5.

Ancillary Studies. Screening tests to evaluate school readiness have established norms and are generally reliable in predicting developmental outcomes. They should be used to consider all areas of readiness (social, behavioral, cognitive) and to provide an explanation of readiness for parents. Test results should be evaluated in conjunction with history, observation, family situation, and previous experiences.

TABLE 7-5	Basic First-Grade School Readiness Skills	

Skills to Assess	Criteria
Language skills	Counts 10 or more objects Uses complete sentences of at least 5 words Uses future tense Gives first and last name Recognizes 4 colors Defines 5 to 7 words Communicates needs Recalls parts of a story Follows 3-part commands Understands number concepts
Personal and social skills	Separates easily from parent Dresses without supervision Plays interactively with other children Has toilet skills Follows instructions Feels support from other adults
Fine motor and adaptive skills	Copies geometric shapes (circle, square, triangle) Draws a person (6 parts with distinct body) Prints some letters Classifies similar objects
Gross motor skills	Hops on one foot Catches bounced ball Walks backward heel to toe Balances on each foot 6 seconds

Management

Preventive strategies for high-risk children begin before the school-age years and include enrollment in preschool, interactive reading with the child from an early age to promote language mastery, increased time for young children to play with peers and engage in creative play activities, and interaction with caring adults (Byrd, 2005).

Ensuring school readiness involves sharing data with school counselors and teachers, parents, and primary care providers, and offering anticipatory guidance in the following areas:

- Teach and encourage parents to assist their child with skills that will be needed for school (e.g., knowing colors and numbers, behavioral expectations).
- Encourage parents to visit the school, meet the teacher, and discuss their child's characteristics with the teacher.
- Instruct parents to rehearse school activities with their child before school begins (e.g., getting to school, finding class, eating meals, going to the bathroom, asking for help, getting home, and following the rules).
- Help parents deal with their own stress of separation. Review the child's expectations for school and identify what will be new and different.
- Provide parents with available community and school resources they may need to access to meet the developmental needs of their child.

- Encourage children to start school with their developmental-appropriate group. Children who are not ready often need extra support at school or home to assist with skill remediation.
- Be an advocate for parents and children with identified deficits to ensure that the school adequately assesses both strengths and weaknesses of children and develops a program of study (e.g., an individual education plan [IEP]) that maximizes children's strengths.
- Counsel parents that deficits in a child's readiness may occur even with the best of parenting.
- Develop a "catch-up" or "tutorial plan" with parents to address deficits in a comprehensive way while preserving the child's self-esteem.
- Monitor the child's progress through the year, advocating as necessary.

LEARNING PROBLEMS
Description

Learning problems can be a hidden handicap that appears during the school-age years. The ability to manage school learning expectations requires growth in four areas: basic processing of information, memorization, increased attention span and recall of important events, and beginning problem-solving skills.

Knowledge (the sum of what children know) rapidly expands as a result of schoolwork, experiences at home, and activities with friends. The organization of knowledge improves as school-age children grow older and integrates knowledge into existing concepts. Self-awareness, reflected by children's ability to predict performance, develops slowly and in areas in which children have the most knowledge.

Although children with learning problems generally have difficulties with basic thinking skills, they may have specific problems in linguistic skills, attention, and organizational skills; higher cognitive functions, such as memory and sensory function; motor capacities; visuospatial analysis and neuromotor function; and social awareness and behavior (Kelly, 2007).

Clinical Findings

History. A complete in-depth history is needed to determine underlying or related issues that may cause or complicate learning difficulties. The history should also examine how a child's learning difficulties affect the child's life. Finally, it should identify areas of strength on which the child and family can build strategies for managing the learning difficulties. The history includes the following:

- *Medical history:* Prenatal history (including exposure to drugs and alcohol and maternal infection), neonatal history, recurrent or chronic medical conditions such as otitis media, allergies, medications (including in utero exposure), hospitalizations, syndromes; congenital, neurologic, metabolic, or endocrine conditions; current illnesses; vision and hearing problems, fetal alcohol spectrum disorder (the leading cause of preventable mental retardation in the U.S. [USDHHS and SAMHSA, 2006]); history of accidents, concussions, or other brain injury
- *Developmental history:* Achievement or regression of developmental milestones, especially in language; experiences for achieving developmental skills at home or in

preschool, daily routines, and preferred play activities; temperament and behavioral concerns of the parents; ability of the child to handle transitions and change; child's initiation of activities versus parent-guided activities; repetitive behaviors
- *Family medical history:* Family history of difficulties in school or school dropout, learning difficulties, attention-deficit/hyperactivity disorder (ADHD) or attention-deficit disorder (ADD), mental retardation, genetic disorders, and overall family members' functioning, substance abuse
- *Family social history:* Problem-solving and decision-making skills, use of community resources, financial resources, family stressors, substance abuse, homelessness, violence, criminal behavior

Physical Examination. A complete physical examination, with special attention to the neurodevelopmental assessment (see Table 7-4) should be performed.

Diagnostic Testing or Evaluations
- *School records:* Information needs to be obtained from the school system to evaluate the child's school performance and standardized testing results. Testing provides a picture of the child's strengths and weaknesses, revealing the cognitive styles that teachers and parents will be most successful in tapping. The Pediatric Examination of Educational Readiness at Middle Childhood (PEERAMID-2), a neurodevelopmental examination for 9- to 14-year-olds, may be administered (see Box 7-1) (Levine, 1995).
- *Psychological testing:* The school may or may not have the capacity for psychological evaluations. Often parents must ask for this, and they may need to seek outside evaluations. Schools are required, under U.S. Public Law 94–142, to provide appropriate education to all children identified with developmental delays.
- *Cognitive testing:* The school's ability to provide cognitive and learning evaluations may be limited, and some school districts do not recognize dyslexia as a learning disorder, requiring the parents to seek outside testing. An evaluation for a learning disorder is not complete without this information.
- *Developmental assessment:* A multidisciplinary developmental evaluation through a developmental program may be needed to provide the most appropriate plan of care for an individual child. Additional testing may be recommended such as genetic testing with chromosome studies, brain scans, or endocrine and metabolic testing.

Differential Diagnosis
The following diagnoses need to be considered in children with learning problems:
- Vision problems
- Hearing problems
- Mental retardation—genetic syndrome, neurologic insult, or malformation
- Cognitive developmental delay
- Speech or language delay
- Depression
- ADHD
- Autism spectrum disorder
- Toxin-related delay (e.g., lead, fetal alcohol syndrome and fetal alcohol effects, other intrauterine substance exposure)

- Medication-related delay (e.g., anticonvulsant, antihistamine)
- Neurologic problems
- Traumatic brain injury
- Dyslexia

Management
Providers can encourage parents to obtain an early diagnosis and identify and access appropriate school programs. Some children qualify for special educational support through IEPs. Parents need to review educational plans, provide an environment rich with experiences for children, and set realistic goals. They also need to act as advocates for their children during every school year because classrooms and teachers change. Parents should work to correct secondary problems, such as poor self-esteem, hopelessness, or depression. Finally, parents need to be encouraged to avoid the use of the many unsubstantiated cures for learning disabilities (see Chapter 15 for further discussion of ADHD and other cognitive-perceptual problems).

SCHOOL REFUSAL (PHOBIA)
Description
School refusal is a generic term that was introduced in the 1970s to describe children's resistance to attending school. The prevalence ranges from 0.4% to 18% of all school-age children. School refusal includes, but is not limited to, separation anxiety disorder, simple and social phobias, and depression (see Chapter 19). Younger children with school refusal are more likely to have separation anxiety disorder, whereas older children are more likely to have generalized anxiety or school phobia. The criteria for a diagnosis include the following: (1) severe difficulty attending school or refusal to attend school; (2) severe emotional upset when attempting to go to school; (3) absence of significant antisocial disorders; and (4) staying at home with the parent's knowledge (Stafford et al, 2007). Children may request to stay home from school with a variety of physical complaints, including stomachaches, headaches, dizziness, fatigue, or a combination of these. The symptoms gradually improve as the day progresses and often disappear on weekends. Unexcused school absences peak with the beginning of school attendance and again at 11 to 12 years old. As many as one third of children who present with school phobia have a comorbid condition such as depressive disorder, ADHD, or conduct disorder (Bernstein, 2008). Recent research suggests that etiologic differences may exist between school refusal and school phobia, establishing the need for distinguishing between these when developing treatment regimens (Dube and Ortinas, 2009; Kearney, 2007).

Clinical Findings
History. Because child, parent, family, and school environmental factors may all play into the causes of school refusal, an in-depth history exploring these areas is needed. Specific areas include the following:
- Frequent somatic complaints or sleep difficulties
- Parents' ambivalent feelings about children's attendance at school, evidence of overindulgence or overprotection
- Difficult home situation (e.g., children may try to stay at home to care for a chronically ill parent or may have a substance-abusing parent who is not attending to the child's academic needs)

- Recent or anticipated loss or separation
- School environment and evidence of bullying, violence, humiliation, lack of privacy (in bathroom especially), mismatch with teacher

Physical Examination. A complete physical examination and any indicated laboratory testing should be done to rule out organic disease.

Diagnostic Testing and Evaluations. Laboratory testing that is symptom specific, noninvasive, and cost effective to rule out organic disease is appropriate to assure child and parents that the problem is taken seriously. Both parent and child may then be more willing to accept the lack of organic disease and work toward addressing the underlying psychological issues and cooperating in the development of a treatment plan.

- Depression and anxiety questionnaires (also see Chapter 19)
- ADHD evaluation tools (see Chapter 15)

Differential Diagnosis

- *Anxiety disorder:* This is the most common reason for school refusal, usually manifesting as an inability to cope with anxiety, especially anxiety stemming from separation.
- *Somatic illness or over response to minor illness:* Avoid provider overresponse with excessive diagnostic testing.
- *Depression:* Isolation from peers, withdrawal from activities, sleep disturbances, erratic moods, poor self-esteem, and decreased activity level
- *ADHD and conduct disorder:* Children who are unsuccessful in school, either academically or socially, may try to withdraw from the school environment.
- *Sexual or physical abuse:* Children who are being abused or who experience violence either at home or at school can feel intimidated to the point that they refuse to attend school.
- Chronic physical illness with poor adaptation
- Learning disability with poor adaptation
- Pregnancy
- Substance abuse in the family
- Parental criminal activity
- Family stressors (e.g., divorce or other significant stressors)
- Family dysfunction
- Truancy

Management

Intervention is generally successful when behavioral measures are combined with supportive counseling of parents. The physical complaints must be reasonably evaluated to rule out organic disease without excessive medical attention or diagnostic testing. Once the possibility of organic disease is set aside (or a plan is established to evaluate somatic problems), children must go to school. Generally, once they are at school, symptoms resolve.

- Support parents in getting children to school and insist on full attendance. Success often follows a calm but firm approach.
- Notify school personnel and encourage them to support and expect children's attendance and intervene to improve any situation related to children's anxiety. Positive reinforcement of school attendance is important (Kearney, 2007).

- Assess home situation and identify issues that must be handled. Provide referrals as needed for family and parent problems for counseling, social service, or other resources. Notify child protection services in the case of threat of harm from parental inability to provide for adequate supervision and needs.
- Refer for psychiatric care if no improvement occurs within 2 weeks.
- Criteria for mental health referral include the following:
  o Unresponsive to pediatric management
  o Out of school for 2 weeks
  o Psychosis
  o Depression
  o Panic reactions
  o Parental inability to cooperate with plan

■ Red Flags for School-Age Children

School-age children have unique personalities and characteristics, differ by ages and developmental stages, and are strongly influenced by the environments in which they live. Because every child and family is different, it can be difficult to say that a particular behavior is "abnormal" or "problematic." Developmentally, school-age children are explorers, and their exploration can lead them to engage in risk-taking behaviors that jeopardize their health (e.g., climbing or playing in unsafe environments or without safety gear; experimenting with smoking or drinking). Research shows that temperament plays a role in risk-taking behaviors, and boys engage in risky behaviors more than girls (Cartland and Ruch-Ross, 2006). Providers need to be aware of these risk-taking behaviors and use opportunities to teach children and their families how to prevent health problems while still encouraging learning and development. Some children demonstrate behavior that is beyond "normal" risk-taking, however, and providers must be alert to "red flags" that place a child at risk for developmental delay and school failure. Table 7-6 outlines red flags in five developmental areas: psychosocial and emotional, cognitive and visual, language and hearing, fine motor, and gross motor for children 6 to 12 years old.

Providers must work with children and their families to identify red flags at an early stage, ensure appropriate and comprehensive evaluation (e.g., medical, psychological, educational), and intervene to prevent further problems. Often the primary care provider's role is one of support and advocacy, whereas special education teachers or psychologists may do actual interventions. In situations in which the child has been referred, the primary care provider has a crucial role collaborating with other professionals to ensure that children and families receive necessary services.

School readiness, learning problems, and school phobia present challenges for school-age children. Assessment of school readiness, screening for early detection of learning problems, and efforts aimed at prevention and/or early detection of issues such as school phobia can best ensure the success of children in school. Once problems are identified, designing interventions through cooperative efforts of providers, families, and school personnel will optimize outcomes of learning and help ensure future success for children.

TABLE 7-6	Developmental Red Flags: School-Age Child				
Age	**Psychosocial and Emotional Skill**	**Cognitive and Visual Abilities**	**Language and Hearing**	**Fine Motor**	**Gross Motor**
6 years	Problems with peer relationships Latchkey: stays home alone Unable to state special quality about self Flat affect, depression, withdrawn Cruelty to animals, friends Interest in fires or fire setting	School problems with grades, behavior, interest in school Unable to sit still in class Unable to give age Watching TV more Unable to name interests	Language partially unintelligible Unable to read simple phrases Unable to relate simple story	Unable to copy "+" Picture of self includes fewer than 8 parts Unable to print name Unable to copy a diamond and square	Unable to catch a ball Unable to walk a straight line
8 years	Lack of hobbies Lack of best friend Cruelty to animals, friends Interest in fires or fire setting Flat affect, depression, withdrawn Defiant attitude	Unable to state days of the week Unable to add and subtract Unable to identify right and left	Problems with reading and math	Unable to tie shoes Picture of self includes fewer than 12 to 16 parts Difficulty holding pencil with penmanship	Poor coordination, endurance, strength
10 years	Lack of team sports or extracurricular activities at school Lacks understanding of rules Poor peer influence, interest in gangs Cruelty to animals, friends Interest in fires or fire setting Flat affect, depression, withdrawn	Lack of operational thinking: cause and effect, relationships of whole and parts, nonegocentric thinking	Problems understanding, following through with verbal instructions	Difficulty with penmanship or cursive writing	Problems throwing or catching
12 years	Risk-taking behaviors: smoking, alcohol, sex Inappropriate for age sexual behavior Cruelty to animals, friends Interest in fires or fire setting Flat affect, depression, withdrawn Defiant, rebellious attitude	Difficulty with school work Lack of organizational skills for homework	Problems with reading comprehension	Difficulties doing paper-and-pencil tasks	Unable to list strengths and physical things he or she likes to do

Developmental Management of Adolescents

DAWN LEE GARZON AND ARDYS M. DUNN

The changes a young person experiences during the transition from childhood to young adulthood are dramatic. The extent of physiologic growth and maturation rivals that occurring during infancy. Social and psychological changes are also extreme and can create a tenuous sense of balance during this phase of development. The common question on the minds of most adolescents is "Am I normal?" Reassurance and information about what to expect as they grow during well-child care are among the most valuable services a health care provider can offer the adolescent. This chapter focuses on the normal physical and psychosocial growth and development of adolescents and provides practitioners with a framework for structuring care of the adolescent client.

■ Development of Adolescents

Puberty is the term for the biologic process that ultimately leads to fertility. The hormonal regulatory systems in the hypothalamus, pituitary, gonads, and adrenal glands undergo major changes between the prepubertal and adult states. Accompanying these changes are rapid growth in height and weight, development of secondary sex characteristics, and onset of fertility (Fig. 8-1) (see Chapters 25 and 35). Normal development can be difficult to define and is, at best, an approximation rather than a precise parameter. However, even though the timing (tempo) of adolescent development is variable, the sequence of events is orderly (Fig. 8-2).

Adolescence refers to the psychosocial and emotional transition from childhood to adulthood. The physical changes of puberty are accompanied by significant cognitive and psychosocial development that affects how adolescents view themselves and how the world views adolescents. Successful development in adolescence culminates in achievement of goals that can provide the basis for a healthy and productive adult life (Table 8-1).

PHYSICAL DEVELOPMENT

Tanner Stages

Pubertal growth and maturation can be divided into five stages ranging from prepubertal (sexual maturity rating [SMR] 1) to adult (SMR 5). These divisions are termed *Tanner stages* (Tanner, 1962) (Figs. 8-3 and 8-4). Pubertal changes occur on a continuum, with individual differences in timing or tempo.

Female Stages. Females enter puberty earlier than males do, and their puberty usually progresses sequentially in the following pattern:

- Ovaries increase in size; no visible body changes occur.
- Breast budding (thelarche) traditionally occurs between 9 and 10 years old, with 95% of normal girls having initial breast development between 9 and 13 years old (Hagan et al, 2008). Evidence indicates that adolescent girls are entering and completing puberty younger than girls did 50 years ago (Euling et al, 2008). Most girls (85%) experience the development of breast buds approximately 6 months before the appearance of pubic hair. Girls of African descent are more likely to develop pubic hair (adrenarche) before or at the same time as breast budding, whereas Caucasian girls typically have thelarche before adrenarche (Herman-Giddens, 2006). The timing of onset of breast development in females has no relationship to breast size at the completion of puberty.
- Rapid linear growth usually begins shortly after the onset of breast budding and reaches its peak about a year later. Most girls experience peak height velocity (PHV) about 6 to 12 months before menarche, generally between 11 and 12 years old, and PHV is completed by about 13 years old. Early developers may experience a height spurt between 9 and 10 years old, whereas late developers may not experience a height spurt until between 13 and 14 years old. Final height is determined by the amount of bone growth at the epiphyses of the long bones. Growth stops when hormonal factors shut down the epiphyseal plates.

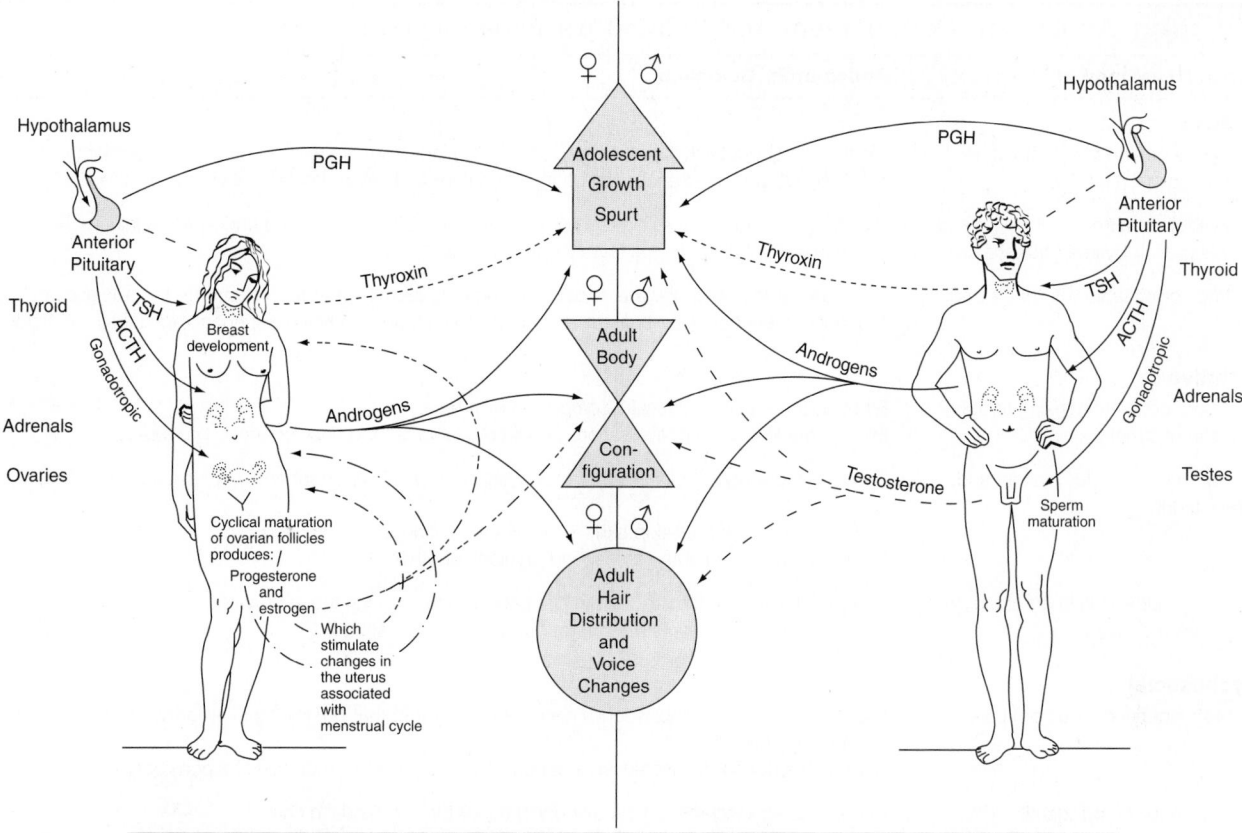

FIGURE 8-1 The endocrine system at puberty. *ACTH,* Adrenocorticotropic hormone; *PGH,* pituitary growth hormone; *TSH,* thyroid-stimulating hormone. (From Valadian I, Porter D: *Physical growth and development from conception to maturity,* Boston, 1977, Little, Brown.)

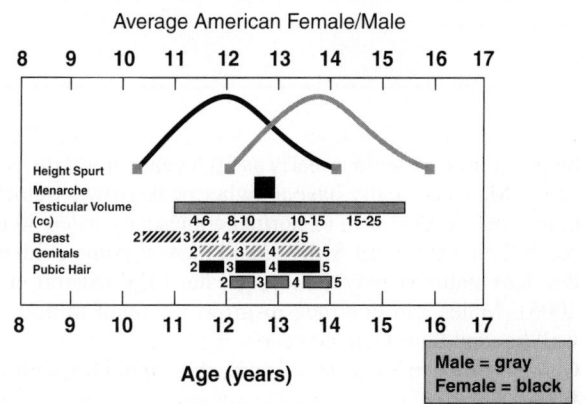

FIGURE 8-2 Sequence of pubertal events. Breast, genital, and pubic hair development indicate Tanner stages 2 to 5. (Adapted from Division of Adolescent Medicine, Children's Hospital Medical Center, Cincinnati, OH, 1995.)

- Appearance of pubic hair (adrenarche or pubarche) commences at about 11.5 years old and is related to adrenal rather than gonadal development, not to thelarche; therefore, it is less valid than other secondary sex characteristics in assessing sexual maturation.
- The first menstrual period (menarche) occurs, on average, at 12.5 years old. More than 95% of girls experience menarche between 10.5 and 14.5 years old. The mean age of

menarche is highly dependent on ethnic, socioeconomic, and nutritional factors. Menarche generally occurs 1.5 to 2.5 years after thelarche. It may be 18 to 24 months after menarche before females establish regular ovulatory cycles. To some degree, menstrual cycles can be affected by the athletic activity of the female. The American Academy of Pediatrics and the American College of Obstetrics and Gynecology recommend that health care providers recognize the menstrual cycle as a "vital sign" because of the need for education regarding normal timing and characteristics of menstruation and other pubertal signs (Hagan et al, 2008).

Changes in the body composition of females occur during puberty, and adolescent girls will benefit from the primary health care provider's reassurance that these changes are normal. Initial breast development usually begins as a unilateral disk-like subareolar swelling, and many adolescents and parents may initially present with concerns about breast tumors. Girls often have asymmetric breasts and need assurance that breasts become more or less the same size within a few years after the onset of breast budding. The female body shape changes as girls progress through puberty, with broadening of the shoulders, hips, and thighs. Girls experience a continuous increase in proportion of fat to total body mass during puberty. They enter puberty with approximately 80% lean body weight and 20% body fat. By the time puberty ends, lean body mass drops to about 75%. Body fat is an important mediator for the onset of menstruation and regular ovulatory

TABLE 8-1   Adolescent Development and Related Anticipatory Guidance

Area of Development	Anticipatory Guidance
Physical	
Experience growth from prepubescence to sexual maturity	Teach child about body functions (e.g., menstruation, nocturnal emissions) of both genders. Teach about the timing and descriptions of primary and secondary sexual characteristics.
Reach adult parameters of height and physical growth by late adolescence	Provide prevention counseling regarding substance abuse, safety, and unintentional injuries (e.g., bicycle helmet use, seatbelts, gun storage).
Become comfortable with one's body	Offer reassurance that physical findings are normal; explain what to expect; listen to adolescents' concerns; encourage exercise, sports participation, and body fitness; encourage healthy nutrition.
Cognitive	
Move from concrete thinking to ability to reason abstractly	Emphasize value of successful completion of school. Engage adolescent in conversation, explain procedures, and answer questions; listen.
Develop personal value system and moral integrity	Encourage discussion of what the adolescent believes is important and what the adolescent finds of value. Help the adolescent develop skills in conflict resolution and prevention. Discuss respect for rights, needs, and opinions of others.
Move from dependence on others to self for risk reduction	Provide information about how to resist peer pressure to engage in risky behavior. Discuss injury prevention strategies at home, work, and school.
Psychosocial	
Establish independence from parents	Explain to parents an adolescent's need for privacy and that not joining in all family activities is not a sign of rejection. Discuss the notion that increased independence also requires increased responsibility.
Develop sense of self-identity	Encourage adolescents to take responsibility for their own health care. Encourage adolescent to take on new challenges; discuss plans for the future (e.g., school, work, family). Help adolescents identify their own personal strengths and joys.
Create new relationships with peers and other adults	Discuss importance of activities with peers; identify healthy ways to be part of a group. Encourage the adolescent to participate in community activities. Provide information and opportunity to discuss questions regarding sexuality, how to differentiate between "love" and "infatuation," how to be sexually responsible, and how to protect against pregnancy and sexually transmitted diseases.

cycles. An average of 17% of body fat is needed for menarche, and about 22% is needed to initiate and maintain regular ovulatory cycles.

Male Stages. Physical body changes of puberty generally occur sequentially in males as follows:

- The initial sign of male puberty is testicular enlargement, on average at age 11 (Hagan et al, 2008). Growth of the testes occurs approximately 6 months before the development of pubic hair in most males. If testicular enlargement does not precede other changes, the provider should consider whether the boy is taking exogenous anabolic steroids. Once puberty begins, the left testis generally hangs lower than the right.
- Pubic hair development follows a pattern similar to that of girls (see Fig. 8-4).
- First release of spermatozoa (spermarche) generally occurs in midpuberty at a mean age of 13.5 to 14.5 years. However, it can occur at any stage of development from SMR 2 to 5.
- Elongation and widening of the penis usually begin in SMR 3 and continue through SMR 5 (see Fig. 8-4).
- Rapid growth in height occurs. The PHV for males tends to occur late in middle puberty to early in late puberty. Boys generally lag about 2 years behind girls, but the

height spurt can begin as early as 10.5 years or as late as 16 years. Males typically have a higher peak growth velocity than females. One fifth of normal adolescent males do not reach their PHV until SMR 5, and there is some evidence that late maturers may achieve greater PHV (Sherar et al, 2005). Males can continue to grow, although minimally, well beyond their teenage years.

- Change in the male voice occurs; this coincides with the PHV.
- Development of axillary, facial, and body hair occurs. Axillary hair generally does not appear before SMR 4 pubic hair. Facial hair appears only after SMR 4 pubic hair and does so in an ordered sequence. It starts at the outer corners of the upper lip and moves inward, then appears on the upper parts of the cheeks and middle of the lower lip, and finally grows along the sides and lower border of the chin. The extent of body hair is determined to a large extent by genetic factors. Body hair develops gradually after facial hair. Body hair changes should not, however, be used to assess pubertal maturation related to changes in the endocrine system.

As with girls, the body composition of adolescent boys changes, sometimes causing great concern for the

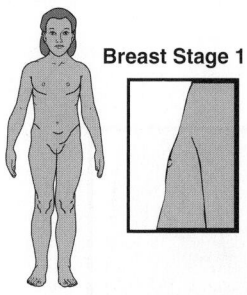

Breast Stage 1

Prepubertal; no noticeable change is seen in the size of the brest.

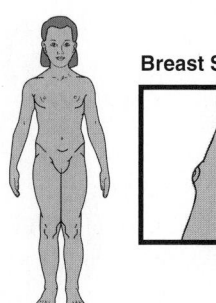

Breast Stage 2

Breast bud stage (thelarche); a small mound is formed by elevation of the breast and papilla, and the areolar diameter enlarges.

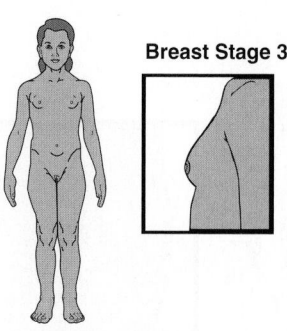

Breast Stage 3

Further enlargement of the breast and areola with no separation of their contours.

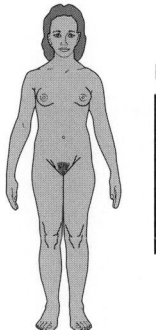

Breast Stage 4

Distinctive projection of the areola, with the papilla forming a secondary mound above the level of the breast. It is important to view the breast both anteriorly and laterally to appreciate this secondary mound.

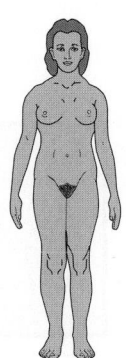

Breast Stage 5

Adult-like; the areola has recessed to the general contour of the breast, and the overall size of the breast is increased. Not all women complete SMR 5.

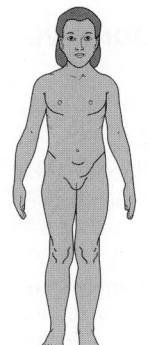

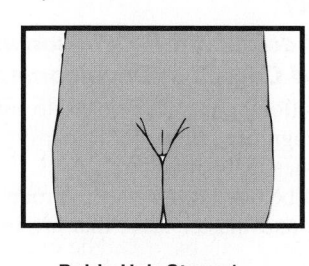

Pubic Hair Stage 1

Prepubertal or child-like; no pubic hair is present.

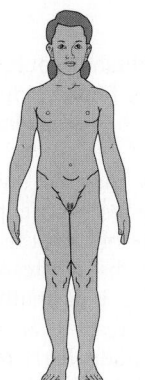

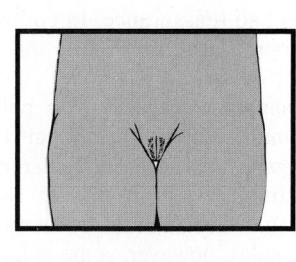

Pubic Hair Stage 2

First appearance of sexual hair (adrenarche or pubarche); pubic hair is sparse, long, slightly pigmented, downy, straight or only slightly curled, and primarily located along the labia.

FIGURE 8-3 Tanner stages: female. *SMR,* Sexual maturity rating. (Adapted from Division of Adolescent Medicine, Children's Hospital Medical Center, Cincinnati, OH, 1995.)

Continued

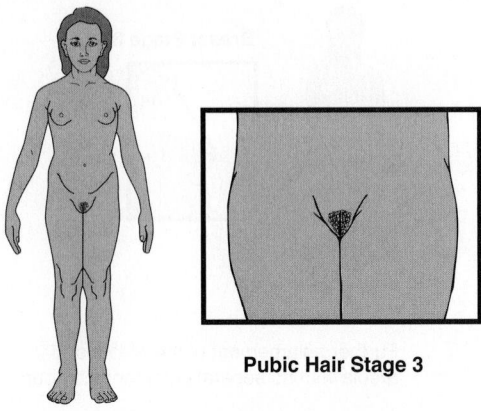

Pubic Hair Stage 3

Pubic hair is coarser, darker, and more curled; spreads over the middle of the pubic bone.

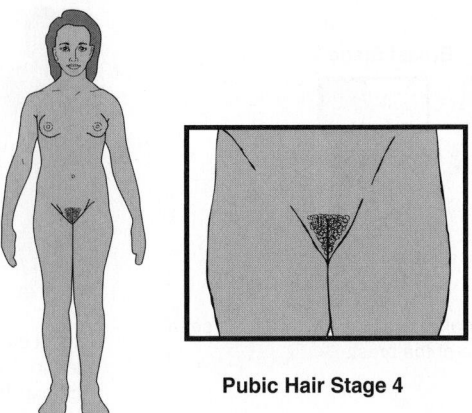

Pubic Hair Stage 4

Pubic hair is adult-like in appearance but not in distribution; does not extend onto the thighs.

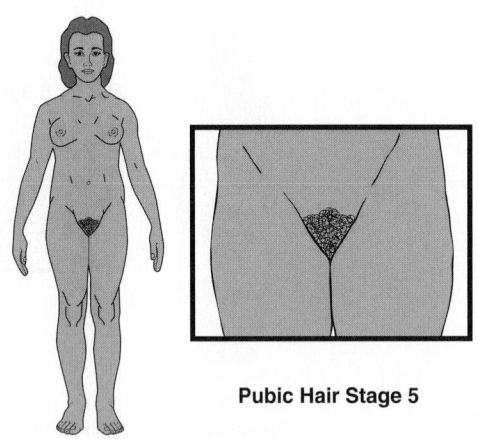

Pubic Hair Stage 5

Pubic hair is adult-like in appearance and extends onto the thighs; may extend in the midline in the shape of a broad-based triangle. Generally, females reach pubic hair stage 5 before reaching breast stage 5.

FIGURE 8-3, cont'd Tanner stages: female.

adolescent. The provider can be an invaluable source of information and reassurance. In contrast to females, males generally increase muscle mass and lose body fat during puberty.

Some changes associated with puberty may be unwelcome. For males, approximately half the population experiences *gynecomastia*, a transient enlargement of breast tissue. Gynecomastia generally lasts 12 to 18 months and resolves completely in nearly all cases by late puberty. In a small percentage of males, however, some palpable breast tissue may persist. Acne starts in early puberty, and by midpuberty many males have moderate to severe acne, which becomes somewhat worse by the end of puberty. Although generally benign, gynecomastia can occur secondary to anabolic steroid or illicit drug use. In cases of persistent gynecomastia or severe acne, the provider should ask questions about the use of alcohol, marijuana, and anabolic steroids, all of which can exacerbate these conditions.

PSYCHOSOCIAL, EMOTIONAL, AND COGNITIVE DEVELOPMENT

Principles of Adolescent Psychosocial, Emotional, and Cognitive Development

Adolescents transitioning from childhood to adulthood should achieve specific cognitive, emotional, and psychosocial developmental milestones that help them:
- Feel a sense of belonging in a valued group
- Acquire skills and master tasks that are important to the valued group
- Develop a sense of self-worth
- Develop at least one reliable relationship with another individual
- Demonstrate cognitive potential

The adolescent's ability to achieve these goals depends in part on brain functioning. Although full sized, the adolescent brain continues to develop functional ability. In particular the prefrontal cortex, which coordinates executive functions of

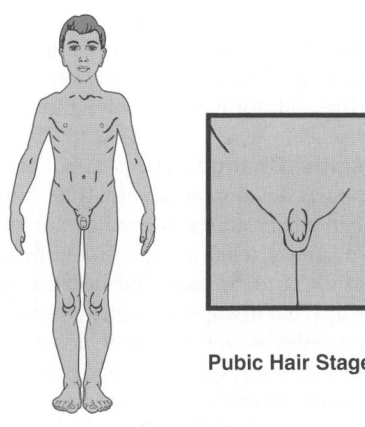

Pubic Hair Stage 1

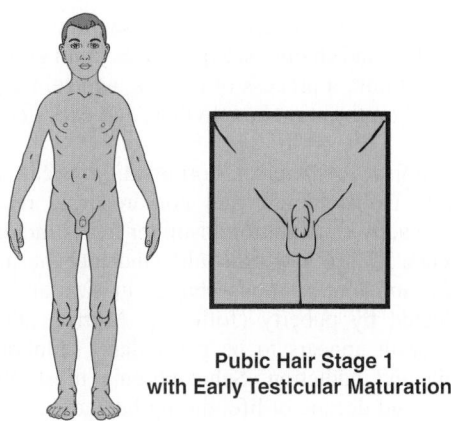

**Pubic Hair Stage 1
with Early Testicular Maturation**

Prepubertal; no pubic hair is present; penis, testes, and scrotum are child-like in size. The prepubertal testis is generally less than 4 mL in volume and less than 2.5 cm in greatest diameter.

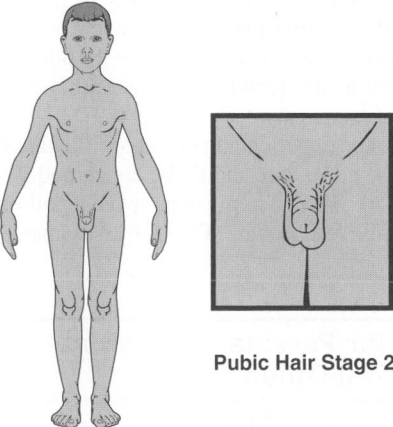

Pubic Hair Stage 2

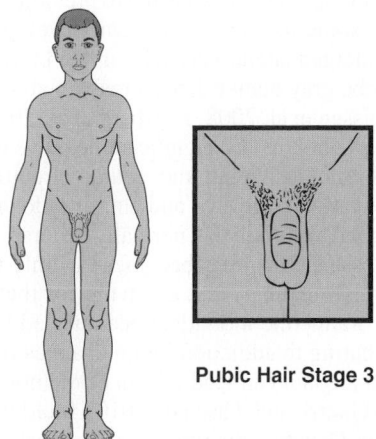

Pubic Hair Stage 3

First appearance of sexual hair (adrenarche or pubarche); sparse growth of fine, downy hair along the base of the penis. Enlargement of the scrotum and testes begins, but the penis usually does not enlarge. The scrotal skin reddens.

Pubic hair is darker, coarser, and curlier and extends over the middle of the pubic bone. Further growth of the testes and scrotum occurs, with enlargement of the penis, mostly in length.

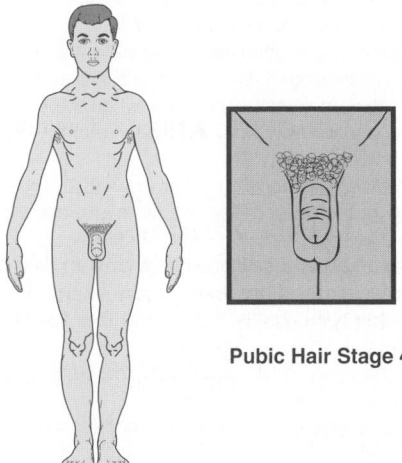

Pubic Hair Stage 4

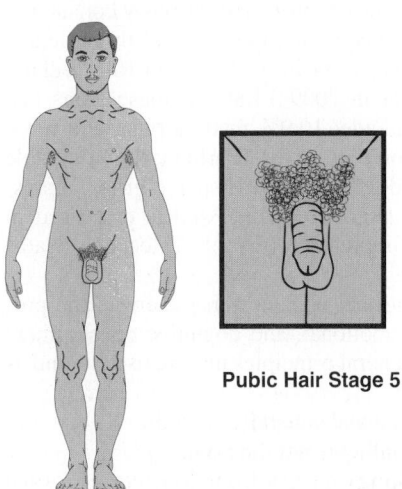

Pubic Hair Stage 5

Pubic hair is adult-like in appearance but not in distribution; does not extend onto the thighs. Growth of the testes (10 to 15 mL) and scrotum continues. The penis increases in size, especially in width, because of growth of the corpora cavernosa in response to testosterone.

Pubic hair is adult-like in appearance and extends onto the thighs; may extend toward the umbilicus. Gentials are adult-like in size. Growth of the penis is generally complete before full development of the testes or pubic hair.

FIGURE 8-4 Tanner stages: male. *SMR,* Sexual maturity rating. (Adapted from Division of Adolescent Medicine, Children's Hospital Medical Center, Cincinnati, OH, 1995.)

abstract thinking, reasoning, judgment, self-discipline, ethical behavior, personality, and emotions, experiences rapid growth. As with the infant brain, a process of pruning and reinforcement occurs, based on the stimuli, activities, and experiences of the teenager.

The brain is subject to chemical, hormonal, physical, and biologic changes. Dopaminergic and noradrenergic receptors become more active and neurotransmitter levels increase during adolescence. Neuroimaging studies indicate the midbrain, amygdala, and hippocampus change in size and are particularly affected by puberty (Joffe and Morris, 2008). The adolescent brain appears to be particularly vulnerable to schizophrenia and addiction. Schizophrenia most often appears in the second decade of life, during late adolescence or early adulthood, and is characterized by disturbances in memory and concentration, a decreased sense of connectedness, and changes in emotional responses. The individual often experiences hallucinations or hears voices. Though its cause is unknown, schizophrenia may be due to previous brain damage, and there is some indication that neurodevelopmental processes (e.g., enlarged lateral ventricles in the brain; left medial and frontal lobe gray matter deficit) may be abnormal with this disease (Janssen et al, 2008; Pagsberg et al, 2007).

Drugs, including alcohol, have a significant negative effect on the adolescent brain, damaging the neural circuitry in the "reward" or motivation pathways and shutting down the body's ability to respond to stimuli that normally generate feelings of pleasure. In essence the drug becomes the only thing that leads to pleasurable feelings, and a craving for the drug is "etched" into the brain—the individual becomes addicted. In addition to contributing to addiction, brain changes resulting from exposure to alcohol can lead to loss of memory and cognitive function (Guerri and Pascual, 2010; Maldonado-Devincci et al, 2010). Genetic structures of individuals vary, however, and not all brains respond to drugs in this way, but the adolescent brain is highly vulnerable.

Suicide and homicide are also risks for adolescents. Although motor vehicle accidents and unintentional injuries are the major causes of adolescent mortality, 14.5% of teens in grades 9 to 12 across the country have seriously considered suicide, and 12% of deaths in the ninth- to twelfth-grade age group are due to suicide. Data from the Youth Risk Behavior Survey indicate that in 2009 13.8% of these teens had seriously considered suicide; 10.9% made a plan, and 6.3% attempted suicide (Eaton et al, 2010). Particularly vulnerable are younger (ninth grade), white and Hispanic girls. Depression is a contributing factor to suicide and is discussed in Chapter 19. Homicide represents 16% of all teenage deaths (Eaton et al, 2010).

A wide variety of normal behavior characterizes the process of psychosocial, emotional, and cognitive development in adolescents. Three general principles may be used to understand the changes seen:

• Transition is continual and generally smooth.
• Disruptive family conflict is not the norm.
• The quality of thinking changes from concrete to formal operational thinking.

Smooth Transition. The first principle of adolescent psychosocial development is that the transition from adolescence to adulthood is continuous and generally smooth. A commonly held myth is that adolescence is a period of "storm and stress." This view was originally described by G. Stanley Hall in 1904 (Hall, 1904). Although his argument was not based on research, this myth continues to be widely believed. It is important to remember that adolescence is only one of many transitional phases in life and, for many people, it may not be particularly difficult.

Family Relationships Change. The second principle of adolescent psychosocial development is that the biologic, cognitive, and emotional changes experienced by adolescents require a reworking of family relationships. Some degree of adolescent-parent conflict is to be expected because of this reworking of relationships, but disruptive family conflict is not the norm. Mundane, everyday issues such as which clothes to wear, hairstyles, household chores, curfew, and friends continue to be the usual sources of parent-adolescent conflict, and negotiation between parent and child is essential. Inexperienced in negotiation, adolescents will often argue a point to excess. It may help to remind parents that this verbal debate, or "arguing," is a normal behavior of teens that reflects their use of more abstract thinking skills. It is a way of practicing abstract thinking and engaging parents. However, the parent should not become too deeply engaged because the adolescent rarely is, and the "arguments" tend to blow over fairly quickly (Box 8-1).

Families should not be experiencing one crisis after another. If family crises are the norm, one should be concerned. When true turmoil exists, it usually represents psychopathology and will not be simply "outgrown." Careful assessment and

---

BOX 8-1 Tips for Parents: Adolescent Survival Guide

• Start with clear rules and expectations before children are teenagers. Work on developing good communication with children early and continue through adolescence. State expectations and future consequences before trouble has occurred (e.g., before the dance, not when the teen comes home late).
• Be firm and follow through.
• Try to be flexible and allow teenagers to negotiate. Discussing principles and negotiating solutions are valuable life skills for the future. Do not negotiate rules that are nonnegotiable.
• Fighting and arguing are typical, often used by teens as they practice their developing reasoning skills. Often teens are engaged more recreationally than emotionally. Therefore, when the parent is tired, disengage and walk away. Try not to take what they say personally.
• Teenagers want parents to be involved, concerned, and ask questions. They just may not know it or know how to express their desire.
• Know who their friends are and call those parents from time to time. Compare household rules if possible.
• Be involved at their school if possible. Try to meet their teachers and stay in contact with them.
• Continue to involve teenagers in family activities, even when they no longer want to. Bringing friends along will help.
• Keep promises made to teens. This builds trust and respect and makes you a role model.
• Model good behavior. Adolescents recognize the hypocrisy of saying one thing and doing another.
• Don't forget that teenagers still need adult supervision at times.
• Keep communication lines open and don't be afraid to start conversations. Adolescents sometimes want to talk to adults but are nervous about speaking first.

treatment are required. Behavior that results in negative consequences is cause for concern (e.g., red hair dye grows out, but being expelled from school has long-term consequences).

Cognitive Changes. The third principle of adolescent psychosocial development is about change in cognitive abilities. Adolescents develop what Piaget referred to as *formal operational thinking*, characterized by the use of propositional thinking and abstract reasoning. The principal difference between concrete and formal operational thinking is the ability to reason using verbal manipulation rather than in terms of concrete objects. In early adolescence, thinking tends to be very concrete. The classic example is an adolescent who when asked, "Are you sexually active?" responds, "No, I just lie there" or when asked, "What brought you here to see me today?" answers, "The bus." Most teenagers acquire increasing sophistication in abstract thought after age 14 years. They learn to conceptualize about past and future events and to relate actions to consequences. During this process, adolescents begin to:
- Consider values. The ones they challenge most are those with which they are most familiar, ones they have grown up with.
- Understand concepts of good and evil and understand human nature (e.g., not all authority figures are good people).
- Be aware of contradictions between what is said and what is done (e.g., adolescents are acutely aware when parents tell their children not to smoke or drink even though they do, or when they tell them to wear their seat belts although the parent does not).
- Understand the significance of their place within the construct of time (past, present, future) and begin thinking about what they will be doing in the future (e.g., college, technical school, job, marriage, and family).

Although most teenagers develop the ability to translate experiences into abstract ideas and think about the consequences of actions, approximately one third do not achieve more fully sophisticated thinking abilities, even as adults. Children who have demonstrated intellectual skill continue to be more successful in academic or intelligence testing as adolescents and adults (Shaw et al, 2006). Neurologic changes underlying the development of executive function, memory, social inhibition, intelligence, and cognition in adolescence are being investigated; additional research is needed to clarify relationships among environment (e.g., drugs, alcohol, noise, etc.), innate traits, and cognitive ability (Blakemore and Choudhury, 2006; Crone, 2009; Luna et al, 2010).

Emotional Changes of Adolescence

Hormones present during puberty cause emotional and physical changes. As with physical growth and development, emotional changes appear differently in males than in females. Some males may experience an association between an increase in testosterone and sad or anxious feelings, acting out, aggressive behavior, or sexual activity.

Some emotional changes that occur are not directly associated with hormonal changes. Research shows that boys with adult-like physiques are given more leadership roles, are more proficient in sports, are perceived as more attractive and smarter than their peers, and are more popular than others in their age group. In general, they demonstrate higher self-esteem in early adolescence. Late-maturing boys who

are short and child-like in appearance until 15 years or older tend to show more personal and social maladjustment over the entire course of adolescence. They can be insecure, suggestible, vulnerable to peer pressure, and subjects of bullying or seen as weak, immature, and less competent than average. Males, as they progress through puberty, typically develop a more positive self-image and mood, whereas females may feel a diminished sense of attractiveness as their bodies mature. Boys tend to be more satisfied with their body image and, depending on their current size, may want to either gain or lose weight, whereas girls are more likely to express a desire to lose weight (Al Sabbah et al, 2009). This dissatisfaction with body image can appear before adolescence (in one study of third graders, 17% of boys and 24% of girls had dieted or were dieting to lose weight [Robinson et al, 2001]), may be related to weight changes in early childhood (Angle et al, 2005), and can continue into the teen years (Al Sabbah et al, 2009).

The emotional affect and behavior of pubescent females differ in other ways from those of boys. Both early-maturing boys and girls demonstrate more risky behaviors than do adolescents who are late maturing, but girls are at greater risk as a result of romantic liaisons. Often these early bloomers get "bumped up" to an older group of peers and become the objects of sexual attention from older males. The developing body of early-maturing females may not match their chronologic age or emotional maturity. This difference can influence their behavior and place them at risk for early sexual involvement, smoking, and drinking (Halpern et al, 2007).

Egocentrism of Adolescents

Changes in the quality of adolescent thinking coupled with physical and emotional changes give rise to a form of egocentrism. This change may result in a rather self-centered, but not necessarily selfish, view of the world. Although there are recommendations that this prototype requires more research for validation and evidence that adolescent egocentrism continues into late adolescence (Schwartz et al, 2008) and adulthood, four major types of egocentrism in the adolescent are generally recognized (Elkind, 1984):
- *Imaginary audience:* Everyone is thinking about them.
- *Personal fable:* They are special.
- *Overthinking:* They make things more complicated than they are.
- *Apparent hypocrisy:* Rules apply differently to them than to others.

Imaginary Audience. Abstract thinking allows teenagers to wonder what others are thinking about. At the same time, adolescents are obsessed by the physical changes brought about by puberty. These changes and their new thinking abilities create the notion that everyone is thinking about the same thing that they are (i.e., them). Teenagers may believe that one can read minds and know what others are thinking. For example, a boy who goes to the pharmacy to purchase a condom may feel that he is "on stage," the object of everyone's scrutiny. An adolescent wearing orthopedic braces may think that everyone is staring at him. A young girl who has a pimple on her nose may feel that it is the first thing others see when they look at her.

Personal Fable. The second type of egocentrism is the personal fable. If everyone is watching you and thinking about you (thanks to the imaginary audience), you must be someone special. The personal fable is the concept that the laws of nature do not apply to oneself and that one's thoughts and feelings are totally unique. The personal fable has a very positive aspect in that it provides adolescents with a sense of importance, purpose, and hope; it helps them to imagine possibilities and opportunities in their lives and futures. Personal fables can also have a negative effect (e.g., when adolescents believe that they will never grow old, cannot get pregnant [especially the first time], cannot get a sexually transmitted infection despite engaging in unprotected intercourse, or will not suffer long-term consequences from substance use).

Overthinking. Overthinking involves making things more complicated than they need to be. An example is an adolescent who attributes complicated motives to simple oversights (e.g., an adolescent boy who thinks that his parents would not have divorced if only he had helped more with the chores around the house or an adolescent girl who breaks up with her boyfriend because she assumes that he does not like her because he did not compliment her on her new red dress).

Apparent Hypocrisy. Apparent hypocrisy is the notion that rules apply differently to adolescents than they do to others. For example, an adolescent girl may believe that she should have free access to her parent's clothes and electronic equipment (such as the MP3 player or home computer), whereas her parents entering her room to borrow a disk constitutes an invasion of privacy.

■ Developmental Screening and Assessment

APPROACHES TO ASSESSMENT OF ADOLESCENTS

Throughout infancy and the preschool and school years, the focus of the health care visit is the parent or caregiver and the child as a unit. This dyad changes with adolescence. Teenagers must be evaluated independently of their parents, and developmental issues must be discussed privately with the adolescents themselves. Nonetheless, parents remain concerned, and it is ideal that they be involved in their child's health care. Adolescents continue to be part of the family system, and providers should work with adolescents to maximize communication with parents around health issues. Some providers believe that involving parents or other significant adults in the adolescent's care is essential. However, that decision is not always the provider's to make, and it may not always be in the best interest of the adolescent. Adolescents must be actively included in decisions about sharing information with others. For many sensitive health issues, providers will need to help the teenager understand and evaluate the risks and benefits of involving family members. They must also provide guidance and support on how to best inform the family, if that is the final choice. This approach can help protect a teen from the parent who may be abusive or unsafe. It can also reduce the problem of parents who are upset if they feel they are denied information about the child they love and for whom they feel responsible.

Effective interviews with adolescent clients are based on the use of good general interviewing techniques: demonstrating respect for the client; establishing parameters of what can be accomplished during the visit; using appropriate body language, active listening, and communication techniques; and working with the client to develop a realistic, individualized treatment plan. The provider gives the message that the teenager and his or her concerns are important, that no judgments will be made, and that the provider and teenager are a team, working together to achieve the healthiest outcome possible.

Preserving confidentiality with the teenager is essential. Adolescents should be reassured that the provider will not share information with the child's parent or caregiver (general confidentiality) unless the adolescent agrees, or unless the health of the child or others may be compromised (e.g., threat of potential suicide, violence, evidence of an eating disorder). Providers must inform the teenager that there are limits to confidentiality (limited confidentiality). As "mandatory reporters," primary health care providers are required by law to report information that puts the child or others in danger (e.g., physical or sexual abuse; some states require reporting teen sexual activity, even if consensual, if an age difference of 3 or more years exists between the couple). If adolescents perceive that their provider will maintain confidentiality, they are more likely to disclose more sensitive, relevant information (Berlan and Bravender, 2009), and it has been found that even when providers tell adolescents there are limits to their confidentiality, teens continue to disclose.

The American Medical Association (AMA) has developed a thorough interview format for teens in their published *AMA Guidelines for Adolescent Preventive Services* (GAPS) program (Elster and Kuznets, 1994), and basic health assessment of adolescents is discussed in Chapter 2. The HEEADSSS technique can be used to assess risk behaviors of adolescents and includes items that reflect the health issues that cause the greatest morbidity and mortality in adolescence (see discussion later in this chapter).

For teenagers who are hesitant to discuss sensitive issues, a questionnaire or checklist may be an effective way to collect information. Questionnaires used to identify adolescent strengths have also been created by the Search Institute and have been used by communities to enhance adolescent self-concept (see Chapter 16).

PHYSICAL DEVELOPMENT

Adolescents should have height, weight, body mass index (BMI), and blood pressure measured at each health maintenance visit. The growth trajectory should be evaluated, using growth grids to identify norms. The Tanner stage (SMR) should be recorded at each visit to evaluate progression of pubertal changes initiated by the endocrine system. Testicular growth can be directly assessed by palpation of the testes in the scrotum and comparison of their size with a standardized orchidometer. Self-assessment is generally reliable, and adolescent males can be asked to evaluate their own level of development if provided with standards against which to compare themselves. Varicocele, or enlarged veins palpable in the scrotum, may develop at sexual maturity and are not cause for alarm unless a discrepancy in testicular size is noted on examination. Gynecomastia in boys should be noted. Scoliosis may develop rapidly at this age, and assessment should be done annually. The thyroid gland should be palpated because goiter may appear in this age group. Additionally, the teen should be questioned about attitudes regarding physical growth and development. Dissatisfaction with body appearance might warrant further probing to elicit unhealthy behavior (e.g., bingeing and purging, steroid use) (see Chapter 19 for information about eating disorders).

COGNITIVE DEVELOPMENT

Assessment should include questions about school attendance, school performance, and educational or career goals. Connectedness to school has been found to be a significant predictor of adolescent well-being; the extent to which a child connects to school depends on characteristics of both the child and the school (Saab and Klinger, 2010; Waters et al, 2010). Children who are behind a grade have a 20% to 30% greater chance of dropping out of school, and school failure can be viewed as "failure to thrive in adolescence" (Reiff, 1998). Chronic absenteeism, class skipping, and other types of school avoidance indicate a problem that may be related to cognitive ability and should be assessed in depth. Objective assessment of cognitive development, as with school-age children, requires formal psychological testing, which is best done through schools.

SOCIAL AND EMOTIONAL DEVELOPMENT

Key areas to assess in relation to social and emotional development include adolescents' emerging independence from family, relationships with peers, and goals for the future (an area that older teenagers should address more specifically than younger adolescents).

Adolescents should be interviewed about school, family, and peer relationships; safety (e.g., use of seat belts); exposure to violence, abuse, or weapons in their home or community; mental health issues such as mood, depression, anger problems, or suicidal ideation; sexuality, sexual activity, and sexual orientation; and involvement in risk behaviors such as tobacco, alcohol, and prescription or street drug use and eating disorders.

PARENT ASSESSMENT

As at other developmental stages of childhood, parents change in response to the adolescent's influence on the family. Parents, too, need advice, support, and encouragement. The normal mood swings of adolescence can trigger strain on family relationships and result in arguments. Parents with balanced approaches that include unconditional love, clear boundaries, and consistent discipline are more likely to have adolescents with less depression and risk-taking and better academic success than parents who are authoritarians (Hagan et al, 2008).

GAPS (Elster and Kuznets, 1994) also recommends health guidance for parents. The parent interview should occur on three occasions during adolescence: early, middle, and late. The interview should consist of parents' concerns about adolescents relating to:

- Health problems
- Physical development
- Social and emotional development
- Parenting issues
- Changing family structures

If problems exist in the parent's view or a discrepancy and potential conflict emerge in the interviews, the provider should bring the teen and parent together to clarify the concern and offer counseling.

■ Anticipatory Guidance During Adolescence

One simple way to understand adolescence is to divide it into three psychosocial developmental phases: early, 11 to 14 years old or junior high school; middle, 15 to 17 years old or high school; and late, 18 to 21 years old or college, work, or vocational-technical school.

Each phase is characterized by certain behavior. Understanding such behavior can assist in identifying behavior of concern to the adolescent or family. Within each developmental phase adolescents deal with issues of autonomy, body image, peer group involvement, and identity development.

EARLY ADOLESCENCE (11 TO 14 YEARS)
Parameters of Normal Development
Early adolescence is the most difficult adjustment period for young people. Rapid changes occur simultaneously in all parts of the adolescent's life; cognitive skills may not keep pace with physical changes; emotional reactions may overwhelm the child's ability to understand and cope. Early adolescents are often confused, even frightened, by the changes they are experiencing. They can be difficult people to be around, and the responses their behavior elicits from parents and other adults may be exactly the opposite of the support, caring, and understanding they desperately need.

Young adolescents begin to renegotiate relationships with parents and other significant adults and develop more intimate contacts with their peers. Because they lack experience and social skills, early adolescents may not yet be a part of an adolescent subculture and can be very lonely. At this stage, teenagers can appear to be anti-adult, preferring to spend more time with friends than with family, and suddenly finding their parents to be an embarrassment. This behavior is a normal and healthy step toward maturity and a first step toward independence. One way of demonstrating independence is to challenge parental authority. The adolescent may become more argumentative and disobedient, refuse to do chores, and want to renegotiate rules (e.g., curfews, allowance, household responsibilities).

Wide mood swings—from euphoria to sadness—can occur within a matter of minutes. Normative fluctuations of mood are linked to adolescent developmental processes and are characterized by their transient nature, commonly measured in hours or days. These emotional fluctuations can and should be distinguished from the unremitting, longstanding mood and behavior changes of serious depressive disorders.

During this period adolescents become extremely conscious of their bodies as they adjust to the physical changes they are experiencing. They begin to spend more time in front of the mirror combing their hair, checking their skin, and putting on makeup. Clothes and appearance become more important for all teenagers, including those with a developmental delay or chronic handicap.

The most important question for an early adolescent is "Am I normal?" Health care providers for adolescents must never lose sight of this concern. Early adolescents often use their friends as the measure by which they determine standards of normal appearance. They become overly sensitive and critical of their own appearance, certain they are too tall, too short, too fat, too thin, too developed, or not developed enough. Health care providers should allay anxiety during an adolescent's examination by actively affirming normalcy.

As their thinking abilities develop, teenagers daydream frequently. Parents and teachers need to be reminded that daydreaming is cognitive work for adolescents and that they need time to participate in this activity. At the same time, adolescents should be given the opportunity to use their growing reasoning skills to actively solve problems, explore values, and examine principles on which they make decisions.

Early adolescents set idealistic goals that change frequently. One day they want to be an engineer and the next day a pilot or a parent who stays home to raise children. Typically these adolescents experience a drop in academic performance in junior high school, which is related to motivation rather than ability. Much of adolescents' time is used in the development of new friendships as a greater number of opportunities become possible.

Adolescents have a desire for greater privacy. They often spend more time in their room alone listening to music or talking on the phone. They magnify their problems and believe that no one could possibly understand what they are feeling.

Early adolescents begin to develop their own value system. They may try value systems other than the one that they have learned from their family, often leaving family members befuddled or even threatened. However, once adolescence is complete, young adults often have a modified value system very similar to the one with which they grew up.

The onset of secondary sex characteristics increases anxieties about menstruation, wet dreams, masturbation, and size of the breasts or penis. This is an opportune time to dispel myths (e.g., masturbation causes blindness and acne) and to provide anticipatory guidance (e.g., a premenarcheal girl often has vaginal leukorrhea, which is generally a clear, mucoid discharge). Same-sex friendships occur, usually with one best friend. These strong friendships may lead to fleeting same-sex experimentation as adolescents further develop their sexual identity. Contact with the opposite sex is usually in groups (e.g., middle school dances with boys on one side of the gym and girls on the opposite side). The peer group serves the purpose of aiding continued identity development.

Sexual feelings emerge, and behavior includes masturbating, telling dirty jokes, making lewd remarks to others, demonstrating interest in watching explicit sexual scenes in the media, or looking at magazines of nude individuals. The type of sexual experimentation may vary greatly, depending on the adolescent's subculture. For example, by this age, some teenagers have already experienced sexual intercourse or pregnancy, whereas others have not even held hands.

Health Supervision

Annual health supervision visits are recommended. Critical components of the visit include developmental surveillance; assessing social and academic progress, including quality of interpersonal relationships and school performance; identifying emotional wellness (e.g., mood, mental health, sexuality); and risk reduction, including injury prevention, substance use prevention, and healthy sexuality (Hagan et al, 2008).

Developmental Anticipatory Guidance

Anticipatory guidance should be an individualized discussion with teenagers that helps them understand, respond to, and take responsibility for their own behavior and development. Separate discussions need to be conducted with parents to help them understand and support their child's maturation and need for independence. In these discussions the provider should clarify what values and expectations parents have for their child and how the teenager perceives those expectations. Some discussion points are outlined here. These topics are not all-inclusive, and they should not be covered exhaustively at each visit. They can be used to apply developmental concepts to the adolescent's daily experiences. Ideas for assessment and management of problems that emerge from these discussions can be found in the following chapters (e.g., sexuality issues are discussed in Chapter 18).

Physical and Sexual Development

- *Rapid physical growth:* Knowing what to expect and understanding the implications of growth (e.g., for injury) help adolescents become more comfortable with their bodies.
- *Physical activity:* Finding ways to enjoy physical activity (e.g., team, club, or individual sports) is an important part of adolescence and sets the stage for lifelong health.
- *Physical health:* Use strategies to support healthy eating despite busy lifestyles. Include the importance of not skipping meals and eating a wide variety of foods. Educate that calcium needs are greater during times of rapid growth and are often insufficient. Also important is a discussion of healthy sleep habits and sleep needs (see Chapter 14).
- *Sexuality:* Discussion should include the following:
  o Menstruation and its management
  o Masturbation
  o Nocturnal emissions
  o Pubertal development of the opposite sex
  o Anticipated sexual changes
  o Beginning awareness of what responsible sexual behavior means physically and emotionally; include abstinence counseling
  o Protection against sexually transmitted diseases and pregnancy

Cognitive Development

- Discuss how meeting academic responsibilities is a priority activity that needs to be integrated with other activities.
- Discuss how changes in cognitive abilities may contribute to "overthinking" or a sense of confusion; encourage him or her to do "reality checks" with a trusted adult.

Social and Emotional Development

- *Family interaction:* Parents should not interpret their child's refusal to join in all family activities as rejection of the family.
- *Feelings:* Discuss how learning to identify feelings is the first step in understanding how "feelings" influence body processes.
- *Peers:* Peer interaction is important for all teenagers.
- *Dating relationships:* Healthy relationships are based on mutual respect.
- *Diversity:* Maturation involves understanding and appreciating multicultural differences.

- *Independence and responsibility:* Developing increased independence and accepting responsibilities at home and school and in the community are essential to maturation.
- *Privacy:* Some privacy within the home should be expected.

Self-Care

- *Injury prevention:* Correct and consistent use of helmets, seat belts, and proper sports equipment should be taught and encouraged.
- *Weapons:* Access to guns and other weapons should be restricted, with emphasis on safety and responsibility.
- *Abusive behavior:* Counseling should be provided on the following:
  - Avoiding gang involvement
  - Bullying, which may be physical, emotional, or sexual
  - Preventing the use of drugs, cigarettes, and alcohol
  - Stopping substance use for those who are using
  - Preventing date rape or other abusive relationships
- *Health care:* Immunization for human papillomavirus (HPV), diphtheria and tetanus toxoids and acellular pertussis vaccine (DTaP), influenza, hepatitis A, and meningococcal meningitis is recommended.

MIDDLE ADOLESCENCE (15 TO 17 YEARS)
Parameters of Normal Development

Parental conflict peaks as middle adolescents continue to argue and renegotiate issues such as curfew, allowance, going to parties or movies, and dating. School and extracurricular activities are often the focus of the middle adolescent's life. Rules and expectations must be clear by this stage. Physical development is nearing completion. Middle adolescents have less concern about body changes, but increased interest in making themselves more attractive. As body attractiveness increases in importance, teenagers spend more time with hairstyles, clothes, and, for some, dieting or activities to build muscle mass. Teenagers with apparent handicaps are equally concerned about their body image and participate in the same activities to improve their appearance. Middle adolescents defy the limits of their bodies, and many have periods of excessive physical activity followed by periods of lethargy.

Middle adolescence is the essence of adolescence and its subculture. Picture in your mind's eye what typical adolescents look like and how they behave (e.g., jocks, nerds, geeks, skaters, druggies, Goths). What are they wearing? How do they act? What language are they using to communicate to adults and to one another? The picture that probably comes to mind is that of a middle adolescent. Middle adolescents stand out for their unique appearance. Peer group involvement is intense and includes the establishment of a dress code, communication style, and code of conduct. They tend to be more nonadult than anti-adult, a characteristic of early adolescents. By this time more than twice as much of adolescents' time is spent with peers as with adults. The need for peer contact is equally important for teenagers with developmental disabilities, chronic handicaps, or both. However, peer involvement may be more limited for this group for any number of reasons (e.g., ostracism by the peer group, parental overprotectiveness, lack of social skills, physical constraints).

Sexual drive emerges, and middle adolescents begin to explore their ability to attract a partner. Dating activity and sexual experimentation and intercourse are beginning at younger ages. Frequently, physical urges precede emotional maturity, and societal pressure to experiment with sex is great. Adolescents of today are much more sexually tolerant than their predecessors. They are more sexually active than their parents were at the same age and may be more sexually active than adolescents of any earlier time, including their older siblings. Ambivalence about desire for pregnancy is not uncommon, especially among adolescents lacking clear future goals.

Intellectual sophistication and creativity increase in middle adolescents. Practicing these skills of reasoning, logic, and decision-making strengthens the adolescent's ability to establish healthy patterns as an adult. They demonstrate increased concern with neighborhood societal issues, such as war or peace and the environment.

Because of the developing egocentrism and the concept of personal fable, with feelings of omnipotence, invulnerability, and immortality, risk-taking and behavioral experimentation intensify. This stage may include smoking, use of alcohol, sexual activity, or drinking and driving.

Health Supervision

Annual health supervision visits are recommended. Critical components of the visit include developmental surveillance; assessing social and academic progress, including quality of interpersonal relationships and school performance; identifying emotional wellness (e.g., mood, mental health); and risk reduction, including injury prevention, substance use prevention, and healthy sexuality (Hagan et al, 2008).

Developmental Anticipatory Guidance
Physical and Sexual Development

- *Physical growth:* Rapid growth and increasing skill allow adolescents to engage in a wider variety of activities.
  - Recommend fitness and sports activities; discuss the dangers of performance-enhancing drugs.
  - Recommend involvement in other activities (e.g., clubs, hobbies, sports).
  - Discuss nutrition and the relationship between good nutrition and health and a positive body image.
- *Physical health:* Use strategies to support healthy eating despite busy lifestyles. Limits are needed on sugary and caffeinated beverages. Often calcium intake is insufficient. Regular physical activity is important. Include the importance of not skipping meals and eating a wide variety of foods. Discuss healthy sleep habits and sleep needs (see Chapter 14).
- *Sexuality:* Provide discussion and counseling about the following:
  - Responsible sexual behaviors
  - Implications of sexual intercourse
  - Encourage abstinence or a return to abstinence
  - Prevention of sexually transmitted diseases
  - Birth control, including emergency methods
  - Breast or testicular self-examination (NOTE: Although the U.S. Preventive Services Task Force [USPSTF] guidelines do not recommend self-examination [USPSTF 2004, 2009], this is common practice and is included in *Bright Futures* recommendations; the USPSTF recommendations are challenged by many (Hendrick and Helvie, 2011).

Cognitive Development

- Discuss the importance of completing schooling and making plans for the future. The transition from middle school to high school can be challenging.
- Acknowledge and validate more abstract reasoning.

Social and Emotional Development

- *Family interactions:*
  - Families should set reasonable limits for adolescents' behavior.
  - Families need to show interest in teenagers' work, interests, and activities.
- *Peers:*
  - Adolescents should establish relationships with peers based on mutual respect, not promiscuous behavior.
- *Independence and responsibility:* Discuss how the adolescent is:
  - Learning to constructively resolve conflicts and manage feelings of anger
  - Learning to identify symptoms of stress and use of stress-reducing techniques

Self-Care

- *Injury prevention:* Encourage correct and consistent use of helmets, seat belts, safe driving (including no talking or texting while driving), and use of proper sports equipment.
- *Weapons:* Emphasis should be on safety and responsibility.
- *Abusive behavior:* Counseling should be provided on the following:
  - Avoiding gang involvement
  - Preventing the use of drugs, cigarettes, performance-enhancing drugs, diet pills, and alcohol
  - Stopping substance use for those who are using
  - Bullying, which may be physical, emotional, or sexual
  - Learning conflict resolution and strategies to manage situations without violence
  - Preventing date rape and other abusive peer relationships
  - Avoiding self-harm (e.g., cutting, bingeing and purging)
- *Health care:* Annual influenza immunization is recommended. Screening for sexually transmitted infections is needed if the adolescent is sexually active. Papanicolaou (Pap) smears should begin within 3 years of onset of sexual activity. Tuberculosis and lipid screening is needed if risk factors are identified.

LATE ADOLESCENCE (18 TO 21 YEARS)

Parameters of Normal Development

Many late adolescents are preparing for high school graduation or entry to college. They work, enter the military, marry, or participate in a vocational or technical training program. These are all examples of normal behavioral autonomy. This period of late adolescence is a time when decisions are made about how to contribute to society as a responsible adult.

By now, adolescents usually relate to the family as adults. Relationships with parents and family are gradually renegotiated to a more adult-adult basis. The role of the parent during late adolescence should be one of support. By the end of late adolescence, this status has optimally progressed to autonomy for adolescents in the context of continuing strong ties of affection to the family.

Late adolescents have attained an adult level of reasoning skills. They are generally capable of understanding the consequences of their actions and behavior and can make complex and sophisticated judgments about human relationships. They no longer base their judgments about people on overt behavior, but have a good understanding of inner motivations, including multiple determinants of an action. Of course, neither teenagers nor adults consistently use this mature level of thinking, and some never reach this level of cognitive maturity.

A substantial number of late adolescents have established their sexuality and entered into an intimate, committed partner relationship. Selection of a partner is based more on individual preferences and less on the peer group's values.

Much of the final shaping of identity centers on adolescents' perceptions of their future options as adults. Among contemporary late adolescents, roughly half attend college, and the other half enter the adult world of work, though increasing cost of higher education is making it more difficult for many young people to afford college. In many significant ways the years in college offer a "moratorium," a time to engage in further consolidation of identity. College life offers both maximal autonomy and a structured, supportive environment in which to complete developmental tasks. In some ways it could be considered a prolonged adolescence. Those adolescents who enter the workforce and leave home immediately out of high school have quite different tasks and experiences. Their identity may be consolidated earlier because they do not have the added time and supportive structures of the college experience. They cannot delay facing the issues of earning a living, forming a family, and accepting other adult responsibilities. For adolescents who are unsuccessful in the educational system or the workplace (underemployed or unemployed), identity may be established by joining peers in gangs or by becoming socially isolated. Some late adolescents opt to join the military and, especially in times of war, face demands that force them to take on adult responsibilities, for which they may not be psychologically or emotionally prepared. Individuals in the military can experience years of posttraumatic stress that jeopardize their sense of self.

Health Supervision

Annual health supervision visits are recommended. Critical components of the visit include developmental surveillance; assessing social and academic progress, including quality of interpersonal relationships and school performance; identifying emotional wellness (e.g., mood, mental health); risk reduction, including injury prevention, substance use prevention, and healthy sexuality; and transitioning to adult health care (Hagan et al, 2008; Sanders et al, 2009).

Developmental Anticipatory Guidance

Physical and Sexual Development

- *Physical health:* Exercise, nutrition, and sleep are important to optimal physical growth; encourage adolescent to incorporate them into lifestyle.
- *Sexuality:* Discussion and counseling should be provided about the following:
  - Responsible sexual behaviors; encourage abstinence or a return to abstinence
  - Implications of sexual activity; sexual feelings for the same or opposite sex should be discussed with a trusted adult or health professional

○ Prevention of sexually transmitted diseases
○ Birth control, including emergency methods
○ Breast or testicular self-examination

Cognitive Development

- Discuss the importance of completing academic work.
- Validate choices made to achieve positive future goals and plan for the future—college, vocational training, military, and job or career.

Social and Emotional Development

- *Family interactions:*
  ○ Closer relationships with and an interest in the family should be reemerging.
  ○ Families need to be supportive of independence efforts.
- *Peers:*
  ○ Intimate relationships are established.
  ○ Respect for the rights, needs, and views of others is a measure of maturity.
- *Independence and responsibility:* Adolescents should be encouraged to do the following:
  ○ Take on new challenges that increase self-confidence.
  ○ Identify talents and interests to be pursued.
  ○ Continue to clarify values and beliefs. Ethical and behavioral role modeling behavior is valued.
  ○ Develop skills in conflict prevention; resolution reflects cognitive growth and maturity.
  ○ Learn to manage stress.
  ○ Find a balance between job and school or vocational training.

Self-Care

- *Injury prevention:* Encourage correct and consistent use of helmets, seat belts, safe driving (including no talking or texting while driving), and use of proper sports equipment.
- *Weapons:* Access to guns and other weapons should be restricted, with an emphasis on safety and responsibility.
- *Abusive behavior:* Counseling should be provided on:
  ○ Avoiding gang involvement
  ○ Preventing the use of drugs, cigarettes, performance-enhancing drugs, diet pills, and alcohol
  ○ Stopping substance use for those who are using
  ○ Bullying, which may be physical, emotional, or sexual
  ○ Learning conflict resolution and strategies to manage situations without violence
  ○ Preventing date rape and other abusive relationships
- *Health care:* Annual influenza immunization is recommended. Screening for sexually transmitted infections is needed if the adolescent is sexually active. Pap smears should begin within 3 years of onset of sexual activity. Tuberculosis screening is needed if risk factors are identified. A fasting lipoprotein analysis is recommended once during late adolescence. Assist the adolescent to learn about health insurance, how to enter and use the health care system, and to take responsibility for self-care.

■ Common Developmental Issues for Adolescents

RISK BEHAVIOR: GENERAL

Description

Risk behavior consists of actions that jeopardize adolescents' physical, psychological, or emotional health. Although health-risk behaviors among adolescents have decreased in the past few years, they continue to be the major cause of morbidity and mortality for adolescents (Eaton et al, 2010). It is a paradox of adolescence that developmental tasks (i.e., gaining independence, developing one's own values, becoming comfortable with one's body, and establishing meaningful relationships) may be achieved (albeit in negative ways) through risk-taking behavior. Adolescents needing peer affiliation and striving for increased autonomy are likely to explore, experiment, and otherwise push the limits of their personal experience—often in ways that put them at risk for health-compromising outcomes.

The most common health risk behaviors among adolescents are tobacco use (discussed later), alcohol use, drug use, behaviors that result in injury or violence, sexual behaviors that result in sexually transmitted infections and pregnancy, poor nutrition, and physical inactivity (Eaton et al, 2010). There is some evidence that the "choking game," or intentional strangulation for the purpose of producing euphoria, is increasing in adolescents. In 2008, the Centers for Disease Control and Prevention (CDC) reported 82 deaths due to the choking game in adolescent males between 11 and 17 years (CDC, 2010). National estimates of the prevalence of sexually transmitted diseases (*Neisseria gonorrhoeae, Chlamydia trachomatis, Trichomonas vaginalis*, herpes simplex virus type 2, and HPV) in adolescent females are 24% of all 14- to 19-year-olds and 34% of sexually active females (Forhan et al, 2009).

However, many adolescents engage in risk behaviors without apparent negative outcomes. Is an adolescent who is sexually active but uses condoms on a regular basis engaged in risk behavior? Is an adolescent who goes to a party on the weekend and has a beer or smokes marijuana at risk? On the other hand, some teenagers who seem at high risk do not engage in risk behaviors. What factors keep them from doing so?

Epidemiology

Although it is normal for behavioral experimentation to occur during this time, adolescents vary tremendously in their ability to think abstractly about the consequences of risky behavior. Their thinking is often characterized by the notion that "it can't happen to me" (personal fable). Although adolescents have an increase in abstract cognitive skills, thinking related to emotionally charged topics (e.g., substance use, sex, school performance, peer pressure) is often less sophisticated. An adolescent who is drinking may be doing so in part to be accepted by friends or to feel a sense of independence and maturity. Because the behavior meets important developmental needs, it may be difficult for the adolescent to look at it objectively and give it up. In addition, the effect of alcohol on brain function further limits the adolescent's reasoning ability.

Environmental factors, both social and physical, can influence adolescents' decisions to take risks. Factors that contribute to the adolescent engaging in risk behaviors include, but are not limited to, the following:

- Poor academic performance or low intellectual function
- Impulsivity or attention-deficit/hyperactivity disorder
- Role models for deviant behavior (e.g., parents who abuse drugs or engage in criminal behavior)
- Lack of constructive support or encouragement from others in social environment

- Low self-esteem
- Sense of hopelessness or helplessness
- Child abuse or other types of early emotional trauma
- Depression or other mental-emotional disorders
- Illiteracy or lack of job skills
- Poverty

Protective Factors

Protective forces may help counter the effects of risk factors and help adolescents make healthier lifestyle choices. Parent monitoring and direction in the child's life has a particularly strong protective influence (Dalton et al, 2006), and community support of positive adolescent behavior appears to minimize risk-taking (see Chapter 17). Examples of adolescent protective factors (Hagan et al, 2008) are:
- High self-esteem
- Sense of future
- Academic success
- Parental engagement
- Positive family environment
- Relationships with caring adults
- Community involvement (e.g., school, religious institutions, volunteering)
- Access to recreation

Adolescents with multiple risk factors and few protective factors are more likely to engage in risk behavior, with potential health- and life-threatening results. These adolescents need prompt attention and assessment to determine the likelihood of negative outcomes. Conversely, resilient adolescents who are doing well, despite multiple risk factors, should be acknowledged and applauded.

Assessment

All adolescents should be assessed for their level of risk-taking behavior. The provider's approach to a discussion of sensitive issues should include ensuring confidentiality, providing privacy, using constructive communication strategies, and establishing rapport.

The HEEADSSS technique is a method of assessing risk behavior. Areas for assessment include **H**ome, **E**ducation and employment, **E**ating, **A**ctivities, **D**rugs, **S**exuality, **S**uicide/Depression, and **S**afety (Box 8-2) (Goldenring and Rosen, 2004). Providers should also be alert for red flags at each developmental stage because delays in development may contribute to negative behavior (Table 8-2).

Clinical Findings

The following are considered examples of risk behavior:
- Substance use or abuse
- Poor academic performance
- Risky sexual activity (including multiple partners, unprotected sexual intercourse)
- Drinking and driving
- Body dysmorphism or eating disorders (see Chapter 19)
- Delinquency or involvement with gangs
- Violence-related behavior, such as carrying weapons

The consequences of such behavior can be addiction, school failure, pregnancy and sexually transmitted diseases, accidents, convictions for driving under the influence,

incarceration, or death. Engaging in chronic risk-taking behavior often arrests developmental progress toward adult emotional maturity.

Management

Interventions should be considered when the adolescent's behavior threatens the accomplishment of developmental tasks or the adolescent's health, safety, and well-being. Generally, when adolescents' behavior supports the achievement of developmental tasks, such behavior should be encouraged. Adolescents who pierce their noses, shave half of their heads, and spend evenings with friends, for example, may be irritating to parents, but their behavior can help them establish their autonomy, identity, and ability to relate to others. On the other hand, such behavior may be an indicator of more serious problems. Tattoos and body piercings, especially among younger adolescents, have been shown to have a strong correlation with risk-taking behaviors (Laumann and Derick, 2006). It is important to understand the meaning of the behavior for the adolescent before making decisions about intervention.

The approach used when providing care to teenagers differs from that used with younger children. Earlier, parents

---

BOX 8-2 Questions for HEEADSSS Assessment

Questions focus on relationships with others, function in school and work, self-efficacy, resilience, and independent decision-making.

- **H**ome: Who lives with you? How are your relationships with the other people with whom you live? Have there been any changes at home? Do you feel safe at home?
- **E**ducation/employment: What do you like/dislike about school? How is school going? How are your grades? Have you ever had trouble at school? Do you work? How many hours do you work? Where do you work? Do you have friends at school? At work?
- **E**ating: Are you comfortable with your body? Are you interested in gaining/losing weight? How do you manage your weight? Tell me about how often you exercise. Tell me about what you normally eat every day.
- **A**ctivities: What do you do for fun? What types of things do you like to do with your friends? What types of things do you like to do with your family? Do you play sports? Are you in clubs or other organizations? How much time do you watch TV? Use the computer? Text? Listen to music?
- **D**rugs: Do you, anyone in your family, or your friends use drugs/tobacco/drink alcohol? Have you ever used performance-enhancing drugs?
- **S**exuality: Do you date? Have you ever had a romantic relationship? What do you consider to be sex? Have you ever had sex? How many partners have you had? Are you interested in males/females or both? Have you ever had someone hurt or threaten you sexually? Do you use birth control/condoms? How often?
- **S**uicide/depression: Do you ever feel like you are all alone or no one cares? Do you feel sad most of the time? Have you ever thought of actually hurting yourself? Do you ever need to use drugs (alcohol, tobacco, street drugs) to make you feel better?
- **S**afety: Have you ever been hurt by or threatened by someone (who)? Have you ever been seriously injured? Do you use sports safety equipment? Do you use seatbelts? Do you text/talk when you drive? Do you ever feel unsafe (where)? Have you ever been bullied?

Adapted from Goldenring JM, Rosen DS: Getting into adolescent heads: an essential update, *Contemp Pediatr* 21(1):64-90, 2004.

were central to the success of interventions. Although parents are still critical to successful intervention, health care providers must recognize that the teenager makes the decisions, and mediation between parent and teen may be necessary at times. The provider's role is to give the adolescent information and guidance to make the best decisions possible. Such information can have a big effect. For example, "brief interventions," two 10- to 15-minute counseling sessions during clinic visits, followed by two nurse-made phone calls reinforcing the advice given by the provider, significantly reduced alcohol consumption and alcohol-related harm (Fleming et al, 2010; Schaus et al, 2009).

TABLE 8-2	Developmental Red Flags: Adolescent		
Age	**Physical and Sexual Development**	**Psychosocial Development**	**Cognitive Development**
Early adolescence (11-14 years)	Difficulty reading close or distant Female kyphosis or scoliosis Less than Tanner stage 2 Female short stature or lack of height spurt Poor nutrition, poor oral health, caries, malocclusion Loss of appetite/ underweight Chronic disease, such as heart disease, hypertension, dyslipidemia, diabetes, or a family member with a chronic or lifelong illness No physical activity; overweight Sleep disturbance Sexual experimentation	*Social habits:* Early experimentation with drugs or alcohol (including tobacco) *Relationships:* Permissive or authoritarian parental style No participation in home chores History of family violence School fights No close or "best" friend Friends or siblings in gangs Cruelty to animals *Sexuality:* Sexual orientation worries *Mood:* Pervasive sad mood, feelings of hopelessness, suicidal thoughts or gestures, history of previous suicide attempt Flattened affect without expressions of joy, sorrow, or excitement Excessive worrying or rumination *Self-concept:* Believes self to be "ugly" or "fat"; is dieting despite normal body size and shape Negative feelings of self-worth Does not fantasize or dream about adult career	Low IQ Behind in grade or failing classes Chronic absenteeism or class skipping Attention problems Lack of organizational skills for homework Disruptive behavior Unable to identify feelings Unable to control own behavior (e.g., anger, impulsivity)
Middle adolescence (15-17 years)	Difficulty reading close or distant Male kyphosis or scoliosis Less than Tanner stage 4 Male short stature or lack of height spurt Male muscular growth without testicular maturation Male persistent gynecomastia and acne Female primary or secondary amenorrhea Poor nutrition, poor oral health, caries, malocclusion Loss of appetite/ underweight Chronic disease such as heart disease, hypertension, dyslipidemia, diabetes, or a family member with a chronic or lifelong illness No physical activity; overweight Sleep disturbance Unprotected sexual intercourse Multiple sexual partners	*Social habits:* Recurrent experimentation or frequent use of drugs or alcohol; blackouts Drinking and driving *Relationships:* Excessively oppositional, defiant of all authority Abusive dating relationships School fights No identified peer group Gang association or involvement *Sexuality:* Sexual orientation worries *Mood:* Pervasive sad mood, feelings of hopelessness, suicidal thoughts or gestures, history of previous suicide attempt Flattened affect without expressions of joy, sorrow, or excitement Excessive worrying or rumination *Self-concept:* Believes self to be "ugly" or "fat"; is dieting despite normal body size and shape Negative feelings of self-worth	Low IQ Behind in grade or failing classes Chronic absenteeism or class skipping Attention problems Disruptive behavior Unable to differentiate emotional states from physical states Unable to control own behavior (e.g., anger, impulsivity) Poor judgment

Continued

TABLE 8-2   Developmental Red Flags: Adolescent—cont'd

Age	Physical and Sexual Development	Psychosocial Development	Cognitive Development
Late adolescence (18-21 years)	Difficulty reading close or distant	No life goals	Low IQ
	Less than Tanner stage 4 or 5	Does not fantasize or dream about adult career	Behind in grade or failing classes
		Social habits:	Dropout
	Poor nutrition, poor oral health, caries, malocclusion	Substance abuse	Attention problems
		Drinking and driving	Disruptive behavior
	Loss of appetite/ underweight	*Relationships:*	Persistent egocentrism
	Chronic disease such as heart disease, hypertension, dyslipidemia, diabetes, or a family member with a chronic or lifelong illness	Lacks intimate relationships	Unable to control own behavior (e.g., anger, impulsivity)
		Abusive dating relationships	Unable to reason or plan based on future and abstract concepts
		Unable to separate from peer groups	Poor judgment
		Unable to separate from parents	Chronic health care seeking for psychosomatic complaints
		Gang association or involvement	
		Unable to keep a job	
	No physical activity; overweight	*Sexuality:*	
		Sexual orientation worries	
	Sleep disturbance	*Mood:*	
	Unprotected sexual intercourse	Pervasive sad mood, feelings of hopelessness, suicidal thoughts or gestures, history of previous suicide attempt	
	Multiple sexual partners	Flattened affect without expressions of joy, sorrow, or excitement	
		Excessive worrying or rumination	
		Self-concept:	
		Believes self to be "ugly" or "fat"; is dieting despite normal body size and shape	
		Negative feelings of self-worth	

Generally, high-risk teenagers require numerous services. Health care providers need to know their state laws regarding adolescent health issues, how to access community resources, and how to use other professionals collaboratively. The following list identifies basic services that at-risk teenagers may need:

- Food resources for teenage parents and their offspring
- Temporary shelters for teenagers
- Counseling and mental health services for teenagers and their families
- Foster care services for teenage parents and their offspring
- Local medical and social work services
- Local juvenile justice system and protective services
- Drug rehabilitation programs for teenagers
- Alternative school and vocational education programs
- Sports, fitness, and community activities for teenagers; after-school programs may be a particularly successful means of preventing risky behavior (Cabral, 2006)
- Support programs for teenagers, such as Big Brothers or Big Sisters

Advocating for children and adolescents at risk; involving their families, communities, and schools; and helping young people identify an individual who cares for them and trusts them are important actions all health care providers can take.

RISK BEHAVIOR: TOBACCO USE

Description

Tobacco use, primarily smoking, appears within a cluster of risk-taking behaviors, and adolescent smokers are more likely than their nonsmoking peers to use marijuana and hard drugs, sell drugs, have multiple drug problems, drop out of school,

and experience early pregnancy and parenthood. These adolescents are also at higher risk for low academic achievement and behavioral problems at school, stealing and other delinquent behaviors, and use of predatory and relational violence (Ellickson et al, 2008). More in-depth discussions of sexuality and substance abuse are found in Chapters 18 and 19.

Many adolescents experiment with tobacco use, but may stop after a short period before becoming addicted to nicotine. Tobacco dependence (addiction) varies from one individual to another and can appear at any time after initiating tobacco use, so prevention and early intervention are essential. High recent cigarette consumption, slow nicotine metabolism, and higher depressive symptoms are related to tobacco dependence in adolescents (Kandel et al, 2007; Karp et al, 2006).

Epidemiology

During the 1990s, cigarette smoking among non-Hispanic black, non-Hispanic white, and Hispanic high school students increased significantly in three assessed areas: lifetime smoking (defined as having ever smoked cigarettes, even one or two puffs), current smoking (defined as smoking on more than one of the 30 days preceding the survey), and current frequent smoking (defined as smoking on more than 20 of the 30 days preceding the survey) (CDC, 2008). Males and Hispanics have the highest cigarette use and Caucasian males have the highest smokeless tobacco use (Eaton et al, 2010). From 1997 to 2009, however, there was a significant decline in smoking among U.S. youth 12 to 17 years old. In 1997, 36.4% of high school students were current smokers and 16.7% were frequent smokers. In 2009, approximately 20.0% were current smokers and 7.8% were frequent smokers (Eaton et al,

2010). In the 2009 survey, 26% of all high school students stated they use some tobacco product (smoking, smokeless tobacco), compared with 28.4% in 2005 (Eaton et al, 2006, 2010). Despite this decline, youth smoking continues to be a serious public health problem, with girls and boys smoking at about the same rates, and increased smoking among youth internationally (Warren et al, 2008).

Smoking is positively related to the tobacco industry advertising cigarettes. Portrayal of smoking in films (Heatherton and Sargent, 2009), parent smoking (Wilkinson et al, 2008), access to cigarettes in the home, close peer or sibling smoking (McLeod et al, 2008), smoking-tolerant schools (O'Loughlin et al, 2009), and stress and lower subjective social status (Wilkinson et al, 2009) are all related to smoking among adolescents.

Clinical Findings

In the clinical setting, adolescents' smoking patterns are best assessed through direct questioning. At every visit, children should be asked whether they or their friends smoke or use other forms of tobacco. Biochemical tests to measure tobacco by-products (e.g., carbon monoxide in serum or expired alveolar air; urine cotinine, a primary metabolite of nicotine; and thiocyanate, a detoxification product of hydrogen cyanide in tobacco smoke) are used primarily in the research setting and are not appropriate as a diagnostic tool in primary care.

Increased incidence of respiratory disease in children, including asthma, is a clinical finding in smokers or in families in which parents smoke (see Chapter 41 for a discussion of environmental tobacco smoke [ETS]).

Management

Management of adolescent tobacco use takes place on two levels: (1) primary, with a goal of preventing the child from starting to use and (2) secondary, with a goal of cessation (Table 8-3).

Educating young people about the actual use of tobacco in their age group may be a means of preventing them from initiating tobacco use. This approach is based on the social norms theory, which states that the perceptions an individual has of group norms of behavior will influence one's own behavior. The social norms approach has effectively reduced alcohol misuse on college campuses and appears to reduce violence against women (Moreira et al, 2009). Applying the social norms approach to tobacco prevention, if young people believe that "everyone is smoking" or even a majority of youth are smoking, they are more likely to begin smoking as well. Informing the child that nearly 98% of very young adolescents and 80% of older adolescents do not smoke can support a personal decision to not smoke.

Prevention may also be facilitated by increasing costs of tobacco products, implementing school-based programs (Botvin and Griffin, 2007), and supporting antismoking messages from parents (Butt et al, 2009). Intervention by dental providers can also prevent initiation or support smoking cessation (Needleman et al, 2010). Although the anti-tobacco messages put out by the industry do not decrease adolescent smoking (Henriksen et al, 2006), state-initiated anti-tobacco advertising seems to be effective (Terry-McElrath et al, 2007).

| TABLE 8-3 | Primary and Secondary Prevention and Tobacco Use Cessation Strategies for Adolescents |

Primary Prevention	Secondary Prevention
Provide multimedia, multisite health information, not limited to schools	Ask at every visit whether adolescent or friends use tobacco
Emphasize skills to avoid peer pressure	Inform adolescent of health risks of tobacco use and process by which one becomes addicted to nicotine; emphasize that it is easier to stop early
Focus on adolescents' developmental need to belong to a social group	Develop mutual understanding of problem
	Determine realistic stop-use date
	Help adolescent identify barriers to stopping and ways to overcome those barriers
	Provide information about self-help and support groups; encourage adolescent to try to stop smoking with a friend
	Provide nicotine patch protocol if adolescent feels this will help
	Schedule follow-up visits to monitor progress; reinforce positive efforts
	Assess parents' tobacco use patterns; provide information and support to stop use

Many children are exposed to nicotine in utero or to secondhand smoke of parents or other caregivers. This puts them at risk for cognitive deficits, low test scores, and poorer school performance (Herrmann et al, 2008); also, children who live in a family with smokers are more likely to become smokers themselves. Although pediatric providers are not the parents' primary caregivers, they can intervene with parents in several ways. Parents can be encouraged to talk to their children about the dangers of smoking; there is evidence that when parents teach their children that smoking is bad, children are less likely to begin, even if the parent continues to smoke (Jackson and Dickinson, 2006). Parents should also be encouraged to stop smoking (see Chapter 41 for "the five As" smoking cessation guidelines for providers from the U.S. Agency for Healthcare Research and Quality [AHRQ]).

In addition, medical practices could implement population-based interventions to help their clients stop tobacco use. These include tracking and monitoring smokers, providing insurance coverage for tobacco-cessation services, educating employees not to use tobacco, and lobbying for public antismoking campaigns and increased taxes on tobacco products.

RISK BEHAVIOR: SELF-INJURIOUS BEHAVIORS

Description

Self-injurious behavior (SIB) is defined as intentionally causing physical harm to oneself for nonsocially sanctioned and nonsuicidal reasons (Whitlock and Knox, 2007). Excluded from this diagnosis are behaviors like piercings and tattoos because these are seen as socially acceptable. SIBs vary widely including cutting, scraping, burning or ripping of skin, subdermal tissue or hair; swallowing toxic substances; breaking bones;

and bruising oneself (Whitlock et al, 2006). The common factor among SIBs is that they are done to relieve distress, as a coping strategy, and to create a sense of calm. Patients often report that the physical pain associated with these acts helps relieve emotional pain (Hicks and Hinck, 2008). These are not suicide attempts, but it is important to note that individuals who engage in SIB are more likely to attempt suicide or to have an eating disorder, a history of abuse or trauma, a mood disorder, or psychological distress than those in the general population and should be assessed for suicide risk (Whitlock and Knox, 2007; Whitlock et al, 2006).

Epidemiology

Most epidemiologic studies indicate that the average age of SIB onset is mid- to late adolescence with a decline in early adulthood (Whitlock et al, 2006). Many believe the prevalence of SIB is increasing, but there are no historical data for comparison, and many studies do not differentiate SIB from suicidal SIB. Data indicate that 17% to 25% of adolescents and young adults report engaging in SIB at least once, with as many as 80% having experimental or mild SIB (Klonsky and Olino, 2008; Whitlock et al, 2006; Williams et al, 2010). Females, Caucasians, and those who identify themselves as homosexual or bisexual are more likely to report SIB. An estimated one half of adolescents and young adults who engage in SIB report a history of physical, sexual, and emotional abuse (Whitlock et al, 2006).

Clinical Findings

History should include focused questions about present and past experiences with self-injury, description of the frequency of these behaviors, and what emotional or mental responses the adolescent gets from self-injury. Given the association of SIB with abuse, adolescents should be assessed for physical and emotional signs of abuse (see Chapter 16). Although these self-injuries can cause a decrease in emotional pain, they often result in guilt. Therefore, adolescents who engage in SIB often hide evidence of their activities, intentionally mask physical marks, and deny or will not disclose their SIBs, thus making diagnosis difficult (Hicks and Hinck, 2008). Suspicion should be raised if adolescents present with hoodies or heavy clothing on hot days, or when there is resistance to allow skin examination. The most common locations for SIB injuries are the arms, legs, and front of the torso. There may be scratches or cuts in various stages of healing or that appear to be in patterns or that form words (Hicks and Hinck, 2008; Williams et al, 2010). Traction alopecia may be present.

Management

Suicide and mental health assessment is needed when adolescents present with suspected SIB. Self-injurers will often accept help during acute phases but lose motivation for help when symptoms are not as acute. The presence of any wounds should be recognized as a call for help (Hicks and Hinck, 2008). Appropriate therapeutic interventions range from cognitive behavioral and family therapy, to antidepressant and psychotropic medications, and even hospitalization. Therapeutic response is usually contingent on the self-injurer feeling recognized by the provider and is achieved when positive

emotional coping skills are learned (Hicks and Hinck, 2008). Prompt referral to a mental health professional is needed if symptoms of psychosis or suicidality are present. However, not all adolescents who use SIB need psychiatric referral. Those who have no other signs of mental illness and who are experimenting with self-injury, or who have engaged in SIB because of peer pressure may not require immediate intervention (Williams et al, 2010).

PRIMARY CARE FOR LESBIAN, GAY, BISEXUAL, TRANSGENDER, AND QUESTIONING YOUTH

Description

One of the major tasks of adolescence is the development of a healthy sexual identity (see Chapter 18). Like their heterosexual peers, lesbian, gay, bisexual, transgender, and questioning (LGBTQ) youth are at risk for medical and social sequelae from their sexual behaviors. Significant social stigma occurs as these adolescents attempt to reconcile their own sexual orientation with social norms. As a result, some LGBTQ young people are at greater risk for depression, substance abuse, suicidal ideation and attempts, family rejection, violence, risky sexual behavior, and school failure (Meckler at al, 2006; Ryan et al, 2009). The American Academy of Pediatrics, the American Medical Association, and the Society for Adolescent Medicine recommend that primary care providers use a nonjudgmental approach to openly discuss sexuality and sexual orientation with adolescents (AAP, 1993; Council on Scientific Affairs, 1996; Emans et al, 1991).

Epidemiology

An estimated 10% of the population is gay, lesbian, bisexual, or transgender (Lee, 2000). Ninety-five percent of LGBTQ adolescents report isolation and estrangement from their peers, usually as a result of feeling different. Up to 40% of LGBTQ adolescents report either having attempted suicide or having seriously thought about suicide; 65% had been verbally insulted, and 25% physically threatened (Dowshen and Garofalo, 2009; Lee, 2000).

Assessment

Only about one third of LGBTQ adolescents report their sexual orientation to their health care provider, and fear of disclosure to parents, friends, and/or family members is one of the most common reasons LGBTQ adolescents do not seek health care (Dowshen and Garofalo, 2009; Meckler et al, 2006). Therefore, it is essential to candidly discuss confidentiality and to use open-ended questions with nonjudgmental language. For example, instead of asking a female adolescent if she has a boyfriend, ask if she dates or is interested in dating. Research indicates that negative health outcomes are associated with family rejection, so evaluation of family responses to the adolescent's sexuality is warranted (Ryan et al, 2009).

Management

The primary care needs of LGBTQ youth are essentially the same as those of any other group: privacy, confidentiality, anticipatory guidance, and health care providers who focus on health and wellness. All adolescent females should receive

HPV vaccination and begin annual cervical cytology within 3 years of initiating sexual intercourse (Dowshen and Garofalo, 2009). Hepatitis A and B vaccination series are part of routine adolescent well care, but are especially important to complete in males who have sex with males. Diagnostic evaluation for human immunodeficiency virus (HIV) and other sexually transmitted diseases is recommended for all adolescents with high-risk sexual activity, regardless of sexual orientation.

Many LGBTQ adolescents do not receive family-oriented primary care (Ryan et al, 2009). It is important for families to keep open lines of communication. Primary care providers should advise parents that negative responses to their child's sexuality may cause negative health outcomes. Referral to community resources and therapy is an effective way to provide adolescents and their families with support and resources that can help improve adolescent health outcomes and family functioning.

Mental health disorders including depression, substance abuse, eating disorders, suicidal risk, and anxiety disorders are more prevalent in LGBTQ youth, although clear indications of the extent of increased risk are not established. Therefore, routine screening for mental health disorders is indicated (see Chapter 19).

Approaches to Health Management in Pediatric Primary Care

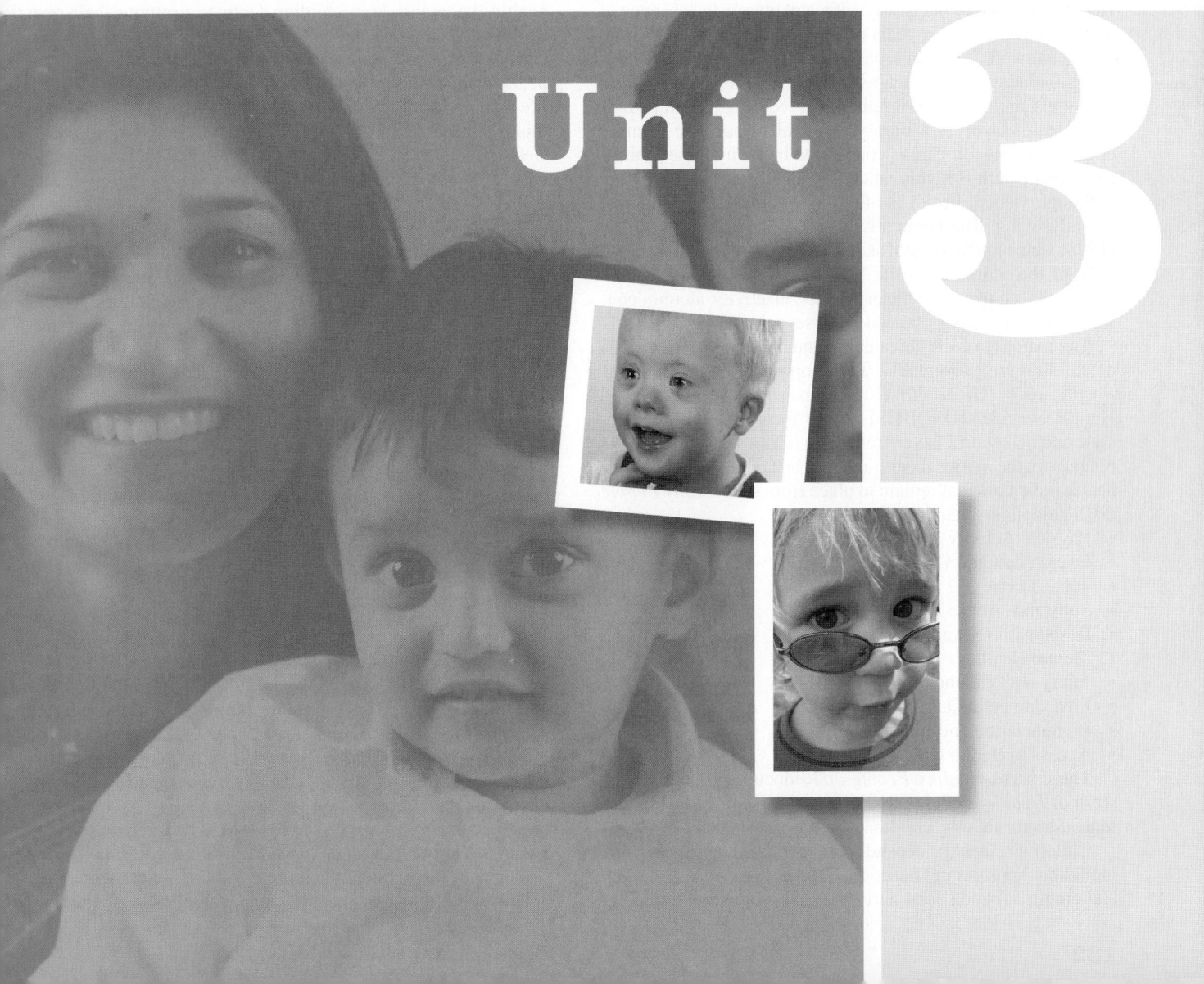

Unit **3**

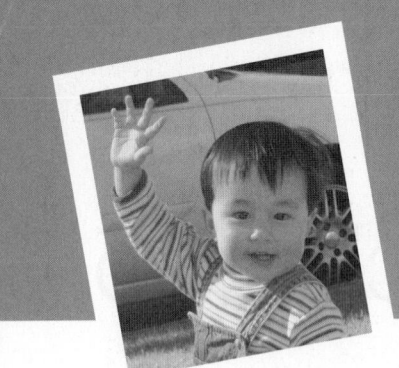

Introduction to Functional Health Patterns and Health Promotion

CATHERINE E. BURNS AND ARDYS M. DUNN

Health is defined in many ways. It is not merely the absence of disease, but includes aspects of physical, mental, social, and emotional well-being. In a positive model of health, the definition includes factors such as strength, resilience, resources, potentials, and capabilities rather than focusing just on pathology. Health involves a biopsychosocial perspective (Pender et al, 2011). Health care is considered by many to be a birthright, and health is highly valued by all cultures in the world. Although valued, health is often compromised by behaviors of daily living. The landmark paper by McGinnis and Foege (1993), since updated by Mokdad and associates (2004), links 50% of the mortality in the U.S. to lifestyle-related behaviors—tobacco use, poor dietary habits, inactivity, alcohol consumption, illicit drug use, and risky sexual practices.

The majority of life-threatening and debilitating conditions of children are preventable. The proposed goals of *Healthy People 2020 (HP 2020)* (U.S. Department of Health and Human Services [USDHHS], 2010) focus on essential lifestyle and behavioral factors related to health with benchmarks related to the above health-related behaviors. The leading health indicators that remain in place from the *Healthy People 2010* guidelines include:
- Physical Activity
- Overweight and Obesity
- Tobacco Use
- Substance Abuse
- Responsible Sexual Behavior
- Mental Health
- Injury and Violence
- Environmental Quality
- Immunization and Infectious Diseases
- Access to Health Care

The current *Healthy People 2020* document expands the work of *Healthy People 2010* by clarifying and adding health indicators for infants, children, and adolescents.

Children's health depends on a multitude of factors, including appropriate nutrition, stimulation, exercise, rest, and emotional and social nurturance. Teaching and modeling healthy behaviors help children learn to promote their own health and, because many health problems of children are carried into adulthood, working with children has long-term health effects on the whole population. In addition to healthy lifestyle behaviors, prevention and management of illness and injury are essential to children's growth and development. Health care providers work with children and their families to ensure that decisions made and actions taken regarding health management are best suited to growing children's needs.

Family health is also important because the child cannot thrive in an unhealthy family. Family health has been defined as a dynamic changing state of well-being, including biologic, psychological, sociologic, spiritual, and cultural factors affecting the family system. Characteristics of healthy families include support for one another, shared responsibilities, shared leisure time, shared religious and core values, respect, trust, and family traditions (Pender et al, 2011).

The skilled clinician must take a broad view of practice and outcomes. Working in an interdisciplinary way at the individual, family, community and health care systems, and policy levels will make more of a difference than working with individual patients alone (Institute of Medicine [IOM], 2001; Williams et al, 2008). A broad array of professionals and citizens must be involved. Nurses, teachers, health educators, city planners, legislators, the industrial community, volunteers, and others from all levels of society need to guide development of an infrastructure that supports individual as well as overall community health. Although this text focuses on management of individual children within families, a broader perspective on community intervention and support for health also needs to be maintained. When opportunities to work with communities on their primary health care issues arise, the provider is strongly encouraged to become involved.

This chapter introduces the functional health patterns unit of the book and examines the first of those patterns: health perception and health management. Within the context of the health perception and health management pattern, models that predict health behavior, factors that influence health promotion behaviors, assessment methods, and specific management strategies for use with children and families are presented. These topics serve as foundations for discussion in the subsequent chapters of this unit, where each of the remaining functional health patterns and its relationship to health are discussed. This chapter emphasizes health promotion and wellness management, specifically looking at how providers can work with children and families to ensure that healthy choices are made. The chapter's goal is to give the reader tools and issues to address to help families change for the better and to help families create environments in which children will thrive physically, mentally, and developmentally.

Functional Health Patterns—The Behaviors of Health

The functional health patterns construct is unique to nursing (Gordon, 1987, 2010) and serve as a framework to organize and analyze all the lifestyle factors that have an effect on children's health. It is a model appropriate to the practice of all pediatric primary care providers. The use of functional health patterns focuses the provider's practice directly on lifestyle and health behaviors and emphasizes the importance of health promotion. It is consistent with the vigorous attention primary care providers apply to the issues of nutrition, activity, coping and stress tolerance, tobacco and drug use, accident prevention, and other lifestyle factors. Lifestyle risk modification has the same or greater effect on health as managing minor illnesses in primary care practice.

The 11 functional health patterns that Gordon (1987, 2010) used to describe the domain of nursing practice serve as the framework for the chapters in this unit. The patterns describe the health-related behaviors in which people engage. These functional health patterns are universal, applying to all humans regardless of age, sex, culture, health status, or other factors. All people need to eat, sleep, and eliminate, for example. Each pattern is described as follows:

- *Health perception–health management pattern:* Describes client perceptions of personal health and health care behaviors, prevention, and compliance with prescriptions for management of health and illness problems. Health management includes the actions taken to deal with these experiences. Health management is based on health perceptions and reflects the judgments of individuals and families, the ways they solve problems, and the decisions or choices they make. Positive health management assumes that wise decisions are made and that resources are available for families to implement these decisions.
- *Nutrition-metabolic pattern:* Describes patterns of food and fluid intake. Includes choice of foods and food supplements, eating habits, and schedules.
- *Elimination pattern:* Describes patterns of bowel and bladder excretion. Includes schedule and habit patterns and use of laxatives or other methods to facilitate excretory functions.
- *Activity-exercise pattern:* Describes patterns of activity and exercise, including type of activity, schedule of participation, vigor, effect on leisure, physical state, and meaning of activity to the client.

- *Sleep-rest pattern:* Describes patterns of sleep and rest, including schedule, habits, aids to sleep, and perceived feelings of renewal, fatigue, or exhaustion.
- *Cognitive-perceptual pattern:* Describes sensory-perceptual and cognitive patterns, including adaptations to hearing, vision, or other perceptual losses; includes the process of finding meaning from environmental stimuli and the effectiveness of efforts to compensate for deficits. Pain perception is a component.
- *Self-perception–self-concept pattern:* Describes patterns of perception and valuing of the self, in addition to evaluation of strengths and weaknesses and sense of self-worth.
- *Role-relationships pattern:* Describes pattern of roles and responsibilities of the client and patterns of relationships with family and others.
- *Sexuality-reproductive pattern:* Describes patterns of satisfaction or dissatisfaction with sexuality and sexual relationships. Involves perception and development of sexual identity, in addition to reproductive expectations, behaviors, and outcomes.
- *Coping-stress tolerance pattern:* Describes patterns of coping with the range of stresses experienced. Includes strategies used, effectiveness, support systems, and perceived ability to control and manage difficult situations.
- *Values-beliefs pattern:* Describes patterns of values and beliefs that influence daily living activities, guide decision-making, and provide meaning to life. Involves religious and spiritual activities and personal values and beliefs.

Health Perception and Health Management Functional Health Patterns

HEALTH PERCEPTION

All people in all cultures make decisions that they believe will positively affect their health and well-being. The primary care provider's job is to assist families to choose lifestyles that will maximize their health using the best evidence available to science. By exploring a family's health perceptions, providers can begin to see reasons behind family health decisions. Components of health perception include: (1) how individuals perceive and feel about their general state of health (past, present, and future); and (2) the belief that there is a relationship between health status and health practices. These factors influence subsequent health behaviors.

Parents', caregivers', and children's perceptions and feelings about children's health status are shaped by several interrelated variables, including:

- Perception of one's susceptibility to the condition
- Severity of the condition
- Extent to which the condition has an effect on one's ability to function
- Knowledge about the condition
- Knowledge about how a child's developmental stage affects his or her responses to illness
- Developmental stage of the child
- Cultural or social cues about the condition and about health and illness in general (see Chapter 3)

The degree to which parents and children believe that they can influence their health status varies. Individuals with an "internal locus of control" believe they can take actions that will make a difference in health outcomes. They are motivated to make change, are active problem-solvers, and are able to more effectively cope with health problems. Those who believe that health outcomes are beyond their control are more likely to be passive and dependent, and may fail to follow through with recommended treatments. The following health behavior prediction models can be used to assess clients' health perceptions to determine the extent to which clients believe they can influence health outcomes. These models can also be used in planning intervention strategies to help families engage in more healthful behaviors.

Assessment Foundations: Health Behavior Prediction Models

Assessment of health perceptions and prediction of health behaviors can be accomplished using a number of different models. Only four of those models are discussed here: the health belief model, the self-efficacy model, the transtheoretical (stages of change) model of behavior change (Prochaska, 1995; Prochaska et al, 1992, 1994), and the health promotion model (Pender et al, 2011). The first three models primarily address issues of motivation, the first step toward action. They provide guidance to assess the client's motivation and strategies to help the client take steps toward positive action. The fourth model is broader in scope.

It is not well understood how the various factors that influence health behaviors develop in children and how and at what age effects will occur. However, these same factors influence parents and health care providers (do providers feel, for example, that they have the requisite teaching and knowledge skills, limited barriers, and the like to influence their clients' health-related behaviors, such as smoking or lack of physical activity), so adult models are important to understand.

Health Belief and Self-Efficacy Models. The health belief model explains behavior used to prevent disease rather than behavior that attempts to promote health. According to this model, people engage in preventive behaviors if they have a reason or motive to do so and if they hold certain beliefs. They must meet the following criteria:

* Feel vulnerable or susceptible to the disease or health problem
* Believe that the disease will have negative consequences for them if they are affected
* Be convinced that taking some action will reduce the risk
* Accept that the benefits of action outweigh the costs

Important factors to this model are the perceived cost-to-benefit ratio of action including:

* Perceived barriers to action
* Perceived self-efficacy
* Activity-related effects or subjective feelings when the person takes on a behavior
* Interpersonal influences such as social norms or personal sources of influence
* Situational influences such as working in a smoke-free environment

For example, this model can be illustrated by assessing the motivation for tooth brushing behavior: the client must believe that caries are possible; that tooth loss, pain, or disfigurement would be an unfortunate consequence of caries; that brushing teeth can prevent caries; and that the benefits of brushing outweigh the inconvenience, time, and costs of maintaining

a supply of toothbrushes and toothpaste over time. This is a simple example. Getting a teenager to change the content in his or her diet after considering the consequences of obesity and perhaps heart disease in later life is not so easy.

Self-efficacy augments the health belief model in predicting when people will make decisions regarding their health behaviors (Bandura, 1997). Bandura explained that expectations of personal efficacy determine whether coping behavior will be initiated, how much effort will be expended, and how long it will be sustained in the face of obstacles and aversive experiences. Bandura thought that two kinds of expectations were important. First, a self-estimate of one's capacity to do what is required to achieve the goal is based on past accomplishments, watching the consequences of other's efforts, and positive verbal persuasion. Emotional arousal provides additional energy for action. Second, the individual needs to believe that if he or she performs as well as expected, the outcome will be favorable—to use the tooth-brushing example, the client believes that he or she can brush adequately to prevent caries. Based on this model, the provider's role is to help clients understand unhealthy conditions, the effects on them if they do nothing, the improved outcomes possible if they take action, and the belief that they are capable of initiating coping behaviors that will be helpful to their health. This is then followed by the provider helping clients master the skills to take effective action or by providing resources to clients.

Stage Model for Behavior Change: The Transtheoretical Model. The transtheoretical model is in wide use. It incorporates elements from health belief and self-efficacy theories to develop a model that can be used to describe the stages of change that individuals go through as they initiate behaviors that promote health. The model describes five stages of change, 10 processes that facilitate movement from one stage to another, and two of the patterns that individuals use to progress through the various stages (Fig. 9-1) (Prochaska et al, 1992). Health providers who understand the stages of change can facilitate movement from resistance to consideration to action for many health behaviors. Motivational interviewing is discussed later as a strategy to help people move through the various stages.

Stages of Change. The five stages are precontemplation, contemplation, preparation, action, and maintenance. Shifts in attitudes and behaviors occur at each stage. The time required in each stage depends on the individual and the task to be attempted.

* *Precontemplation.* At this stage the individual does not acknowledge that a serious problem exists, although a wish to change may be expressed. Resistance to change is the hallmark of this stage, and the reasons not to change are most clear to the individual.
* *Contemplation.* The individual is aware that the problem exists and struggles with the costs and energy required for change. Many individuals remain stuck in this phase.
* *Preparation.* Planning begins in this stage. Small behavior changes may occur in preparation for commitment to the actual plan.
* *Action.* Behaviors to eliminate the problem occur in this stage. These may include initiating new behaviors, accessing resources, modifying the environment, and mitigating barriers.
* *Maintenance.* Plans occur here to prevent relapse, consolidate gains, and establish new behaviors as long-term changes. Maintenance occurs after at least 6 months in the action stage.

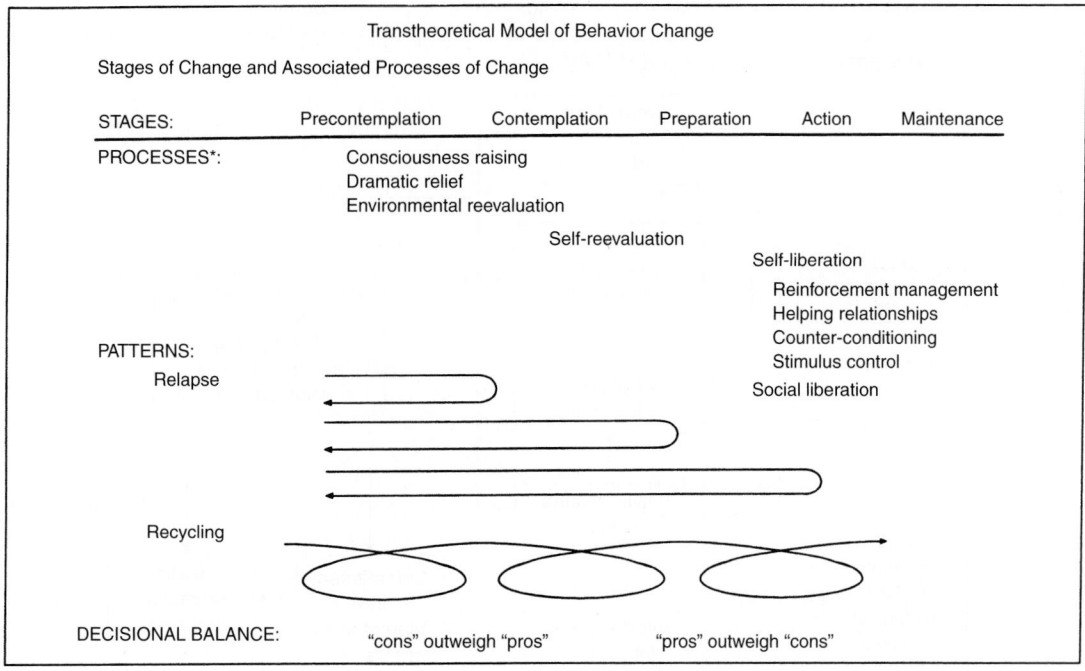

FIGURE 9-1   Transtheoretical (stages of change) model. (Adapted from Prochaska J, DiClemente C, Norcross J: In search of how people change: applications to addictive behaviors, *Am Psychol* 47:1102-1114, 1992.)

Patterns of Change. Most people are not able to proceed through all five stages in a linear way. Rather, there are relapses to the precontemplation stage. Environmental barriers, external pressures to change beyond the individual's own desires, or problems with maintenance of steps not mastered at earlier stages can contribute to relapses. Recycling is a regression to the contemplation or preparation stages. The person spirals through small increments of change, recycling and moving forward again. Success with the change increases with effort, action, and mastery of the tasks of each stage.

Decisional Balance. Another component of the transtheoretical model is the cognitive exercise of weighing the pros and cons of change. In the precontemplation stage, the pros of no change dominate over the pros of change (e.g., "If I stop smoking, I'll gain weight"). To sustain behavior in the action stage and move to the maintenance stage, the pros of change must outweigh the cons of returning to old ways (e.g., "Not smoking is cheaper than smoking"). Because most people at risk for health problems are in a precontemplation stage, programs need to be designed to move them to the contemplative

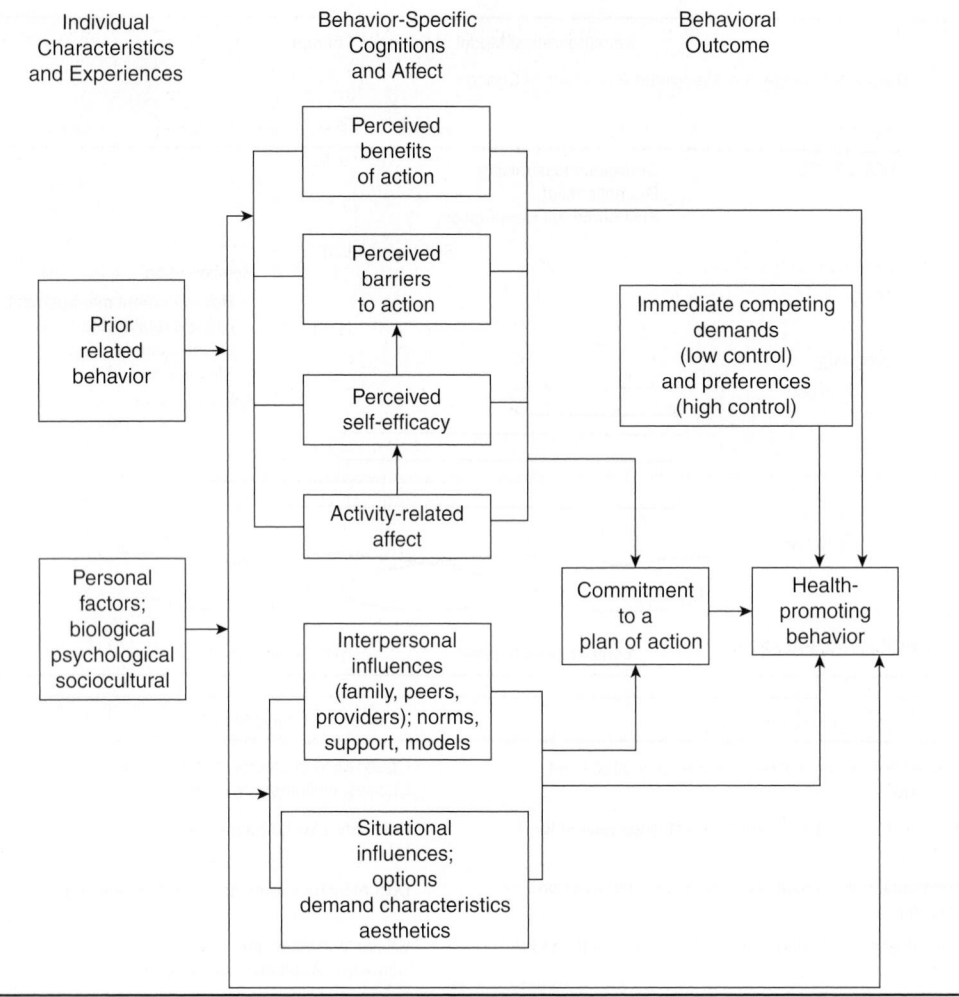

Individual
Characteristics
and Experiences

Behavior-Specific
Cognitions
and Affect

Behavioral
Outcome

Perceived
benefits
of action

Perceived
barriers
to action

Prior
related
behavior

Immediate competing
demands
(low control)
and preferences
(high control)

Perceived
self-efficacy

Activity-related
affect

Personal
factors;
biological
psychological
sociocultural

Commitment
to a
plan of action

Health-
promoting
behavior

Interpersonal
influences
(family, peers,
providers); norms,
support, models

Situational
influences;
options
demand characteristics
aesthetics

FIGURE 9-2 Health promotion model. (From Pender N, Murdaugh CL, Parsons MA: *Health promotion in nursing practice,* ed 6, Upper Saddle River, NJ, 2011, Prentice-Hall).

stage. Also, programs designed to maintain changes are important. Many dieting, smoking cessation, and drug rehabilitation programs fail to initiate and sustain changes because assessment of readiness and readiness training that help individuals move through stages successively are not included in the initial plans. Motivational interviewing, discussed later in the chapter, is a strategy based on the stages of change that appears to have excellent success rates for many health-related behaviors because it helps individuals move to the next stage.

Health Promotion Model. Pender and colleagues (2011) developed a broad model with a focus on health promotion rather than on disease prevention. The model consists of two main domains—*cognitive-perceptual factors* and *modifying factors*—that explain participation in health promotion behaviors (Fig. 9-2). The cognitive-perceptual factors include all the concepts in the health belief and self-efficacy models, locus of control notions, and individuals' definitions of health and their own health status estimates. It adds modifying factors to the model including demographic, biologic, behavioral, and situational factors, in addition to interpersonal influences. Social support structures, the emotional competence of family members, past experience, education and knowledge level (health literacy), values and cultural perspectives, and economic conditions are all modifying factors of importance. Together the

two groups of factors help a person decide whether and when to engage in health promotion behaviors. The model applies to any health behavior.

Commitment to a plan of action is the first step toward behavior change. Immediate or competing demands and preferences influence behavior intentions. The outcome is behavior change to attain a positive health status.

Children's Conceptualizations of Health and Illness

Children's health promotion behaviors are influenced by their own understanding of health and illness, the views and behaviors of their family, and community variables (the last include direct effects of standards and practices in childcare, school, and other community settings, and indirect effects such as cultural and community values related to health). Providers need to understand the health beliefs of their young patients as well as their goals, hopes, priorities, health interests and concerns, perceptions about seriousness of problems, feelings of vulnerability to health problems, and perceptions of benefits and barriers to taking action.

Children's concepts of health and illness must be considered within a developmental framework. One model for understanding children's processing of health information, used more in the 1970s and 1980s, is Piaget's theory of cognitive development. Applying this framework, preschoolers are in Piaget's preoperational stage of cognitive development. They have an egocentric view of health. Children at 3 to 5 years old are just learning about the differences between being sick versus being well for themselves and their family members. They have little understanding of their internal bodies. Their lack of understanding of time and transformations means that the process of healing, for example, is not clearly understood. School-age children are in the concrete operational stage of cognitive development. They list specific acts and rules used to maintain health and generally need overt signs of illness or health to recognize the health status of a person. Adolescents, who are in the formal operations stage, understand the difficulties of defining health (e.g., a person who looks well, but has a cancerous tumor inside versus a person whose mobility is limited but is actually healthy). Teenagers understand the difference between the sick role and actual pathologic conditions, are sensitive to feeling states, and differentiate mental health from physical health. Nevertheless, the provider should not consider all adolescents ready for adult explanations because they vary in their use of formal operations thinking with age and issue.

Koopman and colleagues (2004) studied 158 children in Sweden, 80 with diabetes and 58 healthy classmates. They asked about their understandings of different types of illness (cold, diabetes, infection, and the most and least serious of these). They also asked about illness-related concepts such as pain, becoming ill, and going to the doctor or hospital. They concluded that development of illness concepts is congruent with Piaget's theory of cognitive development. However, they also discovered that the child's perception of illness is based on development of causal thinking about illness. At first, children see causes as *invisible*. Next they see illness from a *distance* perspective, that is, illness comes from external activities, in some cases, magically. In a third phase, children add the notion of *proximity*—one must be close to the people, objects, and events for illness to occur. Later phases are characterized by *contact* and then *internalization* (the causes now are viewed as problems from an unhealthy organ or body part, influenced by something external that was dirty or from an unhealthy body condition such as obesity). Finally, the child describes *body processes* that result in illness and then the child conceptualizes the *mind and body interactions* of illness.

Many developmental theorists are disappointed with the Piagetian framework because they believe it underestimates children's cognitive abilities. Further, they argue that Piaget's theory describes children's logic and capabilities, not their understandings of specific concepts.

Current models assume children are developing their own theories of how things work, including health and illness processes. Research in this area investigates children's understanding of illness and health in light of their understanding of biologic processes. Findings indicate that with more experience and knowledge, children can incorporate more elaborate concepts into theories of how the body works, contagion, and differences between physical and mental well-being, for example. An excellent study by Myant and Williams (2005) explores the understanding of four different conditions—injuries (bruises and broken leg), chickenpox, colds, and asthma—by children at 4 to 5, 7 to 8, 9 to 10, and 11 to 12 years old. The children were asked to describe the condition,

its cause(s), prevention, time course to onset of symptoms, recovery process, and time for recovery. Children had the best understanding at earlier ages for injuries and colds, conditions they experienced in some form. Their understanding became more sophisticated with age. They had the least understanding of asthma, which was neither visible nor commonly experienced. Similarly, adults may be cognitively sophisticated, but demonstrate very elementary understanding of specific conditions based on lack of experience and knowledge rather than inability to process information. Clinicians should provide information based on the child's current base of knowledge and experience. If providers assume, on the basis of age alone, that the child has a certain level of knowledge, experience, or cognitive abilities, they may fail to provide the most useful information to the child.

Children's understandings of mental illness become more refined with age (Wahl, 2002; Watson et al, 2005) (experience, in contrast to age, with mental illnesses has not been studied well as yet). At younger ages children may confuse mental illness with physical illness or learning disabilities. Older children see links between behavior and emotions and cognitive associations. The work of Roose and colleagues (2003) found that by ages 10 or 11 years, youth understood that mental illness is complex and different from physical problems. They saw that emotions, thoughts, and behaviors were all linked in mental illness. From early primary grades, children view deviant behavior negatively, with aggressive behavior causing more rejection than withdrawn behavior. Walsh (2009) suggests that helping children separate the illness from the person may be helpful, especially for those living with a parent with a mental illness. Differences in views of deviant behavior exist among children from different cultures, and the media have a role in children's understanding of mental illness: children will use media stereotypes to structure their thinking about the behavior of people who are mentally ill.

HEALTH MANAGEMENT

Health management is the process of making decisions, taking action, and using resources to maintain and promote health. Health management reflects the underlying beliefs and perceptions that families, parents, and children have about health as discussed previously. The way children's health is managed is also strongly influenced by external factors, including the family, community, environment, peers, their culture, and the degree of health literacy among caregivers. Assessment of these areas, presented here as determinants of health for children, gives the provider invaluable data about health decisions and actions, areas of concern, and appropriate interventions.

Determinants of Health for Children

The Family. The family is the basic unit of health care management for children. The family influences lifestyles and the health status of its members. Child health care is really triadic care, including health care provider, family, and child at every point, which is more complex than adult care. Parents are the primary decision-makers regarding health care of children. Thus, providers need to understand adult and child perspectives on health, decision-making styles, and family dynamics. The psychological characteristics of the family, the belief that members can make a difference, and the role of the family as a natural support system are all important in planning effective health promotion strategies. Knowledge of the family's composition, health, lifestyle, nutrition, economic resources, and recent changes is helpful. Exercise, diet, hygiene, and rest patterns are family routines affecting the health of individual members.

Health Literacy. Health literacy is the ability to read, understand, and apply health information. High health literacy enables individuals to understand their health issues and how they can be treated, know when and where to go when help is needed, take medicines and use other treatments properly, and evaluate the information about health available to them (Betz et al, 2008; Nutbeam, 2000). Although health literacy is defined in broader terms, literacy (reading) and numeracy (arithmetic) are basic factors. An Institute of Medicine (IOM) report, *Health Literacy: A Prescription to End Confusion* (Nielsen-Bohlman et al, 2004) highlights the importance of this issue for the nation's health. The results of low health literacy are costly both in terms of health outcomes and in use of health services (DeWalt and Hink, 2009). Poor health status, adverse health outcomes, and higher disease and disability risks are related to poor health literacy. Those with low health literacy skills use more health services, use more expensive health services such as emergency care, and have greater risks for hospitalization (Mancuso, 2009; Nielsen-Bohlman et al, 2004). Adults with low health literacy are 1.2 to 4 times more likely to exhibit negative health behaviors that affect child health. Teens with low literacy are twice as likely to exhibit aggressive or antisocial behavior. And chronically ill children who have caregivers with low literacy are twice as likely to use more health services (Sanders et al, 2009). Betz (2007) refers to health literacy as the "missing link in the provision of health care for children and their families." Children

of parents with higher literacy skills are more likely to have better health promotion outcomes.

The prevalence of limited health literacy is very high among adults (range 34% to 59%) (Eichler et al, 2009). Downey and Zun (2008) found 20% of adult patients in urban emergency departments and community health clinics had low health literacy levels. A 2009 review article determined that one third of adolescents and young adults had low health literacy, whereas most health information was written above the tenth-grade level. More than 28% of parents had below basic to basic health literacy. Sixty-eight percent were unable to enter names and birthdates correctly on a health information sheet, and 46% were unable to perform at least half of medication-related tasks. Those with low health literacy reported difficulty understanding over-the-counter medication labels and nutrition labels (Yin et al, 2009). Another study found that 75% of the American Academy of Family Physicians (AAFP) educational materials for patients were written above the average reading level (eighth to ninth grade) of the population (Wallace and Lennon, 2004). See Figure 9-3 for a model of the relationship between health literacy and health behaviors and health management.

Community Involvement with Health of Children. The community provides options for health care, an economic base for family survival and prosperity, social norms, and regulation of the environment and behaviors of citizens. It also provides many direct services, including schools, daycare centers, social services, community organizations, and health care centers, that support or impede family efforts to maintain the health of the members.

Family adoption of community standards and health values effectively influences their health behaviors. According to

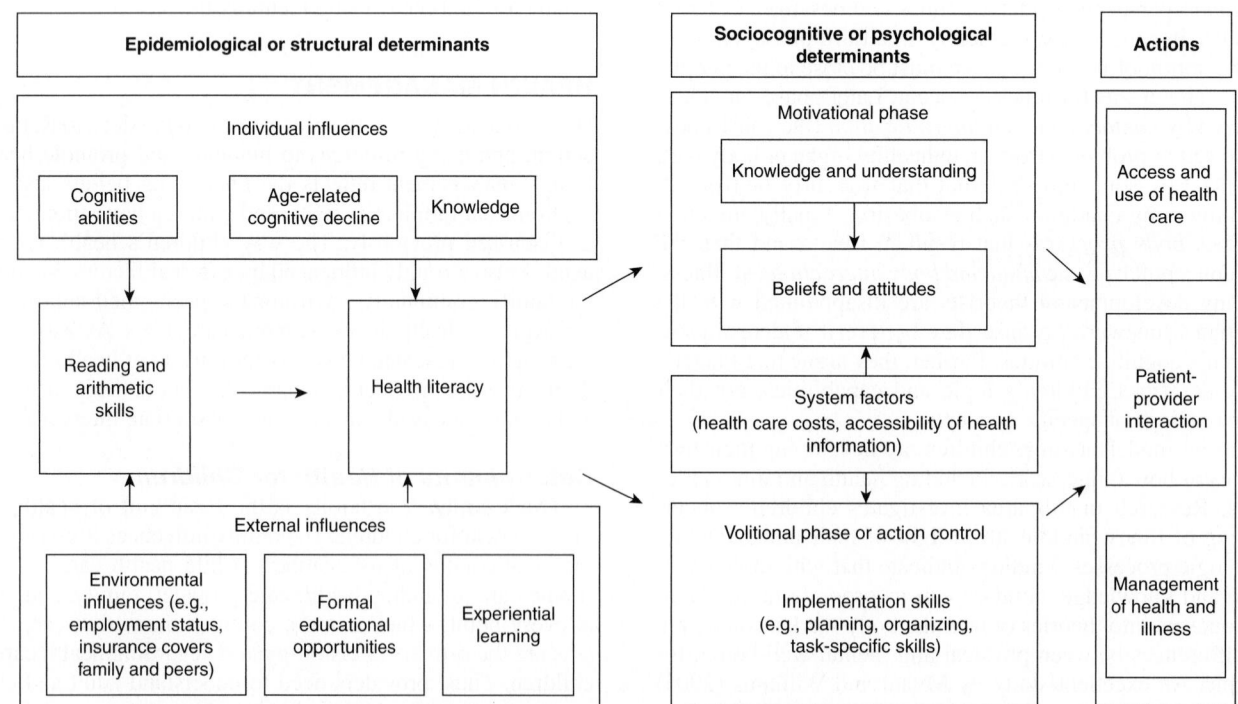

FIGURE 9-3 Health literacy and health actions. (From von Wagner C, Steptoe A, Wolf M, et al: Health literacy and health actions: a review and a framework from health psychology, *Health Educ Behav* 36[5]:863, 2009. Used with permission.)

Rogers's (1983) diffusion theory, innovators are the first to adopt new ideas in a community. They are followed by early adopters, then the early majority, the late majority, and finally the late adopters. When between 10% and 25% of the population adopt an idea, it diffuses through the rest of the population. Thus, for example, when the use of bicycle helmets reaches a critical mass of 10% to 25%, use should become common enough so that the remaining families are persuaded to buy helmets and expect their children to use them.

Community social supports offer a buffer against the stress of daily living, allowing the individual and family to respond more positively to both usual and unexpected events. Families isolated from social networks find it much more difficult to structure health maintenance into their lives or to cope with a child's illness. Connection to a network of community resources (e.g., schools, daycare, recreational facilities) provides structure to support families in daily living activities.

Pediatric providers can help families change lifestyle and behaviors through understanding their health perspectives and being aware of age, sex, health literacy level, and peer and community influences. Figure 9-4 provides a model for use of these many factors to design behavior-change strategies in primary care. It incorporates the community, the practice in a broad sense, and the examination and direct interventions with the individual client. The model is designed to demonstrate strategies for increasing physical activity of adults, but could easily be adapted for use with children and adolescents. Families need economic and material resources for optimal health management. The high cost of health care services and lack of health care insurance coverage are barriers to health care access that contribute to delay or neglect in seeking essential treatment. There must also be a sufficient number of providers and health care services in the community. For many children, economic barriers prevent access to health care, but for others, adequate resources are simply not available in their communities.

Environment. Environmental conditions relate to health management on two levels: first, the nature of the environment affects health status (see Chapter 41). Many children experience unhealthy environmental factors, such as urban crowding, exposure to contaminants, air and noise pollution, streets with heavy traffic, inadequate housing, poor nutrition, lack of playgrounds and recreational facilities, violence, and physical and emotional stress. Second, as noted, resources supporting health may not be present in the physical environment. Frequent moves from one neighborhood, area, or state to another prevent families from establishing ongoing connections with a health care provider, and continuity of care is lost. Rural environments often lack health-related resources, with few providers, clinics, or hospital services easily available. To compound this problem, children living in rural settings are at high risk for injury because of exposure to animals, farm machinery, insecticides, rodenticides, herbicides, unsafe transportation, and other physical hazards.

Peers. Numerous studies support the proposition that peers offer support, influence adherence to treatment regimens, and affect both health promotion and health risk behaviors (Mahat et al, 2008; Nicolas et al, 2009; Reinhardt et al, 2009; Wang et al, 2009; White et al, 2009). Drug use, dental hygiene, safe sex practices, and health-promoting behaviors among African-American adolescent girls have been significantly influenced by peers (Cooper and Guthrie, 2007).

Culture. Culture affects the beliefs that individuals and families hold about the range of health issues they confront: etiologies of diseases, appropriate treatments, proper self-care, preventive activities, and ways of communicating with health care professionals. Culture, language differences, and socioeconomic status can interact and contribute to low

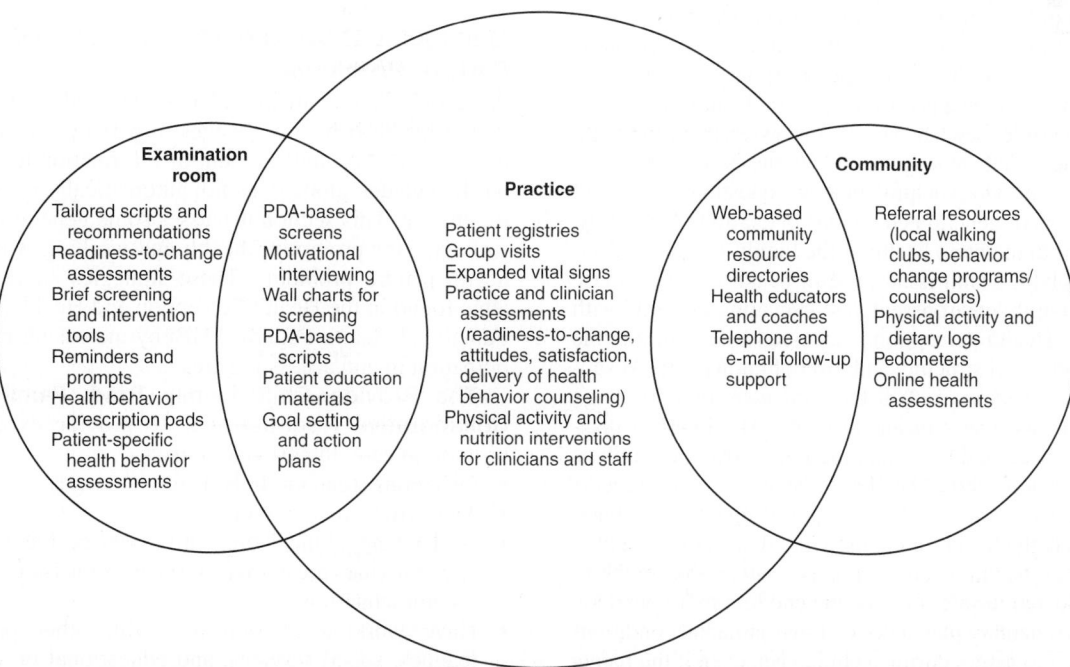

FIGURE 9-4 Integration of health behavior change strategies in primary care. *PDA,* Personal digital assistant (handheld computer). (From Cifuentes M, Fernal DH, Green LA, et al: Prescription for health: changing the health care practice to foster healthy behaviors, *Ann Fam Med* 3:S8, 2005.)

health literacy (Shaw et al, 2009). Health care providers need to accommodate to cultural differences, rather than trying to reshape them (see Chapter 3).

Principles of Screening and Assessment of Functional Health Patterns

Screening methods are used for all children of a given age in the practice, whereas *assessment* is individualized and should yield information about the extent of the problem and a specific client's comorbidities. The goal of screening is to determine if the child falls within the range of normal and if a potential problem exists. The goal of assessment is diagnosis and development of a plan of care to manage the problem effectively and efficiently. As with illness, if an answer to a screening question in the functional health pattern area is atypical, the provider begins the assessment mode to identify the nature, severity, duration, and effects of the problem in order to plan appropriate interventions. For example, if a mother notes that she has not been very happy lately, the Beck Depression Scale might be administered to assess for depression (see Chapter 4 for a fuller discussion of the distinction between screening and assessment).

Lifestyle and health behavior problem screening is a first step. In pediatric practice the majority of screening is done in the clinical interview and consists of more than taking a history of medical problems. It involves learning about concerns and worries, in addition to goals, lifestyle, family life, and cultural background. It produces information to put the child and family into a context necessary to plan for care. For instance, if a family has little money, decisions about care need to factor in the inability to pay for services, medications, or equipment.

Questionnaires have been developed to screen for many kinds of health problems. Among them are instruments that examine diet, smoking, exercise, use of seat belts, and feelings of satisfaction with self and health status. Daily diaries can assist in assessment of food intake, activity, or sleep-wake patterns.

Assessment of the functional health patterns—sleep, nutrition, elimination, play, discipline, use of primary care services, and others—needs to be a part of the general health assessment as much as possible (see Chapter 2). The assessment of health perception and health management patterns is very broad in scope. Table 9-1 provides helpful, practical questions. These fall into the domains of general perceptions of health in the family, strategies used to maintain health of the family members, decision-making about health issues, use of health care resources, health of the family environment, and managing the child with special needs. Health perception is assessed by examining the family's health belief structure and level of knowledge. At subsequent visits, questions look at the particular condition (e.g., "tell me what this illness means to you"). The family's decision-making is assessed by examining how active the family is in making decisions about the child's health care, the process used, and the factors that influence those decisions. The environment affects the health of children and their families and in turn affects their health practices. For example, if the neighborhood is considered unsafe for play, the children may spend too much time in sedentary play indoors. Environmental conditions can be difficult to assess during a clinic visit, even if the parent is open, cooperative, and willing to share information.

After identification of health issues, the provider assesses the family's readiness for change because lifestyle management

is primarily behavioral. Assessment for healthy living uses the same diagnostic reasoning methods that are used to diagnose illness. Critical components of functional health pattern assessment are risk factors, comorbidities, cause, and epidemiology. These findings are then used to form differential diagnoses and options for management that are safe, efficient, effective, and acceptable to the client.

Clinical Findings Indicating Health Perception and Health Management Functional Health Pattern Problems

Families with a positive health management pattern identify, access, and use appropriate social, community, family, and health-related resources effectively and efficiently. When that is not the case, children's health status can be compromised. Some of the clinical findings that indicate problems in this area include:

- No regular health care provider for the child
- History of lack of continuity or fragmented care
- Use of emergency department for nonemergent conditions
- Lack of follow-up care for the child seen in the emergency department
- Failure to adhere to prescribed medical treatment or standards for well-child health supervision after having adequate information for decision-making
- Child at risk for delayed or ineffective treatment, or both
- Poor health status of children as a result of untreated illness or other health problem
- Underimmunization
- Barriers to health care services
- Knowledge deficit about children
- Knowledge deficit related to illness
- Parents' dissatisfaction with health care providers
- Risk-taking behaviors

Management Strategies for Functional Health Pattern Problems

Pediatric primary care providers face the difficult task of facilitating health behavior changes in patients' lives. They may transmit an enormous amount of information to their clients, but knowledge alone does not automatically result in behavior change. This section discusses some general management strategies for promoting health and working with functional health pattern problems. These strategies address the problems found in the Health Perception and Health Management Functional Health Pattern (FHP) by increasing families' participation in and access to care.

The Provider-Child–Family Triad: Family-Centered Collaborative Negotiations. To provide excellent health promotion care, the provider must:

- Give consistent, credible health messages
- Merit trust and confidence
- Understand clinical preventive service recommendations and provide preventive services consistent with those recommendations
- Have working relationships with other provider colleagues, social services, and educational professionals in the community
- Ensure that the clinic setting creates an environment consistent with good health and is developmentally appropriate

TABLE 9-1	Health Perception/Health Management Pattern Screening Questions
Topic	**Questions**
General assessment	How would you describe your child's health right now?
	Compared with other children, how healthy would you say your child is?
	What does it mean for you to say that your child is "healthy"?
	How do you describe good health in your family?
	Do you have any questions or concerns about your child's health, growth, or development?
	How important is it to you to have a regular health care provider?
Belief that health practices affect health status	What do you know about this current condition?
	What caused it?
	What can you do about it?
	What can you do to prevent it?
	Has your child had a problem like this before?
	How do you expect your child to respond when sick? To this particular sickness?
	What have you done for it in the past?
	What do you do or have you done that you believe makes a difference in how your child responds to illness?
	What things can you do to help your child cope with being sick?
	What kinds of feelings do you have when confronted with sudden changes in plans or a disruption of normal routine caused by illness in the family? How do you deal with those feelings?
	How do you think those feelings affect the way you handle your child's health and illness?
Decision-making	What do you do when your child has health problems?
	What makes you decide to call your health care provider or take your child in for an examination?
	Who makes decisions about health care in your family?
	How do you make those decisions?
	Do you talk things over?
	Do you get advice from others?
	Why do you think that you make decisions in that way?
	What are the most important things that you consider when making a decision about your child's health care?
	What is most difficult for you when you have to make decisions related to your child's health?
Health behaviors and use of resources	Do you have a regular health care provider for your child?
	When did you see that person last?
	What health care resources are available to you? Is there a primary care provider you can get to conveniently? Clinics? Pharmacies?
	What immunizations has your child received?
	What have you done to protect your child from injuries?
	There has been much focus on healthy lifestyles, such as eating right and exercising. What does your family do regularly to stay healthy?
	Does anyone in your family (adolescents, you) smoke, drink, or use drugs? How often? What kind? Are there other things that your family does that you think are bad for your children's health?
	Who cares for your child when you are not at home and the child is not in school?
	What helps you learn about health problems and how to take care of them—talking to others, reading, using the Internet, watching videos?
	For this illness:
	• How are you managing household, work, school, and other childcare responsibilities? What is most difficult for you?
	• Having sick children can create a financial strain on families. Is this a problem for your family? What is the most difficult part?
	• How comfortable do you feel managing this illness? Have you had experience in the past that helps you manage?
Environment	Do you use booster seats, seatbelts, or child restraints for your child when riding in a car?
	Where does your child play? Do you believe it is safe?
	Have you gone over personal safety with your child (e.g., "saying no")?
	Is your home childproof? If you have firearms, are they unloaded and locked? Is ammunition locked separately? Are pools fenced and gated?
	How do you heat or cool your home? Is it comfortable?
	Is there any danger of falls?
	Is he or she dressed warmly for cold weather?
	Do you have a working smoke alarm?
	What would you do if your child had a health emergency? Do you have a car, or is there a friend, family member, or neighbor close by who could help you?
	What other conditions in your child's environment do you think could be a health risk?

Continued

TABLE 9-1	Health Perception/Health Management Pattern Screening Questions—cont'd
Topic	**Questions**
Children with special needs	What does it mean for you to say that your child is "healthy"?
	How did you feel when your child's problem was diagnosed? What did you do? What coping strategies do you use as you care for your child?
	How has managing a chronic illness changed your family functioning? How does your family function?
	Who is providing specialty care to your child? Do you believe this is adequate? What other special needs do you believe your child has that require care?
	How comfortable are you in providing home care? What would you need to be more comfortable?
	How are your child's regular health needs met (i.e., those not directly related to the chronic illness, such as immunizations)?
	What resources do you know about that can help you understand and manage your child's illness?
	What special physical arrangements have you made to accommodate your child's illness? At home? In the car? At school or daycare?

- Use motivational interviewing, patient education, and behavioral strategies effectively

Models for interactions between care provider and client (including parent and child) are changing. Parents attending well-child clinics want reassurance and an opportunity to discuss their priorities with providers. They also want greater emphasis on development and behavior, respect for their parental expertise, and positive affect and body language from the provider for themselves and their child. Many indicate a desire for more information in the form of checklists, use of waiting time for presentation of information, visit summaries, e-mail options, information referrals, and community connections (Radecki et al, 2009).

Tyler and Horner (2008) describe a parent-child–based model for interacting with providers that captures the trends in pediatric health promotion care well. Their model is based on essential elements of the Touchpoints program of T. Berry Brazelton (Brazelton and Sparrow, 2003; Brazelton et al, 1997) and the motivational interviewing strategy that is discussed in more detail later in this chapter. Family-centered collaborative negotiation, as Tyler and Horner (2008) describe it, focuses on health concerns defined through the provider-family discussion. Strategies are then identified and adapted to the child's unique issues with a brief motivational interviewing approach. It is the approach of the clinician that is important. In more traditional models of health promotion and prevention, the family and client take passive roles as information is delivered to them through supplemental materials. They are expected to understand and adhere to the clinician's predetermined regimen. However, parents are more likely to accept information or suggestions from providers with whom they have established a high level of rapport and trust (Whitlock et al, 2004), and a great deal of recent research demonstrates that client-centered nonconfrontational approaches effectively minimize resistance to recommendations and promote the client-provider relationship (Suarez and Mullins, 2008). The family-centered collaborative negotiation principles are found in Table 9-2.

For this process to function well, providers must understand the family's health literacy level. Families must be able—or be assisted—to read and communicate effectively, understand abstract health concepts, and mobilize health care resources. Children should be encouraged to participate in the process consistent with their developmental abilities. Adolescents, especially, are at a stage at which they can make many decisions independently of their parents. In any case, collaborative decision-making is preferable.

Helping Families Develop Sound Decision-Making Skills. Providers serve a vital role in helping families and children develop sound decision-making skills by providing information and health education and by giving families an opportunity to explore options for action. The process of making health care decisions includes the following steps and requires mutual contributions from both family and provider, that is, with provider input, the *family* makes decisions appropriate for them:

- Identify problem to be dealt with
- Generate alternative solutions to the problem
- Evaluate the alternatives, looking at feasibility, cost-effectiveness, and so on
- Select a solution
- Develop and implement an action plan based on the solution
- Review outcomes of the decision and change actions as needed

Behavioral Counseling Interventions. Whitlock and colleagues (2004) evaluated behavioral counseling interventions used in primary care. They found rates of behavioral counseling interventions to be far below national targets, though brief interventions integrated into primary care visits are effective for many behaviors including smoking cessation and problem drinking. The term "counseling" implies a cooperative mode of interaction between client and provider rather than a more directive teacher-learner model; behavioral counseling is usually directed at complex behaviors. The goal is self-management of the problem behavior by the client to change and sustain healthy patterns of living.

The Whitlock group (2004) reviewed many studies supporting behavioral counseling. Most of the behavioral counseling interventions are based on the health beliefs, self-efficacy, and transtheoretical models discussed earlier. From their analysis of the studies, they developed several constructs that are useful for providers. First, certain attributes of clients predispose them to successful behavior change:

- There is a desire to change for clear, personal reasons.
- Few obstacles to behavior change are perceived.
- The client has the needed skills and self-confidence for the needed changes.

| TABLE 9-2 | Family-Centered Collaborative Negotiation | | | | |

TOUCHPOINTS COLLABORATION PRINCIPLES AND ASSUMPTIONS			BRIEF NEGOTIATION PRINCIPLES AND APPROACH	
Principles	**Assumptions About Parents**	**Assumptions About PCPs**	**Principles**	**Approach to Practice**
Value and understand PCP-parent relationship.	Parent is the expert on his or her child.	Each PCP is the expert within his or her practice setting.	Be client centered.	Collaborative agenda setting.
Use the behavior of the child as your language.	All parents have strengths.	PCPs want to be competent.	Establish a partnership with client.	Ask permission.
Value passion wherever you find it.	All parents want to do well by their child.	PCPs need to reflect on their contribution to the PCP-parent interaction.	Develop discrepancy between current behavior and lifestyle goals.	Use open-ended questions.
Focus on parent-child relationship.	All parents have something critical to share at each developmental stage.		Explore and resolve ambivalence about engaging in new behavior.	Listen reflectively.
Value disorganization.	All parents have ambivalent feelings.		Elicit self-motivational statements.	Decisions and goals: only the client can decide to change.
Look to support mastery.	Parenting is a process built on trial and error.		Provide no unsolicited advice.	Elicit change talk—interest, confidence, readiness.
Recognize your own biases and beliefs as PCP.			Roll with resistance.	Exchange information—client interprets information provided.
Be willing to discuss matters that go beyond your traditional primary care provider role.			Support self-efficacy.	

PCP, Primary care provider.
From Tyler DO, Horner SD: Family-centered collaborative negotiation: a model for facilitating behavior change in primary care, *J Am Acad NP* 20(4):194-203, 2008. Used with permission.

- The client feels there will be benefits to the change.
- The changes are viewed as congruent with the client's self-image and norms of his or her social group.
- Reminders, encouragement, and social support at key times and from persons and the community whom the client values will support the behavior changes.

A widely used construct that Whitlock and colleagues named "the five A's" describes common elements of various behavioral counseling strategies (Glasgow et al, 2006). They are as follows:

- *Assess:* Ask about behavioral health risks and factors affecting behavioral choices, goals, and methods used.
- *Advise:* Give clear, specific information including harms and benefits of various behavioral options. In many ways, this step comprises models of patient education, assuming that with information, patients will choose to change.
- *Agree:* Find a collaborative plan that provider and client can agree on that is based on the client's goals, interest, and willingness to change.
- *Assist:* Using behavior change techniques, aid the patient to achieve the skills, confidence, and social supports necessary.
- *Arrange:* Schedule follow-up contacts with the client to provide further guidance, support, and encouragement to

continue with the plan or make adjustments as needed. This step might also involve referral to special sources of help.

Motivational Interviewing. Motivational interviewing (MI) is a specific behavioral counseling method to help patients recognize and change risky behaviors. It uses the transtheoretical model discussed earlier. The method was developed by Miller and Rollnick (1991) as they worked with clients with problem drinking behaviors. It fits well with the notions of Whitlock and colleagues (2004) previously discussed. Miller and Rollnick discovered that motivational interviewing is particularly helpful with clients who are reluctant to change or ambivalent about the need to change. In their experience, persuasion rather than coercion, and support rather than argument are more effective. Using the client's intrinsic motivation is most powerful. MI effectively supports change in a variety of behaviors including smoking, drug addiction, inactivity, obesity, diabetic care, and asthma. It works particularly well with adolescents because developmentally they are trying to make their own decisions.

In a meta-analysis of studies comparing motivational interviewing with other strategies, MI outperformed traditional advice in approximately 80% of studies. It is effective in brief encounters of only 15 minutes, though more than one encounter will increase the likelihood of effects. No studies reported it to be harmful (Rubak et al, 2005). Suarez and Mullins (2008) completed an extensive review of MI in pediatric practice and found it to be an effective strategy for decreasing adolescent substance abuse, decreasing health risk behaviors, and increasing adherence to regimens for treatment of various conditions. It also works with parents.

MI uses a stepwise process. One first identifies the patient's readiness for change stage, discussing the pros and cons for change based on that readiness. The discussion needs to match the patient's stage of change, or problems will result. For example, if the provider tries to enter a discussion of pros and cons of various change goals (preparation stage) when the patient is still considering whether behavior change is needed or desired at all (precontemplation stage), the patient will resist. The patient must move through the stages at his or her own pace. The discussions focus on the ambivalence that one feels at each stage and helps the patient come to a decision that motivates action. When using a motivational interview approach, pediatric providers should:

1. Develop rapport with the child and family. Studies support the ideas of active listening, forming a working alliance, and clarifying the patient's views with reflective comments.
2. Set an agenda. "What would you like to discuss today?"
3. Once the agenda is set, ask scaling questions to assess the patient's confidence in making a behavior change and then discover the barriers to confidence improvement. "Why do you feel you are at 4 out of 10 in terms of confidence in yourself to be able to quit smoking? What would help raise your score? Why isn't it lower?" (Sindelar et al, 2004; Suarez and Mullins, 2008).

In the early stages of change, one elicits from the patient advantages and disadvantages of poor adherence and all the possible details regarding the advantages of nonadherence, affirming acceptance of the patient's views and summarizing to be sure the patient has been understood correctly. As the patient moves into a preparation stage, the focus shifts to the equally weighted advantages and disadvantages of adherence; in the action stage, the therapist focuses on the advantages of adherence. See Box 9-1 for some essential features of motivational interviewing. Encounters may last 15 or 20 minutes, but the time spent will be more effective than simply providing quick information or trying to persuade or coerce change, which generally results in resistance to change rather than compliance.

Skilled motivational interviewing is best learned through short training sessions (a couple of hours). It takes at least several days of supervised practice with real patients to become skilled in the use of techniques learned in the classroom. Essential techniques include use of open-ended questions, reflective listening, and double-sided reflection (recognizing pros and cons).

Reframing. Reframing is a counseling strategy in which one changes the context of an experience to give it a new meaning. The goal is to create a frame of reference that focuses on a desired outcome rather than a current problem. It redirects interpretation. Patients who find meaning in their illness may become more invested in self-care. Optimizing one's condition in comparison with others is an example. "I thought I was bad off with condition Y until I talked with a person with condition X. He is much worse off than I am." Support groups are useful in helping people reframe their current condition; clarifying

---

BOX 9-1 | Essential Features of Motivational Interviewing

- Motivation to change comes from within the patient and is not externally imposed by the provider or others.
- Ambivalence must be articulated and resolved by the patient, not the provider. The provider can help facilitate the patient's expressions of both sides of the issue and guide the patient toward a resolution that triggers a desire for change.
- Direct persuasion by the provider will not resolve ambivalence.
- An intervention style that is quiet and eliciting works best.
- Readiness for change is not a patient trait, but a changing product of interpersonal interaction.
- The provider-patient relationship must develop as a partnership rather than an expert-novice or teacher-student relationship.

Adapted from Sindelar H, Abrantes A, Hart C, et al: Motivational interviewing in pediatric practice, *Curr Prob Pediatr Adolesc Health Care* 34(9):322-339, 2004.

---

life values and committing to family or self are all improvements to life. All behaviors are appropriate in some contexts: yelling at a ballgame is OK, but not at home or work; pain is a sign of illness, but may be an indicator that braces on a teen's teeth are beginning to work and move the teeth into a new alignment; surgery is a risk but it is also an opportunity for healing. A child can be viewed as stubborn, but persistence may be a trait that will be helpful during life (Shea, 2006). One needs to be careful, however, not to use reframing to discount, deny, or ignore real problems faced by families. For example, the child who is setting fires should not be described as "demonstrating scientific curiosity."

Overcoming Health Literacy Problems. Screening for health literacy is difficult. Bennett and colleagues (2003) found that having less than a twelfth-grade education, not living with both parents, and not reading for pleasure were collectively a good indicator of a sixth-grade reading level or less. A Rapid Estimate of Adolescent Literacy in Medicine (REALM-Teen) can be used to screen teens in middle school and high school and takes less than 3 minutes to administer (Davis et al, 2006). Helpful programs are available to assess the reading level of written materials such as Emergency Department instructions; an example of their use is found in a paper describing the development of injury prevention materials for people with low literacy skills (Trifiletti et al, 2006). An interdisciplinary organization, Partnership for Clear Health Communication, is working to improve health literacy.

To improve the health literacy of children, health care providers must consider the developmental level and provide materials that are understandable to them—more pictures for younger children, written materials at the appropriate grade level, and use of social support to "scaffold" learning in new areas for the child (Borzekowski, 2009). Improved written materials with brief counseling have been shown to improve adherence (DeWalt and Hink, 2009) (Box 9-2).

Patient Education Strategies. Patient education is the most commonly used strategy for guiding patients to increase health promotion behaviors and manage lifestyle problems. The way in which information is given may be as important as the information itself. Anticipatory guidance as delivered in past years is an outdated model that has been shown to be relatively ineffective (Dworkin, 2007; Mangione-Smith et al, 2007; Moyer and Butler, 2004); nonetheless, it is essential that

BOX 9-2	Goals, Screening, and Interventions for Low Health Care Literacy

Goals

Patients should be able to understand answers to these questions:
- What is my main problem?
- What do I need to do?
- Why is it important for me to do this?

Screening Strategies
- How often do you have someone help you read health materials?
- How confident are you to fill out medical forms by yourself?
- How often do you have trouble learning about health conditions because it is hard to understand written information?

Factors to Consider
- Anxiety, stressors, possible shame or embarrassment
- Language, age, eyesight, hearing, mental status
- Timing related to illness, just given bad news, etc.

Adapted from Mancuso J: Assessment and measurement of health literacy: an integrative review of the literature, *Nurs Health Sci* 11(1):77-89, 2009; Bennett IM, Robbins S, Al-Shamali N, et al: Screening for low literacy among adult caregivers of pediatric patients, *Fam Med* 35(8):585-590, 2003.

BOX 9-3	The Patient Education Process

1. Set the climate for learning—make introductions, provide comfortable environment.
2. Establish a structure of mutual planning—identify mutual goals for learner and provider.
3. Assess the learner's style of learning, level of knowledge and competency, readiness, physical and developmental capabilities, attitudes, and feelings.
4. Plan—provide knowledge, role modeling, practice, discussion. Various aids facilitate teaching—books, pamphlets, diagrams, videos, and models. The plan is formulated with objectives specifying the behaviors that the learner should exhibit to demonstrate learning.
5. Manage the learning intervention—use methods and resources for instruction with the patient or family (or both) to implement the plan.
6. Evaluate the outcomes—judge achievement of objectives and then reformulate the plan to move the learner to the next level.

providers give families and children information about what to anticipate as the child develops as well as ways to best manage these developmental processes. Effective patient education involves providing clients with information about what to expect as their child grows, ways to prevent illness and injury, how to change lifestyle to reduce risks, and strategies to maintain a healthy environment. Within the more current perspectives on helping clients make positive health behavior changes, it could be considered the *assess* and *advise* step of "the five A's" model (the other three are *agree, assist,* and *arrange*) (Whitlock et al, 2004). Patient education is an essential feature to help patients who need to change health behaviors, but is not sufficient in itself unless the patient and family are already motivated and self-sufficient. Patient education is also effective with groups, assuming that providers can also work with individuals to help them implement changes suggested in the group session. In pediatrics, the learner may be the parent, caregiver, or a child or teen who is able to manage some of his or her own health behaviors. One must work to avoid the "top-down" perspective of provider telling client what to do and how.

When working with parents, the provider must keep in mind that parents are experts for their child and home environment, whereas the health care provider has more knowledge about children in aggregate. Thus collaboration between parents and providers produces the best outcomes for the child at hand. Adult education has some unique aspects. First, adults usually want knowledge to help them make decisions for change, not just to gain knowledge per se. Furthermore, they usually have expectations or goals and ideas about activities that will help them. Finally, adults may have to unlearn previous knowledge that is outdated or irrelevant to the situation at hand.

Methods for Patient Education. The core methodology for patient education for individuals and groups is reviewed here and summarized in Box 9-3.

1. *Set the climate for learning.* Patients, families, or groups need to be in an environment that is comfortable, free of distractions, and provides cues that learning activities will occur. Introductions and a mutually agreed-on time limit are helpful. For example, mothers who are worried about being home when the school bus drops off their children attend poorly to teaching, no matter how skilled the provider.

2. *Identify mutual goals of learner and provider.* Learner and provider must reach agreement on what is to be achieved. If learning is to be successful, the client must recognize a need for new knowledge. Getting the client to express questions is the most direct way to identify client needs. The provider can also ask about the client's health goals. Sometimes it is necessary to provide information that alerts clients to potential or emerging problems if lifestyle changes do not occur. In other words, the client does not always come to the provider with preestablished goals or needs; however, the client must agree with the provider that change is necessary for the mutual planning requirement of patient teaching to be met.

3. *Assess the learner.* Assessment includes readiness, attitudes and feelings, style of learning, level of knowledge and competency, and physical and developmental capabilities. Use of one of the health belief models identified earlier provides the necessary information about the readiness, attitudes, and feelings factors. Questions in the following areas are useful:

Readiness
- Does the client ask questions?
- Does the client have multiple stresses in his or her life that inhibit concentration on learning?
- Is the client coping with survival issues, such as chronic poverty, debilitating chronic illness, unemployment, or rehabilitation from substance abuse, that inhibit learning?
- When is the best time to meet with the client, given other daily expectations?

Attitudes and Feelings
- Do health beliefs and perceptions about self-efficacy indicate that the individual feels that he or she has a problem that could be managed through personal involvement?

Style of Learning—Health Literacy
- What are the preferred learning modalities for the client?

- What does the client already know about the subject?
- Judging from the developmental level of the client, how concrete or abstract can the teaching be?

4. *Plan.* The plan is formulated using objectives that specify the behaviors that will demonstrate learning. Objectives need to be realistic, achievable, and relevant to the goals of the client. Both short-term and long-term objectives are written if the goals will not be achieved in one teaching session. The use of both types of objectives helps the client and provider set priorities and stage education in achievable steps. Generally, in routine pediatric visits, objectives are verbally stated, not written, but client and provider should agree on what is to be achieved.

   Various aids facilitate learning such as books, pamphlets, diagrams, videos, and models. The most appropriate learning modalities for the client should be used. Methods for teaching include formal classes, role-playing, demonstration and return demonstration, lecture and discussion, reading, viewing videos, or other activities. The plan should facilitate clear presentation of material to the client, provide for frequent reinforcement and feedback, and include some kind of active involvement of the client. Passive listening does not ensure learning. Health literacy issues must be kept in the foreground.

5. *Advise.* Manage the learning intervention. During the teaching plan implementation, the process is carefully orchestrated to actively engage the client in successful learning. Progress is constantly evaluated, new information added, success reinforced, the pace of feedback assessed, the pace adjusted, and outcomes and achievement of objectives evaluated.

6. *Evaluate the outcomes.* Judge achievement of objectives and then reformulate the plan to move the client to the next level. Evaluate learning using a variety of methods, such as asking questions that require use of new knowledge to answer, watching for new behaviors, and looking for feelings of achievement and expressions of new understanding.

Provide Data. Often providing data about a child's status to the parents or adolescent is a powerful yet easy intervention. The height and weight grid and developmental screening or laboratory test scores with interpretation are often significant motivators or reinforcers for the work that parents have been doing. The key is interpretation of information so that the parents know how their child compares with appropriate norms. Data provided should include both normal outcomes and areas of concern. Radecki and colleagues (2009) found that such data about their child were very important to families attending well-child clinics.

Role Model. Social learning theory suggests that modeling is an effective way for people to learn. Modeling appropriate parenting techniques can be most effective, especially when the parent rehearses the desired behaviors with positive reinforcement. The provider must be careful to create a situation in which parents feel competent—that they are doing a fine job rather than that someone else could do it better. Parents need to feel new confidence as a result of working with the provider and trying out new behaviors. Parenting classes and support groups often provide more time for role modeling and new behavior practice. Several visits are often needed to help parents learn new responses to children's behavior. Part of the developmental process requires that parents make decisions about when to use the new responses they are learning.

Bibliotherapy. Reading material promotion can be an excellent primary care intervention. Books or pamphlets provide information if it is well organized and presented in a manner that facilitates its retention. Furthermore, written materials allow patients or families to pace their learning at their own rate, and serve as a familiar source of reference when needs arise at unexpected times. Redman (1993) refers to printed teaching material as a "frozen language that is selective in its description of reality (which is both a strength and a weakness). It encourages limited feedback, but is constantly available." The good reader uses reading materials efficiently, scanning for important words, stopping to summarize the material learned, and using illustrations to enhance the meanings derived from the text. On the other hand, the unskilled reader either spends an inordinate amount of time trying to master the material at hand or sets aside the task, usually without letting the provider know of the difficulties encountered. Thus the reading levels of the client and the materials must be considered.

Reading provides vicarious role models for both children and parents, acts as a support by acknowledging the feelings and problems encountered by others with similar problems, and expands perspectives on various health-related issues. Stories help children, especially adolescents, explore new ideas, clarify their own feelings and perceptions, and serve as an impetus for change.

The Internet also provides information on many subjects, but readers must be cognizant of the source to sort out reliable information from biased sources. Video libraries provide helpful information with role modeling played out in many cases.

Patient Education With Children and Adolescents. Teaching children includes all the aforementioned steps and careful assessment of the child's developmental level. The concepts children learn vary with cognitive abilities. Children's attention spans are often short; therefore, information needs to be presented in small bites, with frequent reinforcement and opportunities for doing rather than just listening. Reading skills may not be developed, so verbal and demonstration strategies are more effective for younger children. Terminology might need to be adjusted to use simpler words and concepts. Verbal and nonverbal reinforcement and feedback need to be appropriate for the child. The use of star charts is a good way to reinforce behaviors visually and concretely. Such strategies are consistent with school-age children in Piaget's concrete operations cognitive stage.

Developmental level is equally important during adolescence. The young adolescent (13 to 14 years old) understands and engages in learning differently from the 18-year-old. Motivators for teenagers do not include a knowledge of long-term effects. The use of several modalities, such as discussions with peers, reading, reviewing, and viewing audiovisual media, is helpful. Advice needs to be practical. Teenagers do best when they are viewed as decision-makers who need information to make good choices. Identification of strengths and weaknesses is always important. The use of peer groups can be extremely effective.

Preventive Health Care. The use of functional health patterns emphasizes health promotion and the regular clinical visit is an essential management strategy. A clinical preventive services model for health supervision involves regular visits timed to offer periodic screening opportunities. The purpose of the health supervision visit is to assess strengths and weaknesses in health and to intervene to promote the best health possible. Health supervision includes the clinical interview, developmental and educational surveillance, observation of parent-child interaction, physical examination, and screening procedures, such as measuring height, weight, head circumference, body mass index (BMI), vision, hearing, blood pressure, and diagnostic tests like hemoglobin or hematocrit.

Visits with the provider also allow assessment of home, family, and social life, teaching about growth and development, and problem-solving related to issues that affect children's health status. The visits can be used to enhance children's sense of independence and positive self-concept and to encourage children to make healthy lifestyle decisions. As children mature they should be actively involved in the visit, with the provider asking them questions directly and providing appropriate feedback to their responses.

The visits need to be scheduled infrequently enough to be economical, but frequently enough to identify changes in the patterns of growth and development or early physiologic, psychological, or social problems that might be detrimental to the child's health. The American Academy of Pediatrics (AAP) provides a policy, *Recommendations for Preventive Pediatric Care* (2008) that suggests appropriate health maintenance care activities by age. This model is used in *Bright Futures: Guidelines for Health Supervision of Infants, Children, and Adolescents* (Hagan et al, 2008). All pediatric primary care providers should be familiar with its use.

The problem with guidelines for health supervision is that they are too comprehensive to be accomplished within current office schedules. Moyer and Butler (2004) studied gaps in well-child care. They found that 42 preventive service interventions were recommended by two or more of the major pediatric authorities, such as the AAP, *Bright Futures* (Hagan et al, 2008), the American Academy of Family Practice, and *Guidelines for Adolescent Preventive Services* in the behavioral counseling, screening, and prophylaxis domains. Although in 2007 more than 30% of visits to physicians were for well-child care, clinicians were not able to complete all the recommended actions within 20- to 30-minute visits using current patterns of practice. A study by Mangione-Smith and colleagues (2007) found that only 40.7% of the indicated preventive care activities were completed in their study of more than 1500 families over a 2-year period. Moyer and Butler (2004) support the development of recommended health promotion interventions through clinical trials rather than expert opinion. They hypothesize that if it were clear which interventions were most effective, time and costs could be used more efficiently without sacrificing quality through omission of needed guidance, or because of insufficient time, by directing effort toward the most effective activities. Much work needs to be done in this area, and providers need to be alert to research that supports or refutes some of the standard interventions typically recommended in well-child care. In any case, providers are given many ideas for provision of quality care; however, they need to select and prioritize the guidelines to make care realistic and meaningful.

Health System Interventions. Families with children have many complex needs that could often be met by organizations such as governmental agencies; health care services, including clinics, screening programs, health promotion programs, and hospitals; and volunteer programs. A problem in the health management pattern occurs when families lack access to these resources. Strategies to increase parents' ability to access resources occur on two levels: (1) giving parents the information to more easily and appropriately gain access and (2) removing barriers to access.

Referrals should be considered whenever there is need for expertise, a more accessible resource, more time for intervention than is available in the current setting, or special types of intervention, such as a support group, class, or practice opportunities. Managed care settings, in some cases, seem to discourage use of referrals outside the system. However, solving problems efficiently and effectively is cost-effective, even if that means using another resource.

Identifying and using various community resources requires knowledge and skills that some families do not have. Locating services and helping families learn to use them might be necessary. Transportation, financial resources, the process for entering the system, and the services that can be anticipated are all factors to be discussed with families.

Teach Telephone Triage and E-mail Communication. The nature of the telephone interaction between parent and provider is a critical factor in accurately interpreting a child's condition, deciding on appropriate measures of care, and establishing confidence and trust. (See Chapter 21 for a discussion of how pediatric care providers can work with parents to use the telephone in the management of illnesses). Increasingly, health care practices use e-mail communication to assess and give advice or treatment to patients. This trend is just beginning, and many questions remain about safety and appropriate use (Griffiths et al, 2006; Masters, 2008). As with any form of communication, providers who use e-mail should clearly establish with the parent how the technology is to be used (e.g., which types of questions, how quickly can a response be expected, security measures to protect confidentiality).

Identify Resources. Providers serve as advocates by helping families locate local, regional, or national health care resources to meet their health needs. It is important that providers develop and maintain a resource list relevant to their practice. Using a resource list facilitates referrals and recommendations to parents; it gives the clear message that the family is not alone with their concern, that help is available, and that the primary care provider is a knowledgeable ally in the family's effort to maintain good health.

Assist in Contact of Support Networks. As advocates, providers make every effort to encourage independent action and decision-making by families, but if the family's coping abilities are compromised, it is not enough simply to give the name of a resource or contact to the family. In these situations, providers may need to contact the resource themselves or assist the family to make the contact. For some families in crisis, it is appropriate to refer them to a community or mental health professional for help to establish and maintain contact with a supportive network.

Remove Barriers to Care. Financial and insurance issues are key barriers to health care. Providers need to be aware of ways to help parents decrease costs—fewer visits, fewer diagnostic tests, use of community resources, advocacy for needed care with insurance agencies, and creating lower-cost options within agencies whenever possible. Providing clinical services outside normal working hours (i.e., evening and weekend clinics) helps many families access care without losing pay or having to use limited "sick time" hours. Other barriers to health care access are geography and lack of essential infrastructure services, such as transportation and childcare. The lack of primary care resources in rural and isolated areas can prevent families from obtaining regular care. If a family does not have adequate transportation or childcare services, the cost of seeking well-child care or treating minor acute problems that can worsen without medical intervention often outweighs the perceived benefits.

Providers can consult with parents and social workers to identify resources in the community that help overcome some of these barriers. For example, transportation may be available through some managed-care plans or local volunteer organizations (e.g., churches), or a relative may have time to care for other children while the parent takes one child to the clinic. For other barriers, however, the solution lies in making changes in the way health care services are organized and financed. This task goes far beyond the primary care setting, but it is nonetheless the responsibility of all pediatric primary care providers to be aware of and to participate in the process of restructuring and reorganizing the health care system.

Management Strategies for Children with Special Needs

Health management of children with special needs is challenging. Children with chronic illness receive expert illness care from a number of specialists, but their primary care needs may often be neglected. Primary care providers can serve to coordinate health maintenance care with ongoing specialty illness management. Communication and collaboration with the child's specialty physician or care team are essential, as is clear communication with the parents about the role of each provider in the child's care. Providers also need to adapt normal intervention techniques when providing primary care to children with chronic illness. The regular immunization schedule may need to be adjusted, for example, or special techniques for obtaining height and weight or vital signs might be necessary. Parents and children should be assisted to develop ways to meet daily living needs consistent with the child's ability. Children with physical handicaps, for example, require special intervention to meet activity and exercise needs for growth and development.

Evaluating Health Promotion Interventions

The care that many health care providers deliver is rarely evaluated, except in larger organizations. Whitehead (2003) and Pender and colleagues (2011) suggest that evaluation is essential for quality care. The health care team should build evaluation into health delivery services. This begins with identification of goals, program objectives and indicators of success—short term, midterm, and long range. The type of program determines the type of evaluation method used. Evaluations may be quantitative or qualitative or both. Measures should consider program effectiveness, efficiency, efficacy and equity. Program evaluation includes the following questions:

- What knowledge, behavior changes, or outcomes are expected?
- Is the intervention practical and effective in clinical practice?
- How long does it take to become effective?
- How long do the intervention effects last?
- Are there unintended consequences?
- Are clients satisfied?
- What could be done to improve the intervention?
- How much did the intervention cost?

Evaluations assess *outcomes;* for example, how many children were up-to-date on immunizations? How many children lost weight? What was the decrease in use of emergency department services for treatment of asthma? There are short- and long-term outcomes. Program evaluation also assesses the *process* of delivering care; for example, efficiency and time use, or satisfaction with care by staff and clients.

The randomized control trial is considered the best form of outcome evaluation. Mixed methods of data collection are often used. Data should be collected routinely and analyzed as part of the clinic management routines. With the use of automated systems and records in many institutions, the job should be more manageable than in the past. Ultimately the goal is to demonstrate that attention to health promotion and health maintenance activities has benefits to multiple stakeholders, patients, providers, and payers.

Because children change so rapidly, their functional health patterns are stable for only short periods of time. The patterns need continual reassessment in light of developmental progress. Parents also need continuing information and new skills, such as teaching behaviors, to manage their children's evolving health care needs adequately. In addition, a multitude of factors—family practices and attitudes, peer influences, and community effects—shape children's health behaviors. In some ways, health promotion care for children can be more difficult than managing an illness. Developing skill as a manager of health promotion for clients is no easy task, but it is worth the effort. It is in the area of functional health pattern management that the unique contributions of providers to the health care of their pediatric clients are confirmed.

Nutrition

ARDYS M. DUNN

Good nutrition is the foundation for healthy growth and development. Without adequate nutrients, children's physical and mental health can be severely compromised. Children's ability to interact with their environment, to be active and curious, and to explore and learn can be limited. Good nutrition, combined with vigorous exercise, helps children grow and maintain a high level of health. For children with acute or chronic illness, appropriate nutrition can be essential to healing and/or successful management of their condition.

The pediatric primary health care providers' goal is to ensure that children are well nourished. To accomplish this, providers must conduct thorough assessments, provide relevant education, develop clear and appropriate treatment plans, and refer the child and family to nutritional specialists as needed. Interventions aimed at helping children and families meet nutritional requirements and preventing problems related to poor nutrition are based on certain assumptions, including the following:

- Children's nutritional needs vary as they grow.
- Children's nutritional needs are influenced by their state of health.
- A wide range of food choices and feeding behaviors are used to meet nutritional needs.
- Recommended dietary allowances are *guidelines* only.
- Parents and other caregivers are responsible for providing food choices that are nutritionally adequate and for establishing healthy eating patterns; to do so, they must be well informed.
- Family patterns of nutrition and eating are based on social, economic, cultural, and psychological dynamics. Patterns are not related to nutrients alone.
- The primary care provider is a source of information regarding nutrition, feeding patterns, and health.
- The primary care provider works with a network of specialists (e.g., registered dietitians) to manage children's nutrition status.

This chapter looks at the nutritional requirements of children and the ways providers can use nutrition to help children be their healthiest. It begins with the nutritional standards for preventive care recommended by certain professional groups, followed by a review of the functions of specific nutrients in the body and the "recommended daily intakes" for these nutrients. It must be emphasized that these recommendations are just that—recommendations, not requirements—and the

fact that they are often given as a range (e.g., 25% to 35% of energy intake in the form of fat) reinforces the concept that there is latitude in what can be considered healthy nutritional intake.

Approaches to general assessment, diagnosis, and management of nutritional status are then presented. Finally, sections on "normal" and "altered" patterns of nutrition conclude the chapter. The section on "normal" nutrition outlines development of eating habits and age-specific considerations related to food intake, including nutrition for the pregnant teenager and vegetarian diets. In the section on altered patterns of nutrition, several tables summarize nutritional considerations of specific conditions (e.g., diabetes mellitus). It would be impossible within the scope of a general text to discuss nutritional needs of all acute and chronic conditions, so general categories are outlined: conditions that require increased caloric intake, those that require decreased caloric intake, and so on. Obesity has become an epidemic in the United States and other developed countries. This eating problem (epidemiology, etiology, assessment, and management), as currently understood, is discussed.

■ Standards for Preventive Care

The American Academy of Pediatrics (AAP) recommends exclusive breastfeeding until 4 to 6 months old, and continued breastfeeding, supplemented with appropriate foods for infants, until at least 12 months old (AAP, 2005). The AAP also recommends giving 400 International Units of vitamin D to all breastfed infants until 1 year of age and to all children and adolescents with diets deficient in vitamin D (Wagner et al, 2008). The American Medical Association (AMA) supports breastfeeding as the best infant nutrition. It recommends that providers calculate body mass index (BMI) measures in children's routine physical examinations, "recognizing ethnic sensitivities and its relation to stature." The AMA school health advocacy agenda includes attention to healthy eating and exercise in schools and for school-age children (AMA, 2005). The Institute of Medicine (IOM) has published ways to ensure that school food programs meet current dietary recommendations (Committee on Nutrition Standards for National School Lunch and Breakfast Programs et al, 2010). *Bright Futures in Practice: Nutrition* (Holt and Wooldridge, 2011) presents nutritional guidelines, discusses issues and concerns related to pediatric nutrition, and outlines tools for providers to assess and manage nutrition in children. The U.S. Preventive Services Task Force (USPSTF) recommends that children ages 6 years and older be screened for obesity and that they be given, or referred for, comprehensive intensive behavioral interventions to improve weight (USPSTF, 2010). Nutrition standards for children emphasize that:

- Breast milk is the best food for infants.
- Children's diets should include a wide variety of foods.
- Foods should come predominantly from plants, especially:
  - Whole grains
  - Fruits
  - Vegetables
  - Legumes and nuts
- Iron-rich foods are essential, especially for infants and adolescents.
- Fat intake, particularly saturated fats and cholesterol, should be limited. Trans fats should be eliminated from the diet.
- Simple carbohydrates (e.g., refined grains, white bread, sugar, high-fructose corn syrup, sodas) should be limited.
- Extra calcium, iron, and folic acid are important nutrients in adolescent girls' diets.
- Children's diets should include adequate fiber and sodium.

■ Nutritional Requirements and Recommended Daily Intake

The body requires energy, water and electrolytes, and macro- and micronutrients in order to survive. The amounts of these requirements vary greatly. The Food and Nutrition Board (FNB) of the National Academies of Science, IOM, lists dietary reference intakes (DRIs) based on diets consumed in the U.S. and Canada. Developed in 1997, DRIs include the estimated average requirement (EAR), the recommended dietary allowance (RDA), the adequate intake (AI), and the tolerable upper intake level (UL) of foods consumed. DRIs reference parameters of nutrient intake that will meet body needs and prevent adverse effects of excessive intake. They do not, however, set a standard below which the diet is judged inadequate to prevent pathology (basal requirement), or a standard that is sufficient for the body to maintain a healthy body reserve (normative requirement) (FNB, 2005). Based on extensive analysis of scientific evidence on diet and nutrition, and referencing the DRIs developed by the FNB, the U.S. Departments of Agriculture (USDA) and Health and Human Services (USDHHS) publish *Dietary Guidelines for Americans* every five years. These guidelines address questions of nutritional adequacy, energy balance, weight management, and food safety and technology, and make recommendations regarding intake of macro- and micronutrients, water, cholesterol, salt, and alcohol (USDA and USDHHS, 2010). They can assist families and providers to make healthful dietary decisions to meet the nutritional needs of individual children.

ENERGY

An individual's basal metabolic rate and thermoregulation, growth, and activity are the three mechanisms requiring energy intake, measured in kilocalories. The body uses most of its energy for regulatory functions: respiration, digestion, temperature regulation, circulation, and so on. This activity is measured as the body's basal metabolic rate (BMR), or resting energy expenditure (REE). Growth, greatest in infancy and adolescence, is a second source of energy consumption. Finally, activity, exercise, and other metabolic demands, including illness, increase the level of calories needed to support healing and sustain good health. The body meets these energy demands, or estimated energy requirement (EER), by using stored energy sources or calories consumed on a daily basis. EERs for healthy children can vary significantly by age, health status, and activity level. Tables providing a formula to calculate caloric needs of infants and toddlers and children age 2 to 18 years old can be found on the inside cover of this text.

Macronutrients (protein, carbohydrates, and fats) and alcohol are all sources of calories the body uses to meet its energy needs. The body makes no distinction as to the *source* of calories; it will use whichever calories are consumed. It is recommended, however, that caloric intake be distributed among the three macronutrients, with each providing a certain percentage of total daily caloric intake. These recommendations are given as an acceptable macronutrient distribution range (AMDR) and are presented in Table 10-1. They are based on age for children who are of average height, weight, and physical activity level (FNB, 2005; USDA and USDHHS, 2010). If more calories than are required for energy needs are consumed, they will be converted to fat and stored. In addition to energy needs, the body requires essential nutrients for growth and health. If the food a child eats is high in calories (calorie dense) but low in nutrients (nutrient poor, often referred to as "empty calories"), the child will gain excess weight and still be undernourished. Data from the National Health and Nutrition Examination Survey (NHANES) from 2001 to 2004 show that more than 90% of all children ages 2 years and older had intakes of empty calories that exceeded discretionary limits (Krebs-Smith et al, 2010), contributing to overweight and obesity.

WATER AND ELECTROLYTES

Water

Water is the primary component of body tissue, and maintaining fluid balance is essential to good health. Because of the wide variation of healthful intake and output, there is no specific recommended daily requirement for water, though general guidelines are available (Otten et al, 2006). Thirst is generally an adequate indicator of the need to take in more water. Children do not always appreciate the feeling of thirst, however, and may need to be offered water or foods that contain water. Infants present special concerns because they have a large skin surface per unit of body weight, their renal systems are not fully mature to process solutes, they have a high daily water turnover (up to 15% of body weight), and they are unable to express thirst. All these factors make infants uniquely susceptible to rapid variations in water balance.

Water loss is increased by illness, activity, high altitude, high ambient temperature, and dry air. When more than 10% of body weight is lost without replacement, dehydration can become life threatening. If a child is vomiting and has diarrhea, water loss can be significant. Children who exercise strenuously, especially in a warm, dry environment, require

TABLE 10-1   Recommended Daily Allowance or Adequate Intake*of Nutrient by Age for Children of Average Height, Weight, and Physical Activity Level

Nutrient	0-6 mo	7-12 mo	1-3 yr	4-8 yr	Boys 9-13 yr	Boys 14-18 yr	Girls 9-13 yr	Girls 14-18 yr	Pregnant <18 yr
Protein, g/day	9.1*	11	13	19	34	52	34	46	71
Protein (AMDR)	ND	ND	5-20	10-30	10-30	10-30	10-30	10-30	10-35
Carbohydrates, g/day	60*	95*	130	130	130	130	130	130	175
Carbohydrates (AMDR)	ND	ND	45-65	45-65	45-65	45-65	45-65	45-65	45-65
Fats, total, g/day	31*	30*	—	—	—	—	—	—	—
n-6 Polyunsaturated fatty acids (linoleic acid), g/day	4.4*	4.6*	7*	10*	12*	16*	10*	11*	13*
n-3 Polyunsaturated fatty acids (alpha-linolenic acid), g/day	0.5	0.5	0.7	0.9	1.2	1.6	1.0	1.1	1.4
Fats, total (AMDR)			30-40	25-35	25-35	25-35	25-35	25-35	20-35
Vitamin A (RAE), mcg	400*	500*	300	400	600	900	600	700	750
Thiamine (B₁), mg	0.2*	0.3*	0.5	0.6	0.9	1.2	0.9	1	1.4
Riboflavin (B₂), mg	0.3*	0.4*	0.5	0.6	0.9	1.3	0.9	1	1.4
Niacin, mg	2*	4*	6	8	12	16	12	14	18
Pyridoxine (B₆), mg	0.1*	0.3*	0.5	0.6	1	1.3	1	1.2	1.9
Folate, mcg	65*	80*	150	200	300	400	300	400	600
Vitamin B₁₂, mcg	0.4*	0.5*	0.9	1.2	1.8	2.4	1.8	2.4	2.6
Vitamin C, mg	40*	50*	15	25	45	75	45	65	80
Vitamin D, mcg	5*	5*	5*	5*	5*	5*	5*	5*	5*
Vitamin E, mg	4*	5*	6	7	11	15	11	15	15
Vitamin K, mcg	2*	2.5*	30*	55*	60*	75*	60*	75*	75*
Calcium, mg	210*	270*	500*	800*	1300*	1300*	1300*	1300*	1300*
Fluoride, mg†	0.01*	0.5*	0.7*	1*	2*	3*	2*	3*	3*
Iron, mg	0.27*	11	7	10	8	11	8	15	27
Zinc, mg	2*	3	3	5	8	11	8	9	12

*Adequate intake.
†Fluoride supplement is not necessary if the water supply contains ≥0.6 part per million fluoridation.
AMDR, Acceptable macronutrient distribution range; *RAE*, retinol activity equivalents.
Adapted from Food and Nutrition Board, Institute of Medicine (IOM): *Dietary reference intakes for energy, carbohydrate, fiber, fat, fatty acids, cholesterol, protein, and amino acids,* Washington, DC, 2005, National Academies Press; U.S. Department of Agriculture (USDA) and U.S. Department of Health and Human Services (USDHHS): *Dietary Guidelines for Americans, 2010,* Washington, DC, 2010, U.S. Government Printing Office.

additional water intake. After strenuous or prolonged exercise, however, high water intake without electrolyte replacement can lead to water intoxication.

Sodium

Sodium functions primarily to regulate extracellular fluid volume. It also regulates osmolarity, acid-base balance, and the membrane potential of cells and is involved in the cell membrane transport pump, exchanging with potassium in intracellular fluid. Sodium loss occurs with vomiting, diarrhea, and perspiration. Sodium requirements vary with the rate of extracellular fluid expansion, which is most rapid in infants and very young children. It is not necessary to add sodium to the diet, even for children who exercise and perspire heavily. In fact, the typical North American diet far exceeds minimum requirements for sodium intake, with most sodium coming from salt added during food processing and manufacturing. For children 1 to 3 years, 1000 mg per day is considered an adequate intake (AI) of sodium; for children 4 to 8 years,

1200 mg per day; and for children 9 to 18, 1500 mg per day (USDA and USDHHS, 2010).

Potassium

Potassium helps maintain intracellular homeostasis and contributes to muscle contractility and transmission of nerve impulses. Severe potassium deficit (hypokalemia) can lead to cardiac dysrhythmias and death. Excessive potassium (hyperkalemia) can cause cardiac arrest. The urinary and gastrointestinal systems regulate potassium levels, and extreme imbalances are almost always due to disease processes or medication rather than dietary factors. Potassium requirements increase as lean body mass increases and are higher during the rapid growth of infancy and adolescence than during middle childhood. Fruits, vegetables, and fresh meat have high potassium content.

Chloride

Chloride functions with sodium to maintain fluid and electrolyte balance. Loss of chloride occurs through the same routes as sodium loss: vomiting, diarrhea, and perspiration. The major source of chloride is salt (NaCl or KCl) added to foods during processing. There is no recommended daily allowance for chloride, but adequate amounts are ingested with a normal diet.

MACRONUTRIENTS

Protein

Protein is a fundamental component of all body cells. Dietary protein is broken down into amino acids, which are required for the synthesis of body cell protein and nitrogen-containing compounds, some enzyme and hormone activity, cell transport, and tissue growth and development. Ten "indispensable" or essential amino acids are not synthesized by the body and must be provided in the diet (phenylalanine, leucine, methionine, lysine, isoleucine, valine, threonine, tryptophan, histidine, and arginine [arginine is required in diet for infants but not adults]). Depending on their age, children should receive approximately 5% to 30% of daily calories from proteins (see Table 10-1).

Protein and amino acid deficiencies rarely appear alone but follow other dietary deficits. Without sufficient carbohydrate intake, for example, dietary protein cannot be broken down for protein synthesis. Extreme stress and disease can deplete nitrogen, a process that contributes to tissue wasting and creates an increased demand for protein. Growth needs of the premature infant require higher levels of protein intake than those of infants born at term. The demand for protein is not generally increased with normal activity except with some illnesses or to build additional muscle tissue during body conditioning.

Carbohydrates

Carbohydrates are the body's major dietary source of energy. More than half (45% to 65%) of children's body energy requirements should be supplied by carbohydrates (FNB, 2005; USDA and USDHHS, 2010). There are two forms of carbohydrates: simple sugars (the monosaccharides and disaccharides of sucrose, fructose, and lactose found in fruits, vegetables, milk, and prepared sweets) or complex carbohydrates (starches found in cereal grains, potatoes, legumes, and other vegetables). Most dietary carbohydrates should be in the complex form. Refined food products (e.g., products made with white flour, white sugar, white rice, and high-fructose corn syrup) should be limited. Because carbohydrates are essential to facilitate protein synthesis, if carbohydrates are extremely limited or absent from the diet (e.g., with a ketogenic diet used to manage intractable seizures of epilepsy; see Chapter 27), the body utilizes stored triglycerides, oxidizes fatty acids, and breaks down dietary and tissue protein. This process contributes to accumulation of ketone bodies.

Fats

Lipids, fats, and fatty acids are used by the body to provide energy, to facilitate absorption of the fat-soluble vitamins (A, D, E, and K), and to maintain integrity of cell membranes and myelin. Two essential fatty acids are not produced by the body and must be included in the diet. These essential polyunsaturated fatty acids (PUFAs), linoleic acid (LA) and alpha-linoleic acid (ALA), are precursors of omega-6 and omega-3 fatty acids, respectively. LA is found in soy oil, corn oil, and sunflower, safflower, pumpkin, and sesame seeds. ALA is found in large quantities in flaxseed and flaxseed oil and in lesser quantities in walnuts, canola oil, and wheat germ. Adequate amounts of omega-3 and omega-6 fatty acids are produced in the body if there is adequate intake of these two essential fatty acids and the vitamins and minerals necessary to facilitate their conversion.

It is recommended that fat intake for children 1 to 3 years old be 30% to 40% of total caloric intake; children more than 3 years old should gradually adopt a diet of 25% to 35% of total calories from fats, with less than 10% of total calories in the form of saturated fat. Daily diets should have no more than 300 mg of cholesterol. In fact, dietary saturated fats, trans fatty acids, and cholesterol are unnecessary for healthy nutrition, saturated fat and cholesterol intake should be minimal, and there should be zero intake of trans fatty acids (FNB, 2005; USDA and USDHHS, 2010). Numerous studies indicate that diets with high plant fibers, limited saturated fats, low cholesterol, and no trans fats reduce serum cholesterol and LDH levels without affecting normal growth and development (Royo-Bordonada et al, 2006; Ruottinen et al, 2010; Van Horn et al, 2003). When counseling parents about fat in their children's diets, providers should emphasize that a diet with about 25% to 30% of calories from fat easily provides for energy and growth needs; if less than 20% of total is fat, the child can be at nutritional risk.

MICRONUTRIENTS

Vitamins

Recommendations for daily intake of fat- and water-soluble vitamins are listed in Table 10-1. Table 10-2 identifies specific metabolic functions, dietary sources, and signs of deficient or excessive intake of these vitamins.

Fat-Soluble Vitamins. Several characteristics of fat-soluble vitamins (A, D, E, and K) have implications for dietary assessment and management:

- They can be stored for long periods of time in body tissues. As a result, temporary dietary deficiencies may not affect the body's growth and development. If stores are depleted

TABLE 10-2 Vitamins: Function, Dietary Sources, Interactions, Deficiency, and Excess

Function	Dietary Sources	Interactions Affecting Absorption or Utilization	Signs of Deficit	Signs of Excess
Fat-Soluble Vitamins **Vitamin A** Vision, cellular differentiation and growth, reproductive and immune system function	Liver, fish liver oils, fortified milk, eggs, carrots, dark green leafy vegetables	Facilitated by dietary fat, protein, and vitamin E Absorption of vitamin A is hindered by lack of protein, iron, or zinc	Anorexia, dry skin, keratinization of epithelial cells of respiratory tract, night blindness, corneal lesions, increased susceptibility to infections	Headache, vomiting, double vision, hair loss, dry mucous membranes, peeling skin, liver damage Toxic at 10 times the RDA No toxicity with excessive intake of carotenoids (e.g., carrots)
Vitamin D Bone growth and development; regulates intestinal absorption of calcium and phosphorus	Sunlight, artificial ultraviolet light, fortified food products, especially milk	Utilization compromised in patients with renal failure Increased exposure to sunlight increases intake Darker skin and aging skin inhibit synthesis	Inadequate bone mineralization, rickets or skeletal malformations, delayed dentition	Anorexia, nausea, vomiting, diarrhea, weakness, hypercalcemia, hypercalciuria, calcium deposits in soft tissue, permanent renal or cardiovascular damage
Vitamin E Antioxidant, traps free radicals, prevents oxidation of polyunsaturated fats	Vegetable oils, margarine, nuts, wheat germ, green leafy vegetables	Low serum levels have been associated with prematurity and congenital defects of the hepatobiliary system (e.g., cystic fibrosis, biliary atresia)	Macrocytic anemia and dermatitis in infants; neurological defects in severe malabsorption	Unknown, if any
Vitamin K Forms proteins that regulate blood clotting	Green leafy vegetables, milk, dairy products, liver	Inhibited by long-term antibiotic use, hyperalimentation, chronic biliary obstruction, or lipid malabsorption syndromes	Defective coagulation of blood, hemorrhages, liver injury	Vitamin K–responsive hemorrhagic condition, especially if patient is being treated with anticoagulants
Water-Soluble Vitamins **Vitamin C** Essential for collagen formation and function; promotes growth and tissue repair; enhances iron absorption; improves wound healing	Vegetables and fruits, especially citrus fruits, broccoli, collard greens, spinach, tomatoes, potatoes, strawberries, peppers	Vitamin C is easily lost in food storage and preparation with exposure to heat, oxygen, and water Exposure to cigarette smoke increases vitamin C requirement	Scurvy, cracked lips, bleeding gums, slow wound healing, easy bruising	Unknown; excess vitamin is excreted in urine
Thiamine (Vitamin B$_1$) Necessary for carbohydrate metabolism; promotes normal appetite and digestion	Whole grains, brewer's yeast, legumes, seeds and nuts, organ meats, lean cuts of pork	Availability inhibited by presence of thiaminase (found in raw fish); alcohol contributes to thiamine deficiency	Beriberi: muscle weakness, ataxia, confusion, anorexia, tachycardia, heart failure in infants	None by oral intake; excess excreted in urine

Continued

TABLE 10-2 Vitamins: Function, Dietary Sources, Interactions, Deficiency, and Excess—cont'd

Function	Dietary Sources	Interactions Affecting Absorption or Utilization	Signs of Deficit	Signs of Excess
Riboflavin (Vitamin B₂) Necessary for oxidation-reduction reactions; essential for function of vitamin B₆ and niacin; helps maintain integrity of skin, tongue, and lips	Dairy products, meat, poultry, fish; enriched or fortified grains, cereals, and breads; green vegetables, such as broccoli, spinach, asparagus, turnip greens	Positive nitrogen balance contributes to function of riboflavin	Oral-buccal cavity lesions, generalized seborrheic dermatitis, scrotal and vulval skin changes, normocytic anemia, dimness of vision	None known
Niacin (Vitamin B₃) Essential for energy metabolism, glycolysis, fatty acids; maintains nervous system, integrity of skin, mouth, tongue	Meats, fortified grains, legumes Milk, eggs, and meats contain tryptophan	Requires riboflavin for absorption and utilization Grains treated with lime have more biologically available niacin Dietary tryptophan converts to niacin	Pellagra: dermatitis, diarrhea, inflammation of mucous membranes, indigestion	No known toxicity with dietary doses; heat rush and flushing with excessive doses
Vitamin B₆ (Pyridoxine) Essential for metabolism of amino acids, lipids, nucleic acids, and glycogen	Chicken, fish, kidney, liver, pork, red meat, eggs, unrefined rice, soybeans, oats, whole wheat, peanuts, walnuts Processing of foods destroys vitamin B₆	Riboflavin enhances function Increased protein intake increases requirements for vitamin B₆	Seen in combination with other B-complex vitamin deficiencies; dermatitis, anemia, convulsions, neurologic symptoms, and abdominal distress in infants	Ataxia, sensory neuropathy when taken in gram quantities for months or years
Folate (Folacin) Essential for amino acid metabolism and nucleic acid synthesis; red blood cell formation	Liver, yeast, dark green leafy vegetables, legumes, fruits, oranges, brewer's yeast, milk	Only about 25% of folate in foods is directly bioavailable for absorption in intestine; more efficiently absorbed if serum levels are low Boiling milk destroys about 50% of folate present	Poor growth, megaloblastic anemia in severe cases; macrocytic anemia, glossitis, gastrointestinal disturbances; increased risk of neural tube defects in infants of folate-deficient mothers	None known in dietary doses; excessive folic acid supplementation may inhibit uptake of phenytoin and contribute to seizures in epileptic cases controlled by phenytoin
Vitamin B₁₂ Essential for metabolism, adequate red blood cell formation	Animal products: meat, eggs, and milk; shellfish; fortified foods	Absorbed in ileum; intrinsic factor-mediated In strict vegetarians, the vitamin excreted in the bile is reabsorbed	Megaloblastic anemia, neurologic symptoms, sore tongue, weakness	None known

RDA, Recommended dietary allowance.

and nutritional intake is inadequate, signs of vitamin deficiency appear. If intake is excessive, as can occur when supplements are taken, toxic effects can appear.

- They are absorbed in the intestines along with fats and lipids in foods. Low-fat diets and increased intestinal motility or malabsorption syndromes may put individuals at risk for fat-soluble vitamin deficiency.
- They are fairly stable when heated, as in cooking. Food preparation does not destroy fat-soluble vitamins as readily as water-soluble vitamins.

- They require bile for absorption. Conditions that compromise the hepatobiliary system put the individual at risk for decreased vitamin absorption.
- They do not contain nitrogen and do not act as coenzymes in cellular metabolism of nutrients.

Water-Soluble Vitamins. In contrast to fat-soluble vitamins, water-soluble vitamins (C and B complexes) are stored in very small amounts in the body. If water-soluble vitamin intake is more than that needed by the body, absorption (primarily in the jejunum) decreases, and excess vitamins are excreted.

As a result, daily intake of water-soluble vitamins is necessary, and there is little risk of toxicity from large doses. The B vitamins contain nitrogen and serve as essential coenzymes in the body's metabolism of nutrients. Niacin (vitamin B_3) plays a significant role in increasing high-density lipoproteins (HDLs).

Minerals and Elements

Three major minerals—calcium, magnesium, and phosphorus—are present in the body in amounts greater than 5 g. DRIs have been set for boron, calcium, chromium, copper, fluoride, iodine, iron, magnesium, manganese, molybdenum, nickel, phosphorus, selenium, silicon, vanadium, and zinc (FNB,

2005). Table 10-1 identifies recommended allowances for calcium, fluoride, iron, and zinc.

Peak bone density is directly related to calcium intake during the years of bone mineralization, primarily before 20 years of age. Bone calcification continues for several years more, however, so to ensure maximum peak bone density, dietary calcium needs to remain high until about 25 years old. Breastfed infants or those who are fed an approved infant formula receive sufficient calcium and should not be given a supplement. Minerals and essential trace elements, their functions, dietary sources, and signs of deficit or excess are presented in Table 10-3. Foods rich in iron are listed in Table 10-4.

TABLE 10-3 Minerals and Trace Elements: Function, Dietary Sources, Interactions, Deficiency, and Excess*

Function	Dietary Sources	Interactions Affecting Absorption or Utilization	Signs of Deficit	Signs of Excess
Minerals				
Calcium				
Development of bone tissue; vital role in nerve conduction, membrane permeability, blood clotting, and muscle contraction	Milk and milk products, green leafy vegetables, broccoli, kale, and collards, soft bones of fish, sardines, foods processed or fortified with calcium	Absorption enhanced in the presence of vitamin D, adequate protein intake, during periods of rapid growth, and if dietary intake of calcium is low; inhibited by excess sodium or protein	Decreased bone strength, increased risk for fractures	Constipation, increased risk for urinary stone formation; risk for decreased renal function
Phosphorus				
Essential for bone integrity and general metabolism; provides essential energy during the metabolic process	Almost all foods, especially meat, poultry, fish, milk, cereal grains; food additives in processed foods	Absorption inhibited by aluminum hydroxide in antacids, and by excess iron	Bone loss, weakness, malaise, anorexia, and pain	None known
Magnesium				
Activates enzymes, facilitates cell metabolism, maintains electrical potential of cell membranes, enhances transmission of nerve impulses, assists to maintain adequate serum levels of calcium and potassium	Nuts, legumes, whole (unmilled) grains, green vegetables; bananas provide some magnesium	Absorption reduced with high-fiber diet, excess sodium, calcium, vitamin D, protein, and alcohol	Nausea, muscle weakness, irritability	None in healthy individual; with impaired renal function, excess may contribute to nausea, vomiting, hypotension, bradycardia, central nervous system depression
Iron				
Formation of the heme molecule; used in oxygen transport	Meat, eggs, vegetables, cereals, foods fortified with iron additives; Table 10-4 identifies a number of iron-rich foods	Absorption is enhanced if iron stores or daily intakes are low; presence of ascorbic acid increases absorption. Heme iron in meats is more bioavailable than nonheme iron from grains, fruits, and vegetables. Absorption inhibited if the iron-rich food is ingested with milk or caffeine or in presence of phytic acid, oxalic acid, or tannic acid	Anemia. Children are particularly susceptible to iron deficiency during periods of rapid growth combined with low dietary iron intake: from about 6 months to 4 years old and during early adolescence; menstruation puts adolescent girls at risk	Iron poisoning can be fatal; for a 2-year-old, a fatal dose is approximately 3 g; for adolescents and adults, 200 to 250 mg/kg may be fatal

TABLE 10-3	Minerals and Trace Elements: Function, Dietary Sources, Interactions, Deficiency, and Excess*—cont'd			
Function	**Dietary Sources**	**Interactions Affecting Absorption or Utilization**	**Signs of Deficit**	**Signs of Excess**
Zinc				
Cellular metabolism, growth, and repair	Meats, animal products, seafood (especially oysters), eggs	Absorption may be decreased if taken with high-fiber diet, excess iron, copper, folic acid, ascorbic acid	Anorexia, growth retardation, skin changes, immunological abnormalities	Gastrointestinal disturbances, vomiting, acute toxicity, impaired immune response
Iodine				
Production of thyroid hormones	Water, seafood, airborne water from ocean mist, iodized salt, food processing related to milk and bread	None known	Thyroid dysfunction ranging from simple goiter to cretinism and mental retardation	Thyrotoxicosis; goiter, rare and not seen in children with intake up to 1 mg/day; toxic levels not known
Trace Elements				
Selenium				
Unknown	Seafood and organ meats; may be in grains grown in soil containing selenium	Intake linked to vitamin E intake; if vitamin E is adequate, selenium is likely to be also; may need to supplement in lactating women	May be related to muscle weakness and pain, cardiomyopathy (Keshan disease) in young children	Nausea, abdominal pain, diarrhea, fatigue, nail and hair changes or loss; toxic levels not known
		Total parenteral nutrition (TPN) feedings contribute to deficiency		
Copper				
Normal growth	Organ meats, seafood, nuts, seeds; fetus stores copper in liver during gestation	TPN feedings contribute to deficiency; high vitamin C molybdenum, or zinc intake may reduce retention or bioavailability	Bone loss, anemia, neutropenia, growth impairment	Liver disease, gastrointestinal symptoms, diarrhea, vomiting
Manganese				
Unknown, may be related to reproductive health, normal growth	Whole grains and cereals	Increased absorption during third trimester of pregnancy	Unknown, may be related to growth retardation	Unknown, may be related to learning disabilities, anemia
Fluoride				
Prevents dental caries, enhances bone health	Fluoridated water, tea, meat and bones of marine fish, potatoes, wheat germ	Processing foods in fluoridated water or cooking with Teflon increases content; cooking foods in aluminum reduces fluoride	Dental caries, may be related to poor bone health	Mottling of teeth, kidney disease, bone disease, may affect muscle and nerve function
Chromium				
Assists in glucose metabolism	Brewer's yeast, calves' liver, American cheese, wheat germ	TPN feedings can contribute to deficiency	May be related to impairment of glucose tolerance	Unknown, requires further study
Molybdenum				
Enzyme function	Milk, beans, breads, cereals	TPN feedings can contribute to deficiency	Unknown	Related to loss of copper, may lead to goutlike symptoms

*Nearly all trace minerals are toxic in large quantities because many are metals.

TABLE 10-4 Iron-Rich Foods*

Food	High Levels (5 mg/Serving)	Moderate Levels (2-4 mg/Serving)	Low Levels (<2 mg/Serving)
Breads, grains, cereals, seeds†	Almonds (1 cup, whole, oil roasted) Cashews (1 cup, dry roasted) Pumpkin seed kernels (¼ cup, roasted) Fortified cereals Mixed nuts (1 cup, dry roasted with peanuts) Brown glutinous rice (1 cup, cooked) Sunflower seeds (1 cup, dry roasted) Watermelon kernels (1 cup, dried) Wheat germ (1 cup, toasted)	Bagel (1, egg or plain) Bread, Indian fry (1 piece) Breadstick (10, plain, without salt) Filberts (1 cup, dried) Gingerbread (1 piece) Muffin (1 wheat) Peanuts (1 cup, dried) White rice (1 cup, enriched, regular, cooked) Waffles (2 each) Walnuts (1 cup, dried)	Biscuits (1 each) Bread (1 slice, whole wheat) Egg noodles (1 cup, cooked) English muffin (1 each) Pancakes (1 each) Peanut butter (2 Tbsp) Oatmeal (1 cup, cooked)
Fruits†	Apricot (1 cup, dried halves)	Avocado (1 whole) Currants (1 cup, dried Zante) Fig (10 each, dried) Pear (10 each, dried halves) Prune juice (1 cup) Raisins (½ cup)	Apple (1 medium, unpeeled) Apple juice (1 cup) Banana (1 medium) Dried mixed fruit (2 oz) Orange (1 medium) Orange juice (1 cup)
Vegetables†	Kidney beans (1 cup, cooked, fresh) Lentils (1 cup, cooked) Soybeans (1 cup, cooked) White beans (1 cup, cooked) Spinach (1 cup, cooked) Tofu (½ cup, cooked)	Black beans (1 cup, cooked) Garbanzo beans (1 cup, cooked) Refried beans (1 cup, canned) Beet greens (1 cup, cooked) Potatoes (1 medium, with skin, baked) Peas (1 cup, fresh, cooked) Snow peas with pods (1 cup, raw or cooked) Spinach (1 cup, raw) Molasses (2 Tbsp, blackstrap) Spinach (1 cup, frozen, cooked)	Kidney beans (1 cup, canned) Green beans (1 cup, raw or cooked) Broccoli (1 cup) Carrots (1 cup) Corn (½ cup) Lettuce (1 cup) Potato (½ cup, baked, with skin) Sweet potatoes (1 cup, fresh, boiled, mashed) Tomatoes (1 cup fresh) Tomato juice (1 cup, canned) Turnip greens (1 cup, cooked)
Meats, poultry, fish, other protein sources‡	Clams (3.5 oz, 5 each, or 1 cup = 22 mg Fe) Oysters (3.5 oz) Beef heart meat (3.5 oz, cooked) Beef liver (3.5 oz, simmered) Veal liver (3 oz, simmered) Chicken liver (3.5 oz, cooked) Turkey liver (3.5 oz, cooked)	Ground beef (3 oz, cooked lean) Catfish (1 piece, floured, fried) Tuna (1 cup, canned, water packed) Lamb (3.5 oz, cooked)	Roast beef (3 oz, lean) Chicken (1 cup, dark or light meat) Egg (1, whole) Halibut (1 piece, baked or broiled) Ham (1 cup, roasted) Bacon (3 pieces, cooked) Pork (3 oz, lean shoulder roast)

*Cooking in cast iron pans increases iron intake, especially with high-acid foods (e.g., tomatoes).
†Iron in plant foods is better absorbed when eaten with vitamin C or meat products.
‡Iron in meat, poultry, and fish is more bioavailable than iron in other food sources.
Fe, Iron.
Adapted from Hands ES: *Food finder: food sources of vitamins and minerals,* ed 3, Salem, OR, 1995, ESHA Research; and Hands ES: *Nutrients in food,* Philadelphia, 2000, Lippincott Williams & Wilkins.

Use of Vitamin and Mineral Supplements

National surveys reveal that many U.S. children have suboptimal nutrient intakes, especially a deficit of fruits and vegetables that contain many vitamins and minerals. The NHANES data from 2001 to 2004 show that a majority of all Americans, including children, fail to meet federal dietary recommendations (Krebs-Smith et al, 2010). Project EAT (Eating Among Teens) data show a trend toward eating fewer fruits and vegetables as adolescence progresses (Larson et al, 2007), and school-age children are at high risk for vitamin and mineral deficits (Robinson-O'Brien et al, 2010).

In light of these data and when confronted with a "picky eater," parents are justifiably concerned and often ask if they

should be giving their child a vitamin and mineral supplement. Parents should be advised that supplements are not a substitute for food, but may be appropriate in some cases. A child's intake should be assessed over a 3-day period (i.e., DRIs for all foods do not have to be met every day) and strategies to encourage the child to eat a healthful, varied diet put in place. If, after assessment, the provider concludes that the child is at risk for nutritional deficit, multivitamins can be given. Preterm or low-birth-weight babies and children with chronic illness may need supplements, and all pregnant teenagers should receive prenatal vitamins. The AAP recommends a vitamin D supplement in breastfed infants of 400 International Units per day. Children and adolescents whose diet does not include an equivalent amount should also be given a supplement of 400

TABLE 10-5	Healthy Eating Index-2005: Components and Standards for Scoring[1]		
Component	Maximum Score in Points	Standard for Maximum Score	Standard for Minimum Score of Zero
Total fruit (includes 100% juice)	5	>0.8 cup equiv/1000 kcal	No fruit
Whole fruit (not juice)	5	>0.4 cup equiv/1000 kcal	No whole fruit
Total vegetables	5	>1.1 cup equiv/1000 kcal	No vegetables
Dark green and orange vegetables and legumes[2]	5	>0.4 cup equiv/1000 kcal	No dark green or orange vegetables or legumes
Total grains	5	> 3 oz equiv/1000 kcal	No grains
Whole grains	5	>1.5 oz equiv/1000 kcal	No whole grains
Milk[3]	10	>1.3 cup equiv/1000 kcal	No milk
Meat and beans	10	>2.5 oz equiv/1000 kcal	No meat or beans
Oils[4]	10	>12 g/1000 kcal	No oil
Saturated fat	10	<7% of energy[5]	>15% of energy
Sodium	10	<0.7 g/1000 kcal[5]	>2 g/1000 kcal
Calories from solid fats, alcoholic beverages, and added sugars (SoFAAS)	20	<20% of energy	≥50% of energy

[1]Intakes between the minimum and maximum levels are scored proportionately, except for saturated fat and sodium (see note 5).
[2]Legumes counted as vegetables only after meat and beans standard is met.
[3]Includes all milk products, such as fluid milk, yogurt, and cheese, and soy beverages.
[4]Includes nonhydrogenated vegetable oils and oils in fish, nuts, and seeds.
[5]Saturated fat and sodium get a score of 8 for the intake levels that reflect the *2005 Dietary Guidelines*: <10% of calories from saturated fat and 1.1 g sodium/1000 kcal, respectively.
Adapted from Guenther PM, Reedy J, Krebs-Smith SM: Development of the Healthy Eating Index-2005, *J Am Diet Assoc* 108(11):1896-1901, 2008a.

International Units. The dosage is based on the amount used to treat rickets in children (Casey et al, 2010).

Assessment of Nutritional Status

Assessment of nutritional status is done to determine if there is deviation from normal growth and development, whether the child's diet is adequate, and what variables may be influencing the child's dietary intake. When doing nutritional assessment, it is important to remember that eating is a social, cultural, and economic activity; nutritional value of foods is not the only, or often the most important, variable in a child's or family's decisions about what, how, and when to eat.

Much data can be collected in the intake interview, or using a 3-day diet recall. Providers can also use the Healthy Eating Index-2005 (HEI-2005) to assess quality of nutrient intake (Table 10-5). The HEI-2005 is based on *2005 Dietary Guidelines for Americans* and the formerly used MyPyramid model and is a revision of previous Healthy Eating Indices. It lists 12 nutrient categories and gives each a score of 5, 10, or 20, with a maximum score of 100. The HEI-2005 does not require calculation of energy requirements, but measures nutrient units per 1000 kcal, an easier concept for families and children to understand and apply. To analyze individual diets, long-term intake should be assessed; a simple 24-hour recall does not adequately reflect the usual diet and can give a biased HEI number. Ideally a mean daily intake is examined over a period of time, often as long as 1 year. In population studies, HEI scores typically settle around 50 to 60, indicating significant nutritional deficit (Freedman et al, 2010; Guenther et al, 2008a,b).

HISTORY

Questions to elicit a history of nutritional status can be grouped into several categories:
- Nutritional status of mother during pregnancy
- Food and fluid intake of child and of family:
  - Type of feeding method used during infancy: If not breastfed, formula name and preparation. Any problems? When weaned? When solids started? Any allergies or intolerances noted?
  - Current nutritional intake of child (if child is still an infant, ask more specifically about frequency and amounts of feedings in a 24-hour period)
  - Type of foods and fluids
  - Amounts eaten (may use 24-hour recall, 3-day diet history, or length of time and frequency that child is at breast)
  - Additional intake (e.g., vitamin, fluoride, or iron supplements)
  - Is child's intake different from the rest of the family? How?

- Eating patterns:
  - Frequency of eating (nursing, meals, snacks)
  - Bottle feeding: Is bottle propped? Does child take bottle to bed at night or at naptime? Who feeds child?
  - Breastfeeding: On demand or scheduled? How flexible is mother to demands of infant? Is mother working? Is breast milk frozen and fed by someone other than the mother?
  - Feeding patterns or behaviors for both child and family
  - Describe mealtimes: Does family sit down together? Are meals prepared at home? Does child eat at school? How often are "fast foods" eaten? What amount of time is spent eating? How long does it take to feed child?
  - Does family eat out frequently? How many times per week?
- Reactions to and attitudes about foods:
  - Any reaction to particular foods (e.g., vomiting, diarrhea, rash)?
  - Food preferences or dislikes
  - Cultural factors: What beliefs or attitudes does family have about how and what child should eat or how family should eat?
  - What is child's attitude about foods and eating?
  - Feeding abilities of child: For example, does child choke, gag, vomit, have suck or swallow difficulties, or refuse certain foods, perhaps because of texture or smell?
  - Parents' and child's knowledge of foods and nutritional needs
- Management of foods in the family:
  - Who plans, purchases, and prepares food and meals for family?
  - Economic and environmental factors that influence how food is managed: For example, are finances adequate to supply nutritious foods? Is there a refrigerator? Does family have a car to carry larger amounts of food from store? Is there a full-service grocery store in the neighborhood? What is the socioeconomic status of family? Is food shopping budgeted? Are food stamps or other supplemental programs used?
- Health status affected by nutrition:
  - Special considerations for children or family related to food: For example, does child have a chronic condition that requires a special diet, formula, or device for feeding? Are any medications being taken?
  - Elimination patterns
  - Dental status and care of teeth
  - Patterns of wound healing, infections, colds, and mild illnesses
  - Any change in hair, nails, skin, or mucous membranes?
  - Tolerance for hot or cold weather?
  - Growth, activity, and exercise pattern: For example, has child been growing as parent expects? Has there been a history of unusual weight gain or loss? Does child have energy to play? Is the child engaged in strenuous activity such as an athletic training program?
  - Family history: Hypertension, diabetes, hyperlipidemia, obesity, heart disease, allergies, eating disorders?

PHYSICAL EXAMINATION

The physical examination should include the following:
- Body temperature
- Height, weight, and head circumference measurements (see growth charts, Appendix B; also see table on inside cover of this text for average weight and height gains expected during childhood); arm circumference and triceps and subscapular skinfold caliper measurements for children at risk for obesity or malnutrition
- BMI
- Skin condition (clear, smooth, firm, with good turgor)
- Muscle tone, posture, skeletal development (body erect, tone good)
- Hair (smooth, full, shiny; no dryness, broken ends, bare patches, or discoloration)
- Mucous membranes, eyes (moist, shiny, no dark circles, conjunctiva pink)
- Teeth (eruption appropriate to age, gums healthy, no bleeding)
- Neck (thyroid, parotid glands of normal size)
- Abdomen (flat, soft)
- Cardiovascular (no pathologic murmur; normal heart size; skin warm, pink, less than 3-second capillary refill; peripheral pulses equal, strong)
- Neurologic and behavior (alert, active, reflexes present, no complaints of headache, neuritis)

DIAGNOSTIC TESTS

- Laboratory and diagnostic tests are performed as indicated:
  - Hemoglobin or hematocrit
  - Iron and/or ferritin levels
  - Serum levels for various elements: albumin, nitrogen balance, minerals, lipids
  - Bone radiographs for suspected iodine, vitamins C and D, or copper deficiency or to compare bone age with height age (age at which 50% of children reach the patient's height)

■ Management Strategies for Optimal Nutrition

It is the parents' responsibility to provide healthful food that is adequate to meet the child's nutritional needs in an environment that makes eating enjoyable; it is the child's responsibility to decide what and how much of these healthful foods to eat. Critical to this interaction is a parent who knows which foods are healthful and which are not, and who is aware of and responsive to the child's cues around feeding. Also essential is the parents' ability to provide healthful foods; this can be extremely difficult for some low-income families. Food insecurity, even in high-income countries, is common among low-income multiethnic groups, and contributes to health problems (Gorton et al, 2010; Park K et al, 2009). In the U.S., federal programs (e.g., food stamps; Women, Infants, and Children [WIC]) increase families' access to foods.

It is the providers' responsibility to help parents and children make good decisions about nutrition and to facilitate families' access to healthful foods. Providers may know what nutrients are necessary for healthy growth and development, but translating that information into day-to-day diet intake can be complex and confusing. What advice should be given to families when there is such a wide range of "normal" intake? What does it mean, for example, that 35% or less of energy requirements should be in the form of fats? Will it be harmful if a 3-month-old is introduced to commercially prepared fruits and vegetables? What, if any, are the benefits to eating organic foods? Should children avoid sugar or flavored milk? The questions are endless, and often without a clear answer. But the basic message providers should give parents is simple (Pollan, 2007):

- Eat food (versus processed, edible food-products that contain additives, fats, and few nutrients)
- Less of it (i.e., eat appropriate portions, do not overeat)
- Mostly plants
- Exercise

Pediatric providers use nutritional education, counseling, anticipatory guidance, and appropriate referral to ensure that children have optimal dietary intake. MyPlate (formerly MyPyramid) and the HEI-2005 are two tools providers can use to help families identify dietary deficits and make recommendations for change. Cultural issues related to food should be considered in doing an assessment and in planning interventions. Providers may need to refer families to public health nurses for assistance to find adequate food sources and/or to pediatric dietitians for management of special needs diets.

NUTRITIONAL EDUCATION

Education about nutrition should include information about children's age and developmental abilities and characteristics, nutritional requirements, foods that meet children's nutritional needs, and strategies to facilitate the development of healthy eating behaviors. Providers should also explain the relationship between diet and health conditions, including obesity.

MyPlate and MyPlate for Kids

MyPlate is a useful tool for educating families and children of all ages about a healthful diet. Developed by the U.S. Department of Agriculture to implement DRI guidelines of the FNB and reflect the *2010 Dietary Guidelines for Americans,* MyPlate allows individuals to calculate their personal nutrient needs based on age, gender, and activity level. It illustrates the proportions of a healthy diet, emphasizing a foundation of grains, fruits, vegetables, beans, peas, and lean meats, fish, and poultry.

These tools provide in-depth information, resources, and a wide variety of nutrition-related activities to engage individuals in assessing and planning healthy nutrition. School nutrition is also addressed.

Age-Specific Considerations

Healthy eating habits are essential to good nutrition. The role that food plays in the family, the meaning it has for family members, and the way it is incorporated into family dynamics (e.g., parents may use sweets to reward children for good behavior) must be considered as providers counsel families about nutrition. Healthy eating habits begin during gestation and continue throughout the life span. A healthy pregnancy most often leads to a healthy term newborn, ready to learn and master the skills of eating. The toddler and preschool years are critical to establishing lifelong patterns of eating. Many eating problems, including obesity, are in part due to poor

eating habits learned in infancy and early childhood that are reinforced through the school-age and adolescent years. Special considerations related to developing healthy eating habits are presented for each of the age-specific sections that follow. Also covered in this section are specific nutritional needs for children in each age group.

Newborns and Infants

Energy. Rapid infant growth requires high caloric intake. The table found on the inside cover of this text can be used to calculate the energy needs of infants to meet demands of metabolism and growth. Adequate intake of breast milk or infant formula meets all energy needs for infants until 4 to 6 months old.

Fat. For proper myelinization to occur infants must have adequate fat intake. Children younger than 2 years can require more than 30% dietary fat for neural development. The lipids in breast milk and formulas meet infants' dietary requirements. During the second year of life cow's milk can be included in children's diets. The AAP recommends whole milk for children between 12 and 24 months old, although reduced-fat, or 2% milk, is recommended if there is a concern of overweight or obesity, or a family history of obesity or cardiovascular disease (Daniels and Greer, 2008). As part of a varied diet, reduced-fat milk contributes to adequate fat intake and has no negative effect on growth or body composition (Wosje et al, 2001). Fat-free milk is not recommended for children younger than 2 years of age.

Vitamins. Vitamin supplements, except vitamin D, are usually not necessary for healthy term breastfed or formula-fed infants who eat a variety of cereal, fruits, vegetables, and proteins after 4 to 6 months old. Vitamin D supplement (400 International Units daily) is recommended for all breastfed infants and infants who receive an unfortified formula until they are 1 year old. Infants should have an adequate source of vitamin C after 4 to 6 months old. A multivitamin supplement is recommended for infants at nutritional risk.

Iron. Iron deficiency is the leading cause of anemia in children, and iron supplementation is appropriate in some cases. Term infants who are breastfed usually have adequate iron supplies until 4 to 6 months old. Premature or low-birth-weight infants, infants who are exclusively breastfed beyond 4 to 6 months old, and infants who are fed cow's milk before they are 12 months old are at high risk for iron deficiency anemia. Iron-fortified cereals and iron-fortified formulas are excellent sources of dietary iron supplements for infants 6 to 12 months old. Earlier supplementation may be necessary for premature infants, especially those that are breastfed.

Fluoride. The American Dental Association (ADA) recommends fluoride treatment starting at 6 months old (ADA, 2005). (See Chapter 33 for recommended fluoride dosages.) The fluoride level of water used to mix formula should be measured to ensure that infants do not receive excess fluoride. If the water supply is fluoridated, formula-fed infants younger than 6 months old can be given ready-to-feed formula, or nonfluoridated bottled water can be used to prepare formula.

Infant Formulas. Breast milk is the ideal food for newborns and infants and should be promoted unless it is medically harmful to the infant. Most iron-fortified infant formulas provide adequate nutrition and, for some families, may be an appropriate alternative to breastfeeding.

BOX 10-1 Categories of Infant Formulas*

- Premature transitional formulas
  - Higher caloric content more nutrient dense than regular cow's milk–based formulas; 24 kcal/oz
  - Protein source: nonfat cow's milk, whey
- Cow's milk–based formulas
  - Standard formula for healthy term infants; 20 kcal/oz
- Nutrient-dense cow's milk–based formulas
  - Similar to premature formula, but with less phosphorus and calcium; some preparations have up to 27 kcal/oz
- Hypoallergenic formulas
  - Partially hydrolyzed whey-based formulas
  - Soy-based formulas (protein source: soy protein isolate with L-methionine)
  - Extensively hydrolyzed casein–or whey-based formulas
  - Amino acid–based formulas (elemental)
- Formulas with long-chain polyunsaturated fatty acids
  - More closely approximates human milk with content of docosahexaenoic acid (DHA, an omega-3 fatty acid) and arachidonic acid (ARA, an omega-6 fatty acid)
  - May enhance visual and mental development, especially in preterm infants (Fleith and Clandinin, 2005)
- Formulas for feeding beyond 6 months of age (Step-2 formulas), usually calcium fortified, must be supplemented with solids
- Nutrient-dense formulas for older child
  - Caloric content up to 30 kcal/oz; other nutrients increased over regular infant formula
- Specialized formulas
  - Higher caloric content (24-30 kcal/oz); nutrient dense; free amino acid and peptide-based formulas; lactose-free
- Protein supplements
- Nitrogen-free calorie supplements
- Oral electrolyte solutions

*For names of formulas, detailed description of formula content, and links to formula manufacturers for additional information, see *Infant formulas: approximate composition of pediatric formulas*. Available at http://depts.washington.edu/growing/Nourish/Ftable.htm (accessed Sept 24, 2010).

Box 10-1 outlines various types of commercial formulas available.

Occasionally infants demonstrate intolerance to formula, showing irritability, weight loss or slow gain, vomiting, diarrhea, constipation, other gastrointestinal problems, or atopic dermatitis. The provider must work closely with parents to identify a formula tolerated by the infant, being careful to allow sufficient time for the baby to respond to a new formula as it is introduced. This can be a time- and energy-consuming process in which parents need support, reassurance, and encouragement. Referral to a registered dietitian can be helpful.

Introduction of Solids. A number of variables converge at about 6 months that make this an appropriate time to introduce solids into the infant's diet:

- Infants' sucking patterns have changed sufficiently to allow mastery of chewing and swallowing.
- Infants can sit with some support, and they are able to purposefully move their heads.
- Infants are able to grasp, pick up, and bring objects to their mouths.
- Iron stores present at birth are being depleted.
- Growth demands require nutrients other than those provided in milk alone.

BOX 10-2 Principles for the Introduction of Solids into the Infant's Diet

- Introduce one food at a time, waiting 3 to 5 days before offering another to assess for adverse reaction.
- Offer rice cereal, the least allergenic of cereal grains, as the first food.
- Introduce fruits, vegetables, and other cereals in any sequence desired.
- Feed only iron-fortified cereals.
- Prepare food appropriate to child's developmental abilities (e.g., strained, mashed, or finger foods).
- Use home-prepared or commercially prepared foods.
- Provide a variety of foods.
- Help child develop healthy patterns of eating:
  - Be alert and responsive to child's cues when eating.
  - Use a spoon to feed solids.
  - Offer about 1 Tbsp per year of age as a serving for infants; for older children, about one fourth to one half an adult serving.
  - Never force a child to eat.
  - Include the child in family mealtimes.

- Developmental needs (cognitive, sensory, and motor) are stimulated by new foods, textures, smells, tastes, and use of utensils.

Solids can be introduced in whatever sequence the family desires, often based on cultural or family customs, though nonallergenic cereals are usually the first infant foods. Dense proteins should be introduced later to allow for maturation of the renal system. Home-prepared foods, such as grains, mashed bananas, applesauce, pureed squash, cooked vegetables, and blenderized meats, can meet all the child's nutritional needs. Although not necessary, commercial baby foods can provide adequate nutrition, but labels should be examined to determine their content, especially for calories, fats, additives, salt, and sugar. Box 10-2 lists some principles to keep in mind when beginning solids.

Eating Habits. Whether infants are being exclusively breast- or formula-fed, parents need to be alert to cues of satiety. Feeding on demand in early infancy is important, and neonates should not be allowed to sleep for long periods of time without feeding. But feeding primarily to comfort a child should be discouraged; every time a child cries, he or she is not necessarily hungry. Bottle-fed infants, whether formula or breast milk is used in the bottle, can easily be overfed (e.g., the caregiver often urges the infant to take that extra half ounce just to empty the bottle). As a result, infants can learn to ignore feelings of satiety. Self-regulation of intake is evident in young infants, but by the early toddler years, children are influenced by social cues around feeding and can eat more than they need (Fox et al, 2006). Normal-weight term infants who rapidly gain weight in the first months of life are at higher risk for obesity as toddlers and preschoolers (Singhal, 2010). Bottle feeding beyond 12 months old appears to be a risk factor for overweight (Bonuck et al, 2010), and formula-fed infants introduced to solid foods before 4 months are six times as likely to be obese at age 3 (Hah et al, 2011).

Parents should be counseled to respond promptly to a child's feeding cues and to allow the child to initiate and guide the feeding interaction. Do not encourage the child to overeat. A selection of varied, healthful foods gives the older infant a chance to explore textures, smells, colors, and taste. Feeding is also a time when older infants and toddlers learn physical skills of fine motor control, cognitive skills of relationships between action and consequence (the dog *will* eat whatever is dropped on the floor), and skills of social exchange among family members.

Toddlers and Preschoolers

Energy and Protein. The growth rate of toddlers and preschoolers is slower than that of infants, resulting in decreased energy needs per unit of body weight. But because of increased size and activity, these children require an increased number of total calories. Addition of muscle mass also demands a continued high protein intake.

Vitamin and Mineral Supplements. Vitamin supplements are usually not necessary for young children because many foods are fortified and, as noted, supplements should not be considered as a substitute for food. Findings from the Feeding Infants and Toddlers Study (FITS) show that most children who do not use supplements receive adequate amounts of vitamins, and adding a multivitamin supplement can actually place children at risk of excessive vitamin intake; 97% of children who received supplements had more than the tolerable UIL for vitamin A, 66% for zinc, and 20% for folate (Briefel et al, 2006; Fox et al, 2006). Evaluate a child's intake over the course of a week. If children persist with *extremely* limited food choices or picky eating behavior, they might benefit from a children's multivitamin plus mineral supplement.

Eating Habits. Toddlers become more skilled in managing eating, using utensils, joining the family for regular mealtimes, and demonstrating more distinctive food likes and dislikes. They learn how and what to eat by observing adults around them and by responding to the foods adults provide for them. Older infants and toddlers may show an initial aversion to new foods and may demonstrate "food jags," eating only a few kinds of food. With time, guidance, and patience, toddlers will learn to eat a wide variety of foods (see Strategies to Develop Healthy Eating Behaviors). Parents should continue to be responsive to the child's cues for hunger and satiety, providing age-appropriate portions and not insisting on the "clean-plate" approach to nutrition.

School-Age Children

Energy and Protein. Energy and protein needs of school-age children vary greatly, depending on body size, growth patterns, and activity and exercise levels. Protein needs increase in older children as they gain more muscle mass. Active boys from 10 to 18 years old generally need between 2200 and 3200 calories a day, whereas active girls require about 1800 to 2400 calories daily; older children require the higher intake of this range (see table on the inside cover of this text).

Vitamin and Mineral Supplements. Poor eating habits place school-age children at risk for deficiencies in iron, thiamine, vitamin A, and calcium. Teaching children about specific nutrient sources and encouraging healthy eating habits can prevent many problems; supplementation with a daily multivitamin is usually not necessary.

Eating Habits. Food likes and dislikes carry over from the preschool years. There is great variation in appetite and intake as a result of uneven growth and activity levels. School-age children have a tendency to skip meals and are more likely to snack as they become engrossed in activities. This tendency is exacerbated in families with hectic schedules, unstructured

mealtimes, and reliance on fast foods. Parents and children can identify healthful fast foods that fit a busy school-age child's schedule (e.g., homemade burritos, stir-fry chicken, peanut butter sandwiches, an apple, carrot sticks, string cheese, and a bagel on the way to soccer practice). High-fat, high-calorie, low-nutrient snacks, such as chips, soda, and pizza, should be a very small part of a child's diet.

Adolescents

Energy and Protein. The growth rate of adolescents is remarkable (see table on the inside cover of this text), and the description by some parents that their children never seem to stop eating is apt. High levels of energy are needed to support adolescents' rapid growth, and if children participate in sports or other exercise programs, additional caloric intake can be needed. Adequate protein intake is essential to produce muscle mass. The average intake of protein in the U.S. diet is significantly greater than the DRI, so additional supplementation is usually not necessary.

Vitamin and Mineral Supplements. Thiamine, riboflavin, niacin, folate, iron, zinc, and calcium needs increase during adolescence (see Table 10-1). Most adolescents who eat a well-balanced diet need no supplements, but their irregular eating habits put them at risk for deficits. Adolescent girls are at risk for iron deficit when menstruation begins, and children who eat a vegan diet will need vitamin B_{12} supplements.

Eating Habits. Eating habits of adolescents are influenced by their increasing independence and social activity, perceptions of body image, and physical growth patterns. Adolescents often have erratic eating patterns; skip meals; eat high-fat, high-calorie, low-nutrient snack foods; and consume calories late in the day. Skipping breakfast has been associated with obesity in adolescents and young adults; missing this meal is more common among low-income youth, especially African-Americans, living in disadvantaged communities who have no parent at home at breakfast time (Merten et al, 2009). Teens who participate in sports and adolescents who eat a mainly vegetarian diet tend to have healthier eating habits than their nonsports-involved or meat-eating counterparts (Croll et al, 2006; Dunham and Kollar, 2006).

Pregnancy in Adolescence. Pregnancy presents added nutritional demands for growing adolescents. During the pubertal growth spurt, the teenager's body will compete with the fetus for nutrients. This is particularly true of girls younger than 15 years. Infants born to teenage mothers are at higher risk for prematurity, low birthweight, chronic illness, disabilities, and death. Proper nutrition and early prenatal care can increase the chance of a successful pregnancy.

The nutrition needs of pregnant teenagers also are high at a time when the typical teen is likely to have irregular eating patterns that can contribute to poor nutritional status. Calcium; iron; zinc; vitamins A, D, E, and B_6; riboflavin; folic acid; and total calories—all essential to fetal growth—are often found to be inadequate in the diets of female adolescents (Moran, 2007).

When managing the pregnant teenager, providers should carefully assess dietary intake and counsel the adolescent to eat a varied and healthful diet. A prenatal multivitamin and mineral supplement, including iron, calcium, and folic acid, is essential. The pregnant teenager should strive for a total of 1300 to 1500 mg of calcium through diet and supplements each day (Chan et al, 2006). Daily folic acid intake of 0.4 mg is recommended for all girls capable of becoming pregnant, increased to 0.6 mg during pregnancy (FNB, 2005).

Gestational weight gain in adolescents should be carefully monitored using World Health Organization (WHO) growth charts. Adolescents should not gain more than a recommended healthy gestational weight, just because they are adolescents. Healthy teens who are still growing (i.e., less than 4 years after menarche) should gain the amount they would normally gain in 9 months if they were not pregnant plus a normal gestational weight gain. For adolescents who are 4 years past menarche, gestational weight gain should be similar to that of adult women (IOM and National Research Council, 2009). Extra gestational weight gain for normal-weight African-American teenagers has not been shown to be beneficial (Nielsen et al, 2006). Adolescents who begin pregnancy when overweight are at high risk for neonatal and perinatal morbidity (Sukalich et al, 2006). Gestational weight gains of 15 to 25 pounds in overweight and obese adult women and 15 pounds or less in morbidly obese women are associated with fewer adverse outcomes (Crane et al, 2009). There are no data on adolescents to match those of the study by Crane and associates, but weight gain should not be excessive, and all adolescents would benefit from comprehensive prenatal nutrition programs (Nielsen et al, 2006). For those adolescents who meet income guidelines, the federal supplemental food program, WIC, is a valuable resource. In addition to providing nutritious foods, the program offers nutrition education and counseling.

STRATEGIES TO DEVELOP HEALTHY EATING BEHAVIORS

As noted, basic eating patterns are established in the infant, toddler, and preschool years; these patterns tend to continue throughout the child's life.

Parents Decide What Foods to Eat

Children learn eating behaviors by observation and instruction, and parents are the primary teachers in the process. Often that teaching is done without conscious reflection or planning on the part of parents. Studies indicate that children tend to eat what their parents do and that parents who exert overt pressure on their children to eat less fat or more fruits and vegetables—without changing their own habits—actually contribute to poor eating patterns (Spruijt-Metz et al, 2006). The responsibility of parents to provide healthful foods cannot be overemphasized. Parents may rationalize giving their child empty calories rather than nutrient-rich food by stating, "That's all my child will eat, and I know she needs the energy," or "But he cries and carries on if I don't give it to him; I'm just doing it to make him happy." Providers can remind parents that the parent—not the child—decides if an 18-month-old's "treat" is french fries or fruits. Parents have a choice and a serious responsibility to their children's long-term health. If children learn early that healthy, nutrient-filled foods are readily available and that Mom and Dad enjoy them, they might enjoy them as well.

High-fat, high-sugar, and high-salt foods should make up a very small part of the diet, but overly restricting them, especially in children, can contribute to unhealthy attitudes toward food. If these foods are occasionally available, children learn to make better choices about how to fit them into a healthful diet. Intervention by providers in the child's first year of life to teach parents which foods are healthy and encourage them to provide those foods helps establish healthy eating patterns in older children (Vitolo et al, 2010).

Children Decide How Much of These Healthful Foods to Eat

Often parents will try to decide exactly how much their child should eat (e.g., they may make a child sit at the table to finish his vegetables). Appetite fluctuations and preferences are typical of children, and parents should be aware that children may appear to eat less than the parent thinks is sufficient or too much of one particular food to the neglect of others. If parents punish a child for not eating or force a child to eat, they have taken away the child's responsibility to choose. As a result, the child may develop an aversion to certain foods, overeat, or act-out in other ways. Mealtimes can become contests of will between parents and children, creating feelings and patterns of interacting that extend far beyond the dinner table. Parents need to find out what healthy foods their children enjoy (it is perfectly all right to eat only carrots, peas, or broccoli for several weeks in a row!) and make those available. If provided a nutritious variety of foods they like, children tend to select those necessary for their healthy growth, in terms of both amount of calories and other nutrients. A general principle to keep in mind when considering portions is to serve 1 tablespoon of food per year of age. For children younger than 5 years old, one serving is about one fourth to one third of an adult serving; for older children, one fourth to one half of an adult serving. Children's appetites vary, however, and parents should be alert to cues that the child wants more or less of any particular food.

Providers can help parents make the process more positive by having them examine their own values and patterns related to eating, identify and reinforce those they would like to foster in their children, and eliminate those they see as negative. Providers can educate parents about age differences and offer suggestions for effectively managing the eating experience.

Parents should be encouraged to provide the following:
- Positive examples of healthy intake; parents are the child's role model
- An adequate supply of a wide variety of age-appropriate, nutritious foods and snacks
- Limits, but not prohibitions, on consumption of nonnutritious sugars and "sometimes" foods
- Food prepared in a form that stimulates children's appetites
- Regular, structured mealtimes when the family sits down to eat together; this may occur only once a day
- A pleasant, relaxed environment for mealtimes
- Clear, developmentally appropriate expectations for children's behavior at mealtimes
- Developmentally appropriate access to and instruction in the use of utensils
- Appropriate supervision during mealtimes
- Developmentally appropriate opportunities to participate in planning, preparing, and serving meals
- Adequate exercise, sleep, and rest to stimulate appetites

The introduction of new foods can create tension between parents and children, with children refusing to try or rejecting new tastes or textures. Parents should be informed that this is a normal reaction for many children. Children may reject a food up to 15 to 20 times before they become accustomed to it and enjoy eating it, and parents should not be too concerned if a child rejects a particular food. Rather than force the child to try the new food or give in to the child's feeding demands, the food should be removed without comment, then offered again at another meal. With a well-balanced diet, not eating a vegetable prepared at one meal, for example, will not compromise the child's health. However, parents should be encouraged to avoid becoming the child's "short-order cook," preparing a special dish if the child rejects what has been fixed for the family. If a child chooses not to eat much at a particular meal, he or she will be hungrier at the next. Between meals, children should be offered age-appropriate snacks, but snacks should not be a substitute for meals; "grazing" or eating whenever food is available tends to override the child's natural sense of satiety and encourage overeating (Brazelton and Sparrow, 2004).

Strategies that can be used to increase the chances of children accepting a new food include the following:
- Offer the food when children are hungry.
- Allow children to taste a little of the food rather than eating a full portion.
- Expose children to the food by preparing and serving the food without expecting them to eat it.
- Provide an example of parents eating and enjoying the food.
- Prepare the food the way children prefer: few spices, lukewarm, recognizable.
- Associate food with pleasant experiences.
- Never force food on children.

Finally, remind parents that individuals do not need to eat all foods. The parent may not eat some foods because of a personal dislike (e.g., anchovies, sushi, or cilantro); children should be afforded the same courtesy if they have been offered the food numerous times and repeatedly demonstrate dislike. There are many food options for attaining the same nutrients. As children become older, parents can help them master the social skill of politely trying new foods in new situations (e.g., visiting friends or dining in public places).

PHYSICAL ACTIVITY

Physical activity is integrally related to healthy nutrition. It is recommended that children and adolescents engage in 60 minutes of physical activity every day, most of which is moderate- or vigorous-intensity aerobic (exercise that makes them breathe hard); they should do vigorous activity at least 3 days a week and muscle- and bone-strengthening activity at least 3 days a week (USDHHS, 2009). Increased activity creates a demand for more calories and nutrients; more sedentary behavior means the body needs fewer calories, and sedentary lifestyles combined with poor eating habits can contribute to obesity. Figure 10-1 presents an integration of the food guide pyramid with a physical activity pyramid and can be used by providers to proactively counsel children about the importance of being active (see Chapter 13 for suggestions of activities).

VEGETARIAN DIETS

Description

Vegetarian diets are increasingly common, and offer striking health benefits. If vegetarian children continue to follow a plant-based diet into adulthood, they can expect to have lower levels of obesity, high blood pressure, heart disease, diabetes, and perhaps cancer. Vegetarians tend to fall into several categories but are extremely varied as to how much and when plant- or animal-based foods are eaten in their diets:
- Vegans, or strict vegetarians, eat only foods of plant origin, including fruits, vegetables, grains, nuts, seeds, tofu, and legumes (e.g., beans, peas, lentils, and peanuts). Some individuals restrict the type of plants they eat, consuming only nuts and legumes, or no fruit or some other dietary variation. Some macrobiotic diets in which whole grains form the bulk of food eaten are an extreme type of veganism; yet some macrobiotic diets include fish or meat, so would fit in the "sometime" vegetarian category.
- Lacto vegetarians include milk and dairy products in their diet, in addition to all plant-based foods.
- Lacto-ovo vegetarians consume eggs, dairy products, and all plant-based foods in their diet.
- "Sometimes" vegetarians have a diet that consists mostly of plant-based foods, but they occasionally eat fish, chicken, or some seafood, usually avoiding or severely limiting red meat.

Vegetarian and vegan diets can meet all nutritional needs of growing children, including athletes (Jacobs et al, 2009; Craig and Mangels, 2009). For children who are lacto or lacto-ovo vegetarians, or who from time to time eat fish or other meat, it is easy to achieve adequate nutrients needed for proper growth and development. In fact, the diet of these children is often healthier and more likely to meet the *Healthy People 2020* goals than that of their red meat-eating peers (Sabaté and Wien, 2010). However, strict vegan diets may be deficient in some nutrients, specifically protein, vitamin B_{12}, iron, calcium, zinc, riboflavin, and (if exposure to the sun is limited) vitamin D. Attention must also be paid to ensure adequate intake of essential fatty acids (Table 10-6).

Management

Families and children who select vegetarian diets should be supported for their healthy dietary decisions, counseled about potential deficits, educated about alternative sources of nutrients that may be lacking in the diet, and assessed regularly to ensure adequate growth and development is occurring. Nutritional assessment of the child with a vegetarian diet should include regular growth measurements, diet recall and analysis, and laboratory assessment of vitamin B_{12}, zinc, and iron status. Vitamin D supplement (400 International Units daily) may be necessary.

Parents and children should be counseled that some plants have less protein, or less of one kind of protein, than other plants; soy protein more efficiently uses nitrogen than does wheat protein, for example. If the diet is high in one type of protein alone, growth could be affected. Consuming a variety of plants with different configurations of protein can meet the child's needs. This combination has often been called "complementary," one plant providing the protein lacking in another. It is not necessary that these complementary proteins be eaten in the same meal; intake throughout the day is more important (Young and Pellett, 1994). Examples of foods that provide adequate protein intake include combinations of legumes and grains, nuts, or seeds (e.g., peanut butter on wheat bread, beans and rice, lentils and rice, lentils

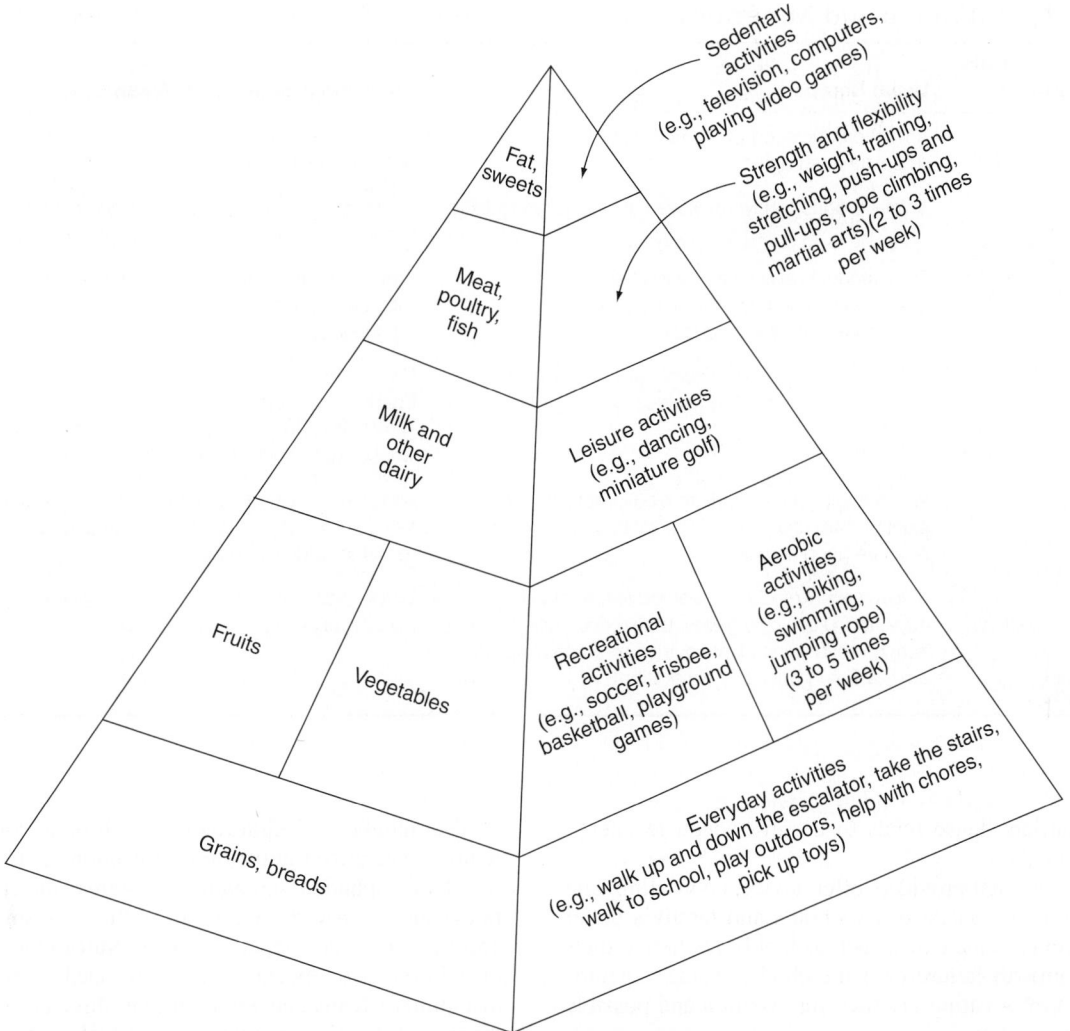

FIGURE 10-1 Physical activity pyramid. (Data from Reinhardt WC, Brevard PB: Integrating the food guide pyramid and physical activity pyramid for positive dietary and physical activity behaviors in adolescents, *J Am Diet Assoc* 102(3 Suppl):S96-S99, 2002; University of Missouri Extension: MyActivity Pyramid for Kids, 2007, Columbia, MO. Adapted from USDA MyPyramid. Available at www.extension.missouri.edu/explorepdf/hesguide/foodnut/00386.pdf [accessed May 11, 2011]).

and sunflower seeds, peas and rye or wheat, or tofu and almonds).

Vitamin B_{12}, in the form of a fortified food (e.g., breakfast cereal, soy milk, nutritional yeast), is required for the child who is a vegan because bioavailable vitamin B_{12} is present only in animal-based foods. Most edible algae (blue-green) used in supplements contains pseudo-vitamin B_{12}, which is inactive in humans (Watanabe, 2007).

Iron needs of vegetarians are calculated to be 1.8 times greater than non-vegetarians because the non-heme iron in plant-based foods is less bioavailable (phytates in grains and legumes also bind with iron to decrease its absorption) (FNB, 2005). Iron absorption can be enhanced by combining intake with vitamin C found in fruits and some vegetables and by processing seeds and grains (e.g., soaking, sprouting, fermenting, or making into bread). Over time, it appears that the absorption of iron from plants improves and most vegetarians in the U.S. are not iron deficient (Craig and Mangels, 2009).

Phytates in grains and legumes also bind with zinc to inhibit its absorption. As with iron, eating zinc-rich foods (e.g., soy, nuts, cheese, legumes, and grains) with organic acids (e.g., citrus) and processing these foods by soaking, sprouting, or leavening with yeast increases zinc absorption. Most vegetarians in the U.S. do not have zinc deficiency. Vegans are at higher risk for zinc deficiency and may need a supplement (Craig and Mangels, 2009).

Because plant-based diets tend to be high in fiber and lower in calories, the child may feel full before consuming sufficient calories and nutrients; and high-fiber macrobiotic diets have resulted in growth retardation in children (Dagnelie and van Staveren, 1994). Children on alternative diets are at risk for nutrition deficits (Kirby and Danner, 2009). Recent research, however, indicates that children with a high fiber intake from a variety of plant-based foods grow well, have adequate energy intake, and experience a reduction in total serum and low-density cholesterol levels (Ruottinen et al, 2010). Like all children, those eating a vegetarian diet should emphasize a wide

TABLE 10-6 Vitamins and Minerals at Risk for Deficit in Strict Vegetarian (Vegan) Diets

Vitamin and Minerals at Risk for Deficit	Usual Sources	Alternative Sources in Vegan Diet
Vitamin D	Animal products: egg yolk, butter, liver, salmon, sardines, tuna; sunlight	Fortified cereals, milk, or margarine; sunlight (20 to 30 min/day, 2 or 3 times per week)
Vitamin B_{12}	Animal products only: meat, fish, eggs, dairy products	Fortified soy milk, fortified soy-based meat substitutes, nutritional yeast, fortified cereals, vitamin supplements
Riboflavin	Dairy products and meat are best sources; also in eggs, dried yeast, grains, dark-green leafy vegetables, avocado, broccoli	Brewer's yeast, wheat germ, beans, almonds, soybeans, tofu, dark-green leafy vegetables, avocado, broccoli, orange juice
Calcium	Dairy products are best source; also in some fruits, nuts, dark-green leafy vegetables	Fortified soy milk, dried fruits, almonds, sunflower seeds, filberts, whole sesame seeds, green leafy vegetables (at same meal, avoid eating spinach, Swiss chard, beet greens, whose oxalic acid hinders calcium absorption)
Iron	Iron in meat sources is more bioavailable than iron in plants; lentils, beans (cooked black, soy, garbanzo, lima) are good sources	All legumes, almonds, pecans, dates, prunes, raisins, fortified cereals, white or brown rice; absorption is enhanced by ascorbic acid–rich foods
Zinc	Meats, animal products, seafood (especially oysters), eggs; found in whole grains, brown rice, nuts, spinach; however, best plant sources also contain phytic acid, which inhibits zinc absorption	Whole grains, brown rice, almonds, wheat germ, tofu, pecans, spinach

variety of nutrient-dense foods to achieve adequate energy and nutrient intake.

It is important that providers offer advice, counseling, and support within the context of the child's and family's belief system. But in extreme cases, such as highly restrictive diets resulting in growth failure or if the child is using vegetarianism as a form of eating disorder, intervention and possible referral are necessary.

Complications

A high incidence of vitamin B_{12} deficiency and suboptimal zinc status has been noted in children who eat a strict vegan diet, and children are at risk for developmental retardation without these nutrients. If girls who are vegetarian become pregnant, the fetus is also at risk for vitamin B_{12} deficiency, with potentially permanent and severe neurologic damage. One study found that adolescents on a vegetarian diet were at risk for binge eating, and former vegetarians were at risk for "extreme unhealthful weight-control behaviors" (Robinson-O'Brien et al, 2009).

■ Altered Patterns of Nutrition

Many children have chronic illnesses, developmental disabilities, developmental special needs, or handicapping conditions that affect their nutritional status. According to the 2005-2006 national survey of children with special health care needs, about 13.9% of U.S. children 17 years old and younger have special health care needs, and some 10% of those children have nutritional problems, specifically swallowing, digesting, or metabolizing food (Data Resource Center for Child and Adolescent Health, 2010).

The number of children with chronic conditions that require specialized nutrition interventions is increasing as a result of expanded screening programs, increased survival rates, and improved prognosis for the very small (less than 1500 g), underdeveloped neonate. Nutritional management of children with special health care needs requires a multidisciplinary team and interventions directed at specifically diagnosed feeding problems. Physical, occupational, and speech therapists, particularly speech pathologists, can assess head and trunk control, positioning, body mechanics, and oral-motor skills. Depending on the child's symptoms and diagnosis, gastroenterologists, allergists, endocrinologists, and other specialists may need to participate in the child's care; surgical and medical intervention may be necessary. For children who are socially or economically deprived, or both, public health nurses, social workers, and psychologists are central to appropriate assessment, counseling, and referral to outside services and agencies. Pediatric dietitians can be critical to success, and the family must be included as an integral component of the team. Primary care providers must carefully assess the nutritional status of this population and make appropriate referrals. Children who meet the criteria outlined in Box 10-3 should be referred to a registered dietitian for comprehensive nutrition assessment and further referral or treatment.

Nutrition and health problems are related in a number of ways: some conditions require more caloric intake (e.g., athetoid cerebral palsy); others require less (e.g., Prader-Willi); some, depending on the individual, may require either more calories or fewer calories (e.g., autism). Some conditions demand special supplements or vitamins and others require special feeding strategies (e.g., the child with cleft palate). The following section outlines principles of care in these categories and highlights several specific conditions.

BOX 10-3 Suggested Criteria for Nutrition Referral

- Markedly overweight or underweight (height or length for weight less than the 5th or more than the 95th percentile)
- Mechanical feeding difficulties or neuromotor dysfunction
- Feeding skills less than those anticipated for developmental level or mental age
- Unusual food habits (e.g., pica or food faddism)
- Inadequate or imbalanced dietary intake, according to dietary history or 24-hour recall
- Nutrition treatment central to medical management (e.g., inborn errors of metabolism, diabetes, malabsorption syndromes, allergy)
- Overt physical signs of nutritional deficiency (e.g., extreme underweight, overweight, anemia)
- Emotional disturbances and associated feeding and nutrition problems (e.g., anorexia nervosa, autism)
- At high risk for compromised nutritional status (e.g., takes stimulant or anticonvulsive drugs, family below poverty level, inadequate housing, pregnant adolescent)

Data from Ekvall SW, Ekvall VK, Frazier T: Dealing with nutrition problems of children with developmental disorders, *Topics Clin Nutr* 8(4):51-57, 1993.

DISORDERS REQUIRING INCREASED CALORIC INTAKE

Description

A common nutrition problem in children with special health care needs is inadequate weight gain and delayed growth. Inadequate caloric intake should be suspected in any child with a weight-to-age ratio below the 10th percentile on standardized growth and BMI charts. For children who are genetically small or have a disabling condition that limits growth, a weight-to-length ratio or weight-to-height ratio below the 10th percentile indicates suboptimal nutrition.

Epidemiology

The actual incidence of children requiring an increased caloric intake is not known, but it occurs commonly.

Caloric needs of children are influenced by multiple factors, and a number of conditions put children at risk for insufficient caloric intake, including the following:

- Conditions in which activity level is increased, either by purposeful or involuntary muscle work, such as athetoid cerebral palsy, attention-deficit/hyperactivity disorder, or chronic lung conditions
- A hypermetabolic state (sometimes complicated by secondary malabsorption), which may be present in the child who has acquired immunodeficiency syndrome (AIDS), cancer, burns, fever, or frequent infections, or who has recently had surgery
- Chronic renal insufficiency
- Psychosocial factors, such as inadequate resources, poor feeding relationship with caregiver, and improper dilution of formula, which can lead to delayed growth and require increased calories for the child's catch-up growth
- Oral-motor impairment or chronic conditions, such as congenital heart disease, which can contribute to fatigue and poor feeding
- Low-birth-weight or premature infants

- Medical treatment (e.g., a child receiving corticosteroid treatment for Crohn disease)
- Conditions in which malabsorption occurs (e.g., cystic fibrosis)

Clinical Assessment and Findings

History. A thorough history should be taken, assessing for the following:

- Type and amount of foods and liquids consumed (e.g., nutrient content and consistency)
- Amount of food that falls from utensils, cups, or bottles during feeding and is not ingested
- Physical effort and time required for meal (the child can sometimes use more calories eating than he or she consumes)
- Any impaired oral functions (e.g., poor suck and swallow, tongue thrust, drooling, difficulty chewing, choking, or aspiration)
- Position of child during feeding
- Family's pattern of feeding child (e.g., time, place, utensils used)
- Child's apparent food likes and dislikes

Physical Examination. Anthropometric measurements are reliable indicators of a child's growth and development, especially if accurately measured and compared over time. Appendix B provides standard growth and BMI charts, in addition to growth charts for premature infants. These charts can be used to determine whether the child is following a consistent growth curve. Growth charts specific to children with Down syndrome, myelomeningocele, Prader-Willi syndrome, sickle cell anemia, and Turner syndrome also have been developed. Anthropometric measurements taken at each visit include the following:

- Height
- Weight
- Weight-to-height ratio
- BMI
- Head circumference
- Arm circumference
- Triceps skinfold measurements

A feeding evaluation can be included in the physical examination, particularly for the child with oral-motor or behavioral problems associated with eating. In this type of assessment parents or caregivers are asked to replicate the home experience, using the same types of foods, utensils, and positioning. If possible, the parents should videotape the child eating at home, and providers should review the video with them. By observing the interaction between the child and the caregiver during feeding, the health care team can more accurately assess feeding success and problems, along with emotional or psychological issues related to feeding.

Diagnostic Tests. Laboratory studies are done as indicated:

- Hematocrit or hemoglobin
- Serum ferritin and transferrin levels
- Metabolic screening (chemistry screen)

Initial basic workup for failure to thrive (FTT) (see Chapter 32) includes the following:

- Complete blood count (CBC) with reticulocytes
- Thyroid studies
- Chemistry screen
- Urinalysis, with culture and sensitivity
- Stool for ova and parasites

- Stool culture for enteric pathogens (e.g., *Escherichia coli*)
- Bone age

Clinical Findings. When a child is malnourished, regardless of cause, the nutritional insult follows a predictable course. In the early stages, the child maintains or begins losing weight. If poor intake continues, the child's linear growth slows or ceases. Finally, head circumference, indicating compromised brain development, levels off.

Other signs of inadequate nutrition include the following:
- Anemia
- Pallor
- Fatigue
- Vulnerability to infections
- Delayed healing
- Behavior problems
- Inactivity
- Irritability
- Poor academic performance, poor vocabulary
- Perceptual difficulties

Management

The management of the child with delayed growth or poor weight gain varies with the underlying cause of the problem and often requires intervention of specialists. Although the primary provider can coordinate the plan of care, a team approach to management is needed.

A child with an increased activity level, a metabolic condition that increases energy requirements, or a condition that decreases the body's ability to absorb nutrients needs to receive caloric- and nutrient-dense meals and snacks frequently, at 2- to 4-hour intervals.

A child with a chronic disease that decreases the appetite (e.g., AIDS, cancer) needs creative approaches that consider food preferences, optimal times of day for snacks and meals, and family dynamics that encourage eating. Some children may be placed on medication to stimulate their appetite.

A child with a condition that affects oral-motor control will need special equipment, specific feeding techniques, proper positioning, and use of foods and liquids with appropriate consistency to improve oral intake.

A child who is not receiving enough food because of neglect, inadequate financial resources, or other psychosocial factors requires referral to appropriate health care professionals and social services. The community health nurse can be an invaluable resource for these children.

Although feeding by the oral route is preferable from a developmental perspective, tube feedings or parenteral feedings may be indicated. Frequently, a medical crisis precipitates the use of supplemental feedings.

Premature or low-birth-weight infants (particularly those with a poor suck) frequently require supplemental feedings. Breastfeeding is both possible and desirable for these infants and ensuring that they receive higher-fat hindmilk is important; pumping may be necessary (see Chapter 11). Human milk fortifiers or premature formulas that increase the caloric density from 20 to 24 kcal/oz can be used. Regular infant formulas can be mixed to increase the kcal/oz ratio from 20 to 24 kcal/oz or 27 kcal/oz, and nutrient-dense formulas for older infants and children are available (see Box 10-1).

Practical suggestions for increasing calories, protein, and nutrients needed for weight gain and growth are outlined in

---

BOX 10-4 Suggestions for Increasing Energy Intake

- Use readily available, economic foods that are familiar to the child.
- Fortify milk by adding 1 cup of nonfat dry milk powder to 1 quart of whole milk. Drink or use to prepare cooked cereals, creamed soups, pancakes, pudding, milkshakes (do not use with children younger than 24 months).
- Add additional margarine or cheese to potatoes, vegetables, casseroles, rice, pasta, cooked cereals, etc.
- Encourage high-calorie snacks, such as fruit juice, dried fruits, nuts, bananas, cheese cubes, pudding or custard, cereal with whole milk, fruit yogurt (alone or as a dip for fruit), cheese or peanut butter on crackers, olives, or sliced or mashed avocado (as a dip for vegetables or crackers).
- Add instant breakfast mixes to whole milk.
- Use commercially prepared formula with high calorie content.
- Use commercial liquid supplements, such as PediaSure for children with lactose intolerance.
- Establish regular times for meals and snacks, 2 to 4 hours apart. Do not allow the child to nibble continually on small amounts of food.
- Keep mealtimes relaxed and pleasant. Avoid scolding, nagging, or forcing the child to eat.
- Allow the infant or child to provide cues regarding hunger and satiety.

Box 10-4. A "complete" multivitamin and mineral supplement is also recommended because it contains the entire spectrum of these nutrients and can usually be chewed or crushed and mixed into soft foods. For children who are underweight or growth retarded, it is not sufficient to simply increase intake of calories, protein, and nutrients to age-specific norms. These children require excess calories and protein for "catch-up" growth until growth is normalized. A method for calculating calories and protein required for catch-up growth is presented in Box 10-5. Calculations for catch-up growth in children with chronic diseases that contribute to poor weight gain (e.g., cystic fibrosis) can be found in more detailed nutrition texts. Some chronic conditions may require more complex treatment, such as growth hormone therapy. Frequent monitoring of the child with inadequate caloric intake is necessary. Infants should be weighed at least weekly, and length and head circumference measured once a month. Children older than 2 years should be measured for height and weight at least once a month.

Complications

Children with a chronic medical condition that requires increased caloric intake are at risk for frequent illness, medical complications, and impaired development, including growth delay. In some cases, restoring nutritional status does not ultimately resolve growth deficits. In the case of environmental deprivation, the success of catch-up growth depends on the timing, length, and severity of the nutritional insult.

Complications secondary to treatment must also be considered for children with caloric deficits. Providers must be alert to negative effects caused by a sudden change to a high-calorie, high-protein diet. The child on a high-protein diet should be counseled to drink adequate fluids. Care must be taken that infants do not receive excess protein in concentrated infant formulas because the breakdown and excretion of protein by the kidneys may place an excessive demand on the renal system. Diarrhea can result

BOX 10-5 Estimating Catch-Up Growth Requirements*

$$\text{Catch-up growth requirement (kcal/kg/day)} = \frac{\text{Calories required dfor weight age (kcal/kg/day)} \times \text{Ideal weight for age (kg)}}{\text{Actual weight (kg)}}$$

1. Plot the child's height and weight on the CDC growth charts.
2. Determine at what age the present weight would be at the 50th percentile (weight age).
3. Determine recommended calories for weight age (see Tables on inside front cover of this text).
4. Determine the ideal weight (50th percentile) for the child's present age.
5. Multiply the value obtained in step 3 by the value obtained in step 4.
6. Divide the value obtained in step 5 by actual weight.
   Estimated protein requirements during catch-up growth can be calculated similarly (see Table 10-1):

$$\text{Protein requirement} = \frac{\text{Protein required for weight age (g)} \times \text{Ideal weight for age (kg)}}{\text{Actual weight (kg)}}$$

*Guidelines are used to estimate catch-up growth requirements. Precise individual needs vary and are mediated by medical status and diagnosis.
CDC, Centers for Disease Control and Prevention.
Adapted from Rathbun JM, Peterson KE: Nutrition in failure to thrive. In Grand RJ, Sutphen JL, Dietz WH, editors: *Pediatric nutrition*, Boston, 1987, Butterworth.

from an abrupt increase in carbohydrate intake. Gradually changing the child's diet can decrease these negative effects.

DISORDERS REQUIRING DECREASED CALORIC INTAKE

Description

Health conditions that contribute to decreased metabolic activity in children can require a decrease in caloric intake. If children's caloric intake exceeds their metabolic needs, excessive weight gain and obesity can occur, placing the child at risk for additional health problems.

Epidemiology

Any disorder or disability that reduces energy output places the child at risk for overweight. Obesity is common, for example, in children with Prader-Willi syndrome, myelomeningocele, or Down syndrome. Excess weight gain occurs in 50% of children with spina bifida.

The child with Prader-Willi syndrome is hypotonic and may demonstrate dysphagia and FTT as an infant. By 3 to 4 years old, the child becomes hyperphagic, lacking the internal regulation responsible for satiety. Children with Prader-Willi syndrome are short in stature.

Most children with Down syndrome have short stature, and before they are 3 years old may have a low weight-to-height ratio. The Down syndrome growth chart should be used to evaluate height and weight. As a result of a lower resting metabolic rate or hypothyroidism, a child with Down syndrome requires fewer calories than a child without the syndrome, and overweight is common, but not inevitable; its incidence can be decreased with healthy eating and exercise habits begun in early childhood.

Clinical Assessment and Findings

History. The history should assess the following:
- Level of physical activity in which child engages
- Diet recall (3 days)
- Mealtime patterns
- Concerns and attitudes of parents and child regarding weight gain

- Previous interventions or attempts to control weight
- Risk for overweight and its complications (e.g., diabetes mellitus, limited mobility, family history of obesity)

Physical Examination. Key components of the physical examination include the following:
- Weight-to-height or weight-to-length ratio. Ratio greater than 75th percentile on growth chart indicates at risk for overweight; greater than 95th percentile indicates overweight
- Triceps skinfold measurement (greater than 85% of norm indicates overweight)
- Midarm circumference
- Body frame type; central adiposity and waist circumference (used more in adults)
- Muscle mass
- BMI in the 85th to 95th percentile indicates overweight; 95th percentile or higher is obese

A child's growth pattern is evaluated over time. A child who is consistently in the 85% weight-to-height ratio may be genetically programmed to be big, whereas a child who suddenly zooms from the 60% to the 90% weight-to-height ratio can be developing a weight problem.

Diagnostic Tests. Laboratory studies include those to rule out metabolic conditions that may cause overweight (e.g., thyroxine [T_4] and thyroid-stimulating hormone [TSH] to rule out hypothyroidism). Because of complications of obesity (e.g., hyperlipidemia, hypercholesterolemia), children more than 4 years old should be monitored annually for risk factors, and laboratory tests should be done as appropriate, including the following (see Chapter 25):
- Hypertension
- Blood glucose
- Complete lipid profile
- Liver function

Management

The goal of nutritional management of children with medical conditions that reduce energy expenditure is to ensure that the child receives adequate nutrients without excessive caloric intake. Families should be referred to a registered dietitian to establish an appropriate caloric level and eating plan individualized to each child's growth needs. A complete multivitamin with mineral supplement is recommended because a restrictive diet can result in nutrient deficiencies. Children should be encouraged to engage in regular physical activity. Though they may not be able to meet the recommended 60 minutes of moderate to vigorous activity each day, the goal is to increase calories used and the child's level of fitness. A team approach, involving a physical or recreational therapist or both, is advised to develop exercise strategies.

In some cases access to food needs to be rigidly enforced (e.g., in children with brain dysfunction affecting hypothalamic control or Prader-Willi syndrome). The family, school, and other care environments need to provide limited access to food, which may include locks on refrigerators, cupboards, and garbage cans.

Frequent monitoring is necessary to assess compliance and devise alternate strategies as indicated; weekly weight and monthly height measurements are recommended.

Support for families and children is essential. Despite the best efforts, many children gain excess weight. Primary care providers can model and encourage a positive, accepting attitude toward the child, independent of weight gain or loss (National Association of Pediatric Nurse Practitioners [NAPNAP], 2006).

DISORDERS REQUIRING RESTRICTED OR SUPPLEMENTAL DIETS

Description

Body metabolism requires hormone, enzyme, or cofactor activity. When there is either too much or not enough of these factors, or when absorption of nutrients is limited, nutritional status is at risk. Under these conditions, nutritional intake must be adjusted by restricting diet or adding supplements (e.g., enzymes) in order to maximize the body's ability to use foods.

A number of metabolic conditions or defects of absorption or transport affect nutritional status in children (Table 10-7). Most are rare, but primary care providers may be part of the team managing the care of a child with inflammatory bowel disease (Crohn disease or ulcerative colitis), short bowel syndrome, celiac disease, or other conditions falling into this category.

Epidemiology

Most metabolic disorders are rare, although in the U.S., type 1 diabetes mellitus affects about 2.8 in 1000 children ages 10 to 19 and 0.76 in 1000 children younger than 9 years. Cystic fibrosis is seen in 1 in 3200 Caucasian infants and 1 in 15,000 black infants. Approximately 1 in 10,000 children are born with phenylketonuria (PKU) (Schulze et al, 2009; Sharma, 2010).

Metabolic disorders may be due to inborn errors of metabolism, genetic conditions other than inborn errors of metabolism, and autoimmune diseases. Surgical intervention, drugs and medications, tumors, and infectious disease also contribute to metabolic dysfunction and problems of absorption or transport. For some individuals a genetic predisposition to the disorder can be triggered by environmental factors, and the disorder appears later in life.

TABLE 10-7	Metabolic Conditions Affecting Nutrition in Children	
Organ Affected	**Excessive Hormone/ Enzyme Production**	**Deficient Hormone/Enzyme Production**
Pancreas	Reactive hypoglycemia Organic or fasting hypoglycemia	Diabetes mellitus Cystic fibrosis
Thyroid	Hyperthyroidism Graves' disease	Hypothyroidism
Parathyroid	Hyperparathyroidism	Hypoparathyroidism
Adrenal cortex	Cushing syndrome Corticosteroid therapy	Addison disease Congenital adrenal hyperplasia
Inborn errors of metabolism		PKU (deficiency of phenylalanine hydroxylase) Maple syrup urine disease Tyrosinemia Galactosemia

Clinical Assessment and Findings

Clinical findings related to specific disorders are discussed in Unit 4. If nutrition is inadequate in children with these chronic conditions, clinical signs and symptoms worsen, pathophysiologic processes of the disorder accelerate, and health is compromised.

Management

Disorders of absorption and metabolism are usually managed with specialized diagnostic tests and treatments and require the efforts of a coordinated health care team. Although not a cure for disease, nutrition is an essential component of treatment plans and can make a critical difference in the child's outcome. The goals of nutritional intervention include the following:

- Provide adequate nutrients for normal growth and development.
- Maintain optimal level of health.
- Prevent or delay development of complications associated with disease progression (e.g., diarrhea, fistulas).
- Prevent or delay need for more aggressive intervention (e.g., surgical bowel resection).

Nutritional intervention in chronic disorders can be extremely complex. Referral to a registered dietitian is necessary, and primary providers should consult frequently with the dietitian.

In some conditions dietary restrictions are lifelong requirements, and success of dietary intervention depends on the child's and family's willingness to adhere to the plan of care. Cooperation is enhanced if the child and family are actively included in decision-making and if meal plans are developed that minimize disruption to the family's lifestyle and maximize flexibility and normalcy for the child. Families and children must be given ample opportunity to express their concerns and frustrations

---

BOX 10-6 Principles for Dietary Management of Diabetes Mellitus

- Individualize diet. There are many types of meal planning systems for those with diabetes; identify what works best for child and family, minimizes conflicts and issues of control and "normalizes" child's intake. Many programs rely most on a liberal diet plan with close insulin coverage.
- Space food intake to account for type of insulin used.
- Structure diet to include foods that everyone else eats; do not be overly restrictive; use insulin coverage to allow child to eat as typical a diet as possible.
- Vary specific nutrient intakes depending on child's age, size, and activity level.

General Guidelines for Nutrients Include:
Energy
- Intake is essentially the same as for child without diabetes; energy demands vary with growth spurts, exercise.
- Maintain plasma glucose as near normal physiological range as possible.

Carbohydrates
- Obtain 55% to 60% of total calories from carbohydrates. Complex carbohydrates are recommended; limit simple sugars; small amounts can be acceptable as part of a mixed meal.
- Emphasize consistent intake of carbohydrates from day to day.

- Include 25 to 40 g/1000 kcal/day of fiber; increase fiber as complex carbohydrates are increased.
- Increase carbohydrates 10 to 30 g/hr (depending on level of exertion) for intensive exercise; best effect if intake is several hours preceding exercise.

Protein
- Same as for child without diabetes.

Fat
- Same as for child without diabetes.

Vitamins and Minerals
- Same as for child without diabetes; if diabetes is poorly controlled, supplements are recommended.

Sweeteners
- Noncaloric sweeteners such as aspartame and saccharine are acceptable but not encouraged; no long-term adverse effects of artificial sweeteners have been noted.
- Caloric sweeteners, such as fructose, sucrose, glucose, sorbitol, and mannitol, can be used (with caution) as a substitute for carbohydrate calories.
- Excess sorbitol intake can contribute to diarrhea.

BOX 10-7 Principles for Dietary Management of Cystic Fibrosis

- Nutrients needed (high protein, high fat, high energy) may cause physical distress; work with family to help them understand the balance between comfort and adequate nutrition sought.
- Small, frequent meals, eaten slowly are better tolerated.
- Consume nutrient-dense foods; avoid "empty calories."
- Increase fluid intake to prevent dehydration and help liquefy secretions.
- Assess intake on a 3- to 5-day diet record rather than daily.

General Guidelines for Nutrients Include:
Energy
- Energy needs are increased as a result of malabsorption of nutrients, extra effort needed for respirations and frequent pulmonary infections. At least 120% to as much as 150% of recommended dietary allowance (RDA) caloric intake is recommended.
- Vary caloric intake for each child, depending on condition, activity, and growth.

Carbohydrates
- Obtain 40% to 50% of total calories from carbohydrates. Simple sugars may be better tolerated than complex carbohydrates.
- Include extra fiber; increase fiber as complex carbohydrates are increased.

Protein
- Higher need than for children without cystic fibrosis; 15% to 20% of caloric intake should be in proteins.

- Breastfed children may need supplements (e.g., casein hydrolysates).

Fat
- Increase to level of tolerance, minimum of 35% and as much as 40% to 50% of total caloric intake.
- Use medium-chain triglyceride oils to enhance absorption and decrease steatorrhea.
- Use corn or soy oil and include absorbable linoleic acid in diet to ensure essential fatty acid intake.

Vitamins and Minerals
- Daily multivitamin supplement and water-soluble preparation of vitamins A, D, and E are recommended; 50 to 100 mcg/day of vitamin K is recommended.
- Daily calcium supplements are necessary to prevent bone loss.
- Normal diet is usually adequate to replace sodium lost through excessive sweat; can use salt tablets (intake is more easily monitored than adding salt to diet) if exercise or fever leads to profuse sweating.

Supplements
- Pancreatic enzymes are indicated.
- Other supplements include casein hydrolysates and powdered or liquid nutrient-dense preparations.

---

regarding the child's condition. Support, empathy, and encouragement from providers can be vital elements in determining how well a family copes with the child's chronic condition.

Certain principles of nutrition related to disorders of absorption and metabolism guide the dietitian, primary care provider, and family as they create diet plans. Boxes 10-6 through 10-9 outline these principles for several specific conditions.

Complications

See Unit 4 for complications of specific disorders. Additionally, fetuses of women with higher than normal phenylalanine levels are at risk for microcephaly, congenital heart defects, and other birth defects. Approximately 1 in 30,000 women in the general population has a phenylalanine level high enough to damage her fetus or contribute to a spontaneous abortion,

---

BOX 10-8 Principles for Dietary Management of Phenylketonuria

- Intervene promptly. Infants who begin treatment before 3 weeks old do not suffer mental retardation secondary to phenylketonuria (PKU).
- All children require phenylalanine in their diet.
- The goal of PKU dietary therapy is to prevent excess phenylalanine accumulation in the body.
- Recommended daily intake of phenylalanine decreases with age. Dietary restrictions continue for life.
- Most foods contain phenylalanine (approximately 5% of all protein is phenylalanine).
- Involve older children in preparation of nutritional supplements.
- Supplements may be more palatable if served as frozen drinks or flavored with juices or fruits.

General Guidelines for Nutrients Include:
Energy, Carbohydrate, Fat, Vitamin, and Mineral
- Basic requirements are same as for child without PKU. Restrictions on high-phenylalanine carbohydrates.
- Daily multivitamin is recommended.
- Nutrient requirements not met by commercial formulas must be supplemented by a phenylalanine-deficient food.
- Supplement with omega-3 docosahexaenoic acid (DHA) may be helpful.

Protein
- Same protein requirements as for child without PKU.
- Phenylalanine intake is restricted. Dietary intake to maintain serum phenylalanine levels between 2 and 10 mg/dL in children. Plasma phenylalanine levels greater than 6 mg/dL should be controlled with dietary therapy.
- Low or minimal phenylalanine medical foods are necessary to meet protein requirements.

BOX 10-9 Principles for Dietary Management of Inflammatory Bowel Disease

- Restrict irritating and poorly absorbed foods (e.g., carbonated beverages, fried foods, spicy foods).
- Decrease intake of foods that stimulate peristalsis (e.g., high-fiber foods) during inflammatory periods. High-fiber foods, especially those that retain water, can be introduced as clinical signs and symptoms decrease.
- Small, frequent meals are better tolerated.
- Vary specific nutrient intakes depending on child's age, size, activity level, and severity of disease.
- Exclusive enteral nutrition early in disease is recommended (Day et al, 2007). Mild disease can require supplemental formulas; severe disease can require enteral elemental nutrition via tube feeding or total parenteral nutrition.
- Condition can be complicated by lactose or gluten intolerance.

General Guidelines for Nutrients Include:
Energy
- Teens need 40 to 50 kcal/kg of ideal body weight per day; younger children need up to 120 kcal/kg of ideal body weight per day.

Protein
- Greater than 1.5 g/kg of ideal body weight per day.

Fat
- Low fat (40 g/day) intake is necessary.
- Emulsified fats or medium-chain triglycerides (commercial preparation) are better tolerated.

Vitamins and Minerals
- Take a 100% to 150% daily multivitamin with minerals supplement.
- May need additional vitamin and mineral supplements (e.g., water-soluble vitamins, vitamin B_{12} intramuscularly), folic acid, iron, zinc, copper, calcium, potassium, and magnesium.

---

but not necessarily high enough to hurt her. All pregnant women should be questioned about a history of PKU or special diets during childhood, and maternal PKU should be considered in any woman who has delivered an infant with microcephaly or has experienced spontaneous abortion.

DISORDERS REQUIRING PHYSICAL ALTERATIONS IN DIET MANAGEMENT

Description
Physical conditions, such as cleft lip or palate, esophageal atresia, cerebral palsy, gastroesophageal reflux, and pyloric stenosis, can create difficulty sucking, chewing, swallowing, or retaining food and liquids in the GI tract.

Epidemiology
Most of these conditions are congenital, and a combination of environment, heredity, and behavior appears to influence their development. Stenoses, atresias, or fistulas can also be secondary to environmental trauma, such as a chemical burn. Incidence varies by condition, with approximately 1 in 750 Caucasian children born with cleft lip and 1 in 2500 with cleft palate in the U.S. each year. Boys are more likely to have a cleft lip with or without a cleft palate, and Asian

children are most likely and African-American children least likely to have clefts. Pyloric stenosis, occurring in about 3 in 1000 births, is four times more common in boys, especially firstborns; it is more frequent in children with Down syndrome and Caucasian children of Northern European heritage. It is rare in Asian children. Esophageal atresia occurs in 1 in about 4000 live births. In more than 90% of cases, it is accompanied by a tracheoesophageal fistula (Orenstein et al, 2007).

Gastroesophageal reflux (GER) is common in normal individuals following a meal and can be exacerbated by increased intraabdominal pressure (as with crying, coughing, defecation, or external pressure from movement or position). GER in infants can occur during, immediately after, or several hours after a feeding. Children with insufficient lower esophageal sphincter tone are especially susceptible to GER. Reflux becomes symptomatic early in life, peaks at about 4 months old, and spontaneously resolves for most children by 12 to 24 months old (Orenstein et al, 2007).

Children with cerebral palsy or other neurodevelopmental problems can have difficulty chewing or maintaining coordinated suck-swallow skills. GER is also a common problem in children with cerebral palsy, and, if the cause for food refusal cannot be determined, GER may be a likely explanation.

TABLE 10-8 Strategies for Feeding in Children With Cleft Lip or Palate

Age	Problem Presented	Management Strategies
Infants	Poor suction when nursing	Individualize position used to feed infant; semi-upright (60 to 90 degrees) position is often most effective.
	Nasal regurgitation	Breastfeed if possible; experiment with nipple position: position nipple toward side of mouth, do not put nipple into cleft.
		Use of longer, soft, or cross-cut nipples and squeezable bottles assists in infants with weak suck.
		Use of prosthetic device may be helpful.
		Wean child by 12 months old.
		Tube or gavage feedings may be necessary in severe cleft.
	Swallows air	Burp frequently.
	Fatigue	Allow sufficient time for feeding; work toward providing adequate nutrients in 30 minutes.
Toddlers	Risk of aspiration	Encourage use of cup, spoon, finger foods as developmentally appropriate.
	Nasal regurgitation	Avoid small, hard, sticky foods that can lodge in palate opening; supervise feeding.
School-age children and adolescents	Malocclusion	Dental referral and treatment are essential.
	Difficulty coordinating chewing, swallowing, and breathing	Teach child how to chew, swallow, and breathe; not to talk and chew at the same time.
		Inform parents that child will chew with mouth open.
	Aspiration	Cut food into small pieces; child can take sips of water while eating.
	Anorexia secondary to decreased sense of taste and smell	Plan diets that stimulate appetite; provide child's favorite foods.

Clinical Assessment and Findings

History. A thorough history of the infant's feeding patterns, incidence of gagging or vomiting, arching and crying during feeding, timing of emesis in relation to feeding, character and quantity of emesis, and associated symptoms is essential. Parents also should be asked about treatments they have tried and whether they have been successful.

Physical Examination. Clinical signs can be present at birth, and a diagnosis of the underlying condition, such as cleft lip or palate, can be made in the delivery room. Roentgenography and endoscopy are diagnostic techniques used to confirm atresias or fistulas. Some conditions, such as pyloric stenosis, occur later in the neonatal period (see Chapter 32).

Management

The treatment goals related to conditions that require biomechanical or physical intervention include the following:
- Provide adequate nutrients for normal growth and development.
- Provide increased calories to add more weight if needed before surgical procedures.
- Strengthen infant's resistance to infection.
- Prepare infant to tolerate stress of surgical procedures.
- Facilitate healing processes postoperatively.
- Ensure correct development and use of oral-facial and oropharyngeal muscles and structures.
- Minimize disruption of family processes.
- Prevent development of feeding problems.

Some conditions require surgical correction of the underlying condition. In many cases (e.g., a simple cleft lip), initial surgical intervention is sufficient, and the child progresses normally. In others, especially for the child with serious or multiple anomalies, long-term treatment is required. However, the treatment itself can lead to problems that require further management. For example, correction of esophageal atresia, tracheoesophageal fistula, or presence of a tracheostomy can result in scarring and strictures, which in turn put the child at risk for impaired swallowing, choking, and aspiration. Table 10-8 lists strategies related to feeding children with cleft lip or palate.

GER usually can be managed in the outpatient setting. All babies "spit up," especially when burped or placed in certain positions directly after a feeding. A small regurgitation of undigested formula or breast milk is usually not of concern, but GER puts the infant at risk for esophagitis, pulmonary infection, and FTT. Table 10-9 lists specific suggestions related to managing GER; and gastroesophageal reflux disease (GERD) is discussed in Chapter 32.

Providers must also support parents emotionally and psychologically as they care for their children. Parents of a child with birth anomalies can suffer shock, loss, guilt, anger, or disappointment and may find it difficult to accept their child. Difficult feeding or uncertainty about the child's long-term prognosis adds additional pressure to parents who are already facing an extremely stressful situation. Creating a positive feeding experience can facilitate a healthy parent-infant bond. Providers can intervene in the following ways:
- Encourage parents to express their feelings.
- Listen without judging, acknowledging those feelings.
- Demonstrate techniques that increase feeding success.
- Explain the child's condition, treatments, and prognoses, both short and long term.
- Emphasize how the parent can be involved in the child's progress.

TABLE 10-9 Strategies for Feeding in Children With Gastroesophageal Reflux

Condition	Management Strategies
Mild	Position infant in flat prone position after feeding if awake and being observed; position in flat supine position if infant will be sleeping. Semisitting position applies abdominal pressure and causes more reflux. Burp frequently during feeding. Thicken formula with rice cereal if formula feeding to decrease episodes of vomiting. May need to use large-hole nipple. One tablespoon of rice cereal per ounce of regular 20 kcal/oz formula increases energy density to 34 kcal/oz, so infant may be at risk for excess intake unless volume per feeding is decreased.
Moderate to severe	Position infant in flat prone position after feeding if awake and being observed; position in flat supine position if infant will be sleeping. Prone or lateral position is not recommended for sleep due to risk of sudden infant death syndrome (SIDS) (Vandenplas et al, 2009). If formula fed, use trial of extensively hydrolyzed or amino acid–based formulas. If breastfed, try removing cow's milk from mother's diet. Reduce volume at each feeding; may need to increase caloric density of feeding to meet infant's energy needs. Consult with pediatric gastroenterologist. Medication may be indicated (see Chapter 32). Surgical referral may be necessary in cases that do not respond to medical management.

- Encourage parents to make decisions related to their child's care; provide suggestions and guidance as the child grows, as treatment is carried out, and as needs change.
- Give positive reinforcement for parents' success.

Complications

Aspiration with damage to lung tissue, FTT, poor parent-child bond, esophagitis, and esophageal strictures are complications of difficulty in feeding.

EATING DISORDERS

An eating disorder is defined as "a situation where the time spent eating (or not eating) in response to an external stimulus is greater than the time spent eating in response to internal hunger cues" (Hahn, 1998). Although problems with feeding (e.g., colic, food refusal, picky eating) are common among children, anorexia nervosa, bulimia, and binge (or out of control) eating are the conditions most frequently identified as eating disorders in the pediatric population (Nicholls and Bryant-Waugh, 2009). These conditions are discussed in detail in Chapter 19.

OBESITY AND OVERWEIGHT

Description

Excessive adipose tissue is the hallmark of obesity and overweight, and may be due to an increase either in the size of fat cells (hypertrophy) or in the number of fat cells (hyperplasia). Childhood-onset overweight that is hyperplastic in nature is especially difficult to control because fat cells can be reduced in size but not in number.

BMI and weight-for-height are used to define parameters of overweight. In adults, normal BMI ranges from 18.5 to 24.9, and an individual is defined as obese if BMI is 30 or greater. In children, the definition of obesity and overweight is less specific. Children are compared with a normative group of peers, and percentiles specific for their age and gender are a more valid indicator of underweight, normal weight, overweight, or obesity than is an absolute BMI (see Appendix B).

The Expert Committee on the Assessment, Prevention, and Treatment of Child and Adolescent Overweight and Obesity (Barlow and Expert Committee, 2007) recommends that children 2 to 18 years old with a BMI greater than or equal to the 95th percentile for age and sex, or those with a BMI greater than or equal to 30 (whichever is lower) be considered obese, not "overweight." Children with a BMI between the 85th and 95th percentiles for age and sex are overweight, not "at risk for overweight." This terminology avoids the confusion of "at risk for overweight" and more clearly categorizes those children who are likely to have health problems as a result of their weight (i.e., those who are obese). There are no BMI parameters for children younger than 2 years; those with a weight-to-height ratio of greater than or equal to the 95th percentile are categorized as overweight. BMI measurements must be used cautiously to assess individual children because some children have a body weight or BMI in excess of the norm for their age, gender, and height without having excess fat. Children who are genetically large-boned may weigh more than their peers, for example, or athletic adolescents may have a higher BMI as a result of heavier muscle mass.

Epidemiology

Overweight and obesity continue to be serious concerns in children and are increasingly common among infants and toddlers. Nearly one third of U.S. children are overweight or obese. NHANES data from 2007 to 2008 indicate that 9.5% of children younger than 2 years old are overweight (≥95th percentile for weight to recumbent height) and data from the Early Childhood Longitudinal Study found 31.9% of 9 month olds and over 34% of 2 yr olds either at risk or obese (Moss and Yeaton, 2011). Nearly 12% of children 2 to 19 years old have BMIs greater than or equal to the 97th percentile, 16.9% have BMIs greater than or equal to the 95th percentile, and 31.7% have a BMI greater than or equal to the 85th percentile (Ogden and Carroll, 2010). The rapid rise in overweight and obesity in the U.S. occurred between the 1960s and 2000, with about 5% of all children 2 to 19 years old being obese in the 1971-1974 NHANES study, and 13.9% in 1999-2000. Since 1999, NHANES data have been collected annually and there appears to be no significant upward trend, except among 6- to 19-year-old boys. There is, however, a significant difference in obesity prevalence by race and gender, with 29.2% of 12- to 19-year-old non-Hispanic black girls and 26.8% of 12- to 19-year-old Mexican-American boys having BMIs greater than or equal to the 95th percentile (Ogden and Carroll, 2010).

Obesity results from a complex relationship of genetics, environment, and the body's response to environmental factors (e.g., neurohormonal regulation). Though studies show a variety of risk factors and predictors for obesity, the specific moderators of excess weight gain vary and the relationship among variables is complex. New discoveries of the factors (e.g., hormones, brown fat, microbes, brain activity) involved in the dynamics of satiety, insulin sensitivity, and weight regulation are being made daily. It may be that most obesity is a function of a genetic predisposition combined with environmental stimuli (Bouchard, 2009). The following discussion outlines what are believed to be major causes or predictors of obesity.

Rapid weight gain in infants from birth to 5 or 6 months old is a strong predictor of overweight in children and puts children at risk for subsequent obesity and metabolic syndrome (Demerath et al, 2009; Goodell et al, 2009; Singhal, 2010; Taveras et al, 2009). "Fat babies" are not necessarily healthy babies; prevention of overweight from birth and early intervention for children at risk for overweight is essential.

A biological imbalance of hormones, peptides, proteins, and other factors may lead to obesity; extensive research is being done in this area, with exciting discoveries that may yield clinical application in the future. Insulin and leptin are two major hormones that normally serve to control satiety and influence weight. Resistance to insulin and to leptin, seen in some racial and ethnic groups, and often found in obese individuals, may contribute to the body's failure to register satiety. Lustig (2006) posits that chronic hyperinsulinemia may be the source of insulin and leptin resistance. Leptin normally stimulates the ventromedial hypothalamus (VMH), sending the message that the body has adequate energy stores. Insulin and leptin share the same "signaling cascade" in the VMH, however, and if insulin levels are high, leptin is prevented from signaling its message of satiety. Hyperinsulinemia thus prevents the message that the body is satiated from getting through; overeating to satisfy hunger can result. Hyperinsulinemia in children has three sources: genetics, epigenetics (small- and large-for-gestational-age infants experience hyperinsulinemia and insulin resistance), and environment. Environmental dynamics contributing to hyperinsulinemia are threefold:

- Increased stress leads to increased cortisol production, which can lead to insulin resistance.
- Decreased physical activity contributes to insulin resistance.
- Diet, especially high levels of fructose and decreased fiber, leads to excess insulin secretion. "High-glycemic" foods (such as soda, sweetened juices, processed breads, pastries, and crackers) are more quickly converted to serum glucose, and stimulate a sharp rise in insulin production. With the high insulin level, glucose is moved quickly into cells, the extra insulin stays in the blood and the resulting hypoglycemia stimulates hormone release that further increases appetite. The end result is overeating and increased fat storage (Otten et al, 2006).

Increasing physical activity and changing diet (eating more low-glycemic foods, such as whole grains, vegetables, and fruits [Reedy and Krebs-Smith, 2010]) can help decrease excess insulin production and restore the body's natural feedback system.

The concept that some people may be "addicted" to certain foods has been proposed and animal and human research in this area is expanding to determine to what extent and by what mechanisms food may be addictive. Some research suggests that the genes and neural pathways characteristic of alcohol dependence may be shared by certain foods, especially sugars (Fortuna, 2010), carbohydrates, fats, and possibly processed salty foods (Corsica and Pelchat, 2010). Others contend that food, per se, is not addictive, but a dietary pattern of restricting and bingeing, especially fats and sweets, leads to a behavioral (in contrast to physiological) addiction (Avena et al, 2008; Corwin and Grigson, 2009).

Decreased physical activity results in decreased energy consumption and, logically, weight gain if dietary intake remains stable; whereas increased physical activity leads to weight loss (Byrd-Williams et al, 2010; Madsen et al, 2009). With the obesity epidemic, it is argued that children have increased the time they spend on sedentary activities (e.g., "screen time"), that many schools have discontinued physical education classes (Brener et al, 2009), that many children are driven to school rather than walking or riding bicycles, and that many neighborhoods are unsafe for outdoor play (Carver et al, 2008, 2010)—all environmental factors that contribute to the problem of excess weight gain. For example, despite the fact that the AAP recommends no television for children younger than 2 years old and 1 to 2 hours per day for older children, about 63% of 0- to-2-year-olds, 82% of 3- to 4-year-olds, and 78% of 5- to 6-year-olds watch television each day (Vandewater et al, 2007). Older children watch about 4.5 hours of television per day, and, with media multitasking, have approximately 10 hours and 45 minutes of media contact in a typical day (Rideout et al, 2010).

The relationship between a more sedentary lifestyle and obesity appears straightforward, but it may not be that simple. Research indicates that since the 1980s, although obesity and overweight have increased significantly among adults, their physical activity has remained essentially the same (Westerterp and Speakman, 2008). Studies of physical activity among children are found to use differing criteria and measurement tools that lack reliability and validity, so data obtained may be less than accurate (Chinapaw et al, 2010). Although most children do not get the amount of exercise recommended by the Centers for Disease Control and Prevention (CDC), it is hard to say how much less active today's children are than those of previous generations. Although, as noted, increased physical activity contributes to weight loss, it may not be lack of physical activity alone that is at the heart of the problem. Changes in eating habits, rather than a decrease in physical activity per se may be more important (Jordan et al, 2008; Strasburger et al, 2010). Watching television replaces active play but it also exposes children to snack-food advertising and increases the likelihood that children will overeat and eat more empty calories (Dubois et al, 2008). This pattern of overweight and poor nutritional intake related to watching television is international in scope (Vereecken et al, 2006).

Temperament may be a risk factor for obesity; in one study, 12-month-old male infants with shorter attention spans and female infants with greater soothability or negative reaction to food were more likely than their counterparts to be overweight at 6 years of age (Faith and Hittner, 2010).

A number of environmental factors put children at risk for being overweight, including having obese parents, maternal smoking during pregnancy, bottle feeding, family stressors, and middle and low socioeconomic status. Research suggests that prenatal exposure to endocrine disruptors, such as bisphenol-A or estrogen, may predispose to overweight and obesity (Hatch et al, 2010; Newbold, 2010).

Psychosocial factors also contribute to the increased incidence of obesity, including family stressors, using food to regulate emotions or to cope with stress, overeating in response to inappropriate body image perceptions, social pressure to be thin, depression, and low self-esteem (Blissett et al, 2010; Dubois and Girard, 2006; Harbaugh et al, 2009; Spruijt-Metz et al, 2006). Children who suffer neglect or abuse or have an overcontrolling parent may turn to food for comfort and solace, with overeating as a result.

Clinical Assessment and Findings

Clinical assessment of obesity is the first step to effectively addressing the problem. Unfortunately many providers do not conduct thorough assessments; in fact, many fail to address the topic of weight in their routine well-child care entirely. In one study, less than 49% of pediatric nurse practitioners (NPs) stated they measured BMI routinely when examining children and adolescents (Small et al, 2009). In a review of data from the National Hospital Ambulatory Medical Care Surveys from 1997 through 2000, Cook and colleagues (2005) found that of nearly 33,000 well-child visits for 2- to 18-year-olds, only 281 (0.78%) had a diagnosis of excess weight gain, obesity, or morbid obesity, despite the fact that approximately 15% of this population reportedly had BMIs greater than or equal to the 95th percentile. This study also noted that if obesity was not a diagnosis, 43.9% of patients were screened for blood pressure; if obesity was a diagnosis, blood pressure screening increased to 61.1% (Cook et al, 2005).

History. Assessment must consider underlying factors and comorbid conditions such as hypothyroidism, polycystic ovary disease, depression, diabetes, and cardiovascular disorders, in addition to examining patterns of eating and exercise for both the child and the family system. The history should include the following:
- Dietary intake, including:
  - Total caloric intake
  - Fat intake as percentage of total calories
  - Carbohydrate intake as percentage of total calories
  - Nutrient adequacy of diet
- Eating patterns, including breakfast, eating outside home, portion sizes, frequency and quality of meals and snacking
- Amount of sweetened beverages and 100% fruit juices consumed
- Exercise pattern
- Hours and types of sedentary activity
- Parental obesity
- Time of onset of excessive weight gain
- Family history of diabetes and cardiovascular disease (hypertension, congenital heart disease [CHD])
- Family or child history of hypothyroidism or other medical conditions that could contribute to overweight

TABLE 10-10 Calculation of Ideal Body Weight from Centers for Disease Control and Prevention Growth Charts*

Ideal Body Weight for Healthy Children	Interpretation
>120%	Overweight
90%-110%	Normal
80%-90%	Mildly underweight
70%-79%	Moderately underweight
<70%	Severely underweight

*% Ideal body weight = Current weight divided by weight at 50th percentile for current stature multiplied by 100.
From Centers for Disease Control and Prevention: *Growth charts* (see Appendix B).

- Episodes of sleep apnea
- Social adjustment, peer group, friends
- Family and child readiness and ability to participate in a weight management treatment program based on healthy eating and activity
- Barriers to exercise and healthy eating (e.g., environmental constraints, physical disability)

Physical Examination. A complete physical examination is necessary to determine the child's level of fitness and anthropometric status, looking especially at the following:
- Blood pressure (measured with cuff that covers 80% of arm)
- Vital signs
- Height and weight (height-to-weight ratio is a better indicator than BMI of overweight in infants and children younger than 2 years old)
- Ideal body weight (Table 10-10)
- BMI
- Triceps skinfold (not recommended in routine assessment by the Expert Committee [Barlow and Expert Committee, 2007])
- Midarm circumference
- Skin (for acanthosis nigricans)

Diagnostic Tests
- Fasting lipid profile
- Fasting glucose tolerance test
- Thyroid screen, TSH, T_4
- Metabolic panel

Differential Diagnosis

The differential diagnoses include medical conditions such as hypothyroidism, polycystic ovary disease, Down syndrome, and Prader-Willi syndrome.

Management

Prevention of overweight and assertive treatment of children who are already overweight should be priorities for care. However, just as they fail to address overweight in their assessments and diagnoses, pediatric providers fall far short in their management of the problem. NHANES data from 2003 to 2006 found that more than 60% of children who were overweight or obese were *not* told by their providers that they needed to lose weight. Less than 38% of overweight children were counseled on healthful nutrition and exercise; adolescents were more likely than younger children to be told they were overweight and counseled on lifestyle changes (Agency for Healthcare Research and Quality, 2010). Regarding prevention, National Ambulatory Medical Care Survey data from 2001 through 2004 indicate that only about one quarter (24.4%) of normal-weight children ages 4 to 18 years received obesity prevention counseling (i.e., diet/nutrition and exercise) during well-child visits. A disturbing finding in this study was that Hispanic children, children on Medicaid, and children seen in hospital-based clinics were significantly less likely than Caucasian, insured children to receive counseling (Branner et al, 2008).

For most children who are overweight or obese, the primary goal of weight management is to normalize, not necessarily reduce weight. Because children are growing and developing, recommendations for treating overweight focus on slowing the rate of weight gain, thereby allowing children to grow into their weight. Restricting fat intake for infants is not recommended because of the rapid neurologic development occurring at this age. If the child is beyond a weight into which he or she will reasonably "grow," weight reduction becomes the treatment goal.

Interestingly, many parents of overweight children perceive their child as normal-weight or even underweight. In a study of 576 child-parent pairs (5- to 12-year-old children), 25% of parents inaccurately stated their child was not overweight. One hundred percent of the parents of children with a BMI equal to or greater than the 95th percentile placed their child in a category other than "extremely overweight," and 75% of the parents of children with a BMI between the 85th and 95th percentiles stated their child was "about right" or "underweight." Parents tended to misclassify boys more often than girls (De La O et al, 2009). This misperception by parents may hinder treatment, especially if the intervention plan requires family lifestyle changes, and may need to be addressed by the provider as a part of treatment.

Panzer (2010) suggests that effective treatment for obesity needs to take into consideration the "subgroups" of obese children: chronically obese (i.e., have never been normal weight), transiently obese (i.e., have significant weight gain and then spontaneous loss without treatment), children with a dual diagnosis or significant comorbidity (e.g., ADHD, depression), and obese children who are "well-functioning."

Lifestyle Changes. If a child's body is able to signal to the brain that it has reached satiety before the child overeats, and if the child responds to the body's cues of satiety, caloric intake will decrease. Research indicates that young infants are highly sensitive to satiety and stop eating when full, but it appears that this natural regulator can be overridden by overfeeding the infant or providing high-calorie foods that are quickly absorbed as glucose (e.g., juice or juice drinks) (Lustig, 2006). In essence, the child no longer knows when he or she is full—when the body has received enough calories. Parents should be encouraged to respond to their infant's cues of satiety by stopping the feeding. As mentioned, infants who experience rapid weight gain in the first months of life are at higher risk for overweight and obesity as toddlers and preschoolers and ultimately for their entire life. Preliminary research suggests that decreasing the protein content of formula in early infancy can bring children back into line with normal growth patterns (Koletzko et al, 2009). Nutrient intake for infants must not be compromised, however. Breastfed infants tend to gain weight more slowly than formula-fed infants, and breastfeeding should be encouraged as a way to prevent overweight.

Children must be monitored for height and weight on a regular basis, but progress should be measured by other parameters as well. Improved dietary habits; increased physical activity, fitness, and strength; and enhanced self-esteem are significant endpoints that should be acknowledged and praised by the family and health care team alike.

Motivational interviewing as described in Chapter 9 may be a helpful strategy when working with adolescents and parents of overweight children. The National Association of Pediatric Nurse Practitioners (NAPNAP) Healthy Eating and Activity Together (HEAT) Initiative (2006) guidelines are consistent with recommendations for developing healthy eating habits and include:

- Educate parents about:
  - Children's growth patterns and nutritional needs
  - Ways children communicate hunger and satiety
  - Strategies for developing healthy eating habits
  - Strategies to encourage physical activity in children
  - Risk factors for overweight
  - Early indicators of overweight
- Implement behavioral change interventions including:
  - Early intervention (in infancy if necessary)
  - Family-centered treatment, with counseling regarding communication and eating habits
  - Increased activity
  - Decreased intake of high-fat, high-glycemic, and high-calorie foods
  - Increased intake of fiber (AAP recommends 0.5 g/kg/day for children older than 2 years [Ruottinen et al, 2010])
  - Appropriate portion sizes
- Provide ongoing support to families

In addition, depending on the child's age, baseline BMI, presence of medical complications, and weight status of parents, treatment can include either weight-loss or weight-maintenance strategies that focus on the following:

- Modify diet to increase fruits and vegetables to five or more per day and eliminate sugared drinks
- Decrease "screen time" to less than 2 hours per day
- Remove television from child's bedroom (if present)
- Emphasize "mindful viewing" of television; TV is never on without attention and thought, never as "background" (Jordan and Robinson, 2008)
- Exercise 1 hour or more per day
- Eat a daily breakfast
- Decrease meals eaten outside home
- Have a family meal at least five or six times a week
- Allow child to self-regulate meals; avoid being overly restrictive. This does not, however, mean the child can eat whatever he or she wants—the parent must provide healthful foods to choose from

The Expert Committee on the Assessment, Prevention, and Treatment of Child and Adolescent Overweight and Obesity (Barlow and Expert Committee, 2007) recommends these strategies in a staged management approach with active monitoring by the primary care provider and involvement of the entire family. If initial efforts are unsuccessful, more rigorous management that may include behavior modification, highly structured monitoring and control, multidisciplinary interventions, medication, or surgery is recommended.

| BOX 10-10 | Guidelines for Managing Childhood Weight Problems |

- Do not put child on a diet. Instead, gradually modify the entire family's eating habits. For example, serve fruit as a substitute for dessert, switch to nonfat or 1% milk, experiment with low-fat recipes and methods of food preparation, and use reduced-fat margarine, salad dressings, and other low-fat condiments. Serve nutritionally dense foods that reflect recommendations of MyPlate, including whole grains, fruits, vegetables, lean-protein foods, and low-fat dairy products.
- Do not force children to clean their plates. They should eat only until they are full.
- Serve age-appropriate portions (e.g., ¼ to ⅓ adult portion for young children).
- Schedule and enforce regular times for meals and snacks. Do not skip meals. Do not allow children to "graze" throughout the day.
- Structure mealtimes to be a family time, eating, sharing, and enjoying food together.
- Have low-calorie, nutritious snacks readily available, such as air-popped popcorn, pretzels, low-fat yogurt, frozen fruit juice bars, skim milk, low-sugar cereals, fresh fruit, and raw vegetables.

- Do not have high-calorie snacks readily available (e.g., potato chips, cookies, cakes, pies, ice cream, candy, soda pop, and doughnuts).
- Promote physical activity. Start slowly, with low-weight–bearing exercise. Set reasonable goals and celebrate achieving them. Make daily exercise a priority. Encourage family participation, individual exercise, and team sports and structured activities with peers as appropriate.
- Limit television viewing to 1 to 2 hours a day or less. Replace television viewing time with family activities, hobbies, chores. Children who watch 4 or more hours of television per day are twice as likely as other children to become obese. Children are more sedentary when they watch television, and frequent food advertising is linked to increased snacking.
- Praise and reward children for the progress they make in reaching nutrition, activity, physical fitness, self-esteem, or weight goals.
- Emphasize the uniqueness of each child, pointing out special talents, abilities, and positive qualities.
- Do not overly restrict children's diets or demand children eat when they are not hungry. This approach actually leads to overeating and subsequent overweight.

Overeating, overweight, and obesity are complex phenomena involving social cues and expectations and physiological dynamics, and their management requires that both the child and family change lifestyle patterns. It may be that a family-based behavior modification approach, using cognitive-behavioral and family therapy will be necessary in most cases for successful weight loss (Panzer, 2010). When the entire family is involved, the overweight child has a much greater chance to normalize weight. Box 10-10 provides suggestions to use when counseling overweight children and their families.

Community Changes. Individual and family interventions may not be sufficient to deal with the causes of obesity. If children cannot safely play outside, for example, it may be impossible for them to get the recommended 60 minutes of moderate to vigorous daily exercise they need. Community change is imperative to support individual and family efforts to lose weight. The CDC recommends community action in six different areas (CDC, 2009):
- Increasing access to affordable healthy foods
- Supporting healthy food choices
- Promoting breastfeeding
- Encouraging physical activity
- Providing safe communities in which to exercise
- Organizing at the grass roots to create and continue health-supportive change

Primary care providers can provide community policymakers with the detailed recommendations presented in the CDC Guidebook, give them information about obesity as a public health problem, and support public policy that creates positive change.

Medications. Lifestyle changes should be the primary treatment for obesity in children and adolescents (Rogovik and Goldman, 2009; Rogovik et al, 2010). Medications should only be used after an intensive, formal trial of lifestyle change has proven ineffective and the child is excessively obese (>95th percentile), or overweight (>85th percentile) with comorbidities present (August et al, 2008). Several medications are used to control weight in adults and adolescents. Orlistat (decreases fat absorption) is the only FDA-approved medication for pediatric use, for children 12 and older. Orlistat is available over the counter and by prescription, so providers should be sure to determine if the family or child is self-medicating. Sibutramine and several appetite suppressants (phentermine, rimonabant, and metformin) are used to treat obesity in adults. Metformin does not have FDA approval for use in treatment of obesity, but has been used experimentally (Park MH et al, 2009). All these medications have potential side effects and it is recommended that, other than orlistat, they not be used with children and adolescents; fiber supplements (e.g., glucomannan) can be used to prevent side effects (e.g., fatty stools) of orlistat.

Surgery. Bariatric surgery (roux-en-Y gastric bypass; laparoscopic adjustable gastric binding; sleeve gastrectomy) has not been widely used as a therapy for adolescents and children, but can be effective in treating morbidly obese adolescents with comorbidities (Brandt et al, 2010). It has been recommended that adolescents be selected for bariatric surgery using criteria set by the National Institutes of Health (NIH) for adult eligibility (Nadler et al, 2009). The Endocrine Society states that adolescents who are morbidly obese (BMI >50) or who have a BMI greater than 40 with comorbidities are candidates for bariatric surgery (August et al, 2008). Some providers believe that having surgery during adolescence (rather than waiting until adulthood) may be more beneficial for individuals with childhood-onset obesity (Inge et al, 2007). But the surgery has potentially serious side effects (Gogakos et al, 2009) and adolescents must be carefully monitored because long-term effects are still unknown (Brandt et al, 2010). It has been used experimentally in younger children (Dan et al, 2010) and more frequently in adolescents, but primary care providers are still cautious about referring patients for surgery; in one study, 48% of providers said they would never refer an obese adolescent for bariatric surgery (Woolford et al, 2010). Table 10-11 summarizes recommendations for both pharmacotherapy and bariatric surgery when treating adolescents.

TABLE 10-11	Recommendations for Pharmacotherapy or Bariatric Surgery	
Expert body	**Recommendations for Pharmacotherapy**	**Recommendations for Bariatric Surgery**
American Academy of Pediatrics	Candidates have (a) attempted comprehensive multidisciplinary intervention; (b) maturity to understand risks; (c) willingness to maintain physical activity	Severe obesity not responsive to behavioral interventions
Endocrine Society	Pharmacotherapy considered if formal intensive lifestyle modification has failed to limit weight gain and severe comorbidities persist after lifestyle modification; BMI must be >95th percentile or >85th percentile with significant comorbidities. Pharmacotherapy should only be offered by clinicians who are experienced in the use of antiobesity agents and are aware of the potential for adverse reactions.	• Tanner stage 4 or 5 and at final or near-final adult height • BMI >50 or BMI >40 and significant, severe comorbidities • Severe obesity and morbidity persists in spite of formal lifestyle modification program, with or without medication trial • Psychological evaluation confirms the stability and competence of the family unit • Access to an experienced surgeon in a medical center capable of providing long-term follow-up, and the institution is participating in a study of bariatric surgery outcomes or sharing research data • The patient demonstrates the ability to adhere to the principles of healthy diet and activity

Data from August GP, Caprio S, Fennoy I, et al: Prevention and treatment of pediatric obesity: an Endocrine Society clinical practice guideline based on expert opinion, *J Clin Endocrinol Metab* 93(12):4576-4599, 2008; Woo T: Pharmacotherapy and surgery treatment for the severely obese adolescent, *J Pediatr Health Care* 23(4):206-212, 2009.

Complications

Children who are overweight are at much higher risk for related conditions, including hypertension, impaired glucose tolerance, sleep apnea, orthopedic problems (e.g., slipped capital femoral epiphysis), social rejection, lowered self-esteem, depression, and suicide. In the child with a physical disability, overweight can further impair mobility and reduce energy expenditure.

ADVERSE FOOD REACTIONS

Description

A distinction is made between *food allergy*, a hypersensitivity to a food or food additive with a reproducible immediate or delayed immune system response (e.g., anaphylactic reaction to ingestion of nuts), and *food intolerance*, a nonimmunologic inability to process or tolerate the food product (e.g., enzyme deficiencies [lactase] or PKU secondary to the body's inability to metabolize phenylalanine) (Fig. 10-2). Food can also be toxic (e.g., food poisoning or toxins from bacteria growing in the food) or create pharmacologic effects (e.g., headaches after eating ice cream). All are considered adverse reactions to food; this section discusses food allergy and intolerance.

Epidemiology

Many individuals believe they have a food allergy or intolerance, with up to 20% changing their diets because of this belief. Actually very few people have true food allergies, and although there have been more food allergies reported, this increase may reflect increased awareness and more frequent use of food allergy codes in recording diagnoses (Branum and Lukacs, 2009). Although there are many studies about food reactions, there are no standard criteria for diagnosing food allergy, which limits the ability to determine prevalence (Chafen et al, 2010). A double-blind, placebo-controlled food challenge is recognized as the gold standard for determining the presence of food allergy, yet many prevalence statistics are by self-report. A 1998 study indicated that only 1% to 2% of individuals met the criteria of a severe immunoglobulin E (IgE)-mediated or anaphylactic reaction or a positive double-blind, placebo-controlled food challenge (Hourihane, 1998). More recently, NHANES 2005-2006 data estimate, based on serum IgE, that 2.5% of the U.S. population has food allergies to four foods (peanuts, cow's milk, eggs, and shrimp), with the rate slightly higher among children (Liu et al, 2010). In another sample of 5300 households, self-reported allergies to peanuts and tree nuts appear to be increasing among U.S. children younger than 18 years old, from 0.6% in 1997 to 2.1% in 2008; peanut allergy reportedly increased from 0.4% to 1.4%, and allergy to tree nuts from 0.2% to 1.1% (Sicherer et al, 2010). Although few children are allergic to foods, one study found food to be the most common cause of anaphylaxis in children seen in an emergency department over a 5-year period (Russell et al, 2010). Factors contributing to adverse food reactions include the following:

• *Heredity.* A child with one parent with a food allergy has a 30% to 35% chance of developing the condition; if both parents have food allergies, the child's chances increase to 65%. Children born with a metabolic disorder can have adverse reactions to specific foods.

• *Immature gastrointestinal tract.* Before 7 months old, the infant gastrointestinal tract is more permeable to large molecules, including most food proteins. Allergies to milk and eggs are more common in younger infants and are often outgrown with age and maturity.

• *Compromised gastrointestinal tract.* As a result of injury or illness, the gastrointestinal system can be more permeable to allergens, such as large proteins.

• *Type of food.* Some foods are more allergenic than others, and some individuals have greater sensitivity to certain foods. Only a few foods—cow's milk, eggs, peanuts, soybeans, wheat, fish, crustaceans, and tree nuts (including almonds and cashews)—account for nearly 90% of IgE-mediated allergic reactions. Commercial baby foods that may appear to be only one fruit or vegetable can have eggs or milk added, sometimes under an unfamiliar name.

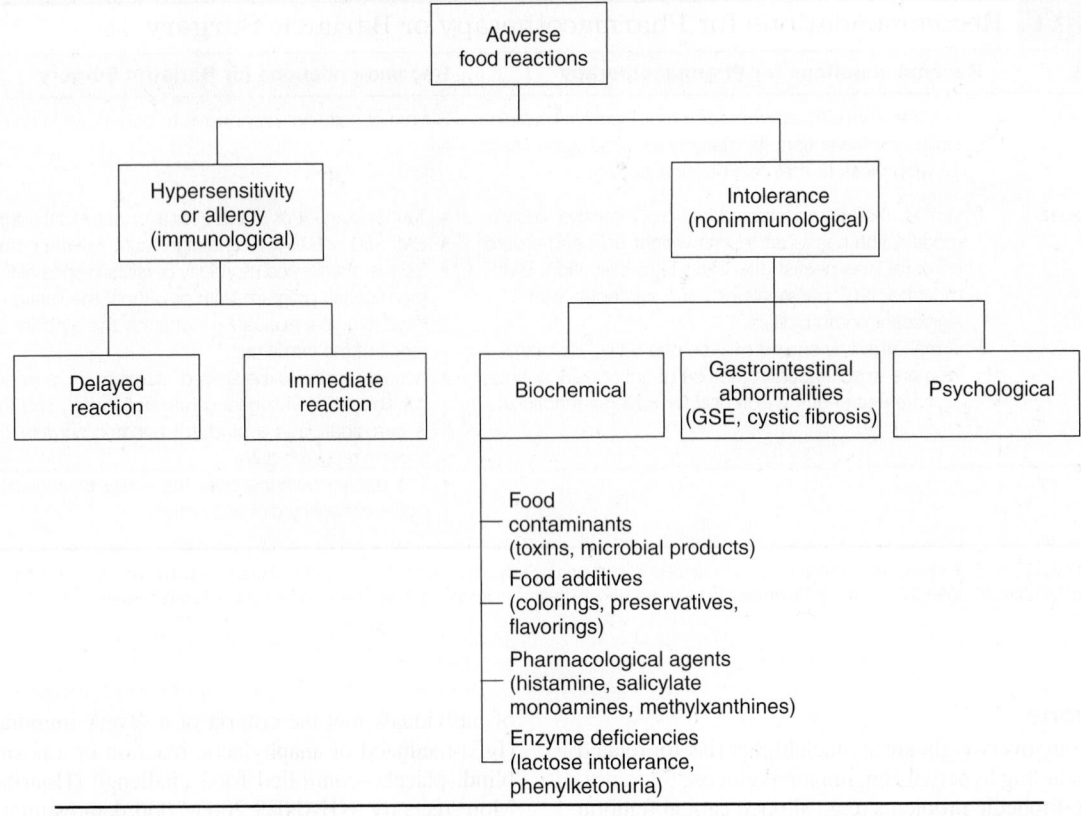

FIGURE 10-2 Adverse food reactions. (From Davis J, Sherer K: *Applied nutrition and diet therapy for nurses*, Philadelphia, 1994, Saunders.)

- *Allergic load or tolerance level.* Conditions such as illness, stress, surgery, or trauma can place excessive metabolic demands on the body. An individual who is susceptible to food intolerance or allergy can have a reaction when these conditions are present. Additionally, individuals may be allergic to more than one food and experience a reaction if more than one allergen is present.
- *Infant diet.* Breastfeeding is protective against allergies, including foods. Solids foods should be introduced between 4 to 6 months of age. Later introduction of solids, including those considered allergenic (e.g., egg whites) may actually increase food sensitization (Anderson et al, 2009; Koplin et al, 2010; Zutavern et al, 2008).

Clinical Assessment and Findings

The goals of clinical assessment are to determine whether an allergic reaction has occurred, whether it is related to food, to which food is it related, and how serious the problem is. This process is extremely challenging and can require referral to a registered dietitian or use of a team approach with primary provider, dietitian, and allergist for a more in-depth diagnostic workup. The basic examination includes the history, physical examination, laboratory studies, and food elimination and challenge.

History. The history should assess the following:
- Age of child
- Suspected food
- Route of exposure: Ingested? Skin touched? Food dust inhaled?
- Amount of exposure

- Onset of symptoms relative to exposure
- Description of symptoms (look, too, for change over the course of the reaction)
- Description of other factors that are present and may contribute to or aggravate an allergic response (e.g., stress, environment, exercise)
- Treatment given and child's response
- Does child have previous history of symptoms following exposure to this food?
- What is the child's diet history? When and what types of foods were introduced into the diet?
- Does the child have a history of symptoms frequently seen in food allergies (e.g., respiratory distress, eczema, urticaria, rashes, colic, vomiting, diarrhea) unaccompanied by other signs of illness or history of exposure to infectious agents?
- Is there a family history of allergies, especially a history of reaction to certain foods?

  Describe the child's usual intake. A food diary is an excellent mechanism for obtaining these data and includes the following:
- All foods and fluids ingested for at least 3 days
- How food is prepared (e.g., commercially, at home, fried, baked)
- How food is stored and fed to the child
- All medications

  A food-symptom diary can also be maintained, listing the child's reactions to foods ingested. This can become a time-consuming, cumbersome task, however, especially if more than one food is involved and requires real commitment on the part of parents.

| TABLE 10-12 | Possible Clinical Manifestations of Food Allergies or Intolerances by Body System | |

System	Symptoms
Respiratory system	Chronic rhinitis Asthma Croup Cough Serous otitis media Bronchitis
Gastrointestinal system	Tingling and swelling of lips, mouth, throat Nausea, vomiting Diarrhea Colic Protein-losing enteropathy Bloating, flatulence Constipation Gastrointestinal blood loss Malabsorption
Integumentary system	Eczema Pruritus Atopic dermatitis Rashes Urticaria
Central nervous system	Headaches (sinus, migraine) Fatigue Drowsiness, listlessness Irritability Depression Excessive sweating
Circulatory system	Hypotension Cardiac dysrhythmias Anaphylaxis Pallor

| TABLE 10-13 | Severity of Allergic Reactions to Foods | |

Severity	Clinical Manifestations
Mild	Localized cutaneous erythema, urticaria, angioedema, oral pruritus
Mild	Generalized erythema, urticaria, angioedema
Mild	At least 1 or 2 (above) plus gastrointestinal symptoms, rhinoconjunctivitis
Moderate	Mild laryngeal edema/mild asthma
Severe	Marked dyspnea; hypotension

Adapted from Clark AT, Ewan PW: Food allergy in childhood, *Arch Dis Child* 88(1):79-81, 2003.

- Serum IgE and eosinophil count (elevated serum IgE and eosinophilia greater than 400/mm^3 are usually related to allergies). This test is done if the child cannot have an SPT done, but it can be expensive, especially if more than one food is suspected. Results must be interpreted carefully by an allergist because findings can reflect exposure to other allergens.
- Atopy patch tests. The atopy patch test (ATP) looks for skin reaction to food, but is not widely used in the clinical setting.
- Radioallergosorbent tests.
- Metabolic screening tests (e.g., PKU).

Food Elimination and Challenge. When a food has been identified as a potential source of the problem, elimination and an oral food challenge (OFC) can be used to confirm the diagnosis. Medical supervision during the elimination and challenge is essential, and the procedure may best be managed by an allergist or immunologist.

The suspected foods are completely eliminated from the child's diet for at least 2 weeks and then gradually reintroduced, one at a time. A single- or double-blind with placebo challenge is most reliable, though an open challenge may be adequate (Bahna, 2007). The initial reintroduction dose should be small, then increased until either the reaction recurs or the amount normally eaten is given. During the elimination and challenge the child should receive no treatment medications for symptoms of reaction (e.g., antihistamines). If exercise is thought to contribute to the initial allergic reaction, exercise must be part of the challenge. An allergy or intolerance is confirmed if symptoms cease when the food is eliminated and then reappear as it is reintroduced. Approximately one-third of individuals are able to replicate signs and symptoms of a problem when challenged (Knight and Bahna, 2006).

If there is a possibility of a severe reaction to a food (e.g., anaphylaxis), the child should be hospitalized with emergency cardiovascular support available for the challenge part of this process. Allergy to peanuts or tree nuts can be lifelong, and children with allergies to nuts should never be challenged.

Physical Examination. Signs and symptoms of adverse food reactions vary by type and severity, from a mild local reaction to life-threatening anaphylaxis, making it difficult to diagnose the condition definitively. Table 10-12 lists possible clinical manifestations of food allergies or intolerances by body system, and Table 10-13 relates clinical features of a reaction to the level of severity of the child's condition.

Height and weight should be monitored closely in children with food allergies because food elimination and use of alternative foods may compromise nutrition and affect growth.

Diagnostic Tests. Laboratory studies can assist in identifying food allergies and intolerances (Lieberman and Sicherer, 2011). They may not be definitive, however, and a good history is often key to diagnosis. Tests include:

- Skin tests. The skin prick test (SPT) is the standard and is very sensitive. Cutaneous response may not correlate with a clinical systemic response, however. Antihistamine medications must be discontinued 3 to 20 days before the test, and the test should be avoided in children who have generalized skin lesions, dermographism, or a severe reaction to food following skin contact or inhalation.

Differential Diagnosis

The differential diagnoses for food allergy and food intolerance include:

- Reactions related to other environmental allergens
- Asthma as a result of other causes

- Immunodeficiency
- Psychological reactions to feeding
- Malabsorption syndromes (e.g., celiac disease), cystic fibrosis
- Lactose intolerance
- Chronic diarrhea
- Heiner syndrome, a milk-induced pulmonary disease with infiltrates, should be suspected in infants and young children who have persistent pulmonary disease without a clear cause (Moissidis et al, 2005).

Management

Care of children with adverse food reactions aims to maintain nutrition levels adequate for normal growth and development, prevent nutritional deficits, avoid exposure to offending food or foods, and respond promptly and appropriately to episodes of exposure. Achieving these goals requires the coordinated efforts of pediatric allergists, dietitians, the primary care provider, and teachers or childcare providers, in addition to children and their families. Once a child has been assessed as to the cause and severity of the condition, a treatment plan can be made.

Elimination Diet. In many cases the offending food or foods must be avoided. Efforts to eliminate the food from the diet raise challenging issues:

- The foods to which most individuals are allergic are very common and very nutritious.
- The food may contaminate other foods or be found in minute amounts in other foods (e.g., processed foods).
- Skin or inhalant contact may occur (e.g., breathing peanut dust) even if food is not eaten.
- Sometimes the individual is allergic to the food in its raw form, but can eat it in a cooked (heat-treated) form; completely eliminating it means unnecessary loss of a good source of nutrients.
- Extensive use of elimination diets can lead to malnourishment; these diets should be used for as short a time as possible.
- Cross-reacting allergens may further limit diets.

Restricted foods need to be replaced with those of equivalent nutrient value in the context of a well-balanced diet. Additionally, the physical problems caused by allergies (e.g., diarrhea, vomiting, dehydration, eczema) can create a need for extra nutrients to maintain health and foster growth. Consultation with a dietitian is recommended. For formula-fed infants allergic to cow's milk, hypoallergenic formula preparations are available. Extensively hydrolyzed cow's milk–based preparations may protect against allergy but can be expensive, and the infant may not accept the taste. Elemental formulas, synthesized free amino acids with vitamin and mineral supplements, can be used. Soy-based formulas are often a first choice alternative for older infants, but as many as 10% of infants allergic to cow's milk are also sensitive to soy (see Chapter 32).

Immunotherapy. Research suggests that in some cases the allergenic food need not be avoided and may be therapeutic in controlling the allergy; there is growing support for the use of oral or sublingual immunotherapy for food allergies (Kim and Sicherer, 2010; Koplin et al, 2010; Scurlock et al, 2010). To date, however, providers are cautioned about applying this approach to routine clinical practice until more research has been done (Scurlock and Jones, 2010). Safety is paramount and children who have a clear reaction to a food allergen should avoid exposure (Prescott et al, 2010).

Food Challenge. The child's allergic status should be reevaluated regularly. Because food allergies and intolerances are often outgrown, the child may be challenged with most offending foods every year or two. Cow's milk allergy is usually outgrown by 2 years; eggs by 4 to 5 years (Fiocchi and Martelli, 2006). Some foods appear to remain allergenic for longer periods (e.g., seafood, peanuts, and tree nuts). If the child's reaction has been serious or even life threatening, the parents may decide to continue to avoid the food; children with allergies to nuts should never be challenged. Many fatalities related to food allergies occur among older children, teenagers, and young adults.

Medication. Self-administered epinephrine is prescribed for children with moderate or severe allergies. Children, their parents, and other caregivers should be educated on intramuscular injection using prepared EpiPens. There is growing evidence that children at risk for food-related anaphylaxis should carry 2 doses of epinephrine (Rudders et al, 2010). Antihistamines are prescribed for children with mild allergies, unless there is a history of a reaction to trace amounts of the allergen or the child has asthma from another cause. In these cases epinephrine is appropriate (Clark and Ewan, 2003). Children with food allergies should wear a medical-alert (MedicAlert) bracelet or necklace. School personnel should be informed of the child's allergy, and a medical plan implemented in the school.

Education. Education of families, children, and adults who are responsible for the child's well-being is critical. The provider can do outreach to teachers, schools, and daycare centers with information about how to understand and safely manage the child's condition, and be an ongoing source of suggestions, support, and advocacy for parents.

Management of food intolerances secondary to metabolic disorders is discussed earlier in this chapter (see Disorders Requiring Restricted or Supplemental Diets).

Complications

Complications of adverse food reactions include the following:
- Anaphylaxis
- Convulsive coughing and sneezing, leading to aspiration or choking
- Asthma
- Malnutrition
- Gastrointestinal dysfunction
- Secondary skin infections
- Disruption of family processes

Prevention

The best treatment for food allergies and intolerances is prevention. Ideally, all infants, but especially those at high risk for allergies, should be breastfed for a minimum of 4 to 6 months, with complementary foods and breast milk until 12 months of age. The first foods introduced should be hypoallergenic (e.g., rice cereal, squash, bananas), and at least 3 to 5 days allowed between each new food so that any adverse reaction has time to occur. Probiotics, in conjunction with breastfeeding or use of hypoallergenic formula, may help prevent allergies (Chafen et al, 2010). As noted, delaying introduction of solids may actually contribute to allergies in susceptible children.

Breastfeeding mothers of infants at high risk for allergies should also avoid allergenic foods (e.g., cow's milk, nuts, fish) because the proteins from these foods may be passed to the infant via breast milk. Garlic, onions, cabbage, and broccoli also have been noted to cause gastrointestinal reactions in infants.

EFFECT OF MEDICATIONS ON NUTRITIONAL STATUS

Description

Medications are designed to alter the body's biochemistry in order to produce a healing effect. These biochemical changes have implications for the individual's nutritional status. Some medications deplete essential nutrients from the body; others interfere with the body's ability to metabolize nutrients; still others have an adverse effect on the appetite or cause nausea. Although a medication can have an immediate effect on an individual, adverse changes in nutritional status are most often seen after prolonged therapy.

Epidemiology

Drug-induced malnutrition results from drug-related alterations in the body's ability to absorb, distribute, metabolize, use, or excrete nutrients and their metabolites (Wynne et al, 2007). Absorption is affected by characteristics of the molecule being absorbed (size, ionization, lipid solubility), gut motility (too rapid as with diarrhea or too slow as with Hirschsprung disease), and environment of the gastrointestinal tract (e.g., gastric pH, lack of intrinsic factor). As medications change gastrointestinal motility or environment, they influence the absorption of nutrients.

Distribution of nutrients is affected by plasma protein-binding capabilities, total body water content, and relative fat content in the body. For example, if a drug that binds highly with plasma protein is taken for long periods of time or if a child has low serum albumin, nutrients have to compete for protein-binding sites.

Metabolism occurs primarily in the liver, and drugs can either inhibit or stimulate hepatic enzyme activity, thus influencing the body's ability to metabolize nutrients for use at the cellular level. The relationship of medications and nutrients in terms of excretion is less marked than with absorption, distribution, and metabolism, but drugs can have an effect on renal function, especially tubular reabsorption, which then affects nutritional status.

Clinical Assessment

Nutritional assessment of children on medication includes the general parameters discussed earlier, such as anthropometric measurements, physical examination, and diet history. Specific attention should be paid to those nutrients for which drug therapy places the child at risk of deficiency.

Management

Management involves ongoing assessment and anticipatory intervention to prevent nutritional problems for children on drug therapy. Referral to a dietitian can be helpful. General interventions include the following:
- Alter dietary intake to include more foods containing nutrients affected.
- Supplement diet with required vitamins or minerals, or both.
- Administer medications in a manner that minimizes their effect on nutrition.
- Consider alternative medications and treatment modalities.

Table 10-14 provides dietary suggestions related to specific classes of medication. This list is limited, and a comprehensive pharmacology reference should be consulted for specific drugs.

Complications

Malnutrition, slowed growth, delayed healing, and drug toxicity are complications of the effects of medication on nutritional status.

TOXIC EXPOSURES IN FOODS

Exposure to toxins and chemicals through the food chain contribute to many health problems in children. Chapter 41 examines the relationship between toxic exposure in foods and children's health.

CONTROVERSIES IN PEDIATRIC NUTRITION

Cow's Milk in Children's Diets

During the first year of life, the use of unmodified cow's milk is not recommended because of its high protein content, its inappropriate nutrient composition, and the risk of gastrointestinal bleeding and allergic reactions. Instead, infants should receive breast milk or an approved iron-fortified infant formula that closely matches the composition of breast milk. Although pediatric providers agree on this recommendation for infants, there is some debate about the use of cow's milk in the toddler's diet.

In most cases, children older than 1 year can safely drink cow's milk, and it can be recommended as a rich source of protein, calcium, riboflavin, and vitamin D. The calcium and vitamin D are present in highly absorbable forms, and the protein is highly bioavailable. Cow's milk is an easy and sure way for children to receive these essential nutrients. For some children, however, true allergy to cow's milk causes gastrointestinal, respiratory, or skin problems; parents may wonder whether the nutritional benefits of cow's milk are worth possible health risks. If the protein and nutrients found in milk are included in the child's diet with other foods, milk may not be necessary.

Lactose intolerance—a condition caused by a lack of the enzyme lactase, normally present in the small intestine—can also limit dairy product intake by children (see Chapter 32). Lactose intolerance is rare in infants but common in older children and adults from Asian, Native American, African American, and Hispanic ethnic groups. Acquired lactose intolerance may follow an episode of viral gastroenteritis in children. The condition causes symptoms of bloating, flatulence, abdominal cramps, and diarrhea from 15 minutes to 2 hours after the consumption of foods containing lactose. Children with low

TABLE 10-14 Nutritional Risks of Selected Drugs

Drug Category or Name	Nutritional Risk	Nutritional Intervention
Antibiotic (e.g., chloramphenicol)	Inhibits vitamin K–producing intestinal microflora Increases excretion of riboflavin Nausea, vomiting, diarrhea Decreases absorption of calcium, fat, and protein Decreases lactase activity Suppresses bone marrow (chloramphenicol) May cause aplastic anemia	Use acidophilus tablets, acidophilus milk, or yogurt to replace gastrointestinal organisms Supplement with vitamin C, B-complex vitamins, vitamin B_{12}, biotin, vitamin K, or well-balanced vitamin and mineral supplement Use lactose-reduced milk
Antihistamine (e.g., cimetidine, diphenhydramine)	Decreases gastric acid secretion, increases pH Decreases absorption of iron, folate, vitamin B_{12} May lead to hyperglycemia May disrupt vitamin D metabolism	
Barbiturate (e.g., phenobarbital)	Breaks down vitamin D May cause calcium deficiency, rickets, or osteomalacia May decrease serum folate, vitamin B_{12}, pyridoxine (vitamin B_6), magnesium May cause nausea, vomiting, constipation	May need vitamin D and calcium supplements Give drug with meals Give high-fiber and high-fluid diet If folic acid supplementation is indicated, administer cautiously
Corticosteroid	Increases protein catabolism and gluconeogenesis; decreases protein synthesis contributing to nitrogen wasting Stimulates appetite May cause hypokalemia, hyperglycemia, acid hypernatremia, hypocalcemia associated with osteoporosis May elevate serum lipids	If edema occurs, restrict sodium intake High doses require calcium and vitamin D supplements Supplement with vitamin B_6, vitamin C, and folic acid Monitor weight and restrict calories if there is excessive weight gain Increase dietary protein
Digoxin	May cause anorexia and nausea, weight loss May cause hypokalemia May increase urinary excretion of magnesium and calcium	Increase dietary potassium Evaluate need to increase dietary magnesium and calcium
Isoniazid	Interferes with enzyme pathway for creation of niacin Increases excretion of vitamin B_6 and folic acid May cause nausea and vomiting Decreases absorption of vitamin E Increases absorption of iron May cause hyperglycemia	Give vitamin B_6 supplement Increase foods high in folate, niacin, vitamin B_6, and magnesium Avoid foods with histamine and tyramine, such as tuna, mackerel, sardines, dry sausages and meats, imitation and hard cheeses, meat and protein extracts, and excessive amounts of caffeine
Methotrexate	Folate antagonist, contributes to folate deficiency May cause stomatitis, anorexia, diarrhea Decreases absorption of vitamins A, D, E, and K, beta-carotene	Give mineral oil Supplement with multivitamin given midway between times mineral oil is administered Give folate
Oral contraceptive	Increases vitamin A and calcium absorption Causes low serum vitamin C; possibly contributes to low levels of vitamins B_1, B_2, B_6, B_{12}, folate, magnesium, zinc	Increase intake of vitamins C, B_1, B_2, B_6, B_{12}, folate, magnesium, zinc
Phenothiazide hydantoin, phenytoin	Increases excretion of riboflavin May cause nausea, vomiting, constipation May cause hyperglycemia Impairs metabolism and absorption of folate; may lead to megaloblastic anemia Inactivates vitamin D; can lead to osteomalacia Decreases serum vitamin K	Supplement with vitamin D, vitamin K, folate, but excessive folate levels can decrease action of anticonvulsants Administer drug with, or immediately after, a meal

TABLE 10-14 Nutritional Risks of Selected Drugs—cont'd

Drug Category or Name	Nutritional Risk	Nutritional Intervention
Supplements		
Calcium	If taken with iron supplement, only calcium carbonate does not affect iron absorption; if taken with fluoride, absorption of both is decreased	
Zinc	>1500 mg/day: decreases copper absorption, possibly leading to anemia-related fatigue	
Iron	Causes nausea, possibly anorexia	
Theophylline	May cause vitamin B_6 deficiency	Give pyridoxine supplements

lactase levels may be able to digest small amounts of milk and other dairy products, especially if eaten with other foods. Yogurt, aged cheese, and fermented dairy products, which are much lower in lactose than milk, are usually better tolerated. Commercial preparations are also available (e.g., Lactaid) that break down the lactose in milk.

Effects of Sugar or Food Additives on Behavior

Food affects the body and its ability to function; just how is often an individual matter, complex and unclear. Many parents, teachers, and even children believe that sugar intake causes behavior problems, primarily hyperactivity. An extensive review of controlled scientific studies failed to find evidence of a causal link between sugar and behavior or cognitive performance (Cruz and Bahna, 2006). But an association between soft drinks and hyperactivity has been demonstrated in teenagers (Lien et al, 2006), and junk food has been associated with hyperactivity (Wiles et al, 2009). Researchers acknowledge the possibility that other components of the soft drink (e.g., caffeine), not sugar, may be the cause of symptoms. The common belief that there is an association between sugar and hyperactivity may stem from the fact that sugar consumption is often related to activities (e.g., birthday parties, Halloween) that result in excited behavior among children. An elimination diet (no sugar) can be tried; if symptoms improve, a double-blind, placebo-controlled challenge can be used to confirm a relationship.

The role of the provider is to educate and reassure parents that moderate sugar consumption in healthy children rarely results in adverse behavior. High-sugar diets are to be avoided, however, because these foods tend to replace more nutrient-dense foods, contribute to overweight and obesity, dental caries, and other health problems. Current dietary recommendations are that 10% or less of calories should come from sugar. In the average child who consumes 2000 calories daily, this amounts to 50 g or the equivalent of 10 teaspoons each day.

Breastfeeding

PAMELA J. HELLINGS

Breast milk is the ideal food for newborns and infants and supports infant nutrition essential for optimal growth and development. In addition to healthy nutrition, breastfeeding gives parents and infants physical, psychological, and emotional benefits that last a lifetime. Breastfeeding should be promoted and supported whenever possible.

Health care providers engage in assessment, education, support, outreach, and advocacy as they promote breastfeeding. Breastfeeding is a learned skill for both the mother and the infant; providers must assess the mother's knowledge level and provide information and guidance to increase the skills of the mother-infant dyad as the breastfeeding experience develops. Providers can educate families about the benefits of breast milk and how to recognize and prevent common problems. As a result, families can make educated choices about infant feeding and quickly find answers to questions and concerns. Breastfeeding is supported when providers take the time to determine the cause of a breastfeeding problem, develop a plan to address the problem, and guide the family through difficulties; these interventions can make all the difference in the decision to continue breastfeeding. Outreach and advocacy for breastfeeding are demonstrated when providers contribute to hospital, clinic, and community committees, advisory boards, and task forces to develop policies that promote and support breastfeeding; when they advise and educate colleagues on breastfeeding issues, teach breastfeeding content to students in the health professions, and serve as expert contacts for the media on issues related to breastfeeding. In all these activities, the health care provider serves an important leadership function in promoting and supporting breastfeeding.

■ Breastfeeding Recommendations

Major health professional organizations, including the National Association of Pediatric Nurse Practitioners (2007), the American Academy of Pediatrics (AAP) (2005), the American Academy of Family Physicians (AAFP) (2008), and the American Dietetic Association (ADA) (James and Lessen 2009) recommend breastfeeding exclusively for the first 6 months of life, then breastfeeding combined with other nutrients for at least the first year.

Proposed breastfeeding goals for *Healthy People 2020* reaffirm those from the *Healthy People 2010* document: 75% of mothers will initiate breastfeeding in the neonatal period; 50% will be breastfeeding at 6 months, and 25% at 1 year of age (U.S. Department of Health and Human Services [USDHHS], 2009). Breastfeeding rates have increased in the U.S. (Table 11-1), and three out of four new mothers initiate breastfeeding, meeting one of the *Healthy People* goals. Exclusive breastfeeding until 3 to 6 months and continued breastfeeding from 6 to 12 months still fall short of desired goals, however (Centers for Disease Control and Prevention [CDC], 2010). In 2011, the U. S. Department of Health and Human Services issued a report entitled *The Surgeon General's Call to Action to Support Breastfeeding* (2011). Twenty actions were identified to support breastfeeding and include:

1. Give mothers the support they need to breastfeed their babies.
2. Develop programs to educate fathers and grandmothers about breastfeeding.
3. Strengthen programs that provide mother-to-mother support and peer counseling.
4. Use community-based organizations to promote and support breastfeeding.
5. Create a national campaign to promote breastfeeding.
6. Ensure that the marketing of infant formula is conducted in a way that minimizes its negative impact on exclusive breastfeeding.
7. Ensure that maternity care practices throughout the United States are fully supportive of breastfeeding.
8. Develop systems to guarantee continuity of skilled support for lactation between hospitals and health care setting in the community.
9. Provide education and training in breastfeeding for all health professionals who care for women and children.
10. Include basic support to breastfeeding as a standard of care for midwives, obstetricians, family physicians, nurse practitioners, and pediatricians.
11. Ensure access to services provided by the International Board of Certified Lactation Consultants.
12. Identify and address obstacles to greater availability of safe banked donor milk for fragile infants.
13. Work toward establishing paid maternity leave for all employed mothers.
14. Ensure that employers establish and maintain comprehensive high-quality lactation support programs for their employees.

TABLE 11-1 *Healthy People 2010* Objectives: Initiation and Duration of Breastfeeding for Children Born in 2007

Healthy People 2010 Objective*	Actual % of Total Population Breastfeeding By Age of Infant	Number of States Meeting *Healthy People 2010* Objective	States That Met All Five Objectives
75% of mothers will initiate breastfeeding (breastfeeding at 7 days)	75%	25	
50% of mothers will be breastfeeding 6-month-old infant	43%	14	
25% of mothers will be breastfeeding 12-month-old infant	22%	15	Alaska, California, Colorado, Idaho, Minnesota, Montana, New Hampshire, Oregon, Vermont, Washington
40% exclusive breastfeeding through 3 months old	33%	17	
17% exclusive breastfeeding through 6 months old	13%	15	

*Reaffirmed as same objective for *Healthy People 2020* (USDHHS, 2009).
Data from Centers for Disease Control and Prevention (CDC): *Breastfeeding among US children born 1999-2007, CDC National Immunization Survey*. Available at www.cdc.gov/breastfeeding/data/NIS_data/index.htm (accessed February 7, 2011).

15. Expand the use of programs in the workplace that allow lactating mothers to have direct access to their babies.
16. Ensure that all child care providers accommodate the needs of breastfeeding mothers and infants.
17. Increase funding of high-quality research on breastfeeding.
18. Strengthen existing capacity and develop future capacity for conducting research on breastfeeding.
19. Develop a national monitoring system to improve the tracking of breastfeeding rates as well as the policies and environmental factors that affect breastfeeding.
20. Improve national leadership on the promotion and support of breastfeeding.

Providers can make a major contribution to breastfeeding's success by supporting these actions.

Hospital-Based Support

THE BABY-FRIENDLY HOSPITAL INITIATIVE

In 1991, the Baby-Friendly Hospital Initiative was developed by the World Health Organization (WHO) and the United Nations International Children's Emergency Fund (UNICEF) to recognize hospitals that provide optimal lactation support. This worldwide initiative continues to train providers and hospitals to promote breastfeeding internationally (UNICEF, 2010a). The 10 criteria to meet a "baby-friendly hospital" standard are outlined in the original joint WHO/UNICEF statement (WHO/UNICEF, 1989) and are used to assess the quality of a lactation program. Every facility that provides maternity services and care for newborn infants should:

- Have a written breastfeeding policy that is routinely communicated to all health care staff.
- Prepare all health care staff in skills necessary to implement this policy.
- Inform all pregnant women about the benefits and management of breastfeeding.

- Help mothers initiate breastfeeding within one half hour of birth.
- Show mothers how to breastfeed and how to maintain lactation even if they are separated from their infants.
- Give newborn infants no food or drink other than breast milk, unless medically indicated.
- Practice rooming-in (i.e., allow mothers and infants to remain together) 24 hours a day.
- Encourage unrestricted breastfeeding.
- Give no artificial teats or pacifiers (also called dummies or soothers) to breastfeeding infants.
- Foster the establishment of breastfeeding support groups and refer mothers to them on discharge from the hospital or clinic.

More than 15,000 facilities have been designated "baby-friendly" internationally, most in developing countries (UNICEF, 2010b). As of May 2011, only 110 hospitals and birthing centers in the U.S. held a baby-friendly designation, so much work remains for U.S. health care providers (Baby-Friendly Hospital Initiative [BFHI] USA, 2011).

Benefits of Breastfeeding

With rare exception, breast milk is the ideal food for a human infant. Each mammalian species provides milk uniquely suited to its offspring, and milk from the human breast is no exception. It is a living fluid rich in vitamins, minerals, fat, proteins (including immunoglobulins and antibodies), and carbohydrates (especially lactose). It contains enzymes and cellular components, including macrophages and lymphocytes, in addition to many other constituents that offer ideal support for growth and maturation of the human infant. As the infant grows and develops, the properties of the breast milk change. The sequence of colostrum, transitional milk, and mature milk meets the changing nutritional needs of the newborn and infant. Thus the milk of a mother of a 9-month-old has different concentrations of fat, protein, and carbohydrate and different physical properties, such as pH, when compared with the milk of the mother of a newborn or 1-month-old. In addition, some of the constituent properties in the milk are different from one time of day to another.

In addition to providing optimal nutrition for growth and development, breastfeeding confers many short- and long-term health benefits to infants. A review of studies examining the effect of breastfeeding on infant health indicates a lower risk of nonspecific gastroenteritis, necrotizing enterocolitis, acute otitis media, severe lower respiratory tract infections, asthma, atopic dermatitis, type 1 and type 2 diabetes, obesity, sudden infant death syndrome (SIDS), and childhood leukemia in breastfed infants (Ip et al, 2009).

In the short term, studies show that breastfed babies have added protection against bacterial, viral, and protozoal illnesses during infancy. Human-milk glycans and immunoglobulins appear to inhibit pathogens from adhering to intestinal mucosa, replicating, and causing disease (Correa et al, 2006). Oligosaccharides in breast milk also support the growth of the infantis strain of *Bifidobacterium longum* in the intestine of the breastfed infant, while suppressing pathological bacteria such as *Escherichia coli*, *Clostridium*, and *Enterococcus* (Marcobal et al, 2010; Zivkovic et al, 2011). Breastfeeding also appears to reduce the incidence of fever after immunization (Pisacane et al, 2010).

The long-term benefits of breastfeeding for 6 months may include a decreased incidence of atopic diseases and an association with lower rates of asthma in young children (Greer et al, 2008). Breastfeeding may also be protective against obesity, has been associated with lower cholesterol in adults (Owen et al, 2008; Singhal, 2010), and may be protective against type 1 and type 2 diabetes in youth (Mayer-Davis et al, 2008).

Initiating breastfeeding is crucial; the infant enjoys health benefits with every day of breastfeeding. Maintaining breastfeeding is also crucial; there is evidence, for example, that infants who are breastfed for 6 months have less risk for infection than those breastfed for 4 months (Chantry et al, 2006). However, exclusive, prolonged breastfeeding may actually contribute to health problems. Pesonen and associates found that infants exclusively breastfed for 9 months or longer had an increased incidence of atopic dermatitis and food hypersensitivity in childhood (Pesonen et al, 2006). Complementary foods should be added to the infant diet by 6 months of age (see Chapter 10). Breastfeeding provides important nutritional and health-related benefits and should be continued to at least 1 year.

There are also benefits for the mother that include more rapid return to her nonpregnant state; establishment of the strong bond associated with successful nursing; decreased risk for breast cancer (De Silva et al, 2010) and ovarian cancer, especially if the lastborn child is breastfed (Titus-Ernstoff et al, 2010); decreased risk for metabolic syndrome (Gunderson et al, 2010); and a variety of other conditions (Stuebe and Schwarz, 2010).

Breastfeeding also provides an economic incentive as a free and plentiful source of excellent infant nutrition. The cost

---

BOX 11-1	World Health Organization Recommendations for Breastfeeding With Human Immunodeficiency Virus

For HIV-positive mothers, the WHO recommends exclusive breastfeeding for the first 6 months unless replacement feeding is:
- Acceptable (socially welcome)
- Feasible (facilities and help are available to prepare formula)
- Affordable (formula can be purchased for 6 months)
- Sustainable (feeding can be sustained for 6 months)
- Safe (formula is prepared with safe water and in hygienic conditions)

Adapted from WHO: *10 facts on breastfeeding*, 2009. Available at www.who.int/features/factfiles/breastfeeding/en/index.html (accessed Aug 9, 2010). *HIV,* Human immunodeficiency virus; *WHO,* World Health Organization.

---

of formula and other necessary supplies easily exceeds $1000 to $1200 each year.

Contraindications to Breastfeeding

In addition to all the beneficial nutrients that are provided to the infant during breastfeeding, certain infections and many drugs or medications can be passed to the infant via breast milk. Although rare, contraindications to breastfeeding occur in some of these situations. In addition, a small number of infant conditions also preclude breastfeeding. Contraindications to breastfeeding include the following:
- Herpetic lesions on the mother's nipples, areolas, or breast
- Maternal diagnosis and treatment of cancer
- Maternal human immunodeficiency virus (HIV) infection, except in some areas (see WHO recommendations [Box 11-1]; breastfeeding for HIV-infected mothers is not recommended in developed countries)
- Infant with galactosemia

SPECIAL SITUATIONS

Additional circumstances require special consideration regarding the advisability or management of breastfeeding. These circumstances include the following:
- Significant maternal or infant illness affecting the ability to feed
- Maternal illness, such as tuberculosis, chickenpox, or hepatitis B
- Invasive breast surgery, in particular breast reduction in which the areola is removed and reattached
- Documented history of milk supply problems

Characteristics of Human Milk
COMPONENTS OF HUMAN MILK

The uniqueness of human milk to support the growth and development of the human infant cannot be overestimated. Scientists continue to find new components and to clarify the purposes of known components. More than 200 constituents of milk have been identified (Lawrence and Lawrence, 2005).

Colostrum

Colostrum production begins at about 20 weeks of gestation. The pregnant woman may notice a small amount of yellow discharge on her nipple or clothing. After delivery of the baby, production of colostrum increases, but is still of low quantity. This thick, rich, yellowish fluid has fewer calories than mature milk (67 versus 75 kcal/100 mL) and is lower in fat (2% versus 3.8%). It is rich in immunoglobulins, especially IgA, and other antibodies. In addition, it is higher in sodium, chloride, protein, fat-soluble vitamins, and cholesterol than mature milk, and it facilitates the passage of meconium. Because of the outstanding contribution to the infant's immunological status, colostrum is often referred to as the infant's "first immunization." Colostrum meets all nutritional needs of a normal term newborn in the first few days of life. No supplementation is necessary.

Transitional Milk

Transitional milk appears several days after delivery. Significant variability is seen in the constituent properties of transitional milk between mothers and within samples from the same mother. However, as a rule, transitional milk has more lactose, calories, and fat and less total protein than colostrum.

Mature Milk

Mature milk gradually replaces transitional milk by about the second week after delivery and provides, on average, 20 kcal/oz.

Water. Approximately 90% of human milk is water. Breast milk can meet all the fluid needs of the infant. Even in tropical and desert climates supplementation is not needed.

Lipid (Fat) Content. Various lipids (fats) make up the second greatest percentage of constituents of human milk. They are also the most variable component, with differences noted within a feeding, between feedings, in feedings over time, and between different mothers. The fat content is approximately 3.8% and contributes 30% to 55% of the kilocalories in human milk. During feeding, fluid in the mammary gland mixes with droplets of fat in increasing concentration. Thus the fat content is higher at the end of the feeding (hindmilk) than it is at the beginning (foremilk). The type and amount of fat in the maternal diet are thought to affect the type of lipid but not the total amount of fat found in the mother's breast milk.

Cholesterol content varies little in human milk and is approximately 240 mg/100 g of fat. Changes in the maternal diet do not produce changes in these cholesterol values. Breastfed infants have higher plasma cholesterol levels than do formula-fed infants. Recent research suggests, however, that breastfeeding may have a protective effect against cardiovascular disease because adolescents and adults tend to have lower cholesterol levels if they were breastfed (Owen et al, 2008; Singhal, 2010; Singhal et al, 2004).

Recent research on how fatty acids, such as docosahexaenoic acid (DHA) and other long-chain polyunsaturated acids (e.g., LC-PUFA), are regulated during breastfeeding and the role they play in brain and retinal growth has shown equivocal results. Early evidence does suggest that DHA has a beneficial effect on an infant's neurobehavioral functioning, especially in preterm infants (Agostoni, 2008; Hart et al, 2006; Heird and Lapillonne, 2005). If infants are not breastfed, formula should be supplemented with DHA.

Protein. Approximately 0.9% of the content of human milk is protein. When milk is heated or exposed to enzymes as in digestion, a clot, or casein, is formed. The clear portion that remains is known as whey. In human milk, 60% to 70% of the protein is whey, which primarily consists of α-lactalbumin and lactoferrin, and 30% to 40% is casein. In contrast, cow's milk is 20% β-lactalbumin and 80% casein, with distinct chemical differences between the casein found in cow's milk and that found in human milk. The curds of human milk are more easily digested by the infant. Other proteins include immunoglobulins, nonimmunoglobulins, and lysozyme—a nonspecific antibacterial factor.

Carbohydrates. The primary carbohydrate of human milk is lactose, which is synthesized by the mammary gland from glucose. Lactose is highly concentrated in human milk (6.8 versus 4.9 g/100 mL in cow's milk) and appears to be essential for growth of the human infant. In addition, lactose enhances the absorption of calcium, a potentially important role because of the relatively low level of calcium in human milk.

Vitamins and Minerals. Human milk has more than adequate amounts of vitamins A, E, K, C, B_1, B_2, and B_6. However, the level of vitamin D intake may not be adequate in breastfed infants who lack exposure to sunlight. Thirty minutes per week of unprotected exposure to the sun while dressed in a diaper only or 2 hours per week clothed (as long as the head is not covered) provides adequate vitamin D for a Caucasian breastfed infant (Konek and Mascarenhas, 2006). Sunscreen blocks vitamin D absorption. The AAP recommends a supplement of 400 International Units/day, beginning shortly after birth for all infants, including those exclusively breastfed, and for children and adolescents (Wagner and Greer, 2008).

Iron is found in low levels in human milk. However, iron absorption from human milk is highly efficient, with 49% of the available iron absorbed in contrast to 4% from formula. A full-term infant who is exclusively breastfed for 4 to 6 months is not at risk for iron deficiency anemia. Zinc is readily available in human milk and has an absorption rate of 41% versus 31% from cow's milk protein formulas and 14% from soy formulas.

■ Anatomy and Physiology

Pregnancy brings about the final stage of mammogenesis—growth and differentiation of the mammary gland and development of the structures to support breast milk production. Estrogen, progesterone, placental lactogen, and prolactin all play a role in mammogenesis. By approximately 20 weeks the breast is capable of milk production. The actual production of breast milk is triggered by the fall in progesterone concentration after birth of the baby. Placental retention inhibits milk production because of the presence of progesterone and other hormones.

Suckling by the infant is essential to establish and maintain lactation. The amount of milk produced depends on stimulation of the breast, removal of milk from the breast, and release of hormones. The concept of "supply and demand" is an important one for providers and parents to understand. Suckling stimulates the hypothalamus to decrease prolactin-inhibiting factor and permits release of prolactin by the anterior pituitary, which leads to a rise in the level of prolactin. Prolactin

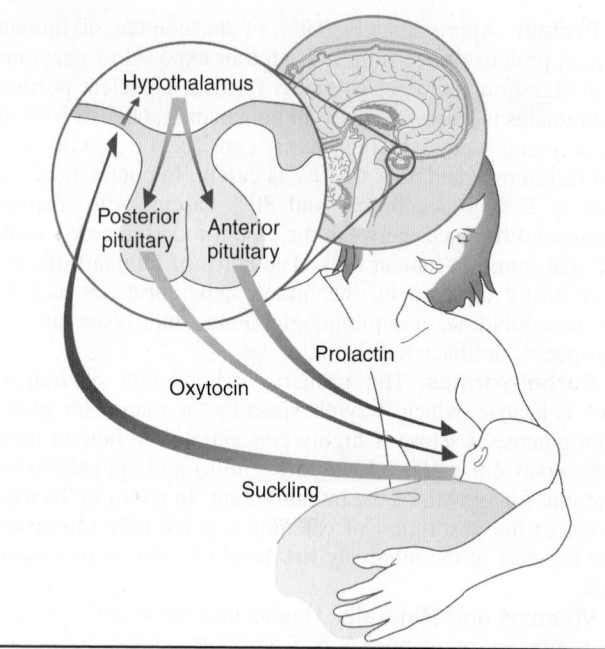

FIGURE 11-1 Neuroendocrine loop.

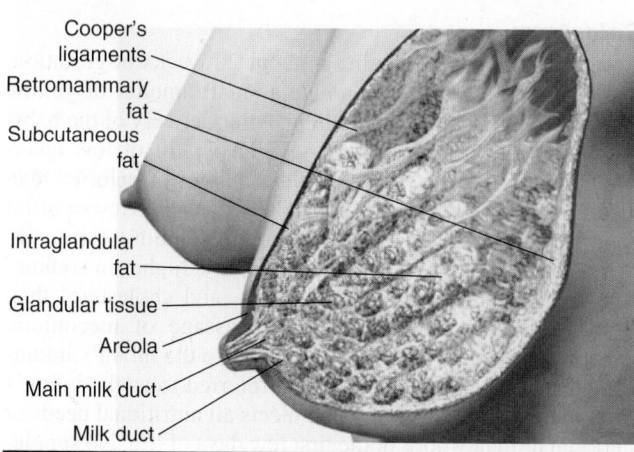

FIGURE 11-2 Anatomy of the lactating breast. (Modified from Medela AG, 2006, Available at http://www.medela.com/IW/en/breastfeeding/research-at-medela/breast-anatomy.html [accessed May 10, 2012]; Ramsay DT, Kent JC, Hartmann RA, et al: Anatomy of the lactating human breast redefined with ultrasound imaging, *J Anat* 206[6]:525-534, 2005.)

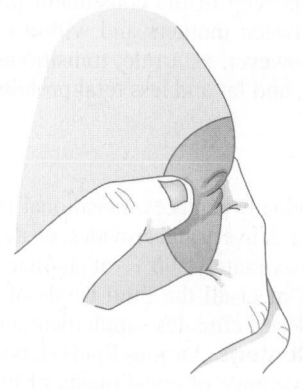

FIGURE 11-3 Pinch test.

levels are directly proportional to the level of suckling by the infant and are more important to initiating than maintaining lactation. The hypothalamus also stimulates the synthesis and release of oxytocin by the posterior pituitary (Fig. 11-1). Oxytocin reacts with receptors in the myoepithelial cells of the milk ducts to initiate a contracting action that results in forcing milk down the ducts. This action increases milk pressure called the *letdown reflex* or *milk ejection reflex.* Oxytocin also aids in maternal uterine involution.

Under the influence of the hormones mentioned previously, the mammary gland undergoes a dramatic change with an increase in size and rapid growth of the lobuloalveolar tissue. The alveoli are the sites of milk production and combine in numbers of 10 to 100 to form lobuli: 20 to 40 lobuli combine into lobes, and 15 to 25 lobes empty into a lactiferous duct. The ducts transport the milk to the nipple (Fig. 11-2).

The nipple and surrounding areola serve as a visual and tactile target to assist with latch-on. The size and shape of the woman's breast and areola vary greatly. Fortunately the size of the breast is not a predictor of breast milk volume. Women with very small breasts can successfully breastfeed. The provider should be alert, however, for the occasional presence of insufficient glandular tissue, which is characterized by the absence of breast changes associated with pregnancy, a unilaterally underdeveloped breast, or conical-shaped breasts.

The size, shape, and position of the nipple also vary among women. The nipple may be everted (protuberant from the breast), flat, or inverted. It is not always possible to detect an inverted nipple by observation only. The "pinch test" may be needed to identify nipples that invert with tactile stimulation to the areola. To do the pinch test, place the thumb and forefinger on opposite sides of the areola about 1 to 1.5 inches back from the nipple-areolar junction. Gently compress as though bringing the two fingers together, causing the nipple to become more everted or inverted. This assessment should be conducted prenatally on every patient (Fig. 11-3). Management of inverted nipples is discussed later in this chapter.

Despite the complexity of the anatomical and physiological processes, the great news is that breastfeeding can proceed for the mother and the baby with little or no awareness on their part of these considerations.

■ Assessment of the Breastfeeding Dyad

Prenatal assessment focuses on maternal expectations for breastfeeding; knowledge about breastfeeding, especially techniques for getting off to a good start; and identification of any contraindications to breastfeeding. A nipple evaluation should be completed. All pregnant women should be assessed, not just primigravidas. In the early postpartum period, assessment focuses on the transition to breastfeeding and should include close observation of a feeding. In addition, signs of progress for successful breastfeeding should be reviewed, and the names and phone numbers of contact persons should be given to mothers for follow-up or questions.

MATERNAL HISTORY

Data should be collected about the following areas:
- Overall health, including documentation of any chronic illnesses or allergies

- Previous breastfeeding experience
- Cultural expectations about breastfeeding
- Routine use of over-the-counter, prescribed, or recreational or street drugs, including tobacco, alcohol, and herbal preparations or supplements
- Surgical interventions, especially to the breast or thoracic region
- Nutritional status
- Family and community support for breastfeeding
- Pregnancy history, especially any complications or need for medications
- Labor and delivery history, including medications, procedures, or complications

INFANT HISTORY

Data are gathered on the infant in the following areas:
- Overall health status
- Congenital conditions, such as cardiac, respiratory, or orofacial conditions
- Trauma or complications during delivery
- Medications received during labor and delivery or in the early postpartum period
- Activities or procedures including circumcision, use of bilirubin lights, or use of bottle, cup, or tube feeding
- Gestational age
- Early responses to feeding attempts

MATERNAL EXAMINATION

Examination of the mother should focus on an evaluation of the breast in the following areas:
- Type of nipples—everted, flat, or inverted
- Presence of surgical scars on the breast or thoracic area
- Any nipple bruising or bleeding

INFANT EXAMINATION

Evaluation of the infant's oral-motor skills and structures is the basis for the examination. The examiner's finger should be inserted beyond the gum line nearly to the soft palate. The infant should be able to suck smoothly and evenly in a wavelike motion of the tongue as the finger is drawn in for suckling. The hard and soft palates should be intact, without palpable clefts or submucosal clefts. The infant should be able to extend the tongue over the lower gum with no evidence of a tight frenulum. In the process of the examination, the infant's state of alertness and readiness for feeding are also observed.

■ Positions for Breastfeeding

Getting off to a good start begins with positioning the baby at the breast in a way that is comfortable for both the mother and baby and that allows for good latch-on. The three most common positions are the cradle, side-lying, and football hold.

PRINCIPLES OF CORRECT POSITIONING

Several principles are common to all of the various positions for breastfeeding, including the following:
- Both the mother and the baby should be comfortable.

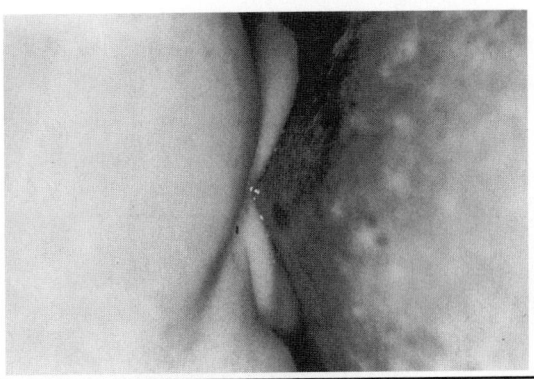

FIGURE 11-4 Lip position.

- The infant should be positioned "face on" at nipple height so that no head turning or tilting is required. The nipple should be directed toward the center of the infant's mouth.
- The infant should be lying on the side, not the back.
- The infant's body should be in good alignment, with a straight line from the ear to the shoulder to the hips.
- The infant's top and bottom lips should be flanged out (Fig. 11-4).
- The infant's tongue should extend forward over the lower gumline and cup around the nipple and areola.
- Good latch-on results in quiet feedings. No "clicking" or "popping" sounds should be heard from the infant. After mother's milk is in, audible swallowing, such as a "glug" or air blowing out the baby's nose, should be heard.

CRADLE POSITION

The cradle position (also called the Madonna or cuddle position) and its variation, the cross-cradle position, begin with the mother sitting upright or leaning slightly forward with her feet on the floor or stool or her legs crossed in front of her. The infant is held with the mouth at nipple height, and the mother and infant are in a tummy-to-tummy arrangement. The mother uses her free hand to support the breast, if needed, while keeping her fingers well back from the areola so that she does not interfere with latch-on. The "cigarette hold," or pinching of the breast tissue, should not be used. In the regular cradle position, the baby's head is supported in the crook of the elbow on the same side as the breast being suckled (Fig. 11-5). In the cross-cradle position, the opposite hand supports the baby's head and shoulders. This position often works well for a premature infant because it provides extra support to the head and trunk.

After positioning the baby, the mother should touch the baby's lower lip with her nipple to stimulate mouth opening. As the mouth opens, the mother should bring the baby close so that the lips come up and over the nipple and back onto the areolar tissue and the nipple rests on top of the baby's tongue. Once the baby appears latched on, the mother can check the lips for a flanged, open placement. At this point the baby is very close to the breast, with the tip of the infant's nose touching it. Mothers often need to be shown that the baby is able to breathe without a need to press down on the breast tissue. If the baby appears to be pushed into the breast, the infant's buttocks should be brought closer into the tummy-to-tummy position. As the mother looks down at her baby, she should see a straight line from the baby's ear to the shoulders to the hips. Once the baby is suckling well, the mother can usually remove the hand that was supporting her breast and

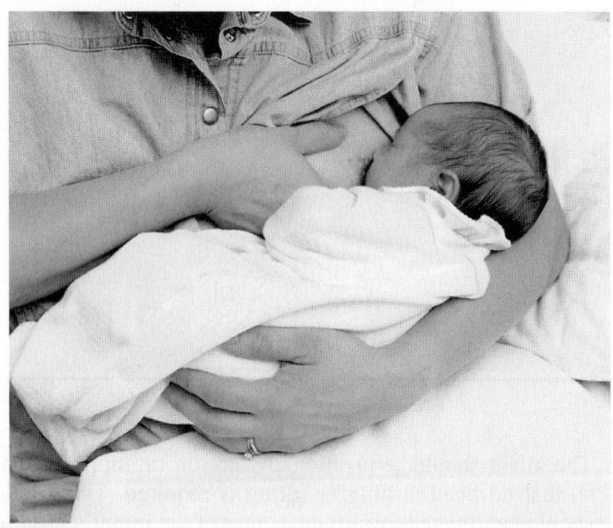

FIGURE 11-5 Cradle hold. The mother positions the infant's head at or near the antecubital space and level with her nipple with her arm supporting the infant's body. Her other hand is free to hold the breast. Once the infant is positioned, pillows or blankets can be used to support the mother's arm, which may tire from holding the baby. (From McKinney ES, James SR, Murray SS, et al: *Maternal-child nursing*, ed 3, Philadelphia, 2009, Saunders.)

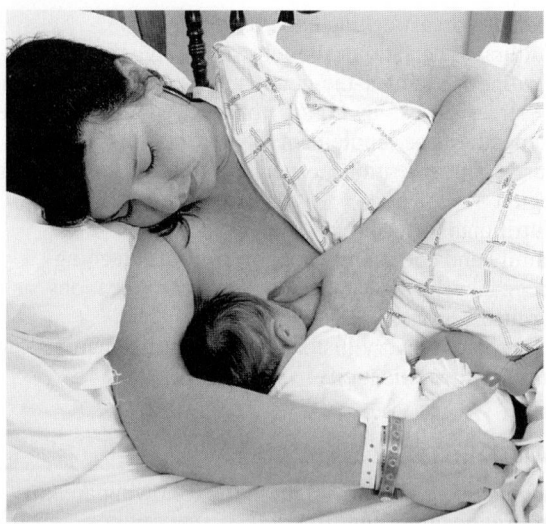

FIGURE 11-6 The side-lying position prevents pressure on episiotomy or abdominal incisions and allows the mother to rest while feeding. She lies on her side, with her lower arm supporting her head or placed around the infant. A pillow behind her back and between her legs provides comfort. Her upper hand and arm are used to position the infant on the side at nipple level and hold the breast. When the infant's mouth opens to nurse, the mother leans slightly forward or draws the infant to her to insert the nipple into the mouth. (From McKinney ES, James SR, Murray SS, et al: *Maternal-child nursing*, ed 3, Philadelphia, 2009, Saunders.)

use it to cradle the baby in her arms. She can also relax back from the forward-leaning position that she used at the beginning.

SIDE-LYING POSITION

The side-lying or other lying-down variations are often helpful when the mother is uncomfortable sitting up or wishes to nap or sleep with her baby. In the early days of learning to achieve latch-on, the side-lying position is not easy to use because the mother cannot see her breast and nipple quite as well. In the hospital, a nurse should be available to help the mother and infant. At home and with practice, the mother and infant can achieve latch-on without assistance.

In the side-lying position, the mother lies on her side, cradles her infant in her elbow, and supports the infant's back and neck. The mother or the nurse should arrange one or two pillows under the mother's head and shoulders and a rolled towel or blanket along the infant's back to keep the infant in a side-lying position. As in the cradle position, the mother may support her breast with her upper hand (Fig. 11-6).

FOOTBALL HOLD

In the football hold the infant is supported off to the side of the mother. This position is often used by a mother who has had a cesarean delivery because it does not require that the infant be positioned along her abdomen or by a mother of multiples when she would like to feed two babies at once. Mothers with flat or inverted nipples are often able to achieve latch-on more easily with this position.

One or two firm pillows should be placed at the mother's side to help support the infant. The baby is in a side-lying position and flexed at the hips, with the buttocks back against the chair or couch. As in other positions, the mother may support her breast to assist with latch-on and remove her hand once the baby is suckling well (Fig. 11-7).

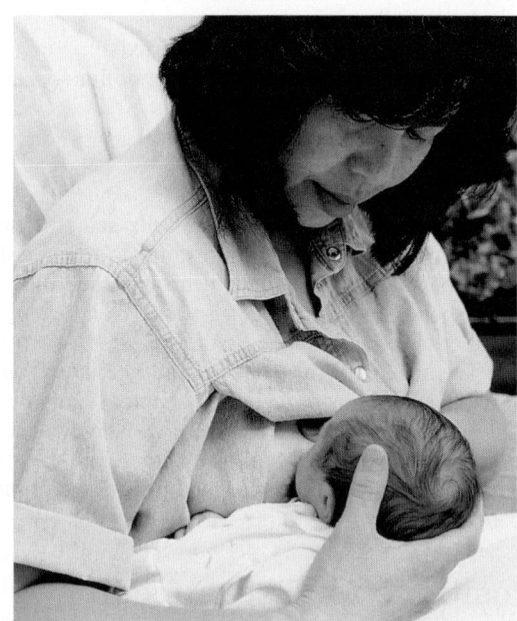

FIGURE 11-7 Football hold. The mother supports the infant's head in her hand, with the infant's body resting on pillows alongside her hip. This method allows the mother to see the position of the infant's mouth on the breast, helps her control the infant's head, and is especially helpful for mothers with heavy breasts. This hold also prevents pressure against an abdominal incision. (From McKinney ES, James SR, Murray SS, et al: *Maternal-child nursing*, ed 3, Philadelphia, 2009, Saunders.)

Dynamics of Breastfeeding

EARLY FEEDINGS

The first breastfeeding should take place as soon after birth as possible. Full-term neonates often have an alert period for 30 to 60 minutes after delivery that is ideal for the first feeding practice. This first feeding can take place in the delivery area, if necessary, and should be encouraged by all in attendance. It will not delay, to any significant extent, any procedures required, such as weighing and measuring the infant, instilling ointment or drops in the infant's eyes, and giving vitamin K injections. These procedures can be done one at a time in the delivery room or at the bedside after return to the room. The mother and infant should remain together as much as possible, with rooming-in preferable. The family's desire to promote close contact and initiate breastfeeding should be made clear to and supported by staff. In addition, the health care provider should advocate changes in institutional policy to support the needs of breastfeeding families.

The infant usually goes into a deep sleep after the initial alertness and is difficult to wake for feeding practice. Parents should be instructed to watch for any awakening behavior, such as opening eyes or movement in the bed. Many newborns will not cry at this point, so parents need to be alert for these signs of feeding readiness. Full-term infants are born with stores of fluid and energy to carry them through this early transition to the nonuterine environment, a time of infrequent feeding and low volume of colostrum. The infant's stomach, liver, and kidneys are gearing up for the larger volumes of higher-fat food that will come in a few days. It is not necessary to provide any supplement, including water, to a healthy full-term neonate. In addition, feeding with a rubber or silicone nipple may lead to nipple confusion because it does not work like the breast in delivering milk.

During this transition time assistance and support from an individual knowledgeable in breastfeeding can be helpful to the mother and infant as they practice latch-on and suckling. The infant should be encouraged to go to each breast for at least 10 to 15 minutes of active suckling, although some infants may spend even longer, up to 20 or 30 minutes. The infant's behavior is much more important during this time than the clock. However, an infant who falls asleep in 5 minutes should be stimulated to continue active suckling. Attention to proper positioning and technique becomes important as the frequency and duration of the suckling behavior increase. A mother is unlikely to get sore or cracked nipples when her infant is latched on correctly. These early feedings are excellent "practice" sessions both for the mother, who gains confidence in her breastfeeding ability, and for the infant, who gets first colostrum and then milk for the efforts at suckling.

The goal of discharge planning is to maintain successful breastfeeding and includes the following:

- Review proper positioning.
- Review signs of good latch-on.
- Review signs of infant progress indicating adequate nutrition (Table 11-2).
- Arrange daily follow-up for 2 to 3 days after discharge.
- Provide a phone contact for questions and concerns.
- Encourage the mother to contact breastfeeding resources whenever she has questions.

These early efforts to provide contact and support during the transition to home can make all the difference in maintaining breastfeeding. Problems encountered during engorgement, sleep deprivation, and times of uncertainty or lack of confidence can be addressed quickly and directly rather than after a bottle has been introduced or the mother's nipples are cracked and bleeding.

FREQUENCY AND DURATION OF FEEDINGS

After the first 24 hours the infant should go to the breast 8 to 12 times (or every 2 to 3 hours) in 24 hours for approximately 20 to 45 minutes at each feeding. Frequent suckling stimulates milk production and establishes a regular routine. Exclusive breastfeeding for the first month should be encouraged to ensure the establishment of adequate milk supply and prevent any nipple confusion. Parents need to be alert for an infant who sleeps for more than 4 hours at a time or who goes to sleep at the breast in 5 minutes. These infants must be actively wakened and stimulated for feeding.

If the mother and infant must be separated for one or more feedings or supplements are medically necessary, they may be given with a dropper, a cup, or a 5-French feeding tube placed at the breast. Proper instructions, close supervision, and follow-up are needed for each of these methods, and they should not be used routinely.

URINE AND STOOL OUTPUT GUIDELINES

Urine

In the first 2 days of life as the volume of breast milk increases, the infant may urinate only 1 to 3 times in 24 hours. By day 3, the infant should have 4 or more wet diapers in 24 hours and then, by day 4, 4 to 6 wet diapers per 24 hours. Over time, the infant should have a minimum of 6 to 8 wet diapers in a 24-hour period. The urine should be light yellow with no strong odor. If the parents are anxious or if they have a question about breastfeeding progress, a diary of wet diapers can be kept to aid in the accurate assessment of progress. Parents need to be alerted, however, to the difficulty of doing accurate diaper counts with disposable diapers and may elect to insert a tissue liner into the diaper or to use cloth diapers for the first few weeks. Ultraabsorbent diapers should be avoided when close monitoring of output is necessary.

Stool

In the first 24 hours after delivery the baby should have at least one meconium stool followed by another on the second day of life. By day 3, stools are beginning to make the transition to the characteristic loose, yellow, seedy stools of breastfeeding, and the infant should begin having 2 or 3 stools in 24 hours. That number may continue to increase in the first few weeks of life. Some infants stool with every feeding. After the first month the pattern may change again because some infants begin to stool less frequently and may go several days to a week between stools. Infrequent stooling, especially in the first month, should stimulate a feeding history and possibly a weight check to make sure that the infant is getting enough breast milk. As long as the infant is healthy and gaining weight, there is no problem.

TABLE 11-2	Signs of Infant Progress: A Handout for Parents						
	First 8 Hours	**8 to 24 Hours**	**Day 2**	**Day 3**	**Day 4**	**Day 5**	**Day 6 On**
Milk supply	You may be able to express a few drops of milk.		Milk should come in between the second and fourth day.			Milk should be in. Breasts may be firm or leak milk.	Breasts should feel softer after nursing.
Baby's activity	Baby is usually wide awake in first hour of life. Put to breast within a half hour of birth.	Wake your baby. Babies may not wake on their own to feed.	Baby should be more cooperative and less sleepy.	Look for early feeding cues: rooting, lip smacking, hands to face. Note that baby swallows regularly while nursing.			Baby should appear satisfied after feeding.
Feeding routine	Baby may go into a deep sleep 2 to 4 hours after birth.	Feed your baby every 1.5 to 3 hours or as often as wanted.	Feedings should be at least 8 to 10 times each day.			May go up to 5 hours between feedings (once in a 24-hour period).	
Breastfeeding	Baby will wake up and be alert and responsive for several more hours after the initial deep sleep.	Nurse at both breasts as long as baby is actively suckling and mother is comfortable.	Try to nurse on both sides at each feeding, aiming for 10 to 15 minutes each side. Expect some nipple tenderness.	Consider hand expressing or pumping a few drops of milk to soften the nipple if the breast is too firm for the baby to latch on.	Nurse at least 10 to 15 minutes each side every 2 to 3 hours for the first few months of life.	Mother's nipple tenderness is decreased or gone.	
Baby's urine output		Baby must have at least 1 wet diaper in first 24 hours.	Baby should have at least 1 wet diaper every 8 hours.	Wet diapers should increase to 4 to 6 in 24 hours.	Baby's urine should be light yellow.	Baby should have 6 to 8 wet diapers per day of colorless or light yellow urine.	
Baby's stools		Baby should have a black-green stool (meconium stool).	Baby may have a second very dark (meconium) stool.	Baby's stools should be changing from black-green to yellow.		Baby should have 3 or 4 yellow seedy stools per day.	The number of stools may slowly decrease after 4 to 6 weeks.

Data from Thilo EH, Townsend SF: Early newborn discharge: have we gone too far? *Contemp Pediatr* 13:29-46, 1996.

PUMPING

Routine pumping is unnecessary for mothers who are available for a feeding every 2 to 4 hours. However, if the mother and infant must be separated for more than 1 or 2 feedings, pumping should be part of the plan to assist with milk production. If the mother and infant are separated right after birth, pumping should begin as soon as possible, within the first 24 hours. The mother should pump 6 to 8 times in 24 hours for 15 minutes if she is using a double-pump setup or 10 minutes per breast if she is using a single-pump setup. She should be encouraged to save even the smallest amounts of colostrum to give to her infant.

Hand expression and manual pumps work well for infrequent or short-duration pumping. However, a hospital-grade piston-style pump that permits pumping both breasts at the same time is ideal for a mother who will have to pump for several weeks or months. No pump works as well as an infant in stimulating production, but frequent pumping goes a long way toward establishing a milk supply and provides the mother with a concrete, healthful contribution to her sick or preterm infant. As the volume of milk goes up over the first few days, the mother can see the success of her efforts. She should be counseled about the increase in production in contrast to the small volume of colostrum produced in the first few days.

COLLECTION AND STORAGE OF BREAST MILK

A mother who is pumping should be reminded to wash her hands well before she begins pumping and to use clean containers for collection and storage. In addition, the pump parts should be thoroughly cleaned after each use. Many of the pump parts can go through a dishwasher, but the directions that come with the pump should be consulted for specific instructions on cleaning.

Milk collected from pumping should be stored in clean plastic bottles or disposable milk bags. It is preferable to store breast milk in small amounts so that only the amount that is needed is defrosted and used. Milk that has been defrosted and not used within 24 hours should be discarded. Pumped breast milk should be refrigerated as soon after pumping as possible and can be stored there for up to 8 days. It can be stored on "blue ice" in a cooler for about 24 hours. If it is not going to be used in that time, it should be frozen. In a refrigerator freezer that maintains a steady temperature, breast milk can be stored for 3 months. Breast milk can be stored for up to 12 months in a freezer where 0° F is routinely maintained (Human Milk Banking Association of North America, 2006). The bottles or bags should be labeled with the date of collection so that the oldest milk can be used first. If the milk must be transported to the hospital or daycare facility, it should be placed in ice or on a blue ice unit to minimize the amount of warming or thawing.

INFANT WEIGHT GAIN

Normal newborn infants lose 5% to 8% of their birthweight in the first few days of life. It is helpful for parents to be aware of both the birth and discharge weights. Once the maternal milk volume increases, the infant begins to gain weight in the range of 0.5 to 1 ounce per day or 4 to 7 ounces per week. Most breastfed infants have regained their birth weight by 2 weeks. One criterion for failure to thrive is lack of return to birth weight by 3 weeks. Breastfed infants usually double their birth weight by 5 to 6 months old and triple it by 1 year old.

There are no growth grids specifically designed for breastfed infants, although WHO standards are based on the growth of an international population of healthy infants, 100% of whom were "breastfed for 12 months and predominantly breastfed until at least 4 months old" (i.e., additional foods were introduced in later infancy) (Grummer-Strawn et al, 2010). The CDC recommends that providers in the U.S. use the WHO growth standards for children up to age 24 months, rather than CDC growth charts (see Appendix B). If CDC growth charts are used, breastfed infants show an apparent decline in growth from 6 to 9 months when compared with formula-fed infants. However, use of the WHO growth standards with the same infants shows breastfed infants to be on target for growth, whereas formula-fed infants have apparent excessive weight gain (van Dijk and Innis, 2009) that may "signal early signs of overweight" (Grummer-Strawn et al, 2010). It is essential to assess developmental progress and other measures of growth (in addition to height, weight, and head circumference) in all infants. Characteristics of a healthy breastfed infant include the following:
- Active and alert state
- Developmentally appropriate progress
- Age-appropriate height and head circumference
- Good skin turgor and color
- Sufficient output of at least 6 wet diapers per day
- Contented and satisfied behavior after feeding

GROWTH SPURTS

Just when parents begin to think that breastfeeding is going well, the first growth spurt occurs and they may become concerned. The term *growth spurt* is used to describe those times during breastfeeding when the baby's growth demands exceed the breast milk supply at that moment. For 2 to 4 days the infant seems to be "hungry all the time" and demands to be fed more frequently. The best response is to increase the number of feedings because increased stimulation of the breast will increase milk production to the amount needed. Once the level of milk production has risen, the infant returns to the normal feeding pattern. However, an inexperienced parent may begin supplementation that can actually lead to a decrease in breast milk production. Growth spurts tend to occur every 3 to 4 weeks, but parents seem to notice them less as time goes on. The behavior becomes an expected part of the breastfeeding experience.

WEANING

The decision about the time for weaning is an individual one. Breastfeeding should be encouraged for at least 1 year, but individual circumstances may dictate a different choice for a family. Sometimes weaning is led by the mother and other times by the infant. A natural weaning process typically occurs as other foods become a part of the infant's diet and the infant begins to participate in self-feeding. When a family inquires about the ideal time to begin weaning, the provider can counsel them to consider factors, such as the following:
- Beliefs and desires of individual family members
- Developmental readiness of the infant
- Nutritional replacements for breast milk
- Social and environmental issues affecting the decision

Whether weaning occurs as a planned or unplanned activity, it is best to implement it gradually. If necessary the mother can use a breast pump to gradually decrease milk production and prevent breast engorgement, blocked ducts, and discomfort. A good approach is to pump when uncomfortable and to pump only to comfort, not to empty. In situations when weaning was not an anticipated or planned event, the health care provider may help the mother deal not only with the act of weaning but also with her feelings about it. Some mothers grieve the early loss of the breastfeeding experience.

In an effort to prevent premature weaning, the providers should maintain close communication with families, especially those who are more likely to wean early. Early identification and support of these families may assist them to continue breastfeeding for a longer period. Factors associated with early weaning include the following (Wijndaele et al, 2009):

- Younger mothers
- Low socioeconomic status
- Low maternal education
- Maternal smoking
- Formula feeding or short duration of breastfeeding sessions
- Lack of information or support from health professionals

Early return to work, lack of support from family, advice from older female family members to wean, and being from a non-Hispanic black cultural group also influence mothers' decisions to introduce solids or wean earlier than recommended.

MATERNAL NUTRITIONAL NEEDS DURING BREASTFEEDING

Maternal nutritional needs increase during lactation. Characteristics of a good diet include the following:

- A minimum of 1800 calories
- An additional 500 calories more than the nonpregnant diet
- Generous intake of fruits and vegetables, whole grain breads and cereals, calcium-rich dairy products, and protein-rich meats, fish, and legumes
- Rich sources of calcium, zinc, folate, magnesium, and vitamin B_6
- Culturally appropriate foods
- Supplementation with calcium or prenatal vitamins or both only if the diet is poor (Lawrence and Lawrence, 2005)

The mother should be encouraged to eat well for her own sake to stay healthy and to meet the energy demands of nursing. In addition, an adequate intake of fluid is necessary, but excessive use of fluids does not increase breast milk production. A good guideline for adequate fluid intake is maternal urine that is light yellow and has no strong odor. Eligible mothers and infants should be referred to the Women, Infants, and Children (WIC) special supplemental food program for nutritional counseling and for food supplements. Most WIC programs offer food supplements for the breastfeeding mother's diet because she does not need formula for the infant. Even with a diet that is adequate in nutrients and calories, a gradual maternal weight loss of 1 to 2 pounds per month usually occurs. In fact, breastfeeding is the ideal way for a mother to return to her prepregnancy weight.

No foods need to be routinely excluded from the maternal diet unless there is evidence that a particular food bothers the infant or the infant appears to be allergic to it. Sometimes the food does not need to be eliminated but merely decreased. For infants with colic, it can be helpful to reduce allergenic foods (e.g., cow's milk, eggs, peanuts, tree nuts, soy, fish, wheat) in the mother's diet (Hill et al, 2005). When a mother has markedly decreased or eliminated cow's milk from her diet, she must add another source of calcium. Certain foods, such as onions and garlic, may change the flavor and odor of the milk, but do not negatively affect its quality. The nutrient characteristics of breast milk are fairly stable. One way to look at the variety of foods in mothers' diets world-wide is to acknowledge that infants are getting early exposure to the foods of their culture.

Increased alcohol intake does not improve lactation performance and intake of an amount more than 0.5 g/kg of maternal body weight (2 cans of beer, 8 ounces wine, or 2 to 2.5 ounces liquor) can impair the milk ejection reflex (Institute of Medicine, 1991). The occasional use of small amounts of alcohol need not be avoided, but regular use should be discouraged.

Large amounts of caffeine from coffee, sodas, or chocolate should be discouraged because caffeine is transmitted via breast milk to the infant and can be associated with jitteriness in the infant and may have a negative effect on the iron content of the breast milk. However, the equivalent of 1 to 2 cups of coffee per day should pose no problem (Institute of Medicine, 1991).

RETURNING TO WORK

Women who return to work outside the home after initiating breastfeeding should be encouraged to continue breastfeeding and be supported in their decision with accurate information about how to manage both work and breastfeeding. The mother can be assisted to investigate her work environment by use of tools, such as a breastfeeding assessment worksheet that reviews type of work performed and where, space for pumping and storing, and individuals and policies that support her intention (Bar-Yam, 1998). The ideal work environment provides the following:

- Breaks or lunchtime (or both) in which the mother can pump or go to the infant
- A private, convenient location for pumping with access to a sink for washing up and a refrigerator for storage
- Supportive colleagues and supervisors

In addition to providing information regarding pumping, storing, and transporting breast milk; introducing the bottle; and handling the challenges of multiple demands (Box 11-2), providers can support community initiatives that promote these conditions in employment settings. Women are more likely to continue breastfeeding if they have workplace support (Mills, 2009), and employers also benefit from breastfeeding mothers whose infants tend to be healthier (Ball and Bennett, 2001).

The National Conference of State Legislatures (NCSL) maintains a database on laws related to breastfeeding including breastfeeding in public and breastfeeding in the workplace. Twenty-four states, the District of Columbia, and Puerto Rico currently have laws specifically related to work and breastfeeding. Individual practitioners can access this website for an update on the laws in their location (NCSL, 2010).

BOX 11-2 Advice for Mothers on Returning to Work

Before Delivery
- Discuss plans with employer before maternity leave.
- Provide employer with information to help in planning (see www. usbreastfeeding.org).
- Discuss options with other employees who have continued to breastfeed after returning to work.
- Gain support of coworkers.
- Investigate pumps, including rental or purchase.
- Identify place to pump and to store breast milk at work.

During Maternity Leave
- Practice method of breast milk expression that will be used at work.
- Begin freezing milk.
- Introduce the bottle after breastfeeding is well established (usually around 3 to 4 weeks).

After Return to Work
- If available use on-site or nearby childcare, so you can go to the infant during the day.
- Ask employer if caregiver for child may bring infant on-site once a day to nurse.
- If possible arrange work hours to maximize times to nurse infant (e.g., arrive at work at 8:30 instead of 8:00).
- Have a picture of your baby at the pump.
- Plan on 15 to 30 minutes to complete pumping.
- Wear clothes for easy access to breasts and to hide leaks.

Feeding Breast Milk
- Warm or thaw milk in warm water.
- Do not use microwave because milk heats unevenly and presents a risk for burns.
- Refrigerate thawed milk for no more than 24 hours; do not refreeze.
- Do not add milk to a bottle that has already been used.

Important Reminders
- Wash hands before and after pumping.
- Rinse pump parts with cool water, then wash with dish detergent and rinse well after each use.

From Tully MR: Working & breastfeeding: helping moms and employers figure it out, *AWHONN Lifelines* 9(3):198-203, 2005.

Medications for Breastfeeding Mothers

Frequently, women question whether they can take certain medications while they are breastfeeding. Concerns relate primarily to two areas—the effect of the drug on maternal milk supply and the effect of the drug on the infant. General guidelines for maternal drug recommendations include the following:

- Give drugs that are normally safe for infants or have been tested in infants.
- Avoid long-acting forms of a drug.
- Schedule feeding at times when the drug level is lowest. Often breastfeeding immediately after taking the drug is the safest time.
- Observe the infant for changes in feeding pattern, fussiness, vomiting or diarrhea, or rash.
- Consider all appropriate options and select the drug with the lowest level in breast milk.

BOX 11-3 Drug References

American Academy of Pediatrics (AAP) Committee on Drugs: The transfer of drugs and other chemicals into human milk, *Pediatrics* 108:776-789, 2001.
Hale TW: *Medications and mothers' milk*, ed 14, Amarillo, TX, 2010, Hale Publishing L.P. Updated and reprinted every other year. Order from 800-378-1317 or www.ibreastfeeding.com.
LactMed: www.toxnet.nlm.nih.gov
Wynne AL, Woo T, Olyaei AJ: *Pharmacotherapeutics for nurse practitioner prescribers*, ed 2, Philadelphia, 2007, FA Davis.

- Avoid drugs that inhibit prolactin release, such as estrogen, antihistamines, and ergot compounds.
- Be cautious about the use of herbal preparations.

A good drug reference should be readily available for providers. Four excellent drug references are shown in Box 11-3. Not all references available to providers offer adequate up-to-date information. Two retail pharmacy databases and the *Physicians' Desk Reference* (PDR), for example, have been found to carry recommendations that inappropriately could interfere with breastfeeding (Akus and Bartick, 2007). Decisions about drug selection are difficult, especially when contraindicated drugs are being considered, but the consequences of weaning and loss of breast milk for the infant must be included in the deliberations.

Common Breastfeeding Problems

FLAT OR INVERTED NIPPLES

Description
A nipple can look as though it is inverted, but a "pinch test" is necessary to determine what happens to the nipple during breastfeeding (see the previous description and Fig. 11-3 for the technique). If the nipple pulls in, it is inverted. If the nipple does not pull in, as happens most often, or everts with compression, it is considered to be flat.

Inverted nipples can make it more difficult for the infant to latch on in the early days because it is harder to pull the nipple into the mouth for suckling. As the baby continues to breastfeed, the nipple tissue elongates; with time the problem usually becomes less severe, and successful breastfeeding is possible. Flat nipples do not generally change over time, but the infant develops a style to more easily latch on successfully.

Epidemiology
Adhesions cause retraction or inversion of the nipples. Flat nipples are often found in women with larger breasts.

Differential Diagnosis
The differential diagnoses for flat or inverted nipples is dimpled, fissured, or unusually shaped nipples.

Management
Prenatal. If the patient is not at risk for preterm labor, breast shells can be used during the third trimester for inverted nipples. The obstetrician or nurse-midwife should be notified before their use. Shells are plastic dome-shaped devices with small

holes for ventilation. An opening in the portion that lies against the skin fits over the nipple, and gentle suction during use helps stretch the nipple tissue. The bra cup holds the shell comfortably in place, and the use of shells during the last trimester generally helps stretch out adhesions in preparation for breastfeeding.

Postpartum. The provider should stay with the mother during early feeding attempts; give extra praise, reassurance, and support; and emphasize the need for extra patience and persistence. Encourage use of the football-hold position during feedings and have the mother lean slightly forward as she latches the baby on.

The mother may find any of the following helpful:
- Wear breast shells between feedings.
- Manually pull or roll the nipple immediately before latch-on.
- Use a breast pump for 1 or 2 minutes before latch-on.
- Put a cold cloth or ice on the nipple for a few seconds before latch-on.
- Avoid pacifiers and bottle nipples until the infant is 4 to 6 weeks old.
- If supplementation is medically indicated, use a syringe, dropper, feeding tube, or supplemental nutrition system.

Complications
Complications of flat or inverted nipples include the following:
- Frustration
- Loss of self-confidence
- Inadequate infant nutrition and its sequelae
- Severe maternal engorgement, plugged ducts, or mastitis
- Discontinued breastfeeding

SORE NIPPLES
Description
Soreness of the nipples is pain caused by irritation or trauma to the nipples and areola, often accompanied by a breakdown in skin integrity.

Epidemiology
Sore nipples have many causes, including the following:
- Improper latch-on and positioning at the breast
- Prolonged negative pressure
- Inappropriate suction release from the breast
- Use of or sensitivity to nipple creams and oils
- Incorrect use of breastfeeding supplies (e.g., pumps, shells, shields)
- Thrush (candidiasis)
- Leaking nipples that are not properly air-dried

Clinical Findings
The nipples, areolae, and breasts are tender, bruised, raw, cracked, bleeding, blistered, discolored, swollen, or traumatized.

Differential Diagnosis
The differential diagnoses for sore nipples include the following:
- Mild tenderness, which is sometimes described by new mothers as they are getting used to the infant's suckling

- Breast or nipple trauma from another cause
- Thrush (candidiasis)
- Mastitis
- Abscess
- Milk plugs at the nipple pores

Management
The following measures can be taken to manage sore nipples:
- Assess breastfeeding at an early feeding. Prevent the problem by demonstrating and reinforcing the proper latch-on technique and positioning of the infant.
- Counsel mothers to seek help early for more than mild tenderness. Nipples can be damaged by constant high negative pressure and do not "toughen up" as breastfeeding progresses. Cracking and bleeding are not normal.
- Rub a few drops of colostrum or hindmilk onto the nipple and areola after every feeding and let it air-dry.
- Expose the nipples to air for short periods several times a day.
- Use breast shells to prevent the bra or clothing from rubbing against the nipple.
- Nurse from the least sore side first.
- Use short, frequent feedings.
- Pump the affected breast if pain is too severe to allow nursing.
- Use mild analgesics, as necessary.
- Refer to a lactation specialist as appropriate.

SEVERE ENGORGEMENT
Description
Severe engorgement is characterized by extremely full, sore, and swollen breasts, beyond the normal fullness experienced as the milk comes in.

Epidemiology
Engorgement is caused by milk stasis in the breast from inadequate emptying.

Clinical Findings
The following are seen in severe engorgement:
- Painful, hard, lumpy, swollen breasts
- Breasts usually warm to the touch
- Nipples flattened by the swelling
- Bruising or trauma to the nipples and areolae

Differential Diagnosis
The differential diagnosis for severe engorgement is bilateral mastitis.

Management
The following measures can be taken to manage engorgement:
- Take a hot shower or wrap the breasts with warm, wet compresses for 5 to 10 minutes before nursing. Disposable diapers can be wet with hot water and then wrapped around each breast and "tabbed" to hold them in place. The plastic liner holds the heat in longer than an ordinary washcloth or towel does.

- Gently massage the entire breast or use an electric pump with intermittent suction on the minimal setting for several minutes after using wet heat.
- Manually express milk before feeding to soften the areola and make it easier for the infant to latch on properly.
- Nurse frequently and make certain that latch-on and position are correct, and audible swallowing is heard.
- Avoid long stretches between feedings in the early weeks as the milk supply is being established. Pump the breasts if a feeding will be missed.

MASTITIS
Description
Although rarely seen in the postpartum hospital setting, mastitis is an infection of the breast that can occur at any time during lactation. Occasionally it has been identified during the third trimester of pregnancy.

Epidemiology
Staphylococcus aureus, streptococci, and *Corynebacteria* are most commonly associated with mastitis (Arroyo et al, 2010). Predisposing factors include:
- Stress, fatigue
- Cracked nipples, plugged ducts
- Constricting, improperly fitting bra
- Inadequate emptying of the breast
- Sudden weaning or a significant decrease in the number of feedings
- Using a manual pump

Clinical Findings
The following are seen in mastitis:
- Malaise
- Breast tenderness or pain
- A reddened, warm lump in any quadrant, sometimes associated with red streaking
- Flulike symptoms, including fever, chills, and body aches
  An old adage is that the "flu" in a breastfeeding woman is mastitis until proved otherwise.

Management
Recommendations for treatment of mastitis include the following:
- Empty the breast. Nurse frequently, or if pain is severe, pump milk carefully from the affected breast. Breast milk is not infected and is fine for the infant.
- Use analgesics as necessary.
- Although more studies are recommended to determine the appropriate role of antibiotics to treat mastitis (Jahanfar et al, 2009), antibiotic therapy has been a mainstay of treatment for mastitis. Administer oral antibiotics such as penicillinase-resistant penicillin or a cephalosporin that covers *S. aureus.* Treatment should be maintained for 10 to 14 days. Dicloxacillin is often used, and amoxicillin-clavulanic acid and cefuroxime have been found to be effective with few adverse effects (Benyamini et al, 2005).
- Administration of oral *Lactobacillus fermentum* CECT5716 or *L. salivarius* CECT5713, probiotics isolated

from human milk, has been found to be as effective as antibiotic therapy (Arroyo et al, 2010).
- Rest (extremely important).
- Do not wean abruptly because of the possibility of mastitis progressing into an abscess.
- Take warm showers or use warm wet compresses.
- Increase fluids.

Complications
Abscess and septicemia are complications of mastitis.

NIPPLE CONFUSION
Description
Nipple confusion can occur when an infant is accustomed to nursing from a bottle and is introduced to the breast. When offered the breast, these babies use the same sucking pattern as with a bottle, which makes it difficult to obtain adequate nourishment and may contribute to maternal sore nipples. Infants may cry, fuss, or push away with their arms during attempts to nurse.

Epidemiology
Different oral-motor skills are used in breastfeeding and bottle feeding, and infants who have been given a bottle or pacifier sometimes attempt to breastfeed as though they were bottle feeding. Thus unless absolutely necessary, early bottle feeding and pacifier use should be avoided in the breastfeeding infant.

Clinical Findings
The following are seen in nipple confusion:
- Ineffective suckling at the breast
- Breast refusal
- Sore, red, or bruised maternal nipples

Differential Diagnosis
The differential diagnoses for nipple confusion are other causes of fussiness and refusal to feed.

Management
The following are recommended to manage nipple confusion:
- Avoid all baby bottle nipples and pacifiers for the first 4 to 6 weeks or until the infant is breastfeeding successfully.
- Retrain the infant to suck correctly at the breast by correct positioning at the breast, proper latch-on technique, suck training to repattern tongue movements, and supplementation via alternative methods if required.
- Consult with a lactation specialist as indicated.
- If supplements are medically indicated, give with an eyedropper, spoon, syringe, or cup or through a 5-French feeding tube (attached to a 20- or 30-mL syringe) taped to the areola or breast. The end of the tubing protrudes slightly past the end of the nipple so that the tube, nipple, and areola are in the infant's mouth.
- Use of a thin silicone nipple shield may help the infant successfully latch on and suckle, especially with the preterm infant (Eglash et al, 2010) and using nipple shields can encourage continued breastfeeding (Chertok, 2009).

Cleansing and drying both the shields and breast after feeding are important to prevent skin breakdown and infection.

Complications

The following are complications of nipple confusion:
- Failure to thrive
- Hyperbilirubinemia
- Colic and crying
- Prolonged feedings
- Sore and cracked nipples
- Plugged ducts
- Mastitis
- Frustration

BREAST MILK JAUNDICE

Description

Breast milk (late onset) jaundice is an elevated serum indirect bilirubin concentration with the peak level occurring on or after the seventh to tenth days of life in an infant drinking an adequate amount of breast milk with no other signs of liver abnormality.

Epidemiology

The exact cause of breast milk jaundice is unknown; however, an enzyme may be present in some mothers' milk that inhibits the action of glucuronyl transferase and increases intestinal absorption of bilirubin. Breast milk jaundice is more common in Asian and Native American infants. Siblings with the same mother are often affected. True breast milk jaundice is uncommon and estimated to occur in less than 1 in 200 births (Lawrence and Lawrence, 2005; Preer and Philipp, 2010).

Clinical Findings

Physical Examination. The following are seen with breast milk jaundice:
- Healthy and thriving infant
- Adequate stooling and voiding
- Appropriate weight gain
- Appearance of elevated bilirubin levels between the seventh and tenth days of life
- Bilirubin peaks around day 10 to 15
- Persistence into the third month of life
  Diagnostic Studies. The following tests are usually indicated:
- Serum bilirubin
- Urine and other cultures, which are sometimes necessary to rule out infection

Differential Diagnosis

The differential diagnosis for breast milk jaundice is pathological jaundice.

Management

Continue breastfeeding unless clinical signs of pathological jaundice are observed. See Chapter 38 for a discussion of pathological jaundice. The family should be reassured that breast milk jaundice is not harmful.

THRUSH

When oral candidiasis is diagnosed in the infant or found on the nipple or areolae of the nursing mother, both members of the dyad should be treated. See Chapter 36 for a discussion of candidiasis.

POOR WEIGHT GAIN

Description

Problems associated with poor weight gain occur at two different times and represent different challenges for management. During the newborn period, initiation of breastfeeding may not proceed normally, and the infant may actually continue to lose weight or, at best, gain very slowly. After the newborn period, infants may gain weight more slowly than expected given normal parameters for their age.

Epidemiology

Poor weight gain has a number of contributing factors, including the following:
- Infrequent or inadequate feeding because of poorly managed breastfeeding or environmental or social circumstances in the family system
- Inadequate milk production
- Genetic predisposition
- Infection
- Organic disease
- Physical anomaly that prevents good suckling or swallowing

Clinical Findings

The following may be seen in poor weight gain:
  Infant Factors
- Continued weight loss after 5 to 7 days old
- Failure to regain birthweight by 2 to 3 weeks old
- Failure to maintain an ongoing weight gain of 0.5 to 1 ounce per day
- Weight below the third percentile for age (this finding can be a pattern over time or a sudden change)
- Lethargic, sleepy, inactive, unresponsive infant
- Newborn or young infant sleeping longer than 4 hours between feedings, although one 5-hour stretch at night can be normal
- Dry mucous membranes
- Poor skin turgor
  Technique Factors
- Ineffective latch-on or sucking
- Short time at the breast (the infant is removed before nursing is finished, thus reducing access to hindmilk and total consumption)
- Infant kept on a preset schedule despite cues for more feeding
- Infant given water between feedings to "get through" to the next feeding
- Infant encouraged or allowed to sleep through the night before 8 to 12 weeks old
- Fewer than eight feedings in 24 hours
- Infant fed in a distracting environment
- In older infants, breastfeeding offered after solids are given
- Infant in a daycare setting that does not facilitate breastfeeding

Maternal Factors
- Does not initially respond to infant's cues for feeding or does not recognize that waking is needed to establish feeding
- Hectic schedule with limited time for breastfeeding
- Recent illness or significant weight loss
- Uses oral contraceptives or other hormones

Differential Diagnosis

The differential diagnoses for poor weight gain are a pattern of slower but normal weight gain in healthy breastfed infants and failure to thrive.

Management

The following measures should be taken to manage poor weight gain:
- Complete a thorough history to elicit information regarding infant and maternal factors.
- Conduct a thorough assessment of breastfeeding techniques to accurately determine the extent to which mismanagement is a cause.
- Provide instruction, encouragement, and reinforcement for correct breastfeeding techniques.
- Refer for treatment of physical or organic causes.
- Be alert for any infant who has lost too much weight and is unable to feed with vigor at the breast; such infants require an immediate infusion of calories for energy.
- Use a supplemental system at the breast if supplementation is required.
- Encourage and reassure the parents.

Complications

Complications of poor weight gain include developmental delay, poor bonding, and severe dehydration. In situations of early failure to establish breastfeeding, some infants may appear to be in a septic state and require hospitalization for rehydration and further evaluation.

Elimination Patterns

ARDYS M. DUNN

Gastrointestinal (GI), renal, urinary, and integumentary systems function to eliminate metabolic by-products and body wastes. This chapter discusses normal bowel and bladder function, normal developmental activities such as toilet training, and behaviors that are often self-limited in young children but can require intervention (e.g., encopresis and enuresis). Problems related more directly to GI and renal pathology are presented in Chapters 32 and 34. Dermatologic conditions are discussed in Chapter 36.

Healthy children demonstrate an extremely wide range of elimination patterns, and primary care providers (PCPs) have a responsibility to help parents understand what is "normal" behavior and what constitutes a problem. This can be a challenge because cultural and social expectations about elimination vary greatly, causing some parents to believe that their child has a problem when none exists. Also, developmental processes, such as toilet training, can lead to problems if not appropriately managed. Providers must conduct thorough and accurate assessments, provide anticipatory guidance for parents about what to expect as their child develops, help parents facilitate healthy bowel and bladder function, and refer for more complicated conditions.

■ Standards

The American Academy of Pediatrics (AAP) and the U.S. Preventive Services Task Force (USPSTF) do not recommend routine urinalysis for asymptomatic children; screening urinalysis should be conducted based on a specific clinical symptom or condition (AAP and *Bright Futures*, 2007; USPSTF, 1996). The AAP recommends that toilet training begin when the child is ready, which is not before 18 to 24 months of age (Wolraich and Tippins, 2003).

■ Normal Patterns of Elimination: Bowel and Urinary

INFANTS

Bowel Patterns

Bowel patterns of infants are related to the frequency and amount of feeding and differ between formula-fed and breastfed babies. Breastfed infants commonly have many small stools per day in the first weeks of life; frequent stooling in the neonate is an indicator of adequate breast milk intake (Shrago et al, 2006). During the second month of life infant stooling decreases markedly, from a median of six stools to one stool per day; nearly 40% of infants do not stool every day (Bekkali et al, 2009a; Tunc et al, 2008). Some older breastfed infants may stool as infrequently as once every 8 to 14 days. In exclusively breastfed infants, infrequent stooling is not a problem; if the infant is thriving, happy, and has no clinical signs (e.g., abdominal distention, irritability, vomiting), parents can be reassured that it is transient. The stools of breastfed infants are usually soft, sticky, or watery with a curdlike texture, light yellow, and have a "sour" but not unpleasant odor. Iron supplements can darken the stool and make it firmer.

Formula-fed babies have two to four stools each day in the first month. As patterns become established, the number of stools decreases and older formula-fed infants may have one to three soft semiformed stools each day. Stools of formula-fed infants are firmer, darker, and smellier than those of breastfed infants. They may be brown, greenish, or dark yellow depending on the type of formula and whether it is iron-fortified or if the child is given iron supplements. The stools of both breastfed and formula-fed babies become firmer, darker and more predictable as solid foods are introduced.

Urinary Patterns

Urination is associated with fluid intake, increasing as infants take more fluids. Healthy, well-hydrated infants, whether breastfed or formula-fed, should urinate a minimum of 6 times a day but can void in small amounts as many as 15 to 20 times a day. Fever in infants can quickly lead to dehydration, with less frequent urination.

Voluntary bowel and bladder control depends on myelination of the pyramidal tracts in the spinal cord, a process probably completed between 12 and 18 months of age. Infants 9 to 12 months old generally have regular patterns; they may have a bowel movement early in the morning or after feeding or stay dry for several hours and urinate immediately after waking from a nap. Parents may use these regular patterns to begin introducing the toddler to toilet training, and some parents will place the younger child on the "potty" when the child shows elimination cues.

TODDLERS AND PRESCHOOLERS
Bowel Patterns
Toddlers and preschoolers usually have a regular pattern of elimination. Although they typically have one to three stools a day, it is not unusual for children in this age group to defecate every other day or every third or fourth day. It is a myth that healthy children must have a bowel movement every day. Normal stools have an unpleasant odor and are soft, formed, and various shades of brown, depending on the child's diet.

Urinary Patterns
By the time children are 2 years old, renal function is fully developed. The urinary pattern of toddlers and preschoolers is influenced by fluid intake, environmental conditions, perspiration, fever, and diarrhea with significant fluid loss. They typically urinate 8 to 14 times a day. Cold weather, excitement, and stress lead to increased frequency. Children generally do not void during sleep after 18 months (Jansson et al, 2005).

SCHOOL-AGE CHILDREN
Bowel Patterns
Elimination patterns in school-age children approximate those of adults. Depending on intake, a child may have bowel movements from one to three times a day to once every 2 to 3 days. Stool is soft, formed, and brown and has an odor. School-age children should be completely toilet trained, although occasional soiling of underwear occurs as a result of poor hygiene or because children do not respond quickly to defecation cues. During the school-age years it is important to be cognizant that children increasingly need independence and privacy; these needs extend into the arena of toilet management.

Urinary Patterns
School-age children have essentially the same capacity as adults to produce urine—between 650 and 1500 mL in a 24-hour period—but the kidneys are still small and accommodate a smaller urine volume at any one time than those of adults. Children normally void 5 or 6 times a day. Girls appear to have slightly larger bladder capacity than boys. Dysfunctional voiding (too little means 1 to 3 times a day; too much means 8 to 12 times a day), daytime incontinence, or nocturnal enuresis warrants further evaluation, especially because these conditions can be associated with infection, dehydration, constipation, or sexual abuse.

ADOLESCENTS
Bowel and Urinary Patterns
GI and renal functions are at adult levels in adolescents, and patterns of elimination are similar to those of adults. Abnormal variation can occur in teenagers who have eating disorders. Adolescents are also susceptible to the demands of schedules, stress, and irregular eating patterns. The need for privacy, safety, and personal space can inhibit normal elimination in public places, such as school or dormitory restrooms (Kistner, 2009). Sexual activity can contribute to changes in bowel or bladder function, including infections or constipation.

■ Assessment of Patterns
Assessment of elimination patterns begins with a thorough health history with questions being asked of the parent or the child, depending on the child's age and ability. As variations of normal behavior become evident, relevant follow-up questions should be asked to clarify and complete the health picture.

HEALTH HISTORY
Description of Current Status
The patient's current elimination status can be assessed with the following questions:
- How often does your child urinate? How many wet diapers does your baby have in a 24-hour period?
- How often does your child have a bowel movement? Describe what the stools look and smell like. How does your child act when having a bowel movement?
- Describe anything unusual about your child's elimination habits. Does your child resist going to the bathroom?
- Describe your child's toileting habits. For example, at what time of day does your child have a bowel movement?
- Do you use any medications, including over-the-counter preparations or home remedies, to help your child with bowel movements?
- How do you think the process of toilet training will happen (ask of parents of a 9- to 12-month-old child)?
- Is your child toilet trained? When did training begin? Describe the process. How often do "accidents" happen? How do you (parent) feel toilet training is progressing?
- What names do you use in your family for stool and urine, for body parts, and for the process of using the toilet?

Birth History
Determine whether any problems with the child's urine or stool were present at birth. For example, did the baby pass a meconium stool within 48 hours after birth? How soon after birth did the baby urinate?

Review of Systems
The review of systems should include the following questions:
- Has your child ever been constipated or had diarrhea? How does the parent define constipation and diarrhea? (Box 12-1 summarizes the Rome III criteria for functional constipation. See Box 12-2 for the Bristol Scale of stool quality that reflects colonic transit time.) Is it chronic or occasional? Did it start after a particular incident (e.g., illness, during toilet training, with a certain food or change in diet)?
- Has your child ever had a urinary tract infection (UTI)? Describe. Any workup (e.g., ultrasonography [US], urethrogram), findings, treatment, and follow-up?
- Has your child had any illness, elinjury, or operation related to the bowel or bladder? Describe.

BOX 12-1 Rome III Criteria for Functional Constipation: Infants and Children

Child must have at least two of the following criteria, at least once a week, for at least 1 month (infants to 4 years old) or for at least 2 months (children over 4 years old); with no evidence of structural, metabolic, or endocrine disease:

- Two or fewer defecations per week
- At least one episode of fecal incontinence per week (after child is toilet trained)
- History of excessive stool retention, retentive posturing in children 4 or more years old
- History of painful or hard bowel movements
- History of large-diameter stools, could obstruct toilet
- Presence of large fecal mass in rectum

From Rome Foundation: *Rome III diagnostic criteria for functional gastrointestinal disorders.* Available at www.romecriteria.org/criteria (accessed Aug 9, 2011).

BOX 12-2 Bristol Stool Form Scale

Type 1	Separate hard lumps, like nuts	Slow colonic transit
Type 2	Sausage-shaped but lumpy	Slow colonic transit
Type 3	Sausage or snakelike but with cracks on surface	Normal colonic transit
Type 4	Sausage or snakelike, smooth and soft	Normal colonic transit
Type 5	Soft blobs with clear-cut edges	Normal colonic transit
Type 6	Fluffy pieces with ragged edges, mushy stool	Fast colonic transit
Type 7	Watery, no solid pieces	Fast colonic transit

Adapted from Choung RS, Locke GR 3rd, Zinsmeister AR, et al: Epidemiology of slow and fast colonic transit using a scale of stool form in a community, *Aliment Pharmacol Ther* 26(7):1043-1050, 2007.

- Does your child have a physical condition or chronic illness that affects voiding or bowel movements?
- Is there a history of bed-wetting; at what age did it resolve?

Family History

Determine whether any family members, including parents, have had problems with urination or bowel movements and describe them (e.g., chronic constipation or diarrhea, bed-wetting). Has the child or family traveled or lived outside the U.S.? Does the family residence use well water?

Environment and Psychosocial Issues

Environmental and psychosocial issues should be assessed, using questions such as:

- How do you, as a parent, feel about the issue of toileting?
- How do you interact with your child around toileting issues?
- How do you deal with toileting "accidents" (including bed-wetting)?

- What plans do you have for managing toilet training?
- Describe your child's typical diet.
- Tell me about the toileting facilities at your child's house, daycare, and school. How do you think they affect your child's toileting habits?

PHYSICAL EXAMINATION

The physical examination includes external examination of the perineum, anus, and urinary meatus and auscultation and palpation of the abdomen for bowel sounds, softness, masses, peristalsis, and tenderness.

LABORATORY AND DIAGNOSTIC TESTS

- Urinalysis (with or without urine culture) as indicated based on symptoms
- Stool specimen, as indicated by history and symptoms
- Diagnostic imaging as indicated after above initial laboratory workup and assessment/management considerations (see Chapters 32 and 34)

■ Management Strategies for Normal Patterns

TOILET TRAINING

Toilet training occurs in the toddler and preschool years and is usually complete by 4 years of age. Successful toilet training requires sensitivity, understanding of development, good communication, hope, humor, and patience. In addition to becoming self-sufficient in their toileting, children should also learn that elimination is a natural and necessary process. As self-toileting is mastered, parents and children should experience pride and satisfaction in having worked together to accomplish an important developmental task.

The health care provider plays an important role in providing anticipatory guidance to parents. Introduce the topic of toilet training at the 9-month visit and again at 12, 15, and 18 months; assess parents' expectations and plans and provide ample opportunity for discussion of realistic toileting outcomes.

When to begin toilet training is a perennial question of parents. Providers can emphasize that every child is unique, and readiness cues should ultimately be used to decide when to begin training. Physiological readiness develops by about 18 months. True voluntary sphincter control is a function of psychological and social development as well, so most children are not usually ready for independent toilet training until 24 months or even older. Guidelines for assessing toilet-training readiness include physical, cognitive, interpersonal or psychological, and parental skills (Table 12-1).

Over the past 4 decades, the median age to begin toilet training in the U.S. has increased from less than 18 months to between 21 and 36 months; some studies show no benefit to beginning training before 27 months (Choby and George, 2008). Internationally, the age of initiating toilet training has also increased (Mota and Barros, 2008; Vermandel et al, 2008). In the U.S., race and socioeconomic status may influence the decision about when to begin toilet training, with one study showing that higher-income Caucasian parents view 25.4 months as an appropriate age in contrast to

TABLE 12-1	Guidelines for Assessing Readiness to Toilet Train

Skills to Assess	Criteria
Child's physical skills	Has voluntary sphincter control Stays dry for 2 hours, may wake from naps still dry Is able to sit, walk, and squat Assists in dressing self
Child's cognitive skills	Recognizes urge to urinate or defecate Understands meaning of words used by family in toileting Understands what the toilet is for Understands connection between dry pants and toilet Is able to follow directions Is able to communicate needs
Child's interpersonal skills	Demonstrates desire to please parent Expresses curiosity about use of toilet Expresses desire to be dry and clean
Parental skills	Expresses desire to assist child with training Recognizes child's cues of readiness Has no compelling factor that will interfere with training (e.g., new job, move, family loss or gain)

BOX 12-3 Management of Toilet Training

- Keep child as clean and dry as possible:
  - Change diapers frequently.
  - Use training pants or underwear when child stays dry for several hours during the day; use diaper at night.
- Talk to child about toilet training:
  - Praise child for asking to have diaper changed.
  - Explain connection between being clean and dry and using toilet.
  - Provide opportunity for child to use toilet, especially before going out to play, going on a trip, before naps, and at bedtime; set an example with adult behavior.
  - Do not constantly remind child to use the toilet; avoid "nagging."
- Teach child how to use toilet:
  - Allow child to observe while parents or older siblings use toilet.
  - Demonstrate how to sit on toilet, use toilet paper, flush, and wash one's hands.
- Provide practice time for child:
  - Provide a potty chair or portable toilet seat.
  - Allow child to sit on potty chair with clothes or diaper on.
  - Encourage child to use potty chair while parent uses regular toilet.
  - Have child sit on potty chair without diapers for 5 to 10 minutes at a time.
  - Practice at times the child usually urinates or defecates.
- Provide a comfortable, safe-feeling environment:
  - Seat child facing backward on a regular toilet or provide a footstool to rest the feet on.
  - Never flush the toilet when child is sitting on it.
  - Stay with child for safety reasons.
- Give consistent, positive feedback:
  - Praise child for trying and for success.
  - Be understanding of child's refusal to use toilet.
  - Never demand performance.
  - Never make child sit on toilet if child resists.
  - Ignore or minimize undesired behavior.
  - Never scold or punish if a child wets or soils.
  - Use star chart or other reward for success.
  - Do not praise excessively.

African-Americans (18.2 months) and other racial groups (19.4 months) (Horn et al, 2006). In some cultures, early *assisted* toilet training (in contrast to *independent* toilet training in which the child learns self-management) may be the norm, with some Asian and African-American families beginning toilet training between 1 and 3 months old. This method requires that the caregiver be highly motivated to note and respond to infant elimination cues; initially the caregiver takes responsibility for placing the child on the toilet when necessary. As the child matures, he or she takes more self-responsibility (Rugolotto et al, 2008; Sun and Rugolotto, 2004). As families from various cultural groups immigrate to the U.S., health care providers need to understand these practices and be open to developing mutually agreed-on approaches to toilet training.

If begun too early, toilet training can be very stressful, contributing to enuresis, encopresis, and refusal to toilet (Mota and Barros, 2008). Late training may also be a problem. A large study by Joinson and associates (2009) found that children who started toilet training after 24 months had more problems with incontinence than children who initiated training earlier. According to Wu (2010), however, no controlled clinical trials support the hypothesis that late toilet training contributes to incontinence.

Children are typically trained first for nocturnal bowel control, then daytime bowel control, daytime bladder control, and finally nocturnal bladder control. Average times for being fully trained are around 3 to 4 years old, with a normal age variation of up to a year for individual children. In a population of U.S. Caucasian children, the average ages for girls and

boys to accomplish other tasks of toilet training were as follows (Schum et al, 2002):

- Showing an interest in using the toilet: girls, 24 months; boys, 26 months
- Telling parents of their need to use the toilet: girls, 26 months; boys, 29 months
- Staying dry for at least 2 hours: girls, 26 months; boys, 29 months
- Staying dry during the day: girls, 32.5 months; boys, 35 months

There is little evidence regarding which toilet training strategy (e.g., early assisted; Brazelton's child-oriented approach [Brazelton and Sparrow, 2004]; operant conditioning such as Azrin and Foxx's *Toilet Training in Less Than a Day* [1974]) is most effective. When children and parents are ready to begin toilet training, several management techniques can be helpful (Box 12-3). If children resist training, the effort should be put on hold for a few weeks before trying again. If toddlers seem to be toilet trained for a brief period and suddenly regress to wetting and soiling consistently, they should be placed back in diapers and the process begun again within a few weeks. It is extremely important that parents and children do not become engaged in a "battle for control" over toilet training. Ultimately it is the child's responsibility to control bowel and urinary function, and toilet training is only one of the many tasks toddlers master on their way to independence. Parents have the responsibility to assist in the process by providing a positive environment and opportunities, teaching the techniques, and setting a positive example. It appears that a structured yet flexible approach that is responsive to the child's cues is likely to be most successful.

Parents can become extremely frustrated if their expectations do not match the abilities and performance of their children, and child abuse related to toilet training may occur. Berkowitz (2000) asserts that issues around toileting are the second most prevalent factor precipitating fatal child abuse. Health care providers can play a crucial role in making the experience a positive one and preventing abuse by giving parents information about child development, techniques for managing the training process, and support and encouragement for their efforts.

■ Altered Patterns of Elimination

DYSFUNCTIONAL ELIMINATION SYNDROME

Dysfunctional elimination syndrome (DES) is any abnormal pattern in bowel or bladder function at an age when an individual is developmentally capable of control. A number of factors contribute to DES, and the close relationship between bowel and bladder function is key to understanding this complex and varied condition; it is, in reality, a set of conditions. The child may actively try to prevent bowel movements or urination (e.g., the school-age child who has restricted access to bathroom facilities). An illness may lead to dehydration, constipation, painful bowel movements, and subsequent stool withholding by the child. Trauma or disruption of the child's life may contribute to developmental regression, with bed-wetting or inappropriate stooling. A large longitudinal study indicates that developmental delay, difficult child temperament, and maternal depression in the first 2 years of life may contribute to problems with bladder or bowel control in the school-age child (Joinson et al, 2008). Any of these factors could lead to elimination problems.

Urgency, frequency, and incontinence are common in DES, and the child may have difficulty initiating urination or completely emptying the bladder. Persistent problems with incomplete emptying of the bladder can lead to UTI. Constipation can exacerbate bladder dysfunction by applying pressure to the bladder wall or restricting urinary flow. The child may experience stool incontinence (encopresis), with or without constipation. Elimination problems also contribute to family difficulties, bullying, social isolation, emotional problems, and antisocial behaviors in families of children with fecal soiling (Joinson et al, 2006; Kaugars et al, 2010; Lottman and Alova, 2007; van Dijk et al, 2010).

The following sections discuss bowel dysfunction (fecal incontinence [encopresis] and stool toileting refusal) and urinary dysfunction (dysfunctional voiding and enuresis) in the healthy child who has no neurological or structural defect that could cause the problem. These conditions are considered here as developmental problems of normal urinary and bowel habits, improving for most children as they mature. If assessment indicates a pathological condition may be present, further investigation and different management, including referral, are necessary.

ENCOPRESIS

Description

Encopresis is defined as fecal incontinence after an age when the child should be able to control bowel movements, usually 4 years old; fecal incontinence occurs at least once per month for at least 2 months prior to diagnosis. Primary, or continuous, encopresis is present in children who have never been toilet trained. Secondary, or discontinuous, encopresis is seen in those who were previously trained but who begin to soil. There are two subtypes of encopresis: encopresis with constipation, associated with stool retention, constipation, and incontinence overflow (functional retentive fecal incontinence); and encopresis without constipation, or functional nonretentive fecal incontinence.

In encopresis with constipation, stool retention over time leads to distention of the colon and stretching of the rectum, ineffective peristalsis, decreased sensory threshold in the rectum, and weakened rectal and sphincter muscles. Stool becomes dry, hard, and difficult to evacuate (can be impacted), and bowel movements can be painful. Soft, semiformed, or liquid stool from higher in the colon leaks around retained stool and passes uncontrollably through the rectum, causing soiling. The child is often unaware of the incontinence. Children with encopresis with constipation may either refuse or be willing to use the toilet.

Children with encopresis without constipation (functional nonretentive fecal incontinence) are not constipated, but have overflow incontinence or voluntary bowel movements in their clothing or other inappropriate places.

Epidemiology

Encopresis may be more common than believed because many families hesitate to inform their health care provider about it. In the school-age child, it is more common among boys than girls (Boris and Dalton, 2007a). The cause of encopresis is unclear, may be multifactorial, and appears to differ among children. Both physiological and psychosocial factors are involved. Often children with encopresis with constipation have a history of an acute stool problem that was not adequately managed (e.g., the child had an illness that caused dehydration and constipation), leading to a cycle of constipation—painful defecation—stool retention—more severe constipation—more painful defecation—more stool retention and so on.

Children with nonretentive encopresis appear to have more behavioral problems and externalizing behavior than children with retentive encopresis or those without stooling problems, though it is unclear which causes which (Burgers and Benninga, 2009). Some of these children may also have a developmentally delayed or faulty perception of the need to stool and will soil as a result (Pakarinen et al, 2006).

Physiological. Physiological factors related to encopresis with constipation include the following:
- Inadequate fluid intake
- Dehydration caused by illness and fever or during active play in hot weather
- A change in diet, such as the introduction of solids or increased carbohydrates and decreased fiber
- Inappropriate use of laxatives, suppositories, or enemas by parents who do not understand normal bowel patterns in children and infants
- Secondary stool retention and constipation due to:
  ○ Painful bowel movements
  ○ Anal fissures
  ○ Paradoxical constriction of the external anal sphincter muscle during attempted defecation
  ○ Neurogenic conditions (e.g., aganglionic colon [Hirschsprung disease], cerebral palsy, myelomeningocele)
  ○ Endocrine and metabolic conditions (e.g., hypothyroidism)
  ○ Medications (e.g., opioids, iron supplements)

Psychosocial. Psychosocial factors related to constipation and encopresis include the following:
- Major family or life adjustments, such as loss of a parent, sibling, or other significant person
- Inappropriate toilet-training techniques leading to a power struggle; children who are pushed might rebel in the only way they can, by refusing to cooperate
- Irregular toileting patterns, often caused by travel, unfamiliar or unpleasant bathrooms, lack of regular routine, or child being absorbed in play or activities
- Physical and/or sexual abuse

Clinical Findings

History. The history can include the following:
- Stained underwear
- Report of fewer than three bowel movements per week
- Difficult or painful defecation
- Large-caliber or hard stool
- Child suddenly becoming still during play, attempting to hide when urge to defecate is felt
- Child attempting to retain stool (e.g., crossing legs, grimacing, or shifting from one foot to another)
- Reports of a bloated sensation, abdominal pain, or both
- Odor of stool from leakage into underwear
- Streaks of bright blood on toilet paper or underwear
- Enuresis
- UTIs
- Anorexia
- Avoiding using the toilet at school or other public places

Physical Examination. The physical examination should assess for the following:
- Overflow soiling
- Abdominal distention
- Abdominal tenderness on palpation
- Impactions felt on digital rectal examination (rectal examination may be deferred if the history and other signs allow for a clear diagnosis because it can be traumatic for the child)
- Mass felt at the midline in the suprapubic area (descending colon); ropey loops of bowel may also be palpated in right and left lower guadrants
- Anal fissures

- Sacral dimple or hair tuft
- Neurological signs: absent or diminished abdominal, cremasteric, anal wink reflexes, and deep tendon reflexes (DTRs) in lower extremities may indicate a neurological cause

Laboratory and Diagnostic Tests. X-rays and laboratory tests to identify structural or organic causes of constipation are not routinely necessary, but can be appropriate if clinical suspicion is high or primary treatment for encopresis is unsuccessful. Results of an abdominal flat plate radiograph can indicate accumulation of stool in the sigmoid colon (see Chapter 32).

Differential Diagnosis

The differential diagnoses for encopresis with constipation are as follows:
- Anorectal stenosis
- Spina bifida occulta, spinal cord dysplasia, tethered cord, spinal cord tumor
- Hirschsprung disease
- Mental retardation
- Hypothyroidism
- Hypercalcemia
- Cerebral palsy
- Other organic causes of constipation (e.g., cystic fibrosis)
- The normal red-faced grunting and straining of infants on defecation

Management

Treatment of children with encopresis differs depending on whether they have impactions, are constipated, or have normal bowel movements but defecate in places other than the toilet. In all cases, the goals of treatment are to establish a regular bowel routine, "demystify" the problem, alleviate blame, and gain cooperation for treatment plans.

Treatment approaches for children with constipation have followed a pattern of (1) bowel evacuation using laxatives and/or enemas; (2) bowel retraining to establish a regular pattern of stooling; and (3) ongoing maintenance with diet, exercise, and regular toileting hygiene to prevent recurring constipation. It has been argued, after reviews of research literature, that treatment of constipation in children has been based largely on empirical trial and anecdote, rather than evidence-based research, and that more extensive work is needed to determine specific causes and best treatment practices (Pijpers et al, 2009).

The emphasis in treating nonretentive fecal soiling is on behavioral therapy, educating the child and parent about normal stooling, and establishing a structured pattern of toileting. Box 12-4 outlines approaches to treating a child with encopresis without constipation (also see Stool Toileting Refusal, Management).

Children who have encopresis with constipation present a greater challenge. Education of parents and children is equally vital to successful treatment (Philichi, 2008). A clear message to children and parents should be that the dynamics of encopresis (retention, colon stretching, decreased peristalsis, impaction, leaking) are not voluntary—no one is to blame; they can, however, be reversed through bowel rehabilitation. Correcting them will take hard work, cooperation, and time, and the provider will work with the family to ensure success. Figure 12-1 can be used to educate parents and children about the bowel rehabilitation process involved in the treatment plan.

Figures 12-2 and 12-3 present algorithms that PCPs can use to manage constipation in children younger and older than 1 year. Table 12-2 provides guidelines for treating a child with encopresis with constipation, including appropriate medications. Research indicates that polyethylene glycol 3350 (PEG) may be more effective than lactulose (Lee-Robichaud et al, 2010) and that enemas may be as effective as laxatives (Bekkali et al, 2009b). Retentive encopresis

without impaction may not require such extensive intervention; PEG and mineral oil may be used for catharsis in children younger than 7 years or those who are unable to tolerate enemas or suppositories.

Management of encopresis is often multidisciplinary. Psychological counseling of both the child and family may be necessary in some cases, with referral to a psychologist or behavioral pediatrician. Adding formal behavioral therapy may reduce incontinence slightly more than medical treatment alone (Brazzelli and Griffiths, 2006). However, in one study, conventional medical treatment that included education about symptoms, encouraged the child to respond to defecation cues, and emphasized positive feedback was as effective as an approach that combined behavioral therapy and laxatives (van Dijk et al, 2008). Because encopresis often occurs in school-age children, medical providers may need to consult with the school nurse to ensure that the child receives appropriate medications, hygiene management (may include access to a more private toilet), and essential psychological and emotional support in the school setting.

BOX 12-4 | Management of Children With Mild Encopresis Without Constipation

- Monitor diet:
  - Ensure adequate fiber and water intake (cereals, oatmeal, breads, fruits, and vegetables).
  - Decrease milk to 16 oz/day; limit cheese, rice, applesauce, bananas.
  - Provide 2 to 4 oz prune juice daily (high-sorbitol content).
- Avoid use of stool softeners or laxatives.
- Give child all responsibility for own toilet habits. Stop parental reminders to use toilet. Stop all urging and criticisms.
- Use incentives or rewards to reinforce positive behavior. Give incentives immediately after child defecates in toilet. Put time limit on use of incentive (e.g., can watch a video for 30 minutes, can ride a bike for 15 minutes).
- Establish a regular toileting routine.
- Encourage daily physical exercise.

Complications

Persistent encopresis is an unpleasant condition, and children with encopresis often experience ridicule and shame. Age-group peers frequently treat children with scorn, hostility, and rejection. Teachers and other adults might be disgusted by children with encopresis, and parents, dealing with anger, guilt, embarrassment, and helplessness, find their children and the condition extremely difficult to manage. Social, interpersonal, and family relations are at grave risk.

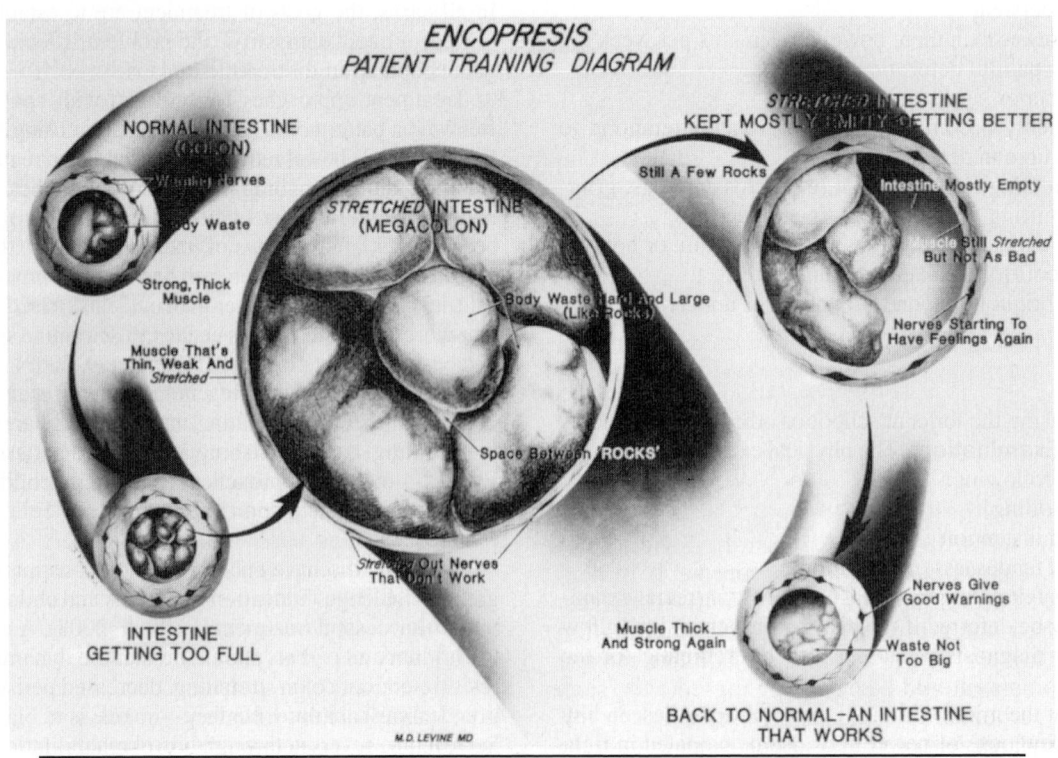

FIGURE 12-1 Encopresis: patient training diagram. (From Levine MD, Carey WB, Crocker AC: *Developmental-behavioral pediatrics*, ed 4, Philadelphia, 2009, Saunders.)

ALGORITHM

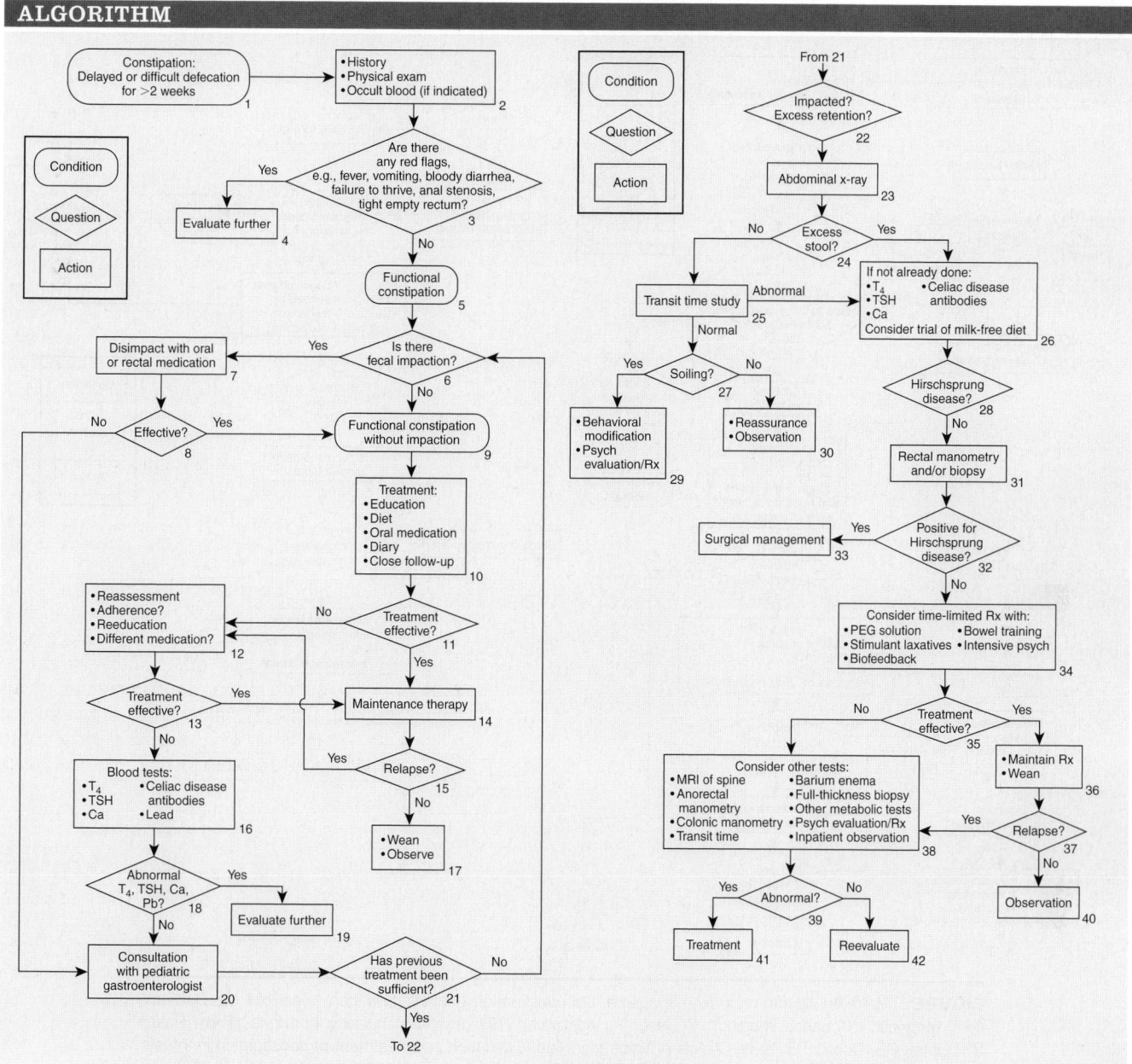

FIGURE 12-2 An algorithm for the management of constipation in children 1 year and older. *Ca,* calcium; *MRI,* magnetic resonance imaging; *Pb,* lead; *PEG,* polyethylene glycol electrolyte; *psych,* psychological management; *Rx,* therapy; *T4,* thyroxine; *TSH,* thyroid-stimulating hormone. (From Baker SS, Liptak GS, Colletti RB, et al: Clinical practice guideline evaluation and treatment of constipation in infants and children: recommendations of the North American Society for Pediatric Gastroenterology, Hepatology and Nutrition, *J Pediatr Gastroenterol Nutr* 43:e1-e13, 2006.)

Patient Education and Prevention

The best treatment of encopresis is prevention. If constipation or encopresis is caused by an underlying anatomic or organic cause (e.g., Hirschsprung disease, spina bifida occulta, hypothyroidism), early diagnosis and referral are essential. It is important for the pediatric provider to understand the relationship between constipation and encopresis, recognize conditions that may contribute to each, and provide parents with anticipatory guidance related to dietary and toileting management of their children to prevent their occurrence. It is equally important to provide support during treatment. Although parents should be informed that treatment may be required

for months or years, providers should emphasize that by following a clear, consistent, aggressive treatment protocol the condition can be managed. Finally, providers, parents, and the child must work together to prevent recurrence of symptoms after successful treatment.

STOOL TOILETING REFUSAL

Description

Stool toileting refusal (STR) is present when a strates a pattern of successfully using the toilet refuses to use the toilet for bowel movements. The

ALGORITHM

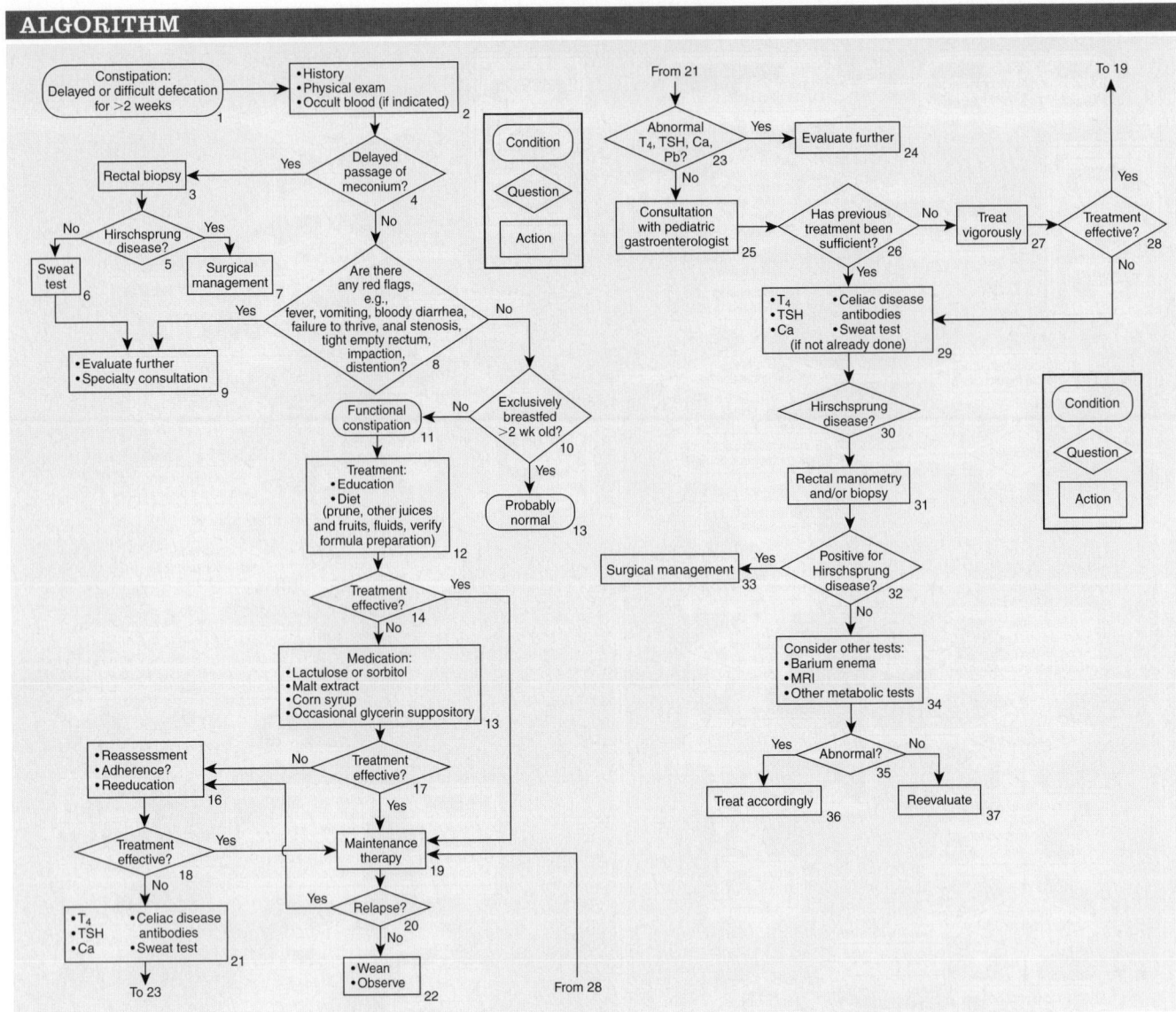

FIGURE 12-3 An algorithm for the management of constipation in infants less than 1 year old. *Ca,* Calcium; *MRI,* magnetic resonance imaging; *Pb,* lead; *T₄,* thyroxine; *TSH,* thyroid-stimulating hormone. (From Baker SS, Liptak GS, Colletti RB, et al: Clinical practice guideline. Evaluation and treatment of constipation in infants and children: recommendations of the North American Society for Pediatric Gastroenterology, Hepatology and Nutrition, *J Pediatr Gastroenterol Nutr* 43:e1-e13, 2006.)

will usually defecate in a diaper, training pants, or "pull-ups." In some cases, children will retain stool or defecate outside the toilet. Encopresis without constipation also fits this description: the child defecates outside the toilet when beyond the age of expected training. Children who hide when they defecate are more likely to show STR than children who do not hide (Taubman et al, 2003a).

Epidemiology

The incidence of STR has not been recently documented. Taubman (1997) found that 22% of healthy children between 18 and 30 months old experienced at least 1 month of STR. In a study of children who were trained at early ages (some as early as the first 6 months of life), there was a nearly 12% incidence of STR (Lugolotto et al, 2008). The cause of STR is unknown, but the

presence of younger siblings in the household and the parents' inability to set limits for the child may be related. Although children who displayed STR tended to have "a more difficult temperament" than did children who were toilet trained, they did not have any more behavior problems (Blum et al, 1997). Constipation and painful bowel movements appear to precede rather than follow the problem (Blum et al, 2004).

Clinical Findings

History. Parents or caregivers report that the child demonstrates the following:

- Bladder control but refusal to defecate on the toilet
- A regular pattern of bowel movements
- Signs that a bowel movement is imminent
- May have a history of hiding when defecating, either before or after toilet training begins

TABLE 12-2	Management of Children With Encopresis With Constipation	
Treatment Phase	**Treatment Program**	**Comments**

Phase I: Catharsis (bowel clean-out)	Oral administration:
	• Polyethylene glycol (PEG) 3350: 1 to 3 g/kg/day in two to four divided doses
	or
	• Magnesium citrate:
	 <6 years, 1 to 3 mL/kg/day
	 6 to 12 years: 100 to 150 mL/day
	 >12 years: 150 to 300 mL/day *plus* (if desired)
	• Stimulants such as bisacodyl (Dulcolax) once a day as tolerated
	or
	• Enema clean-out (infrequently used)
	 ○ Sodium phosphate (Fleet) enema:
	  2 to 11 years: 6 mL/kg/day per rectum; may give up to 135 mL once a day in older children
	  >11 years: an adult enema or 135 mL per rectum once a day
		Home treatment is preferred. Catharsis should take 3 to 5 days or until stool output is runny diarrhea.
		Mix 17 g PEG 3350 (about 4 level tsp Mira-LAX) in 8 oz of fluid to equal approximately 2 g/oz; can be stored in refrigerator for 48 hours.
		Catharsis may need to occur in the hospital if:
		• Retention is severe
		• Home compliance is poor
		• Parents prefer admission
		• Child needs enema for clean-out and parent should not administer
		Pediatric enema is 67.5 mL; adult enema is 135 mL.
		The child may have watery or soft stools for several days after clean-out. Child and parents should be informed that this does not indicate cure, but that ongoing maintenance and bowel retraining are essential for the bowel to return to normal functioning (see Fig. 12-2).

Phase II: Maintenance (regular bowel movements over 4 to 12 months)	Oral laxatives • PEG 3350 0.5 to 1 g/kg/day orally in two divided doses • Lactulose 1 to 3 mL/kg/day orally in two divided doses • Magnesium hydroxide 1 to 3 mL/kg/day orally in two divided doses Behavioral training • Establish daily toilet sitting 15 to 20 minutes after meals two or three times a day for 5 to 10 minutes • Provide positive reinforcement for toilet sitting and stooling • Keep a diary of bowel movements, recording time and amount • Increase physical exercise; have child be active in the 15 to 20 minutes between mealtime and sitting on toilet Dietary changes • Increase dietary fiber • Ensure adequate fluid intake	Adjust daily medications to achieve one to three soft, mushy stools per day. PEG has been shown to be effective when used alone and more effective than lactulose (Candy and Belsey, 2009; Lee-Robichaud et al, 2010). Use of senna is not recommended. Plan on 6 months of treatment before bowel regains normal function.
Phase III: Weaning and long term follow-up (normal stool function over time)	• Gradual tapering of laxative • Regular visits (about every 4 to 10 weeks) depending on severity and need of family • Telephone availability to discuss progress and adjust doses • Counseling or referral as appropriate for psychosocial and developmental issues • Continued education regarding normal bowel function	Goals of follow-up visits: • Monitor compliance. • Provide encouragement and support. • Detect and treat relapse early if it occurs.

Adapted from Kehoe TD: The constipated 8-year-old. In Burns CE, Richardson B, Brady MA, editors: *Pediatric primary care case studies*, Sudbury, MA, 2010, Jones and Bartlett.

Physical Examination. The physical examination will be unremarkable if the child has a pattern of regular bowel movements.
• Examine the anus for fissures or irritation that may cause a child to refuse to defecate.
• Check for signs of stool retention:
 ○ Abdominal distention
 ○ Abdominal tenderness on palpation
• Palpate for a mass in the sigmoid colon or at the midline in the suprapubic area (impaction).

Differential Diagnosis
The differential diagnoses include stool withholding, constipation, and encopresis.

Management
When parents refrain from expressing negative messages about stooling or fecal matter and praise the child for defecating in the diaper, the duration of STR appears to shorten (Taubman et al, 2003b). Behavioral management is appropriate for

younger children. Return them to diapers and reintroduce toilet training in about a month or when the child indicates interest. Some children prefer not to wear diapers all the time but will ask to have one put on when they feel the urge to defecate. After having a bowel movement they ask to be changed and return to wearing training pants. This pattern may continue for several weeks or months. For older children, schedule daily times for the child to sit on the toilet for 5 to 10 minutes; have these times be positive, never punitive or forced. Never flush the toilet while the child is sitting on it. Provide incentives and give positive feedback when the child successfully uses the toilet for bowel movements (e.g., the parent can use star charts). If the child has constipation, fecal impaction, or both, initial bowel clean-out is necessary, in conjunction with increased fiber and fluid in the diet. Mineral oil, suppositories, or medication may be useful. Table 12-2 outlines the management of a child with encopresis with constipation.

Complications

Refusal to use the toilet for bowel movements may lead to stool withholding, constipation, and impaction, conditions that result in primary encopresis. Psychological complications include embarrassment, shame, conflict, and stress between children and parents, especially as the child becomes older. Child maltreatment can be a significant complication.

Patient Education and Prevention

Prevention through appropriate toilet training is key (see Box 12-3). If a child refuses to defecate on the toilet, use of punishment or force can complicate the problem. Parents should be alert for signs of constipation (see Box 12-1) and should encourage fluids, fiber, and exercise to facilitate bowel movements and prevent encopresis.

DYSFUNCTIONAL VOIDING

Description

Dysfunctional voiding is defined by the International Children's Continence Society (ICCS) as dysfunction during voiding in which the child contracts the external urethra in a "staccato pattern" resulting in intermittent flow, prolonged micturition time, and often incomplete emptying of the bladder. Dysfunctional voiding is not a problem of bladder filling but of bladder emptying. Either detrusor overactivity or underactivity may be present; a long-standing pattern of incomplete emptying can lead to overextension of the bladder and subsequent underactive detrusor function. As a result, UTI, symptoms of urgency, frequency, and overflow incontinence can occur (Chase et al, 2010).

Epidemiology

The cause of dysfunctional voiding is unknown, but it is believed to be multifactorial, and may be related to maturational delay, learned behavior, retention of infantile patterns, and genetic or congenital factors. Constipation, UTI, structural abnormalities, stress, and abuse must be considered. It is more common in girls and is usually seen in children 4 to 8 years old, after toilet training but before puberty.

Clinical Findings

History. Because of the varied problems associated with dysfunctional voiding, children have a history of differing symptoms, including the following:
- Infrequent voiding
- Sudden daytime incontinence after having been dry
- Urgency
- Frequency
- Inability to stop the voiding stream
- Occasional nocturnal enuresis, but usually daytime wetting
- Enuresis after giggling
- Incontinence after voiding
- Constipation
- UTI
- Presence of local factors (e.g., bubble bath, tight underclothes)

The history should also include information about the child's general development (achievement of developmental milestones), pattern of toilet training and elimination (frequency and volume of voiding and timing of episodes of incontinence), any stressors experienced following toilet training, family history of problems with voiding, and the child's behavioral patterns, including the child's and family's emotional response to the condition.

Physical Examination. A complete physical examination should be done (including checking females for labial adhesions and males for meatal stenosis). Consider, particularly, the possibility of constipation.

Laboratory and Diagnostic Tests. Urodynamic diagnostic procedures are not routinely done. The following tests may be indicated:
- Urinalysis
- Urine culture and sensitivity
- Repeat uroflowmetry with electromyography (EMG) of perineal muscles (if the test is available)
  - Uroflow measurement should be done three times on a well-hydrated child in a nonstressful setting.
  - A staccato flow pattern with prolonged flow time and reduced maximal flow rate is diagnostic (Chase et al, 2010).
- Measurement of postvoid residual urine volume using US
- Renal and bladder US if structural abnormalities are suspected; an abnormal US can show a normal upper renal system and a thick-walled bladder, a compensation to resistance caused by external sphincter contractions
- Voiding cystourethrogram (VCUG) in boys and radionuclide cystogram in girls if:
  - There is a history of recurrent or febrile UTI; with first UTI in boys
  - Thickened bladder wall on US
  - Boy is more than 5 years old and has both nocturnal and diurnal enuresis
  - Child at puberty has persistent enuresis (Feldman and Bauer, 2006).

Differential Diagnosis

The differential diagnoses for dysfunctional voiding include:
- UTI
- Structural abnormality, such as abnormal sphincters, ectopic ureter, duplicated urethra, or urethral valves
- Neurogenic bladder

Education for Dysfunctional Voiding

The provider should explain:
- How the bladder works: describe filling and emptying process, especially as it is related to problem of external sphincter contraction during voiding
- Relationship between abdominal, pelvic floor, and external sphincter muscles; how to be aware of and to relax muscles to allow complete voiding
- Relationship of bladder and bowel function
- Complications of inadequate bladder emptying
- What parents and child can do to correct the problem (bladder retraining):
  ○ Establish a consistent, structured regimen of toileting: set a timed-voiding schedule, usually every 2 to 4 hours during the day; try to hold urine if there is urgency before the minimum time; void before going to bed and immediately on rising in morning
  ○ Keep an ongoing voiding and stooling diary
  ○ Ensure adequate fluid intake; drink most liquids earlier in the day, decrease intake in late afternoon and evening; no more than 6 oz in the evening
  ○ Practice good toilet hygiene: correct wiping, skin care, changing wet linens and clothing
  ○ Use correct toilet posture: sit comfortably with hips slightly abducted and feet and buttocks well supported
  ○ Void with relaxation; have child take a deep breath and relax the sphincter when exhaling; can use a straw to breathe through
  ○ Void to completion; teach child to use Credé maneuver or manual pressure over suprapubic area to complete voiding
  ○ Double void (void shortly after one voiding session, or stay on toilet for a few minutes and void again)
- Treatment expectations and timeline for treatment

- Nonneurogenic neurogenic bladder (Hinman syndrome)
- Vesicoureteral reflux
- Trauma or abuse
- Urethritis (may be caused by chemicals in soaps, bubble baths)

Management

The goal of management is to prevent or break the cycle of urinary dysfunction and its complications. Intervention includes the following:
- Treat any UTI if present (see Chapter 34).
- Treat constipation if present. This may eliminate the entire problem, but can take months to adequately correct (see Encopresis). Parents must be aware of the possible need for long-term treatment.
- First-line treatment should involve behavioral "urotherapy" including:
  ○ Education of child and family of the urodynamics of dysfunctional voiding (Box 12-5)
  ○ A structured regimen of timed voiding (Allen et al, 2007) to "retrain" the bladder (see Box 12-5)
  ○ Treatment of pelvic floor dysfunction, if appropriate (e.g., increasing awareness of pelvic floor muscle function and using biofeedback). Urotherapy combined with biofeedback has been shown to be more effective than urotherapy alone (Kibar et al, 2010).

- Second-line treatment combines urotherapy with pharmacotherapeutics. The ICCS has noted, "Currently there are no approved pharmacological therapies to our knowledge for dysfunctional voiding in children..." and use of medications is "an off-label method" (Chase et al, 2010, p 1301). Anticholinergics are used if an overactive bladder is present, but have no effect on underactive detrusor function. Of the anticholinergics, oxybutynin chloride is not recommended for use in children younger than 5 years old. Tolterodine has been used effectively and with fewer side effects than oxybutynin in children with detrusor instability (Kilic et al, 2006). For the child with a refractory overactive bladder, a combination of oxybutynin and tolterodine or solifenacin may be effective (Bolduc et al, 2009), and for children who do not respond to oxybutynin or tolterodine, solifenacin alone has shown success (Bolduc et al, 2010). Botulinum-A toxin to inhibit acetylcholine release and alpha-blockers to relax the smooth muscles of the external urethra have also been used, again, off-label. Such use of botulinum-A toxin in children is investigational (Chase et al, 2010).
- Teach parents or child to perform intermittent catheterization if appropriate. Self-catheterization has been effective in decreasing dysfunctional voiding and promoting continence (Pohl et al, 2002).
- Treat skin breakdown if present.

Patient Education and Prevention

Effective toilet training can prevent urinary retention, especially if children learn to be sensitive and responsive to cues to urinate. Parents should be instructed to be alert to signs of dysuria. If urination is painful, children often struggle to retain urine or void incompletely. Early treatment for UTIs is essential to prevent renal dysfunction.

ENURESIS
Description

Enuresis is defined as voluntary or involuntary urination into bed or clothes at an age when toilet training should be complete. Children who have never established control have primary enuresis. Secondary enuresis is present when children have been dry for more than 6 to 12 months and begin wetting. Nocturnal enuresis, also called monosymptomatic nocturnal enuresis (MNE), is incontinence during sleep. Diurnal enuresis, daytime wetting, occurs during waking hours. There is no consensus on what frequency of wetting justifies a diagnosis of enuresis. The *Diagnostic and Statistical Manual of Mental Disorders, 4th Edition* (DSM-IV) specifies two wet nights per week, and the International Classification of Diseases (ICD) specifies one night per month as the threshold for enuresis. Parents may ask for help if their child has as few as one to three wet nights per month, a number that some use as a standard for "cure or full response to therapy" (van Gool, 2002).

Epidemiology

The age at which urinary continence is normally achieved varies greatly. As a result, the prevalence of enuresis is difficult to assess. Generally enuresis is not considered to be

| BOX 12-6 | Voiding Frequency and Volume Chart |

		Days							
Measure for 2 to 3 Days	**Measure for 1 Week**	**1**	**2**	**3**	**4**	**5**	**6**	**7**	**Comments**
Intake									
Voided volume	Voided in toilet (#)								
	Wet during day (#)								
	Wet during sleep (#)								
	Quality of urination (check if present):								
	Weak stream?								
	Interrupted stream?								
	Urgency?								
	Dribbling?								
	Wets a little, wakes and stops?								
	Bowel movements (#)								
	Bowel movements (quality)								

outside the range of normal limits before 5 to 6 years old. Boys are more likely to have nocturnal enuresis than girls, and African-American children have a greater incidence of enuresis than Caucasian children. Approximately 7% of 5-year-old boys and 3% of 5-year-old girls have enuresis; 3% of 10-year-old boys and 2% of 10-year-old girls. At 18 years old, 1% of boys have enuresis, but it is rarely seen in girls (Boris and Dalton, 2007b). Although the numbers of children with enuresis decrease with age (suggesting that most children "grow out" of the problem), for those who continue, the problem can be severe. In one large study, nearly half of the affected 19-year-olds were wet seven nights a week (Yeung et al, 2006).

The cause of enuresis varies among children and can be difficult to determine. A number of factors have been found to be associated with enuresis, including the following:

- Familial disposition. Chromosomal studies suggest a genetic linkage for enuresis, with genes probably located on chromosomes 12 and 13 (Elder, 2007) but the exact placement is unclear (Schaumburg et al, 2008). It is estimated that 77% of children with enuresis have two parents with a history of enuresis; 50% of children have one parent with a history of enuresis; and for 15% of children with enuresis, neither parent has a history of enuresis.
- Neurological developmental delay (von Gontard et al, 2006).
- Behavioral comorbidities (e.g., externalizing behaviors) (Zink et al, 2008). There appears to be a high association between enuresis and attention-deficit/hyperactivity disorder (ADHD) (Shreeram et al, 2009).
- Small bladder capacity. A bladder capacity of 300 to 350 mL is necessary for a child to sleep through the night without incontinence. In some children bladder capacity appears normal during the day, but is functionally reduced at night (Yeung et al, 2002).
- Sleep disorders. Obstructive sleep apnea and disordered sleep patterns are associated with increased incidence of nocturnal enuresis (Barone et al, 2009; Dhondt et al, 2009; Nevéus, 2009). Preliminary studies indicate a possible connection with sleep-related breathing disorders and facial patterns (Carotenuto et al, 2011), and obstructive sleep apnea-hypopnea syndrome (Yue et al, 2009) leading to nocturnal polyuria.

- Stress and family disruptions, such as a divorce, move, or a new member.
- Detrusor instability, in which the child has learned to inhibit sphincter relaxation and prevent complete emptying of the bladder, combined with delayed arousal from sleep and polyuria can be a factor in nocturnal enuresis (Chandra et al, 2004).
- Hormonal regulation. Some children with enuresis may have lower levels of antidiuretic hormone (ADH), contributing to nocturnal polyuria (Yue et al, 2009).
- Abnormal circadian rhythm for diuresis, sodium excretion, and glomerular filtration, leading to nocturnal polyuria (De Guchtenaere et al, 2007).
- Chronic constipation or fecal impaction.
- Stress incontinence.
- Inappropriate toilet training, especially when parents are overly demanding or punitive of the child.

Clinical Findings

The goals of assessment are to: (1) determine if there are comorbid or underlying conditions that require referral for further evaluation and/or treatment; and (2) establish the best approach to treating this particular child's condition (Nevéus et al, 2010).

History. Parents should be asked about the following, and use of a bladder function diary that notes frequency and volume may be invaluable (Box 12-6):

- Voiding characteristics (findings marked with an asterisk(*) warrant referral to a pediatric urologist (Nevéus et al, 2010):
  - Urgency, dysuria, or dribbling
  - Retentive behaviors, holding pubis, crossing legs
  - Number of voids per day; nocturia present?
  - Volume voided
  - Frequency of wetting
  - Type of urinary stream: weak? interrupted?*
  - Need to use abdominal pressure to urinate*
  - Daytime incontinence and nocturnal enuresis combined*
- Fluid intake
- UTI
- History of enuresis, treatment, and age of resolution for other family members, including parents
- History of toilet training; age began, how handled. Was child ever dry? For how long?

- Effect of enuresis on child and parents
- Manner in which family deals with the enuresis (e.g., is child punished? Who changes the bed? Any previous medical treatment?)
- Bowel patterns; fecal incontinence? Quality of stool (see Box 12-2)
- Sleep patterns
- General health:
  ○ Prenatal and perinatal history
  ○ Is child tired? Does child have weight loss, excessive thirst or hunger? (e.g., diabetes)
  ○ Has the child been diagnosed with a neuropsychological condition? (e.g., ADHD)
- Presence of other behavior problems
- Changes in the home, family, or school environment

Physical Examination. The physical examination includes the following:

- Assess the external genitalia for signs of irritation, infection, labial fusion, meatal stenosis.
- Assess for bladder capacity; parents can collect and measure urine over 3 days.
- Observe the size and velocity of the urine stream.
- Check for fecal impaction.
- Examine the abdomen for masses, especially at the suprapubic midline and in the left lower quadrant.
- Examine the lower back for dimples, hair tufts.
- Assess for neurologic function, DTRs.

Laboratory and Diagnostic Tests. A urinalysis, with culture, is recommended in all children with enuresis. More sophisticated testing is usually not necessary, although an US to assess bladder wall thickness may indicate severity of the problem.

Differential Diagnosis

The differential diagnoses include daytime, or extraordinary, urinary frequency, a benign condition of excessive (more than 8 to 12 per day, often as frequent as every 15 to 30 minutes) urination seen in previously toilet-trained children. Daytime urinary frequency syndrome has no known cause, but may be associated with viral cystitis or urethritis, stress, and hypercalciuria. Considered self-limited because it does not typically respond to medication, daytime urinary frequency syndrome can persist for months or even years, but typically lasts about 6 months (Bergmann et al, 2009).

Organic causes of enuresis must be identified. The most common organic cause is a UTI that may be related to encopresis. A child with enuresis should be examined for fecal impaction and a history of soiling. Other organic causes to consider are listed below. Worsening incontinence, development of neurological signs (e.g., weakness in legs), and increased urine volumes or dilution warrant referral to specialists for further evaluation.

- Diabetes mellitus
- Diabetes insipidus
- Sickle cell disease, in which treatment by means of forced fluids may lead to increased urine output
- Chronic renal failure, in which the kidneys are unable to concentrate urine
- Structural anomalies such as vesicoureteral reflux, ectopic ureter (constant leakage is noted)
- Neurological abnormalities, including neurogenic bladder
- Hypercalciuria

- Obstructive uropathy
- Vaginitis
- Sleep apnea

Management

A thorough examination to distinguish between organic and nonorganic causes is the first crucial step. Treatment is then based on the underlying cause and involves behavioral modification, medication, treatment of comorbid or organic conditions, or a combination of these modalities. The goals of treatment are to establish normal bladder function and prevent physical and emotional or psychological complications. Outcomes of treatment are categorized as full response (greater than 90% reduction in wet nights), partial response (50% to 90% reduction in wet nights), or no response (less than 50% reduction in wet nights). A cure is a full response that continues 6 months or longer after treatment has ended (van Gool, 2002). Referral to a pediatric urology specialist may be necessary.

Because functional enuresis is largely self-limited, there is consensus to delay aggressive treatment until the child is 6 to 8 years old. Treatment strategies for children 6 years old or older include the following:

- *Enuresis alarm.* Use of an enuresis alarm is effective in about two thirds of cases (Glazener et al, 2005) and is a first choice for therapy. Behavioral modification results when an electric alarm with a bell or buzzer is triggered as the child begins to wet. Reflexively, urination stops and the child must then use the toilet. Initially, children may not rouse, and parents must take them to the toilet, even though the child may not be fully awake. Wet bed linens and pajamas are then changed and the alarm is reset. Subsequently, as the alarm is triggered and the child is roused, the child learns to associate a full bladder and the beginning of urination with waking and toileting. Once the child has achieved 2 consecutive weeks of dryness, the alarm is used every other night. If the child remains dry for another month, the alarm can be discontinued. After an initial 2 weeks without wetting, the effect of alarm therapy is reinforced if the child "overlearns" (is given extra fluids 1 hour before bedtime) and has "dry bed training" (is taken to toilet repeatedly and changes his or her own sheets if they get wet). Use of alarms takes longer than medication to have an effect (on average, 12 weeks, but can be as long as 6 months), but has no serious side effects, and shows a significantly lower relapse rate over time than treatment with medication (Glazener et al, 2005). Low functional bladder capacity and difficulty arousing the child have been found to limit the success of alarms (Butler and Robinson, 2002). Some children, especially older children, may object to continued use, others may relapse without the external stimulus, and parents must be committed to getting up with the child for up to 3 months of treatment.
- *Bladder control training (urotherapy).* Because many children with enuresis have low functional bladder capacities, the goal of urotherapy is to increase children's awareness of the need to urinate and to give them more control of the urination process. Establishing a regular voiding schedule is imperative (see Box 12-5); children should void before going to bed and again immediately upon waking in the morning. Urotherapy involves increasing daytime urination by encouraging children to urinate on schedule and not waiting until the micturition urge is felt. Urotherapy trains

children through visualization exercises to imagine what it feels like to have the urge to urinate and encourages them to practice urinating. Proper posture (sitting upright, feet on floor; standing erect) while urinating is important to be more sensitive to cues of a full bladder and to control urination. This approach has been used effectively for children with diurnal incontinence (Mulders et al, 2011).

- *Motivational therapy.* This strategy assumes that children will take responsibility for the problem and for learning how to resolve it. The family is expected to provide supportive reinforcement for positive behavior such as use of a "star chart," rewards, and praise. Children are taught to be increasingly sensitive to their body's cues to urinate, encouraged to void in the toilet, and reinforced, either emotionally, materially, or both, for success. This therapy is emotionally time-consuming and requires a high level of healthy communication between parents and children. Provider support of both parents and children is essential, and the provider should see children every 2 weeks.
- *Drug therapy.* Drug therapy (Table 12-3 lists dosing and comments) is second-line therapy and not curative. It is often used in conjunction with other strategies and usually has high initial success rates. Unfortunately, it can be expensive and high relapse rates can occur when the drug is discontinued. However, it can be very useful for overnight stays (e.g., camp) when staying dry is important to the child. Medications used for children with MNE include antidiuretic analogs (desmopressin), muscarinic acetylcholine receptor blockers (oxybutynin, tolterodine, solifenacin), and tricyclic antidepressants (imipramine). Medications used for adults may be found to have pediatric application as well, including botulinum toxin and alpha-adrenergic blockers (Duel, 2009), but are not approved for treatment of enuresis. An exploratory study indicates that ibuprofen (12.5 mg/kg in the experimental group studied) may be useful in treating MNE (Gelotte et al, 2009).

Children taking medications on a regular basis should have a drug "holiday" every 3 to 6 months to assess the need for continued pharmacotherapy. If wetting recurs, medication can be continued at the effective dosage for another 3 to 6 months. After 1 month without wetting, medications can be tapered over a 2- to 4-week period, decreasing the dose (e.g., from 0.6 to 0.4 mg/day of desmopressin), decreasing dosing by 1 day a week, then to every other day.

Desmopressin has an antidiuretic effect and appears to be most effective in children with large nocturnal urine production and normal nocturnal bladder capacity. Its effect is immediate and the drug can be taken only on nights the child wants to be sure to stay dry (Nevéus et al, 2010). A combination of desmopressin and alarm therapy appears to be effective (Vogt et al, 2010), especially for children with nocturnal polyuria (Kamperis et al, 2008); and a recent study indicates desmopressin may be as effective as alarm therapy alone (Evans et al, 2011). Desmopressin has also been used in combination with anticholinergics with success (Austin et al, 2008). There is a high relapse rate associated with short-term therapy, but long-term oral therapy has been found to be safe and effective (Lottmann et al, 2009). Desmopressin nasal spray has led to hyponatremia, has a black box warning from the U.S. Food and Drug Administration (FDA), and is not recommended for routine use (Robson, 2009). Controlled studies suggest, however, that if properly administered, there may be few side effects. Providers must be certain that the appropriate dose is prescribed. Patients should be cautioned to avoid high fluid intake with the medication, to be sure that the correct dosage is given, and to discontinue the medication if headache, nausea, or vomiting occurs (Robson et al, 2007; Van de Walle et al, 2010).

Oxybutynin chloride is an anticholinergic drug that relaxes the smooth muscle of the bladder, allows increased urine retention, and reduces frequency. It is sometimes used in conjunction with desmopressin, and it appears to be most effective as a treatment for MNE if the child also has daytime incontinence (Robson and Leung, 2006). Anticholinergic

---

TABLE 12-3 Drug Therapy for Children with Monosymptomatic Nocturnal Enuresis

Medication	Dosing	Comments
Desmopressin acetate	Oral: one 0.2-mg tab once daily at bedtime; can be adjusted up to maximum of 0.6 mg/day If effective, continue use for 3 to 6 months then taper	Effective in children with nocturnal polyuria and normal bladder volume Not recommended in children younger than 6 years Nasal spray not recommended Caution must be used with patients who are hypertensive or have a potential for fluid-electrolyte imbalance (e.g., children with cystic fibrosis susceptible to hyponatremia). Use least amount effective. Try lower dose for 1 week before increasing if child is still wetting. Take on empty stomach; avoid caffeine, chocolate, aspartame, and carbonated beverages. Children must be wakened to urinate within 10 hours of taking the medication.
Oxybutynin chloride, immediate or extended release	5 mg once daily at bedtime; increase as tolerated or needed to achieve dryness in 5-mg increments to maximum of 20 mg daily	Effective in children with daytime enuresis. Use least amount effective. Not recommended in children younger than 6 years of age. Extended release form must be swallowed whole without chewing, crushing, or breaking capsule.

drugs are indicated in children only if standard treatment fails, take effect after about 2 months, and require the provider to be sure the child has no postvoid residual urine that could contribute to UTI (Nevéus et al, 2010).

Imipramine is a tricyclic antidepressant whose action related to enuresis is not entirely clear. Because of serious side effects, most significantly cardiac death, high failure rate when the drug is discontinued, and a low long-term response rate, imipramine is not considered a first-line medication and is not used by most providers. It should not be used in children less than 5 years old. The ICCS recommends use of imipramine only in select cases when other treatment has been ineffective and only as therapy in tertiary treatment centers (Nevéus et al, 2010); daily dosage should not exceed 2.5 mg/kg (Long, 2010).

A "full-spectrum" treatment plan, combining alarms, behavioral and motivational therapy, and medication is highly effective (Van Kampen et al, 2009). Successful treatment has been correlated to age, motivation, and family functioning and requires committed involvement of both parents and children. Families should be active in deciding what treatment is most appropriate and when it should be implemented.

Nontraditional or experimental measures have also been used to treat enuresis. Hypnosis, self-hypnosis, and acupuncture may have promise, but require more clinical research (Gold et al, 2007; Jindal et al, 2008; Libonate et al, 2008). Although not yet approved for use in pediatrics, sacral nerve stimulation may be appropriate for children with severe voiding dysfunction that has not responded to aggressive medical or behavioral treatment (Humphreys et al, 2006; Roth et al, 2008).

Complications

Enuresis contributes to poor self-esteem and disrupted family interactions and threatens the child's ability to establish strong peer relationships. Parents of children with nocturnal and diurnal enuresis rate those children as having more problem behaviors than do parents of children without enuresis; these parents also rate their own stress level as higher (De Bruyne et al, 2009). Effective treatment improves behavior and self-concept, suggesting that enuresis precedes behavior problems (Rocha et al, 2008).

Patient Education and Prevention

Supportive education of parents and positive reinforcement of children's efforts can help prevent enuresis. For 3- to 5-year-old children, a nonjudgmental attitude of "benign neglect" in the face of accidents is the best approach. For older children with enuresis, aggressive long-term interventions are appropriate; wetting is a common phenomenon, and parents should be reassured that it rarely indicates disease. Dealing with a child who wets frequently can be frustrating, however, and parents need to know that the provider is committed to working closely with them until the child is dry.

13

Physical Activity and Sports for Children and Adolescents

MAXINE FOOKSON AND CATHERINE G. BLOSSER

"Regular physical activity is essential for health and quality of life."

Physical Activity Collaborative, 2008, p 1

The importance of physical activity during infancy, childhood, and adolescence cannot be overstated. Maintaining a healthy level of activity in combination with eating a healthy diet are the two most important factors in preventing chronic disease (USDHHS, 2008a). And yet, nationally and internationally, populations fail to meet recommended physical activity goals at all ages. Research has revealed that the medical costs in the U.S. due to factors directly resulting from lack of physical activity are more than $188 billion per year (Physical Activity Collaborative, 2008).

This chapter gives health care providers (HCPs) the information and tools necessary to promote physical activity in the clinical setting and to become advocates in the larger public health arena to champion the importance of physical activity in the lives of youth. The chapter covers physical activity guidelines, recommendations for all age ranges and abilities, the preparticipation examination, and medical concerns and conditions specific to the student athlete that need to be considered before recommending the most healthy and safe sport.

■ Physical Activity: Definition and Surveillance Data

According to the Centers for Disease Control and Prevention (CDC):

"Physical activity is defined as any bodily movement produced by skeletal muscles that results in energy expenditure. The energy expenditure can be measured in kilocalories. Physical activity in daily life can be categorized into occupational, sports,

household, or other activities. Exercise is a subset of physical activity that is planned, structured, and repetitive and has as a final or an intermediate objective the improvement or maintenance of physical fitness" (Thompson et al, 2003, p 3109).

Because maintenance of physical activity is such an important health behavior, it is one of the topics monitored in the CDC's biannual Youth Risk Behavior Surveillance System (YRBSS) (Eaton et al, 2010). The YRBSS monitors health risk behaviors of high school youth, grades 9 through 12; data are collected every 2 years. None of the YRBSS data show that physical activity goals set by *Healthy People 2010* (USDHHS, 2008b) are being met in terms of:

- High school students doing any kind of physical activity that increased heart rates more than usual for 60 or more minutes per day at least 5 days per week
- Attending school physical education (PE) class at least 1 to 5 days in a school week
- Percentages of middle or junior high schools or high schools requiring daily PE

Further data analysis reveals that:

- Physical activity rates decreased for all students as they progressed through high school (i.e., rates of physical activity were highest for ninth graders and decreased through twelfth grade). This was true in 2007 and 2009 (Eaton et al, 2010).
- Attendance in a PE class was higher for males than for females (USDHHS, 2008b).
- In 1969, approximately 42% of American children walked or cycled to and from school, compared with only about 16% in 2001 and about 14% in 2008. Concern with vehicular speed and other safety issues were cited by parents as reasons they discouraged such active transportation by their children, even when they lived within less than two miles of the school (U.S. Department of Transportation [USDOT], 2008, 2010).

- Between 2003 and 2009 there was a significant linear rise in the amount of recreational computer/video game hours; between 1999 and 2009, there was a significant linear decrease in television time (Eaton et al, 2010).
- Between 2007 and 2009, there have been no statistically significant increases in physical activity behaviors; females remain less likely to have been physically active than males (Eaton et al, 2010).

Physical activity rates are also decreasing across the globe, with 60% of the world's population failing to meet the minimal physical activity recommendations required to promote health (World Health Organization [WHO], 2010a). In developing and developed nations urban poverty, concern about crime, structural barriers in the environment (e.g., lack of safe recreational areas, high traffic density, overcrowding), increase in sedentary jobs, increased reliance on passive forms of transportation, and poor air quality contribute to inactivity. The WHO concludes that this lack of physical activity is a contributing factor to the major health problems caused by noncommunicable diseases in many nations (WHO, 2009, 2010a).

■ Promoting Physical Activity: Guidelines and Standards

Each of the following guidelines addresses physical activity from a somewhat different viewpoint. All the guidelines and recommendations are complementary to one another.

2008 *PHYSICAL ACTIVITY GUIDELINES FOR AMERICANS*

The 2008 *Physical Activity Guidelines for Americans* (USD-HHS, 2008a) provide specific clinical recommendations that address and promote physical activity and are applicable for ages 6 and older. Recommendations include:

- Children and adolescents should strive for 60 minutes of physical activity daily; the minutes do not necessarily need to be contiguous.
- Physical activity should be of moderate to vigorous levels.
- Physical activity should include each of the following on 3 or more days per week:
  - Aerobic activity for cardiovascular and respiratory fitness
  - Resistance activities for muscular strength
  - Weight loading for bone strength
- Physical activity should be enjoyable to the child/adolescent and developmentally appropriate.
- In becoming more physically active, a child or adolescent who was previously inactive should increase time and intensity gradually.
- Any level of physical activity is better than none at all.

A full summary of the guidelines and other online resources can be accessed over the Internet. (See Resource list.)

HEALTHY PEOPLE 2010 AND *2020*

Healthy People 2010 and the newer *Healthy People 2020* are broad-based collaborative efforts to address 10 high-priority public health issues; physical activity is one of these indicators. The wording of the *Healthy People 2020* document refers

clinicians to the 2008 *Physical Activity Guidelines for Americans* for specific clinical intervention recommendations. The following objectives relate to physical activity and fitness in children/adolescents (USDHHS, 2009):

1. Increase the proportion of the nation's public and private schools that require daily physical education for all students.
2. Increase the proportion of adolescents who spend at least 50% of school physical education class time being physically active.
3. Increase the proportion of the nation's public and private schools that provide access to their physical activity spaces and facilities for all persons outside of normal school hours (that is, before and after the school day, on weekends, and during summer and other vacations).
4. Increase the proportion of adolescents that meet current physical activity guidelines for aerobic and for muscle-strengthening activity.
5. Increase the proportion of children and adolescents who meet the guidelines for television viewing and computer use.
6. (Developmental objective) Increase the proportion of trips made by walking.
7. (Developmental objective) Increase the proportion of trips made by bicycle.
8. Increase the proportion of states and school districts that require regularly scheduled elementary school recess (new objective for 2020) (the 2008 *Physical Activity Guidelines for Americans* recommend a minimum of 20 minutes per day recess in addition to PE class while in school).
9. Increase the proportion of physician office visits for chronic health diseases or conditions that include counseling or education related to exercise (new objective for 2020).

AMERICAN ACADEMY OF PEDIATRICS GUIDELINES

The American Academy of Pediatrics (AAP) endorses the 2008 *Physical Activity Guidelines for Americans*. The organization's own policy statement includes the following recommendations (AAP, 2010a):

1. Physicians and health care professionals should participate with schools in implementing and setting goals to develop wellness policies for healthy nutrition, physical activity, and other strategies that promote wellness of students.
2. Advocate for school curricula that emphasize the health benefits of regular physical activity and for recreational programs that promote the use of community and school facilities after hours by children and youth at reasonable costs.
3. Advocate for the reinstatement of compulsory, quality, daily PE classes for K through 12 that are enjoyable and help students develop attitudes and skills for lifelong active lifestyles; maintain school recess, and promote extracurricular physical activity programs before and after school hours.
4. Promote recreational facilities, parks, playgrounds, bicycle and walking paths, sidewalks, and marked crosswalks.
5. Providers should inquire about nutritional intake, plot body mass index (BMI), promote healthy eating and physical activity, and note and discuss the limitation of sedentary activities.

6. Encourage a culture of family physical activity by advocating that parents act as role models, incorporate physical activity in to their own lives, and support their children in age-appropriate sports and recreational activities.

7. Suggest that overweight children initially participate in activities that place less stress on weight-bearing joints, such as swimming, water polo, strength training, and cycling.

■ Health Benefits of Physical Activity

Activity patterns become long-term lifestyle habits that either promote or compromise the health of the individual in the future. Physical activity promotes physical health as well as motor and cognitive development and psychological well-being, and is essential for optimal functioning of body systems.

In a literature review, Strong and colleagues (2005) reviewed the health benefits of physical activity for children and adolescents. Most of the studies reviewed were based on the benefits achieved by moderate to vigorous physical activity for 30 to 45 minutes per day on 3 to 5 days per week. The authors concluded that for the average child or adolescent not involved in such intensity of exercise, more time in intermittent or less rigorous physical activity would be required in order to achieve the same benefits. Their findings are the basis for some of the provisions in the 2008 *Physical Activity Guidelines for Americans*. The physical and psychological benefits of physical activity include:

- Prevention of overweight and obesity (reduced body fat) For obese youth, moderate to vigorous physical activity done at a minimum of 3 days per week for a minimum of 30 minutes' duration each session, reduces adiposity
- Improved cardiovascular health, including increased endurance and improved aerobic capacity
- Reduced risk of metabolic syndrome (type 2 diabetes)
- Improved muscular strength and endurance
- Improved skeletal health including increased bone mineral content and bone mineral density
- Improved general self-concept
- Reduction in depression and anxiety symptoms
- Improved academic performance (measured in better grades, higher standardized test scores, better memory and concentration)

Newer studies have demonstrated that increased aerobic fitness in children is correlated with larger basal ganglia in the brain. This helps maintain attention and better coordinate actions and thoughts ("executive function"); the greater hippocampal volumes lead to enhanced cognitive control (Chaddock et al, 2010).

HEALTH CONDITIONS BENEFITING FROM PHYSICAL ACTIVITY

For some individuals, regular physical activity is an even more crucial component of preventing and treating chronic health problems. The following highlight the major findings of the effect and benefits of physical activity on several important health conditions.

- *Obesity.* Inadequate physical activity and energy-dense, nutrient-poor foods are the largest contributors to the staggering rise in childhood obesity rates, not just in the U.S.,

but internationally. Although reduction of obesity is a national health goal as stated in *Healthy People 2010* and *2020*, little progress has been made to reduce that epidemic (see Chapter 10 for a discussion on obesity).

The increase in global chronic disease rates caused by poor diet and inactivity is a major public health concern of the WHO, which reports that more than 42 million children younger than 5 years are obese (WHO, 2010b). In 2004, the WHO developed a population-wide global strategy on diet, physical activity, and health and later published a framework for member countries to implement and monitor their progress to increase physical activity (WHO, 2004). The U.S. has the highest rate of obesity in males 15 years and older of all member WHO countries (WHO, 2010c).

○ Obesity in childhood or adolescence greatly increases the risk that the person will remain obese as an adult. A study in England showed that the propensity to gain weight was related to lower self-esteem in childhood. This weight gain was more likely to occur in children who felt less in control of their lives and who worried (Ternouth et al, 2009). Studies have also demonstrated that a lower body satisfaction in adolescents is related to lower physical activity and more hours of TV watching (Neumark-Sztainer et al, 2004).

- *Hypertension.* For hypertensive youth, regular aerobic activity helps reduce blood pressure. Studies have shown that the most beneficial type of activity to lower blood pressure is aerobic exercise at a level that improves one's aerobic fitness for a minimum of 30 minutes, 3 days per week. Resistance training coupled with aerobic exercise has also been shown to be beneficial in terms of maintaining blood pressure within the normal range once the hypertension is resolved (AAP, 2010a; Strong et al, 2005).

- *Metabolic syndrome.* For individuals with metabolic syndrome, engaging in moderate to vigorous regular physical activity has the positive effects of increasing high-density lipoproteins (HDLs) and reducing triglycerides and insulin levels. Exercise has not been shown to reduce total cholesterol or low-density lipoproteins (LDLs). In the studies reviewed by Strong and colleagues, 40 minutes of moderate to vigorous exercise on 5 days of the week is required to have measurable effects on reducing lipids and insulin level (Strong et al, 2005).

- *Reactive airway disease.* Children with asthma who do regular aerobic physical activity have been shown to experience improved aerobic and anaerobic fitness. There is no evidence that physical activity improves pulmonary function status (Pianosi and Davis, 2004).

- *Special needs children.* Children and youth with disabilities require special focus in order to ensure that they have access to the means to be physically active and at levels that offer health benefits. Due to higher levels of physical inactivity, youth with physical disabilities experience poorer cardiovascular health, lower levels of muscular endurance and higher obesity levels than do children without disabilities (Murphy et al, 2008). Benefits of physical activity for children and adolescents with disabilities are physiological and psychological—improved self-esteem, greater independence, and improved social skills. Recommendations for providers to promote physical activities for children having special needs include (Murphy et al, 2008):

○ Being aware that participation in sports and being physically active is important for children with disabilities

TABLE 13-1	Socioecological Model for Effective Promotion of Physical Activity by Providers
Level of Intervention	**Examples**
Individual Level Address physical activity during patient visits.	• Discuss physical activity recommendations as anticipatory guidance during well-child examinations and as part of healthy lifestyle counseling in obesity prevention and treatment. ○ Assess physical activity level as "vital sign" at all patient visits. • Use motivational interviewing techniques in patient visits to address and promote behavioral change for increasing physical activity. Base intervention on "stages of change" theory as a collaborative patient/provider model. See Chapter 9 for a discussion of these techniques.

Organizational Level
Promote activities on an institutional level that encourage physical activity.
	• Promote activities that encourage organizational physical activity promotion, for example:
	  ○ School programs such as walk or bike to school days
	  ○ Screen time awareness week
	  ○ Intramural programs
	  ○ Advising child care centers about ways to increase physical activity for children and staff
	  ○ Advising schools and parents about importance of recess and physical education
	  ○ Encouraging schools to *not* withhold recess as a punishment for misbehavior

Community Level
Encourage local projects that promote physical activity.
	• Promote activities that help communities structure public space and promote physical activity.
	  ○ Ensure safe and easily accessible park and playground space.
	  ○ Ensure affordable organized activities (e.g., scholarships to pay for team sports or after-school activities for low-income youth).
	  ○ Advocate for bike lanes and walking trails in the community.
	  ○ Advocate for vehicular speed control along major routes to schools to encourage walking/cycling safety (see CDC, Kids Walk-to-School website).
	  ○ Promote programs that teach bike safety and distribute low-cost helmets.
	  ○ Advocate for keeping school buildings open after school for supervised physical activities.

Public Policy Level
Involve public bodies (e.g., school boards, local/state government) to ensure laws and policies promote physical activity.
	• Advocate for changes in public policy by:
	  ○ Addressing hearings on importance of maintaining physical education in schools
	  ○ Addressing zoning issues to maintain or increase green spaces such as parks, bike trails, walking trails
	  ○ Working with planners to ensure that communities are designed to promote family friendly physical activity (e.g., adequate sidewalks and crosswalks, residential areas within waking distance to neighborhood schools, adequate lighting at playfields and parks)

CDC, Centers for Disease Control and Prevention.

○ Performing preparticipation examinations to identify the individual's strengths as well as areas where adaptation is required
○ Communicating with PE teachers, coaches, and trainers to ensure that adaptations are available
○ Being aware of resources for youth and families that advocate for sports inclusion for children with special health care needs

Strategies to Support Physical Activity for Children and Adolescents

MOTIVATION AND BARRIERS TO MAINTAINING PHYSICAL ACTIVITY

A number of factors affect an individual's motivation to become and/or maintain a physically active lifestyle. Physical activity, like any behavior, operates on a socioecological model. Table 13-1 describes the different levels of influence a clinician can engage in to promote physical activity. The effect

of socioeconomics, race/ethnicity, and culture is important to be aware of in order to effectively and equitably address the barriers and resources for physical activity (Brennan Ramirez et al, 2008). A midcourse review of *Healthy People 2010* (USDHHS, 2006) describes some local, state, and federal level community health approaches (and the extent of their effectiveness) to decreasing disparities.

Can Health Care Providers Influence Lifestyle Behaviors?

Kant and Miner's study showed that 51% of adolescents with a BMI equal to or greater than 95% were counseled by their providers (only 17% with a BMI between 85% and 95% were similarly counseled). In the group that received counseling, dietary changes were made by the youth, but they did not make changes in their physical activity levels (Kant and Miner, 2007). Another study found that exercise and restricting intake were preferred methods of weight loss after receiving counseling (Klein et al, 2006).

Surveys have also reported that physicians doubt their ability to influence lifestyle behaviors, feel they lack formal education needed to counsel effectively, and are not reimbursed for this time-consuming endeavor (Howe et al, 2010; Sesselberg et al, 2010). Although the most recent U.S. Preventive Services Task Force (USPSTF) review concluded that the "evidence is insufficient to recommend for or against behavioral counseling in primary care settings to promote physical activity" (USPSTF, 2002, p 2), others believe that counseling about the health benefits of physical activity is an efficacious use of time and produces results (AAP, 2010b). The *MyActivity Pyramid for Kids* is a distinctive and fun handout for engaging children and adolescents in efforts to increase their activity levels (see University of Missouri Extension website).

Familiarity with the theories of James Prochaska and Carlo DiClemente about change, motivation, and motivational interviewing will provide practitioners with clinical skills to collaboratively work with patients to support behavioral change. See Chapter 9 for a discussion regarding techniques for motivational interviewing.

COUNSELING FAMILIES ABOUT ORGANIZED SPORTS FOR THEIR CHILDREN

Being physically active is best achieved as a lifelong habit when it is encouraged from infancy. Guidance to parents and other caregivers is important so that youth can benefit and thrive from athletic endeavors without experiencing psychological or physical harm.

More and more, organized sports are taking the place of children's casual and informal play times (AAP, 2007a). It is now more common to see preschool sports training and teams. When done in an age or developmentally appropriate manner, these activities allow children to benefit from the safety of coaching, proper equipment use and playing facilities, and adult guidance.

Table 13-2 provides guidance for a developmentally appropriate approach to sports activities. The following are some basic concepts to keep in mind when counseling parents, guardians, and youth about athletic participation (AAP, 2007a):

- Regardless of age, the goals of sports participation should be to have fun, to develop skills, and to form a foundation for lifelong fitness.
  - The clinician should always be alert for youth athletes who appear to be stressed or pressured by adults (parents, coaches) to achieve a certain level of competition. Explore motivation for participation because there may be pressure to perform in order to get recognized by professional scouts, receive athletic scholarships, or make a varsity team. One study (Savage et al, 2009) showed that perceived encouragement from fathers (but not mothers) for physical activity was a significant factor in mid-adolescence.
- For the young child entering sports (preschool through school-age), the goals should be healthy activity, learning basic skills, and rules of the game. The skills of several children of the same age can be widely discrepant.
  - Up to the age of puberty, any organized athletic activities should complement rather than replace less structured physical activity that focuses on fun and playfulness (e.g., free play, "pick up" games, and school PE).
  - In general, preschool children have limited attention spans and can be distractible. It is advised that structured exercise sessions be short (no longer than 15 to 20 minutes), that there be 30 minutes of free play, and that activities be playful, creative, and allow exploration of movement (AAP, 2007a).
- About 7 years old children are generally ready for organized noncontact sports, but involvement should be guided by the individual child's cognitive and motor development and interest. It is important to keep the focus on participation rather than on winning.
  - Even with team sports for young children (up through about the age of 10 years), it is advisable to maintain enthusiasm through noncompetitive means (praise, fun experiences, team and leadership building activities). Such things as score-keeping, trophies for performance, awards for "best player," although well intentioned, may be detrimental to positive self-esteem and one's future interest in sports for this age group.
  - Clinicians are in an excellent position to be sure parents and coaches for the younger child understand the developmental level of this age group.
- About age 10, children become more ready to master complex skills such as rules and strategies for competitive sports. It should always be a goal to keep the focus on skill development, personal improvement, and individual positive strides, rather than on competition, embarrassment, or unnecessary regimentation or stress.
- The child who is an exceptional athlete may still have maturation difficulties in social and psychological areas. Finding a balance in supporting the development of an athletically gifted child can be difficult given the stress this child may face in the competitive arena.
- Parents and coaches should always role model best athletic practices for injury prevention and sportsmanship (e.g., wear bicycle helmets when riding with their children, pre- and postgame handshakes with opposing team members).
- Children with handicaps should be encouraged to participate in sports that best fit their abilities and that are safe.
- Children with academic problems should not be denied participation in sports. Studies have concluded that an increase in PE time at school does not negatively affect academics (CDC, 2010a). Sports can be the best arena for boosting self-esteem for the child who does not experience success in the classroom. Helping the child find a balance between academic work and sports participation is essential.
- Boys and girls can play together, especially in the prepubertal years. Differences in height and weight can make it unsafe for smaller girls to compete in contact sports with boys after puberty.
- Children should not focus on sports specialization until puberty (Brenner, 2007). Prior to that age, it is recommended that children play varied sports, enabling them to maintain their energy and interest for a longer time.
- Sports specialization at a young age and/or overtraining can cause overuse injuries (microtrauma damage to bone, muscle, or tendons that occurs from repetitive overuse without sufficient rest and healing time) and/or "burnout" (symptoms include repeated overuse and other injuries, general fatigue, psychological stress, and decreased athletic performance; participation becomes a chore; and a lack of joy and enthusiasm are expressed) (Metzl, 2003; Smith and Link, 2010).

TABLE 13-2 Appropriate Fitness Activities by Age Group

Age Group	Strengths/Development Factors	Fitness Activities	Family Fitness Fun
Infant-toddler	<ul><li>Enjoys playing with family and others</li><li>Enjoys moving</li><li>Enjoys playing with objects</li><li>Is curious and explores environment</li><li>Moves in new ways when challenged with interesting activities</li><li>Mastering basic motor milestones</li></ul>	<ul><li>5 minutes of "tummy time" for young infants; provide safe spaces to crawl, roll, pull, stand, cruise, climb, walk, run, and explore.</li><li>Place objects slightly out of reach.</li></ul>	<ul><li>Walking, playing, running</li><li>Avoid overuse of strollers and walkers</li><li>Play "patty-cake," "peek-a-boo"</li></ul>
2 to 3 years	<ul><li>Participates in and enjoys many physical activities</li><li>Enjoys playing with family and others</li><li>Fundamental skills developing: throwing, catching, running, jumping, skipping, hopping, balancing, self-confidence</li></ul>	<ul><li>Unstructured play that focuses on participation, not competition: hopping, running, dancing, tumbling, throwing, rolling, swinging, climbing, playing in sandbox, supervised water play, tumbling, tag, going down toddler-sized slides, chasing bubbles, digging in soil.</li><li>Most children are not ready for organized or competitive sports.</li></ul>	<ul><li>Walking, playing, and running in the backyard</li></ul>
4 to 5 years	<ul><li>Mastering more complex motor activities—running, jumping, skipping, throwing, climbing, kicking, balancing</li><li>Enjoys sharing activities with parents</li></ul>	<ul><li>Roll large balls, play catch, ride bike with training wheels away from traffic, swimming, dancing, jumping rope, skiing, skating, hopscotch, Frisbee, walking, kickball.</li><li>Judgment, safety awareness, and coordination skills are limited.</li><li>Enroll in swimming lessons.</li><li>Encourage activities needing short bursts of energy within an hour per day to help reduce or prevent excessive weight gain.</li></ul>	<ul><li>Walking, playing, running, tennis, skiing, dancing, scavenger hunts, supervised water play, ice-skating, hiking, bike riding</li><li>Emphasize variety over one particular activity</li></ul>
6 to 12 years	<ul><li>Participates in and enjoys many physical activities</li><li>Develops a positive attitude toward physical activity</li><li>Wants to improve motor skills</li><li>Is developing a sense of responsibility for own health</li><li>Has positive role models for physical activity</li><li>Has opportunities for participation in physical activities; activities should be fun and for the purpose of building skills rather than muscles</li><li>5-6 years: mastering fundamentals of skilled movements</li><li>7-9 years: refining skills such as distance throwing and accuracy</li><li>10-11 years: beginning complex skills (e.g., basketball); integrating cognitive skills with motor skills for sports (e.g., rules, strategy, team roles)</li></ul>	<ul><li>Abilities developed sufficiently for participation in organized sports; balance and postural control reached.</li><li>Noncompetitive sports include swimming, cycling, netball, gymnastics, dance, and martial arts.</li><li>Competitive sports: netball, baseball, tennis, table tennis, soccer.</li><li>Avoid sports specialization until >10 years.</li><li>Strength training at age 7 or older (with supervision) helps build muscles to minimize later injury. Examples include push-ups and sit-ups/crunches; can use elastic bands, weight machines designed for children, dumbbells.</li><li>Monitor eating disorders for those in gymnastics, wrestling, or dance.</li><li>Number of pitches should be limited (80 per game or 200 per week); proper training, preseason conditioning, and throwing mechanics are crucial.</li><li>Continue with strength-training program as long as supervised and employs full-range, multi-joint exercise two or three times weekly with 6 to 15 repetitions per set, no more than three sets.</li></ul>	<ul><li>Walking, bike riding, camping, hiking, tennis, skiing, dancing, ice-skating, swimming</li><li>Counsel against use of trampolines</li></ul>

Continued

TABLE 13-2	Appropriate Fitness Activities by Age Group—cont'd		
Age Group	**Strengths/Development Factors**	**Fitness Activities**	**Family Fitness Fun**
13 to 18 years	• Participates in physical activities • Enjoys physical activities • Wants to improve skills but still feels competent • Takes responsibility for own health • Has positive role models for physical activity • Mastering complex skills for some sports or recreational activities	• Any activity, including competitive sports, skateboarding, inline skating, power walking, rock climbing, snowboarding, rowing, weight training (with supervision), running. • Strength training especially good for females younger than 16 years to increase bone mineral density. • Exercise at least 60 minutes, three times a week.	• Walking, cycling, camping, hiking, tennis, skiing, dancing, ice-skating, swimming

Data from American Academy of Pediatrics, Committee of Sports Medicine and Fitness: Policy statement: risk of injury from baseball and softball in children, *Pediatrics* 107(4):782-784, 2001; Faigenbaum AD, Micheli LJ, for American College of Sports Medicine: Current comments, report on youth strength training, *Sports Med Bull* 32(2):28, 2007. Available at www.acsm.org/AM/Template.cfm?Section=Current_Comments1&;Template=/CM/ContentDisplay.cfm&ContentID=8657 (accessed Nov 28, 2010); Gunner KB, Atkinson PM, Nichols J, et al: Health promotion strategies to encourage physical activity in infants, toddlers, and preschoolers, *J Pediatr Health Care* 19:253-258, 2005.

• Suggestions for preventing overtraining and burnout (Brenner, 2007) include:
  ○ Keep practices interesting, varied, and fun.
  ○ Take 1 or 2 days a week off from organized activity, allowing the body to rest (okay for the athlete to do recreational physical activity if desired on the days off).
  ○ Schedule breaks from training every 2 to 3 months (after a season is completed). During this time the athlete can cross-train or participate in other physical activity to stay in shape.
  ○ Discourage competing in multiple sports during the same season.
  ○ Adhere to sport-specific guidelines (e.g., number of pitches per game for baseball/softball, safe increases in distance training for runners).

STRENGTH TRAINING

Strength training refers to the use of resistance methods (such as free weights, weight machines, elastic bands, or body's weight) to increase muscular strength and endurance. Strength training can be used for several reasons: to enhance performance in a particular sport, as a component of rehabilitation after some injuries, and, for some, to enhance muscle mass for appearance.

The safety of strength training for children and young adolescents had been questioned in the past due to possible detrimental effects of such training on immature skeletons. The concern was that the lack of sufficient circulating androgens (needed for muscular strength and mass) could lead to damage of open growth plates, causing premature closure of epiphyses (Young and Metzi, 2010). However, more current consensus is that strength training is advantageous, even for young athletes, provided that it is done in a safe and supervised manner (AAP, 2008a; Faigenbaum and Micheli, 2007). Strength training must be differentiated from weight training, weight lifting, powerlifting, or bodybuilding, which are still not recommended for prepubescent children and young adolescents due to concerns of safety on immature skeletons (AAP, 2008a; Young and Metzi, 2010).

Benefits of strength training include improved cardiovascular fitness, strength, flexibility, body composition, bone mineral density, blood lipid profile, and mental health. Additionally, strength training is an important component to weight management programs because it produces metabolic rate increases without having to do high-impact activities (AAP, 2008a). Additionally, as a component of a well-rounded conditioning program, it has been shown to reduce blood pressure in hypertensive youth; when included in the preseason conditioning and training program for many sports, it correlates with a decrease in sports injuries (Young and Metzi, 2010).

Strength training for young athletes needs to be supervised; there are fewer injuries from strength training than from the sports themselves (notably lower back strains). Box 13-1 lists general guidelines for strength training by the preadolescent.

Restrictions on who can safely do strength training include youth with severe hypertension; anyone who is receiving chemotherapy with anthracyclines or any other potentially cardiotoxic medication; youth with some forms of cardiomyopathy (particularly hypertrophic cardiomyopathy); individuals with moderate to severe pulmonary hypertension (at risk for acute decompensation with a sudden change in hemodynamics); and those with Marfan syndrome with a dilated aortic root. Youth with seizure disorders should be withheld from strength training programs until clearance is obtained from a neurologist (AAP, 2008a).

PRESEASON CONDITIONING AND INJURY PREVENTION

A variety of strategies can be used to reduce the incidence and severity of injuries and heat-related illnesses and dehydration (see also Chapter 39). Some of the more typical injury conditions that can be avoided with simple prevention strategies are included in Table 13-3. Readiness can be addressed from two perspectives, developmental readiness and preseason conditioning readiness. Developmental readiness has been previously discussed.

BOX 13-1	Safe Practices for Strength Training for Youth Athletes

- Children who are ready to play in organized sports (e.g., Little League baseball, soccer) are ready to participate in some form of strength-related activity, even if it consists of only push-ups and sit-ups for young children.
- Strength training should be only one component of a well-rounded fitness program.
- Prior to starting a formal strength training program, the child should ideally have a physical examination, especially if he or she has any known or suspected health condition.
- Athletes and families should be advised of the dangers of using performance-enhancing drugs to increase strength and muscle mass.
- Training should be done under the supervision of a coach or trainer who is familiar with the appropriate training regimens for different age groups and knowledgeable about the equipment and its use.
  - Training should be progressive—start at zero or low weight with few repetitions; when able to perform sets of 6 to 15 repetitions

with ease, gradually increase weight increments by 5% to 10%. Avoid maximal lift weight and powerlifting until Tanner stage 5 has been reached to avoid potential injury to long bones, growth plates, and back (Hatfield, 2010).
  - Begin with one set each of upper and lower body exercises to allow focus on major muscle groups.
  - Train no more than two or three times a week, on nonconsecutive days to allow for recovery and to produce the greatest gains in strength building.
  - Emphasize proper technique and safety rather than amount of weight lifted.
- Exercises should be balanced among all muscle groups, including core muscles.
- Ensure adequate fluid intake during training.
- All training sessions should begin and end with a period of warm-up/cool-down exercises that include stretching and dynamic movement, such as a slow jog, jumping, or skipping.

Data from American Academy of Pediatrics, Committee on Sports Medicine and Fitness: Policy statement: strength training by children and adolescents, *Pediatrics* 121(4):835-840, 2008a; Faigenbaum AD, Micheli LJ: *Preseason conditioning for young athletes*, 2000. Available at www.acsm.org/AM/Template.cfm?Section=Search&;SECTION=Updated_single_page&CONTENTID=8685&TEMPLATE=/CM/ContentDisplay.cfm (accessed Aug 26, 2010); Hatfield D: *Strength training for children: a review of research literature.* Available at www.protraineronline.com/post/jun1_01/children.cfm (accessed Aug 26, 2010); Young WK, Metzi, JD: Strength training for the young athlete, *Pediatr Ann* 39(5):293-299, 2010.

Preseason conditioning (examples: preparatory muscle conditioning and plyometric training [exercises that combine strength with speed of movement to enhance power, such as hops and jumps; the central nervous system becomes conditioned to react quickly to stretching and shortening]) is a method for decreasing overall injuries. One study showed a 51% decrease in knee and ankle injury incidence and the severity of injuries due to conditioning (Olsen et al, 2005). Conditioning also lessens overuse injuries (stress fractures, bursitis, tendinopathies) and the amount of time needed for rehabilitation, helps strengthen bone, facilitates weight control, enables the nervous system to react more quickly to the stretch-shortening cycle, improves balance and coordination, adds muscle mass, and improves performance. When started in players as young as 10 to 12 years old, warm-up programs help them establish overall motion patterns. Such conditioning is not sport specific, but entails activities geared toward improving strength, flexibility, and endurance; it is not to be confused with weight lifting or bodybuilding. Coaches and fitness instructors should be certified and be knowledgeable about age-specific training techniques and safety; adult training techniques should never be applied to children.

Use of Helmets for Cycling and Winter Sports

More children and adolescents visit emergency departments for cycling injuries than for any other recreational activity (U.S. Consumer Product Safety Commission [USCPSC], 2006). Two thirds of all brain injury fatalities result from such incidences (American Association of Neurological Surgeons, 2010). Ninety-one percent of bicyclists who died in a crash were not wearing a helmet (Insurance Institute for Highway Safety, 2008). Despite preventing approximately 85% of head injuries and 88% of brain trauma, only 45% of children 5 to 14 years old reported wearing a helmet in states with helmet laws, whereas 39% did so in states without such laws (Safe

Kids USA, 2004; USCPSC, 2006). Valuable information about bike safety for children is available from the National Highway Traffic Safety Administration. Proper use starts with proper fitting.
- Try on several sizes and models to find the best fit that:
  - Places the helmet low on the forehead
  - Positions the brim so that it is parallel to the ground when the head is upright (child should be able to see the brim when looking up). This may require removing or installing inside pads to enable a snug fit, or adjusting sizing ring
  - Securely fastens the chin strap to the point where the helmet will not shift over the eyes, rock side to side, or come off when the child shakes the head
- Helmets should carry a USCPSC sticker.
- A helmet should be thrown away if it has been involved in any substantial blow that resulted in marks on the outer surface; do not purchase secondhand helmets.
- Replace helmets every 5 years or sooner, depending on the manufacturer's recommendations.
- Children are more likely to wear helmets if a parental rule exists about its unconditional use, if parents wear helmets during cycling activities, and if there is a mandatory state helmet law, although these usually only apply to children younger than 16 years.

The efficacy of helmet use for young recreational skiers is controversial. A USCPSC (1999) study estimated that 44% of head injuries (53% for children younger than age 15) and 11 deaths could have been prevented by the use of helmets. The USCPSC study also referred to a Swedish study that found a 50% decrease in head injuries in those using helmets versus those without. Shealy's (2010) study of head injuries on ski slopes, though, found an increase in injuries when a helmet was used. He conjectured that the use of a helmet was seen as a license to ski faster or take chances (like skiing among trees). The helmeted skiers also suffered more serious head injuries than those unhelmeted.

TABLE 13-3 Common Injuries and Prevention Strategies

Medical Condition	Prevention Strategies	Comments
Muscle soreness	• Warm up body temperature before gentle stretching to maintain flexibility. • Start with lighter weights and fewer repetitions when starting a new regimen.	• Soreness should be minor, resulting from microscopic muscle or connective tissue damage; it is a normal result of muscles that are adapting to a new exercise program. • Clinicians should explain this soreness ahead of time so that new exercisers do not use this condition as an excuse to stop their fitness regimen.
Strains and sprains	• Do preseason stretching. • Tape site of previous injury. • Warm up body temperature before stretching. • Maintain playing surfaces. • Use proper footwear. • Limit practice time.	• These injuries are mostly related to pivoting sports, such as basketball, football, volleyball. • Knee braces do not have sufficient scientific evidence to recommend or prescribe them for pediatric athletes. However, their use seems to provide subjective relief, and they are often prescribed clinically. There are four categories of knee braces: sleeves (worn during sports if swelling occurs); prophylactic braces (protection of knee ligaments during contact sports); functional (intended to prevent reinjury after torn knee ligaments; not for prophylaxis); and postoperative or rehabilitative. They should not replace rehabilitation and surgery, if required (Martin and AAP, 2001).
Fractures	• Do strength-conditioning exercises. • Use proper techniques. • Take safety precautions. • Use protective gear that fits well, such as wrist guards.	• These injuries most commonly involve the upper extremities, as when falling on an outstretched hand. Lower-extremity fractures can occur with such sports as soccer.
Stress fractures	• Use soft running and playing surfaces. • Use proper footgear. • Do strengthening exercises. • Stop activity when pain occurs.	
Lacerations/contusions/abrasions	• Protective equipment is essential.	• These injuries are mostly related to baseball (contusion/abrasion), soccer, cycling, and ice hockey (lacerations).
Anterior leg pain syndrome (shin splints)	• Stretch before and after activity. • Pronate and supinate feet while standing. • Use soft playing surface. • Use proper footwear: proper fit, impact-absorbing sole, support for hindfoot. • Avoid sudden increase in activity. • Limit forceful, extensive use of foot flexors.	
Plantar fasciitis	• Use proper footwear (cushioned with fitted heel counters or lifts). • Stretch calf and Achilles tendon. • Do ice massage after event. • Correct biomechanical errors. • Limit hills and speed work; increase soft-surface running.	
Blisters	• Wear socks. • Wear properly fitted shoes. • Use powder, petroleum jelly, or a product such as Second Skin on reddened or at-risk areas.	
Head and neck injuries	• Have appropriate supervision and coaching that teaches proper skills, such as tackling. • Adhere to safety rules of the game. • Strengthen neck muscles. • Use appropriate equipment: helmets, face and mouth gear. • Follow concussion guidelines for return-to-sport after injury (see Table 13-9 and 13-10).	• Greatest risks for these injuries are from cycling, diving, equestrian sports, football, gymnastics, ice hockey, wrestling, trampolines, football, rugby, and cheerleading. • Risks increase with age (Safe Kids Worldwide, 2007).
Eye trauma	• Wear headgear and protective glasses.	• Eye injuries are most commonly related to baseball and ice hockey.

TABLE 13-4	Nutrition Recommendations for Athletes
Nutrient	**Recommendations**
Calories from carbohydrates/fat/protein	• Maintain same as for all people: 55% to 75% carbohydrate, 25% to 30% fat, 15% to 20% protein. • Do not decrease caloric intake during sports season. • May need 1500 to 3000 kcal more than recommended dietary allowance to meet activity requirements. • Allow appropriate vegetarian diets.
Vitamins and minerals	• Same as for all people, unless an increase is medically indicated. • Adolescent girls may need to bring calcium (1200 mg/d) and iron intake up to recommended range. • Do not take salt tablets, as hypernatremia and delayed gastric emptying can result.
Carbohydrates	• 6 to 8 g/kg body weight • Use nutritious foods such as fruits, vegetables, grains, and milk sugars. • Carbohydrate intake during prolonged activity may increase performance. • Carbohydrate intake of 75 g in first 30 min and 100 g every 60 min for 2 hours after performance is recommended to promote muscle glycogen resynthesis and rapid reloading.
Protein supplements	• None needed; hypercalciuria with calcium loss and dehydration can occur if protein intake is too high.
Fluids	• Plain water before, during, and after activity if physicial exertion lasts no more than an hour. • Athletic drinks containing electrolytes may be helpful for endurance athletes, those who sweat heavily, and when exercise lasts 1 hour or more; avoid carbonated drinks (can delay gastric emptying and intestinal absorption). • Fluid every 15 to 20 min (5 oz in those weighing <40 kg; 9 oz for 60 kg; 10 to 12 oz if >60 kg) • Replace water loss after activity: 1 liter per kg (16 oz or 0.5 L/lb) of weight lost (determined by prepractice and postpractice weights). • Avoid caffeine drinks because they can increase diuresis.

Data from American Academy of Pediatrics Committee on Nutrition: Guidelines for pediatricians: nutrition and sports, *Sports Shorts*, issue 6, 2001. Available at www.aap.org/sections/sportsmedicine/PDFs/SportsShorts_06.pdf (accessed Sept 16, 2010).

At a speed in the range of 25 to 40 mph, whether one is wearing a helmet or not, a helmet is not viewed by Shealy as providing the protection needed to prevent serious head trauma. Helmets are highly advocated by the National Ski Areas Association and such winter sports programs as Lids on Kids.

Basic Metabolic and Nutritional Needs and Abuses in Athletes

Growing children and adolescents have higher basal metabolic rates than do adults, and they require sufficient caloric intake to both sustain growth as well as to provide energy and nutrients for sports. Youth athletes are also less energy efficient when physically active than adult athletes, thus, their caloric needs are 20% to 30% greater when doing comparable activities (Baker, 2009). Nutrition recommendations are summarized in Table 13-4.

CALORIES

Depending on the sport, calorie requirements for active teenagers exceed baseline needs by 1500 to 3000 calories. The recommended diet for the athlete is the same as for all people. The daily energy and micronutrient requirements for athletes at various ages can be found in Chapter 10.

CARBOHYDRATES

Short-term, high-intensity activities (e.g., high jumping or diving) involve using anaerobic fuel sources, whereas longer-term activities involve use of aerobic sources (e.g., running or cross-country skiing). Carbohydrates are used in both anaerobic and aerobic metabolic states, but fats and proteins are used only aerobically. Complex carbohydrates (e.g., fruits, nuts, cereals, grains, pasta, dried beans) are preferable to simple carbohydrates (such as cookies, sugary foods, ice cream, some crackers). Simple carbohydrates should not exceed 10% of daily carbohydrate intake (Nemet and Eliakim, 2009). Complex carbohydrates, although providing readily available energy, do not cause the rapid rise in blood glucose levels with resultant insulin rebound that simple carbohydrates do. Hypoglycemia can result from insulin excess, which is counterproductive to the energy needed in the sport.

In general, carbohydrates will be most effectively converted into the needed energy if they are consumed several hours before the athletic event or practice. Approximately 300 g of carbohydrate-rich food, 2 to 3 hours prior to exercise is recommended. Ingesting carbohydrates just before activities has no effect on performance. Carbohydrate loading has not been studied in children and is generally not recommended. If an athlete is participating in long-endurance events, carbohydrate loading may be appropriate once or twice during an entire season, and only with the guidance of a coach, trainer, or nutritionist with experience in the age group (Baker, 2009). Carbohydrate intake (30 g/hr) during physical activity lasting more than 1 hour improves performance. After competition, carbohydrate intake is again important to improve muscle glycogen resynthesis, which is most rapid in the first few hours after exercise. During the 2 hours after performance, consuming carbohydrates (approximately 75 g) in the first 30 minutes and 100 g every 60 minutes will achieve this resynthesis. This can be in the form of snacks or liquids.

PROTEIN

Protein provides energy when stored glycogen and fat are depleted during endurance exercise. Amino acid/protein supplements do not increase muscle mass or decrease body fat. Hypercalciuria with calcium loss and dehydration can occur if protein intake is too high because the excess nitrogen, and hence water, is excreted. Additionally, eating too much protein may lead to an underconsumption of adequate carbohydrates and fats, causing the excess protein to be stored as fat.

FATS

Dietary fats serve as high-calorie sources of energy. Emphasis should be on polyunsaturated fats, with saturated fats not exceeding about 10% of the total fat calories. Athletes who are restricting nutritional intake of fats may under-consume them, thus becoming deficient in fat-soluble vitamins (A, D, E, and K).

INTENTIONAL WEIGHT LOSS

Weight loss by adolescent athletes can be a dangerous practice. Wrestlers may try to lose weight to be eligible to compete in a lower weight class; runners sometimes vomit to run lighter; and female gymnasts may practice significant nutritional control to maintain weight and size. Dancers, divers, figure skaters, and cheerleaders also control weight for appearance advantages. Bodybuilders, rowers, distance runners, and swimmers often try to control their weight. Starvation can lead to suppressed growth hormones, can interfere with pubertal gonadal hormone changes, and may result in eating disorders. Nutritional counseling is essential, including a reminder that muscle weighs more than fat, and that during adolescent growth, weight gain is normal.

Wrestlers often engage in repeated bouts of excessive weight loss or weight cycling. Such transient weight cycling can deplete electrolytes, decrease glycogen stores, affect hormones, diminish nutritional status, impair mental and academic performance, reduce immune function, alter hormonal status, and lead to pulmonary emboli and pancreatitis. This temporary weight cycling may adversely affect or alter growth patterns in weight and height and performance (Housh and Johnson, 2007). This practice is to be discouraged because of the risk for long-term dysfunctional eating and short-term effects discussed earlier. Measurements of body composition before and during the wrestling season can help coaches and parents stay alert to risky behavior; any planned weight loss should involve appropriate dietary changes and exercise training. Wrestlers, coaches, and parents may elect to sign a contract requiring that the child eat three meals a day, that fluid be available at all times, and that no artificial means be used to remove fluids from the body (e.g., sauna or sweatsuit, laxatives, diuretics, diet pills, licit or illicit drugs, nicotine, prolonged fasting, over-exercising, or vomiting).

SPORTS DRINKS

Sports drinks are among the most popular supplements used by youth athletes. More than 7 million adolescents in the U.S. are estimated to consume them (Nemet and Eliakim, 2009). Some may contain dangerously high levels of caffeine and should be discouraged. See the discussion later in this chapter about performance-enhancing drugs and "energy drinks." The ingredients in these widely available drinks contain 6% to 8% carbohydrates (glucose, sucrose, and fructose). Some formulations also contain complex carbohydrates (e.g., maltodextrin) and amino acids. Other ingredients maintain fluid electrolyte balance (sodium, potassium, and magnesium). In studies, young athletes have reported positive effects after consuming these drinks at recovery; however, no objective effect on physical performance or recovery has been found. There may be a place for electrolyte replacement drinks in high-endurance athletes. However, there is no sufficient evidence to show that carbohydrates or electrolytes in these beverages are needed in a typically active young athlete who maintains a balanced diet (Nemet and Eliakim, 2009). In addition, for nonathletic youth, sports drinks add a considerable number of unnecessary calories.

■ Health Care for Young Athletes

An estimated 35 million children, adolescents, and young adults participate in some manner of sport, whether organized or recreational. Approximately 7.4 million students in the U.S. participate on an organized sports team (Krajnik et al, 2010). Though relatively safe in children, athletic participation by adolescents becomes more high risk for serious injury. A holistic approach to health care for young athletes involves preventive care (preparticipation physical examination, anticipatory guidance about safe athletic participation, and guidance on any adaptations needed for specific health concerns), care for sports-related injuries, and care for any psychological issues that may arise.

Children with special health care and developmental needs deserve special mention in order to encourage healthy and appropriate sports participation and fitness. Many children and adolescents with intellectual and developmental disabilities (e.g., those with Down, fragile X, Turner or Klinefelter syndromes, autism) are capable of performing exercise or strenuous activities (Pitetti et al, 2009). The goals of physical exercise are to reduce any deconditioning (a result of immobility and prior levels of physical activity), to improve physical functioning, and to improve self-esteem and well-being. These children are at particular risk for obesity, which in turn leaves them susceptible to developing chronic diseases, including heart disease, stroke, hypertension, and diabetes. With regular exercise muscle strength, flexibility, and joint structure and functioning can be better maintained (Murphy et al, 2008). Although the Special Olympics has highlighted global competitive games, the enduring focus has been to educate those with disabilities to make healthy lifestyle choices that will improve their overall long-term health. The Special Olympics provides guides for healthy nutrition; lifestyle choices and ways to increase one's level of physical fitness; sponsors health screening clinics for people with disabilities; and serves as a resource for community professionals to learn about the physical activity opportunities for children with disabilities that will enable them to participate and compete at high levels.

THE PREPARTICIPATION PHYSICAL EXAMINATION FOR SPORTS

For many youth, the preparticipation physical examination (PPE) is their only health assessment for several years. It may serve as an entry into health care and enable the provider to schedule a follow-up visit to address other health risks and concerns. However, because PPEs are not required for many of the recreational activities in which youth engage, there is a recommendation by a consensus group (consisting of sports medicine practitioners and consultants from the American Academy of Family Physicians [AAFP], the AAP, the American College of Sports Medicine [ACSM], the American Medical Society for Sports Medicine, and the American Osteopathic Academy of Sports Medicine) that a PPE serve as an additional opportunity for a well-child examination for *all* children. In this way, health and fitness will be promoted and assessed in all children (Editorial Staff, 2010). Included in this examination should be the use of a health questionnaire that targets certain cardiac health issues and the use of standard PPE forms. The PPE monograph contains the recommended questionnaire, PPE, and clearance forms; they are available for downloading from the AAFP. The complete monograph also contains guidelines for clinicians evaluating children with special needs and the female athlete; it is available for purchase (AAFP, AAP, ACSM et al, 2010).

The PPE historically served as a vehicle to provide liability protection, satisfy insurance regulations, and detect cardiovascular risks for sudden death. Over the years, other objectives have been identified that include the following (DeBerardino and Owens, 2009):

- Evaluating health status, including fitness level
- Detecting injuries, conditions, and illnesses that might limit competition and lead to significant morbidity or mortality and require further evaluation and treatment
- Recommending alternative sports activities, as appropriate, or excluding the person from certain sports
- Identifying lifestyle risk factors and promoting healthy choices
- Documenting an athlete's age, grade-level eligibility, and emotional maturity level
- Collecting medical data for emergencies
- Recommending ways to improve athletic performance
- Interacting with youth on a variety of health-related issues

The American Heart Association (AHA) recommends an initial comprehensive examination and then another PPE every 2 years for high school students with an interim history review in intervening years. The National Collegiate Athletic Association stipulates an initial comprehensive examination on entry into college level athletics, with interim questionnaires done in subsequent years. The AHA recommends both history and examination prior to entry into playing college sports and an interim history and blood pressure in the subsequent 3 to 4 years of college (DeBerardino and Owens, 2009).

Following a comprehensive PPE, an annual "screening" PPE may be requested, such as for high school students. Salient areas to cover include review of the complete health history with special addition to any interval history of syncope, chest pain, hypertensive symptoms, seizures, palpitations, injuries (orthopedic, neurological [concussions], eye), pulmonary and skin conditions, menstrual irregularities, and risky behaviors (including drug use). The physical examination itself should particularly assess cardiac (including checking femoral pulses), neurological, abdominal (palpating spleen, liver, kidneys), and musculoskeletal systems; as well as height, weight, and blood pressure (Chelminski, 2010).

Studies indicate that between 0.3% and 1.3% of athletes are disqualified from participation based on the findings of the PPE. Between 3.2% and 13.9% require further evaluation in order to be cleared (Greydanus and Patel, 2009). The majority of findings that disqualify a potential athlete or that give cause for further evaluation are musculoskeletal, followed by cardiovascular and then neurological complaints (Hergenroeder, 2008). Any positive cardiac findings on the history (personal or family) or on the physical examination warrants a referral for more in-depth cardiac evaluation prior to sports clearance (AAFP, 2010).

Table 13-5 provides recommendations and guidance on safe sports for various medical conditions and can be a useful reference for complex decision-making. In addition, consultation with the appropriate specialist working with the patient's particular health condition may be needed before giving athletic clearance or recommending any specific modification or adaptation to a fitness regimen.

To avoid any malpractice liability, it is important that the PPE be done according to customary and standard practices for this type of examination; all history and physical findings must be fully documented, particularly cardiovascular in cases of sudden death. Should the athlete, athlete's family, or guardian disagree with the provider's advice against participation in a certain chosen sport, the provider needs to obtain the athlete's, parent's, or guardian's signed informed consent statement acknowledging understanding of the advice and potential dangers of participation. Counseling about more appropriate alternative sports should occur and be documented. In addition, the patient and parents should be counseled that (Chelminski, 2010):

- Even though the examination appears to be "normal," data on the exact risks of a known sport are often limited. Providers must exercise their best assessment skills using such data as that provided in this chapter and/or in consultation with a sports medicine specialist.
- Sudden cardiac death is rare.
- Injury (versus medical diseases) is a more common cause of morbidity and mortality; safety and conditioning are paramount for prevention.
- Use of performance-enhancing drugs and sports nutritionals and drinks are potentially dangerous or ineffective.

Ideally the sports physical examination should be an individually scheduled appointment with the child's primary care provider. This allows for the best exchange of personal information and enables follow-up of concerns. Scheduling the examination at least several weeks prior to the beginning of the sports season allows time for any subsequently indicated medical follow-up, consultation, or referral. However, mass screenings are common in many school districts as an efficiency measure or because some youth may not be able to afford the examination or have difficulty getting to an appointment. However, with mass screenings there is a loss of continuity from history to physical examination, lack of privacy for consultation, lack of provider and patient familiarity, and minimal opportunity to use the visit for health-promotion purposes. Communication with parents, coaches, and trainers is essential; they need to be aware of the athlete's health status in case problems arise during participation.

The AAP has classified the most common sports activities into three types: contact and collision, limited contact,

Text continued on p. 234

TABLE 13-5 Medical Conditions and Sports Participation	
Condition	**May Participate**
Atlantoaxial instability (instability of the joint between cervical vertebrae 1 and 2)	
Explanation: Athlete (particularly if he or she has Down syndrome or juvenile rheumatoid arthritis with cervical involvement) needs evaluation to assess the risk of spinal cord injury during sports participation, especially when using a trampoline.	Qualified yes
Bleeding disorder	
Explanation: Athlete needs evaluation.	Qualified yes
Cardiovascular disease	
• Carditis (inflammation of the heart)	No
Explanation: Carditis may result in sudden death with exertion.	
• Hypertension (high blood pressure)	Qualified yes
Explanation: Those with hypertension (>5 mm Hg above the 99th percentile for age, gender, and height) should avoid heavy weightlifting and power lifting, bodybuilding, and high-static component sports. Those with sustained hypertension (>95th percentile for age, gender, and height) need evaluation. The National High Blood Pressure Education Program Working Group report defined prehypertension and stage 1 and stage 2 hypertension in children and adolescents younger than 18 years of age.	
• Congenital heart disease (structural heart defects present at birth)	Qualified yes
Explanation: Consultation with a cardiologist is recommended. Those who have mild forms may participate fully in most cases; those who have moderate or severe forms or who have undergone surgery need evaluation. The 36th Bethesda Conference defined mild, moderate, and severe disease for common cardiac lesions.	
• Dysrhythmia (irregular heart rhythm)	Qualified yes
○ Long-QT syndrome	
○ Malignant ventricular arrhythmias	
○ Symptomatic Wolff-Parkinson-White syndrome	
○ Advanced heart block	
○ Family history of sudden death or previous sudden cardiac event	
○ Implantation of a cardioverter-defibrillator	
Explanation: Consultation with a cardiologist is advised. Those with symptoms (chest pain, syncope, near-syncope, dizziness, shortness of breath, or other symptoms of possible dysrhythmia) or evidence of mitral regurgitation on physical examination need evaluation. All others may participate fully.	
• Heart murmur	Qualified yes
Explanation: If the murmur is innocent (does not indicate heart disease), full participation is permitted. Otherwise, athlete needs evaluation (see structural heart disease, especially hypertrophic cardiomyopathy and mitral valve prolapse).	
• Structural/acquired heart disease	Qualified no
○ Hypertrophic cardiomyopathy	Qualified no
○ Coronary artery anomalies	Qualified no
○ Arrhythmogenic right ventricular cardiomyopathy	Qualified no
○ Acute rheumatic fever with carditis	Qualified no
○ Ehlers-Danlos syndrome, vascular form	Qualified yes
○ Marfan syndrome	Qualified yes
○ Mitral valve prolapse	Qualified yes
○ Anthracycline use	
Explanation: Consultation with a cardiologist is recommended. The 36th Bethesda Conference provided detailed recommendations. Most of these conditions carry a significant risk of sudden cardiac death associated with intense physical exercise. Hypertrophic cardiomyopathy requires thorough and repeated evaluations, because disease may change manifestations during later adolescence. Marfan syndrome with an aortic aneurysm also can cause sudden death during intense physical exercise. An athlete who has ever received chemotherapy with anthracyclines may be at increased risk of cardiac problems because of the cardiotoxic effects of the medications, and resistance training in this population should be approached with caution; strength training that avoids isometric contractions may be permitted. Athlete needs evaluation.	
• Vasculitis/vascular disease	Qualified yes
○ Kawasaki disease (coronary artery vasculitis)	
○ Pulmonary hypertension	
Explanation: Consultation with a cardiologist is recommended. Athlete needs individual evaluation to assess risk on the basis of disease activity, pathologic changes, and medical regimen.	

TABLE 13-5	Medical Conditions and Sports Participation—cont'd	
Condition		**May Participate**

Cerebral palsy

Explanation: Athlete needs evaluation to assess functional capacity to perform sports-specific activity.

Qualified yes

Diabetes mellitus

Explanation: All sports can be played with proper attention and appropriate adjustments to diet (particularly carbohydrate intake), blood glucose concentrations, hydration, and insulin therapy. Blood glucose concentrations should be monitored before exercise, every 30 min during continuous exercise, 15 min after completion of exercise, and at bedtime.

Yes

Diarrhea, infectious

Explanation: Unless symptoms are mild and athlete is fully hydrated, no participation is permitted, because diarrhea may increase risk of dehydration and heat illness (see fever).

Qualified no

Eating disorders

Explanation: Athlete with an eating disorder needs medical and psychiatric assessment before participation.

Qualified yes

Eyes

- Functionally 1-eyed athlete
- Loss of an eye
- Detached retina or family history of retinal detachment at young age
- High myopia
- Connective tissue disorder, such as Marfan or Stickler syndrome
- Previous intraocular eye surgery or serious eye injury

  Explanation: A functionally 1-eyed athlete is defined as having best-corrected visual acuity worse than 20/40 in the poorer-seeing eye. Such an athlete would suffer significant disability if the better eye were seriously injured, as would an athlete with loss of an eye. Specifically, boxing and full-contact martial arts are not recommended for functionally 1-eyed athletes, because eye protection is impractical and/or not permitted. Some athletes who previously underwent intraocular eye surgery or had a serious eye injury may have increased risk of injury because of weakened eye tissue. Availability of eye guards approved by the American Society for Testing and Materials and other protective equipment may allow participation in most sports, but this must be judged on an individual basis.
- Conjunctivitis, infectious

  Explanation: Athlete with active infectious conjunctivitis should be excluded from swimming.

Qualified yes

Qualified no

Fever

Explanation: Elevated core temperature may be indicative of a pathologic medical condition (infection or disease) that is often manifest by increased resting metabolism and heart rate. Accordingly, during athlete's usual exercise regimen, the presence of fever can result in greater heat storage, decreased heat tolerance, increased risk of heat illness, increased cardiopulmonary effort, reduced maximal exercise capacity, and increased risk of hypotension because of altered vascular tone and dehydration. On rare occasions, fever may accompany myocarditis or other conditions that may make usual exercise dangerous.

No

Gastrointestinal

- Malabsorption syndromes (celiac disease or cystic fibrosis)

  Explanation: Athlete needs individual assessment for general malnutrition or specific deficits resulting in coagulation or other defects; with appropriate treatment, these deficits can be treated adequately to permit normal activities.
- Short-bowel syndrome or other disorders requiring specialized nutritional support, including parenteral or enteral nutrition

  Explanation: Athlete needs individual assessment for collision, contact, or limited-contact sports. Presence of central or peripheral, indwelling, venous catheter may require special considerations for activities and emergency preparedness for unexpected trauma to the device(s).

Qualified yes

Qualified yes

Heat illness, history of

Explanation: Because of the likelihood of recurrence, athlete needs individual assessment to determine the presence of predisposing conditions and behaviors and to develop a prevention strategy that includes sufficient acclimatization (to the environment and to exercise intensity and duration), conditioning, hydration, and salt intake, as well as other effective measures to improve heat tolerance and to reduce heat injury risk (such as protective equipment and uniform configurations).

Qualified yes

Continued

TABLE 13-5	Medical Conditions and Sports Participation—cont'd
Condition	**May Participate**
Hepatitis, infectious (primarily hepatitis C) *Explanation*: All athletes should receive hepatitis B vaccination before participation. Because of the apparent minimal risk to others, all sports may be played as athlete's state of health allows. For all athletes, skin lesions should be covered properly, and athletic personnel should use universal precautions when handling blood or body fluids with visible blood.	Yes
HIV infection *Explanation:* Because of the apparent minimal risk to others, all sports may be played as athlete's state of health allows (especially if viral load is undetectable or very low). For all athletes, skin lesions should be covered properly, and athletic personnel should use universal precautions when handling blood or body fluids with visible blood. However, certain sports (such as wrestling and boxing) may create a situation that favors viral transmission (likely bleeding plus skin breaks). If viral load is detectable, then athletes should be advised to avoid such high-contact sports.	Yes
Kidney, absence of one *Explanation*: Athlete needs individual assessment for contact, collision, and limited-contact sports. Protective equipment may reduce risk of injury to the remaining kidney sufficiently to allow participation in most sports, providing such equipment remains in place during activity.	Qualified yes
Liver, enlarged *Explanation*: If the liver is acutely enlarged, then participation should be avoided because of risk of rupture. If the liver is chronically enlarged, then individual assessment is needed before collision, contact, or limited-contact sports are played. Patients with chronic liver disease may have changes in liver function that affect stamina, mental status, coagulation, or nutritional status.	Qualified yes
Malignant neoplasm *Explanation*: Athlete needs individual assessment.	Qualified yes
Musculoskeletal disorders *Explanation*: Athlete needs individual assessment.	Qualified yes
Neurologic disorders • History of serious head or spine trauma or abnormality, including craniotomy, epidural bleeding, subdural hematoma, intracerebral hemorrhage, second-impact syndrome, vascular malformation, and neck fracture. *Explanation*: Athlete needs individual assessment for collision, contact, or limited-contact sports.	Qualified yes
• History of simple concussion (mild traumatic brain injury), multiple simple concussions, and/or complex concussion *Explanation*: Athlete needs individual assessment. Research supports a conservative approach to concussion management, including no athletic participation while symptomatic or when deficits in judgment or cognition are detected, followed by graduated return to full activity.	Qualified yes
• Myopathies *Explanation*: Athlete needs individual assessment.	Qualified yes
• Recurrent headaches *Explanation*: Athlete needs individual assessment.	Yes
• Recurrent plexopathy (burner or stinger) and cervical cord neuropraxia with persistent defects *Explanation*: Athlete needs individual assessment for collision, contact, or limited-contact sports; regaining normal strength is important benchmark for return to play.	Qualified yes
• Seizure disorder, well controlled *Explanation*: Risk of seizure during participation is minimal.	Yes
• Seizure disorder, poorly controlled *Explanation*: Athlete needs individual assessment for collision, contact, or limited-contact sports. The following noncontact sports should be avoided: archery, riflery, swimming, weightlifting, power lifting, strength training, and sports involving heights. In these sports, occurrence of a seizure during activity may pose a risk to self or others.	Qualified yes
Obesity *Explanation*: Because of the increased risk of heat illness and cardiovascular strain, obese athlete particularly needs careful acclimatization (to the environment and to exercise intensity and duration), sufficient hydration, and potential activity and recovery modifications during competition and training.	Yes

TABLE 13-5	Medical Conditions and Sports Participation—cont'd	
Condition		**May Participate**

Organ transplant recipient (and those taking immunosuppressive medications)
Explanation: Athlete needs individual assessment for contact, collision, and limited-contact sports. In addition to potential risk of infections, some medications (e.g., prednisone) may increase tendency for bruising. — Qualified yes

Ovary, absence of one
Explanation: Risk of severe injury to remaining ovary is minimal. — Yes

Pregnancy/postpartum
Explanation: Athlete needs individual assessment. As pregnancy progresses, modifications to usual exercise routines will become necessary. Activities with high risk of falling or abdominal trauma should be avoided. Scuba diving and activities posing risk of altitude sickness should also be avoided during pregnancy. After the birth, physiological and morphologic changes of pregnancy take 4 to 6 weeks to return to baseline. — Qualified yes

Respiratory conditions
- Pulmonary compromise, including cystic fibrosis — Qualified yes
  Explanation: Athlete needs individual assessment but, generally, all sports may be played if oxygenation remains satisfactory during graded exercise test. Athletes with cystic fibrosis need acclimatization and good hydration to reduce risk of heat illness.
- Asthma — Yes
  Explanation: With proper medication and education, only athletes with severe asthma need to modify their participation. For those using inhalers, recommend having a written action plan and using a peak flowmeter daily. Athletes with asthma may encounter risks when scuba diving.
- Acute upper respiratory infection — Qualified yes
  Explanation: Upper respiratory obstruction may affect pulmonary function. Athlete needs individual assessment for all except mild disease (see fever).

Rheumatologic diseases
- Juvenile rheumatoid arthritis — Qualified yes
  Explanation: Athletes with systemic or polyarticular juvenile rheumatoid arthritis and history of cervical spine involvement need radiographs of vertebrae C1 and C2 to assess risk of spinal cord injury. Athletes with systemic or HLA-B27-associated arthritis require cardiovascular assessment for possible cardiac complications during exercise. For those with micrognathia (open bite and exposed teeth), mouth guards are helpful. If uveitis is present, risk of eye damage from trauma is increased; ophthalmologic assessment is recommended. If visually impaired, guidelines for functionally 1-eyed athletes should be followed.
- Juvenile dermatomyositis, idiopathic myositis — Qualified yes
- Systemic lupus erythematosus
- Raynaud phenomenon
  Explanation: Athlete with juvenile dermatomyositis or systemic lupus erythematosus with cardiac involvement requires cardiology assessment before participation. Athletes receiving systemic corticosteroid therapy are at higher risk of osteoporotic fractures and avascular necrosis, which should be assessed before clearance; those receiving immunosuppressive medications are at higher risk of serious infection. Sports activities should be avoided when myositis is active. Rhabdomyolysis during intensive exercise may cause renal injury in athletes with idiopathic myositis and other myopathies. Because of photosensitivity with juvenile dermatomyositis and systemic lupus erythematosus, sun protection is necessary during outdoor activities. With Raynaud phenomenon, exposure to the cold presents risk to hands and feet.

Sickle cell disease
Explanation: Athlete needs individual assessment. In general, if illness status permits, all sports may be played; however, any sport or activity that entails overexertion, overheating, dehydration, or chilling should be avoided. Participation at high altitude, especially when not acclimatized, also poses risk of sickle cell crisis. — Qualified yes

Sickle cell trait
Explanation: Athletes with sickle cell trait generally do not have increased risk of sudden death or other medical problems during athletic participation under normal environmental conditions. However, when high exertional activity is performed under extreme conditions of heat and humidity or increased altitude, such catastrophic complications have occurred rarely. Athletes with sickle cell trait, like all athletes, should be progressively acclimatized to the environment and to the intensity and duration of activities and should be sufficiently hydrated to reduce the risk of exertional heat illness and/or rhabdomyolysis. According to National Institutes of Health management guidelines, sickle cell trait is not a contraindication to participation in competitive athletics, and there is no requirement for screening before participation. More research is needed to assess fully potential risks and benefits of screening athletes for sickle cell trait. — Yes

Continued

TABLE 13-5	Medical Conditions and Sports Participation—cont'd	
Condition		**May Participate**
Skin infections, including herpes simplex, molluscum contagiosum, verrucae (warts), staphylococcal and streptococcal infections (furuncles [boils], carbuncles, impetigo, methicillin-resistant *Staphylococcus aureus* [cellulitis and/or abscesses]), scabies, and tinea *Explanation*: During contagious periods, participation in gymnastics or cheerleading with mats, martial arts, wrestling, or other collision, contact, or limited-contact sports is not allowed.		Qualified yes
Spleen, enlarged *Explanation*: If the spleen is acutely enlarged, then participation should be avoided because of risk of rupture. If the spleen is chronically enlarged, then individual assessment is needed before collision, contact, or limited-contact sports are played.		Qualified yes
Testicle, undescended or absence of one *Explanation*: Certain sports may require a protective cup.		Yes

This table is designed for use by medical and nonmedical personnel. "Needs evaluation" means that a physician with appropriate knowledge and experience should assess the safety of a given sport for an athlete with the listed medical condition. Unless otherwise noted, this need for special consideration is because of variability in the severity of the disease, the risk of injury for the specific sports, or both.

From Rice SG, American Academy of Pediatrics Council on Sports Medicine and Fitness: Medical Conditions Affecting Sports Participation, *Pediatrics* 121(4):841-848, 2008. Copyright American Academy of Pediatrics, 2008. Used with permission.

and noncontact (Box 13-2). The provider can make specific recommendations as to which sports are appropriate for young people with identified health problems using Table 13-5.

Components of the Preparticipation Physical Examination

Health History. The previously mentioned history form, available from the AAFP, is recommended. Generally, the following areas should be included:
- General medical history
- Prior surgeries and any sequelae
- Previous trauma, especially musculoskeletal or central nervous system injuries (notably head injuries)
- Family history of cardiac risk factors, including unexplained drowning or unwitnessed car accidents (these can indicate an undiagnosed heart problem)
- Specific cardiovascular disease questions (Box 13-3)
- Prior heat-intolerance episodes
- Asthma or other allergic reactions
- Loss of function or absence of any paired organs (eye, testes, kidneys)
- Seizure disorder or any other unexplained loss of consciousness
- Infectious mononucleosis
- Skin infection
- Anatomic abnormalities, Down or Marfan syndrome, or history of Marfan syndrome in the family
- Obesity
- Medications including supplement use, herbal remedies
- Immunization status
- Nutritional history—rapid weight changes, dieting, body perception
- In females—menstrual history

When performing the history portion of the PPE, providers should assume a more holistic view about the planned activity by asking about the following:
- The particular sports activity planned
- Extent of participation

- Level of competition
- Training schedule
- Coaching and supervision—is there a team HCP?
- Hazardous playing and field conditions
- Plans for the activity in the future
- Health promotion and preventive strategies planned
- Planned nutrition
- Preparticipation conditioning
- Risk behaviors, such as increased alcohol consumption, driving while intoxicated, lack of seatbelt use; lack of helmet use during extreme recreational sports activities (e.g., inline skating, skateboarding, snowboarding); use of drugs or performance-enhancing substances (including steroids [dehydroepiandrosterone (DHEA), androstenedione], creatine, gamma-hydroxybutyrate [GHB], gamma-hydroxybutyrolactone [GBL], 1,4-butanediol [BD]); smoking; and sexual history
- Family involvement and support (athletes participating in extreme sports who do use protective equipment do so because of parental and peer influence, rules, and requirements [ACSM, 2005])
- Psychological issues
- Stress management during the competitive season
- Measures for success
- Recent life changes
- Strategies to maintain schoolwork

Physical Examination. The physical examination should consist of two parts: the musculoskeletal examination and the general head-to-toe physical examination (see also Chapters 7 and 8), with particular focus on cardiovascular and neurological systems. The 90-second musculoskeletal screening examination is recommended (Fig. 13-1). It is standardized to detect 90% of significant injuries and has 51% sensitivity and 97% specificity (McCarthy, 2006). The examination focuses on musculoskeletal alignment, flexibility, and proprioception, which are effective measures of abnormalities and injury sequelae. Table 13-6 describes the components that should be included for different organ systems, including elements of the cardiovascular examination

BOX 13-2 Classification of Sports According to Contact

Contact	Limited Contact	Noncontact
Basketball	Adventure racing[a]	Badminton
Boxing[b]*	Baseball	Bodybuilding[c]
Cheerleading	Bicycling*	Bowling
Diving	Canoeing or kayaking	Canoeing or
Extreme sports[d]	(whitewater)	kayaking (flat
Field hockey	Fencing	water)
Football, tackle*	Field events	Crew or rowing
Gymnastics*	High jump	Curling
Ice hockey[e]*	Pole vault*	Dance
Lacrosse*	Floor hockey	Field events
Martial arts[f]*	Football, flag or touch	Discus
Rodeo	Handball	Javelin
Rugby*	Horseback riding	Shot-put
Skiing, downhill	Martial arts[f]*	Golf
Ski-jumping	Racquetball	Orienteering[g]
Snowboarding	Skating*	Powerlifting[c]
Soccer*	Ice	Race walking
Team handball	Inline	Riflery
Ultimate frisbee	Roller	Rope jumping
Water polo	Skiing	Running
Wrestling	Cross-country	Sailing
	Water	Scuba diving
	Skateboarding	Swimming
	Softball	Table tennis
	Squash	Tennis
	Volleyball	Track
	Weight lifting	
	Windsurfing or surfing	

*Most hazardous for head and spinal injuries (Cantu RD, Cantu RV: Head injuries. In DeLee JC, Drez D Jr., Miller MD, editors: *DeLee and Drez's orthopaedic sports medicine: principles and practice*, ed 3, Vol. 1, Philadelphia, 2009, Saunders.
[a]Adventure racing has been added since the previous statement was published and is defined as a combination of two or more disciplines, including orienteering and navigation, cross-country running, mountain biking, paddling, and climbing and rope skills.
[b]The American Academy of Pediatrics opposes participation in boxing for children, adolescents, and young adults.
[c]The American Academy of Pediatrics recommends limiting bodybuilding and powerlifting until the adolescent achieves sexual maturity rating 5 (Tanner stage 5).
[d]Extreme sports has been added since the previous statement was published.
[e]The American Academy of Pediatrics recommends limiting the amount of body checking allowed for hockey players 15 years and younger, to reduce injuries.
[f]Martial arts can be subclassified as judo, jujitsu, karate, kung fu, and tae kwon do; some forms are contact sports and others are limited-contact sports.
[g]Orienteering is a race (contest) in which competitors use a map and a compass to find their way through unfamiliar territory.
From Rice SG, American Academy of Pediatrics Council on Sports Medicine and Fitness: Medical conditions affecting sports participation, *Pediatrics* 121(4):841-848, 2008. Used with permission.

(also review Box 13-3). It is important for the provider to include a genital exam. This examination provides information with regard to sexual maturity (Tanner stage or sexual maturity rating [SMR]) and provides an opportunity for counseling about general development. The SMR level may be important in certain sports in which weight and strength are of consideration as the adolescent achieves greater maturity. Adolescents also may have greater muscle mass in comparison with a less mature, but equal weight teen at a lower SMR. In addition, sexually transmitted infections, testicular cancer, and varicoceles are important topics to consider and discuss (McCarthy, 2006).

BOX 13-3 Cardiovascular Screening and Examination for Competitive Athletes on the Preparticipation Physical Examination

Medical History Risk Factors
Personal History
- Exertional chest pain/discomfort
- Unexplained syncope or near-syncope (differentiate between vasovagal; of greater concern if syncope occurs with exertion)
- Excessive exertional and/or unexplained dyspnea or fatigue, associated with exercise
- Prior recognition of a heart murmur or history of congenital heart disease
- History of illnesses with possible cardiac complications (rheumatic fever, Kawasaki infection)
- Elevated systemic blood pressure (see "hypertension" guidelines)

Family History
- Premature death (sudden and unexpected, or otherwise) before age 50 years due to heart disease or other unexplained cause, in any relative
- Disability from heart disease in a close relative less than 50 years of age
- Specific knowledge of certain cardiac conditions in family members: hypertrophic or dilated cardiomyopathy, long QT syndrome or other ion channelopathies, Marfan syndrome, or other clinically important dysrhythmias

Physical Examination Elements Related to Cardiovascular Screening
- Auscultate for heart murmur (auscultate with patient in sitting, lying down and standing positions, or during Valsalva maneuver to detect murmurs of dynamic left ventricular outflow tract obstruction)
- Femoral pulses to exclude aortic coarctation
- Physical stigma of Marfan syndrome
- Check blood pressure (preferably in both arms)

Adapted from Maron BJ, Thompson PD, Ackerman MJ, et al: Recommendations and considerations related to preparticipation screening for cardiovascular abnormalities in competitive athletes: 2007 update: a scientific statement from the American Heart Association Council on Nutrition, Physical Activity, and Metabolism. Endorsed by the American College of Cardiology Foundation, *Circulation* 115(12):1643-1655, 2007. Used with permission of the American Heart Association.

Diagnostic Studies. Although the following can be useful for evaluation of a specific disease, there is no true indication from a health screening perspective to include them in the PPE, unless otherwise indicated:
- Urinalysis: Not recommended. Certain elite amateur or professional organizations may require urine drug screening.
- Hematocrit or hemoglobin are not recommended for males; in adolescent girls, iron deficiency anemia is common enough that it may be appropriate to screen.
- Human immunodeficiency virus (HIV) testing: Encouraged if the athlete has any risk factors. Certain elite amateur or professional organizations may require screening.
- Noninvasive tests such as electrocardiogram (ECG), echocardiogram, or exercise stress tests are not recommended as a universal part of the PPE (AAFP, 2010).
- Test for sickle cell trait in high-risk groups (see following discussion).

• Appropriate for interscholastic, intramural, and extramural sports activities.

• A screening evaluation created to direct attention to problems but not evaluate the problems.

• Identifies the following conditions that might be adversely affected by athletic participation:

a. Congenital problems

b. Acquired problems

Questions such as the following are to be answered by the athlete and signed by BOTH the athlete and parent:
• Have you ever had an illness, condition, or injury that required you to go to the hospital, either as a patient overnight or in the emergency room or for x-rays; required an operation; caused you to see a doctor; caused you to miss a game or practice?

• Are you now or have you been under the care of a physician for any reason?

• Do you currently have any medical problems or injuries?

• Have you ever had a broken bone, joint sprain or ligament tear, muscle pull, head injury, neck injury or nerve pinch, dislocated joint, back trouble or problems?

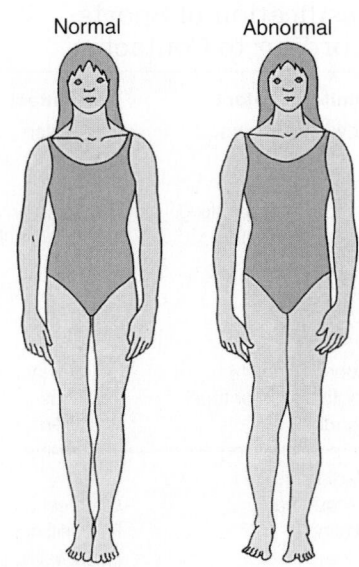

ACTIVITY 1

Normal   Abnormal

Instructions to patient:
"Stand up straight and face me."

What is screened:
Acromioclavicular joints, symmetry of extremities

ACTIVITY 2

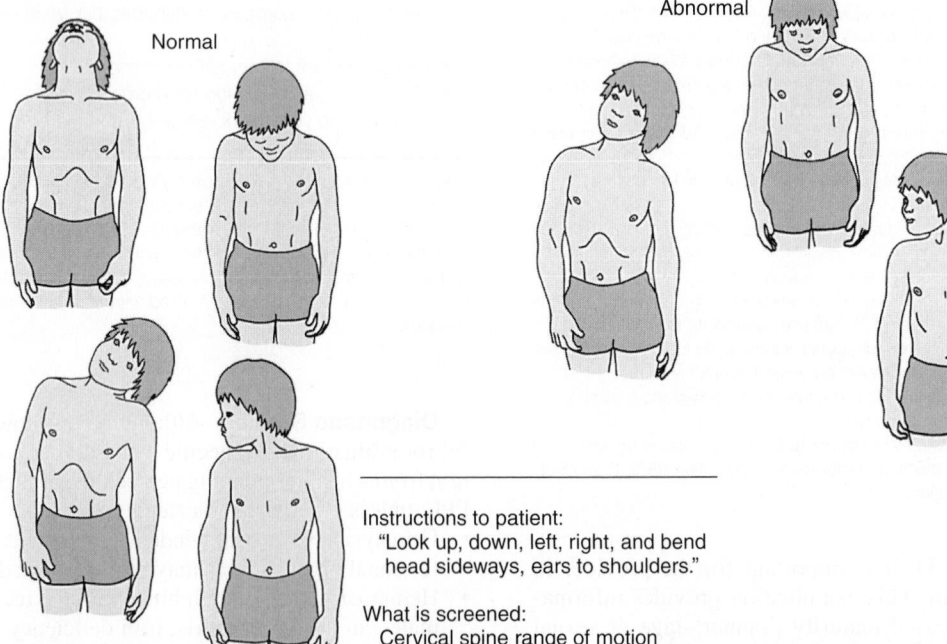

Normal

Abnormal

Instructions to patient:
"Look up, down, left, right, and bend head sideways, ears to shoulders."

What is screened:
Cervical spine range of motion

FIGURE 13-1 Illustration of the 90-second sports musculoskeletal examination (Adapted from Ross Products Division, Abbott Laboratories, Columbus, OH 43216. From *For the practitioner: orthopaedic screening examination for participation sports.* © 1981 Ross Products Division, Abbott Laboratories. Text adapted from Garrich JG: Sports medicine, *Pediatr Clin North Am* 24:737-747, 1977.)

ACTIVITY 3

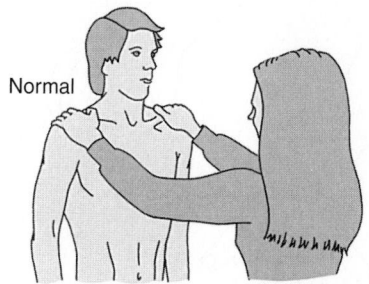

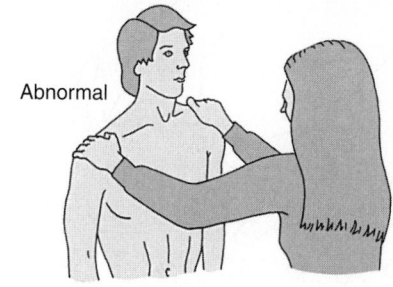

Instructions to patient:
"Shrug your shoulders." (Against resistance by examiner)

What is screened:
Trapezius strength

ACTIVITY 4

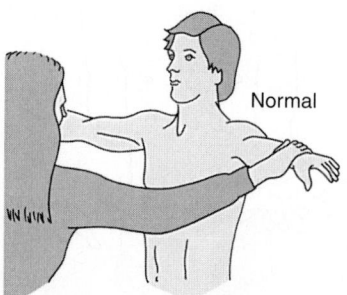

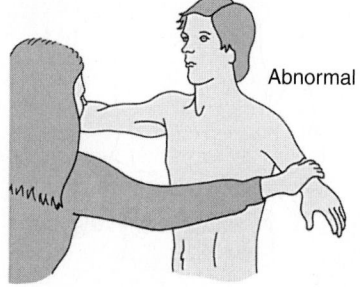

Instructions to patient:
"Hold arms outstretched from your sides and lift them." (Against resistance as examiner pushes down)

What is screened:
Shoulder range of motion

ACTIVITY 5

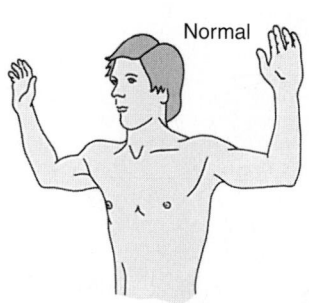

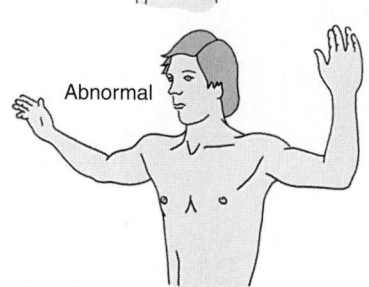

Instructions to patient:
"Raise your elbows at your sides 90 degrees. Rotate your hands backwards."

What is screened:
Deltoid strength
Shoulder rotation

ACTIVITY 6

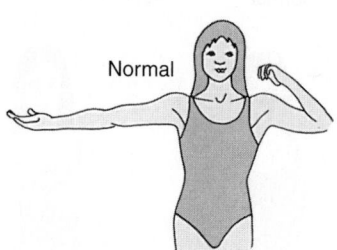

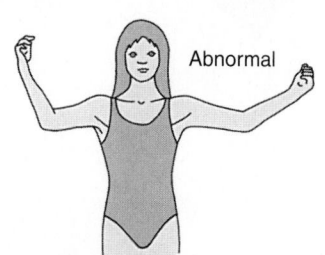

Instructions to patient:
"Hold arms straight out from sides, palms up. Flex and extend your elbows."

What is screened:
Elbow range of motion

Continued

FIGURE 13-1, cont'd

ACTIVITY 7

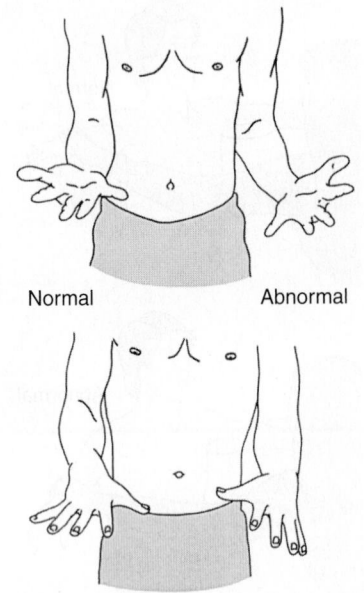

Instructions to patient:
"Let your arms down again. Flex your elbows so that your hands reach straight out. Rotate your wrists, palms facing up, then down."

What is screened:
Wrist range of motion (pronation/supination)

ACTIVITY 8

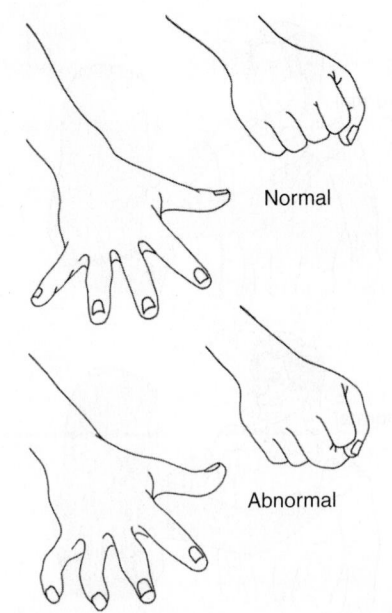

Instructions to patient:
"Show me your hands. Spread your fingers out (examiner resists spreading). Make a fist and squeeze."

What is screened:
Hand/finger range of motion and strength

ACTIVITY 9

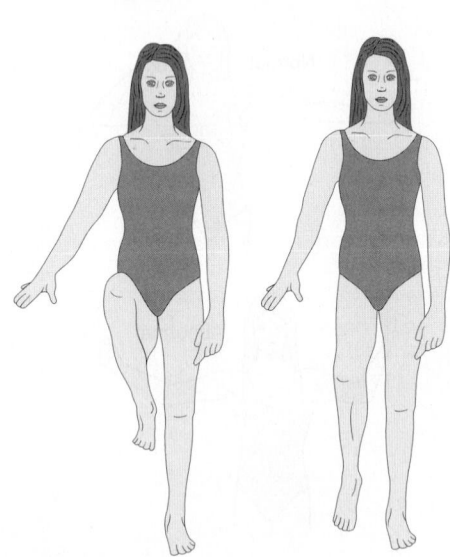

Instructions to patient:
"Lift your right leg up, bent at the knee. Repeat using the other leg."

What is screened:
Leg symmetry, knee or ankle effusion

ACTIVITY 10

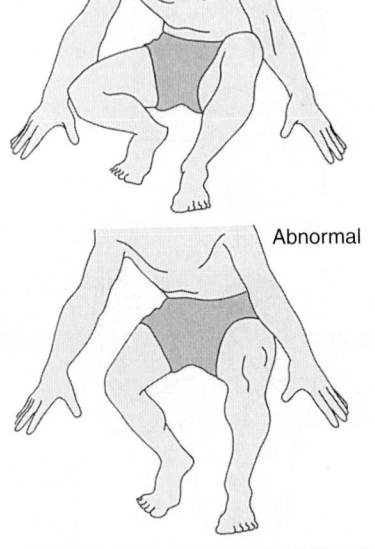

Instructions to patient:
"Squat like a duck, and walk four steps away from me."

What is screened:
Hip, knee, and ankle range of motion

FIGURE 13-1, cont'd Illustration of the 90-second sports musculoskeletal examination.

ACTIVITY 11

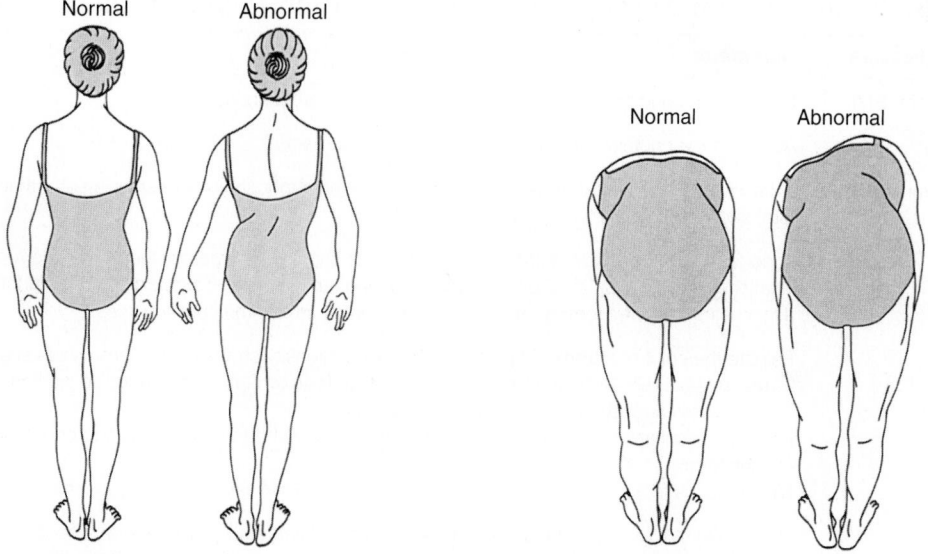

Instructions to patient:
"Stand up straight. Keep your knees as straight as you can, and try to touch your toes. Straighten slowly."

What is screened:
Shoulder symmetry, scoliosis, hip range of motion, hamstring tightness

ACTIVITY 12

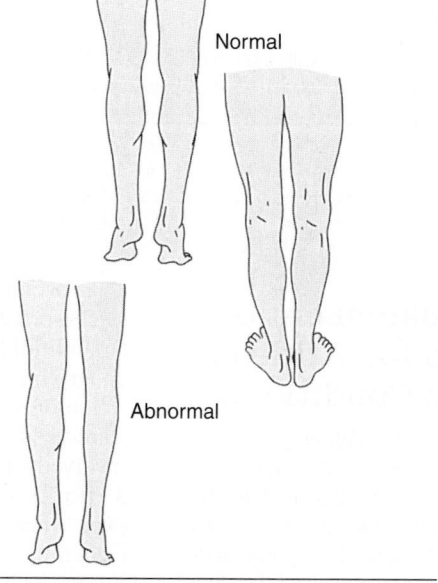

Instructions to patient:
"Stand up on your tiptoes."

What is screened:
Calf symmetry, leg strength

FIGURE 13-1, cont'd

TABLE 13-6　Example of an Appropriate Preparticipation Physical Examination

Examination Feature	Comments
Height and weight; BMI	Establish baseline and monitor for eating disorders, steroid abuse.
Blood pressure	Assess in the context of participant's age, height, and sex.
General appearance	Excessive height and excessive long-bone growth (arachnodactyly, arm span greater than height, pectus excavatum) suggestive of Marfan syndrome.
Eyes	Important to detect vision defects; one of the eyes should have greater than 20/40 corrected vision. Lens subluxations, severe myopia, retinal detachments, and strabismus are associated with Marfan syndrome. Note any anisometropia for the record. Absence of one eye will limit some sport choices.
Cardiovascular (see also Box 13-3)	Palpate the point of maximal impulse for increased intensity and displacement, which suggest hypertrophy and failure, respectively. Note heart rate, rhythm. Check for murmurs. A murmur that worsens with standing or Valsalva maneuver suggests hypertrophic cardiomyopathy. Perform auscultation with the patient supine and again with the patient standing or straining during Valsalva maneuver. Simultaneous femoral and radial pulses; femoral pulse diminishment suggests aortic coarctation.
Respiratory	Observe for accessory muscle use or prolonged expiration, and auscultate for wheezing. Exercise-induced asthma will not produce manifestations on a resting examination and requires exercise testing for diagnosis (refer to Box 13-4 for clinic exercise challenge procedure).
Abdominal	Assess for masses, tenderness, or organomegaly (especially liver and spleen). In females assess for any pain, enlargement over hypogastric area or pelvis that might suggest pregnancy or gynecological problem; proceed with further workup as indicated.
Genitourinary	Hernias and varicoceles do not usually preclude sports participation. Check for single, undescended testicle, masses. Discuss testicular cancer and provide information about the self-testicular exam.
Musculoskeletal	Use the 90-second orthopedic examination (see Fig. 13-1). Consider supplemental shoulder, knee, and ankle examinations as indicated specific to the chosen sport's injury prone areas.
Skin	Evidence of molluscum contagiosum, herpes simplex, impetigo or lesions suggestive of MRSA, tinea corporis, or scabies would temporarily prohibit participation in sports where direct skin-to-skin competitor contact occurs (e.g., wrestling, martial arts).
Neurological	Gross motor assessment with attention to equality of strength, especially with a history of recurrent stingers/burners, head injury. Usually sufficiently grossly assessed during the 90-second musculoskeletal exam.

MRSA, Methicillin-resistant *Staphylococcus aureus.*
Data from American Academy of Family Physicians, American Academy of Pediatrics, American College of Sports Medicine, et al: Preparticipation physical evaluation form, 2010. Available at www.aap.org/sections/sportsmedicine/PDFs/PPE-4-forms.pdf (accessed Sept 16, 2010); DeBerardino TM, Owens BD: The team physician: the preparticipation examination, on-field emergencies, and ethical and legal issues. In DeLee JC, Drez D Jr., Miller MD, editors: *DeLee and Drez's orthopaedic sports medicine: principles and practice,* ed 3, Vol 1, Philadelphia, 2009, Saunders.

■ Evaluation and Management of Sports Participation for Athletes with Specific Health Conditions

Table 13-5 summarizes the AAP's recommendations regarding sports participation for youth with specific health conditions. The clinician's recommendations should be communicated to the youth and their parents and recorded in the student's permanent record; the form should be returned to the school or sports facility. Several high-risk conditions are discussed in the following text in terms of their influence on the clinician's decision-making and for the purposes of counseling and health management.

CHRONIC MEDICAL CONDITIONS

Asthma

Comprehensive management of intermittent and persistent asthma is discussed in Chapter 31. The goal is to achieve adequate asthma control so that the individual can fully participate in recreational or organized competitive sports.

Exercise-Induced Asthma

Description and Epidemiology. Exercise can act as an additional trigger for bronchospasm in individuals with underlying reactive airway disease, or exercise may serve as the only trigger for bronchospasm in some people. Most studies suggest that release of inflammatory mediators is involved in the etiology (USDHHS, 2007). Approximately 8% to 15% of the general population (20% in elite athletes) experience exercise-induced asthma (EIA) (Eichner, 2008). Generally, the prevalence is higher for those participating in cold weather sports (e.g., ice hockey, figure skating, cross-country skiing) when the environment is dry and cold, in comparison to those participating in sports in warmer weather or in warm/humid environments (American Academy of Allergy, Asthma, and Immunology [AAAAI], 2008). Sports with the highest risk of triggering EIA are those that require continuous activity (e.g., basketball, soccer, or long-distance running).

Up to approximately 90% of children with diagnosed asthma may experience EIA symptoms (ACSM, 2008). Conversely, some patients who present with EIA symptoms actually represent undertreated persistent asthma. In one study of 263 potentially asthma-related sports deaths, 61 were actually found to have died from their asthma, and 90% of those athletes had a known diagnosis of asthma; only 5% were on a controller medication (Eichner, 2008).

Two other studies may serve as additional diagnostic nuggets when assessing and managing asthma symptoms: the more overweight the child, the greater the likelihood of developing asthma (Sheerin, 2005), and asthma symptoms worsen and require an increase in bronchodilator use in female athletes when in the midluteal phase of their menstrual cycles (i.e., day 21 of a 28-day cycle) (Stanford et al, 2006).

EIA usually occurs during or minutes after vigorous activity, reaches its peak 5 to 10 minutes after stopping the activity, and resolves after another 20 to 30 minutes. Some reports indicate that there is a refractory period of up to 1 hour after an EIA episode that allows for an asthma symptom-free interval after warm-up exercises (USDHHS, 2007). This period either allows the person to exercise without recurrence or to experience a lessened EIA event.

Diagnostic Studies. Spirometry is the gold standard test for EIA (USDHHS, 2007). History alone is suggestive, but probably underdiagnoses EIA. Box 13-4 explains the procedure for an office-based exercise challenge.

Management. Management includes using both pharmacological and nonpharmacological regimens.

Nonpharmacological management includes (AAAAI, 2008; Homnick, 2009):

- Perform warm-up drills to maintain airway warmth and moisture, just to the point of wheezing; then cool down to an asymptomatic state before vigorous exercise. This can help athletes use the refractory period to resume vigorous exercise without experiencing EIA. Covering the mouth and nose with a scarf or mask when exercising in cold air achieves the same purpose.
- Participate in athletic conditioning to help improve muscle and exercise efficiency.
- Warm down, or gradually decrease exercise at the end of a session. This seems to help decrease the magnitude of the attack.
- Try to exercise indoors during peak allergy, pollen, and air pollution times.
- In the rare event that treatment modalities are not helpful, choose a sport that takes place in warm, humid air or that does not involve continuous activity, such as swimming, water polo, diving, walking, leisure cycling, hiking, free downhill skiing, wrestling; team sports requiring short bursts of energy (baseball, football, wrestling, golf, gymnastics, short-distance track and field).

Pharmacologic management should be considered in a step-wise approach, adding each medication as needed to gain control. Manage underlying asthma appropriately following recommendations discussed in Chapter 31. Additionally, consider adding (USDHHS, 2007; Saglimbeni, 2009):

- A short-acting inhaled β_2-agonist (SABA) 15 to 30 minutes before the sports activity. An SABA will help up to 90% of EIA and duration is up to 3 to 6 hours. Long-acting β-agonist use is discouraged in treating EIA because it may not provide immediate or adequate coverage or its use may disguise persistent asthma that would be better treated with an inhaled steroid.

BOX 13-4 Office Free-Run or Exercise Challenge to Diagnose Exercise-Induced Asthma

1. Get baseline heart rate (HR) and spirometry* (FEV$_1$/FVC).
2. Have patient exercise by running around, doing the usual sport, or running on a treadmill.
   a. Exercise to get HR up to 70% to 80% of maximum predicted HR and maintain for 6 to 10 minutes
3. Repeat postexercise spirometry.
   a. Do readings every 2 to 10 minutes for 15 to 30 minutes; compare with baseline
4. Interpretation of results based on percent reduction in PEF or FEV$_1$ from baseline:
   a. 10% to 20% reduction: mild EIA
   b. 20% to 40% reduction: moderate EIA
   c. >40% reduction: severe EIA

*If spirometry (gold standard) is not available, a handheld peak flowmeter is acceptable to obtain peak expiratory flow rate (PEFR).
EIA, exercise-induced asthma; *FEV$_1$,* forced expiratory volume in 1 second; *FVC,* forced vital capacity; *PEF,* peak expiratory flow.
Data from Saglimbeni AJ: *Exercise-induced asthma: differential diagnoses and workup,* 2009. Available at www.emedicine.medscape.com/article/88849-diagnosis (accessed Nov 28, 2010).

- A leukotriene receptor agonist (montelukast or zafirlukast) daily for incompletely controlled EIA when used with other agents. These medications do not offer immediate action but can help EIA with regular use over time; they are not advised for individuals with intermittent EIA.
- A mast cell stabilizer (inhaled cromolyn or nedocromil) before exercising; the use of cromolyn and an SABA in combination can be helpful in more than 70% to 80% of individuals when administered 30 to 45 minutes preexercise.

Teachers and coaches should be aware of the youth's asthma or EIA. A written school sport management plan should be in place.

Cardiac Conditions

The goal for the primary care provider (PCP) is to recognize athletes who are at risk of significant morbidity or mortality from preexisting cardiac conditions. The degree of maximal oxygen update (dynamic component) as related to the need for increased cardiac output and blood pressure (static component) varies by sport. Additionally, the provider needs to consider the effect of the athlete's emotional involvement (stress load) during competition, as well as demands placed upon the cardiovascular system due to decreases in available oxygen (high elevation competition or an underwater sport) or extremes in temperature (Mitchell et al, 2005). Mitchell and colleagues (2005) developed a diagram showing the interrelationship of the two components; it is a valuable aid for making a clinical decision regarding the eligibility or disqualification of an athlete based upon the cardio demands of the particular sport they desire to play and their preexisting cardiovascular condition (available for access at www.onlinejacc.org/cgi/content/figsonly/45/8/1364).

Cardiac Murmurs. Because cardiac murmurs are a common finding in children, it is important to distinguish between benign and pathological murmurs. See Chapter 30 regarding the auscultation of heart sounds and describing murmurs. For the PPE specifically, perform the following:

- Evaluate heart sounds and listen for murmurs in each of five areas of the heart (see Fig. 30-2 in Chapter 30). Auscultate the chest with the patient supine and standing. A useful way to further differentiate a benign from concerning murmur is to have the patient do a Valsalva maneuver, or squat then stand, during auscultation. Squatting increases venous return to the heart, thus increasing left ventricular size and stroke volume. Standing or doing Valsalva, on the other hand, decreases venous return and stroke volume. Increased stroke volume usually causes murmurs to be louder with squatting and quieter when the person stands or does Valsalva. If the reverse is heard, that is, softer with squatting and louder with standing or doing a Valsalva, then hypertrophic cardiomyopathy or mitral valve prolapse must be ruled out (Giese et al, 2007; Patel, 2009a).

Concerning features of murmurs that require further evaluation include diastolic murmurs or systolic murmurs (grade 3 or greater); radiation of the murmur; or wide or fixed splitting of S_2.

Diabetes Mellitus

The goal for children and adolescents with both type 1 and type 2 diabetes mellitus (DM) is to support athletic participation consistent with the individual's goals and desires. Type 1 and type 2 DM are discussed separately because management and monitoring issues differ between the two types.

Type 1 Diabetes Mellitus. Participation in sports is encouraged for the child or adolescent with type 1 DM. Any restrictions placed on an individual athlete would only be necessary when optimal glycemic control cannot be maintained or if complications or comorbidities are not compatible with the activity. Youth with DM should follow the same physical activity guidelines as all children—striving for 60 minutes of physical activity daily (Silverstein et al, 2005).

Control of the athlete's blood glucose level during rigorous exercise is a challenge. During physical exercise the body's oxygen demands increase greatly. In order to meet these energy needs, skeletal muscle relies on stores of glycogen, triglycerides, free fatty acids, and glucose production, largely from the liver. For the nondiabetic athlete, hormonal mediators maintain normal blood glucose levels even under high athletic conditions. In these individuals, exercise leads to decreased plasma insulin levels and increased glucagon that triggers hepatic glucose production. However, in the type 1 diabetic person, this hormonal pathway is interrupted. Thus, for diabetic individuals who have too little insulin in their system exercise can trigger release of high levels of glucose and ketone bodies, leading to hyperglycemia and eventually, if unchecked, to diabetic ketoacidosis. Conversely, if too much exogenous insulin is administered, the feedback loop for increased glucose mobilization is interrupted and hypoglycemia results (Silverstein et al, 2005).

It is generally recommended that athletes with type 1 DM have a medical team participating in their health care. This team ideally includes an endocrinologist and nutritionist who specialize in DM and who are familiar with the energy requirements of the individual's sport. Depending on the level of athletic endeavor, a trainer may also be part of the team. There is a useful reference for health providers and trainers managing the type 1 diabetic athlete written by the National Athletic Trainers' Association (NATA); recommendations are consistent with American Diabetes Association (ADA) guidelines (Jimenez et al, 2007).

Glycemic control requires periodic blood glucose monitoring, careful planning of meals and carbohydrates, snacks around the time of exercise, and adjustments in insulin dosing. It is essential that coaches, trainers, or other athletic staff be aware of the young athlete's diabetes care plan and be trained in aspects of care as outlined in the recommendations found in Box 13-5.

Type 2 Diabetes Mellitus. Young people with type 2 DM should be strongly encouraged to be physically active. Inactivity and the increasing obesity epidemic are directly related to the increasing incidence of type 2 DM in young people. Physical activity is not only one of the major type 2 DM prevention messages, but also a critical component in treatment.

The benefits of regular physical exercise for this disorder include increased insulin effectiveness due to improving insulin-receptor sensitivity, weight control, reduced risk of cardiovascular disease, reduced dyslipidemia risk, and improved self-confidence and self-esteem. Glycemic control during exercise is generally not difficult to maintain. In addition, physical activity and regular exercise are critical for

---

BOX 13-5 Recommendations for the Care of the Athlete With Type 1 Diabetes Mellitus

Key safety recommendations for the young athlete with type 1 diabetes mellitus (DM) include:

- Always wear medical alert identification.
- Never exercise alone (use the "buddy system").
- Maintain adequate hydration before, during, and after exercising.
- Avoid injecting insulin into the limb that is most active in the exercise performed (i.e., inject at a distant site) to avoid overly rapid insulin absorption.
- Avoid extreme heat (sauna, moist heat pack, thermal ultrasound) or extreme cold (ice) to area of recent insulin injection.
- Always have diabetic supplies available.
- Be aware that trauma (injury) can affect blood glucose levels (usually toward hyperglycemia) and be prepared to manage.

Restrictions or special considerations for young athletes with the following complications from DM include:

- Retinopathy—avoid strenuous static activities in which Valsalva-like maneuvers may increase intraocular pressure and precipitate hemorrhage.
- Severe hypertension—see Tables 13-5 and 13-7.
- Nephropathy—no specific guidelines exist; individualize considering youth's level of stamina; low to moderate intensity may be tolerated if monitored closely.
- Neuropathy—rare in young diabetics, but need to monitor for loss of sensation; preventive care is recommended (good footwear, care of blisters and sores).

Data from Jimenez CC, Corcoran MH, Crawley T, et al: National Athletic Trainers' Association position statement: management of the athlete with type I diabetes mellitus, *J Athl Train* 42(4):536-545, 2007.

weight loss, which also helps to improve the type 2 diabetic individual's glycemic control (Kamboj and Draznin, 2009).

The PPE for the young athlete with type 2 DM should include all recommended screenings at the recommended intervals for long-term glycemic control (e.g., HbA_{1c}) and comorbidities (dyslipidemia and cardiovascular risks). These are discussed further in Chapter 25.

At the time of sports or exercise, young type 2 DM athletes who are diet controlled do not require glucose monitoring and often do not need any additional snacks or calories. The exception would be if they are participating in a prolonged or exceptionally rigorous sport, in which case additional calories may be needed (e.g., soccer, running). Consultation with a nutritionist is advised to ensure that these athletes are getting adequate calories from carbohydrates and an appropriately balanced and low-fat diet. For adolescents who are taking oral hypoglycemic medication or insulin for type 2 DM, the benefits of improved insulin sensitivity through regular exercise participation may enable them to reduce medication. Glucose monitoring, both through self-monitoring of serum glucose as well as HbA_{1c} levels, are performed at the following times in order to provide important data for any medication adjustment (Clarke, 2008):

- At least twice yearly in those meeting treatment goals and with stable glycemic control
- Quarterly in those whose therapy has changed or who are not in stable glycemic control

Insulin therapy should be considered for those whose HgA_{1c} levels are greater than 8% (American Association of Clinical Endocrinologists [AACE], 2007).

The obese person with type 2 DM may initially be in poor physical condition with regard to sports endurance. Therefore, activity and exercise plans should allow for a gradual and safe buildup in intensity and length. Additionally, a nutritionist can be helpful in ensuring adequate calories for performance needs as well as for safe weight loss.

Hypertension

Hypertension is the most common cardiovascular condition seen in competitive athletes (AAP, 2010c). Table 13-7 summarizes the recommendations. Additionally, the athlete must:

- Be counseled to avoid anabolic steroids, growth hormone, illicit drugs (especially cocaine), nonprescribed stimulants, over-the-counter medications (e.g., pseudoephedrine and ephedra [ma huang], alcohol, tobacco, caffeine, energy and sports drinks [see also section on performance-enhancing drugs] and high-sodium foods.
- Be aware that with strenuous exercise and excessive sweating a total-body sodium deficit can occur. Therefore, care must be taken to rehydrate with the intake of salt-containing fluids and foods to ensure greater body water retention and distribution to all fluid compartments. A sports nutritionist or trainer can assist with proper rehydration.
- Be aware that for some athletic governing bodies, use of diuretics and beta-blockers is prohibited. These drugs have been shown to possibly decrease athletic performance in some individuals. Medication adaptations and registration of medications with the sport governing body may be required.

Seizures

Generally, all children and adolescents with seizure disorders should be encouraged to participate in the majority of sports. If well controlled, few restrictions are placed on the sports. If the seizures are poorly controlled there needs to be an individualized decision, but generally the person should be excluded from contact, limited-contact, or collision activities or hazardous sports until controlled. Contact sports have not conclusively been shown to provoke seizures, although head injury is always a risk (especially in football) (Fountain and May, 2003). Additionally, individuals may need to be restricted from the following noncontact sports: archery, riflery, swimming (discourage

TABLE 13-7	Recommendations for Sports Participation by Athletes With Hypertension	
Hypertensive Status	**Sports Activity Limitations**	**Management**
Normotensive	No limitations to competitive sports	Counsel to adopt healthy lifestyle behaviors: regular physical activity, healthy diet, avoidance of drugs, tobacco, and alcohol.
Prehypertensive	No limitations	Blood pressure checks every 6 months; counsel as above
Stage 1 hypertension—without end-organ damage, including left ventricular hypertrophy (LVH) or concomitant heart disease	No limitations or restrictions	Recheck blood pressure in 1 to 2 weeks, or sooner, if symptomatic. Refer to a specialist if patient is symptomatic, has any signs of cardiovascular disease, or has persistently elevated blood pressure on two additional occasions. Counsel on healthy lifestyle as above.
Stage 2 hypertension—no end-organ damage, including LVH or concomitant heart disease	Restrict from sports with high static and dynamic components—until blood pressure is in the normal range.	These athletes must be evaluated by a specialist immediately if symptomatic, or within 1 week, even if asymptomatic.
Hypertensive with concomitant cardiovascular disease	Eligibility is usually based on the type and severity of the other cardiovascular disease.	Management dependent upon recommendations of cardiac specialist

Data from American Academy of Pediatrics (AAP) Council on Sports Medicine and Fitness: Policy statement: athletic participation by children and adolescents who have systemic hypertension, *Pediatrics* 125(6):1287-1293, 2010c; Mitchell JH, Haskell W, Snell P, et al: 36th Bethesda Conference: Task Forces 8: classification of sports, *J Am Coll Cardiol* 45(8):1364-1367, 2005.

or closely supervise), weight lifting, powerlifting, and sports that involve heights (rock climbing, bungee jumping, hang-gliding, skydiving) (Rice and AAP, 2008). Flotation devices should always be worn when participating in rowing, fishing, or boating activities. Other water sports (scuba diving, underwater swimming, and diving) and motor sports (many state laws prohibit such activity) should be avoided or warrant considerable discussion. Exclusion is based on the rationale that having a seizure would put the individual or others at significant risk.

The psychological benefits of sports participation generally outweigh risks caused by acute stress, hyperventilation, or the occasional altered pharmacokinetics of seizure drug therapy that may occur during activity. Benefits of participation include some evidence of a reduction in a number of seizures (Fountain and May, 2003).

A decision about participation in a specific sport should be made with information about the type of seizure, likelihood of having a seizure, and presence of any comorbid conditions. Discussions ought to include the participant, parents, coaches or trainers, and neurologist (Howard et al, 2004). In addition, consideration must be given to possible side effects (notably sedation, ataxia, dizziness, or others) from anticonvulsant medication that could impair performance or put the individual at risk.

Sickle Cell Trait

Sickle cell trait (SCT) is discussed in Chapters 26 and 40. Though typically asymptomatic under most circumstances, it can have implications for competitive athletes. Under conditions of intense exertion during sports, an athlete with SCT can experience sickling of the red blood cells. Small vessels supplying vital organs become blocked, resulting in ischemia and muscle breakdown (rhabdomyolysis); the athlete collapses, and death can occur unless treatment is begun immediately. Acute rhabdomyolysis from sickling is one of the top four causes of sudden death in young athletes (NATA, 2007).

Athletes with SCT can participate in all sports, but it is important to know who they are in order to ensure safety in training and in all aspects of participation. In 2010, the National Collegiate Athletic Association (NCAA) Legislative Council announced a protocol stipulating that all athletes participating in NCAA Division I sports must have sickle cell testing performed; show proof of sickle cell testing; or sign a waiver demonstrating that they understand the importance of testing for sickle cell, decline testing, and thereby release their institution from any liability related to declining testing (Hosick, 2010). Although this legislative rule only addresses the NCAA member colleges and universities, it would be efficacious to recommend that youths in a high-risk group be tested and know their SCT status.

Preventive measures to reducing risk of a sickling crisis include (Casa and Csillan, 2009; Patel, 2009b):

- Build up slowly in training, allowing for periods of rest and recovery between repetitions. Allow the athlete with SCT to self-pace in training.
- Follow preseason heat acclimatization guidelines for training and for any changes in climate or altitude during competitions.
  - Adjust athletes' work and rest cycles on an individual basis accounting for climate and altitude.

- Ensure preseason strength and conditioning training.
- Athletes with SCT should avoid performance tests in such things as mile runs and serial sprints.
  - Activities such as repetitive high-speed sprints or interval training that produce lactic acid buildup should be accompanied by extended recovery periods.
- Ensure adequate hydration.
- Athletes with SCT should not train or compete when ill.
- Stop the workout *immediately* at onset of symptoms of muscle cramping, pain, swelling, weakness, tenderness, fatigue, or inability to catch one's breath.
- Educate the athlete, trainers, and coaches about how to handle a sickle cell emergency.
- Have an emergency medical plan written and onsite.
- A sickling collapse is a medical emergency. Field-side first aid includes monitoring vital signs, emergency respiratory and cardiac support as needed, cooling the athlete if overheating has occurred, and administering oxygen. Emergency care/transport (911) must be called promptly.

ACUTE INFECTIONS

Infectious Mononucleosis

The peak age groups affected by infectious mononucleosis (IM) are adolescents and young adults. IM is covered in more depth in Chapter 23.

With regard to athletes, splenomegaly (which occurs in 50% to 100% of cases of IM), is the most concerning clinical issue. There is a 0.1% to 0.5% risk of splenic rupture in those playing sports with this condition. The risk of rupture increases when participating in a contact or collision sport or a sport in which there is an increase in the intraabdominal pressure (e.g., rowing and weightlifting requiring Valsalva maneuvers).

Diagnosing splenomegaly can be a challenge. Athletes often have well-defined and firm abdominal musculature, making palpation of the spleen difficult. Studies have questioned the validity of palpation in diagnosing splenomegaly (Putukian et al, 2008). However, imaging is not recommended as a routine diagnostic measure or in making return-to-play decisions because there is great variance in normal spleen size (the only way to accurately diagnose splenomegaly on ultrasound is to get baseline and serial images over time). Recommendations to the clinician for return-to-play for the athlete with IM are as follows:

- Advise the athlete to avoid any form of exertion, including all sports during the first 3 weeks (minimum) after onset of symptoms when the spleen is more likely to enlarge.
- At 3 weeks after symptom onset, assuming the athlete is afebrile and symptom-free, he or she may return to light, noncontact activities. No sports should be played if there is risk of chest or abdominal contact or if it involves increased intraabdominal pressure or Valsalva maneuvers.
- Fully returning to play should be made on a case-by-case basis and is generally considered safe at 4 weeks after symptom onset, assuming the patient's physical stamina has returned and all symptoms have resolved. If the sports involved increases intraabdominal pressure, a longer recovery time is suggested (ACSM, 2008; Putukian et al, 2008).

BOX 13-6 Prevention of Transmission of Communicable Skin Infections Among Athletes

Prevention at an Individual Level

- Perform frequent handwashing using good technique (with soap or nonwater alcohol hand sanitizer with an ethanol content of at least 60%) by all athletes and trainers.
- Shower after each practice and game (preferably with antimicrobial soap, especially if doing a body contact sport such as wrestling, rugby, football).
- Regularly launder clothing, uniforms.
- Regularly clean all personal equipment (e.g., helmets, body pads, knee/ankle sleeves and braces, etc.).
- Refrain from cosmetic body shaving.
- Never share personal care items such as razors, towels, cosmetics.
- Report and seek professional care for all skin rashes, lesions, sores.
- Never get into a common hot tub, sauna, or whirlpool if athlete has any type of skin lesion that may be draining, open, or known to be infected.

Institutional or Sports Organizational Preventive Measures

- Coaches and training staff must be knowledgeable about communicable disease issues for their sport. Many sports organizations have such guidelines on their websites.
- Coaches should educate athletes about infectious disease guidelines including exclusion-from-play; return-to-play; handwashing and showering expectations; bagging up and uniform laundering expectations.
- Institutions and sports clubs must follow guidelines for cleaning and disinfecting all commonly used equipment. See CDC web page for information about cleaning common equipment (www.cdc.gov/features/mrsainschools).
- Institutions/recreational clubs, etc. must allocate adequate resources to purchase any necessary cleaning materials and to have volunteers/staff trained in proper cleaning and disinfecting procedures.

CDC, Centers for Disease Control and Prevention.
Data from Centers for Disease Control and Prevention: *Questions and answers about methicillin-resistant* Staphylococcus aureus (MRSA) *in schools,* 2007. Available at www.cdc.gov/features/mrsainschools (accessed Aug 11, 2010).

TABLE 13-8 Recommendations for Return-to-Play for Athletes With Communicable Skin Conditions

Condition	Return-to-Play Guidelines
Tinea corporis	• Minimum 72-hours on a topical fungicide • Lesions must be covered with a gas-permeable dressing followed by underwrap and stretch tape
Tinea capitis	• Minimum 2-weeks systemic antifungal therapy
Herpes simplex (primary)	• Free of systemic symptoms of viral infection, fever, malaise, etc. • No new lesions for at least 72 hours • No moist lesions; all lesions must be covered with a firm, adherent crust • Minimum 120 hours on a systemic antiviral therapy, if prescribed (fully formed, ruptured, crusted-over lesions will not be affected by antiviral therapy) • Active lesions cannot be covered to allow participation
Herpes simplex (recurrent)	• No moist lesions; all lesions must be covered with a firm, adherent crust • Minimum 120 hours on a systemic antiviral therapy, if prescribed (fully formed, ruptured, crusted-over lesions will not be affected by antiviral therapy) • Active lesions cannot be covered to allow participation
Molluscum contagiosum	• Lesions must be curetted or removed • Localized lesions may be covered with a gas-permeable dressing followed by underwrap and stretch tape
Furuncles, carbuncles, folliculitis, impetigo, cellulitis, or methicillin-resistant *Staphylococcus aureus*	• No new lesions for at least 48 hours • Minimum 72 hours of antibiotic therapy (see also Chapter 23) • No moist, exudative, or draining lesions • Active lesions cannot be covered to allow participation

Data from Vasily DB, Foley JJ: Guidelines for disposition of skin infections. In Halpin T, editor: NCAA 2004 Division I Wrestling Championships Handbook, Indianapolis, 2004, National Collegiate Athletic Association.

Skin Infections

Communicable dermatological conditions are a common concern in sports. Many sports involve close body-to-body (skin-to-skin) contact, involve sharing training equipment, or have the potential of compromising skin integrity from abrasions and injuries. Prevention of infection is key. Box 13-6 lists the most effective measures to prevent transmission of common skin infections among athletes. Table 13-8 outlines return-to-play recommendations for athletes with several of the more common communicable skin infections.

Human Immunodeficiency Virus and Other Blood-Borne Viral Pathogens

The health care provider must consider the effect of playing a sport on the well-being of not only the individual athlete with an infectious blood-borne pathogen but also of other athletes with whom that person may come into contact. HIV and hepatitis B virus (HBV) and C virus (HCV) are discussed here.

HBV is more stable and, therefore, there is a slightly higher risk of transmission than with HIV. There has been only one documented case of HBV spread (between sumo wrestlers) in sports. The chance of transmission is considered extremely low, and no exclusion is recommended. However, it may be prudent to exclude HBV carriers from intense contact sports, such as wrestling (NCAA, 2009). There is no epidemiological evidence of transmission of HIV infection through sports contact—even in collision and high-impact sports (CDC, 2010b).

Deciding whether the HIV-, HBV-, or HCV-infected athlete can play sports should be made on an individual basis depending on the person's overall health status, immune function, and general stamina (NCAA, 2009). There is no evidence that moderate intensity physical activity or the stresses of athletics are detrimental to the athlete with HIV. If the student-athlete is asymptomatic and without evidence of deficiencies in immunological function, then the presence of HIV infection alone does not preclude participation. Athletes with acute hepatitis B or C may participate in sports once they are symptom-free and physically well.

Athletes, trainers, coaches, or anyone with possible exposure to blood or other body fluids should adhere to universal infection control procedures. Refer to Box 13-7 for a summary of preventive measures for trainers and coaches.

High-Risk Conditions for Sports Participation

SUDDEN CARDIAC DEATH IN YOUNG ATHLETES

Sudden cardiac death (SCD) in young athletes is a relatively rare, but tragic occurrence. In young athletes (i.e., less than age 35) SCD is most commonly caused by underlying, often congenital, cardiac disease. When the athlete is under exertion, this cardiac condition can produce malignant ventricular dysrhythmias (ventricular tachycardia or ventricular fibrillation) (SCD is more often a result of coronary artery disease in those over age 35). Because many athletes are totally asymptomatic until the one traumatic event occurs, screening for risk factors or subjective or objective signs of heart disease are essential components of the PPE. See Chapter 30 for a discussion about the major underlying cardiac conditions that put one at risk for SCD. See Box 13-3 for screening questions that highlight worrisome signs and symptoms in individuals possibly at risk of sudden death during exertion. For specific recommendations about sports participation and restrictions for each of the various cardiac conditions, the reader is referred to the 36th Bethesda Conference Report (American College of Cardiology, 2005). Other potential causes of SCD include:

- Anabolic steroids: Reports of myocardial damage and infarction (McDevitt and Brown, 2009)
- Commotio cordis: A rare situation in which an athlete suffers a direct blow to the precordium by a projectile object such as a ball, hockey puck, or a fist. If this happens at a vulnerable period of the cardiac cycle it can trigger ventricular fibrillation (Patel, 2009a).
- EIA: Although EIA may produce symptoms described as chest pain or chest discomfort, this can also be a sign of left ventricular outflow tract obstruction or coronary artery anomalies and should be further evaluated if the history and physical examination are not clear for EIA.

MUSCULOSKELETAL

All musculoskeletal injuries require individual assessment and decision-making. Sprains, subluxations, dislocations, muscle contusions, and overuse injuries can result in pain and changes to joints, ligament stability, range of motion, strength, and endurance. Referral to an orthopedist or physical therapist may be required. Immediate referral is predicated on vascular or nerve compromise and open fracture. Before returning to

BOX 13-7 Recommendations for Trainers and Coaches to Prevent the Transmission of Blood-Borne Pathogens in the Sports Environment

HIV
- No restriction on sports participation by athletes with HIV
- Universal screening of athletes for HIV status is not recommended. HIV screening recommendations are the same as for all adolescents—on a case-by-case basis as a general health guideline for sexually active youth or if other risk behaviors are disclosed.
- The health status of all athletes with regard to HIV should be held in confidence (as is all other health-related information).
- Health care providers who perform PPEs do not have to disclose an athlete's HIV status on the PPE form.
  - Reduce risk of transmission by counseling an HIV-positive individual on safety and personal responsibility with regard to care and minimizing exposure risks for themselves and others.

Hepatitis
- Ensure that all athletes are fully immunized against HBV.
- Hepatitis B– and hepatitis C–positive athletes—slightly higher (although small) risk of infection transmission possible:
  - Educate about transmission
  - Encourage participation in a sport in which transmission risk is low

General Guidelines
- For athletes, coaches, trainers:
  - If bleeding occurs during the sport, the participant needs to cease playing until the bleeding has stopped.
  - Follow universal precautions with regard to handling of bodily fluids, equipment, or clothing that becomes contaminated with all possibly infectious materials.

HBV, Hepatitis B virus; *HIV*, human immunodeficiency virus; *PPE*, preparticipation physical examination.
Data from National Collegiate Athletic Association (NCAA): Guideline 21: blood borne pathogens, *2009-2010 NCAA sports medicine handbook*, Indianapolis, 2009, National Collegiate Athletic Association, pp 66-71; Patel DP, Kumar A, Feucht C: Infectious and dermatologic conditions. In Patel DP, Greydanus DE, Baker RJ, editors: *Pediatric practice: sports medicine*, New York, 2009, McGraw Hill, pp 196-199.

sports participation, the athlete must be able to demonstrate the following (Magee, 2005):
- Minimal swelling or joint effusions; some mild discomfort, swelling, and/or stiffness can be expected during initial reentry into activity, which should respond to icing
- Pain-free full range of motion
- At least 90% to 95% of normal strength
- Ability to perform all motions and actions of the required sport
- Confidence in ability to do the activity at requisite level for the sport

If these conditions are not met, repeated injury can be anticipated from residual musculoskeletal deficiencies (e.g., instability, loss of strength, tissue compromise). Successfully returning to sports participation does not solely depend on the absence of pain; correct rehabilitation, which includes regaining strength and coordination of the injured area, is an important factor. A progressive trial of sports activities may be necessary before full return-to-play is accomplished.

BOX 13-8	Recognizing a Concussion (Signs and Symptoms)

Physical	**Cognitive**	**Emotional**	**Sleep**
• Headache (persistent, mild) • Nausea • Vomiting • Balance problems • Dizziness • Visual problems • Fatigue • Sensitivity to light and/or noise • Numbness/tingling • Dazed or stunned (befuddled facial expression) • Seizure (transport to hospital in order to differentiate between seizures due to concussion,* posttraumatic brain injury, convulsive syncope, drug-related epilepsy [e.g., cocaine], or idiopathic primary epilepsy)	• Feeling mentally "foggy" • Feeling slowed down (slurred, incoherent speech; disjointed or incomprehensible statements) • Difficulty concentrating (cannot recall words, numbers; unable to follow through with normal activities) • Difficulty remembering time, place, date • Forgetful of recent information or conversations • Confused about recent events • Delayed verbal and motor responses (slower to answer questions or follow instructions; walking in wrong direction) • Repeats questions • Gross incoordination (stumbling, unable to walk tandem or in a straight line)	• Irritability (low frustration tolerance) • Sadness • More emotional (appears distraught, crying for no apparent reason) • Nervousness	• Drowsiness • Sleep disturbance (sleeping less or more than usual) • Trouble falling asleep

*_Concussive seizure_ is characterized by short, initial tonic stiffening, often followed by a short period of myoclonic jerks, after which the athlete may ambulate to the sideline without a significant postictal period (DeBerardino and Owens, 2009).
Adapted from American Academy of Neurology Quality Standards Subcommittee: Practice parameter: the management of concussion in sports (summary statement), _Neurology_ 48:581-585, 1997; Centers for Disease Control and Prevention: _Heads up: facts for physicians about mild traumatic brain injury (MTBI)_. Updated March 18, 2010. Available at www.cdc.gov/concussion/headsup/physicians_tool_kit.html (accessed Aug 20, 2010).

NEUROLOGICAL

Head Injury: Mild Traumatic Brain Injury and Concussion

It is estimated that concussions occur in 1.6 to 3.6 million young athletes annually (Lovell and Fazio, 2008). Head and neck injuries cause 70% of sports-related traumatic deaths and 20% of permanent disabilities (CDC, 2007). The sports posing the highest risk for head injuries are football, bicycling, basketball, soccer, and trauma on playground equipment. One study found that a child was six times more likely to acquire a severe concussion during an organized sport than from other recreational activities (Browne and Lam, 2006).

Central nervous system trauma is important to assess because repeated concussions are often progressively more serious or can result in _second-impact syndrome_. The symptoms from a concussion may affect four domains (physical, cognitive, emotional, and sleep). Symptoms may appear in all domains or in just one. If any symptoms are present, a concussion should be suspected; symptoms may appear even several hours after the injury. Numerous studies show that children and adolescents often take longer to recover from concussions than do adults (McCrory et al, 2009). If severe enough, the injury may precipitate a seizure lasting 1 to 2 minutes. The incidence of posttraumatic epilepsy is less than 10% after a concussion or contusion (Cantu and Cantu, 2009).

Various factors have been identified that may modify or intensify concussion severity and lengthen recovery (McCrory et al, 2009). These include:
- Increased number, severity and duration of symptoms (especially if lasting >10 days)
- Prolonged loss of consciousness (LOC) >1 minute, amnesia

- Concussive convulsions
- Repeated concussions; recent past concussion; second-impact syndrome (this second blow may have seemed minor but can cause massive brain swelling and herniation with risk of mortality or morbidity within minutes; occurs in an athlete who has not fully recovered from a previous concussion)
- Age less than 18 years
- Comorbidities: migraines, depression, ADHD, learning disabilities, sleep disorders
- Use of some psychoactive medications or anticoagulants

Physical Examination. A sideline evaluation of any player with a head injury should be performed, using a standardized tool such as the Standardized Concussion Assessment Tool 2 (SCAT2) (available at www.thinkfirst.ca/documents/SCAT2_000.pdf). All the domains possibly impaired by a head injury should be evaluated (Box 13-8). Additionally, note:
- Pupils: Symmetry and reaction
- Coordination: Finger-nose-finger; tandem walk
- Sensation: Finger-nose with eyes closed; Romberg test
- Physical: Test for the appearance of symptoms listed in Box 13-8 by having the youth do a 40-yard sprint, five push-ups, five sit-ups, and five knee bends

Diagnostic Studies. Generally, computed tomography (CT) imaging is negative in a concussion; imaging is needed if there is suspicion of an intracranial hemorrhage. Magnetic resonance imaging (MRI) with magnetic resonance angiogram is indicated if carotid dissection or stroke is suspected; positron-emission tomography (PET) is used in cases in which the individual has persistent symptoms (Cantu and Cantu, 2009).

TABLE 13-9	Recommendations for Management of Concussion* in Sports		
Definition	**First Concussion**	**Second Concussion**	**Third Concussion**
Grade 1 No LOC; transient confusion; PTA, PCCS† <30 minutes	• Athlete may return to play that day in select situations if clinical examination results are normal at rest and with exertion; otherwise return to play in 1 week • Athlete should be taken to the emergency department if mental status abnormalities last more than 1 hour	• Return to play in 2 weeks if asymptomatic for 1 week	• Terminate season‡; may return to play next season if asymptomatic
Grade 2 LOC <1 minute; duration of PTA ≥30 minutes but <24 hours; PCCS† >30 minutes but <7 days	• Athlete may return to play in 2 weeks if asymptomatic at rest and with exertion for 7 days	• Minimum of 1 month without playing; after that may return to play if asymptomatic at rest or with exertion for 1 week; consider terminating season‡	• Terminate season‡; may return to play next season if asymptomatic
Grade 3 LOC >1 minute; PTA >24 hours; PCCS† >7 days	• Athlete may return to play in 1 month if asymptomatic at rest and with exertion for 7 days	• Terminate season‡; may return to play next season‡ if asymptomatic	• Terminate contact sports for 1 year; RTP in noncontact sports after that

LOC, Loss of consciousness; *PCCS,* postconcussion signs/symptoms other than amnesia; *PTA,* posttraumatic amnesia; *RTP,* return to play.
*A concussion is defined as head trauma-induced alteration in mental status that may or may not involve loss of consciousness. Concussions are graded in three categories. Definitions and treatment recommendations for each category are presented.
†Mental status abnormalities include impairment in orientation, memory, concentration, or delayed recall.
‡Season refers to a playing season, not a year. For example, football season is one season; if followed by a baseball season, that is the second season, etc.
Data from Cantu RC: Posttraumatic retrograde and anterograde amnesia: pathophysiology and implications in grading and safe return to play, *J Athl Train* 36(3):244-248, 2001; Cantu RC, Cantu RV: Head injuries. In DeLee JC, Drez D Jr., Miller MD, editors: *DeLee and Drez's orthopaedic sports medicine: principles and practice,* ed 3, Vol 1, Philadelphia, 2009, Saunders.

Management. Management requires physical and cognitive rest until symptoms resolve. Cognitive recovery may lag behind physical symptom resolution, and this domain plays an important part in return-to-play decisions. Table 13-9 lists management recommendations. Once symptoms resolve, the athlete can progress through steps to gradually return to play. Table 13-10 describes the recommended step-wise return-to-play protocol.

Neck

After neck injuries, the athlete should be free of neck and arm pain, have full range of neck motion, and have full neck strength before returning to play. Neck radiographs and MRI, if done, should not reveal abnormal position, disk disease, or spinal stenosis.

Burners and Stingers

Burners and stingers are nerve root or brachial plexus compression or traction injuries and generally cause unilateral symptoms. This is a common injury in contact or collision sports, notably football and wrestling. The names derive from the sensation of a burn, stinging, electric, or "lightning bolt" sensation down an arm to the hand. The sensation can last seconds to minutes, but up to 10% can last hours, days, or longer. They may require a more extensive evaluation if:
• Weakness lasts more than a few days.
• There is a symptom of neck pain, or burners or stingers occur in both arms.
• There is prior history of recurrent burners or stingers.

Youth with mild to moderate burners or stingers must be free of all symptoms before given sports clearance; they should not be allowed to play if any neck pain or arm weakness remains.

Transient Quadriplegia

This condition is a much more significant problem and generally appears with bilateral symptoms. It is a contraindication for contact and collision sports until fully evaluated or if any objective structural problems are found. All transient quadriplegia muscle function and strength must have returned prior to clearance to resume play. Rehabilitation may be needed to achieve this.

HERNIA

Hernias should be repaired. However, the teen with a hernia need not be restricted from sports participation, but should be aware of the symptoms of incarceration.

ABSENCE OF PAIRED ORGANS

Sports that involve objects, sticks, or racquets, or aggressive play, such as football or basketball, have greater risks for eye injuries. Baseball is the most dangerous eye sport. Face shields are now required for hockey, and the incidence of serious injuries in this sport has dramatically decreased. Eyewear is available for all sports except boxing and full-contact martial arts.

The child with one eye or best-corrected vision in one eye worse than 20/40 should be required to wear molded polycarbonate sport frames with 3-mm-thick polycarbonate lenses

TABLE 13-10	Graduated Return-to-Play Protocol	
Rehabilitation Stage*	**Functional Exercise at Each Stage of Rehabilitation**	**Objective of Each Stage**
1. No activity	Complete physical and cognitive rest	Recovery
2. Light aerobic exercise	Walking, swimming, or stationary cycling keeping intensity <70% MPHR No resistance training	Increase HR
3. Sport-specific exercise	Skating drills in ice hockey, running drills in soccer. No head impact activities.	Add movement
4. Noncontact training drills	Progression to more complex training drills (e,g., passing drills in football and ice hockey) May start progressive resistance training	Exercise, coordination, and cognitive load
5. Full-contact practice	Following medical clearance, participate in normal training activities	Restore confidence and assess functional skills by coaching staff
6. Return to play	Normal game play	

*Stay at each stage for 24 hours before progressing to next stage, as long as asymptomatic. If symptoms evolve at any stage, drop back to prior stage.
HR, Heart rate; *MPHR,* maximum predicted heart rate.
Used by permission from McCrory P, Meeuwisse W, Johnston K, et al: Consensus statement on concussion in sports: the 3rd International Conference on Concussion in Sports, 2008, *J Athl Train* 44(4):434-448, 2009.

for all sports involving rapidly moving objects, bats, or racquets. For collision sports involving headgear, such as football, hockey, or lacrosse, the same frames and lenses should be worn under the cage shield or mask. These individuals should not participate in sports in which the use of eye protection is not possible. A history of detached retina is significant, and participation should be limited to nonstrenuous sports until consultation with an ophthalmologist is complete (see also Table 13-5).

Young men with a single testicle can be adequately protected with the use of a hard-cup athletic supporter for contact and collision sports and those in which objects are projected at high speed. Females with one ovary would not be restricted (NCAA, 2010). A signed letter of understanding and waiver release by the student, parent, or guardian for the athlete's record are indicated.

ATLANTOAXIAL OR ATLANTO-OCCIPITAL INSTABILITY

About 15% of children with Down syndrome can have an anomaly of the cervical vertebrae at the space between C-1 and C-2 known as atlantoaxial (or atlanto-occipital) instability (AAI) (Patel and Greydanus, 2009). Under certain circumstances—with sudden or extreme flexion or hyperextension of the head and neck—subluxation and spinal cord compression can occur as a result of the vertebral anatomy and lax ligaments.

Asymptomatic cases of AAI are screened by obtaining lateral radiographic views of the cervical spine in flexion, extension, and neutral position; those with atlantoaxial separation greater than 4.5 mm or a neural canal width less than 14 mm are excluded from certain sports. The most recent AAP policy statement (2007b) recommends radiographic screening once during the preschool years (between 3 and 5 years). However, studies have not found the approach of universal screening effective or necessary because the risk of injury is very small unless the individual playing certain sports is symptomatic. For that reason, many now advise a PPE plus radiological imaging of the cervical spine only for youths with Down

syndrome wanting to participate in sports (Koutures et al, 2008). An MRI is done if instability is detected by radiograph. The risk of spinal cord injury cannot be minimized.

Clearance for Special Olympics requires such screening. Unless two physicians and the athlete (or parent/guardian, if a minor) sign a waiver, Special Olympics excludes those with AAI from the following sports: swimming butterfly stroke and any dive starts, pentathalon, high jump, equestrian sports, gymnastics, soccer, alpine skiing, and warm-up exercises that put stress on the head and neck (Special Olympics, 2010). All athletes with known problems in the cervical area should not engage in contact or collision sports, limited contact or impact sports, or in diving (see Box 13-2). They may, however, engage in most of the listed noncontact sports.

SPECIAL CONSIDERATIONS FOR THE FEMALE ATHLETE

Injuries and the Female Athlete

The female athlete has a four to six times greater risk of injury to the knee than does a male athlete (Cincinnati Children's Hospital, 2010). This injury typically occurs to the anterior cruciate ligament (ACL) during deceleration, landing, pivoting, or contact with another athlete. Sports that increase this risk are basketball, field hockey, lacrosse, skiing, and soccer. It is theorized that the increased risk is due to several factors including biomechanical, greater joint laxity in females, and hormonal effects on connective tissue (Groeger, 2010). ACL injury prevention conditioning programs are effective in reducing injury risk two- to fourfold (Quinn, 2008). Many girls' sports teams are incorporating some version of an ACL injury prevention training as part of their warm-ups. Components of such training include muscle strengthening, balance, proprioception, landing techniques, and body and joint awareness.

Other injuries common in the female athlete include those of the patellofemoral joint and shoulder (sustained during diving, gymnastics, swimming, throwing, and volleyball)

BOX 13-9 | The Female Athlete Triad: Recommendations for the Clinician

1. Screen for all elements of the triad at the PPE and at annual physicals.
2. If one component of the triad exists, screen for the others.
3. Treatment of female athlete triad should be multidisciplinary, potentially including mental health professional, nutritionist, and coach or trainer.
4. Athletes with a suspected eating disorder should also be referred to a nutrition professional and a mental health professional for screening/treatment (if necessary).
5. Diagnosis of amenorrhea—screen for other causes (see Chapter 18). Functional hypothalamic amenorrhea (from the events of the triad) is a diagnosis of exclusion.
6. Screen bone mineral density:
   • After a stress or low-impact fracture
   • After a total of 6 months of amenorrhea or oligomenorrhea
   • As part of the assessment of a disordered eating pattern
7. The initial goal of treatment is to increase energy intake and decrease energy expenditure.
8. Preventive counseling for all athletes should include nutritional (energy) needs for sports; importance of bone mineralization during child and adolescent years, including bone health throughout life, stressing importance of physical activity, calcium, and vitamin D.

PPE, Preparticipation physical examination.

(ACSM, 2003). Stress fractures must be suspected in female athletes with low body weight and/or amenorrhea (see following discussion regarding the female athlete triad). The female athlete who is amenorrheic has a four times greater risk of stress fracture than does the athlete with normal menses (Groeger, 2010).

Intensive sport training does not appear to delay the growth and sexual maturation of young female athletes. This concern has been repeatedly raised at every world Olympics in regard to female gymnasts. However, summaries of studies conclude that the differences in growth and maturation are more likely due to genetics and physique preselection rather than to extended, intensive training (AAP, 2010d).

The Female Athlete Triad

The *female athlete triad* consists of three entities: a disordered eating pattern, menstrual dysfunction (amenorrhea or oligomenorrhea), and osteopenia or osteoporosis. At the root of this triad is the emphasis (either real or perceived by the athlete) on a lean body, maintaining a low weight, and/or retaining one's prepubertal physique. Girls who participate in sports that emphasize leanness are at the greatest risk of the triad of disorders. These sports include distance running, gymnastics, dance/dance team, figure skating, and cheerleading. It is estimated that the incidence of having all three components of the female athlete triad is 4.3% (Pantano, 2009). The symptoms of the triad occur along a continuum rather than in unison; therefore, the identification of the early existence of an eating disorder, weight loss, or menstrual irregularities from a PPE history or examination should alert the provider to take a more thorough history and initiate early treatment. Eating concerns and menstrual cycle disorders occur far more often and should

be addressed to prevent development of the full triad (Nattiv et al, 2007). Inadequate bone mineralization during the critical adolescent years puts the teen at lifelong risk of osteoporosis, which increases the risk of stress fractures during adolescence and throughout life and further increases the potential for skeletal problems at menopause.

Disordered eating patterns can be due to either intentional caloric restriction (an eating disorder that may or may not encompass all the criteria for an anorexia or bulimia diagnosis) or an inadvertent insufficient intake in calories to meet the athlete's metabolic demands of her sport. Disordered eating, whatever the cause, leads to low energy availability. It is thought that when one's energy deficit reaches a critical low threshold, a cascade of hormonal and biochemical events occur that negatively affect the menstrual cycle and skeletal integrity (Nattiv et al, 2007). Box 13-9 lists recommendations for evaluating and managing an individual identified as having the female triad.

HEAT AND HUMIDITY

Core body temperature is a balance of heat generation and heat dissipation (see also Chapter 39). A major contributor to core body temperature is the heat generated by muscle contractions. Exercising muscle generates 10 to 20 times the amount of heat of resting muscle; approximately 75% of this energy generation is converted to heat, but only 25% actually goes into muscle work (AAP, 2000). Under ideal conditions this can result in an increase of core body temperature of 1.8° F (1° C) in 5 minutes. When environmental heat or humidity excesses are added to the equation, the body must dissipate the heat at increased rates. Unless the usual heat dissipation mechanisms are properly working, heat stroke can result within 15 to 20 minutes. Heat is dissipated through evaporation (20% to 25%), convection (15%), and radiation (60%). It is dissipated only through evaporation when environmental temperature exceeds body temperature and, thus, only when humidity is 75% or less. There is no evaporation at 90% to 95% humidity. Thus, the combination of high heat and high humidity greatly taxes the body's ability to effectively lower core temperature.

Children have a higher metabolic rate at a given submaximal walking or running speed so they produce more heat per mass unit. This higher metabolic load, in addition to several other pediatric physiological factors (poor sweating capacity, larger surface-to-mass ratio, and an immature cardiovascular system), results in a shorter tolerance for exercising in hot climates and greater susceptibility to heat stress. Children also dehydrate sooner and have higher core temperatures than do adults; adolescents are somewhere in the middle in terms of this ability. Inadequate heat acclimatization, heavy uniforms and gear, certain chronic illnesses, and specific sports put the young athlete at further risk of heat-related injury. Athletes who are poorly conditioned, obese, dehydrated, have poor nutritional status (e.g., eating disorders), or who are ill with a mild acute illness or fever are at greater risk. Individuals with the chronic diseases and special needs previously discussed in this chapter (including cystic fibrosis) are notably at risk. Additionally, decreased sweat production may occur with spina bifida, quadriplegia, scleroderma, severe eczema, and sunburn among other conditions. These individuals need particular supervision because they might not recognize early warning signs of heat effects and may not hydrate adequately.

Certain drugs can also increase heat production or decrease sweating (e.g., amphetamines, lysergic acid diethylamide [LSD], alcohol, thyroid hormone, antihistamines, anticholinergics, haloperidol, phenothiazines, diuretics, laxatives, monoamine oxidase inhibitors, tricyclic antidepressants). Caffeine and alcohol also reduce the body's ability to deal with heat.

Data from a limited survey of 100 high schools showed that football players had a 10 times higher risk of heat-related illness (the highest number occurring in August) than athletes who participated in eight other sports (CDC, 2010c).

Heat Illnesses (Hyperthermia)

Heat illness occurs in a gradual sequence from less to more serious. Generally, if an athlete recognizes the symptoms of the earlier stages and takes appropriate action, progression can be stopped. It is essential that coaches, parents, or others on the field be aware of symptoms of heat-related illnesses and assist the athlete to take appropriate measures even if it means dropping out of an event.

Heat Cramps. Prickly heat, heat edema of hands and feet, and heat syncope are early indicators of the body's responses to excessive heat. Heat cramps are one of the mildest forms of heat illness and occur most commonly when athletes are not adequately conditioned for participation at high temperature or humidity and fail to hydrate properly. Symptoms include painful muscle spasms, usually of the calf and hamstrings (can occur in the abdomen, shoulders) during or after strenuous exercise with profuse sweating. The cramps are brief (less than 1 minute), intermittent, and painful. They may occur after intense exercise and are thought to be related to electrolyte depletion. The person generally feels thirsty but remains well oriented and alert. Oral rehydration with an electrolyte solution (a sports drink, or 0.5 to 1 teaspoon of salt in 1 quart of water), gentle stretching, and resting in a cool area are generally sufficient. Intravenous saline solution may be needed in more severe situations.

Heat Exhaustion. Heat exhaustion is the most common heat illness of athletes. It occurs with excess sweating in a hot, humid environment. It is a reversible condition, whereas heat stroke causes irreversible damage to tissues. Symptoms include headache, fatigue, weakness, dizziness, orthostasis, nausea, anorexia, and possibly syncope and diarrhea. The core temperature may range from 100° F (37.7° C) to over 103° F (39.4° C) (Landry, 2007). Mentation is generally normal; dry tongue and mouth and weight loss may occur. Cardiovascular symptoms may result from volume loss and include tachypnea and orthostatic hypotension. Malaise, myalgias, vertigo, chills, visual disturbances, and cutaneous flushing may also occur. The skin is ashen, cold, and clammy because of sodium depletion or hot and dry from water depletion. Mild shock may be present, but there are no major central nervous system dysfunctions. Management includes rest in a cooler environment; cooling measures, such as removing clothing, fanning, spraying and sponging the skin with water, applying ice to the groin and axillae; and oral or intravenous fluids. The child should be allowed unrestricted access to salty foods. Emergency department monitoring is

recommended. If the athlete is confused or refuses to drink, intravenous fluids are needed. A patient with the latter symptoms may need hospitalization.

Heat Stroke. Heat stroke is a medical emergency with a mortality rate of 50% (Landry, 2007). It can occur over several days, as with a heat wave, or rapidly with exertion. In either case, rapid cooling is essential because the high body temperature damages tissues and alters heart, lung, brain, kidney, and other organ system functions. Persons participating in intense exertion experience the symptom of excessive sweating. High core temperature (greater than 104° F [40° C] and can be greater than 107° F [41.6° C]), shock or coma, circulatory abnormalities, disseminated intravascular coagulation, rhabdomyolysis (due to acute or chronic compartment syndrome), dysrhythmias, and seizures can result. Sweating may or may not be present depending on the degree of depletion of fluids that has occurred. Rapid transport to an emergency department is essential. While waiting for transport, the patient should be placed in a cool environment, clothing should be removed, and water should be applied to the body with fanning to increase evaporation. Fluids should be given orally if the athlete is alert; antipyretics are not useful. The patient may need cardiopulmonary resuscitation until emergency transportation arrives.

Preventive Measures. Heat-related illnesses are totally preventable. *Heat-acclimatization* is the process in training by which athletes are exposed gradually to high-temperature environmental conditions. This training requires a minimum of 14 days. By adhering to a carefully proscribed schedule, athletic performance improves, and the risk of later exertional, heat-related illness is reduced. For that reason many sports associations at both the high school and collegiate level require heat-acclimatization periods in their initial training schedules (Casa and Csillan, 2009). Specific heat acclimatization guidelines for athletic training are available from the National Athletic Trainers' Association. The AAP (2007c) offers a guideline for determining the restraint on activities at different levels of heat stress, as measured by a psychometer (commercially available apparatus with three thermometers for use in the athletic environment). See Box 13-10 for strategies to prevent heat illnesses.

Dehydration

The young person can prevent dehydration by drinking cool water before, during, and after activities. Performance and normal thermoregulation can decrease with as little as 1% dehydration. Thirst should not be the guide to hydration needs (Landry, 2007). After competition, rehydration is important. Small amounts of sodium and carbohydrates, such as are found in sports drinks, enhance rehydration; additional sodium supplements are not recommended. Drinking fluids with caffeine should be avoided because these beverages increase urine output, causing further dehydration (see discussion and warning that follows about energy drinks). Use of separate fluid containers for each child participating may help monitor the intake of each while decreasing the risk of disease spread (see Box 13-10 for fluid intake recommendations for athletes). Scheduling fluid breaks and rotating players more frequently may also help prevent dehydration.

BOX 13-10	Strategies to Prevent Heat Illnesses

- Athletes should be gradually acclimatized to heat over the first 14 days of practice if hot weather is present. Heat acclimatization refers to length, frequency and level of practice, protective equipment that is worn, and prescribed rest periods and days off. Recommendations for a 14-day heat acclimatization practice schedule can be found at www.nata.org/consensus-statements.
- Athletes should wear lightweight, dry, permeable clothing. Protective gear that may add or trap heat should be added gradually throughout the acclimatization period.
- Athletes should be fully hydrated before activity begins.
  - Preexercise hydration recommendations: 500 to 600 mL (17 to 20 oz) of water or sports drink 2 to 3 hours before exercising; 200 to 300 mL (7 to 10 oz) 10 to 20 minutes before starting exercise.
- Rehydration fluids should be readily available at all athletic practices and events. Athletes should drink cool water or sport drink (more efficiently absorbed than warm beverage) every 10 to 20 minutes at a rate of 150 mL (5 oz) if less than 40 kg; 270 to 300 mL (9 to 10 oz) if 60 kg; 300 to 360 mL (10 to 12 oz) if more than 60 kg in weight.
- In extremely warm weather, consider pre- and postpractice game weigh-ins. The athlete should not lose more than 2% of body weight during the athletic session. Postpractice fluid replacement should take place within 2 hours of the session.
- Water is adequate if exercise lasts less than1 hour; if available, oral rehydration solutions should be used if activities exceed 1 hour.
- Athletes should have scheduled rest periods in the shade every 20 to 30 minutes, with helmets and other warm gear removed.
- Athletes at greater risk should be observed carefully. Risk factors include cystic fibrosis, hyperthyroidism, cardiovascular conditions, sickle cell trait, obesity, previous heat stroke, general health problems, poor conditioning, diabetes, kidney disorders, and medications (e.g., diuretics, antihistamines, antidepressants, and others).
- Activities should be scheduled in early morning or evening to avoid direct sunlight and the hottest time of day; preseason full practice in late summer for sports involving larger players is risky (start workouts slowly in early summer and work up to full practice).
- Activity should cease if any signs and symptoms of heat illness develop.
- Salt tablets should not be used.

Data from AAP: Guidelines for pediatricians: exertional heat-related illness, *Sports Shorts,* issue 2, 2000. Available at *www.app.org/sections/sportsmedicine/SportsShorts.cfm* (accessed Sept 3, 2010); AAP Committee on Sports Medicine and Fitness: Climatic heat stress and the exercising child and adolescent, *Pediatrics* 106(1):158-159, 2000, reaffirmed 2007; AAP Healthy Children: Exertional heat-related illness, 2010. Available at www.healthychildren.org/English/health-issues/injuries-emergencies/sports-injuries/pages/Exertional-Heat-Related-Illness.aspx accessed Sept 3, 2010); Casa DJ, Csillan D: National Athletic Trainers' Association Consensus Statement: Preseason heat-acclimatization guidelines for secondary school athletes, *J Athl Train* 44(3):332-333, 2009; Casa DJ, Armstrong LE, Hillman SK, et al: National Athletic Trainers' Association position statement: fluid replacement for athletes, *J Athl Train* 35(2):212-224, 2000; Joy E, American Medical Society for Sports Medicine: Sports medicine tip sheet—heat illness. Available at www.amssm.org/MemberFiles/Heatillness.pdf (accessed Sept 3, 2010); Mueller FO, for the Ohio High School Athletic Association: Heat stress and athletic participation. Available at www.ohsaa.org (accessed Sept 3, 2010).

USE OF PERFORMANCE-ENHANCING ERGOGENIC DRUGS AND SUPPLEMENTS

Ergogenic drugs refer to legal and illicit substances used to enhance athletic performance. Athletes use these substances because they are purported to have a variety of effects, such as increasing energy; prolonging sports endurance; increasing lean body mass; decreasing adipose tissue; increasing or decreasing weight; improving cardiovascular status; and enhancing overall performance in a given sport. Such claims and beliefs about these substances serve as powerful enticements to young athletes. The steroid precursors, growth hormone, and ephedra substances have not been proven to enhance performance, yet they can have serious side effects of which youth are often unaware. Street names include gym candy, pumpers, weight trainers, stackers, roids, juice, and Arnolds.

There are a number of issues regarding the safety and moral questions that arise from use of ergogenic substances. These include concerns about the nonregulation and monitoring of the components of these substances, many of which may have potential and dangerous side effects, and disrespect for the value of nondrugged performance based on a regimen of committed training, good coaching, a balanced diet, and a healthful lifestyle, all of which are principles of team and individual athletics (AAP, 2008b).

The preponderance of ergogenic drug use can be attributed to many modern influences. These include the message by top athletes and sports icons that ergogenic drugs are acceptable because of their own use; the emphasis and status placed on sports by society; canvassing ever younger players by sports scouts; and pressure to fund college education via sports scholarships. Impressionable youngsters are manipulated by an aggressive media and product industry. Alluring advertising techniques, such as flashy, catchy labels on supplements and "used-by-the-pros" proclamations, capitalize on immature developmental levels (that make youth more vulnerable to peer pressure) and the need for success and self-esteem. The written information that discusses the warnings and side effects of ergogenic aids are often above the reading levels of middle schoolers (Calfee and Fadale, 2006).

Recognition and Prevention of Performance-Enhancing Drug Use

All high school and collegiate sports associations have strongly worded policies prohibiting the use of performance-enhancing substances. They issue and actively enforce no-tolerance policies and endorse the U.S. Anti-Doping Agency regulations and world antidoping code. It is important for clinicians to be aware of and communicate these positions to young athletes and their parents. Anticipatory guidance and education are essential in this area. Education needs to include both benefits and risks, and the educator needs to be well informed to be credible. "Clean" team members can provide leadership by disavowing performance-enhancing drugs and emphasizing the integrity (fair play) of sports competition. Parents and coaches should intervene whenever necessary. The Adolescents Training and Learning to Avoid Steroids program (Goldberg et al, 1996) continues to be a model for such interventions. Nutrition and strength-training techniques, as previously discussed, are important aspects of "natural" athletic performance enhancement programs.

Given the prevalence of these drugs, clinicians must be alert to recognizing their use in patients. Athletes at highest risk for use include those in sports requiring high levels of strength, speed, size, power, and endurance. One should be alert to use in athletes who express frustration with having reached a plateau in their sport and are looking for a way to "get over a wall" or "break through." The athlete who uses

---

BOX 13-11 Assessing Patients for Use of Performance-Enhancing Substances*

1. Are you using any substances or supplements to improve your performance in your sports(s)?
2. Do you use any substance to improve your body's appearance, weight, or strength?
3. How do you feel you are doing at your sport? Is your performance where you would like it to be? Are you satisfied with how you are doing? If not, how are you planning to improve?
4. What are your goals with regard to your sport?
5. Are there people in your life (coaches, parents, self) who are pressuring you to improve your performance?
6. Do you know of any athletes or other peers who are using performance-enhancing substances?
7. What questions do you have about drugs or supplements or other things athletes might use to enhance performance?

*Be sure to include questions about all drug and alcohol use and needle use as per general adolescent health guidelines.

Adapted from Holland-Hall C: Performance-enhancing substances: is your adolescent patient using? *Pediatr Clin North Am* 54(4):651-662, 2007.

---

other illicit drugs, tobacco, or alcohol may be at increased risk as well (Holland-Hall, 2007). Box 13-11 suggests several interviewing questions to assess the use of performance-enhancing substances.

Anabolic-Androgenic Steroids

The term *anabolic* refers to the drug's ability to stimulate protein synthesis; *androgenic* refers to the stimulation of male secondary sexual characteristics. Anabolic-androgenic steroids (AAS) react with a variety of receptors in the body including glucocorticoids, progestin, estrogen, and androgen. Endogenous anabolic steroids start adolescent development in the prepubertal male. The exogenous drug used by both sexes for performance enhancement or appearance is derived from testosterone. This produces changes in the endocrine/reproductive, cardiovascular, hepatic, musculoskeletal, and neurological systems. The AAS drugs are Class III controlled substances. Steroids are often taken from 1 to 100 times the normal therapeutic dose.

The prevalence rates among high school students in the U.S. range from 2.1% to 7.5% across state surveys with more males than females reporting usage (Eaton et al, 2010). Calfee and Fadale (2006) found that up to one third of those taking anabolic steroids were nonathletes who used them to enhance their appearance. Athletes in the following sports have been shown to be at most risk of using/abusing these substances: football, wrestling, bodybuilding, sprinting, shot-putting, discus throwing, and weight lifting (Greydanus and Feucht, 2009). Twenty-five percent to 33% who use the injectable form report sharing needles, which puts them at risk for HIV, HBV, and HCV (Calfee and Fadale, 2006).

Clinical effects can be irreversible and extremely serious in males and females. Up to 30% of users experience some mild subjective effects, which can include acne, seborrhea, weight gain, deepening voice, precocious puberty, gynecomastia in males, or premature balding. With sustained use, some of the more serious side effects include cardiac failure, impotence,

edema, testicular atrophy, liver dysfunction and possibly malignancy, and tendon or muscle injuries (as a result of the development of dysplastic collagen fibrils). Premature epiphyseal closure can leave the immature athlete shorter than expected. Hepatotoxicity is most related to the 17-alkylated derivatives. In females AAS use can cause irreversible menstrual irregularities and breast atrophy, virilization (enlargement of the clitoris, hirsutism, male pattern baldness, deepening of the voice with larynx changes), and amenorrhea (may be partially reversible after termination of use). Approximately 50% of steroid users meet the mental illness standards for drug dependence or abuse. Mood swings, violent behavior, heightened aggression, and depression severe enough to be linked with suicide have been described (Calfee and Fadale, 2006; Jenkins and Adger, 2007).

Steroid users may use the substance in three preparations: oral, injected, or transdermal. The oral forms are shorter acting and excreted over days; the injectables are longer acting and can take months to eliminate from the body. Withdrawal effects can occur up to a year or more after ceasing use. Generally used in the off-season (to gain strength and prevent detection), these drugs are taken in cycles of use lasting 4 to 12 weeks each. Sometimes more than one type of steroid is used at a time ("stacking"), or the steroids are dosed incrementally and used in both the oral and injectable forms and then tapered at the end of a cycle ("pyramiding"). Newer, "designer" synthetic steroids (Tetrahydrogestrinone [THG], gestrinone, and trenbolone) have been produced in an attempt to prevent detection by doping tests; tests have since been devised. Drugs used to mask the detection of steroids may include uricosuric agents (probenecid), diuretics (spironolactone, furosemide), and epitestosterone.

Androstenedione and Dehydroepiandrosterone

Androstenedione ("andro") and related dehydroepiandrosterone (DHEA) are prohormones that are converted to either testosterone or estrone. Androstenedione is the more potent of the two and is a Class III controlled drug. DHEA may be purchased over the counter. Usage data is scant, but studies have shown that up to 4% of high school athletes and nonathletes used precursors, and 5.3% of college athletes reported use (Calfee and Fadale, 2006).

Steroid precursors are used because of the mistaken belief that they will increase testosterone and produce the same effects on muscles and performance as seen with anabolic steroids. Studies, however, have demonstrated no convincing measurable changes in athletic performance (Jenkins and Adger, 2007). Rather than show increases in testosterone levels, steroid precursors significantly increase estrone and estradiol levels to the point of causing adverse changes in lipid levels and endogenous testosterone over time; male gynecomastia; virilization in females; priapism; and possible hyperplastic prostatic changes. Additionally, potential impurities in the products can produce positive drug screens (Calfee and Fadale, 2006).

Growth Hormone

Human growth hormone (HGH) (available in a biosynthetic, injectable form) is often used one or more times a month and is banned by sporting leagues. It is taken in the mistaken belief that it will enhance athletic performance through anabolic mechanisms of increasing lean body mass and decreasing fat mass. It can, however, produce premature epiphyseal closure, jaw enlargement, hypertension, insulin resistance, slipped capital femoral epiphysis, and (rarely) papilledema with intracranial hypertension. Athletes who take it report a "feel-good" sensation (probably caused by fluid shifts within tissues) and decreases in subcutaneous fat for a fit appearance. There is risk of HBV, HCV, and HIV because of needle-sharing practices. One study showed an incidence rate of 5% in high school students; half of them were combining HGH with steroids. An NCAA study revealed an incidence use of HGH at 3.5% (Calfee and Fadale, 2006).

Creatine and Other Supplements

Creatine is involved in the production of energy for muscular contraction and is found in fish, meat, milk, and other foods in small amounts. Synthetic creatine is an over-the-counter supplement used in the belief that it enhances athletic endurance by improving muscular contraction strength and performance. It increases (by approximately 20%) stores of muscle phosphocreatine that in turn release initial energy for muscle contraction in short, high-intensity activities (e.g., wrestling), quickening phosphocreatine replenishment during recovery, and delaying fatigue onset. The exercise must be maximal and anaerobic and last long enough to deplete the stores nonusers would have. If the duration of the activity is too long (more than 60 seconds), however, other sources of energy supplant the creatine effects, and benefit is not seen.

Athletes generally take a cycle of 5 g, four times daily for 4 to 6 days and then a maintenance dose of 2 g per day for the following 3 months. A month of abstinence then is practiced. It is important for those taking creatine to drink 6 to 8 ounces of water to prevent dehydration. Carbohydrate-rich fluids increase the absorption, and caffeine impairs uptake.

Side effects of creatine supplementation can include weight gain due to water retention, poorer performance, anxiety, fatigue, headaches, rashes, dyspnea, muscle cramps, mild gastrointestinal distress, and elevated serum creatinine and renal disease (rare). There are no data showing the effects of long-term use, the effect of supplementation on the other creatine storage organs (brain or heart), or effects in those younger than 18 years old. Additionally, there are no studies that show any improvement in long-term endurance sports with creatine supplementation, and most studies show no ergogenic effects at all (Greydanus and Feucht, 2009).

Creatine supplementation is not recommended in those less than 18 years old. However, incidence studies have reported a usage range of 5.6% to 8.2% in 10- to 18-year-olds; the majority did not know how much they consumed or that they were, in fact, consuming beyond the recommended amounts. The use in twelfth graders (44%) and college athletes (25% to 78%) is similar (Calfee and Fadale, 2006).

Ephedra

Ephedrine has a chemical structure similar to amphetamine. It enhances the release of norepinephrine and stimulates the central nervous system. The herbal form is ma huang. Ephedra was banned as an energy enhancer and diet aid in 2004 by the U.S. Food and Drug Administration (FDA); a nationwide effort in 2006 focused on curbing the retail sale

of pseudoephedrine. However, some products that contain ephedra were not banned. These continue to include traditional Chinese herbal medicines, herbal teas, and medications that contain chemically synthesized ephedra (Kapner, 2008). Dietary supplements for bodybuilding and weight loss are readily available over the Internet and can include ephedra as an ingredient or as an unlisted one. The ephedra may be combined with a botanical source of caffeine, notably guarana *(Paullinia cupana),* Kola nut *(Cola nitida),* or yerba mate.

Athletes use ephedra to provide quick energy and help in losing body fat, thereby enhancing speed and appearance. However, no actual boost in endurance or weight loss is seen when the drug is used alone. When combined with caffeine, there is some improvement with endurance, and there can be weight loss in the obese on dietary restrictions (this weight loss is not seen in lean athletes) (Jenkins and Adger, 2007).

Adverse reactions include tachycardia (most often), hypertension, dysrhythmias, anxiety, tremors, insomnia, seizures, paranoid psychoses, stroke, myocardial infarction, and sudden death. The incidence is variously reported to be as high as 26% in high school females, 12% in high school males (Calfee and Fadale, 2006), and 2.5% in college athletes; ice hockey athletes reported the highest use rates (Kapner, 2008).

Energy Drinks

Energy drinks are promoted as energy-enhancing substances and are heavily promoted without offering much information about their potential side effects. Advertisements for these drinks promote improved physical and cognitive performance, "fun," and their psychoactive and stimulant drug effects. They are loaded with caffeine, sugar, and other ingredients (e.g., ginseng, taurine, guarana, B-complex vitamins). When combined with alcohol (a popular drink), one study of college students revealed that there was more sexual assault, driving with an intoxicated driver, and being physically hurt or injured and requiring medical treatment. Twenty-four percent reported consuming this combination drink over the prior 30-day period (O'Brien et al, 2008). When used in this combination, the stimulating effect of the energy drink deceives imbibers into thinking they are less intoxicated than they are. Another study showed a consumption rate of the energy drink alone at 51% of college students in an average month (Malinauskas et al, 2007). Reports of use rates in youth 11 to 18 years old range from 30% to 42.3% (Heneman and Zidenberg-Cherr, 2007; Pennington, 2010). Many European countries have imposed restrictions on where the energy drinks may be sold, banned them, or required they carry a health warning about the high caffeine content.

When consumed in large amounts, the high caffeine content combined with after-exercise physiological recovery mechanisms and/or alcohol consumption, can result in side effects including dehydration, insomnia, headaches, increased systolic blood pressure and heart rate, nervousness, nosebleeds, vomiting, seizures, heart dysrhythmia, and even death (Kapner, 2008).

Nutritional Supplements

Nutritional supplements are readily available to aspiring athletes who believe that they will perform better if using them. They generally are composed of one or more of the following: a vitamin, a mineral, an herb or other botanical, an amino acid, a dietary supplement that raises the total daily intake or a concentrate, metabolite, constituent, extract, or a combination of the last four ingredients. The concern with these products is that studies have shown a broad inconsistency in the accuracy of labeling ingredients and amounts; contamination; and the inclusion of dangerous substances (e.g., steroids). They are to be discouraged (Calfee and Fadale, 2006).

Recreational Activities: Safety Issues

Recreational activities play a key role in maintaining and promoting physical activity and health. Health care providers should ask children and youth about all of their physical health activities and update this information regularly. Some activities may be important for independent transportation (e.g., skateboarding, cycling), may serve as a cross-training method for another sport, and be relatively inexpensive versus organized sports. Many of these activities involve mortality (from spinal cord or head trauma) and morbidity (e.g., general body trauma, fractures, torn ligaments, concussions) unless undertaken safely. The following guidelines should be offered to parents of children and to youth who participate in these recreational activities:

- *ATVs and golf carts.* The AAP and ATV industry recommendations differ as to the age of the rider and size of the ATV. The AAP (2007d) steadfastly advises that no children under 16 years of age should ride regardless of the engine size; engines ≥90 cc are acceptable for those 16 years and older. They should not be driven on public or paved roads, only on designated trails, and at safe speeds. Drivers should take an ATV safety course; not carry passengers; wear motorcycle helmets, safety glasses, reflective outerwear, and other protective gear; have flags, reflectors, and lights on vehicles; install seatbelts; and not ride at night (Enoch, 2008). New safety guidelines proposed for golf carts include premarket seatbelts, speed control, and slower braking mechanisms (Watson et al, 2008).
- *Golfing.* Supervise children at all times who have a golf club in hand; educate about the rules of golf (standing at least four club lengths away from a swinging club; "stop-look-and-swing" before swinging), and store golf clubs out of the reach of children (Brian and Glazer, 2005).
- *Playground equipment.* Playground surfaces should be regularly inspected for hazards (sharp protrusions, detached matting, no exposed concrete footings), and be constructed out of shock-absorbing, single-unit materials (e.g., rubber mats, shredded tires, and loose fill [double-shredded bark mulch, wood fibers, sand, fine/medium gravel]) with a minimum thickness of 9 inches (American Academy of Orthopedic Surgeons [AAOS] [2009a]; Horn et al, 2010). Under no circumstances should children be allowed on equipment that is placed over a hard surface (concrete, asphalt, grass and soil [soil can become hard packed]). Playgrounds should be properly designed for safety, with swings placed away from sandboxes, separate areas for preschoolers and older children, widely spaced for popular activities, good sight lines for supervision, and barriers between playground and street.
- *Roller sports and cycling.* Skateboards are not to be ridden by children under 5 years of age; 6- to 10-year-olds should be closely supervised by knowledgeable adults or adolescents (AAP, 2009). Preventive measures (many apply to general cycling safety) include riding in skateboarding parks; riding on smooth surfaces away from traffic; using quality skateboards (shorter decks are best for beginners; fit to weight of child); keeping all equipment in proper shape (inspect for broken, cracked parts, sharp edges; slippery board top with nicks/cracks; lubricate parts); learning basic skills of slowing, turning, and falling safely; practicing tricks/jumps only in controlled parks; keeping in good physical shape by stretching and conditioning before and after activity; not wearing headphones while riding; not putting another rider on the same skateboard, bicycle, or scooter; knowing rules of the road (stopping at stop signs, etc.); knowing what to do in emergencies; not riding at night; and wearing proper safety equipment (properly fitting helmet, wrist guards, knee and elbow pads, shoes). (See helmet guidelines discussed earlier in this chapter.)
- *Swimming.* All children should learn to swim; most deaths occur at times of inadequate supervision or due to an overestimation of swimming ability (Healthy Children, 2010). Children are judged to be water safe at 4 years of age, if trained (Brent and Weitzman, 2004).
- *Trampolines.* They cannot be recommended for home use; however, some advice to parents and those using equipment (USCPSC, 2000) includes allowing children on the trampolines only under the close instruction and supervision of adults who are prepared to respond to medical emergencies; netting around the trampoline perimeter will help keep the jumper confined to the jumping surface (will not reduce accidents due to the surface itself); not allowing jumpers to jump onto the trampoline from a higher level/object/surface; padding the entire frame, hooks, and springs; only one person on trampoline at any given time; if the trampoline is over 20 inches off the ground, no one under 6 years of age should use it; no ladders should be attached to the trampoline; and not allowing somersaults or stunts (acrobatic maneuvers).
- *Winter sports.* Safety measures include taking lessons; fitness training to reduce fatigue; going slower; choosing terrain that fits skills level; making 2 to 3 warm-up runs when skiing or snowboarding; checking snow conditions; wearing helmets; staying within the boundaries of the ski areas; knowing that bindings are more important than boots (bindings should be no greater than 3 to 4 years old); using sunscreen; skiing with a buddy; wearing layers; knowing the rules; adhering to storm warnings; knowing the signs of hypothermia; not skiing if tired or in pain; and staying alert and in control (AAOS, 2009b). Cross-country/backcountry skiers need to be prepared to assume risks related to environmental factors (e.g., avalanches, hypothermia).

14

Sleep and Rest

LYNNE A. FROST AND CATHERINE E. BURNS

Every child needs adequate sleep for good health. Without it, serious health and developmental problems may appear. Sleep disturbances may manifest as bedtime resistance, inability to fall asleep, nighttime waking, arousal difficulties, or excessive daytime sleepiness.

Sleep problems represent one of the most common concerns of parents, and children's sleep is receiving much needed attention, both clinically and in research. Sleep will be an extremely frequent topic for discussion with parents. A variety of studies highlight some of the issues and significant prevalence of sleep problems in children. In the review of sleep studies, it is commonly noted that 20% to 30% of young children experience some form of sleeping difficulty (Boergers et al, 2007; Jenni et al, 2007). Frequent night waking was reported to occur in more than 35% of 2.5-year-olds, decreasing with age to approximately 13% of 6-year-olds (Petit et al, 2007). Similarly, this study found that the number of children having difficulty falling asleep decreased with age as well, from 16% at 3 years to 7.4% at age 6. Canadian researchers Touchette and colleagues (2005) found that 23.5% of 5-month-old children did not sleep 6 consecutive hours. Furthermore, 33% of children who did not sleep 6 consecutive hours at 5 months or 17 months continued to be unable to sleep 6 hours at 2.5 years old. Sleep problems have been identified in greater than 35% of school-age children and adolescents (Rodriguez, 2007). It is estimated that 15 million U.S. children are affected by some form of sleep inadequacy, with a surprising 40% at a moderate or severe level of impairment (Smaldone et al, 2009). On the other hand, sleep disorders are underdiagnosed, with only 3.7% of children with an International Classification of Diseases, 9th revision (ICD-9) sleep disorder diagnosis (Meltzer et al, 2010).

Insufficient sleep affects and is affected by many areas of child and family well-being, including physical and mental health issues. As noted in Box 14-1, many behavioral, mental health, and family problems can be related to sleep problems (Smaldone et al, 2009). Pediatric sleep problems may also produce sleep deprivation and stress in the caregiver(s). As with all other primary care problems in pediatrics, the provider must be vigilant for a myriad of potential causes.

Attention to cultural definitions of normal sleep habits also is essential. Sleep can be considered a biologically driven behavior that is strongly shaped and interpreted by cultural values and beliefs of the parents. Not all cultures expect children to sleep in separate beds or rooms, nor is it expected that most sleep will occur during the nighttime hours in an uninterrupted fashion (Dewar, 2008a). The hours of sleep, methods of helping the child to initiate the sleep cycle, and expectations for normal sleep behavior are also culturally driven.

◼ Normal Sleep Stages and Cycles

The essential functions of sleep are not fully understood. Sleep is traditionally considered a time of renewal for the mind and body, but it is not simply a state of rest. At times the brain is more active in sleep than in wakefulness and, because infants and young children spend the majority of their time in sleep, it is considered a time for essential brain development. Growth and healing, learning and processing information, and many other functions are facilitated by the sleep state. Fewer studies have been done with children, but sleep deprivation in adults has negative effects on concentration, cognition, and emotional functioning (Davis et al, 2004).

CIRCADIAN RHYTHMS AND ESTABLISHMENT OF NORMAL SLEEP PATTERNS

Many biological activities are set on a 24-hour cycle. These include sleep and wakefulness, body temperature regulation, hormonal activity, respiratory, cardiac, renal, and intestinal functions. Circadian rhythms are not established in the newborn, and homeostatic mechanisms are also poorly developed. Thus, sleep can occur around the clock with ease although patterns are irregular. Circadian rhythms emerge at about 2 to 3 months old (Sheldon, 2004).

Melatonin secreted by the hypothalamus is responsible for the timing of physiological processes, including the sleep-wake cycle. Light suppresses melatonin production, and darkness is associated with the highest melatonin levels. In normal humans melatonin begins to rise when the sun sets, peaks at 2 AM, and falls to almost undetectable levels in the daytime. The day-night melatonin cycle is established between 4 and 6 months old. Levels peak at ages 1 to 3 years and then decline with age. Maternal melatonin crosses the placental barrier and is secreted in breast milk. Prolactin, growth hormone, and testosterone are also on circadian rhythm patterns with maximal

BOX 14-1 Etiology of Sleep Problems in Children

Sleep problems may result from a variety of other problems, including the following:

- Physical factors
  - o Ear infections
  - o Neurological disorders
  - o Hypothyroidism
  - o Obesity
  - o Tonsillar and adenoid hypertrophy
  - o Pain
  - o Blindness
  - o Orofacial anomalies
  - o Asthma
  - o Down syndrome and other genetic conditions
  - o Chronic diseases, such as cystic fibrosis
- Psychological factors
  - o Developmental stage
  - o Stress, depression, separation and other anxieties, or other mental health problems
  - o Attention-deficit/hyperactivity disorder (ADHD), learning and behavior problems
  - o Mental retardation
  - o Autism
- Family factors
  - o Parental mismanagement of sleep routines
  - o Family conflict and violence
  - o Parental physical and emotional health
  - o Maternal depression
- Environmental and temperamental factors
  - o Temperament characteristics, including low sensory threshold, negative mood, and decreased adaptability
  - o Environmental factors, including sleeping arrangements, altered daily routines, and feeding practices
- Caffeine, medications, toxins, or substance abuse

secretion at night (Stevens, 2008). Growth hormone appears to be secreted in larger amounts during stages III and IV of sleep (Rodriguez, 2007).

SLEEP CYCLE

Normal sleep can be divided into two distinct phases: rapid eye movement (REM) sleep and nonrapid eye movement (NREM) sleep. Each phase has distinctive levels of arousal, autonomic response, brain activity, and muscle tone. NREM sleep can be further divided into four distinct stages as defined by changes in electroencephalographic (EEG) patterns. Newborn sleep cycles are discussed separately in this chapter.

Rapid Eye Movement Sleep

REM sleep is considered to be the dreaming phase. EEG waves are similar to those of the awake state, suggesting that higher levels of brain activity are at work; however, the function of REM sleep is unclear. Although nerve impulses to the spinal cord and muscles are blocked, leaving the body paralyzed except for minor twitching, the respiratory, eye, and middle ear muscles remain active. The child may smile in a transitory way or make short utterances. Breathing and heart rates become irregular and relatively rapid. Reflexes, kidney function, hormonal secretions, and auditory sensitivity are all

altered. The rapid eye movements of this phase are of particular interest. People awakened during REM sleep may report dreams at the time. Children as young as 2 years old have reported dreams during REM sleep. Because REM sleep is associated with arousals and is preponderant in the first year of life, infants are likely to have problems with maintaining sleep. Some mothers are concerned about their infants' restless sleep when it is only REM sleep that they are observing.

REM sleep occurs in approximately 90-minute periods with the longest REM episode occurring just after the body temperature reaches its lowest point during the night, around 5 AM. Thus in older children and adults, most REM sleep occurs later in the night. The proportion of REM sleep decreases from 55% in infancy to about 25% by the time the child is 5 years old.

Nonrapid Eye Movement Sleep

The four stages of NREM sleep become distinguishable within 6 months of birth. In the preschool and school-age years, NREM stages III and IV are preponderant. These stages end with a REM phase. The parasomnias, including nightmares and sleepwalking, which are related to this transition from NREM to arousal or REM phases, occur most commonly in children in these age groups (Rodriguez, 2007).

Stage I. Stage I sleep is a state of drowsiness and transition to sleep. There may be eye-rolling movements, decreased body movements, and perhaps opening and closing of the eyelids. Individuals may believe that they are awake, but they cannot report accurately events that occurred during this time. In mature individuals, stage I accounts for about 5% of sleep.

Stage II. Stage II sleep is somewhat deeper than that of stage I, although the person can still be easily aroused. Eye movements, breathing, and heart rate slow. Muscles weaken, although the child can reposition. If aroused, the person may report thinking about things and may report dreams. Mature sleepers spend about 50% of their sleep in this stage, generally in the last half of the night.

Stages III and IV. These two stages are nearly identical and sometimes called delta, deep, or slow-wave sleep. Stage III sleep is deeper than that of stage II. The body is deeply relaxed, breathing is shallow, and heart rate is slow. Stage IV is defined by the EEG pattern it produces. When the delta waves occupy 50% of the EEG pattern, stage IV sleep has begun.

During stages III and IV the sleeper is hard to arouse. If awakened, the individual feels confused and disoriented. About 15% to 20% of sleep takes place in stages III and IV, occurring earlier in the night. Stages III and IV sleep seem to develop at about 3 to 4 months old; by 4 months, stages III and IV comprise more than half of the total sleep.

In neonates three types of sleep are recognized: quiet, active, and indeterminate sleep. These correspond to NREM sleep, REM sleep, and a period that is neither of these as measured by polysomnography. REM sleep represents a larger proportion of the overall sleep duration in neonates than it does in adults (Stevens, 2008).

Sleep Cycle Processes

Two main processes are theorized to regulate sleep and wakefulness. The circadian process dictates sleep and wakefulness based on an internal rhythm related to a light-dark

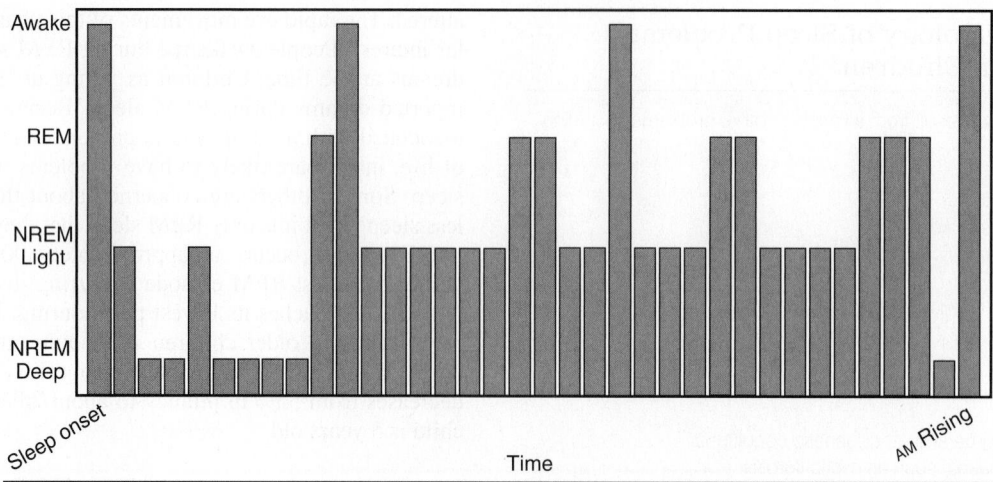

FIGURE 14-1 Schema of typical night sleep pattern with sleep states and stages.

cycle. The homeostatic process requires the body to build a need for sleep while awake and as the sleep need is satisfied through sleeping, to build a need for wakefulness. The longer one is awake, the greater the drive for sleep and vice versa.

Sleep onset is the time when the person enters stage I NREM sleep. The sleep period begins with sleep onset and continues until full arousal occurs. The sleep cycle includes the repeated episodes of NREM and REM sleep of the sleep period. Waking involves full alert and recall after the sleep period. Semi-wakefulness or alerting to the immediate environment occurs easily in REM sleep or stages I or II in NREM sleep. The REM phase becomes more pronounced later in the evening (Fig.14-1).

In the first weeks of life the sleep cycles consist of equal periods of active and quiet sleep with active sleep initiating each cycle, but by 6 months, NREM sleep occurs first. As the infant matures, consolidation of sleep cycles occurs and awake periods lengthen during the day. REM sleep decreases and social cues, such as feeding and nighttime routines, begin to influence sleep cycles. Because young infants have more sleep cycles per night than older individuals do, each cycle with a brief waking that precedes the next sleep period, and because infants often have more difficulty returning to the next sleep cycle from this normal waking episode, more opportunities for sleep disturbances can arise with infants. In a classic study, Anders (1979) found that on average infants less than 12 months of age awaken three times from their sleep cycles per night regardless of whether their parents are aware of these awakenings.

After 6 months of age most of the NREM deep sleep occurs in the early night, so associated problems, such as night terrors and sleepwalking, occur then. Most REM sleep occurs in the second half of the night, so problems associated with REM sleep, such as nightmares, occur more in this phase. The short periods of wakefulness throughout the night are when problems of night waking or difficulty entering the next sleep cycle may occur. In older children and adults, the periods of semi-wakefulness may last for a few seconds to a few minutes. It may be the time when one turns over, looks at the clock, or adjusts the covers. Both total amount of sleep and proportion of REM sleep decrease with age.

DURATION OF SLEEP

Children need more sleep time than adults but gradually achieve adult sleep patterns the older they become (Rodriguez, 2007). Sleep requirements over a 24-hour period vary widely and change as children mature. The typical neonate sleeps 16 hours each day, but some may require up to 18 hours of sleep per day. One third of this is daytime sleep. The longest neonate sleep period is 2.5 to 4 hours and can occur at any time during the 24-hour day (Dewar, 2008c). By 3 months, the baby sleeps almost 15 hours, but the sleep times are more clearly organized into daytime wakefulness and nighttime sleep with a 5-hour period of consistent nighttime sleep (Jenni et al, 2006). Most 6-month-old infants sleep through the night and have morning and afternoon naps. At 1 year most children sleep about 13.9 hours. The morning nap is generally given up between 12 and 24 months, but the afternoon nap may persist until the child is 4 or 5 years old. By 2 years the child is probably sleeping 11 to 12 hours at night with a 1- to 2-hour nap after lunch. Five-year-olds sleep 11 hours per night on average. Four- to 6-year-olds generally have an 8 PM bedtime and 7 AM wake time on weekdays and slightly later bedtimes on weekends (Touchette et al, 2008). The average sleep requirement for adolescents is believed to be about 8 to 9 hours per night (Table 14-1) (Dewar, 2008b,c; Jenni et al, 2007; Rodriguez, 2007).

■ Sleep Issues

CO-SLEEPING ISSUES

Sleep habits are strongly influenced by culture. Co-sleeping is common in many cultures and has been the human norm for thousands of years. Co-sleeping by family members is probably more common worldwide than is separate sleeping as advocated in the U.S. Warmth, protection, and a sense of well-being are undoubtedly facilitated by having babies sleep with their mothers or siblings (Dewar, 2008a,b). One of the greatest advantages of co-sleeping is the facilitation of breastfeeding. Parents of co-sleeping infants report that not only is breastfeeding improved, but parental sleep and parent-infant bonding is as well, and there is a decrease in nighttime infant crying (Goldberg and Keller, 2007). It is most common in

TABLE 14-1 Average Sleep by Age

Age	Nighttime Sleep (hr)	Daytime Sleep (hr)
1 week	8.25	8.25
1 month	8.5	7
3 months	10	5
6 months	11	3.4
9 months	11.2	2.8
12 months	11.7	2.4
18 months	11.6	2
2 years	11.4	1.8
3-5 years	12.5	
5-11 years	11	
12-17 years	8-9	

Adapted from Dewar G: *Baby sleep requirements: a guide for the science-minded parents,* 2008b. Available at www.parentingscience.com/baby-sleep-require-ments.html (accessed Jan 10, 2010); Dewar G: *Newborn sleep patterns: a guide for the science-minded parents,* 2008c. Available at www.parentingscience.com/newborn-sleep.html (accessed Jan 10, 2010); Jenni O, Molinari L, Caflisch J, et al: Sleep duration from ages 1 to 10 years: variability and stability in comparison with growth, *Pediatrics* 120:769-776, 2007; Rodriguez A: Pediatric sleep and epilepsy, *Curr Neurol Neurosci Rep* 7:342-347, 2007.

African-American and Hispanic families. Co-sleeping is also common with absence of one parent from the home. Co-sleeping is not in itself a reason for sleep problems. However, some families allow the child to sleep with the adults because of problems with enforcing bedtimes, anxiety about leaving the child alone, problems with the quality of daytime interactions, or a desire to avoid the spouse. Sexual abuse of the child also needs to be considered (see Chapter 17 for further child abuse discussion). In these cases, intervention may be helpful to the family (Howard and Wong, 2001).

Although studies have shown that co-sleeping facilitates breastfeeding as well as maternal-infant bonding, the American Academy of Pediatrics (AAP) Task Force on Sudden Infant Death Syndrome (SIDS) states that bed sharing should not be considered as a strategy to reduce SIDS risk (AAP, 2005). The task force recommends "a separate but proximate sleeping environment" in which the young infant sleeps in the same room but in a separate bed, crib, bassinet, or cradle. There is some conflicting evidence as to whether bed sharing is actually a risk factor for SIDS. Some studies have concluded that co-sleeping alongside a parent is not the specific increased risk factor for SIDS, but rather an infant sleeping alongside a non-parent that is the actual threat for SIDS (Goldberg and Keller, 2007). Some leading pediatric sleep, medical, and breastfeeding experts caution that the AAP's recommendation may cause problems with bonding, quality of sleep, and enhancement of breastfeeding practices (Eidelman and Gartner, 2006; Gessner and Porter, 2006; Pelayo et al, 2006). Richard Ferber (2006), a pediatric sleep expert and longtime critic of co-sleeping, now believes there are benefits to this arrangement when practiced safely. Care should be taken to avoid using soft sleep surfaces such as quilts, blankets, pillows, comforters, or other similar materials. The bed sharer should not smoke or use substances that impair arousal. Parents should understand that safety standards are in place for the design of infant cribs. There are no standards for adult beds, so entrapment may be a possibility. Parents who plan to co-sleep should have an "exit plan," such as ending the practice at 6 months, before the child will

protest excessively (Sobralske and Gruber, 2009). School-age children who want to co-sleep with parents may have significant emotional problems, such as separation anxiety, which may require counseling.

SLEEP POSITIONING

Studies have provided strong evidence that positioning young infants on their backs significantly decreases the incidence of SIDS. The AAP (2005) recommends that all infants sleep in a supine position unless there is some specific medical contraindication to that position. Side sleeping is not recommended. The AAP also recommends use of a crib and avoidance of soft materials in the sleep environment, bed sharing, smoking during pregnancy and afterward, and overheating the infant. Offering a pacifier at sleep times seems to have some effect in reducing SIDS risks (AAP, 2005). SIDS is also discussed in Chapter 38.

The AAP (2005) recommends that parents place the baby on its stomach while awake to encourage upper body motor development and to prevent positional plagiocephaly. Parents seem to understand the "Back to Sleep" guidelines more than they do infant positioning with "tummy time" during awake times (Koren et al, 2010).

■ Assessment

Assessment of sleep patterns requires an understanding of the developmental progression of sleep patterns, a comprehensive history, and a complete physical examination. Assessment of sleep patterns should be included in all well-child visits. Before a decision is made that a sleep problem exists, the provider must be sure to determine whether the child's sleep pattern is problematic for the caregiver and/or results in daytime sleepiness with disruption to the child's health and well-being. The clinician must be careful not to impose his or her ideas of the best sleep habits onto the family and remember that cultural patterns are very strong in this area of childrearing. Late bedtimes, early rising, night waking, and co-sleeping may be upsetting to some parents but not to others. Of course, preventive counseling is always in order.

INDICATORS OF SLEEP PROBLEMS IN CHILDREN AND ADOLESCENTS

Sleepiness in infants is especially difficult to notice because they sleep so many hours normally. They should not have sleepiness that is severe enough to interfere with feeding. Toddlers and preschoolers may show signs of hyperactivity, emotional lability, irritability, and aggressiveness when sleepy. Alternately, the child may fall asleep during activities when alertness would be expected, such as at mealtimes.

School-age children are usually considered to be good sleepers. Taking naps or sleeping at school are not normal behaviors. Other concerning symptoms may include inattention, restlessness, emotional lability, or daydreaming at school. There is considerable overlap of these symptoms with attention-deficit/hyperactivity disorder (ADHD), and indeed the two problems are often related.

Adolescents have many problems with sleep that may manifest as excessive sleepiness, difficulties with mood regulation,

BOX 14-2	Sleep Screening Tool

1. Does your child attend daycare or school?
   Starts at_____AM/PM; ends at_____AM/PM
2. In the past week, has your child taken a medication, alcohol, or herbal remedy for sleep?
   If yes, list name_____, frequency of use_____.
3. Rate your child's sleep quality.
   _____ Good (sleeps through the night most nights)
   _____ Poor (has problems sleeping most nights)
   _____ Very bad (has problems sleeping every night)
4. Bedtime routine and child response:
   • What time does your child typically go to bed?
     weeknights_____, weekends_____.
   • Where does your child sleep?
   • How difficult is it for your child to settle and fall asleep after bedtime rituals?
     _____Not difficult
     _____Somewhat of a struggle
     _____A constant struggle
   • Length of time between going to bed and sleep onset?
     _____minutes
   • Does your child fall asleep by himself or herself? yes/no. If no, what is the child's routine? (Needs body contact, bottle or pacifier, TV or radio noise, or other stimuli to induce sleep)
5. What is the nap(s) routine?
   • What are typical hours for naps? AM:_____, PM:_____
   • Repeat other questions for bedtime routine: place, difficulties, routines.

6. How difficult is it for the child to get up in the morning?
   _____Not difficult
   _____Somewhat of a struggle (15-30 minutes some mornings)
   _____A constant struggle (more than 30 minutes every morning)
7. Night waking: In the past week, how many times did your child wake up during the night?
   _____never or once,_____ 2 or 3 times,_____4 or more times
   What was the main reason for waking?_____thirst, _____bladder,_____other reason (please describe)
   How much time does the child spend awake between 10 PM and 6 AM?_____hour(s) _____minute(s)
8. In the past week, how sleepy was your child during the day?
   _____Not at all sleepy
   _____Naps or falls asleep some days
   _____Naps or falls asleep most days
   _____Falls asleep in class most days
9. Risk factors for sleep problems: Does your child:
   _____Have other behavioral or emotional problems?
   _____Have health or developmental problems?
   _____Take substances that might affect sleep: medicines, caffeine, street drugs, cigarettes?
10. Do you consider your child's sleep to be a problem? _____yes, _____no
    _____Serious problem
    _____A small problem
    _____Not a problem at all

Data from Howard B, Wong J: Sleep disorders, *Pediatr Rev* 22:327-341, 2001; Lee K, Ward T: Critical components of a sleep assessment for clinical practice settings, *Issues Ment Health Nurs* 26:739-750, 2005; and Sadeh A: A brief screening questionnaire for infant sleep problems: validation and findings for an Internet sample, *Pediatrics* 113:e570-e577, 2004.

impaired academic performance, and increased risk for accidents and obesity. These may be related to adolescent changes in sleep physiology and lifestyle habits of the teen years. Chronic sleep deprivation is a common reason for sleepiness in adolescents (Noland et al, 2009). Sleep loss or disturbances have been associated with increased risk of future depression and anxiety in adolescents (Alfano et al, 2009). Noland and associates (2009) identified the risk of adolescent obesity to increase by 80% due to each hour of chronically lost sleep. Sleep deprivation in adults causes poorer high-order cognitive functioning; accidents and poor judgment are outcomes (Stevens, 2008).

HISTORY

Pediatric sleep has become a topic of interest with increasing research and attention to sleep issues in children with a variety of health problems. Several child sleep screening tools can be used by clinicians in everyday practice to assess sleep hygiene (Box 14-2) (Lee and Ward, 2005; Sadeh, 2004). Because sleep problems are so common and tend to persist, it is recommended that sleep be addressed at well-child visits, as a component of care of sick children when sleep is likely to be interrupted, and with all children with chronic conditions because so many have associated sleep problems. The normal sleep pattern, the general health history, sleep habits of the parents and family, and the sleep environment are assessed for factors that may affect sleep and rest. Significant sleep problems need to be referred to sleep centers or other specialists.

Normal Sleep Pattern

1. Nighttime and daytime sleep hygiene patterns include the following:
   • Quality of sleep
   • Sleep hours, including naps and awake time when parents are also awake. Number and frequency of feedings (for infants less than 3 months old), day and night.
   • Description of the state changes of the child, moving from wakefulness to sleep and then to waking again
   • Cues given by the infant or child to indicate need for sleep or rest
   • Daytime sleepiness indicators—napping, falling asleep in class, inattention, behavioral problems, accidental injuries in adolescents
   • Factors that might mask daytime sleepiness including sensory input, exercise, psychoactive substances such as caffeine, emotional state, motivation, or competing physiological needs, such as hunger
   • The routines used for getting the child to sleep and the child's behavior at these times, especially sleep resistance and sleep latency
2. Sleep problem history questions generally focus on normal sleep habits and then sleep onset, maintenance of sleep through the night, arousal, and daytime sleepiness issues. Factors that might affect sleep need to be identified. For each problem, the clinician needs to know:
   • Age when problem began and circumstances
   • Aggravating and relieving factors
   • Effects on daily living for child and family
   • Effects on the child's health and well-being

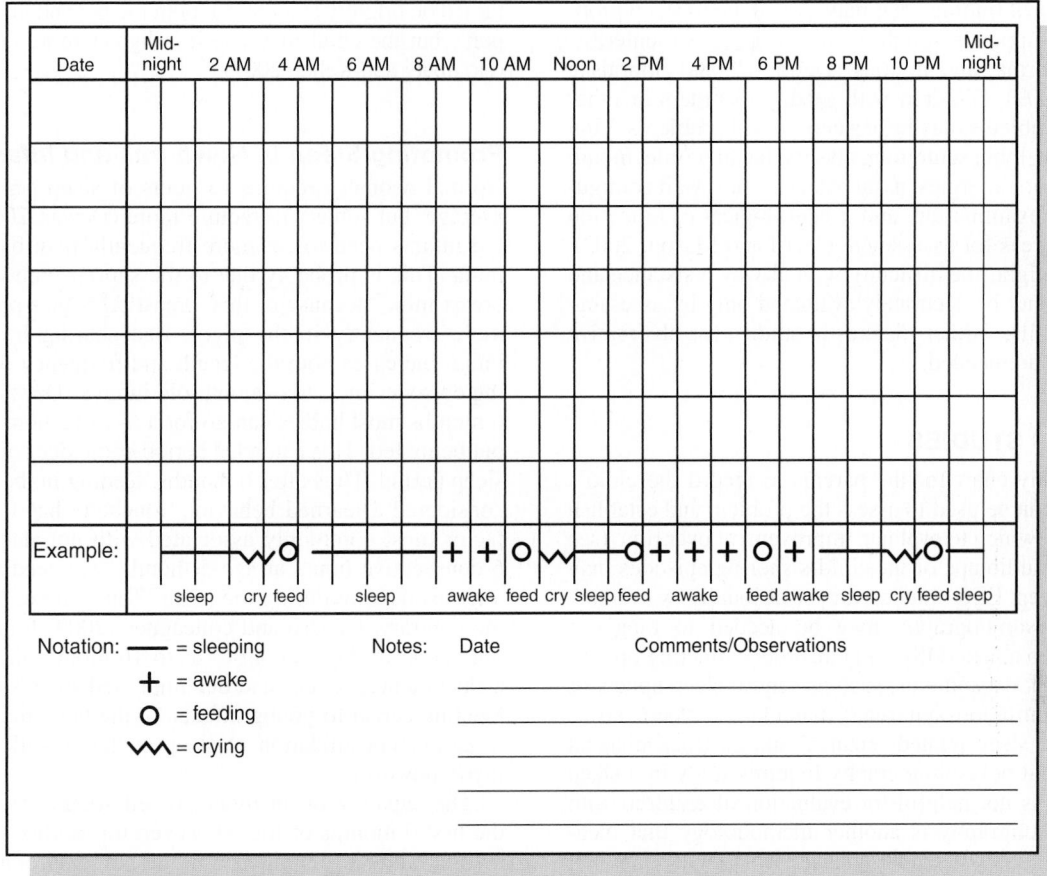

FIGURE 14-2 Example of sleep-activity-feeding record.

Additionally the environment should be assessed for noise, light, temperature, safety, and co-sleeping pattern. Schedules that affect sleep are also assessed (e.g., shift-work, school hours, night work, childcare schedules). A sleep activity record (Fig. 14-2) may be helpful to clarify any problems.

General Health History

- Indicators of the health and well-being of the child: Energy and alertness for daily activities need evaluation. The child with chronic inadequate sleep may appear to the parents to be functioning well. However, with more sleep, the parents will notice a decrease in irritability and better performance in many arenas.
- Past medical history and review of systems: Medical problems of the child are often associated with sleep difficulties. Ear infections; medications, such as bronchodilators; neurological problems, such as ADHD, seizures, Rett syndrome, and cerebral palsy; respiratory conditions; atopic conditions; gastroesophageal reflux; cardiac conditions; or anything that causes pain can affect sleep. Consider all the physical factors identified earlier in this chapter.
- Developmental problems can affect the child's ability to learn appropriate sleep behaviors.
- Depression, anxiety, or other psychiatric problems may be significant in older children with sleep problems.

- Psychoactive substance/medication/tobacco use, including caffeine drinks and alcohol, can affect sleep.
- School performance or peer relationships can contribute to disrupted sleep.

Parental and Family Assessment

- Indicators of the health and well-being and rest of the caregiver: Maternal depression has been clearly associated with children's sleep disruptions.
- Parental knowledge and beliefs about infant and child sleeping patterns: Parental understanding of the relationships between illness, temperament, and sleep should be explored.
- Parental ability to modulate the child's sleep and rest state and stress experienced in doing so
- Family sleep routines and expectations
- Recent changes in family living arrangements
- Divorce, separation, or other family stresses
- Extent of the disparity of the problem with family's cultural expectations
- Family history of sleep disorders

PHYSICAL EXAMINATION

It is important that a general physical examination be performed to detect signs of illness or pain. Signs of fatigue, irritability, or inattention may be associated with lack of adequate rest. Other clinical findings that may contribute to sleep problems include upper respiratory infection, gastroenteritis, teething, pinworms, and injuries (Dewar, 2008a; Sobralske and Gruber, 2009). Children with seizure disorders or other neurological problems may have sleep-related problems. Vital signs, oxyhemoglobin saturation, obesity, facial profile, mouth breathing, signs of allergies, nasal patency, chest wall configuration, cardiac examination, and a neurological examination are important areas for assessment (Ward and Mason, 2002). The degree of nighttime difficulty with airway resistance and obstruction cannot be accurately evaluated only by assessing the size of tonsils; further diagnostic studies for obstructive sleep disorders are needed.

DIAGNOSTIC STUDIES

A 24-hour, 7-day chart for the parents to record the child's sleep patterns can be used to assess the problem and establish a baseline from which to evaluate improvement over time (see Fig. 14-2). An audiotape of the child's snoring episodes may be helpful. Sleep EEG studies are occasionally warranted. Nocturnal polysomnography may be needed to diagnose obstructive sleep apnea (OSA) and disorders affecting breathing during sleep; dyssomnias, such as central sleep apnea, or central hypoventilation syndrome; narcolepsy; sleep movement disorders; sleep-related seizures; and gastroesophageal reflux. Nocturnal polysomnography requires study in a sleep laboratory and is not helpful for evaluation of children with parasomnias. Actigraphy is another methodology that measures the child's state of activity. It is helpful in understanding patterns of sleep-wake activity over time. The child wears a wrist or ankle bracelet for several days that monitors movement patterns. Other diagnostic studies may include EEG, surface electromyograms, electrocardiogram, CO_2 measurements, and pulse oximetry (Rodriguez, 2007).

■ Strategies for Prevention and Management of Sleep Problems

PREVENTION OF SLEEP PROBLEMS

Prevention of sleep problems is always best. *Sleep hygiene* is a term used to define healthful sleep behaviors. Good sleep hygiene requires an environment that is dark, quiet, and slightly cool; a regular schedule for waking, naps, and bedtime; and sleep-conducive activities in the child's life (National Sleep Foundation, 2009).

Setting the Sleep Cycle

People use a variety of cues to set the cycle, including daylight, darkness, meals, and activities. Parents need to make these cues clear to infants and children to help them establish healthful bedtime and sleep patterns. The cues of darkness and cool temperature should enhance sleep.

Exposure to bright light for even 1 minute at night will suppress melatonin production for at least 40 minutes. Use of aspirin, ibuprofen, and other nonsteroidal antiinflammatory drugs during the night also suppresses melatonin synthesis. These drugs inhibit the lowering of body temperature during the night, another factor in melatonin production. Lights should not be turned on brightly at night (for both mother and infant sleep support), but the child may nap in a lighter room during the day (Goldberg and Keller, 2007).

Promoting Sleep in Newborns and Infants

Normal neonates require 16 hours of sleep per 24 hours on average, but some will require more (Dewar, 2008c). Breastfed infants need to eat more frequently than babies fed formula. This is probably due to the shorter emptying time for breast milk. Because of this, breastfed babies probably wake more frequently in the night. Bed sharing by mother and infant increases both the length and frequency of breastfeeding episodes in 3- to 4-month-old infants (Dewar, 2008c). By 6 months most babies can go for a 6- to 12-hour period without being fed. This extended period coincides with the longest sleep period. Thus after 6 months, feeding in the night can be considered a learned behavior. Touchette has found that the factor most commonly associated with not sleeping at least 6 consecutive hours at age 5 months was feeding the infant after awakening during the night (Touchette et al, 2005). On the contrary, Cubero and colleagues (2009) found that feeding cereal in the evening to 8- to 16-month-old infants with a documented sleep disorder improved their sleep patterns. Feeding cereal to young infants, in the hope that it may lead to earlier consolidation of sleep cycles is still considered a myth, however.

The capacity of an infant to self-soothe develops within the first 3 months of life. However, this ability varies greatly across cultures, families, and home environments. Many authors believe that children from earliest infancy should be put into bed awake so that they learn to put themselves to sleep with self-soothing behaviors, such as thumb sucking. Others believe that self-soothing does not emerge until 3 months or later; until that time, the caregiver needs to provide soothing. Bringing an inanimate transitional object to bed is a sleep aid for many children from 3 months on. The transitional object may change from time to time, at least among infants (Sobralske and Gruber, 2009). Some sleep problems, such as trained night feeding and trained night crying, are learned. For instance, the child who is always rocked to sleep in the mother's arms and then moved to the crib when asleep learns that the place to go to sleep is in the mother's arms. During arousals in the night, the child then looks for those arms and not the sides of the crib to move into the next sleep cycle.

The provider needs to be respectful for nighttime interactions between caregiver and infant, temperament, breastfeeding patterns, and factors such as working parents and daycare when planning an individualized approach to sleep habits with parents that is nonthreatening and nonjudgmental (Owens, 2008). Providing information to parents about the development of normal sleep patterns in children and sleep hygiene patterns they need to teach their children is often helpful to them.

Promoting Sleep in Older Children and Adolescents

Sleep needs steadily decrease with the child's age. Nighttime sleep should increase somewhat when naps are eliminated from the child's schedule. The circadian timing system changes with puberty (Rodriguez, 2007). These changes, including phase, period, melatonin secretory pattern, light sensitivity, and phase relationships, have the potential to alter sleep patterns substantially, putting the adolescent at risk for sleep problems. After the neonatal period, for most infants and children, establishing a bedtime routine is probably the most important thing that parents can do. Often this routine includes "stepping-down" activities to provide cues for sleep: a bath (if this can be a quiet activity), changing into pajamas, brushing teeth, and sharing a story, song, or prayer. Getting ready for nighttime should be a pleasant time that the child looks forward to. Many children like to take a comfort object to bed with them. If the child responds to the bedtime routine with a tantrum, the pleasant activities are stopped, and the child is immediately put to bed. It may be difficult for parents to maintain consistent responses.

The room temperature should be less than 75° F. Lights should be turned out, although a hall light or nightlight may be reassuring to the child. Establishing consistent wake-up and naptime routines and schedules are also useful strategies. The wake-up time is the most powerful time for setting the sleep-wake cycle. Avoidance of stimulating drugs and foods, such as caffeine, coffee, and chocolate during the afternoon and evening is important (Noland et al, 2009). Other sleep hygiene principles include avoiding hunger and excessive fluids at bedtime or during the night.

Sleep and Television Viewing

In a study of more than 2000 children 4 to 35 months old, Thompson and Christakis (2005) found that 34% had irregular naptime schedules and 27% had irregular bedtime schedules. The number of hours of television watched per day was positively correlated to both the irregular nap and bedtime schedules. Another study by Noland and colleagues (2009) found that teens who watched television before bedtime, particularly while in bed were at greater risk for frequent sleep problems. Reducing their television viewing to less than 1 hour per day may significantly reduce subsequent sleep problems across the pediatric age range.

MANAGEMENT OF SLEEP PROBLEMS

Managing sleep problems is not easy. Clinicians need to be aware of their own cultural biases and avoid assumptions about family sleep values and practices before deciding that a problem exists. If the family identifies sleep as a problem or the child's health and well-being are affected, then a sleep problem diagnosis may be made. Usual management strategies include counseling parents, modifying diet, ignoring nocturnal crying, and scheduling awakenings. Deeper fears, depression, or family stresses may require counseling. Parenting tips for managing the infant's state changes are helpful, and successful parenting strategies should be supported (Table 14-2).

For sleep disorders, both parental and child behavioral approaches are discussed with each condition. Parental compliance is essential to management of sleep problems in children.

Sleep Management for Difficult Children

Helping parents to understand their child's temperament can be a useful intervention. A variety of studies have associated intense or difficult temperament patterns or behavioral issues

with sleep difficulties (Sobralske and Gruber, 2009). For example, for the child who is less adaptable or who has tendencies to withdraw from new situations, changing the sleep routine in any way may be particularly difficult. For children who are "difficult" (irregular, intense, with frequent negative moods), parents should be informed that sleep schedules and needs will be unpredictable, and reactions to parental interventions may be intensely resistant. Strategies parents have used with success in the past should be identified, and similar parenting activities adapted for managing sleep difficulties. Children with low sensory thresholds also have more problems with night waking because they are more sensitive to light, sound, temperature, and tactile stimulation (Carey, 1974). All these stimuli must be considered by parents who are trying to promote sleep onset and maintenance behaviors in their children.

Family Issues

Family stressors need to be recognized and dealt with. Posttraumatic stress disorder, abuse, domestic violence issues, or other psychological problems in children may also be factors requiring family and individual counseling.

Comorbidities

The outcomes of sleep problems, such as poor school performance and behavioral problems, need to be addressed as do precursors, such as chronic pain. As many as 50% of children with ADHD have been reported to have sleep problems (Goodlin-Jones et al, 2009). Sleep-disordered breathing, restless legs syndrome (RLS), and medication effects may be associated with difficulties falling asleep. Comorbid psychiatric conditions, such as depression and anxiety, have been correlated with sleep problems as well (Alfano et al, 2009). Liu and colleagues (2007) report that 72% of adolescents diagnosed with depression report insomnia (53%), hypersomnia (9%), or both.

Medications

Medications are not generally recommended for childhood sleep problems. The *Pharmacologic Management of Insomnia in Children and Adolescents: Consensus Statement* specifically notes that the treatment of pediatric insomnia is an unmet medical need. However, "before appropriate pharmacologic management guidelines can be developed, rigorous, large-scale clinical trials of pediatric insomnia treatment are vitally needed to provide information to the clinician on the safety and efficacy of prescription and over-the-counter agents for the management of pediatric insomnia" (Mindell et al, 2006, p e2). Hypnotic drugs, such as benzodiazepines, are discouraged because of the problems with dependence and because they are used for their sedative adverse effects rather than for primary effects on sleep-wake cycles or hyperarousal. Antihistamines have not been studied for effectiveness when used for long periods. Tricyclic drugs are sometimes used, especially for arousal disorders when other treatments are inadequate. Clonidine, antidepressants, mood stabilizers, and antihistamines are being used for children with ADHD but without data related to efficacy or safety (Mindell et al, 2006).

Ineffective management strategies include use of diphenhydramine medication, which will provide moderate

TABLE 14-2	Prevention of Sleep Problems: Highlights for Parental Counseling

Newborn

During the night	Put the baby to bed while drowsy but still awake.
	Feed the baby at the parents' bedtime and then let the baby awaken for feedings and feed with little stimulation, dim lights, no play.
	Avoid bringing the baby into the parents' bed, but sleeping in the same room is recommended.
	Put the baby to sleep on his or her back with head clear of blankets or soft items.
	Encourage nighttime sleep.
During the day	Respond to crying; hold the baby when fussy.
	Hold the baby frequently to prevent fussy episodes.
	Schedule feedings at least 2 hours apart.

Ages 2 to 4 Months

During the night	Move the baby to a separate bedroom unless this is not the cultural norm for the family.
	Try to delay and then discontinue middle-of-the-night feedings.
	No bottles in the crib.
	Continue to keep middle-of-the-night feedings (if they are still occurring) as nonstimulating occasions.
	Encourage self-soothing.

Ages 6 to 12 Months

During the night	Keep soft toy animal, doll, or blanket in the crib for snuggling.
	Leave the bedroom door open and respond to any fears quickly and with reassurance.

Age 1 Year and Older

During the night	Keep bedtimes friendly and predictable occasions. Establish a routine.
	Always respond to nighttime fears with reassurance and comfort.
	Allow the child to take increasing responsibility for self-management of body functions, including sleep.
	Expect the child to remain in bed during the night.
	Do not send the child to bed hungry.
	Keep the bedroom quiet, cool, and dark.
During the day	Avoid products containing caffeine for at least several hours before bedtime.
	Be sure the child has had some active play time, preferably outdoors, every day.
	Keep television out of the child's bedroom.
	Do not use the bedroom for timeout punishment.

Adolescents

	Keep wake-up and sleep times about the same every day.
	Avoid sleeping-in on weekends.
	Naps should be short.
	Spend some time outdoors every day for daylight exposure.
	Exercise regularly.
	Use the bed for sleeping only.
	Have a quiet down time before trying to sleep.
	Don't go to bed hungry.
	Avoid caffeine from dinnertime on.
	Do not use alcohol.
	If smoking, do not smoke at least 1 hour before bedtime.
	Do not use sleeping pills, melatonin, or other over-the-counter sleep aids unless prescribed by a health care provider.

Adapted from Owens JA: Sleep medicine. In Kliegman R, Behrman R, Jenson H, et al, editors: *Nelson textbook of pediatrics,* ed 18, Philadelphia, 2007, Saunders, pp 91-99.

improvement, but the sleep problems can be expected to return when medication is stopped. This medication may also result in paradoxical hyperactivity.

Common Sleep Problems

The line between normal and problematic sleep may be somewhat fuzzy. The clinician needs to determine that the child's sleep patterns are problematic for the caregivers and family or are resulting in problems for the child's health and well-being. The *International Classification of Sleep Disorders, Revised* (ICSD-R) (American Academy of Sleep Medicine [AASM], 2001) is more complex than the system used in this chapter and refers to both adult and child sleep problems. It classifies sleep problems as dyssomnias, or problems of insufficient, excessive, or inefficient sleep; parasomnias, or problems that intrude on the sleep state; and medical or psychiatric sleep disorders. This section discusses the problems summarized in Table 14-3.

TABLE 14-3   Summary of Common Pediatric Sleep Problems and Interventions

Sleep Problem	Clinical Findings	Differential	Intervention
Dyssomnias			
Night waking	Needs help during the night to enter the next sleep cycle	Medical problem, pain, hunger, trained night feeder Depression	Always put the child to bed while still awake; keep day and nighttime cues very clear; do not reinforce calling out or crying behavior; try scheduled wakening technique
Sleep refusals	Toddler or preschooler refuses to settle down when put to bed	Fears, separation anxiety, sleep needs less than parents' expectations Temperament irregular or low sensory threshold Emotional stress	Maintain consistent sleep routine and expectations; use transitional objects
	Infant awakens predictably to be fed after 4 months old	Night wakening, pain, medical problem, feeding needs	Move the child onto a 3- to 4-hour feeding schedule in the day; at first feed the infant only once after the parents' bedtime; then either eliminate the feeding or progressively decrease the volume of that feeding
Delayed sleep phase	Child goes to bed late and awakens late	Sleep refusal, depression	Have the child awaken progressively 15 minutes earlier until appropriate bedtimes and waking times result
Advanced sleep phase	Child goes to bed early and awakens early		Progressively have child stay up later; awakening will occur later
Unpredictable schedule	Child goes to bed and awakens at random times	Erratic schedule; inconsistent parent expectations; excessive naps	Keep predictable eating, activity, and sleeping schedules for the family; maintain consistent expectation for bedtime and awakening but allow child to stay awake in bed if not disruptive to others
Parasomnias			
Nightmares	Child awakens in fear, crying, has memory of event; is interactive while upset; occurs in latter half of the night; slow return to sleep	Night terrors; seizures; stress if nightmares occur frequently	Soothe and reassure the child; a nightlight or flashlight may help if child is afraid of the dark
Night terrors and sleepwalking (variant)	Child awakens screaming, crying, but is not interactive with the parent at the time; has no memory of the event; occurs in the first third of night; rapid return to sleep; sleepwalking is variant	Nightmares; seizures; physical exhaustion	Protect the child from injury if he or she is thrashing about or walking; help the child to lie down to return to sleep; protect child from stairways and other unsafe places sleepwalker might go
Medical/Psychiatric Problems			
Depression	Insomnia or hypersomnia or both with other symptoms of depression	Other psychiatric disorder; dyssomnia or parasomnia disorder	Manage the psychiatric condition first
OSA	Snoring with apneic periods against increased respiratory efforts, restless sleep, daytime sleepiness, fatigue	Central apnea; benign snoring; seizure disorder	Refer to sleep studies and then to ENT for possible adenotonsillectomy if OSA is diagnosed

ENT, Ear, nose, and throat; *OSA,* obstructive sleep apnea.

■ Dyssomnias

Dyssomnias are disorders of sleep related to the process of going to sleep, putting oneself back to sleep from an arousal, and sleeping on a regular basis at a reasonable time. Causes may be intrinsic, such as narcolepsy, OSA, RLS, or extrinsic, such as adjustment to a new environment (Petit et al, 2007).

SLEEP-ONSET ASSOCIATION DISORDER (NIGHT WAKING)

Description

The child is unable to enter the sleep cycle easily unless a particular routine is carried out. For an infant the problem results in frequent night waking and crying, most often between midnight and 5 AM.

Epidemiology

This is most commonly a learned behavior, often seen in infants who fall asleep while being rocked or fed and who are then put into their beds. For the child older than 6 months who feeds at night, night feeding in volume, frequent daytime feedings (grazing), feeding until asleep, and leaving a bottle in the bed are causes of this sleep disturbance.

Sleep-onset association problems are common and steadily decline with age. It is estimated that approximately 25% of children 6 months to 5 years of age have difficulty with falling asleep or remaining asleep throughout the night. Nighttime waking decreased from 36.3% at 2.5 years old to 13.2% by the time the child was 6 years old (Petit et al, 2007). As many as 95% of infants cry after a nighttime awakening and require parental help to return to sleep. This number falls to 30% to 40% by the time the child is 1 year old (Ward and Mason, 2002). Touchette and colleagues (2005) found that the most strongly associated factor with not sleeping at least 6 consecutive hours at 5 months was feeding the child after an awakening, and parental presence until sleep onset was the factor most associated with not sleeping 6 consecutive hours or more at ages 17 months and 29 months.

Clinical Findings

The history reveals a baby or child who has frequent night awakenings. When the parent goes to the child and repeats a particular intervention, the child falls asleep promptly. The history needs to assess why the child has difficulty falling asleep or awakens during the night, in addition to the parental response and bedtime routine. With this disturbance, middle-of-the-night feedings occur in a child older than 4 months.

Differential Diagnosis

Pain or a medical condition affecting sleep, fear in an older child, inappropriate expectations related to the amount of sleep the child needs, day-night reversal and gastroesophageal reflux are possible differential diagnoses. OSA, nightmares, RLS, and mood disorders can cause night waking.

Management

The infant or child must learn to independently transition from the arousal phase into the next sleep cycle throughout the night. The parent must learn to change the responses given during the night. Two strategies have been recommended in the literature:

- Extinction and graduated extinction. Put the child down to sleep at night while he or she is awake. When the child awakens and cries in the night, the parent should go to him or her briefly to give comfort and reassurance but not to hold, rock, or feed. The parent's response must be supportive and comforting but should not reinforce a return to old patterns of infant behavior or parental response. This technique is termed extinction. Going "cold turkey" (not going to the child at all from the very beginning) is difficult for parents to do, although children learn to return to sleep alone within a few nights, crying for shorter periods each time. Results should be seen in 3 to 5 days and will be maintained over time for extinction. With extinction,

a mild increase in problem behaviors may recur 15 to 30 days after treatment begins. Parents must maintain the extinction behaviors at this time (Meltzer and Mindell, 2004). Waiting for progressively longer intervals before going to the child over several nights may work if the parents can maintain compliance (graduated extinction). Parents' behaviors, such as the amount of touch, the proximity to the child, the duration of time between and the duration of the check-in are faded (Meltzer and Mindell, 2004). Graduated extinction results will be evident in a few days to a few months.

- Scheduled awakenings. Alternatively, use a planned or scheduled awakening approach. The first night, the parent should go to the child 15 minutes before night awakening is expected. The child is awakened, rocked for a few minutes, and then left again. When spontaneous awakenings stop, scheduled awakenings are gradually delayed 15 to 30 minutes more each night. If the child then awakens spontaneously, he or she learns to wait for the parents to come, knowing it will happen, and gradually learns to return to sleep (Meltzer and Mindell, 2004). Difficulties with this method include the requirement that parents waken their child once or several times during the night. Also it can take several weeks for effects to be seen. The awakenings do not address bedtime resistance or independent sleep initiation (Meltzer and Mindell, 2004). It may be easier to work on development of self-sleep during naps first and then transfer this behavior to nighttime. Most infants use sleep aids, such as a blanket or stuffed animal, to assist with self-soothing (Burnham et al, 2002).

Complications

Night feedings should not be withheld from children who are not thriving for other reasons and who need the nutrition of another nighttime feeding.

SLEEP REFUSAL (BEHAVIORAL INSOMNIA)

Description

In toddlers and preschoolers the problem is often one of difficulty with bedtime settling. A child needs to learn to sleep alone and put himself or herself to sleep. The child may experience an inability to make the transition from daytime activities to nighttime sleeping.

Epidemiology

A variety of studies report that approximately 20% of children between 15 and 48 months old engage in bedtime resistance. Bedtime resistance was identified in 25% of patients 2 to 13 years old, with 29% of preschoolers experiencing the problem (Archbold et al, 2002). Separation anxiety is a problem for some, as are nighttime fears.

Clinical Findings

The child makes repeated attempts to obtain parental attention (e.g., demanding snacks, asking for a drink, requesting another story, leaving bed to return to family activities, watching activities from afar).

Differential Diagnosis

Infant: Sleep association problem, hunger, circadian rhythm disorder

Preschooler: Sleep association problem, circadian rhythm disorder, limit setting, bedtime fears

School age and adolescent: Sleep association problem (TV or radio on); circadian rhythm disorder; anxiety at bedtime related to daytime stresses, exposure to violence, chaotic household, family stresses, sexual or physical abuse

Management

For the toddler or preschooler who exhibits sleep refusal, try the following regimen:

1. Use a sleep log to chart the child's pattern initially. It can then be used to mark progress toward the goal.
2. Maintain the bedtime routine and use transitional objects and a quiet environment for sleep. The routine should not be longer than 30 minutes (Mindell et al, 2006).
3. Positive routines may be helpful for children having difficulty falling asleep at bedtime. The parents develop a set of bedtime routines that the child enjoys. Four to seven activities are included. If a tantrum occurs, the routine is terminated, and the child is told that it is time for bed (Meltzer and Mindell, 2004).
4. Set limits on the child's demands for attention. The parent should leave the room at the end of the bedtime routine, expecting good behavior. If the child arises, return the child to bed, saying, "It is time for bed," each time the child gets up. Tantrums of up to 45 minutes may occur the first night and perhaps longer the second night but then should decrease on succeeding nights (Meltzer and Mindell, 2004).
5. Be sure that the child is not being expected to sleep earlier or for longer periods than expected for his or her age.

For children older than 3 years, positive rewards, such as sticker charts, may help. Payoffs need to occur frequently.

Stresses and fears must be addressed. If the child has bedtime fears, leaving may increase the problem. In these cases, the parent may sit quietly in the room until the child falls asleep. When the child can fall asleep easily this way, the parent should move to the bedroom door and eventually out of sight. The child needs to understand that the parent will only remain in the room if there are no tantrums and the child stays in bed.

INSOMNIA AND HYPERSOMNIA AND COMORBID CONDITIONS IN ADOLESCENTS

Adolescents may have problems with difficulty falling asleep, sleeping less than usual, sleep quality, waking up with difficulty, sleeping more than usual, napping during the day, and trouble waking up. These conditions are considered significant if they persist more than 2 weeks.

For adolescents with insomnia, there is a significantly increased risk of developing an anxiety or depressive disorder (Alfano et al, 2009; Smaldone et al, 2009). Sleep problems should be considered a marker of more significant depression. Some of the associated mental health symptoms may include greater depressed mood, irritability, sadness, psychomotor agitation, fatigue, anhedonia, inappropriate guilt, weight loss, diurnal variation, and anxiety disorders (Liu et al, 2007).

In addition to the effects on mental health, research is linking inadequate sleep to pediatric obesity (Noland et al, 2009). The risk of developing obesity may be increased as much as 80% for a 1-hour deprivation in adolescent's regular sleep requirements.

■ Sleep-Cycle Problems (Circadian Rhythm Disorders)

DELAYED SLEEP PHASE

Description

The sleep cycle begins at a late hour and is followed by a late awakening. This is commonly an adolescent problem.

Etiology

The child's internal clock for sleep and rest is not consistent with appropriate hours for sleep. Excessive naps or late morning waking may be related factors, especially for school-age children and adolescents.

Differential Diagnosis

The differential diagnoses are prolonged bedtime routine and oppositional disorder, which both involve active resistance to going to bed rather than inability to fall asleep.

Management

Three approaches are suggested:

1. Keep the nighttime routine in place but awaken the child earlier each morning in 15-minute increments.
2. For the adolescent or older child who is off schedule by many hours (e.g., at the end of summer, when beginning the school year will require getting up earlier), it could take weeks to back up the cycle appropriately using 15-minute increments. In this case it is better to go forward in time. In other words, have the child remain awake until the next evening and then go to bed at the desired hour, beginning the desired routine from that point.
3. Have the child or family keep a sleep log to document gradual change (Howard and Wong, 2001).

ADVANCED SLEEP PHASE

Description

The sleep cycle begins too early with correlated early rising.

Management

Meals, naps, and bedtime should be delayed until the desired times. The early waking resolves itself.

INAPPROPRIATE OR UNPREDICTABLE SCHEDULES

Description

Some people have a poorly organized sleep-wake cycle. This is described by some as a temperament problem of rhythmicity.

Management

The routines of eating, activities, and sleeping should be kept as regular as possible. The older child may need to learn to play quietly in bed until others awaken or until a clock radio begins to play. At night the child may need to learn to read or listen to music in bed when bedtime comes.

■ Parasomnias: Night Terrors, Sleepwalking, and Nightmares

In parasomnias, behaviors intrude on ongoing sleep rather than representing disruptions of the sleep process, such as going to sleep, waking in the night, or sleeping on an inappropriate schedule. Parasomnias are divided into arousal disorders, sleep-wake transition disorders, REM parasomnias, and miscellaneous parasomnias. The arousal disorders include sleep terrors and sleepwalking. A nightmare is a REM parasomnia, and enuresis and bruxism are miscellaneous parasomnias. Parasomnias usually do not result in excessive daytime sleepiness or insomnia but are disruptive to a sleeping household.

Positive family histories are common. In general they are more common in males, and children with one type of parasomnia are more likely to exhibit symptoms of another at some point. Parasomnia prevalence rates vary depending on the specific sleep disorder, the child's age—generally between 5% and 35% (Meltzer et al, 2010).

AROUSAL DISORDERS

NIGHT TERRORS OR SLEEP TERRORS

Description

Night terrors are defined as a partial awakening during the transition from NREM sleep stage III or IV in which the child is not fully conscious and aware of surroundings. Confusional arousals are similar to night terrors although the child does not express fear, terror, or panic. Rather the child has marked mental confusion (Ward and Mason, 2002).

Epidemiology

These disorders are related to the transition from the stage IV NREM sleep to the REM sleep cycle and are not psychological or developmental problems. Excessive fatigue or unusual daytime stresses may precipitate attacks in some children, but they are not considered mental health problems. A full bladder, fever, pain, and environmental factors, such as noise, are also considered trigger factors. Family history is often positive. Night terrors are most common in 3- to 6-year-olds, although they occur in children from 18 months to adolescence. Incidence has been reported at 3% of children, mostly from 18 months to 6 years. The median age is 3.5 years (Connelly, 2005).

Clinical Findings

Episodes occur 60 to 90 minutes after onset of sleep and may last from less than a minute to 5 minutes but the child may remain inconsolable for 5 to 30 minutes after the episode

(Connelly, 2005). The child usually sits up screaming but cannot be reasoned with or consoled. Indeed, the child does not even seem to hear the caregiver. The child can have pallor, pupil dilation, piloerection, tachycardia, and sweating, all symptoms of an autonomic discharge (Connelly, 2005). The child may speak incoherently and may thrash about. The child is not awake or aware of the surroundings and does not remember the episode in the morning. It is the caregiver who is disturbed, not the child. Episodes do not occur every night, and there is a strong family history of these episodes (Rodriguez, 2007).

Differential Diagnosis

The differential diagnoses are nightmares or seizures with stiffening, jerking, or drooling. Consider sleep-disordered breathing as a secondary sleep disorder.

Management

Reassurance that the child is mentally and developmentally normal should be provided. Interventions should focus on preventing injury and guiding the child back to bed. Emptying the bladder at bedtime should be routine. Waking the child 30 minutes before the expected episode each night for about a week may interrupt the pattern. The child should be protected from injury, and babysitters should be prepared for these episodes. An afternoon nap may change the sleep stages at night (Connelly, 2005; Howard and Wong, 2001).

If sleep-disordered breathing is identified through polysomnography, referral to an otolaryngologist for consideration of tonsillectomy with or without adenoidectomy and/or turbinate treatment. In one study an amazing 100% of children with parasomnias and sleep-disordered breathing treated surgically were cured of their parasomnia postoperatively and showed significant academic improvement compared with children that had not undergone surgical intervention (Rodriguez, 2007).

For severe cases (frequent or with safety problems), benzodiazepines are the most commonly prescribed medication. Clonazepam, lorazepam, or diazepam can be effective in small doses. However, prolonged use can result in significant side effects (Sheldon, 2004).

SLEEPWALKING (SOMNAMBULISM)

Description

Sleepwalking is a variation of night terrors in which the manifestation is walking rather than sitting up and screaming. It occurs with arousal from stage IV sleep, usually 1 to 2 hours into sleep. Episodes usually last less than 15 minutes and vary in frequency.

Epidemiology

The cause is the same as that for night terrors; it is an arousal disorder in stage IV. It can be triggered by excessive fatigue, changes in routines, or daily stress. Consider sleep-disordered breathing as a secondary sleep disorder (see Night Terrors or Sleep Terrors, earlier). Family history is often positive. Sleepwalking is more common in boys and tends to be outgrown.

It occurs in 17% of children at one time or another. It is most common in children between 8 and 12 years of age.

Clinical Findings

The child arises and walks about without being fully alert and responsive. The child may fall or bump into things, wander in illogical places, or urinate outside the toilet. He or she does not remember the incident in the morning.

Differential Diagnosis

The differential diagnoses are dissociative state and seizure.

Management

The child needs to be led back quietly to bed. A gate may need to be placed across the bedroom door if the sleepwalking becomes frequent. Doors may need to be secured to ensure that the child does not wander into unsafe areas. Stairways are particularly dangerous to the sleepwalking child as well as open windows (AASM, 2006b). An afternoon nap may also be helpful in altering the stage IV pattern.

As with sleep terrors, consider tonsillectomy for children with associated documented sleep-disordered breathing.

RAPID EYE MOVEMENT PARASOMNIAS

NIGHTMARES, MONSTERS, AND OTHER NIGHTTIME FEARS

Description

A nightmare is classified as a REM parasomnia disorder. Nightmares occur as the child awakens from REM sleep, remembering dreams that are disturbing. This is most prominent in 5- to 10-year-olds. Occasional nightmares are normal and benign. The child is awake, frightened, and able to describe the fears (Schredl et al, 2009). They are rare before 3 years of age. Certain drugs, such as antidepressants, may trigger nightmares (AASM, 2008).

Differential Diagnosis

The differential diagnosis for nightmares is night terrors, in which the child is not fully conscious. The significance and severity of other nighttime fears need to be assessed. Separation anxiety in toddlers, domestic violence, or a scary event may make nighttime frightening.

Management

Parents should give comfort, reassurance, and a sense of security and not dismiss the fear as imaginary. The child may need to have the parent lie down with him or her for a period of time, or the child may even get into bed with the parent. However, this should not become habitual. Monsters may be kept away by keeping on a nightlight, by using a flashlight, or pantomiming actions to "sweep them away," or by keeping the bedroom door open. Behavioral strategies or counseling may be required if nighttime fears are frequent or the degree of fear is exceptionally severe or associated with daytime behavioral or performance problems (Sheldon, 2004).

SLEEP-WAKE TRANSITION DISORDERS AND MISCELLANEOUS PARASOMNIAS

RESTLESS LEGS SYNDROME AND PERIODIC LIMB MOVEMENTS

Description

RLS has long been identified as a parasomnia in adults. RLS is a sensory and motor disorder characterized by an uncontrollable sensation in the legs accompanied by an irresistible urge to move the legs, usually with immediate resolution of the noxious sensations. The syndrome is clinical and difficult for children to describe and thus has been considered to be underdiagnosed. Children with RLS have been shown to frequently have aggression, inattention, hyperactivity, and daytime sleepiness caused by an inability to sleep or difficulty maintaining sleep (Picchietti et al, 2007). The following criteria must be met for diagnosis:
1. An urge to move the legs, usually accompanied by unpleasant sensations in the legs that:
   - Begin or worsen with rest or inactivity, such as lying or sitting
   - Are worse or only occur at night
   - Are partially or totally relieved by movement, such as walking or stretching, at least as long as the activity continues
2. If the child cannot describe the sensations, the child should meet at least two of the following criteria:
   - Sleep disturbance not typical for age
   - Biologic parent or sibling with documented RLS

Periodic limb movements (PLMs) are repetitive jerks, typically of the legs, that are found by polysomnography to occur every 5 to 90 seconds. They occur most often during stages I and II of NREM sleep. RLS and PLMs usually occur together, but PLMs may occur without RLS.

Epidemiology

Altered brain acquisition of iron has been identified as a major factor in RLS (Connor et al, 2011). Central dopaminergic systems are involved because dopaminergic medications improve symptoms. There is an inherited tendency. Iron deficiency is a common cause of secondary RLS. Peripheral neuropathy and uremia are also causes of secondary RLS. Medications, such as antidepressants, selective serotonin reuptake inhibitors (SSRIs), sedating antihistamines, and dopamine receptor antagonists may worsen or precipitate cases. PLMs are related to RLS. Picchietti and associates (2007) determined the prevalence in 8- to 17-year-olds to be approximately 2%, with a positive family history in 70% of cases.

Differential Diagnosis

Other differential diagnoses include pain for an identifiable physiological reason, sleep-disordered breathing, such as OSA, growing pains, muscle tics, ADHD, muscle pain, leg cramps, Osgood-Schlatter disease, chondromalacia patellae, and arthralgias (Maheswaran and Kushida, 2006).

Management

No medications have been approved for children with RLS. Clonidine (Catapres) and clonazepam have been used, but it is recommended that these be managed by a sleep specialist because clonazepam may exacerbate problems of children with sleep-disordered breathing (including respiratory collapse). Dopaminergic agents and benzodiazepines have been used (AASM, 2006a). Reducing conditions that worsen the RLS should be tried, including management of iron deficiency, good sleep hygiene practices, and limiting medications that make it worse. Ropinirole (Requip) is the first U.S. Food and Drug Administration (FDA)–approved drug for RLS in adults.

HEAD BANGING AND BRUXISM

Sleep-wake transition disorders include sleep talking, nocturnal leg cramps, and rhythmic movement disorders, such as head banging and body rocking, which usually occur with sleep onset. Rhythmic sleep disorders are common and reported in two thirds of normal children, with a male-to-female ratio of 4:1 (Sheldon, 2004). Most of these disorders disappear by 4 years of age. No interventions are considered necessary aside from ensuring the child's safety and parental reassurance (Owens, 2007).

Sleep bruxism is stereotypic grinding or clenching of the teeth during sleep. There may be some relationship to stress. It frequently appears between 10 and 20 years old, although there is a short-lived infant version. Seizure disorder would be a differential diagnosis. A dental referral may be useful. Bruxism is seen in 8.2% of the population (Wills and Garcia, 2002).

■ Sleep-Disordered Breathing

OBSTRUCTIVE SLEEP APNEA AND OTHER DISORDERS

Description

Sleep-disordered breathing includes a wide range of disorders varying in intensity, from simple snoring to more significant OSA, which can be a serious problem for some infants and children because it is an indicator of severe airway obstruction. These disorders of breathing during sleep can be characterized by prolonged partial upper airway obstruction and/or intermittent complete obstruction (obstructive apnea) that disrupts normal ventilation during sleep and normal sleep patterns despite normal respiratory effort and chest wall expansion. This may result in frequent sleep arousals, hypoxemia, or hypoventilation (Owens, 2008). Sleep-disordered breathing is considered to be a continuum of problems ranging from partial obstruction of the airway (snoring) to increased upper airway resistance syndrome to continuous episodes of complete upper airway resistance (Szuhay and Rotenberg, 2009). The conditions without obstructive apnea, frequent arousals from sleep, or gas exchange abnormalities are not of concern.

Etiology

Collapse of the pharyngeal airway with increased airway resistance above the collapsing segment causes sleep apnea. The child makes repeated vigorous attempts to breathe. Snoring is associated with these efforts, but will not be heard if obstruction is complete. Arousal may occur, and with it upper airway muscle tone improves. The cycle may repeat many times during the night. The condition may also be partial, called obstructive hypoventilation. Other causal factors may include the following (Owens, 2008):
- Large adenoids or tonsils or both
- Nasal deformities
- Abnormally small oropharyngeal structures as in Pierre-Robin syndrome
- Craniofacial structural problems, such as midface hypoplasia
- Factors affecting neural control, such as generalized hypotonia, central nervous system injury, and brainstem dysfunction, which includes cerebral palsy and muscular dystrophy (these conditions relate to incoordination of upper airway muscles)
- Idiopathic or genetic cause—Prader-Willi syndrome, sickle cell disease, mucopolysaccharidosis, Down syndrome
- Obesity

Epidemiology

Prevalence estimates for sleep apnea in children are approximately 3%, with a peak age between 2 and 8 years of age (Szuhay and Rotenberg, 2009). Sleep-disordered breathing among adolescents has been estimated at 20% with snoring at least a few nights per month, 6% with snoring every or nearly every night, and 2.5% to 6% of adolescents with apnea-like symptoms. Rates are higher among African-Americans and those with a higher body mass index (BMI) (Johnson and Roth, 2006).

Clinical Findings

History. Sleep screening should be a part of all routine health care visits. The following signs and symptoms are associated with OSA:
- Disrupted sleep patterns (timing, restlessness, positions, diaphoresis, behavior while asleep)
- Snoring (pitch, periods of silence, intensity, onset, frequency, duration)
- Observed increased breathing effort (rib cage retraction, paradoxical chest wall movement) or apnea
- Decreased alertness and functioning when awake
- Associated conditions (e.g., craniofacial syndromes, tonsillar hypertrophy, atopy)
- Impaired growth and development
- Factors indicating a high-risk patient: infant, patient with craniofacial disorder, Down syndrome, cerebral palsy, neuromuscular disorder, chronic lung disease, sickle cell disease, central hypoventilation syndromes, or genetic-metabolic storage disease
- Cognitive problems at school (Barone et al, 2009)
- Overweight and obesity have been associated with children with OSA undergoing testing more than 50% of the time (Owens et al, 2008)

Physical Examination. The physical examination should include the following:
- Vital signs, including evaluation for hypertension
- Height and weight for failure to thrive or obesity, as well as BMI measurements
- Complete ear, nose, and throat examination, including tonsils and adenoids, midfacial hypoplasia, retrognathia or micrognathia, patency of nasal passages, tongue size, signs of cleft palate
- Cardiac functioning for evidence of cor pulmonale, to include increased pulmonic component of the second heart sound indicating pulmonary hypertension

- Observation for digital clubbing, pectus excavatum
- Muscle tone

Laboratory Evaluation. Tape-recording the apneic episodes may be helpful in assessing the problem. The child needs to be referred for a variety of sleep studies, in addition to electrocardiogram and echocardiogram if the problem is severe. Nocturnal pulse oximetry, videotaping, and daytime nap polysomnography are useful if the results are positive, but they do not rule out OSA syndrome if negative. Nocturnal polysomnography is the gold standard diagnostic technique and should be used initially or if the pulse oximetry, videotaping, and daytime nap polysomnography results are negative. Radiographs of the neck may demonstrate upper airway narrowing as a result of adenoid hypertrophy (Barone et al, 2009).

Differential Diagnosis

The differential diagnoses are seizure disorder and central apnea, which are characterized by no airflow and no respiratory effort. Central apnea is a brainstem problem that is more commonly seen in premature or newborn infants. Primary snoring (without obstruction) also needs to be considered.

Management

An American Academy of Pediatrics clinical practice guideline (Marcus CL, Brooks LJ, Draper KA, et al: Clinical practice guideline: diagnosis and management of childhood obstructive sleep apnea syndrome, *Pediatrics,* Aug 27, 2012. [Epub ahead of print.]) recommends that all children be screened for snoring. Those with snoring and symptoms of obstructive sleep apnea syndrome (OSAS) should receive polysomnography. Adenotonsillectomy is the treatment of choice for children with adenotonsillar hypertrophy with postoperative evaluation for further treatment needs. Continuous positive airway pressure (CPAP) is recommended for those in whom adenoids and tonsils were not removed or if OSAS persists. Weight loss for overweight/obese children is recommended in addition to other therapy. Intranasal corticosteroids can be used for children with mild OSAS and contraindicated adenotonsillectomy or for mild postoperative OSAS. Avoidance of indoor pollutants may help. Oxygen therapy is not helpful and may worsen hypoventilation. High-risk children need to be referred to a pediatric specialist because they are at increased surgical risk and require more complex management (Szuhay and Rotenberg, 2009).

Complications

Cardiac problems, including cor pulmonale resulting from hypoxic episodes, right ventricular hypertrophy, pulmonary hypertension, heart failure, systemic hypertension, and polycythemia can occur. Neurological problems, including failure to thrive, developmental delay, learning problems, hyperactivity, excessive daytime sleepiness, and morning headache, have been reported (Szuhay and Rotenberg, 2009).

■ Special Considerations for Children with Chronic Disorders

Chronic health conditions such as ADHD, asthma, diabetes, and obesity have been associated with increasing sleep difficulties. This in turn may ultimately have a greater effect on the quality of life and morbidity associated with the underlying pathological process. Children with neurodevelopmental difficulties or delays are also at greater risk for such complications. Research in autistic and autism spectrum disorder has clearly identified chronic sleep disturbances that affect the diagnosed child as well as family members or caretakers (Johnson and Malow, 2008; Krakowiak et al, 2008). As many as 66% of children ages 4 to 10 years with pervasive developmental delays, including autism and Asperger disorder, had documented moderate sleep disturbances, generally insomnia (Souders et al, 2009).

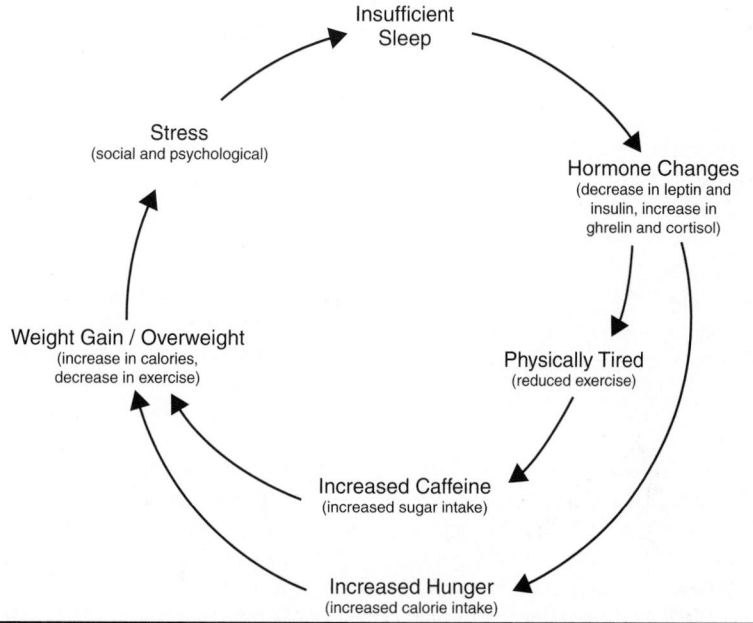

FIGURE 14-3 Reduced sleep duration–overweight cycle. (From Noland H, Price JH, Dake J, et al: Adolescents' sleep behaviors and perception of sleep, *J Sch Health* 75[5]:224-230, 2009. Used with permission.)

Careful consideration needs to be taken when evaluating core components of underlying conditions to determine if exacerbations are related to poor quality of sleep versus poor sleep being an indication of worsening of symptoms, such as seen in asthma (Kieckhefer et al, 2009). It is of equal importance to obtain a history of symptom severity in correlation with nighttime waking from both the parent and child because this may vary in opinion. From a clinical standpoint it is often difficult to discern a worsening of daytime symptoms, such as seen with ADHD, as a result of sleep disturbance or failure of medication treatment to produce desired effects in behavior modifications (Owens et al, 2008). Furthermore, it is imperative to evaluate the nature of medications that may have rebound effects that stimulate arousal when nighttime sleeping is expected. This is a common concern with many ADHD stimulants used to reduce daytime symptoms.

A variety of neurological conditions such as epilepsy, cerebral palsy, brain tumors, and peripheral nervous system disorders such as spinal muscular atrophy greatly increase the likelihood of developing OSA. These children may have other sleep disturbances also. Special consideration for these children will need to be provided by the practitioner to avoid further complications in these children's lives (Szuhay and Rotenberg, 2009). Careful consideration of the underlying disease process, repeated hospitalizations, family dynamics, and concurrent medication regimens will document a comprehensive view of compounding factors that may lead to disordered sleep as well as deterioration from baseline status as a result of chronic sleep disturbance (Owens, 2009). A multispecialty team approach for these patients may prove to be significantly useful for overall patient care outcomes. The first-line of approach should be sleep hygiene—providing an optimal environment, scheduling, sleep-practice, and physiological sleep-promoting factors such as minimizing light and temperature (Jan et al, 2008). Some special measures are helpful to these children.

There is a negative relationship between sleep duration and obesity (i.e., children sleeping 10.5 to 11 hours per night were more likely to be obese than children sleeping 12 to 13 hours per night) (Chaput et al, 2006; Owens et al, 2008) (Fig. 14-3). Studies have also shown that obese children with sleep apnea also experience more behavioral problems (47%) and ADHD (23%). The clinician needs to weigh the relative contributions of being overweight, insufficient sleep, and comorbid sleep disorders in managing these children's behavior (Owens et al, 2008).

Cognitive-Perceptual Disorders

Attention-Deficit/Hyperactivity Disorder, Learning Problems, Sensory Processing Disorder, Autism Spectrum Disorder, Blindness, and Deafness

NANCY BARBER STARR, MAXINE FOOKSON, CATHERINE E. BURNS, AND CRIS ANN BOWMAN-HARVEY

Cognitive development is the foundation for intelligence (Wilks et al, 2010), and cognition and perception affect a child's ability to learn, comprehend and use information to understand and follow directions, retain information, make decisions, and solve problems. Cognition and general knowledge represent the accumulation and reorganization of experiences that result from participating in a rich learning setting with skilled and appropriate adult interventions. From these experiences children construct knowledge of patterns and relations, cause and effect, and methods of solving problems of everyday life.

Gordon (2010) describes the cognitive-perceptual functional health pattern to include the adequacy of sensory modes, such as vision, hearing, taste, touch, or smell, as well as the cognitive functional abilities such as language, memory, and decision-making. Sensory experiences such as pain (see Chapter 22) and altered sensory input may also be identified.

Piaget's theory of cognitive development is probably the most classic (see Chapter 4). Newer theories and ideas related to the development of cognition and sensory awareness are emerging and being developed. *Neurodevelopmental functioning* of the brain uses a model of a tool kit full of basic instruments (functions) with different functions working in clusters (like tools) in different kinds of learning. The concept of *multiple intelligences* was introduced to describe different ways a child may be hard-wired to process information. *Information processing* looks at human learning with a computer as a model. *Social cognition* looks at the spectrum of social behaviors and affiliation with others.

Perception is the child's ability to receive information from the internal and external environments through the senses: vision, hearing, touch, taste, and smell. Traditionally it was thought that learning occurs as a child receives visual or auditory input. The *sensory processing* theory, also referred to as sensory integration, refers to the way the nervous system responds to, processes, and organizes information through the senses in order for learning and physical and emotional development to occur. This theory expands sensory input to include vestibular and proprioception (Miller et al, 2009). Epigenetics provides a link between genetic and environmental factors affecting development. Wegner (2009) proposes a societal-familial-individual matrix as a clinical means of evaluating these factors.

Facilitating and monitoring cognitive-perceptual developmental progress as well as ensuring the maximum function of all the senses should be an integral part of primary care. Screening hearing and vision is a recognized standard of care. Following cognitive development in infancy and early childhood is primarily done by monitoring language and problem-solving domains integral to the other developmental parameters and should ideally be performed with standardized screening tools. As the child enters school, monitoring the adaptation to and performance in school becomes the key. Soliciting information about school performance from preschool through high school shows interest in the child's mastery of educational tasks and managing academic challenges. Primary care providers may be consulted for guidance about appropriate timing and school placement for a child, performance more or less than expectations, problems, and the need for further assessment. As developmental experts, primary care providers need to be able to identify problems; advise, counsel, and educate parents; participate on interdisciplinary teams for diagnosis and management; and mediate and advocate for children and their learning needs.

■ Standards for Care

Healthy People 2020: Health Promotion and Disease Prevention Objectives for the Year 2020 supports the need for visual and hearing screening in children (U.S. Department of Health and Human Services [USDHHS], 2010). New objectives for 2020 include "increase the proportion of children who are ready for school in all five domains of healthy development"; "increase educational achievement of adolescents and young adults"; and "increase the percentage of young children with autism spectrum disorder (ASD) and other developmental delays who are screened, evaluated, and enrolled in early intervention services in a timely manner" (USDHHS, 2010).

The U.S. Preventive Services Task Force's (USPSTF) (2010) *Child and Adolescent Recommendations for Development and Behavior* states that there is "insufficient evidence to recommend for or against routine, brief, formal screening instruments in primary care to detect speech and language delays in children up to 5 years of age."

Bright Futures: Guidelines for Health Supervision of Infants, Children, and Adolescents (Hagan et al, 2008) addresses health promotion to ensure physical, cognitive, and socioemotional health, supporting the healthy development of the child. This includes surveillance and screening for early identification and intervention of any problems. Specific cognitive skills in infancy, early childhood, middle childhood, and adolescence are identified in the Child Development section. Screening for vision and hearing is recommended and considered effective.

■ Theories of Normal Cognitive-Perceptual Development

PIAGET: COGNITIVE DEVELOPMENT

Piaget's learning model is discussed in detail in Chapter 4, but key concepts include *assimilation* (taking in information through any and all the senses), *accommodation* (taking one's current abilities/understanding and modifying them to adjust to the new circumstance or challenge), *schema* (organizing this into a new mental structure or physical action), and *equilibrium* (a new level of cognition).

NEURODEVELOPMENTAL FRAMEWORK

A neurodevelopmental framework is a model of learning based on a synthesis of research from neuroscience, cognitive psychology, and child and adolescent development explaining how the brain functions and how these functions affect student learning and performance. Every person has strengths and weaknesses that influence learning, as well as particular affinities—subjects, ideas, and pursuits they're drawn to. "Collectively, these strengths, weaknesses, and affinities shape both how we learn and what engages us—which, in turn, influence how much we actually learn and thrive in a given situation" (All Kinds of Minds, 2010).

There are eight constructs to the neurodevelopmental framework, which are listed in Table 15-1. Identifying a child's strengths and weaknesses by using these constructs provides a method to describe, organize, and address individual students' learning needs.

MULTIPLE INTELLIGENCES

In 1983 Dr. Howard Gardner, a professor of education at Harvard University, developed the theory of multiple intelligences to account for the broad range of human potential in children and adults. Gardner believed the traditional measure of intelligence, based on IQ testing, was inadequate and left many talented and intelligent children and adults floundering (Smith, 2010). He identified eight different intelligences (Table 15-2) that many educational systems have begun to use.

INFORMATION-PROCESSING THEORIES

Information processing (IP), which is thinking or problem-solving, looks at information presented, processes used to transform information, and memory limits that constrain the amount of information that can be represented and processed. A child's ability to encode—identify and use critical information to create internal representations—is critical. If children fail to identify or comprehend critical elements, or do not know how to encode them efficiently, they do not learn from potentially useful experiences.

Structural components include sensory register with visual and auditory registers (like input devices for a computer), short-term storage/memory (like the central processing unit of a computer), and long-term storage/memory (like hard drive storage).

Process components include rehearsal activity—used to keep information in the short-term store, the working memory; automatic processing—transforms information outside the direct control of the individual to retain information not consciously remembered; and the task environment or the context of the child—for example, a particular solution to a problem may create moral conflicts and thus alter the child's options. Figure 15-1 illustrates an information-processing model.

SOCIAL COGNITION

Social cognition, also called intuition or common sense, is the ability to interpret behavior and emotions of self and others. It is not well documented and difficult to measure or assess, so exists on a spectrum. There is a neural overlap with intellectual cognition, but social cognition also has distinct processes. Components of social cognition include the ability to:
- Understand thoughts, intentions, and emotions of self and others
- Follow the rules of social play, to regulate one's own responses to unstructured or ambiguous social environments
- Understand/anticipate how peers feel (empathy)
- Communicate and comprehend social meaning; understand body language and perceive faces

A spectrum of developmental skills for each age cluster has been identified (Hansen and Ulrey, 2009), but in general includes:
- Infancy—eye contact, social smile, reaching, emerging joint attention, use of others' emotions to regulate self
- Toddler/preschool—emerging empathy, understanding social rules, constructing narratives and reciprocity in play
- School age—functioning successfully and flexibly in both structured and unstructured situations; "street smart"
- Adolescence—forming social group affiliations and emerging sexual identity; social testing and teasing

TABLE 15-1	Constructs of the Neurodevelopmental Framework
Attention	A series of control mechanisms through which the brain regulates learning and behavior. Components include: • Mental energy related to CNS arousal, mobilization and distribution of mental effort • Processing and regulation of incoming stimuli • Production, or the output of work, behavior and social activity *Executive functions* are loosely related cognitive processes that enable self-regulation, problem-solving, and goal-oriented actions including inhibition, flexibility (ability to shift between activities or thoughts), emotional control, working memory, and monitoring.
Memory	Organized storage and recall • Short-term memory: initial registration of information or skill • Active working memory: ability to keep in mind components of a task while working to complete it • Long-term memory: occurs in non-REM sleep; five main systems of consolidation • Retrieval: recall of data or skill on demand • Delayed automatization: ability to access what has been learned
Language	• Phonology: processing, retaining, and manipulating language • Semantic deficits: understanding word meanings • Syntax: understanding and formulating complex sentences • Discourse: processing and retention of language delivered in large amounts • Receptive and expressive language
Spatial ordering	• Mostly processed through visual pathways • Awareness of shape, position, relative size, foreground and background relationships, and form constancy
Temporal sequencing ordering	• Awareness and application of time and sequence • Used to manage time, process multistep explanations and procedures, register lengthy sequences
Neuromotor function	• Graphomotor function/dyspraxia (eight subtypes) • Fine motor function • Gross motor incoordination
Higher-order cognition	• Sophisticated thinking skills • Formation/acquisition of concepts • Critical thinking • Problem-solving • Understanding and formulating rules • Brainstorming and creativity • Metacognition (the ability to think about thinking)
Social cognition	• Awareness of interaction with and effect on others • Ability to enter smoothly into new relationships • Capacity to time and stage interactions effectively • Sensitivity to social feedback cues • Knowledge of how to resolve social conflict without aggression • Adaptive use of language/verbal pragmatics • Ability to establish truly reciprocal (sharing) relationships • Inclination to overcome egocentricity to praise or nurture others

CNS, Central nervous system; *REM,* rapid eye movement.

SENSORY PROCESSING

All humans receive information from their environment through their senses: vision, hearing, touch, taste, smell, position (proprioception), and movement (vestibular). Sensory processing, also known as sensory integration, has to do with how individuals respond to, process, and/or organize sensory information for use in functional daily life routines and activities. Three processes of sensory integration have been described (Miller et al, 2009): sensory modulation—the regulation of responses to sensory stimulation; sensory discrimination—interpreting the specific characteristics of sensory stimuli (intensity, duration, spatial and temporal elements); and sensory-based motor, which include balance and core stability, as well as motor planning and sequencing movements.

THE SOCIETAL-FAMILIAL-INDIVIDUAL MATRIX OF SCHOOL ACHIEVEMENT

Wegner (2009) proposes a matrix of societal, family, and individual elements that affect a child's ability to achieve academically. Success can be defined as "successful attainment of skills commensurate with the child's cognitive profile" and is often measured by passing all grades in school. This matrix offers a way to examine the interplay of a child's individual profile, family factors, and community characteristics.

TABLE 15-2	Multiple Intelligences
Intelligence	**Description**
Linguistic	Sensitivity to language; language-based function (word smart)
Logical-mathematical	Abstract reasoning, manipulation of symbols, detection of patterns, logical reasoning (number/reasoning smart)
Musical	Detection and production of musical structures and patterns; appreciation of pitch, rhythm, musical expressiveness (music smart)
Spatial	Visual memory, visual-spatial skills, visualization (picture smart)
Body-kinesthetic	Representation of ideas, feeling in movement; use of body, coordination, goal-directed activities (body smart)
Naturalistic	Classification and recognition of animals, plants (nature smart)
Social/interpersonal	Sensitivity and responsiveness to moods, motives, intentions and feelings of others (people smart)
Personal/intrapersonal	Sensitivity to self, feelings, strengths, desires, weaknesses and understanding of intention and motivation of others (self smart)

Individual characteristics affecting academic performance include: (1) cognition—often considered the predictor of academic success; (2) developmental skills—play a role in contributing to intelligence; (3) resilience—contributes to a child's motivation to succeed or ability to persevere through failure; and (4) desire for education—a personal belief that education is important and contributes to the future.

Family factors that influence student educational achievement include: (1) community acceptance of varied types of family structures; (2) family values at odds with the larger community causing missed opportunities for the child; (3) performance expectations out of line with a child's capabilities, either too high or too low; and (4) parental academic abilities that not only genetically influence a child's capability but also affect the home support a child may receive.

Societal factors that influence educational systems include: (1) economic—the affluence of the community affects resources and experiences as well as, potentially, the quality of teachers attracted; (2) political—politicians may be hesitant to promote tax increases to provide needed resources for schools; (3) religious—a preponderance of a specific religious group may exert influence on a school's curricula, policy, and procedures; and (4) cultural—as with religion, ethnic and cultural groups may exert pressure on a school.

■ Effects of Cognitive-Perceptual Problems on the Child and Family

Although most children develop according to normal patterns, developmental delays, specific deficits, and alterations in cognitive-perceptual development sometimes occur. Delays from environmental deprivation or neglect are frequently reversible, once identified.

Feedback provides information to the child, positive reinforcement for correct responses to stimuli, and negative reinforcement for behaviors that are not appropriate. Parents, peers, and others provide important feedback to the child. For some children with perceptual problems, not only is the initial cue missed but also the feedback cues. This feedback is an essential component of the learning process.

Knafl and colleagues (1996, 2001) identified the following family management styles when a child has a chronic or disabling condition: thriving, accommodating, enduring, struggling, and floundering. Each management style described how parents perceived the child (normal, problematic, tragic), the parenting philosophy and view of illness, and their perception and approach to managing the illness. For example, parents who embraced a thriving family management style viewed the condition from a "life goes on" perspective and normalized the child's illness as best they could. They had a parenting philosophy that was able to accommodate the condition into parenting activities and a confident mind-set, and they were proactive in their management approach.

Other typologies have been described for families with children with other cognitive-perceptual problems. Kendall (1998) described four types of families of children with attention-deficit/hyperactivity disorder (ADHD) along a trajectory: the chaotic family, the ADHD-controlled family, the surviving family, and the reinvested family. Other studies of families living with ADHD indicate considerable disruption to family routines and an inability to achieve some sense of "normalcy." Some families describe family life as a "nightmare," despite outward indicators (intact marriage, stable residence, adequate income, resources to manage the ADHD, etc.) that the family is doing well (Shelton, 2001). Families of learning-disabled children have been described as healthy, split, chaotic, and blaming (Ziegler and Holden, 1988).

■ Cognitive-Perceptual Development Problems and Primary Care

ASSESSMENT

Assessment of cognitive-perceptual development should be incorporated at every well-child visit from birth through young adulthood. Assessment of a child's cognitive-perceptual development includes consideration of risk factors and current performance as elicited by history, actual assessment via screening tools, direct observation of the child and caregiver, as well as review of school data.

History

The provider should be alert to risk factors related to problems in cognitive-perceptual development.
- Genetic elements—any disorder, condition, or malformation with identifiable cognitive effect (e.g., trisomy 21, velocardiofacial syndromes)
- Prenatal factors—risk factors such as maternal/paternal age at conception; maternal use of tobacco or alcohol; maternal hypertension and other complications; fetal hypoxemia or suboptimal growth

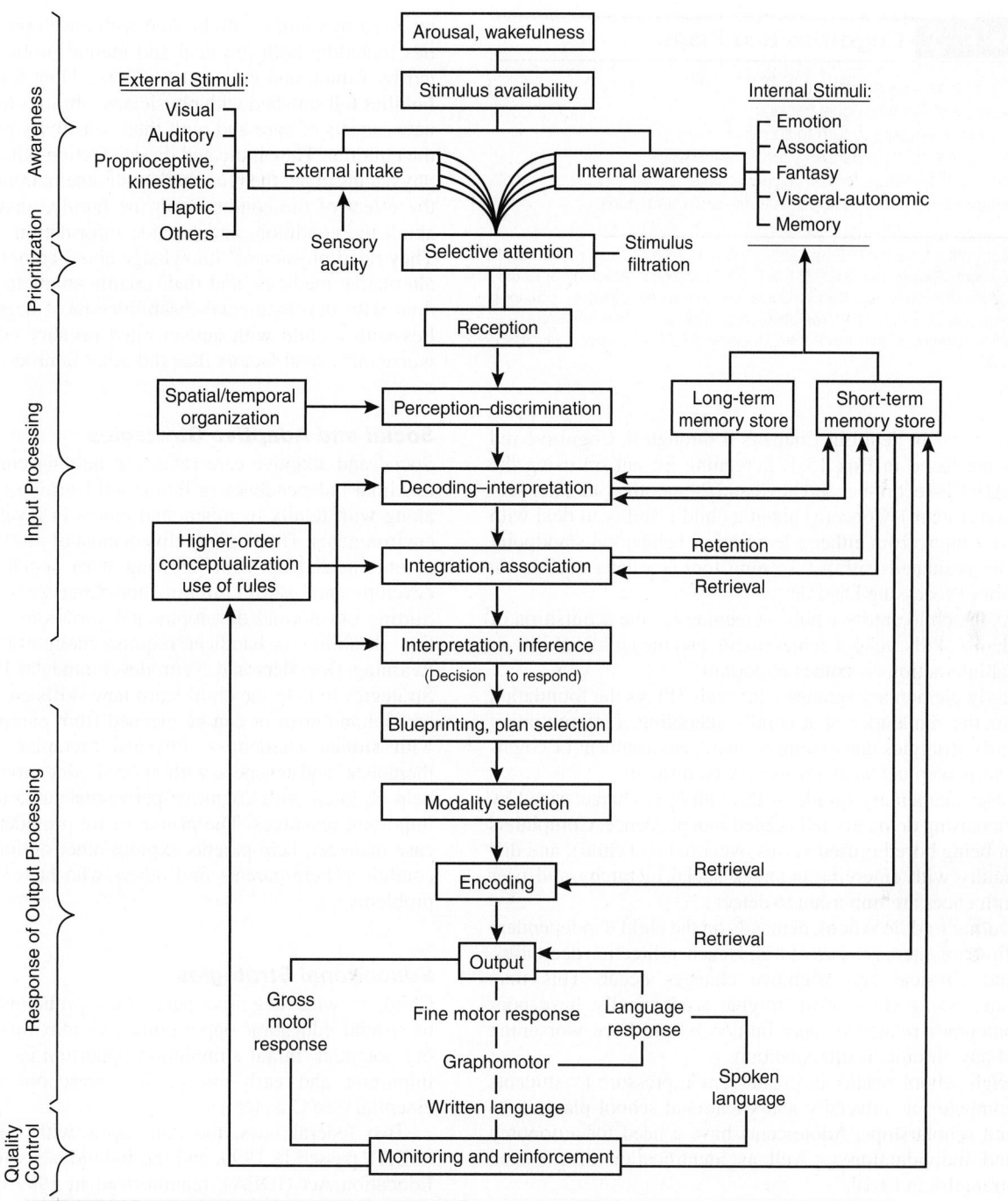

FIGURE 15-1 Information-processing model. (From Levine M, Brooks R, Shonkoff J: *A pediatric approach to learning disorders,* New York, 1980, Wiley, p 480.)

- Birth and perinatal events—adverse events during delivery; prematurity; prolonged neonatal complications
- Infancy to 3 years—maternal depression; family wellness indicators; parental literacy, child deprivation, neglect, or abuse
- Three years through kindergarten entry—child interaction difficulties in larger group settings; lack of independent play or sustained interest in preferred activity, lack of expanding conversation and interactions with adult

- School age and adolescence—difficulties in academic settings, problems with interactions with peers or in large group settings

Screening

A developmental screening tool should be used consistently throughout the first 6 years of life to monitor children for any delay or lagging performance. Developmental screening

BOX 15-1	Cognitive Red Flags

- 2 months—lack of fixation
- 4 months—lack of visual tracking
- 6 months—failure to turn to sound or voice
- 9 months—lack of babbling consonant sounds
- 24 months—failure to use single words
- 36 months—failure to speak in three-word sentences

Data from Wilks T, Gerber R, Erdie-Lalena C: Developmental milestones: cognitive development, *Pediatr Rev* 31(9):364-367, 2010; American Academy of Neurology and the Child Neurology Society: *Guideline summary for clinicians: screening and diagnosis of autism,* 2010. Available at http://aan.com/professionals/practice/guidelines/guideline_summaries/Autism_Guideline_for_Clinicians.pdf (accessed Jan 5, 2011).

is discussed in detail in Chapters 4 through 8. Cognitive red flags are listed in Box 15-1. Screening for autism using the M-CHAT is recommended at 18 and 24 months (see later section on Autism). Concerns about a child's ability to deal with sensory input from either a learning or behavioral standpoint can be evaluated with a screening tool (see later section on Sensory Processing Disorder).

As the child enters school, screening for the acquisition of academic skills, school achievement, and the child's ability in social interactions becomes important.

- Early elementary (grades 1 through 3) lays the foundation for the remainder of a child's schooling. Differentiating early struggles due to temperament, environment or cognitive-perceptual weaknesses may be difficult.
- Later elementary (grades 4 through 6) is characterized by increasing demands and needed independence. Complaints of being bored (gifted versus overwhelmed child); and difficulty with emerging complex social hierarchy and peer influences are important to detect.
- During middle school, demands on the child's independent direction increase, parental and teacher direction decreases, and physical and cognitive changes occur. This may cause some children to struggle academically, have poor outcomes related to peer influence, and have worsening of any chronic health condition.
- High school results in greater grade pressure as students compete for university and vocational school placements and scholarships. Adolescents have a need for autonomy and individuation as well as identification of personal strengths and goals.

If any problems or concerns are identified, further evaluation should be undertaken. This is discussed later in the chapter.

Monitoring *hearing and vision* is the first step in assessment of perception. It is of note that children with cognitive-perceptual variations may achieve motor milestones on time, but experience delays in speech, social, and emotional areas of development.

MANAGEMENT STRATEGIES

Children and families with problems in this domain generally need support in four areas: social and adaptive skills, education, family support, and multidisciplinary health care team consultations. Many families find this support lacking from their primary care providers. Satisfaction with primary care

received by families of children with developmental disabilities including both physical and mental problems was studied by Liptak and colleagues (2006). They found that most families felt satisfied with physicians' abilities to keep up with new aspects of care and with their sensitivity to the needs of the children. They indicated dissatisfaction with the ability of physicians to put them in touch with other parents, understand the effect of the condition on the family, answer questions about the condition, and provide information and guidance. They rated physicians' knowledge about complementary and alternative medicine and their qualifications to manage children with developmental disabilities most negatively. Families with a child with autism rated primary care physicians worse on several factors than did other families.

Social and Adaptive Strategies

Social and adaptive care relates to helping children achieve maximal independence in living and learning in order to get along with family members and others in a variety of social environments. The family delivers most of this care, but some parents need help with knowing what social and adaptive developmental steps children should master at various ages. Sorting out normal developmental variations from dysfunction, disability, or handicap requires thoughtful analysis (see Learning Disorders and Neurodevelopmental Dysfunctions). Strategies to help the child learn new skills are often learned by trial and error or can be gleaned from parents of children with similar challenges. Physical therapists, occupational therapists, and teachers with special education and skills to help children with cognitive-perceptual impairments can be important resources. The primary care provider can serve as case manager, help parents explore other options, or act as a conduit to help parents find others who have solved similar problems.

Educational Strategies

Children with cognitive-perceptual problems are entitled to special education opportunities to maximize their learning potential. Infant stimulation opportunities are extremely important and early-intervention preschool programs are essential (see Chapter 4).

Two federal laws, the Americans with Disabilities Act (ADA), passed in 1990, and the Individuals with Disabilities Education Act (IDEA), reauthorized in 1997, provide mandates for reasonable accommodations that schools must provide to help children with disabilities to achieve meaningful, equal opportunity to benefit from educational services. Free and appropriate public education (FAPE) and least restrictive environment (LRE) are ideas that are built into the special education system. A response to intervention (RTI) approach is a tiered response to determining if a child has a disability and qualifies for special education. It is more effective in identifying students with learning disabilities than the traditional IQ discrepancy model. Once a child has been identified with special learning needs, an Individualized Education Plan (IEP) or a 504 plan are two means of delineating help for the child. Table 15-3 provides a differentiation of services.

- The IEP originates from the IDEA and is designed for children who demonstrate a gap between learning potential and actual academic performance. An IEP is a written plan

TABLE 15-3	504 and Individualized Educational Plan (IEP) Evaluation and Educational Plans
ADA/504	**IDEA/IEP**
Which is right?	
• For simple accommodations or minor changes • Easier, faster, more flexible	• Needs a wide range of services or protections • More involved with mandated parental participation
Eligibility	
• Based on identification of psychological or physical disorder that "substantially limits" a "major life activity" (learning and/or behavior)	• Must meet criteria of qualified disability (ADHD not included); often other health impairments (OHI); developmental delays, emotional disturbances or specific learning disability (SLD) that seriously affect learning or behavior and "by reason thereof" needs special education and/or related services
Evaluation	
• An evaluation (not formalized testing) compiled by the school from a variety of sources to confirm assumption • No money to cover evaluation or support/sustain accommodation • Can occur without parental knowledge or participation	• A complete evaluation compiled by a team of professionals including testing and information from a variety of sources • Federally funded • Must have written consent to perform
Provisions	
• A plan with individualized accommodations (not a listing) such as extra time to complete assignments, a copy of notes, providing a quiet place to take tests, or assistive technologies • No legal requirements for what is included in a 504, for parent involvement or for mandated reevaluation	• An individualized IEP describes the child's learning problems, details services to be provided, sets annual goals, and defines how progress will be measured • Changes made only in meeting and in collaboration • Special provisions if suspended or expelled • Reevaluation mandated every 3 years

ADHD, Attention-deficit/hyperactivity disorder; *IDEA,* Individuals with Disabilities Education Act; *IEP,* Individualized Educational Plan.

defining the child's disabilities, current level of educational performance, educational needs, and specific annual goals developed by a multidisciplinary team with parent involvement. An IEP includes specific academic, communication, motor, learning, functional, and socialization goals.

• The Section 504 plan specifies "reasonable accommodations" to help children with disabilities benefit from their education. Eligibility is based on the existence of an identified physical or mental condition that "substantially limits a major life activity" (learning). Each school district handles 504 plans differently, but there should be a 504 coordinator that oversees the process. Many children with ADHD and learning disabilities who do not have cognitive deficits but do have learning weaknesses, or behavioral or emotional problems that interfere with learning are eligible for a 504 plan.

When children reach school age, decisions are made collaboratively between parents and school personnel about the best placement of the child (mainstream classroom, special classroom, or combination of settings). A wealth of information about these legal rights and provisions can be found on the Internet.

Family Support Strategies

Living with a child with a cognitive-perceptual problem generally requires an environment that offers consistency for the child. The family must also develop a structure with organization to support the child without becoming overprotective or intrusive.

Social support has been shown to provide significant benefits to families with children with health problems of all sorts. National organizations provide information and expert advice, and local groups can facilitate direct help.

Multidisciplinary Team Strategies

The use of a variety of specialists can provide the best resources for children with special needs. Generally, these include medical specialists, physical and occupational therapists, social workers, and specially educated teachers. The primary care provider helps families identify appropriate teams, serves as a case manager among the parties, and ensures that primary health care needs are integrated with the special services provided.

◼ Cognitive-Perceptual Problems of Children

ATTENTION-DEFICIT/HYPERACTIVITY DISORDER

Description

ADHD is one of the most commonly diagnosed behavioral disorders in childhood. It is considered a neurobiologic condition because it has a clear neurologically based etiology with symptoms that profoundly affect the behavior of individuals across many settings in their lives (Pliszka and American Academy of Child and Adolescent Psychiatry [AACAP], 2007). The symptoms of ADHD can affect cognitive, educational, behavioral, emotional, and social functioning in individuals with ADHD.

The core symptoms of ADHD are *inattention, hyperactivity, and impulsivity.* In ADHD these symptoms occur at a developmentally inappropriate level. There is a range of severity of symptoms from one individual to the next. Also, the scope and severity of behaviors may change within an individual as maturation occurs. The criteria defining ADHD were

TABLE 15-4	*DSM-IV-TR* Criteria for Attention-Deficit/Hyperactivity Disorder
Domain	**Criteria**
Essential features	• Some symptoms that caused impairment were present before age 7 years • Some impairment from the symptoms is present in two or more settings (e.g., at school [or work] and at home) • There must be clear evidence of significant impairment in social, academic, or occupational function • The symptoms do not occur exclusively during the course of a pervasive developmental disorder, schizophrenia, or other psychotic disorder and are not better accounted for by another mental disorder (e.g., mood disorder, anxiety disorder, dissociative disorder, or personality disorder)
Inattention traits	Six or more of the following symptoms of inattention: • Often fails to give close attention to details; makes careless mistakes in schoolwork, work, or other activities • Often has difficulty sustaining attention in tasks or play activities • Does not seem to listen when addressed directly • Often does not follow through on instructions and fails to finish schoolwork, chores, or duties in the workplace (not due to oppositional behavior or failure to understand instruction) • Often has difficulty organizing tasks and activities • Often avoids, dislikes, or is reluctant to engage in tasks that require sustained mental effort (such as schoolwork or homework) • Often loses things necessary for tasks or activities (e.g., toys, school assignments, pencils, books, or tools) • Is easily distracted by extraneous stimuli • Is often forgetful in daily activities
Hyperactivity/ Impulsivity traits	Six or more of the following symptoms of hyperactivity-impulsivity: • Often fidgets with hands or feet or squirms in seat • Often leaves seat in classroom or in other situations in which remaining in seat is expected • Often runs about or climbs excessively in situations in which it is inappropriate (in adolescents or adults may be limited to subjective feeling of restlessness) • Often has difficulty playing or engaging in leisure activities quietly • Is often "on the go" or acts as if "driven by a motor" • Often talks excessively • Often blurts out answers before questions have been completed • Often has difficulty waiting turn • Often interrupts or intrudes on others (e.g., butts into conversations or games)

From American Psychiatric Association: *Diagnostic and statistical manual of mental disorders,* fourth edition, text revision, Arlington, VA, 2000, American Psychiatric Association.

established by the American Psychiatric Association (APA) in the *Diagnostic and Statistical Manual of Mental Disorders,* fourth edition (DSM-IV) (APA, 2000) (Table 15-4).

ADHD has three different diagnostic subtypes depending on the number of positive symptoms in each category (Box 15-2).

ADHD is now understood to be a chronic condition with persistence in many individuals into adolescence and adulthood (Van Cleave and Leslie, 2008). Approximately 60% to 85% of children with ADHD continue to have symptoms into adolescence (Pliszka and AACAP, 2007). Factors that increase the risk of ADHD persisting into adolescence and adulthood include a strong family history of ADHD and the comorbidities of aggression and other conduct problems. Multiple studies cited by Spencer and colleagues (2007) show that untreated adults with ADHD struggle with a great many social difficulties including higher rates of marital discord and divorce, lower socioeconomic status, higher unemployment rates, higher rates of substance abuse, poor self-esteem, and higher rates of traffic violations and motor vehicle accidents.

Etiology

Prevalence in the U.S. ADHD prevalence rates vary depending on the source, criteria used to make the diagnosis, and the ages sampled. Overall, the rate of ADHD diagnosis is increasing at a higher rate among teenagers than among

BOX 15-2	Attention-Deficit/Hyperactivity Disorder (ADHD) Diagnostic Subtypes

ADHD, Combined Type
• Six or more symptoms from each of the categories (inattention and hyperactivity/impulsivity) are present
• Accounts for 50% to 75% of ADHD cases
• Coded as 314.01

ADHD, Predominantly Inattentive
• Six or more of the inattentive symptoms are identified, but fewer than six in hyperactivity/impulsivity
• Accounts for 20% to 30% of ADHD cases
• Coded 314.00

ADHD, Predominantly Hyperactive/Impulsive
• Six or more of the hyperactivity/impulsivity symptoms are identified, but fewer than six in inattention category
• Accounts for approximately 15% of ADHD cases
• Coded 314.01

Data from Lollar DJ: Function, impairment, and long-term outcomes in children with ADHD and how to measure them, *Pediatr Ann* 37(1):28-36, 2008.

younger children (Centers for Disease Control and Prevention [CDC], 2010b; Pastor and Reuben, 2008). There is a 9.5% prevalence for children between 4 and 17 years (5.4 million children), based on parental report of their child having been diagnosed with ADHD (CDC, 2010a). Rates by age are cited as 4- to 10-year-olds, 6.6%; 11- to 14-year-olds, 11.2%; and 15- to 17-year-olds, 13.6%. In 2007, 4.8% of children diagnosed with ADHD were being treated with medication for this condition. ADHD has always been more prevalent in boys than in girls. Current rates show the prevalence in boys at 13.2% and in girls at 5.6% (CDC, 2010a). Girls are more likely than boys to have the symptoms of ADHD, predominantly inattention. This subtype also has greater academic difficulty than ADHD, predominantly hyperactive/impulsive. About 4% of children with ADHD also have a diagnosed learning disability (Pastor and Reuben, 2008).

Cross-Cultural Considerations. In the U.S. the incidence of ADHD in Hispanic children is 5.6%, compared with 10.5% among non-Hispanic children (CDC, 2010a). Those most to least likely to be diagnosed with ADHD are multiracial, African-American, and Caucasian. ADHD has been well documented outside of the U.S. Studies show a similar range of rates of ADHD incidence occurring in children internationally (Buitelaar et al, 2006; Faraone et al, 2003). Although there is agreement across cultures about the presence of ADHD, perceptions often vary by culture, with a paucity of ADHD research from developing countries.

Although ADHD is a condition with a proven neurobiologic basis, it occurs within a sociocultural framework. This is an important consideration for providers in giving sensitive care to families. Perceptions about parenting and childrearing, beliefs about medication and the health care system in general, family and social networking roles in managing child behavior problems, and parents' own experiences with school are all factors that shape the approach to seeking care, diagnosis, and treatment. Families may have differing understandings of what constitutes behavior problems. Studies show that providers who are most sensitive and successful in working with families are open and honest in the discussion of diagnoses and all treatment options, include key family members in collaborative decision making, and strive to become more aware of the community and cultural values of the populations with which they work (Olaniyan et al, 2007).

Effect on Individuals, Families, and Communities. Because ADHD symptoms cross over so many settings and are chronic, often into adulthood, this condition has a major effect on the individual as well as on his or her family and community. Table 15-5 summarizes impairments across the life span. In families in which ADHD is present, significantly higher levels of stress (than in the general population) are reported. Individuals with ADHD (with and without comorbid conditions) have six times greater difficulty in the areas of friendship with peers, and emotional, and conduct problems than their nonaffected peers. There is a nine times greater likelihood of family stress; problems with classroom learning and conduct; and difficulties with leisure activities (e.g., playing with friends or participating on a sports team) (Strine et al, 2006).

The injury rates among children with ADHD are higher than in the general population. Emergency department admissions rates for children and teens with ADHD are

| TABLE 15-5 | Summary of ADHD Impairments Across the Life Span |

Life Stage	Impairment
Childhood	• Academic difficulties including: ○ Needs for special education (high comorbidity with learning disabilities) ○ Grade retention ○ Classroom behavior management issues ○ Difficulties with friendships and peer relationships ○ Behavioral difficulties at home and other settings (childcare, sports, after-school programs) ○ High comorbidity with other childhood psychiatric problems ○ Associated difficulties (at higher rates than non-ADHD children) with sleep disorders, enuresis, encopresis
Adolescence	• Academic difficulties including: ○ Needs for special education (high comorbidity with learning and emotional disabilities) ○ School failure and dropout ○ Social difficulties with peer relationships ○ Substance abuse (in untreated ADHD) ○ High comorbidity with other psychiatric disorders (depression, anxiety, conduct disorder) ○ High-risk behaviors leading to greater accident rates ○ Involvement in juvenile criminal activities
Adulthood	• Fewer employment possibilities and higher rates of unemployment • Higher risk of tobacco, drug, and alcohol abuse • Higher risk of motor vehicle accidents • Marital discord and higher divorce rates • Increased incidence of criminal involvement

ADHD, Attention-deficit/hyperactivity disorder.
Adapted from Pliszka S, American Academy of Child and Adolescent Psychiatry (AACAP) Work Group on Quality Issues: Practice parameter for the assessment and treatment of children and adolescents with attention-deficit/hyperactivity disorder, *J Am Acad Child Adolesc Psychiatry* 46(7):894-921, 2007; Spencer TJ, Biederrman J, Mick E: Attention-deficit/hyperactivity disorder: diagnosis, lifespan, comorbidities and neurobiology, *Ambul Pediatr* 7(3):73-81, 2007.

81% compared with 74% in the general population. Serious accidents such as motor vehicle accidents occur at a higher rate for individuals with ADHD. Adolescents with ADHD also have a greater incidence of traffic violations and driving while under the influence of drugs or alcohol (CDC, 2010a).

ADHD is a chronic health condition and has significant direct and indirect costs at all levels of society. On an individual level ADHD significantly affects self-esteem, peer relationships, educational achievement, and prospective employment possibilities. ADHD, primarily the combined and hyperactive/impulsive subtypes, are predictors of substance abuse, criminal behaviors, marital difficulties, and divorce. Thus the condition can be seen as having indirect costs to society and the legal and criminal justice systems.

ADHD is also a significant cause of family stress and financial burden. Parents of children with ADHD report days of missed work due to the child's school and medical appointments. Many of the services required for adequate evaluation and treatment of ADHD are not covered by health insurance (e.g., psychological testing, mental health care, or educational testing beyond that done at the school). The average annual direct health care costs for an individual with ADHD are $1,574 compared with $541 for a matched control without ADHD (CDC, 2010a).

Pathophysiology

ADHD is an extremely heterogeneous disorder, meaning there is a wide spectrum of symptoms and severity. Increasingly, neurobiologic research provides strong evidence that ADHD is primarily a genetic, inheritable disorder. There also appears to be a number of environmental factors that may play into the disorder by modulating (i.e., increasing or decreasing) one's predisposition to underlying biochemical vulnerability (Krull, 2010a; Singh, 2008).

Complex neurobiologic activity that takes place in the prefrontal cortex (PFC) is called "executive functioning." The PFC is a highly specialized region where organization and regulation of information and stimuli occur. Executive functioning refers to the interwoven processes continually occurring in the PFC: organizing and making sense of input received, sustaining focus on relevant stimuli, suppressing irrelevant stimuli (distractions), drawing on memory to understand stimuli, planning and organizing for future goals and consequences of actions, and regulating emotional and behavioral responses. The PFC in turn transmits information to, and receives input from, other brain areas such as the sensory cortices, basal ganglia, and cerebellum (for attention regulation and motor response) and to the amygdala, hypothalamus, and brainstem nuclei (where emotions and attention/arousal maintenance are regulated) (Arnsten, 2009; Krull, 2010a; National Resource Center on ADHD, 2009).

Genetics and Neurobiologic Pathophysiology. ADHD appears to be caused by deletions or duplications in a number of genes. The genes that are affected are those that regulate the manufacturing of the catecholamine (noradrenergic) neurotransmitters noradrenaline and dopamine in the brain (Arnsten, 2009). The net result of the genetic irregularities is that these neurotransmitters are less available in certain brain regions in individuals with ADHD. Both dopamine and noradrenaline (dopamine more strongly in ADHD) are known to be essential for healthy brain function, especially for alerting to and maintaining attention, maintaining an appropriate level of internal arousal, and inhibiting external distraction. Attention is a complex and multilayered neurologic activity requiring the function and interconnection of a number of different areas of the brain.

Brain imaging shows structural and chemical differences in the temporal and parietal cortices and the PFC in individuals with ADHD compared with those without this condition. The temporal and parietal regions of the brain are responsible for sensory awareness—recognizing and perceiving incoming information, orienting in time and space. Structurally, imaging has shown the brains of individuals with ADHD have smaller prefrontal cortical volumes. Neurochemically, there is also reduced catecholamine activity, particularly in the areas of the basal ganglia and the PFC. It is now felt that these "under-activated" brain regions and the pathways interconnecting them account for the symptoms of ADHD.

Environmental Factors. In many areas the research on environmental factors that contribute to ADHD is inconclusive. Some of the areas that have been or are being researched include:

- *Prenatal maternal tobacco use.* Prenatal maternal tobacco use is associated with a 2.4-fold increased risk of ADHD (Froehlich et al, 2009).
- *Prenatal alcohol use.* Direct association with ADHD is not as well established in the literature (DynaMed Database, 2010).
- *Lead exposure.* Froehlich and associates (2009) report a direct correlation between early lead exposure and later ADHD diagnosis even with low lead levels (<10 mcg/dL).
- *Prematurity and low birthweight.* Prematurity and low birthweight increase ADHD risk by 2.64-fold (DynaMed Database, 2010).
- *Food additives (artificial colors and flavors).* There have been a number of studies in this area and none have shown a causal connection between food additives and ADHD. Elimination of food additives is not a recommended part of any ADHD practice guidelines (Krull, 2010b).
- *Refined sugar.* Although some children respond to excessive sugar with an increased activity level, reviews of many studies fail to show an association with sugar and ADHD (Krull, 2010b).
- *Essential fatty acids (omega 3 and omega 6).* These nutrients are integral in the development and functioning of neuronal membranes. Three studies showed no benefit to fatty acid supplementation for children with ADHD, although benefits were found in one study (Krull, 2010b).
- *Iron deficiency.* Low serum ferritin is associated with learning difficulties. One study showed that children with ADHD had lower serum ferritin levels than matched non-ADHD children. Another study (Krull, 2010b) showed that iron supplementation in children with low serum ferritin levels improved ADHD symptoms.
- *Zinc.* Limited research has demonstrated zinc deficiency in children with ADHD and/or a benefit from zinc supplementation on ADHD symptoms (Krull, 2010b).

Environmental factors such as family adversity and stress, violence in the home, parenting style, and poverty have been studied with regard to how they may contribute to the etiology of ADHD. There is no clear evidence about these factors causing ADHD. However, any of these factors can be seen as modifying or modulating ADHD, as well as other childhood psychiatric conditions (Spencer et al, 2007).

Clinical Findings

Often the patient presents to the provider after having been referred by a child care provider, the school, or the parent/guardian for concerns about excessive energy and activity, fidgety behavior, distractibility, poor school performance, poor relations with peers, aggressive behavior, failure to organize or complete tasks, or some variation of these symptoms. ADHD symptoms can affect the very domains of life where children and adolescents are working on developmental mastery—school, peers, family life, sports, and recreational activities. If the presenting complaint/visit is not specifically about school or behavioral concerns, it is important for the provider to inquire about those areas of the patient's life.

TABLE 15-6 Clinical Tools and Evidence-Based Guidelines for ADHD Assessment and Treatment

Name of Tool or Guideline	Age Applicable	What Is Included
National Initiative for Children's Healthcare Quality (NICHQ) and American Academy of Pediatrics (AAP): *Caring for children with ADHD: a resource toolkit for clinicians* (www.nichq.org/resources/ADHD_toolkit.html)	School-age children and adolescents	Materials for ADHD diagnosis and management based on the DSM-IV criteria for school-age children and adolescents; Vanderbilt ADHD assessment tool and scoring information
AAP Clinical Practice Guideline: *Diagnosis and evaluation of the child with attention-deficit/hyperactivity disorder*, 2000 *Clinical Practice Guideline: Treatment of the school-aged child with attention-deficit/hyperactivity disorder*, 2001 (http://pediatrics.aappublications.org)	Ages 6 to 12 years	Algorithm and practice recommendations for assessment, diagnosis, and treatment
The American Academy of Child and Adolescent Psychiatry (AACAP): *Practice parameter for the assessment and treatment of children and adolescents with attention-deficit/hyperactivity disorder*, 2007	Ages 3 through 17 years	Recommendations about assessment, diagnosis and treatment
Institute for Clinical Systems Improvement (ICSI) Health care guideline: *Diagnosis and management of attention-deficit/hyperactivity disorder in primary care for school-age children and adolescents*, March 2010 (www.icsi.org)	School-age children and adolescents	Algorithms for diagnosis and treatment, background on ADHD, tables about ADHD medications, table of the full DSM-IV-TR diagnostic criteria

ADHD, Attention-deficit/hyperactivity disorder; *DSM-IV, Diagnostic and Statistical Manual of Mental Disorders, fourth edition.*

Assessment

The diagnosis and management of ADHD can be made in the primary care pediatric office, but involves working with the child's school and other domains where the child regularly spends time (e.g., after-school or childcare programs, sports activities, etc.). There is no "one" assessment tool to diagnose ADHD though there are a number of tools and evidence-based practice guidelines that are available to help clinicians develop an organized, efficient, and safe practice in assessing, diagnosing, and caring for children and adolescents with ADHD. Table 15-6 provides resource information for the four main guidelines.

The components of the ADHD assessment include:
- Interview of parent and child or adolescent for history gathering
- Physical examination
- Gathering information about symptoms on standardized ADHD behavioral assessment scales from several different sources (parents, caregivers, teachers, sports coaches)
- Gathering other pertinent evaluations (if done) such as school testing and psychological or other mental health evaluations

History. Table 15-7 outlines many of the areas for assessment and suggested topics to explore in taking a history when evaluating for ADHD.

Physical
- Vital signs—weight, height, blood pressure, pulse
- General observation of child's behavior (may or may not present with ADHD symptoms in a structured clinical setting); observations of parent-child interaction
- General—dysmorphic stigmata suggestive of genetic syndrome or prenatal exposure to drugs or alcohol
- Skin—café au lait spots; signs of abuse
- Ear, nose, and throat (ENT)—signs of past recurring otitis media (scarring of tympanic membranes), signs of respiratory allergies, enlarged tonsils

- Cardiovascular—heart sounds and rhythm, murmur, pulses
- Neurologic—general screening exam—mental status, general cognition and mental process as appropriate for age, speech and language, and motor skills

Other Studies. In general, no other studies are indicated in the workup of ADHD, although occasionally vision and hearing screen (if not up-to-date with normal results at school), screening for anemia, lead screening, and thyroid screening are indicated.

ADHD Standardized Assessment (Behavior) Scales. Evidence-based practice guidelines recommend use of ADHD-specific behavior rating scales (American Academy of Pediatrics [AAP], Committee on Quality Improvement, Subcommittee on Attention-Deficit/Hyperactivity Disorder, 2000; Institute for Clinical Systems Improvement [ICSI], 2010; Pliszka and AACAP, 2007). These scales, which should be completed independently by individuals who know the child or adolescent from at least two different domains of life (e.g., home, school, daycare), provide the most objective data to assess the scope and severity of the symptoms. It is essential to include school data in the evaluation process. As children get older, and attend middle or high school, it is appropriate to obtain information from various teachers who work with the student throughout the school day. This information provides valuable insight into symptom variation at different hours of the day as well as clues to possible learning difficulties in specific subjects.

There are a number of different behavioral scales developed to evaluate ADHD. Some cost money and others are available to download at no charge. It is generally recommended that a provider become familiar with one scale and its scoring and interpretation in order to be efficient. Additionally, many of the scales screen for the common comorbidities that often accompany ADHD. Behavioral rating scales are extremely useful to assist in diagnosis and to monitor change

TABLE 15-7 Attention-Deficit/Hyperactivity Disorder History

Assessment Area	Suggested Topics to Explore
Chief complaint and history of present problem	Major areas of concern First awareness of problem Beliefs about causation of problem Previous evaluations and results Medication history for behavioral, emotional, or learning problems
Birth history*	Prenatal history; maternal health; use of medications, recreational drugs, alcohol, and tobacco during pregnancy Prematurity, low birthweight or IUGR Birth and postpartum complications, anoxia, difficult delivery, birth defects Neonatal behavior: feeding, sleep, temperament problems
Medical history	Chronic diseases, ongoing medications Hospitalizations, prolonged illness Trauma history (head injury, frequent injuries) Poisoning or lead or environmental exposures Neurologic status, seizures, tics, habit spasms, uncontrolled twitches, outbursts of uncontrollable sounds or words Environmental allergies Cardiovascular history (see section about cardiovascular risks with stimulants)
General health*	Vision, hearing
ADHD history	Attention: paying attention, sustaining attention, listening, following through, organization, reluctant to engage in activities that need sustained attention, loses things, distracted, forgetful Activity: fidgets, leaves seat, runs or climbs when inappropriate, has difficulty with quiet games, talks excessively, has problems waiting turn, interrupts, "on the go"
Developmental history*	Milestones: motor, personal-social, language, cognitive Strengths (e.g., personality, activities, friendliness) Weaknesses
Behavioral history*	Frequency with which child complies when told to do something Methods used at home to improve behavior and effectiveness Parenting skills and style, cultural beliefs Parental agreement about child management Counseling history for child or family (or both)
Academic history	Child's progress at each grade level (strengths seen) Adjustment problems at school, child's history with peers, friendships Difficulties with specific skills: reading, writing, spelling, math, concepts Performance problems: attention, grades, participation, excessive talking, disturbing others, fighting, bullying, teasing, abusive language, not completing work School assistance: tutoring, counseling, special help

Functional Health Patterns

Feeding	Not able to sit through a complete meal Messy and clumsy with utensils, dishes, and glasses Inadequate caloric intake can be result of symptoms and further exacerbated by medications used to treat ADHD Gastric distress may be a side effect of stimulant medication
Elimination	Enuresis, encopresis
Sleeping	Difficulty falling asleep, night waking, needs less sleep than other family members Complains about fatigue interfering with completion of tasks
Activity	Difficulty maintaining routines for activities of daily living
Cognitive	Level of performance is below potential for achievement Tends to miss the point of conversations and activities Often does things the hard way in absence of established routines
Self-concept	Struggles with low self-esteem, moodiness
Role relationships	Births, deaths, deployment Marriage and family transitions: separation, divorce, remarriage Violence: domestic, current or past abuse of parent or child; problems with the law; weapons in the home Inadequate social and relational skills Lies, steals, plays with fire, hurts animals, is aggressive with other children, talks back to adults

TABLE 15-7	Attention-Deficit/Hyperactivity Disorder History—cont'd
Assessment Area	**Suggested Topics to Explore**
Coping and stress tolerance	Family stress and coping patterns Stressors: parent job loss or change, financial problems Outbursts of temper, low tolerance for frustration Moody, worried, sad, quiet, destructive, fearful or fearless, self-deprecating Somatic complaints
Social and environmental history*	General family relationships (child and parents/siblings) Home, daycare, and school environments Family social risk factors: recent moves, financial stress, parental job losses, births, deaths, divorces, remarriages, alcohol and drug use, involvement with law enforcement, weapons in the home
Family history*	ADHD, neurologic problems, learning difficulties Mental health history of close family members, health or behavior problems in other family members Genetic disorders: cognitive disabilities, growth disorders, neurofibromatosis Drug or alcohol abuse (current and/or past)
Teacher history	Obtain information from school about child's problems, strengths, weaknesses, academic management of issues

*These must be included in the assessment.
ADHD, Attention-deficit/hyperactivity disorder; *IUGR,* intrauterine growth retardation.

once treatment has begun. Table 15-8 has information on several of the commonly used ADHD behavioral rating scales.

Differential Diagnosis and Comorbidities

ADHD has a high frequency of comorbidities with other psychiatric or learning disorders. Approximately 25% to 35% of children and adolescents with ADHD also have a learning disorder (Pliszka and AACAP, 2007). The most common learning difficulties coexisting with ADHD are in the areas of reading, speech, and language. More than half (54% to 84%) of children and teens with ADHD also meet the diagnostic criteria for oppositional defiant disorder (ODD) (Pliszka and AACAP, 2007). Approximately one third of children and teens with ADHD have comorbid conduct disorder (CD) (Krull, 2010a). Both ODD and CD are more frequent in those who have ADHD, combined or predominantly hyperactive/impulsive subtypes. The comorbidities of ODD and CD are also more common in boys than in girls. Fifteen to 19% of adolescents with ADHD develop a substance disorder or use tobacco (Pliszka and AACAP, 2007). In general, children and adolescents with ADHD combined type have the highest rate of psychiatric comorbidities and suffer the greatest impairment (Spencer et al, 2007). Anxiety disorders coexist with ADHD approximately 33% of the time. Depression comorbidity is also seen at a rate of about 33% (Krull, 2010a). Other conditions that occur more often with ADHD than in the general population include enuresis, encopresis, sleep difficulties, tics, and difficulty with motor coordination (Adesman, 2003). When considering comorbidities, it is important to assess if the symptoms being reported are ADHD with comorbidity, or the comorbid disorder masquerading as ADHD (seen commonly with substance abuse, especially tobacco).

Management

Once the evaluation is completed, the provider reviews and synthesizes all the data—including the complete history, physical examination findings, behavioral rating scales from the various domains, and any other evaluations that may have been done (school reports, psychoeducational testing, mental health assessment), assessing the onset, duration, and pervasiveness of symptoms, and determining the level that symptoms are impairing daily function. Although the discussion of ADHD is often one of identifying difficulties in many dimensions of a young person's life, it is imperative for clinicians to also identify the strengths that exist and to build on those during the entire diagnostic and treatment process. When planning for treatment, both pharmacologic and nonpharmacologic approaches should be included in the plan of care.

Pharmacologic Management

Stimulants. The first-line medications for ADHD treatment are the stimulant medications—methylphenidate (MPH) and amphetamines (AMPs) (both available in a variety of forms) (Table 15-9). The other ADHD-specific medication is atomoxetine, a norepinephrine site-specific drug. The pharmacologic action of the stimulants occurs in the dopaminergic and noradrenergic pathways in key areas of the brain where ample bioavailability of these compounds is essential but decreased in individuals with ADHD. These medications increase the availability of these neurotransmitters at the neuron synapses. Numerous studies conclude that medication is the most effective treatment for ADHD (Krull, 2010b; Pliszka and AACAP, 2007). The most comprehensive medication studies to date are the Multimodal Treatment Study of Children with ADHD (MTA study) and the Preschool ADHD Treatment Study (PATS). The MTA study has data from 8 years of treatment research on school-age children. The PATS has been ongoing for 3- to 5-year-olds since 2006 (Krull, 2010b; Lerner and Wigal, 2008; Pliszka and AACAP, 2007).

Overall findings about medication treatment for ADHD summarized from the MTA and PATS (AAP, Committee on Quality Improvement, Subcommittee on Attention-Deficit/Hyperactivity Disorder, 2001; Krull, 2010b; Lerner and Wigal, 2008; Pliszka and AACAP, 2007) concluded that the two groups of stimulants, MPH and dextroamphetamine (AMP) are equally efficacious in treating ADHD. Individual patients may have a more favorable response to one group over the

| TABLE 15-8 | Commonly Used ADHD Behavior Rating Scales |

Name of Scale and Principle Author	Comments
Vanderbilt Attention-Deficit/ Hyperactivity Disorder (ADHD) Diagnostic Rating Scale (Wolraich, 2005) (Available in the NICHQ/ AAP ADHD clinician toolkit)	• Parent and teacher forms • Screens for comorbid conditions • Normed by age and sex • Separates inattention and hyperactive/impulsive factors • Follow-up version has questions about medication side effects • Available in English and Spanish • May be used free of charge
ADHD Rating Scale IV: Checklists, Norms, and Clinical Interpretation (Dupaul GJ, Power, TJ, Anastopoulos A, Reid R, 1998)	• Based on DSM-IV-TR/DSM-PC criteria for ADHD • Normed by age and sex • Separates inattention and hyperactive/impulsive factors • May be used free of charge
Child Attention Profile (Barkley RA, Murphy KR, 2005)	• Based on inattention and overactive items from the Achenbach Child Behavior Checklist • Normed by sex • Separates inattention and overactive factors • May be used free of charge
Conners Parent and Teacher Rating Scale (Conners, 2010)	• Multiple scales assessing conduct, learning, psychosomatic, impulsive/hyperactive, and anxiety dimensions • Some concern over few items focusing on cognitive (inattention) versus behavioral (hyperactive/impulsive) features of ADHD • May be used for a fee • Available in English and Spanish

DSM-IV-TR, Diagnostic and Statistical Manual of Mental Disorders IV-TR, text revision; *DSM-PC, Diagnostic and Statistical Manual of Mental Disorders for Primary Care.*
Adapted from Institute for Clinical Systems Improvement (ICSI): *Health care guideline: diagnosis and management of attention deficit hyperactivity disorder in primary care for school-age children and adolescents,* March 2010. Available at www.icsi.org (accessed Oct 30, 2010); National Initiative for Children's Healthcare Quality (NICHQ): *Caring for children with ADHD: a resource toolkit for clinicians.* Available at www.nichq.org/resources/ADHD_toolkit.html (accessed Nov 28, 2010).

other. If treatment at the highest tolerated dose of one group of stimulants does not help, the recommendation is to try the second group. There is no predictor as to which stimulant will work better for any individual patient (Pliszka and AACAP, 2007). The studies also found that 65% to 75% of individuals will get significant benefit from the stimulant medications and that a 65% to 75% response rate increases to approximately 85% having a favorable response if both groups of stimulants are tried (i.e., moving to the second group if the patient is a nonresponder to the first group). Benefits have been seen at long-term follow-up, but the positive response to medications seems to diminish over time (Pliszka and AACAP, 2007). Other findings include that long- and short-acting forms of each of the medications are equally efficacious, with long

acting preferred because no midday school dosing is required; improved compliance is seen with the long-acting stimulants; long-acting medication lessens the stigma of having to take a medication at school; it is safe to begin treatment with a long-acting medication unless dosage titration or side effects are of concern; and side effect profiles are the same for the short- and long-acting forms of each of the medications.

When dosing stimulants for school-age children and adolescents:

• The dose response is very individualized for each of the medications.
• Dose is not weight based, but rather follows the recommended dose ranges.
• Begin at the low end of the dose range and titrate up every 1 to 3 weeks. During the titration the patient should be monitored for symptom improvement and side effects at each dose change.
• It is recommended that providers consider the full range of possible therapeutic doses because approximately one third of individuals respond at the low dose, one third at mid-dose range, and one third require the higher doses for maximum benefit.
• The dosing goal is maximum reduction of ADHD core symptoms with minimal side effects.
• If the patient arrives at the top of the dose range without benefit or experiences side effects, it is recommended that he or she be changed to the alternative stimulant group or atomoxetine.

When titrating dose conversion from MPH to AMP, use 2 mg MPH: 1 mg AMP and 1 mg MPH immediate release equals 2 mg MPH extended release.

Pharmacologic Approaches at Different Ages. Most medication testing has been done with children ages 6 to 12 years. In general, most providers are less enthusiastic to put younger children on a stimulant medication. A few guidelines have emerged from the PATS and other research of medication use and preschool-age children.

• Both MPH and AMP are effective in preschool-age children (ages 3 to 5 years).
• A lower dose range is recommended in young children due to the increased incidence of side effects.
• The most common side effects in preschool-age children are emotional lability (crying, moodiness) and social withdrawal.
• Methylphenidate is metabolized more slowly in younger children, thus the lower dose range (0.3 to 1.1 mg/kg/day) should be used.
• In preschool-age children, dose titration upward should move slowly and more conservatively than for older children.
• Be sure to offer careful instructions on monitoring of side effects and for benefits so the lowest effective dose can be recognized.

Atomoxetine. Atomoxetine is the only noncontrolled, nonstimulant medication approved as a first-line medication for ADHD. It is approved for use in children older than age 6 years (ICSI, 2010). Atomoxetine is a norepinephrine reuptake inhibitor. It works to increase norepinephrine availability in key areas of the brain. Unlike the stimulants, the effects of atomoxetine are not immediate; patients need to be advised that it may take up to 6 weeks of regular use before effects are noted. Atomoxetine can be dosed once or twice daily (usually once daily). Although not as effective as either MPH or AMP,

| TABLE 15-9 | Stimulant Medications Used to Treat ADHD Symptoms |

Medication	Dosing Form/ Units	Duration and Pattern of Release	Starting Dose (Max Dose)	Approved Age	Comments
Amphetamines					
Adderall XR (mixed amphetamine salts)	Daily 5-, 10-, 15-, 20-, 25-, 30-mg capsule	8-12 hr; 50% immediately released; 50% released 4 hr later	10 mg; increase 10 mg weekly (40 mg)	6+	May sprinkle on applesauce and swallow without chewing
Adderall (mixed amphetamine salts (amphetamine-dextro-amphetamine)	bid or tid 5-, 7.5-, 10-, 12.5-, 15-, 20-, 30-mg scored tablet	4-6 hr; 100% released immediately	5 mg daily or bid; increase 2.5 mg/wk (40 mg)	3+	
Dexedrine (dextroamphetamine)	bid or tid 5-, 10-mg tablet	4-5 hr; 100% released immediately	5 mg daily or bid; increase 5 mg/wk (40 mg)		For 3-5 yr old, 2.5 mg daily with increase of 2.5 mg/wk
Dexedrine spansules (dextroamphetamine)	bid 5-, 10-, 15-mg spansule	6-8 hr; 40% released immediately; 60% released continuously	5 mg daily; increase 5 mg/wk (40 mg)	3-16	May sprinkle on applesauce and swallow without chewing
Vyvanse (lisdexamfetamine)	Daily 20-, 30-, 40-, 50-, 60-, 70-mg capsule	Up to 12 hr; released continuously	20 mg daily (70 mg)	6-12	May sprinkle contents in glass of water; needs to be drunk immediately
Methylphenidates					
Concerta (methylphenidate)	Daily 18-, 27-, 36-, 54-mg tablet	9-12 hr; 22% released immediately; 78% released continuously	18 mg daily; increase 18 mg/wk (72 mg)	6+	Noncrushable; must be swallowed whole
Daytrana patch (methylphenidate)	Daily 10-, 15-, 20-, 30-mg transdermal patch	9-12 hr; released continuously	Apply 2 hr before desired effect (30 mg)	6+	Remove after 9 hr (may remove earlier) Skin hypersensitivity especially if patch not removed after 9 hr
Focalin (dexmethylphenidate HCl)	bid or tid 2.5-, 5-, 10-mg tablet	4-6 hr; 100% released immediately	2.5 mg bid; increase 2.5-5 mg increments (20 mg)	6-17	
Focalin XR (dexmethylphenidate HCl)	Daily or bid 5-, 10-, 15-, 20-mg capsule	6-10 hr; 50% released immediately; 50% released in 4 hr	5 mg; increase 5 mg/wk (20 mg)	6+	May sprinkle on applesauce and swallow without chewing
Ritalin (methylphenidate HCl)	bid or tid 5-, 10-, 20-mg tablet	2-4 hr; 100% released immediately	5 mg (60 mg)	6+	Rapid onset, rapid termination of action
Ritalin LA (methylphenidate HCl)	Daily 10-, 20-, 30-, 40-mg capsule	8-10 hr; 50% released immediately; 50% modified release	10 mg daily; increase 10 mg/wk (60 mg)	6+	May sprinkle on applesauce and swallow without chewing

Data from Albury R, Rousseau L, So T, et al: Caring for individuals with ADHD throughout the lifespan: pharmacologic treatment strategies for children, adolescents, and adults with ADHD, *Counsel Points* 1(2):1-14, 2009. Available at www.delmedgroup.com (accessed Jan 5, 2011); Floet A, Scheiner C, Grossman L: Attention-deficit/hyperactivity disorder, *Pediatr Rev* 31(2): 56-68, 2010; Pliszka S, American Academy of Child and Adolescent Psychiatry (AACAP) Work Group on Quality Issues: Practice parameter for the assessment and treatment of children and adolescents with attention-deficit/hyperactivity disorder, *J Am Acad Child Adolesc Psychiatry* 46(7):894-921, 2007; Vierhile A, Robb A, Ryan-Krause P: Attention-deficit/hyperactivity disorder in children and adolescents: closing diagnostic, communication, and treatment gaps, *J Pediatr Health Care* 23(1S):s5-s21, 2009.

atomoxetine is about 70% effective (ICSI, 2010). Atomoxetine may be a preferable first choice in the following conditions:

- Family preference for nonstimulant medication
- Substance abuse concerns in the family
- ADHD with anxiety or if the patient has difficulty with sleep initiation, according to several studies (ICSI, 2010)
- Patients who have had side effects from the stimulants, including tics

Second-Line or Adjunct Medications. Second-line or adjunct medications include bupropion, the tricyclic

antidepressants, alpha-agonists (clonidine, guanfacine) and are only considered if a child fails to respond to medication trials at appropriate doses for an adequate length of time. Referral to psychiatry usually occurs at this point for careful review of the diagnosis, for accuracy, and to ensure identification of any undetected comorbidity.

Medication Monitoring. During the initiation (titration) phase of medication treatment, monitoring should be done as each dose change occurs. Once the individual is stable on an effective dose, medication monitoring should occur at a minimum of every 6 months (ICSI, 2010). Visits should include:

- Vital signs including height, weight, blood pressure, and pulse
- Review of ADHD behavior rating scales (see Table 15-8). The Vanderbilt scale has a follow-up version for parents and teachers that collects information about the core ADHD symptoms and level of impairment, and evaluates potential side effects.

Medication Side Effects. Often the minor side effects from the medications are transient and resolve spontaneously after several weeks. Sometimes a dosing adjustment, timing of medication dose, taking the medication with food, or an adjunctive medication to treat symptoms can help. MPH and AMP have about the same rate of side effects. Minor side effects of the stimulants include decreased appetite, weight loss, insomnia, gastric upset or abdominal pain, and headaches. Minor side effects of atomoxetine include headaches, gastric upset, decreased appetite, and sedation.

Many of the minor side effects can be minimized by having patients eat a healthy meal before taking their medication, taking the medication with food, or eating soon after the dose. Advising about sleep hygiene or considering a safe medication (e.g., melatonin) at bedtime, and/or use of a mild analgesic such as acetaminophen for headache complaints are also helpful strategies.

A preexisting *tic disorder* used to be considered a contraindication for stimulant use. About 60% to 70% of children with Tourette syndrome or chronic tic disorder have comorbid ADHD. It is felt that low to moderate doses of MPH may improve behavior without making the tics worse (in fact, there may be some improvement) (Krull, 2010b). About 15% to 20% of children who are treated with stimulant medication develop tics. Many of these are transient or disappear once the medication is stopped. The recommendation is that if the tics are not severe or disturbing to the child or adolescent and if the medication is having a net benefit, it is acceptable to continue treatment with the stimulant (Krull, 2010b). If the tics worsen, switching to atomoxetine is an option.

Some children taking stimulants experience "rebound" moodiness as the medication wears off. This often happens in the afternoon after school. It is felt to be due to medication effects waning, tiredness, and the post–school day stresses. This symptom can be treated by including a low dose in the afternoon of the same short-acting stimulant that the child is taking.

Findings show that the stimulant medications have a mild effect in decreased *height velocity.* Studies have found that the effect is greatest during the first 3 years of medication use and that the overall net decreased effect on adult height is not significant (Krull, 2010b). It is recommended that the weight and height of all children and adolescents taking ADHD medication be monitored at least every 6 months. If there is a decrease across two percentile lines, in either height or weight, consider a drug holiday or change in medication (Krull, 2010b).

Usual *cardiovascular* side effects of stimulant medications are a clinically insignificant increase in heart rate and blood pressure (Lerner and Wigal, 2008). This minor variation should not pose any risk to children and adolescents who do not have underlying heart disease (see the following section on cardiac risk).

Cardiovascular Side Effects. The U.S. Food and Drug Administration (FDA) continuously monitors the possible connection between the use of stimulants for ADHD and reports of sudden cardiac deaths in children. The FDA's conclusion is that stimulants and atomoxetine do not increase the risk of sudden cardiac death for children with *normal* cardiovascular history and physical examination (Krull, 2010b; Lerner and Wigal, 2008). Stimulant medications generally should not be used on anyone with preexisting heart disease or symptoms that suggest a possible cardiovascular problem. Recommendations for cardiovascular screening for all children and adolescents prior to initiating treatment with any of the first-line ADHD medications follow.

- A cardiac history should be taken for any previously detected cardiac problems, palpitations, seizures, syncope, exercise intolerance not explained by poor conditioning, chest pain, hypertension, heart murmur, and dysrhythmias (Perrin et al, 2008).
- A family cardiac history should be taken for early cardiac deaths or any rate, rhythm, or structural cardiac problems in the family (Perrin et al, 2008; Pliszka and AACAP, 2007).

If the cardiac history and examination are negative, the AAP recommends no further tests prior to starting ADHD medication. If there are any positives in the history or examination, a consultation with a pediatric cardiologist is necessary before initiating medication.

Suicidal Ideation or Attempts. In 2005, a boxed label warning was added to atomoxetine following reports of suicidal attempts by children or adolescents taking this medication. Although the risk is considered small, it is imperative that the practitioner carefully review this risk with patients and families and have a careful plan for monitoring. Parents and patients should be advised that if there is any change in mood—depression, mood lability, agitation, suicidal thoughts or gestures—this constitutes an emergency and they must get care immediately (Krull, 2010b). Preexisting and development of suicidal thoughts, hallucinations, psychosis, or mania are absolute contraindications to the use of medication. These children need referral to a qualified mental health clinician (Krull, 2010b).

Liver Toxicity. In 2004 the FDA issued a boxed warning about liver toxicity from use of atomoxetine. This was based on an idiosyncratic reaction that caused liver toxicity in six patients taking this medication. One patient died from liver failure, and all the other affected patients recovered after the atomoxetine was stopped. Currently, there is no recommendation to do liver studies prior to initiating treatment. Patients should be warned to stop their medication and call their provider immediately if symptoms of dark urine, flulike illness, fatigue, abdominal pain, or nausea occur.

Nonpharmacologic Management. Although studies have shown that psychosocial treatment modalities are not as powerful as medication to reduce core ADHD symptoms, these treatments are clearly effective and important (Evans et al, 2008; Krull, 2010b; Pliszka and AACAP, 2007). Pediatric providers are in a position to implement psychosocial strategies as well as to refer patients to mental health providers. Psychosocial treatment modalities for ADHD should be used especially if:

- ADHD symptoms are mild.
- There is a poor response to medication alone.

- There is a presence of psychosocial stressors.
- Younger children are involved (see medication issues in preschool-age children).
- There is family preference.
- There is concurrent medication, especially with significant comorbidities (Evans et al, 2008; Pliszka and AACAP, 2007).

Regular follow-up of the child and family with ADHD is essential for medication monitoring, but it is also important to assess the child and family functioning and need for family support or other resources. Education about how normal growth and development interacts with the symptoms of ADHD should be updated as children move through developmental stages.

Family and Patient Psychoeducation. Families need to be well educated about the disorder because a large part of the treatment for ADHD involves parent-management techniques. The chronic nature of ADHD has a tremendous effect on family functioning. Conversely, family factors play a part in the outcomes for children with ADHD. Parents often have to educate others about the special needs of their child. Because children with ADHD manifest a great variety of behaviors, parents become the experts who ultimately manage the problems and affect the outcome for their child.

There are many excellent resources for reliable patient education about ADHD. It is important to consider education of the child or adolescent, the parents, teachers and other caregivers. It is suggested that providers have several resources with which they are familiar and comfortable recommending to families.

Family Support. It is necessary initially to help parents understand the complexity of the diagnosis, to deal with feelings of shock or confusion, and to cope with guilt. The diagnosis of a child is often the first clue to the eventual diagnosis of an older sibling or a parent who is experiencing similar difficulties. ADHD symptoms can impact the already complex relationships within a family, so ongoing support is equally important.

- *Behavior training* for parents and children can be helpful. There are a variety of parenting programs that help parents learn to give differential attention to positive behavior, set up rewards and reinforcement for positive behavior, give clear and effective commands and structure, and establish safe and consistent discipline strategies.
- *Family meetings* provide opportunity to discuss structure, rewards and consequences as well as plan and problem solve.
- *Support groups* can offer understanding and specific expertise in managing daily problems that come from living with a diagnosis of ADHD.
- *Family therapy or counseling* is frequently used short term with goals specific to the family's situation. It is especially helpful if there is aggressive behavior or problems related to anxiety, self-esteem, and depression or if other family members (especially siblings) are in need of psychological assessment or support.

Home Management
- *Environmental management.* A calm, predictable home with clear, consistent morning and evening routines is extremely helpful for the child with ADHD. An organized place for everyday things to go is another way to provide structure.
- *Homework support* is essential (Box 15-3). Mental fatigue should be monitored.

BOX 15-3 | Tips for Homework Success

1. Provide a quiet location where work will be done with minimal distractions.
2. Set up a work station equipped with necessary materials.
3. Establish a homework time as early as possible to prevent the child from being too tired.
4. Establish a homework plan: review assignments and make a schedule for completion.
5. Structure time for breaks as often as every 15 minutes if needed.
6. Permit time for editing so as not to lose points due to editing errors.
7. Use a timer to help with time management.
8. Provide incentives to help motivation.

Data from Lambros KM, Leslie LK: Management of the child with a learning disorder, *Pediatr Ann* 34(4):259-261, 2005.

- *Exercise.* Daily time to be active and expend energy is extremely important in helping children with ADHD stay regulated. Tai chi and karate, which demand discipline and self-control, can be very helpful.
- *Downtime or senseless fun.* Children with ADHD need more time than most children for normal activities of childhood, including time to do nothing and daydream.
- *Nutrition.* Saltine crackers offered with the morning dose of stimulant medication can decrease complaints of stomachaches. Providing instant breakfast drinks and other high-calorie foods to supplement calories when the child has low calorie intake because of difficulty sitting through meals or side effects of medications may be helpful.
- *Sleep.* Many children and adults with ADHD do not require as much sleep as other people or have trouble initiating sleep or staying asleep. It is important to periodically ask if the child is sleeping well and staying in bed the entire night. Ritualized bedtime routines are important to ADHD families; detailed instruction in massage, deep breathing, and relaxation techniques is sometimes helpful.
- *Patience, unconditional love, and support* are especially important for children with ADHD because they face so many challenges in getting through their day. Plan a daily "time in" for 15 to 20 minutes with undivided parent attention focused on a child-selected activity.

School Management
- Provide or work with the school to develop suggestions for *classroom adaptations* that are helpful to the student (Box 15-4). Multiple adaptive technologies may be considered.
- Build *home and school communication* through such means as daily progress notes or behavioral report cards.
- When ADHD affects a student's academic performance, schools have a role in establishing *educational plans* for the management of ADHD. An IEP or 504 plan offers opportunities for special accommodations at school (see earlier section in this chapter). These plans can include academic learning and behavior modification objectives.

Activities, Friends and Self-Esteem
- Children with ADHD have a constant struggle with self-esteem as they strive to meet expectations placed on them. It is crucial to identify their areas of strength and pleasure and provide opportunities to develop those areas rather than constantly focusing on remediating areas of weakness (see Chapter 16 for more information regarding self-esteem).

BOX 15-4   Suggestions for Classroom Adaptations for Children with Attention-Deficit/Hyperactivity Disorder

Memory and Attention

- Seat the child close to the teacher away from heavy traffic areas (e.g., doorways).
- Keep oral instructions brief with repetitions.
- Provide written directions.
- "Walk" the child through assignments to be sure they are understood.
- Break tasks and homework into small tasks.
- Use visual aids, hands-on, and experiential teaching methods rather than strict lecture style.
- Teach active reading with underlining and active listening with note taking.
- Provide remedial help in small sessions.
- Teach subvocalization to aid memorizing.
- Establish a hand gesture that reminds the child to focus and return to task.
- Allow nondistracting motor activity during tasks requiring concentration (e.g., squeezing a ball or fingering Velcro to replace pencil tapping).

Impulse Control

- Allow for freedom of movement as much as possible (e.g., classroom helper).
- Never punish the child by taking away physical education, recess, or other physical outlets.
- Teach the child to monitor quality of work before turning it in.

Classroom Atmosphere

- Provide a structured classroom with clear expectations.
- Use moderate, consistent discipline.
- Rely on positive reinforcement for good behavior.
- Provide a quiet place to work in the classroom (headsets with select music may block out distractions).

Organizational Skills

- Establish a daily checklist of tasks.
- List homework assignments in a special notebook with the due date and needed resources.
- Follow up on homework not turned in.
- Allow extra time for gathering necessary items, packing backpack, etc.
- Provide an extra set of textbooks for use at home.
- Teach strategies for time management and basic study skills.

Productivity Problems

- Divide worksheets into sections.
- Reduce the amount of homework and written classwork.
- Cut down on the number of math problems to be completed.

Written Expression

- Give extra time to complete written tests and assignments.
- Provide help with handwriting.
- Allow child to dictate reports and take tests orally.
- Reduce the quantity of written work required.
- Do not reduce grades for untidy work, spelling errors, or poor handwriting.

Self-Esteem

- Reward progress.
- Encourage performance in areas of child's strength.
- Avoid humiliation.
- Give hand signals only the child can see as private reminders of appropriate behavior.

Social Relationships

- Provide feedback about behavior involving other children.
- Make sure other children do not believe that the child is doing less or is allowed unacceptable behavior; change the rules for all children, if necessary.

Adapted from Baren M: Managing ADHD, *Contemp Pediatr* 11:33, 1994; Connors S: *Catalog of accommodations for students with Tourette's syndrome, attention deficit hyperactivity disorder, and obsessive compulsive disorder*, Bayside, NY, 2005, Tourette's Syndrome Association.

- *Activities* of the child's choosing or developmentally appropriate work can help build peer relationships and self-esteem.
- *Friendships* may come more easily if structure is provided (going to a movie or a sporting event) and time frame consistent with what the child can handle.
- *"Coaching"* is a slightly different approach to assisting a child or adolescent develop skills that are difficult for him or her. Problem solving, time management, and organization are skills that are often identified. Learning strategies are another area in which coaching is successful. These skills include, for example, how to be an active learner, learning how to learn, and learning how to organize learning.
- *Social skills training.* Although the research on the efficacy of teaching social skills to children with ADHD has been disappointing, there is some promise to programs that generalize what children learn in the clinical setting to the classroom and other peer settings (Evans et al, 2008). The difficulty seems to be that there is not a lack of knowledge of what behavior is appropriate, but rather a lack of ability to act on what is known.

Advocacy and Case Management. Families often need assistance in accessing educational services and primary care providers are often in a position to exercise some influence in the local schools when services are not forthcoming. Additionally, primary care providers may be able to offer case management services to ADHD families—coordination of medical supervision, school programs, and family therapy or parent training programs—in order to help families to manage ADHD successfully.

Patient Referral

It is important for primary care practitioners to know when to refer a child or adolescent to a mental health specialist or psychiatrist. Reconsider accuracy of diagnosis and refer if a child or adolescent:

- Is a nonresponder to trials at therapeutic dose levels with at least two of the first-line medications
- Has side effects or preexisting conditions that would be contraindications to ADHD treatment with any of the first-line medications
- Has high levels of comorbidities that may be more challenging to treat and may require mental health and/or educational specialists

Complications

Children with ADHD can develop depression, problems with self-esteem, and failure to meet school educational expectations. Medication interactions and side effects are also potential complications, especially in children with concurrent diagnoses of emotional disorders and chronic illness. With different physicians prescribing medications, side effects can be missed because they mimic symptoms already present in a confusing and complicated disorder. A cumulative effect can be seen when relationships at home, school, and in the community deteriorate, putting the child or adolescent with ADHD at risk for engaging in delinquent or socially unacceptable behaviors.

Prognosis With Long-Term Treatment

Based on the findings of the MTA study and other research, over the long term (8 years for the MTA study group), some decreased benefit is gained from medication treatment and from decline in medication adherence. Those more likely to experience greater decrease in treatment benefit are individuals with higher baseline comorbidities, especially aggressive behaviors, conduct disorder, and oppositional defiant disorder (Gilchrist and Arnold, 2008; Krull, 2010b). Some promising findings are summarized in the review by Krull (2010a):

- Adolescents who are adequately treated for their ADHD are less likely to abuse drugs or alcohol than nontreated peers with ADHD.
- Adolescents being adequately treated have a lower dropout rate and are more likely to report success in setting and completing goals.

More research is needed in looking at the long-term effects of ADHD treatment on affected children's academic improvement and overall social and peer successes.

LEARNING DISORDERS AND NEURODEVELOPMENTAL DYSFUNCTIONS

Description

In the world of learning disorders, the terminology can be confusing and consensus on definition lacking. Learning disabilities are neurologically based or "hard-wired" and should be suspected when there is discrepancy between aptitude (intelligence) and achievement (learning output) on standardized tests, or when measured achievement falls below a set standard. Neurodevelopmental dysfunction, evaluating how the brain works, is another way to look at areas of difficulty in a child's functioning. This process looks at a child who is struggling in school as an individual with a unique profile of neurodevelopmental strengths and weaknesses across the eight constructs (see Table 15-1). When neurodevelopmental dysfunctions are disruptive of learning, these problems are referred to as learning disabilities. Neurodevelopmental status can be described according to a hierarchy (Box 15-5).

Most children with academic struggles have more than one dysfunction that results in delayed or difficult acquisition and reduced productivity. The disorders may occur with other handicapping conditions, such as sensory impairment, mental retardation, or emotional disturbance; cultural differences; or educational deficits, but are not caused by those conditions or influences.

The theory of multiple intelligences (see Table 15-2) begs us to remember that although schools focus primarily on linguistic and logical-mathematical intelligence, and American culture esteems highly articulate or logical people, there are other types of intelligence. Unfortunately many children with other intelligences don't receive much reinforcement in school and, in fact, may end up being labeled "learning disabled" or underachievers, when in actuality their unique ways of thinking and learning aren't addressed by the typical classroom.

Learning disabilities (LDs) are manifested by consistent, significant difficulties in acquiring and using reading, writing, listening, speaking, reasoning, math, and social skills. They can be broadly grouped as follows:

Language-Based Learning Disorders

- Basic reading disabilities (Glascoe and Hamilton, 2010)
  - Difficulty with sound-symbol association (dyslexia)—difficulty sounding out words; phonologic awareness
  - Difficulty with acquiring sight word vocabulary—orthographic disability, difficulty memorizing written words, lack of fluency
  - Difficulty with reading comprehension—hyperlexic disability, difficulty with content-focused subjects, applied math (work problems)
- Written expression disability
  - Difficulty with forming letters and words
  - Difficulty with organizing thoughts on paper

Nonverbal Neurodevelopmental Dysfunctions

- Mathematics disability
  - Semantic—retrieval of math facts
  - Procedural—working memory
  - Visual-spatial—mastering concepts
- Motor learning disabilities—delays or difficulty performing expected fine and gross motor activities (6%) (Clayton and Dodd, 2005)

Executive Functions. This group of related mental processes and behaviors enables self-regulation and metacognition. Executive function disorder can occur independently but often occurs with ADHD, LD, and ASD as well as with medical conditions such as prematurity, prenatal drug and alcohol exposure, and traumatic brain injury (Miller, 2005).

- Self-regulation components include:
  - Inhibition—ability to stop or delay a first response, interrupt an inappropriate behavior, resist interference by distracting thoughts or stimuli
  - Flexibility—ability to shift or transition between activities or thoughts
  - Emotional control—ability to modify emotional expression to most adaptive

---

BOX 15-5 Hierarchy of Neurodevelopmental Status

- Variation—an unusual pattern of neurodevelopmental function (e.g., a higher divergent mind)
- Dysfunction—a distinct weakness within a neurodevelopmental function (e.g., a weak retrieval area)
- Disability—a performance deficiency caused (at least in part) by a neurodevelopmental dysfunction (e.g., trouble throwing a ball)
- Handicap—a disability occurring in a much-needed or critical performance area (e.g., a significant reading problem)

Data from Levine MD: Differences in learning and neurodevelopmental function in school-age children. In Carey WB, Crocker AC, Coleman WL, et al, editors: *Developmental-behavioral pediatrics*, ed 4, Philadelphia, 2009, Saunders, pp 535-546.

- Metacognition is used to self-manage and self-monitor in order to reflect, plan, and execute as well as organize, be insightful, make logical decisions, and complete complex activities. Components include:
  - ○ Working memory—verbal (self-talk, blending and organization) and nonverbal (mental representation and manipulation of visual-spatial information) deficits described as forgetful or careless
  - ○ Problem-solving
  - ○ Monitoring—task or self

Epidemiology

Learning disorders may result from a variety of genetic, constitutional, or neurodevelopmental factors. Any factor that disrupts central nervous system function may result in a learning disorder. The incidence is thought to be 10% to 15% of the population. About 15% to 20% of people in the U.S. (1 in 7) have a language-based disability (NICHHD, 2010); 80% of children identified with LDs have reading disabilities (Glascoe and Hamilton, 2010; LD Online, 2010; Levine, 2009).

Clinical Findings

Language processing, visual and auditory processing, memory, motor coordination, and spatial and temporal orientation difficulties are hallmarks of the condition, although a child will probably not have difficulties in all areas.

- Reading—difficulty decoding unfamiliar words, poor comprehension and retention, slow reading rate
- Mathematics—difficulty remembering number facts, solving practical problems
- Writing—poor and labored handwriting, faulty spelling, grammar and syntax errors
- Struggles to keep up with class peers and fails to acquire the foundational skills in core academic subjects necessary for continued learning

Assessment

Assessment includes identification of risk factors, observation for characteristics of learning disorders, and consideration of other causes for the learning problems.

History

- Family history
  - ○ Dyslexia or other learning disability (frequently familial) and level of academic achievement
  - ○ Attention deficits
  - ○ Grade retention or school dropout
- Medical history
  - ○ Prematurity, low birthweight
  - ○ Head injury or seizure disorder
  - ○ Chronic health condition
  - ○ Early developmental concerns or delays
- Patient assessment
  - ○ Child's connectedness to school (feels accepted, valued, respected, included)
  - ○ Child's description of the problems
  - ○ Child's perception of the cause of the problems
  - ○ Child's experiences at school with teachers, peers, homework

---

BOX 15-6 Level I School Performance Prescreening Questionnaire

1. Do you have any concerns about your child's learning or school performance?
2. Do you have any concerns about your child's attention, concentration, impulsivity, and/or overactivity?
3. Do you have any concerns about how your child is doing in certain subjects at school? If yes, is it reading? Writing? Math? Other?
4. Do you have any concern about how much your child is enjoying school compared with friends or classmates?
5. Does your child have any problems completing homework?

Data from Kelly D, Aylward G: Identifying school performance problems in the pediatric office, *Pediatr Ann* 34(4):259-261, 2005.

- Parent interview
  - ○ Functioning at home versus school
  - ○ Coping with school; psychological, behavioral, and stress responses to the problems
  - ○ Ability to attend to and complete tasks
  - ○ Strengths and weaknesses of the child
- Teacher feedback/school review
  - ○ Teacher's report of academic performance, absences, engagement, behavioral information
  - ○ Results of any educational testing
- Red flags (Lambros and Leslie, 2005)
  - ○ Previous speech delay (50% meet criteria for reading disability) (Glascoe and Hamilton, 2010)
  - ○ Difficulty developing phonemic awareness
  - ○ Discussion about possible retention
  - ○ Child/adolescent "hates school" and does not like subjects involving significant reading
  - ○ Parent senses that something is just not right

Physical Examination

- Behavioral observations
- Hearing and vision evaluation; sensory processing screening
- Physical examination, especially for neurologic problems, dysmorphic features, minor congenital anomalies

Screening. Developmental surveillance is an ongoing part of routine health care in the preschool years. It is equally important once a child reaches school age, to continue surveillance of school performance to identify difficulties that may not arise until the child faces the challenges of school. The goal of screening is to identify children who are having problems and need further evaluation.

- School performance prescreening questionnaire (Box 15-6)—a five-item instrument that can be administered at every well-check. If the prescreening questionnaire shows no evidence of school problems, screening should occur at the next routine visit. If school problems are suspected, a school performance screener should be administered.
- School performance screener (Box 15-7)—a more comprehensive assessment tool for follow-up of positive prescreening questionnaires; used in conjunction with samples of school work, report cards, and previously administered tests

A helpful tool is the National Center for Learning Disabilities' *Learning Disabilities Checklist* (available online), which is organized by skill set and age group.

BOX 15-7 Level II School Performance Screener

1. In what area(s) does your child have problems in school performance? Learning/achievement? Attention/concentration/memory? Behavior?
2. Subjects/activities of difficulty: Reading? Math? Spelling? Writing? Speaking? Listening? Remembering? Science? Social studies? Language/grammar? Following directions? Inconsistency? Transferring knowledge from one situation to another? Organizing?
3. Current grade? What grade did problems become evident? Did child repeat a grade? Ever in danger of repeating a grade?
4. Grades on report card? Performance on standardized testing? Is excessive amount of help needed to do homework? Is excessive amount of homework due to child not completing in school? Would grades be lower without a great amount of extra work being done at home with parents? Is homework a battle each night?
5. Stressors? None? Current? At time of onset of school problems? With family? Peers? At school?
6. Medical concerns? Frequent ear infections? Hearing problem? Vision problem? Pre-/perinatal problems? Allergies? Loss of consciousness? Sleep problem? Describe.
7. Strengths? Reading? Math? Spelling? Writing? Speaking? Listening? Remembering? Science? Social studies? Language/grammar? Other? Learns better by seeing versus hearing? Learns better by hearing versus seeing?
8. How does the child get along with peers? Involved in extracurricular activities? Type? If so, how does he or she do?
9. Emotional issues: Lack of motivation? School avoidance? Homework avoidance? Seems "lazy"? Irritable? Anxious? Volatile? Down on self? Aggressive? Gives up easily? Refuses to work in class? Doesn't turn work in? Oppositional? Angry?
10. Tested by school system? If yes, eligible for services? Receives services (types)? Found ineligible? Has received services, but they have been discontinued?

Data from Kelly D, Aylward G: Identifying school performance problems in the pediatric office, *Pediatr Ann* 34(4):259-261, 2005.

Differential Diagnosis

Behavioral problems (especially ADHD and oppositional behavior) and problems with social interactions may be associated but are separate conditions. Visual or hearing problems, school absence, environmental deprivation in preschool, ADHD, fetal alcohol syndrome, lead or other toxic exposure, mental retardation, fragile X syndrome, and emotional disturbance are included in the differential diagnosis.

Management
Primary Care Provider's Role
- Monitor child's development from birth through adulthood.
- If concerns arise, support the family through the assessment process, which is often lengthy and emotional (see Educational Support).
- Once diagnosed, help parents and children understand the implications of a particular LD:
  ○ Identify the child's strengths, affinities, and interests in order to develop passions and areas of expertise.
  ○ Help parents understand how a LD affects interactions with peers and everyday life.
  ○ Link children and families to reliable resources.

BOX 15-8 A Parent's Response to a Learning Disability

How to respond:
1. Know your child's strengths.
2. Collect information about your child's performance.
3. Have your child evaluated.
4. Work as a team to help your child.
5. Talk to your child about learning disabilities.
6. Find accommodations that can help.
7. Monitor your child's progress.
8. Know your legal rights.
9. Organize information about your child's learning disability—a folder with letters and material, copies of school files, samples of work that demonstrate difficulty as well as strengths, keep a contact log; keep a log of own observations.

Data from LD Online: *LD basics: how to respond*, 2010. Available at www.ldonline.org/ldbasics/respond (accessed Nov 23, 2010).

  ○ Not all children with learning disorders qualify for special resource services.
  ○ Serve as case manager; help parents explore other ideas and act as a conduit to help parents find others who have solved similar problems.
Social and Adaptive
- Assistive technologies: Read-aloud devices from text and computer programs to help remediate deficiencies may be helpful. Calculators and word processors may help circumvent handwriting problems.
- Accommodations as discussed in the introductory section of this chapter.
Educational support
- Psychoeducational evaluation should include identification of strengths and weaknesses, determination of cognitive ability, assessment of perceptual strengths and weaknesses, examination of communicative ability, and assessment of social and emotional adaptation (Dworkin, 2009).
- Development of an IEP or a 504 plan (see Educational Strategies)
Family support
- Help parent devise an organized approach to responding to struggles the child is having (Box 15-8).
- Provide homework help (see Box 15-3).
- Encourage parental involvement—Epstein model (Lambros and Leslie, 2005).

Complications

School avoidance, acting-out, disengagement, or alienation are areas of concern. Lowered self-esteem and coexisting mental health problems (up to 50%) such as anxiety and depression can be experienced (Dworkin, 2009).

Prevention

Student engagement in school is defined as participation, performance, and identification with the school. Research supports the fact that attendance, completion of school work, and participation in extracurricular activities leads to positive school performance.

Starting early in life, children need to be exposed to language—reading and talking. The Reach Out and Read program, in which health care providers give and encourage reading, has proven successful.

SENSORY PROCESSING DISORDER

Description

Sensory processing, also called sensory integration, refers to the way central and peripheral nervous systems manage incoming sensory information in order to create appropriate motor and behavioral responses for effective learning, motor skill development, social interaction, and regulation of energy levels and emotions. Sensory processing disorder (SPD) results when there is difficulty with the detection, modulation, discrimination, and/or sensation of sensory input that is chronic and disrupts everyday life. Sensory systems include touch, vision, hearing, taste, smell, vestibular (movement), and proprioception (muscle and joint position). Children with SPD do not have cognitive delays and may even be intellectually gifted; their brains are just wired in a different manner.

Sensory processing problems fall into two main diagnostic clusters: (1) sensory-based motor disorders like vestibular-based postural disorder and dyspraxia, and (2) sensory modulation disorders like sensory defensiveness, sensory under-responsivity, and sensory seeking. Vestibular-based postural disorder involves impaired balance secondary to an altered sense of the physical body. Children with dyspraxia have difficulties discriminating tactile stimuli. Sensory modulation disorders affect one's ability to regulate sensory input and may result in hypo- or hyperresponsiveness to external stimuli or in sensory seeking. Children who are sensory defensive tend to be loud and respond to stimuli in a more intense way or for a longer time. Children who are under-responsive tend to be socially withdrawn with low activity levels. Children who are sensory seeking crave sensory experiences, often in socially unacceptable ways. The net result of sensory modulation disorders is that stimuli that may be considered to be pleasurable or positive in most individuals will be painful, irritating, and unpleasant.

Etiology

Like many sensory-processing and neurodevelopmental disorders, specific causes have not been identified. SPD research suggests that it is often inherited (genetic). Prenatal and birth complications (especially in infants less than 32 weeks of gestation and with birthweight less than 1500 g, or those who have been exposed to alcohol and drugs) have also been implicated. Environmental factors may be involved, especially institutionalization (overseas adoptees), severe physical or sexual abuse, poverty, related risks, lead poisoning, and newborn hospitalization for medical conditions (Miller, 2006).

Clinical Findings

Children with SPD face many challenges in everyday life. Motor clumsiness, behavioral problems, and difficulties with abilities needed for school success are not uncommon. Children who are over-responders have difficulties with clothing, physical contact, light, sound, and food. Children who are under-responders have little or no reaction to stimulation, pain, and extreme hot or cold and can risk injuring themselves. Children who are sensory seekers are on perpetual overdrive and often in trouble with friends and family. When there is muscle and joint impairment (postural disorder), posture and motor skills are affected (floppy babies, klutz, spaz). These children have difficulty with changes in ground surfaces, may appear to be uncoordinated, or may have delayed oculomotor control. Children with dyspraxia do not do well when asked to recognize and distinguish shapes and textures, may have poor handwriting, or present with altered ability to do things like tying shoes, using buttons, or dressing themselves.

Sensory problems in infants become behavioral problems in preschoolers often caused by others' negative reactions to their behaviors. Adolescents and adults may have difficulty with close relationships, with recreation, and with performing routines and activities involved in school or work (Case-Smith and Ratliff-Schaub, 2009).

Assessment

History

- Look for relationships between behaviors and specific sensory experiences.
- Infants may be colicky or fussy babies, with difficulties eating and sleeping; fearful of movement; resist being held or comforted.
- Preschoolers may not engage in purposeful interactive play; feeding, dressing, skill development may be delayed; defiant, irritable, stubborn; resist transitions and certain activities; sleep and eating problems continue.
- School age—trouble with handwriting, figuring out steps in a game, organizing school work, and spontaneous play interaction; trouble with handling change and transition; easily frustrated.
- Adolescence—trouble with social interaction, learning in classroom and physical skill development.

Physical Examination. Evaluation is usually conducted by an occupational therapist with sensory integration and praxis (motor planning) tests.

Screening. Screening should take place for any differences in development that are significant enough to warrant suspicion or are concerning enough to the parents. Red flags for SPD are found in Box 15-9, and a complete list for each subtype is listed in Miller (2006). Screening should result in one of three findings: (1) no further evaluation needed; (2) watch and re-screen; or (3) complete evaluation recommended. An SPD Checklist and Sensory Profile, Short Sensory Profile, and/or Sensory Processing Measure can be found at www.spdfoundation.net.

Differential Diagnosis and Comorbidities

There is a much higher prevalence of SPD in children who are gifted, have ADHD, ASD and Fragile X syndrome (Sensory Processing Disorder [SPD] Foundation, 2010). ADHD and ASD are considered unique disorders with distinct symptoms. However, somewhere between 40% and 60% of children with ADHD also have SPD and vice versa. Up to 75% of children with ASD have SPD, but the reverse is not true. Differential diagnoses include other developmental delays, cognitive delays including Down syndrome, anxiety, aggression, and other mental illness.

Red Flags for Sensory Processing Disorder

If more than a few of the symptoms listed here fit your child, refer to the complete Sensory Processing Disorder (SPD) Checklist. A Spanish-language copy of the Red Flags is available on the SPD's website.

Infants and Toddlers
____ Problems eating or sleeping
____ Refuses to go to anyone but me
____ Irritable when being dressed; uncomfortable in clothes
____ Rarely plays with toys
____ Resists cuddling, arches away when held
____ Cannot calm self
____ Floppy or stiff body, motor delays

Preschoolers
____ Overly sensitive to touch, noises, smells, other people
____ Difficulty making friends
____ Difficulty dressing, eating, sleeping, and/or toilet training
____ Clumsy; poor motor skills; weakness
____ In constant motion; in everyone else's face and space
____ Frequent or long temper tantrums

Grade Schoolers
____ Overly sensitive to touch, noise, smells, other people
____ Easily distracted, fidgety, craves movement; aggressive
____ Easily overwhelmed
____ Difficulty with handwriting or motor activities
____ Difficulty making friends
____ Unaware of pain and/or other people

Adolescents and Adults
____ Overly sensitive to touch, noise, smells, and other people
____ Poor self-esteem; afraid of failing at new tasks
____ Lethargic and slow
____ Always on the go; impulsive; distractible
____ Leaves tasks uncompleted
____ Clumsy, slow, poor motor skills or handwriting
____ Difficulty staying focused at work and in meetings

From Sensory Processing Foundation. Available at www.spdfoundation.net/redflags. html.

Management

Early diagnosis and treatment increase the chance of successful intervention especially as related to acquiring skills for school. It also minimizes the secondary issues that develop when children receive inappropriate labels and begin to feel like they are "failing." Occupational therapists trained in using a sensory integration approach do the initial evaluation and treatment with the goal of developing automatic and appropriate responses to sensation so that the child can function competently in play, at school and in daily living and self-care routines. Therapy includes the use of sensory stimuli in one domain to affect performance in another, usually taking place in a sensory-rich gym or environment providing what is called sensory nourishment or a "sensory diet." Over time new neurologic connections are established allowing regulation of arousal and attention, formation of attachment and social relationships, and organization of actions in the physical world.

It is helpful for families with children with SPD to know that these children often hold it together in school, but fall apart when they come home; are often controlling in an attempt to manage what is happening inside their brains; can sometimes accomplish something if they put 100% effort into it, but can't always perform at 100%; often have trouble with transitions, family gatherings, parties, vacation (things considered fun); do best with an environment that is predictable and routine and the same from day to day; and may be sensitive to touch and pull away from hugs and cuddling.

Complications

Inability to make friends, poor self-concept, academic failure, being labeled clumsy, uncooperative, belligerent, disruptive, and out of control leads to anxiety, depression, aggression, or other behavior problems. Parents may be blamed or criticized for the child's behavior.

AUTISTIC SPECTRUM DISORDERS: AUTISM, ASPERGER SYNDROME, PERVASIVE DEVELOPMENTAL DISORDER

Description

Autism is a complex neurodevelopmental disorder. The AAP (2010) describes "autism spectrum disorders (ASDs) as a group of related developmental disorders caused by a problem in the brain that affects a child's behavior, social and communication skills." ASDs include autistic disorder, pervasive developmental disorder-not otherwise specified (PDD-NOS), and Asperger syndrome. ASDs cause lifelong disability that usually becomes apparent in the first 3 years of life. Development is uneven, with occasional talent in a limited area such as music or mathematics, coupled with severe deficits in other areas. Many autistic children have other impairments, such as mental retardation (60% to 75%) or seizures. The disorder varies considerably in severity.

Autistic disorder describes a child who meets full diagnostic criteria in terms of language, social interaction, and repetitive, restricted behavior. The diagnostic criteria for autism require the presence of six symptoms from three categories (Box 15-10 lists the criteria). In general, they encompass problems with social interactions, communication, and language skills with abnormal ways of relating to people, objects, and events; abnormal responses to sensory stimuli, usually sound; and restricted, repetitive, or stereotyped behaviors and echolalic speech. Sleep disturbances are also common among children with autism.

Milder forms of ASD are Asperger and PDD-NOS. Butter and Mulick (2009) describe these disorders as follows: Asperger disorder is diagnosed when typical language development is present in the context of impaired social interactions and repetitive, restricted behaviors. There are qualitative impairments in the development of social interactions, language is not as severely impaired as it is with autism, and there are repetitive movements and restricted, obsessional interests. The person with Asperger syndrome may appear "eccentric" to others. The diagnosis of PDD-NOS is reserved for cases in which the central features of language delay, impaired reciprocal social interaction, or restricted, repetitive behaviors are present but not in the degree that would warrant a more specific diagnosis. Whether PDD-NOS is a distinct diagnosis or a milder form of autism with higher functioning is unknown at this time. Box 15-11 lists "red flags" for autism screening.

BOX 15-10 Diagnostic Criteria for Autistic Disorders

A. A total of more than six items from the following criteria with at least two from criterion 1 and one each from criteria 2 and 3:
  1. Qualitative impairment in social interaction as manifested by at least two of the following:
     a. Marked impairment in the use of multiple nonverbal behaviors, such as eye-to-eye gaze, facial expression, body posture, and gestures to regulate social interaction
     b. Failure to develop peer relationships appropriate to developmental level
     c. Lack of spontaneous seeking to share enjoyment, interests, or achievements with other people (lack of showing, bringing, or pointing out objects of interest)
  2. Qualitative impairments in communication as manifested by at least one of the following:
     a. Delay in or total lack of development of spoken language (not accompanied by an attempt to compensate through alternative modes of communication, such as gesture or mime)
     b. In individuals with adequate speech, marked impairment in the ability to initiate or sustain a conversation
     c. Stereotyped and repetitive use of language or idiosyncratic language
     d. Lack of varied, spontaneous make-believe play or social imitative play appropriate to developmental level
  3. Restricted, repetitive, and stereotyped patterns of behavior, interests, and activities as manifested by at least one of the following:
     a. Encompassing preoccupation with one or more stereotyped and restricted patterns of interest that is abnormal either in intensity or focus
     b. Apparently inflexible adherence to specific, nonfunctional routines or rituals
     c. Stereotyped and repetitive motor mannerisms (e.g., hand or finger flapping or twisting, or complex whole-body movements)
     d. Persistent preoccupation with parts of objects
B. Delay or abnormal functioning in at last one of the following areas with onset before 3 years old:
  1. Social interaction
  2. Language as used in social communication
  3. Symbolic or imaginative play
C. Disturbance not better accounted for by Rett disorder or childhood disintegrative disorder

From American Psychiatric Association: *Diagnostic and statistical manual of mental disorders,* text revision, *(DSM-IV/TR),* Washington, DC, 2000, American Psychiatric Association.

BOX 15-11 Red Flags for Autism

- Does not respond to his or her name by 12 months of age
- Does not point at objects to show interest (pointing at an airplane flying over) by 14 months
- Does not play "pretend" games (pretending to "feed" a doll) by 18 months
- Avoids eye contact and wants to be alone
- Has trouble understanding other people's feelings or talking about their own feelings
- Has delayed speech and language skills (no babbling or gesturing by 12 months old; no single words by 16 months; no two-word [not echolalic] phrases by 24 months old)
- Repeats words or phrases over and over (echolalia)
- Gives unrelated answers to questions
- Gets upset by minor changes
- Has obsessive interests
- Flaps their hands, rocks their body, or spins in circles
- Has unusual reactions to the way things sound, smell, taste, look, or feel
- Fails to meet childhood developmental milestones
- Has a sibling with autism
- Has loss of any language or social abilities at any age

Data from Centers for Disease Control and Prevention (CDC): *Autism spectrum disorder: signs and symptoms.* Available at www.cdc.gov/ncbddd/autism/signs.html (accessed Nov 3, 2010c); American Academy of Neurology and the Child Neurology Society: *Guideline summary for clinicians: screening and diagnosis of autism,* 2010. Available at http://aan.com/professionals/practice/guidelines/guideline_summaries/Autism_Guideline_for_Clinicians.pdf (accessed Jan 5, 2011).

Etiology

There is good evidence of genetic links for some types of autism (10%). The CDC (2010e) reports that through family studies among identical twins, if one child has autism, the other is affected 60% to 96% of the time. The risk decreases to about zero to 24% for nonidentical twins. In addition, parents who have a child with an ASD have a 2% to 8% chance of having a second child who is affected. Other possible causes include prenatal infections, such as congenital rubella or cytomegalovirus, neonatal infections, and the environment. The cause is unknown for most cases.

There has been a great deal of negative and high-profile media attention (not supported by evidence) concerning a risk of autism associated with vaccination despite overwhelming evidence that no such association exists. See Chapter 23 for a full discussion of vaccine controversies.

The incidence rate for autism is about 1:100 children. The ratio of male-to-female children is 4.5:1 (CDC, 2010e).

Clinical Findings by Age

Infants. An autistic infant may be a passive, nonengaging, quiet, floppy infant or a difficult, colicky, stiff baby with poor eye contact. Attachment problems appear. There is failure to respond to name or gestures. Autism is usually not identified in infancy although some developmental problems, especially in the social arena, are emerging.

Toddlers. During the toddler stage, parents are convinced that something is wrong with their child. Language delays, lack of social relatedness, and severe behavior problems are common. Expressive language is delayed. Socially the child exhibits detachment, decreased eye contact, a lack of fear, and poor creative play skills. Tantrums that persist; repetitive movements; a preference to line, stack, or spin toys; and insistence on routines are commonly observed behaviors. Use of echolalia is persistent. Children have relative strengths in visual-motor problem-solving and delays in language. The Modified Checklist for Autism in Toddlers (M-CHAT) (available at www.firstsigns.org/downloads/m-chat.pdf) is one of several scales developed to identify autism in 24-month-old children.

Preschoolers. Language delays include lack of meaningful speech, decreased gestures, and gaze disturbances. Social interaction disturbances, such as lack of fear of strangers, invasion of the territory of others, preference to be alone, and lack of social awareness, are often seen. Persistent and insistent behaviors are common. Symbolic play is limited. The child may have precocious or average development of rote memory skills but often without comprehension of concepts.

School-Age Children. School-age children with autism often lack reciprocal friendships and continue with language, social, and behavioral problems. Transitions from place to place and activity to activity are difficult. Behaviors are ritualistic.

Adolescents. Adolescents usually continue with similar behaviors. Rote learning is possible, but comprehension lags. It should be noted, however, that some high-functioning autistic children are mainstreamed and do very well in regular classrooms. Mildly affected persons may have social relationship problems.

Assessment

If there is a concern that a child has an autism spectrum disorder, a comprehensive diagnostic assessment is needed. Assessments should be done by a multidisciplinary team, addressing core symptoms, cognition, language, and adaptive, sensory, and motor skills (Levy et al, 2009). Early identification is important because intervention services may be more effective if started early in the child's life.

History. Developmental history is essential. A family history may reveal other members with pervasive developmental disorder, autism, speech delay or language deficits, mood disorders, or mental retardation. The review of systems should investigate seizures, hearing loss, head injury, and meningitis.

Physical Examination. The child should be checked for general appearance of genetic syndromes and neurologic findings of focal abnormalities.

Other Tests. Evaluation of the child for autism is best done at a specialty center. It is a diagnosis by exclusion. Testing should include the following:
- Developmental and IQ testing
- Behavioral assessment
- Audiologic evaluation
- Periodic lead screening because these children have a high prevalence for putting things into their mouths (pica)
- DNA analysis for Fragile X syndrome, tuberous sclerosis, and high-resolution chromosome analyses for various cytogenetic abnormal findings, especially those with mental retardation, dysmorphic features, congenital anomalies, or a family history of autism or mental retardation. Fluorescence in situ hybridization (FISH) testing for specific chromosome problems should follow if first DNA analyses are negative.
- Metabolic testing if there is a history of developmental plateauing or deterioration, decompensation with illnesses, unusual odors, food intolerances, failure to thrive, seizures, cyclic vomiting, questionable newborn screening results, or other indicators of metabolic disease
- Electroencephalogram (EEG) if needed for seizures (Barbaresi et al, 2006)
- Computed tomography scans and magnetic resonance imaging are not routinely indicated (Butter and Mulick, 2009).

Differential Diagnosis

Children who fail routine developmental screening should begin an early identification process. Assessments should use DSM-IV diagnostic criteria and standardized methods to assess core and comorbid symptoms. The primary care provider should analyze familial and provider concerns, descriptions of behavior, medical history, and questionnaires like the M-CHAT (Levy et al, 2009).

Once early identification is complete, experts in the field finalize diagnosis differentiating between autism and other developmental disorders such as gifted child, elective mutism, obsessive-compulsive disorder, Tourette syndrome, schizophrenia of childhood, conduct disorder, mental retardation, Rett syndrome, hearing impairment, lead poisoning, phenylketonuria, tuberous sclerosis, and Fragile X syndrome. Asperger syndrome includes characteristics of mild autism but without language or developmental delays. Children with ADHD may appear poorly focused, whereas children with autism may seem rigid in attitudes and behavior.

Management

Management of children with ASD is complex and requires a multidisciplinary approach. A focus on interactive patterns is the mainstay of management of autism. Children need educational classrooms that range from full- to part-time special education as well as the availability of resource rooms. Social skills training, one on one or in small groups, early and intense developmental work, and most recently, parenting strategies are part of management. The parenting role has come to the forefront with a focus on parents being important collaborators at all stages—from assessment through goal development and treatment delivery (Levy et al, 2009). Early intervention programs offer diverse approaches for autistic children, but it is important that each program independently looks to each child's needs for the utmost success.

Behavior. The most important aspect of autism management is behavioral training. The target behaviors vary according to age, developmental level, and disruptiveness of behaviors. The applied behavior analysis (ABA) approach to development of appropriate behaviors in autistic children is considered an optimal strategy and is the most well researched. ABA requires extensive parental education and is very time intensive and expensive, thereby limiting its use by many families. Another well-researched model is TEACCH (Treatment and Education of Autistic and Communication related Handicapped CHildren), although TEACCH has relatively less well-documented outcomes (Barbaresi et al, 2006).

Education. Extensive assessment and early, intense intervention are necessary to maximize educational abilities and enhance learning for children with autism. Planning for care requires cognitive testing to identify the child's strengths and weaknesses, in addition to social, behavioral, and language assessment. Early intervention programs for preschoolers, school-based special education, and information and assistance for school personnel are essential. Specific components for effective educational intervention have been identified (Myers, 2009).

When special abilities are discovered in children with autism, attempts should be made to encourage opportunities for success in these areas. Accommodations to advance children in these areas are necessary, and parents and school personnel need to become skilled advocates for the child. Protection from unrealistic expectations of social competence is often necessary to help the child with autism to succeed. The long-term goal should be to permit the child to function as effectively and comfortably as possible in the least restrictive environment.

Medication. Although there is no medication available for the treatment of the core symptoms of autism, medications used to treat behaviors associated with autism has shown moderate success. The most common comorbid symptoms addressed by pharmacotherapy are attentional difficulties, hyperactivity, affective difficulties (e.g., anxiety or depression), interfering repetitive activity, irritability, aggression, self-injurious behavior, and sleep disruption (Levy et al, 2009). Usually, autistic children do not benefit from stimulant medications unless they also suffer from an attention deficit. Serotonin reuptake inhibitors (fluoxetine) may be helpful as studies have shown abnormal serotonin function for some if they are depressed or anxious. Because 25% of autistic children also have seizures, they may be given anticonvulsants. Atypical antipsychotics, such as risperidone, are sometimes used for aggression, irritability, and other difficult behaviors (FDA, 2006). Citalopram, after several studies, is not recommended for repetitive behaviors in autism. Medication should never be used in isolation to treat autism.

Diets. There are no significant results from any special diets, though it is important to attempt to ensure that children are getting necessary nutrition. This is difficult for some autistic children due to sensory limitations; sometimes these children will eat very few foods, sometimes fewer than five. Several nutritional strategies have been suggested, including restriction of food allergens, probiotics, yeast-free diet, gluten- and casein-free diet, and dietary supplements such as vitamins A, C, B_6, and B_{12}, and magnesium, folic acid, and n-3 fatty acids. Most of these interventions have little evidence-based research to support them (Marcason, 2009). Additionally there are several drawbacks to specialized diets. Not only are cost, time to prepare such meals, and effects on other family members things to consider, but also some studies have shown amino acid depletion and bone loss due to specialized diets. Further information on nutritional intake, interventions, and therapies in autism is available in articles by Geraghty and coworkers (2010a,b).

Family Counseling and Support. Families need a great deal of support and training to manage children with autism. They may benefit from assistance from members of the Autism Society of America or other resources.
- The family and siblings may need supportive counseling and referral because of the considerable stress found in families with children with autism.
- Long-term care needs to be addressed because few autistic children become fully independent, employed adults, although the prognosis for children with autism is highly variable and very difficult.

Complementary and Alternative Therapies. There is no scientific evidence that supports CAM treatments. This includes biologically based treatments such as supplements, specialized diets, immune therapies, gastrointestinal treatments, chelation, and withholding immunizations as well as nonbiologic treatments such as manipulative and body-based treatments (e.g., craniosacral manipulation and auditory integration), mind-based and body-based therapies (e.g., yoga), and energy medicine (Levy et al, 2009).

There is no support for mercury causation from vaccines, bacterial or fungal contamination, and the pancreatic enzyme, secretin, has not been shown to be effective in treating autism. Clinicians should counsel parents that they will be confronted with some of these theories and many of these therapies have not been studied well or at all. Parents should be sure that they only consider evidence from randomized, double-blind, placebo-controlled clinical trials published in peer-reviewed journals and realize that "such treatments may take time, effort, and financial resources away from effective, evidence-based interventions" (Barbaresi et al, 2006, p 1173). Practitioners should try to teach and support families in their decisions for care while assessing the effectiveness, risks, and monitoring for possible side effects of such treatments.

DEAFNESS

Description

Deafness as a cognitive-perceptual problem is discussed in this chapter. Other information related to hearing screening and ear problems is found in Chapter 29. Deafness is classified as conductive or sensorineural. The hearing threshold in decibels is used to classify hearing loss as mild (20 to 40 dB), moderate (41 to 60 dB), severe (61 to 90 dB), and profound (>91dB). Conductive deafness is caused by a mechanical interruption of the sound waves from the external ear to the inner ear. It can sometimes be corrected through medical or surgical management. Hearing aids can be useful in assisting transmission of sound waves. Sensorineural hearing loss (SNHL) indicates inability of the inner ear or nerve to respond to sound waves. Sensorineural deafness can involve some frequencies more than others, resulting in a distortion of sound that may not be helped by amplification. Central deafness or auditory neuropathy is the least common hearing condition seen in children and is a problem between the brainstem and cortex in which sounds are heard but not understood. Mixed types also occur. Newborn hearing screening is now resulting in much earlier identification of children with hearing loss. This screening is discussed in Chapter 29.

Etiology

The prevalence rate of newborns and infants with sensorineural hearing loss greater than 35 dB is estimated to range between 1.3 and 3.8 per 1000 live births (Kelly, 2009). An additional 1-2 per 1000 may have milder or unilateral involvement (Haddad, 2007). The prevalence of SNHL increases to 2.7 per 1000 at age 5 years and 3.5 per 1000 by adolescence (Morton and Nance, 2006). As many as 13 per 1000 school-age children have a unilateral hearing loss greater than 26 dB and 1 or 2 per 1000 have SNHL greater than 45 dB (Haddad, 2007). More than 300 genetic conditions that have deafness as one component have been identified. There are now more than 100 chromosomal loci and 65 genes associated with hearing loss (Kelly, 2009). Approximately 50% of hearing loss is due to genetic factors (Haddad, 2007). Acquired hearing loss may result from maternal infections such as toxoplasmosis, rubella, cytomegalovirus, and herpes simplex; exposure to toxins such as alcohol and mercury; extreme prematurity with risks of hypoxia, acidosis, hypoglycemia, ototoxic drugs, and others.

Hyperbilirubinemia is considered a risk for hearing loss but neonatal infections are more dangerous. Nine percent of postnatal meningitis cases result in SNHL. Prolonged exposure to loud noise may also result in hearing loss (Vogel et al, 2007).

Conductive losses may occur due to interference with or destruction of the mechanisms for hearing; otitis media, cholesteatoma, tympanosclerosis, otosclerosis; and other conditions must all be considered (Kelly, 2009). In one study, neurodevelopmental comorbidities were identified in 48% of children with severe or profound SNHL. Cognitive, behavioral-emotional, and motor disorders were most frequent. Thirty-seven percent of children had brain malformations and white matter abnormalities (Chilosi et al, 2010).

Clinical Findings and Developmental and Behavioral Effects

Factors affecting the behavioral and developmental outcomes include the degree of hearing loss, the etiology of the loss (which may result in comorbidities), the age at onset of deafness, the family environment, and the timing and appropriateness of educational interventions. Most hearing-impaired children have some usable hearing. Table 15-10 outlines developmental milestones for the deaf child.

Language Effects. Children who do not hear have difficulties in language development. This, in turn, affects their ability to communicate their needs and thoughts and also their inner language development, the ability to translate experiences into verbally mediated thoughts and memories. To compensate, they may use more visual-spatial short-term memory than temporal-sequential (Kelly, 2009).

Cognitive Developmental Effects. Children who are deaf generally do well on nonverbal and performance measures of intelligence but fall short wherever abstract concepts and language abilities are required. Because early schooling focuses on development of communication, these children may have less time focused on instruction in other areas. It is common for deaf children to score lower on reading comprehension and mathematical tests.

Social and Emotional Development. Some studies have shown that deaf children may manifest more behavioral and emotional problems than do normal-hearing children (Barker et al, 2009; Wake et al, 2004). Impulsivity and aggression are common. Hearing-impaired children at ages 18 months to 5 years seem to have more language, attention, and behavioral difficulties and spend less time communicating with their parents than do normal-hearing children (Barker et al, 2009). Unless their families focus on methods for joint

TABLE 15-10	Developmental Milestones of Blind and Deaf Infants and Children	
	Blind (Without Associated Handicaps)	**Deaf**
Infants (0-1 yr)	• Tends to lie quietly in crib. Attachment problems possible as a result of decreased social cues and visual following. • Decreased use of hands and bringing hands to midline, decreased prone position, decreased facial expressions. • Gross motor: Head control 3-6 mo, sit 10.3 mo, pull to sit 15.6 mo, creep 15 mo, stand 15.3 mo, and walk independently 19.8 mo. Creeping delayed until "reach on sound" cue is achieved. • Fine motor: Hands to midline 4.8 mo, reaches 5.5 mo, ulnar grasp 6 mo, transfers 8.5 mo, pincer grasp 12.6 mo. • "Reach on sound": Turns toward sound 6 mo, tries to reach 9.1 mo, reaches for sound nearby 12.2 mo. Uses sound for orientation 18.2 mo (Eliza et al, 2002). • Social: Increased separation anxiety may begin by 6 mo. Increased echolalia (Ryan, 1988). • Cognitive: Sensorimotor delays common. Delayed object permanence.	• Sensorimotor stage normal • Language development: Deaf children exposed early to sign language develop language similarly to hearing children exposed to spoken language (Meadow-Orlans, 1990). • Deaf children exposed to both spoken and sign language learn both and progress as hearing children (Meadow, 1980). • Deaf children exposed only to spoken language have language delays (Gregory and Mogford, 1981). • Language output decreased around 6-9 mo
Toddlers (12 mo-2 yr)	• Decreased aggression but increased tantrums and motor behavior when frustrated. • Continued delayed object permanence. • Walks at 17 mo on average. • "Blindisms" appear—rocking, swaying, head turning (Phillips and Hartley, 1988).	• Sensorimotor stage normal • Language output decreased
Preschoolers (3-5 yr)	• Decreased social skills, decreased self-help skills. • "I" sense of self delayed to 4 yr (Phillips and Hartley, 1988).	• May have preoperational delays (Quigley and Kretschmer, 1982) • Symbolic play may be delayed if language skills are decreased.
School-age children (6-12 yr)	• Reading and mobility delays. • Conservation delayed to 9 yr (Tobin, 1972).	• May have concrete operations delays (Quigley and Kretschmer, 1982) • Decreased self-concept
Adolescents (13-19 yr)	• Delays may continue or adolescent may finally achieve developmental level with achievement in academic and social maturity areas.	• Increased adjustment problems and decreased social maturity (Meadow, 1980) • Decreased self-concept • May have formal operations delays

communication, children with hearing loss may not receive the same nurturing and social support as their hearing cohorts may receive from their parents. For example, if a child learns American Sign Language but his or her parents do not, that communication opportunity is lost.

Comorbidities. Hearing-impaired children often suffer from comorbidities, such as genetic conditions with multisystem problems, cerebral palsy, visual problems, and intellectual disabilities.

Family Effects. Parents of children who have hearing loss and undergo cochlear implantation express stresses in their everyday lives in several domains: implant drawbacks, communication difficulties, child's behavior and character, socialization, habilitation demands and parenting role, financial difficulties, services, educating others and/or advocacy, and academic concerns (Zaidman-Zait, 2008).

Assessment

The AAP (1999) recommends universal hearing screening of all neonates. Methods may include evoked otoacoustic emissions (EOAEs) and auditory brainstem response (ABR), either alone or in combination (Haddad, 2007). Because health care professionals treat infants and toddlers on multiple occasions, there are many opportunities for screening and paying close attention to parental concerns about their child's hearing. Early identification and intervention in children with hearing impairments significantly affects the child's development, language acquisition, and academic achievement. For children with possible deafness, the provider should do a thorough assessment for hearing loss as described in Chapter 29.

- Vision screening should be done because deaf individuals need good sight. Usher syndrome, which includes deafness and later retinitis pigmentosa, may need to be identified.
- Development needs to be monitored regularly, especially in linguistic and cognitive areas.

Differential Diagnosis

Cerumen impaction, otitis media with effusion, and chronic suppurative otitis media with perforation of tympanic membrane are differential diagnoses for conductive loss. Consider tumor with sensorineural loss. For the child with significant hearing loss, comorbidities may exist, including developmental and communication problems, family disruptions, depression, genetic disorders, and others.

Management

- Full hearing, developmental, and language assessment must be completed once a hearing loss is identified. Referral to a pediatric otolaryngologist is important.
- Newborn screening with identification of children with hearing loss and subsequent early intervention do better on a variety of developmental outcomes than children identified at age 9 months or later (Korver et al, 2010).
- The most important factor in management of children with hearing loss is to expose them to good language models in both visual and auditory modalities as soon as the hearing loss is detected and throughout the child's life to ensure adequate cognitive, emotional, social, and educational development.

- Parents may be confronted with many choices and, due to a variety of factors including depression, may defer decisions regarding treatment for a period of time. Primary care providers need to encourage them to move ahead with language and communication strategies from early infancy on (Kushalnagar et al, 2010).

Multidisciplinary Team. The use of a multidisciplinary team working with the family provides the best support for the child with a hearing impairment. The team should include a primary care provider, a physician, an audiologist, a speech and language pathologist, a sign language specialist, a teacher of the deaf, and others as needed. From an information-processing perspective, much of the management of the deaf child is directed at providing stimuli that the infant and child can use to understand and interact with the environment. Visual stimuli are used as the primary substitute for auditory deficits. Language serves not only as a communication device but also as a system for storing and using information.

Amplification Devices and Their Care. Identification and amplification at very early ages makes a significant improvement in speech and language abilities of hearing-impaired children (Haddad, 2007; Sininger et al, 2010). The age at fitting, degree of hearing loss, and cochlear implants were important factors in best auditory development outcomes. Different types of hearing aids have different purposes. The body box is used for children younger than 3 years old and for those in need of more powerful or durable amplification. Postauricular devices are used for older children. Ear molds need a good fit (sometimes revised every 3 to 6 months with growth) and careful cleaning to avoid clogging. By 4 to 6 years old, ear molds are changed yearly.

External otitis media can be avoided with use of petroleum jelly to decrease friction and adjustment of molds to reduce irritation. Ear molds should be washed with soap and water each night. If an infection occurs, it can usually be managed by using an antibiotic ointment and leaving the molds out for 1 to 2 days. For fungal infections, antifungal drops should be used and the molds left out for 3 to 5 days.

Cochlear implants are used with many children who will not benefit from traditional hearing aids. They help children access some sounds in the environment, but positive outcomes involve multidisciplinary teams of specialists. Cochlear implants provided to infants who had exhibited normal hearing, even if only for a brief period in life, can result in better speech and language proficiency at 5 years old (Kelly, 2009). Children with cochlear implants have been found to have better motor development, verbal development, and attention at 5 to 9 years old (Schlumberger et al, 2004). More long-term studies are showing educational achievement and employment levels similar to their normal-hearing peers (Venali et al, 2010).

Family Support. Often there is stress for the family when the diagnosis is made. Parents of deaf children also report stress with different stages of their child's life (e.g., education causes more stress in parents of children who were diagnosed more than 5 years earlier than in those with children diagnosed less than 2 years earlier) (Meinzen-Derr et al, 2008). Siblings may also need support as they cope in a family with a child who has a disabling condition (Kelly, 2009). Parents often need counseling, support, and information related to their acceptance and parenting of the identified child. Grandparents and extended family also need information and support.

Those receiving social support report lower levels of stress (Asberg et al, 2008).

Education. Early education for deaf children should begin in infancy. Children identified with hearing loss by 6 months old who received early intervention services had better language development than children identified later. Deaf children need opportunities to learn by using their strongest modalities. Language and communication needs are paramount. There are several schools of thought related to education of the deaf. Oralists focus on amplification, speech reading, and speech training. They do not support exposure to sign language. Those who believe in the total communication approach counter that the use of sign language links the deaf to the deaf community and increases their acquisition of language and functioning in adulthood. Total communication methods include amplification, sign language, finger spelling, speech reading, and speech training. American Sign Language (ASL) is the language the deaf use with one another, and it provides the strongest link with the deaf community for the child. The use of cochlear implants, however, is rapidly changing the perceptual environment of deaf children so that older arguments may be less relevant currently. Parents are sometimes pressured by professionals or other deaf people to accept one approach over the other. Educational services need to be family centered and culturally sensitive.

Interpreter Services. If children sign, they should be provided with an interpreter during health care visits. Deaf children may have inadequate health care information and knowledge because of poor communication between provider and child.

Genetic Counseling. Refer families for genetic counseling if the problem is inheritable.

Habilitation Services. Many technologic advances help those who have hearing impairments. Free-field amplification systems may be used by the teacher to amplify his or her voice for deaf students. Alerting and warning devices such as strobe lights, vibrating wake-up alarms, text messaging, e-mail, closed-captioned television and movies, phones with captioning capabilities, hearing guide dogs, and social networking sites on the Internet are helpful advances.

BLINDNESS

Description

Blindness varies from inability to distinguish light from darkness to *partial vision,* defined as visual acuity between 20/70 and 20/200 best corrected. *Legal blindness* is defined as distant visual acuity of 20/200 in the better eye or a visual field that includes an angle not greater than 20 degrees. *Amaurosis* is the medical term for partial or total loss of vision.

Children with visual impairments experience developmental delays (see Table 15-10). Children with blindness plus other handicapping conditions have greater developmental delays. Blindness affects bonding, wakefulness, balance, gross and fine motor functions, spatial concepts, language, and learning. Children with blindness have a tendency to develop stereotyped motor behaviors. In one study, all 9 children with blindness alone walked independently at a mean of 19.8 months old, whereas only 1 of 11 children with blindness and associated handicaps walked independently. The remaining 10 of that group displayed an absence of almost all neuromotor skills (Fazzi et al, 2008).

Etiology

Approximately 33% of blindness is due to genetic conditions, 27% to prenatal causes such as optic nerve hypoplasia and structural anomalies, 26% to perinatal causes, and 5.7% to childhood causes. Congenital cataracts, congenital glaucoma, high refractive errors, retinopathy of prematurity (ROP), detached retina, neurologic conditions involving cranial nerve II, cortical blindness, and optic atrophy are included among these categories. Retinoblastoma, trauma, infection, hydrocephaly, and genetic conditions are also etiologic factors. Increased risks also exist for low birthweight, small-for-gestational age and large-for-gestational age babies. One study of children in Sweden showed that 97% of infants born before 25 gestational weeks had ROP (Jacobson et al, 2009), although the number of children who lose vision due to ROP has been decreasing owing to early diagnosis and treatment. Abruptio placentae, preeclampsia, and breech deliveries also increase risks (Tornqvist and Kallen, 2004). See Chapter 28 for more information.

About 1 in 500 children in the U.S. has partial vision; about 35,000 children are legally blind (Olitsky et al, 2007). More than 50% of children with blindness or significant loss of vision have comorbid chronic or neurologic conditions. Mental retardation, autism, cerebral palsy, seizure disorders, hearing loss, chronic lung disease, cardiac conditions, and metabolic disorders are among these conditions (Teplin et al, 2009).

Clinical Findings and Developmental and Behavioral Effects

Vision triggers curiosity, helps integrate information, and invites exploration more than any other sense (Teplin et al, 2009). Children who have significant visual loss need more hands-on experiences. One cannot assume that sensory compensation is automatic but must be aggressive in helping children to make compensations as needed. Many strategies can be developed and taught. Communication is less affected than adaptive motor skills, and language serves as a main bridge toward helping the child understand the world in which he or she lives. The age at which vision is lost is important because children with even a short time of visual experience perceive the environment as a place with different dimensions (Teplin et al, 2009). Blindness interferes with social interactions and may delay bonding. Parents may find that smiles in infants are muted or fleeting so they must identify other signs that their baby wants and needs them. They need to learn to respond to other social cues such as reaching out to touch. Blindness affects the development of motor skills because the child is not sure of his or her environment.

Signs and Symptoms. Signs and symptoms of blindness may include the following:

- History of failure of the infant to follow a moving object or wandering eyes
- Poor visual acuity, reduced visual fields, and poor depth perception
- Poking the eyes or waving the hands in front of the face
- Nystagmus
- Failure to blink at a camera flash in front of the face
- Failure to fix and follow by 6 weeks
- Photophobia or chronic tearing
- History of prematurity with diagnosis of ROP

- Fixed strabismus or intermittent strabismus persisting longer than 6 months of age
- Lack of smiling in response to visual stimuli
- Timidity, clumsiness, or behavioral change may be initial signs in young children.
- Deterioration in school performance and indifference to school activities may be clues in the older child who may be either hiding the disability or unaware of deteriorating vision.

Assessment

Primary care providers need to remember that the blind child needs special cues to understand the environment. Talk softly to the infant or child before touching and look for a variety of body cues rather than visual or facial signals. Be gentle in touching because the child has no warning that contact is coming. For older children, address the child by name, describe what you plan to do and how, warn the child of contacts or discomforts anticipated, and let the child touch or examine instruments when possible.

The following should be assessed:

- Prenatal and birth history
- Family history of genetic visual impairments
- Family issues and environment
- General medical history
- Developmental history (attachment, midline play, reaching, gross motor skills, language skills)
- Sleep patterns

Physical Examination. The physical examination should include a search for the following:

- Enlarged or cloudy cornea
- Abnormal or absent red reflex
- Lack of pupillary reflex
- Nystagmus
- Neurologic disorder

Other Tests. Regular ophthalmologic examinations and developmental testing are recommended.

Differential Diagnosis

See the etiologic factors discussed earlier. Complex ophthalmologic studies are often needed to diagnose the cause of blindness. These are best done by specialists.

Management

As with other disabling conditions, parents want to be told as soon as possible about their child's visual impairment. Parents want not only the diagnosis but also resources and direction about where to get more information. For parents of school-age children, information regarding education for their child is especially important. Other comorbid conditions that children may have often receive more attention from health care providers, yet visual deficits affect the child's life and development significantly and must be addressed.

Primary Care Provider Role Expectations. The primary care provider is expected to:

- Provide emotional support and help to parents.
- Provide information about relevant parent support groups and national/local organizations.
- Encourage discussion of development.

- Assess the effect on siblings.
- Share knowledge related to school-based and community resources; eligibility requirements for special services.
- Communicate regularly with the specialists also serving this child and family.
- Help the family with developmental transitions such as beginning school, adolescence, and independent living.

Multidisciplinary Team. The primary care provider, ophthalmologist, special certification teacher, and orientation and mobility specialist are among important team members for visually impaired children and their families. Genetics counselors, social workers, and other specialists can also be useful.

Family Support. As noted, families with blind children adapt in a variety of ways. Because visual cues are so important in language and social interactions, the family of the blind child may experience difficulties with attachment resulting from failure of eye contact and facial expressiveness. Families of children with visual impairment may benefit from specialized anticipatory guidance designed to facilitate development throughout childhood. One hospital found that designating a health care worker to accompany families and patients to key diagnostic visits and serve as a first contact person with support and information about educational, social, and multidisciplinary health care services had positive outcomes for families (Rahi et al, 2004).

Parent support groups are valuable, and national organizations provide reading materials that are very helpful. Sometimes families benefit from counseling.

Education. Public school educational programs for the visually impaired child include several distinct models. Infant early education and developmental preschool programs are essential. When children are ready to enter elementary school, full-time classes for blind children are sometimes available. These are taught by teachers with special certification to work with the blind. Some schools have resource-room programs in which the child spends part of the day with a specially trained teacher and the remainder of the day in a regular classroom. Some school districts provide itinerant programs in which a specially trained teacher works with several teachers in regular classrooms, consulting with them about the learning needs of the visually handicapped children involved. Schools for the blind are generally reserved for children with multiple handicaps.

IEPs or 504 plans need to be developed annually, with input from parents and school officials. When the child enters school, psychological assessments need to be done using tests designed for blind children to ensure correct educational placement and appropriate educational support systems.

Educational programs for visually handicapped children need to include some extra components. Blind children begin learning Braille when sighted children learn to read. They learn to write Braille in the early elementary grades by using a special keyboard. By fourth grade, blind children should also learn to use a regular keyboard. Developing additional listening skills and gaining proficiency in the use of computers with aids are also essential skills. The Optacon is a handheld device that translates printed text into tactile displays. Children are ready to use this device at about 10 years old. The ViewScan can be used by partially sighted individuals to enlarge type size for reading text on a screen.

Habilitation. Sleep patterns are likely to be disturbed in visually impaired children. They may take longer to get to sleep and have longer and more frequent night wakings than their normally sighted peers (Fazzi et al, 2008). Daily living skills that may be affected include dressing, eating, hygiene, use of the telephone, and handling money. An orientation and mobility specialist teaches the visually handicapped child to travel with a sighted guide, use a cane, and use public transportation. Physical education and fitness are as important to visually impaired children as to other children. Generally, individual sports, such as gymnastics and swimming, are more successful endeavors for a blind child than team sports, even if the child is partially sighted.

Developmental Interventions. Some strategies that parents can use to promote development in their visually impaired infant or child are found in Table 15-11.

TABLE 15-11	Developmental Interventions for Visually Impaired Infants and Children		
Age	**Psychosocial**	**Cognitive**	**Motor**
Infancy	Hold and talk to the infant to promote recognition through tactile and auditory modalities. Respond to other social cues from the infant besides smiling.	Stimulate the hands and mouth. Provide a cradle gym so that reaching and touching give feedback. Provide toys with feedback, such as sound, interesting textures, or tastes.	Encourage the prone position at times while awake, a position that blind children do not generally like because they have no reinforcement visually for lifting the head. Also encourage head turning. Bring the hands into midline. Exercise the legs and massage during baths and diaper changes. Put bells on booties.
5-8 mo	Stranger anxiety occurs early. Parents need to be available. Provide predictable routines.	Provide finger foods. Provide new temperatures, textures, toys with various sounds and sensations. Talk to the child. Call attention to music and other sounds in the environment. From infancy, provide labels for objects because this helps them form semantic knowledge of object perceptions (Gliga et al, 2010).	Encourage play outdoors and on the floor. Dance and move the child actively. Sleepy behavior may be an indicator of insufficient sensory stimulation.
9-12 mo	Provide predictable routines. Touch and voice are important. Cuddle.	Encourage reaching to find a sound source. Provide toys that respond to the actions of the child to develop cause-effect concepts. Name and describe the activities and items in the environment.	Encourage creeping about which will occur after the child can reach for a sound. Help to stand and cruise. Touch and name body parts.
Toddler	Stranger anxiety continues. Reassure toddler of return. Regression and tantrums are frustration responses. Guide behavior into more appropriate responses. Reduce frustrations when possible.	Continue to work on object permanence concept, which is delayed. Noncontingent sounds, such as television or radio, are not helpful. Articulation may be normal but the child may not easily progress to meaningful sentences. Pair lessons with hands-on activities.	Walking should begin. Crab walking is a common problem that needs to be eliminated. Walking with the child's feet on the adult's can help develop the reciprocal pattern. "Blindisms" may appear and can be altered with teaching. Walk together both indoors and outdoors.
Preschool	Interactions with peers and sighted children. Establish behavioral limits as with sighted children. Teach self-help skills: hygiene, feeding, dressing.	Teach games with directional concepts. Provide experiences in a variety of settings: park, grocery, etc. Give verbal descriptions of play areas and activities of other kids in the space.	Develop motor skills: walking, climbing, swimming.
School age and adolescence	Continue to develop social skills and develop self-esteem through opportunities to be successful in activities. Provide opportunities to be with other children. Continue to develop self-help skills.	School with additional supports for the visually impaired in the following areas: • Orientation and mobility • Social interaction skills • Independent living skills • Recreation/leisure skills • Career education • Use of assistive technologies • Self-determination	Specific mobility training with balance, coordination, strength, visual-motor control and finger dexterity content.

Data from Lewis V: *Development and disability*, Philadelphia, 2003, Blackwell; Teplin S: Visual handicaps. In Green M, Haggerty R, editors: *Ambulatory pediatrics*, Philadelphia, 1999, Saunders; Teplin SW, Greeley S, Anthony TL: Blindness and visual impairment. In Carey WB, Crocker AC, Coleman WL, et al, editors: *Developmental-behavioral pediatrics*, ed 4, Philadelphia, 2009, Elsevier, pp 698-716.

Self-Perception Issues

NANCY BARBER STARR AND SARA D. DEGOLIER

All people—children and adults—have mental pictures of themselves that steer the course of their lives. This mental picture, or self-perception, begins to develop at birth, emerges in childhood, and is refined and crystallized in adolescence, but it continues to evolve throughout life. Self-perception is often used as an indicator and even a predictor of mental health (U.S. Department of Health and Human Services [USDHHS], 2010a; Wang and Veugelers, 2008; Wang et al, 2009). Multiple factors influence self-perception (Fig. 16-1). Self-perception has to do with how individuals act, think, and feel about themselves, their abilities, and their bodies. It is also influenced by the response of others to them. This perception, in turn, influences the attitudes each person takes and the choices each person makes throughout life. Children's self-concept powerfully affects their happiness, academic performance, relationships, creativity, healthy risk-taking, perseverance, resilience, and problem-solving (Neifert, 2005). A positive self-perception is a precious gift that provides the confidence and energy to take on the world, to withstand crises, and to focus outside oneself. It enhances the building of relationships and giving to others. Adolescents (in particular) with a positive self-perception have a significant protective factor to minimize the risk of suicide (Sharaf et al, 2009). Positive self-esteem is protective because it enhances children's abilities to deal with risk and learn to cope effectively (Riesch et al, 2006). People with a negative self-perception tend to focus on their own needs, trying to get and prove their self-worth. Children and adolescents with low self-perception have limited ability to respond to daily and developmental challenges (Wang and Veugelers, 2008). A negative self-perception drains energy, interferes with building relationships, and often leaves the person feeling like a victim. People with poor self-perception are more likely to participate in negative behaviors such as school absence, smoking, drinking, drug use, and delinquency, and are more likely to experience eating disorders, anxiety, depression, and suicidal behaviors (Slattery, 2008; Wang and Veugelers, 2008). Poor self-esteem can be a symptom of a mental health disorder or emotional disturbance (USDHHS, 2010a).

When children and adolescents are asked to give a self-description, they use physical, social, and psychological dimensions referring to home, school, sports, or activities that they are involved in (Dixon and Stein, 2006). Scharf and Mayseless (2009), in a study evaluating social leadership in elementary students, showed the socioemotional characteristic of positive self-perception as an important quality. This positive self-perception can be in any of six domains: scholastic, peer acceptance, athletic, physical, conduct, or self-worth. Self-esteem is enhanced by linking praise to correction and emphasizing improvement and lifelong learning (academically, socially, culturally, and occupationally).

Assessment of self-perception is not a straightforward task but is interwoven with other data that the provider collects. It may be helpful to think of self-esteem as including cognitive, affective, and behavioral aspects (Reasoner, 2002). The *cognitive* element emerges as an individual thinks about the discrepancy between the ideal self and the perceived self. The *affective* component refers to the feelings that emerge when considering the discrepancy between the two selves. The *behavioral* aspect is seen in traits, such as assertiveness, resilience, and being decisive and respectful of others. Routine anticipatory guidance, education, and counseling, individualized to the child and family, give the provider the opportunity to facilitate the development of positive self-perception and to assist in preventing potential problems. Self-perception problems are often hidden within somatic complaints, and treating these problems requires an awareness and sensitivity to the child or adolescent to identify and deal with them. If done successfully, the child's life can be significantly affected.

■ Standards of Care

Bright Futures: Guidelines for Health Supervision (Hagen et al, 2008) does not specifically address self-perception, but interweaves it throughout the approach to health supervision. *Bright Futures in Practice: Mental Health* (Jellinek et al, 2002) focuses on prevention of psychosocial problems and early recognition of mental disorders. The comprehensive practice guide and toolkit have a section in each developmental chapter that focuses on self-functioning and its appropriate assessment and management. Both the *Healthy People 2020* objectives (USDHHS, 2010b) and the *Guide to Clinical Preventive Services* (U.S. Preventive Services Task Force [USPSTF], 2010) address the need to screen for depression and potential suicide. Depression and suicide are potential complications of negative self-esteem and should be considered

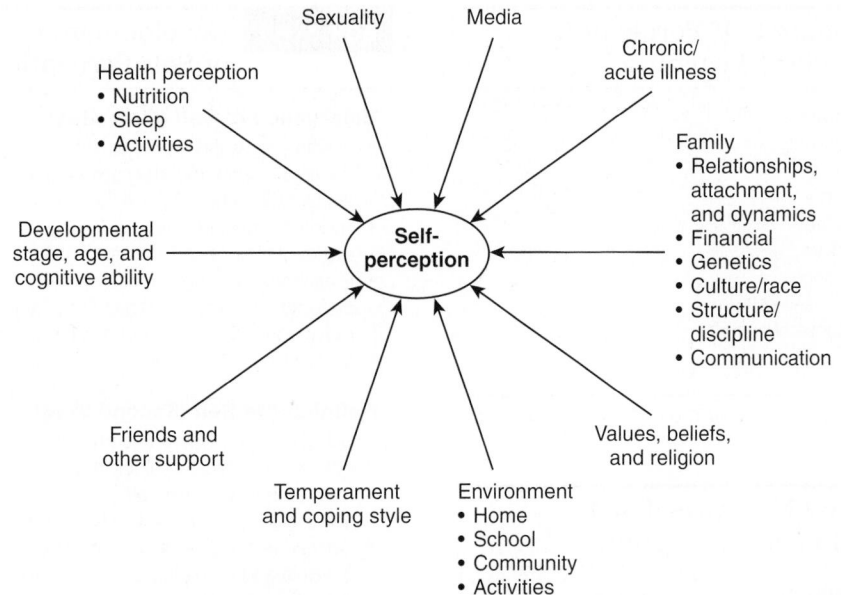

FIGURE 16-1 Factors that influence self-perception.

by the provider working with children and adolescents (see Chapter 19 for an in-depth discussion of these topics).

Normal Patterns of Self-Perception

COMPONENTS OF SELF-PERCEPTION

The term *self-perception* may be used interchangeably with terms such as *self-concept*, *self-esteem*, and *self-image*. The term *body image* refers to one's picture of and feelings regarding one's body.

Self-perception, being personal and subjective, includes both a description of the self and an evaluation of that description. The description a person draws and the evaluation a person makes come from thoughts and feelings, beliefs and convictions, observations, understanding, insight, and awareness received both from the self and from others. The three key components of self-perception are significance, worthiness, and competence (Box 16-1). *Significance* comes from having a sense of belonging; feeling loved and lovable; feeling secure, cared for, and supported; and being accepted and understood unconditionally for whom one is, not what one does. This is the most important component in developing and maintaining a healthy self-esteem. Females are more likely to channel their self-perception into feeling desirable especially through relationships (Slattery, 2005).

Worthiness comes from understanding that as an individual you have a purpose in life. It is feeling valuable, acceptable, meeting personal moral standards, and respecting and feeling good about oneself. It also has to do with being respected and accepted by others. Feeling unconditional love, "no strings attached," is the cornerstone of self-worth.

Competence comes from feeling capable, confident, adequate, in control, and able to approach new tasks and deal with life optimistically, hopefully, and with courage. Males are more likely to channel their self-perception into feeling capable

especially through significance and achievement (Slattery, 2005). Competence is one part of resilience—the inner strength to cope with any challenge one faces in life (Brooks, 2010). Competence is measured in terms of cognitive, physical, or social skills.

Children who feel significant, worthy, and competent confidently initiate activities, explore the environment, take risks, and rebound from disappointments. Appreciating themselves, they are able to reach out to and interact with others, accepting and offering love, respect, and encouragement. Perry (2001) describes an active learning process beginning with a child's natural curiosity that leads to mastery and accomplishment, thereby growing a child's self-esteem and resilience (Box 16-2).

Children who do not feel significant, worthy, and competent look increasingly to *external measures*, such as those listed in Box 16-3, to try to create a positive self-perception. Physical attractiveness, socioeconomic status, and intelligence (academic achievement) are three measures frequently used in society to evaluate people. State of physical health, temperament, coping style, and an overly protective environment are other factors that affect self-perception. However, undue or excessive emphasis on external measures causes children to compare themselves with others, adopting the description and evaluation others make of them. Most of us are what we think others think we are (Dobson, 1999), or "If you think you can't, you can't" (Neifert, 2005). Children whose self-perception is based on a comparison of themselves with others

---

BOX 16-2 Enhancing Self-Perception: The Cycle of Learning

- Curiosity results in exploration.
- Exploration results in discovery.
- Discovery results in pleasure.
- Pleasure leads to repetition.
- Repetition results in mastery.
- Mastery results in new skills.
- New skills lead to confidence.
- Confidence contributes to self-esteem.
- Self-esteem increases sense of security.
- Security results in more exploration.

From Perry BD: Creating novelty, *Scholas Parent Child* 9:67-68, 2001. Copyright © 2001 by Scholastic Inc.

BOX 16-3 External Measures Used to Build Self-Perception

Physical appearance or attractiveness: How do I look?
Intelligence: What do I know?
Performance: How do I do?
Importance: Whom do I know? Who knows me?
Financial status: What and how much do I have?
Control: What and whom do I control?

BOX 16-4 Red Flags for Self-Perception Problems

- Constantly asking for reassurance: Do I look OK? Am I fat?
- Constantly showing bravado: Do you know I know so and so? Do you know I'm involved with such and such?
- Depression or suicide: You are better off without me.
- Obsessive disorders, such as eating disorders, alcohol or drug use

Data from Slattery J: Self-esteem. In *Discovery years, focus on your child*, CD, 2005.

BOX 16-5 Developmental Stages of Self-Perception

Emergence of Self (First Stage)

- Infants—view the world as responsive or unresponsive to their needs and learn that they are separate individuals who affect others by their behavior.
- Toddlers—explore their capabilities and limits and make others aware of their needs, desires, and concerns.
- Preschoolers—begin to use personal pronouns and pretend play, become aware of discrepancies in abilities, discover their bodies, move from seeing themselves as the center of the world, describe themselves categorically.

Refining the Self (Second Stage)

- School-age children—become more confident of their own self-evaluation, evaluate self on the basis of external evidence, compare themselves with others, increasingly depend on peers for self-evaluation, criticize and ridicule deviations from normal.
- Early adolescents—"try-on" images, finalize body image, focus on physical and emotional changes with peer acceptance determining self-evaluation, use interpersonal self-description.
- Late adolescents—refine and crystallize self-perception (physical, social, spiritual) with values, goals, and competencies guiding their future in place.

---

feel and describe themselves as insecure, inferior, and inadequate. Attempting to prove themselves, they often become both bossy and aggressive, or people pleasers and approval seekers. Red flags for self-perception are listed in Box 16-4.

DEVELOPMENTAL STAGES

The development of children's self-perception is closely tied to normal growth and development. Each stage of growth and development provides opportunities to learn about the self and interact with and observe others and the environment. Transient periods of low self-esteem are a normal part of development and can occur when a child is working on mastering new skills or sets new goals. Self-perception can change as a result of relationships or experiences or can be maintained in spite of contrary evidence (e.g., the adolescent cheerleader who is loved and is successful in school and relationships, yet is anorexic and feels she is never "good enough").

One theoretic perspective that can be useful clinically is to view the development of self-perception as occurring in two stages (Box 16-5). The first stage, *emergence of the self*, occurs in infants, toddlers, and preschool-age children.

Parents and caretakers play a key role during this stage. Infants as early as 4 months old learn that they are separate individuals who affect others by their behavior, thus laying the foundation for self-development (Rochat and Striano, 2002). This is best accomplished in a supportive environment where infants come to view the world (their parents and caretakers) as responsive to their needs, both physical and emotional.

Toddlers, with their new motor, cognitive, and language skills, learn to explore their capabilities and limits and make others aware of their needs, desires, and concerns. They thrive with positive acceptance, praise, and guidelines that set limits while allowing them to make choices.

As preschoolers' feelings of competence begin to emerge, and with better self-recognition, they demonstrate increasing use of personal pronouns and pretend play (Lewis and Ramsay, 2004). At this age children become aware of discrepancies in abilities and discover their whole body, including the differences in sexes. Preschoolers internalize parents' demands and move away from seeing the self as the center of the world. Parents and teachers can begin to coach the preschooler in early problem-solving skills. Siblings and peers play an increasingly important role in the preschooler's life. When 4- to 7-year-old children are asked to describe themselves, they give categorical identification, describing themselves according to basic features with concrete, often external facts (Dixon and Stein, 2006).

Refining the self, the second stage of self-development, occurs in school-age children and adolescents as they developmentally become more self-aware. Friendships, peers, and the time spent in various activities play increasingly larger roles in shaping the child's character and personality and thus self-perception. As early as 5 to 10 years old, children will cite themselves, not adults, as the authority on self-knowledge (Burton and Mitchell, 2003). Cultural stereotypes, such as those found in magazines, television, billboards, and the Internet, influence the child's perception of society's "ideal" self.

School-age children are preoccupied with evaluating themselves on the basis of external evidence: cognitive and physical skills, achievements, physical appearance, social abilities and acceptance, and a sense of control. They are particularly prone to comparing themselves with others, making them more vulnerable to social pressure. Any deviation from what society considers "normal" is subject to criticism and ridicule.

From 8 to 11 years old, when asked to describe themselves, school-age children give comparative assessments detailing linear, often rigid and rule-based descriptions that compare themselves with peers (Dixon and Stein, 2006). Research stresses the importance of assessing peer perception hand-in-hand with self-perception in determining social functioning (Salmivalli et al, 2005; Troop-Gordon and Ladd, 2005).

Self-perception continues to be refined during early adolescence, and solidifies in later adolescence. Adolescents are defining who they are; where they are going; and how they are getting there. Early adolescents, from 12 to 15 years of age, provide descriptions of themselves with *interpersonal implications* that lack flexibility and detail their sense of self based on relationships, with personal characteristics as the basis and reason for relationships (Dixon and Stein, 2006). Early adolescents are still highly dependent on cultural stereotypes and peer acceptance, with physical and emotional changes being the main focus of self-evaluation. Self-concept may decline across late childhood and early adolescence and then become increasingly differentiated as the child matures. Body image formation, a crucial element in shaping identity, is finalized at this stage and is derived more from peers than parents (Putnick et al, 2008). Any defect, disability, or discrepancy between what is seen and what is visualized as ideal is magnified and significant in the adolescent's eyes.

Middle adolescents, not yet comfortable with their bodies, spend much time focused on their appearance, trying on various looks. Part of the development of body image includes developing a sense of sexual self or becoming comfortable with one's sexuality, assuming culturally defined sexual roles, behaviors, and activities (Dixon and Stein, 2006). Self-esteem, shown to have low stability during childhood, is increased throughout adolescence (Trzesniewski et al, 2003).

In the late adolescent years (15 to 19 years), as older teens mature behaviorally, emotionally, and cognitively, they are able to integrate family, peer, education, social, cultural, and community into their self, and establish an independent self with vocation, relationships and values (Dixon and Stein, 2006). At this stage adolescents may begin to develop their own life story with important memories that help to make sense of their past, present, and future (McLean, 2005).

It is important, especially in adolescence, to evaluate self-concept over multiple domains (Putnick et al, 2008). Areas to be evaluated in the adolescent include academic achievements (scholastic competence), athletic achievements, peer (social) acceptance, physical appearance and attributes, interpersonal acceptance (close friendships, romantic appeal), moral behaviors as compared with internal standards, sense of control over personal accomplishments, relationships, and participation in activities.

A study by Putnick and colleagues (2008) showed the way a child perceives parenting behaviors can indirectly influence the child's self-concept. This is especially true during the stress of the transition to adolescence. Teenagers had positive self-concept when they perceived their parents as being accepting (parent involved), with some degree of strictness (supervision), and granting of psychological autonomy. Donaldson and Ronan (2006) showed that participation in sports and perceived competence had a positive effect on self-concept, resulting in confidence and greater social skills. Another study of adolescent self-esteem examined eight domains identified across a number of instruments: personal security, home and parents, peer popularity, academic competence, attractiveness, personal mastery, psychological permeability, and athletic competence (Quatman and Watson, 2001). Of the eight domains, only peer popularity and academic competence showed no significant difference between genders, although boys still exceeded girls in all eight. Parents and home life, personal security, academic competence, and personal mastery were the four domains that strongly influenced global self-esteem. Low priority was assigned to athleticism. The authors concluded that boys seem to have an "at homeness" in the world, both in the home and outside, where they feel confident and masterful, not undone by adversity. In contrast, girls felt significantly less confident and masterful and more psychologically vulnerable.

DEVELOPMENTAL ASSETS, THRIVING, AND "SPARKS"

Developmental assets are positive experiences, relationships, opportunities, and personal qualities that are building blocks to help children and adolescents grow into healthy, caring, and responsible adults. In 1990, based on extensive research studies, the Search Institute identified 40 assets related to child and adolescent development, risk prevention, and resiliency (Search Institute, 2010a). The assets are found in eight areas of human development and are grouped into external and internal assets. External assets are factors in the environment (home, school, community) that (1) support, (2) nurture and empower, (3) set boundaries and expectations, and (4) speak to constructive use of time. Internal assets are attitudes that include: (1) a commitment to learning, (2) positive values, (3) social competencies, and (4) positive identity. The assets are described in the asset checklist (Fig. 16-2).

Assets are applicable to all young people regardless of gender, ethnic heritage, economic situation, or geographic location. Research shows that the more assets a young person has, the more likely he or she is to make wise decisions and choose positive lifestyles while avoiding harmful or unhealthy choices. Most children and adolescents have fewer than 20 assets, and boys experience 3 fewer than girls (Search Institute, 2010b,e). Developmental assets promote positive attributes and behaviors, including exhibiting leadership, maintaining good health, valuing diversity, and working to succeed in school. The assets have also been shown to be protective against high-risk behaviors such as problem alcohol use, violence, illicit drug use, and sexual activity. Evidence shows positive protective effects on tobacco use, depression and attempted suicide, antisocial behavior, school problems, driving and alcohol, and gambling (Search Institute, 2010d).

Building on the initial research done with adolescents, the Search Institute has now created Developmental Asset Lists for Adolescents (ages 12 to 18), Middle Childhood (ages 8 to 12), Grades K-3 (ages 5 to 9), and Early Childhood (ages 3 to 5). The asset lists have been translated into 14 different languages. All of these are accessible

an asset checklist

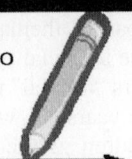

Many people find it helpful to use a simple checklist to reflect on the assets young people experience. This checklist simplifies the asset list to help prompt conversation in families, organizations, and communities.
NOTE: This checklist is not intended nor appropriate as a scientific or accurate measurement of developmental assets.

❑ 1. I receive high levels of love and support from family members.

❑ 2. I can go to my parent(s) or guardian(s) for advice and support and have frequent, in-depth conversations with them.

❑ 3. I know some nonparent adults I can go to for advice and support.

❑ 4. My neighbors encourage and support me.

❑ 5. My school provides a caring, encouraging environment.

❑ 6. My parent(s) or guardian(s) help me succeed in school.

❑ 7. I feel valued by adults in my community.

❑ 8. I am given useful roles in my community.

❑ 9. I serve in the community one hour or more each week.

❑ 10. I feel safe at home, at school, and in the neighborhood.

❑ 11. My family sets standards for appropriate conduct and monitors my whereabouts.

❑ 12. My school has clear rules and consequences for behavior.

❑ 13. Neighbors take responsibility for monitoring my behavior.

❑ 14. Parent(s) and other adults model positive, responsible behavior.

❑ 15. My best friends model responsible behavior.

❑ 16. My parent(s)/guardian(s) and teachers encourage me to do well.

❑ 17. I spend three hours or more each week in lessons or practice in music, theater, or other arts.

❑ 18. I spend three hours or more each week in school or community sports, clubs, or organizations.

❑ 19. I spend one hour or more each week in religious services or participating in spiritual activities.

❑ 20. I go out with friends with nothing special to do two or fewer nights each week.

❑ 21. I want to do well in school.

❑ 22. I am actively engaged in learning.

❑ 23. I do an hour or more of homework each school day.

❑ 24. I care about my school.

❑ 25. I read for pleasure three or more hours each week.

❑ 26. I believe it is really important to help other people.

❑ 27. I want to help promote equality and reduce world poverty and hunger.

❑ 28. I can stand up for what I believe.

❑ 29. I tell the truth even when it's not easy.

❑ 30. I can accept and take personal responsibility.

❑ 31. I believe it is important not to be sexually active or to use alcohol or other drugs.

❑ 32. I am good at planning ahead and making decisions.

❑ 33. I am good at making and keeping friends.

❑ 34. I know and am comfortable with people of different cultural/racial/ethnic backgrounds.

❑ 35. I can resist negative peer pressure and dangerous situations.

❑ 36. I try to resolve conflict nonviolently.

❑ 37. I believe I have control over many things that happen to me.

❑ 38. I feel good about myself.

❑ 39. I believe my life has a purpose.

❑ 40. I am optimistic about my future.

FIGURE 16-2 An asset checklist. (This list of 40 Developmental Assets® is reprinted with permission from Search Institute®.)

without charge at the Search Institute website (www.search-institute.org). Common threads and unique features for each developmental age group are reflected in the asset lists. The middle childhood assets include the transition toward emerging self-hood and self-regulation. The early-childhood assets respond to early childhood issues with essential ingredients that relate to school readiness, school success, and a happy productive life.

The latest research coming from the Search Institute has to do with the concepts of thriving and sparks (Search Institute, 2010c,d). Thriving "focuses on how an individual is 'doing' at any given point in time as well as the path that he or she is taking into the future." Thriving indicators are "constructive behaviors, postures, and commitments that societies value and need in youth." *Sparks*, as identified by Benson (2008), are "something inside your teenager that gets him excited.

BOX 16-6 The Ten Most Common Sparks Identified by American Teenagers

Creative arts
Athletics
Learning (e.g., languages, science, history)
Reading
Helping, serving
Spirituality, religion
Nature, ecology, environment
Living a quality life (e.g., joy, tolerance, caring)
Animal welfare
Leading

Data from Search Institute: *Sparks.* Available at www.search-institute.org/what-kids-need-sparks (accessed Oct 19, 2010c).

TABLE 16-1 Positive Parenting Behaviors and Psychosocial Risk Factors Affecting Child Development and Self-Perception

Positive Parenting Behaviors and Perceptions	Psychosocial Risk Factors
• Talk frequently with children • Modeling and expanding children's utterances • Actively teaching new words • Sitting down to meals • Talking together • Describing to children what they are seeing and doing	• Three or more children in family • Two or more household moves in the past year • Elevated scores on depression screening • Limited English facility

Data from Glascoe FP, Leew S: Parenting behaviors, perceptions, and psychosocial risk: impacts on young children's development, *Pediatrics* 125(2):313-319, 2010.

Sparks are the thing that gives teenagers (and actually all people) meaning." Sparks are "an interest, talent, skill, asset, or dream that truly excites young people and helps them discover their true passions." Using sparks help young people develop positive self-perception and discover and cultivate talents and interests that shape the rest of their lives. The 10 most common sparks identified by American teenagers are listed in Box 16-6.

ENVIRONMENTAL INFLUENCES

A variety of factors influence the development of self-perception. Some of the more noteworthy ones include significant relationships, attachment, temperament, heredity, health, race, ethnicity and culture, social experiences, stress and trauma, and media and technology.

Significant relationships include parents or parent figures, siblings and other family members, and ongoing caretakers. Parents contribute significantly to a child's self-evaluation and feelings of self-worth through parental acceptance and psychological control exerted over their child (Putnick et al, 2008). If parents are struggling and divorce occurs, a negative effect on the child's self-esteem may occur (Dalgas-Pelish, 2006). Perceived social support and feelings of connectedness with family (or other caring adults) are protective of and associated with high self-perception. That support can buffer adolescents from feelings of loneliness and social isolation (Sharaf et al, 2009).

As self-esteem develops there are some differences between boys and girls. Boys tend to focus more on achievement, whereas girls look to relationships. Girls look to their mothers as role models, and boys look to their fathers. At the same time, a father's positive interaction with his daughter helps her to feel cared for, protected, and respected. A mother's positive interaction with her son helps him to build confidence, believe in himself, and set his own goals (Slattery, 2008).

Studies have shown that first-born children have higher levels of self-worth (Shebloski et al, 2005). As children get older, peers and authority figures also have an influence. Constant unconditional acceptance and love, empathy, and an attitude of understanding, coupled with appropriate limits and boundaries, are the most important interactions these significant others offer. Time spent with and encouragement given to the child, both in being together and in doing things, in addition to sharing life's happenings (listening, talking, and problem-solving), are also essential ingredients (see the

Parenting Pyramid discussed in Chapter 4). A key component in children's development of positive self-perception is the sturdy base built by positive relationships. By feeling, seeing, and hearing these continual reinforcements, children internalize or know that they are significant, worthy, and competent.

Glascoe and Leew (2010) identified six positive parenting behaviors and perceptions that predicted average to above-average development in young children. Children with developmental assets that prepare them for school are less likely to have low self-esteem. Additionally, Glascoe and Leew (2010) identified four psychosocial risk factors. The parenting behaviors and risk factors are listed in Table 16-1. Riesch and colleagues (2006) reviewed individual, family, and environmental factors that predict poor self-esteem. Improving the parent-child communication process may reduce the risk of low self-esteem. In contrast, Neifert (2005) has identified six common errors that parents unintentionally make that chip away at their child's self-esteem (Box 16-7). A study of French-Canadian children who experienced verbal aggression from parents (e.g., rejection, demeaning, terrorizing, criticizing, or insulting) showed significantly lower self-esteem. These children perceived themselves as less competent, less comfortable, less worthy, and more prone to depression (Solomon and Serres, 1999). In general, peers and authority figures serve to confirm or deny what is taught at home.

Attachment. Neurobiologic studies of brain development are confirming and expanding the important role that attachment plays in a developing child's brain, mind, and emotions. The right brain specifically deals with self-awareness, self-recognition, and processing "self-related material" (Schore, 2005). Attachment and right-brain development in turn have a significant effect on the development of a child's self-perception. Rees (2005) describes attachment as observed patterns of relationships. A child's attachment may be described as follows (Rees, 2005; Zuckerman et al, 2005):
- *Secure*—These children value relationships, but are independently confident of their own self-worth.
- *Insecure avoidant*—These children appear emotionally independent, but often have difficulty relating to peers and a poorly developed sense of self; these children's skills lie with inanimate objects rather than personal and social interactions.

BOX 16-7 | Common Errors That Erode Self-Esteem

Although no parent deliberately undermines his or her child's self-esteem, many unintentionally chip away at a youngster's self-worth by committing the following common errors.

- **Negating a child's feelings.** Children's feelings are an important part of their identity and when parents reject their children's emotions it feels like the parent is rejecting them.
- **Frequent criticism and dwelling on negatives.** Disappointment in children makes them disappointed in themselves. Whereas parents may forget their critical remarks, children often take such comments literally and internalize them.
- **Using put-downs and derogatory labels.** Negative labels damage a child's self-image and often become self-fulfilling prophecies. Parents should choose positive nicknames that convey affection and their high opinion of their child: "Ace, champ, precious, pal."
- **Typecasting or stereotyping.** Although children enjoy having a unique identity, typecasting can restrict their sense of possibility and narrow their expectations.
- **Expecting too much.** Unrealistic expectations create excessive pressure and feelings of inadequacy. "Just a little bit better" gets translated as "not good enough." Praise a child for what he does well instead of focusing on what could be better.
- **Tying children's character or personal worth to their performance or behavior.** Verbal blasts such as "I'm so disappointed in you" make the parent's love feel conditional and subject to cancellation when the child's behavior does not measure up. Focus on the problem behavior rather than criticizing your child. Unconditional love means that nothing your child could ever say or do would cause you to withdraw your love.

From Neifert MA: Self-esteem and emotional health, *A Dr Mom Presentation,* Denver, 2005.

- *Insecure anxious*—These children often depend on the attention and approval of others for their self-worth, use physical symptoms for attention, and become uncertain and anxious in social situations.
- *Insecure ambivalent or resistant*—These children depend on relationships and are fairly organized in life circumstances, but may also be wary of their safety.
- *Insecure disorganized*—These children are neither effectively self-sufficient nor able to use relationships; they tend to have more associated social and emotional developmental problems.

Insecure attachment is not in and of itself pathologic but is on a continuum of attachment styles that may or may not present a problem (Rees, 2005). Lee and Hankin (2009) found insecure attachment with dysfunctional attitudes predictive of lowered self-esteem, which in turn was related to higher depression and possibly anxiety. Because attachment has to do with a secure, confident, basic connection to a caring adult and the adult's ability to foster a positive attachment to his or her child, the role of the adult or parent's attachment must also be considered. Assessment of adult attachment has as high as an 85% predictive correlation with the actual parental attachment to his or her children. Four categories of adult attachment identified by Zuckerman and colleagues (2005) are:

- Free or secure—in adult relationship and attachment extending to their children
- Dismissive of early attachment—minimizing the importance of attachment with subsequent emotional disconnection from their own children

- Preoccupied with their own early attachment—past issues interfere with current functioning and often lead to ambivalent attachment of parent and child
- Disorganized with unresolved trauma or loss—overwhelming issues from the past intrude unpredictably often causing disorganized attachment in the child

Temperament. A child's temperamental traits play a role in the development of self-perception. This is particularly the case when there is a mismatch of temperaments, especially between parent and child, or when a child has traits that are labeled difficult or challenging. If these traits are understood and managed correctly, the child's self-esteem can be positively affected. However, if temperament is not understood, the child may carry negative perceptions and labels that adversely affect his or her self-perception (see Chapters 4 and 19 for further discussion of temperament).

Heredity contributes to the development of self-perception due to family traits over which the child has no control. Appearance, intelligence, and family characteristics, including alcoholism, mental illness, and disfiguring disease, are to be considered. Conditions such as poverty and homelessness also are important (Costello et al, 2003).

Health or chronic conditions can also affect self-perception. Children with disabilities may have emotions or beliefs about their capabilities that can negatively affect their self-perception (Dahlbeck and Lightsey, 2008). It has been long thought (and not much studied in children) that obesity has a negative effect on self-perception. A longitudinal study done in Canada by Wang and colleagues (2009) showed that low self-esteem did not predict excess weight, but that over a 4-year period, excess body weight did predict low self-esteem. Other factors such as physical activity, diet quality, and lifestyle choices may actually play a larger role in a child or adolescent's self-perception (Ozmen et al, 2007; Schmalz et al, 2007; Ternouth et al, 2009; Wang and Veugelers, 2008; Wang et al, 2009). Lemeshow and associates (2008) evaluated self-esteem by looking at self-perception of social status in school as a factor contributing to weight gain in teenage adolescent girls. They found that girls who perceived themselves as having a higher social standing in school were protected from an increase in weight as measured by body mass index (BMI) over a 2-year period. Teasing that occurs when a child is obese is consistently associated with low self-esteem, depression, and potential suicide (Eisenberg et al, 2003).

Race, ethnicity, and cultural identity are factors that have been studied over the last 50 years. Sanders-Phillips and colleagues (2009) investigated risk factors for health disparities in children of ethnicity. Racial socialization is an important goal in raising children who develop cultural pride and well-being and learn to cope with racial discrimination. When parents are stressed by their own experiences and reactions, they are less able to parent with warmth and caring, which in turn affects a child's self-esteem. Adolescence is a critical time for racial-ethnic identity (REI) formation, and success in establishing an identity is positively associated with self-esteem. In addition, this becomes a protective factor and translates to doing well in school (Altschul and Oyserman, 2006; Hitlin et al, 2006; Quintana et al, 2006; Supple et al, 2006). Phillips and associates (2008) conducted a study on multi-heritage children in the United Kingdom who are considered at risk for multiple problems, including a lower self-esteem. The program, including group work and mentoring, had a positive effect on the children overall (as measured by self-esteem, well-being, and behavior) but interestingly not a significant effect on self-esteem itself as measured either by self-report or by parental perception. In spite of social exclusion, high levels of family breakdown, underachievement in school, and distinct patterns of racism, the children did not suffer from low levels of self-esteem as measured either before or after participation. Gray-Little and Hafdahl (2000) performed a meta-analysis of 261 studies on self-esteem. Comparisons based on more than one-half million respondents showed that African-American children, adolescents, and young adults had higher self-esteem scores than their comparable Caucasian counterparts. The authors, however, caution against using race as an independent variable in assessing self-esteem.

Social experiences. Children's social experiences provide opportunities to observe the world, test skills and abilities, interact with others, and try various roles. Positive experiences, such as success in solving problems, working out difficulties, and learning to carry on after setbacks, contribute to significance, self-worth, and competence, encouraging further exploration and risk-taking. The school setting (from preschool through late adolescence) is a prime place for these experiences. Confidence and motivation are provided by successful school performance (Wang and Veugelers, 2008). However, clubs, sports, and community and religious avenues also offer opportunities for success and alternate experiences. Friendships (having a best friend) and extracurricular activities are experiences that have been shown to increase self-esteem (Dalgas-Pelish, 2006). Negative experiences cause children to retreat or attempt to compensate through other means.

Stress and trauma. Studies over the past two decades have consistently shown that stress and trauma affect the development of the brain. Trauma is defined as "any stressful event that is prolonged, overwhelming, or unpredictable" (Post, 2010, p 12). Children who are chronically stressed or have experienced trauma often become fearful and stress-sensitive, resulting in difficult behaviors that affect their interactions with others. If interactions are consistently negative, the child's self-perception is affected. Schmidt and associates (2008) studied adolescents who were born very preterm and found a significant effect on social and affective development that resulted in reduced self-esteem in some adolescents most likely due to a lower level of social competence and difficulties in psychosocial functioning (see Chapter 19).

Media and technology. The use of various forms of media and technology consumes more of a teenager's time than any other activity except sleeping (Strasburger, 2006). Media and technology include television, movies, music, radio, video games, the Internet (including networking sites), cell phones, text messaging, and MP3 players. Strasburger (2006) states, "Virtually every concern that they (teenagers) and their parents might have about that young person has some potential basis in the media" (p 317). The American Academy of Pediatrics (AAP) (2009) released a statement regarding the effect of music, music lyrics, and music videos on children and youth. The statement recommends that providers be familiar with the role of music in their patients' lives; be familiar with the effects of that music; and encourage parents to take an active role in monitoring the type of music that is listened to. Strasburger (2006) states that many teenagers use the Internet to learn more about their sexuality as a part of their growing identity. Girls' body image is often negatively affected by the bombardment of images of models and movie stars, whereas boys may be influenced to use products to try to improve their muscular appearance. Use of networking sites can have a positive effect on self-esteem if adolescents receive positive feedback on their profile, but a negative effect if feedback is negative (Finn, 2010; Valkenburg et al, 2006). Video game playing, which typically occurs more commonly in males, tended to show a lowering of self-esteem and self-concept (Jackson et al, 2009). Some benefits that have been identified include forging a sense of identity apart from one's family, experience of a virtual community, amelioration of social anxiety and loneliness, and "trying on" of new identities (Allison et al, 2006). These benefits must be weighed against the addictive, all-consuming nature of games that interfere with an adolescent's interaction with the real world.

■ Assessment of Self-Perception

The goal of assessing self-perception is to know how children describe and evaluate themselves and to identify the sources that provide the input they use to develop their sense of self. These assessments then lay the groundwork for planning interventions for the child and family. Corresponding assessments of the parents', caretaker's, and peer's perception of the child is important.

Assessment of self-perception is not a simple task. It cannot be observed directly or obtained from questioning alone but must be inferred from observed behavior, self-statements, and other relevant information. Self-rating, observational scales, draw-a-person tests, and puppet interviews are other means of assessment. The puppet interview is an indirect interview with a large hand puppet for 5- to 7-year-olds (Verschueren et al, 2001). The draw-a-person test, used with younger children, asks the child to draw a picture of himself or herself and a picture of another child. A comparison of the two drawings often gives an idea of the child's self-perception. Somewhere between fourth and sixth grades, self-esteem inventories can be considered. A comprehensive meta-analysis of measures of self-esteem for young children is available (Davis-Kean and Sandler, 2001) as are a variety of measures for adolescents (Schott and Bellin, 2001).

HISTORY

It is very helpful to routinely ask children to describe themselves during health supervision visits. At younger ages questions may be focused, gradually becoming more open-ended as children mature. Asking parents questions is also beneficial. The following questions may be helpful when assessing a child's self-perception in the clinical setting.

General Questions
- What do you like about yourself?
- What are your best qualities?
- What do you do well? What are you better at than most people? What are you proud of?
- How do you respond to failure? How do you respond to new challenges?
- Do you have close friends?

- How does your (parent's) own style (e.g., personality, patience, energy level, talents) compare with your child's?
- Are you (parent) setting reasonable or attainable expectations for your child?

Components of Self-Perception

The wording in these questions is for parents but may be adjusted to address the children/adolescents as they are able to answer for themselves.

Significance

- Does the child feel loved, lovable, cared for, secure, supported, accepted, and understood?
- Is this love conditional or unconditional? Is this based on who the child is or what the child does?

Worthiness

- Does the child feel valuable, acceptable?
- Are self-respect and self-liking evident?
- What beliefs or convictions does the child have about himself or herself? Are these beliefs or convictions realistic? Do they match the child's lifestyle?

Competence

- Does the child feel capable, adequate, optimistic overall?
- Does the child approach new tasks with confidence?
- What are the child's cognitive, physical, and social strengths?

Developmental Stage

Infant

- Does the infant recognize self as separate from others?
- Does the infant realize his or her effect on others?

Toddler

- Does the toddler explore capabilities and limits?
- Does the toddler make others aware of needs, desires, and concerns?

Preschooler

- "How do you describe yourself in two or three words?"
- Does the child use personal pronouns? Participate in pretend play? Describe activities? Discover his or her body?
- Is the child internalizing parental demands? Moving away from self as center of the world?
- Are siblings and peers increasingly important? How does the child think, feel, and act about self?

School-Age Child

- "How do you describe yourself in two or three words?" (Home, sports, school, activities may be clue words.)
- How does this view compare with the child's perceptions of peers' evaluation of him or her?
- What cognitive and physical skills and achievements are described?
- What friends, social abilities, and activities are described?
- Is there a sense of control over life? Confidence in self?

Early Adolescent

- "How do you describe yourself in two or three words?" (Home, sports, school, activities may be clue words.)
- What role do peers play in how the adolescent feels about himself or herself?
- How are physical attributes described (body image)?
- What are academic, physical, and social activities and achievements?
- How do moral behaviors compare with internal standards?
- Is there a sense of control over personal activities, accomplishments, and relationships?

Late Adolescent

- "How do you describe yourself in two or three words?" (Home, sports, school, activities may be clue words.)
- What lifestyle choices are being made? What values, goals, and plans are expressed? Is there a sense of optimism about that direction?

Developmental Assets

To determine how many and what assets a child has, the appropriately-aged (Early, K-3, Middle, or Adolescent) asset list can be used (available at www.search-institute.org). It is suggested that parents and children complete the lists separately, then sit down and share each other's responses. These checklists become helpful tools for parents and children to compare their perceptions, identify strong and weak areas, and plan for areas of growth.

Environmental Influences

Family Structure

- Who makes up the family? Significant others? Caretakers? What is the family like?
- What is the family's social and financial status?
- What is the physical living situation?
- Does anyone in the family have any physical disease? Any mental or social problems (e.g., mental illness or retardation, alcoholism)?

Parental Influences

- Who is primarily responsible for parenting the child? How do parents describe themselves? Perceive their role?
- How does the parent describe the child? How valued is the child? How is that shown?
- What are parental expectations for the child? Is the child given age-appropriate guidance, responsibilities, and freedoms?

Significant Others Outside Family

- Who are they? Peers? Teachers? Neighbors? Authority figures? Social supports? Networks? Mentors?
- What are the relationships like?

Attachment

- "How does the child relate to adults?" (Rees, 2005)
  - Secure—seeks closeness and attention appropriately?
  - Insecure, avoidant—seeks closeness and attention too little?
  - Insecure, anxious—seeks closeness and attention too much?
  - Insecure, ambivalent—seeks closeness and attention, but is not calmed by it? Seeks closeness and attention inconsistently?
  - Insecure, disorganized—interpersonal behavior chaotic and ineffective?
- What is the parental attachment style? Free? Dismissive? Preoccupied? Disorganized?

Temperament Issues

- What temperament traits does the child have?
- How does the parent describe the child? React to the child? Interact with the child?

Environment

- What is the child's environment like? What experiences or opportunities are there? Within the family? In the neighborhood? More formal activities (e.g., play groups, extracurricular activities)?

- What experience or opportunities are there within the family and in the community to test skills and abilities? Interact with others? Try new roles? Is this encouraged?
- How protected is the child?
  Discipline
- How is the child disciplined? What methods are used? Is guidance given?
- Are limits and consequences clear?
- Is the child allowed to try without unrequested assistance provided too soon and not be rescued?
  Communication
- What messages is the child receiving (e.g., "you are a helper," or "you are a bad boy")?
- Is he or she listened to? Are feelings acknowledged?
- What does the child say about himself or herself (e.g., describes self as "good" or "bad," "smart" or "dumb")?
- What and how much media are the child viewing?

OBSERVATIONS DURING THE HISTORY AND EXAMINATION

Direct questioning about all the areas previously listed gives the provider information about the child. However, equally important is observation of the child and interactions between the child and the accompanying person(s) throughout the office visit.

- What is the relationship between the two?
- What actual words are said? With what tone of voice?
- What kind of nonverbal interaction occurs? What kind of physical interaction?
- Is the child encouraged to answer questions and perform tasks? Is rescuing occurring? Is guidance given?
- What expectations are voiced?
- How is discipline conducted within the examination setting? What limits are set?
  Box 16-8 lists risk factors for low self-perception.

◼ Management Strategies for Developing Positive Self-Perception

Anticipatory guidance, education, and counseling are strategies the provider uses to guide and direct the family, child, and adolescent in developing healthy self-perception. If problems

---

BOX 16-8	Risk Factors for Low Self-Perception

Physical alterations, including body image: chronic illness (visible or not), disfiguring disabilities, sensory disabilities, obesity, anorexia
Mental and emotional alterations: school problems, such as slow learner, semiliterate, underachiever, culturally deprived, late bloomer, difficult temperament, emotional or mental illness or abuse
Environmental and relational alterations: disrupted families and family relationships or inability to meet basic needs, unrealistic expectations or faulty thinking, temperament or personality misfits, attachment disorders, social disorders, stress, past experiences of failure, rejection, criticism

---

are significant and the child or family is in distress, refer for more in-depth counseling (see Chapter 19).

When working with the child and family, specific strategies to improve self-perception are chosen, keeping in mind that familial, generational, ethnic and cultural practices, stress, trauma history, and chronic illness influence the choice and use of strategies. A multitude of books on developing children's self-esteem are available, a few of which are included in the reference list at the end of the book.

FACILITATE GOOD PARENTING

- Know yourself. Parental self-perception, either positive or negative, has a significant effect on the child's self-perception. "If Mama ain't happy, ain't nobody happy." Parents should be encouraged to understand and accept themselves, acknowledge their strengths and accept their uniqueness, take care of themselves, treat themselves with respect, and be aware of their own feelings.
- Know your child/children. See what they see; feel what they feel; hope what they hope. This provides needed empathy. Children have their own personality, temperament, dreams, and opinions and need to be known, loved, accepted, and respected for who they are.
- Value your child/children. Appreciate and praise who they are rather than what they do. Show belief in their ability to learn, improve, and grow. Look in their eyes when you talk to them. Recognize their unique means of self-expression. Delight in their discoveries. Contribute to their collections. Identify their strengths, focus on their efforts, structure situations for success, and offer thanks for what they do. Avoid shame, criticism, and humiliation.
- Avoid comparing children. Children are individuals who grow and develop in their own way and at their own rate. Celebrate their accomplishments. Tell them how terrific they are. Their individuality needs to be respected, and comparisons with siblings or peers should be avoided.
- Be available to the child both physically and emotionally, teaching the child, modeling behavior, and helping the child learn to relate to others. A sense of security and belonging occurs as you meet basic needs and spend time together, enjoying the child, having fun, touching, talking, and watching.
- Make them believe you are always on their team. Do things with them, not just for them. Show up at their concerts, games, and events. Visit their schools. Presence endorses the child's involvement and reinforces the importance of their efforts.
- Take time; avoid being hurried, especially during times of transition. Schedule times to be together. Play with your children, and let them choose the activity and set the pace. Spend at least 20 minutes each day giving them undivided attention. Consider whether dawdling, acting out, or feeling bad may be related to being hurried and feeling lack of emotional support.
- Know their friends. Encourage positive involvement with friends and activities. Help find the right niche (e.g., length of time, type of activity) that fits the child. Show an interest in friends (e.g., host a sleepover, take a group to the zoo). Steer them away from less constructive friends and activities.

- Let go. Empower them to make decisions. Trust them. Give them responsibility. Develop a gradual, planned granting of freedom and responsibility, beginning in infancy and ending in late adolescence. Letting go offers trust, provides opportunities, gives choices, instills confidence, and refrains from rushing to aid a struggling child. As part of this process, each year the child should make more decisions and assume more routine responsibilities than during the prior 12 months.

MAINTAIN APPROPRIATE EXPECTATIONS OF THE CHILD

- Keep expectations involving tasks, toys, and roles appropriate to the child's age. Expectations that are too high lead to pressure on children and a constant feeling of failure even when children are doing their best. Expectations that are too low diminish children's value and make them feel as if the parent has no faith in them. Expecting their best can be overly demanding because no one can consistently "do their best" all the time.
- Set expectations that are appropriate to the child's unique qualities. Each child's individual personality, temperament, strengths, and weaknesses must be considered. Parent-driven versus child-driven expectations need to be identified. Although this is a sensitive issue, knowing where expectations begin (with parent or child) and how they fit the child and family is important. Recognize differences between the parent's style and abilities and the child's.
- Clearly stating expectations so that both the child and parent understand can prevent frustration, distrust, and further problems.
- Develop resilience in children by learning to view failure or mistakes as chances to learn. Mistakes are accepted and expected. Realistically assessing performance, emphasizing strengths, and discussing strategies that could lead to success prepare children to approach future obstacles and disappointments.

USE DISCIPLINE TECHNIQUES THAT ENHANCE SELF-PERCEPTION

- The goal of discipline is to teach children, not punish them. The manner and intent of providing discipline are as important as the techniques used (see Chapter 4).
- Identify limits and consequences clearly and follow through. Knowing clearly what is expected provides security for the child. Encourage flexible limit setting (e.g., "You have to wear a coat, but you may choose the blue or red one").
- Help the child learn to choose acceptable behaviors and learn self-control. Establish house rules. Catch the child being good and offer praise. Be sincere.
- Foster problem-solving to build confidence. Begin by providing opportunities to make choices and decisions. Teach the steps to problem-solving (stating the problem, expressing needs, considering alternatives, agreeing on a solution, and implementing and following through with the agreed-on solution). Take time and let the child work through the process.
- Provide guidance, but avoid rescuing children. Respect their choices, allowing them to persevere, learn, and work through frustration. This helps them learn independence and empowers them for further success. Rescuing

(providing unrequested assistance too soon) must be differentiated from guiding, encouraging, and being an ally to the child. Guidance helps children understand themselves and the surrounding world, develop a conscience, and steer clear of potential problems.

COMMUNICATE POSITIVELY AND WITH RESPECT

- Listen to children. Good listening means taking them seriously, being interested, and letting them finish what they are saying. Show love in the way the child most appreciates. This may be through touch (giving hugs and back rubs), verbally (encouraging words and tone of voice), or nonverbally (positive facial expressions or high-fives). Say "I love you" often and in a variety of ways.
- Be aware of the words used, in addition to the tone of voice, the intent of the words, and body language. Avoid negative messages that are sent in comparisons, put-downs ("You are such a baby"), humiliation ("You can't do anything right"), labeling ("You're such a slob"), and fault-finding.
- Praise and encourage children often, especially as they undertake new challenges or roles. Say "thanks" for their cooperation. Catch them doing well (e.g., "I like the way you..."). Acknowledge their help (e.g., "I appreciate..."). Love their person (e.g., "I love being with you...").
- Use communication techniques that convey respect. Ask open-ended questions to encourage dialogue. Listen with empathy. Apologize and ask forgiveness when appropriate.
- Help children identify, handle, and express their feelings by accepting and acknowledging them. Avoid statements that deny children's feelings (e.g., "You don't really hate your sister") or that give false reassurance (e.g., "You'll get over it in a few minutes. Stop complaining"). Instead, use reflective statements (e.g., "Your sister really upsets you when she gets into your things" or "It's hard having to wait your turn, isn't it?") Listen. Parents should share their own feelings and failures. Intervention may take place at the thought and behavior level after feelings are brought forward.
- Use "I" statements, not "you" judgments. This separates performance from worth and validates children's behavior while still allowing the behavior to be modified. "I like your drawings *and* I need you to color on the paper, not on the wall." Use "and," which tends to connect words instead of "but," which tends to negate what was said before.
- Be aware of children's "self-talk." What children say to themselves not only reflects what they believe, but also gives further definition to who they are. Positive statements enhance self-perception and minimize stress children feel. "Stinkin' thinking" (Hart, 1990) or negative statements reflect low self-perception and require intervention.
- Nurture curiosity and exploration to encourage mastery of new skills and help children reach their potential.

PROVIDE HELPFUL STRATEGIES FOR THE CHILD, ADOLESCENT, AND PARENT

- Support early and ongoing self-assertions as means of children expressing themselves. For example, allow a preschooler to wear the outlandish outfit chosen unless it is totally inappropriate (a bathing suit in November) or a school-age child to create the menu one night a week.

- Offer genuine encounter moments (GEMs) (Hall, 1998). A GEM is a mutually agreed-on time that is set apart for 100% attention and love, focused attention, or direct involvement. The child takes the lead in how the time is spent.
- Assume the best in your child and focus on the positives. Make a list of positive attributes and strengths, and let your child hear you speak positively about him or her.
- Encourage a healthy connectedness. Children need to belong to and feel that they are a part of their family and groups outside their family through social activities and links within their community, ethnic group, or geographic area.
- Use the 10-20-10 strategy (spending 10 uninterrupted minutes in the morning, 20 uninterrupted minutes after school or in the afternoon, and 10 uninterrupted minutes in the evening) (Forbes and Post, 2006) to give one-on-one undivided attention.
- Find and build on the "island of competence" (Brooks, 2010). Every child has interests and abilities that can be developed and displayed to provide the child with a sense of success and a defense from failure. Identify what the child is interested in and good at and encourage and praise those skills, talents, efforts, and achievements. Seven kinds of intelligence have been identified: linguistic, mathematic, spatial, musical, bodily, interpersonal, and intrapersonal, and any or all can be used to build and affirm the child's island of competence.
- Help your child compete (Dobson, 1999). A child needs encouragement to develop skills, opportunities to use the skills, and second chances when failure occurs. A child is empowered by having an ally in these endeavors.
- Help your child develop a sense of purpose, knowing that he or she can affect the outcome of events in life. Children feel more effective and less bored and resentful if they feel they are contributing. Provide opportunities to make choices, solve problems, and develop responsibilities.
- Promote a sense of ownership. Children who are given responsibility for themselves and their actions are also given a sense of control over their life.
- Keep a close eye on the classroom. Problems in the classroom are often symptoms of other problems in a child's life. Temporary rough spots are normal and must be distinguished from more pervasive problems that require intervention.
- Defuse feelings of inferiority (Dobson, 1999). Throughout the school years and adolescence, comparisons are the norm, and feelings of inferiority often result. Children aware of this fact who have learned to compete and compensate are more likely to believe in themselves despite feelings of inferiority.
- Prepare for adolescence. A special time set aside to talk with preadolescents about the coming physical, social, and hormonal changes helps prepare them to handle the transitions with greater ease.
- Affirm that good lifestyle choices (physical activity, healthful diet) are boosters to self-perception.
- Encourage parents to act as "coach" for their children rather than being authoritarian. Encourage building life skills and increasing parent-child connection—communication, support, problem solving, help-seeking—especially in the adolescent years or with children or adolescents struggling with low self-perception.

ENCOURAGE ASSET BUILDING, THRIVING, AND DEVELOPMENT OF SPARKS

- Foster identification and building of developmental assets.
- Adopt a thriving perspective.
- Help preteens and teens recognize their own spark(s).
- Relationships are critical and the process is ongoing.
- Involve everyone (child, parents, teachers, health care providers, and community members) in asset building.
- Use intentional redundancy because hearing the same positive messages over and over again from many different people is important.
- Refer to the wealth of information available from the Search Institute.

■ Specific Self-Perception Problems in Children

SELF-ESTEEM PROBLEMS

Description

When a child's sense of *significance* is disturbed, self-esteem problems arise. The child has a loss of confidence, and feelings of insecurity are evidenced, and the child may question "Am I loved?"

Etiology

Self-esteem problems arise when children are unsure of belonging and of being loved, cared for, and accepted. Low self-esteem often results when love is conditional, with acceptance coming for what they do rather than who they are. Attachment problems may be found in the family system. Child maltreatment, especially emotional and physical abuse, has been shown to interfere with the development of a healthy self-esteem (Kim and Cicchetti, 2006); emotional maltreatment (abuse or deprivation) is an extreme example of this (see Chapter 17). Self-esteem problems may be situational, transient, or chronic. Girls with low self-esteem are three times more likely to initiate sexual intercourse than girls with high self-esteem (Spencer et al, 2002). A relationship between acne and poor self-esteem (probably because of the effect on body image) has been demonstrated (Hedden et al, 2008).

Assessment

The child with self-esteem problems seeks attention, importance, and security. There may be a history of rejection or a dysfunctional family. Parental insensitivity, fatigue and time pressure, guilt, and rivals (e.g., siblings) may all contribute. Self-destructive behaviors (e.g., suicide, eating disorders, teen pregnancy) may be present. Self-absorption or obsession with external markers of self-worth may be evident (see Box 16-3).

Because of the desire for acceptance and love, these children are often people pleasers. Position and status are attempts to prove importance. Counterproductive coping strategies may be used (Table 16-2). Disruptive behavior, social withdrawal, poor academic achievement, anxiety, depression, and delinquency are associated with poor self-esteem. Attention-seeking may be extreme, causing aggression and leading to behavior problems.

TABLE 16-2	Counterproductive Coping Strategies: Signs of Low Self-Esteem
Behavior	**Example**
Quitting	Ending a game before it is over to avoid losing
Avoiding	Not even trying something for fear of failure
Cheating	Copying answers from someone else on a test
Clowning around	Acting silly to minimize feeling like a failure
Controlling	Telling others what to do
Bullying	Putting others down to hide feelings of inadequacy
Denying	Minimizing the importance of a task
Rationalizing or making excuses	Blaming the teacher for failing a test

Differential Diagnosis

Differential diagnoses include personal identity problems, role performance problems, and body image problems.

Management

Unconditional love, acceptance, belonging, and security are needs that are not being met. Refer to the management strategies section for specific ideas to achieve these, especially "parental roles," "know your children," "limits and consequences," and "10-20-10 strategy." Children with chronic illness may be helped by participating in groups with others dealing with similar issues. Providing education and treatment for adolescents with acne may be a relatively simple way to boost self-esteem.

Complications

Anxiety, attachment disorders, behavior problems, cutting, depression, suicide, eating disorders, teen pregnancy, aggression, and violence are complications of self-esteem problems.

PERSONAL IDENTITY PROBLEMS
Description

When children are uncertain of their *worth*, personal identity is shaky, and feelings of inferiority are manifested. Children may feel confused about who they are and may question, "Am I OK?"

Etiology

Personal identity problems arise when children do not receive respect as individuals and are not valued for who they are. This results in their questioning their worth and makes them wonder if they truly are OK. The child relies on others to define self, never knowing for sure who he or she is. This leads to internalizing others' negative perceptions. Potential parental

factors that contribute to these feelings of inferiority include insensitivity to the child in words or attitude, fatigue and time pressure, guilt, and rivals for love. Attachment problems may be found in the family system.

Assessment

Children with personal identity problems do not feel good about themselves and often lack evidence of self-respect and self-liking, feeling as if they have not lived up to adult expectations. They may talk about themselves in degrading terms. There is a struggle to prove "I am OK." Coping may take the form of withdrawal, fighting, clowning, denying there is a problem, or striving for conformity. There may be a history of the child being criticized, embarrassed, shamed, or humiliated, or of familial mental illness or abuse.

Differential Diagnosis

Self-esteem problems, role performance problems, and body image problems are differential diagnoses for personal identity problems.

Management

Self-respect, self-value, and feeling good about oneself are aspects of self-perception that are not developed. (See the section on management strategies for specific ideas to work on these aspects of self-perception, especially "value children," "maintain appropriate expectations of the child," and "defuse feelings of inferiority.") Helping the child learn to compensate can conquer low self-esteem (see section on finding the "island of competence"). The "10-20-10 strategy" to ensure one-on-one interaction can be especially helpful with these children.

Complications

Anxiety, depression, guilt, anger, and hostility are complications of personal identity problems.

ROLE PERFORMANCE PROBLEMS
Description

When children are unable to perform expected activities or behaviors because of physical, mental, or cognitive disability or if they feel *incompetent*, role performance problems emerge. Feelings of inadequacy often result, and the child may think, "I can't do it." A typical scenario involves a child with school problems.

Etiology

Role performance problems arise when children do not feel adequate, confident, and in control and can occur in cognitive, social, and physical arenas.

Assessment

Children with role performance problems may retreat and be hesitant to approach new opportunities and experiences, or they may be perfectionists, always striving to prove competence. A history of failure, or being a slow learner, semiliterate, an underachiever, a late bloomer, or culturally deprived may be found.

Differential Diagnosis

Self-esteem problems, personal identity problems, body image problems, and actual physical, mental, learning, or cognitive problems are differential diagnoses for role performance problems.

Management

Because the child has feelings of incompetence, inadequacy, and lacks confidence and a sense of control, strategies to develop these skills are needed. See management strategies section for specific ideas to work on these aspects of self-perception, especially "find and build on the 'island of competence'" (a key) and "help your child compete." Working with the school and the parents to achieve these goals is helpful.

Complications

Complications of role performance problems include anger and aggression, anxiety, behavior problems, depression, withdrawal, and somatic complaints.

BODY IMAGE PROBLEMS
Description

When there is a discrepancy between how children perceive their bodies, how they actually are, and how they want them to be, the result is body image problems. The discrepancy may be temporary or permanent, seen or unseen, and occurring in terms of size, function, appearance, or potential. Attitudes, feelings, and fantasies play a role in body image. Sexuality, especially in female adolescents, is a part of a teenager's developing body image that is very vulnerable to the influence of media (Gurian, 2010; Strasburger, 2006). Eating disorders are one manifestation of a body image problem (see Chapter 19).

Etiology

Disturbance in body image arises from sources as varied as physical illness or disability, chronic illness, emotional disturbances, abuse, attitudes conveyed by others, or perception of what is "normal" from the media. Body image problems are most common in adolescence, when teenagers are most concerned about physical appearance in comparison with that of their peers, but they also occur in younger children. An example of a younger child's body image disturbance can be seen when a child suffers a fractured bone, is immobilized, and is unable to cope with not being able to master his or her environment.

Assessment

Children with disturbed body image may have concerns related to body size, function, appearance, or potential. These may be noted by questioning or techniques such as the puppet interview or draw-a-person. A body esteem questionnaire for adolescents is available (Mendelson et al, 2001).

Possible behaviors include the following:
- Lack of maternal identification (aspiring to be like one's mother). Maternal identification positively correlates with self-esteem and negatively correlates with eating problems and body dissatisfaction in girls (Hahn-Smith and Smith, 2001).
- Refusing to look at or touch an altered or missing body part
- Preoccupation with the loss or change
- Feeling shame and embarrassment
- Distorted perception of a normal body
- Fear of rejection or unwanted attention from others
- Overexposure or hiding of body part
- Actual or perceived change in structure and function of body or body part

Differential Diagnosis

Self-esteem, personal identity, or role performance problems are differential diagnoses for body image problems.

Management

The discrepancy between the real and the desired body, in addition to the cause of the discrepancy, must be identified. Severity and cause of the discrepancy guide the intervention. If the discrepancy is developmental and not severe, education and counseling should help. If the problem is significant, referral for mental health care is often necessary.

Practices to develop appropriate ideas about appearance and value include the following:
- Explore parental feelings about their child's appearance. Look for ways to broadcast healthy attitudes.
- Prompt children to determine where attitudes originate. Appreciate concern about physical appearance, but discuss extremes. Favorite television shows or movies are good starting points.
- Teach that happiness and beauty do not go hand in hand. Discuss feeling beautiful (outward changes) and being beautiful (inward growth).
- Stress the need to celebrate each family member's uniqueness. Focus on personality traits and attitudes about life, school, and people, not on externals.

Other helpful interventions include the following:
- Encourage regular physical activity, especially with other family members. Developmentally focused youth sports programs (*Girls on the Run* and *Girls on Track*) showed positive self-esteem and body image findings (DeBate et al, 2009). Ransdell and associates (2001) found improved physical self-perception in adolescent girls and their mothers when they participated in a physical activity intervention together.
- Point out ways the child or adolescent is on target developmentally and identify what can be expected over the next year. Emphasize the fact that there is a high degree of variability in development.
- Make family connections—look for features similar to other family members; include talents and internal characteristics as well.
- Play the appreciation game—name body parts and say something nice about that part (e.g., "Thanks, ears, for letting me listen to my iPod").
- Go to the *Don't Buy It: Get Media Smart* website (see http://pbskids.org/dontbuyit).

- Stay positive—don't make or allow disparaging comments and give yourself a compliment often.
- Identify areas where assistance is needed.
- Refer to counselors, dietary therapy, occupational therapy, or physical therapy as appropriate.
- Collaborate with the school nurse or teacher to plan for the child's return to school.
- Involve the child in a peer group with similar problems.
- Verbalize acceptance.
- Use play therapy to encourage verbalization.

- Teach new ways of handling situations to accommodate for loss or change.
- Discuss ways to camouflage areas of concern (e.g., wig or scarf for hair loss).
- Compliment behaviors that indicate acceptance.
- Provide ongoing support and encouragement as a primary care provider with focus on positive aspects of body and functioning.

Role Relationships

JOY S. DIAMOND, DENISE C. ABDOO, MARGARET A. BRADY, AND ARDYS M. DUNN

Understanding family dynamics and role relationships is essential to the delivery of health care services to children and adolescents in all pediatric settings. However, pediatric primary care providers carry the major responsibility for advising parents on how to effectively handle relationship issues with children at home, in school, and in the community. Parents and other family members are solely responsible for the health and welfare of their young children and must learn key communication and interaction skills to effectively rear their child. The pediatric provider must be sensitive to the roles that parents or caregivers, siblings, extended family members, and peers have in shaping the developing child. Likewise the community is an extension of the family and serves as a major component in the widening circle of influence that affects the lives of children and adolescents. Chapter 2 outlines important considerations and appropriate tools to be used when assessing family systems. This chapter discusses the family life cycle and family variations. In addition, it covers the assessment and management of situations or events that the provider is likely to encounter in a primary care setting related to family relationship problems, sibling rivalry, violence, and child maltreatment or neglect. Preventive interventions for role-relationship problems directed at specific individuals or groups at risk (selective interventions) as well as at the population as a whole (universal interventions) are identified. Advice about securing safe, nurturing, and developmentally appropriate childcare is also discussed.

■ Standards of Care

Healthy People 2020 addresses issues of violence and abusive behavior and their negative effect on children, families, and society (U.S. Department of Health and Human Services [USDHHS], 2010a). Recommendations include:

- Reduce bullying, dating, and sexual violence.
- Decrease the percentage of public middle and high schools with a violent incident.
- Reduce physical assaults and physical fighting among adolescents.

Child maltreatment is recognized as a significant public health problem. The target goal of *Healthy People 2020* is no more than 2.2 child maltreatment *deaths* per 100,000 children younger than age 18. The goal for reducing nonfatal child maltreatment is 8.5 per 1000 children younger than the age of 17 years. National, state, and local efforts must be dedicated to reducing preventable death and disability and to enhancing the quality of life for all children. Health professionals in their individual practice settings and as a collective group must commit to improving the quality of life by incorporating health promotion and disease prevention as integral components of health care for children and their families. Identification of at-risk families and referral for intervention must always be viewed as priorities.

■ Family Relationships and Dynamics

FAMILY LIFE DYNAMICS

The family is a dynamic social system that is usually the most powerful and constant influence of a child's development and socialization. The family provides emotional connections, behavioral constraints, and modeling that affect the child's development of self-regulation, emotional expression, and expectations regarding behaviors and relationships (Coley, 2009). Changes in one family member's behavior affect everyone else in the family unit.

Healthy families are cohesive and adaptable, with positive communication patterns. *Family cohesion* is an indication of the strength of the emotional bonding between family members and can range from the extremes of very low (disengaged) to very high (enmeshed) bonding, with moderate to high (connected) bonding representing the middle ground. *Family adaptability* is the ability of a family system to change its power structure, role relationships, and relationship rules in response to situational and developmental stress. The range of adaptability varies from very rigid (very low) to chaotic (very high), with a middle ground between structured and flexible. A key element in adaptability is the ability to change as appropriate in a given situation. *Communication patterns* range from positive communication skills that convey messages such as empathy, reflective listening, and supportive

---

BOX 17-1 Six Key Dimensions Affecting Family Functioning

- *Resources* that are available to the family include a social support network of extended family members, friends, and community, in addition to financial and other material assets. Families with limited resources or social support networks are more vulnerable to stressful life events than are families with resources and support systems in place.
- *Stresses and changes* the family faces are numerous and can include financial strains, illness, marital strain, family transitions, losses, and lack of effective coping strategies. Life brings transitions that necessitate change. Many transitions are normal, some are anticipated, and others are unexpected; all can have a significant effect.
- *Childrearing styles* are composed of parenting behaviors and beliefs that influence the environmental milieu in which the child learns about the world. Certain childrearing styles (e.g., an uninvolved, permissive, or strict authoritarian parenting style) are ineffective and have dire consequences for the emotional health of a child.

- *Values* shared by family members provide a framework to guide, explain, and understand events being experienced and within which to find comfort, joy, and solace. Spiritual beliefs are one example of values that can support a family in its everyday life and in times of challenge.
- *Roles and structures* vary greatly from one family to another, within an individual family, and as family members grow and develop. Role responsibilities and structures often change in response to external demands experienced by the family; shifts in the role of one family member can affect the role functions of other family members.
- *Coping style* of the family speaks to the ways that demands are met, transitions handled, and concerns resolved. Positive or effective coping is characterized as a creative response to a change or stressor that results in a new behavior or attitude. Coping styles reflect habitual patterns of action. Over time, coping effort develops into a coping style.

---

comments, to negative communication skills that reflect double messages, double binds, criticism, and minimize opportunities to share feelings. Communication is one of the most crucial elements within an interpersonal relationship. Family cohesion and adaptability are threatened and thwarted with negative communication patterns. The result of negative communication is a chaotic household marked by high levels of family distress.

Each family has its own unique pattern of growth and development, and family systems evolve and change, demonstrating different dynamics depending on the stage of the family's life cycle. Just as a child goes through stages of development, so do family units. Family life with young infants and preschool children is vastly different from family life with school-age children, with early versus late adolescents, or with young adults. Also different types of family units—nuclear, single-parent, divorced, or blended—express different styles or patterns of family life.

DIMENSIONS OF FAMILY FUNCTIONING

Common themes exist within all families, and six key dimensions have a significant effect on family functioning, contributing to cohesiveness, adaptability, and positive communication (Box 17-1). To assist parents and children across the family life cycle and especially during times of stress, the provider must carefully assess these elements.

THE INTERACTIVE FAMILY

A family is interactive, both within the family circle and between the family and its community. Within the family each member influences all other family members and is likewise affected by them. Maladaptive patterns of interaction among family members can place a child and family at risk for negative outcomes. For example, if the family unit does not provide a protective, interactive, supportive, and loving environment to nurture the child or fails in its responsibility to help the child learn self-discipline and the ability to socialize with others, the child often develops maladaptive behaviors.

Authoritative parents closely monitor their children with warmth and emotional support while maintaining firm boundaries. An authoritative style grants autonomy that is age-appropriate and permits the child to make decisions based on readiness factors; encourages the expression of feelings, thoughts, and desires; and promotes joint decision-making when appropriate as the young child matures and develops throughout childhood and adolescence. Research has demonstrated that parents with authoritative parenting styles have a positive influence on eating habits, teenage driving, and risk-taking behaviors (Ginsburg et al, 2009; Montgomery et al, 2008; Ventura and Burch, 2008).

There are factors that are protective and foster resiliency. Certain temperaments, a caring relationship and/or social support outside the immediate family, community resources and opportunities, and effective parenting can counter the negative effects of adverse risk factors and contribute to a child's positive mental health. The degree of satisfaction as a couple and as parents is an important outcome measure of how well the family is functioning as a family unit. Single-parent households may face many challenges that can have a negative effect on the family unit, but can be enhanced by developing nurturing relationships in both the parent's and the child's life. Children are at risk for developing mental health problems as a result of environmental factors, such as living in poverty, living in a community with a high crime rate, living in a home marked by marital conflict or domestic violence, living in a home in which they or their siblings are the victims of child maltreatment or neglect, or having a parent who abuses alcohol or other substances, or has a mental illness.

■ Assessment of Family Relationships and Dynamics

In addition to stressful issues that may arise with "typical" family relationships, providers are likely to encounter not only parent- or child-initiated concerns, situations, and events related to relationship problems, but also violence, child maltreatment, or neglect. Families and children who are experiencing or who are at risk for stressful situations must

---

BOX 17-2 Significant Factors for Assessment of High-Risk Family Relationships and Dynamics

Child Factors
- Chronologic age and developmental level
- Present or past history of physical, emotional, or cognitive problems
- Personality traits, characteristics, and temperament
- Prior maltreatment or significant negative life events
- Special care needs
- School performance

Parent/Caregiver Factors
- Physical, intellectual, or emotional functioning, illnesses, or limitations
- Level of involvement in childcare and life events of child
- Level of parenting skills, childrearing style, and communication skills
- Beliefs about discipline and corporal punishment
- Parental role and supports
- Parental history of experienced dysfunctional childrearing practices or any maltreatment or neglect
- A victim or perpetrator of domestic violence
- Current or previous history of substance abuse
- Financial resources, especially if poverty or limited finances are an issue

Social and Environmental Factors
- Sibling assessment
- Type and strength of family social support network or social isolation
- Peer group relationships
- Stresses, crises, or conflicts in the home environment
- Cultural belief system
- Environmental condition of home and surrounding community
- Stresses in the neighborhood environment
- Availability and accessibility of community support systems and partnerships

---

be identified. Assessment of families is also discussed in Chapter 2.

Family strengths and attributes that sustain and help families effectively deal with any level of stress are important factors to evaluate. In an assessment of family dynamics, the health care provider must investigate the relationships between the child, parent, or caretaker, as well as the social and environmental factors. Each factor must be analyzed separately, with its various components identified. The interactive effect of these factors must then be explored. The goal of assessment is to determine factors that have a positive or negative effect on the child's growth and development.

Though the list is not exhaustive, Box 17-2 includes significant child, parent or caregiver, and social and environmental factors that can be used to alert the provider to areas that need further investigation.

Management for Health Promotion and Disease Prevention

Primary care providers are often approached by parents with concerns about developmental or role-relationship issues that can be managed with healthy parenting and good communication (see Chapters 4 through 8 and 19). A supportive health care professional is in a strategic position to prevent problems and empower parents and children by providing anticipatory guidance, education, motivational support, resources, and opportunities for counseling.

Providers are typically involved in universal preventive interventions related to both physical and mental health issues. Universal preventive interventions are directed at enhancing the parent-child relationship. Universal interventions address the population as a whole and stress promoting wellness, improving communication, and strengthening relationships. Selective preventions are directed at individuals or groups at risk for the development of mental health and/or relationship problems. Indicated preventions are for high-risk individuals who are experiencing symptoms or who have biologic markers for mental illness. Selective and indicated

preventions often use a multidisciplinary approach, with community resources and other professionals from various social fields joining together. The provider must develop a plan of action with goals and outcome measures and specific criteria that indicate when there is need for referral to a mental health or other professional.

Family Relationships and Challenges

TWO-PARENT FAMILIES

Two-parent families include married couples with children, unmarried couples with children, remarried couples with blended families (or stepfamilies), and gay or lesbian couples. Two-parent families experience the same stressors as do single-parent families, but children in two-parent families tend to have social, economic, and health advantages. Parent educational levels, economic status, and health status are generally higher in two-parent families than in single-parent families (Annie E. Casey Foundation, 2010). Parents often cite, although this is seldom researched, that even when the division of labor is uneven, it is still a relief to have another adult with whom to share the work of raising children. Several studies, however, show that children's well-being depends on composition of the household and not just the number of adults present.

WORKING PARENTS AND CHILD CARE

In 2009, more than 59% of mothers with preschool-age children (younger than 6 years) were employed and 76% of those worked full-time. During the same year, 72% of women with children between 6 and 17 years old were employed (Bureau of Labor Statistics, 2010). According to the Children's Defense Fund fewer than 10% of child care centers and fewer than 1% of family child care homes are accredited. Additionally the annual cost of child care in a center for a 4-year-old child is more than annual in-state tuition at a public four year college; in five states it is at least twice the cost (Children's Defense Fund, 2010).

When a single parent works outside the home or both parents in a two-parent family work outside the home, the two roles of working parents need to be coordinated to promote positive family outcomes. Carter (1999) identified three unresolved problems related to work and families that can affect parenting: men's unequal contributions to housework, workplace inflexibility, and the increasing number of hours both men and women are spending outside the home. Many studies have explored the effect of maternal employment on children. The outcomes are complex and depend not just on whether a mother is employed, but on the family circumstances, daycare, home environment, marital status, consistency of employment, work stress, and other variables (Halpern, 2005). Consistently shown, however, is that poverty operates to create negative outcomes for children and families; maternal employment may mitigate this factor. Research findings show that, generally, children can develop equally well regardless of the employment status of their parents; the home environment is more important (Halpern, 2005).

SEPARATION AND DIVORCE

Description

Divorce or the separation of parents has a profound effect on all family members. Divorce is an emotionally stressful and complex transition for families. It can lead to significant emotional disruption and disequilibrium in the lives of children who perceive divorce as a dramatic, painful, and challenging event in their lives. Behavioral changes are an expected reaction as the child attempts to adjust to the changing family situation. Custodial and visitation arrangements for children are variable. Joint custody is an option that allows both parents the opportunity to participate in mutual decision-making about their child's life and welfare. Various living arrangements and visitation rights are possible with joint custody. There are instances in which single custody is in the best interest of the child, however, and the noncustodial parent may have limited contact and involvement in the child's life.

Taking a developmental-behavioral perspective of understanding divorce as an ongoing process rather than a concrete event is key. Each child has a unique history and resultant possible new family life. Regardless of the parents' perspective, divorce is a loss of family as the child knows it and therefore the child will experience grief. Important parent factors include a stable parenting foundation provided in early years and parental warmth and praise for the child through the divorce. Children with behavior problems and more difficult temperaments before the divorce tend to have more difficulty adjusting to divorce than children with an easy temperament, above-average intelligence, who are physically attractive, and have a sense of humor and better self-esteem (Tanner, 2009).

Research studies that investigate the psychological consequences of divorce on children have reported varying data about its negative effect. Although children from divorced families have more adjustment problems and depressive symptoms than children whose parents do not divorce (Ge et al, 2006), those problems may arise from the conflictive relationships existing before the divorce, rather than the divorce per se. Children whose parents were cooperative reported better relationships with their parents, grandparents, and siblings (Ahrons, 2007).

Divorce can also be positive when parents are able to develop a more civil relationship with each other that focuses on what is best for the child. The child may also gradually adopt roles that support self-reliance, awareness of needs of others, and an increase in responsibility (Tanner, 2009).

Epidemiology

The rate of divorce in the United States has been fairly stable for the last 20 years (Tanner, 2009). The Centers for Disease Control and Prevention (CDC) reported a provisional divorce rate of 3.4 per 1000 marriages in 2009, down slightly from the 3.5 per 1000 in 2008 and 3.6 in 2007. The marriage rate was 6.8 per 1000 in 2009 (down from 7.1 in 2008 and 7.3 in 2007) (CDC, 2009). Roughly 48% of all new marriages end in divorce within 20 years. Approximately 50% of the divorced adults remarry within 4 years (Tanner, 2009).

Assessment

The goal of assessment of the family experiencing separation or divorce is to determine both the needs and strengths of the family in order to assist the family with healthy coping. Child-related factors to consider include the developmental stage of the children and common psychosocial reactions to divorce likely at that stage. Additionally the psychosocial effect of the divorce on the parents and the economic consequences of divorce on the family unit must be determined (Box 17-3).

Management

Anticipatory guidance given to parents who are in the process of separating and divorcing is outlined in Table 17-1.

BOX 17-3 **Assessment Factors in Divorce**

Developmental Stage of Children
- Age and developmental stage of children greatly affect their response to separation and divorce of parents.
- Common reactions of children to divorce by age group:
  - 2-5 years: Regression, irritability, sleep disturbances, aggression
  - 6-8 years: Open grieving and feelings of rejection or being replaced; whiny, immature behavior; sadness; fearfulness
  - 9-12 years: Fear and intense anger at one or both parents
  - >13 years: Worried about own future, depressed, or acting-out behaviors (e.g., truancy, sexual activity, alcohol or drug use, suicide attempts)

Common Issues for Children of Divorcing Parents
- Continued tension, conflict, and fighting between parents
- Litigation disputes over custody and visitation arrangements
- Abandonment by one parent or sporadic visitation (decreased availability) vs. denial of visitation
- Diminished parenting resulting from such factors as availability issues or emotional inaccessibility, distress, or instability
- Limited social support system outside nuclear family
- Feelings of loneliness or emotional abandonment, or both

Economic Consequence of Divorce
- Often devastating economic hardships and decline in living standards (especially for women)
- Nonpayment or delinquency in payment of child support

TABLE 17-1 Key Anticipatory Guidance Issues for Families Experiencing Divorce or Separation

Anticipatory Guidance Issue	Discussion Points With Parents
Advise parents to prepare the child for the impending breakup.	If possible tell the child in advance of the breakup. Children who are appropriately prepared may cope better with the separation and change in family structure. Discussions should focus on supporting the child's needs for reassurance and stability, not on blame, recriminations, or the parent's needs.
Explain to parents the need to discuss the following key issues with their children.	Assure children they will continue to see the departing parent when possible. Explain what divorce means in language appropriate to the child's cognitive and developmental level; offer an explanation of reasons for the divorce in the same terms. Reassure children that they did not cause the divorce or separation, that they cannot correct their parents' unhappiness in the marriage, and that the divorce is the parents' decision. Explain what the family structure will look like afterward and what changes will be necessary in the way the family functions. Explain the visitation arrangements as soon as they are established. Reassure children that they will be cared for, and they are not being abandoned by either parent, unless a parent has disappeared or refuses involvement. Tell children that feelings of sadness, anger, and disappointment are normal; encourage them not to "take sides," but love both parents.
Discuss the need for consistency.	Parents should strive to maintain consistent daily routines between the two households; encourage the use of security items that the child may depend on or carry familiar items between the homes during the transitional period. Be consistent in disciplinary practices.
Suggest self-help measures.	Children and parents may benefit from attending divorce recovery workshops, classes about families in transition, or peer support groups. School counselors, religious groups, or community and social service agencies may be helpful resources.
Acknowledge grief.	Providers should acknowledge the grief that both the parent and child are experiencing, and provide support.
Discuss when referral for mental health counseling might be indicated.	Children often demonstrate internalized or externalized psychosocial problems in response to divorce. Counseling may be indicated for the family members.

Patient Education and Prevention

The goal of health education for children and parents experiencing divorce is to help restore a sense of wholeness and integrity in children's lives. Providers must stress those factors that have been shown to significantly affect whether the child will experience a healthful adjustment to the divorce (Box 17-4). Successful efforts implemented during initial periods of disequilibrium and reorganization will strengthen normal development and prevent future psychological trauma. In an early research study, Wallerstein (1983) identified six psychological tasks that children of divorce must master beginning from the time of parental separation and culminating in young adulthood (Box 17-5). These tasks continue to be relevant for children whose parents are divorced. If these psychological tasks are not achieved, the child's mastery of normal developmental tasks associated with growing up is negatively affected. Long-range and preventive interventions need to focus on helping the child achieve these tasks or goals.

It may be a good idea to schedule additional visits or telephone contacts with the family to monitor their adjustment. Support can be provided by focusing on the family's positive strengths and ability to be resilient.

BOX 17-4 Factors Affecting a Child's Ability to Achieve Healthy Adjustment to Divorce in His or Her Family

- The opportunity for continued participation of the noncustodial or visiting parent in the child's life on a regular basis
- Custodial parent attempts to make visits with the other parent a routine event so there is consistent contact (phone, visiting, e-mail)
- The ability of the custodial parent to handle and successfully parent the child
- The ability of parents to separate their own feelings of anger and conflict and resolve their own hostility toward each other so that the child's need for a relationship with both parents is met; divorced parents do not put the child in the middle
- The child does not become involved in parental conflict and does not feel rejected
- The availability of a social support network
- The ability of parents to meet the child's developmental needs and to help the child master the developmental tasks before him or her
- The child's overall personality and personal assets and deficits

BOX 17-5	Six Psychological Tasks Children of Divorce Must Master

- Acknowledge the reality of the marital breakup.
- Disengage from parental conflict and distress and resume customary pursuits.
- Resolve loss of familiar daily routine, traditions, and symbols and the physical presence of two parents.
- Resolve anger and self-blame.
- Accept the permanence of the divorce.
- Achieve realistic hope regarding relationships—the capacity to love and be loved.

Data from Wallerstein JS: Children of divorce: the psychological tasks of the child, *Am J Orthopsychiatry* 53:230-243, 1983.

SINGLE-PARENT FAMILIES

Description

Numerous circumstances lead to single-parent households, including unemployment, divorce, births to unmarried mothers, abandonment of the family by a parent, incarceration of a parent, or death of a parent. Although the vast majority of single parents are women, increasingly fathers are raising their children in single-parent homes. Single-parent households may be headed by a divorced parent or by a parent who has never been married. Today single parents may range from adolescents enrolled in welfare programs to company executives with live-in nannies. In general, children living with a divorced parent have an advantage; divorced parents tend to be older, with more years of completed schooling, and with higher levels of income than do parents who have never been married. Children in single-parent families benefit when both parents are involved in their lives, regardless of marital or living arrangements. Clearly, understanding the family context is fundamental to assessing these families.

Single parents across socioeconomic parameters all experience the demands and burdens of raising a child alone. Even with help, the weight of responsibility is felt and exacerbated by lack of time and role strain. Single mothers who are employed experience more distress than partnered employed women but factors such as income adequacy, psychological work quality, and work-family conflict also affect the outcomes (Dziak et al, 2010). Single parents sometimes have difficulty accessing health care. Research suggests that affordability is a more significant issue than time pressures or workplace demands (Kneipp, 2002). The relatively large proportion of single parents who are classified as "working poor" puts them above the income level for subsidized care and below the level where they could realistically afford health insurance.

Studies demonstrate higher levels of depressive symptoms and problematic substance use in children living in single-parent families compared with mother-father families (Barrett and Turner, 2005). Barrett and Turner report that this relationship probably is linked more with exposure to stress and association with deviant peers. Likewise, living in a single-parent household is strongly associated with poorer child health, largely as a factor of an associated accumulation of social disadvantage (Bauman et al, 2006). Cohabitation of a parent and a nonparent is considered to be more detrimental to children than a single parent living alone. Rates of divorce are higher among those who later marry, and breakups occur during the cohabitation period. More children experience child abuse, and poverty rates tend to be higher than with married families.

Single-parent families are distinguished from multigenerational families, which are defined as families with a single parent or a married couple living with their children, their parents, their in-laws, or their grandchildren.

Epidemiology

About 22.6 million children (32%) lived in single-parent households in 2008. African-American children are more likely (65%) to live in a single-parent than a two-parent household unlike children from all other racial groups (Annie E. Casey Foundation, 2010). Single mothers are overrepresented among the very poor and those needing social assistance. The incidence of single-parent families varies by geographic, racial, and ethnic demographics.

Assessment

Several key areas are important to assess when working with single parents and their children. They can be divided into parent- and child-related factors.

Parent-related factors include the following:
- Emotional and physical well-being of the parent
- Availability of emotional support from their social network
- Living situation, presence of financial difficulties, insurance coverage
- Availability of financial and emotional support from a noncustodial parent
- Availability and quality of child care for parents who must work
- Opportunities for the single parent to have a social life and relationships or personal time
- Ability of the parent to maintain consistency in discipline, in addition to a positive outlook and commitment to parenting

Child-related factors include the following:
- Role of the child in the family; responsibilities for taking care of siblings
- Relationship with custodial parent
- Location of and relationship with the noncustodial parent
- Availability of emotional support from his or her social network
- Availability of opportunities to accomplish age-appropriate developmental tasks (e.g., is child doing well in school? Does he or she have friends? Is child participating in sports or club activities?)
- Signs of problem behavior at school, at home, or with social activities
- The presence of children in the home with special needs (e.g., developmental disability, cognitive delay, or chronic illness)

Management

Resiliency in single-parent families is associated with individual characteristics of optimism, perseverance, faith, expressions of emotions, and self-confidence (Greeff and Ritman, 2005). Many single families cope well with the demands they face, benefiting from advice, anticipatory guidance, encouragement,

BOX 17-6 Significant Determinants for Successful Childrearing in a Single-Parent Home

- Support persons in the child's life who:
  - Collaborate with the single parent
  - Develop quality relationships with the child
  - Are available for the child
- Adults in child's community who provide support, including teachers, school officials, health care providers, and support person(s) for the parent
- Capacity of parent to communicate with child in open, direct, and understanding manner
- Ability of parent to recognize child's need for opportunities for enjoyment and accomplishment outside the home and to provide for the child
- Economic stability and well-being that is adequate to meet family's needs

and support of the provider. On an individual level, several critical factors promote successful childrearing in single-parent homes. The availability of a social support network and positive communication patterns are key (Box 17-6). Social organizations such as Big Brothers Big Sisters offer a supportive role model for children in single-parent families. Parents Without Partners is a national organization that offers social activities and support for single parents.

Single parents commonly seek advice about dating situations and explaining money problems to their children. Suggest that the parent meet his or her date outside the home until a decision is made as to the direction of the adult relationship. Young children tend to quickly attach to individuals who are kind and spend time with them, whereas an older child may become jealous or see the individual as a threat. Financial concerns frequently are issues in single-family homes. Urge the parent to explain the family's money situation in a way the child can understand based on age. When money is limited or tight, the child can be told simply and briefly that the family may have to wait to buy or limit buying "extras" or that some activities may have to be curtailed. The child can be helped to learn about the value of saving money for special treats.

If parents request specific help or demonstrate signs of being exhausted, depressed, overwhelmed, burdened, or socially isolated, a referral for more specialized services such as counseling may be appropriate. Similar signs in children plus deviant behaviors, emotional adjustment problems, or school disciplinary, academic, or behavioral problems can be indicators for mental health referral.

Patient Education and Prevention

Although individual families may be helped to gain better coping skills, significant positive change in the quality of life of single-parent families depends on restructuring and increasing economic, educational, and family support resources in the community. Primary care providers should be informed about the effect that social service legislation has on the families they serve and be willing to advocate for policy changes.

REMARRIAGE: THE BLENDED FAMILY
Description

A blended family is one in which two adults create a reorganized family by joining with their children from previous relationships. Although this term usually refers to families created by remarriage after divorce, it is also used to describe families created by remarriage after the death of spouses. The introduction of a stepparent and possibly stepsiblings can be beneficial for a child or can be a time of difficult adjustment. The majority of children within blended families gradually adjust well to their new family situations.

Epidemiology

Approximately 50% of women and men who divorce or are widowed remarry within 4 years (Tanner, 2009). With remarriage, children become members of blended families. Blended families can present unique parenting challenges in family adaptation, cohesiveness, coping, and role relationships.

Assessment

Assessing how the children are coping with the significant changes in their lives and realignment of family roles can help both the provider and the parents direct their attention (Box 17-7).

Management

The goal of primary care interventions is to foster positive parenting behaviors, protect the development of the children, and enhance family functioning. Some counseling tips are listed in Box 17-7. Carefully assess any behavioral concerns. Whether the family is given guidance and followed closely by the primary care provider or given a referral to mental health services depends on the presence of significant behavioral or mental health problems. Providers should investigate community services that assist blended families, such as a self-help group for stepparents or a parenting group. Written information including telephone numbers of community resources should be maintained in a handbook or resource guide kept in the practice setting.

Patient Education and Prevention

Before remarriage, counseling and guidance that looks at coping with transition in a blended family should be explored with parents. Many children go on to develop strong and meaningful attachments to their stepparents if the relationship is cultivated over time with careful sensitivity to the needs of the child.

ADOPTIVE PARENT FAMILIES
Description

Adoption is the legal process that gives individuals who are not birth parents legal and permanent parental responsibility for children. Birth parents terminate their rights, and the adoptive parent(s) are awarded legal custody. Thus a new nuclear family is created.

Adoptive parents come in every variety—married couples, single parents, intrafamily adoption, subsidized adoption of

BOX 17-7	Assessment of and Counseling Tips for Children in Blended Families

Assessment

Developmental Stage of Child

- Age and developmental stage of child greatly affect child's response to the remarriage and ability of child to cope with change and new family relationships.
- Early adolescence is often a time of greatest difficulty in adjustment to remarriage.
- A mother's subsequent pregnancy is often a time of increased frequency and intensity of problems with young children.

Common Issues for Children in Blended Families

- Complex relationship with new family members
- Altered relationships with own family members and possible feelings of betraying other biologic parent or being torn between parents
- Possible relocation and separation from family members and friends
- Continued or new tensions between parents and tensions between stepparents; rivalries between parents and stepparents
- Jealousy among stepsiblings
- Establishing new family traditions and values
- Continuing to respect earlier family history, traditions, and loyalties that may be in conflict with new family ties
- Unrealistic expectations by child of stepparent
- Unrealistic expectations by stepparent for instant love, respect, and obedience from child
- Tensions within blended family household, creating anxiety and fear of another family breakup

Characteristics of Problem Behaviors in Blended Families

- Problems can occur at home and at school.
- Children in divorced and blended families experience more behavioral, social, emotional, and educational problems than do children from nondivorced families.
- Parental conflict more than family structure is the critical factor that influences both marital and family adjustment.

Counseling Tips

- Discuss upcoming changes with your child before remarriage and address possible fears, feelings, and expectations.
- Keep the marriage strong by a nurturing husband-and-wife relationship.
- Blended-family parents need to agree on discipline issues, how to set limits, and type of discipline; remembering to be consistent.
- Start new family traditions, such as weekly family meetings.
- Be patient and as flexible as possible; do not expect your child(ren) to have an immediate positive relationship with the new stepparent.
- Spend quiet, alone time with your child as much as possible and preferably every day.
- Do not force your child to align with the new parent and remember that a second parent does not replace the first; support and help maintain the relationship of your child with the other birthparent.

children with special needs, gay and lesbian parents, grandparents, or other extended family members. Independent, identified, and international adoptions; surrogacy arrangements; and open adoptions are examples of various forms of adoption. Public and private agencies, independent adoption through attorneys, and foreign adoption services are potential avenues to assist in the placement of children.

Epidemiology

Since 1975, with the dissolution of the National Center for Social Statistics, there have been no federal agencies or nonprofit organizations collecting data on the annual number of total adoptions in the U.S. The Adoption and Safe Families Act of 1997 requires states to collect information about the adoptions of children in public foster care, but these are the only adoption-related statistics regularly reported by governments. Beyond that, most statistics kept today are kept by private agencies. The Adoption History Project (AHP) (2010) reports that even at the height of their popularity in 1970 when 175,000 adoptions were reported, adoption is rare, with 125,000 adoptions per year in the U.S. However, as adoption has become more visible with growing numbers of transracial and international adoptions producing families in which parents and children look nothing alike, attention attracted by these adoptive families has led many Americans to believe that adoption is increasing.

Assessment

Assessment of these families includes asking about the legal status of the adoption, the timing of the adoption in the child's life, arrangements regarding involvement of the birth parents or other family members, decisions about how and when to

tell the child about being adopted, and potential health concerns related to the birth parents or family, if known.

Important information that the provider should attempt to ascertain when assisting adoptive families includes the following:

- Legal arrangements and circumstances surrounding adoption process
- What, if any, contact will the birth parent or parents have with the child
- Timing of finalization of the adoption and length of waiting period
- Support services available for the adoptive family if an agency is arranging the adoption
- Knowledge of medical and psychosocial history of birth parents and child
- Any known or suspected medical (including growth and development) problems
- Information about the pregnancy, delivery, and neonatal period or subsequent medical problems
- Children adopted from foreign countries can be at risk for medical problems. Routine recommended screening tests are outlined in Box 17-8. If the reliability of prior vaccination history is questionable, an acceptable practice is to repeat the vaccinations (AAP, 2009).

Management

Often parents request a preadoption consultation. This is an ideal time to review any identified issues. Other families may be in a foster care situation and considering adoption. Support through this process, before adoption is finalized, is crucial because there may be many hurdles with which to contend. Once adoption is finalized, close monitoring and support by

---

BOX 17-8 Recommended Screening Tests for Children Adopted from Foreign Countries

- Newborn metabolic screening panel (all infants)
- Complete blood count with differential, platelet count, and indices
- Iron studies (ferritin, serum iron, iron saturation)
- Vitamin D (250 A total vitamin D), calcium, phosphorus
- Thyroid stimulating hormone, free thyroxine
- Urinalysis
- Lead level
- Tuberculin skin test, despite any previous BCG vaccination; if positive result, obtain chest x-ray (see Chapter 23)
- Stool for ova and parasites, *Giardia* antigen, and *Cryptosporidium*
- Hepatitis B panel, including surface antibody and antigen and core antibody
- Hepatitis C antibody
- Syphilis serology
- HIV elisa
- Developmental, dental, hearing, and vision screening
- Hemoglobin electrophoresis (Asian, Latin-American, and African children)
- G-6-phosphate dehydrogenase assay (Asian, Mediterranean, and African children)
- Malaria (PCR) (children from tropical or subtropical regions and those with fever of unknown origin)
- Rickets (radiograph) (Chinese children)
- Lactose intolerance (black, Latino, American-Indian, and Asian children)

BCG, Bacille Calmette-Guérin; *HIV*, human immunodeficiency virus; *PCR*, polymerase chain reaction.

---

the primary care provider during the initial adoption period are important. Scheduling of additional or more frequent health supervision visits is appropriate even when all appears well, but especially if high-risk situations or conditions are identified. If problems arise, prompt referral to specialty medical services, mental health, or social service agencies is imperative. Children with known special needs who are adopted are often eligible for federal and state financial support and services. The presence of a social support network is important. Adoptive parents face the same parenting challenges as biologic parents do when their child passes through the various developmental stages of childhood. In addition, adoption is a lifelong commitment that can present special challenges for parents. Excellent books about adoption for adults and children are available.

Families adopting children with special needs may require extra assistance with family bonding, behavioral, mental health, and physical needs. Such families seek social support when experiencing emotional pain, using informal social support systems first and then looking for professional help when other interventions have been found inadequate, often as a crisis intervention. These families need preventive resources, reassurance of competence, and encouragement to strengthen social support networks before child placement.

Patient Education and Prevention

When considering adoption, parents often benefit from a preadoption visit to the health care provider who will take care of their child. Parents often have many questions about the

initial adoption period and the establishment of a family relationship. Issues that the provider should address with parents include the following:

- There should be a gradual disclosure of the adoption to the child. Such disclosure should be done earlier rather than later, and children should always be told the truth about where they came from and why they were adopted.
- Discussions of the adoption should be open, keeping in mind the child's developmental stage, cognitive abilities, and emotional needs. It is important for adoptive parents to reassure the child in words and actions that he or she is loved, and the adoptive parents will always be there for the child.
- Discussions with the parents should address any myths, concerns, or fears that the parents might have about adoption and their adopted child.
- Parents need to understand that their child's wish to know about or seek out the biologic parents is not a rejection of them.
- Adolescence can be difficult for adoptive children as they seek their own identity and deal with the fact that they are adopted. If teenagers wish to seek out their biologic parents, states usually will not release information until after the child is 18 years of age.
- Adoption of an older child may present an extra challenge, especially if the child has been shuffled between homes or emotionally scarred by abuse or neglect. Telling parents about such challenges can help them to be better prepared to handle some of the difficulties that may lie ahead for their family and seek counseling early if needed.

■ Variations in the Family Unit

There are a number of variations in the family unit. Some reflect changes in American family life and the diversity of parental experiences. Each situation is unique and requires a thorough assessment. Discussion regarding key issues related to some of these variations follows.

ADOLESCENT PARENTS
Description

Adolescents who become parents generally face the problems inherent when a major role is assumed before the adolescent is developmentally ready. Adolescent parents have developmental needs of their own and, not infrequently, their needs are in conflict with those of their children. Adolescent pregnancy is marked by lower self-esteem, poorer educational and vocational outcomes, and socioeconomic disadvantages for the mother. Often adolescent mothers feel isolated, exhausted, and depressed. Children of adolescent mothers are more likely than children of older mothers to have a low birth weight, to have ongoing health problems during childhood, to grow up in homes without fathers, and to be raised in poverty or near poverty. They are also at high risk for cognitive delays, behavioral problems, and difficulties in schooling (Hoffman, 2008). Some teens can successfully parent their infant if given support. However preexisting family and individual factors that lead a teenager to become a mother before completing the educational and developmental tasks necessary for adult life are more relevant predictors of successful parenting.

Epidemiology

The birth rate for U.S. teenagers ages 15 to 19 fell 6 percent to 39.1 per 1,000 in 2009, a record low for the nation. Birth rates for younger and older teenagers and for Hispanic, non-Hispanic white, non-Hispanic black, American Indian or Alaska Native, and Asian or Pacific Islander teenagers all reached historic lows in 2009 (National Center for Health Statistics, 2010).

Assessment

Questions that can help formulate an idea about the environment in which a child will be raised include exploring the adolescent parent's own support system, attitudes toward parenting, and source of parenting advice. In addition, it is helpful to understand the adolescent's school status, child care arrangements, financial situation, and plans for the future. Assessment of at-risk status varies depending on the stage of the teen. Addressing issues that arise during pregnancy, at birth, and in infancy can contribute to a more successful pregnancy outcome and prevent problems from appearing later in the child's or teen parent's life.

Before Pregnancy

- Adolescent sexuality is an issue that should be discussed routinely at every health care encounter (see Chapter 18). Early identification and targeting of at-risk teens (both female and male) for intervention is an important role of the provider. Predictors of teen motherhood are listed in Box 17-9.

Pregnancy

- Disclosure of pregnancy to family, the baby's father, peers, or other significant people. Who has the teen told about the pregnancy? Are they supportive?
- Access to prenatal care and adherence to pregnancy health supervision guidelines; referral to Women, Infants, and Children (WIC) program and community health nurse
- Support for remaining in school during pregnancy
- Adjustment to the emotional and physical changes of pregnancy
- Preparation and plans for the delivery and after the baby is born: current living arrangements; plans for future living and childcare arrangements, returning to school or work, and financial support; identifying primary care provider for child; identifying and applying for health care insurance for infant and mother.

Birth and Postpartum

- Preparation for childbirth and postpartum care
- Identification of people available to give emotional support and physical help

---

BOX 17-9 Predictors of Teen Motherhood

- Sexual molestation as a child
- Abuse or neglect in childhood
- Being a child of an addicted parent
- Family history of mental illness
- Lack of family involvement; an intolerable home situation as defined by the teen
- Poor academic achievement or school dropout
- Loss of a parent by death, separation, divorce, or foster placement
- Living in an impoverished social environment where adolescent pregnancy is commonplace and accepted
- Confusion about own sexual orientation

Infancy

- Adolescent mother-infant attachment. Is there evidence of healthy attachment or emotional or physical neglect?
- Confidence and ability of teen mother to care for her infant.
- Conflicts between the teen's needs and those of her infant. Is the mother more interested in reestablishing her adolescent lifestyle or caring for her infant?
- Living arrangements: with whom and where are the teen mother and baby living?
- Plans for birth control
- Degree of involvement of the social support network in the mother's and infant's life. Is the baby's father invested in the child? Support from extended family?
- Return to school or the workforce. What are the child care arrangements?
- Adequacy of financial resources

Later Years. Toddler years are challenging, particularly for teens who themselves are survivors of abuse or neglectful parenting. Typically the teen mother and young child, if living with family, move out on their own or move in with the mother's partner. The provider needs to assess the following:

- Mother's ability to cope with the variety of toddler behaviors
- How well the family unit is functioning
- Progress made by the mother toward reaching her life goals

As the child gets older the teen mother is thought of as a young mother. Children of these mothers, especially those who are poor and living in urban settings, are more likely than their peers to have behavioral problems. When their own children are adolescents, they find this a particularly difficult period, and often they become young grandmothers as the teen pregnancy circle is perpetuated.

Management

Key points in management include the following:

- Maintain regular and frequent contact with the teen mother during her pregnancy and during the child's infancy and early childhood.
- Refer to a community health nurse for home visits early in pregnancy and postpartum. This intervention has proven most successful in delaying subsequent pregnancy and improving healthy parenting and family life.
- Provide referrals for resources and community agencies that can assist teen mothers (e.g., parenting classes or literature; support groups; special clinic programs that see both infants and teen mothers; WIC program; early child intervention programs provided by school districts and Head Start).
- Remember that the teen mother and the infant or child has their own separate needs for health supervision and guidance.
- Provide a supportive environment for the teen mother. Have a plan for follow-up so that teen mothers do not get lost in the system.
- Involve other family members (e.g., grandparents, the father) in discussions about child-rearing issues depending on the teen's wishes.
- Emphasize the strengths of the teen mother and praise her positive efforts.
- Intervene early when warning signs of potential neglect or abuse are evident.
- Facilitate further education to minimize effects of poverty on child rearing.

CHILDREN LIVING WITH GRANDPARENTS OR EXTENDED FAMILY MEMBERS

Of the 2.8 million children living with someone other than their parents in 2009, 54% of them lived with grandparents. Thirty-four percent were under five years of age, 48.6% were ages 6 to 14, and 17.4% were 15 to 17 years of age (Forum on Child and Family Statistics, 2009). The reasons why grandparents assume parenting responsibility for their grandchildren vary, but they rarely do so unless the parent is unable or unwilling to parent. In the U.S., substance abuse (40%) and child neglect are primary reasons (Goodman et al, 2004). Death of a parent, parental immaturity, and incarceration also are reasons for placement with grandparents.

Grandparents face significant legal issues around custody, adoption, guardianship, and foster care. Trying to enroll a grandchild in school can lead to a minefield of legal issues. In addition, although some states provide financial assistance to grandparents, others do not. Grandparents may have difficulty accessing and paying for health care. For example, some insurance carriers do not allow grandchildren as dependents. More than 90% of grandparents do not receive social security and 85% do not receive public assistance. Only a few have foster family status, which would provide some help with child care, remuneration, developmental assessments, and tutoring. Grandparents may be in their 30s or their 80s, and may have boundless or flagging energy. They may still be active in a job they love, or they may have looked forward to enjoying their retirement and new challenges. They may be thrilled to be parenting again, or they may be clinically depressed. There is no "one size fits all" template.

The incidence of diabetes, hypertension, depression, and coronary heart disease is greater among caregiving grandparents than it is for noncaregiving grandparents (Hayslip and Kaminski, 2005). Compounding the practical economic and health issues are the psychological and emotional responses of all involved. Grief, anger, confusion, resentment, and depression can describe reactions of grandparents and their grandchildren. At the same time, relief that the grandchildren are safe, loved, and nurtured can be present. Sensitivity and openness to grandparents can allow them to express their ambivalence and concerns. Expressed respect and appreciation can help form a working partnership.

Knowledge of resources can be especially helpful. The AARP has a website for grandparents, which lists excellent resources, including information for grandparents parenting grandchildren. The site includes information about financial assistance, including the Temporary Assistance to Needy Families (TANF) program, online and community-based support groups, books and other literature, and a wide range of other resources. Support groups have been shown to be helpful in reducing the stress of raising grandchildren.

Providers should be alert to the following as they work with grandparents who are caregivers:

- Often children have lived with one or two biologic parents before either voluntary or court-ordered placement with the grandparent.
- Children can be involved in continuing conflict with their biologic parent or parents and may experience emotional reaction to separation from or abandonment by the parent(s).
- Children can experience the loss of friends, schoolmates, and familiar surroundings.
- Children need a supportive environment and consistency in discipline.
- Families may need significant support from social service agencies, the educational system, and health care providers.

CHILDREN LIVING WITH TWO PARENTAL FIGURES WHO ARE UNMARRIED—COHABITATION

Children can be the biologic children of two adults who decide not to marry but live together (cohabitation), the biologic children of one of the adults but not the other, or children who live with their guardian and the guardian's unmarried partner. In each of these family situations, the development of a high-quality parent-child relationship, consistency in discipline, and a continued commitment to the child are hallmarks of successful parenting and childrearing.

- Children face significant developmental risks if they sense a lack of permanence or certainty in their lives; if family life is characterized by conflict or poverty; or if there is inconsistency in who lives in the home, frequent breakups, new adult relationships, or frequent changes in living arrangements.
- Children can be torn emotionally if other significant adults in the children's lives (other biologic parents, grandparents, or other extended family members) express distress about the relationship between the unmarried adults.
- Cohabitation tends to be a short-term arrangement with about 55% of couples marrying and 40% dissolving in 5 years (Garfield, 2009).
- Many families who cohabitate live with higher levels of stress, conflict, and ambiguity as well as fewer economic resources that have the potential to negatively affect the children involved (Garfield, 2009).

CHILDREN LIVING IN FOSTER OR GROUP HOMES

Children are generally placed in protective custody because of concerns of neglect, physical abuse, sexual abuse, or other forms of child maltreatment or because their parents are unable to care for them. Some children are placed in foster care because they need specialized medical, psychiatric or mental health, and developmental assistance beyond the ability of their biologic parents to provide. The children may need to be removed from a chaotic and unsafe family environment. They may have been abandoned or orphaned. These children, first and foremost, are at risk for deep-seated feelings of insecurity, loss, and anger. They often perceive themselves as different; they must learn coping strategies; they encounter difficulties with the foster care system and must cope with transitions between foster homes and the lack of a medical home (Ellerman, 2007).

The number of children in foster homes is increasing, and meeting their psychosocial needs is a growing problem in the U.S. About half of all foster children live in family foster homes with nonrelatives; about 25% live with relatives. Only 52% of the 285,000 who exited foster care were reunited with their families (Child Welfare Information

Gateway, 2010). Data collected by the Administration for Children and Families (ACF) noted that as of July 29, 2010, there were 424,000 children in foster care placements in the U.S. compared with 523,000 children at the same time in 2002. These foster care numbers are more meaningful when analyzed more fully. There were 276,000 children who exited foster family placement, 57,000 who were adopted (54% adopted by their foster parents), 255,000 who entered care that year (a decreasing number), 115,000 waiting to be adopted, and 70,000 whose parental rights had been terminated (USDHHS, 2010b).

Assessment of these families includes exploration of the child's history that resulted in foster family placement, identification of health issues that precipitated or resulted from separation from the birth parents, and evaluation of the foster parent.

Foster parents have a difficult role in society. They want to be treated with respect and to have their care and knowledge of the foster child acknowledged. They want to have the assistance they need to provide the best care possible to the children in their care. They report feeling great loss with relinquishment and death, and find parenting a child with a chronic or complex medical need to be a life-changing experience (Lauver, 2008). Often they report that their concerns and needs often are not recognized by health care professionals (Pasztor et al, 2006). Exploring concerns the foster parent has with his or her parenting, with attention not only to the child's needs, but also to the foster family's needs, may help establish a working relationship that can benefit all (Lauver, 2008; Pasztor et al, 2006). Again, providing resources can be helpful. The Child Welfare League of America's website has excellent information and resources about and for family foster care providers. In addition, the National Foster Parent Association provides support and caregiving information for foster families.

- Children frequently have a history of significant stress, hardship, and emotional turmoil in their family life.
- Children can experience multiple placements and separation from siblings—40% of children in foster care placement for more than 1 year experience three or four placements (Christian and Blum, 2006).
- Foster children are often involved in family reunification programs and are placed back with their parents under the supervision of the child protective services.
- Foster children are placed under legal mandates in foster homes that mirror the children's ethnic, racial, and cultural identities as much as possible.
- Foster children often receive disjointed health care; a medical passport can be used as a means to keep track of medical problems, treatments, and special needs. However, a complete past medical history often requires extensive inquiry of past services delivered by emergency departments and other care providers (obtain release-of-information confirmation from the state agency who has legal custody of the child).
- Foster children have special needs, should be followed closely, and should receive preventive health services.
- Children are emancipated from the foster care system at 18 years old and need to be prepared for this major life change. It is reported that a high majority of these adolescents end up on the streets if they are not ready for living independently (National Coalition for the Homeless, 2009).

CHILDREN LIVING WITH HOMOSEXUAL PARENTS

Children living in families headed by a gay or lesbian parent or a same-sex couple have similar family lives and developmental outcomes of children of heterosexual couples (Tasker, 2005). Gay and lesbian parents face the same problems as all parents do, with an added concern about societal attitudes and behavior that add stress to their lives and the lives of their children (Weber, 2008).

- Children living with homosexual parents may be the "biologic products" of former heterosexual relationships; they may have been adopted, or they may have been conceived by assisted reproduction (i.e., egg or sperm donation, artificial insemination). These families reflect every ethnic, racial, and socioeconomic group in the U.S.
- Many studies have demonstrated that children of homosexual parents show no significant differences in their emotional and social adaptation, self-esteem, gender identity, sexual behavior, or sexual orientation than their counterparts raised by heterosexual parents (Garfield, 2009).
- Children can experience problems because of social stigmatization, secrecy of parents, isolation from extended family, or negative reaction of the noncustodial, biologic parents (Garfield, 2009).
- Children do well if the homosexual relationship is healthy, and if the stepparent is supportive of the other parent and the child or children.
- Children find it easier to deal with questions posed about their parents if they learn about their parents' sexual orientation during childhood rather than during adolescence.
- Children are not at risk to develop a homosexual identity based on their living situation.

■ Other Challenges to the Family Unit

Premature births, multiple births, and children with chronic illness or special needs are challenges to the family unit that can cause periods of disequilibrium. Seeking appropriate childcare and dealing with sibling rivalry are other typical concerns.

PREMATURE INFANT

Low-birthweight and premature infants present special issues for new parents. There may be an extended time between the birth of the child and being able to bring the child home. Concerns about the child's physiologic vulnerability may arise. Almost certainly, costs and time commitments around the care of the infant will be increased. Parents may have the same concerns as parents of a full-term newborn, but their fears and anxieties about being responsible for a seemingly fragile newborn may be close to overwhelming. Similar to the situation of a multiple birth, exploring who is caring for the child and who is helping the parents is a priority.

MULTIPLE BIRTHS

A family faced with caring for newborn twins, triplets, or more, even while delighted, can be quickly overwhelmed by the responsibility and amount of work involved. Assessing

| BOX 17-10 | Characteristics Unique to Multiple Birth Children |

- Develop a special sibling relationship marked by loyalty and cooperative play
- Have periods in which they get along well or quarrel with each other just as other siblings do
- Work out relationships among themselves
- Function more independently, needing less parental attention
- Develop their own language among themselves as young children
- Display sibling rivalry, especially if they are fraternal rather than identical twins

parents' level of fatigue, ability to seek and accept support, and plans for ongoing care is useful to both the provider and the parents. Behavioral challenges and the children's own unique relationships can be a challenge (Box 17-10).

Advise parents who have multiple births to do the following:

- Breastfeed if possible. Twins can be breastfed at the same time or one right after the other. Develop a plan to rotate breastfeeding if the mother has more than two infants.
- Organize the home for daily activities and plan ahead to have sufficient supplies and toys.
- Attempt to get twins or triplets on the same schedule (awake, sleep, feeding) as much as possible.
- Schedule daily activities to accomplish all that needs to be done.
- Take time out for themselves and as a couple.
- Keep a sense of humor.
- Promote individuality of each child. Spend individual time with each child.
- Seek out support people to help (e.g., enlist the aid of extended family members) during early infancy when the tasks of physically caring for multiple infants can be overwhelming.
- Contact support groups.

When the children are school age, there is no exact recommendation for classroom placement for multiples. Children of multiple births may find it easier to develop a sense of self and make their own friendships if in separate classrooms. If there are older siblings, encourage parents to be cognizant of their needs and feelings.

CHILDREN WITH CHRONIC ILLNESS OR SPECIAL NEEDS

Children with special needs have been defined by the government as "those who have or are at risk for a chronic physical, developmental, behavioral, or emotional condition and who also require health and related services of a type or amount beyond that required by children generally" (McPherson et al, 1998, p 138). Almost 14% of U.S. children have special needs.

Parents caring for a child with a significant medical or developmental challenge, whether it is a chronic illness, a disabling condition, or a developmental disability, are responsible for their child's daily medical care, monitoring, and management. The care can be minimal or consume hours of every day and night. The monitoring can be casual or meticulous; the management, routine or complex. Survival may be a realistic concern. Parents become medical experts, care coordinators, and systems advocates (Kratz et al, 2009).

Chronic illness in children is relatively rare and widely heterogeneous; nevertheless, it has profound implications for the organization of children's health services, and providers have the challenge of identifying and treating a myriad of conditions (Wise, 2007). National surveys suggest that approximately 30% of all children have some form of chronic condition. The most common chronic illness is asthma, with 13% of children having been diagnosed at some time in their lives; half of these children reported to have experienced asthma symptoms in the previous 12 months. Approximately 8% of children (boys 50% more likely than girls) have been diagnosed with attention-deficit/hyperactivity disorder (ADHD). Obesity (body mass indexes [BMIs] greater than the 95th percentile) affects nearly 17% of all children ages 6 through 19. The incidence of type 2 diabetes is increasing. Although there are not reliable national data regarding mental illness, it is estimated that approximately 5% of children 6 to 19 years of age suffer from depression. Increasing survival rates for children who were premature, have congenital anomalies, or have genetic disorders also contribute to the increased numbers. Of note, as reported in 2008, approximately 6.6% of all children had no health insurance, potentially negatively affecting their overall health status. About 2 million children were unable to get needed medical care because the family couldn't afford it (3%), and medical care for 3.5 million children was delayed because of worry about the cost (5%) (Bloom et al, 2009).

The physical and psychological health of the caregiver is essential to that person's ability to care for the child and family. Raina and colleagues (2005) found that the best predictors of caregiver well-being for 468 families with a child with cerebral palsy were: (1) child behavior, (2) caregiving demands, and (3) family functioning. A study of 36 families caring for technology-dependent children found that time demands around the clock, a lack of trained respite care providers, and limits on school, employment, and social life were significant problems (Heaton et al, 2005). Families "live worried" and are often overwhelmed but feel the need to stay in the struggle on behalf of their child. They also worry about how to survive as a family (Coffey, 2006).

The effect of a chronic illness or disabling condition on a family, including the child, parents, siblings, and extended family, is influenced not only by the diagnosis and its sequelae, but also by the meaning it has for the family and individual members. Families experience grief, both at the time of diagnosis and as a chronic state, perceive a lack of information, and experience inadequacy of relationships with some providers (Kepreotes et al, 2010). Themes of challenge for families of children with disabilities can be grouped into four areas: access to information and services, financial barriers, school and community inclusion, and family support (Resch et al, 2010). Families of children with a developmental disability rated primary care physicians low on understanding the impact of the child's condition on the family (Liptak et al, 2006).

All developmental levels present challenges and opportunities for these families; however, the interface between families and schools around developmental and health issues can be particularly difficult. Parents generally want their child to be placed in a situation in which he or she has the maximal opportunity to be successful.

Parents also want their child to be as "normal" as possible. The process of normalization is important to their health. Parents acknowledge the condition and potential effect, redefine

---

BOX 17-11 Guidelines for Selecting a Childcare Provider: A Four-Step Approach

Step 1: Interview Potential Childcare Providers and Observe the Program or Setting

Start early in your search for an appropriate childcare facility.

Ask questions about:

1. Cost—cost calculation per hour, daily, weekly, monthly; any late fees; policy about fee structure and rules (e.g., if the child is absent)
2. Enrollment—number of children enrolled in the program, the maximum daily capacity of setting, adult-to-child ratio, number of children in a group
3. Child factors—age of the children served in the setting or program
4. Daily activities or program plan—structured vs. unstructured activities
5. Accreditation and licensing regulations related to the provider or setting; review copy of any license or certificate
6. Caretaker issues—credentials and experience and turnover rates (e.g., academic degrees, coursework, staff have current CPR certification)
7. Policies—open visiting, illness in the child requiring school exclusion, emergency care, nutrition and feeding policies, discipline, adult supervision of children at all times
8. Illness prevention—cleanliness of setting, handwashing, immunization requirements for child and staff

Carefully observe the environment:

1. Look at provider-child interactions—check for evidence of nurturing, responsive, comforting interactions.
2. Look at safety issues of the physical environment—the play areas, toileting and diaper changing areas, outdoor environment, napping and eating areas.
3. Assess the quality of the learning materials and toys.

Step 2: Check References

1. Talk to parents with children enrolled in the program or being cared for by the provider; ask about their experience, whether they were nurturing to the children and responsive to parents; ask about reliability and consistency of the providers.
2. Talk to local childcare resource and referral program or licensing office; Child Care Aware provides information about the nearest childcare resource and referral programs.

Step 3: Make a Decision Based on Specific Criteria

1. The child will be happy with this care provider and have a safe, nurturing, and developmentally appropriate environment.
2. If the child has special needs, these will be met.
3. The values of the provider and parents are compatible.
4. The childcare is affordable.

Step 4: Be an Involved Parent

1. Regularly talk to the provider about how the child is doing.
2. Talk to the child daily about activities and experiences at the facility.
3. If possible visit the setting unannounced and observe at various times of day.
4. Communicate with other parents and become involved in childcare events as much as possible.
5. Join in special events (e.g., field trips, holiday activities).

Data from Child Care Aware: 5 steps to choosing quality child care. Available at www.childcareaware.org/en/5steps.

(or adapt) their definition of normal to fit their family, engage in behaviors that fit the definition of normal, develop a treatment regimen that also fits, and interact with others based on the view that the child and family are normal (Knafl et al, 2001). Promoting normalization can be a powerful intervention.

Often parents become medical experts in their child's diagnosis and management as well as in their child's idiosyncratic responses. They expect to be treated seriously and with respect, and set high standards for their child's health care providers. In a classic paper, Thorne and Robinson (1988) described three phases of the relationship between health care providers and health care recipients or family caregivers. *Naive trusting* is the first stage, a time when the family assumed that its perspective is shared by the professionals who care for their family members, the family members' involvement as caregivers is respected and acknowledged, all professionals would be highly knowledgeable and skilled, and that communication would be honest and direct. As ongoing interactions with health care professionals teach families that these assumptions are not always valid, a second phase, characterized by *disenchantment,* occurs. Anger reflects the loss of trust in health care providers, and family members move toward trying to protect their family member. Finally, but not inevitably, family members move to a phase called *guarded alliance.* The no longer naive family members are able to reconstruct trust on a more sophisticated level, sharing it only with individual professionals who earn it.

Providers working with families of children with chronic illness should assess family systems for the risk of emotional

and financial stress and its consequences, most notably maltreatment of the child. Chapter 21 provides a discussion of issues for care providers to consider when working with children who have chronic illness and their families.

CHILD CARE

Parents are challenged with selecting a qualified child care provider who provides a safe, nurturing, and developmentally appropriate setting. The individual needs of the child together with parental needs for work coverage and flexibility must be matched with the philosophy and constraints of the child care setting. The primary care provider is often called on to advise parents about how to select a suitable provider. A four-step approach developed by Child Care Aware (2010) is recommended as a guideline for parents (Box 17-11).

SIBLING RIVALRY

The birth or adoption of a sibling is a life-changing experience for the older sibling. Many parents voice concerns about the potential challenges with the older siblings, especially transient behavioral regressions occurring after a new infant is brought home. The developmental stage of the older sibling at the time of the new sibling's arrival is an important consideration in helping parents prepare their older child for the new sibling and in dealing with rivalry behaviors afterward. For example, the 2-year-old who is working on developing autonomy often feels highly vulnerable with the appearance of a new sibling.

Additionally, many school-age children experience feelings of sibling rivalry, which may continue in varying degrees as the children grow and develop. Sibling rivalry involves the realization by the child that he or she must share his or her parents' attention and affection. The child may feel threatened or displaced.

Assessment

To assess sibling rivalry after the arrival of a new infant, ask the parent whether the older child has:
- Manifested regressive behaviors since the new sibling arrived (e.g., bed-wetting, return to the bottle, temper tantrums, separation issues)
- Made negative comments about the new sibling or has demonstrated verbal or physical aggression toward the parents or new sibling
- Voiced psychosomatic complaints

To assess sibling rivalry at any point, ask parents to:
- Describe sibling behaviors that concern them—fighting, verbal abuse, bickering.
- Identify any precipitating events or situations that seem to elicit negative behaviors between the siblings.
- Identify how rivalry behaviors between siblings were handled in the past and encourage the siblings to resolve the issues between them rather than the parents trying to resolve issues.

The provider should also ask parents to describe how they have reacted to the behaviors or verbal comments and if and how they have disciplined the child.

Management

Anticipatory guidance about this common challenge is critical. The provider needs to prepare parents before the arrival of the new sibling for the possibility of sibling rivalry and guide them in managing this situation. Before delivery or adoption:
- Explain to parents that at the time of the arrival of the new baby the other sibling(s) may exhibit regressive behaviors.
- Encourage parents to do the following:
  - Tell the child about the pregnancy or adoption of the new baby, using a time frame and language appropriate to child's developmental stage.
  - Investigate the possibility of sibling preparation classes for older siblings.
  - Prepare the child for changes in the daily routines and change in the time he or she will have with the parents; give children realistic expectations of their interactions with the baby.
- Include an older child in preparations for new baby and in the excitement of the event (e.g., have the child visit the mother and baby in the hospital if possible.)

After the infant or child comes home:
- Encourage parents to consistently spend time with the older sibling to include the older sibling in the care of the new baby.
- Explain the need for tolerance when a child exhibits regressive behaviors, knowing the behaviors are not permanent.
- Educate parents about teaching children to distinguish between acceptable and unacceptable behaviors as well as accountability for negative behaviors.

BOX 17-12 | Managing Sibling Rivalry

Do

Allow children to vent negative feelings.
Encourage children to develop solutions for problems with siblings.
Anticipate problem situations.
Foster individuality in each child.
Spend time with children individually.
Compliment children when they are playing together.
Tell children about the conflict you had with your siblings when you were a child.
Define acceptable and unacceptable behaviors for sibling interactions.

Do Not

Take sides.
Serve as a referee.
Foster rivalry by comparing siblings or their accomplishments.
Use derogatory names.
Permit physical or verbal abuse between siblings.

Literature in general encourages nonintervention for minor squabbles, encouraging child-centered articulation of more significant arguments, and parental intervention if physical or verbal abuse occurs (Anderson, 2006). Box 17-12 has other strategies to help siblings learn to live together.

■ Circumstances Affecting Families

Poverty, homelessness, military deployment and death are challenges to the family unit that can cause periods of disequilibrium.

CHILDREN LIVING IN POVERTY

Families are facing poverty in increasing numbers, and children are the most at risk. Thirteen million children (18%) lived in poverty in 2008, living in two-parent, single parent, employed or unemployed households; 32% of children living with their single-parent mother were classified as living in poverty; 27% of children lived in households where no parent had full-time, year-round employment (Annie E. Casey Foundation, 2010). These figures precede the recession and job losses of 2008-2011. African-American and Native American families are especially affected.

In some states welfare reform has resulted in the working poor, who make too much to qualify for subsidized health care, having to choose between keeping a job that helps feed their family or meeting their children's health needs (Annie E. Casey Foundation, 2010). Impoverished women enrolled in the Temporary Assistance for Needy Families (TANF) program, which was intended to bring welfare mothers back into employment, have faced significant problems in many places. Immigrant women in the country for less than 5 years are not eligible for the TANF program. The low-wage jobs most TANF recipients are prepared for do not pull them out of poverty. Further, they face the conflict of working to pay for food and shelter versus overseeing the health, safety, and education of their children. Few have employer health insurance, few can pay for quality daycare, and many work two jobs to make ends meet, further separating them in time, place, and energy from their children. If women terminate from the TANF program, they have neither work nor welfare support. Greater than 60% report mental and physical health problems in themselves and at least one of their children (Hildebrandt and Stevens, 2009).

DISPLACED OR HOMELESS CHILDREN AND THEIR FAMILIES

The number of homeless children in the U.S. is growing, with substance abuse and poverty as prime reasons for this increase. Homeless children and their families have difficulty with the most basic needs of food, shelter, and clothing. Accessing education and health care may be difficult to impossible. The health care visit may be in response to a crisis that could not be denied, but assessment should include well-child care, including immunizations, on the operating principle that every child should receive the maximum care possible. About 1 in 50 children (1.5 million) were homeless in the United States in 2008 (National Center on Family Homelessness, 2010). According to the National Coalition for the Homeless (2009), 41% of the homeless population is comprised of families. Seventy-one percent of cities surveyed reported an increase in the number of families with children seeking assistance (National Coalition for the Homeless, 2009; U.S. Conference of Mayors, 2007). Rural and suburban communities are increasingly plagued by the problem.

Characteristics of these homeless children include:
- Living in poverty because of limited employment opportunities, low wages, lack of affordable housing, no medical insurance, and inadequate social support services
- Living in families with a history of substance abuse, domestic violence, mental illness, or unexpected family or economic crisis
- The majority of these children are younger than 5 years old
- Runaway adolescents who are often victims of physical or sexual abuse and neglect or teens alienated from their parents for multiple reasons
- Living in a variety of environments, such as a car, motel, makeshift shelters, or homeless shelters; often children and parents in families are separated
- Poor school attendance: only 77% of homeless children attend school regularly
- Health care problems (Box 17-13)

MILITARY DEPLOYMENT

Since 2001, 1.5 million active duty and reserve forces have been deployed around the world, with one third of them having served at least two tours in a combat zone (Johnson et al, 2007). Approximately 2 million children are living in military families—41% of the children are birth to age 5 years, 31.4% are 6 to 11 years, 23.8% are age 12 to 18 years, and 3.8% are ages 19 to 23 (Lemmon and Chartrand, 2009; Perou, 2010). Having a parent sent to an active combat zone with an undetermined return date may rank as one of the most stressful events of childhood. Children in such situations may be vulnerable, especially as the coping resources of the remaining parent (or guardian) may be compromised by his or her own distress and uncertainty. Most of what children and adolescents experience and comprehend is based on their developmental level or mental age (Lincoln et al, 2008). A study conducted by Chandra and associates (2010) revealed several interesting findings about the experience of children in military families. They found that children had more emotional difficulties compared with their peers; older youth and girls of all ages reported significantly more school, family, and peer-related difficulties with parental deployment; and the length of parental deployment and the poorer the nondeployed caregiver's mental health, the greater number of challenges for children both during deployment and deployed-parent reintegration (e.g., children experienced greater role-shifting during deployment and reintegration). Protective and risk factors have been identified. Protective factors include resilience, family preparedness, mental health status of at-home parent, and active coping style. Risk factors include history of rigid coping styles, family dysfunction, young families (especially first military separation), families recently moved to a new duty station, foreign-born spouse, families with young children, families without unit affiliation, pregnancy, and dual-career or single parents (Perou, 2010). Primary care providers are in a unique position to recognize the psychological strain on these children and their families, initiate referrals to mental health providers when indicated, and provide support and resources.

DEATH IN THE FAMILY

Death in families is traumatic and disruptive. It is discussed in Chapter 19 as a grief and bereavement issue.

■ Role-Relationship Problems
VIOLENCE
Description
Violence is the outcome of aggressive behavior that becomes destructive and results in physical injury to people or damage to property. Violence has been acknowledged as a major social and public health problem, and it has become a way of life for many of today's youth, who are either perpetrators, victims, or

---

BOX 17-13 Health Care Problems for Which Homeless Children Are at Risk

- Tuberculosis
- Multiple caries
- Impetigo
- Social isolation at school because of an unkempt appearance
- Poor hygiene
- Substandard living conditions leading to possible unsanitary conditions
- Mental health problems, including social isolation at school (e.g., due to unkempt appearance)
- Early initiation of and sustained substance abuse
- Sexually transmitted infections (STIs) for runaway teens and for those who prostitute themselves; pregnancy
- Abuse due to increased vulnerability in multifamily/people habitation and family stress

witnesses of violent acts. Characteristic features of violence are listed in Box 17-14.

Five main categories of violence can have an effect on children and their families:
- Domestic violence, including child abuse, corporal punishment, sibling violence, and spousal abuse
- Predatory violence (e.g., a crime or assault)
- Peer violence, such as fighting, gang violence, and bullying (that can become violent)
- Sexual assault and rape
- Dating violence including date rape

There is no one cause of violent behavior. Violence has certain antecedents, such as a situational crisis, and risk factors have been identified that increase the likelihood of violent behavior (e.g., abuse of alcohol). Developmental and environmental factors contribute to violence (e.g., impulsivity in young children; poverty and limited resources); however,

not all individuals exposed to such factors resort to violence. Violence is, in large part, a learned behavior, and what children are taught, by example and instruction, becomes part of their methods of social interaction. Effective management of violence in families and communities depends on understanding major influences and key risk factors that contribute to or sustain violence (Box 17-15).

Bullying can be considered aggressive behavior and can be an antecedent to violence. Bullying, as defined for research purposes is "repeated negative behavior by one or more individuals aimed at a person who is perceived as being weaker or more vulnerable" (Glew et al, 2010, p E68). Physical threats, verbal humiliation, malicious rumors, and social ostracism are types of bullying.

Epidemiology

Bullying is common among elementary school children, even being considered a normal developmental phenomenon comparable to toddler tantrums or sibling rivalry. Self-reported grade school bullying is reported as 12% to 19% with increased levels occurring through eighth grade. Playground observation revealed rates as high as 77% in third through sixth graders. Bullying becomes a problem when it is rewarded or ignored or the child doesn't move to more mature ways of influencing others (Glew et al, 2010).

Homicide and injury are typically the end results of violence. Although murders of children have decreased significantly in the past few years (the good news), they continue to be the second leading cause of death for all children ages 10 to 24 years and the leading cause of death for African-Americans. In 2009, 32% of high school students reported being in a physical fight over the previous 12 months; and nearly 6% of high school students reported taking a gun, knife, or club to school 30 days prior to being surveyed. Additionally, 20% of

---

BOX 17-14 | **Key Features Characteristic of Violence**

- Continuity: Once it is used as a coping mechanism, violence becomes a habit that is hard to break.
- Reciprocity: Violence generates violent behavior in others, increasing tension and eliciting negative responses.
- Sameness: One form of violence becomes as acceptable as another. As its use becomes more common, violence permeates all of one's life.
- Addiction: Violence gives a sense of power and control that, although temporary, is addictive.
- Limitations of options or alternative actions: Reasoning is difficult in violent situations, and problem-solving abilities are not used.
- Escalation: Violence begets more frequent and more intense violence, with potential for serious sequelae.

BOX 17-15 | Major Influences That Contribute to or Sustain Violence

Family Influences	**Individual Influences**	**Economic Influences**	**Societal and Environmental Influences**
• Authoritarian childrearing attitudes	• Low IQ	• The child poverty rate in the U.S. is among the highest in the developed world, with approximately 18% of children living in poverty (Annie E. Casey Foundation, 2010)	• Exposure to violence in the media and at school
• Harsh, lax, or inconsistent disciplinary practices	• Poor behavioral control		• Easy access to weapons, alcohol, and other drugs
• Low parental involvement and/or education	• Deficits in social, cognitive, or information-processing abilities		• Lead poisoning
• Low emotional attachment to parents or caregivers	• Attention deficits, hyperactivity, learning disorder, easily frustrated, difficulty making transitions	• Great disparity in the poverty rates based on ethnic group with black children and Native American children especially affected	• Diminished economic opportunities
• Poor family functioning or high levels of family disruption	• Antisocial beliefs and attitudes		• High level of transience
• Poor monitoring and supervision of children	• High emotional distress, history of early aggressive behavior or treatment for emotional problems	• Factors associated with poverty:	• High concentration of poor residents
• Parental substance abuse or criminality	• Exposure to violence and family conflict	◦ Poor housing	• Low levels of community participation
	• Involvement with drugs, alcohol, or tobacco	◦ Malnutrition	• Socially disorganized neighborhood
	• History of violent victimization or involvement (e.g., history of date rape)	◦ Transience	
	• No sense of a future or hope for a better life	◦ Lack of connectedness to schools and community	

high school students reported being bullied on school property (National Center for Injury Prevention and Control, 2010).

Boys are more likely to perpetrate violence and are more often victims of violence, except for sexual assault. Girls engage in silent and indirect aggressive behaviors (Christian and Blum, 2006; Simmons, 2002).

Although there are major differences in rates of violence-related injuries and death by ethnic groups, the majority of homicides involve people who know each other and are of the same race. The typical scenario is played out as follows: an argument occurs, alcohol or drugs have been consumed, a weapon is available and used, and a homicide is the end result. The direct and indirect costs in medical expenses, loss of productivity, and decreased quality of life are immense.

Assessment

The assessment of youths who are victims or perpetrators of violent crime should focus on certain key pieces of historical information and the presence of risk factors to help determine the potential for future violence (Table 17-2). If possible, the youth and parent(s) should be interviewed separately.

- History of the episode
  - What seemed to cause the incident?
  - Did the child or family know who was involved, or was this a random event?
  - Were alcohol and/or drugs involved?
  - Did either the victim or the perpetrator have or threaten to use a weapon? If yes, what type of weapon?
- Past history
  - Have there been incidents of violence or assault?
  - What is the usual pattern of drug or alcohol use?
  - Does the child have a history of mental health problems, or was the youth a victim of child abuse?
  - Does the youth have a criminal or police history?
  - Is he or she a loner with weak social ties? Do the youth's friends engage in antisocial or delinquent behavior?
  - Is there gang involvement or membership, or do friends carry weapons?
  - Does the youth have access to or carry a weapon or weapons?
- Family and social history
  - Does the youth feel safe at home and in his or her neighborhood? How is the youth supervised by his or her parent(s)?
  - Is there a family history of child abuse, substance abuse, domestic violence, mental illness, fighting at home, or a criminal record?
  - Are there handguns or rifles in the home?
  - Does anyone in the home use drugs or have a problem with alcohol?
  - Is the youth attending school? If yes, have there been any academic or behavioral problems?
  - Does the youth have a job? How is free time spent? Are the youth's friends in gangs or in trouble with the law? Gang involvement and association with antisocial delinquent peers are major risk factors for involvement in violent behavior.
  - Are siblings involved in gangs? Do they have criminal histories? Have any family members ever been victims, witnesses, or perpetrators of crime?

TABLE 17-2	Risk Factors for Serious Youth Violence	
Factor	**Early Onset (<12 years old)**	**Later Onset (>12 years old)**
Individual	Male Substance use* General offenses* Low IQ Antisocial behavior and attitude Aggression and dishonesty (males only) Hyperactivity Exposed to TV violence or video games	Male Aggression (males only) General offenses Low IQ Substance abuse Criminal activity (directed at people) Risk-taking behaviors
Family	Low SES or poverty Antisocial parents Single-parent home Poor parent-child relationship Abusive, neglectful parents Access to guns	Low SES or poverty Antisocial parents Single-parent home Antisocial or abusive parents Lack of parental involvement Access to guns
School	Poor attitude and performance	Poor attitude and performance Academic failure
Peer	Weak social ties (the loner) Antisocial peers	Weak social ties* Antisocial delinquent peers* Gang membership*
Community		Neighborhood crime, drugs, violence, and disorganization

*Factors with strongest effect.
SES, Socioeconomic status.
Adapted from Christian CW, Blum NJ: Violence. In Kliegman RM, Marcdante K, Jenson HB, et al, editors: Nelson essentials of pediatrics, ed 5, Philadelphia, 2006, Saunders, p 125.

Management

The primary care provider is likely to become involved with (1) the health care management of minor trauma resulting from assault, (2) counseling after an incident of violence or threat of violence, and (3) the prevention of youth violence. In brief, the following are the key points in the management of minor assaults:

- Treatment of minor trauma or referral
- Alcohol and drug screening
- Reporting the incident to law enforcement
- Referral to social worker or mental health professional and to community programs as appropriate

Protective factors and resilience identified with decreased violent behaviors in youths includes frequent shared activities with parents; the ability to discuss problems with parents; connectedness to family or adults outside of the family; perceived parental expectations for school performance that are high; religiosity; positive social orientation; commitment to school and involvement in social activities with peers; and consistent presence of parents during one of any of the following times—when

- Do not carry a weapon; instead, "fight clean" (i.e., discuss the issue in conflict). Carrying weapons only makes one less safe; pulling out a weapon begins a cycle of retaliation.
- Do not go into harm's way. Avoid being around fights because the cycle of escalation and retaliation often involves innocent people.
- Avoid being caught alone; stay with friends.
- Do not be provoked into fighting. Words are said and names are called, not because the names are true, but rather to provoke anger and a fight.
- If one becomes involved in a fight, try to end the incident on equal ground; that way anger is more likely to be diffused. The person who wins often takes on the aggressor role; the loser then becomes the scapegoat. Thus violence continues and becomes cyclic.
- Suggest discussions with friends about ways to handle potential situations in which a gun or knife might be brandished.
- Do not join gangs or associate with individuals who turn to violence as a way of settling differences.
- Report threats of school violence to adults.

BOX 17-17 Talking With Teens About Date or Gang Rape

- Males as well as females can be victimized.
- Alcohol intoxication or the use of drugs is a major factor in date rape. Prevention includes not placing oneself in harm's way by using such substances.
- Manipulative verbal threats and physically trapping the victim are common tactics used by perpetrators.
- Reluctance to report gang or date rape is common. However, keeping the rape a secret only leads to self-doubt and delays healing. The teen should report the rape immediately and seek professional counseling.

awakening, arriving home from school, at evening mealtime, or bedtime (AAP, 2009; Cowell et al, 2009; Jellinek, 2007). Providers should discuss how parents can incorporate such protective factors in to their family life.

Prevention of Youth Violence. Prevention of youth violence requires use of a public health model that addresses the complexity of causes and risk factors behind the problem. Some issues can be addressed in the primary care setting, while others require more active involvement in the community as a child and family advocate.

Primary Prevention
- Strengthen families
  - Provide parents with skills for effective parenting (see Chapters 4 through 8 and 16).
  - Support parents to be actively involved with their children, to supervise youths and their activities, and to monitor the child's peer group (having friends who engage in conventional, nonviolent behaviors is a protective factor).
  - Connect families to needed community service resources.
  - Educate parents about the effect of violence on their children (media and technology); discuss ways to minimize exposure; teach about gun safety.
- Strengthen developmental competencies of youth
  - Educate youths about violence at an early age.
  - Teach anger management and strategies for preventing a fight (role-playing).
  - Promote self-defense strategies, such as learning a martial art.
  - Discuss ways to manage a difficult or potentially violent situation (Boxes 17-16 and 17-17).
- Improve the environment:
  - Support diversity training and bullying prevention programs in public schools.
  - Support after-school programs for youth and work for community commitment to youth programs.
  - Make neighborhoods and schools safe places for youth.

  - Involve the community in a commitment to preventing violence.
  - Address the issues of media violence and of condoning violence as a way of life.
  - Regulate alcohol sales to and use by youth.
  - Support legislation to control handguns.
  - Limit access to and carrying of weapons.

Secondary Prevention
- Care for children exposed to or threatened by violence
  - Address any physical or emotional problems resulting from violence in the primary care setting. Early intervention can prevent more serious problems later; referral may be necessary.
  - Refer to community programs that make home visits to mothers of new babies, especially those in low-income and teen-mother families.
  - Advocate for support groups for children who have suffered trauma or loss (e.g., school counseling for traumatic experiences).
  - Refer families to community support programs, such as Big Brothers Big Sisters of America.
- Screen for potential problems
  - Assess for violence risk factors at all health supervision and illness visits.
  - Screen for alcohol abuse problems.
  - Ask about weapons in the home—their presence, use, storage, and access.

Tertiary Prevention. Treatment and rehabilitation programs for offenders and treatment for victims and their families can be difficult and costly and yield only mixed results. The National Center for Victims of Crime has a Teen Victim Project website that offers help for this population (www.ncvc.org/ncvc/main.aspx).

CHILD MALTREATMENT

Description

Child abuse is an all too common pediatric problem. Until the late twentieth century, the issue of child abuse and neglect was often unrecognized or even ignored due to antiquated notions of the child as "property" and ineffective social services. Since the 1962 publication of *The Battered Child Syndrome* by C. Henry Kempe and Brandt Steele, great strides have been made in our medical, legal, and social approaches to child maltreatment.

Child maltreatment is defined as the physical or mental injury, sexual abuse, or exploitation, negligent treatment, or maltreatment of a child by a person who is responsible for the child's welfare under circumstances that indicate harm or threatened harm to the child's health or welfare (Federal Child Abuse Prevention Treatment Act 42, U.S. Code 5106g [4]). Child abuse and neglect can be broken down into four subcategories: physical abuse, sexual abuse, emotional maltreatment, and neglect.

The role of the primary care provider in caring for a child victim is to recognize the signs and symptoms of the four subcategories of abuse. A complete medical evaluation should be performed to identify all abusive injuries as well as to exclude all other possible etiologies. The provider should know when and how to refer families and victims for further assessment, treatment and therapy when needed, as well as to perform anticipatory guidance and prevention in the general office setting.

Children who are maltreated are at risk for revictimization and are prone to psychological and behavioral difficulties across their life span. This is especially true for children who are sexually abused or experience physical abuse and aggression (Wekerle et al, 2006). The importance of early identification and intervention cannot be emphasized enough. It has been pointed out that the philosophy "I am not my brother's keeper" should never be applied to children. Children are a vulnerable, easily traumatized, powerless group, and it is the responsibility of all those who work with them to provide protection and care and to be our children's keepers.

Epidemiology

In 2009 there were 3.6 million total referrals in the United States to child protective services involving approximately 6 million children. Of these referrals 62% were screened for response by social services. Children less than 1 year of age had the highest rate of victimization, with a rate of 20.6 per 1000 children. More than half of the child victims were girls (51.1%), and 48.2% were boys. Nearly one half of all maltreatment victims were Caucasian (44%), 20.7% were Hispanic, and 22.3% were African-American. When stratifying the data, as in prior years, the most common form of abuse is neglect (78.3%), followed by physical abuse (17.8%), sexual abuse (9.5%), and emotional maltreatment (7.6%). A child may suffer from multiple forms of abuse (USDHHS, 2010c).

In 2009, 1770 children were the victims of fatal abuse (2.34 per 100,000). Of these children, nearly 80% were less than 4 years of age, with a similar incidence in girls and boys. Child physical abuse was a major contributor, and nearly 40% of all child fatalities were caused by multiple types of maltreatment. The perpetrator of the abuse is most commonly a biologic parent of the child (80.9%) with women more often responsible (53.8%) than men (44.4%), and 83.2% were less than 49 years of age (USDHHS, 2010c).

General Assessment Guidelines

Box 17-18 lists behavioral signs that should be investigated in a child suspected of having been abused. Pitfalls for which pediatric providers must be alert include (Stirling, 2006):
- Missing significant injury or findings by not doing a complete evaluation
- Failing to consider the possibility of child abuse as one of the differential diagnoses
- Not recognizing abuse or neglect as the source of a behavioral problem

---

| **BOX 17-18** | Behavioral Signs Associated With Child Maltreatment |

- Overly compliant or exhibits exaggerated fearfulness
- Clingy and indiscriminate attachment
- Extremes in behavior (aggressive or passive)
- Apprehensive when other children cry
- Wary of physical contact with adults
- Frightened of parents and/or of going home
- Exhibits drastic behavioral changes in and out of parental or caregiver presence
- Depressed, hypervigilant, withdrawn, apathetic, antisocial; exhibits destructive behavior
- Suicidal (suicide attempts or plans) or engages in self-mutilation
- Overprotective of parents or caregivers
- Displays sleep or eating disorders

- Assuming that a family is not abusive (i.e., "a good family")
- Keeping inadequate records of the encounter and evaluation

General Management Strategies

Pediatric primary care providers are in a unique position to identify children who are maltreated and to institute strategies for primary prevention aimed at high-risk families. All categories of child abuse endanger the child's physical or emotional health and development. Although the severity of injury is always an important consideration in treatment and disposition of the child, it does not determine, per se, whether intervention will occur. The burden to report minor injury or emotional maltreatment is just as great as the burden to report significant trauma resulting in grave bodily injury.

All states have mandatory reporting laws that require health care professionals to report *suspected or known* child maltreatment to the appropriate agencies. Both civil and criminal immunity is ensured to mandated reporters who are acting within their professional role in making a required or authorized report. If the history or physical examination is suspicious for child abuse, the provider should report to either child protective services (also known as social services or department of family and youth services) or law enforcement. If the child is in imminent danger, a report should be made to both child protective services and law enforcement. Because each state has its own reporting laws and procedures, providers should contact the department of social services or the office of the attorney general in their state for written guidelines about individual state reporting laws and procedural policies related to child abuse. The telephone number for reporting suspicion of abuse should be readily available in each practice setting. All clinic personnel (including unlicensed) need to be aware of their role in reporting possible abuse (may be observed in the waiting or examination rooms). If in doubt about the need to file a formal report regarding a particular situation, consultation with staff at the local abuse reporting agency is appropriate and encouraged.

PHYSICAL ABUSE

Description

Any act that results in nonaccidental physical injury to a child is physical abuse. Physical abuse often occurs when the parent or caregiver is frustrated or angry. In these instances the injury is frequently a result of shaking, striking, or throwing the child and can involve unreasonably severe corporal punishment or unjustifiable punishment. Physical injury also can represent intentional, deliberate assault, such as burning, biting, cutting, poking, twisting limbs, or torturing.

Assessment

Determining the presence of physical abuse can be difficult. A child or parent may disclose a history of an inflicted injury, or there may be suspicious behavioral or physical findings. Behaviors are not definitive signs of physical abuse but are important areas to investigate for additional information. Specific physical findings are often the key to a diagnosis of non-accidental injury resulting from physical abuse. The provider should have a high level of suspicion if there are discrepancies in the history of the injury, the child's age and developmental capabilities, and the type and severity of injury. For example, infants who do not cruise should not bruise.

History. The history should assess for the following:
- Child states that injury was caused by abuse.
- Injury is unusual for a specific age group.
- Injuries are unexplained or implausible (e.g., parent or caregiver cannot explain injury, is vague about how the injury occurred, gives discrepant accounts of what happened, or blames someone else); explanation does not match the type or mechanism of injury; or child is not developmentally capable of reported injurious behavior.
- Parent or caregiver delays seeking care for child, seeks inappropriate care (e.g., for something other than the true issue), or age of injury is inconsistent with the history.
- Child, parent or caregiver, or both, hides injury (e.g., child wears excessive layers of clothing), or child is kept out of school.
- There is presence of triggering behaviors, such as inconsolable colicky infant, toilet-training accidents, or sleeping or discipline problems that may have led to a violent response by a caregiver.
- There is a report of a crisis or stressful time for the family (e.g., financial difficulties) or domestic violence.
- There is a problem with substance abuse in the family.
- Family history of von Willebrand disease, hemophilia or clotting disorder, or osteogenesis imperfecta.

Physical Findings. Tables 17-3 and 17-4 describe common sites of injury and common characteristics of physical abuse by type of injury. Key considerations of abuse that should guide the physical examination include the following:
- Location of the injury
- Type of injury: bruising, burns, inflicted fractures, or head trauma
- Pattern of bruises, abrasions, lacerations (i.e., does it resemble a known object?)
- Presence of multiple injuries, particularly in different stages of healing
- Multiple mechanisms of injury (burns, fractures, bruises)
- Signs of concurrent medical, hygienic, supervisory, or nutritional neglect (Hymel and Hall, 2005)
- Most infant falls do not result in head injury. Falls from beds or sofas do not cause skull fractures, and less than 1% of infants in a large study suffered concussion or skull fracture because of a fall (Warrington et al, 2001).

TABLE 17-3	Common Sites of Injury in Physical Abuse of Children
Location of Injury*	**Common Physical Finding**
Head area	Eyes—bilateral black eyes Earlobe—pinch and pull marks Cheek—slap marks, squeeze marks Upper lip and frenulum— lacerations or bruises Scalp—bare and broken hair, bruises
Neck	Choke marks
Trunk	Trunk—bite marks, fingertip encirclement marks, hand slap, pinch mark, belt mark Buttocks and lower back—paddling and strap marks
Anogenital	Pinch marks, penile wrapping with constrictive materials
Extremities	Upper arms—grab marks Ankles or wrists—tethering, friction burn marks Feet—pin or razor tattoo marks

*The shins elbows, and knees are the most typical sites of accidental, non–child abuse injuries where bruises, cuts, and abrasions are most commonly seen. The back surface of the body, from knees to neck, is the most common site of intentional, abusive injuries.
Data from Harris TS: Bruises in children: normal or child abuse? *J Pediatr Health Care* 24(4): 216-221, 2010.

- Falls less than 5 feet (1.5 m) in vertical height have a less than one in a million chance of death (Chadwick et al, 2008).

Diagnostic Studies. These should include:
- Blood coagulation studies: platelet count, bleeding time, prothrombin time, partial thromboplastin time, disseminated intravascular coagulation (DIC) panel on any child who is severely bruised or has a history of "easy bruising" and suspicious bruises
- Serum calcium, phosphorus, and alkaline phosphatase levels are useful measurements if bone disease is suspected
- Radiographic studies
  - A child with limited range of motion or bony tenderness on examination should have a local radiologic evaluation. A radiologic skeletal survey should be ordered for any child with soft-tissue findings who is nonverbal, immobile, or unable to give a clear history (usually younger than 2 years of age). Table 17-5 gives the details of a complete skeletal survey.
  - Bone scans, computed tomography scan, and a magnetic resonance imaging study should be ordered on the basis of physical findings or symptoms.
- Ultrasonography is useful if visceral injury is suspected. Other studies are ordered depending on physical findings.

Differential Diagnosis

Differential diagnoses are identified by type of intentional physical injury:
- Soft-tissue injuries
- Normal bruising from accidental injuries that typically involve the knees, anterior tibia, and forehead
- Mongolian spots

TABLE 17-4	Common Characteristics of Physical Abuse by Type of Injury

Type of Injury	Key Considerations
Bruises—surface and soft tissue	Pattern, shape, outline or image of the object (e.g., handprint, cord or buckle shapes) Location—sites other than over bony prominence (knees, shins, elbows, forehead) Number—more than one body surface or plane Multiple bruises with various stages of coloring
Burns—superficial or deep	Location: burns on palms, soles, flexor surface of thighs or perineum are pathognomonic for abuse; positive image of the shape of the object used to burn the child (e.g., curling irons, cigarette lighters, cigarettes, irons) Patterns, such as sharply demarcated or circumferential (e.g., sock, glove, zebra, branding, doughnut or cigarette shape) Cigarette burns—7.5- to 10-mm round lesion, raised edges and deep eschar
Human bite marks	Oval-shaped pattern, such as doughnut or double-horseshoe shape; adult >3 cm between canine teeth; can be on any part of the body; can have discrete tooth marks within the arcs or central ecchymosis between the arcs
Abrasions and lacerations	Location Number "C" or "U" shape typical of belt buckle mark
Ligature marks	Typically, around neck or extremities; linear image at site where tool placed
Central nervous system trauma	Radiographic findings (e.g., subdural hematomas, subarachnoid hemorrhages, skull fractures, suture spread), retinal hemorrhages; head trauma can have symptoms of irritability, lethargy, seizures, apnea, or coma
Shaken infant syndrome	Retinal hemorrhage, subdural hematoma, posterior rib and metaphyseal fractures
Internal organ trauma	Liver, bowel, spleen, pancreas, kidney damage consistent with blunt-force trauma May be no visible marks or bruises on abdomen May have symptoms of shock Internal injury is second leading cause of death in child abuse
Skeletal fracture	Spiral fractures of long bones, avulsion of metaphyseal tips, multiple rib fractures in different stages of healing, subperiosteal proliferation reaction, unexplained fracture, especially in a young, nonambulatory child; fractures from birth injuries heal by 4 months
Poisoning or ingestion of medication	Deliberate poisoning or exposure to substance abuse via breast milk, passive inhalation of marijuana
Munchausen syndrome by proxy	Creates a fictitious illness or induces illness in child; signs and symptoms stop when perpetrator no longer has unsupervised contact with child

TABLE 17-5	Skeletal Survey

Area of Body	X-Ray View Requested
Skull	AP and lateral views
Spine	AP and lateral views
Chest/ribs	AP, lateral, and oblique views
Pelvis	AP views
Long bones	AP and lateral views
Hands	Oblique views
Feet	AP views

AP, Anteroposterior.

- Cultural practices, such as coining (cao gio) or spoon rubbing (quat sha), sometimes practiced by Southeast Asian groups
- Burns: impetigo, bullous impetigo, or toxic epidermal necrolysis (scalded skin syndrome)

- Fractures: osteogenesis imperfecta and rare bone diseases, such as rickets, scurvy, congenital syphilis, and neoplasms
- Head injuries: bruising from falls
- Bruising or bleeding (hematologic disorders, such as vitamin K deficiency, von Willebrand, hemophilia)

Management

Medical treatment of specific types of injuries is discussed in Chapter 39 of this text under the appropriate illness-related heading. If physical abuse is suspected, certain general management strategies should be followed. The provider must:

- Report suspicions of child maltreatment to child protective services or law enforcement agencies, or both; this protects the provider against any charges of nonreporting.
- Carefully document findings and any statements made by parent or caregiver or child, or both.
- Secure photographic documentation of soft tissue injury or burn injury; this may be done by law enforcement personnel or health care providers, as appropriate.

- Refer for appropriate medical treatment of injuries depending on type and severity of injury.
- Refer for psychological counseling; this is generally handled by child protective services. The need for long-term or intermittent therapy often depends on the individual child, the severity of the physical and emotional injuries, and other life events.

Patient Education and Prevention

At-risk families have certain characteristics. A key to education and prevention is to identify families that have:

- A parental history of abuse during childhood or a history of domestic violence. Pursue affirmative responses with further questions as to what, if any, intervention(s) were taken.
- A history of child maltreatment including child death (categorized as extremely high risk), drug abuse, violent behavior, or serious mental illness
- A mother who does not show attachment to her infant, makes negative remarks about the child, or lacks basic parenting knowledge, skill, and motivation
- Evidence of spanking of young infants
- A lack of social support networks: is the parent isolated?

The following interventions are efficacious for at-risk children and families:

- Make early referrals for supportive services, including social service referrals, parenting classes, self-help groups (e.g., Parents or Alcoholics Anonymous plus battered women's services), respite care, public health nurse visits, or a combination of these.
- Provide close primary care supervision and ill-child follow-up visits.
- Use a multidisciplinary team approach to manage at-risk or high-risk families. A team approach gives objectivity to a situation.
- Report immediately to child protective services if abuse is suspected.
- Use the services offered by community child abuse prevention programs.

NEGLECT

Description

Physical neglect refers to the negligent treatment or maltreatment of a child that can harm or threaten harm to a child's health or welfare. Neglect by the parent or caregiver can be severe or more subtle in its effects. Severe neglect includes instances in which the parent or caregiver fails to protect the child from dangers, such as severe malnutrition (may be seen clinically as medically diagnosed nonorganic failure to thrive [FTT]); willfully places the child in a situation in which the child's health is endangered (e.g., exploitation requiring a child to witness or engage in criminal behavior); or intentionally fails to provide adequate clothing, shelter, education, or medical care. General neglect refers to failure to meet the child's basic needs, such as adequate food, clothing, shelter, medical care, or supervision in which no obvious physical injury to the child occurred as a result. A key factor in neglect is the extreme or persistent presence of these conditions in the child's environment.

BOX 17-19 | General Indicators of Neglect: Child, Home, Supervision Factors

Child
Dirty, malnourished, poor hygiene, inadequately dressed for weather
Inadequate medical and dental care (has multiple caries)
Always sleepy (chronic fatigue) or hungry
Exhibits food insecurity behaviors (hiding, bingeing, stealing)

Home
Fire hazards or other unsafe conditions
No heating or plumbing
Nutritional quality of the food inadequate
Meals not prepared; food spoiled in refrigerator or cupboards

Supervision
Child has history of repeated physical injuries or ingestion of harmful substances with evidence of poor supervision by adult caregiver
Child cared for by another child
Child left alone in the home, car, or anywhere without supervision (typically defined as a child younger than 12 years old who is left unsupervised during the daytime or a child 16 to 18 years old left unsupervised by an adult at night)

Assessment

Assessment should focus on the key issue of whether the child's safety and welfare are threatened. General indicators of neglect are divided into child, home, and supervision factors (Box 17-19). In the primary care setting, providers can more accurately assess child factors than they can assess home factors or the degree of adult supervision provided. Questions and discussion about the home situation, however, can be included in the history (e.g., report of child food bingeing, stealing, or hoarding; young children taking care of younger children; young children being responsible for getting their own meals; history of eating only fast foods).

Referral to a community health nurse for home assessment may be available and efficacious, and a report of child neglect to child protective services may lead to an investigation. If the child is attending Early or regular Head Start, the home health staff can help with the home assessment. However, if the provider even suspects neglect, a call to the local child protective service provides needed guidance. Child protective workers look at home factors with a focus on a safe and sanitary environment. To determine degree of adult supervision, factors such as the child's age and level of functioning, the length of time the parent was away, where the parent went, whether the parent left a plan of supervision (e.g., relative or adult living next door or nearby who was readily available to the child), and how often the child has been left alone, are investigated. Most child protective services hold parents to the standard of a "reasonable or prudent" parent. Economic factors are also considered when making judgments about parents' efforts to provide adequately for their children.

Differential Diagnosis

Differentiating willful neglect from neglect resulting from poverty, mental retardation, or mental illness is necessary. Educational neglect (parent makes no provisions for the child to attend school) differs from truancy or elopement (i.e., child is sent to school, but never arrives).

Management
Referral to child protective services is needed in cases of neglect. Additionally, providers can also refer families to community health and social service agencies, including Head Start.

EMOTIONAL MALTREATMENT
Description
Emotional maltreatment or mental injury is harm to a child's ability to think, reason, or feel. It may take two forms: emotional abuse or emotional deprivation. Emotional abuse is also perpetrated by parents who subject children to cruel statements and acts or who reject, terrorize, ridicule, isolate, and corrupt the child. Torture, confinement, exposure to violence (witnessing domestic violence), and deprivation of food and water are extreme examples.

Failure to adequately nurture children with support and affection so that the child can develop a healthy personality is an example of emotional deprivation. Parents or caregivers who do not provide the normal experiences necessary for a child to feel loved, wanted, secure, or worthy are depriving their child of the emotional security that is critical for positive self-esteem.

Emotional maltreatment may contribute to psychological FTT, speech or sleep disorders, or a wide range of behavioral and emotional problems in children (e.g., withdrawal, aggressiveness, neediness, conduct and/or attachment disorders). Consistency or recurrence of negative parental behaviors and willful cruelty or unjustifiable emotional punishment are key indicators of emotional maltreatment.

Parents or caregivers can ignore or reject their child for any number of reasons, including drug use, psychiatric disturbances, personal problems, or other preoccupying situations. Poor coping skills, high stress levels, a history of emotional maltreatment, and poor parenting can contribute to the parent's behavior. Children with chronic illness or those who are "different" than their siblings may become scapegoats in the family system.

Assessment
A range of behavioral and physical (e.g., psychosocial FTT) indicators can lead to a suspicion of emotional maltreatment, but the signs and symptoms can also be due to other causes. Therefore, a careful history is important. It is essential to interview parents, caregivers, and any child older than 3 years.

History. The history can include the following:
- Past health history—might be suggestive of neglect (e.g., little or no health care supervision, immunizations not up-to-date, earlier removal of a sibling for neglect)
- Interview with mother—might reveal mother's negative feelings toward child, a state of feeling overwhelmed or depressed, plus feelings of being deprived or unloved; mother may be cognitively delayed
- Behavior problems with child in school, among peers (e.g., bullying, being picked on, withdrawal)
- Feeding and dietary history should be obtained, but may not be truthful—can be helpful in distinguishing formula-preparation error from neglect

- Inquire about financial hardships related to inability to provide for basic needs, especially food

Physical Findings. Physical assessment of emotional maltreatment can be difficult. Assessment of psychosocial or nonorganic FTT is one means of assessing emotional maltreatment. FTT can be related to physical and psychosocial factors, and both should be considered because they may be concurrent. Assessment of FTT is discussed in Chapter 32. Assessment should include:
- *Child's behavior:* child may avoid eye contact, resist being cuddled, or have an expressionless face.
- *Mother-child interaction:* parent may indicate a lack of attachment or presence of anger or dislike of child; may belittle, tease, or verbally abuse child.
- *Associated developmental delays:* results from little psychosocial stimulation.

Differential Diagnosis
Intentional mental injury should be distinguished from that caused by parental deficits, such as cognitive, psychological, and economic limitations. Psychopathology in the child resulting from other causes is also in the differential diagnosis.

Management
Because emotional maltreatment is generally difficult to prove, the provider must carefully document what was said in the interview and what behavioral indicators were found. Referral to a community health nurse for in-home assessment is appropriate if the provider has concerns. Referral to a mental health professional for evaluation should be considered to determine whether the behaviors or psychopathology, or both, in the child are due to parental emotional abuse or deprivation. Reporting concerns to the appropriate child protective services agency is essential, as is close supervision of these families. Family therapy may be necessary, and parents can benefit from parenting support and education, in addition to social service support to cope with demands on the family system (e.g., childcare, nutritional education, access to economic resources, Early Head Start). The child may need to be placed in foster care.

If a child has FTT, the condition must be treated clinically (see Chapter 32). Close and long-term health care supervision and follow-up plus psychosocial intervention and local case management by child protective services are needed.

Patient Education and Prevention
Prevention of emotional maltreatment and psychosocial FTT generally involves the same prevention strategies as identified in the section on physical abuse and neglect. Early recognition and intervention are key to preventing subsequent mental health problems. Frequent health visits to monitor the height and weight of infants who are falling behind is essential to prevent significant growth and development problems.

SEXUAL ABUSE
Description
Sexual abuse or *sexual maltreatment* is defined to include acts of sexual assault or sexual exploitation of minors, or both. These acts can occur over an extended period of time

or involve a one-time incident; they may or may not involve force; they can involve threats of physical harm to a child or others in the family or involve emotional entrapment of the child, and they can often involve a secret between the victim and the perpetrator. The perpetrator is usually known to the child and is often a "trusted" adult. A growing group of perpetrators are adolescents who commit sexually aggressive acts on young children.

Sexual assault of children includes a range of acts including rape, rape in concert, incest, sodomy, lewd or lascivious acts on a child younger than 14 years old (e.g., fondling or touching of genital areas and breasts or inappropriate kissing), oral copulation, and penetration of genital or anal openings by a foreign object. Sexual exploitation includes activities, such as pornography depicting minors and promoting prostitution by minors. The percentage of sexual abuse cases increases with age with reported abuse among girls (10.8 per 1000) slightly more prevalent than among boys (9.7 per 1000) (USDHHS, 2010c). Multigenerational abuse is common in cases of child sexual abuse.

Assessment

Chapter 35 discusses the examination of the genitalia in girls. The child or adolescent who has been sexually assaulted by a stranger usually discloses the abuse and comes in for an immediate evaluation. This type of assessment is straightforward and involves the usual taking of a history and performing the medical examination with collection of possible evidence.

If the incident occurred within 72 hours, evidence (e.g., saliva, semen, nail scraping, and head and pubic hair) is collected, and testing for sexually transmitted diseases should be done. These children are often seen in the emergency department of a local hospital or, ideally, at a special center that treats victims of child sexual abuse.

The pediatric primary care provider is likely to become involved in a child sexual abuse case in any of the following circumstances: there is a spontaneous disclosure by the child; a parent voices concerns about the possibility of abuse or reports a disclosure by the child; there are suspicious physical or historical findings, or both; or laboratory tests indicating sexually transmitted infections (STIs) are positive. In many instances, sexual abuse occurs over several years before the child discloses.

An expert in the medical examination of children suspected of being sexually abused should evaluate the child if the incident or incidents occurred more than 72 hours before the disclosure. The assessment of a child who has been molested in the past but whose molestation has only recently been disclosed, or who is suspected of being sexually abused, should focus on three areas: behavioral indicators, physical indicators, and the interview of the child (Box 17-20).

Interview of the Child. The purpose of the health provider interview with the child is to collect adequate information to decide whether to report, or at least consult about, the case. A social worker, psychologist, or law-enforcement person with experience in evaluating sexually abused children will conduct a detailed forensic interview after the case is reported.

BOX 17-20	Behavioral and Physical Indicators of Sexual Abuse

Behavioral Indicators	**Physical Indicators— Nonspecific**	**Physical Indicators—Specific**	**Lack of Significant Physical Findings**
• Loss of bowel and bladder control	• Pain on urination; vaginal or penile discharge; vaginal, rectal, or penile bleeding	• Blunt-force trauma (lacerations, bruising, abrasions, tears) to the genital or rectal areas, or both, that is inconsistent with the history or these same findings with a history of sexual contact or penetration	• Most child victims of sexual abuse do not have any significant physical findings.
• Regressive behaviors, such as newly manifested clinging and irritability in young children, thumb sucking, renewed need for a security object	• Enuresis and encopresis • Urethral or lymph gland inflammation; genital or perianal rashes; labial adhesions	• Commonly encountered STIs:	• Lack of findings is often the result of delayed disclosure and the nature of the abuse.
• Night terrors, inability to sleep alone, bed-wetting after having been dry at night	• Pain in anal, gastrointestinal, pelvic, and urinary areas	○ Diagnostic of sexual abuse— gonorrhea (by culture) and syphilis if not perinatally acquired, nondelivery-related or nonpregnancy-related chlamydia (culture is the only reliable diagnostic method), HIV, and herpes type 2	• Most sexual abuse of young children does not involve penetrating trauma.
• Overeating or lack of appetite; compulsive behaviors or unusual fears and phobias	• Genital injuries or signs, such as bruising, scratches, bites, grasp marks, swelling of the genitalia that are unexplained or inconsistent with history	○ Probably diagnostic—condyloma acuminatum (appearing after 3 years old and not perinatally acquired) and *Trichomonas vaginalis*	• "It's normal to be normal" examination. Even in cases in which a perpetrator was convicted for sexual abuse and perpetrators report penile-genital contact, a majority of victims had normal or nonspecific examinations.
• Change in school performance; loss of concentration or easy distractibility		○ Possible—herpes type 1 and nonvenereal warts (may be due to autoinoculation in the genital or anogenital area)	
• Sexualized behavior or play inappropriate for developmental level (see Table 18-2)		○ Uncertain—bacterial vaginosis and *Mycoplasma*	
• Depression or inactivity, poor peer relationships, poor self-esteem, acting-out, excessive anger		• Pregnancy, sperm, and semen are certain indicators of sexual abuse in young children	
• Runaway, suicide attempts, prostitution or promiscuity, substance abuse, teen pregnancy, psychosomatic, gynecologic, and gastrointestinal complaints			

HIV, Human immunodeficiency virus; *STI,* sexually transmitted infection.

When talking with a child who is disclosing sexual abuse, or whom you suspect was or is being sexually abused, the provider needs to be nonjudgmental, use language that the child understands, identify the words the child uses for the genital and rectal areas, have the child report what happened in his or her own words, and ask open-ended questions. Leading questions should not be used.

If the child gives a spontaneous or clear disclosure of sexual abuse during a primary care visit, report the case. Consider separate questioning of the child and parent or caregiver if the child is 4 years or older.

Recanting a disclosure of sexual abuse is not uncommon because of fear of what disclosure can bring to the family or child.

Diagnostic Studies. Any sexual abuse of children that involves oral, genital, rectal, or penile contact or penetration within the previous 72 hours requires that appropriate forensic specimens be collected. It is best to discuss what types of diagnostic testing should be done with a child abuse expert prior to obtaining samples. Testing for *Neisseria gonorrhoeae, Chlamydia trachomatis,* and syphilis should be considered. Cultures are still the gold standard in testing for STIs in victims of child sexual abuse; however, research suggests that nucleic acid amplification tests (NAATs) on urine might be adequate to use for diagnosing *N. gonorrhoeae* and *C. trachomatis* in child victims of sexual abuse. It is important to check with your local forensic experts to ensure that NAATs will be recognized as legal proof of infection (Black et al, 2009; Girardet et al, 2009).

Testing for STIs in children who were molested in the past (more than 72 hours previously) is based on the history provided and physical findings (i.e., genital discharge). Recent exposure and the possibility of penile contact are key indicators for whether specimens need to be collected. Testing for *N. gonorrhoeae, C. trachomatis,* and syphilis should be considered in all children with a history of sexual abuse. A colposcopic examination of the genital and rectal areas by an expert in the field is often requested by law enforcement agencies to determine whether there is evidence of acute traumatic or past healed injury to the genital or rectal areas.

Differential Diagnosis

Differential diagnoses include straddle injury to the genitalia or rectal area, which produces labial ecchymosis, abrasions, or tears; penetrating vaginal trauma from accidental injury, such as jumping from dresser onto bedpost (needs careful investigation and should have an easily identifiable history); perinatally acquired STIs or STIs acquired through close contact but not sexual abuse; lichen sclerosus, poor hygiene, and pinworm infestation, resulting in vulvar skin irritation; and foreign body (frequently toilet paper) and other nonsexually transmitted bacteria causing vaginal discharge.

Management

An immediate forensic examination for a chain of evidence is required if trauma is present or the child gives a history that sexual abuse, including ejaculation, occurred within 72 hours. Specimen collection for semen, STI, pregnancy, and other evidence is done according to the local law-enforcement protocol for child or adolescent rape.

If the primary care provider is the first health care provider to see the child, he or she is likely to become involved in the following management issues:

- Careful documentation of the history and physical examination findings for medical-legal purposes
- Reporting of the case to law enforcement and social service agencies as required by law
- Referral for medical and psychosocial evaluation by experts in the field of child sexual abuse
- Referrals for crisis counseling of the child and other family members as needed
- Treatment of STI; consider postexposure prophylaxis; follow-up STI cultures or blood work as indicated (e.g., human immunodeficiency virus [HIV] screening at the appropriate timelines)
- Referrals for therapy, in addition to support and encouragement, for the child and family

Patient Education and Prevention

Prevention of later psychological problems related to child sexual abuse and revictimization is key. Prevention of sexual abuse involves the following steps:

- Instruct parents and caregivers about the need for early and consistent education of their children regarding:
  - Good, bad, and secret touching of private parts
  - How to say no or the use of self-defense techniques (e.g., yelling, kicking, or fighting back) if someone inappropriately touches them
  - To tell a responsible adult
  - Not to keep secrets
- Parents should again bring up this subject as their child progresses through the various developmental stages. Young children who have been molested by a trusted adult often do not disclose for many years because they were threatened not to tell anyone or they interpreted the sexual activity (if it is not painful) as a sign of affection from the trusted adult and not as molestation. Later feelings of guilt, fear, and betrayal can emerge when children realize they were molested.
- Emphasize to parents that they must not place their child in high-risk situations (e.g., a parent who was abused by her father may have kept this a secret, blaming herself for what happened; she may erroneously believe that the perpetrator will not sexually abuse her child and leaves her daughter with him). Counsel that children are never safe around a pedophile.
- Provide families with information and educational reading materials about the topic of sexual abuse of children. Teaching should be tailored to the child's cognitive and learning abilities.
- Report promptly any suspicion of sexual abuse.
- Support efforts to target high-risk groups for intervention to prevent the continued spread of child abuse (e.g., children who have exhibited sexual curiosity beyond the bounds of normal or have experimented with but not yet victimized other children [see Chapter 18 regarding normal sexual exploration and activities]; hence they become a juvenile perpetrator acting out the sexual activity or violence done to them).
- Support public education efforts and community child sexual abuse prevention programs.
- Educate parents about the need to talk to their children about their daily activities, especially what their children did during the time they were not with the parents.

Sexuality

TERAL GERLT, CATHERINE G. BLOSSER, AND ARDYS M. DUNN

Sexuality is a multidimensional process that begins at birth. Despite what parents may think, children will become sexual people "with or without their involvement" (Thornton and Collins, 2004, p 802). The primary care provider can play a crucial part in educating parents to anticipate, recognize, and guide their children through the stages of sexual development. At age-appropriate times, the primary care visit provides children and adolescents with opportunities to explore questions they have about their sexuality. Much of the literature on sexuality deals with problems. This chapter focuses on health promotion, emphasizing that sexual development is a normal and healthy part of human growth.

Standards

Bright Futures: Clinical Guide to Performing Preventive Services, developed by the American Academy of Pediatrics (AAP, 2010), and the still-used *Guidelines for Adolescent Preventive Services* (GAPS), developed by the American Medical Association (AMA, 1997), offer the most comprehensive evidence- and consensus-based strategies concerning clinical preventive counseling and screening for adolescents. Together, these guidelines include many interventions that address the promotion of healthy adolescent sexual development and the prevention of negative consequences of sexual behaviors. Additionally, the updated Centers for Disease Control and Prevention (CDC) *Sexually Transmitted Diseases Treatment Guidelines* recommend high-intensity behavioral counseling for all sexually active teens at risk for STIs and HIV (Workowski and Berman, 2010). Strategies include:

- Ensuring a confidential environment in which the adolescent and health provider can freely exchange information
- Assessing and providing guidance toward the healthy accomplishment of physical, sexual, social, moral, cognitive, and emotional developmental tasks
- Supporting parental behaviors that promote healthy adolescent adjustment
- Health guidance that promotes wellness and healthy lifestyles, such as responsible sexual behaviors (e.g., abstinence, limiting the number of sex partners, and the modification of sexual practices)

- Education about the use of latex condoms to prevent sexually transmitted infections (STIs), including infection with human immunodeficiency virus (HIV), and appropriate methods of birth control with instructions on how to use them effectively
- Annual interviews about involvement in sexual and other lifestyle behaviors (e.g., alcohol and drug use) that may result in unintended pregnancy and STIs, including HIV infection
- Questions that explore the adolescent's sexual orientation, number of sex partners in the previous 6 months, if the individual has exchanged sex for money or drugs, pregnancy, and STI history
- Assessing sexual maturity stages for normal progression
- Educating about breast and testicular self-examinations
- Screening sexually active adolescents for STIs (chlamydia and gonorrhea) and pregnancy and partner notification and referral for treatment. Those initiating sex early in adolescence, those residing in detention facilities, those who attend STI clinics, young men who have sex with men, and those using injection drugs are particularly at risk (Workowski and Berman, 2010).
- Confidential HIV and syphilis screening of adolescents at risk for infection
- Routine cervical cytology screening at age 21 (The American Congress of Obstetricians and Gynecologists (ACOG)); or 3 years after the onset of sexual activity (AAP et al, 2010)
- Annual interviews about any history of emotional, physical, and/or sexual abuse by caregivers, friends, or intimate partners
- Initiating the series of hepatitis B vaccinations for those 11 years and older if series not already completed
- Human papillomavirus (HPV) vaccination (either Human Papillomavirus Bivalent [Types 16 and 18] Vaccine, Recombinant [Cervarix] or Human Papillomavirus Quadrivalent [Types 6, 11, 16, and 18] Vaccine, Recombinant [Gardasil]) for females to prevent cervical cancer and Gardasil for males 9 to 26 years old before their first sexual encounter, if possible. Only Gardasil protects against the HPV types that cause most genital warts in males and females (CDC, 2010).

■ Normal Patterns of Sexuality

HISTORICAL AND CULTURAL CONTEXT OF SEXUALITY

The term *psychosexual* development is often used to describe the continuum of sexual development from infancy to adulthood. Historically, however, Freud first used this term as an integral concept in his theories of personality development—and eventually psychoanalysis. His concern was focused on the "sexual desires" he believed were intrinsic formative drives, instincts, and appetites that led to one's behaviors and beliefs. The interplay between expressing these sexual desires and the perceived need to repress them led to his five psychosexual stages of normal sexual development (oral: 0 to 18 months old; anal: 18 to 36 months old; phallic: 3 to 6 years old; latency: 6 years old to puberty; genital: puberty and beyond). The developmental characteristics and the ages at which he assigned the stages varied as Freud advanced his theory throughout his career.

Among others, Erik Erikson furthered the discussion of sexual development by maintaining that children developed in predetermined stages. The stages were based on socialization and the effect this had on a child's personality, interactions with others, and self-esteem. Unsuccessfully fulfilling one stage prevented one from progressing to the next, until resolved. Successful completion of Erikson's stages related to the eventual healthy development of sexuality in terms of one's gender-role socialization, body image, social relationships, attitudes, values, and self-esteem.

Societal socialization norms and values provide males and females with rules about how they should behave. In Western cultures (although this is becoming less absolute), a person's sexual orientation has often been used to define the entire personality and identity. Other cultures and societies differ markedly on this last point. They may allow for greater gender diversity, viewing sexual roles, sexual assignment, and sexual behaviors on more of a continuum or have strict laws (cultural or religious) against the practice of anything other than heterosexuality (Ahmed et al, 2004; Sison and Greydanus, 2007). Global internet technology is also changing the way world views are disseminated, and individuals now have increasing opportunities to communicate their current social realities with others regarding sexual values, norms, relationships, and behaviors (Sison and Greydanus, 2007).

Contemporary Definitions

Sexuality has been defined by the Sexuality Information and Education Council of the United States (SIECUS, 2010, p 1) as encompassing:

> the sexual knowledge, beliefs, attitudes, values, and behaviors of individuals. Its various dimensions involve the anatomy, physiology, and biochemistry of the sexual response system; identity, orientation, roles, and personality; and thoughts, feelings, and relationships. Sexuality is influenced by ethical, spiritual, cultural, and moral concerns. All persons are sexual, in the broadest sense of the word.

Murphy and Elias (2006, p 398) summarize that:

> sexuality extends beyond genital sex to include gender-role and socialization, physical maturation and body image, social relationships, and future social aspirations.

Both definitions illustrate the multidimensional process of sexual development. The complexity of sexuality hinges on the key notion of gender. The following contemporary definitions explore this notion more fully:

- *Gender identity:* The knowledge of oneself as being male or female. It is believed to evolve from a combination of genetic, prenatal and postnatal endocrine influences, and postnatal psychosocial and environmental experiences (Hines, 2009; Meininger and Remafedi, 2008; Murphy and Elias, 2006). It usually relates to anatomic sex, but not always (e.g., transgendered persons). One's gender identity develops in stages according to age stage and cognitive development, which are discussed later. Many theorists argue that gender identity is not fully established until a child has mastered the concept of gender permanency (5 to 7 years old). Others believe gender identity is achieved in the toddler and preschool years. Research of children with complex genital anomalies suggests that genital appearance alone may not be a crucial determinant in the formation of gender identity. In males, genital appearance does not necessarily predetermine their gender identity. In females, prenatal androgen exposure, rather than the degree of evident virilization, proved to be more causal in atypical gender identity (Ahmed et al, 2004; Hines, 2009).
- *Gender role:* The outward expression of maleness or femaleness; it usually relates to anatomic sex, but not always, such as with transvestites (Frankowski, 2004). This process begins at preschool age and continues into adulthood. It is characterized by the emergence of behaviors, attitudes, and feelings that are labeled as male, female, or neutral. Ahmed and colleagues (2004) suggest that gender role behavior is dependent on testosterone and estradiol exposure. Testosterone levels, measured in amniotic fluid, appear to predict male-typical behavior in childhood. Other behaviors that have been linked to the amount of testosterone exposure prenatally include core gender identity, physical aggression, and empathy (Hines, 2009).
- *Gender assignment:* Gender assignment generally occurs at birth, based on genital appearance and is the keystone, in many societies, for future gender socialization (i.e., gender identity). In most cases, genital appearance is determined from conception and is based on the 46XX and 46XY chromosome karyotypes and the appropriate masculinization effect of prenatal steroid exposure (testosterone and dihydrotestosterone). In approximately 1 in 4500 births, gender assignment may be difficult to assign at birth as a result of complex genital anomalies. In these cases, chromosomal analysis may be only one step in the process of assigning gender because gonadal dysgenesis can lead to karyotype variations. Also in these cases, gender assignment is done after careful consideration of the pathological conditions of the clinical syndrome (fetal exposure to prenatal steroids and degree of masculinization), long-term psychosexual and psychosocial functional outcome of surgical correction, and androgen support (see Chapter 25).
- *Gender attribution:* This is a subjective perception of person based on a number of cues (e.g., manner of dress, hairstyle, gait, mannerisms, and choice of occupation).
- *Gender, or sexual, orientation:* ("Whom do I love?") refers to an individual's feelings of sexual attraction and erotic

potential. Meininger and Remafedi (2008, p 554) define sexual orientation as:

an individual's attractions to the same or opposite sex. Sexual orientation is not dichotomous, and individuals tend to fall along a continuum of sexual expression and desires rather than into exclusive categories. The phrase *sexual preference* implies choice and should not be used in reference to sexual orientation.

Heterosexuality, homosexuality, and bisexuality are part of the normal spectrum of human sexuality and are equally valid and healthy developmental outcomes for youth (American Psychological Association [APA], 2008; Bidwell, 2009). Sexual orientation is not known to be caused by any particular factor or factors. Possible genetic (neuroanatomic), hormonal (neurophysiologic), developmental, social, and cultural influences have been postulated but have not been definitively identified. Most people have little or no sense of choice about their sexual orientation (APA, 2008; Remafedi, 2011). Adolescents may express different sexual behaviors, including short-term homosexual experiences. Teens may actually not be sexually active, but label themselves gay, lesbian, or bisexual because of to whom they are physically or emotionally attracted.

Sexual Health

A new working definition of sexual health has been put forth by a group of international experts (Glasier et al, 2006, p 3):

Sexual health is a state of physical, emotional, mental, and social well-being in relation to sexuality; it is not merely the absence of disease, dysfunction, or infirmity. Sexual health needs a positive and respectful approach to sexuality and sexual relationships, and the possibility of having pleasurable and safe sexual experiences that are free of coercion, discrimination, and violence. For sexual health to be attained and maintained, the sexual rights of all individuals must be respected, protected, and satisfied.

Sexual function incorporates the biological component of the human sexual response cycle and refers to the ability to give and receive sexual pleasure. *Sexual self-concept* is the psychological component of sexuality, the image one has of oneself as a man or a woman, and the evaluation of one's adequacy in masculine and feminine roles. *Sexual relationships* refer to the social domain of sexuality and include the interpersonal relationships in which one's sexuality is shared with others.

STAGES OF DEVELOPMENTAL PATTERNS OF SEXUALITY

The primary care provider is in a unique position to incrementally educate parents about their child's sexual maturation starting from infancy and to distinguish between normal and problematic sexual behaviors. Anticipatory guidance will not only enable parents to accurately understand their child's normal sexual development but also provide a structure for healthy parent-child sexual discussions in an ongoing open manner throughout the child's life. Table 18-1 discusses the components of development and behavior related to sexuality.

Infancy to 2 Years Old

Newborn infants are reflexive beings, responding to their physical environment without hesitation or cognition. Sexual reflexes are present prenatally and are easily stimulated in the infant. It is not uncommon to observe a penile erection in prenatal ultrasounds or in the nursing child, for example. Just as infants are fascinated by and explore their hands and feet, they explore their genitalia. Touching the genitalia—even masturbating—is pleasurable and soothing, is a natural part of exploring their environment, and begins as early as 3 to 5 months old. The provider should point out the spontaneity of this reflexive behavior so that a parent does not assign an adult sexuality interpretation to it.

Healthy parent-infant bonding requires physical contact and social interaction. Parents must hold, cuddle, stroke, talk to, look at, and respond to children if children are to develop a sense of trust, on which intimacy will be based in later years, and a positive self-image.

By the end of the first year, the child can differentiate between the sexes; some may even discriminate between sex-assigned toys. As society furthers its influence, children form their identities early and learn about their gender roles from the reinforcement of behaviors expected of males and females.

Two to 5 Years Old

Toddlers are able to recognize and pronounce themselves "I'm a girl" or "I'm a boy," but they can easily confuse gender in others and sometimes in themselves. Changing one's style of clothes, for example, can be perceived as a change in gender. Children cannot integrate gender identity into their self-concept until they understand that gender is a permanent condition. The age at which this notion occurs is around 4 or 5 years old. Theorists argue that gender identity is fully attained between 5 and 7 years old, at which time this identity truly motivates sex-appropriate gender behavior (Ahmed et al, 2004).

Children in this age group are extremely curious about their environment; they love to explore and experiment. Up to the age of 5 years, the variety and frequency of sexual behaviors increase, then start decreasing (Kellogg, 2009). Children have a cognitive awareness of the pleasure self-stimulation gives them and frequently masturbate, but, as with infants, they attribute no erotic or sexual meaning to their actions. They lack the concept of personal space and how their behavior may be misinterpreted as being sexual or improper. This is a good time for parents to discuss the notion of "private parts" and begin to teach the child that self-stimulation is acceptable, but done in private. Parental redirection is usually all that is required (Kellogg, 2009).

The combination of curiosity and lack of self-consciousness characteristic of toddlers can contribute to embarrassing social incidents for their parents. They may be curious about what others look like under their clothes, they may touch other children's bodies, "play doctor," pretend to be Mommy and Daddy, and may enjoy running around naked. By 4 years old children may attach themselves more to the parent of the opposite sex.

Parents should be encouraged to use the appropriate names for body parts and bodily functions, even though they may also be using slang words. This will enable children to better comprehend discussions with health providers, teachers, or health educators when the anatomical and physiological terms are used.

TABLE 18-1 Sexual Behaviors, Self-Concept, and Relationships During Childhood Through Young Adulthood

	Normal Sexual Behaviors	Sexual Self-Concept	Sexual Role and Relationship
Infancy (birth through 1 year)	• Orgasmic potential present • Erectile function present • May explore genital area during diaper changes	• Gender identity reinforced	
Toddler	• Genital pleasuring and exploration • Sensual activity (e.g., hugging, stroking mother's breasts or other body parts)	• Association of sexuality and good and bad • Distinction between self and others	• Sex role differences learned • Discrimination between male and female role models • Sexual vocabulary learned
Preschool	• Sex play—exploration of own body and those of playmates; taking clothes off; showing genitals to other children or adults • Self pleasuring (masturbation) especially when tired	• Gender identity understood as a permanent condition	• Sex roles learned • Parental attachment and identification
School age (5 to 11 years)	• Masturbation (may occur more in public) • Sex play between peers (playing "house" or "doctor"); exploration through looking at and touching genitals • Asking questions and talking about sex • Dressing up as the opposite sex as part of dramatic play	• Curiosity about sex • Sexual fears and fantasies • Interest in aspects of sexual development • Self-awareness as sexual being	• Same-sex friends • Off-color humor related to sexuality
Adolescence, prepubertal	• Menarche (female) • Seminal emissions (male)	• Concerns about body image	• Same-sex friends • Sexual experiences as part of friendship
Adolescence, early	• Awkwardness in first sexual encounter • Masturbation, petting • May or may not be sexually active • May be aware of or question sexual orientation	• Anxiety over inadequacy, lack of partner, virginity	• Appropriate sex friendships • Dating
Adolescence, late	• May or may not be sexually active • May be aware of or question sexual orientation	• Responsibility for sexual activity	• Intimacy in relationships learned
Young adult	• Experimentation with sexual positions, expressions • Exploration of techniques	• Responsibility for sexual health (e.g., contraception, STI prevention) • Development of adult sexual value system, tolerance for others	• Giving and receiving; pleasure learned • Long-term commitment to relationship developed

STI, Sexually transmitted infection.

Data from Hillman JB, Spigarelli MG: Sexuality: its development and direction. In Carey WB, Crocker AC, Coleman WL, et al, editors: *Developmental-behavioral pediatrics,* Philadelphia, 2009, Saunders.

Because children at this age interpret statements literally and have "magical" thinking, their understandings of the physical self can be distorted, and lengthy explanations about body functions can be misunderstood. Parents should help children understand that they and their bodies come in different shapes, sizes, and colors; that all of these are equally important; that boys and girls also share the same parts, but different genital parts; and that sharing and respect are important aspects for developing friendships. It is appropriate for parents to introduce the notion of germs and hygiene, such as washing hands. This will help establish a framework for parents to advance the discussion to include sexually transmitted infections later in life.

Friedrich and colleagues (1998) noted that children who spend more time in childcare environments demonstrate a larger number and frequency of observed sexual behaviors. Other situational factors can induce an increase in observed sexual behaviors in this age group, such as the birth of a new sibling, watching their mother breastfeed, and viewing another child's or adult's nudity (Kellogg, 2009).

Five to 9 Years Old

School-age children continue to have a high level of curiosity about sexuality, their bodies, and their environment. They are aware of the pleasure stimulation gives and continue to actively seek autoerotic arousal for enjoyment. Again, reassure parents that this behavior is not associated with sexual fantasies. Contacts with other children may give them new ideas about sex, and sex games are typical (e.g., playing house or doctor) between same-age children, either of the same or opposite sex. This is normal behavior as long as a child is not emotionally distraught by the encounter or if it involves one child who is older than the other. Parents should avoid being overly alarmed if they witness this play. It is appropriate for parents to redirect the play to other activities. They should then discuss the situation later with their child to explore the experience, ascertain if the child was uncomfortable, and again emphasize the notion of privacy and respect for one's body. Box 18-1 discusses sexual actions beyond self-stimulation and sex play that can indicate possible sexual abuse.

By 5 to 7 years old, the use of sexual or "potty" language becomes evident, often to test parental reaction. Children at this age identify more with the same-sex parent; they tend to cluster into same-sex groups if given the opportunity. They are curious about where babies come from.

By the time children are about 8 years old they begin to understand the significance of sexuality. They learn more about their body and body functions, "giggle" with children of their same sex when talking about sexuality, perhaps because they conceive that sex is a secretive topic. Unless parents actively communicate with their children, sexual lessons will be learned from peers, the media, jokes, and movies.

Some children may begin pubertal changes during this time and may be embarrassed by them. Acne, oily skin, and sweating may occur. As their bodies change they become curious and want to see others' bodies. Masturbation is still a normal way for them to explore their bodies. Sexual language is often used more to insult others or appear smart in front of their friends.

Parents and teachers are in key positions to teach children that their sexual curiosity and feelings are normal, to help boys and girls better understand how sexual development is an integral part of growing up, to use respectful language, and to reinforce that they are always available for questions. Simple discussions about the body can introduce further discussions about hormones and reproductive systems. Establishing a good history of communication about sexuality and other subjects lays the groundwork for being accessible to update information as the child matures. This is also a good time for parents and others to reinforce the notion that there is diversity in families within which parents and adults love and care for children.

Preadolescence

Preadolescence is marked by the onset of pubertal changes. About this time, children understand sexuality as a normal part of life. Both males and females understand the changes that are occurring in each others' bodies and by 10 to 12 years of age are ready to discuss sexual behavior and reproduction. Self-stimulation as a result of sexual reflexes may now become connected to sexual fantasies, sexual behavior, and sexual relationships. It is still common for preadolescents to socialize and develop close relationships mostly with members of the same sex. Both sexes often become uncomfortable or embarrassed about the changes in their bodies, particularly girls because breast development is more obvious to others. Privacy becomes more important.

Parents should discuss menstruation before it occurs so as not to cause undue alarm and have the child be caught "off guard." Being mindful of their values and beliefs, parents should discuss abstinence, STIs (including HIV), birth

---

BOX 18-1	Signs That Sexual Play May Go Beyond Normal*

- The behavior is not age-appropriate.
  Example: A 5-year-old walks around the house with his or her hands in his or her underwear.
- The behavior is prolonged.
  Example: Child frequently engages in sexual play and rarely moves on to other activities.
- The child looks anxious or guilty or becomes extremely aroused.
- Child is being forced into sexual play through bribes, name-calling, physical force.
- Child knows more about sexual matters than age-appropriate.
  Example: Mimicking sexual intercourse.

*Most sexual play is accompanied by laughter and lightheartedness (the little girl who giggles when lifting her skirt; the little boy who laughs when he shows you his penis wrapped in a towel).
Adapted from Todd CM: Responding to sexual play, *Child Care Center Connect* 3(5):1-3, 1994, University of Illinois Cooperative Extension Service. Available at www.nncc.org/Guidance/cc35_respond.sex.play.html (accessed Sept 3, 2010).

control, the human papillomavirus immunization for both sexes, consequences of early sexual activity (including teen pregnancy), and the influence of peer pressure. This is also a good time to discuss sexual orientation.

Adolescence

Adolescence is a period of rapid physical, emotional, and social change that presents a developmental challenge to both children and parents. In terms of sexuality, adolescents fit their sense of sexual being into their evolving self-image and personal identity; they learn about their bodies' (sometimes unexpected and embarrassing) sensual and sexual responses to stimulation, and they develop a sense of the moral significance of sexuality. Recent studies provide differing ages when adolescents report experiencing their first sexual intercourse in the U.S. (at 14.2 years [Tu et al, 2009] or at about 17 years [Guttmacher Institute, 2011]). Seventy percent of both sexes will have had sexual intercourse by the time they reach their 19th birthday (Guttmacher Institute, 2011).

Privacy is essential for the adolescent to explore this emerging self. Activities such as group social functions, dating, participation in sports, and interactions at work and school provide opportunities to learn social and interpersonal skills of intimacy.

Learning how to communicate about sex, how to set limits, how to prevent misunderstandings, and how to say yes or no are important skills for adolescents. Equally important is the process of developing a set of sexual values. Whether the adolescent practices abstinence, has a double standard for men's and women's sexual behavior, or is exploitative or nurturing in close personal relationships is a reflection of the adolescent's sexual values.

Sexuality in Individuals With Intellectual and Developmental Disabilities

The sexual development of youth with intellectual and physical developmental disabilities (I/P/DD) is the same as those without such physical or cognitive limitations. The clinician needs to focus on the developmental level rather than chronological age when determining appropriateness of sexual behavior. For example, an individual with a cognitive level of a preschooler will normally exhibit sexual behaviors consistent with that developmental level.

The provider must also recognize that I/P/DD individuals have the same desires to make decisions and foster fulfilling relationships with others. Their abilities to develop healthy sexual identities and engage in sexual behaviors often largely hinge on society's comfort and proactive support concerning their right for healthy sexual expression, rather than on their disability itself. Individuals with I/P/DD may be viewed by society (including health providers, teachers, and parents) as being childlike, asexual, sexually inappropriate, having uncontrollable sexual urges, or being sexual deviants. Institutional isolation, overprotection, lack of awareness by others of their sexual needs, and pessimism about their potential often ends up inhibiting the healthy sexual and psychosocial development of these individuals. As a consequence, many people with disabilities are vulnerable to sexual abuse and exploitation by those who house, employ, and take care of them. A person with a disability is three times more likely to be a victim of physical and sexual abuse; those with intellectual and mental disabilities are more vulnerable (WHO and United Nations Population Fund [UNPF], 2010). This victimization can lead to low self-esteem, anxiety, depression, and adjustment disorders (Murphy and Elias, 2006).

People with I/P/DD largely acquire their sex education from formal educational programs and the media rather than from family or friends. Females may obtain such education in the form of abuse. These individuals are less likely to share their thoughts, feelings, and experiences with family and friends (Ailey et al, 2003). Unless healthy sexuality is taught and supported, unhealthy and abusive sexuality can occur. Sex education can be effective for those with I/P/DD, and topics should include those listed in Box 18-2. The depth and length of discussion should vary depending on the type of disability (e.g., sex education taught to a child with autism would have a different focus than that taught to a child with Down syndrome). Excellent resources and books for parents, teachers, and clinicians can be accessed from Planned Parenthood, SIECUS, and the National Dissemination Center for Children With Disabilities (NICHCY).

FACTORS THAT CAN ALTER SEXUAL BEHAVIORS

Other factors can influence the frequency and number of different sexual behaviors exhibited by children. These include exposure to family nudity; co-bathing; limited privacy; exposure to readily accessible pornographic materials; exposure to sexual acts; extent of adult supervision; stressors (violence, parental absence due to incarceration, criminal activity, death, illness); sexual and physical abuse; neglect (can result in indiscriminate affection-seeking or interpersonal boundary problems); and psychiatric diagnoses (conduct disorder, attention-deficit/hyperactivity disorder [ADHD], oppositional defiant disorder) (Kellogg, 2009).

■ Assessment of Normal Patterns of Sexual Development

Sexual development, questions, and concerns are present throughout childhood, although for many children the onset of their first sexual intercourse is the cornerstone of their

---

BOX 18-2 Sexual Education Topics for the Individual With Intellectual and Physical Developmental Disabilities

Body parts
Concepts of privacy and choice
Masturbation
Sexual abuse prevention
Menstruation
Homosexuality
Marriage
Sexual interaction
Dating and intimacy
Appropriate social behaviors
Birth control, pregnancy
Sexually transmitted infections (STIs)
Self-esteem
Attitudes and values
Sexual responsibility and privileges, and consent

Data from Ailey SH, Marks BA, Crisp C, et al: Promoting sexuality across the life span for individuals with intellectual and developmental disabilities, *Nurs Clin North Am* 38:229-252, 2003.

"sexuality." Assessment of sexuality and sexual maturation should be integrated into the health history, interview and discussion, and physical examination at all health maintenance visits. A useful tool for the clinician is the Child Sexual Behavior Inventory (available at www4.parinc.com). This tool is completed by parents and can help evaluate normal and age-appropriate sexual behaviors for those 1 to 12 years of age. It was developed to aid in evaluating whether a child has been or may have been sexually abused. However, it can provide assistance to the provider dealing with a parent who is concerned about their child's sexual behavior.

CONFIDENTIALITY

Research has shown clear evidence that sexuality education leads to a reduction in early onset of sexual intercourse and risky sexual behaviors (Kirby, 2007).

The AMA (1997), AAP, Society for Adolescent Medicine (SAM), ACOG, Association of Women's Health, Obstetric and Neonatal Nurses (AWHONN), National Medical Association, and the American Academy of Family Physicians (AAFP) have endorsed policies advocating confidential medical visits for adolescents (AAFP, 2008; AAP, 2007; AWHONN, 2009; SAM, 2004). The National Association of Pediatric Nurse Practitioners (NAPNAP) supports confidentiality regarding sexual orientation and gender identity in accordance with state regulations regarding confidentiality of minors (NAPNAP, 2006). Despite these outstanding policies, many adolescents are not seeking health care due to concerns for confidentiality. Lehrer and associates (2007) found a strong correlation between youth concerns about confidentiality and certain risk characteristics. The odds of avoiding medical care due to confidentiality concerns increased in the presence of poor parental communication, high depressive symptoms, and suicidal ideation and/or attempt in the last year for both sexes. Females also had a significant correlation between foregoing medical care due to confidentiality concerns when their histories included sexual intercourse, no birth control used with last sexual encounter, prior STI, or any alcohol use in the past year.

Health providers need to be clear about their policy of confidentiality with both the youth and parent before the need arises. This discussion needs to include confidentiality boundaries (i.e., severe mental health issues and safety) and billing statements that may be sent to parents.

HISTORY

Functions of the Sexual History

The sexual history achieves several purposes. Not only is it a tool to collect information, but the process itself gives permission to the child, adolescent, or parent to ask questions and receive reliable information regarding issues of sexual concern. It sets the stage to incorporate accurate, sexuality-specific education as a normal component of anticipatory guidance.

Types of Sexual Histories

The sexual history can be either comprehensive or problem-oriented. The comprehensive sexual history is detailed, encompassing all aspects of sexual information about individuals, their family of origin, siblings, and peer relationships. A comprehensive history is lengthy and may not be accomplished at the first visit or in a single interview; it can be anxiety producing to have the client disclose such a level of detail during early visits, and clients can become fatigued by one lengthy interview (Box 18-3).

In contrast, the problem-oriented sexual history usually focuses on the current complaint or assessment of specific behaviors, such as the risk of exposure to pregnancy or the acquisition of STIs. Problem-oriented sexual histories are shorter, more direct, and specific to the issue at hand (Box 18-4).

Approach to Taking a Sexual History

The interviewer should do the following when taking a sexual history:

- Reassure the client that asking sexual questions is a normal part of clinical practice: "I'm going to ask you a few questions that I ask all my young adult patients about their health and relationships" (Monasterio et al, 2007).
- Give appropriate, factual information; use medical-sexual terminology rather than slang, unless the client cannot relate to medical terms.
- Use language that validates the client's understanding of terms and concepts. For example, when talking with adolescents, the question "Are you sexually active?" seeks information regarding current activity on a planned and regular basis. The adolescent who has concrete cognitive abilities may respond negatively. However, the question "Have you ever had a romantic relationship with a boy or a girl?" allows for a more inclusive description of sexual activity. Define "sex" as oral, vaginal, or anal.
- Use open-ended questions. Questions that contain "why" can require a level of analysis beyond the capabilities of children operating at a concrete level of cognition.

- "When you think of people to whom you are sexually attracted, are they males, females, both, neither, or are you not sure yet?" is a useful question that opens up a conversation for youth struggling with their sexual orientation (Murphy and Elias, 2006).
- Phrase questions that may be emotionally laden in a way that lets clients know that their experience may not be exceptional (e.g., "Many people have been sexually abused or molested as children; did this happen to you?").
- When asking sensitive questions, phrasing the question in a way that normalizes it makes answering the question easier: "How often do you masturbate?" is better than "Do you masturbate?" (Monasterio et al, 2007).

PHYSICAL EXAMINATION

The physical examination serves to identify normal variations of sexual anatomy, the stage of sexual development (Tanner stages), and any pathological condition. The physical examination should include examination of the breasts, pattern of body hair growth, and external genitalia. In sexually active adolescents or when an abnormality is suspected, a pelvic and/or rectal examination may be indicated. Laboratory studies are performed as needed, which may include a Papanicolaou (Pap) smear (see Chapter 35 for current guidelines); cervical, urethral, rectal, and/or pharyngeal cultures; urine-based nucleic acid amplification test (NAAT); blood work for STIs (see Chapter 35); or genetic studies if indicated.

The physical examination should be performed with care and sensitivity to the child's or adolescent's feelings. Very young children and toddlers make no distinction between examination of external genitalia and other body parts; young school-age children can be extremely modest, act embarrassed, and resist taking off their clothes for the examination. Older school-age children and adolescents can misinterpret the examination procedures and may feel violated or abused. The child needs to feel an element of control during the examination. By taking the time to provide clear explanations of procedures, using straightforward techniques, and involving the child in the examination (e.g., asking if the child wishes to have the parent or another adult present), the clinician can better achieve the fine balance necessary to perform a thorough, respectful examination.

■ Management Strategies of Normal Patterns

The health provider has two primary goals related to management of sexual development in children: first, to help children achieve a healthy sexual identity and function and second, to provide support for parents to enable them to guide their children through the process. By counseling parents about children's sexual development, both goals can be achieved. Anticipatory guidance about sexual development and maturation that is age-appropriate should be provided to parents and their children as a matter of course. In particular the provider must:

- Assess the parent's level of understanding regarding normal physical and psychosocial sexual development in children.
- Provide or clarify information as needed.

BOX 18-3 Comprehensive Adolescent Sexual and Reproductive History

Background Data

Adolescent
  Age (birth date)
  Sex
  History of risky behaviors (e.g., drug history: onset, duration, and frequency of use of cigarettes, alcohol, other illicit drugs)
Parents
  Ages
  Religions
  Educational levels
  Occupations
  Marital status
  Affectional relationship (parent to parent)
  Child's feelings toward parent(s)

Childhood Sexuality

  What were your parents' attitudes about sexuality when you were a child?
  How did your parents handle nudity?
  When do you first recall seeing a nude person of the same sex? Opposite sex?
  Who taught you about sex, sex play, pregnancy, intercourse, masturbation, homosexuality, STIs, birth?
  How often did you play doctor or nurse or have other sex play with another child?
  Tell me about any other sexual activity or experience that had a strong effect on you.

Adolescent Sexuality

Girls
  Onset of breast development?
  When did pubic hair appear?
  Onset of menstruation (age, regularity of periods [initially, now])?
  When was your last normal menstrual period (LNMP)?
  What hygienic methods are used (pads, tampons)?
  How were you prepared for menstruation? By whom?
  What were your feelings about early periods? Later periods?
  Have you had unusual bleeding or pains?
Boys
  How were you prepared for adolescence? By whom?
  Age of first orgasm (ejaculation)?
  What were "wet dreams" like? How did they make you feel?
  When did pubic hair appear?
Body image
  How do you feel about your body? Breasts? Genitals?
  How much time do you spend nude in front of a mirror?
Masturbation
  How old were you when you began?
  What are others' reactions to your masturbation?
  What methods do you use?
  What are your feelings about it?
Necking and petting
  How old were you when you began? How often?
  How many partners do you currently have?

Intercourse
  How often have you had intercourse?
  How many partners?
  How often do you initiate sex?
  How often do you currently have sex?
  How often have you had oral sex?
  Are your partners male, female, or both?
  Type of intercourse: penile-vaginal, orogenital, penile-anal, oral-anal.
Contraceptive use
  What kinds of contraceptives have you used?
  What are you using now?
  Do you have any problems with contraceptives?
  Do you use condoms?
  How do you communicate about contraception with your partner?
Gender identity and expression
  What does it mean to be lesbian, gay, bisexual, or transgender?
  Do you think you might be lesbian, gay, bisexual, or transgender?
  Do you think you need to have sex to find out?
  Have you known any homosexual or transgender individuals?
  How long have you had homosexual or transgender feelings?
  How often have you been approached?
  How often have you had homosexual experiences? What kinds of experiences? What were the circumstances?
Seduction and rape
  When have you seduced someone sexually?
  When has someone seduced you?
  Have you been raped?
  Have you raped someone? How often have you forced someone to have sex?
Incest and abuse
  What kinds of touching did you receive in your home?
  From your mother? Father? Brother(s)? Sister(s)? Other relatives? Others?
Prostitution
  What feelings do you have about prostitution?
  Have you ever accepted money for sex?
  Have you ever had sex with a prostitute?
STIs
  How old were you when you learned about STIs?
  Have you ever had an STI? Gonorrhea? Syphilis? Chlamydia?
  Do you have any signs or symptoms now of STIs?
Pregnancy
  Have you ever been pregnant? At what age?
  How was it resolved—miscarriage, abortion, adoption, marriage, single parenthood?
  Do you think there is a chance you are pregnant now?
  Have you caused a pregnancy?
Abortion
  What are your feelings about abortion?
  Have you (or a partner) had an abortion? If yes, at what age? What were your feelings?
  What about your feelings now? What about your feelings immediately afterward? What about your feelings after 1 year?

STIs, Sexually transmitted infections.
Adapted from Laube HH: The use of a sexual history with adolescents. In Blum RW, editor: *Adolescent health care: clinical issues,* New York, 1982, Academic Press; Neinstein L, editor: *Adolescent health care: a practical guide,* Philadelphia, 2008, Lippincott Williams & Wilkins; Olson J, Forbes C, Belzer M: Management of the transgender adolescent, *Arch Pediatr Adolesc Med* 165(2):171-176, 2011.

| **BOX 18-4** | Problem-Oriented Adolescent Sexual History |

Describe the sexual concern, problem, issue, or difficulty that you have. Include:

History:
- Type of sex—oral, anal, and/or vaginal
- Condoms—consistency of use, for which sexual practices
- Previous STIs; medication allergies
- Most recent sexual encounter; number of partners in past 2 months
- Use of illegal drugs and alcohol by self and partner (include which drugs, frequency, route)
- Does patient and/or partner have sex with men, women, or both?
- Recent travel and location
- Any symptoms of dysuria, frequency, hematuria; adenopathy; fatigue; weight loss; night sweats; unexplained diarrhea; fever; rectal discharge, bleeding, constipation, pain?
- Women only: additional symptoms of:
  - Vaginal discharge, bleeding, color of discharge; skin rashes, lesions, sores and location; pruritus (vulvar, anal, oral, other); pain (abdominal, vaginal, vulvar, anal, headache, joints)
  - LNMP, description, changes
- Birth control method(s), consistency of use
- Men only: symptoms of:
  - Penile discharge; lesions and/or pruritus (penis, scrotum, urethra, oral cavity); pain in testes
- How do you feel about discussing this problem?
- How long have you had it? When did this problem begin?
- What do you think caused you to have this problem?
- What might be contributing to this problem?
- What kinds of things have you done to treat or solve this problem?
- What health professionals have you seen?
- What, if any, medication have you taken or are you taking?
- Have you talked to a friend or relative?
- Have you read any books to solve this problem? What books?

STI, Sexually transmitted infection; *LNMP*, last normal menstrual period.
Adapted from Laube HH: The use of a sexual history with adolescents. In Blum RW, editor: *Adolescent health care: clinical issues,* New York, 1982, Academic Press. Additional information from Buttaro TM, Trybulski J, Bailey PP, et al: *Primary care: a collaborative practice,* ed 4, Philadelphia, 2012, Mosby.

- Provide strategies and support for teaching children about sexuality.
- Assist the parent to connect to community-based resources.

"Normal sexual behavior" is not always clear and the range is especially wide in the 2- to 6-year-old. Tables 18-1 and 18-2 provide information to help distinguish between the more common, uncommon, and abnormal displays of sexual behavior.

SETTING THE STAGE

When working with children, the provider focuses on establishing and maintaining a positive relationship based on mutual trust and respect. The child needs to feel validated and comfortable revealing concerns and asking questions. In addition to using a constructive approach to taking a sexual history, a positive relationship can be achieved by:

- Asking questions to give the message that the child is expected to be changing and is aware of and curious about those changes (e.g., "How are you feeling?" "How's your body?" "Do you notice that you're getting taller?" "Have you noticed your breasts getting any bigger?" "Boys' penises begin to get longer and wider as they become teenagers. Have you noticed any changes in yours?")
- Listening thoughtfully and carefully to the child's input
- Responding positively by answering the child's questions as fully as possible; being nonjudgmental, calm, friendly, and open; and having a sense of humor, yet taking the child seriously
- Using appropriate teachable moments during the health visit (e.g., when examining a 3-year-old for inguinal hernia, the clinician can discuss appropriate and inappropriate touching with the child and his or her parent)
- Providing accurate information and referral resources as appropriate
- Respecting the child's need for privacy (e.g., knocking before entering the examination room, providing appropriate gowns, examining the child semiclothed)
- Maintaining confidentiality as appropriate, especially with an adolescent; however, children of any age may give information that need not be shared with the parent

SEX EDUCATION

For a child, developing healthy sexuality means gaining knowledge about physical changes; shaping a positive gender identity; clarifying one's sexual identity as a boy or a girl; establishing close, intimate relationships with others; and demonstrating the ability to make healthy judgments about sexuality and sexual activity. The questions a child asks and the behaviors displayed can embarrass some parents, who may respond in a manner that frightens, shames, or confuses the child. Children are born as sexual beings, and parents, whether or not they are aware of it, are constantly providing lessons in sex education. The way parents respond to a child's innate sexuality (innocent curiosity about sex, gender, and body parts and functions) and allow it to unfold is the core of a child's sex education. This response does more to mold that child's mature sexual behavior than all the information or misinformation parents may provide.

Parents should be encouraged to take advantage of teaching opportunities in normal childhood sexual play and to answer questions simply and directly at the child's level of understanding (Box 18-5). Box 18-6 outlines what children should know about sexuality at different ages.

Research has shown clear evidence that comprehensive sexuality education leads to a reduction in the early onset of sexual intercourse and risky sexual behaviors (Kirby, 2007; Suellentrop, 2010). Yet, sex education in the schools remains controversial and subject to federal, state, and local mandate as to content. With the passage of the Patient Protection and Affordable Care Act (health reform), signed into law in March 2010, there are now funds available for comprehensive sex education. States may apply for grants from the State Personal Responsibility Education Program (PREP) but must use evidence-based elements in the curriculum (National Campaign to Prevent Teen and Unplanned Pregnancy, 2010). See Box 18-7 for criteria of effective curriculum-based comprehensive programs.

The SIECUS (2004) has published *Guidelines for Comprehensive Sexuality Education: Kindergarten–12th Grade.*

TABLE 18-2	Red Flags for Abnormal Sexual Behavior of Children and Adolescents	
Age	**Can Occur in Normal Children but Require Assessment of the Child's Environment (Violence, Abuse, Neglect)**	**Red Flags**
12 years or younger	• Asking peer/adult to engage in sexual act(s)* • Simulating foreplay with dolls/peers (e.g., petting, French kissing) • Inserting objects into genitals* • Imitating intercourse* • Touching animal genitalia*	• Preoccupied with sexual play • Engaging in sexual play with children who are 4 or more years apart • Attempting to expose others' genitals (e.g., pulling another's pants down) • Precocious sexual knowledge • Sexually explicit proposals or behaviors that induce fear/threats of force or that are physically aggressive (including written notes, graffiti) • Compulsive masturbation; interrupts tasks to masturbate • Chronic peeping, exposing self, using obscenities, exhibiting pornographic interests • Simulating intercourse with dolls/peers/animals with clothing on or off • Oral, vaginal, anal penetration of dolls, peers, animals • Sexual behaviors that are persistent and cause anger in child if they are distracted
Older than 12 years	• Pornographic interest • Sexually aggressive themes/obscenities; may embarrass others with these • Sexual preoccupation/anxiety interferes with daily activities • Single occurrences of peeping, exposing self, simulating intercourse with clothes on	• Chronic, public masturbation • Degrading or humiliating self or others with sexual themes • Grabbing or trying to expose others' genitals • Chronic occupation with sexually aggressive pornography • Sexually explicit talk or sexual behaviors with children 4 or more years younger (sexual abuse) • Making sexually explicit threats (including written) • Obscene phone calls, voyeurism, exhibitionism, sexual harassment • Performing rape or bestiality • Genital injury to others

*Uncommon but can occur in normal children 2 to 6 years (Kellogg, 2009 [reference below]).

Data from Hillman JB, Spigarelli MG: *Sexuality: its development and direction.* In Carey WB, Crocker AC, Coleman WL, et al: *Developmental-behavioral pediatrics,* Philadelphia, 2009, Saunders; Kellogg ND for the American Academy of Pediatrics, Committee on Child Abuse and Neglect, 2008-2009: Clinical Report—the evaluation of sexual behaviors in children, *Pediatrics* 124(3):994-998, 2009; Rich P: *Child sexual behaviors: what is considered "normal" sexual development and behavior.* Updated 2008. Available at www.selfhelpmagazine.com/article/child_sexual_behavior (accessed Oct 15, 2010).

BOX 18-5	Approaches to Teaching Your Child About Sex

• Find out what your child already knows.
  ○ Understand the question before answering.
  ○ Check to be sure your answer is understood. Make sure you answer the question that is asked, and give your child a chance to ask more questions.
• If your child asks a question about sexuality at an inconvenient time, set a time and place as soon as possible to answer the question.
• Discuss sex in a matter-of-fact way.
• Use correct terminology when talking about body parts; use dolls and books as guides.
• Keep the topics short and to the point, remembering the child's attention span.
• Do not worry about telling children too much about sex. They tune out what they do not understand.
• Encourage questions. Never embarrass children or tell them they are too young to understand or that they will learn that when they grow up.

• Include values, emotions, feelings, and decision-making in your discussion. Do not focus only on biological facts.
• Let your child know that people have different beliefs about sexuality.
• Bring up topics of STIs, including HIV/AIDS.
• Discuss anticipated changes of puberty before they occur. Do not wait until your child is a teenager.
  ○ Discuss menstruation with both girls and boys.
• If you do not know the answer to your child's question, say so, and then look it up. Ask your pediatric primary care provider.
• If your child is masturbating in public or engaging in sex play, redirect him or her to other activities. At a later time, discuss where a more appropriate private place is for the child to masturbate.
• When your child uses obscene or derogatory words calmly explain what they mean, why it is not appropriate to use them, and that use of certain words can be insulting (e.g., "gay"). Do not laugh or joke about your child's use of such words because this can serve as encouragement.

AIDS, Acquired immunodeficiency syndrome; *HIV,* human immunodeficiency virus; *STI,* sexually transmitted infection.

Data from Dunn J, Myers-Walls JA: *Tips for providers.* Written for Provider-Parent Partnerships, Purdue University. Available at www.extension.purdue.edu/providerparent /Health-Safety/Sexuality.htm (accessed Sept 3, 2010); Masters WH, Johnson VE, Kolodny RC: *Human sexuality,* ed 5, New York, 1995, HarperCollins College Publishers.

BOX 18-6 Sexual Development: What Should Children Know?

By 5 Years Old, Children Should:
- Use correct words for all sexual body parts.
- Be able to understand what it means to be male or female.
- Understand that their bodies belong to themselves, and they should say "no" to unwanted touch, having their private parts touched (except for hygiene purposes by a parent), and during physical examinations by their healthcare provider when accompanied by a parent.
- Know where babies come from; how they "get in" and "get out."
- Be able to talk about body parts without feeling "naughty."
- Be able to ask trusted adults questions about sexuality.
- Know that "sex talk" is for private times at home.

Elementary School Children (6 to 9 Years Old) Should:
- Be aware that all creatures grow and reproduce.
- Be aware that sexuality is important at all ages, including at their parents' and grandparents' ages, and that it changes over time.
- Know and use proper words for body parts—their own and those of the opposite sex.
- Understand that there are many kinds of caring family types so that they do not see a single model of family as the only possible one.
- Be aware that sexual identity includes sexual orientation: lesbian, gay, heterosexual, bisexual, transgender.
- Understand the basic facts about how an individual acquires HIV/AIDS.
- Take an active role in managing their body's health and safety.

Nine- to 13-Year-Olds Should:
- Be informed about human reproduction.
- Be aware of changes they can expect in their bodies before puberty (9 to 11 years old).

- Know how normal developmental changes begin, including normal differences and when those events occur for males and females.
- Know how male and female bodies grow and differ.
- Understand the general stages of the body's growth.
- Understand the facts about menstruation and wet dreams.
- Know that emotional changes are very common during this time.
- Understand that human sexuality is a natural part of life (12 to 13 years old).
- Be aware of how behavior can be seen as sexual and how to deal with sexual behavior (by 12 to 13 years old)
- Be aware that sexual feelings are normal and okay.
- Know how to recognize and protect themselves against potential sexual abuse, and how to react to such dangers.
- Be able to recognize male and female prostitution and its dangers.
- Know how babies are made and what behaviors are likely to lead to pregnancy.
- Know that it is possible to plan parenthood.
- Understand that having a child is a long-term responsibility, and every child deserves mature, responsible, loving parents.
- Be aware that contraceptives (birth control methods) exist (and should be able to name some).
- Know what abortion is.
- Know what STIs are.
  - Understand how a person can get STIs.
  - Be aware of how a person can protect himself or herself from STIs.
  - Know how STIs are treated.

Look for more detailed information and information about what older teens should know and understand about sexuality at www.plannedparenthood.org/parents/human-sexuality-what-children-need-know-when-they-need-know-it-4421.htm.
AIDS, Acquired immunodeficiency syndrome; *HIV,* human immunodeficiency virus; *STIs,* sexually transmitted infections.

The guidelines are organized around six key concepts, and content is divided into four developmental levels (human development, relationships, personal skills, sexual behavior, sexual health, and society and culture) (see www.SIECUS.org).

Many professional nursing and medical organizations have policy statements or position papers that support comprehensive sex education in the schools and at home (AAFP, 2010; AAP, 2007; ACOG, 2005; American Nurses Association [ANA], 1991; SAM, 2004; Santelli et al, 2006; Society of Pediatric Nurses, 2004). They encourage abstinence as the adolescents' best choice to prevent pregnancy and STIs; they also encourage parental involvement. However, all state that counseling and education on contraception, STIs, and HIV/AIDS are essential.

COUNSELING OF THE ADOLESCENT

Today's adolescents face multiple influences, including societal expectations that are at odds with the media's portrayal of sexuality; cultural norms, beliefs, and attitudes of the family of origin; peer group pressure to conform; and the individual's own values and belief system (Brown and Brown, 2006). All these influences need to be considered and addressed when counseling.

BOX 18-7 Criteria of Effective Curriculum-Based Comprehensive Sexuality Education Program

- Focus on clear health goals.
- Focus narrowly on specific types of behavior leading to the health goals.
- Address sexual psychosocial risk and protective factors that affect sexual behavior.
- Create a safe social environment.
- Include multiple activities to change each of the targeted risk and protective factors.
- Use instructionally sound teaching methods that actively involve participants, help them personalize information, and are designed to change the targeted risk and protective factors.
- Use activities, methods, and messages that are appropriate to the teens' culture, developmental age, and sexual experience.
- Cover topics in a logical sequence.
- Select educators with the ability to relate to young people and then train and support them.

Data from Kirby D: *Emerging answers: research findings on programs to reduce teen pregnancy and sexually transmitted diseases,* Washington, DC, 2007, National Campaign to Prevent Teen Pregnancy. Available at www.thenationalcampaign.org/EA2007/EA2007_full.pdf (accessed Sept 2, 2010).

The health care provider should use the answers given by the adolescent in the sexual history to further guide the counseling and educational needs of that individual. It may take several visits for the trust relationship to grow before the adolescent is willing to divulge certain aspects of his or her sexual self. The provider's job is to assure the adolescent of the confidential nature of the relationship and provide opportunities for trust to develop.

Adolescents should be counseled that abstinence is the most effective strategy for the prevention of pregnancy, STIs, and HIV/AIDS. Further, they need to know that it is a choice to remain abstinent and a choice to become sexually active, not just something that happens; with that choice comes responsibilities. Open communication and respect for self and their partner will lead to choices that include protection from STIs and pregnancy.

When counseling adolescents, the provider's approach needs to be appropriate for the psychosocial developmental stage of the teen. Using Piaget's stages of development as the basis, counseling may be tailored accordingly. Early adolescents (12 to 14 years old) are concrete thinkers and cannot get to the abstract thought of "what if." Counseling language needs to be in simple concrete terms. Using pictures and direct questions and statements will help facilitate this. Middle adolescents (15 to 17 years old) are starting to understand abstract concepts, but will often regress to concrete thinking in stressful situations. An adolescent at this age may demonstrate mature thought processes at one point in time yet revert to concrete thinking at another. The provider needs to adjust the approach to middle adolescents accordingly, help them to identify the inconsistencies in their thought processes, and guide them through to the logical consequences. Late adolescents (18 to 21 years old) generally have abstract thought more firmly established and are future oriented. However, this ability will vary, as with the general adult population.

CONTRACEPTIVE AND SAFER SEX COUNSELING

It is important to use gender-neutral phrasing when discussing safer sex and contraception and not assume heterosexuality. Providers who provide contraceptive and safer sex counseling to adolescents should understand that the successful use of any method requires a complex process of knowledge, decision-making skills, and public behaviors. To use contraceptives and/or protective barriers successfully, an individual must master the following:

- *Knowledge.* For most adolescents, this means mastery of a barrier method (such as male or female condoms) to prevent an STI, in addition to a variety of hormonal methods for contraceptive purposes.
- *Ability to plan for the future.* Planning for the future requires self-admission that the adolescent will have sex in the future and the ability to take the steps necessary to use a method consistently and correctly.
- *Willingness to acquire needed contraceptive and/or barrier methods publicly.* The adolescent must be willing and able to be public with requests for contraceptive and/or protective devices (e.g., to purchase condoms at a local pharmacy or to seek services at the local clinic, school-based health facility, or private practice) (see Chapter 35 for more in-depth information on contraceptive methods).

- *Communication skills.* Adolescents must have the ability to communicate with another person, such as their partner, healthcare provider, pharmacist, or salesperson, about their individual contraceptive and/or protective barrier needs.

■ Special Counseling Needs

Children's sense of self; personality; relationship to others and to the physical world; cognitive, emotional, and spiritual abilities; perceptions; and expressions are all influenced by and, in turn, influence their sexual development. If children experience difficulties with sexuality, all other aspects of development are affected. Issues of major concern include child sexual abuse (see Chapter 17) and adolescent pregnancy (see Chapter 35). The counseling and support needs of gay, lesbian, bisexual, transgendered, and questioning (GLBTQ) youth is another issue.

GAY, LESBIAN, TRANSSEXUAL, AND QUESTIONING YOUTH
Description and Epidemiology

The concept of sexual orientation includes at least three distinctive components: sexual imagery (fantasies or attraction), actual sexual behavior responsiveness, and the person's self-identification as heterosexual, bisexual, or homosexual. Transgender individuals identify themselves as the gender opposite of their biological sex. Their sexual orientation may be heterosexual, homosexual, or bisexual.

Adolescent-specific data on sexual orientation are sparse. Remafedi and colleagues (1992) surveyed a representative sample of 34,706 Minnesota junior and senior high school youths and reported that 10.7% were unsure of their sexual orientation, 88.2% described themselves as exclusively heterosexual, and 1.1% described themselves as bisexual or primarily homosexual. Garofalo and coworkers (1999) used the Youth Risk Behavior Survey data from 1995 and reported that 3.8% of students self-identified as gay, lesbian, bisexual, or not sure of sexual orientation. Random-probability nationally based survey data on adolescent sexual orientation are absent.

Möller and colleagues' study of children exhibiting cross-gender behavior showed a prevalence rate of 2.6% to 6% in young males and 5% to 12% in young females. The majority of children outgrew this behavior by puberty; those with a pattern of extreme cross-sexual identification from toddlerhood on identified themselves as transsexual in adolescence. There are no good systemic, epidemiological studies documenting prevalence rates (Möller et al, 2009).

The etiology of sexual orientation is unknown, and the sequential developmental phases from childhood to adulthood are debated (Bidwell, 2009). Sexual orientation tends to unfold with an awareness of same-sex attraction by the child's prepubertal years (Remafedi, 2011). As mentioned earlier, the development of sexual orientation is probably multifaceted and the result of a combination of genetic, biologic, and environmental factors that may affect males and females differently (Remafedi, 2011). Some postulate that it is a purely biological phenomenon, largely determined in utero, as evidenced by the high concordance of homosexuality among monozygotic twins (especially in males). Researchers have studied prenatal androgen exposure, loci on the X chromosome, and neuroanatomical differences in the brain (especially in females) (Remafedi, 2011; Gooren, 2006). The work of Bell and colleagues (1981) served to rule out many psychosocial components when the researchers concluded that homosexuality does not result from a cold, distant father; poor peer relationships; sexual abuse; or sexual experimentation in childhood.

Assessment

The development of a minority sexual orientation involves a process of acknowledging and integrating one's sexual identity. The gold standard model of homosexual identity formation includes (Troiden, 1988):

- *Sensitization* occurs during childhood when individuals identify themselves as feeling different from others of the same gender. Girls describe themselves as "unfeminine," whereas boys often report feelings of disinterest in sports and a proclivity for artistic endeavors. Boys state that they are often called "sissies."
- *Identity confusion* usually occurs during adolescence when individuals begin to question whether they may be homosexual. On average, this occurs for males at 17 years old and for females at 18 years old. Feelings of inadequacy, insecurity, self-deprecation, poor self-esteem, and depression can result from unresolved identity confusion.
- *Identity assumption* is the stage at which the child assumes a homosexual identity that is shared with others. The age at which this occurs varies by gender (males at an average age of 19 to 21 years and females 21 to 23 years). Exploration of the homosexual role can lead to multiple sexual experiences with accompanying risks of acquiring STIs and HIV. In contrast, close long-term relationships can develop. The same relationship problems as his or her heterosexual counterpart can occur.
- *Commitment* is an internalized pledge to live as a homosexual and enter into a same-sex relationship. This process can be referred to as "coming out." External disclosure to others who are not homosexual may vary, depending on what is perceived to be safe to the individual. A stigma management strategy of blending, or acting in a "gender-appropriate" manner, may be adopted in an attempt to be safe in environments that are not tolerant or accepting of homosexuality.

Many transgender youth wish to undergo phenotypic transitioning. This process involves three phases: reversible, partially reversible, and irreversible (Olson et al, 2011).

Management

The goal of the provider working with adolescents who are GLBTQ is the same as with any adolescent: promote healthy sexual development, assess social and emotional well-being, and encourage physical health through healthy lifestyle choices. It is important to support and validate the adolescent throughout the process of developing his or her awareness of and commitment to a sexual orientation and provide a safe environment in which to access health care (Frankowski, 2004; Garofalo and Katz, 2001). These adolescents have indicated that there are qualities of the primary care provider that they find most helpful, including cleanliness, confidentiality, respect, competence, honesty, good listener, and having a nonjudgmental attitude (Ginsburg et al, 2002).

The counseling needs of GLBTQ youth are much the same as with any adolescent. Specific interventions include the following: ensuring confidentiality, using gender-neutral nonjudgmental language, displaying information that is important to GLBTQ youth, and providing information about available resources for support. Encourage abstinence, promote safer sex for those who are sexually active, and counsel about the association between substance abuse and unsafe sexual practices (Frankowski, 2004). Transgender youth and their families need to be encouraged to learn about and engage in phenotypic transitioning (i.e., social transitioning and hormone therapy at about 16 years old or Tanner stage 2 or 3) (Olson et al, 2011).

For many GLBTQ youth the process unfolds without event, whereas others have a more rocky transition and engage in risky behaviors and experience complications (Busseri et al, 2008; Garofalo and Harper, 2003; Mustanski et al, 2007; Remafedi, 2011; Russell and Toomey, 2010). Refer to mental health counseling as indicated (especially necessary for transgender youth). Maturity, access to accurate information, positive role models, and social support influence the GLBTQ youth's self-acceptance and success with intimate relationships (Remafedi, 2011).

Complications

Garofalo and Harper (2003) list the top ten threats to the health and well-being of gay and bisexual male youth; many are applicable to all GLBTQ youth:

- HIV/AIDS
- Stigma and heterosexism
- Depression, suicide
- Club drugs and circuit parties
- STIs
- Cigarettes, alcohol, and substance abuse
- Body image and disordered eating
- Homelessness
- Violence and victimization (ridicule, prejudice, hate crimes, physical and sexual abuse)
- Access to care (lesbians are less likely to seek preventive health services) (Rakel and Rakel, 2011)

It is beyond the scope of this text to do justice to the many management issues facing the primary care provider working with sexual minority youth. Several professional resources are available to guide the clinician, including those cited by Frankowski (2004), Garofalo and Harper (2003), Meininger and Remafedi (2008), NAPNAP (2006), Rakel and Rakel (2011), and Remafedi (2011).

Coping and Stress Tolerance
Mental Health and Illness

DAWN LEE GARZON

The term "mental health disorder" describes conditions that affect behavioral, emotional, and neurological development, psychiatric illnesses, and circumstances that result in stress and altered coping (Committee on Psychosocial Aspects of Child and Family Health and Task Force on Mental Health, 2009). There are many reasons for mental health problems in children, including exposure to environmental toxins, such as lead and mercury; genetic inheritance; caregiver neglect or abuse; and exposure to violence. Anxiety and depression stem from genetic predispositions, neurohormonal influences, and the stresses and strains of modern family life. An increasing body of evidence indicates that epigenetics, or the role of nongenetic influences in gene expression, may be a significant contributor to mental illness. Known epigenetic influences include trauma, parenting style, nutrition, hormones, stress, social support, drugs, and family interactions (Stufferin-Roberts et al, 2008). Common childhood stressors include parental divorce or separation, domestic violence, child abuse or neglect, natural disasters, familial mental illness, exposure to media reports of traumatic events, school problems, interpersonal conflict, and military deployment of a loved one (American Academy of Pediatrics [AAP], 2009).

The 2009 America's Children's Report of Leading Health Indicators for Children 4 to 17 years old (Forum on Child and Family Statistics, 2009) showed that 5% of responding parents identified their children as having definite or severe emotional or behavioral problems. Significant problems were identified for 6.4% of males and 3.9% of females and were more likely to occur for children living in families with incomes at 100% of the federal poverty level (7%) than those with incomes at or above 200% of the federal poverty level (3.9%). Children without parents (11.5%) or those living with their mother only (7.1%) were more likely to have significant problems compared with children living in two-parent families (4.2%). National estimates indicate that between 13% and 20% of American children require mental health services, and that most children with diagnosed psychiatric disorders have severe impairment. Yet only half of the children and adolescents who meet diagnostic criteria for a mental health disorder have visited a health care provider for treatment of their condition in the past year and less than 20% receive the treatment they need (Forum on Child and Family Statistics, 2009; Hagan et al, 2008; Merikangas et al, 2010; Report on Healthy Development, 2009).

As of 2009 there were only 7400 child psychiatrists and an estimated 15 million children and adolescents who required their services (American Academy of Child and Adolescent Psychiatry [AACAP], 2009b). The availability of child psychiatrists is especially limited in rural counties and in areas of high poverty (AACAP; Thomas and Holzer, 2006). In addition, health insurance coverage for mental health services has declined, and cost control results in more restrictions on access to mental health care. Consequently, primary care providers must take active roles in the identification, and early intervention of children and adolescents with mental health disorders (Foy et al, 2010; National Association of Pediatric Nurse Practitioners [NAPNAP], 2007). However, primary care providers often do not appropriately recognize, treat, or refer children with significant psychopathology. Additionally, studies show that when primary care providers do use psychopharmacotherapeutic approaches, they often do not leave patients on these medications long enough to get the desired therapeutic benefit (Kelleher and Stevens, 2009). Barriers to the creation of a mental health medical home include insufficient provider education, time constraints, limited reimbursement for services provided, provider lack of familiarity with screening methods, and social stigmas that affect the child, family, and providers (Foy et al, 2010; Jellinek et al, 2009).

■ Mental Health Influences
NEUROBIOLOGICAL CONTEXT

Early mental health influences include the child's genetic composition and the intrauterine environment's effects on the developing fetus. Maternal nutrition, especially B_{12} and folic acid intake, and stress hormone levels are among the most documented influences on the structure and function of the evolving central nervous system (Beydoun and Saftlas, 2008). Severe prenatal nutritional deficiency is associated with the development of schizophrenia, schizoaffective disorders and congenital central nervous system abnormalities (Tottenham et al, 2010). Genetic disorders with behavioral components, like Prader-Willi, are more common in children born through in vitro technologies, raising the concern that suboptimal embryonic nutrition can alter brain development and differentiation (Stufferin-Roberts et al, 2008).

Risk and protective factors for psychopathological conditions emerge from the interaction of genes and environmental experiences. The protective effect of nurturing parenting is evident in animal research that demonstrates that rats who receive lots of maternal attention have a weaker hypothalamic-pituitary-adrenal (HPA) stress response (Szyf et al, 2005). Children exposed to physical abuse, sexual abuse, verbal abuse, or neglect are more likely to have altered white matter development than their nonabused peers (Choi et al, 2009). The number and combinations of risk and protective factors for any individual are likely to determine behavior patterns, comorbidities, severity, and course of psychopathological conditions during childhood, adolescence, and adulthood.

Functional magnetic resonance imaging (fMRI) and positron-emission tomography (PET) scans allow the identification and description of patterns in brain structure and function in normal children and adolescents. These imaging techniques also document altered patterns of structure and function in children and adolescents diagnosed with psychopathological conditions. From infancy through early adulthood, changes in the limbic system, specifically the amygdala and hippocampus, influence emotional development and the emergence of affective disorders, substance abuse, and high-risk behaviors (Stufferin-Roberts et al, 2008). However, none of these brain differences appear to be necessary or sufficient for psychopathological conditions to occur. Rather, environmental strengths and vulnerabilities, and cumulative life experiences influence the number and severity of symptoms and the adaptive competencies the child displays at any age (Burt, 2009).

Research demonstrates the profound effects of stress and environmental deprivation on the young child's brain development (Carmody and Bendersky, 2006). Activation of the HPA axis triggers release of cortisol, feeding the fight-or-flight response. Elevated serum cortisol levels act as a toxin on neurons in the central nervous system, inhibiting the growth of dendrites and neurons and causing the death of neurons. Research also demonstrates the profound effects of the use-it-or-lose-it phenomenon on the number of neurons and dendritic growth and interconnections. In the final phase of brain growth, known as differentiation, the brain prunes away unused neurons and dendritic connections. Brain imaging of children exposed to the chronic stress of emotionally and materially deprived environments shows reduced brain volumes compared with the brain size of age- and sex-matched children from nondeprived environments (Tottenham et al, 2010). In short, all forms of material and interactive experiences actively shape children's brain architecture.

Chronic triggering of the HPA stress response hones the speed and intensity of a neurological response. Chronic stress leads to swift, strong expressions of distress to even minor stressful stimuli. For example, preterm infants respond with a strong cry to even minor chilling or discomfort. Infant and child crying has profoundly negative effects on normal adults, triggering the adult's own stress response. Thus excessive and prolonged crying is a significant risk factor for child abuse and the development of problems in the parent-child relationship.

Normal developmental changes add an important layer of influence and complexity to the interaction between the genetically driven biology of the child and his or her interaction with the environment.

Mental Health in Primary Care

Child and adolescent mental health has profound effects on child development, family functioning, and society as a whole. Primary care providers, as medical home providers, are ideal mental health advocates because of their:

- Established therapeutic relationships with children and families
- Capacity to engage in mental health promotion and anticipatory guidance
- Familiarity with normal child development and healthy parenting
- Experience coordinating care with other health care specialists
- Familiarity with chronic care principles and practice improvement (Committee on Psychosocial Aspects of Child and Family Health and Task Force on Mental Health, 2009; NAPNAP, 2007).

According to the *Report on Healthy Development: A Summit on Young Children's Mental Health* (2009), the following strategies can be used to ensure optimal mental health. First, parents need to know that when they provide for their child's social and emotional needs, their child is more likely to have healthier behavior, improved school performance, and better interpersonal relationships. Second, responsive and stable caregiving positively influences brain development. Next, parents should be educated about normal child development, with special emphasis on developmental stress points and transitions. Parents need to know that predictable home, childcare, and school routines are essential to a child's mental health. Anticipatory guidance related to healthy prenatal care, diet, and exposures should be a part of routine wellness care. Lastly, parents need support of healthy parenting skills, and they need to know that early mental, verbal, and emotional abuse is particularly toxic to the developing child. The following discussion details strategies that can be used to foster childhood mental wellness.

PREVENTION

Primary Prevention

Primary prevention of mental health problems occurs through positive, nurturing parent-child relationships. Children need to experience a secure attachment relationship and a sense of self-worth and being worthy of love. This serves as a foundation for developing social, emotional, and cognitive competence (Lieberman and Van Horn, 2009). Additional protective factors that promote resilience and mental wellness include:

- Responsive, thoughtful caregivers
- Supportive families
- Clear behavioral standards
- Parental recognition of individual achievements, efforts, and improvements
- Healthy peer relationships
- High-quality preschool, elementary, and secondary schools

- Faith
- Sense of control over one's life
- Sense of one's purpose, and clear self-identity
- Opportunities to interact with positive peers and adults
- Freedom from racism, sexism, discrimination, and poverty (Foy et al, 2010)

Pediatric providers must consistently screen for parent depression at health visits beginning with the prenatal visit because parental depression threatens healthy parenting (Hagan et al, 2008). A large body of research supports the significant negative effects of maternal depression, including prenatal depression, on the behavior and development of infants and young children (Pfefferle and Spitznagel, 2009). The U.S. Preventive Services Task Force (USPSTF) (2006) states that the two-question depression screen (i.e., persistent feelings of sadness or the blues and lack of pleasure in things previously enjoyed) is as effective as longer screening tools to identify maternal depression.

Healthy parenting strategies result in parents who are positive in tone and regard for the child, responsive to the child's autonomy and individuality, neutral in response to unwanted behavior, and attentive to the child's needs (Box 19-1 and see Chapters 4 and 16). Parents who have not experienced this type of nurturing often need education and coaching in positive parenting behaviors from a pediatric provider (McDonough, 2005).

The development of trust and a sense of security in the world begins with effective, timely parental response to the infant's needs. Contrary to popular belief, responsive parenting results in children who are able to self-regulate their behavior and who are confident and competent rather than clingy. As children become more mobile and autonomous late in the first year, parents should begin to use limit-setting strategies that include reasoning, explanations, and distractions. Effective use of discipline and a teaching-based style enhance the development of self-regulation and foster a strong self-concept and social competence (see Chapters 4 and 16). Through anticipatory guidance, pediatric providers assist parents to handle predictable life events that are likely to influence children, such as changes in daycare, moves, or changes in schools. Increasing the parent's awareness of the child's developmental and temperamental needs can facilitate the identification of strategies to effectively facilitate transitions. Providers should assist parents to find ways to help their children use developmentally appropriate coping strategies. For example, parents can encourage symbolic play in preschoolers, or use discussion about developmentally appropriate books or movies with older children to help them express feelings and worries and gain control of their situation.

Secondary Prevention

Secondary prevention, or early detection and intervention, addresses unanticipated life events. Social, emotional, or behavioral problems may emerge even in the context of positive parenting approaches. Early recognition of pediatric mental illness is easier when parents have a realistic understanding of their child's development and primary care providers actively screen for developmental red flags. Secondary prevention involves working collaboratively with parents to identify and implement appropriate management strategies or to explain and reinforce the value of mental health recommendations.

Medication may be necessary to manage some pediatric mental health problems. However, most mental health problems require a combined approach of psychotherapy and medication. Studies show medication combined with psychotherapy is superior to medication alone.

Use of medication to treat mental health problems in children is increasing, but there are concerns about pharmacological interventions of which primary providers must be aware. There are few randomized control trials involving children that demonstrate pharmacotherapeutic safety and efficacy. Existing research shows that medications that are effective in the management of adult mental health conditions are less effective or may be completely ineffective in children with similar diagnoses, likely due to differences in the organization and function of the developing brain of children at different ages. Many drugs used to treat mental health conditions have serious adverse side effects and require ongoing physiological monitoring (Table 19-1). Primary care providers assess for interactions between medications used in treating mental health conditions and commonly prescribed medications also used in primary care, such as antibiotics and contraceptives, which may result in impaired drug effectiveness or toxic side effects.

Tertiary Prevention

Tertiary prevention and intervention address major losses and trauma (e.g., victimization through sexual or physical abuse, parental marital problems, divorce, substance abuse, and

---

BOX 19-1 Positive Parenting Strategies

Attend to the Child Individually

Allow the child to make reasonable choices.

Respond to child's bids for attention with eye contact, smiles, and physical contact.

Comment on child's appropriate and desirable behavior frequently and positively throughout the day.

Provide guaranteed special time daily: no interruptions, no directions, no interrogations.

Prevent secondary gains for the child's minor transgressions by having no discussion, physical contact, perhaps even eye contact; be neutral and simply state the preferred behavior.

Listen Actively

Paraphrase or describe what the child is saying.

Reflect the child's feelings.

Share the child's affect by matching the child's body posture and tone of voice.

Avoid giving commands, judging, or editorializing.

Follow the child's lead in the interaction.

Convey Positive Regard

Communicate positive feelings (e.g., love) directly.

Give directions positively, firmly, and specifically.

Provide notice before requiring the child to change activities.

Label the behavior, not the child.

Praise competency and compliance; say thank you.

Apologize when appropriate.

Avoid shaming or belittling the child.

Strive for consistency.

| TABLE 19-1 | Evidence-Supported Drug Therapy for Common Mental Health Conditions in Childhood |

Drug Class and Examples	Conditions Treated	Primary Care Drug Interactions	Common Side Effects
SSRIs			
Fluoxetine (FDA approved)	Anxiety; major depressive disorder, OCD, selective mutism	Multiple drug interactions Contraindicated drugs: MAOIs, tryptophan, St. John's wort, thioridazine, and TCAs	Headache, nervousness, insomnia or sedation, fatigue, nausea, diarrhea, dyspepsia, appetite loss Diet: avoid tryptophan supplements, grapefruit juice, and alcohol
Escitalopram (FDA approved)	Depression, anxiety	Same as above but better drug interaction profile	
Fluvoxamine (not approved for children younger than 18 years old)	OCD	Increased risk of bleeding: NSAIDs, aspirin, warfarin	
Sertraline (only approved for OCD)	OCD		
Mood Stabilizer			
Lithium	Bipolar disorder CD	Multiple drug interactions Risk for toxic drug levels: NSAIDs, metronidazole, and a wide range of antihypertensives	Weight gain, acne, sedation, tremors, gastrointestinal upset, hair loss Diet: limit caffeine, alcohol; ensure good fluid intake; maintain salt intake
Anticonvulsants Used as Mood Stabilizers			
Carbamazepine	Bipolar disorder	Multiple drug interactions Decreased effectiveness: corticosteroids, oral and subdermal contraceptives, and doxycycline Risk for toxic drug levels: clarithromycin, cimetidine, erythromycin, ketoconazole, itraconazole, and loratadine	Drowsiness, restlessness, nausea, vomiting, diarrhea, dyspepsia, tremor Diet: avoid alcohol and grapefruit juice
Valproic acid	Bipolar disorder	Multiple drug interactions Risk for toxic drug levels: aspirin-containing products	Drowsiness, irritability, restlessness, headache, ataxia, dizziness, nausea, vomiting, diarrhea, dyspepsia, weight gain, pancreatitis, thrombocytopenia, carnitine deficiency, tremor, liver failure, diplopia, blurred vision Diet: increase foods high in carnitine (red meats and dairy products)
Second-Generation Antipsychotics			
Risperidone (FDA approved)	Aggression CD ODD Schizophrenia Tourette syndrome	Multiple drug interactions Avoid: St. John's wort Potentiates: antihypertensives	Hypotension, syncope, tachycardia, insomnia, agitation, headache, dizziness, seizures, rash, weight gain, nausea, vomiting, diarrhea, polyuria, weight gain, elevated lipids, hyperglycemia, rhinitis, sedation Diet: oral solution not compatible with cola or tea
Olanzapine	Bipolar disorder		
Quetiapine (FDA approved)	Bipolar disorder Schizophrenia		

CD, Conduct disorder; *FDA,* U.S. Food and Drug Administration; *MAOIs,* monoamine oxidase inhibitors; *NSAIDs,* nonsteroidal antiinflammatory drugs; *OCD,* obsessive-compulsive disorder; *ODD,* oppositional defiant disorder; *TCAs,* tricyclic antidepressants; *SSRIs,* selective serotonin reuptake inhibitors.
Information in the table drawn from:
American Academy of Child and Adolescent Psychiatry (AACAP): Practice parameter for the assessment and treatment of children and adolescents with anxiety disorders, *J Am Acad Child Adolesc Psychiatry* 46:267-283, 2007.
American Academy of Child and Adolescent Psychiatry (AACAP): Practice parameter for the assessment and treatment of children and adolescents with bipolar disorders, *J Am Acad Child Adolesc Psychiatry* 46:107-125, 2007a.
American Academy of Child and Adolescent Psychiatry (AACAP): Practice parameter for the assessment and treatment of children and adolescents with depressive disorders, *J Am Acad Child Adolesc Psychiatry* 46:1503-1526, 2007b.
American Academy of Child and Adolescent Psychiatry (AACAP): Practice parameter for the assessment and treatment of children and adolescents with oppositional defiant disorder, *J Am Acad Child Adolesc Psychiatry* 46:126-141, 2007c.
Garzon D: Childhood depression: diagnosis and management in an era of black-box warnings, *Adv Nurs Pract* 15(2):35-48, 2007.
Taketomo CK, Hodding JH, Kraus DM: *Pediatric dosage handbook,* ed 17, Hudson, OH, 2010, Lexi-Comp.

parental psychopathological conditions). Even in the absence of behavioral manifestations of distress, a referral to a mental health specialist for further assessment and intervention is suggested because of the short- and long-term problems that result from traumatic experiences. In these cases, parents may not understand the need for referral. It is most helpful for the pediatric provider to frame the behavior problem as a "normal response to an unusual or stressful situation" with the goal of referral being to maximize the child's development and growth. A release of information allows direct contact with the consultant to ensure follow-through. Ongoing follow-up is essential with children, families, and other professional providers.

APPROACHES TO CHILDREN BY DEVELOPMENTAL LEVEL

Special Approaches from Infancy Through Early Childhood

The early child years are the most critical for mental wellness. It is important for infants, toddlers, and preschoolers to have nurturing, supportive environments with ample opportunities for physical, emotional, and social growth. Healthy attachment is critical to the development of healthy, happy, and self-confident children. Infants and young children with good attachments develop the confidence to explore their world and learn cognitive and social skills. Parental strategies that foster good attachment include using loving verbal and nonverbal communication, providing consistent routines, having frequent "fun" and play time, accurately reading child signals, and providing timely response to the child's needs (Report on Healthy Development, 2009).

By early infancy, attentive parents describe their baby's likes and dislikes, sensitivities, and signals. Many babies comfort themselves for brief periods. Babies who receive prompt responses to their needs typically provide less intense distress signals and develop the ability to wait for care (Hagan et al, 2008). Parents face the challenge of becoming effective, adaptive teachers for their changing baby.

Parents should provide older infants, toddlers, and preschoolers the opportunity to develop an "emotional IQ." This can be achieved by allowing the child to express and recognize the full spectrum of human emotion, from good to bad, and to develop skills to cope with negative emotions. Children learn empathy when the child receives sensitive empathic care. By this stage, signs of parenting that impede mental wellness include difficulty with limit setting, frustration and negativity with toddler behavior, limited or absent verbal communication with the child, hurtful teasing, and multiple bruises and injuries suggesting inadequate supervision, abuse, or neglect of the child (Hagan et al, 2008).

Physical, emotional, and verbal abuse are especially toxic to the young child who is developing self-identity and learning how to relate to others (Report on Healthy Development, 2009). Therefore, it is important for primary care providers to educate parents about strategies that can be used when they are overwhelmed, and how to communicate with their child in a developmentally appropriate manner. Nurse home visitation programs are effective for improving parenting skills, enhancing parental social support, and improving parent-infant attachment in at-risk families (Council on Community Pediatrics, 2009).

Special Approaches During the School-Age Years Through Adolescence

Normal children at this age have significant abilities to control their emotions, behavior, and attention. The child's social roles and behavior expectations change dramatically at home, at school, and among peers. The child's self-concept and self-esteem face daily challenges in comparisons with peers' performance in academics, sports, and social interactions. Parents should support their child's self-esteem and exploration of a wide range of interests, and protect the child from early engagement in competition for which he or she is not emotionally ready (Hagan et al, 2008).

Stress is a known risk factor for mental illness. It is important to allow older children and adolescents opportunities for "downtime" and relaxation. Healthy parenting during these ages involves modeling and teaching healthy ways to deal with stress. Primary care providers can improve coping by using strategies to improve resilience and communication skills (AAP, 2009). Special care should be paid to avoid child "overscheduling." All children and adolescents need time to relax and to mentally recharge from the stresses of school, work, and extracurricular activities. Family interventions that improve communication and foster healthy coping include family game nights and shared, sit-down meals.

It is important for parents to recognize that although adolescents' cognitive skills are nearly at adult levels, their ability to make good decisions under the influence of strong emotions is not as developed. Girls are especially vulnerable to affective disorders. Social roles and behavior expectations change dramatically with sexual maturation. On the positive side, altruism and idealism emerge, leading many adolescents to significant achievements. Parents are challenged to provide accurate and timely information, sensitive support, and appropriate limits to their adolescent.

High-risk adolescent behaviors include sexual activity, alcohol and drug use, driving while intoxicated, tobacco use, aggressive or hostile behavior, depressed mood, and school absenteeism or academic failure (Hagan et al, 2008). Failure to set appropriate limits and expectations, lack of pride in the adolescent's achievements, negative affect toward the adolescent, frustration or anger with the normal level of adolescent mood lability, and failure to support the adolescent's positive engagement in the community and school signal problems in the parent-adolescent relationship.

■ Temperament Influences on Mental Health

Temperament is a foundation for coping. Temperament involves an individual's characteristic style of emotional and behavioral response across situations and has generally come to be accepted as inborn. Although biological in origin, temperament characteristics evolve and develop over time and are influenced by and patterned in significant ways by the social environment. This view of temperament is clinically important because both short- and long-term psychosocial adjustments are shaped by the goodness-of-fit between the individual's temperament and the social environment. (Goodness-of-fit refers to the congruence of a child's temperament with the expectations, demands, and opportunities of the social environment, including those of parents, family, and daycare or school setting.) (See Table 4-2 for information about temperament types.)

TABLE 19-2	Strategies to Help Parenting of Children With Different Temperaments
Temperament Characteristic	**Strategy**
Activity	Recognize the child's activity level and plan high-energy activities (such as long walks, family outings) with naps and child's energy levels in mind. Plan for activities to keep high-energy children busy in situations when quiet is required (such as during religious services).
Rhythmicity	Take the child's normal sleep, wake, and feeding schedule in mind when planning activities and outings. Avoid activities during "normal" naptimes. Use normal elimination patterns as a guide during toilet training.
Approach or withdrawal	Help teach young children skills to deal with discomfort felt while meeting new people or having new experiences. Provide opportunities for children with approach/withdrawal problems to experience new situations and to meet new people in a supporting and loving environment. Recognize that new situations may be stressful.
Adaptability	Teach young children how to deal with disappointment. Provide reassurance when things don't go as planned.
Threshold of response	Recognize that not all children require the same amount of stimulation for calming. Adapt redirection strategies to the child's personal response threshold. Modify approaches to the situation, i.e., serious situations require a more firm approach (e.g., when the child is in danger) and use care to not overrespond to more mild situations (e.g., when juice spills or things break).
Intensity of reaction	Help children to recognize their responses to positive and negative emotions. When an overresponse occurs, teach children how to modify their behavioral response to their feelings. Do not avoid situations in which frustrations may occur; part of developing emotional maturity is experiential.
Quality of mood	Use positive reinforcement for good mood responses to situations. Ignore negative mood responses.
Distractibility and attention span/persistence	Take a child's development and distractibility into consideration when doing tasks that require concentration (i.e., homework, quiet time). Teach the child strategies to help stay on track. Help parents set realistic expectations of the child's attention span.

TEMPERAMENT TYPES

Three temperament types are clinically significant and cross-culturally generalizable: difficult, easy, and slow to warm up. Children with difficult temperaments tend to have an intense and negative mood, slow adaptability, withdrawal from new situations, and irregular biological functions. Children with easy temperaments typically exhibit a positive mood, low intensity, easy adaptability, and regular and predictable biologic and behavioral patterns. These children are often described as being easygoing. Children with slow-to-warm-up temperaments are characterized by initial quiet alertness and subdued emotionality. Although reserved in new situations and with new stimuli, once the initial novelty wears off, slow-to-warm-up children demonstrate behaviors similar to children with easy or difficult temperaments. There is no absolute standard for any of these classifications, and all features of temperament must be considered in the context of the parents' evaluations.

TEMPERAMENT AS A RISK FACTOR

Difficult temperaments are most often associated with behavior disorders, although temperament alone is not a risk factor for maladjustment. Rather, temperament exerts an influence on children's psychosocial adjustment by affecting caretaker-child interactions. Difficult temperamental features tend to engender parental criticism and irritability, power struggles, and restrictive parenting. Critical mediators of the role of temperament in the development of behavioral disorders include parental psychological functioning, marital adjustment, child-rearing attitudes and practices, and social support factors.

Although temperament is unrelated to intelligence quotient (IQ), it affects academic outcomes, and some children are clearly disadvantaged by their more difficult temperaments in the majority of school environments.

TEMPERAMENT MANAGEMENT

The goal for the primary care provider is to help parents achieve goodness-of-fit for their children. Specific strategies for intervening with temperament issues have been developed for parents (Table 19-2). Those who care for children (e.g., parents, teachers, other caregivers) should:

- Recognize the child's innate behavioral qualities as expressions of temperament. This recognition can be facilitated by interview about child responses (e.g., changes in activities, new situations, changes in routines, new people) or by completing a standard temperament questionnaire.
- Understand how temperament is related to behavior and is not amenable to change. Allow parents to express their feelings about their child or their child's behavior and assisting them to reframe their assessment more positively. Members of the extended family who often advise parents may need to be included to help alleviate parental feelings of failure.
- Develop temperament-based management strategies, especially ways to deal with the more challenging areas of temperament. Such strategies can be applied to new situations as the child develops and becomes more autonomous, including those that occur in toddlerhood and preschool, such as mealtime and bedtime, or during school-related activities, such as doing homework.

Assessment and Management of Mental Health Disorders

The definition of a mental health disorder is a sustained behavior change that results in functional impairment. Because mental health problems cover a broad range of behavioral, emotional, and psychological disorders, many of which include genetic influences, the accurate identification of emotional, social, behavioral, and mental health status requires a thorough history and a physical examination. The physical examination detects underlying physical conditions that can result in behavioral or emotional changes. Primary care providers must recognize that common illness symptoms, such as fever, can change a child's behavior because of malaise, arthralgias, or other physical symptoms. A series of laboratory, developmental, and psychological tests may also be required. Suggested areas to explore with relation to mental health problems (or coping/stress problems as defined by Gordon's Functional Health Patterns) are reviewed below.

ASSESSMENT

Approaches to Children of Different Ages

During all health visits the primary care provider should assess the quality of the verbal and nonverbal exchanges between infants, children, and adolescents and their parents and the health care provider (Hagan et al, 2008). Specific attention should be paid to assess the emotions and energy the child displays, and the presence or absence of interaction among those present in the examination room. Additionally, *Bright Futures* and the AAP call for assessment of the family psychosocial functioning at all routine health supervision visits and routine screening for mental health issues using validated instruments (Foy et al, 2010; Hagan et al, 2008).

The manner in which the provider conducts the history and physical examination is as important as the information obtained. Many parents share their concerns only after a long period of trying to solve the problem themselves. They may be upset, worried, or frustrated. Many people are reluctant to discuss symptoms because of social stigmas against mental illness.

Providers are more likely to get a clear picture of what is happening and gain the family's trust if they take the time to sit down and actively listen at length to both the parent's and child's concerns and perceptions. It is critical to avoid rapidly firing questions, restricting the history to a preprinted schedule of questions, or taking notes that detract from giving full attention to the child and family. Sufficient time should be scheduled for the history and physical. If a potentially significant but nonemergent problem is uncovered in the course of an episodic visit, a lengthier appointment should be scheduled to avoid hurrying the assessment and potentially missing important data. It is essential to obtain information from the child's perspective and to use age-appropriate strategies.

Infants. Observations of babies and toddlers with their parents in structured and unstructured situations offer valuable clues to the strengths and limitations of each partner in the interaction. Understanding each partner provides guidance in developing a plan of care for any identified problems and is a way to follow progress in the relationship over time. Even unstructured observations allow the observer to appreciate the emotional exchanges and the presence or absence of sensitive and contingent interactions between the infant and parent.

Toddlers and Young Preschoolers. Playing with figures, dolls, and toys gives older toddlers and young preschoolers a way to express their feelings and emotions. Having a variety of dolls and toys on hand and allowing the child to play spontaneously provide the opportunity for the professional to ask questions within the nonthreatening context of play. This also helps to direct probing with parents. If the parent has already identified situations or people who provoke troubled behavior, the provider may select toys that are likely to elicit the child's story in play. For example, if the concerning behaviors began shortly after the birth of a new sibling, a baby doll, mother and father dolls, and a doll the age and gender of the child could be selected.

School-Age Children. Older preschoolers and young school-age children can be assessed by offering them the opportunity to draw a picture of themselves and their family, and asking them to tell a story about their picture. This allows the professional the opportunity to evaluate the child's feelings and emotions and, if problems and concerns become apparent, clarify details from the child's perspective in a nonthreatening and familiar way.

Adolescents. The primary care provider should separately interview the school-age child and adolescent. Allow 20 to 30 minutes for the school-age child and 30 minutes or more for the adolescent to share their perspectives and feelings. Most children are comfortable talking about their feelings and experiences if they have a supportive listener. It is important to clarify issues related to confidentiality with both the adolescent and caregiver prior to initiating a mental health assessment. Tailor questions to the child's or adolescent's level of understanding, keeping questions simple and providing examples to younger children. Sample questions include:

- "Tell me about some of the things you do very well. What types of things do you have a hard time doing?"
- "You look very sad to me. Would you share with me what is making you sad?"
- "Many children have things they worry about. What worries you most?"
- "How are things going in your family?"
- "How is school going?"
- "How are your relationships with other people? Do you feel like other people understand you and see you for who you really are?"
- "Everyone feels angry at times. What makes you angry? What do you do when you are angry?"
- "If you could change one thing in your life, what would it be?"
- "Tell me what you think the problem is from your point of view."

History

Correctly pinpointing mental health disorders requires a more thorough history than does the diagnosis of many physical health problems. Following the comprehensive health history model found in Box 2-2 will be helpful as daily living (functional health), disease, developmental, and family domains must all be addressed.

The Symptom Analysis: Behavioral Manifestations. Parents are keen observers of their children, so it is wise to listen carefully to their observations and concerns. Behaviors that concern a parent may include those that are developmentally normal for the child, or they may represent extremes of the range of normal behavior. By obtaining a clear idea of the parent's concerns, the provider can assess the parent's level of knowledge about child development and behavior, clarify which behaviors are developmentally normal (but distressing to the parent), and confirm which behaviors fall outside the range of normal. Eliciting information from teachers and other caregivers reinforces parental reports and provides a contextual understanding of child behavior.

Family Domain: Common Family-Related Stressors. Common stressors that should be identified through the history are discussed in this section. Questions and specific examples of stressors are found in Table 19-3.

- **Recent Changes.** When inquiring about recent changes in the child's life, it is helpful to specifically ask about changes in the family, work, school, and other settings because parents may not perceive some changes as sources of stress for their child. For example, parents may welcome a job promotion that includes the need for travel and a significant pay increase. However, this same change may stress the child, who is old enough to worry about how life will change with a traveling parent. Most recognize that the addition of a new family member is life changing for children already in the home, but other family changes like having a grandparent move in or an older sibling move out can be equally stressful. It is important to consider the developmental context of events and whether most children of a similar age would find the incident threatening or upsetting.

- **Contextual Changes in the Family.** Contextual changes are more enduring changes in life circumstances, either for better or worse, which provoke changes in the child's perception of self, family, or feelings of relationship security. These changes may result in self-blame or stem from the actions of other family members, especially parents, creating a sense of betrayal.

- **Parent Stress and Mental Illness.** All parents face stress and feelings of being overwhelmed. It is important to assist parents to identify situations in which they know risk of stress is greatest. For example, certain developmental stages are commonly more taxing than others and many young children have increasing behavioral problems in the late afternoon hours as fatigue increases and energy levels lag. Primary care providers provide anticipatory guidance to develop interventions to help parents predict and minimize these "at-risk" times. Parents with mental illness are at risk for increased role strain and parenting difficulties because of how their condition affects their perceptions and coping skills.

- **Impaired Parenting.** Impaired parenting occurs when there is a mismatch between parenting behaviors and a child's developmental or situational needs. This may result in inappropriate stimulation, inconsistent care, inappropriate supervision, developmentally inappropriate behavioral expectations, harsh words, child abuse or neglect, or child rejection. It is important to explore parenting influences. Parents face a tremendous challenge to adapt their parenting skills to the individual development and behavior of each child in their family. This may be evidenced by parental verbalization of dissatisfaction with their role, exacerbation, or inappropriate communication with the child. Child behaviors that may indicate impaired parenting include acting-out, developmental regression, and other aberrant behaviors.

- **Parents' Personal History of Being Parented.** A significant body of research confirms the effect of the parents' personal history of being parented on the quality of parenting provided to children. Parents' recollections of how they were parented are powerful influences on parental perceptions of child behavior, beliefs about children and childrearing, and ultimately the parenting behaviors used in the home (Lieberman and Van Horn, 2009). It is important to have the parents share memories, good and bad, of their childhood and what they liked and disliked about the parenting they experienced (see Table 19-3).

- **Family Health History.** A thorough history of mental and developmental disorders in family members should be conducted, including school failure, delinquency, substance abuse, learning disorders, reading problems, mood disorders, personality disorders, schizophrenia, attention-deficit/hyperactivity disorder (ADHD), autism, genetic syndromes, and birth defects.

Disease Domain

- **Prenatal and Birth History.** Was the pregnancy planned and wanted; maternal illnesses and discomforts during the pregnancy; problems with the pregnancy; when prenatal care began; maternal alcohol, drug, and tobacco use; occupational or environmental exposures; results of prenatal testing; maternal weight gain during pregnancy; response of significant others to the pregnancy; presence of social support during the pregnancy; and maternal depression during pregnancy. Also, spontaneous or induced labor, length of labor, complications or medical conditions arising during labor, type of delivery, and delivery complications.

- **Postnatal History.** Gestational age, birthweight and length, problems after delivery (including hypoglycemia and hyperbilirubinemia), problems in the first 2 weeks of life, difficulty feeding, excessive irritability or lethargy, maternal postpartum depression, and results of newborn screening.

- **Past Medical History.** Childhood illnesses and traumatic injuries, especially neurological injuries and soft neurological signs of developmental significance (e.g., delayed speech).

Developmental Domain: Developmental Progress. Achievement of milestones, level of social skills, relationships with peers, emotional maturity (e.g., ability to deal with the full spectrum of emotions)

Daily Living Domain. All areas of the daily living domain need to be explored because behavior may affect all areas of daily life—nutrition, elimination, sleep, activities, relationships with others, communication patterns, sense of self, cognitive perceptual behaviors, and so on.

Physical Examination

The practitioner should complete a thorough physical examination with particular attention to recognition of physical anomalies and neurological system evaluation. Also important is evaluation of affect, cognition, and mental status.

Diagnostic Studies

Laboratory Studies. Pertinent laboratory tests (hemoglobin, ASO titer, blood lead level, serum electrolytes, drug tests for alcohol or illicit substances, or urinalysis) can rule out physical health problems with behavioral manifestations.

TABLE 19-3 History Taking: Areas for Assessment of Mental Health

Topic	Sample Question	Potential Stressors
Behavioral manifestations: symptom analysis	"Please describe your child's behavior. What seems to make it better or worse? How have you tried to help your child? How does the behavior make you feel? How do think your child feels?"	• Unrealistic parental expectations for child behavior
Recent changes	"What events or changes have occurred in your family in the past year?"	• Increasing frequency or severity of behavior • Unpredictable situational context that elicits or maintains problem behavior (setting, timing, who is present, triggers) • Behavior negatively affects relationships or child functioning • Negative peer and/or teacher responses to and consequences of problem behavior • Parents' feelings hurt by the behavior • Parents unable to empathize with how the child feels • Parents unsure about what the parent needs and what the child needs to improve the situation
Contextual changes within the family	"Who lives in your home? Have there been any recent changes at home or changes in family relationships?"	• Changes in household composition (e.g., births, expansion of household to include elders) • Risk of loss or loss of attachment figure(s) • Changes in family relationships (e.g., death, separation, divorce, older sibling moving away) • Separation from the parent for foster care or care by others • Return to the biological family from kinship care or foster care • Family violence • Witness to trauma or violence • New role or responsibilities presenting a psychological challenge (e.g., birth of a sibling) • Sibling with special health care needs • Mental health problems of parents, especially maternal depression • Child's chronic illness or handicap
Recurring experiences	"Tell me about the things you find difficult or stressful as a parent, especially in caring for this child."	• Parental overprotection or neglect • Restrictive or overpermissive parenting • Control struggles • Ineffective conflict resolution • Lack of effective parental supervision • Parental failure to protect child in risky situations • Ineffective limit-setting strategies • Use of harsh discipline practices • Parental mental or physical illness • Reliance on the child by the parents for emotional comfort and support
Parents' personal history of being parented	"Tell me about your most favorite and least favorite memories of growing up. How is your parenting similar to and different from the parenting you received as a child? What are your expectations for your child?"	• Parent abused or neglected as a child • Parent adopted or in foster care as a child • Unhappy parent childhood, poor role models • Poor family communication patterns in family of origin • Any indicators of parental psychopathological condition, particularly maternal depression • The parents' perception of the child, especially temperament, poor fit with parent • The parents' knowledge and beliefs about harsh discipline or coercive parent-child interactions • The parents' knowledge and beliefs about the development of autonomy and self-esteem, especially in relation to parenting strategies (e.g., praise and affection) and conflict resolution • Parental strategies to facilitate the child's coping, given developmental level and temperament • Unrealistic academic, athletic, or social expectations of the child

The family history and findings on the physical examination may warrant chromosomal studies.

Imaging Studies. Imaging of the central nervous system may be recommended depending on family history, developmental, and neurological findings.

Behavioral/Developmental Screening and Assessment Tools. A structured developmental screening or assessment should be included in the assessment. If warranted by suspicious or ambiguous findings, a referral for a thorough developmental evaluation by a skilled psychologist or multidisciplinary developmental assessment team is appropriate. Behavioral rating scales or checklists are valuable screening tools, especially those with established reliability and validity that provide norms as a basis for comparison. Screening instruments with sound reliability and validity include the Ages & Stages Questionnaire for developmental screening; the Ages & Stages Social-Emotional Screen for social and emotional concerns; the 10-minute Brief Infant-Toddler Social-Emotional Assessment (BITSEA) screen and its companion in-depth assessment, Infant-Toddler Social-Emotional Assessment (ITSEA), for use as a follow-up assessment if problems arise on the BITSEA screen. The Achenbach Child Behavior Checklist has excellent reliability and validity and has been used successfully with a wide variety of clinical populations. Available in English and Spanish, it provides separate checklists for assessment of children 1.5 to 5 years old and 6 to 18 years old, with norms provided by age and gender, and separate report forms for parents and teachers. Other checklists with clinical utility include the Pediatric Symptom Checklist (PSC) for children at least 11 years old (Hagan et al, 2008). Even if children's scores do not reach a clinical level by normative standards, attention must be paid to notably high scores, stable problem behavior, and attending circumstances.

Maternal postpartum depression (PPD) can negatively affect infant development, so routine screening for symptoms of PPD is merited during episodic health visits in early infancy (Hagan et al, 2008). Standardized screening tools like the Edinburgh Postnatal Depression Scale (EPDS) are easy to use in the clinical setting. Mothers with positive screens should be referred to adult mental health professionals for further evaluation and treatment.

Temperament assessment can be useful for infants, toddlers, preschoolers, and school-age children. Parent reports of temperament reflect the parents' perception, which may not accurately reflect objective reality. However, accurate or not, the parents' perceptions influence their behavior and feelings toward the child and must be taken seriously.

A behavioral diary or log kept by parents, by the school-age child or adolescent, and by the teacher informs the practitioner and family about the situational context for and severity of the behavior. Often this monitoring process itself serves as an effective intervention.

MAKING MENTAL HEALTH AND BEHAVIORAL DIAGNOSES

Making mental health diagnoses is often difficult. One must decide whether behaviors are within normal limits for age, temperament, family, health, and other factors. Comorbidities are common. In practice, several diagnoses may need to be addressed: the behavior, the family effects, nutrition, sleep, and other interrelated issues. In many cases, a mental health specialist such as a clinical psychologist or psychiatrist may be required to assist in diagnostic decision-making.

STRATEGIES FOR MANAGEMENT

After the diagnostic list is made, the primary care provider will need to decide how to manage and/or co-manage problems with other pediatric specialists. Pediatric primary care providers manage more mental health problems than ever before, largely because the scarcity of mental health services or inadequate insurance coverage makes mental health care out of reach for many families. However, many primary care providers lack adequate education to manage complex problems. In addition, it is financially difficult for many busy primary care practices to offer the extended appointments needed for high-quality mental health care.

As a rule, if the cause of the problem is a life event with acute, short-term consequences, such as the death of a pet or a friend moving away, or a common developmentally normal but troublesome behavior (e.g., temper tantrums or sibling rivalry), it can be managed in the primary care setting. More enduring problems, such as loss of a parent or major depression, require referral to or consultation with a pediatric mental health specialist.

Appropriate care of pediatric mental illness always requires an interdisciplinary approach. Pharmacotherapy alone is never appropriate, nor should it be used without a thorough mental health evaluation (AACAP, 2009a). Clinical practice guidelines further emphasize the need for treatments to be evidence-based and inclusive of short- and long-term follow-up plans. All ethical issues regarding consent and assent are especially important in mental health care. Parents and patients should be aware of treatment risks, benefits, and alternative options (AACAP, 2009a).

Common Mental Health Problems

Special Problems of Infancy and Early Childhood

For many years it was believed that infants and young children could not have mental health problems. It was as though pediatric health care providers believed that young children were protected from even the most adverse experiences. Research since the 1940s clearly demonstrates that this is not the case. Today, despite a growing body of knowledge about children's mental health problems, frameworks used to identify and treat disorders in older children, adolescents, and adults still provide little guidance in the care of the very young. The *Diagnostic Classification of Mental Health and Developmental Disorders of Infancy and Early Childhood* (DC:0-3R) defines conditions that affect the youngest children (Zero to Three, 2005).

At first glance the diagnoses seem to address familiar issues in infant and early childhood development, and are commonly addressed in pediatric primary care. Closer examination of the diagnostic criteria demonstrates that these diagnoses address more serious degrees of maladaptive behaviors, often with a significant parental dysfunction and distress. These issues are beyond the management abilities of most primary care providers who do not have extensive preparation in the field of infant mental health. One of the most common classifications (feeding disorders) is presented here, while regulation disorders are discussed in Chapter 15. The purpose of including them is to increase the primary care provider's awareness of the range of conditions that are best treated by the infant mental health specialist.

FEEDING DISORDERS

Feeding the infant and young child is a key parental task. Parents feel successful and competent when their infant or young child feeds vigorously and grows well. Conversely, feeding problems result in parental frustration and failing child growth and can provoke feelings of failure in many parents. Feeding problems are among the most stubborn challenges primary care providers encounter (see Chapter 10). A serious problem exists when an infant or young child fails to establish a regular feeding pattern based on hunger and satiety. The potential diagnoses cover problems in:

- State regulations that interfere with the infant's ability to feed well
- Lack of reciprocity between the caregiver and infant during the feeding
- Infantile anorexia associated with a very active infant or young child who refuses food
- Sensory food aversions that are so numerous and extreme they result in nutritional deficiencies (Zero to Three, 2005)

REGULATION DISORDERS OF SENSORY PROCESSING

These disorders are discussed in Chapter 15.

THE SHY CHILD
Description
Shyness is a pattern of social inhibition with unfamiliar people, with novel objects, or in unfamiliar situations. Inhibition is evident in infancy as an inborn bias to respond to unfamiliar events with anxiety, distress, or disorganization. Many toddlers are shy, but this diminishes normally by school age. Although most shy children do not develop later internalizing disorders, extremely shy toddlers may be at risk for social withdrawal in later childhood and for developing an anxiety disorder in adolescence.

Epidemiology
Shyness is caused by a rather stable temperamental disposition toward withdrawal that is linked to family factors. Shyness is common. Behavioral inhibition in social situations may be adaptive if handled effectively by the parent and can be indicative of optimal self-regulation and development of conscience.

Clinical Findings
Retreat and withdrawal from social stimulation are noted in infancy. In toddlerhood, general inhibition persists, evidenced by irritability, withdrawal, and clinging to the mother in new situations. Shy children are slower to approach peers or initiate play with an unfamiliar child and often spend more time observing the situation and other children in play before engaging. School-age shy children continue to make fewer social approaches. They usually "warm up slowly" or may engage in solitary but appropriate play. Viewed by their peers as likable but shy, these children may be neglected by their peers. One or both parents usually identify themselves as shy (Rubin et al, 2010).

Differential Diagnosis
Children with social withdrawal rather than shyness have a lower rate of social interaction overall and do not warm up to social situations.

Management
Parenting strategies that provide warmth, sensitivity, and responsiveness to the child's inhibition and shyness will foster security in attachment relationships and facilitate social competence. In preschool and school-age children, insensitivity and a lack of responsiveness foster a sense of insecurity and predict social withdrawal, with associated internalizing disorders, including depression and adolescent anxiety. It is helpful to have parents prepare shy children for new situations by visiting new settings, identifying a sensitive adult to whom they may turn with requests or concerns, and negotiating for them to be allowed to watch and observe before engaging in play or other activities.

BEREAVEMENT
Description
Grief is a feeling of distress, sorrow, and loss, whereas *bereavement* is the process of dealing with loss. Many people use grief and bereavement terms interchangeably. *Mourning* is the psychological process set in motion by loss of a loved one. The death of someone important to a child is considered one of the most stressful events to be experienced. For children and adolescents, death of a parent or sibling is the most profoundly disturbing loss.

Epidemiology
The clinical picture of bereavement and grief depends, to some extent, on the concept of death. In infancy and toddlerhood, death is perceived as separation or abandonment, with no real cognitive understanding of death or the emotional resources to deal with loss; the central issue is the sense of loss or abandonment that can be due to temporary causes (e.g., parental travel, sibling hospitalization, natural disaster), long-term causes (e.g., parental separation, foster care placement), or permanent (e.g., death) (Serwint, 2007). Family member loss is particularly difficult because it results in the loss of the love and support from that person, significant effect on family functioning and resources, and changes in routines. Preschoolers, up to 6 years old, tend to perceive death as a continuation of life under different circumstances. Death is personified and perceived as a punishment (AAP, 2000). From 6 to 11 years old, children grasp the irreversibility and finality of death, akin to the adult concept,

although they struggle with understanding the specific loss of the loved one. Preadolescents and adolescents are able to be more abstract and philosophical about death. At any given developmental stage, a child can resolve the effect of the death only at that developmental level. Thus bereavement resurfaces, and the significance of the loss needs to be reworked at each subsequent developmental stage. It is expected that most children and adolescents experience at least one significant loss before they reach adulthood. It is estimated that 5% of children lose one or both parents to death before 15 years old.

Clinical Findings

Infants and toddlers cry out or search for the absent caregiver, refuse the attempts of others to soothe them, withdraw emotionally, appear sad, and no longer engage in age-appropriate activities. Sleep and feeding are disturbed; they display developmental regression and demonstrate extreme reactions to reminders of the missing caregiver through apathy, anger, or crying.

For a preschool and older child, grief is a process that unfolds over time. Initially children may seem emotionally unmoved, but the initial shock and denial give way to depressive symptoms that can last for weeks or months. A normal reaction to loss, depressive symptoms include sadness, feeling depressed, vomiting, bed-wetting, poor appetite, weight loss, insomnia, crying, internalizing symptoms (e.g., headache and stomachache), anxiety, guilt, and idealization of the person who died. Rage is a common reaction to the death of a parent, typically directed at the surviving parent and others in the immediate family. Angry behavior may be directed at peers as well, compounding a sense of inferiority and alienation. Fears of dying, disease, and growing old are often stimulated. Identification with the deceased is common and needs to be assessed to determine whether this furthers or inhibits development. Similarly, a fantasy connection to a dead parent can develop and may be helpful. Guilt and responsibility are typical issues for children but are less problematic for adolescents. Adolescents often manifest a sudden "maturity" along with numbness, regrets, disorganization, and despair before closure and reorganization are achieved. It is not unusual for adolescents to develop stronger ties with friends and to distance from family while grieving.

Differential Diagnosis

Children at high risk for pathological bereavement or depression generally have a previous history of individual and family problems. Symptoms of bereavement that should concern the provider include the following:
- Long-term denial and avoidance of feelings
- Suicidal wishes
- Preoccupation with death
- Distressing guilt about actions taken or not taken
- Preoccupation with worthlessness
- Persistent anger
- Decline in school performance
- Social withdrawal
- Persistent sleep problems
- Hallucinations beyond transitory experience of hearing the voice of, or seeing the image of, the deceased

Management

Parent education facilitates effective bereavement management in children and adolescents. A first question is whether children and adolescents should attend the funeral or memorial service. Children need to participate in the rituals around death as much as they choose. Such services and rituals provide even young children with an important way to grieve, especially if such involvement is supportive, appropriately explained, and congruent with the family's values.

Children need parental help to understand the facts of death and to correct misunderstandings as they develop; children cannot understand, however, beyond their cognitive level. Parents often need to be reassured that showing their own feelings (e.g., disbelief, guilt, sadness, anger) is normal and helpful to children; sharing feelings about and memories of the family member who died is helpful as well. Sensitivity to the child's reactions of grief and restlessness is important, as is support for the child's assimilation and mastery of the loss and emotional experience. Children need to express and work through feelings and fantasies related to the loss; communication is a must.

There are many books about death, loss, and grieving for children and adolescents that are geared to the various developmental levels. It is critical for children to have an attachment to an adult who can be an effective source of support and involvement, as well as a focus for reactions to loss (Serwint, 2007). The child must be sensitively prepared for any changes occurring at the same time as the death, with the family advised to minimize these as much as possible. Any parental loss before 5 years old probably warrants treatment. Because bereavement resurfaces at subsequent developmental phases, early parental loss should be determined and current symptoms assessed as a possible manifestation of recurring bereavement issues.

■ Fears, Phobias, and Anxieties

FEARS AND PHOBIAS

Description

Fear is the occurrence of various avoidance responses to particular stimuli; it is a state of apprehension in response to a threatening situation. In contrast, a phobia is a persistent, extreme, and irrational fear triggered by the presence or anticipation of the presence of a specific person, object, or situation. The onset of fears occurs normally during late infancy and early toddlerhood and manifests as separation anxiety and stranger anxiety.

Epidemiology

Childhood fears are a part of normal development. Fears have a developmental function, and the nature of predominant fears varies with age. Specific phobias occur in about 5% of the population and in 15% of children referred for anxiety-related problems. Phobias are determined by multiple factors including genetic influences, temperament, parental mental health problems, and individual conditioning histories.

Clinical Findings

Infants typically react fearfully to loss of support, height, and unexpected stimuli. Toddlers experience separation anxiety and fear physical injury and strangers. Preschoolers fear imaginary creatures, animals, darkness, and being alone; they also demonstrate some persistent separation anxiety. Fear of animals and darkness extends into school age, but safety, natural events, and school- and health-related fears dominate. In preadolescence and adolescence, fears of bodily injury, economic and political catastrophes, and social fears are central. Fear and phobic reactions typically involve symptoms of autonomic arousal. In phobias, the symptoms of autonomic arousal may evolve into panic attacks or phobic-avoidant reactions.

Differential Diagnosis

Distinction must be made between abnormal fears and normal developmental fears. Clinical phobias are defined on the basis of persistence, magnitude, and maladaptiveness.

Management

Most fears are short-lived, are not serious, and do not predict adult mental health problems. Parents must be cautioned against using fears as a form of behavioral control (e.g., threats of abandonment with toddlers, or threatening a school-age child with an immunization) or as a discipline strategy (e.g., leaving a preschooler alone in a dark room). When the fear negatively affects the child's functioning, developmental progress, learning experiences, and level of comfort, referral is necessary. Treatment for fearful and phobic infants, toddlers, and preschoolers focuses on improving parent mental health, parental–child behavior management skills, and the quality of the marital relationship. Various management strategies are available for treatment of phobias in children older than 5 years, including systematic desensitization, contingency management, cognitive-behavioral procedures, and family interventions (AACAP, 2007).

ANXIETY

Anxiety is a diffuse apprehension in response to less specific stimuli; fear stimuli are more specific. It is a normal developmental phenomenon that is experienced by every person at some point. Anxious responses include somatic symptoms mediated by the autonomic system. These responses include physiological changes, such as increased heart rate and blood pressure, tremor, sweating, and enhanced vigilance and reactivity. Anxiety that persists at high levels and is reflected in maladaptive behavior warrants diagnosis and treatment. Anxiety disorders include conditions associated with childhood, like separation anxiety, and those also associated with adulthood like generalized anxiety disorder, obsessive-compulsive disorder (OCD), and posttraumatic stress disorder (PTSD). Children diagnosed with anxiety disorders tend to have multiple problems, are impaired in important areas of social functioning, and live with parents who experience symptoms of anxiety or mood disorders. Anxiety disorders typically appear in the preschool years. The earlier the onset of these disorders, the greater the impairment in social and personal development thus leading to a much greater likelihood of poor subjective views of their personal mental and physical health, social relationships, career satisfaction, and home and family relationships (Olantunji et al, 2007).

Risk factors include: (1) genetics, (2) temperamental disposition for behavioral inhibition, and (3) social environment or life circumstances (e.g., parental distress or dysfunction or trauma), especially during vulnerable developmental periods (e.g., attachment or separation-individuation) (Stafford et al, 2007). Youngsters with anxiety disorders are at high risk for subsequent anxiety disorders, for comorbid mood disorders, and for adolescent substance abuse. Anxiety disorders distinctly cluster in families (AACAP, 2007).

SEPARATION ANXIETY DISORDER

Description

The essential feature of separation anxiety disorder is an abnormal reaction to real or imagined separation from major attachment figures, home, or familiar surroundings (Hanna et al, 2006). Separation anxiety is a normal developmental phenomenon from about 7 months old through the preschool years. However, some infants and toddlers experience excessive levels of distress with separation from the major caregiver. These children cry persistently and cannot be comforted or refuse to be cared for and comforted by a competent, substitute caregiver. Alternatively, older infants, toddlers, and preschoolers may act aggressively toward the substitute caregiver or intentionally injure themselves (Zero to Three, 2005).

Separation anxiety disorder, in which reactivity to separation interferes with daily activities and developmental tasks, manifests from 5 to 16 years old; the mean age for clinical presentation is 9 years (Hanna et al, 2006). This diagnosis can be a precursor for panic disorder in adolescence or adulthood (Stafford et al, 2007).

Epidemiology

Separation anxiety disorder evolves from a poor attachment relationship or the interaction among physiological, cognitive, and overt behavioral factors in response to life events that threaten safety or primary relationships, or both. It is probably the most common anxiety disorder from older infancy through the school-age years and the most common mental health reason for referral (Zero to Three, 2005). Among infants and young children, only about 10% of those affected by separation anxiety are referred for care despite the concerns of the majority of parents. Older children are usually brought to the health care provider when the disorder results in school refusal or somatic symptoms. About 80% of children with school refusal are thought to have separation anxiety disorder, many of these with comorbid depression (Stafford et al, 2007).

Clinical Findings

The following are found in separation anxiety disorder:
- Developmentally inappropriate or excessive anxiety about separations
- Unrealistic worry about harm to self or attachment figures or about abandonment during periods of separation
- Reluctance to sleep alone or sleep away from home
- Persistent avoidance of being alone
- Nightmares about separation
- Physical complaints and signs of distress in anticipation of separation
- Social withdrawal during separations
- Environmental stress, parental dysfunction, and maternal depression are risk factors for separation anxiety disorder, especially with panic disorder or agoraphobia

The Spielberger State-Trait Anxiety Inventory for Children (STAIC) is a 20-item, self-report scale useful with children 9 to 12 years old; it can also be used with high reading-skill younger children and low reading-skill adolescents.

Differential Diagnosis

Anxiety disorder not associated with separation is a differential diagnosis. Anxiety may occur as a response to trauma or a manifestation of PTSD (AACAP, 2007). It is essential to attend to cues that a traumatic experience or situation (e.g., sexual or physical abuse) is the source of the symptoms of anxiety. From 30% to 70% of children and adolescents with an anxiety disorder have a depressive disorder, and 15% to 25% of children and adolescents with an anxiety disorder also meet the diagnostic criteria for ADHD (AACAP, 2007). Common comorbidities with separation anxiety include social phobia and overanxious disorder (Stafford et al, 2007).

Management

Anxiety disorder is best treated as a family system or relationship-based problem (Stafford et al, 2007). Relief of symptoms is the first priority in school-age children. Identifying and treating the sources of the problem is the first line of treatment for infants through preschoolers and a secondary focus of treatment for school-age children. Note the role of attachment figures and refer the child to a child therapist for early intervention. Among school-age children, psychoeducational, behavioral, and cognitive-behavioral approaches have been effective (In-Albon and Schneider, 2007). In general, pharmacotherapy is used only if the child fails to respond to nonpharmacological intervention and considerable impairment in function is experienced.

Before beginning a medication regimen, it is a good idea to refer the patient to a child psychiatrist or child and adolescent mental health care provider for a medication evaluation. Selective serotonin reuptake inhibitors (SSRIs) are the first-choice medications in separation anxiety disorder, in part because of their limited adverse effects (Stafford et al, 2007).

GENERALIZED ANXIETY DISORDER

Description

Generalized anxiety disorder is cognitive and obsessive in nature. The child experiences excessive anxiety, worry, and apprehensive expectations generalized to a number of events or activities. These anxieties do not focus on a specific person, object, or situation, nor are they the result of a recent stressor. Children with generalized anxiety disorder are characterized as "worriers." The exact onset is not known, but the diagnosis occurs most often among older children and adolescents 9 to 18 years old.

Epidemiology

Generalized anxiety is one of the most prevalent psychiatric disorders, affecting approximately 1% to 2% of children, and is responsible for approximately one third of mental health service utilization (Chueng and Jensen, 2009; Merikangas et al, 2010). There is a familial association for generalized anxiety disorder that suggests a genetic vulnerability to anxiety; twin studies suggest that shared environment is far less important than genetic factors (AACAP, 2007).

Clinical Findings

Major symptoms of generalized anxiety disorder are:
- Worry about future events
- Poor-quality sleep
- Irritability and tantrums in young children
- Preoccupation with past behavior
- Overconcern about competence
- Marked preoccupation with performance
- Significant self-consciousness
- Restlessness
- Difficulty concentrating
- Somatic complaints without a physical basis
- Unexplained fatigue
- Unusual need for reassurance
- Comorbidity with other anxiety disorders or mood disorder, which is common

Differential Diagnosis

Differential diagnoses are separation anxiety, adjustment disorder associated with a specific stressor, and attention-deficit disorder. It is important to attend to cues that might point to traumatic experiences or conditions as the source of anxiety symptoms. It is important to rule out the presence of pediatric autoimmune neuropsychiatric disorders associated with streptococcal infection (PANDAS) (see Obsessive-Compulsive Disorder).

Management

The treatment of preschool children and toddlers generally focuses on behavioral and family interventions. Preschoolers may benefit from play therapy. Although clinicians administer SSRIs and other psychotropic medications to children as young as 2 years old, there are no efficacy data, and long-term developmental sequelae of these treatments are unknown. Refer the older child or adolescent to a pediatric mental health therapist for treatment of symptoms using relaxation techniques or cognitive-behavioral therapy (CBT). Individual and/or family counseling can be used to identify the source of anxiety. Treatment outcomes are more positive when parents are involved in interventions that target familial contextual processes. Younger school-age children especially seem to benefit from a combination of cognitive-behavioral strategies and family intervention (AACAP, 2007). Individual and group treatments or child- and family-focused treatments are equally effective, and follow-up data demonstrate that treatment gains are maintained up to several years after treatment (In-Albon and Schneider, 2007).

Pharmacological intervention is advisable, especially if there is comorbid social phobia or separation anxiety disorder. Evidence points to the safety and efficacy of the SSRIs, especially fluvoxamine and fluoxetine, and other medications like buspirone (Isper et al, 2009). Benzodiazepines have not been shown to be superior to placebo in randomized controlled trials and potentially cause tolerance and dependency (AACAP, 2007).

OBSESSIVE-COMPULSIVE DISORDER

Description

Obsessions are recurrent thoughts, images, or impulses that are disturbing to the child and difficult to dislodge. They often involve a sense of risk or fear of harm to the child or family members; concerns about contamination are common. Compulsions are repetitive behaviors or mental acts that the child feels driven to perform with the aim of reducing the anxiety associated with obsessions and include behaviors such as washing (e.g., hands, objects, or body), counting, or arranging objects. Recurrent worries, rituals, and superstitious games are common in children at various stages of development. These behaviors result in mild anxiety but do not cause distress. OCD differs from normal child behavior in that it results in marked distress, is time consuming (individuals often spend a minimum of 1 hour a day engaged in the behavior), and interferes with the child's social, familial, or academic function. Abnormal compulsive behavior is distinguished by a sense of urgency or a profound discomfort until the ritual is completed. Children often deny the fear and lack recognition of the "senselessness" of the ritual and seem to hide their illness. Obsessive thoughts are intrusive, recurrent, and disturbing and, unlike anxious worries, are generally unrelated to events or situations.

Epidemiology

OCD is more common than previously thought and national estimates indicate a prevalence of 1% to 4% (Sturm, 2009). OCD is more common in males (3:2) prior to adolescence, but gender-based differences disappear after puberty. OCD can be diagnosed as young as 2 years of age, especially in children with play or interests that have a compulsive or ritualistic quality (e.g., playing with objects in only one certain sequence, with interruption producing intense distress), but the mean age of symptom onset is 10.3 years (Sturm, 2009). Research indicates that as many as one third to one half of adults with OCD had initial symptoms before age 15 (Gilbert and Maalouf, 2008). Like most psychiatric conditions, OCD is a chronic disease, and research demonstrates as many as 40% of children continue to have the disease 2 to 7 years later, despite undergoing treatment (Leckman et al, 2009).

Multiple theories suggest neurobiological causes of OCD that include alterations in serotonin and abnormalities in the basal ganglia and functionally related cortical structures (Lewin et al, 2005). There are strong familial patterns of transmission, and the link between genetics and OCD is strongest for early-onset disease (Sturm, 2009). Lastly, a subgroup of pediatric patients with OCD is diagnosed with PANDAS, which is believed to be the result of autoimmune responses following group A beta-hemolytic streptococcus (GABHS) or *Mycoplasma pneumoniae* infections (Leckman et al, 2009). PANDAS diagnostic criteria include dramatic onset of OCD or tic disorder in children between 3 years and puberty shortly following GABHS infection and symptom exacerbation (Sturm, 2009).

Clinical Findings

OCD is a chronic condition, with high rates of comorbidity, typically other anxiety disorders, major depression, or substance abuse disorder. Disruptive behavior disorders and learning disorders are also common comorbid diagnoses. OCD is characterized by obsessions and compulsions, as previously defined. Children may not recognize that their obsessions or compulsions are excessive or unreasonable, so determination of insight into the behaviors is important. They derive no pleasure from their ritualistic activity. The obsessions and compulsions are time consuming and may significantly interfere with the child's or adolescent's normal routine, academic performance, and social functioning. The most common obsession is fear of contamination that results in compulsive washing and avoidance of "contaminated" objects. Other common obsessive worries include fears about safety (their own or their parents'), exactness or symmetry, and religious sinfulness (scrupulosity). Common compulsions include repetitive counting, arranging or touching patterns, and compulsive rechecking (doors, homework, exam items) (Gilbert and Maalouf, 2008; Sturm, 2009). Often children express the need to repeat a behavior "until I get it right."

Differential Diagnosis

In order to assess context and severity of symptoms, primary care providers should obtain information from the child, parents, family members, and teachers (Sturm, 2009). A diagnosis of OCD is warranted if the content of the obsessions and compulsions is unrelated to another mental health disorder (e.g., social phobia, trichotillomania, pervasive developmental disorder, body dysmorphic disorder). Medical conditions that mimic OCD include carbon monoxide poisoning, tumors, encephalitis, traumatic brain injury, Prader-Willi (compulsive eating), drug side effects (stimulants), and rheumatic fever. Providers should assess developmental history to determine delays and/or difficulties. School performance may be impaired and OCD may mimic learning disorders when children have compulsions to reread or rewrite, or have pathological perfectionism (Sturm, 2009). Parents of children with secretive rituals may bring their child to primary care with complaints of skin rashes (dermatitis, chapped hands), temper tantrums, declining school performance, or sudden food or activity aversions. Individuals with self-injurious behavior (see Chapter 8) physically harm themselves in order to decrease mental anguish; however, this disorder is distinct from the rituals of OCD.

Assessment should include symptom description and context, frequency, and effect on daily functioning. The National Institute for Health and Clinical Excellence guidelines indicate that six screening questions can be used to determine OCD pathology (Box 19-2). Children with suspected PANDAS and unclear history of recent upper respiratory tract infection should

---

BOX 19-2 Quick Screening Questions for Obsessive-Compulsive Disorder

- Do you wash yourself or clean more than most people?
- Do you feel the need to check or double-check things often?
- Do you have thoughts that bother you that you would like to get rid of but can't?
- Do you find yourself spending a lot of time doing things (brushing teeth, getting dressed)?
- Does it bother you when things are not lined up or are not in order?
- Do these problems bother you?

Data from NICE guidelines (National Institute for Health and Clinical Excellence, 2005).

have confirmation of streptococcal infection either by throat culture or ASO titer. Clinical findings that differentiate PANDAS from classic OCD are urinary frequency, hyperactivity, impulsivity, and worsening handwriting (Bernstein et al, 2010).

Management

OCD is a chronic condition that includes persistent symptoms in 60% of those with subthreshold disease, and 41% of those with full clinical disease (Gilbert and Maalouf, 2008). Decisions regarding treatment of OCD should center on the degree of child impairment. If the child's symptoms do not interfere with the child's life and do not cause undue distress, treatment can be deferred (Sturm, 2009). Optimal treatment involves an individualized and developmentally appropriate approach that centers on child and family therapy to help the child learn to manage his or her anxiety and distress (Mancuso et al, 2010). Drug therapy results in an average of 25% decrease in symptoms severity. Evidence suggests that SSRIs (sertraline, fluoxetine, and fluvoxamine) provide the best pharmacological effects with the greatest drug safety margin (Mancuso et al, 2010). Clinical and empirical evidence suggests that CBT, alone or in combination with pharmacotherapy, is an effective treatment for OCD in children and adolescents. Anxiety management training and OCD-specific family interventions may play an adjunctive role, especially in preventing the avoidant behavior that is a complication of OCD (AACAP, 2007). Recent findings support the efficacy of CBT with a structured family component. SSRIs are second-line pharmacological agents and have demonstrated effectiveness and improvement in quality of life in randomized controlled trials (Isper et al, 2009; Reinblatt and Riddle, 2007).

Research indicates that antibiotic treatment can help rapidly diminish tics in a subgroup of children with PANDAS; however, routine penicillin prophylaxis is not recommended (Sturm, 2009). Individuals with severe symptoms may benefit from plasma exchange and immunoglobulin administration, but this treatment combination remains controversial (Mancuso et al, 2010).

TIC DISORDERS

Description

Tic disorders are characterized by repetitive, fast, unconscious movements or vocalizations. Tourette syndrome results in motor and verbal tics that persist for more than 1 year. All children have some repetitive habits such as finger sucking or hair twirling, and many of these are adaptive behaviors that help decrease stress or provide a sense of calm. Habits are considered pathological when they have no clear purpose and when they result in physical or social impairment. Common pediatric tic disorders include trichotillomania (pulling out hair), bruxism (tooth grinding), skin pulling, and nail biting (Blum et al, 2009; Gleason et al, 2007). The disorders cause significant anxiety for affected children and often result in impaired self-esteem, bullying, and emotional or academic problems.

Epidemiology

Transient tics are fairly common and occur in 12% to 24% of school-age children, whereas chronic tics, those that last for more than 1 year, occur in 1% to 2% of the population. Half of all motor tics begin by age 7 and half of all vocal tics begin by age 9 (Blum, 2009). There is some evidence that children with developmental disorders have greater risk of developing tics than their nonaffected peers (Gleason et al, 2007). There are clear genetic influences to Tourette syndrome. The prevalence of Tourette syndrome is approximately 10% to 15% in children with affected first-degree relatives (Blum, 2009).

Clinical Findings

Motor tics can be simple (involving a single muscle group) or complex (complicated movements like jumping or a series of simple tics). Common simple tics include blinking, twitching of hands or limbs, shoulder shrugging, tongue thrusting, or squinting. Verbal tics include vocalizations or pushing air through the nose. The most common verbal tics involve grunting sounds or clearing the throat. Obscene gestures and swearing are rare (Blum, 2009). Symptoms generally worsen during periods of stress, fatigue, or anxiety.

Differential Diagnosis

There is considerable diagnostic overlap between tic disorders, learning disorders, and OCD. Differential diagnoses include OCD, PANDAS, attention-deficit disorder, seizure disorders, and dyskinesias.

Management

Mild tics do not require treatment. Children with moderate to severe tics that disrupt their self-esteem or impair their socialization best respond to psychotherapy, specifically CBT (Blum, 2009; Gleason et al, 2007). The focus of treatment is to extinguish the tic, to increase children's awareness of the behaviors, and to teach another behavior to engage in when they feel they are about to have a tic behavior. Best responses are often obtained with older children and adolescents. Common reminder strategies include using an elastic bandage over a digit to discourage thumb sucking, using an elastic hair band to make it difficult to grasp hair, or placing a rubber band that can be gently pulled when a child is aware of engaging in a tic behavior. Positive reinforcement is another effective extinguishing strategy. It is important to note that tics cannot be extinguished when the child is not interested in stopping the habit (Blum, 2009). When used, common psychopharmaceuticals include SSRIs, atypical antipsychotics, and anticonvulsants (Parraga et al, 2010).

RESPONSES TO TRAUMA: POSTTRAUMATIC STRESS DISORDER

Description

PTSD describes a characteristic set of symptoms that develops following exposure to a severe stressor or trauma. The trauma may result from a single event ("one sudden blow" trauma) or variable, multiple long-standing events, such as ongoing maltreatment. According to the *Diagnostic and Statistical Manual of Mental Disorders,* Fourth Edition (DSM-IV-TR), the criteria for PTSD include:

- Witnessing or experiencing a traumatic event(s) that resulted in risk of death or serious injury to oneself or a loved one

- Event(s) that resulted in fear, helplessness, horror, agitation, or disorganized behavior (the latter two are more common in children)
- Symptoms that cause increased arousal, emotional numbing, and intrusive thoughts
- Symptoms that last at least 1 month and cause significant impairment in social, cognitive, or school functioning
- Acute symptoms that last less than 3 months and chronic symptoms that last more than 3 months (American Psychiatric Association [APA], 2000)

Epidemiology

Exposure to trauma is a key feature of the diagnosis of PTSD. Unfortunately there are those who are skeptical about whether children suffer from PTSD. Parents and teachers frequently minimize traumatic effect, perhaps to relieve themselves of vicarious distress or to reassure themselves that their children have not suffered harm. Others, including mental health professionals, rationalize that children are too young to remember the trauma or too immature to be affected. However, the clinical descriptive and empirical evidence documents PTSD symptoms and other psychological difficulties experienced by children in various catastrophic situations and in situations of maltreatment.

Substantial PTSD rates are documented for children in foster care who were sexually or physically abused. This evidence leads to a better understanding of the clinical manifestations of PTSD in children. Three factors consistently influence the severity of the response: severity of the trauma exposure, parental distress related to the trauma, and temporal proximity to the event.

Retrospective reports of adults with mental health problems indicate that PTSD is more common than previously believed. Prevalence rates of 0.1% to 6% for children exposed to traumatic stressors are reported (Meiser-Stedman et al, 2008). The rate of PTSD is high among those who have been physically and sexually abused, with estimates ranging from 25% to 75% of sexual abuse victims. The closer the perpetrator is in relation to the victim, the greater the trauma (e.g., PTSD is more likely when the perpetrator is a member of the immediate family as opposed to an extended family member, family friend, or stranger) (Zero to Three, 2005).

Clinical Findings

A diagnosis of PTSD requires that the child demonstrate specific behaviors following trauma, as follows:
1. The child repeatedly reexperiences a set of symptoms from each of three categories (APA, 2000), including the following:
   - Recurrent and intrusive memories of the trauma
   - Nightmares of monsters or threats to self or others or distressing dreams about a specific event
   - Distress caused by cues that symbolize or resemble an aspect of the trauma, including physiological reactivity
2. The child demonstrates three of the following symptoms reflecting avoidance of stimuli associated with the traumatic event(s) and numbing of general responsiveness. These symptoms must not have been present before the trauma:
   - Avoidance of reminders of the trauma
   - Efforts to avoid thoughts, feelings, or conversations linked to the trauma

- Amnesia for an important aspect of the trauma
- Detachment or estrangement from others
- Emotional constriction (restricted range of affect)
- Diminished interest in or participation in usual activities
- A sense of a foreshortened future

3. Two persistent symptoms of increased arousal must be new to the child, present for at least 1 month, and cause clinically important distress or negatively affect functioning. These symptoms include the following (Stafford et al, 2007):
   - Sleep disturbances
   - Hypervigilance
   - Difficulty concentrating
   - Exaggerated startle response
   - Agitated or disorganized behavior
   - Irritability or angry outbursts, extreme fussiness or tantrums

Among infants, toddlers, and preschoolers, symptoms must be understood within the context of the trauma itself, the child's temperament and personality, and the caregiver's ability to support the child and provide a sense of safety and protection. There is significant research that indicates that the algorithms to diagnose infants and preschool children with PTSD should have a smaller number of avoidance symptoms and a removal of the diagnostic criteria that emotional response be present at the time of trauma (Meiser-Stedman et al, 2008). Table 19-4 includes a listing of PTSD symptoms by age group.

Assessment

PTSD assessment in children requires careful and direct clinical interviews with the child and parents. If the identified traumatic event involves a parent as the perpetrator of child

TABLE 19-4	Posttraumatic Stress Disorder Symptoms by Age Group
Age Group	**Common symptoms**
Infancy	Feeding problems, failure to thrive, sleep problems, irritability
Preschool age	Sleep problems, nightmares, developmental regression, aggression, extreme temper tantrums, anxiety symptoms, sudden worsening of fears, irritability, avoidance symptoms
School age	Sleep problems, nightmares, developmental regression, repetitive themes in play, social withdrawal, may have partial amnesia of events, new onset anxiety or fears, panic attacks, impaired concentration, impaired school performance, avoidance symptoms or hypervigilance
Adolescence	"Acting-out," nightmares, insomnia, extreme startling, social withdrawal, fears, anxiety, panic attacks, depression, anger or rage, internalizing, suicidal ideation, impaired concentration, impaired school performance, hypervigilance

Data from Cheung A, Jensen P: Major disturbances of emotion and mood. In Carey WB, Crocker AC, Coleman WL, et al, editors: *Developmental-behavioral pediatrics*, Philadelphia, 2009, Saunders, pp 461-473; Stafford B, Boris N, Dalton R, et al: Anxiety disorders. In Kliegman R, Behrman RE, Jenson H, et al, editors: *Nelson textbook of pediatrics*, Philadelphia, 2007, Saunders, pp 117-120; Zero to Three: *Diagnostic classification of mental health and developmental disorders of infancy and early childhood: revised edition (DC:0-3R)*, Washington, DC, 2005, Zero to Three Press.

maltreatment or domestic violence, the nonoffending parent or other caretaker should be interviewed. During assessment do not use prompting or leading questions. Instead ask questions about whether someone has invaded the child's privacy, how it may have happened, and how the injuries came to be. Assessment should ascertain that a trauma has occurred, the nature of the trauma, and the consequent symptom pattern.

Differential Diagnosis

The stressor must be of an extreme nature to warrant a diagnosis of PTSD. However, the stressor can be of any severity in an adjustment disorder (e.g., moving, starting a new school, birth of a sibling, divorce). Acute stress disorder is distinguished by the symptom pattern occurring and resolving within a 4-week period after the traumatic event. Recurrent intrusive thoughts occur in OCD but are experienced as inappropriate and are not related to an experienced trauma as they are in PTSD. Flashbacks also connect to the event and involve a feeling of reliving the event in PTSD, whereas hallucinations and other perceptual disturbances are unrelated to exposure to trauma. Memory is intact and psychic numbing and dissociation are absent with depression or externalizing disorders, such as conduct disorder (CD) unrelated to trauma. Anxiety disorders, the most common differential diagnosis, are distinguished by not being precipitated by a traumatic event.

Comorbid conditions in preschoolers differ from those of adults and older children. Oppositional defiant disorder (ODD) is most common, followed by separation anxiety disorder and ADHD. Major depressive disorder is very unlikely.

Management

A report to social service agencies is essential for children younger than 18 years. Referral to a pediatric mental health specialist is crucial. There is emerging evidence that betablockers like propranolol may be effective at decreasing somatic symptoms (e.g., racing heart rate and hyperpnea) associated with posttraumatic stress responses. Anxiety and depressive symptoms respond well to SSRIs (Delahanty and Ostrowski, 2008).

Crisis intervention is often necessary for the child as well as the parents. The primary care provider should educate parents about trauma and PTSD. Most pediatric psychiatrists use medications to treat PTSD, preferring SSRIs and alpha-adrenergic agonists. Child psychiatrists tend to prefer psychodynamic or cognitive-behavioral approaches, and nonmedical therapists tend to prefer the modalities of cognitive-behavioral, family, and nondirective play therapy. Symptom patterns persist, so consistent follow-up assessment is important. Early intervention and management are associated with the best long-term outcomes.

■ Mood Disorders

DEPRESSION

Description

There are three categories of depression that occur during childhood and adolescence: major depressive disorder, dysthymic disorder, and adjustment disorder with depressed mood (APA, 2000). Major depressive disorder (MDD) is defined as a depressed or irritable mood or a markedly diminished interest and pleasure in almost all of the usual activities for a period of at least 2 weeks, or both. A dysthymic disorder is characterized by depressed or irritable mood for the majority of days in the past year that is less intense but more chronic than major depressive episodes. Adjustment disorder with depressed mood typically occurs within 3 months after a major life stressor, involves less-severe symptoms, and is relatively mild and brief.

MDD in turn has three subclassifications: psychotic depression, seasonal affective disorder, and atypical depression (AACAP, 2007b). Children and adolescents with psychotic depression (e.g., affected individuals have hallucinations or delusions) have a greater incidence of adverse long-term outcomes, resistance to psychopharmacotherapy, and a much higher risk of developing bipolar depression. Atypical depression affects approximately 15% of children with depression and is characterized by hypersomnia, increased appetite, psychomotor retardation, and weight gain (Garzon, 2007). Seasonal affective disorder is most common during the fall and winter months when there is less daylight.

Epidemiology

Depression rates increase with age. Although depression occurs in children younger than 5 years, the true incidence is unknown given the limits of cognitive and language skills to communicate feelings. Depression is estimated to affect 1% to 3% of school-age children; the rate increases up to 5% by late adolescence. Twenty percent to 50% of adolescents report significant, subsyndromal levels of depression (Hankin, 2006). This rate increase for adolescents is thought to be linked to biology (e.g., sexual maturation and the influence of the sex hormones), social environment (e.g., greater social and academic expectations, greater exposure to negative events), and developmental factors (e.g., increased autonomy and abstract thinking). Vulnerability to depression involves an interplay of genetic, biological, biochemical, and psychosocial forces. Genetic factors underlie the risk for major depression, especially for childhood onset. The offspring of depressed parents are three times as likely to be diagnosed with depression, with a peak incidence at 15 to 20 years old (Boris et al, 2007a).

Three biological theories of depression are used to understand the psychopharmacology of depression: impaired neurotransmission, endocrine dysfunction, and biological rhythm dysfunction. Given a biological predisposition, certain life events may trigger the onset of depression. These include loss of a parent or significant other, losses that attend a disability or injury, family dysfunction, and physical or sexual abuse. There is a high risk of recurrent depression persisting into young adulthood. Cognitive vulnerabilities are implicated as factors related to depression. These include negative inferential styles about causes, consequences and the self, the tendency to ruminate in response to depressed mood, and self-criticism (Hankin, 2006).

An important feature of early-onset depressive illness is the potential for the condition to switch from unipolar depression to bipolar depression. As many as one third of preadolescent children who meet criteria for major depression develop bipolar depression (Garzon, 2007). Psychiatric comorbidity with depression is to be expected. The most common comorbidity with depression is an anxiety disorder (up to 70%)

that occurs two or three times more often than conduct disorder. Other comorbid conditions include dysthymia, disruptive behavior disorders, eating disorders, substance abuse and/or dependence, learning disorders, stress disorders, and ADHD (AACAP, 2007b). Comorbid conditions may also occur with a variety of medical conditions, especially those with a neurological component, such as brain injury, learning disorder, migraine headaches, and epilepsy.

Clinical Findings

Older children and adolescents with depression usually present with symptoms similar to those of adults. However, many children with depressed mood actually do not admit to feeling sad, but rather present with irritability, fluctuating mood, temper tantrums, social withdrawal, somatic complaints, agitation, separation anxiety, or behavioral problems (AACAP, 2007b). Males are more likely to have externalizing symptoms (e.g., aggression, acting-out, anger) and females are more likely to have internalizing symptoms (e.g., somatic complaints, feelings of sadness). Major depression symptoms represent a persistent change that occurs across settings, activities, and relationships and causes the child distress, impaired functioning, or developmental alteration. Infants and young children may present with failure to thrive, speech and motor delays, repetitive self-soothing behaviors, withdrawal from social interaction, poor attachment, and loss of developmental skills. Infants may not respond to extra efforts to soothe or engage them.

Toddlers and preschoolers may lack energy, be too eager to please others, be excessively or unusually clingy or whiney, and have problems with separation, with a persistence and intensity atypical for toddlerhood (Cheung and Jensen, 2009). Common symptoms of major depression in preschoolers include sad or grouchy mood (98%), lack of pleasure in play or activity (98%), poor appetite and weight loss, sleep problems (80%), low levels of energy and activity (80%), low self-esteem (78%), and increased death or suicide play or talk (74%).

School-age children may manifest irritability, anger, or hostility in addition to externalizing behavior, such as hyperactivity, difficulty handling aggression, or reckless behavior. Frequent absences from school, perhaps because of school phobia, or poor performance and other school problems are common. On the other hand, school-age children may have internalizing symptoms, such as boredom, lack of interest in playing with friends, social withdrawal, somatic complaints (e.g., stomachaches, headaches, muscle aches, or tiredness), eating or sleeping disturbances, enuresis, or encopresis. Some children with depression describe themselves in negative terms, whereas others, in an effort to compensate for feelings of poor self-worth, become preoccupied with attempting to please others.

Depression symptoms in adolescents include impulsivity, fatigue, hopelessness, antisocial behavior, substance use, restlessness, grouchiness, aggression, hypersexuality, and problems with family members or at school. Social withdrawal, manifested as shyness, boredom, or a lack of motivation is common (Garzon, 2007). Substance abuse is a problem for about 20% of adolescents.

Talking directly with the child or adolescent is essential because it is thought that half of depression cases are missed when only parents are interviewed. The following depressive symptoms are common:

- Depressed mood: sad, "blue," down, angry, bored
- Loss of interest and pleasure in usual activities
- Change in appetite or weight (loss or increase)
- Insomnia or hypersomnia
- Low energy and fatigue
- Difficulty concentrating; indecision
- Feelings of worthlessness or inappropriate or excessive guilt
- Recurrent thoughts of death or suicidal ideation

A diagnosis of major depressive disorder is made if there have been at least 2 weeks of depressed mood or loss of interest and at least four additional symptoms of depression. The symptoms cause considerable distress and impairment in social and academic functioning and cannot be caused by bereavement. Therefore, it is important to assess the following:

- Recent life events and losses
- Family history of depression or other psychiatric disorders
- Family dysfunction
- Changes in school performance
- Risk-taking behavior, including sexual activity and substance use
- Deteriorating relationships with family
- Changes in peer relations, especially social withdrawal

Undiagnosed and untreated/undertreated depression can be fatal. Suicide is the third leading cause of death for 14- to 24-year-olds (Centers for Disease Control and Prevention [CDC], 2007). Possible warning signs for suicide are listed in Table 19-5.

Depression Scales

Both patient self-report and clinician-completed rating scales are available. Table 19-6 contains a listing of these scales.

Differential Diagnosis

Some medications and certain chronic illnesses (hypothyroidism, adrenal insufficiency, epilepsy, metabolic disease, sleep disorders, hepatitis, multiple sclerosis, inflammatory bowel disease, and type 1 diabetes) predispose children and adolescents to depression. If a substance (e.g., medication, toxin, or drug of abuse) is related to the mood disturbance, a substance-induced mood disorder is diagnosed. Medications commonly causing depressive symptoms include beta-blockers, benzodiazepines, nonsteroidal antiinflammatory drugs (NSAIDs), stimulants, clonidine, corticosteroids, oral contraceptives, and isotretinoin. Infections, lead intoxication, anemia, eating disorders, mitral valve prolapse, premenstrual syndrome, and neurological disorders can mimic depression in children and adolescents. In general, a physical examination and screening laboratory tests are necessary to rule out organic causes. Suggested diagnostic testing for an individual with new symptoms of depression include complete blood count (CBC), pregnancy testing, Epstein-Barr titers, thyroid panel, liver function testing, urinalysis, and drug screening.

Depressive symptoms in response to a psychosocial stressor are diagnosed as adjustment disorder, which has a good short-term prognosis and does not predict later dysfunction. With separation anxiety disorder, depressive symptoms usually arise only in the context of separation and resolve quickly

TABLE 19-5	Warning Signs for Suicide

Area of Functioning	Signs*
Changes in behavior	Accident prone or risk taking Drug and alcohol abuse Physical violence toward self, others, or animals Loss of appetite Sudden alienation from family, friends, coworkers Worsening performance at work or school Putting personal affairs in order Loss of interest in personal appearance Disposal of possessions Writing letters, notes, or poems with suicidal content; talking about suicide Buying a gun
Changes in mood	Expressions of hopelessness or impending doom Explosive rage Dramatic swings in affect Crying spells Sleep disorders Talking about suicide
Changes in thinking	Preoccupation with death Difficulty concentrating Irrational speech Hearing voices, seeing visions Sudden interest (or loss of interest) in religion
Major life changes	Death of a family member or friend (especially by suicide) Separation or divorce Public humiliation or failure Serious illness or trauma Loss of financial security

*These signs must be interpreted in context. Many of them are common outside the realm of presuicidal behavior.

TABLE 19-6	Diagnostic Rating Scales for Depression Diagnosis

Scale	Appropriate Ages
Child Behavior Checklist (CBCL)	1.5 to 5 and 6 to 18 years
Children's Depression Rating Scale-Revised (CDRS-R)	6 to 12 years
Reynolds Child Depression Scale (RCDS)	6 to 12 years
Children's Depression Inventory (CDI)	6 years to adolescent
Beck Depression Inventory (BDI)	Adolescents
Reynolds Adolescent Depression Scale (RADS)	Adolescents
Center for Epidemiologic Studies-Depression Scale (CES-D)	Adolescents
Depression Self-Rating Scale	Adolescents
Pediatric Symptom Checklist (PSC)	4 years to adolescent

with reunion; however, concomitant depressive disorder is not uncommon. A depressive episode with irritable mood can be difficult to distinguish from a manic episode with irritable mood; careful evaluation of the presence of manic symptoms (e.g., excessive activity, inflated self-esteem, little need for sleep, talkativeness) is required. Many adolescents and adults who develop mania had preponderantly depressive symptoms in childhood. Family history of bipolarity is an important risk factor. Depression can be differentiated from the irritability and inattention of ADHD in that children with MDD are not usually impulsive. In addition, they typically have a normal attention span before the onset of symptoms.

Management

The first goals of management are to determine suicidal risk and intervene to prevent suicide. Suicidal risk is greatest during the first 4 weeks of a depressive episode. Patients with acute suicidal intent that includes a plan, psychosis, risk of abuse, and unstable behavior require immediate psychiatric

evaluation. Cumulative suicidal risks—prior suicidal behavior or attempts, depression, and alcohol, tobacco or drug abuse/dependence—require psychiatric intervention as well, and immediate referral must be made (Meyer et al, 2010). Attention must also be paid to establish a safe environment (e.g., removal of firearms, knives, and lethal medications [including tricyclic antidepressants (TCAs)]). Families of adolescents with depression may be noncompliant with recommendations to remove guns from the home in spite of compliance with other aspects of treatment. Vigilant follow-up in this regard is crucial. Other management strategies by the primary care provider include referral to community resources, such as hotlines, and commitment to a no-suicide agreement by which the adolescent agrees to refrain from harming himself or herself and promises to notify the caretaker or health care professional if suicidal ideation returns. It is important to note that suicidal ideation often increases during the treatment phase known as emergence. Emergence occurs in the first week to month of treatment when the patient's energy levels increase, but feelings of hopelessness and helplessness have not yet receded.

A major depressive episode requires intervention by a mental health specialist. Unfortunately only about half of individuals with depression achieve full remission of their symptoms. Therapies typically include CBT in a group or individual psychotherapy format. Group CBT may help adolescents. Often, family therapy or psychoeducation is indicated.

A central issue in psychopharmacological approaches is that children and adolescents are not usually included in clinical drug trial research; safety and efficacy data from the literature about adults are often extrapolated to children. Available studies do not support the efficacy of TCAs for depression in young children, and they may actually be harmful. Although the 2004 "black box" warning for SSRIs occurred because of concerns of increased suicidality with use of these medications, randomized controlled trials of pediatric depression consistently demonstrate that best treatment responses come from combinations of CBT and SSRIs (Garzon, 2007). CBT appears to have a protective effect against suicide. Currently, fluoxetine and escitalopram are the only SSRIs with U.S. Food and Drug Administration (FDA) approval for use in children 12 years and older. The FDA recommends specifically against the use of paroxetine in children and adolescents because of the 3.5-fold increased risk for suicide. Activation (e.g., elevated energy without mood change) and mania can occur in patients secondary to treatment with antidepressants. Therefore, it is critical that parents be taught about symptoms that merit immediate evaluation including decreased impulse control, marked elevated mood, acting-out, fearlessness, and risk taking (Garzon et al, 2009). For children with psychosis, child psychiatrists often add antipsychotics like risperidone or olanzapine to the therapeutic drug plan (Cheung and Jensen, 2009).

Close follow-up is recommended for all children and adolescents with depression, especially when symptoms are significant enough to merit pharmacotherapy. Providers should make phone contact with the patient and/or family within 3 days and see the patient weekly until stable. Maintenance visits can occur at 3-month intervals. Again, close communication during the first 4 weeks of treatment is critical.

Prognosis

MDD is a chronic condition with a high rate of recurrence. Although most children and adolescents will recover from a MDD episode, the probability of recurrence is 60% within 2 years and 75% by 5 years. Poor long-term outcomes are associated with severe disease, frequent disease, and in patients with significant family dysfunction, low socioeconomic status, and history of abuse or family strife (AACAP, 2007b).

BIPOLAR DISORDER

Description

Bipolar disorder (BPD), formerly known as manic depression, is characterized by unusual shifts in mood, energy, and functioning and may begin with manic, depressive, or a mixed set of manic and depressive symptoms. The majority of adults with bipolar disorder report their initial symptom was depression, with bipolar disorder developing in 20% to 40% of depressed children and adolescents (AACAP, 2007a). It is a recurrent disorder in which nearly all of those (90%) who have a single manic episode will have future episodes. Approximately 2.6% of children younger than age 18 meet the diagnostic criteria for BPD. The risk of suicide in bipolar depression is the highest of all the psychiatric disorders (AACAP, 2007a). Up to one third of all children with BPD will attempt suicide (Demeter et al, 2008).

A characteristic pattern usually evolves for a particular person, with manic episodes preceding or following major depressive episodes. Most individuals with bipolar disorder return to a full level of functioning between episodes; 20% to 30% experience persistent mood lability and interpersonal difficulties (APA, 2000). Sometimes psychotic symptoms develop after several days or weeks of manic symptoms. Such features tend to predict that the individual with subsequent manic episodes will again experience psychotic symptoms.

Epidemiology

Multiple theories explain the cause of BPD, but no definitive cause is known. Imaging studies reveal that there are structural changes commonly found in the third ventricle, the white matter, the prefrontal cortex, the amygdala and the basal ganglia (DelBello et al, 2006). Genetic factors (specifically, defects on chromosomes 1, 6, 8, and 22) account for almost 60% of bipolar cases. There is evidence of a genetic influence for bipolar disorder from twin studies and adoption studies; bipolar disorder tends to cluster in families. Parents who are bipolar are at greater risk for having bipolar children (AACAP, 2007a). Fifty-nine percent of adults with bipolar depression report onset of symptoms during childhood or adolescence, but the onset of symptoms before age 10 is rare (0.5%) (AACAP, 2007a). The most common onset of symptoms occurs between 15 and 19 years. There is no differential incidence based on race, ethnicity, or gender. Children with ADHD seem to be vulnerable to bipolar illness, or it may be that attention-deficit disorder or ADHD is a misdiagnosed early sign of the mania to come (Zepf, 2009). If children are also bipolar, treatment of ADHD with psychostimulants or antidepressants may precipitate a manic episode. Antidepressants in depressed children (6 to 12 years old) may also precipitate mania and the onset of bipolar illness.

Clinical Findings

Bipolar disorder in childhood or early adolescence appears to be a different, more severe form of the illness than occurs with late adolescent or adult onset. The early-onset form is characterized by irritability and continuous, rapid-cycling, and mixed-symptom state that may also co-occur with disruptive behavior disorders (e.g., ADHD or CD); features of ADHD or behavior disorder are often early symptoms. Prepubertal and early adolescent bipolar disorder is a fairly homogeneous phenotype, with no differences according to gender, puberty, or comorbid ADHD. In the late adolescent or adult form, the hallmark features include classic manic episodes, episodic patterns of mania and depression, and relative stability between episodes. Symptoms include the following:

- Severe mood changes—extreme irritability or overly elated and silly
- Inflated self-esteem or grandiosity
- Increased energy
- Decreased need for sleep (sleeps few hours or no sleep for days without tiring)
- Talkativeness or compulsion to talk; frequent topic changes or cannot be interrupted
- Distractibility, with attention moving constantly from one thing to another
- Increase in goal-directed activity (socially or at school)
- Physical agitation
- Risk-taking behaviors or activities; taking "more dares"
- Hypersexuality in talk, thoughts, feelings, or behaviors
- Suicidal thoughts and behaviors in 76% of cases and suicidal attempts in 31% of cases (Chang, 2009)

More than half of adolescents experience depression as their initial symptom (Chang, 2009). The most common symptoms of mania include irritable mood and grandiosity (80%), elevated mood (70%), decreased sleep (70%), racing thoughts (70%), poor judgment (70%), flight of ideas (50%), and hypersexuality (33%) (Kowatch et al, 2005).

The child or adolescent who has depression but also manifests symptoms of ADHD that seem severe (e.g., extreme temper outbursts and mood changes) should be evaluated by a child psychiatrist with experience in bipolar disorder. Symptoms are manifested in relatively age-specific ways (AACAP, 2007a).

With mania, children appear to be the happiest of people, but the happiness and laughter do not match the situation or context. Grandiosity may manifest in efforts to correct teachers or critique their efforts, seeing themselves as above rules and laws, or devoting time to an activity for which they have no talent. Children's sleep difficulties (a hallmark sign) are reflected in high activity levels before bed (e.g., rearranging the furniture), whereas adolescents need little sleep at all. Risk-taking behavior ranges from children climbing excessively high trees or hopping between rooftops to adolescents driving recklessly and speeding. In adolescents, manic episodes are more likely to include psychotic features and may be associated with school truancy, school failure, substance use, or antisocial behavior. No laboratory findings diagnostic of a manic episode have been identified, so a careful history and a thorough assessment are crucial.

Assessment for comorbid conditions is important (AACAP, 2007a). Anxiety disorders, including panic disorder, affect about 30% of prepubertal patients and 10% of adolescent patients with bipolar disorder. Other common comorbidities include conduct disorder, substance abuse, oppositional defiant disorder, disruptive behavior disorder, and personality disorders (AACAP, 2007a).

Differential Diagnosis

A manic episode must be distinguished from a mood disorder caused by a medical condition (e.g., brain tumor) and a substance-induced mood disorder (e.g., laughing fits with marijuana, amphetamine highs followed by withdrawal "crashes," perceptual distortions or hallucinations of hallucinogens). Distinguishing BPD from ADHD can be a challenge. ADHD, like mania, is characterized by excessive activity, poor impulse control and judgment, and denial of problems. However, ADHD lacks a clear onset or episodes, mood disturbances, and psychotic features. Recent evidence suggests that children with ADHD are vulnerable to bipolar disorder and that pharmacological treatments may precipitate manic episodes, so providers should carefully evaluate and refer any child treated for ADHD who does not respond to therapy or who experiences a sudden worsening of agitation while using ADHD medications.

Management

Referral to a child psychiatrist or child mental health care provider is critical. Current recommendations for pharmacological treatment include the use of mood stabilizers, such as lithium, alone or in combination with antiseizure medications (e.g., valproate, divalproex) and atypical antipsychotics (e.g., risperidone). Neither antidepressants nor stimulants have proven effective. Antidepressant use may potentiate manic responses. The use of lithium must be carefully monitored. Data strongly support long-term maintenance on lithium to prevent relapse of bipolar symptoms (AACAP, 2007a).

The best clinical responses occur when pharmacotherapy is combined with individual and family psychotherapy (Chang, 2009; Miklowitz et al, 2008). Therapy should focus on minimizing comorbidities, enhancing problem-solving and communication skills, and reducing negative self-thoughts. Other nonpharmacological interventions with proven effectiveness include stress reduction, healthy diet, routine exercise, and developing good sleep hygiene.

■ Attention-Deficit/Hyperactivity Disorder

ADHD is the most common of all child and adolescent behavioral disorders, affecting approximately 8% of the population (Merikangas et al, 2010). Discussion of this condition is found in Chapter 15.

■ The Aggressive Child

SOCIAL AGGRESSION

Description

Social aggression is a pattern of social behavior with the intent to harm others (Leff et al, 2009). Onset may occur as early as toddlerhood. It can be overt (e.g., hitting or pushing) or covert (e.g., gossiping or socially ostracizing).

Epidemiology

Approximately 5% to 6% of U.S. children have behavioral problems with aggression and 1% to 10% of children meet criteria for ODD (Barbaresi, 2009; Copeland, 2006). Males are more likely to be aggressive than females, and aggression peaks during adolescence (Leff et al, 2009). Females are more likely to be socially or covertly aggressive, whereas males are more likely to be overtly aggressive. Acute, stressful life events or transitions can precipitate a brief period of social aggression. Significant risk factors include a history of maltreatment; inconsistent or harsh discipline, or both; lack of maternal responsiveness; separations from parents, shifts in parent figures, or parental rejection; and other enduring circumstances. Social aggression can be a precursor to CD or oppositional disorder. Research indicates that there is a inherited pattern of susceptibility to be aggressive (Leff et al, 2009).

Clinical Findings

During preschool, social aggression manifests as oppositional or defiant behavior and is considered clinically significant if it interferes with normal developmental functioning. The pervasiveness, intensity, and persistence of irritable, argumentative, defiant, and easily annoyed behaviors identify a pathological condition and may be precursors to ODD. In the preschool period, children have a beginning understanding of the effect of their behavior on others and can control their behavior on the basis of internalized norms and developing self-regulation. When social aggression becomes a pattern, peer rejection is common. Aggressive behavior involves the following:
- Destruction of property
- Name-calling
- Physical pestering and deliberately annoying others

- Hitting, biting, kicking, fighting
- Frequent conflict with peers
- Temper tantrums
- Carrying expectations of others' hostility
- Misinterpreting social cues and responding aggressively
- Lack of problem-solving in social situations
- Use of bad language, swearing, obscene language and gestures
- Arguing for long periods
- Inappropriately suggestive or aggressive sexual behaviors

Differential Diagnosis

ODD is a pattern of open defiance and noncompliance toward authority figures. ODD symptoms emerge during the preschool years and persist for a minimum of 6 months. CD is a clear pattern of behavior established over a 6-month period, typically diagnosed at school age. CD differs from ODD in that it involves serious aggression toward people or animals, willful destruction of property, or theft (Leff et al, 2009). However, there is growing evidence that preschool children manifest clinically significant disruptive behavior problems, and valid diagnoses of ODD and CD can be made even in young children. Typical and atypical problems can be differentiated, and with a developmentally based DSM-IV framework, children with these problems can be identified (Boris et al, 2007b).

Management

It is important to ascertain whether a difficult temperament underlies the behavioral difficulty, especially in conjunction with a lack of fit with parental temperament. A difficult temperament may account for a child's being harder to discipline, having social behavior problems in school (e.g., poor fit with the teacher), or having poor academic achievement. In these situations the use of positive parenting strategies does not have to change, but supportive counseling for the parents should be provided regarding temperament, its manifestations, and strategies for managing transitions and other difficult times or behaviors. A conference with the teacher may provide similar information and explore strategies to facilitate the child's learning and positive behavior.

When social aggression is a response to acute stress, the problem usually resolves if parents use positive parenting strategies and facilitate developmentally appropriate coping efforts. If peer relationship development is hampered, close monitoring of and intervention with peer interactions by daycare, preschool, and school personnel, especially with the parents present for observation, enhances appropriate social behavior and competence. Changing schools in an effort to ameliorate problems is not advised because children carry their social difficulties with them and assume the same roles in new groups. Teachers need to be supportive and facilitative.

When social aggression becomes a pattern of social behavior, referral for intervention is critical. Negative behavior in preschool playgroups is predictive of externalizing behavior problems in kindergarten. Substantial research literature supports the stability and persistence of disruptive behavior and aggression from toddlerhood to school age. Early intervention is essential. Parental education should focus on reestablishing positive parent-child interactions, use of consistent limit setting, and teaching parents to use effective discipline (Barbaresi, 2009).

CONDUCT DISORDER

Description

CD is a repetitive and persistent pattern of behavior in which the basic rights of others, or major age-appropriate societal norms and rules are violated (APA, 2000). The onset of aggressive behavior is observed in toddlerhood. Early-onset conduct problems are diagnosed from 4 to 6 years old; a formal diagnosis is typically made when the child is 7 years or older.

Epidemiology

The cause of the disorder rests in chronic negative circumstances, as described for social aggression. CD is frequently associated with a history of harsh discipline, abuse, or neglect. Prevalence rates range from 1% to 10% (Leff et al, 2009). Conduct disorder is more common in males than females (3:1). However, it is thought that the prevalence data do not accurately reflect the occurrence of CD for females because the diagnostic criteria emphasize physical aggression.

Behavioral dysregulation tends to become notable during the transition from early to middle childhood and is mediated by changes in the structure and demands of the social environment—peers and school settings. There is a high rate of comorbidity with major depression, and the joint presence of CD and depression increases the risk for substance abuse and suicide. ADHD is found to influence the development, course, and severity of CD.

Clinical Findings

Clinical features fall into four main subgroups: aggressive behavior that threatens or results in physical harm to other people or animals, nonaggressive behavior that causes property damage, lying or stealing, and serious violation of rules or laws. Several factors are relevant to practitioners for their prognostic importance: how atypical the behaviors are for age or gender, how overt versus covert the behaviors are, the nature of any aggression, and the presence of early antisocial or psychopathy-related symptoms. Most commonly, referrals for clinical treatment are for aggressive behavior patterns. Physical aggression toward others includes the following:

- Hitting, kicking, fighting
- Physical cruelty to animals or people
- Physical destruction (including fire setting)
- Frequent temper tantrums
- A high rate of annoying behavior, such as yelling, whining, or threatening
- Disobedience to adult authorities
- Lying, cheating
- Covert stealing
- Truancy and running away from home
- Blaming others for mistakes
- Use of or selling illegal drugs
- Engaging in deviant sexual behaviors (e.g., sexual assault)
- Academic problems

There is growing evidence that preadolescent and adolescent girls manifest CD more indirectly through verbal and relational aggression, including alienation, ostracism, and character defamation directed at the relationships between friends. With CD, social role functioning tends to be impaired, with poor academic performance, poor family and peer relationships, and poor self-management.

Differential Diagnosis

Oppositional defiant disorder is characterized by more disobedience than aggressiveness and is evidenced in preschool or early school age. ADHD is characterized by inattention, impulsiveness, and hyperactivity but willful destruction is uncommon. CD is distinguished from isolated acts of aggressive behavior by degree of aggression exhibited, the presence of willful defiance, and by the persistence of symptoms for a minimum of 6 months (Leff et al, 2009). A thorough physical examination is essential to rule out organic causes of behavior and to identify evidence of abuse, neglect, and substance abuse disorders.

Management

If aggressive behavior is identified before a CD develops, preventive efforts can be implemented. Successful programs are multifaceted, including a parent-directed component (e.g., parent education and support for positive parenting strategies and healthy, consistent approaches to discipline), social-cognitive skills training, proactive classroom management and teacher training, and group therapy (Leff et al, 2009). Effective education includes conflict resolution strategies and development of coping and resiliency skills. Once a CD is evident, referral for child and family intervention is crucial.

Safety is a priority in caring for children with aggressive and oppositional disorders. Because of the strong association of child abuse and neglect with CD, it is critical to determine if the child is in safe living conditions. If there is evidence of abuse or neglect, prompt referral to child protective agencies is mandatory. The practitioner must also determine whether other family members are safe from the child's or adolescent's aggressive behavior. Potential interventions when family safety is at risk include referral for inpatient psychiatric evaluation, notification of the police of criminal activity, supporting the family to petition the juvenile court for services, and referral to community health services.

Family therapy can be helpful for adolescents with CD. Collaboration between the family and the school is of critical importance, and the primary care provider can assist with strategies. Isolated individual treatment is not superior to parent intervention programs. Education about problem-solving skills may also be effective.

Psychopharmacological intervention is reserved for explosive aggression and includes mood stabilizers, typical and atypical antipsychotics, clonidine, and stimulants. Given the high risk for substance abuse in those with CD, caution should be exercised in prescribing medications.

Prognosis

CD in childhood may predict antisocial personality disorder in adulthood. Poorer prognoses are associated with increased severity of symptoms.

OPPOSITIONAL DEFIANT DISORDER

Description

ODD is a pattern of negative, hostile, and defiant behavior that is excessive compared with other children of the same age (AACAP, 2007c). Symptoms often occur in early childhood, from 3 to 7 years old. The disorder typically begins by 8 years old (Barbaresi, 2009).

Epidemiology

Etiological factors include many of the parenting and family dysfunctions identified for social aggression (AACAP, 2007c). Precursors to the disorder are common in early childhood, especially defiance and negativism. More common in boys before puberty, the gender distribution is approximately equal thereafter. Estimates range from 10% of girls and 14% of boys 10 to 13 years old to 12% of 17- to 20-year-olds. Some studies report slightly higher rates of ODD in males, whereas others do not.

Clinical Findings

The essential feature of ODD is a recurrent pattern of behavior that is negative, defiant, disobedient, and hostile toward authority figures. Behavior is typically directed at family members, teachers, or peers whom the child knows well. The child manifests the following behaviors to an extent that leads to impairment:

- Actively defies or refuses adult requests or rules
- Is argumentative, angry, resentful, touchy, or easily annoyed
- Easily loses temper
- Blames others for own mistakes or difficulties
- Deliberately does things to annoy others
- Children often see their own behavior as justifiable, not oppositional or defiant (APA, 2000)

Differential Diagnosis

CD involves more serious violations of the rights of others and a more willful disregard of authority.

Management

Attend to the early signs of defiant and oppositional behavior or aggression, or both, by educating parents about positive parenting strategies and by exercising consistent, healthy discipline, as with the management of CDs. Because these children typically do not perceive themselves as having a problem and the cause rests with the family system, referral for intervention is indicated. As described for CD, parent training programs are more successful, especially if they include information about child behavior in multiple environments (e.g., school and home) and target dysfunctional family processes. Child training groups provide added benefit if combined with parent training groups. Again, collaboration with the school is important. These multiple approaches, conducted simultaneously, are most effective.

■ Autism Spectrum Disorder

The diagnostic cluster referred to as autism spectrum disorder (ASD) includes the following diagnoses: Asperger syndrome, pervasive developmental disorder, and autism. These complex disorders are diagnosed using DSM-IV-TR criteria, result in significant interpersonal alterations, and are discussed in Chapter 15.

Eating Disorders

Description

Eating disorders cause abnormal eating behaviors that are secondary to altered body image (dysmorphism). Anorexia nervosa (AN) and bulimia nervosa (BN) are the primary eating disorders of concern; however, there are other conditions in this diagnostic cluster including eating disorder not otherwise specified, rumination disorders, pica, and feeding disorders of infancy. Some believe obesity should be classified as an eating disorder because of the correlation between self-soothing and eating, and because many obese individuals have feelings of loss of control over their eating and symptoms of body dysmorphism. Eating disorders are complex conditions that are very difficult to treat and are associated with significant medical and mental health comorbidities. Anorexia has the highest mortality rate of all the mental health conditions. The 5-year mortality rate for AN is 15% to 20%, and the majority of these deaths are caused by electrolyte imbalance, malnutrition, and suicide (Miller and Golden, 2010). Due to the complexity of these disorders, specialty care is needed; however, primary care providers play a critical role through detection and early intervention, case coordination, and monitoring for complications.

Epidemiology

Lifetime prevalence rates for AN and BN are approximately 1% each (Miller and Golden, 2010). Both disorders affect females at much greater rates than males (9:1). Symptom onset usually occurs during mid- to late adolescence, but preadolescent cases do occur and are associated with significantly higher morbidity and mortality. Athletes are more likely to develop eating disorders, especially those who compete in sports that are based on weight divisions (e.g., wrestling), long distance running, and those with emphases on aesthetic lines and flexibility (e.g., dancers, gymnasts, ice skaters). Other individual risk factors include middle to high socioeconomic status, divorced families, chronic disease (e.g., diabetes mellitus, cystic fibrosis, depression, obesity, substance abuse), recent weight loss in a previously obese person, personality disorders (e.g., borderline, narcissistic, antisocial), strong will, and history of child abuse. Children and adolescents with eating disorders are more likely to have parents who have a weight or fitness focus, are substance abusers, have high achievement expectations, who comment on their child's physical appearance, have difficulty expressing emotions, or who are overprotective or enmeshed with their children. Like most mental illness, there is an increasing body of evidence suggesting a strong genetic component to AN and BN that results in altered serotonin and dopamine receptors (Gowers, 2008).

Clinical Findings

Diagnosing anorexia or bulimia can be difficult. Some clinical findings characteristic of these disorders occur in the healthy adolescent. For example, it is not uncommon for a 14-year-old girl who is neither anorexic nor bulimic to express concern about her body appearance, stating that she is too fat or ugly. Additionally, anorexic or bulimic adolescents and their families commonly hide their condition and actions, deny problems, or present a mature, self-sufficient, and successful facade. Early in the disease process the family system may appear to be coherent, making it difficult to collect accurate data about family relations and behavior patterns that contribute to eating disorders.

Many consider anorexia and bulimia to be part of a disease continuum with categories that are more arbitrary than actual. Clinical presentations vary depending on the disease severity. Both AN and BN are associated with disordered eating and body dysmorphism with or without purging (e.g., laxative abuse, enemas, diuretics, induced vomiting). Generally there is no loss of appetite or sense of hunger. Affected individuals often link feelings of self-worth with weight or the ability to restrict food intake despite being hungry (Gowers, 2008). Diagnostic criteria for anorexia are:
- Refusal to maintain body weight at least 85% expected for age and height or failure to gain weight during growth periods so that weight drops below 85% expected
- Intense fear of weight gain and "being fat"
- Body dysmorphism
- Amenorrhea for at least three cycles (menstrual disorders are the leading reason for presentation at primary care offices) (Gowers, 2008)
- Binge eating/purging subtype, which is associated with frequent purging although bingeing episodes are rare Diagnostic criteria for bulimia are:
- Consuming large quantities of food in a short period of time (within 2 hours)
- Loss of control during binge episodes (e.g., can't control the amount of food they eat or are shocked at amount consumed)
- Engaging in repeated behaviors to lose weight including purging, excessive exercise, or fasting
- Bingeing or purging behaviors that occur at least twice a week for at least 3 months

Individuals with AN are underweight, but children and adolescents with BN are often average weight or overweight. In addition to the regular primary care monitoring of weight and growth, it is important to include routine screening to detect the red flags and treatment signs listed in Table 19-7. Also helpful is the SCOFF questionnaire. This five item screen asks the following questions:
- Do you make yourself **S**ick because you feel uncomfortably full?
- Do you worry that you have lost **C**ontrol over what you eat?
- Have you lost **O**ver 10 pounds in the last 3 months?
- Do you believe you are **F**at when others say you are thin?
- Would you say **F**ood dominates your life? (Kirkby and Brown, 2007)

Patients with suspected eating disorders need a thorough history and physical examination, and evaluation for comorbid depression, anxiety, suicidality, and risk of physical harm. Common history findings include:
- Menstrual irregularity
- Altered body perception, may manifest as feelings of being fat even though not overweight
- Preoccupation with food; often fixes elaborate meals but does not eat; has rituals associated with food

TABLE 19-7	Red Flags and Signs That Indicate Need for Eating Disorder Treatment

Red Flags	Needs Treatment Signs
Reads diet books or clips dieting articles	Regularly fasts or skips meals
Visits pro-anorexia or bulimia websites (pro Anna or pro Mia)	Stops eating with family or friends
Intense focus on diet or regular dieting	Misses two or more periods during weight loss
Sudden desire to be a vegetarian	Reports binge eating
Sudden picky eating	Reports purging
Visits bathroom regularly during or after meals	Parents find laxatives or diet pills
Showers multiple times a day	Excessive exercise
Skips meals because "I ate at school" or other place away from home	Refuses to eat non-diet foods
Large amounts of missing food	Refuses to eat meals prepared by others Extreme calorie counting or portion controls

- Desire to lose weight, and history of dieting or food rituals
- Weight fluctuation or loss
- Guilt about eating
- Hides eating or lies about having eaten or amount eaten
- Displays social isolation and mood changes: irritable, sullen, hostile, introverted, unhappy, intolerant of others, can have suicidal ideation
- Has fixed, highly structured schedule, inflexible to change
- Cold intolerance
- Fatigue
- Myalgias
- Constipation, diarrhea
- Abdominal bloating, gastrointestinal (GI) distress
- Sleep deprivation
- Sore throat
- Dizziness, syncope
- Other destructive behaviors: shoplifting, substance abuse, self-harm
- Family history of chaos, abuse, sexual abuse
  Common physical findings that may indicate an eating disorder are:
- Altered growth
- Round face with parotid gland enlargement
- Fluid retention
- Facial edema
- Thin body type
- Hypotension
- Low body temperature
- Bradycardia, orthostatic hypotension
- Shallow respirations
- Dental enamel erosion, dental caries
- Russel sign (e.g., knuckle cuts/calluses/abrasions from inducing vomiting)

- Thinning hair, alopecia, decreased deep tendon reflexes
- Abdominal distention, altered bowel sounds
- Lanugo, dry skin
- Muscle atrophy
- Mental torpor

Laboratory Studies

Laboratory testing is done to ascertain the degree of electrolyte imbalance and malnutrition, and to rule out other causes of weight loss and amenorrhea. Suggested diagnostic testing for an individual with a newly diagnosed eating disorder includes CBC (anemia), serum electrolytes (potassium, sodium, and acid-base imbalance), fasting glucose (diabetes), electrocardiogram (ECG) (premature ventricular contractions and QT elongation), thyroid studies (hyperthyroidism), bone density (if amenorrheic to look for osteopenia), urinalysis, liver function testing, follicle-stimulating hormone (FSH), and luteinizing hormone (LH).

Differential Diagnosis

Inflammatory bowel disease and peptic ulcer disease result in chronic pain and microscopic or gross bleeding. Central nervous system lesions cause focal neurological signs. Hormonal and metabolic diseases cause symptoms like polyphagia, polydipsia, polyuria, abnormal hair growth, and goiter. Immune disorders are associated with frequent, rare, and opportunistic infections. Other mental health differential diagnoses include OCD, substance use disorder, and major depression.

Management

Management of children and adolescents with anorexia nervosa or bulimia is difficult, in part because the child, family, and even the health care provider often deny the significance of the problem. Even though early detection and treatment are helpful in reducing physical complications, diagnosis can be delayed and treatment may be inadequate. Because the issue is not food, but rather sociopsychological dynamics of control in the child's life, effective treatment is complex and long term (American Dietetic Association, 2006). Eating disorders are managed with a multifaceted approach with emphasis on nutritional rehabilitation, pharmacotherapeutics (e.g., antidepressants, atypical antipsychotics), and individual, family, and group therapy. Intensive, in-patient management is warranted for medical instability, psychosis or self-destructive behavior, and failure to improve with outpatient therapy. The evidence for cognitive behavioral therapy is strong, and family therapy clinically improves weight gain and parental control of renutrition (Sigel et al, 2009).

Many children and adolescents with eating disorders require in-patient management, especially if there are fluid and electrolyte imbalances, cardiovascular instability, or significant mental illness. Individual and family therapy is critical. Pharmacological approaches include antidepressants and atypical antipsychotics, but their use is controversial in many cases. The role of the primary care provider in the management of eating disorders is primarily that of screening and early identification. Weight gain during refeeding is expected to occur at 1.1 pounds (0.5 kg) per week (Sigel et al, 2009). Close monitoring for refeeding syndrome is warranted. This is a rare, potentially life-threatening condition that occurs in the first days of enteral or parenteral feeding, and results in severe fluid and electrolyte imbalance (Gowers, 2008). Symptoms include confusion, severe irritability, organ dysfunction, and seizures.

Complications

AN has the highest mortality rate of all mental health disorders. The complications of AN or BN include:

- Death, usually secondary to cardiac arrhythmia, hypokalemia, congestive heart failure, or suicide
- Altered metabolism (chronic)
- Alcohol and drug addictions
- Osteoporosis
- GI disturbance: ulcers, motility disorders
- Fertility problems
- Gynecological problems related to prolonged amenorrhea
- Growth retardation
- Dehydration

■ Substance Abuse

Description

Substance use is a precursor to abuse or dependence, and regular use clearly increases the risk for developing a substance use disorder (SUD). However, the use of substances per se is not sufficient for a diagnosis of SUD. Substance abuse is a maladaptive pattern of the use of alcohol or drugs manifested in significant impairment or distress. The criteria for substance dependence in adults include tolerance, withdrawal, and compulsive drug use. For children and adolescents tolerance and loss of control are not good indicators for a diagnosis. Instead, alcohol-related blackouts, craving, and impulsive sexual or risk-taking behavior tend to be more important criteria (AACAP, 2005). Tobacco use is discussed in the environmental health chapter.

Epidemiology

Twenty-five percent of students drank alcohol for the first time before 13 years old, and about 21% reported episodic heavy drinking in the 2009 Youth Risk Behavior Surveillance report (Eaton et al, 2010). However, nearly half of problem drinkers are thought to have tried alcohol by 10 years old and two thirds by 13 years old. The percentage of students reporting lifetime use of alcohol, marijuana, steroids, methamphetamines, and hallucinogenic drugs has decreased in the last decade, although the percentage of those reporting current use of cocaine and amphetamines has not changed significantly (Eaton et al, 2010).

The cause of SUD is multifaceted. Many contributing factors exist, including the following:

- Genetic vulnerability (family history)
- Parental substance use
- Dysfunctional family relationships, such as rigidity, distant relationships, neglect, or lack of supervision
- Negative life events
- Psychiatric conditions (e.g., CD, ADHD, depression)
- Low self-esteem, poor body image
- Ineffective coping (poor emotional regulation, poor problem-solving skills)

- School failure
- Rigid, non–alcohol-using, ultraconservative family
- Latchkey child
- Poor sleep hygiene
- Low religiosity
- Sexual activity
- Homosexuality, bisexuality
- Competitive athleticism

Precipitating life events tend to center around loss of relationships (e.g., parental separation, divorce, or death; death of a close friend) and chronic negative circumstances (e.g., parental substance abuse, maltreatment).

Data from the Youth Risk Behavior Survey indicate that 40% of teens reported drinking alcohol and 20% reported using marijuana within the previous month. Approximately 24% of high school students binge drink (Eaton et al, 2010). The majority of adolescents who use drugs do not progress to abuse or dependence. Peer influence seems to be less significant to the cause of substance abuse than previously thought. Boys tend to be more involved in use of both alcohol and drugs of all kinds than girls are at the same age. It is estimated that for both boys and girls abuse of alcohol and other drugs is negligible from 10 to 13 years old, but doubles between mid-adolescence (12 to 16 years old) and late adolescence (17 to 20 years old), peaks between 18 and 25 years old, and declines thereafter (Eaton et al, 2010).

Clinical Findings

Identifying an adolescent's problem with substance abuse requires a careful assessment, conducted with an accepting, nonjudgmental, nonthreatening, matter-of-fact attitude. The covert nature of substance abuse and the dynamic of denial make it crucial to avoid a critical tone (see Chapter 8 for discussion of adolescent risk behavior).

History. Interviewing the adolescent with the parents is a key strategy for obtaining information about etiological factors and behavioral, cognitive, emotional, and physical changes they have observed in the adolescent. However, it is essential that the adolescent also be interviewed alone at every visit to assess mental health and family issues.

When talking about substance use with an adolescent, it is important to begin with general questions that are not overly personal. Begin by asking the adolescent about acquaintances or friends who smoke, drink, or use drugs; whether anyone in the family has had problems with these; and what the adolescent does with friends when they get together. It is helpful to ask about experimentation, under what circumstances it occurs, and the adolescent's feelings about it. To obtain a chronological history of tobacco, alcohol, or drug use it may be helpful to approach the subject by inquiring about prescription drugs and moving to illicit substances. The key is to remain nonjudgmental to elicit information that will indicate whether the adolescent is experimenting, a regular user, or dependent on substances. Ask about the adolescent's source of drugs or alcohol; the adolescent who uses substances provided by a friend or acquaintance is less advanced than one who purchases them directly. The practitioner should ask, "What? How much? How often? When? How? Where? With whom? Does the patient use substances at parties, home, school, alone, or with friends?"

The CRAFFT questionnaire is an appropriate screening instrument for substance abuse in the primary care setting

(Knight et al, 2007). This questionnaire involves the following questions:

- C - Have you ever driven or ridden in a *car* or other moving vehicle when you or someone else has been drinking or using drugs?
- R - Do you ever use drugs or alcohol to *relax*, feel better about yourself, or fit into a group?
- A - Do you ever use alcohol or drugs when you are *alone*?
- F - Do you ever *forget* to do things when you are drinking or using drugs?
- F - Has anyone (*family or friends*) ever told you that you drink or use drugs too much?
- T - Have you ever gotten into *trouble* because of your drinking or drug use?

Positive responses to two or more items indicate a high likelihood for substance abuse and merits further evaluation and treatment (Knight et al, 2007).

Significant behavioral changes that may reflect drug use include the following (Foy et al, 2010):

- Infants and young children
  - Excessive crying
  - Poor feeding or failure to thrive
  - Irritability, jitteriness, or excessive lethargy
  - Poor eye contact
  - Sleep disorders
- Older children and adolescents
  - Decreased school performance
  - Lethargy, hyperactivity or agitation, hypervigilance, decreased attention
  - Disinhibition; deviant or risk-taking behavior
  - Repeated absences from school; suspensions from school
  - Loss of interest in previously enjoyed activities
  - Withdrawal from family and usual friends, or change in friends to those involved in drugs and alcohol
  - Irritability, fighting or acting-out
  - Hypersexuality
  - Exaggerated mood swings
  - Change in sleep patterns, nightmares
  - Altered menstruation
  - Change in appetite (from anorexia to unusual hunger)

Mood changes include swings from depression to euphoria, nervousness, unreasonable anger, and frequent expressions of hopelessness or failure. Low self-esteem typically characterizes those who abuse substances.

Physical Examination. Physical signs that indicate a substance use problem include the following:

- Weight loss
- Red eyes, associated with marijuana use
- Hoarseness, chronic cough, wheezing with use of inhalants and cocaine
- Frequent "colds" or "allergy" symptoms, epistaxis, and perforations of nasal septum with cocaine and inhalant use
- Accidents, trauma, injuries
- Intoxication
- Complete or partial amnesia for events during intoxication with alcohol and date rape drug use
- Dilated or constricted pupils
- Gynecomastia, irregular periods, small testes with marijuana
- Needle tracks occur with intramuscular (IM) steroids or IV heroin use

- Generalized pruritus with opiate use
- Reflux, diarrhea, gastritis, and constipation with opiate and alcohol use
- Perioral sores or pyodermas from huffing and bagging

Laboratory Studies. Urine toxicology can be helpful to verify adolescent truthfulness, although a positive drug screen result does not indicate substance abuse or dependence, but only indicates substance use. A negative drug screen result does not rule out an SUD. The approximate duration that drugs can be detected in the urine is as follows (AACAP, 2005):

- Stimulants—1 to 2 days
- Cocaine and its major metabolite—1 to 3 days
- Sedative-hypnotics—1 day to 1 week
- Barbiturates—2 to 4 weeks
- Quaaludes—2 to 3 weeks
- Opiates—1 to 2 days
- Marijuana—up to 30 days

Duration of detection from last substance use varies according to the laboratory and type of test used. The AACAP recommends that to obtain a valid result, a positive result on immunoassay should be followed by confirmation with a more sensitive method, such as gas chromatography or mass spectrometry.

Differential Diagnosis

Substance abuse is distinguished from social drinking or non-pathological substance use by the presence of compulsive use, craving, or substance-related problems (AACAP, 2005). SUDs are comorbid most often with CD, depression, and anxiety.

Management

Exposure to tobacco and alcohol and illicit substances begins in early childhood. The pediatric primary care provider should discuss parental modeling for the use of alcohol, tobacco, and other substances in early childhood during routine well-child visits. It is important to educate school-age children and their parents about substance use and its consequences. For adolescents, a direct assessment and an interview about substance use are essential. Parents should be advised not to involve their child in their own substance use. Something as seemingly innocuous as "getting Dad a beer from the refrigerator" gives the child practice in alcohol use.

Substance abuse must be treated, and referral to a substance abuse program is crucial. The initial goal is to help adolescents take positive steps toward changing their substance use and abuse behavior. If the adolescent denies any problem, efforts should focus on helping the adolescent acknowledge problems. Clarifying reported negative consequences, creating doubts about substance use, and raising awareness of the risks related to current use are motivational interviewing strategies that may be helpful. It is important to remain empathic and yet emphasize the adolescent's responsibility to make healthy choices. If the adolescent has not reached a level of chronic use, prevention of harm is the goal of the intervention. Guide the adolescent to examine his or her substance use responsibly and identify ways to prevent harmful consequences.

If the adolescent progresses to chronic substance use, a number of options exist. Outpatient or day treatment programs are effective for those who can live and be managed at home. For adolescents with more serious addiction, comorbid psychiatric conditions, or suicidal ideation, residential treatment or hospitalization may be necessary. Given the prominence of family dysfunction and family life events in the cause of the problem, family-based treatment programs are essential. Family treatment, rather than family psychoeducation or family support groups, has been shown to be superior to other

modalities. Follow-up assessments should include substance use issues and other predictors of use: stress or negative life events, depression or negative affect regulation, and the presence of positive support within or outside of the family. Self-help or 12-step groups are thought to be an essential element in the recovery process.

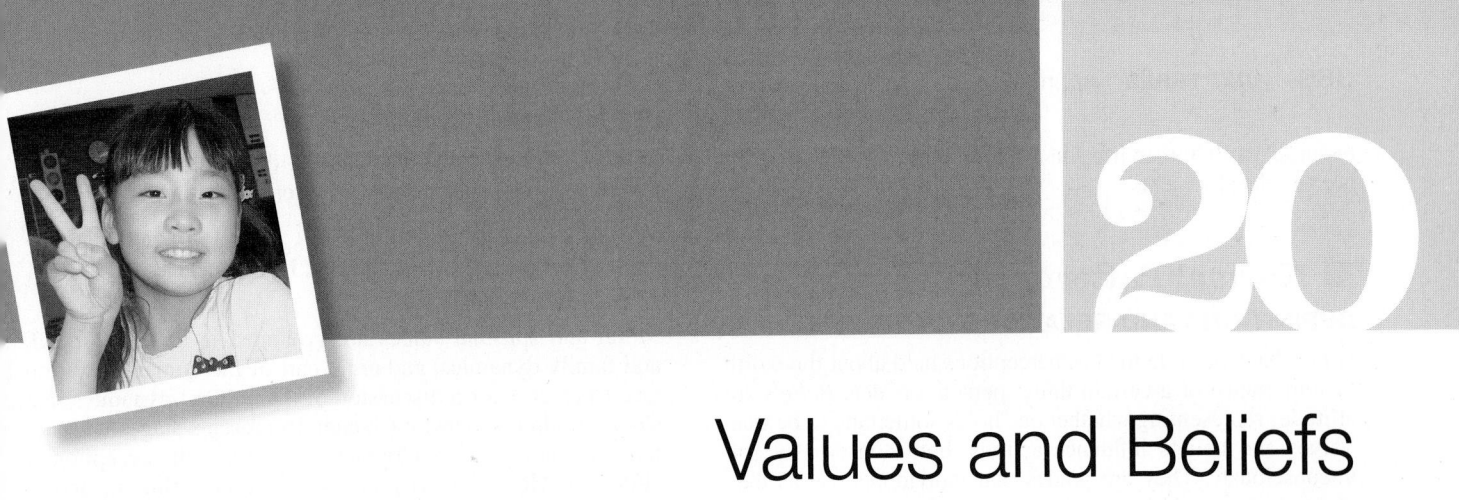

Values and Beliefs

ARDYS M. DUNN

Children's health and well-being are not determined by physical measures alone. As discussed in previous chapters, being part of a family and community, being valued and nurtured by others, and belonging and *mattering* to other individuals give children a strong sense of self and the foundation to establish healthy relationships and face life's challenges positively. The child's values and beliefs and expression of spirituality and faith are integral to this process of development. Pediatric primary health care providers must be aware that beliefs, faith, religion, and spirituality affect children's health. The use of meditation, prayer, relaxation, and other mind-body therapies is known to facilitate healing, and there is growing recognition of the importance of attending to matters of spirituality, morality, and religion in health care. Holistic pediatric care includes assessment of social, cultural, and spiritual dimensions. It considers the effect of values and beliefs on health care decisions and explores ways to support values, beliefs, and subsequent actions that promote health. Pediatric providers who incorporate spiritual care into their practice offer children and their families an invaluable resource to find meaning, comfort, and healing.

Standards of Practice

Health care in the U.S. has tended to focus on physical health and illness rather than the integration of mental, emotional, and spiritual health. When individuals have received care in the spiritual realm, they have traditionally been referred to chaplains, pastors, or other religious leaders in their faith community. However, the importance of health care providers being able to address the spiritual element of care has become more widely acknowledged. This is particularly true in end-of-life and palliative care, but guidelines related to spiritual issues in all areas of health care are also being developed.

The Society of Teachers of Family Medicine has published spiritual care competencies for the family resident education program that focus on knowledge, skills, and attitude. Health care providers should have a conceptual framework of spirituality in their clinical care; understand the differences between spirituality and religion, the influence of beliefs on patient care, and ethical issues between patient and provider;

and know where and how to access resources for spiritual care (e.g., chaplains). They should be skilled at assessing spiritual components of client systems, listening with attention to spiritual needs, and providing a therapeutic, compassionate presence to support healing. Finally, they should demonstrate respect for patients and colleagues, and develop a mindfulness to personal spiritual beliefs and perspectives, caring for the self and using practices that strengthen their healing intention as providers of patient care (Anandarajah et al, 2010). Courses such as The Healer's Art, taught in many medical schools across the country, can provide the framework for developing such competencies (Pearson, 2009).

The Joint Commission (TJC) requires spiritual assessments of patients admitted to tertiary care hospitals (TJC, 2010), and clinical guidelines for palliative care have been developed by the National Consensus Project for Quality Palliative Care (NCPQPC, 2009). Depression may have a spiritual connection, and the U.S. Preventive Services Task Force (2009) recommends screening adolescents (ages 12 to 18) for major depressive disorders; there is not sufficient evidence to warrant screening of younger children (ages 7 to 11).

The spiritual and child health initiative developed by the Department of Pediatrics, Boston Medical Center and Medical Anthropology (Barnes et al, 2000) articulated guidelines for general pediatric practice, suggesting that providers:
- Anticipate patients will have spiritual or religious concerns.
- Develop a self-awareness of one's own spiritual and religious history and perspective.
- Become broadly familiar with the religious worldview of the patient groups for whom they care.
- Work with individual families and children to learn their specific values and beliefs.
- Develop strategic interviewing skills.
- Develop a resource list and network of local consultants.
- Refer patients to appropriate spiritual care providers.

Much of the focus on spiritual needs of children and families has been related to critical care or end-of-life decisions, and addressing spiritual beliefs may be particularly important for families facing life-threatening illnesses that seem unfair or that have no reasonable explanation. However, these discussions should be part of well-child visits as well as care of children who are acutely or chronically ill. Spirituality is essential to all human life and is a critical part of every child's healthy development.

■ Normal Patterns of Behavior

DEFINITIONS AND RELATIONSHIP TO BEHAVIOR

Values have been defined as perceptions held about the worth or importance of a certain thing, person, or idea. *Beliefs* are attitudes representing whether one holds something to be true. Values and beliefs influence actions, both consciously and unconsciously. They are guides that individuals use as they make decisions. Values and beliefs are learned phenomena, and recognition and acceptance of shared values and beliefs are fundamental to the integrity of the individual, the family, and the social group (see Chapter 3). Although perceptions, attitudes, values, and beliefs are transmitted from one generation to another, they remain open to change and are responsive to social contexts and situations. Values clarification is the process by which one examines behavior in light of values and changing circumstances and asks why a certain action is taken or whether that action is consistent with the values one claims to have. Change in values, beliefs, and behavior can result from the process of values clarification. *Faith,* according to Fowler and Dell, is the basis for developing beliefs, values, and meaning. Faith "(1) gives coherence and direction to persons' lives; (2) links them in shared trusts and loyalties with others; (3) grounds their personal stances and communal loyalties in a sense of relatedness to a larger frame of reference; and (4) enables them to face and deal with the challenges of human life and death, relying on that which has the quality of ultimacy in their lives" (Fowler and Dell, 2004, p 17). In this broad conceptualization, faith encompasses a wide range of religious and spiritual expression.

Spirituality has been defined as an awareness of and commitment to a sacred, unifying force that gives meaning to life; the recognition of a nonmaterial higher power that encompasses all of life's affairs and is mediated through the individual's relationships to others, to the community, and to the environment (McLeod and Wright, 2008). Although integral to religion, spirituality and religion should not be confused. Religion is the organized expression of values and beliefs through religious activities, rituals, and behaviors. Characteristics of spirituality are listed in Box 20-1.

EXPECTED PATTERNS OF BEHAVIOR RELATED TO VALUES AND BELIEFS

Children's values and beliefs are related to their developmental stage and are reflected in different behaviors at different ages. In general, "adaptive, competent functioning" reflects positive values and development (Kochanska et al, 2010a). In particular, the development of moral integrity (or conscience) and spirituality (or faith) is expected of the healthy child. As they develop moral and spiritual values, healthy children achieve a positive sense of self, learn to value themselves and their contribution to the family and larger social system, and feel a sense of understanding and belonging to their community. Children's expression of faith depends on their experiences with faith language, ritual, and organization; those children raised in families where prayer, discussion of religious beliefs, and participation in religious rituals and events

is the norm will express their faith differently than children raised in a more secular family system.

DEVELOPMENT OF MORAL INTEGRITY OR CONSCIENCE

Moral and spiritual values are grounded in cultural, social, and family dynamics, and are a part of the human condition (see Chapter 3 for a discussion of the cultural dynamics that shape children's growth; Chapter 16 presents stages and factors influencing the development of healthy self-perception in children). Moral integrity involves demonstrating an understanding of right and wrong (moral cognition); engaging in reflection on ethical issues of justice and fairness (moral judgment); expressing a sense of responsibility to oneself, others, and the environment (moral sensitivity and emotions); and taking action based on one's moral values (moral character). Moral virtues include things such as honesty, openness, fairness, self-control, constancy, unity, and dedication. Empathy, a fundamental moral emotion, is the ability to understand the perspective or condition of another and to experience a visceral or emotional reaction to that condition.

The development of moral integrity is an evolutionary process, influenced to a degree by prenatal and genetic factors and continuing into adulthood. It is difficult to say at just what age or stage, with what degree of complexity, and as a result of which variables children will demonstrate moral integrity. Kohlberg (1969) claims that mature moral reasoning does not appear until postconventional stages 5 and 6 (middle to late childhood and adolescence). Fontaine and colleagues (2009) found that the ability to assess the moral value of behaviors and make moral decisions (the Response Evaluation and Decision [RED] process) was rudimentary before middle childhood. Gibbs and associates (1992) argue that mature moral reasoning can appear as early as stages 3 and 4 (early school-age children), as children develop friendships, learn to

---

BOX 20-1 Characteristics of Spirituality

Inner Resources and Identity

Those who possess inner resources have a sense of wholeness, competence, and direction. They are capable of responding to crises or turmoil and draw on inner strengths to maintain a sense of stability and control. They have values that give them courage and hope.

Interconnectedness

Interconnectedness is the sense of being an integral part of the world and attached to others, to one's environment, and to a universal or supreme being.

Purpose or Meaning of Life

A sense of direction and meaning and a reason for existence are developed in the relationships individuals have with others and their world.

Transcendence

The ability to go beyond, or transcend, the experiences of daily life is evident in the expression of hope, meaning, and direction when an individual is faced with fear, inability to effect change, uncertainty, and ambiguity.

From Howden J: Development and psychometric characteristics of the Spirituality Assessment Scale, *Dissertation Abstracts Int* 54:166, 1993.

care about others, and understand rights and responsibilities as essential to societal functioning. Other research suggests that preschool-age children "attempt to construct moral self-consistency," making efforts to present themselves as "good" in their stories (Gutzwiller-Helfenfinger et al, 2010); that "children's early conscience, a system that comprises self-regulated conduct and moral emotions...begins to emerge in the toddler years" (Kochanska et al, 2010a, p 1320); and that even very young children demonstrate a moral awareness, though it is primarily experiential rather than reflective (Johansson, 2001). Ongoing research continues to identify specific characteristics, dynamics, and determinants of the process of developing moral integrity.

- *Developmental theories:* Research on the ways children gain moral integrity has primarily been based in developmental theory. Kohlberg's notion that moral development proceeds sequentially through phases related to intellectual development and social interactions is probably the most well known of these theories (Kohlberg, 1969), although other developmental perspectives have been offered. Freud, for example, asserted that children develop a conscience through identification with a significant caregiver mediated by the processes of guilt and shame. Piaget claimed that children's moral development parallels their intellectual development and ability to reason. And social learning theory (e.g., Vygotsky) states that positive role modeling and active social engagement with others teaches moral behavior. These theories are discussed more fully in Chapter 4.

- *Attachment, temperament, and reciprocity:* Kochanska and colleagues have conducted extensive research on how toddlers and preschool children develop a moral identity, a sense of their "moral self" that guides their future conduct. Secure attachment to the primary caregiver early in life is a critical determinant; this attachment supports an "eager, willing stance" toward the parent, and facilitates internalization of parental rules and standards as well as a sense of empathy with others (Kochanska et al, 2010b). In fact, secure attachment may override genetic effects as children develop the ability to self-regulate (Kochanska et al, 2009). Temperament can affect the child-parent interaction and the development of conscience in two ways: first, the natural temperament of the child may lend itself to internalization of parental values. Children with a naturally fearful temperament tend to more quickly internalize their parents' message and, as a result, require gentle parenting with "subtle discipline" for healthy development. Second, temperament may be difficult or conflictive between parent and child and require more directive socialization strategies. Children who demonstrate a "fearless" temperament appear to function best when there is a "mutually positive, responsive, binding, and cooperative orientation between parent and child" (i.e., reciprocity) (Kochanska and Aksan, 2006). When the parent is responsive to the child, the child's cooperation is enhanced; children actively engaged in a supportive, reciprocal relationship with their parent more likely want to do what the parent suggests (Kochanska et al, 2004, 2010a).

- *Gender:* Some theorists contend that gender plays a significant role in the way children interpret situations and make choices based on moral judgment (Gilligan, 1990), and there is evidence that girls are likely to be more empathic and more highly skilled in emotional judgments than boys (Fumagalli et al, 2010; Malti and Buchmann, 2010).

The relationship among genetics, neurobiology, and environment (including socialization) as determinants of this gender difference remains to be explained.

- *Neurobiology:* Recent research explores the role of neural development on moral behavior (Shirtcliff et al, 2009). Empathy, it appears, is grounded in the brain. Three primary areas of brain circuitry process emotions, memory, and the cognitive functions that integrate behavioral responses:
  - The limbic system (amygdala, thalamus, and hypothalamus in particular) stores emotional memory, transmits messages of stress (fight or flight), and appears to enable emotions of bonding, affiliation, and (their negative counterpart) separation. Activity in the amygdala (emotional memory) in particular stimulates activity in the orbital frontal cortex and ventromedial prefrontal cortex, centers of emotional learning, judgment, and decision-making.
  - The mirror neuron system functions to encourage imitation and is activated when pain is experienced; imagining or anticipating pain, or observing others' experience of pain also activates this system.
  - The paralimbic system (insula and anterior cingulate cortex [ACC]) connects the limbic and mirror neuron systems with peripheral physiologic stimuli, both physical and emotional. The insula is activated by negative arousal, for example, pain, bad smells or taste, or fear. Conflict activates the ACC, which works with the insula, connecting physical arousal to emotions and engaging the memory of the limbic system to evaluate, judge, and (ultimately) act, all in an effort to relieve distress. Real and imagined arousal activates the paralimbic system, as does the perception of arousal in others.
  - Functional deficits in these areas of the brain limit the individual's ability to feel emotion—in self or others, to make good judgments or decisions, and to demonstrate empathic, morally integrated behavior (Shirtcliff et al, 2009). Responsive parenting and positive physical experience (e.g., gentle touch, nurturing, comfort) early in childhood appear to strengthen these areas of the brain, stimulating positive vagal nerve function, and contributing to feelings of calmness and compassion (Eisenberg and Eggum, 2008; Narvaez, 2010).

- *Epigenetics:* Findings of early research in the area of epigenetics suggest that epigenetic changes may mediate the effect of prenatal and infant environment on mental health and disease in older children and adults (McGowan and Szyf, 2010). In animal studies, behavior of a high-nurturing parent stimulates the gene that encodes glucocorticoid receptor proteins and relieves stress. A study of suicide victims who were abused as children revealed that they had decreased levels of this marker, suggesting that child abuse may have an epigenetic effect that leads to prolonged stress and mental disorders (McGowan et al, 2009).

DEVELOPMENT OF SPIRITUALITY

Although it has been argued that children are intrinsically spiritual, the development of spiritual expression in children is largely seen as paralleling cognitive and moral development (Fowler, 1981; Stilwell et al, 1998; Walker et al, 2000; Wolf, 2000). Table 20-1 presents a developmental perspective of faith and outlines age-specific interventions to enhance healthy growth. Infants and toddlers are engaged in the processes of

TABLE 20-1 Developmental Outcomes and Appropriate Interventions Related to Values and Beliefs

	Infant (0-12 months old)	Toddler and Preschooler (1-5 years old)	School-Age Child (6-12 years old)	Adolescent
Moral integrity and conscience (right and wrong; sense of responsibility to oneself, others, and the environment)	Develops sense of trust in caregivers (Erikson, 1963); learns to adjust to family routine (e.g., sleeping, eating)	Believes rules are absolute; behaves well for fear of punishment or to receive rewards (Kohlberg, 1969); develops sense of autonomy, initiative, and purpose; differentiates self from others (Erikson, 1963)	Believes rules exist to keep order and protect people and that everyone benefits from them; behaves well to please others, to avoid guilt, and to maintain status of "good" child (Kohlberg, 1969); develops sense of industry, faith in self-competence; explores, creates, collects; understands cause and effect (Erikson, 1963); begins to understand and manage strong feelings, and develop and express moral decision-making	Rules are based on ethical judgment; believes individual answers to personal conscience, has moral obligation to a social contract; behaves to maintain respect of self, peers, and larger community (Kohlberg, 1969); integrates personality and develops sense of identity, loyalty to group and significant others (Erikson, 1963)
Faith development (Fowler, 1981 as cited in Mueller, 2010)	Undifferentiated faith based on trust in relationships with parents and caregivers; infant develops object permanence, sense of trust, attachment, and sense of being nurtured	Intuitive-projective faith based on images, feelings, and symbols; children use imagination to make meaning of their world; egocentric thinking may contribute to misconceptions; child begins to participate in family's religious practices and rituals	Mythic-literal faith, with more concrete beliefs, a more rigid system of order and activities; faith as assent, as child learns to master the environment and become competent; child begins to explore ultimate issues, develop understanding of the meaning of life	Synthetic conventional faith—ideas about spirituality are synthesized through interpersonal relations with peers, parents, other significant adults, and life experiences; adolescent explores identity and personal meaning of faith; faith becomes source of identity as child seeks understanding of self in the world (Quinn, 2008); adolescent demonstrates self-reflection, insight, sense of inner spiritual process and presence in the world, and continues to more fully develop understanding of ultimate questions, life's meaning
Experienced faith (infancy through early adolescence) Affiliative faith (late adolescence)	Children experience faith through relationships with others and others' faith traditions			Adolescent actively participates in a faith community, feels a sense of belonging, awe, and wonder; acknowledges authority of faith community
Parental Interventions to Foster Healthy Development	Respond to infant's physiologic and emotional needs promptly and adequately; demonstrate loving, gentle approach in communication and interaction	Treat child with respect and acceptance; provide security, love, and companionship; set realistic limits on behavior, using positive discipline rather than punishment; remove temptation from environment; provide positive role model; provide guided opportunities to interact with adults and other children and active play alone; be patient; involve child in family religious practices; begin to establish regular tasks for child in family activities	Treat child with respect and acceptance; set realistic limits on behavior; provide opportunities for active play alone and with other children; encourage peer group activity; allow children to make decisions as appropriate, helping them to explore meanings of feelings, events, and interactions; choose narrative stories related to children's experience of moral dilemmas to explore right and wrong and to help child develop values; establish regular tasks for child as member of family; help child be successful in the family; teach family values and standards; encourage continued participation in family religious practices	Treat adolescent with respect and acceptance; set realistic limits on behavior; model and encourage family's moral standards; encourage involvement in family activities; allow children to make more of own choices regarding values and beliefs; allow appropriate experimentation in dress, hair, makeup as child develops sense of self; do not overreact to adolescent "crises"; provide opportunities to discuss values, ethics, and moral behavior; provide support and encouragement for successes and failures in school, social, athletic, and work activities; encourage continued participation in family religious practices

gaining trust and establishing autonomy or separateness of self from the parent. They are becoming a part of a bigger culture (i.e., the family). Preschool and early school-age children gain an understanding of the meaning of life through fantasy play, active engagement with their environment, strong attachments to their parents, and growing relationships with their peers. Although they have achieved the task of defining themselves as separate individuals, the thinking and behavior of preschool and early school-age children in relation to faith issues are expressions of the family's faith and practice. School-age children and adolescents define life's meaning within the context of their self-sufficiency, competence, and role differentiation and in their relationship to both peers and adults. Exploring their understanding of the ultimate questions in life, adolescents are interested in issues such as life, death, war, evil, good, and creation, and develop increasing wisdom as they discuss and think about these important matters.

■ Assessment of Normal Patterns

The goals of assessing values and beliefs include the following:
- Determine the nature of the child's and family's belief system.
- Identify ways that the family interacts (internally and with the larger community) to support these beliefs.
- Clarify how beliefs affect decisions and behaviors related to health care.
- Develop an understanding of how this particular illness or health issue challenges the child's and family's belief system.
- Determine how the provider can best address values, including spiritual or religious issues when giving care.

Because children are in the process of developing values and beliefs and because much of their development depends on their interaction with the parent or caregiver, assessment questions are often directed to the parent or caregiver. This can yield a wealth of information, but it may not accurately or completely assess the child's needs or understandings. Children may not be able to understand what is happening to them; they cannot always express themselves clearly or use the words or symbols related to values, beliefs, faith, or spirituality that are more familiar to adults. Interpreting and understanding the emotional and spiritual meaning a given experience has for a child is a significant challenge to even the most skilled health care provider.

HISTORY

Moral Integrity or Conscience

The following points can guide the assessment:
- How does the child define right and wrong? How does the child's behavior reflect his or her moral understanding? How does the child demonstrate moral reasoning?
- What are family attitudes or beliefs about what is right and wrong?
- How are parents teaching their child about right and wrong?
- What other influences affect the child's concept of right and wrong (e.g., daycare, teachers and counselors, peer group)?
- How do parents set limits on the child's behavior?
- How does the child respond to discipline and limits?

- What messages do parents give about the value and importance of the child's contribution to the family and the community?
- What messages do parents give about the value of respecting other people, ideas, property, and the environment?
- What opportunities do parents give the child to make independent, age-appropriate decisions?
- What traditions and family-centered activities does the family have? How is the child included in these activities?

Spirituality

An initial screening can determine if more in-depth assessment or pastoral intervention is appropriate. Grossoehme (2008) developed such a tool to be used by chaplains when initially interviewing hospitalized children or adolescents. Use of the screening tool appears to generate productive "deeper conversation with the patients" (Fig. 20-1).

Most spiritual assessment tools have been developed for use with adults in critical care. Some, however, have been used with children and families, and providers are encouraged to find the set of questions that best suits their practice, constructed with the assessment goals listed previously in mind (Table 20-2). Use of a broad framework, including culture, religion, and spirituality is recommended. The following information should be identified in relation to spirituality:

General. Tell me about your religious or spiritual beliefs related to the following issues:
- Family relations, gender roles, and children's and parents' responsibilities
- Sexuality issues (e.g., responsible sexuality, male and female roles, homosexuality, premarital sex)
- Dietary restrictions
- Rituals (e.g., prayer at mealtime, bedtime, or during times of crisis)
- Use of drugs, alcohol, or tobacco
- Medical treatment

Inner Resources and Identity
- What are your child's goals in life? Your family's goals?
- What are your child's strong points? Your family's strong points?
- What do you like about yourself? Your child? Your family?
- How important is faith or spirituality in your child's life? In your life?
- What brings you, your child, and your family joy and peace? Where do you find hope and comfort?

Interconnectedness
- How do you feel about your child? About yourself? About your family?
- What do you do as a family to show love for each other?
- Who are significant people in your child's and your family's life?
- Whom do you ask for support when your family needs help?
- How do members of your family share feelings with others?
- Do you feel that you and your family are part of a community? Of a larger world or universe?
- Does the family belong to a religious or spiritual group?

Purpose or Meaning of Life
- What are your family's religious, spiritual, and cultural beliefs? What ethics or values are important in your family's life?
- What gives life meaning? What is the most important thing in life?

Child/Adolescent Spiritual Screening Tool

Name: _____ Age:_____

Please draw a circle around the answer below each statement.

How often do you think that...

1. A good God watches over me.
    Never   Rarely   Sometimes   Often   Always

2. I have to live with God's punishment.
    Never   Rarely   Sometimes   Often   Always

3. I feel God's love in my life.
    Never   Rarely   Sometimes   Often   Always

4. Embarrassment plays a big role in my life.
    Never   Rarely   Sometimes   Often   Always

5. My hope tells me life's got to get better.
    Never   Rarely   Sometimes   Often   Always

6. I wish my family were with me more right now.
    Never   Rarely   Sometimes   Often   Always

7. I have friendships with kids in church.
    Never   Rarely   Sometimes   Often   Always

8. My loneliness makes life hard.
    Never   Rarely   Sometimes   Often   Always

9. Prayer helps me.
    Never   Rarely   Sometimes   Often   Always

10. God feels very far away from me.
    Never   Rarely   Sometimes   Often   Always

11. Having my parents nearby helps me when life is hard.
    Never   Rarely   Sometimes   Often   Always

12. My religion tells me my sickness (or my problem) is my fault.
    Never   Rarely   Sometimes   Often   Always

13. People show their love for me.
    Never   Rarely   Sometimes   Often   Always

14. My God is an angry God.
    Never   Rarely   Sometimes   Often   Always

15. I love who I am.
    Never   Rarely   Sometimes   Often   Always

16. Betrayal is part of my life story.
    Never   Rarely   Sometimes   Often   Always

17. I have lost a lot in life.
    Never   Rarely   Sometimes   Often   Always

FIGURE 20-1 Spiritual screening tool for children and adolescents. Odd numbered items 1 through 15 indicate spiritual strengths; even items 2 through 16 and item 17 indicate spiritual needs. Extent to which needs outweigh strengths may be one indication of how much an individual needs spiritual counseling. (From Grossoehme DH: Development of a spiritual screening tool for children and adolescents, *J Pastoral Care Counsel* 62(1):71-85, 2008.)

TABLE 20-2 Spiritual Assessment Tools			
HOPE (Anandarajah and Hight, 2001)	**BELIEF (McEvoy, 2000)**	**SPIRIT (Highfield, 2000)**	**FICA (Puchalski and Romer, 2000)**
• Where does client find **H**ope, peace, and comfort? • Does client participate in **O**rganized religion? • What are **P**ersonal spiritual practices? • What **E**ffect do these behaviors have on the client's health decisions?	• What is client's **B**elief system? • **E**thics or values? • **L**ifestyle behaviors (e.g., diet, rituals)? • **I**nvolvement in a spiritual community? • Religious **E**ducation and knowledge? • **F**uture events and decisions about health that will be affected by religious beliefs?	• **S**piritual belief system (religious affiliation)? • **P**ersonal spirituality (beliefs that child/family accept)? • **I**ntegration and involvement with a religious community? • **R**ituals and restrictions? • **I**mplications for medical care (beliefs provider should take into consideration when discussing medical care)? • **T**erminal events planning (e.g., advance directives, contacting clergy)?	• **F**aith and belief: Do you consider yourself religious? What gives your life meaning? Helps you cope with stress? • **I**mportance: How important is your faith or beliefs? How do they influence your health or how you have managed this illness? • **C**ommunity: Are you a part of a spiritual or religious community? Does this support you? Is there a group of people you love and who are important to you? • **A**ddress: How would you like me, as your health provider, to address these issues in giving you care?

• How does your family express religious, spiritual, and cultural beliefs? How is your child involved?
• What rituals or practices contribute to a sense of spiritual fulfillment or peace?
• How do you teach your child about values and beliefs? How else does your child learn about values and beliefs?
• Are you comfortable talking about your beliefs with your child?

Transcendence
• How do members of your family deal with spiritual distress during a crisis?

PHYSICAL EXAMINATION

Objective assessment of values and beliefs is largely based on observation, and, though subject to interpretation, these observations can indicate the child's sense of valuing others, self, and the environment. Observe the child's behavior, especially noting interaction with parents, other adults, and peers. The child exhibits the following behaviors:
• Appears at ease, although behavior may vary (e.g., shy, quiet, active, talkative, engaging) depending on developmental level and temperament
• Engages actively, spontaneously, and affectionately with parent or caregiver
• Responds to parent or caregiver cues; follows directions and conforms to limits set without demonstrating guilt or fear of punishment
• Shares toys, depending on age
• Respects people and property
• Is not physically aggressive, depending on age
• Is able to articulate moral reasoning (older child)
• Is able to articulate a faith statement, depending on spiritual, religious, and cultural background (older child)

■ Management of Normal Patterns

The goals of management are to facilitate the development of moral integrity (including moral identity, judgment, and conduct) and a sense of spiritual self within the major areas of spirituality: self-awareness as a spiritual being, and relationships with others, the environment, and with a sacred or transcendent entity.

Parents can encourage their child's development of moral integrity in the following ways:
• Be a loving, responsive, and accepting presence in their children's lives. This responsibility cannot be overemphasized; children's understandings and expressions of self-concept, spirituality, and moral integrity derive in large part from the quality of their interactions with significant adults.
• Set realistic standards or limits for right and wrong behavior.
• State what is acceptable and what is unacceptable behavior.
• Provide a rationale for limits set; the explanation varies depending on the cognitive and developmental level of the child.
• Articulate personal values, beliefs, and faith statements for the child. Give clear, age-appropriate explanations and spiritual lessons.
• Be a role model for constructive and positive behavior.
• Reinforce positive behavior and attempts at positive behavior.
• Hold children accountable for negative behavior; use "consequences" that are age-appropriate and that fairly suit the behavior being sanctioned.
• Teach children strategies to avoid misbehavior; teach constructive coping skills.
• Use creative parenting strategies (e.g., distraction, diversional activities) to help children avoid misbehavior.
• Provide a developmentally appropriate environment to minimize children's misbehavior. It is easier to remove a breakable object from a table than to keep saying no or to punish a child for breaking it.
• Provide opportunities for children to make age-appropriate decisions independently.
• Praise children in front of others.
• Do not give false praise.
• Articulate and reinforce messages that children belong and are valued for themselves, not just for their behaviors.
• Establish family traditions and projects that actively involve children (e.g., family outings or family value sessions, during which family members share a meal with directed conversation). Do not expect perfection.

- Involve children in the family's religious and cultural practices.
- Provide and encourage opportunities for children to engage with the larger community in activities that support the child's interests and reinforce family values.
- Engage the child in nature-based activities (e.g., walks, visits to parks, outdoor camps) that strengthen a sense of ecologic connection and responsibility.
- Provide opportunities for the child to explore moral and ethical dilemmas and to develop possible solutions.
- Discuss moral and spiritual implications of events in the child's life (e.g., death of a grandparent, birth of a sibling, sharing, stealing, violence portrayed in media).
- Listen to and answer the child's questions.
  Primary health care providers should do the following:
- Be aware of their own values and beliefs.
- Distinguish between moral and medical advice. Be willing to offer both, while recognizing that personal proselytizing is inappropriate in the provider-patient relationship.
- Recognize and respect differences between their values and client's values.
- Provide an opportunity for parents to express values and beliefs and to discuss their child's moral and spiritual development.
- Provide information about parenting strategies, discipline, and effective communication between child and parents.
- Assist parents and child in values clarification as appropriate.
- Provide a role model of positive behavior.
- Offer an understanding, compassionate, and accepting presence.
- Listen and respond to the unique condition of each individual.
- Modify the treatment plan as appropriate to meet spiritual and religious needs.
- Refer the family for religious or spiritual counseling as indicated or requested.

■ Altered Patterns

LACK OF MORAL INTEGRITY OR CONSCIENCE

Description
Although lack of moral integrity is not a clinically defined condition, some children demonstrate a lack of an age-appropriate capacity to respect others or the environment, to judge behavior as right or wrong, and to express empathy or remorse. They frequently engage in antisocial behaviors (see Chapter 19 for a fuller discussion of social aggression, conduct disorder, and oppositional defiant disorder).

Epidemiology
An estimated 5% to 7% of children continue to demonstrate externalizing behaviors, act aggressively, and engage in antisocial behaviors as they move into middle childhood (Fanti and Henrich, 2010). A multitude of factors contribute to poor moral reasoning and antisocial behaviors, including temperament, negative experiences in infancy and childhood (e.g., maternal depression, unresponsive parenting, abuse), and environmental damage to neurologic systems.

Assessment
See Assessment of Normal Patterns.

Clinical Findings
Many behaviors seen are typical of normal children, depending on age, developmental, and cognitive levels (e.g., lying, hitting, refusing to share), but the child expresses little or no remorse for negative behavior; demonstrates no internalization of a sense of justice, fairness, or right and wrong; fails to develop an ability to self-regulate behavior; and continues antisocial behaviors beyond the expected developmental age.

Differential Diagnosis
Attention-deficit/hyperactivity disorder, social aggression, conduct disorder, oppositional defiant disorder, and depression are differential diagnoses.

Management
Early and assertive intervention can help many children develop a more healthy sense of their moral self and decrease antisocial behaviors (Shirtcliff et al, 2009), especially, it appears, if treatment emphasizes developing moral judgment and correcting "self-serving cognitive distortion" (Barriga et al, 2009). In addition to strategies listed here, see the discussion of management strategies for normal moral development in this chapter and for social aggression, conduct disorder, and oppositional defiant disorder (Chapter 19). In extreme cases, referral for psychiatric management may be necessary.

- Use storytelling, especially the personal narrative (the child's own story), to explore moral and ethical issues (Bennett, 2008; Gutzwiller-Helfenfinger et al, 2010).
- Encourage interaction with older children who demonstrate higher levels of moral reasoning (Leman, 2002).
- Watch films, television, videos, and DVDs together with children, and discuss books with adolescents.
- Monitor, discuss, and limit child's access to Internet and computer games.
- Assist child in values clarification process.

Complications
Antisocial behavior and delinquency are behavioral disorders in which lack of moral integrity is a key component.

SPIRITUAL DISTRESS

Description
Spiritual distress is an "impaired ability to experience and integrate meaning and purpose in life through connectedness with self, others, art, music, literature, nature, and/or a power greater than oneself" (North American Nursing Diagnosis Association [NANDA], 2009, p 208).

Epidemiology
Because of the complex nature of spirituality, spiritual distress can result from a number of factors. For children issues of death and dying and serious illness are major causes of

spiritual distress, but any crisis can threaten the sense of meaning that is fundamental to spiritual integrity. For infants and very young children, the simple fact of being hospitalized and removed from the routine and comfort of family life can lead to spiritual distress. Factors that can contribute to spiritual distress include the following:

- Trauma or violence, to self or to significant others
- Loss of significant other, especially parent or sibling
- Debilitating disease
- Chronic disease
- Separation of child from his or her family
- Isolation
- Homelessness
- Recommended medical therapies in conflict with child's or family's religious or spiritual beliefs (e.g., Christian Scientist)
- Barriers in the health care setting to practicing spiritual rituals (e.g., hospital routines that ignore patient's need to worship)
- Beliefs of health care providers, family members, or peers that conflict with those of child or parent

Assessment

See Assessment of Normal Patterns.

Clinical Findings

The following may be seen in spiritual distress:
- Depressive behavior
- Suicidal ideation
- Withdrawal
- No participation in usual religious practices
- Disparaging family's spiritual beliefs and values
- Questioning one's own value, meaning, and purpose of life
- Expressions of anger, resentment, fear of God
- Expressions of fear of suffering or death
- Expressions of inner conflict and doubts about beliefs
- Expressions of sense of spiritual emptiness
- Sleep disturbance
- Somatic complaints
- Behavior changes with mood swings
- Request for spiritual assistance

Differential Diagnosis

Depression, poor coping mechanisms, conduct disorders, antisocial behavior, and posttraumatic stress disorder are differential diagnoses for spiritual distress.

Management

Spiritual integrity is fundamentally a sense of meaning and purpose: one has a direction, control, and promise in a future. Health crises can easily undermine this integrity. Management goals for spiritual distress focus on helping children and families make sense of the events they are experiencing, and, if not to regain control, to better understand what is happening to and with them. McLeod and Wright (2008) present a model of spiritual care practice using conversations to generate new understandings that ultimately relieve suffering and help families live with "unanswered" and "unanswerable" questions.

This model assumes an open-ended, evolving interaction, with questions, dialogue, and reflection to explore difficult issues about the meaning of life. It assumes that each family system is unique and must be met with honor and respect. The process includes:

- "Calling forth and gathering" the family's and child's story of the illness; what has happened to them, how it has affected their faith or belief system
- "Opening space" in which feelings, ideas, thoughts can be examined and interpreted, and where reflection is invited
- Using imagination and metaphor to hear and express meaning; this is often accomplished by telling stories, especially the patient's or similar stories, and offering hypothetical beliefs
- Listening with "open silence" so the patient and family can express themselves freely
- Providing rituals that lead to conversation about the suffering being experienced (e.g., doing a genogram; asking the "one-question question" ["If you could have just one question answered in our work together, what would that question be?"]) (McLeod and Wright, 2008, p 126)

Meaning is generated in the conversations, in the interaction of questions, reflection, and answers, and clients express comfort even if the health outcome is ultimately beyond their control (McLeod and Wright, 2008).

In the process of developing a spirituality screening tool, Grossoehme (2008) found that adolescents identified several critical spiritual strengths and needs when they were confronted by a health problem:

- Strengths: talking with parents, the presence of parents, and believing in a loving God
- Unfilled needs: feeling isolated from one's family, feeling betrayed, and lacking a sense of purpose in life

Other management strategies can draw on these strengths, address these needs (and others), and ease distress:

- Identify and change situational factors that exacerbate distress.
- Assist parents to help their child process experiences contributing to distress. Engaging the child in conversation can be helpful. Referral may be necessary in cases in which the child is experiencing significant psychological trauma. An integrated team composed of psychologist, clergy, and parish nurse can be appropriate. Hospital chaplains can be especially helpful to some families (Robinson et al, 2006), and crisis therapy (e.g., response play therapy) can be effectively used when children are not able to verbally express their distress (McPherson, 2004).
- Provide comfort and security to allay fears and reassure child. With hospitalized infants and toddlers, ensure that they have the same staff caregiver and have parents stay with them as much as possible.
- Encourage child to participate in spiritual practices as desired. Adolescents who have a relationship with a religious institution, in particular, tend to have healthier attitudes and behaviors (Wong et al, 2006).
- Encourage child to express feelings about what is happening to him or her.
- Encourage child to talk about beliefs and understandings of stressors such as death and illness.
- Answer questions honestly, according to the child's age and developmental level.

- Work with parents to help them process the experience from their perspective (see previous model of conversations: what is the parent's answer to the "one-question question"?)
- Advocate for the child and parent when they express beliefs in conflict with those of other health care providers or other family members.
- If parents refuse treatment for their child:
  o Consider use of alternative methods of care.
  o Provide opportunity for parents to discuss implications of their decision.

o Provide opportunity for parents to express negative feelings.
o Obtain a court order for care or temporary guardianship if necessary to treat the child.

Complications

Depression, suicide, and conduct disorders can be complications of spiritual distress.

Approaches to Disease Management

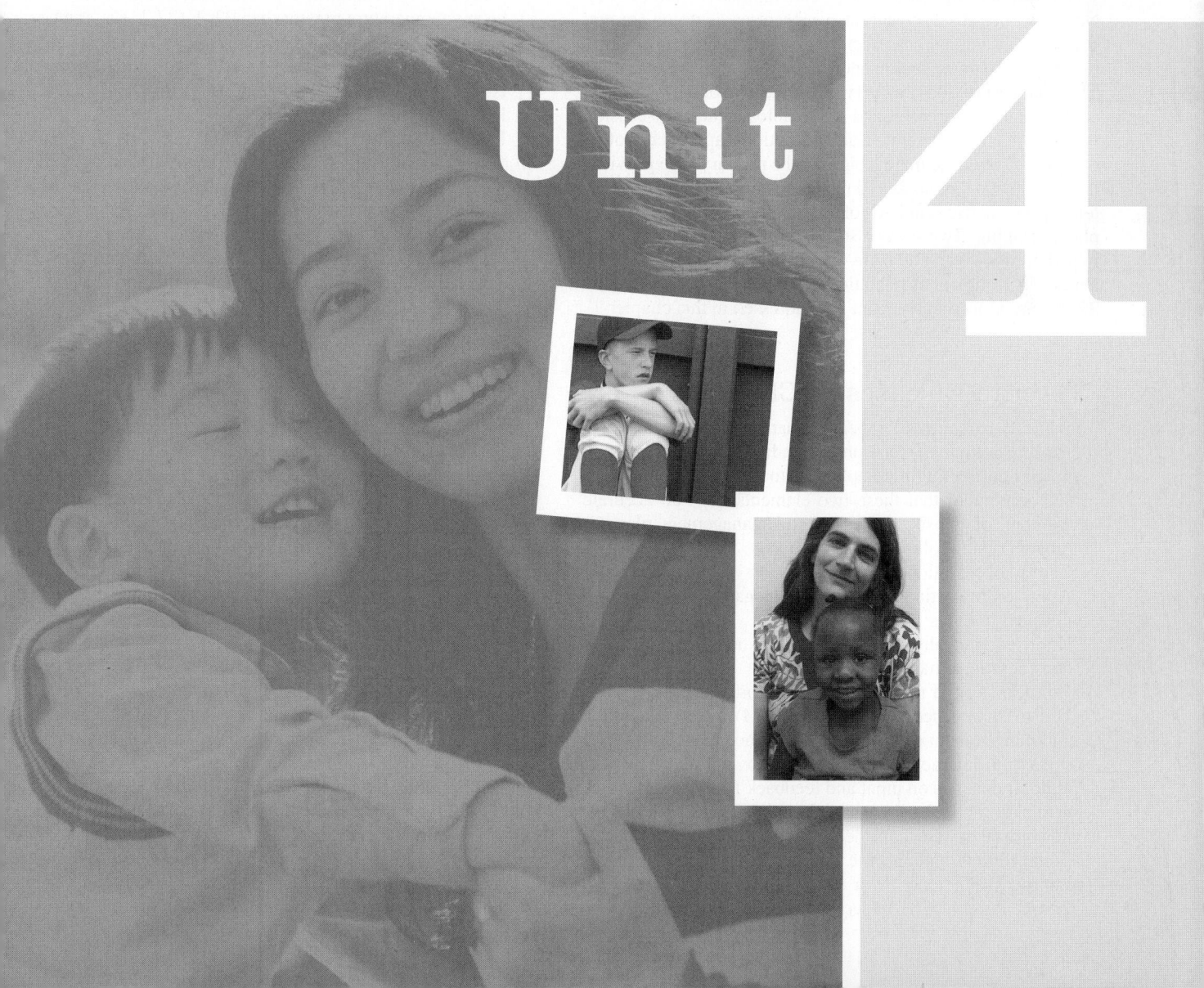

Unit

4

Introduction to Disease Management

RITA MARIE JOHN AND MARGARET A. BRADY

Respiratory and gastrointestinal infections are the most common illnesses seen in pediatric practice settings and may present as minor or life-threatening acute illnesses (Smith, 2011). Noninfectious diseases can also present as acute or chronic conditions, such as those seen with inflammatory or allergic responses, trauma, malignancies, or autoimmune diseases. This chapter provides an overview of the care of the child with acute or chronic diseases, and moves into a general discussion on assessment, management, and educational approaches of all diseases. One of the major roles for the primary care provider is to arrive at a diagnosis and management plan that is consistent with pediatric standards of practice; this may involve telephone triaging. Two areas also deserve special consideration in pediatrics—fever and pain—because these problems can be a part of the clinical presentation. Pain is addressed in Chapter 22; fever and its management are addressed in this chapter.

■ Acute Diseases in Children

The health care provider begins management of an acute illness by getting a clear understanding of the presenting complaint and taking a complete history. The provider must always remember that these two elements, plus an accurate assessment, diagnosis, and successful management plan are contingent on the following six factors:
1. Careful observation of the child
2. Attention to pertinent positive and negative historical and physical findings
3. Knowledge of physiological functions and developmental considerations that vary by age
4. Consideration of the trajectory of the problem over time
5. Use of shared decision making (SDM) in the evaluation and management of the child. This concept is crucial for a successful interaction between the provider and family or child. It depends on input and feedback from the parents or caretakers and, if appropriate, the child. This resulting partnership takes into consideration culture, patient choices, social milieu, and specific patient needs, and, as a result, improves adherence to a management plan (Butz et al, 2007; Fiks et al, 2010) (see Shared Decision-Making).

6. Use of health literacy concepts. It should not be assumed that any medical term used by the parent means the same to providers. For example, a parent's definition of fever may be any temperature greater than 99° F (37.2° C), or wheezing to a parent may in fact be rhonchi. A parent who is told that the management needed for the child's problem is some "tincture of time" may go to the local pharmacy looking for that "medication."

Feedback from the family and child needs to be obtained in order to ensure that there is understanding and agreement about the management plan and what was told to the parent about the diagnosis and etiology of the problem if known. When satisfied that these six parameters have been given adequate attention, an action or management plan is formed that is acceptable to the parent or guardian, child, and provider.

SHARED DECISION-MAKING

The shared decision-making partnership varies with different situations and requires different levels of involvement from the provider; the goal is to jointly make decisions consistent with the patient's wishes (Kon, 2010). Many parents are interested in helping to make decisions and want support and information in the evaluation of options (Jackson et al, 2008). Other families prefer provider-driven decisions. It is not always possible to have parent or patient input into decisions (e.g., emergency intervention after a life-threatening accident), but some providers assume a paternalistic approach to patients and families in all of their interactions. This approach is one in which the provider tells the family and child about the plan without giving them options. At the other end of the spectrum, all options are presented and discussed with the family or child, and the decision is left up to the family members without any provider input. The shared decision-making approach is somewhere in the middle; the provider, family, and child jointly decide the course of action. A good example of SDM might involve the decision to order diagnostic testing by a primary care provider. The decision needs to consider family, child, and provider preferences because there are many courses of action that can lead to the same end. Parents of a 6-year-old may pressure the provider to order blood work and imaging studies when the diagnosis is clearly primary enuresis and not related to a kidney abnormality. In this situation ordering extensive laboratory and other diagnostic tests would not be the best course of action for the child. Similarly, if the diagnosis appears to be systemic lupus erythematosus, the child would be better served by being referred to a pediatric rheumatologist for confirmation of the initial diagnosis, ordering of laboratory tests, and treatment.

The use of SDM is supported by research findings that show improved health outcomes when the family agrees to the management plan (Hirsch et al, 2010; Merenstein et al, 2005). And yet Cox and colleagues' study (2007) showed that passive involvement in decision-making by parents and children is more the norm, occurring in 65% of visits. A recent Cochrane review failed to come to any firm conclusion on how best to encourage professionals to adapt SDM into their practice (Légaré et al, 2010). Shared decision-making is a key point in the management of both acute and chronic illness.

PATIENT EDUCATION AND PREVENTION

Primary care providers' effectiveness is enhanced by their ability to educate children and their families about the prevention of disease and the management of common acute illnesses. The patient-parent educational component of the management plan must be individualized and include the following essential points:

- Information about the length of time it can take before the child improves and symptoms wane; description of what the course of the disease or illness is likely to be and signs of improvement
- Written information about specific signs and symptoms that indicate worsening of the illness, the need for immediate medical attention or for a return visit sooner than planned (e.g., a newborn with a fever of 100.4° F [38° C]; a child with severe lethargy, tender abdomen, labored breathing, stiff neck, bluish lips, purple "dots" on the skin, severe pain, inability to walk, or fever greater than 104° F [40° C])
- Specific, written instructions about when to return for any necessary follow-up or when to be available for a scheduled telephone conference. With electronic medical records, a recall system should be set up to ensure successful follow-up is completed. If the electronic medical record does not allow for a recall, a clinic tickler file is particularly useful for tracking patients whose diagnostic studies or follow-up appointments are crucial to successful management or treatment. This tickler file can be a simple card file, divided by months. For example, a card would list the patient's name, date, clinic number, medical problem, and contact information and be placed in the file in the month when follow-up is needed.
- Written instructions using key concepts of health literacy to make sure that families truly understand special treatment or therapy, how to use adaptive devices, and how to perform home monitoring tests (see Health Literacy later in this chapter)
- Careful instructions about the proper dosing of medication, the potential for the need to switch medications during treatment, and the side effects of both prescription and over-the-counter (OTC) drugs (see Appendix A and Pharmacological Agents and Patient Education later in this chapter)

- Issues related to administration of medications at school. All appropriate forms must be completed and school personnel instructed on key issues related to pharmacological therapy.
- Specific information about any dietary needs or changes, special hydration needs (i.e., electrolyte solutions or increase in fluid intake), plus any changes in eating patterns that can be expected
- The rationale for and procedures involved with diagnostic testing, including laboratory (e.g., blood, urine, or cerebrospinal fluid [CSF] cultures; skin testing; antibody titers; or rapid antigen testing for preliminary diagnosis), radiographic, or imaging tests and the meaning of results
- Estimations of the length of time or time frame before laboratory or imaging results are available, especially when there will be long waiting periods (these are particularly frustrating for parents)
- Information about the cause, if known, and epidemiology of infectious or noninfectious illnesses or medical conditions, communicability issues, and prevention guidelines, if applicable
- Information about prevention and recurrence risk
- Determination of impediments that prevent the parent or child from complying with the management plan (e.g., limited financial resources, inability to read, dysfunctional family, transportation problems) and discussion about steps to correct these difficulties
- Recognition and discussion of cultural practices and beliefs about illnesses. Discuss the potential benefit or harm from specific folk medicine or complementary and alternative medicine (CAM) practices (including herbal, dietary supplements, or botanical preparations) if used either alone or concurrently with prescribed or OTC medications.
- Information for the working parent about resources for sick care in the community that are convenient (accessible) and affordable

When discussing the management plan with parent(s) and/or child, sit down and make eye contact with them. It is a sign of respect and should be a standard of care. The parents' or caregivers' understanding of instructions should always be assessed by asking them to repeat what they have been told. By doing this any misunderstandings can be addressed. One of the ways to obtain this feedback is by using the three questions in the "Ask me three" plan (Abrams et al, 2009; Partnership for Clear Health Communication, 2010):

- "What is my main problem?"
- "What do I need to do?"
- "Why is it important for me to do this?"

It is important to allow time for the body's natural defense system to fight disease. Premature and excessive pharmacological therapy can result in needless iatrogenic disease and resistance to antimicrobial agents and often confuses the clinical picture. The drug of first choice—the one that is least harmful—should be given time to work. Prematurely changing to a new drug, adding additional drugs, and using more toxic drugs are dangerous practices and can decrease confidence in the provider (Ledford et al, 2010).

For the most part, parents are alert to subtle changes in their children, so it is important to listen attentively when parents voice their concerns. A sick child who is medically considered high risk due to physical or social problems merits closer observation and follow-up than does the average thriving child who becomes ill. If the child returns and is not significantly improved or is more symptomatic, the initial evaluation and diagnosis should be revisited by carefully analyzing the symptoms, investigating problems related to compliance or adherence, repeating the physical examination, reviewing likely differential diagnoses, and confirming the diagnosis before deciding on another management plan. Be sure to have the family's current or contact telephone number in case a telephone contact needs to be made regarding the results of diagnostic tests that come back or to monitor the course of the child's condition.

The number of infants and young children in group daycare is expanding as the number of women in the workforce increases. This phenomenon creates several issues:

- The disease pattern in this cohort of children is often related to group exposure to illnesses.
- The issue of multiple caregivers can complicate history taking. It is critical to get as much information as possible from as many sources. When the person bringing the child is not the caregiver, the provider should use the phone to communicate with the actual caregiver.
- Sometimes parents express feelings of guilt because they must work and their child is exposed to various communicable illnesses at daycare. Simply explaining that children do get sick during childhood may help relieve stress for parents.

With the diversity of dialects spoken in the United States, language issues can be barriers to providing optimal health care. If a practice setting does not have access to an interpreter or native speaker, interpreter services can sometimes be obtained from local telephone services. It is important that both the health care provider and the parent or caretaker can communicate with and understand each other (see Chapter 3).

Emergency department (ED) visits are often used for the treatment of minor illnesses by families without insurance or by those whose employment precludes visits to a primary care provider during regular clinic or office hours. Data about ED visits in 2007 revealed that 18.6% of children younger than 15 years of age went to pediatric EDs with the most common reason being fever, cough, and vomiting. There were 121 per 10,000 visits for asthma in children younger than 5 years of age (Niska et al, 2010). Health care providers working in EDs must adhere to illness assessment and management protocols and provide critical documentation outlining their physical examination and diagnostic findings, assessment, and management strategies, including education and needed follow-up.

■ Chronic Diseases in Children

The types and characteristics of chronic diseases in children are varied and include a spectrum of rare conditions and genetic or prenatal conditions. Some chronic conditions are not permanent, serious, or obvious, whereas others are irreversible, involve acute exacerbations and remissions, and are readily apparent. The number of children with chronic conditions also varies depending on the definition and methods used to classify a chronic condition (Allen, 2010).

Children with special health care needs (CSHCN) are defined as "those who have or are at risk for a chronic physical, developmental, behavioral, or emotional condition and who also require health and related services of a type or amount beyond that required by children generally" (McPherson et al, 1998, p 138). This definition remains the guiding principle to identify children eligible for federal and state assistance because of their chronic health condition. The need for services, rather than medical diagnosis, is the key factor or criterion that labels a child as having special needs. Using this criterion, about 18% of the pediatric population younger than the age of 18 years has a physical, developmental, behavioral, or emotional condition that requires additional services beyond that required by children generally (Levine, 2011). These children make up nearly 25% of pediatric outpatient visits (Hing et al, 2010).

The number of children reaching young adulthood with severe long-term illness continues to grow with advances in medical and surgical technology, requiring more coordinated care (Stille, 2009), and the percentage of children with certain chronic conditions, such as asthma and obesity, is escalating (Wise, 2007). If the definition of a chronic condition is limited to those with conditions lasting or expected to last longer than 3 months and that limit social functioning or recreational activities, then approximately 6% of children have chronic illnesses. These figures do not include children with speech defects, visual and hearing disabilities, chronic ear infections, chronic skin conditions, and dental decay. Approximately 6% to 7% of children experience illness or disability that interferes with the child's usual daily activities (Wise, 2007).

There can be great variability in the presentation and the course of illness among children with special needs. They and their families often face a range of problems that are as diverse as the conditions that cause these difficulties. A variety of genetic, congenital, and acquired conditions can lead to permanent or persistent problems that have a significant effect on the child's and family's lifestyle. Health care providers must remember that family members are the ones who bear the major daily burden of care. There are several key points to keep in mind when working with these children and their families:

- Integrate clinical practice guidelines as part of the care for patients with special health care needs. These are available at www.guidelines.gov and include guidelines published by the National Association of Pediatric Nurse Practitioners (NAPNAP) and the American Academy of Pediatrics (AAP).
- Prevention of special health problems is a primary goal of care and includes the following:
  - Early prenatal care for all pregnant women
  - Genetic counseling as indicated
  - Elimination of environmental triggers or toxins
  - Early identification of the condition or disease is of paramount importance
- Early intervention from the time of birth and afterward to prevent secondary psychosocial difficulties is crucial; the developmental aspects of long-term illness must be addressed.
- Counseling may be needed for the child and family to handle psychosocial and behavioral problems or to discuss their emotions and feelings.
- The child, the family, and school personnel must be consulted to ensure that the child is able to attain realistic developmental milestones.
- Appropriate educational support in school is a right.
  - Public Law 94-142, the Education of All Handicapped Children Act of 1975, mandates an appropriate education for all school-age children with developmental disabilities in the least restrictive environment.

○ Public Law 99-457 (1986) provides states with the opportunity to extend benefits of Public Law 94-142 to children from birth to 2 years old.

○ Prevention of discrimination is a right and is mandated under legislation related to individuals with disabilities. The Americans with Disabilities Act (1990) is a law that provides federal protection in the areas of employment, transportation, public accommodations, and communication for individuals with disabilities. The scope of protection covers both private and public sectors. The Individuals with Disabilities Educational Improvement Act (IDEIA) has been amended several times since the original act was passed to bridge the gap between what children with disabilities learn and what is required in a regular curriculum (IDEA-Public Law 105-17, 1997). It provides for the least restrictive environment for educating all children with disabilities. This act was reauthorized and amended in 2004 and 2008.

○ Section 504 of the Rehabilitation Act of 1973 for students with disabilities in regular education/inclusive settings prevents discrimination and provides safeguards and support for reasonable accommodations in the school settings, such as ramps, use of assistive technology, special seating arrangement, and permission to hand in assignments late due to illness (Sadof and Nazarian, 2007).

• Each state has programs (Title V) to assist CSHCN with medical care and to provide links to social services, state vocational rehabilitation programs, and state school-to-work projects.

• Social service support is essential to help determine financial eligibility for Supplemental Security Income (SSI) or state program benefits (e.g., Medicaid) for individuals with physical, mental, and developmental disabilities, or specific chronic diseases.

• Advocacy for children with chronic conditions and their families includes assisting them to secure coordinated and comprehensive health care and community-based services as needed.

• Provision of primary care services—regular health maintenance supervision and anticipatory guidance—must not be overlooked.

EMOTIONAL SUPPORT

Helping parents and children more effectively handle the emotional stress associated with a chronic illness and condition is a major focus of care. Key points to be cognizant of include:

• The time of diagnosis and periods of exacerbations of illness are viewed as times of crisis and added stress. *Chronic sorrow* is a phenomenon that involves feelings of sadness, anger, guilt, or failure. Parents of a child with a chronic condition may experience these feelings at various times during their child's life. The term was coined by Olshansky in the 1960s to describe cyclical, recurring feelings of sadness during one's lifetime that are of differing degrees of intensity. It involves grieving without finality. It is not pathological and does not occur uniformly within families (Hobdell, 2004; Roos, 2002; Shepard and Mahon, 2002).

• Developing a trusting relationship with these children and their families involves being respectful and accepting of their varied emotional needs.

• Engaging parents and their children in the treatment plan is a major and essential task (see Shared Decision-Making earlier). Self-management of their disease whenever possible empowers the child, parents, or both.

• Research has demonstrated that more paternal involvement in illness-related support is associated with better family and maternal outcomes in families of children with chronic illness; hence in a two-parent household, participation by both parents in their child's care and health care visits should be encouraged (Gavin and Wysocki, 2006).

• Partial or poor adherence to complex treatment regimens should be addressed. Motivational interviewing techniques can be a useful tool. Nonadherence issues should be dealt with in a collaborative, "blame-free" problem-solving approach.

• Parents of children with chronic diseases are more likely to think about using, or are using, CAM practices. Respecting their reaching out for additional treatments is important. However, it is not common for parents to reveal this to their conventional pediatric providers, so it is important that the health care provider ask about such practices. Some of these treatments may be harmful or ineffective. (See Chapter 42 for a full discussion on engaging the parents in a discussion about CAM, for being an advocate for the patient, and for becoming a collaborative agent with the family.)

FAMILY-CENTERED CARE

Family-centered care is a key concept that should be used to empower the family. Parents who have infants and young children with chronic conditions should be viewed as therapeutic partners in the management plan. Communications with parents should be open and honest. They should be treated with respect and dignity and allowed to vent their emotions and to use coping mechanisms that work for them. Likewise as the older child and adolescent mature, their partnership role emerges. Relapses in adherence behavior are problematic but not unusual in situations involving complex treatment plans. Problems of adherence to the management plan can lead to serious medical complications, increased rates of hospitalization, greater length of hospital stay, and increased health care costs. Therefore, the provider should explore with parents and children what can help them become more adherent using motivational interviewing (Schwartz, 2010; Suarez and Mullins, 2008). Box 21-1 outlines categories and key factors to consider when addressing concerns about adherence. Training in motivational interviewing, in which the interviewer seeks to ascertain the individual's level of readiness to change, is a promising technique to use in situations of less than optimal adherence. The key tenets of motivational interviewing are to establish and express empathy; to provide the choice to change or not; to work with patients and families to identify their own personal treatment goals; to work with resistance; to assist in the removal of barriers to change; to provide feedback; and to advocate for the development of patient self-efficacy (Fielding and Duff, 2006) (see Chapter 9 for more information).

Family support groups are often beneficial; they offer an opportunity to interact with others who have experienced many of the same challenges, difficulties, sorrows, and triumphs. The provider must address sibling issues and feelings, such as

---

BOX 21-1 Key Factors That Affect Treatment Adherence in Children and Adolescents With Acute or Chronic Diseases

Illness
- Severity of the illness and its predictability
- Length of illness and prognosis
- Effect of illness on functional and social activities of daily living

Management
- Complexity of treatment plan
- Length of time for each treatment, how often, and for what length of time treatments must continue
- Visibility of assistive equipment

Family
- Support network and size of family
- Financial resources; knowledge base and the understanding of illness or condition; overall cognitive skills; communication style
- Coping ability and skills; problem-solving skills
- Family's belief system and spiritual base

Patient
- Age
- Cognitive, social, and emotional level of development; temperament
- Peer group; coping ability

Health Care Provider and Environment
- Communication style of health care providers with child, family, and other health care providers; belief in patient empowerment
- Organization of clinic or office setting to be child-, teen-, and family-friendly; need for adaptive modifications in their environment
- Number of health care providers involved in the child's care; team member collaboration and partnership among themselves and with the family
- Open and "blame-free" approach when adherence issues arise

---

anger or embarrassment; a sense of being overwhelmed with added responsibilities; or believing they need to be the protector for their brother or sister. These groups can be face-to-face or Internet based depending on patient preferences.

ESTABLISHING A MEDICAL HOME

Children with chronic diseases have unique health and psychosocial needs. The health care provider may give care to a child with a rare disease or disorder or be involved with the management of a child with a much more common chronic condition, such as asthma or cerebral palsy. Of note, an increasing number of primary care providers are involved in the specialty care of children with chronic conditions. Each child with a chronic illness deserves a medical home where they, as unique children and families, can receive comprehensive, culturally effective, community-based, family-centered coordinated health care (McAllister et al, 2009).

The critical issue in health promotion and disease management for children with special health needs is to ensure an organized and coordinated approach to provide appropriate treatment for the child's specific chronic disease

or condition and to ensure that the child's primary health care needs are met. The goal of the medical home should be to: (1) provide family-centered care; (2) provide clear, unbiased information about medical care, management, and community resources; (3) provide all-encompassing primary care that is available on an in-patient and outpatient basis 24 hours a day throughout the year; (4) provide care over an extended period of time that allows for transitions to adult care; (5) provide appropriate referrals to subspecialists and care coordination with the team; (6) maintain a record of pertinent information; (7) interact with educational systems including early intervention programs; and (8) provide developmentally appropriate and culturally competent counseling to ensure optimal outcomes (Medical Home Initiatives for Children With Special Needs Project Advisory Committee, 2008).

Health care management for children with special health needs includes: (1) assessing their needs; (2) planning comprehensive health care to provide for physical and psychosocial needs; (3) facilitating and coordinating services; (4) following up and monitoring services given and the child's progress; and (5) empowering the child and family through education, counseling, and support. Addressing issues up front about quality of life should always be part of the assessment process in chronic pediatric illness management. Child and parent perceptions about quality of life issues, such as physical and emotional pain and discomfort, may not be the same as those held by the health care provider. Child, parent, and health care provider may each have different perceptions. It is vitally important to determine how the child and the parent feel—physically, emotionally, and socially—by listening to them and asking for their input, rather than assuming that all is going well based on outward appearances. Health care management of children with chronic disease is about empowering them to live their lives to the fullest potential.

Providing quality care requires screening patients with chronic conditions who are at risk for other medical problems. For example, patients with Down syndrome have a 3% to 5% risk for hypothyroidism and should receive yearly screening for thyroid disease (AAP and Committee on Genetics, 2001). Prevention of further disability by ensuring that screening and clinical practice guidelines for chronic disease management are meticulously adhered to is a key component of the medical home.

The level or type of involvement in the treatment and management of a child with a specific chronic disease may vary depending on the unique situation of the child and family and the health care provider's subspecialty training and education. Strategies related to fostering the child's psychosocial development should be addressed at each health care encounter. A holistic approach to care is a major tenet of the medical home model. Certain situations may require additional advocacy when children with special needs and their families are in a particularly vulnerable position (e.g., if the parent of a child with special needs loses his or her job or suffers significant illness or injury and cannot adequately provide for the child). Children with chronic conditions do well when family functioning is high and there is positive family adaptation. The philosophy underlying the medical home model is to provide for open communication between parents and providers and to advocate for effectively and efficiently coordinated health care services.

Although chronic illnesses are diverse in their severity and effect on the child, certain issues are often common concerns for children with chronic conditions and their families and their health care management. By using a medical home model, members of the health care team can communicate about a variety of issues (Stille, 2009). They include the following:

- The high cost of treatment—the potential need for financial assistance
- Lack of, or difficulties and barriers in, acquiring health care insurance
- Family lifestyle alterations that may be required of parents, siblings, or both, in caring for the child
- The need to overcome system barriers that families may face navigating through the maze of agency paperwork
- The need for supervised care by multiple health care providers and the frequent lack of coordination of services in providing continuity of care
- Unpredictability of the condition and the potential for complications, frequent medical visits, hospitalizations, and death
- The desire to be kept informed of their child's condition and progress
- Treatments or procedures that may be embarrassing, painful, or time consuming
- The developmental effect that chronic disease can have on a child, especially during adolescence and early adulthood (periods of increased vulnerability)
- Longevity concerns—ability to live and function independently as an adult, including the need for career and vocational counseling
- The level of knowledge parents need about the pharmacological management of pain and the disease process or other therapeutic treatments, including nutritional support for the at-home care of the child
- The effect of stress on emotional and psychological well-being of the child and family members—parents or caregivers, siblings, and possibly the extended family support network
- Acceptance by peers
- Parental striving to successfully normalize their child's life by acknowledging the child's condition and its effect on family lifestyle while actively engaging in accommodations to focus on the child and not the condition
- Dealing with feelings (e.g., anger, sorrow) while attempting to cope with chronic illness
- Developing advocacy skills for these children to access services through schools, state and community agencies, or special federally sponsored programs
- Securing special illness-related equipment (e.g., movement and mobility aids, such as walkers, wheelchairs, or braces) or acquiring communication aids, such as hearing aids or special computers with voices
- Finding respite care or transitional care for the dependent adult child
- Legal conservatory issues and the concern about who will care for the child as an adult when parents are no longer capable of providing physical care or are deceased

Pediatric health care settings should work to establish a medical home with a multidisciplinary team model and care coordination. These teams offer the expertise of many individuals in a united approach. In ideal situations the involvement of a clinical social worker, a community health nurse, or a nurse case manager is important to secure essential community resources for the child and family. Parents or guardians are a crucial part

of the team. All team members must remember to respect the knowledge that parents or caregivers have about their child, their child's condition, and how the child is likely to respond physically and emotionally to new therapeutic interventions or treatments, situational changes, or exacerbations of illnesses. Other principles coming out of the medical home model are to:

- Develop a database for CSHCN who require additional contact time outside of the typical scheduled time frame for either sick or well visits and be sure to flag their charts. An electronic medical record system may provide a function for this. This will help in scheduling additional visit time and alert the office staff when scheduling visits.
- Designate a care coordinator for each special care needs patient and train the staff about the medical home concept.

■ Assessment

HISTORY AND PHYSICAL EXAMINATION

Chapter 2 discusses the complete history and physical examination of children from infancy through adolescence. In addition, each of the pediatric disease management chapters in this unit focuses on key questions to ask in history taking and highlights significant findings to be alert to if found on physical examination. Careful attention must be given when analyzing the signs and symptoms of a child's illness, including the presentation of clinical findings, the course of the disease process, and its associated manifestations. A clear history of the illness is essential and requires a comprehensive description of any symptom or sign of illness.

The physical examination is often a challenge when a young child is ill and uncooperative. Patience is important when examining children who are sick. The sick child should be carefully assessed so that significant physical findings are not missed during a hurried or cursory examination. The parts of the physical examination that are especially bothersome or frightening to a child, based on either historical information, observation, or age factors, should be performed last. Often examining the child on the parent's lap can be helpful in these situations. Repeating parts of the examination or observational reassessment is sometimes useful (e.g., after a febrile child is given acetaminophen and the fever abates).

To help assess the severity of illness in infants and young children, careful attention must be given to judging key indicators during the history and the physical examination (Box 21-2). These indicators are an important part of the assessment and judgment when determining management, and include level of consciousness, hydration, color, respiratory status reaction to stimulation, sleep-to-awake or awake-to-sleep state, and response to social cues. The child should be noted to have either a normal (NL), moderately impaired (MI), or severely impaired (SI) response in each of the key areas (McCarthy, 2007; National Institute for Health and Clinical Excellence, 2007).

DIAGNOSTIC STUDIES

Laboratory Studies

Chapter 26 contains a detailed discussion of the complete blood count (CBC) and provides insight as to the information that can be gained from a CBC, in addition to indications for ordering this basic laboratory study. Coagulation studies are also discussed. Chapter 23 discusses the laboratory workup for young

---

BOX 21-2 Indicators for Assessing Severity of Illness in Pediatric Patients and a Scoring Guide

1. Level of consciousness or quality of cry
   - Strong cry with normal tone or content and not crying (NL)
   - Whimpering or sobbing (MI)
   - Weak or moaning or high pitched cry (SI)
2. Hydration
   - Skin normal; eyes and mouth moist (NL)
   - Skin and eyes normal and mouth slightly dry (MI)
   - Skin doughy or tented and eyes may be sunken; dry eyes and mouth (SI)
3. Color
   - Pink (NL)
   - Pale hands, feet, or acrocyanosis (MI)
   - Pale or blue or ashen gray or mottled (SI)
4. Respiratory status
   - Normal
   - Nasal flaring, tachypnea, oxygen saturation of ≤95%, crackles (MI)
   - Grunting, tachypnea with more than 60 breaths/minute, moderate or severe chest in-drawing (SI)
5. Reaction to stimulation by parent or health care provider (HCP)—how a crying child reacts when held, patted on back, jiggled on lap, or carried
   - Strong cry and normal tone or content and not crying (NL)
   - Crying on and off (MI)
   - Cries continuously or minimal response (SI)
6. Sleep-to-awake or awake-to-sleep state
   - If awake then stays awake or, if asleep and stimulated, wakens quickly (NL)
   - Eyes close briefly then awakens or awakens but needs prolonged stimulation (MI)
   - Not able to arouse or falls to sleep (SI)
7. Response to social cues (being held, kissed, hugged, touched, quietly talked to, or comforted)—for infants 2 months or less use alert ratings
   - Smiles or alerts (NL)
   - Either briefly smiles or alerts to cue (MI)
   - No smile, face anxious, dull look, expressionless, or no alerting (SI)

MI, Moderately impaired; *NL,* normal; *SI,* severely impaired.

Data from McCarthy PL: Evaluation of the sick child in the office and clinic. In Kliegman RM, Behrman RE, Jenson HB, et al, editors: *Nelson textbook of pediatrics,* ed 18, Philadelphia, 2007, Saunders; National Institute for Health and Clinical Excellence (NICE): Feverish illness in children, 2007. Available at www.rcpch.ac.uk/Research/ce/Guidelines-frontpage/Guideline-Appraisals-by-Organisation/National-Institute-for-Health-and-Clinical-Excellence-NICE (accessed Nov 5, 2010).

children with a fever of undetermined origin. All disease entities or conditions addressed in this text include information about diagnostic studies and laboratory tests. Diagnostic studies and tests can be valuable, but it should be remembered that no diagnostic test is 100% sensitive and specific. False positives and false negatives occur; therefore, these tests are only one part of the entire database. Tests should be ordered only when the results are necessary to guide clinical decision-making.

Imaging Studies

When deciding whether to order diagnostic imaging studies, the provider should keep the following goals in mind: order only those tests that give the most information for the least money, are the least invasive, are crucial in the establishment of a concrete diagnosis, and are critical elements in the development of the treatment plan. There are several useful points to remember about common imaging tests:

- Conventional radiographs
  - Useful diagnostic tools if correctly ordered (e.g., the type of view[s] needed)
  - Least expensive of the imaging tests
  - Readily available
- Computed tomography (CT) imaging
  - Best for detecting calcifications and fresh blood; shows greater bone detail than magnetic resonance imaging (MRI) (Smith, 2011)
  - Can be used with contrast material (taken by mouth, rectum, or injected via vein) for special evaluations, such as abnormalities affecting blood vessels; check for allergies to iodine or seafood, kidney disease, or prior reaction to contrast materials
  - Shows relationships well; images can be presented in the frontal, transverse, or sagittal planes or obtained in three-dimensional imaging
  - May require sedation or anesthetic for infants and young children
  - Requires radiation exposure, which increases cancer risk (Brenner and Hall, 2007; Brenner et al, 2001); it is therefore important that CT examinations be performed only when absolutely necessary (Cohen, 2009).
  - Costly
- MRI
  - Detects neuronal migrations, soft-tissue lesions, and abnormalities of brain structure, ventricular size, as well as chronic subdural effusions
  - Provides excellent images of soft tissue without exposure to ionizing radiation; MRI shows greater tissue detail than CT (Smith, 2011)
  - Often requires sedation or anesthetic in infants and young children because immobilization is necessary
  - Advanced MRIs include diffusion MRI, magnetization transfer MRI, fluid-attenuated inversion recovery (FLAIR), magnetic resonance angiography, magnetic resonance gated intracranial CSF dynamics (MR-GILD), magnetic resonance spectroscopy, functional MRI (fMRI), real-time MRI, and interventional MRI; usually ordered by specialists
  - Expensive
- Ultrasonography
  - Gives two-dimensional images and measurements of internal organ systems; however, air-filled lungs and gas-filled bowel loops are impenetrable to ultrasound
  - With Doppler ultrasound blood flow direction and velocity can be measured; a still picture of the image can be recorded as a permanent record, or sonography can be viewed as the image is being projected onto a video screen
  - Highly dependent on operator skill and experience
  - No sedation required
  - No radiation exposure; noninvasive

DETERMINING A DIFFERENTIAL DIAGNOSIS

Following the history and physical examination, possible diagnoses need to be generated. The management plan will be the direct result of the working diagnosis and the differential. Diagnostic errors are more common than realized. Elstein (2009) estimated diagnostic error at 15%; Berner and Graber's 2008 review of diagnostic error rate for specific conditions was 10% to 69%. They concluded that the rate of diagnostic error is unacceptably high (Berner and Graber, 2008). The Harvard Medical Practice Study reported a rate of diagnostic error of 17% after reviewing 30,195 records (Leape et al, 1991). It is imperative that providers consider all possibilities to avoid reaching a premature conclusion. Diagnostic errors remain a leading cause of malpractice claims (Berner and Graber, 2008). With increasing time constraints in clinical practice, difficulty in keeping track of patients in large group practices, and the development of the full clinical picture that may only become evident over time, it is important to use every available resource to elucidate difficult diagnoses.

Strategies to assist health care providers in overcoming diagnostic errors include improving education, practice, and training and getting feedback on diagnostic errors (Berner and Graber, 2008). Whereas a complete review of the various methods to reduce error is outside the scope of this chapter, an essential point to remember is that reflective practice leads to improvement over time. On a systems level, consulting with or referring difficult patients to a more experienced health care provider or using a computerized diagnostic decision support may be helpful. Data suggest that computerized diagnostic systems may give useful suggestions providing that all symptoms are entered correctly into the database. Internet-based decision support systems, such as DXplain, Gideon, Isabel, Lifecom, and VisualDx, allow providers to consider a wider variety of differential diagnoses and formulate an appropriate plan. Diagnostic decision support systems do not make a diagnosis but provide differentials based on age, gender, geographic area, symptoms, and signs.

MANAGEMENT

Acute Illnesses

Chapter 23 identifies specific infectious diseases and assessment criteria for illnesses or problems commonly seen in childhood. It also discusses an overall assessment and management plan for sick, febrile children. In general, with infectious diseases, the age of a child is a significant factor to consider when doing an assessment and creating a management plan. The immune response in infants from birth to 90 days old, for example, is particularly poor because of their immature immune system. Infants and young children are at increased risk for overwhelming bacteremia with any infection.

Management of an ill child can include a short stay in an outpatient clinic, private office, or emergency or urgent care department for intravenous hydration, pulmonary therapy, medication, and/or close observation. The neonate between 0 and 28 days is generally hospitalized when the fever is greater than 100.4° F (38° C) because the physical examination cannot always predict serious bacterial infection at this age. Between 1 and 2 months admission depends on the results of diagnostic studies and whether the infant can be adequately followed up within 24 hours (Ishimine, 2007). Administration of ceftriaxone can be considered in these patients on a case-by-case basis. After 2 to 3 months of age and before 3 years of age, admission again depends on history, symptomatology, and laboratory results (e.g., an abnormal

chest x-ray). Typically children in this age group have more frequent outpatient management and close follow-up than younger children. Before sending an ill infant or child home from the office (rather than admitting the child to the hospital), the provider must carefully assess the parent's ability to cope with a significantly ill child and recognize signs and symptoms of worsening illness.

The plan of care following a sick visit is organized according to diagnostic studies, medications prescribed, education, follow-up, and referrals. Each visit plan needs to consider the patient's or parent's desires, the most appropriate, if any, diagnostic test needed to evaluate the presenting problem, the follow-up needed, and whether referral is needed.

■ Pharmacological Agents and Their Use

PRESCRIPTIVE AUTHORITY FOR NURSE PRACTITIONERS

Nurse practitioners (NPs) must be knowledgeable about the individual state regulations that govern their prescription-writing privileges. Some states do not use the term *prescribe* to identify what NPs do when writing medication prescriptions for patients. For example, in California the term *furnish* is used to describe this activity. The individual state board of registered nursing identifies the terminology to be used for this activity and regulates (either as a single state regulatory entity or jointly with medicine or pharmacology state boards) the activities and procedures related to this particular function. Regulations about prescriptive activity vary from state to state. NPs are legally obliged to follow all state regulations and mandates related to any prescriptive authority granted to them.

PRESCRIBING PHARMACOLOGICAL AGENTS

When prescribing pharmacological agents or recommending OTC drugs, it is important to be knowledgeable of the pharmacodynamics and pharmacokinetics of the drug, the usual dosage, adverse reactions, drug interactions, and the indications and contraindications for its use in children (see Appendix A). The provider must have a clear purpose in mind for using a particular drug and should not prescribe or recommend agents because of pressure from a parent or any other individual. Keep the following points in mind when prescribing drugs or OTC medications:

- Lack of compliance or adherence in taking medications can be a major problem. Factors that affect compliance include:
  - The more often a drug must be given per day the greater the chance that a dose or doses will be missed.
  - Drugs that have a bitter or repulsive taste are difficult and sometimes impossible to get a child to take. For an extra cost, some pharmacies sell flavoring products that increase palatability (e.g., FLAVORx).
  - The greater the number of drugs that a child is given, the greater the potential for a drug dose to be missed, drug interactions, or the wrong drug to be taken.
  - Waking a child to take a medication is difficult for parents; prescribe round-the-clock dosing only when it is essential to maintain tight therapeutic drug levels.

- Poorly given or inadequate instructions increase the risk that the prescribed agent will be misused.
- Children with renal or hepatic dysfunction require dosing adjustments.
- Use clinical practice guidelines, if available, to enhance or optimize outcomes for patients.
- Be aware of the influence of advertising in prescribing practice. The newest agent may be much more expensive and there may be no evidence that use of the agent leads to better patient outcomes.
- Use a decision support system to investigate the possibility of drug interactions and side effects. Such support systems may be part of the electronic medical record (EMR) or can be used via a smart phone application like CheckRx from Skyscape or Epocrates or accessed via an online program, for example, drug interaction checker on Medscape or Epocrates. Be sure to check for interactions between pharmacological agents and any herbal, botanical, or dietary supplements.

PREVENTION OF ALLERGIC AND ADVERSE REACTIONS

Pediatric patients are at increased risk for adverse drug reactions for numerous reasons such as the need for individualized doses based on patient's age, weight, and clinical condition and changing pharmacokinetic parameters at various ages and stages of maturational development. Selecting the appropriate pharmacological agent to adequately treat an illness or condition and minimizing the risk of medication errors are important. Lists of current medications and dosages for prescription and OTC drugs, herbals, dietary supplements, and botanical preparations should be in a standard place in the patient's chart. Allergies to medications, with the identified adverse response, should be highlighted in a place that is easily visible. Advise the parents to have their child wear an Allergy Alert bracelet or necklace if they are subject to a life-threatening allergy (e.g., a severe peanut allergy).

SAFE PRESCRIPTION-WRITING PRACTICES

In order to prescribe, the provider must take a history and conduct a physical examination as well as document the encounter. Prescriptions should be written in a manner that conveys accurate information to the pharmacist and the patient or parent. The following suggestions are made to ensure safe prescription writing for children (AAP, 2007; Taketomo et al, 2011):
- Avoid the use of a terminal 0 to the right of the decimal point (e.g., use 5 rather than 5.0) because the decimal point might not be read correctly and result in 10 times the desired dose (e.g., 3.0 mL can be mistaken for 30 mL).
- Place a leading 0 (zero) before fractions less than 1 (one). For example, write 0.3 mL rather than .3 mL, which can be confused with 3 mL if the decimal point is inadvertently missed.
- Insert a space between the last number and its units (e.g., 15 mg, not 15mg). Do not place a period after mL or mg when writing a prescription.
- Write out dosage units rather than using abbreviations (e.g., milligram or microgram rather than mg or μg)
- Never use dangerous abbreviations, such as q.d. or qd (daily), qod (every other day), μg (microgram), or U or u (unit), which may be misinterpreted for q.i.d. or qid

(4 times daily) or 0 (zero), respectively. Write out in full the words "daily" or "unit." The abbreviation O.D. means right eye; never use O.D. as an abbreviation for once daily.
- Do not use abbreviated drug names such as MS or MTX.
- Use the metric system only.
- Write legibly.
- Make sure that the patient's weight is correct in kilograms and that the weight-based dose does not exceed recommended adult dose. Check all calculations (AAP, 2007).
- Make sure to specify exact dosage strength to be used.
- Be specific with instructions (e.g., "take 2 tablets each night at bedtime"), avoiding vague instructions (e.g., "take as directed").
- Review the prescription with the parent and/or patient: name of the medication, the reason for its use, and direction for its use. Have the patient or parent repeat information back to you; a return demonstration (see Pharmacological Agents and Patient Education) may be appropriate.
- Issue a complete prescription that contains all of the following:
  o Patient's full name, age (date of birth), address, and weight (for infants and young children)
  o Name of the drug, dosage, and strength
  o Instructions if a brand name drug is to be used rather than the generic drug option
  o Total amount or quantity (number of pills, milliliters of liquid) to be dispensed
  o Route of administration (e.g., take by mouth, instill in both ears, insert in rectum, instill in right eye)
  o General instructions to the patient or parent about indications for or the purpose of taking the medication, how frequently, and for how long (e.g., take three times a day until completed, take every 4 to 6 hours as needed for pain for 3 days). Consider writing the times of drug administration with the parents having their input as to times that would work into their schedule.
  o Special instructions to the patient or parent about the drug (e.g., give with food, do not give with dairy products) or other instructions (e.g., translate to the primary language of the parent if English is not spoken or read)
  o Number of refills
  o Instructions to fill with a measuring device or other essential delivery devices (e.g., spacer or nebulizer for an aerosolized medication)

The Institute for Safe Medication Practices (ISMP) website is an excellent source of information about error-prone abbreviations (www.ismp.org/Tools/errorproneabbreviations_pdf). In addition, some prescription plans or health care settings may require that a diagnosis and allergies to medication be listed on the prescription form. Do a SCRIPT analysis after you have written a prescription for any medication. This will help the provider review the pharmacological management plan and evaluate whether all five points have been considered and adequately covered. SCRIPT is a useful acronym to remember and stands for the following:
- Side effects
- Contraindications
- Right medication, dosage, frequency, route, and duration
- Pediatric considerations
- Transmittal of all necessary information on the prescription

Write the prescription only in the name of the child being seen. Depending on state law, a health care provider can be charged with a criminal act for writing a prescription in a person's name with insurance when the prescription is meant for someone without insurance (John, 2007). Writing for nonpatients—family and friends—or writing outside one's scope of practice could result in a sanction by the provider's licensing board and should not be done.

PHARMACOLOGICAL AGENTS AND PATIENT EDUCATION

Before patients and their parents or caregivers leave the health care setting, they should have a basic understanding about the pharmacological effect of any medication, OTC drug, or medicinal product that is prescribed or recommended. Points of information that should be emphasized include the following:

- The purpose of the drug, how much should be given, and the frequency of administration
- Instructions about the indications for using a drug that is given on an "as necessary" basis or under specific circumstances (e.g., a rescue plan for the child with asthma whose symptoms are worsening)
- Signs or symptoms that indicate that a drug is either effective or not producing the desired effect or effects
- Possible drug-drug or drug-nutrient interactions, precautions, or adverse reactions that can occur
- Information about drug stability, such as the need for refrigeration or storage and compatibility issues (not exposed to light or mixing with foods or other drugs)
- If applicable, any monitoring parameters that are required for safe administration of the drug or to maintain effective therapeutic blood levels
- Pregnancy risk factor of a drug (refers to the U.S. Food and Drug Administration's [FDA] A, B, C, D, or X categories that indicate the potential of a systemically absorbed drug causing birth defects) and the need to screen for pregnancy when giving specific drugs to female teenagers
- For children who take multiple medications, the importance of always carrying with them an up-to-date list of medications (prescription, OTC, herbal products, vitamins, and minerals), their strengths and dosages, in addition to a list of medications the child cannot take in case of an emergency or if the child is seen by another health care provider
- Tips to help parents administer medications that may be difficult to get the child to take (e.g., how to hold an infant or small child when administering a medication)
- Some medications can be safely mixed to mask the flavor of unpleasant medications. However, be sure to counsel about any medication that may have untoward interactions with foods or that should be administered on an empty stomach. The following is a listing of liquids or solid foods that may be suggested: chocolate or strawberry syrup, ice cream, applesauce, frozen juice concentrates (orange, grape, lemonade), chocolate pudding, regular or frozen yogurt, and jelly. Other suggestions are to have the child eat peanut butter crackers before taking a medicine, eat part of a flavored ice popsicle before and after taking medications, or chew on ice chips before or after the dose. Be sure to tell parents that they need to check with the pharmacist to determine whether the medication can be taken with food.

Return demonstration can be a useful adjunct to evaluate the ability of the parent or child to administer a drug or drugs in the desired fashion. Return demonstration is a desired teaching tool in many situations. Examples of such circumstances include the following:

- Administering oral suspensions to infants and young children
- Measuring small or exact dosages (e.g., when a syringe is needed to measure amounts)
- Giving injectable, intravenous, gastrostomy, or nasogastric tube medications
- Instilling ophthalmic drops or ointments or nasal sprays or drops
- Using a metered-dose inhaler (MDI), spacers, or inhalation equipment
- Ensuring that parents with limited cognitive abilities can safely administer medication to their children
- Administering multiple medications to ensure that the correct dose of the correct medication is given (e.g., 3 mL of amoxicillin suspension and 1 mL of metoclopramide syrup and not the reverse)

■ Parent and Child Educational Considerations

Education should be directed to the guardian and/or parent as well as the child. The families' ability to understand the health plan needs to be considered in designing educational strategies. The severity of the illness or disease and the child's age, maturity, and cognitive level are key factors that determine the child's degree of involvement in self-care activities related to acute illness and chronic disease management. Children should be taught basic health promotion and disease prevention behaviors (e.g., handwashing) from early childhood. Likewise they should be involved in the management of their illness to the fullest extent possible considering their developmental capabilities. Children should be consulted regarding their responsibilities for self-care. The pediatric provider also might be called on to be a liaison with school district personnel about the child's illness or medical condition in order to optimize the child's educational and social experience at school.

■ Health Literacy

The population of the United States is changing with diverse cultures and languages (see Chapter 3). A cross-sectional study of U.S. parents showed that 28.7% had below-basic to basic health literacy (Yin et al, 2009). In order to deliver high-quality care for both acute and chronic care management that closes health disparity gaps, information must be developed for clients with low health literacy, often in languages other than English.

Written instructions and easy-to-read handouts with simple illustrations are useful for parents, caregivers, and children. Simply giving oral or written instructions is not enough; the provider needs to make sure that the receiver understands them. In designing handouts, using plain, conversational language, simple words and short sentences without medical jargon increases comprehension. To obtain the reader's attention, fonts larger than 12 points with bullets, white space between sections to separate ideas, and drawings next to related text facilitate the understanding of the information (Miller, 2001; The Joint Commission, 2007). In addition, avoid using double negatives; consistent word usage avoids confusion, and a table of contents is useful for lengthy handouts (Miller, 2001). Whether a practice setting develops its own instruction sheets or uses information sheets from other resource texts, it is important that the instructions be written in the family's native language and at a reading level appropriate for the individual family. Several different tools assess reading level and ease of readability of material such as a patient handout (e.g., Fog Index, SMOG, Flesch-Kincaid Test). The best tool to estimate reading level is the SMOG, and a level no higher than fifth grade is best for patient materials (Wilson, 2009).

A number of books written for the lay public are excellent resources to suggest to parents. The care providers should develop a list of appropriate books and websites to give to parents based on the literacy level and unique characteristics. Select books that offer guidance about common infections of childhood, preventive pediatrics, common behavioral problems, and other frequently encountered pediatric concerns. Each practice setting should have its own list of books and supply of handouts, brochures, pamphlets, and other printed resources to share with families in their practice. The Centers for Disease Control and Prevention (CDC) offers health education information through their "Ounce of Prevention Campaign" that addresses common pediatric infectious diseases and their prevention (www.cdc.gov/ounceofprevention).

Illness Prevention

Prevention of illness and communicable diseases is a significant goal when providing primary health care services for children or managing the care of children with chronic diseases or conditions. Health care providers must be vigilant in their practice settings to prevent or reduce the possibility of exposure to communicable diseases and to control the spread of infectious diseases that are a threat to infants, children, and youth. Using the following guidelines can further the goal of prevention:

- All children should be appropriately immunized against vaccine-preventable diseases according to the recommendations of the Advisory Committee on Immunization Practices (ACIP), the AAP, and the American Academy of Family Physicians (AAFP). See Chapter 23 for the recommended immunizations and schedules.
- Communicable diseases need to be identified and treated appropriately and reported in a timely fashion to public health departments as required by law.
- Develop practice setting policies about the following: segregate infected children from well children as quickly as possible; avoid crowded waiting rooms, shorten waiting times, and minimize sharing of toys; wash hands before and after each patient contact; wipe the body of otoscopes or ophthalmoscopes regularly with alcohol; clean ear curettes after each use or use disposable ones, and disinfect with bleach solution or alcohol or sterilize any nondisposable tool if used between patients or contaminated with blood or other body secretions.
- Health practices to prevent or control the spread of infectious disease must be carried out in home care programs, out-of-home child care programs, schools, health care settings, and hospitals. Daycare in a small daycare home is

associated with less spread of infectious disease than is daycare provided in a larger center. Key practices include the following:
  - ○ Use effective personal hygiene—handwashing procedure should take 40 to 60 seconds (World Health Organization, 2009). Teach parents and children the importance of washing their hands, especially after toileting, blowing their nose, and before eating. The CDC has excellent materials that can be used with families.
  - ○ Ensure appropriate environmental sanitation—disposing of waste (e.g., blood, urine, feces, vomit, saliva) together with proper cleaning and disinfection of equipment, toys, toilets, eating areas, and diaper-changing surfaces. There should be a regular schedule of cleaning, in addition to cleaning when contaminated.
  - ○ Personnel should be regularly updated regarding blood-borne pathogen guidelines.
  - ○ Reduce respiratory spread of disease—cough into one's sleeve and minimize use of handkerchiefs; cover mouth when sneezing or coughing, dispose of tissue after wiping nose, and wash hands immediately; discourage habits of touching the mouth, nose, and eyes; eliminate passive smoke and provide adequate ventilation.
  - ○ Do not serve raw or undercooked eggs or meats.
  - ○ Promote appropriate handling, preparation, sanitation, and storage of food.
  - ○ Reduce exposure to communicable disease by separating sick children from well children.
- Educate youth about the prevention of sexually transmitted infections.
- Educate young children and teenagers to not share food, liquids, personal hygiene products, cosmetics, hair coverings, grooming products, or towels with others.
- Discourage children from kissing pets and playing in areas of animal fecal contamination (e.g., sandboxes).
- Provide preventive health guidance about avoiding second-hand smoke.

Caring for Our Children: National Health and Safety Standards: Guidelines for Out-of-Home Child Care Programs outlines preventive health practices to promote a safe environment for infants and children. It addresses the issues of disease prevention and management in family and group daycare homes and childcare centers (The American Public Health Association and AAP, 2002). In addition, several out-of-home daycare resources are listed in Box 21-3. Preventing and controlling the spread of illness in these group settings are important issues in maintaining health.

Referrals and Consultative Services

On many occasions primary care providers identify clinical or behavioral problems that they are uncomfortable with or unprepared to manage. In these instances patients should be referred to other providers for assessment and management. In other situations the primary care provider may wish to continue to manage the patient's care but seek consultation with other experts in the field about particular aspects of the case. Whether the primary care provider refers the patient and family to, or consults with, another health care expert, certain information must be shared with the referral or consultant

---

BOX 21-3 Organizational Resources for Illness Prevention and Out-of-Home Daycare

Early Education and Childcare Initiative (www.healthy childcare.org/index.html)
- Programs for teaching care providers how to administer medications
- Quality childcare
- Quarterly newsletter for health care providers, teachers, and providers

Healthy Kids, Healthy Care (www.healthykids.us)
- Parent-friendly information for children
- Helps parents talk with providers about providing a safe and healthy home for children

National Resource Center for Health and Safety in Childcare and Early Education (http://nrckids.org)
- Goal is to help foster health and safety in out-of-home educational settings

Child Care Aware (www.childcareaware.org)
- Helps parent identify childcare resources

---

provider in an organized, logical fashion. Guidelines for presenting this information are as follows:
- Give the patient's name, age, tentative or actual diagnosis, and what you want the consultant to do (e.g., "newly diagnosed type 1 DM; needs initial insulin control and diet recommendations").
- In a sentence or two briefly discuss why the patient or family is being referred or the reason that a consultation is being requested.
- Give a synopsis of the patient's history, clinical findings, prior management plan, and outcome of treatment if applicable.
- Identify any pertinent past medical history, such as chronic illnesses or conditions.
- Provide pertinent family, educational, or social information, including insurance coverage if this is problematic.

If the primary care provider is referring the patient for problem-focused care, this should be made clear to the referral provider. In addition, the primary care provider and the referral specialist must coordinate their services, being clear on who is responsible for which services (e.g., follow-up testing, monitoring, and treatments); clear communication and shared information between the two providers is essential. The primary care provider should maintain a listing of specialty providers in the local area who take referrals from the primary care provider's work setting. If the provider is employed in a large health maintenance organization, there should be a list of pediatric specialty providers within the organization. The child's insurance coverage is often a major factor in referral, and often prior authorization from an insurance carrier is needed for a referral. Important information to gather about specialty providers includes their specialty or subspecialty practice area, evaluation of their effectiveness (can be an informal notation, such as "great resource person"), and, if applicable, their fees for service (e.g., full fee or sliding scale) and which insurance plans will reimburse for their services.

Whether consulting formally or informally with another provider about the care of a particular patient, the primary care provider should present information about the patient, as listed previously, and discuss potential management options. At the end of the consultation, the primary care provider should summarize in the patient's chart the key areas that were discussed and the recommendations that were agreed on.

Often overlooked sources of free consultation are state and local public health departments or agencies, health-related professional organizations, and some major medical centers that provide telephone consultation for providers in their service area. Again a notation should be placed in the child's chart if the case is discussed with a consultant in such an agency. Connecting with colleagues on the Internet is another option. Real-time chat sessions and e-mail exchanges are possible sources of consultation; however, information secured from unknown sources or not documented or referenced should be verified for accuracy.

When a patient is referred to another provider, the primary care provider must explain the reason for the referral to the child and parent, how the transfer of care will be managed, and when the patient is to return to see the primary care provider. The information should be presented in such a manner as to dispel fears of abandonment or giving up. The bond between the child, the parent, and the primary care provider is a strong relationship that individuals rely on. If the primary care provider plans to seek a consultation, the child and parent should be informed by explaining the need for a second opinion or the desire to collaborate with others to ensure that nothing has been missed. After the consultation parents should be informed about what was decided. Finally, the parent may seek consultation with another health care provider. If so, treat this as the parent's need to collaborate in the child's care and listen to the recommendation by this consultant. Be sure that the consultant's reports are filed in the child's chart.

■ Referral to National and Local Organizations and Resources for Chronic Medical Issues

Parents and their children with specific disease entities or health conditions can benefit from the educational materials, resources, and support that national health organizations provide. Learning to live with a chronic disease or handicapping condition presents a special challenge to families. Most national organizations provide written materials that parents and children can easily understand about the cause, management, and treatment of the particular disease in question. These materials also help parents explain their child's condition to teachers and others. Many of these national organizations can guide parents and children to support groups with other families and children who are similarly challenged and to health professionals and other related groups who specialize in the treatment of a particular disease entity. Likewise these organizations can assist parents in accessing unique services to benefit their children (e.g., enrolling in special camps and sports activities, learning about the various legal rights of children with disabilities or handicapping conditions, and acquiring special adaptive equipment).

Many national and local health organizations and foundations provide educational materials and valuable information designed for health professionals about a variety of subjects related to their target population of children. For children with rare disorders, the National Organization for Rare Disorders (NORD) may be able to assist parents and offer information about the child's condition or disease (www.raredisease.org). Often these national organizations can provide up-to-date information about new treatment modalities or management strategies. Health care providers should take advantage of the services that these organizations offer. In addition, every clinical or practice setting should have a listing of local community resources. One can make up a personal local resource guide and keep this information along with a listing of national organizations.

Tips Regarding Documentation: Patient Visit and Follow-Up

There are several important rules for the primary care provider to remember regarding documentation when charting. Many malpractice claims against care providers are due to a lack of documentation. The old adage, "If it isn't in writing, then it wasn't done" has been used more than once to find care providers liable and render a judgment in favor of the plaintiff. Good documentation practices include:

- Being alert to a complaint or combination of complaints that are red flags for more serious illness (e.g., abdominal or chest pains, headache, syncope). Be sure to note pertinent positive and negative history and physical findings relative to these complaints when charting.
- Identifying differential diagnoses and ruling out the worst possible illness first. Be sure to gather enough data to either rule in or out the diagnosis based on history, physical findings, or diagnostic studies. If you put "rule-out" on your assessment, you have to include a management plan to do so (i.e., it cannot be listed as a diagnosis or a differential diagnosis if you don't plan to do anything about "ruling it out").
- Conveying the seriousness of the issue to the family or caretaker if there is the probability of a serious illness and the patient needs to return for additional visits or have diagnostic studies done. Be sure to document that conversation.
- Knowing patient or family risk factors and screening for them through diagnostic tests or history.
- Ensuring that there is a system in place in the practice setting to follow up and secure the results of diagnostic tests that were ordered. There should be a mechanism to ensure that the test or procedure was done and that the provider was given the results and documented reviewing them.
- Following up all abnormal test results. There should be a note placed in the patient's chart that the abnormal results were discussed (and with whom) and the plan of action.
- Following up on referrals to other health care professionals or agencies and documenting the recommendations or treatments implemented from these referral sources.
- Making sure that results of newborn screenings are in the chart.
- Revisiting an unresolved problem until it is resolved. This can be accomplished by:
  - Rescheduling a follow-up examination.
  - Telephone contact with the family to determine if the complaint or illness has been resolved.

Chart audits should be a regular part of practice quality improvement. Look for such things as omissions of information, whether problems identified in earlier visits were addressed at subsequent visits until resolved, compliance with routine health maintenance screenings, and adherence to evidence-based practice guidelines.

Telephone Management of Illnesses

TELEPHONE TRIAGE SYSTEMS

All primary care providers should ensure that their practice settings have a standardized approach to telephone triage. Triage protocols classify problems into one of several categories. These include life-threatening, emergent, urgent, nonurgent, recurrent, or mildly ill. Protocols may vary slightly, but the major aim is to provide safe advice while avoiding unnecessary visits to an urgent care center or ED. Protocols may use a standardized algorithm in order to obtain history, leading to a patient disposition to manage specific health concerns (Black, 2007). Several excellent resources address telephone triage management of illnesses in children (Briggs, 2006; Poole, 2003; Schmitt, 2010). Telephone triage can also be called telehealth, telephone advice services, telephone consultations, or telenursing. Many insurance companies offer telephone triage services as part of the benefits to the insured to avoid unnecessary ED visits. Patients have reported satisfaction with nurse-run telephone advice services (Mayo et al, 2002), and the safety of such advice using protocols has been documented in the literature (Kempe et al, 2006).

A major benefit of telephone triage is to provide convenient access to health care professionals and health care advice. Management-by-telephone protocol in an individual practice setting should accomplish the following objectives:

- Allow the telephone triage person to manage ill-child calls safely; prevent harmful triage or recommendations.
- Provide a standard of care.
- Prevent omissions resulting from forgetfulness or fatigue.
- Improve quality of care.

The method of interaction, screening questions to ask, expressing concern, and reflective listening are all important points. The individual doing the telephone triage must be receptive to the parent's call, stressing that the call is as important to the provider as it is to the parent. Parents can be anxious and find it difficult to calmly state the problem. Additionally, the triage person needs to be a perceptive, conscientious, and calm individual who carefully listens to the caller; asks questions as dictated by protocol and by judgment; processes the information; determines the correct management protocol to use for a particular situation; gives the necessary instructions to parents; offers comfort and understanding to help the parent manage the illness; and documents the encounter. In addition, all these activities must be performed in a relatively short period of time.

Steps of an Effective Triage System

The major difficulty in providing telephone advice is the difficulty of accurately assessing a situation without visual input. The sequence of steps that one must go through in using telephone protocols includes the ability to do all of the following:

- Collect data about the symptoms through open-ended and direct questioning.
- Identify the problem or main symptom.
- Develop a working assessment.
- Decide on a triage category for the patient.
- Select the correct protocol.
- Correctly advise the patient about the course of action.

Questions should be asked in an effort to narrow the problem clinically and to assist the parent to be clear and focused. In addition, questions should be clustered by area of concern, should move from most to least serious, and should follow a logical sequence based on initial data obtained. When using protocols, the nurse needs to make sure that each question is asked but can add additional questions if needed. Screening questions that should be asked of parents include the following:

- Duration: How long has the problem been present?
- Description: Tell me about the problem. What signs and symptoms are present?
- Clinical changes: How has the child's behavior or activity level changed (e.g., eating, sleeping, playing, interaction with peers and family members)?
- Appetite: Has there been a change in the child's drinking or eating habits?
- Elimination: Has there been associated changes in bowel or bladder habits?
- Sleep pattern: Has there been a change in the child's normal sleeping habits?
- Environmental problems: Has there been any recent exposure, change, or stress in the child's environment?
- Cause: What does the parent believe is contributing to or causing this condition?
- Management: What has the parent done for the condition, and with what effect?
- Feelings: Does the parent feel anxious about how the child is behaving?

Keep in mind that protocols are a tool and should not override one's own professional judgment. If the provider feels that the patient needs to be seen despite what the telephone triage advice protocol states, then the patient should be seen. The provider's preference needs to be made clear to those triaging.

If the office or clinic is not using a standardized telephone triage reference source (such as that by Schmitt as mentioned above), office protocols should be developed to ensure an effective telephone management system. Office protocols may be prewritten and should be regularly reviewed and modified by the physician or NP. There is also a wide variety of telephone triage programs that are Internet-based and will record the answers as the questions are asked. In the future, telephone advice may be supplemented by Internet webcam via programs like Skype that allow the patient to be viewed by the person giving the advice.

Nonemergent calls to a practice about a sick child during the day are usually routed through a telephone receptionist, who can make an appointment, if appropriate, or transfer the call to a triage nurse or primary care provider, who in turn can determine the urgency of the need to see the child, give home care advice, or refer to the primary care provider for care. If home care advice is given, the triage person should use standards of care or telephone advice protocols discussed previously. It is extremely useful to have the triage notes automatically routed to the appropriate primary care provider so that the provider can be alert to any significant issues with the child (e.g., increasing calls indicating exacerbation and poor control of asthma).

After-hours or call centers are another avenue that pediatric practices use for handling sick calls after office hours. These centers employ nurses and NPs who use telephone protocols to guide parents in the management of their child's illness until their regular health provider is available. Call centers alleviate the burden of night call and are set up to use telephone protocols and a software program for documentation. It is incumbent on the pediatric health care providers within their practice setting to evaluate whether such a center would effectively meet their standards of care for after-hours management of children.

DOCUMENTATION OF TELEPHONE CALLS

Documentation of telephone triage calls and their disposition is an important element in a successful system for managing telephone calls for sick children. A documentation system may be part of the EMR, be a separate log, or a sticky label that is included in the patient's medical record. Written or electronic documentation accurately records the information so that other providers know about a child's problem. Such documentation also ensures a medicolegal defense; a method to review medical records for quality improvement and assurance purposes; an avenue to assist in complaint resolution if parents are upset about the advice given to them; and a tool to use when making follow-up calls to the family. Important items to include in any telephone log are:

- Date and time
- Patient data—name, age, sex, telephone number—and history of chronic disease or condition
- List of medications and their dosage if prescribed by the health care providers
- The chief complaint and a brief list of symptoms and signs, including their duration and frequency
- Documentation of sleeping pattern; activity level, appetite; and bowel and bladder elimination
- Diagnosis or working assessment
- Triage category (life-threatening, emergent, etc.)
- Instructions given about follow-up
- An "other" section for any additional comments that are deemed important information

When using telephone protocols in a practice setting, training is essential and ensures consistency in the use of the system. Staff sessions, designed to review the written or electronic documentation, are also useful teaching tools and should be encouraged. Perhaps the most important point to emphasize about the use of any telephone management system is the need to assess the comfort of the parent with the advice given. Parents should be asked at the end of the telephone contact whether they are comfortable with the advice and plan. If the parent is not satisfied or is uneasy about the plan, primary care provider consultation should be an option. Finally, parents should be told to call back if their child's condition worsens or the problem persists too long.

BOX 21-4 General Guidelines for Parents When Calling the Primary Care Provider

- When calling for **nonurgent** matters, such as well-baby advice, prescription refills, or appointments, call during office hours whenever possible.
- When calling for an **emergency,** tell the receptionist or answering service that your call is an emergency call.
- Give the following **information on every call:** your child's name, age, sex, major problem, and telephone number where you can be reached.
- Be ready to give **information related to your child's problem** as briefly and clearly as possible:
  - What are the signs and symptoms?
  - How long has the problem existed?
  - What have you done for the problem?
  - How did your child respond to what was done?
  - How do you feel about your child's condition? What is your intuition? Is your child getting better or worse?
- Be ready to give information about your child's general health.
  - Does your child have any chronic illnesses that need to be considered?
  - Is your child receiving medications for this problem or another problem? Has your child recently received immunizations?

- Does your child have any allergies?
- If you do not talk to your provider directly, before hanging up, ask when your call will most likely be returned.
- If you do not receive a return call within a reasonable amount of time, call back to make sure your message was taken correctly.
- If your provider decides not to examine your child, before hanging up make sure you determine the following:
  - The most likely cause of your child's condition
  - Which medicines or treatments should be given
  - What signs or symptoms to watch for
  - When you should call back for more advice or to report changes in your child's condition
  - If you do not understand the instructions, ask to have them repeated or call back for clarification.
  - If you are instructed to come to the office or go to an emergency department, make sure you have clear directions on how to get there. If you are too anxious to drive, ask a friend or neighbor to drive or call a taxi. If an ambulance is necessary, the provider may be able to call it for you.

EDUCATING PARENTS ABOUT HOW TO USE THE TELEPHONE AND ELECTRONIC MANAGEMENT SYSTEMS

Practice settings should have an electronic messaging or telephone call policy about sick calls and should acquaint parents with this policy. The policy should cover basic information about the office protocol for handling calls, requests for advice sent electronically about sick children, or other child-related concerns during office hours such as well-child questions, prescription refills, nighttime (after-hours) calls, and weekend and holiday calls. Who screens calls, when calls are returned (e.g., during the noon hour or from 4 to 5 PM), and after-hours coverage are points to cover in the policy. Likewise, a policy about staff's role in answering electronic messages should be in place.

Parents should be encouraged to handle minor illnesses at home without unnecessary calling in for advice. Home instruction sheets for managing fevers (including dosage charts) and common childhood illnesses or books on common pediatric illnesses designed for parents are excellent resources to provide to parents (Schmitt, 2005). Pamphlets can be given to parents at anticipatory guidance visits. In addition, NAPNAP has several handouts that can be accessed from its website, and there is also a parent section on the AAP website, which is an excellent resource. During illness visits, parents should be told what to expect when their child is ill, preparing them for the increasing temperature, vomiting, or diarrhea, in addition to what to do if they occur.

Parents need to know what type of situations require a call for emergency medical services or the poison control center. If sick care is necessary after scheduled office hours, parents will need to give the following information about their child:

- The main symptoms
- Any chronic disease or health problem
- Temperature (and route it was taken)
- Approximate weight
- Names and dosages of current medications

- Type of insurance coverage
- Preferred name of pharmacy and phone number

Box 21-4 provides general rules for parents when calling a health care provider. Box 21-5 gives parental guidelines for deciding when to call.

■ Fever in Children

Fever is a common phenomenon seen in children and is a complex systematic inflammatory response that involves modification of the body's thermoregulatory center (hypothalamus) set point. The pathophysiology of fever is a result of an alteration in the thermoregulatory center of the preoptic nuclei of the anterior hypothalamus. Within the center is a group of neurons that maintain the body temperature. These neurons are sensitive to cytokine-mediated responses as well as acute phase reactants such as toxins and products of viral or bacterial metabolism. Antigen-antibody complexes and complement components also act as pyrogens, causing monocytes to activate to become macrophages and other inflammatory cells to release cytokines. Cytokines are a critical factor in the fever and the inflammatory response, releasing prostaglandin E that raises the thermoregulatory set point (Avner, 2009). In addition, heat production is caused by increased cellular metabolism, involuntary shivering, autonomic responses such as vasoconstriction, and behavioral responses such as covering oneself.

The differential diagnosis in a febrile child includes infectious and noninfectious causes (Ishimine, 2007). However, viral infections are responsible for most children's fevers. The differential for fever includes bacterial infection, malignancy, reaction to immunizations, and connective tissue disease.

Body temperature as well as the measurement of that temperature varies. The measurement of fever can be done in several ways. Most pediatric sources define *fever* as a rectal temperature higher than 100.4° F (38° C) (Ishimine, 2007). Rectal temperature remains the gold standard unless it is contraindicated for a medical reason. A rectal temperature more

BOX 21-5 Guidelines for Parents for When to Call the Primary Care Provider

When to call immediately for an infant younger than 3 months:
Baby has the following symptoms:
- Is lethargic (very sleepy or difficult to arouse), has poor color, or appears limp and unresponsive
- Has a rectal temperature of 100.4° F (38° C) or higher
- Refuses to eat three or four times in a row
- Has repeated bouts of diarrhea or vomiting
- Has a labored, wheezing, or grunting breathing pattern that lasts longer than half an hour
- Has an illness associated with a rash that looks like bleeding under the skin
- Baby's eyes, hands, or feet have a yellow, jaundiced color or the baby develops pumpkin-colored skin
- You feel very nervous about your baby's illness or general condition

When to call immediately for an older child (child has the following symptoms):
- Seems unresponsive, does not make eye contact with you, or has cold and clammy skin that is not associated with vomiting
- Looks much sicker than usual with a routine illness
- Has an illness with a rash that looks like bleeding under the skin (purple blotches or spots)
- Has any symptom that you believe to be unusual or frightening; this includes trouble breathing, stiff neck, severe headache, or very high fever

When to call immediately after trauma or injury:
- Child has struck his or her head and has either lost consciousness, has nausea or vomiting, or complains of severe headache; also call if there is mental confusion, unbalanced walking, poor coordination, loss of memory, or a discharge coming from one or both ears

- There is continued swelling, tenderness, or a strange look to the injured part
- Child refuses to use an injured extremity for more than half an hour
- There is a deep puncture wound, a cut longer than 0.5 inch, or your child has not received a tetanus shot within the past 5 to 10 years
- There is injury to an eye that causes redness, pain, or tearing for more than 15 minutes
- Child has been bitten by an animal, and the bite has gone through the skin
- You need first aid instructions to control bleeding or other problems
- You believe that your child may have swallowed a toxic or poisonous substance

When to call about symptoms:
- You are concerned about how your child looks
- Symptoms seem to be getting worse or last longer than expected
- Fever of more than 101° F (38.3° C) has lasted longer than 24 hours
- Cough, cold, sore throat, or runny nose has lasted longer than 48 to 72 hours
- Vomiting has lasted longer than 8 hours or diarrhea longer than 24 hours or when there is blood in the stool or vomit
- Child has severe stomach pains lasting longer than 4 hours
- Symptom seems more severe than it has in the past
- Child has a rash or other problem, and you are not sure what is causing it
- You are not certain whether the child needs to be seen by the health care provider

closely approximates body core temperature readings than do axillary, oral, temporal, or tympanic measurements. The poorest correlation with core temperature is the axillary method (ranging in error between 27.8% and 33%) (El-Radhi and Barry, 2006; Haddadin and Shamo'on, 2007). Axillary temperatures are recommended in the neonatal period but after this period, the method is not effective and is influenced by sweating. An oral temperature is more comfortable for children more than 5 years of age and is more accurate than axillary measurement. The results of oral readings are slower and influenced by tachypnea, hot and cold drinks, exercise, mouth breathing, and thermometer position.

While both the tympanic membrane and hypothalamus share the same blood supply from the internal and external carotid arteries, the reading can be affected by poor positioning, cerumen, and otitis media. When the thermometer tip is not securely fitted in the canal, the reading measures the temperature of the ear canal, skin, or cerumen. However, with proper use the reading is rapid, clean, convenient, and risk-free (Avner, 2009; El-Radhi and Barry, 2006). The newest method for measuring temperature is the temporal artery route, but more studies are needed to confirm its accuracy (Titus et al, 2009). The method is controversial in children less than 36 months (Holzhauer et al, 2009).

Physiologically the child's heart rate increases 10 to 15 beats per minute and respiratory rate increases three to five breaths per minute for each elevation of degree centigrade (C) (Avner, 2009). There is a normal diurnal variation in body temperature with a low point between 4 and 8 AM and a peak later in the day at 4 to 6 PM. Body temperature also varies by age (younger infants have a higher temperature), gender,

physical activity, and surrounding air temperature. Environmental conditions (e.g., swaddling an infant) may produce transient elevated temperatures, and it may be necessary to take several readings to verify whether an elevated temperature is due to an environmental or a pathological cause.

Although fever can be related to an infection, clinical appearance is the more accurate way of evaluating a child with a fever (Avner, 2009; Ishimine, 2007). Parents with "fever phobia" need reassurance because they may believe that temperatures cause brain damage or, if not treated, will go higher. Cellular damage does not occur until temperatures reach more than 105.8° to 107.6° F (41° to 42° C). Fevers less than 105.8° F (41° C), per se, are not associated with brain damage. Parents need to know that except for temperatures more than 104° F (40° C), fevers are a body defense mechanism. Fevers are thought to impart a beneficial effect by enhancing immunological responses, such as increasing phagocytosis and leukocyte migration, and interfering with viral replication and virulence of some microbes. However, there are potential adverse effects from fevers, including increased metabolic rate with associated fluid loss, oxygen consumption, and increased caloric needs. High temperature can precipitate seizures in up to 5% of susceptible infants and young children (Major and Thiele, 2007). Although the associated symptoms of headache, malaise, anorexia, and irritability are uncomfortable for the child, the overall state of the child needs to be determined by complete history and physical and prompt follow-up.

Health care providers generally treat fevers depending on the severity of the fever or to provide comfort to the child. Parental concern can be a factor in a decision to use an antipyretic. Likewise, suppressing a fever in a young child who is ill can also assist in clinical decision-making if the irritability, tachypnea, and tachycardia associated with a fever resolve after administration of an antipyretic. However, a febrile child's response to antipyretics should not be the sole criterion used to decide whether a pediatric patient is bacteremic. Many health care providers treat fever to provide comfort to a child and use pharmacological agents when a temperature exceeds 101° F (38.3° C). Some clinicians use temperatures greater than 101.5° F (38.6° C) as their guide to treatment. However, the overall appearance of the child determines management. A reduction in fever after antipyretic administration is not the deciding factor of whether a child is sick. Rather it is the clinical appearance of the child after fever reduction that is the guiding factor. The appearance of a child who has a benign illness and a high fever usually is better (i.e., does not appear as ill), whereas a child with a serious infection will still appear ill after fever reduction (Avner, 2009).

Since the widespread introduction of pneumococcal vaccine into pediatrics, the risk of pneumococcal bacteremia has been greatly reduced, particularly in the child from 3 to 36 months (Carstairs et al, 2007; Herz et al, 2006). Therefore, the use of a CBC and blood culture in this age group is less likely to reveal information about the cause of illness. However, urine cultures should be considered in febrile children less than 6 months, uncircumcised males less than 12 months, and all females less than 24 months who present with fever of greater than 101° F (38.3° C) for more than 2 days without another source (Ishimine, 2007).

FEVER MANAGEMENT

Management strategies for fever control include the following:
- Nonpharmacological measures:
  - Provide adequate hydration.
  - Provide reassurance to parents and advice that not all fevers need to be treated.
  - Provide appropriate clothing; do not bundle in additional clothing or coverings.
  - Provide ambient environment temperatures of around 72° F (22° C).
  - Sponge with tepid water for temperatures greater than 104° F (40° C). Sponging should be stopped if the child starts to shiver. Ice-water baths and alcohol sponging should not be done.
- Pharmacological measures include antipyretic agents (Taketomo et al, 2011) (Table 21-1):
  - Acetaminophen, PO, 10 to 15 mg/kg/dose every 4 to 6 hours, not to exceed five doses in 24 hours; temperature generally is reduced by 1° to 2° C within 2 hours. At an oral dose of 15 mg/kg/dose, it is as effective as ibuprofen at 10 mg/kg/dose. Acetaminophen is the drug of first choice.

TABLE 21-1	Antipyretics: Infants and Children (≤12 Years of Age)	
Drug	**Dose**	**Comments***
Acetaminophen	10 to 15 mg/kg every 4 to 6 hours PO (not to exceed 5 doses/24 hr); or 10 to 20 mg/kg every 4 to 6 hours per rectal suppository as needed	Temperature reduced by 1.8° to 3.6° F (1° to 2° C) within 2 hours; 15 mg/kg/dose as effective as ibuprofen at 10 mg/kg/dose; drug of choice
Ibuprofen	For temperatures <102.5° F (39° C): 5 mg/kg/dose every 6 to 8 hours as needed For temperatures ≥102.5° F (39° C): 10 mg/kg/dose every 6 to 8 hours as needed	Use in children 6 months to 12 years; maximum daily dose of 40 mg/kg; temperature stays lower for a longer period of time with ibuprofen vs. acetaminophen. Use with caution if decreased liver function, asthma, or coagulation disorder.

*Educate parents that the goal of antipyretics is to make the child more comfortable.

  - Ibuprofen in children 6 months to 12 years old: for temperature less than 102.5° F (39.2° C), 5 mg/kg/dose every 6 to 8 hours; for temperature greater than or equal to 102.5° F (39.2° C), 10 mg/kg/dose every 6 to 8 hours with a maximum daily dose of 40 mg/kg/day. The duration of fever response with ibuprofen may be longer than with acetaminophen. Thus the temperature remains lower for a longer time with ibuprofen.
  - Naproxen sodium is marketed as a "fever reducer." However, it has not been well studied as an antipyretic in children and should not be used for this purpose.

Acetaminophen and ibuprofen work in the same manner by inhibiting prostaglandin synthesis without affecting the baseline body temperature (Taketomo, 2011). Alternating these antipyretics remains a controversial practice, with studies varying in quality and showing varying effectiveness (Erlewyn-Lajeunesse et al, 2006; Hay et al, 2008; Kramer et al, 2008; Nabulsi et al, 2006; Sarrell et al, 2006). Because of the lack of solid clinical evidence and the risk of overdosing, the practice of alternating these drugs is not recommended (Nabulsi, 2006) and is not endorsed by the AAP.

Pediatric Pain Management

JENNIFER NEWCOMBE AND MARGARET A. BRADY

Health care providers must be familiar with the assessment and effective management of pain in the pediatric and adolescent populations as many children undergo painful operative and diagnostic procedures. For example, in 2006 over 1.1 million circumcisions were performed on male newborns born in the United States (Buie et al, 2010). This procedure is associated with acute pain.

Pain results from injury or disease or as a side effect of diagnostic or therapeutic procedures or surgery. Preterm infants are a particularly vulnerable population who must undergo numerous painful procedures (Zeltzer and Krell, 2007). These early painful experiences are significant events, and pain studies document that unrelieved pain has negative physiological and psychological consequences. Early pain stimuli and experiences can produce long-term consequences for the child. It is thought that early and prolonged pain may affect the child's pain systems, stress response and behavior, and learning resulting in increased pain sensitivity (Palermo and Zeltzer, 2009; Weisman et al, 1998; Zeltzer and Krell, 2007). Inadequate pain control during initial procedures can decrease the effectiveness of analgesia during subsequent procedures. Neonates and pediatric oncology patients who have inadequate analgesia experiences suffer long-standing alterations in their pain perceptions and later responses to painful procedures (Zempsky et al, 2004). Accordingly, best practice standards for pediatric care necessitate that pain management be part of all treatment plans, from minor painful procedures to more serious illness or injury. Therefore, all health care management plans should include the elimination of preventable pain and reduction of unpreventable pain.

The importance of effective pain management in children cannot be overemphasized. To this end, a joint statement was issued by the American Academy of Pediatrics (AAP) and the American Pain Society (APS) (2001) reinforcing the need for health care providers to treat pain and suffering in all infants, children, and adolescents. This statement continues to be a relevant document today. Also, that same year, The Joint Commission recognized pain as "the fifth vital sign" and established standards requiring the assessment of pain in all patients (Phillips, 2000).

The focus of this chapter is minor pain assessment and management in primary and emergency care settings. The pediatric provider should seek other references for more in-depth discussions of chronic pain treatment in pediatric patients.

■ Pain in Children

Key factors that influence effective pain management in children include the following:

- Established pain is difficult to control; therefore, essential goals of pain management are prevention of and quick action in response to pain.
- Pediatric and adolescent patients and their families should be involved as much as possible in pain education—its assessment and management. Parents must be educated about their role in engaging and providing distraction and comfort to their child during and after painful procedures (e.g., needlesticks, ear examinations, vaccinations).
- Culture and family learning patterns must be considered (e.g., beliefs about pain, folk remedies, how pain is expressed verbally, and language barriers).
- Genetic stressors may be responsible for differing levels of neurotransmitters or medication responses.
- Children's pain perceptions are influenced by individual, physiological and psychological differences, memories, and prenatal and perinatal stressors.
- Chronic pain is rarely associated with sympathetic nervous system arousal. Therefore children with chronic pain may not appear to be in pain. This may negatively affect their evaluation and treatment. To effectively treat chronic pain in children, physical and psychological manifestations of chronic pain must be considered.
- Developmental issues (e.g., cognitive, emotional, and physical), age, and temperament significantly affect how pain is interpreted, expressed, and controlled. Therefore, pain management must be tailored to the child's age and developmental level.
- Cognitive issues that influence pain perception include the child's memory and level of understanding, ability to control what will happen, attachment of meaning to a situation with regard to pain, and expectations of the intensity of pain.
- Emotional issues that affect a child's pain perception include anxiety, fear, frustration, anger, and depression.
- Social issues, such as how others react to the child in pain, influence the treatment plan. Likewise, family harmony or conflict influences a child's pain.
- Pain perception involves complex neural interactions that send out impulses or noxious stimuli generated by tissue

damage. Melzack and Wall's gate control theory of pain (1965) explains the four processes necessary for pain to occur (Golianu et al, 2000; Wendel, 2009):

- o Transduction—painful or noxious stimuli are translated into electrical signals at sensory nerve endings and forwarded to the spinal cord via A-delta fibers and C fibers. The A-delta fibers are myelinated and when activated result in sharp, stinging sensations. In contract, C fibers are unmyelinated and their activation results in vaguely located dull or burning pain.
- o Transmission—the electrical impulses are forwarded through the sensory nervous system through both the peripheral and central nervous systems.
- o Modulation—alteration of information by endogenous mechanisms results in lessening or amplification of the initial signal.
- o Perception—the emotional and physical experience of pain.
- Health care provider's fear of severe adverse events from pain medications, such as central nervous system and respiratory depression related to their use, often results in inadequate pain control (Kraemer and Rose, 2009).
- For a variety of reasons (e.g., fear of getting a shot), some children do not report pain to health care providers.

The goal of acute pain management in pediatrics is to effectively control pain with minimal therapy and side effects. Positive outcomes of effective pain control are decreased suffering, increased satisfaction for the child and parents, an enhanced recovery process, and a positive script learned by the child related to pain and its management that can be used in the future. In some situations (e.g., after surgical procedures, severe burns, or with chronic pain issues), complete "freedom" from pain is not possible; however, much can be done to alleviate pain in these situations through the use of analgesic agents and other adjunctive therapies.

BARRIERS TO TREATMENT OF PAIN IN CHILDREN

The AAP Committee on Psychosocial Aspects of Child and Family Health and APS Task Force on Pain in Infants, Children, and Adolescents recognize the following barriers in the assessment and management of acute pain (2001):

- Myth that children, especially infants, do not feel pain the way adults do, or if they do, there is no consequence
- Lack of assessment and reassessment for the presence of pain
- Misunderstanding of how to conceptualize and quantify a subjective experience
- Lack of pain treatment knowledge
- The notion that addressing pain in children takes too much time and effort
- Fears of adverse effects of analgesic medications, including respiratory depression and addiction
- Personal values and beliefs as health care professionals about their meaning and value of pain

Health care providers must be cognizant of these issues and the negative effect that these barriers exert on their pain management strategies. Effective management of pain is the responsibility of all health care providers, whether one is the sole manager of pain or one who refers the child out to a specialized pediatric pain management team.

■ Overview of Pain

Pain perception develops early in fetal life. By the end of the second week of gestation, fetal skin and mouth sensory neurons develop and these structures mark the foundations of neural pain transmission. At approximately 32 weeks of gestation, the beginning of the neuronal pain inhibiting mechanism appears and continues developing until the newborn period. It is postulated that newborns who are subjected to repetitive acute pain events experience central neural changes that program them to later pain vulnerability, cognitive effects, and opioid tolerance (Zeltzer and Krell, 2007).

Pain is an acute or chronic phenomenon. Acute pain often is associated with an identifiable injury that resolves in a predictable and expected time frame. Physiological changes in the nervous system are responsible for chronic pain that results from untreated or undertreated persistent acute pain. Factors not necessarily related to the initial cause of the pain may perpetuate it. Pain is further classified as nociceptive or neuropathic. *Nociceptive* pain is subdivided into two subcategories that describe the physiological structures associated with nociceptive pain—somatic and visceral. *Somatic* pain is well localized in skin and subcutaneous tissues but does not encompass bone, muscle, blood vessels, and connective tissue. Somatic pain is typically described as dull or aching. In contrast, *visceral* pain involves the internal organs of the body, is poorly localized, and is typically described as a continual aching sensation or a deep, crampy or sharp, squeezing pain. Visceral pain may result in referred pain that involves distant dermatomal or myotomal sites. The mechanisms associated with visceral pain include distention, stretching, compression and/or infiltration of an organ. *Neuropathic* pain is associated with injury to the peripheral nerves, spinal cord, or brain. This painful sensation is characterized as a shooting or stabbing pain that is superimposed on a backdrop of aching and burning. Key features are poor localization, paresthesias, and dysesthesia (Wendel, 2009).

■ Pain Assessment

A systematic approach to the assessment of child and adolescent pain begins by obtaining a pain history from the child or the parent. When talking with younger children, ask the parent what words the child uses for pain (e.g., "owie," "boo-boo," "ouchie," "hurting," "uncomfortable," "warm," or "stinging") and use these words with the child. Behavioral observations and physiological findings provide additional information to the comprehensive pain assessment. Pain evaluation in children needs to be multidimensional. The provider must collect data about what children say about their pain, assess for physiological and emotional manifestations of pain, and investigate other pertinent factors that contribute to the child's pain as listed earlier.

CLINICAL FINDINGS
History

A careful history is necessary and requires a systematic approach. An interval history and examination are needed when pain does not abate as expected or there is a change in quality, intensity, duration, or location. Pain has a sensory and emotional component. Because pain is a subjective phenomenon, it is measured best by self-report (Zeltzer and Krell, 2007). The following information should be obtained during pain assessment:

- Pain history (symptom analysis)
  - Intensity (mild, moderate, severe, overwhelming)
  - Location (including areas of radiation and referral)
  - Quality—how pain is described by child or parent (e.g., stinging, burning, "big ouchie") and any pain behaviors noted
  - Pain duration
  - Temporal features or chronology (when and how the pain started, precipitating factors, any variations in intensity and quality)
  - Previous treatments or procedures
  - Aggravating or alleviating factors
  - Other associated symptoms, such as anxiety, tachycardia, diaphoresis
- Past pain experience, including the child's memory of the painful experience and the pain treatment
- Cultural beliefs about pain and its causes and treatment
- Self-reports of pain in the verbal child (if possible obtain pain history as noted). Use age-appropriate language. The lower age limit for successful use of a self-report pain scale is generally 3 or 4 years old (Hicks et al, 2001; Wolraich et al, 2008; Wong and Baker, 1988). Between the ages of 3 and 7 years, children's ability to describe the location, intensity, and quality of their pain increases. Introduction to the pain scale includes an explanation that this is one way for children to express how they hurt (Wolraich et al, 2008). Providers should select reliable, valid, sensitive, and easily understood instruments that can be used consistently. The use of self-report tools, patient pain journals, and other objective pain measures help quantify pain before treatment and serve to evaluate the outcome of treatment. Selected common pain scales are shown in Table 22-1.
- Factors that influence self-report of pain include (Marie, 2009; Wolraich et al, 2008):
  - Situational influences may modify children's pain scores (i.e., setting, person asking, or what they expect to happen as a result of their answer).
  - Children may underreport pain if they lack knowledge that pain can be treated or if they fear their complaint may upset their parents.
  - Some children may overstate their pain in order to receive increased attention.
  - Various factors and perceptions affect a child's report of pain including nausea, anxiety, or fears such as receiving an injection, talking to a health care provider, disappointing or bothering others, getting a medication, or a need to be rehospitalized. Younger children may confuse fear with pain.
- Children with developmental delays may have difficulty reporting pain, may be less precise in their communications, or may be unable to verbally communicate their pain. Their pain expressions may be less precise, resulting in slower reporting of pain (Wolraich et al, 2008). However, if self-report is possible, it is always preferred over observational tools.
  - Children with developmental delays are no less sensitive to painful stimuli than children with normal development. Those with autism spectrum disorder may be both hyposensitive and hypersensitive to sensory stimuli (Overlander et al, 1999; Wolraich et al, 2008).
  - The revised FLACC scale is also valid for children from 4 to 19 years with cognitive impairment (Malviya et al, 2006). This pain scale focuses on five behavioral components and is commonly used in children less than 3 years. The acronym FLACC stands for assessment of the child's **F**acial expression, **L**eg movements, **A**ctivity level, **C**ry, and **C**onsolability.
- Few scales are valid for intubated children. However, some intubated children are still able to self-report by using a faces pain tool, writing notes, and so on.
  - The COMFORT scale (Bear and Ward-Smith, 2006) has established validity and reliability for use in mechanically ventilated children. It combines six behavioral and two physiological measures.
  - Monitor physiological parameters such as increases in heart rate, blood pressure, respiration, and decreased oxygen saturation in intubated children.

Pediatric pain assessment can be challenging given developmental and cultural considerations that influence pain expression. These include whether distressed behaviors manifested by either verbal or nonverbal children of various ages indicate pain, or how other causative factors such as anxiety, fear, stress, or hunger in the infant and young child affect pain and its expression. A detailed pain history is often essential and necessary.

There are various types of pain: acute, chronic persistent, recurrent, nociceptive, neuropathic, and psychogenic (Table 22-2). Choice of treatment depends on the type of pain, in addition to its intensity: fair, moderate, or severe. Table 22-3 provides management guidance using pharmacological drugs.

Behavioral Indicators

Displayed nonverbal cues are important indicators of pain (Craig and Korol, 2010). Behavioral observations include vocalizations (e.g., crying, whimpering, whining); social withdrawal; changes in sleep patterns (more or less); verbalizations; facial expressions of guarding, grimacing, tightly closed eyelids, vigilance, or anger; motor responses; body posture; and activity, such as rubbing or touching the painful site, avoiding the painful site, or guarding the affected area (e.g., not letting anyone touch the abdomen or withdrawal of an injured limb). These may be the only cues of pain in preverbal or nonverbal children. Infants in pain sleep less, are irritable and agitated, do not feed well or refuse to feed, and have increased muscle tone (Schechter, 2006). It is important to remember that behaviors in cognitively impaired children are often very individualized and may not be those typically associated with pain.

Physiological Indicators

Physiological parameters (e.g., alterations in heart rate, oxygen saturation, respiratory rate and pattern, and blood pressure) are neither sensitive nor specific indicators of pain, particularly in children who experience chronic pain. Other physical indicators include findings such as diaphoresis and pallor. Pulse-oximetry readings may decrease due to increased oxygen consumption. Other physiological

TABLE 22-1 Common Pain Rating Scales Used to Measure Pain in Pediatric and Adolescent Patients

Pain Scale/Description	Instructions	Recommended Age/Comments
FACES Pain Rating Scale* (Wong, 1996; Wong and Baker, 1988): Consists of six cartoon faces ranging from smiling face for "no pain" to tearful face for "worst pain."	*Original instructions:* Explain to the child that each face is for a person who feels happy because he has no pain (hurt) or sad because he has some or a lot of pain. Face 0 is very happy because he does not hurt at all. Face 1 hurts just a little bit. Face 2 hurts a little more. Face 3 hurts even more. Face 4 hurts a whole lot. Face 5 hurts as much as you can imagine, although you do not have to be crying to feel this bad. Ask the child to choose the face that best describes how he or she is feeling. Record the number under the chosen face on the pain assessment record. *Brief word instructions:* Point to each face, using the words to describe the pain intensity. Ask the child to choose the face that best describes his or her own pain and record the appropriate number.	Children as young as 3 years Using original instructions without affect words, such as "happy" or "sad," or brief words resulting in same pain rating, probably reflecting child's rating of pain intensity. For coding purposes, numbers 0, 2, 4, 6, 8, 10 can be substituted for 0 to 5 system to accommodate 0 to 10 system. The FACES Pain Rating Scale provides three scales in one: facial expressions, numbers, and words.
Oucher scale (Beyer, 1989): Consists of six photographs of child's face representing "no hurt" to "biggest hurt you could ever have"; also includes a vertical scale with numbers from 1 to 100; scales for African-American and Hispanic children have been developed (Villarruel and Denyes, 1991).	*Numeric scale:* Point to each section of scale to explain variations in pain intensity: "Zero means no hurt." "This means little hurts" (pointing to lower part of scale, 1 to 29). "This means middle hurts" (pointing to middle part of scale, 30 to 69). "This means big hurts" (pointing to upper part of scale, 70 to 99). "100 means the biggest hurt you could ever have." Score is actual number stated by child. *Photographic scale:* Point to each photograph on Oucher scale and explain variations in pain intensity using the following language: first picture from the bottom is "no hurt," second is "little hurt," third is "a little more hurt," fourth is "even more hurt than that," fifth is "pretty much or a lot of hurt," and the sixth is the "biggest hurt you could ever have." Score pictures from 0 to 5, with the bottom picture scored as 0. *General:* Practice using Oucher scale by recalling and rating previous pain experiences (e.g., falling off a bike). Child points to number or photograph that describes pain intensity associated with the experience. Obtain current pain score from the child by asking, "How much hurt do you have right now?"	Children 3 to 13 years Use numeric scale if child can count to 100 by ones and identify larger of any two numbers or by 10s (Jordan-Marsh et al, 1994). Determine whether child has cognitive ability to use photographic scale; child should be able to seriate six geometric shapes from largest to smallest. Determine which ethnic version of Oucher scale to use. Allow the child to select a version of Oucher scale or use the version that most closely matches the physical characteristics of the child.
Poker chip tool† (Hester et al, 1989): Uses four red poker chips placed horizontally in front of the child.	Say to the child: "I want to talk with you about the hurt you may be having right now." Align the chips horizontally in front of the child on the bedside table, a clipboard, or other firm surface. Tell the child, "These are pieces of hurt." Beginning at the chip nearest the child's left side and ending at the one nearest the right side, point to the chips and say, "This (first chip) is a little bit of hurt and this (fourth chip) is the most hurt you could ever have." For a young child or for any child who may not fully comprehend the instructions, clarify by saying, "That means this one (first chip) is just a little hurt, this (second chip) is a little more hurt, this (third chip) is more yet, and this one (fourth chip) is the most hurt you could ever have." Do not give children an option for zero hurt. Research with the poker chip tool has verified that children without pain will so indicate by responses, such as "I don't have any." Ask the child, "How many pieces of hurt do you have right now?" After initial use of the poker chip tool, some children internalize the concept of "pieces of hurt." If a child gives a response, such as "I have one right now," *before* you ask or before you lay out the chips, record the number of chips on the pain flow sheet. Clarify the child's answer by words, such as, "Oh, you have a little hurt? Tell me about the hurt."	Children as young as 4 years

TABLE 22-1	Common Pain Rating Scales Used to Measure Pain in Pediatric and Adolescent Patients—cont'd	
Pain Scale/Description	**Instructions**	**Recommended Age/Comments**
Word-Graphic Rating Scale‡ (Tesler et al, 1991): Uses descriptive words (may vary in other scales) to denote varying intensities of pain.	Explain to the child, "This is a line with words to describe how much pain you may have. This side of the line means no pain and over here the line means the worst possible pain." (Point with your finger where "no pain" is and run your finger along the line to "worst possible pain," as you say it.) "If you have no pain, you would mark like this." (Show example.) "If you have some pain, you would mark somewhere along the line, depending on how much pain you have." (Show example.) "The more pain you have, the closer to worst pain you would mark. The worst pain possible is marked like this." (Show example.) "Show me how much pain you have right now by marking with a straight, up-and-down line anywhere along the line to show how much pain you have right now." With a millimeter rule, measure from the "no pain" end to the mark and record this measurement as the pain score.	Children 4 to 17 years
Numeric scale: Uses straight line with endpoints identified as "no pain" and "worst pain" and sometimes "medium pain" in the middle; divisions along line are marked in units from 0 to 10 (high number may vary).	Explain to the child that at one end of the line is a 0, which means that a person feels no pain (hurt). At the other end is usually a 5 or 10, which means the person feels the worst pain imaginable. The numbers from 1 to 5 or 10 are for a very little pain to a whole lot of pain. Ask the child to choose a number that best describes his or her pain.	Children as young as 5 years, as long as they can count and have some concept of numbers and their values in relation to other numbers. Scale may be used horizontally or vertically. Number coding should be same as other scales used in a facility.
Visual analogue scale (Cline et al, 1992): Defined as a vertical or horizontal line that is drawn to a certain length, such as 10 cm, and anchored by items that represent the extremes of the subjective phenomenon, such as pain, that is measured.	Ask the child to place a mark on a line that best describes the amount of his or her own pain. With a centimeter ruler, measure from "no pain" end to the mark and record this measurement as the pain score.	Children as young as 4.5 years, preferably 7 years. Vertical or horizontal scale may be used.
Color tool (Eland, 1993): Uses markers for child to construct own scale that is used with body outline.	Present eight markers to the child in random order. Ask the child, "Of these colors, which color is like …?" (the event identified by the child as having hurt the most). Place the marker (represents severe pain) away from the other markers. Ask the child, "Which color is like a hurt, but not quite as much as…?" (the event identified by the child as having hurt the most). Place the marker next to the marker chosen to represent severe pain. Ask the child, "Which color is like something that hurts just a little?" Place marker with the others. Ask the child, "Which color is like no hurt at all?" Show the four marker color choices to the child in order from worst to the no-hurt color. Ask the child to show on the body outlines where he or she hurts, using the markers. After the child has colored in the hurts, ask if they are current hurts or hurts from the past. Ask if the child knows why the area hurts if it is not clear to you why it does.	Children as young as 4 years, provided they know their colors, are not color blind, and are able to construct the scale if in pain.

*Wong-Baker FACES Pain Rating Scale Reference Manual, describing development and research of the scale, is available from the Mayday Pain Resource Center, City of Hope National Medical Center, 1500 East Duarte Road, Duarte, CA 91010; phone: (626) 301-8941.
†Developed in 1975 by NO Hester, University of Colorado Health Sciences Center, School of Nursing, Denver, CO 80262. Also available in Spanish and French.
‡Instructions for Word-Graphic Rating Scale from Acute Pain Management Guideline Panel: *Acute pain management in infants, children, and adolescents: operative and medical procedures; quick reference guide for clinicians,* AHCPR pub no 92-0020, Rockville, MD, 1992, Agency for Health Care Policy and Research (now the Agency for Healthcare Research and Quality [AHRQ]), Public Health Service, U.S. Department of Health and Human Services.
Word-Graphic Rating Scale is part of the Adolescent Pediatric Pain Tool and is available from Pediatric Pain Study, University of California, School of Nursing, Department of Family Health Care Nursing, San Francisco, CA 94143-0606; phone: (415) 476-4040.
From Hockenberry-Eaton M, Wilson D, Jackson C: *Wong's nursing care of infants and children,* ed 7, St Louis, 2007, Mosby, pp 210-212.

TABLE 22-2	Origins and Classifications of Pain		
Type	**Description/Characteristics**		**Examples**
Origin			
Acute	Brief; associated with tissue damage or inflammation; intensity steadily diminishes over days to weeks Often identifiable cause, predictable and expected time frame		Surgical pain, burns, fractures, infection (e.g., cellulitis), trauma (e.g., puncture wound)
Chronic persistent	Persistent or near-persistent pain lasting 3 months or longer with changes in the nervous system		Arthritis, joint pain (e.g., juvenile arthritis, sickle cell crisis)
Recurrent	Repetitive painful episodes alternating with pain-free intervals		Headache; abdominal, chest, or limb pain
Classification			

Nociceptive
  Somatic
  Visceral
	Pain due to stimulation of nociceptors in the peripheral nervous system
	Well localized, throbbing, aching, or dull
	Poorly localized; deep, crampy, or sharp, squeezing pain; persistent aching feeling
			Laceration or sunburn
			Appendicitis, dysmenorrhea

Neuropathic	Persistent pain related to persistent or abnormal excitability in the peripheral or central nervous system with no ongoing tissue injury; often described as "burning," "strange," or "pins and needles" Shooting, stabbing over a background of aching and burning; not well localized		Amputation pain syndromes, plexus injuries, reflex sympathetic dystrophy; postherpetic neuralgia
Psychogenic	Persistent pain that is a manifestation of a psychiatric disease		Somatization disorder, somatoform pain disorder, conversion disorder

From Betz CL, Sowden LA: *Mosby's pediatric nursing reference,* ed 6, Philadelphia, 2007, Mosby.

responses to pain include changes in metabolic functioning (e.g., hypermetabolism, hyperglycemia, or lipolysis), decreased gut motility, sodium and water retention, and cytokine production.

■ Management

Pain type and intensity (e.g., fair, moderate, or severe) guide pain management decisions. Table 22-3 provides management guidance using pharmacological drugs. If pain is secondary to a known etiology or underlying disease, the health care provider must treat its underlying causes. Other measures may be needed to control pain symptoms. Principles of effective office-based pain management include the use of a combination of pharmacological and nonpharmacological measures. Other elements that contribute to anxiety and affect child pain perception should be considered. The environment should be child-friendly, calming, and have colorful walls with pictures, together with a collection of toys and games to minimize fear associated with an unfamiliar setting.

ACUTE PAIN MANAGEMENT

Common nonpharmacological measures used with acute pain include the following:

Infants

- Sensorimotor techniques for infants, such as pacifiers, swaddling, holding, singing, calming music, and rocking
- Sucrose solution via pacifier or gloved finger. Administer 2 minutes before a procedure is started. Analgesic effect may

last for 8 minutes and another dosing of additional sucrose solution may be repeated (Tsao et al, 2008). Sucrose loses its efficacy by age 4 to 6 months (Schechter et al, 2007).

Children and Adolescents

- Cognitive-behavioral strategies, such as relaxation procedures (controlled breathing and progressive muscle relaxation), music, play therapy, and preparatory information before painful procedures or surgeries. To be effective, cognitive and behavioral strategies should appeal to the child's imagination, sense of play, and attention. It is important to consider the child's age as well as developmental abilities and preferences (Sinha et al, 2006).
- Physical strategies, such as application of heat (if muscle spasm) or cold (if swelling, bleeding, or pain), pressure, massage, acupuncture, exercise, rest, or immobilization; physical therapy can be a useful modality especially for children with musculoskeletal pain or children who are deconditioned from inactivity; transcutaneous electrical nerve stimulation (TENS) is an effective treatment for localized pain (Zeltzer and Krell, 2007).
- Distraction techniques have proven effectiveness. These include having the child watch a video, practice imagery, perform self-hypnosis, look out the window, or play with a toy; praising the child; giving the child a party blower, bubbles, or pinwheel and asking the child to blow the pain away; providing stickers or stamps; or gently stroking the child.

Pharmacological measures used in primary care settings for acute pain include the following (see Table 22-3):

- Analgesic for mild to moderate pain (Taketomo et al, 2011): acetaminophen 10 to 15 mg/kg every 4 to 6 hours

TABLE 22-3	Common Oral Pain Medications and Doses Used With Children (<50 kg)		
Pain Medication	**Dose (mg/kg)**	**Frequency**	**Comments**
Acetaminophen	10-15	Every 4-6 hr (do *not* exceed five doses/24 hr)	Nonopioid No inflammatory activity 24-hr maximum limit: term neonates less than 10 days (60 mg/kg); term neonates greater than 10 days (90 mg/kg)
Ibuprofen	4-10	Every 6-8 hr; max daily dose 40 mg/kg/day	Nonsteroidal antiinflammatory drug (NSAID) use in children >6 mo
Codeine	0.5-1	Every 4-6 hr; max dose for children 60 mg/dose	Opioid Decreased incremental analgesic effect with doses higher than 65 mg; 10% of individuals cannot metabolize this drug, so does not always work well
Naproxen	5-7	Every 8-12 hr	NSAID Oral liquid available
Acetaminophen with codeine	0.5-1 (of codeine) and a safe dose of acetaminophen	Every 4-6 hr; max dose, 60 mg/dose	
Acetaminophen with hydrocodone (moderate pain)	Dose in children has not been well established. Dose is limited by appropriate dose of acetaminophen and hydrocodone (usual initial dose: 0.2 mg/kg).	Every 3-4 hr	Used for moderate pain; preferred over acetaminophen with codeine because it causes fewer side effects; consider if acetaminophen or ibuprofen is not effective
Oxycodone	0.05-0.15	Every 4-6 hr	Opioid This is a high-alert medication with risk of harm if used in error
Acetaminophen with oxycodone	10-15 (of acetaminophen) or 0.05-0.15 mg/kg/dose up to 5 mg/dose (of oxycodone)	Every 4-6 hr	This is a high-alert medication with risk of harm if used in error
Methadone	Initial: 0.1 mg/kg/dose every 4 hours for 2-3 doses, then 6-12 hours as needed or 0.7 mg/kg/24 hours divided every 4-6 hours	Max dose: 10 mg/dose	Opioid Half-life is up to 96 hr; useful in chronic pain and with opioid-tolerant people. Patients need to be weaned off, not abruptly stopped in order to avoid withdrawal symptoms.
Aspirin	10-15	Every 4-6 hr; max dose 4 g/day	NSAID Association with Reye syndrome Inhibits platelet aggregation; may cause postoperative bleeding; do not administer to children with suspected or confirmed viral infection—used only in limited conditions

Data from Taketomo CK, Hodding JH, Kraus, DM: *Pediatric dosage handbook*, ed 17, Hudson, OH, 2011, Lexi-Comp.

as needed not to exceed five doses in 24 hours. Adolescent and adult dosage is 325 to 650 mg every 4 to 6 hours or 1000 mg/dose three or four times a day; maximum daily amount is 4 g. Antiinflammatory agents are more effective if inflammation is a key factor causing pain because acetaminophen has limited peripheral antiinflammatory action. Acetaminophen is potentially hepatotoxic, so avoid its use in children with hepatic disease or dysfunction. Because it is a component in many over-the-counter (OTC) preparations, be alert to the potential for overdose if several drugs with acetaminophen are taken by the patient.

- Oral nonsteroidal antiinflammatory drugs (NSAIDs): The usual pediatric dosage for children weighing less than 50 kg and dosages for children and adolescents 50 kg or more are listed in pediatric drug texts (Schechter, 2006; Taketomo et al, 2011). Consult a pharmacology text for additional information about drugs, such as availability in liquid, tablet, or gel form and the corresponding concentration (milligrams per dose) of the various preparations:
  - Aspirin 10 to 15 mg/kg/dose every 4 to 6 hours as needed up to a maximum of 4 g/day for children. However, because its use is contraindicated in children younger than 18 years of age because of its association with Reye syndrome, it should only be used in the management of selected pediatric conditions (e.g., juvenile arthritis and Kawasaki disease). Due to bleeding issues, aspirin should be discontinued 10 to 14 days before major invasive procedures or surgeries.

○ Ibuprofen 4 to 10 mg/kg every 6 to 8 hours as needed for infants >6 mos and children with a maximum daily dose of 40 mg/kg/day; adolescent and adult: 200 to 400 mg/dose every 4 to 6 hours as needed with 1.2 g/day maximum. Avoid if there is an aspirin allergy, anticipated surgery, bleeding disorder, hemorrhage, gastritis, or renal disease. Use with caution in children not eating solids.

○ Naproxen, older than 2 years: 5 to 7 mg/kg every 8 to 12 hours; adolescents and adults for mild to moderate pain or dysmenorrhea: initial 500 mg dose and then 250 mg every 6 to 8 hours or 500 mg every 12 hours, maximum 1250 mg/day initially and then maximum daily dose 1000 mg/day. This medicine requires similar cautions as ibuprofen. Delayed-release preparations are not recommended for acute pain management.

• Opioid agonists are used for moderate to severe pain. All opioids produce a range of side effects including constipation, nausea and vomiting, pruritus, sedation, respiratory depression, and urinary retention. Side effects should be anticipated and treated aggressively (Greco and Berde, 2005). Consideration in dosing is needed for opioid-naïve children. Common opioid side effects and management are listed in Table 22-4 and as follows (Taketomo et al, 2011):

○ Codeine—oral, 0.5 to 1 mg/kg every 4 to 6 hours with 60 mg dose maximum. For younger patients it is typically given as an acetaminophen and codeine elixir. It is a highly constipating drug and associated with nausea, gastrointestinal distress, and vomiting. Usual adult dose is 30 mg; range per dose is 15 to 60 mg every 4 to 6 hours as needed.

○ Hydromorphone—oral, young children: 0.03 to 0.08 mg/kg/dose every 3 to 4 hours as needed; children more than 50 kg and adolescents: 1 to 2 mg/dose every 3 to 4 hours as needed for opioid-naïve children; those with prior opioid exposure may need a higher dose up to adult dosage of 2 to 4 mg/dose every 4 to 6 hours with a maximum of 8 mg/dose. The use of hydromorphone by primary care providers in the ambulatory management of pediatric pain is limited.

○ Methadone is a synthetic opioid that has a long duration of action (12 to 36 hours). Traditionally it is used with opioid-dependent patients (e.g., neonatal abstinence syndrome). Methadone is being increasingly used in cases of acute pain to provide stable levels of opioid analgesia. Methadone has a high bioavailability (85%) making it an attractive oral analgesic. Children: 0.1 mg/kg/dose orally every 4 hours initially for two or three doses and then every 6 to 12 hours as needed; it can also be dosed at 0.7 mg/kg per 24 hours divided every 4 to 6 hours. The maximum dose is 10 mg/dose. Methadone dosing must be individualized. Prior opioid exposure and withdrawal symptoms are key factors to consider. Patients must be carefully monitored to avoid overmedication with repeated doses. Abrupt discontinuation after prolonged use may result in withdrawal symptoms or seizures. Methadone has the potential to increase the QTc interval (the QT interval corrected for heart rate) so a baseline electrocardiogram is usually obtained (Kraemer and Rose, 2009).

○ Hydrocodone (commonly combined with acetaminophen)—dose has not been well established in children.

TABLE 22-4	Management of Common Opioid Side Effects	
Side Effect	**Comments**	**Drug Dosage**
Nausea	Exclude other processes such as bowel obstruction. Consider switching to different opioid. Use antiemetics.	Metoclopramide: 0.1-0.2 mg/kg/dose/IV every 6-8 hr as needed Ondansetron: refer to a pediatric pharmacology text
Pruritus	Exclude other causes, such as drug allergy. Consider switching to different opioid. Use antipruritics.	Diphenhydramine: 0.5 mg/kg PO/IV every 6 hr Hydroxyzine Child: less than 6 years: 50 mg/day PO in divided doses Child: 6 years and older: 50-100 mg/day PO in divided doses
Constipation	Regular use of stimulant and stool softener laxatives	Docusate Child: 5 mg/kg/day PO in 1-4 divided doses Bisacodyl Child: 5-10 mg PO as a single dose

IV, Intravenous; *PO*, per mouth.
Data from Greco C, Berde C: Pain Management for the hospitalized pediatric patient, *Pediatr Clin North Am* 52:995-1027, 2005; Taketomo CK, Hodding JH, Kraus, DM: *Pediatric dosage handbook,* ed 17, Hudson, OH, 2011, Lexi-Comp.

The Agency for Healthcare Research and Quality dosing guidelines for opioid-naïve children less than 50 kg who are in moderate or severe pain are as follows: usual initial dose based on hydrocodone is 0.2 mg/kg/dose orally every 3 to 4 hours; for those more than 50 kg, the usual initial dose is 10 mg every 3 to 4 hours. Typically adolescents and adults may require 1 to 2 tablets or capsules every 4 to 6 hours as needed. Hydrocodone is available in fixed combinations with acetaminophen. If given with acetaminophen, the maximum recommended dose of acetaminophen, for a child or adult, cannot be exceeded.

○ Oxycodone—oral, 0.05 to 0.15 mg/kg every 4 to 6 hours (available in liquid and in varied concentrations) for children as needed. Initial dose is 5 mg every 6 hours for children greater than 50 kg and adults. For moderate to severe pain, the usual initial dose is 10 mg every 3 to 4 hours as needed for those more than 50 kg. It comes in 5 mg tablets and a controlled-release product and is available alone or in fixed combinations with acetaminophen.

○ Morphine—oral, a dose of 0.3 mg/kg is recommended as an initial dose for the child in severe pain with subsequent recommended dosing of 0.2 to 0.5 mg/kg/dose every 4 to 6 hours as needed; intravenous (IV) bolus, 0.05 mg/kg/dose initially, then at 0.1 to 0.2 mg/kg/dose every 2 to 4 hours (recommended maximum doses by age: infants, 2 mg/dose; child 1 to 6 years, 4 mg/dose; 7 to 12 years,

8 mg/dose; adolescents, 15 mg/dose. Adult dosage is 10 to 30 mg orally (prompt release) every 4 hours or 15 to 30 mg (controlled release) every 8 to 12 hours as needed. IV, intramuscular, or subcutaneous 2.5 to 20 mg/dose every 2 to 6 hours as needed; typically 10 mg/dose every 4 hours as needed. This drug is not used commonly in primary care settings for the management of acute pain. IV use necessitates close monitoring of vital signs and pulse oximetry with infants younger than 3 months old as they are more susceptive to respiratory depression.

- Topical analgesic creams, such as eutectic mixture of local anesthetics (EMLA) and iontophoresis delivery of drugs, are used with procedures involving skin punctures. Topical liposomal 4% lidocaine creams (LMX4) provides effective analgesia in 30 minutes, whereas EMLA takes 1 hour for full effectiveness. Lidocaine iontophoresis provides anesthesia in 10 minutes, but about 5% of children view the sensation as unpleasant (Zempsky et al, 2004). Subcutaneous injection of combinations of local anesthetics, such as lidocaine, epinephrine, and tetracaine (LET), are useful in suturing lacerations. Never use epinephrine-containing local anesthetics for digits or the penis because of end artery adverse effect.
- Benzodiazepines may play a role in the treatment of pain if spasms are a contributing factor to the pain experienced by a child (Schechter, 2006). Again check for drug and herbal interactions with benzodiazepines (see Table 42-3).

Pharmacological Considerations

There can be interactions between herbal preparations and common pain relievers and anesthetics (see Table 42-3). Stop herbal supplements at least 1 week before any scheduled surgical procedure to prevent any alterations in coagulation or interactions with anesthesia (see Table 42-3 for specific examples). Should the provider and family or patient wish to consider nonpharmacological management of pain as an option, Table 42-5 provides some guidance.

An essential consideration in administering analgesics is whether there is a need to maintain certain serum concentration levels. In situations that require a steady-state serum concentration for pain relief (e.g., following same-day surgery, fractures), around-the-clock dosing of pain medications for 48 to 72 hours is preferable to "as needed [prn]" dosing, which is associated with drops in serum concentration levels. When the child is then given a prn dose of medication, a significant period may elapse before adequate analgesic effect occurs.

Factors That Produce Age-Related Differences in Analgesia Responses

- Neonates and young infants have delayed hepatic enzyme maturation resulting in altered drug metabolic inactivation. Analgesics metabolized in the liver, such as opioids, have a prolonged elimination half-life in newborns and young infants. Rates of maturation of individual enzyme functions vary, but most mature by approximately 6 months of age (Greco and Berde, 2005).
- Glomerular filtration is reduced in the first few weeks of life, which results in slower elimination of opioids and their active metabolites (Greco and Berde, 2005).
- Toddlers and preschool children's renal clearance of analgesics is greater than that of adults (Zeltzer and Krell, 2007).

- Neonates and young infants have decreased plasma protein binding for many drugs, which results in greater concentrations of pharmacologically active unbound drug (Greco and Berde, 2005).

CHRONIC PAIN MANAGEMENT

Surveillance of the pediatric population estimates that approximately 15% of children are living with chronic pain (Thompson et al, 2010). Children and adolescents with chronic pain are at greater risk for both emotional and functional problems including more depressive symptoms. As many as 40% of these patients report that chronic pain negatively affects their school attendance, participation in hobbies, appetite, and quality and quantity of sleep and results in increased health service use (Guite et al, 2009). A gender difference is noted after puberty with females reporting higher pain intensity, longer lasting pain, and more frequent pain than do males. Girls are also more likely to experience more severe pain problems compared with boys (Palermo and Zeltzer, 2009). It is not always feasible to eradicate the pain; return of function is often then the goal.

Chronic pain is differentiated from acute pain when the duration of pain is 6 months or longer. A diagnosis of pain disorder is made when the primary complaint is severe pain. A diagnosis of a pain disorder involves five key features: pain in one or more anatomical sites that is the predominant focus; significant distress involving social or other important functions; psychological factors implicated in either the onset, severity, exacerbation or maintenance of the pain; the pain is not due to malingering or a fictitious illness; and a mood, anxiety, or psychotic disorder is not related to the etiology of the pain. Chronic and recurrent pain disorders in children typically involve complaints of abdominal, limb, or chest pain and headache (Scheffer, 2011).

Health care providers may worry that they will miss an organic cause when dealing with a child with recurrent or chronic pain whose etiology may be in question. A comprehensive evaluation that includes a thorough history of the pain with questioning about the possibility of comorbid conditions such as depression, anxiety disorders, and contributing psychosocial factors and a focused physical examination are the first key steps in the evaluation. If warranted by historical and physical data, selected laboratory and/or radiographic testing can then be conducted. There is no standard laboratory workup for the evaluation of chronic pain. Extensive laboratory investigations are neither always needed nor recommended and can be harmful. Having cautiously collected and evaluated the data, the primary care provider is then ready to explain what is thought to be causing or adding to the child's pain and has set the stage for a child, parent, and provider partnership to develop a comprehensive treatment plan that will effectively manage that child's pain (Box 22-1).

Pharmacological measures and nonpharmacological techniques are used in the primary care setting for chronic pain management. Pharmacological measures include:

- NSAIDs, acetaminophen, and tricyclic antidepressants (TCAs) are the primary treatments used to treat chronic pain unrelated to disease or trauma. Assess the efficacy of the pharmacological therapy as follows:
  - Have the child or parent use a pain intensity rating scale and keep a diary of the child's activities and pain.
  - On follow-up visits, question whether symptoms improved.

BOX 22-1 Key Strategies in the Evaluation and Treatment of Chronic Pain

Evaluation

History Key Points

- Actively listen to the parent's and child's description of the pain experience; listen to their pain story.
- Be sure to talk to the adolescent alone.
- Ask questions related to the presence of psychosocial and developmental comorbidities or contributing psychosocial-developmental factors (e.g., school issues, family dysfunction, negative coping strategies, depression).
- Question about onset of pain; time of day; duration; frequency of pain episodes and if sudden or gradual onset; location and radiation; associated symptoms; description of the pain; what started the pain and/or keeps it going; what has been used to control the pain (medications, CAM, other modalities); how is pain affecting the child's and family's life (sleep, activities, appetite); what decreases the pain or makes it worse

Physical Examination Focus Points

- Note the child's appearance, posture, and gait.
- Carefully examine areas of hypersensitivity and tender points in muscles or tendon insertion sites.

Laboratory and Imaging Studies (Limit Testing to Only What Is Needed)

- Only tests needed based on history and physical examination and if not done recently

- Consider such routine tests as complete blood count (CBC) with differential, sedimentation rate, obtain a urinalysis if child's physical examination suggests the need for such tests.

Treatment

- Educate child and family about the nature of chronic pain and the reason for the child's pain.
- Focus efforts on helping the child enhance his or her coping skills.
- Identify a plan with the child and family on how to improve child's functional ability, emphasizing:
  - Sleep: improving sleep hygiene using psychological strategies and pharmacologic agents if needed
  - Cognitive-behavioral therapy: biofeedback, hypnotherapy, relaxation techniques
  - School: talk with the parents, child, and school personnel to develop a plan to help child reach potential in the school setting in academic, social, and physical activities
  - Physical therapy and mental health referral if indicated
  - Other treatments to reduce stress: massage; art, aroma, music therapy; acupuncture, yoga
- Medication: as needed while remembering that nonpharmacological strategies and interventions are also essential management tools

CAM, Complementary and alternative medicine.
Modified from Palermo TM, Zeltzer LK: Recurrent and chronic pain. In Carey WB, Crocker AC, Coleman WL, et al, editors: *Developmental-behavioral pediatrics,* ed 4, Philadelphia, 2009, Saunders.

- Selective serotonin reuptake inhibitors (SSRIs), opioids, certain anticonvulsants, muscle relaxants (e.g., cerebral palsy), and other selected medications may be needed. TCAs are used for phantom limb, peripheral neuropathy, migraine headaches, radiation-induced nerve injury or tumor-associated nerve damage (Palermo and Zeltzer, 2009). Use of tricyclics is contraindicated in patients with cardiac conduction disturbances. The pain dosage for TCAs (more commonly used in children with chronic pain) is lower than the dosage prescribed in the treatment of depression. The U.S. Food and Drug Administration (FDA) has not approved the use of these drugs for depression in pediatric patients (Taketomo et al, 2010); therefore, the primary care provider's role would be to refer to the appropriate pain management specialist for the initial assessment for such drugs and assist in the monitoring of children on TCAs. Tricyclics have significant adverse effects such as sedation, orthostatic hypotension, dry mouth, constipation, and urinary hesitancy. These side effects typically subside as the child develops tolerance to the medication. Patients treated with antidepressants require close monitoring and observation for worsening of depression, suicidality, and unusual behavior, especially during the first few months of therapy. Family members must be educated to closely observe the patient and communicate the patient's condition frequently with the health care provider (Taketomo et al, 2011). Gabapentin is the anticonvulsant most frequently used to treat neuropathic pain associated with burning, stabbing, or aching. Due to few adverse effects it is often considered a first-line therapy. Children requiring these agents for the management of their chronic pain are best handled by referral to pain management specialists. The Lidoderm patch, a topical agent, is also used for the treatment of focal neuropathic pain.

Nonpharmacological techniques and considerations include:

- Physical therapy, relaxation, massage, guided imagery, biofeedback, hypnosis, heat and cold, distraction, TENS, music therapy, acupuncture, and psychological therapy, which are frequently used as adjuncts to pharmacological therapy of chronic pain. Invasive techniques, such as neuroablative procedures and spinal cord stimulation, are occasionally used as a last resort. Hypnotherapy and biofeedback may be beneficial in the treatment of chronic pain.
- Critical factors in chronic pain assessment include level of child and family distress (including their level of anxiety, depression, and feelings of hopelessness), cultural beliefs, and pain perception.

Parental strategies to encourage optimal coping with chronic pain issues include (Palermo and Zeltzer, 2009):

- Not giving excessive attention, special privileges, or treats when the child complains of pain
- Encouraging normal activities, within reason, during pain episodes (e.g., going to school, doing chores)
- Spending time during the day doing quiet, low-key activities when the child cannot go to school or participate in other events. Activities such as playing games all day and excessive time spent watching television or videos may reinforce the child to not want to participate in "well" activities.
- Lessen the focus on pain by not repeatedly asking about the child's pain. Children typically will let their parent know when they are in pain.

TABLE 22-5 Common Pediatric Pain Problems and Pain Relief Strategies	
Pediatric Pain Problems	**Pain Relief Strategies**
Otalgia	Acetaminophen or ibuprofen Antipyrine and benzocaine otic drops Warmed compresses pressed against the ear
Pharyngitis	Acetaminophen or ibuprofen Antibiotics if GABHS Saltwater gargles Anesthetic lozenges for older child
Stomatitis	Ibuprofen Bland diet Saline mouth rinses for older children Benadryl-calcium carbonate (Maalox) (in a 1:1 preparation) to coat the mucous membranes Viscous lidocaine (remember the potential for aspiration and toxicity) Sucralfate
Musculoskeletal injury	RICE—**R**est, **I**ce, **C**ompression, and **E**levation Immobilization of affected area Cold for the initial 48 to 72 hours NSAIDs
Fractures and sprains	NSAIDs Narcotic analgesics if severe fracture or sprain Topical ibuprofen, ketoprofen, and felbinac give relief in soft tissue trauma, strains, and sprains; however, studies have involved only adults
Injection pain (e.g., immunizations)	Distraction and relaxation techniques EMLA cream (maximum recommended dose based on application area; is also age and weight dependent)* Ice Spot pressure (press down into muscle where shot is to be given) Vapocoolants
Neonate and infant procedural pain	Sucrose orally Sucrose pacifier Acetaminophen
In emergency department or urgent care settings: Intravenous line placement or venipuncture, lumbar puncture, abscess drainage, joint aspiration	EMLA/LMX4 (prevent mucous membrane contact or ingestion)†
Laceration	Lidocaine, epinephrine, and tetracaine (LET) Procedure: Use on open wounds that are simple lacerations of head, neck, extremities, or trunk that are <5 cm in length; use 3 mL max; place LET mixed with cellulose on open wound and cover with occlusive dressing or place two cotton balls soaked with LET in the wound. Contraindications: Allergy to amide anesthetics, gross contamination of wound Do not use on mucous membranes, digits, genitalia, ear, or nose.

*EMLA (eutectic mixture of local anesthetics) is contraindicated in patients with congenital or idiopathic methemoglobinemia or in infants less than 12 months old who are being treated with sulfas, acetaminophen, benzocaine, chloroquine, dapsone, nitrofurantoin, phenobarbital, phenytoin, or quinine.
†EMLA/LMX4 (liposomal 4% lidocaine cream) contraindicated with nonintact skin, allergy to amide anesthetics, or in emergent situations.
GABHS, Group A beta-hemolytic streptococcus; *NSAIDs,* nonsteroidal antiinflammatory drugs.
Data from Taketomo CK, Hodding JH, Kraus DM: *Pediatric dosage handbook,* ed 17, Hudson, OH, 2011, Lexi-Comp; Zempsky WT, Schechter NL: Office-based pain management, *Pediatr Clin North Am* 47:601-615, 2000; Zempsky WT, Cravero JP, Committee on Pediatric Emergency Medicine and Section on Anesthesiology and Pain Medicine: Relief of pain and anxiety in pediatric patients in emergency medical systems, *Pediatrics* 114:1348-1354, 2004.

- Based on developmental appropriateness, reinforce the child's role in pain self-management through the use of nonpharmacological strategies. When the child reports pain, ask, "What do you think you can do to help lessen your pain?" Then talk about the nonpharmacological strategies. However, give breakthrough pain medication if the child requests it.

Chronic pain is most successfully treated by a coordinated, planned, interdisciplinary approach. It is essential that all team members are giving the same message in an integrated team approach format.

Table 22-3 identifies common oral pain medications used in pediatrics and their dosages. Table 22-5 outlines specific pain problems commonly seen in pediatrics, in addition to pain relief strategies. The health care provider should be familiar with clinical practice guidelines that address pain management related to common chronic pediatric conditions. Sickle cell anemia and JA are examples of chronic conditions marked by acute, chronic, and mixed (acute superimposed on chronic) pain. The National Heart, Lung, and Blood Institute published a key document titled *The Management of Sickle Cell Disease* (2002) that addressed a variety of disease-related issues including pain management. This landmark document tackled the misconceptions about pain in children with sickle cell anemia and provided guidelines for the proper use of analgesia. It is available for historical reference. Pain is a critical feature of this disease and can have significant negative effects on quality of life. There are also guidelines available from the American Pain Society for the management of pain in children with JA (http://www.ampainsoc.org/pub/arthritis.htm). Knowing appropriate pain management resources and using pain control protocols are key elements in optimizing the care of children with chronic diseases and improving their quality of life. Specific disease-related pain management is discussed in subsequent chapters of this text.

■ Patient and Family Education

Several key principles related to pain management and administration of pain medications must be emphasized to parents and children. They include:
- Pain medication should be taken exactly as prescribed.
- Myths related to addiction and the use of opioids for pain control should be discussed when these agents are needed for pain control.

- The use of other methods of relieving pain should be used because they are essential components of the pain management plan. Medication alone is not sufficient to manage chronic pain; similarly, cognitive-behavioral therapies are helpful in acute pain situations.
- Teens should be warned about drinking alcohol with opioids.
- The health care provider needs to be kept apprised of all prescribed, OTC, and herbal medications being taken.
- Pain medication taken over a long time may need to be tapered and not abruptly stopped.
- Pain medication works most effectively if taken before severe pain is experienced.
- Common side effects such as constipation, dizziness, nausea, drowsiness, sweating, and flushing occur with the administration of pain medications. The health care provider should be made aware of these problems so appropriate interventions can be suggested.

■ Partnership in Care

A child, parent, and health care provider partnership is essential for effective pain management. Follow-up assessment determines whether optimal pain control is achieved, evaluates whether pharmacological side effects are minimized or being managed effectively, and ensures the causative factor for pain was correctly identified. Follow-up assessment may be conducted via phone contact or appointment. The time frame for follow-up contact needs to be individualized depending on the severity of pain, underlying health condition, and parent-child socioemotional factors.

Infectious Diseases and Immunizations

CATHERINE G. BLOSSER, MARGARET A. BRADY, AND ROBERTA BENTSON ROYAL

Infections are among the most common reasons for children to be taken to their health care provider for a sick visit. Although viruses are the most frequent cause of childhood infectious illnesses, bacterial infections (particularly of the skin and mucosal surfaces) are also common. The ability to distinguish serious infections from those that resolve with minimal or no intervention is an important skill for primary care providers. Nearly as important as the medical care provided to the sick child is the ability to effectively communicate with, educate, and support the often frustrated and anxious parents. Additionally, the provider must include preventive education, including vaccinations, in the routine delivery of primary health care.

■ Pathogenesis of Infectious Diseases

Bacteria are the dominant life form on earth and are found virtually everywhere in the environment. They are often controlled by viruses. Humans become colonized with bacteria on the skin and mucosal surfaces (including the upper respiratory and gastrointestinal tracts) shortly after birth. These bacteria are generally harmless and may be beneficial because many normal flora can minimize colonization by potentially pathogenic organisms (Table 23-1). Infectious agents cause disease when the balance between harmless colonization and protective immunity is disrupted in favor of harmful proliferation of a microorganism. Dangerous viruses are rare, fortunately, because of their inability to meet all three criteria at once: inflicting serious harm, going unrecognized by the immune system, and being able to efficiently spread.

The human immune system is complex and provides many layers of protection from disease. Skin and mucosal surfaces provide a barrier to invasion by microorganisms, and antibodies and immune cells allow the body to defend itself in general and specific ways against invasion by pathogens. Microorganisms may breach the immune barrier provided by skin and mucosa by binding to cell surface structures; for example, influenza virus uses its hemagglutinin protein to attach to cell membranes and invade respiratory mucosa. Disease caused by microbial pathogens can result from destruction of infected cells and tissues and from disruption of normal cell functions. Some disease symptoms are caused by the immune system response to infection, which can result in local or systemic inflammatory responses.

■ Clinical Findings

Most infectious illnesses in pediatrics are diagnosed solely based on history and physical examination. Laboratory testing is generally reserved for unusual, serious, or difficult to diagnose cases.

HISTORY

The goal of a comprehensive history is the generation and prioritization of differential diagnoses for that particular individual based on symptomatology and history. Crucial aspects of the history that help distinguish infectious illnesses from other types of diseases or assist in determining the responsible pathogen include:

- *The history of present illness with a careful analysis of the presenting symptoms.* When did the symptoms start? What other symptoms were associated with the illness? Were there periods when the patient seemed improved or even back to normal? Details about the presenting history are critically important and can help narrow the differential diagnosis from a broad list of possibilities. As an example, fever is most commonly associated with infectious illnesses, but also occurs with rheumatologic or oncologic diseases.
- *A comprehensive past medical history.* Careful questioning makes certain diagnoses more or less likely. A history of asthma in a teenager with fever and cough, for example, is suspicious of atypical pneumonia. Determine place of birth.

TABLE 23-1 Common Distribution Sites of Normal Microflora* Found in Humans

Bacterium	Very Commonly or Commonly Found in These Locations	Notes
Aerobic Bacteria		
Gram Positive		
Staphylococcus aureus	Skin, hair, naso-oropharynx, lower GI, cerumen	Rarely found in the vagina and conjunctiva; trachea, bronchi, lungs, and sinuses are normally sterile; has potential for being a pathogen New study shows that high levels of MRSA bacteria in the nose are indicative of MRSA colonization in the axilla, groin, perineum; if screening cultures are done, culturing the nose will produce reliable results of colonization in other areas (Mermel et al, 2011)
Staphylococcus epidermidis	Skin, hair, naso-oropharynx, adult vagina, urethra, conjunctiva, ear (including cerumen), lower GI	Occasionally found in the vagina of prepubertal females; found in low numbers in "normal" urine, probably as result of contamination from urethra and skin areas
Streptococci		
• Streptococcus saprophyticus	Skin, hair, naso-oropharynx, lower GI, cerumen, mouth, nasal passages, nasopharynx	Occasionally found in urethra and conjunctiva; group B uncommonly found in oropharynx and postpubertal vagina
• S. mitis	Skin, conjunctiva, nasopharynx; less commonly in adult vagina and urethra	Uncommon in GI tract
• S. mutans	Mouth; less common in pharynx	Has the potential of being a pathogen
• S. pneumoniae (Pneumococcus, Diplococcus)	Nasopharynx, mouth; rarely found in conjunctiva, ear, vagina	Has the potential of being a pathogen
• S. pyogenes (group A)	Mouth, pharynx; rarely skin, conjunctiva, ear, adult vagina	Has the potential for being a pathogen
• S. viridans	Nasopharynx, mouth, skin	
Bifidobacterium bifidum	Lower GI	
Enterococcus faecalis	Lower GI, postpubertal vagina; occasionally found in mouth, urethra	Rarely found in pharynx; has potential of being a pathogen
Propionibacterium acnes	Skin	
Gram Negative		
Acinetobacter johnsonii	Skin, urethra, adult vagina	
Corynebacterium	Skin, cerumen, naso-oropharynx, mouth, lower GI, urethra, adult vagina	
Citrobacter diversus	Lower GI	
Enterobacter	Lower GI, prepubertal vagina, mouth, axillary area	Has the potential of being a pathogen
Escherichia coli	Lower GI, vagina, mouth, urethra	Has the potential of being a pathogen
Haemophilus influenzae	Nasopharynx, but not commonly; rarely conjunctiva, ear	Has the potential of being a pathogen
Kingella kingae (formerly referred to as Moraxella kingae)	Pharynx	Has the potential of being a pathogen (cause of invasive infections in young children)
Klebsiella pneumoniae	Nose, colon, axillary area	
Lactobacillus spp.	Pharynx, mouth, lower GI, adult vagina	
Moraxella catarrhalis	Nasopharynx	
Morganella morganii	Lower GI	
Mycobacterium spp.	Skin, lower GI, urethra; rarely nasopharynx, mouth	

TABLE 23-1	Common Distribution Sites of Normal Microflora* Found in Humans—cont'd	
Bacterium	**Very Commonly or Commonly Found in These Locations**	**Notes**
Mycoplasma	Mouth, naso-oropharynx, lower GI, vagina; rarely urethra	
Neisseria spp. (e.g., *N. mucosa*)	Nasopharynx (90%-100% of population); less commonly in conjunctiva, mouth, urethra, vagina	*N. meningitidis* occurs in nearly 100% of the population as normal flora in the pharynx; less commonly in nose, mouth, vagina; *N. meningitidis* has the potential for being a pathogen
Proteus spp.	Lower GI, vagina, skin, nasopharynx, mouth	
Pseudomonas aeruginosa	Lower GI, but not commonly; rarely in pharynx, mouth, urethra; lungs of patients with cystic fibrosis (CF)	Has the potential of being a pathogen
Anaerobic Bacteria		
Bacteroides spp.	Lower GI, urethra; rarely adult vagina	Has the potential of being a pathogen
Clostridium spp.	Lower GI; rarely mouth	Less commonly found in adult vagina, skin; can be found in small numbers in urine, but is probably a contaminant. Has the potential for being a pathogen.
Streptococcus spp	Mouth, colon, adult vagina	
Spirochetes (a distinct form of bacteria)	Pharynx, mouth, lower GI	
Fungi		
Actinomycetes spp.	Pharynx, mouth	
Candida albicans	Skin, conjunctiva, mouth, lower GI, adult vagina	Can be found in voided urine, but is a contaminant
Cryptococcus spp.	Skin	
Protozoa	Mouth, lower GI, adult vagina	
Viruses		The role of viruses as normal flora is undetermined.

*Normal microflora in humans consist of indigenous microorganisms that colonize human body tissues and live in a mutualistic state without producing disease. An individual's microflora depends on genetics, age, sex, stress, nutrition, and diet. A pathogen is a microorganism (or virus) than can produce disease. Normal flora can become pathogens when a host is compromised or weakened (endogenous pathogen); other microorganisms can invade a host during times of disease only (obligate pathogens) or lowered resistance (opportunistic pathogens). More than 200 species of bacteria are known to comprise the normal microflora. Skin microflora can also include yeast (*Malassezia furfur*), molds (*Trichophyton mentagrophytes* var. *interdigitale*), and mites (*Demodex folliculorum*). The spinal fluid, blood, urine, and tissues are normally sterile; the cervix is normally sterile, but can demonstrate flora similar to those in the upper area of the vagina. Antibiotics can have a minor to major effect on the microflora (e.g., ampicillin has a major effect; erythromycin a moderate effect; and sulfonamides and penicillins have minor effects).
GI, Gastrointestinal; *MRSA,* methicillin-resistant *Staphylococcus aureus.*
Data from Burton GR, Engelkirk PG: *Microbiology for the health sciences,* ed 5, Philadelphia, 1996, Lippincott Williams & Wilkins, p 177; Mikat DM, Mikat KW: *A clinician's dictionary guide to bacteria and fungi,* ed 4 (revised), 1983, distributed by Eli Lilly and Company, pp 60-64; Mermel LA, Cartony JM, Covington P, et al: Methicillin-resistant *Staphylococcus aureus* (MRSA) colonization at different body sites: a prospective, quantitative analysis, *J Clin Microbiol* 2011 Jan 5. [Epub ahead of print]; Tannock GW, editor: *Medical importance of the normal microflora,* Boston, 1999, Kluwer Academic Publishers, pp 3-5; Todar K: The normal bacteria flora. In Todar, K, editor: *Todar's online textbook of bacteriology,* 2008. Available at www.textbookofbacteriology.net/normalflora.html (accessed Dec 12, 2010).

- *Current and recent medications.* Recent antibiotic use may affect the provider's ability to interpret negative culture results or be important information to know in the case of methicillin-resistant *Staphylococcus aureus* (MRSA) tissue infection. Include any nonprescription, herbal, or natural health products that may have recently been used.
- *Immunizations.* Adherence to recommended vaccine schedules (including age and spacing of vaccines) is an important consideration if the child's symptoms suggest a disease usually prevented by vaccines.
- *Family history, particularly regarding infectious illness.* Important information includes a history of any relative (first or second degree) with a known immune deficiency, with

numerous infections or difficulty recovering from infections, or with a history of recurrent miscarriages. Any of these may raise suspicion for an immune deficiency. A strong history of autoimmune disease in the family may suggest possible rheumatologic diagnoses as opposed to an infectious process.
- *Social history.* Attendance at daycare or school or living in a crowded setting is associated with increased exposure to viral infections. A history of travel to areas with endemic illnesses is important to elicit (e.g., area endemic for Lyme disease, malaria, or parasitic illnesses). A sexual history obtained under confidential conditions is very important for accurate assessment of the adolescent and for males who have sex with males.

- *Exposure history, including any known contacts with individuals with similar symptoms.* In addition to suggesting a presentation consistent with epidemic illness (e.g., as occurs with viruses, such as influenza or enterovirus), a comprehensive, in-depth exposure history can provide important clues in diagnosis of infections that might otherwise not be considered. Specific questions include any contact with individuals with known illnesses or at high risk for certain illnesses, such as tuberculosis (TB) or human immunodeficiency virus (HIV) or contact with animals or animal by-products (e.g., hides, waste, blood). Other exposures of importance include environmental tobacco smoke or mold.
- *Complete review of symptoms.* Some presenting features of the illness may be discounted or forgotten by parents or patients and are recalled only when direct questions are asked.
- *Diet history.* Any ingestion of raw milk or undercooked or raw meats and/or fish; history of pica.

PHYSICAL EXAMINATION

A complete physical examination is necessary; however, the differential diagnoses generated during the process of taking the history can stimulate the examiner to provide extra focus on certain aspects of the examination.

Physical findings that may be encountered with infectious diseases include:

- Abnormal vital signs (e.g., fever, tachypnea, low blood pressure [concerning for dehydration and/or septic shock]).
- Irritability is nonspecific in ill children, but may raise concern for meningitis or Kawasaki disease. Lethargy raises concern for meningitis (particularly in infants and younger children).
- A stiff or painful neck (suggestive of meningitis).
- A new murmur (may herald the possibility of endocarditis or rheumatic fever).
- Refusal to walk (can be a manifestation of deep tissue infections [e.g., pyomyositis], osteomyelitis, septic arthritis, or meningitis).
- Skin or mucous membrane changes (exanthema or enanthema, respectively) are common with viral illness, and characteristic rashes are typically associated with specific illnesses (e.g., chickenpox).

■ Diagnostic Aids

LABORATORY STUDIES

In selected circumstances, laboratory evaluation can help clarify a diagnosis or rule out a serious illness that may be under consideration. When in doubt, consulting with knowledgeable laboratory personnel not only can aid in the appropriate test(s) being ordered, but can save valuable resources and time. The following factors should be considered when determining which diagnostic tests to order if an infectious disease is suspected:

- The quality of the specimen sent to the lab strongly affects the reliability of the results. For example, pus aspirated from a skin infection is generally more likely to grow the pathogen of concern than is a surface swab and has the added advantage of allowing the specimen to undergo a Gram stain. The collection site of the microbiologic specimen needs to be appropriately cleansed to minimize possible skin contamination.
- The timing of sample collection affects the degree to which the results help in diagnosis. Bacterial cultures collected after the administration of antibiotics may remain negative, even with active infection. Acute and convalescent titers or certain blood chemistries can help in a diagnosis or monitor response to treatment.
- The amount of any specimen can affect the laboratory's ability to process the sample correctly.
- Microbiologic samples can require special handling and should be transported to the laboratory promptly. The laboratory should be contacted if there is any question regarding the collection and transport of samples.
- Be prepared to prioritize test requests when only a limited quantity of specimen can be collected.

Complete Blood Count

A complete blood count (CBC) provides information on the relative amount of different cell types in the circulation. From an infectious disease standpoint, the white blood cell (WBC) count is generally the most useful piece of information obtained from the CBC. It is often elevated (*leukocytosis*) in bacterial infections and may be decreased (*leukopenia*) in some viral infections. A differential WBC count is often obtained along with a CBC; bacterial infections often (but not always) cause increases in the neutrophil (or polymorphonuclear cell) count and may cause an elevation in bands (immature neutrophils). Normal values for total white cell count and the differential vary with age (see Appendix C, Table C-1). Medications may also commonly affect the WBC count. Steroids can increase the white count, for example, and the long-term use of certain medications can decrease the white count. The clinical state of the patient may also need to be considered in the interpretation of the white count (e.g., overwhelming bacterial sepsis can lead to decreased WBCs).

Although acute infection generally does not affect the hemoglobin or hematocrit levels, chronic inflammatory disease processes commonly cause low red cell levels (*anemia*). The platelet count is often elevated (*thrombocytosis*) during acute infection.

C-Reactive Protein

The C-reactive protein (CRP) is among the serum measures known as "acute phase reactants," referring to parameters found in blood that increase in the setting of acute inflammation. Serious bacterial infections are more likely to lead to an increased CRP than other types of infections (Maheshwari, 2006). Although the optimum value above which CRP is most highly predictive of bacterial rather than viral infection has not been established, it is generally uncommon for a viral infection to result in a CRP more than about 10 mg/dL in young children (Hsiao and Baker, 2005). In addition, CRP is sometimes a beneficial tool for monitoring the body's response to treatment in certain infections. For example, the CRP often is elevated in osteomyelitis before antibiotic treatment, but usually falls rapidly with effective therapy.

Inflammatory processes other than infection may lead to an elevated CRP, including trauma, rheumatologic diseases, and oncologic diseases. Persistent elevations of CRP may be related to adiposity (Puder et al, 2010). Of note, different laboratories may report CRP in different units (usually either mg/L or mg/dL; 10 mg/L equals 1 mg/dL).

Procalcitonin

Along with CRP and WBC, serum procalcitonin (Pro-CT) is considered a promising biomarker for differentiating certain viral infections from serious bacterial infections; in some cases it has proven to be a better marker of sepsis than the erythrocyte sedimentation rate (ESR), WBC, CRP and interleukin-6 (IL-6) (Tasabehji et al, 2008). Procalcitonin is a protein that has activity similar to a hormone and a cytokine. It is produced by several cell types and many organs in response to proinflammatory stimuli, particularly due to bacteria (Hatzistilianou, 2010). Pro-CT levels tend to rise and fall more quickly than CRP during onset and control of bacterial infections (Long and Nyquist, 2008). It may prove to be a valuable tool when the ability to draw and process blood cultures is limited (Fan et al, 2010; Galetto-Lacour and Gervaix, 2010). Its usefulness has been studied for bacterial pneumonia; fever without origin in children 1 week or less of age or 1 month to 36 months of age; bacterial infection in febrile neutropenic children with cancer; diarrhea-associated hemolytic-uremic syndrome; bacterial causes of acute hepatic disease; septicemia versus systemic inflammatory response syndrome; bacterial versus aseptic meningitis; and various diseases that involve inflammatory processes (e.g., Crohn disease, systemic lupus erythematosus [SLE]) (Long and Nyquist, 2008).

Erythrocyte Sedimentation Rate

The ESR is another measure of inflammation and reflects the observation that red blood cells (RBCs) settle more rapidly when acute phase proteins (such as fibrinogen) are present in serum than when they are not. Although the ESR is not a specific test for infection, it is useful in helping evaluate fever of unknown origin and, like CRP, can be used to monitor response to therapy. A low sedimentation rate (<10 mm/hr) is unlikely if the cause of prolonged unexplained fever is a bacterial infection. *Bartonella* infection, mycobacterial infection, or abscesses are typically associated with an elevated ESR. Similarly, viral infections result in mean ESR values around 20 mm/hr (90% <30 mm/hr), with the exception of adenovirus, which may be associated with values higher than 30 mm/hr. The ESR can be more than 60 mm/hr in children with fever of unknown origin who have bacterial or mycobacterial infection, collagen vascular disease, or inflammatory pseudotumor (Long and Nyquist, 2008).

During the waxing and waning period of infection, the ESR tends to increase and resolve more slowly as compared with CRP values. ESR is considered a useful marker to evaluate the effectiveness of therapy when long-term antibiotics are needed. Thus, it is used when managing diseases (such as osteomyelitis) whereby effectiveness of treatment is judged, in part, by the normalization of the ESR. Like CRP, the ESR is often elevated in noninfectious conditions, causing inflammation, particularly rheumatologic diseases, for which ESRs greater than 100 mm/hour are common. Anemia also causes a nonspecific increase in the ESR.

Cultures, Stains, and Antimicrobial Susceptibility Testing

The usefulness of microbiologic testing is absolutely dependent on the quality of the sample obtained for evaluation and on the correct choice of test for the given clinical situation. Details of appropriate tests for given infections are discussed in the sections about the infectious agents.

Bacterial infections occurring in an otherwise normal child typically result in migration of WBCs to the site of infection, especially neutrophils. The presence of pus can assist in the diagnosis of some infections.

Staining methods can be useful in certain clinical situations, such as when fungal or other infections are suspected. Antigen detection immunofluorescence or antibody assays (e.g., complement fixation tests [CFTs], immunofluorescence [IF] techniques, enzyme-linked immunosorbent assays [ELISAs]) are often used in the diagnosis of viral infections. There are many diagnostic staining methods available (certain commonly used staining tests are covered in more detail under specific infections).

Specimens from fluids or tissue can be sent for bacterial, viral, or fungal cultures; however, the laboratory may need to be notified in cases of certain suspected pathogens to provide specific instruction for the most accurate evaluation of the sample. Additional testing of bacteria may be done on cultured samples to evaluate susceptibility to the more common antibiotics that could be used. Of particular importance is the growing emergence of MRSA, and providers need to know the resistance patterns within their communities. In some communities, MRSA may be susceptible to doxycycline, trimethoprim-sulfamethoxazole (TMP-SMX), or clindamycin; however, susceptibility testing for a given isolate is needed to be sure that an appropriate antibiotic has been chosen (see later discussion about MRSA and *Klebsiella* resistance).

Deoxyribonucleic Acid Testing

Deoxyribonucleic acid (DNA) testing has become increasingly common in the in-patient setting and is being used more frequently in clinical practice. These tests generally rely on polymerase chain reaction (PCR) to amplify pathogen-specific DNA, followed by detection using labeled DNA or ribonucleic acid (RNA) probes. Specimens of fluid or tissue may be evaluated by PCR. Pathogens that are commonly detected by PCR include *Neisseria gonorrhoeae*, *Chlamydia trachomatis*, HIV, *Bordetella pertussis*, herpesviruses, and enteroviruses.

Serologic Tests

For some infections, diagnosis by culture is difficult or impractical. In specific situations, tests that rely on the generation of an antibody response may be useful. Various methods can be used to detect the presence of antibodies to specific infectious organisms, though cross-reactivity may cause false-positive and false-negative test results. Specific organisms that often rely on serologic diagnosis include HIV, West Nile virus, *Bartonella henselae*, and *Mycoplasma pneumoniae*.

Imaging Techniques

Plain Films. Radiographs remain a common modality to assist in the diagnosis of many infections including bone, sinus, and lung infections.

Computed Tomography Scans. Deeper infections, such as abscesses, often require evaluation via computed tomography (CT) scanning.

Magnetic Resonance Imaging. Magnetic resonance imaging (MRI) is the most sensitive imaging modality used in the evaluation of osteomyelitis. It is also often used for brain imaging in cases of encephalitis.

Ultrasound. Ultrasonographic imaging can be used to evaluate the visceral organs, including the liver, spleen, and kidney, for fluid collections suspicious of abscess. It is also commonly used in evaluating kidney anatomy in patients with initial urinary tract infections (UTIs). Echocardiography is a specialized ultrasonographic technique used in the diagnosis, evaluation, and monitoring of endocarditis or Kawasaki disease.

Nuclear Imaging. Several nuclear imaging techniques have been used in evaluating possible infections, including indium-labeled WBC scans ("tagged white cell scans"), gallium scans, bone scans, and positron-emission tomography (PET) scans. Some of these techniques may have limited use in pediatrics, although the bone scan remains useful in the diagnosis of osteomyelitis (Lee and Worsley, 2006).

■ General Management Strategies

PREVENTING THE SPREAD OF INFECTION

Thorough and frequent handwashing is the most effective means of preventing the spread of infection. In addition to educating parents and patients on the importance of proper handwashing, it is crucial that health care providers demonstrate proper handwashing during the care of their patients. There is no excuse for not properly cleaning hands before the examination of a patient. Alcohol-based hand rubs may be substituted for soap and water in most cases as long as the ethanol content is at least 40% but preferably at least 60% or more (Reynolds et al, 2006). Such gels are ineffective against controlling the spread of *Clostridium difficile*. The Centers for Disease Control and Prevention (CDC) recommend using gloves and washing hands with soap and water after being in contact with individuals with *C. difficile*–associated disease (CDC, 2010a).

Specific guidance that should be given to children and parents includes:

- Hands should be washed after using the bathroom, before meals, and before preparing foods. The proper technique includes scrubbing with soap and water for at least 20 seconds (the time it takes to sing "Happy Birthday" twice), rinsing with warm water, and drying completely.
- Avoiding finger-nose and finger-eye contact, particularly if exposed to someone with a cold.
- Using a tissue to cover the mouth and nose when coughing or sneezing may help prevent the spread of pathogens. If a tissue is unavailable, the upper sleeve should be used (not the hands).

USE OF ANTIBIOTICS

It is generally known that antibiotics are often prescribed for conditions that do not require their use and that such inappropriate prescribing patterns are likely to contribute to the emergence of resistant bacteria. The CDC has a task force dedicated to tracking the emergence of drug-resistant pathogens and preventing their spread (www.cdc.gov/drugresistance/actionplan/taskforce). One of the risk factors associated with inappropriate prescriptions in children is pressure from the parents to prescribe antibiotics. Providers are encouraged to educate patients and parents about the role and efficacy of antibiotics and to assume a more "targeted therapy" approach when prescribing. The CDC provides brochures, posters, and information sheets that may be helpful in explaining the importance of judicious use of antibiotics. Knowledge about emerging resistance patterns, local epidemiology, and susceptibility patterns of bacterial agents within their practice communities will better arm the provider to appropriately prescribe. An unexpected benefit found from the flu vaccine has been that the number of antibiotic prescriptions written for respiratory infections has decreased. This in turn ultimately has resulted in lowered overall rates of antibiotic-resistant bacteria (Kwong et al, 2009).

■ Prevention of Infection Through the Use of Vaccines

Immunization is the process by which the body is artificially induced to mount a defense against certain foreign antigens. In this way the immune system is primed to provide future protection with the next exposure to these same antigens. This is achieved by either (1) *active immunization* that involves introducing either a vaccine or toxoid (inactivated toxin) or by (2) *passive immunization* that involves administering an exogenous antibody, such as an immune globulin (IG). The specific agents employed in each type of immunization are discussed in the following sections.

Childhood immunization is not only a mainstay of preventive disease control but it is also cost effective. However, continued efforts must be maintained and strengthened (Pickering et al, 2009; Rongkavilit, 2010). Active immunization has been achieved by the administration of live attenuated and inactivated forms of vaccines. Vaccines exist to combat infections from *Haemophilus influenzae* type B (HiB), meningococcus, diphtheria, pertussis, tetanus, polio, measles, mumps, rubella, human papillomavirus (HPV), hepatitis A and B (HA and HB), influenza, varicella, rabies, typhoid, zoster, Japanese encephalitis, rotavirus, yellow fever, and pneumococcus; all but five are on the routine recommended vaccine schedule for all or specific populations of children and adolescents. Primary care providers may still encounter children with these illnesses because not all routine vaccines have been given as part of preventive health care during childhood or adolescence (see following discussion on parental refusal to vaccination).

Providers must continue to educate parents and patients about the need to keep immunizations current; parents may question this need because many of these diseases have low rates of occurrence in the U.S. Furthermore, the high incidence of global travel leaves underimmunized populations vulnerable to reintroduction of preventable diseases from endemic countries. Preventable epidemics may result.

BARRIERS TO VACCINATION

Primary care providers are frequently faced with immunization issues: shortages of vaccines, vaccine refusal, vaccine schedule changes, and unique immunization needs of special populations. Shortages of vaccine have resulted from manufacturing pitfalls. Recent efforts by the U.S. Department of Health and Human Services (USDHHS) include increasing manufacturing capacity to respond to both seasonal and pandemic influenza vaccines by securing adequate egg supplies year-round; providing better guidance for and contracts with vaccine manufacturers; and focusing on cell-based vaccines. In cases of shortages, the CDC provides tiered guidelines for priority administration.

Product recalls, new vaccines, changing immunization schedules, program funding issues, and provider confusion can lead to inadequate immunization rates and levels of disease protection. Medical providers also report inadequate reimbursement, storage and stocking issues, documentation hassles, language barriers, counseling issues, and safety concerns as reasons for not offering vaccinations onsite (Riley, 2006). System barriers such as vaccine costs, a lack of centralized vaccine registry and universal vaccination records, and the complexity of the immunization schedule may also affect immunization rates (Stevenson, 2009).

Several demonstration and research projects have had success in raising immunization rates including community partnerships that involve school-based immunization programs. Such programs reach a large population of underimmunized children. They also bypass difficulties, such as lack of adequate insurance (Rodewald and Orenstein, 2006) or lack of priority on the part of families for preventive care measures (Rusk, 2006).

Parents refuse vaccinations for their children based on many issues: concerns of vaccine safety, including safety of vaccine ingredients; inadequate safety testing; concerns that they may cause learning disabilities; and concerns that they are painful. Some parents express a cynical belief that vaccines are recommended for the profit of pharmaceutical companies, medical providers, and government agencies. The success of vaccine programs has decreased the incidence of disease leaving many people with no experience or awareness of the seriousness of vaccine-preventable diseases. Some parents believe that vaccine-preventable diseases are not very serious and that natural immunity is superior to immunity from a vaccine. Some cite religious reasons for avoiding vaccinations, and others believe that the number of vaccines given overloads or weakens a child's immune system. There has been a great deal of negative and high-profile media attention concerning a risk of autism (not supported by evidence) associated with vaccination despite overwhelming evidence that no such association exists (Chatterjee and O'Keefe, 2010; National Network for Immunization Information, 2009; Price et al, 2010).

Some helpful points to keep in mind when discussing immunizations with parents include (Amer, 2009):
- Listen: Understand that parents may not use the same decision-making processes that medical providers use.
- Be familiar with common myths regarding the dangers of vaccines and be prepared to address them. Inform concerned parents that all childhood vaccines are available in thimerosal-free forms.
- Be honest and respectful when discussing the known risks and benefits of vaccination and attempt to correct misperceptions or misinformation.
- Emphasize the balance between risks and benefits of vaccination and that the risk associated with disease is far greater than the risk of a serious adverse vaccine reaction.
- Provide parents with printed educational materials from a reliable source, such as the local health department, and encourage parents to visit reputable websites for more information (e.g., the Immunization Action Coalition, the National Network for Immunization Information, the CDC, and the American Academy of Pediatrics [AAP]).

Some medical providers have explored the option of dismissing patients from their practice because of parental refusal of vaccinations. Dismissal may adversely affect access to care and health outcomes for a child (Phillips, 2010). Over time, with subsequent visits, the opportunity for education, the development of respectful communication and an ongoing relationship may help parents to reconsider their choices about immunization. When parents decline immunization it is important to document vaccine discussions and ask parents to sign a vaccine refusal form (available at www.cispimmunize. org/pro/pdf/RefusaltoVaccinate_2pageform.pdf). The AAP discourages patient dismissal but supports it when there is a substantial level of distrust, notable differences in the philosophy about care, or poor communication between provider and patient or family. Advanced notice is requisite (Diekema and AAP Committee on Bioethics, 2005).

VACCINES FOR CHILDREN PROGRAM

The Vaccines for Children (VFC) program enables medical providers to obtain all or most Advisory Committee on Immunization Practices (ACIP)-authorized vaccines without cost. These vaccines are provided free to children younger than 19 years of age who are Medicaid eligible, are uninsured, are Native American or Alaska Native. To date the VFC program pays for 50% of all vaccines administered to children in the U.S. under the age of 6 years (Smith, 2010). In addition, children whose insurance does not cover immunizations (underinsured) are eligible to receive vaccines at federally qualified health centers and rural health clinics. All states receive a set level of federal VFC funds. Some states augment that amount to cover more vaccines.

Providers wishing to participate need only to contact their local state Medicaid office to enroll; they need not be a Medicaid-participating provider. Free vaccines plus their shipping costs and an administrative fee, which varies from state to state, are included in this incentive package; there is a minimum of paperwork for the provider.

VACCINE SHORTAGES

The Vaccine Management Business Improvement Project is in charge of addressing all problems related to vaccine shortages including vaccine procurement, ordering, distribution, and management. In addition, federal legislative proposals are underway to ensure federal-private sector partnerships to provide necessary incentives and protections to quickly bring additional and better vaccines to market. Ongoing information regarding vaccine shortages and expected procurement data are available at the National Center for Immunization and Respiratory Disease website (www.cdc.gov/vaccines/vac-gen/shortages).

Medical providers should develop their own tracking system to recall patients whose vaccinations were delayed because of supply shortages. During such times providers should check with the websites of AAP, ACIP, and National

Immunization Program recommendations regarding vaccine deferrals, prioritization of high-risk children, and suspensions of school and childcare entry requirements.

VACCINE SAFETY AND RESOURCES FOR PROVIDERS

Informed consent is critical when discussing the benefits and risks of vaccination. The National Childhood Vaccine Injury Act of 1986 (Public Law 99–660, amended by Public Law 101–239) calls for standardized consent forms (Vaccine Information Statement [VIS]). All practitioners are required to use these forms to fulfill their duty to warn the public about possible adverse events. VIS forms are available in 30 different languages on the CDC website. The act also requires that the vaccine lot number, site of inoculation, and name of the person administering the vaccine be included in the medical record. Some state laws require a parental signed consent form. People administering vaccines should be knowledgeable about the signs and symptoms of an allergic reaction and be prepared to treat such a reaction.

The National Childhood Vaccine Injury Act also requires health care providers to report vaccine-related adverse events that occur after immunization so that unexpected patterns and safety concerns can be addressed. The suspected events are to be reported to the USDHHS Vaccine Adverse Event Reporting System (VAERS), using their standard confidential form. Information on which vaccine-associated injuries are reportable as well as official report forms can be downloaded from www.vaers.hhs.gov or from the U.S. Food and Drug Administration (FDA) website.

In 2001 the CDC established the Clinical Immunization Safety Assessment (CISA) network in response to the realization that many adverse events became evident only after completion of prelicensure studies of vaccines and that many primary care providers would not necessarily be privy to such events. CISA develops research protocols around any given adverse event; helps understand the adverse event at the possible genetic, population, or subpopulation level; establishes risk levels; and serves as a referral source for clinicians. Providers can receive vaccine safety information, including how to manage postvaccine adverse events from the CDC.

VACCINE CONTROVERSIES

As reported in the Institute of Medicine (IOM) Immunization Safety Review Committee's intensive review (IOM, 2004) and reaffirmed by the AAP (2010a), there has been no substantiated evidence of a causal relationship between thimerosal-containing vaccines or measles, mumps, rubella (MMR) vaccine and "pervasive developmental disorders," such as autism, attention-deficit/hyperactivity disorder (ADHD), speech/language delays, childhood disintegrative disorder, Asperger syndrome, or Rett syndrome. They also reported finding no general connection, no biologic mechanism consistent with a relationship between immunization or an adverse event, or insufficient causal evidence between hepatitis B and demyelinating diseases of the central nervous system (CNS) and peripheral nervous system (multiple sclerosis, acute disseminated encephalomyelitis, optic neuritis, transverse myelitis, Guillain-Barré syndrome [GBS], and brachial neuritis [Stratton et al, 2004]). The IOM also investigated the role

that multiple vaccines might play in causing type 1 diabetes or serious infections. After a review of dozens of scientific research studies, a causal relationship was dismissed. However, there was some mixed evidence among studies regarding a possible connection between multiple vaccines and asthma. The Immunization Safety Review Committee concluded that further research in all these areas was warranted given the public concern with vaccine safety, the threat of increased populations going unvaccinated because of these fears, and the resulting resurgence of preventable diseases. The AAP, IOM, and CDC are good resources for tracking these ongoing studies and their findings.

Vaccines that are thimerosal-free or contain trace amounts are on the CDC's recommended list for childhood immunizations with two exceptions. Multidose vials of inactivated flu vaccine and multidose vials of one of the meningococcal vaccines contain thimerosal. There are thimerosal-free alternatives available for each of these products.

VACCINES ON THE HORIZON

Modern vaccinology research is addressing new vaccine development including *Shigella* conjugate vaccine for children; vaccines for herpes simplex virus types 1 and 2; cytomegalovirus (CMV) (to prevent congenital CMV); Marburg virus (a hemorrhagic fever disease); dengue fever; hantavirus; HIV; West Nile virus (WNV); Lassa fever; drug-resistant pneumococci and staphylococci; enterococci (for traveler's diarrhea prevention); severe acute respiratory syndrome (SARS); Ebola; and urinary tract infections. Several different types of cancer vaccines are under investigation. Other studies are ongoing to develop a conjugate group B streptococcus vaccine for pregnant women to provide passive immunity to their fetuses, a vaccine to cover more serotypes of *Haemophilus influenzae,* and live and subunit parainfluenza type 3 vaccines.

New vaccine delivery systems are being investigated that include skin-patch vaccines (undergoing human trials against the flu and traveler's diarrhea), edible vaccines, and needle-free injections. DNA technology is also being explored for use in encoding host immunogenic antigens.

ACETAMINOPHEN PROPHYLAXIS AFTER VACCINATION?

Research is questioning the wisdom of recommending prophylactic administration of acetaminophen prior to or following vaccines. Significantly lower antibody responses were detected in infants and children vaccinated with a 10-valent pneumococcal nontypeable *H. influenzae* protein D-conjugate vaccine (PHiD-CV) coadministered with the hexavalent diphtheria/tetanus-3-component acellular pertussis/hepatitis B/inactivated poliovirus-types 1, 2, 3/HIB (DTaP-HBV-IPV/HIB) combination and oral rotavirus vaccines given at the recommended scheduling for primary and booster doses. The antibody responses were compared against a group of children who had not received prophylactic acetaminophen (Prymula et al, 2009). Further, an earlier study showed no efficacy to acetaminophen prophylaxis for the prevention of febrile responses following booster vaccination for the DTP vaccine in those 15 to 20 months old (Yalçin et al, 2008).

ACTIVE IMMUNITY

General Principles

Inoculating a child with all or part of a modified product from a microorganism evokes an immune response. Whole organisms (live, attenuated, or killed), modified proteins, and/or sugars are used to prepare certain vaccines. The response to a live attenuated vaccine is often as protective as the natural infection. Antiinvasive, antiadherence, antitoxin, neutralizing antibodies, or other protective responses can be found soon after the vaccination is given. Live attenuated vaccines usually confer broader and longer-lived immunity than the inactivated types that require booster vaccines. Killed and inactivated vaccines can provide systemic protection (IgG antibodies), but may fail to provide local mucosal antibody (IgA). Thus, although protected from systemic illness, a recipient of a killed vaccine can have local colonization or infection that can be a problem during an epidemic. The active and inert vaccine ingredients differ among manufacturers. One must be aware of these components (such as antimicrobials) because of a patient's possible hypersensitivity to the ingredients.

The ACIP of the CDC, the AAP, and the American Academy of Family Physicians (AAFP) annually approve a new unified recommended childhood immunization schedule so U.S. providers can download the most recent immunization schedules at the beginning of each calendar year (http://www.cdc.gov/vaccines/recs/schedules/child-schedule.htm). There are three schedules covering the recommended immunizations: for those 0-6 years old; for those 7-18 years old; and a catch-up schedule for individuals 4 months to 18 years who start their vaccines late or who are delayed. Other countries may follow the same schedule or determine their own recommendations (World Health Organization [WHO] can be consulted at www.who.int).

Maternal antibodies neutralize certain vaccines, so some are delayed until the child is 1 year old (e.g., measles). Infants vaccinated in the first year of life require more inoculations than older children. Children who are not immunized in the first year of life should be vaccinated according to the most recent catch-up immunization schedule previously mentioned. Missed vaccinations should be given as soon as possible, and the entire series does not need to be repeated.

Vaccines given outside the U.S. are acceptable as long as there is reliable written evidence of administration (including dates and number of doses), and the age and spacing are the same as CDC recommendations. If in doubt, antibody titers can be checked or the child reimmunized. Generally most vaccines used worldwide have been produced with adequate quality control and are reliable, but vaccine handling can be suspect (Pickering et al, 2009). If in doubt, immunize. Children adopted from overseas generally need all immunizations repeated to account for any inaccuracies in reporting or vaccine potency questions. Proper storage of vaccines and correct immunization technique are critical for optimal results. The manufacturer's package inserts provide this information.

Research is ongoing regarding the effect of environmental pollutants on the body's immune responses to vaccinations. Increased levels of prenatal and/or postnatal polychlorinated biphenyls (PCBs) have been correlated with lowered antibody response to tetanus and diphtheria vaccines in children at 18 months and 7 years old (Heilmann et al, 2006), but not at 6 months (Jusko et al, 2010). Early postnatal exposure to this agent was the primary predictor of decreased response in the formerly cited study.

The ACIP offers some general vaccination guidelines including (Pickering et al, 2009):
- Vaccine doses may be given 4 days prior to or later than minimum intervals or ages to provide some schedule flexibility.
- If two live virus parenteral vaccines are given less than 28 days apart, the vaccine given second should be disregarded; repeat this second vaccine at least 4 weeks later.
- Do not aspirate the syringe before injection (unproven necessity); do not recap the needle after use.
- When multiple vaccines are given on the same extremity, the sites of injection should be at least 1 inch apart; the anterolateral aspect of the thigh is the preferred site for this.
- Parent or guardian recollection of a child's immunization status may not be reliable; use only written, dated records.
- Reimmunization of an immune individual is not harmful.
- Reduced or divided doses of vaccines should not be given.
- Techniques to decrease the pain of immunizations include applying pressure to the injection site for about 10 seconds before vaccination; putting sucrose on the tongue or pacifier of an infant; having children blow a pinwheel or bubbles during the procedure.
- Those administering vaccines should know how to recognize and respond to syncope following immunization and severe allergic reactions, including anaphylaxis. Individuals with severe allergy to latex should not be administered vaccines that come from vials or syringes that contain latex (vial stoppers, syringe plungers can contain latex; see package insert).
- Failure to transport and store vaccines correctly can lead to vaccine failure; there should be designated personnel to daily monitor and document storage requirements (temperature, safety precautions).
- In some circumstances (imminent travel, delayed immunizations) an accelerated schedule is available from the ACIP.
- The major contraindication for any vaccine is anaphylaxis with a prior dose or to a vaccine component.

Considerations When Choosing Inactive Vaccines

Information about side effects, precautions, contraindications, and special case considerations of the various attenuated or killed vaccines is available from the CDC, from the manufacturers' package inserts, or from a current AAP *Red Book* (Pickering et al, 2009). Some of the more general side effects from these vaccines include (Pickering et al, 2009):
- Fever and local reactions (swelling, pain, erythema), usually within the first 24 to 72 hours (diphtheria/tetanus/acellular pertussis [DTaP]; hepatitis A virus [HAV]; *Haemophilus influenzae* type b conjugate [Hib]; hepatitis B virus [HBV]; pneumococcal conjugate [PCV-13]; and meningococcal [can include headache and irritability] vaccines).
- Sterile abscesses due to a hypersensitivity response to the vaccine itself or to an adjuvant (notably alum) (DTaP).

Some general contraindications for these vaccines include (Pickering et al, 2009):
- Anaphylaxis: To a prior dose; to neomycin, polymyxin B, or streptomycin (IPV); to alum or 2-phenoxyethanol (Havrix only for HAV).

- Pregnancy (human papilloma virus vaccine [HPV]), or used cautiously (IPV)
- Allergies to vaccine components or yeast (HBV and HPV vaccines)
- Moderate to severe acute infection (HPV and Hib vaccines)

Inactivated Vaccines

Diphtheria and Tetanus Toxoids with Pertussis Vaccine. Diphtheria and tetanus toxoids with acellular pertussis vaccine (DTaP) are used in the U.S. for children less than 7 years old; the whole-cell product, diphtheria and tetanus toxoids with pertussis vaccine (DTP), no longer available in the U.S., may be available in other parts of the world. Tdap is given to those 7 years of age or older. The DTaP has fewer side effects than the whole-cell vaccine. If given in another country, DTP is an acceptable alternative to DTaP; once in the U.S., DTaP would be given to complete a primary series. Combination vaccines are available that include DTaP, HiB, and other vaccines; however, single DTaP products cannot be mixed with any other vaccine.

Universal immunization with DTaP (or DTP) is the only effective control measure for these illnesses and are given to children under the age of seven. The duration of immunity after pertussis infection has not been established, but it is believed to be short (Pickering et al, 2009). Diphtheria and tetanus toxoids are highly effective vaccines as proven by the rarity of these diseases in the U.S. All of the available vaccines are equally effective, but differ slightly in their components.

Evidence from research studies suggests that controlling pertussis in young infants may depend on older children and adults receiving a booster with Tdap rather than with Td. This is the reason behind the newest recommendation that those needing a booster (or for wound management) be given a single dose of Tdap. This includes 7-10 year olds who may be underimmunized or whose immunizations history is incomplete (replaces the prior 11-12 year old adolescent booster dose recommendation), adolescents, those pregnant, and adults (including if ≥ 65 years and older in contact with infants under 12 months of age and health care workers of any age) (AAP, 2011a). Tetanus prophylaxis as part of wound management (Table 23-2) is based on age, nature of the wound, type of prior tetanus-diptheria toxoid vaccine, and vaccine reaction history.

Polio Vaccine. Prior to January 2000 the live oral trivalent polio vaccine (OPV) was the vaccine of choice. However, as the incidence of wild-type polio decreased and the cases of vaccine-associated paralytic polio (VAPP) outnumbered wild virus cases, the recommended vaccine for polio changed to inactivated polio vaccine (IPV). IPV is the only polio vaccine available in the U.S.; seroconversion to each of the three serotypes of polio ranges from 99% to 100% after three doses. If mass vaccination is needed to control wild polio outbreaks of paralytic polio, OPV would be considered a public health intervention because IPV does not protect against intestinal infection with wild virus. The need for booster dosages of enhanced IPV has not been determined; immunity is believed to possibly be lifelong. The CDC provides guidelines for when polio vaccinations should be considered for those immunocompromised or at risk of imminent exposure from travel or outbreak, including adults.

Haemophilus influenzae Type B Vaccine. Of the six serotypes of *H. influenzae*, type B is the most virulent, accounting for pneumonia, bacteremia, meningitis, epiglottitis, septic arthritis, cellulitis, otitis media, purulent pericarditis and other less common infections, notably in those under the age of 4 years. Until the advent of the first Hib polysaccharide vaccine in 1987, it was the most common cause of bacterial meningitis in children in the U.S. The issuance of this vaccine resulted in a phenomenal 99% decrease in the incidence of HIB disease in children less than 5 years. Most new cases in the U.S. now occur in those underimmunized or in infants who have not completed their primary series (Pickering et al, 2009). It continues to be a problematic pathogen in countries that do not have this vaccine routinely available.

Guidelines for chemoprophylaxis are available for exposed, unimmunized household contacts younger than 4 years of age who are at risk of invasive HIB disease.

Hepatitis A Virus Vaccine. The primary HAV vaccine initiatives have focused on children in order to prevent transmission to adults in whom the illness is likely to be serious. Current guidelines include universal vaccination for those 1 to 18 years old and for other subsets of the population (discussed later).

TABLE 23-2 Tetanus Prophylaxis in Wound Management

Previous Tetanus Immunization	Clean, Minor Wounds	Other Wounds (Contaminated By Dirt, Feces, Soil, Saliva; Burns, Avulsions, Punctures; Due to Missiles, Crushing, Frostbite)
Uncertain or fewer than three doses	Td or Tdap only*	Td or Tdap* and TIG† within 3 days
Three or more doses	Td or Tdap* *only* if last dose >10 years ago	Td or Tdap* if last dose >5 years ago

*In those ≥7 years old, (including adolescents, those pregnant, adults, those ≥65 years in contact with infants >12 months old and healthcare workers of all ages), Tdap is preferred for prophylaxis as a booster dose if not given prior (applies if Td has been previously given; there is no minimum interval necessary between Td and Tdap); any subsequently needed prophylaxis or catch-up doses would be given as Td per catch-up schedule or every 10 years if caught-up. In children younger than 7 years old, use DTaP (DT if pertussis is contraindicated).

†If tetanus immune globulin (TIG) is not available, intravenous immunoglobulin (IVIG) can be substituted.

TIG, tetanus immune globulin.

Data from Academy of Pediatrics, Committee on Infectious Disease: Policy statement: additional recommendations for use of tetanus toxoid, reduced-content diphtheria toxoid, and acellular pertussis vaccine (Tdap), Pediatrics 128(4):809-812, 2011; Pickering LK, Baker CJ, Kimberlin DW, et al: *Tetanus. Red book: 2009 report of the committee on infectious diseases* ed 28, Elk Grove Village, IL, 2009, American Academy of pediatrics, p 657.

The two inactivated HAV vaccines licensed in the U.S. have seroconversion rates of greater than 99% after the second vaccine. They are conjectured to provide immunity for up to 14 to 20 years in children and for a minimum of 25 years in adults (Fiore et al, 2006). A recommendation for a booster dose has not been determined.

HAV vaccine can be administered simultaneously with other childhood vaccines, but should be given at a separate injection site (intramuscular [IM] injection in the deltoid). The risk of vaccination to a pregnant woman is considered low to nonexistent. Seroconversion of immunocompromised patients (including those with HIV) may be suboptimal.

Recommendations also target the following groups of individuals (Fiore et al, 2006):

- Those traveling to countries where HAV is endemic (notably Central or South America, Mexico, Asia [except Japan], Africa, and eastern Europe [see www.cdc.gov/travel])
- Children and adolescents residing in and in contact with others from communities with a high incidence or outbreak of HAV
- Children in diapers in daycare centers with high rates of HAV
- Men who have sex with men
- Severe illness (e.g., chronic liver disease)
- Illicit-drug users (using injectable or noninjectable drugs)
- Those with blood-clotting disorders (e.g., hemophiliacs)
- Healthy persons who are older than 1 year who are household members and close contacts, including baby sitters, during the 60-day period after the arrival of an international adoptee (AAP, 2011b).

The use of postexposure IG versus a single dose of HAV vaccine shows equal efficacy for preventing symptomatic disease if given within 14 days of exposure (Pickering et al, 2009).

Hepatitis B Virus Vaccine. Two recombinant HBV vaccines, composed of HBsAg protein, are licensed in the U.S. They are equally immunogenic and interchangeable when used as directed according to manufacturer's guidelines. The seroconversion rate is 90% to 95%. Immunogenicity appears to be 20 or more years. Routine booster doses are not recommended except for patients receiving hemodialysis or for other immunocompromised patients whose annual anti-HBs levels have fallen to less than 10 milli-international units/mL. Pregnancy and lactation are not contraindicated for vaccination. (See Table 23-3 (under Comments) on the immunoprophylaxis management of the newborn whose mothers are HBV surface antigen [HBsAg] positive.)

Although recommendations call for universal immunization of all newborns weighing equal to or more than 2000 g prior to hospital discharge (those preterm weighing <2000 g should wait a month), young children, and adolescents not previously vaccinated, there are also specific individuals who should receive HBV immunization (Pickering et al, 2009):

- Hemophiliac patients and other recipients of certain blood products
- Intravenous (IV) drug users
- Heterosexual persons with a history of multiple sex partners in the previous 6 months or with recent sexually transmitted infections
- Men who have sex with men
- Household and sexual contacts who are chronic carriers of HBV or who are HBsAg positive

- Adoptees from foreign countries despite their immunization history; household members of adoptees and those foreign born from HBV-endemic, high-risk countries or children born to first-generation immigrants from such endemic areas
- Alaska Native and Pacific Islander children
- Specific infants, children, and other household contacts in populations of high HBV endemicity
- Staff and residents of residential institutions for the developmentally disabled
- Staff and attendees of nonresidential daycare and school programs for the developmentally delayed if an identified HBV carrier is known to attend or poses risk of infecting others
- Hemodialysis patients
- Health care workers and others with occupational risk
- International travelers who travel to areas of high or intermediate HBV endemicity and who otherwise may be at risk
- Inmates in juvenile detention and other correctional facilities

Either HBV vaccine plus HBIG or HBV vaccine alone can be used effectively for postexposure immunoprophylaxis if given within 12 to 24 hours of exposure (Pickering et al, 2009).

Human Papillomavirus Vaccine. Gardasil (referred to as HPV4) is a quadrivalent vaccine that protects against the two primary oncogenic strains types 16 and 18, as well as types 6 and 11. The efficacy rate is greater than 99% after a series of three doses with antibody responses greater for females 9 through 15 years as compared with those older than 15 years or age. It is unclear about the cross-protection against cervical intraepithelial neoplasia types not included in the vaccine. There is no protection for HPV oncogenic types acquired prior to the vaccine.

Cervarix (referred to as HPV2) targets HPV types 16 and 18 and is encouraged for use in females 9 through 26 years. It has shown some cross-protection against incident infection of other HPV vaccine types that also cause cancer; its efficacy rate is greater than 99% after a series of three doses for types 16 and 18 (CDC, 2010b).

Preadolescent females (11 or 12 years; as early as 9 years) and all sexually active women (through 26 years old) are encouraged to routinely receive the vaccine because there is benefit before they have been exposed to any and all of the different HPVs included in the vaccine. The vaccines should not replace routine cervical cancer screening. The vaccine is offered under the VFC program for females.

The FDA has approved Gardasil for males ages 9 through 26 years to prevent genital warts and male HPV-associated cancers; the CDC has not recommended Gardasil be made part of a male's routine immunizations (CDC, 2010c). Males at greatest risk for infection and associated disease include men who have sex with men.

Duration studies have only been done up through the first 5 years post-vaccination, and no waning of protection has been seen (Pickering et al, 2009). Prevaccine Papanicolaou (Pap) or pregnancy tests are not warranted; providers are encouraged to report any exposure to these vaccines during pregnancy to the manufacturer.

Influenza Vaccine. The ACIP recommends universal vaccination for those more than 6 months of age, including all adults, unless contraindicated. Influenza disease rates are highest among children less than the age of 2 years, in those equal to or older than 65 years, and in those with high-risk medical conditions. Children serve as a major vector for influenza transmission because of their own high rates for contracting the virus; they also shed the virus at higher rates and for longer periods than adults. After even one influenza illness, people remain susceptible to other influenza strains; severe epidemics have occurred historically. See the discussion regarding influenza later in this chapter.

Two multivalent vaccines are available; each contains three virus strains (influenza A [H3N2 and seasonal H1N1], and B). The trivalent inactivated vaccine (TIV) is available IM for those 6 months or older, whereas the live-attenuated inactivated vaccine (LAIV) is restricted to healthy, nonpregnant individuals 2 years to 49 years. The LAIV is only available as an intranasal prefilled spray for these age groups (further information about restrictions is available from the CDC). The number of dosages depends on the age and vaccine history during any prior influenza season. The vaccine should be given yearly.

The influenza vaccine is formulated yearly based on epidemiologic forecasts. Usually one or two influenza A virus strains are changed based on the anticipated dominant influenza strain(s) projected to infect the population in the approaching flu season. Major changes in viral antigens generally occur at 10-year intervals. This process is called *antigenic shift*. Minor variations that occur are called *antigenic drift*. These changes within the virus can prevent the body's immune system from recognizing the altered strain and mounting an immunologic response.

Because other common childhood viral agents can cause diseases that look like influenza, the effect of the vaccine is less likely to be evident in children. The efficacy rate ranges from 50% to 95% for TIV in healthy children older than 2 years (higher if the vaccine strain closely matches the circulating wild strain); the efficacy is lower in children less than 24 months of age. LAIV has shown an efficacy rate of between 86% and 96%. Some studies have shown that LAIV has a greater relative efficacy when compared with TIV in younger children (Pickering et al, 2009).

The vaccine should be given as soon as it becomes available before the onset of the yearly influenza season. It can be given any time until the anticipated end of the infective season to cover intermittent peaks (including April). Different preparations of the vaccine have different recommendations for administration as to site and concurrent use with live vaccines. The CDC provides an algorithm for determining the dosage; providers can sign up for vaccine updates from the CDC as the influenza season progresses.

Meningococcal Vaccine. Of the 13 serotypes of *Neisseria meningitidis*, serogroups B, C, Y, and W135 are most often associated with meningococcal disease. Serogroups B, C, and Y each cause one third of the diseases in the U.S., whereas serogroup A is rare. Most infections in children younger than the age of 1 year are attributed to serogroup B, whereas C, Y, and W135 cause three fourths of infections in those 11 years and older. There is no vaccine for serogroup B, whereas the other four serogroups are covered by current vaccines. Meningococcal disease is associated with high morbidity and mortality in those who are infected, though only 1400 to 2800 infections are diagnosed annually in the U.S. (Cushing and Cohn, 2008).

Three vaccines are available and have some age restrictions. These include two quadrivalent conjugate meningococcal

vaccines (MCV4) (meningococcal [Men] ACWY [Groups A, C, Y and W-135]-D [Menactra] and meningococcal [Groups A, C, Y and W-135] oligosaccharide diphtheria CRM_{197} conjugate vaccine [MenACWY-CRM, Menveo]) and meningococcal polysaccharide vaccine (MPSV4). They are given to those high risk for contracting meningococcal infection, including all adolescents; college freshmen living in dormitories; military recruits; those with functional asplenia or persistent deficiencies (and including infants 9-23 months); and travelers to hyperendemic or epidemic countries.

MenACWY-D can be given to infants as young as 9 months and up through the age of 55 years if at high risk; MenACWY-CRM is given to those 2 to 55 years of age; and MPSV4 is only used if MCV4 is unavailable and for those older than 55 years of age. Either MenACWY-D or MenACWY-CRM is indicated for routine vaccine for those 11-12 years old with a booster given at age 16 years or at age 13-18 years if not previously vaccinated. Individuals with prior GBS infection should not receive MCV4. Any possible cases of GBS following vaccination should be reported to VAERS; as an alternative, MPSV4 can be considered (Pickering et al, 2009). Depending on when an individual was initially vaccinated with MCV4 or MPSV4 and his or her risk factors, reimmunization may be recommended every 5 years if risk remains (see CDC website for further information) (CDC, 2009a).

Pneumococcal Vaccines. There are 91 known serotypes of pneumococcus, and there has been a shift in the pneumococcal strains responsible for illness. As a result, more illness is ascribed to the serotype 19A, which was not covered by the previous pneumococcal conjugate vaccine, PCV7. Pneumococcal conjugate vaccine 13 (PCV13), covering 6 additional serotypes, became available in 2010. This vaccine provides protection against serotype 19A and has replaced PCV7 (CDC, 2010e). Children under 5 years of age who have completed the four-dose PCV7 series should receive a single PCV13 dose. Children who have not completed their PCV7 series should complete with PCV13. Older children and adolescents (6 to 18 years) with certain medical conditions may benefit from PCV13 vaccine even if they have previously completed a series of PCV7 or the 23-valent pneumococcal polysaccharide vaccine (PPSV23) (Hayden, 2010). Refer to the CDC website for specific recommendations during the time of transition between PCV7 and PCV13 vaccine formulations.

23-Valent Polysaccharide Pneumococcal Vaccine (PPSV23). PPSV23 confers broader coverage against 23 pneumococcal serotypes rather than the 13 in PCV13. PPSV23 is administered to children 2 years and older and adults at high risk or presumed high risk of pneumococcal disease (see the CDC website for specific recommendations). The number of doses varies according to the number of prior PCV7 or PCV13 vaccines given and the age of the child. Children younger than 2 years of age have shown poor immunogenicity to this vaccine; duration of protection is regarded as relatively short (Pickering et al, 2009).

Live Vaccines
Precautions Regarding Administration of Live Vaccines. It is important for providers to consult with infectious disease experts and authoritative reference resources when contemplating administering live vaccines to immunocompromised individuals. Recommendations may differ according to the individual's degree and type of compromise. If individuals cannot produce antibodies, they are

unlikely to respond to a vaccine; if a live vaccine is given while on IGIV, the virus will be neutralized by antibodies in the IGIV product. An individual with a low T-cell count or a cellular immunodeficiency can be seriously compromised if given a LAIV. A child with DiGeorge syndrome, HIV infection, cancers, immunosuppression, or other cellular immune problems should not receive such viral vaccines until the T-cell function is within an appropriate range.

Bacille Calmette-Guérin Vaccine. Bacille Calmette-Guérin (BCG) live vaccine was developed in the early part of the twentieth century to prevent the spread of TB. The vaccines in use worldwide differ in composition and efficacy because of the differing attenuated substrains of *Mycobacterium bovis* from which they are derived. Two BCG vaccines are licensed for use in the U.S. The WHO does not recommend any particular BCG over another (WHO, 2009). The vaccine is widely recommended at birth as a public health measure in more than 100 countries in order to prevent disseminated and other potentially fatal effects from *Mycobacterium tuberculosis* disease (meningitis and miliary) in infants and children. The efficacy of BCG in this population is approximately 75%. For all populations worldwide, the efficacy is closer to 50% (WHO, 2009). The vaccine does not protect against primary or reactivation of latent infection. Countries have their own immunization schedules regarding BCG vaccination. The vaccine is ideally given to infants at birth. Until 2 months of age, healthy infants may be given BCG without having a tuberculin skin test (TST), unless suspected of having congenital infection; after that, a TST is required prior to vaccination with BCG. In infants who are exposed to smear-positive pulmonary TB shortly after birth, 6 months of prophylactic isoniazid should be given prior to receiving the BCG vaccine (WHO, 2010). New recombinant BCG and live attenuated TB vaccines are currently under development using state-of-the-art technology.

In the U.S., BCG use is not generally recommended. BCG is considered in special circumstances for infants and children with negative TST who: (1) live with persons with infectious pulmonary TB who are untreated or ineffectually treated; cannot be removed from those persons; and are without a source of long-term primary treatment; or (2) live with persons who have drug-resistant forms of TB (to isoniazid and rifampin) and cannot be separated from those persons.

Before administering BCG in the U.S., pediatric TB experts should be consulted. Health care workers in high-risk settings also may be candidates for BCG (Pickering et al, 2009). A complete guideline for the use of BCG is available from the WHO.

Tuberculin Skin Testing. BCG vaccine can produce a mild to severe hypersensitivity reaction, giving a false-positive reaction in children who receive the Mantoux skin test. However, children with prior BCG vaccination should receive the skin test. The size of the reaction can vary depending on several factors: the age of the BCG vaccine itself, its quality, the strain of *M. bovis* used, the number of past doses of BCG vaccine received, nutritional status, immunologic factors, infection with environmental mycobacteria, and the frequency of skin testing (boosts the response). The degree of positivity decreases over time, depending on the age at vaccination. The role of the skin test is limited in TB-endemic countries (WHO, 2004).

Measles-Mumps-Rubella Vaccine. MMR is a trivalent vaccine; this combination is also offered as a quadrivalent vaccine with varicella (MMRV). It is still possible, but often difficult, to obtain measles, mumps, and rubella vaccines individually.

The ACIP recommends that health care personnel demonstrate evidence of immunity to each of these diseases. Proof of immunity is based on having received the vaccines (measles: two doses; mumps: two doses; rubella: one dose), or laboratory confirmation/evidence of disease, or born prior to 1957 (ACIP, 2009).

Measles. A live further-attenuated vaccine using a chick embryo cell culture is licensed for use in the U.S. The seroconversion rate is greater than 99% for those receiving two appropriately spaced doses (Pickering et al, 2009). Children who do not receive the second dose at kindergarten should be revaccinated at the earliest possible time. Persons vaccinated with killed vaccine, live vaccine and IgG, and those vaccinated before 12 months old should be revaccinated twice more. In children receiving synagis, MMR vaccine can be given on schedule.

The measles component is responsible for almost all the adverse reactions to the MMR vaccine. Transient rashes (about 2%) and fever of 103° F (39.4° C) (up to 15%) occur approximately 5 to 12 days after vaccination. Those with fever usually have no other symptoms, and the fever generally resolves within 1 to 2 (up to 5) days. Febrile convulsion is an infrequent occurrence in children; however, the risk increases 8 to 14 days after primary vaccination with MMR (1 per 3000 to 4000 children). Allergic reactions to trace amounts of one of the components (e.g., neomycin, gelatin) and thrombocytopenia have been reported, but they are very rare occurrences.

Newer studies have shown that when the combination MMRV vaccine is given for the primary dose, the risk for febrile seizures increases twofold (one additional seizure in 2300 to 2600 children over MMR alone when varicella is given at the same time in a different site) in children between 12 and 23 months. The ACIP recommends that health care providers discuss this increase in risk with parents and offer either the MMR and varicella separately as the primary dose for this age group or the combination (MMRV). The MMRV given as the second dose between 4 and 6 years is not associated with the same increased risk for a febrile seizure (Marin et al, 2010).

The contraindications to measles vaccine should be reviewed prior to administering the vaccine to those also needing a TST; who are pregnant or planning to become pregnant within the next 28 days; who have had an anaphylactic reaction to gelatin, egg, neomycin, or prior MMR vaccine; or who have a febrile illness. There are selected recommendations for giving MMR to those with compromised immune systems and for those who have received immunoglobulins and blood products. Guidelines are available from manufacturer package inserts or from the CDC. Encephalopathy and encephalitis are rare complications of the vaccine, and they occur at a much lower rate than after the natural disease.

Measles Exposure or Epidemics. In cases of exposure to measles infection, the measles vaccine can provide some protection if given within 72 hours. IG can be used within 6 days of exposure to measles infection and prevents or modifies the infection in susceptible people (children and adolescents with HIV infection and children born to HIV-infected women whose own HIV infection status is unknown). During measles outbreaks, immunization can begin as early as 6 months of age. Two more doses of the vaccine are then given at the routine recommended ages.

Mumps. The live-attenuated mumps vaccine is given in combination with MMR or MMRV. It is estimated to achieve an 88% to 95% seroconversion rate after the two appropriately spaced doses (Pickering et al, 2009). The length of protection is being monitored and may be shorter than once anticipated. Fever, parotitis, and orchitis have been rarely reported as side effects; causality has not been established for other effects such as febrile seizures, rash, pruritus, nerve deafness, encephalopathy, encephalitis, purpura, or paralysis. These side effects occur at a much lower rate than they do after the natural disease. Contraindications and the use of IG are the same as for measles.

Rubella. The live-attenuated rubella vaccine is given in combination with measles and rubella (MMR) or with added varicella (MMRV). The seroconversion rate is greater than 95%. Mild reactions to the vaccine include fever (5% to 15%), lymphadenopathy, rash (5%), joint pain (less than 1%) and arthralgia (usually seen more in unvaccinated postpubertal females; onset 7 to 21 days after vaccine), small peripheral joint pain, and paresthesias. Contraindications are the same as for the measles vaccine. If inadvertently given to a pregnant woman, it does not serve as an indication for termination of the pregnancy. However, the woman should be informed that the fetus is at a maximum theoretic risk of 1.3% to exhibit signs of infection rather than congenital defects (CDC, 2001). Refer to the AAP *Red Book* or CDC for information regarding special vaccination precautions for children who are immunocompromised.

Females less than 13 years of age without documentation of rubella immunity (documented second dose of MMR or laboratory confirmation) should be the focus for vaccination. Postpubertal females should be evaluated for rubella susceptibility and given the vaccine if indicated; routine prenatal screening is warranted.

Measles, Mumps, Rubella, and Varicella. Combination MMR and varicella vaccine is as effective as when MMR and varicella vaccines are given separately, avoids potentially missing the administration of one of these vaccines, allows fewer vaccinations, and has excellent immunogenicity. See the prior discussion under measles side effects regarding the increased risk of febrile seizures with the MMRV versus when MMR and varicella are given at the same time in different injection sites.

Varicella Vaccine. This LAIV from the Oka strain of varicella-zoster virus (VZV) is well-tolerated and immunogenic. Postlicensure studies have shown seroconversion rates ranging from 70% to 90% after one dose; a second dose raises the rate to greater than 95% (Marin et al, 2007). Two vaccines are licensed for use in the U.S: a single-antigen vaccine and quadrivalent vaccine with measles, mumps and rubella (MMRV).

A small percentage of vaccinees (20%) develop localized pain, erythema, and tenderness. Others (3% to 5%) may develop a mild, generalized maculopapular rash or a varicelliform eruption (3% to 5%, with a few lesions that are generally nonvesicular) after vaccination. The varicelliform rash generally occurs within 2 weeks of vaccination, and wild-type varicella-zoster virus has been isolated from these lesions. A short period of fever may also occur 5 to 12 days after the vaccine. Given the low risk of secondary transmission, immunocompromised household contacts do not need to be isolated from recently vaccinated individuals. Those that contract varicella infection after being immunized usually have minimal fever, fewer than 50 lesions, and recover more rapidly than if they had not been vaccinated.

When to Consider Postexposure Prophylaxis for Varicella Disease. Postexposure varicella-zoster immune globulin (VariZIG) is available to those for whom exposure poses significant risk. It is available 24 hours per day from FFF Enterprises (1-800-843-7477), and participation requires strict compliance to forms and protocols. As a substitute, IGIV, acyclovir, or varicella vaccine (given within 72 hours [and possibly up to 120 hours] after exposure) can be considered (Pickering et al, 2009). The indications for prophylaxis are included in Table 23-3. Other individuals are also considered for prophylaxis if significant exposure to varicella or zoster occurs; guidelines are available from the CDC or current AAP *Red Book*.

There are limited data on acyclovir as a postexposure prophylaxis measure for healthy children.

The varicella vaccine should be given 5 months after VariZIG, unless varicella disease occurred despite VariZIG administration. Serologic testing to determine vaccine-induced antibody response may be unreliable and should not be used to determine susceptibility. The test is more reliable for diagnosing natural infection, but not in those who are immunocompromised (Pickering et al, 2009).

Rotavirus Vaccine. An estimated four out of five children are likely to be infected with a rotavirus before 5 years old. There are two rotavirus vaccines licensed in the U.S., oral human-bovine reassortant pentavalent rotavirus (RV5) and oral human attenuated rotavirus (RV1). They are both effective vaccine formulations; contraindications include a history of intussusception or severe combined immunodeficiency disease. Dosing differs between the two. Both vaccines demonstrate similar safety and efficacy profiles; the AAP has no preference (Pickering et al, 2009). Ideally the same vaccine should be used, but this is not absolute given extenuating circumstances (vaccine name unknown or unavailable). Children with immune deficiencies may be those with the greatest need for disease protection and those at highest risk for serious effects from a live virus vaccine. Refer to the CDC website or AAP *Red Book* for information on contraindications, warnings and precautions, and immunization of children with specific health conditions prior to administration. Consultation with an immunologist may be helpful in particularly complex situations.

Smallpox Vaccine. There is one smallpox vaccine licensed in the U.S. containing a live vaccinia virus to protect against variola major and variola minor. Smallpox vaccine should not be routinely given. In the case of a smallpox outbreak, high-risk individuals will be vaccinated per CDC guidelines issued at the time. Containment of an outbreak is discussed later in this chapter under Infectious Agents Used in Bioterrorism, Smallpox.

PASSIVE IMMUNITY: THE IMMUNOGLOBULINS

Passive immunization entails immunizing an individual with a solution of preexisting antibodies to prevent or amend an infectious disease. These antibodies are derived from sera of pooled human IG, illness-specific human IG, antibodies formulated from animals, or monoclonal antibodies. Passive immunization is reserved for patients who suffer from immunodeficiencies in whom a live or attenuated vaccine could be dangerous or who have a problem making antibodies. IG is also indicated for nonimmunized or underimmunized patients who have been exposed to an infectious disease and whose incubation period is not long enough to allow complete active immunization. Patients at high risk for developing severe complications from an infectious disease should receive passive immunization when exposed. Some patients who suffer from disease-produced toxins benefit from antitoxin passive immunization. A poisonous snakebite, tetanus, diphtheria, and botulism are examples of this. IG manufactured in the U.S. is screened for HIV-1 and HIV-2, syphilis, human T-lymphotropic viruses (HTLV-1, HTLV-2), WNV, hepatitis B and C, most for *Trypanosoma cruzi* (Chagas disease), and selected ones for CMV. Additionally, the U.S. requires manufacturers of IGIV and other preparations administered IV or IM to undergo procedures to inactivate or remove viruses (Pickering et al, 2009).

IGs are given either IM or IV (IGIV). Most adverse reactions from IG involve localized pain at the injection site but can also include flushing, headache, chills, sweating, and shock. It should not be given to people who have had prior adverse reactions to IG. Systemic reactions may occur, so administering personnel should be prepared to handle acute reactions and, in specific individuals, vasomotor or cardiac complications (e.g., elevated blood pressure, cardiac failure, or both).

Some hyperimmune globulin preparations from human donors provide "superimmunity" because of their high antibody levels to certain infectious diseases. Such products include those for HB (HBIG), rabies (RIG), tetanus (TIG), varicellazoster (VariZIG), botulinum antitoxin (BIG), and cytomegalovirus (CMV-IGIV). Equine-derived antisera are available for botulism, tetanus, diphtheria, and rabies. These can have more severe adverse reactions (including fatal anaphylaxis). They should be used with caution and only after hypersensitivity testing to animal sera is completed by a specialist.

IGIV was originally used to provide immunogenicity to individuals with primary immunodeficiencies. Its use has proven effective, and it is FDA-approved for children with Kawasaki disease, HIV, immune-mediated thrombocytopenia, secondary immunodeficiency from chonic lymphocytic leukemia, and stem cell transplantation. IGIV has also been used with varied efficacy in low-birth-weight (LBW) infants, GBS, toxic shock, severe anemia caused by parvovirus B19 infection, and unresponsive neonatal alloimmune thrombocytopenia. Off-label use is discouraged. Some of the more routine passive immunizations given to pediatric patients are listed in Table 23-3.

Respiratory Syncytial Virus Prophylaxis

One product is on the U.S. market for use in infants at high risk for adverse outcomes after RSV infection: palivizumab. Palivizumab, a humanized mouse monoclonal antibody, has the benefit of being administered IM rather than IV. It is given in five monthly IM injections during RSV season (usually November through March or April depending on the region) and is generally well-tolerated. Palivizumab has been shown to be safe and effective in reducing RSV hospitalizations in high-risk infants by 39% to 82%. Recurrent RSV infection can occur in the same child—even if he or she has received palivizumab—due to more than one RSV circulating within any given community. It has a high cost-to-benefit ratio. Consider RSV prophylaxis for the following children (Pickering et al, 2009):

- Infants born at or before 28 weeks of gestation during RSV season until they are 12 months old
- Premature infants (from 29 weeks to 32 weeks of gestation) if they will be younger than 6 months old during RSV season.

- Children younger than 2 years old with chronic lung disease (CLD) who required treatment for their CLD within 6 months of the onset of RSV season (including oxygen therapy)
- Infants born between 32 and 35 weeks of gestation if RSV season occurs before they are 3 months old, and they are either in group childcare or have siblings less than 5 years of age.
- Children younger than 2 years of age with hemodynamically significant cyanotic or complicated congenital heart disease
- Infants born less than 35 weeks of gestation with neuromuscular disorder or congenital anomalies that compromise handling of respiratory secretions

Consult the AAP *Red Book* (Pickering et al, 2009) for more specific and latest recommendations, including the length of prophylaxis. Adverse reactions may include otitis media, rhinitis, upper respiratory tract infection, apnea, rash, and injection site reaction; alanine aminotransferase (ALT) and aspartate aminotransferase (AST) lab levels may increase and hemoglobin/hematocrit levels may fall. Once opened, a vial of palivizumab must be used within 6 hours (there is no preservative). It can be given concurrently with other vaccines.

Infections in Children in Child Care Settings

In the U.S., approximately 15.6 million preschoolers (41% infants; 53% toddlers) with working parents spend significant "care time" in settings outside of their homes (Schwartz, 2010; Sosinsky and Gilliam, 2007; Waggoner-Fountain, 2007). This population is more immunologically susceptible to illness because of their ages, hygiene habits, dietary factors (including nutritional deficits that may be a result of hunger) (Schwartz, 2010), chronic disease status, and close proximity to one another. Transmission depends on the prevalence in the population, infectivity, and survival characteristics of the organism. The environment enhances easy exposure to many infectious agents, whether spread from diapers, airborne, or from play surfaces. Although any illness can present and spread in a childcare setting, the diseases are primarily respiratory and gastrointestinal in nature. Children in such settings are 2 to 18 times more likely to suffer from a myriad of infectious diseases; receive two to four times more antibiotic treatments; and acquire antibiotic-resistant organisms more frequently than children not in childcare (Waggoner-Fountain, 2007). Infections typically spread in childcare settings are listed in Table 23-4. With the increase in drug resistance, these infections are eliciting great concern.

In addition to educating parents about ways to decrease the incidence and transmission of infectious diseases, including the vaccination of children, health care providers can be a valuable resource for helping establish written policies for childcare settings in their communities. These policies should address prevention and control of infectious agents and include:

- Current immunization records of children and staff
- Provisions for exclusion of ill children and staff
- Instructions on cleaning potentially contaminated areas
- Procedures for changing diapers and their disposal; those primarily handling food should not change diapers
- Procedures regarding the handling of food and pets
- Guidelines for identifying and reporting infectious diseases

TABLE 23-3   Immunoglobulins Used in Children

Immunoglobulin	Reference Name	Indications for Use	Comments
Botulism immune globulin intravenous	BIG-IV	• Botulism toxin A or B in infants <1 year old	• Available as BabyBig from California Department of Health Services (510-231-7600). A trivalent equine antitoxin may be indicated for life-threatening food-borne botulism (other than infant botulism) but risk must be weighed against side effects (fever, serum sickness, anaphylaxis); only available from CDC.
Cytomegalovirus immune globulin intravenous	CMVIG	• For organ transplants. Studies ongoing to evaluate use for: CMV pneumonia, CMV in children with HIV infection, and CMV transmission to newborns	• Used in combination with IV ganciclovir to treat CMV pneumonia
Diphtheria immune globulin (from equine sera)		• Life-threatening *Corynebacterium diphtheriae* disease	• Only available from CDC to treat life-saving diphtheria; anaphylaxis and delayed serum sickness are possible adverse reactions and need to be weighed against risks of disease
Hepatitis B immune globulin	HBIG	Prophylaxis for those unvaccinated or incompletely vaccinated; who have discrete identifiable exposure to blood; or body fluids that contain blood: • Newborns whose mothers are HB surface antigen (HBsAg) positive • Household contacts <12 months old who have received only one prior HBV vaccine and the second dose is not due • Sexual partners of known HBsAg-positive cases, including sexual assault or abuse victims • People accidentally inoculated with a contaminated needle • Individuals with percutaneous or permucosal exposure to body secretions of known cases	• Newborns receive HBIG and hepatitis B virus (HBV) vaccine within 12 hours after birth at different injection sites. If mother's HBV status not known before delivery, infants should receive HBV vaccine; HBIG is given within 7 days of delivery if mother tests positive for HBsAg postpartum. Preterm infants less than 2000 g would receive HBIG if mother's HBsAg is unknown or cannot be quickly determined. • Sexual partners of known cases: HBIG and HBV vaccine up to 14 days after last exposure; repeat vaccine at 1 and 6 months • Household contacts <12 months: HBIG and three doses of HBV vaccine. If >12 months: follow index case's antibody profile (if a carrier, vaccinate all household members). If children and adolescents have documented HBV series and unknown seroconversion status, a booster dose is indicated. • HBV vaccine can also be used for postexposure prophylaxis if given within 12-24 hours after exposure.
Immune globulin	IG	Hepatitis A prophylaxis: • Household contacts and sexual partners of known cases • Persons accidentally inoculated with a contaminated needle • Newborn infants of infected, jaundiced mothers • People with open lesions directly exposed to body secretions of known cases • Children in schools where more than one case is reported • All children and employees of daycare centers where a case is reported • Custodial care residents and staff in close contact with an active case • Persons traveling to developing countries for less than 3 months • HAV vaccine can be given concurrently with the IG, if warranted, for those traveling internationally.	• Given IM • Is given within 2 weeks of exposure; can be used in children <2 years old; is thimerosal free; >85% effective; dosage for those with continuous exposure to hepatitis A virus (HAV) differs from that given for short-term exposure • HAV vaccine can also be used for postexposure prophylaxis if given within 14 day of exposure
		Measles prophylaxis: • To prevent or modify infection in unvaccinated children <1 year old, pregnant women, and the immunocompromised who have been exposed to measles • IGIV can also be used	• Given IM • Not indicated in those who have had one dose of vaccine at ≥12 months old, unless immunocompromised • Given within 6 days after exposure; the dose for those immunocompromised differs according to the degree and type of immunodeficiency, if IGIV has been given, and prior dosage amounts of IG

TABLE 23-3 Immunoglobulins Used in Children—cont'd

Immunoglobulin	Reference Name	Indications for Use	Comments
		Rubella prophylaxis: • Modifies or suppresses the clinical manifestations of the disease, urine shedding, and decreases the rate of viremia. For use in: ○ Early pregnancy after confirmed exposure and only if termination of pregnancy is not an option ○ Infants after maternal exposure ○ Older children not vaccinated with known exposure or at serious risk (immunocompromised)	• Given IM • If pregnant woman is exposed to wild rubella or as a result of being accidentally vaccinated within 3 months of conception, a blood specimen should be obtained as soon as possible. The presence of serum antibodies suggests that the fetus is not at risk (1.4%-2% theoretic risk). If no antibody is detected, a second maternal sample should be obtained 2-3 weeks later: ○ A positive test indicates recent maternal infection. ○ A negative test requires a third sample 6 weeks later. A positive test then indicates recent maternal infection. ○ A negative test at 6 weeks after exposure indicates that maternal rubella infection has not occurred. • Administration of IG and the absence of clinical manifestation of maternal rubella infection do not guarantee the infant will be born without congenital rubella syndrome. IgM antibody (not IgG) after IG can be used to determine maternal infection after exposure.
Immune Globulin Intravenous	IGIV	• FDA approved for treating primary immunodeficiencies, chronic lymphocytic leukemia, bone marrow transplantation, HIV in children, ITP, Kawasaki disease; IGIV contains measles antibodies sufficient for measles prophylaxis.	• Off-label use has created shortages. Off-label use with limited results includes treatment for toxic shock, preterm infant to boost immunity, parvovirus B19 infection, immune-mediated anemia and neutropenia, Guillain-Barré.
Mumps immune globulin		• Ineffective in preventing infection after exposure	• No longer available in the U.S.
Polio	Polio-IGIV	• Used for virulent polio outbreaks in the immunocompromised and those with debilitating illnesses	• An accelerated IPV schedule is indicated during outbreaks for those underimmunized or unimmunized.
Rabies immune globulin	RIB; RIB-HT (heat treated)	• For postexposure prophylaxis for rabies; used in conjunction with rabies vaccine	• Prior to use, consult with local health authorities.
Respiratory syncytial virus	RSV-IGIV (no longer available)	• Reduces risk of RSV bronchiolitis or pneumonia in high-risk children	• Palivizumab, a monoclonal antibody, is used. See section in chapter that discusses RSV.
Tetanus immune globulin	TIG	• For individuals with tetanus-prone wounds who are undervaccinated (fewer than three tetanus toxoid vaccine doses) or whose vaccination status is unknown • For individuals with tetanus infection in combination with antibiotics (metronidazole or penicillin G) • For immunodeficient patients, including those with HIV; they should be considered undervaccinated regardless of actual tetanus toxoid status	• Tetanus-prone wounds include those contaminated with dirt (especially if around horses), feces, or saliva; puncture wounds; avulsions; wounds acquired as a consequence of missiles, burns, crushing, or frostbite • In infants <6 months old without the initial three-dose series, decision to use TIG depends on mother's tetanus toxoid immunization history at the time of delivery and if the wound is tetanus prone • TIG is given IM plus a dose of tetanus toxoid vaccine • If TIG not available, IGIV may be considered (though not licensed for this use in the U.S.); equine tetanus antitoxin (TAT) is another alternative to TIG (not available in the U.S.)— hypersensitivity testing required before use of TAT • Smaller dose is administered for tetanus neonatorum
Vaccinia immune globulin intravenous	VIG-IGIV	• Being held in reserve to prevent or manage complications of smallpox should vaccinia be used as an agent of bioterrorism; can be used in individuals receiving an experimental vaccine that involves a vaccinia carrier virus	• Only available from CDC

Continued

TABLE 23-3	Immunoglobulins Used in Children—cont'd		
Immunoglobulin	**Reference Name**	**Indications for Use**	**Comments**
Varicella immune globulin	VariZIG	Given to those exposed to varicella infection who are most susceptible to varicella and most likely to develop the disease and in whom complications of the infection would result: • Household contacts • Playmates with face-to-face contact (5 minutes to 1 hour) • Infant whose mother had varicella onset 5 days or less before delivery or within 48 hours after delivery • Immunocompromised children and adolescents without history of varicella, varicella immunization, or known to be susceptible • Hospitalized preterm infants 28 weeks or more gestation whose mother lacks history of varicella or serologic evidence of protection • Hospitalized preterm infants less than 28 weeks' gestation or less than 1000 g birthweight regardless of mother's history or varicella-zoster virus serologic evidence* • Other conditions: see CDC guidelines	• Available from FFF Enterprises 24 hr/day (1-800-843-7477) • Administered no longer than 96 hours after exposure • Not indicated in infants whose mothers had zoster infection • In the absence of VariZIG and within 96 hours of exposure, IGIV can be considered; if over 96 hours of exposure, acyclovir may be considered.* • Varicella-zoster immune globulin (VZIG) not available in the U.S.

*Consult with an expert in infectious disease or the CDC.
CDC, Centers for Disease Control and Prevention; *CMV,* cytomegalovirus infection; *HIV,* Human immunodeficiency virus; *IG,* immune globulin; *IgG,* immunoglobulin G; *IgM,* immunoglobulin M; *IM,* intramuscular; *IV,* intravenous; *RSV,* respiratory syncytial virus; *ITP,* idiopathic thrombocytopenia purpura; *IVIG,* intravenous immunoglobulin.
Data from Goldman DC: Passive immunization. In Long SS, Pickering LK, Prober CG: *Principles and practice of pediatric infectious diseases,* ed 3, Philadelphia, 2008, Churchill Livingstone; Pickering LK, Baker CJ, Kimberlin DW et al: *Red Book: 2009 Report of the Committee on Infectious Diseases,* ed 28, Elk Grove Village, Il, 2009, American Academy of Pediatrics.

Some general guidelines for exclusion are included in Box 23-1. Children should not be excluded for (Pickering et al, 2009):
• Yellow or green nasal discharge
• Nonpurulent conjunctivitis without fever or behavioral change
• Exanthem without fever or behavioral changes; erythema infectiosum (fifth disease) in an otherwise healthy individual
• Fever of less than 101° F (38.5° C) without other illness symptoms
• HB carrier status
• Most viral infections (e.g., CMV, mononucleosis)
• Nits, if being treated
• HIV infection
• Scabies, after treatment started

■ Specific Viral Diseases

ENTEROVIRUSES

NONPOLIO ENTEROVIRUSES
Epidemiology
Of the more than 90 serotypes of nonpolio RNA enteroviruses (e.g., coxsackieviruses and echoviruses), 10 to 15 serotypes account for most diseases. They are grouped into four species—human enteroviruses (HEVs) A, B, C, and D.

Hand-foot-mouth, herpangina, pleurodynia, acute hemorrhagic conjunctivitis, myocarditis, pericarditis, pancreatitis, orchitis, and dermatomyositis-like syndrome are manifestations of infection. These enteroviruses are also the most common cause of aseptic meningitis; they have also been associated with paralysis, neonatal sepsis, encephalitis, and other respiratory and gastrointestinal symptoms. The specific serotype may not be unique to any given disease (Abzug, 2007).

As evidenced by the name, enteroviruses concentrate on the gastrointestinal tract as their primary invasion, replication, and transmission site; they spread by fecal-oral contamination, especially in diapered infants. They are also transmitted via the respiratory route and vertically either prenatally or in the parturition period. They have a worldwide distribution, occurring in temperate climates during the summer and fall, and in tropical climates year-round. Transplacental transmission can occur due to exposure to maternal blood or secretions during delivery in a mother infected with HEV and who lacks antibodies to that particular serotype. Transplacental infection can lead to serious disseminated disease in the neonate that involves multiorgan systems (liver, heart, meninges, and adrenal cortex).

Nonpolio enteroviral infection is not a reportable disease nor is it routinely tested for in the clinical setting, so the overall incidence rate is not known (CDC, 2006a). The National Enterovirus Surveillance System (NESS) of the CDC has an ongoing

TABLE 23-4	Pathogens and Modes of Transmission in Daycare		
Modes of Transmission	**Bacteria**	**Viruses**	**Parasites, Fungi, Mites, and Lice**
Respiratory	*Haemophilus influenzae* type B *Neisseria meningitidis* Group A streptococcus *Streptococcus pneumoniae* *Bordetella pertussis* *Mycobacterium tuberculosis* *Kingella kingae* (also known as *Moraxella kingae*)	Adenovirus Coronavirus Influenza A and B Measles Mumps Rubella Varicella-zoster Metapneumovirus Parainfluenza Parvovirus B19 Respiratory syncytial virus Rhinovirus	
Fecal-oral	*Campylobacter jejuni* *Salmonella* spp. *Shigella* spp. *Clostridium difficile* *Aeromonas* *Plesiomonas* *Escherichia coli* O157:H7	Enteroviruses Hepatitis A virus Rotavirus Calicivirus Astrovirus Norovirus (Norwalk) Enteric adenovirus	*Cryptosporidium parvum* *Giardia lamblia* *Enterobius vermicularis*
Person-to-person via skin contact	Group A Streptococcus *Staphylococcus aureus*	Herpes simplex Varicella-zoster Molluscum contagiosum	*Pediculus capitis* *Sarcoptes scabiei* *Trichophyton* spp. *Microsporum* spp.
Contact with blood, urine, or saliva		Cytomegalovirus Hepatitis B Hepatitis C Herpes simplex Human immunodeficiency virus (HIV)	

Data from Clements DA: Infections in daycare environments. In Burg FD, Ingelfinger JR, Polin RA, et al, editors: *Current pediatric therapy*, ed 18, Philadelphia, 2006, Saunders; Pickering LK, Baker CJ, Kimberlin DW, et al: Children in out-of-home child care. In *Red Book: 2009 Report of the Committee on Infectious Diseases*, ed 28, Elk Grove Village, IL, 2009, American Academy of Pediatrics, p 126.

BOX 23-1 Recommendations for Excluding Children from Daycare

- Illness prevents the child from participating in program activities.
- Illness results in greater care need than the childcare staff can provide without compromising the health and safety of the other children.
- Child has fever, unusual lethargy, irritability, behavioral changes, persistent crying, difficulty breathing, intermittent abdominal pain, or other signs of possible severe illness.
- Diarrhea (defined as an increased number of stools in comparison with the child's normal pattern, with increased stool water or decreased form) that is not contained by diapers or toilet use; blood or mucus in stool.
- Persistent abdominal pain lasting more than 2 hours
- Vomiting more than two times in the previous 24 hours
- Mouth sores associated with an inability to control drooling of saliva
- Rash or known methicillin-resistant *Staphylococcus aureus* infection with fever or behavioral changes
- Purulent conjunctivitis with fever and/or behavioral changes
- Scabies prior to starting treatment

Data from Pickering LK, Baker CJ, Kimberlin DW, et al: *Children in out-of-home child care.* In *Red Book: 2009 Report of the Committee on Infectious Disease,* ed 28, Elk Grove Village, IL, 2009, American Academy of Pediatrics.

---

surveillance system and encourages practitioners to test for enterovirus in patients diagnosed with aseptic meningitis.

In known cases, infants less than 12 months have the highest prevalence rate (>25%), and HEVs account for 55% to 65% of hospitalizations for suspected infant sepsis. In addition to younger age, illness occurs more frequently in males, those living in crowded, unsanitary conditions, and in those of lower socioeconomic status (Abzug, 2007). Infection can range from asymptomatic to undifferentiated febrile illness to severe illness. Young children are more likely to be symptomatic.

Incubation Period

Incubation period is 3 to 6 days (less for hemorrhagic conjunctivitis). After infection, the virus is shed from the respiratory tract for up to 3 weeks and fecally for up to 7 to 11 weeks; it is viable on environmental surfaces for long periods (Abzug, 2007).

Clinical Findings

History. General symptoms include:
- A mild upper respiratory infection (URI) is common and may include complaints of sore throat, fever, vomiting, diarrhea, anorexia, coryza, abdominal pain, rash, and headache.

- Nonspecific febrile illness of at least 3 days: In young children, there is an undifferentiated abrupt-onset febrile illness (101° to 104° F [38.5° to 40° C]) associated with myalgias, malaise, irritability; fever may wax and wane over several days.
- Onset of viral symptoms within 1 to 2 weeks after delivery for neonates infected transplacentally (risk of severe disease is higher than for those acquiring the virus postnatally) (CDC, 2008a).

Physical Examination. *General findings:* Mild conjunctivitis, pharyngeal infection, cervical adenopathy. Other findings include (Abzug, 2007; CDC, 2008a; Pickering et al, 2009):

- *Skin:* Rash may be macular, macular-papular, urticarial, vesicular, or petechial. May imitate the rash of meningitis, measles, or rubella.
- *Herpangina:* There is a sudden onset of high fever (up to 106° F [41° C]) lasting 1 to 4 days. Loss of appetite, sore throat, and dysphagia are common, with vomiting and abdominal pain in 25% of cases. Minute vesicles (from 1 to more than 15 lesions of 1 to 2 mm each) appear and enlarge to ulcers (3 to 4 mm) on the anterior pillars of the fauces, tonsils, uvula, and pharynx and the edge of the soft palate. The vesicles commonly have red areolas up to 10 mm in diameter. The entire course usually lasts 3 to 7 days with complete recovery.
- *Acute lymphonodular pharyngitis:* This manifests as an acute sore throat lasting approximately 1 week.
- *Hand-foot-mouth disease:* This is a clinical entity evidenced by fever, vesicular eruption of the buccal mucosa of the mouth, and a maculopapular rash involving the hands and feet. The rash evolves to vesicles, especially on the dorsa of the hands and the soles of the feet, and lasts 1 to 2 weeks (see Color Plate).
- *Aseptic meningitis:* There are the usual signs of fever, stiff neck, and headache. Altered sensorium and seizures are common. Most cases appear in epidemics or as unique cases; most patients recover completely.
- *Paralytic disease:* A Guillain-Barré–type syndrome has been described.
- *Congenital or neonatal infection:* The neonatal infection often manifests as a sudden onset of vomiting, coughing, anorexia, fever or hypothermia, rash, jaundice, irritability, cyanosis, tachycardia, and dyspnea. It is often mistaken for pneumonia. The later three symptoms can progress to myocarditis and congestive heart failure. Infants can go into cardiac collapse, have hepatic and adrenal necrosis, suffer intracranial hemorrhage, and die. For those who survive severe disease, the recovery can be rapid.
- *Acute hemorrhagic conjunctivitis:* Characterized by sudden eye pain, photophobia, blurred vision, tearing, and conjunctival erythema and infection. Most patients recover in a few weeks.
- *Pleurodynia* (Bornholm disease or devil's grip): This condition usually occurs in epidemics, but some isolated cases can occur. It is most often caused by type B disease, but echoviruses have been implicated. There may be a prodrome before the onset of chest pain ushered in by headache, malaise, anorexia, and myalgia. The onset of chest or upper abdominal pain can be sudden, is pleuritic in nature, and is aggravated by deep breathing, coughing, or sudden movements. The pain occurs in waves of spasms that last several minutes to several hours and is described by patients as feeling like being stabbed with a knife or being squeezed in a vise. It can be mistaken for coronary artery disease, pneumonia, or pleural inflammation. Low to high fever occurs, and a pleural friction rub often is heard. The disease generally lasts from 3 to 6 days (up to a few weeks).

- *Orchitis:* This type B infection is clinically similar to mumps.
- *Myocarditis or pericarditis:* HEVs are associated with 25% to 35% of cases of myocarditis and pericarditis of identified cause. Symptoms can range from mild to severe (sudden death), and male adolescents and young adults are particularly vulnerable (Abzug, 2007).
- *Respiratory* symptoms are frequently reported before the onset of fatigue, dyspnea, chest pain, congestive heart failure (CHF), and dysrhythmias. Wheezing, asthma exacerbation, apnea, respiratory distress, pneumonia, otitis media, bronchiolitis, croup, parotitis, and paroxysmal thoracic pain may be seen.

Diagnostic Studies. PCR is highly sensitive for all enteroviruses, results can be available in hours, and the test is more sensitive than cell culture. Cultures can be obtained from throat, stool, rectum, cerebrospinal fluid (CSF), and blood; sensitivities range from 0% to 80% (Pickering et al, 2009). CBC is usually normal. Serology for serotype-specific IgM antibody or other testing is less useful than culture or PCR.

Differential Diagnosis

The differential diagnosis includes other causes of the aforementioned conditions (e.g., viral or bacterial infections [pneumonia, meningitis, sepsis], or connective tissue diseases).

Management

There is no specific therapy available. IGIV has been used and proven helpful in some cases. Antiviral therapy is being developed. The antiviral, pleconaril, is being studied for use in neonates with life-threatening disease (CDC, 2008a).

Prevention

Enteric precautions and good handwashing are the only efficient control measures.

POLIOMYELITIS VIRUS
Epidemiology

The poliovirus is an enterovirus with three serotypes (types 1, 2, and 3). The disease ranges from an asymptomatic illness to severe CNS involvement. Humans are the only documented source of infection. Transmission is through fecal-oral and respiratory routes. Almost all cases in North America occur in individuals most likely exposed to children who had received oral poliovirus vaccine in another country (Pickering et al, 2009). There have been wild-type poliovirus importations into countries previously deemed polio-free (Europe, Africa and Asia); polio has not been eliminated in Pakistan, India, Nigeria, and Afghanistan (CDC, 2010f). However, the incidence worldwide remains low—1291 cases reported in 2010 (WHO, 2011).

Poliomyelitis should be considered in any unimmunized or underimmunized child who has a nonspecific febrile illness, aseptic meningitis, or paralytic symptoms (occurs in from 0.1% to 2% of infections). Asymptomatic disease occurs in 95% of those infected (Pickering et al, 2009); symptomatic but nonparalytic illness occurs in approximately 5% of cases (Simoes, 2007).

The diagnostic test of choice is a viral culture from stool and throat (two samples taken 24 to 48 hours apart) as soon as polio is suspected and at least within 14 days of onset of symptoms. The wild-type virus needs to be differentiated from the vaccine-acquired type. The CSF may be normal or show changes based on the degree of CNS involvement. Antibody titers vary from the acute phase and those taken 3 to 6 weeks later.

Differential Diagnosis, Management, and Prevention

Polio is rare. Differential diagnoses include other conditions causing flaccid muscular weakness and/or paralysis: GBS, peripheral neuritis, transverse myelitis, encephalitis, VAPP, rabies, tetanus, botulism, demyelinating encephalomyelitis, tick-bite paralysis, WNV, spinal cord tumors, familial periodic paralysis, myasthenia gravis, and hysterical paralysis. Conditions that cause decreased limb movement or pseudo-weakness are also differential diagnoses and include unrecognized trauma of the sciatic nerve, toxic synovitis, acute osteomyelitis, acute rheumatic fever, scurvy, and congenital syphilitic osteomyelitis.

Management is supportive and directed at minimizing skeletal deformity in the paralytic form of the disease. Both nonparalytic and mild paralytic cases can be managed on an outpatient basis, but otherwise individuals should be hospitalized. During the early stages of the disease, individuals should be advised against increasing their physical activity, exercising, or becoming fatigued because these factors may increase the risk of paralytic disease (Simoes, 2007).

Prevention measures include active and passive vaccination; the CDC provides guidelines for vaccination in individuals traveling to endemic countries.

HEPATITIS A VIRUS
Epidemiology
HAV is an RNA-containing virus belonging to the Picornaviridae family; it causes a primary infection in the liver. It is a highly contagious infection and commonly spreads through person-to-person contact and fecal-oral contamination of food and water; rarely is it transmitted by contaminated blood transfusion. It accounts for most of the acute and benign viral hepatitis in the U.S. and worldwide. There is no seasonal or geographic variance.

Transmission occurs readily in households and daycare centers; risk factors also include personal contact with an infected individual, international travel, recognized foodborne outbreak, men who have sex with men, and illicit drug use (Pickering et al, 2009). In children less than 6 years old, about 30% are symptomatic, with less than 10% having jaundice (CDC, 2010g). This high anicteric incidence allows considerable spread of disease to adult caretakers in childcare settings. Infants are protected by maternal antibodies during the first few months of life. Older children and adults tend to have more symptomatic disease. The incidence rates are similar across all age groups and geographic regions; rates decrease dramatically in the 5-14 year age ranges after the advent of the HAV vaccine program for children that targeted high-risk communities in the U.S. (Pickering et al, 2009).

Incubation Period
The incubation period is 15 to 50 days (average 25 to 30 days). The period of contagion is as long as the patient sheds virus and usually lasts 1 to 3 weeks. The patient is most contagious from up to 2 weeks before the onset of illness until 1 week after the onset of jaundice.

Clinical Findings
The following two phases may be seen:
1. *Preicteric phase:* This phase manifests as an acute febrile illness. Malaise, nausea, anorexia, vomiting, digestive complaints, and occasional abdominal complaints occur. This phase goes unnoticed in many children. There can be dull right upper quadrant pain during exercise.
2. *Jaundiced phase:* Jaundice appears shortly after the onset of symptoms (70% incidence in older children and adults) (Pickering et al, 2009) and can last from a few days to almost a month; it may be subtle in children. Urine darkens, and stools become clay colored. Often these are the only apparent signs of the illness. Diarrhea is common in infants, whereas constipation is more common in older children and adults. Patients feel sick. Infants have poor weight gain during the icteric phase.

Fulminant disease is rare. There is no chronic disease. Complete recovery can be expected within 1 month with occasional relapses lasting up to 6 months.

Diagnostic Studies. Serologic testing is widely available. IgM-specific antibodies indicate recent infection. These are replaced by IgG-specific antibodies 2 to 4 months later and serve as indicators of past infection. Changes in liver enzymes indicate the degree of injury. There is elevation of serum transaminases (serum glutamic-oxaloacetic transaminase [SGOT], AST, serum glutamate pyruvate transaminase [SGPT], ALT). Prothrombin time can be elevated.

Differential Diagnosis
Any cause of jaundice is in the differential diagnosis of HAV.
- *Infancy:* Physiologic jaundice, hemolytic disease, galactosemia, hypothyroidism, biliary metabolic disorders, biliary atresia, alpha 1-antitrypsin deficiency, and choledochal cysts. Hypervitaminosis A causes a yellow pigmentation (carotenemia) of the skin often mistaken for jaundice in children. Infections, such as toxoplasmosis, rubella, CMV, and herpes (TORCH) also cause hepatitis.
- *Older infants, children, and adolescents:* Hemolytic-uremic syndrome, Reye syndrome, malaria, leptospirosis, brucellosis, chronic hemolytic diseases with gallstone development, Wilson disease, cystic fibrosis (CF), Banti syndrome, collagen-vascular disease (e.g., SLE), infectious mononucleosis syndrome (IMS), CMV, coxsackievirus, toxoplasmosis, Weil disease, yellow fever, acute cholangitis, amebiasis, and hepatitis B, C, and D. Drugs and poisons such as pyrazinamide, isoniazid, valproic acid, acetaminophen overdose, zoxazolamine, gold, cinchophen, phenothiazines, and methyltestosterone also cause hepatitis.

Management

Therapy is supportive. Good hand hygiene after diaper changes is a crucial preventive measure, especially for daycare personnel. The use of gamma globulin or HAV vaccine within 2 weeks of exposure is discussed earlier in this chapter (see Table 23-3). Those with acute infections who work as food handlers or in schools/childcare settings should be excluded for 1 week after onset of symptoms.

Complications

Although patients can become very ill, most cases of HAV resolve completely. Fulminant hepatitis with liver failure is rare.

Prevention

HA vaccine for those 12 months and older and improved sanitation.

HEPATITIS B VIRUS

Epidemiology

HBV is a DNA-containing hepadnavirus. It is highly contagious and causes severe liver disease. The most common method of transmission is percutaneous or mucous membrane exposure to contaminated blood, wound exudates, semen, vaginal secretions, or saliva (lesser so); it is not spread by the fecal-oral route. HBV can survive in a dried state for more than 1 week, but is highly susceptible to common household disinfectants. Prolonged percutaneous contact with contaminated fomites can be a source of infection.

The major reservoirs for HBV are healthy chronic carriers and patients with acute disease. Approximately 1.2 million people have chronic HBV in the U.S. and approximately 350 million worldwide (CDC, 2010g; WHO, 2008). Unimmunized children who have immigrated to the U.S. from China, Southeast Asia, Africa, and other high endemic areas pose the highest infection risk. However, because of the high HB immunization coverage in children within the U.S., transmission is rare. Highest rates of infection across all age ranges are reported in men from 24 to 44 years old (CDC, 2009b). Perinatal transmission is highly efficient during the birthing process (in utero transmission is rare) from female carriers (HBsAg positive or HBeAg positive, or both) to their newborn children. The infection rate is 70% to 90% if both maternal antigen markers are positive, and 5% to 25% if the mother is HbsAg positive but HBeAg negative (Pickering et al, 2009).

Whether one eventually develops chronic infection depends on the age one is infected and the rate of loss of HBeAg. More than 90% of untreated newborns develop chronic infection after exposure. From 25% to 50% of children, who acquire the infection between 1 and 5 years old, (versus 6% to10% who are exposed as older children and adults) develop chronic HBV infection (CDC, 2010g). Individuals who abuse IV drugs or who engage in sexual activity with multiple partners or have male-to-male sex have the greatest risk of acquiring HBV. Health care workers who are exposed to blood, blood products, or blood-contaminated body fluids (includes those working with the developmentally disabled) are also at a high risk, as are chronic renal dialysis patients. Tattooing or body piercing with contaminated instruments is another route of infection. Breastfeeding is not contraindicated. Adolescents who missed the birth dose of HBV should be screened, especially if their parents were born in regions of high-HBV endemicity.

Incubation Period

The incubation period is 45 to 160 days (average of 120 days).

Clinical Findings

HBV has a range of illness from asymptomatic seroconversion to fulminating disease and death. HBV usually has a gradual onset. Most children who acquired HBV at an early age are asymptomatic. Some have minimal nonspecific constitutional complaints such as fever, nausea, and minimal hepatomegaly. Arthralgia and skin problems, such as urticaria or other rashes, can be the first apparent signs. Papular acrodermatitis has been described in infants. Acute HBV infection is somewhat similar to the icteric phase of HAV, but it is usually more severe. Skin, mucous membranes, and sclerae are icteric. The liver is enlarged and tender.

Diagnostic Studies. Serologic tests include HBsAg, hepatitis B core antigen (HBcAg), HBeAg, and antibodies to these antigens; the results can be useful in determining the stage of infection (Table 23-5). Positive HBsAg and HBcAg assay results indicate active infection. Changes in liver enzymes indicate the degree of injury. There is elevation of serum transaminases (SGOT, AST, SGPT, ALT). Prothrombin time can be elevated, especially in fulminating disease. Hybridization assays, nucleic acid amplification testing, and gene amplification techniques (e.g., PCR) are also available.

Differential Diagnosis

Any cause of jaundice is included; refer to the section on differential diagnosis of HAV.

Management

A specialist in hepatitis B in children should be consulted. Therapy is supportive. The use of active and passive vaccination has been discussed. Interferon-alfa and lamivudine are FDA-approved drugs for children. Those with chronic infection should receive yearly liver ultrasound and testing of liver function and alpha-fetoprotein concentration, and vaccinate for HAV. Liver biopsies may be done to accurately monitor the effects of liver involvement. HBIG and corticosteroids are not useful.

Complications

Approximately 15% to 25% of those chronically infected will develop hepatic and extrahepatic complications (liver failure, cirrhosis, hepatocellular carcinoma) (CDC, 2010g).

Prevention

The initial infection can be prevented with HB vaccination; transmission in utero or during labor to newborns and postexposure prophylaxis is covered in Table 23-3.

TABLE 23-5 Interpretation of the Hepatitis B Serologic Panel

HBsAg*	Anti-HBs	Anti-HBc IgM†	Anti-HBc IgG	Interpretation	Comments
+	−	−	−	Early acute infection	First indicator to appear as early as 1-2 weeks after infection but before clinical symptoms. Usually persists throughout the illness. Ensure household and sexual contacts are vaccinated.
+	−	+	+	Acute infection	Highly infectious, active replication of virus. Ensure household and sexual contacts are vaccinated.
+	−	−	+	Chronic infection	Low replication of the virus, low infectivity, or HbsAg carrier.
−	−	+	−	"Window period" following acute infection	Patient probably not infectious.
−	−	−	+	Remote infection with loss of detectable anti-HbsAg; remote infection with possible low-level HbsAg; possible false-positive test	Patient is not infectious to household, sexual, needlestick exposures.
−	+	±	+	Resolved infection	Patient is immune, not infectious.
−	+	±		Healed infection	Patient is immune, not infectious.
−	+	−	−	Immune following vaccination; resolved infection with loss of detectable anti-HBc	Patient is immune, not infectious.

*The presence of HBsAg alone is insufficient for a diagnosis of acute infection.
†Anti-HBc IgG may also be reported as simply anti-HBc (or HBcAb) and can persist indefinitely.
See text for definitions of abbreviations.
Adapted from Centers for Disease Control and Prevention (CDC): *Interpretation of the hepatitis B panel.* Reviewed 2005. Available at www.cdc.gov/ncidod/diseases/hepatitis/b/Bserology.htm (accessed Dec 12, 2010); State of Alaska Epidemiology Bulletin: *Serologic test for viral hepatitis, part 2.* Available at www.epi.hss.state.ak.us/bulletins/docs/b1991_31.pdf (accessed Dec 12, 2010).

HEPATITIS C VIRUS

Epidemiology

Hepatitis C virus (HCV), a single-stranded RNA virus with seven genotypes in the Flaviviridae family, causes the chronic form of what used to be called non-A, non-B hepatitis. From 75% to 85% of infected individuals develop chronic infection. The incidence in the U.S. is approximately 1.3% and remains fairly stable (CDC, 2010g). The risk factors associated with HCV are illicit IV drug use (75%, with an estimated one third of injection drug users between 18 and 30 years old infected), imprisonment, occupational (1%) or sexual exposure (1% to 10%), and transfusions or organ recipients prior to 1992 (rare now). Hemophiliacs treated with inadequately screened blood products are at high risk; those on chronic hemodialysis have moderate risk (10% to 20%). Perinatal transmission by non–HIV-infected women is approximately 5% to 6%; HIV-positive mothers have a greater likelihood of transmitting the virus to their infants. Vaginal birth and breastfeeding do not contribute to higher rates of transmission, and women with HCV alone should not be discouraged from experiencing either (Pickering et al, 2009). Studies demonstrate an increased incidence of transmission to female infants. It is postulated that this may be a reflection of hormonal or genetic differences in susceptibility or response to the infection; there is greater mortality in utero for males infected with the virus than for females (Beasley, 2005).

Incidence of persistent hepatitis infection in children is from 50% to 60%, typically asymptomatic. HCV infection has the highest rate of developing into chronic infection than all of the other hepatitis infections; 70% to 80% of adult cases are characterized by chronic infection and liver disease, whereas the incidence of these complications in children is thought to be lower (Pickering et al, 2009).

Incubation Period

HCV has an incubation period ranging from 2 weeks to 6 months (average 45 days).

Clinical Findings

Onset of symptoms is often insidious, and most children are asymptomatic. Flulike prodromal symptoms followed by jaundice occur in 20% to 30% of cases (CDC, 2010g). Chronic hepatitis with cirrhosis is a late occurrence, often 20 to 30 years later. Fulminant infection is uncommon.

Diagnostic Studies. There is no serologic marker for acute infection. Confirmation of HCV using IgG antibody enzyme immunoassay for anti-HCV or nucleic acid assay to detect HCV RNA are diagnostic. False-negative results can occur, however, early in the infection. The majority of individuals seroconvert within 15 weeks postexposure or within 5 to 6 weeks after the onset of illness symptoms. A newborn can be anti-HCV positive from maternal transfer for up to 18 months, so testing should ideally be done after that time. Liver function tests are indicated; liver biopsy is confirmatory.

Differential Diagnosis

Differential diagnoses include HAV and HBV and other causes of chronic hepatitis. See section on differential diagnosis of HAV.

Management

Treatment of acute HCV is supportive; there is no effective treatment to prevent the progression to cirrhosis, liver failure, or hepatocellular cancer. Chronic HCV infections in children respond to therapy with nonpegylated interferon alfa-2b therapy and ribavirin (for use in children 3 to 17 years). HAV and HBV vaccines should be given to prevent further liver complications. Liver damage can be exacerbated by comorbid conditions such as cancer, iron overload, thalassemia, or HIV. Drugs such as acetaminophen or antiretroviral medications need to be closely monitored; patients should have serum hepatic transaminases monitored closely. Breastfeeding by an HCV-positive mother is not contraindicated unless she has cracked or bleeding nipples. Children with HCV infection need not be excluded from daycare facilities (Pickering et al, 2009). Individuals with HCV should be discouraged from using alcohol (to prevent further liver injury) and from sharing razors and toothbrushes; condom use should be encouraged.

Prognosis

The course of HCV is generally mild even with cirrhosis. Liver transplantation is an option, although reinfection is common and gradually progressive. The outcome of chronic HCV disease in children is less known.

Prevention

IG is not recommended for prophylaxis after exposure. There is no HCV vaccine.

HEPATITIS D VIRUS

Hepatitis D virus (HDV) is caused by an RNA virus that is structurally different from HAV, HBV, and HCV. HDV infection is uncommon in children but must be considered in cases of fulminant hepatitis or hepatic failure. It cannot cause infection unless the patient also is infected with HBV, which it needs to replicate. Transmission is through parenteral, percutaneous, or mucosal contact (including sexual) with infected blood and can be acquired either as a coinfection with or superinfection in an individual with chronic HBV. Incubation is 2 to 8 weeks. In the U.S., it is diagnosed most commonly in drug users, individuals with hemophilia, and immigrants from southern Italy and parts of Eastern Europe, South America, Africa, and the Middle East. Mother-to-newborn transmission is uncommon (Pickering et al, 2009). Infection is detected using IgM antibody to HDV. There is no vaccine against HDV. However, HBV vaccine is preventive of HDV because HDV

requires comorbidity with HBV to be infective. Those with chronic HBV should take precautions against being infected.

HEPATITIS E VIRUS

Hepatitis E virus (HEV) is an RNA virus in the family Hepeviridae; certain strains can also have zoonotic hosts (e.g., swine, nonhuman primates). It is passed via the fecal-oral route. Contaminated water is the most common reservoir. It is an acute infection whose symptoms resemble those of other viral hepatitis. Symptomatic individuals are usually older adolescents and young adults; pregnant women are particularly vulnerable to more serious illness (notably in the third trimester). Children are either asymptomatic or experience mild symptoms. If symptoms appear, they do so within 15 to 60 days (mean 40 days) after exposure. Endemic areas include India, the Middle East, parts of Africa, Southeast Asia, and Mexico. Most cases in the U.S. are found in immigrants or visitors from these locations. Clinical symptoms (jaundice, malaise, anorexia, fever, abdominal pain, arthralgia) are similar to HAV, but often more severe. Laboratory studies include IgM and IgG anti-HEV, but these can be unreliable. Definitive diagnosis is determined by the detection of viral RNA in serum or stool using reverse transcriptase-PCR assay. Treatment is supportive; there is no approved vaccine in the U.S. Good hand hygiene is crucial. Chronic infection is rare, and recovery is usually complete. The overall mortality rate is 4% or less; however, in pregnant women the mortality rate ranges from 10% to 30% (CDC, 2009c).

■ Herpes Family of Viruses

The herpes family of viruses is large. They have several features in common: all infect humans, the infection is lifelong, the viruses establish latency, and reactivation is controlled by immune function. Most active infections are self-limited. Infection becomes serious and dangerous when the cellular immune system is not working properly or when it is naïve (newborn). This family of viruses includes herpes simplex virus (HSV), VZV, Epstein-Barr virus (EBV), CMV, roseola (human herpesvirus 6 and 7 [HHV-6 and HHV-7, also known as exanthema subitum or sixth disease]), and human herpesvirus 8 (HHV-8, also known as Kaposi sarcoma–associated herpesvirus). HSV, VZV, and roseola are discussed in the following sections. The reader should consult other resources for a discussion about herpesvirus 8.

HERPES SIMPLEX VIRUS
Epidemiology

HSV is among the most widely disseminated infectious agents in humans; it is a double-stranded DNA virus. HSV has two antigenic types. HSV-1 is associated chiefly with nongenital infections of the mouth, lips, eyes, and CNS. HSV-2 is most commonly associated with genital and neonatal infection (accounts for 75% of neonatal cases; the rest are attributed to HSV-1). Both types are equally devastating to a newborn. There can also be mixing and matching of both HSV types in different mucus membrane locations. Type 1 strains can be found in the genital tract (autoinoculation or oral-genital contact). Type 2 lesions found in the mouth or pharynx usually result from oral sexual activity.

Primary infection with type 1 virus typically is the causative agent in those 6 months to 5 years old and most often presents as gingivostomatitis. Distribution is worldwide, but the infection is more frequent in crowded environments. It is spread by intimate, direct contact usually by an adult with or without symptoms. There is no seasonal variation.

Type 2 infections usually occur as a result of sexual activity. Sexual molestation must always be ruled out when the infection is found in non-neonates; for this reason determining the type of virus is always important. Neither type is transmitted by inanimate objects, such as toilet seats (Pickering et al, 2009).

Neonatal HSV-2 infection is primarily transmitted from the mother as the infant passes through an infected birth canal with viral migration via the neonate's conjunctiva, nose and/or mouth mucosa, or broken skin (e.g., from forceps or a scalp electrode). Infection can also occur with cesarean births. Risk of infection for an infant born to a mother with a primary genital infection is 25% to 60%. The risk for infants born to mothers with recurrent HSV genital infection is approximately 2%. The incidence is 1 in 3000 to 20,000 live births. However, about 75% of infants with congenital HSV infection are born to women without a history or clinical findings of active infection during pregnancy (Pickering et al, 2009). Postnatal transmission is described, but is less common. Mothers can inoculate their babies from oral, breast, or skin lesions. Fathers also can inoculate infants with nongenital lesions from their mouths or on their hands. There can be lateral transmission from an infected baby in the nursery due to inadequate hand hygiene by hospital personnel.

Incubation Period

Period of communicability for types 1 and 2 (when not in the neonatal period) is 2 days to 2 weeks (Pickering et al, 2009). Some cases of congenital infection occur more than 6 weeks after birth. Infection can be transmitted during either primary or recurrent infections, whether symptomatic or asymptomatic.

Clinical Findings

Manifestations are determined by the port of entry of the host, age, state of health, and immune competence. Eczema alone or in combination with other manifestations is also a complicating factor. Specific clinical findings, diagnosis, and treatment of gingivostomatitis, neonatal herpetic infection, eczema herpeticum, herpes vulvovaginitis, and herpes keratoconjunctivitis are discussed in other chapters.

Neonatal Infection. The neonate is always symptomatic. Infection is evidenced by skin vesicles or scarring, eye findings (chorioretinitis, keratoconjunctivitis), microcephaly, or hydranencephaly at birth. Those with skin, eye, and mouth (SEM) involvement usually are symptomatic by 5 to 11 days after birth, with 80% to 85% having skin lesions; if left untreated the disease can progress to encephalitis or disseminated disease. Infants with CNS (encephalitis) disease generally show symptoms suggestive of bacterial meningitis at 8 to 17 days after birth; about 60% will have skin lesions. With untreated CNS disease, half will die; those that survive generally demonstrate neurologic sequelae. Infants with disseminated infection are symptomatic at 5 to 11 days after birth. Symptoms are similar to that of bacterial sepsis, with 75% having skin lesions; the mortality rate is 90% if untreated

(20% if treated) with severe neurologic sequelae in survivors (Stanberry, 2007) (see also Chapter 38).

Traumatic Herpetic Infection. This is a localized infection that occurs in a susceptible child because of an abrasion, teething, laceration, or burn that is inoculated with herpesvirus by an orally infected parent who kisses the "booboo." Vesicles appear at the site of the lesion. There may be fever, constitutional symptoms, and regional lymph node involvement.

Acute Herpetic Meningoencephalitis. After the neonatal period, infection with HSV-1 is a leading cause of intermittent, nonepidemic encephalitis in children and adults in the U.S. Encephalitis can be focal, mimicking a mass lesion. Diagnosis is made by brain biopsy. In contrast, HSV meningitis is usually a relatively benign disease most often caused by HSV-2.

Recurrent Infections. The body does not truly eradicate the virus; the virus lies dormant, and recurrent infections are common. Recurrent infections occur either as herpes labialis (aka "fever blister") or genital herpes. Some incidence of recurrent aseptic meningitis can be attributed to HSV infection.

Diagnostic Tests. If suspicious for neonatal infection, intrapartum cultures from mother and child should be obtained on the day of delivery at 12 and 24 hours or earlier. Tests may include viral culture, cytology-Pap smears, Tzanck stains, ELISA, fluorescent techniques, glycoprotein G assay, blood or CSF PCR in neonates, or histologic evaluation and viral culture from a brain biopsy in cases of encephalitis. Cultures in neonates need to be taken from skin vesicles, mouth, nasopharynx, eyes, blood, rectum, and CSF. Serologic tests are not helpful in neonates. If encephalitis is suspected, an electroencephalogram (EEG) and MRI of the brain are performed. In disseminated disease, elevated transaminase and/or radiographic evidence of HSV pneumonitis may be seen.

Differential Diagnosis

The diagnosis is usually not a problem if vesicles are present. Coxsackievirus can cause a vesicular stomatitis.

Management

Treatment is supportive except in life-threatening illness, neonatal infection, or disease in immunocompromised patients, at which time parenteral acyclovir is the treatment of choice. The role of long-term suppressive or intermittent acyclovir for neonatal HSV is unknown and under study (Pickering et al, 2009). Any lesion found should be cultured. In a woman with *primary* genital infection, cultures and empiric parenteral acyclovir for the newborn are often given. Infants born to women with active *recurrent* genital infection are generally not given empiric antiviral medication, but instead are closely monitored by parents, caregivers, and providers over the following 6 weeks. Careful hand hygiene before and after handling newborns and refraining from kissing or nuzzling (masks can be worn until lesions have crusted) by those with active infection are basic preventive measures.

Complications

Usually the infection is mild. Major problems have been discussed. Bacterial superinfection is always a problem. There is an increased incidence of cervical cancer in women with HSV-2 infections.

Prevention

- All pregnant women must be asked about HSV infection in themselves and all sexual partners.
- Signs and symptoms of HSV should be carefully monitored throughout pregnancy.
- During labor all women must again be questioned about HSV and carefully examined for signs and symptoms of infection. Cesarean delivery is indicated in women with apparent infection unless membranes are ruptured for more than 4 to 6 hours. Scalp monitoring should be avoided.
- Toddlers and infants with primary gingivostomatitis who are drooling should be excluded from childcare centers if they cannot control their saliva. Children with recurrent "fever blisters" may attend school. Covering recurrent HSV lesions with a bandage is appropriate for children with active nonmucosal involvement.
- Wrestlers should be excluded from competition until lesions have healed (Pickering et al, 2009). (See also Table 13-6).

INFECTIOUS MONONUCLEOSIS SYNDROME

Epidemiology

IMS is caused by the Epstein-Barr family of herpesvirus in more than 90% of cases; the remaining cases are attributed to acute CMV, *Toxoplasma gondii*, adenovirus, viral hepatitis, HIV, and possibly rubella. Its distribution is worldwide, with more than 95% having been infected (Jenson, 2007). Older children and adolescents in poor urban settings or developing countries are seropositive for EBV. In these children primary infection tends to produce only mild symptoms and is subclinical. Exposure occurs in infancy or early childhood. In more developed countries infection in those less than 4 years of age is rare; one third of cases occur during adolescence or young adulthood (Jenson, 2007). The mode of transmission is personal contact, usually from deep kissing; by penetrative sexual contact; or from the exchange of saliva among children. The virus can live outside the body in saliva for several hours (Pickering et al, 2009). About 20% to 30% of healthy immune individuals shed EBV at any one time. From 60% to 90% of EBV-infected individuals on immunosuppressive therapy, including those on steroids, shed virus (Jenson, 2007).

Incubation Period

Because IMS virus is found in the saliva and blood of both clinically ill and asymptomatic infected persons for many months, the period of communicability is difficult to assess. The period of incubation is thought to be from 30 to 50 days. It is only mildly contagious.

Clinical Findings

IMS is the "great impostor" and can mimic any disease imaginable. It is a disease of the primary lymphoid tissue and peripheral blood. Lymphoid tissue—regional lymph nodes, tonsils, spleen, and liver—is enlarged. Atypical lymphocytes are seen in the peripheral blood. Almost all body organs are involved, including but not limited to the lungs, heart, kidneys, adrenals, CNS, and skin. Symptoms are variable and can last up to 2 to 3 weeks. Clinical presentation can include the following (Jenson, 2007; Johannsen and Kaye, 2009):

- *Fever:* Moderate to high fever (<103° F [39.4° C]) is common (>90%). In severe cases, fever can reach 104° to 105° F (40° to 40.6° C). Fevers usually wane over a 10- to 14-day period.
- *Sore throat:* Usually begins a few days after the fever with an average incidence of about 80%. The throat is very painful for 7 to 10 days. There is marked tonsillar enlargement, grayish exudates (in approximately 30% of cases), ulceration, and pseudomembrane formation. Petechiae are found on the palate (in approximately 25% to 60% of cases). The airway can be compromised (<5% of cases) and is an indication for hospitalization.
- *Lymphadenopathy:* Anterior and posterior cervical and submandibular nodes are more commonly involved, less so the axillary and inguinal nodes. Epitrochlear lymphadenopathy is highly suggestive of the disease. Nodes are firm but usually nontender, are discrete, and range from 1 to 4 cm in size (up to 90% incidence).
- *Splenomegaly:* Occurs typically 2 to 3 cm below the costal margin in approximately 50% of cases. Rupture is rare.
- *Hepatomegaly:* 10% to 15%; jaundice occurs in about 5% of cases.
- *Skin rash:* Occurs in 3% to 15% of cases, usually on the trunk, arms, and palms. It can be maculopapular, urticarial, scarlatiniform, hemorrhagic, or nodular (rarely petechial, vesicular, or hemorrhagic) and usually occurs during the first few days of symptomatology onset and lasts 1 to 6 days. The rash occurs more frequently in patients taking ampicillin (up to 100%); probably represents a form of arteritis or vasculitis rather than hypersensitivity to ampicillin, and typically starts 5 to 10 days after the drug has begun. A symmetric rash of erythematous papules with or without coalescence on the cheeks, extremities, and buttocks (looks like atopic dermatitis) is associated with EBV infection as well (the Gianotti-Crosti syndrome).
- *Vision:* Perceptual distortions in size, shapes, and spatial relationships can occur. Periorbital edema has been reported in 30% of cases.

Other systemic manifestations can include myalgia, arthralgia, headache, chest pain, nausea, anorexia, vomiting, ocular pain, photophobia, conjunctivitis, gingivitis, abdominal pain, orchitis (rare), diarrhea, cough, pneumonia, myocarditis, pericarditis, rhinitis, epistaxis, bradycardia, aseptic meningitis, GBS, Bell palsy, Reye syndrome, and acute cerebellar ataxia (Johannsen and Kaye, 2009).

Diagnostic Studies. The CBC has a classic picture of more than 10% atypical lymphocytes and lymphocytosis; elevated liver enzymes are typical. Monospot and the serum heterophile test are positive in 85% of infected patients older than 4 years (often negative in those less than 4 years of age). Children older than 4 years usually must be ill for approximately 2 weeks before seroconverting. Viral culture and Epstein-Barr–specific core and capsule antibody testing are usually used for diagnosis if the primary screening test results are negative, and there is continued suspicion of IMS (e.g., in younger children). Depending on the specific EBV antigen system tested, levels can be detectable for years after infection.

Differential Diagnosis

IMS is in the differential diagnosis of almost every infectious disease. Conditions and infections typically associated with a mononucleosis-like syndrome are gram-positive alpha-beta hemolytic streptococcal pharyngitis, leukemia, lymphoreticular malignancies, adenoviruses, toxoplasmosis, CMV, rubella, HIV, hepatitis, SLE, drug reactions, and diphtheria.

Management

Treatment is supportive with adequate bed rest (for debilitating cases), over-the-counter pain relievers, fluids, and calories. Corticosteroids and acyclovir are not recommended for routine uncomplicated disease; penicillin products should not be given. Contact sports and strenuous exercise should be avoided for 4 weeks and especially in those with hepatosplenomegaly. (See Chapter 13 for return-to-play sports participation after hepatosplenomegaly.) Symptoms generally resolve within 2 to 4 weeks; fatigue and weakness may persist for up to 6 to 12 months after severe infection. Complete recovery can be expected in more than 95% of cases without any specific treatment (Johannsen and Kaye, 2009).

Complications

Clinically healthy patients experience few sequelae. Rare complications include splenic rupture, neurologic complications (from aseptic meningitis, encephalitis, myelitis, optic neuritis, cranial nerve palsies, GBS), thrombocytopenia, agranulocytosis, hemolytic anemia, orchitis, myocarditis, or chronic IMS. The virus also seems to increase the risk for Hodgkin disease. Death is rare. There is no convincing evidence that supports an association between EBV infection or reactivation to chronic fatigue syndrome (Johannsen and Kaye, 2009).

Prevention

Persons with a recent history of IMS or an infectious mononucleosis-like disease should not donate blood or organs.

ROSEOLA INFANTUM (EXANTHEM SUBITUM)

Epidemiology

Roseola infantum is also known as exanthem subitum or sixth disease; it is one manifestation of infection caused by HHV-6 (less commonly, HHV-7 that causes infection later in life). Humans are the only natural reservoir. The method of transmission is not completely understood but is probably spread via the oral, nasal, and conjunctival routes of other family members, caregivers, or close contacts. Transmission either prenatally or during or after parturition is suspected. The disease is most commonly acquired by children between 6 and 24 months old (peaks by 15 months), after protective maternal antibodies have waned. It is rare in children younger than 3 months old or older than 3 years, but has been documented in infants as young as 8 weeks old (typified by a febrile illness without localized symptoms). Most children are HHV-6 seropositive by 4 years of age, and about 85% are seropositive for HHV-7 by adulthood (Pickering et al, 2009). This shows that there is asymptomatic illness or roseola without rash; in the U.S. the rash is evidenced in about 25% of cases (in Japan rates reach 75%) (Cohen, 2009). Reactivation of infection can occur in those immunocompromised. Visits to emergency departments are common as a result of the associated fevers, toxicity, and/or seizures associated with this disease in infants.

The disease occurs worldwide, year-round, and shows no gender preference.

Incubation Period

The incubation period has a mean of 9 to 10 days. The period of communicability is probably greatest during the fever phase before the rash erupts.

Clinical Findings

There is a sudden onset of fever from 101° to more than 103° F (38.3° to more than 39.5° C) for 3 to 7 (commonly 3 to 4) days, but the child does not seem particularly ill. There may be signs of a URI; lymphadenopathy in the cervical and posterior occipital areas; lethargy; infected palpebral conjunctiva; eyelid edema; gastrointestinal complaints; reddened TMs (without bulging or effusion); and, occasionally, a febrile convulsion (10% to 15% of cases) (Pickering et al, 2009). As the fever breaks, a diffuse, nonpruritic, discrete, rose-colored maculopapular rash, 2 to 3 mm in diameter, appears (Fig. 23-1). It fades on pressure and rarely coalesces. The roseola exanthema is similar to the rash of rubella. The rash lasts hours to 2 to 3 days, begins on the trunk, and spreads centrifugally. In the rare case of CNS involvement, the anterior fontanelle may bulge.

Diagnostic Studies. The WBC count is distinctive, showing a decrease for age initially, dropping further by the third or fourth day, and then returning into the normal range. It tends to follow the fever pattern. Serologic testing involves isolating HHV-6 for peripheral blood mononuclear cells and documenting a significant rise in antibody titer; however, test results can vary widely so diagnosing unequivocal acute infection is problematic. Serial titers 2 to 3 weeks apart are more reliable. Fourfold increases in HHV-6 or HHV-7 IgG antibodies suggest active infection. Virus cultures can be helpful. A rapid HHV-6 culture is available. A reverse transcriptase-polymerase chain reaction (RT-PCR) assay can distinguish between the acute and latent infection.

Differential Diagnosis

The clinical course usually makes this illness easy to diagnose. Most viral rashes, scarlatina, and drug hypersensitivity are included in the differential diagnoses. A roseola-like

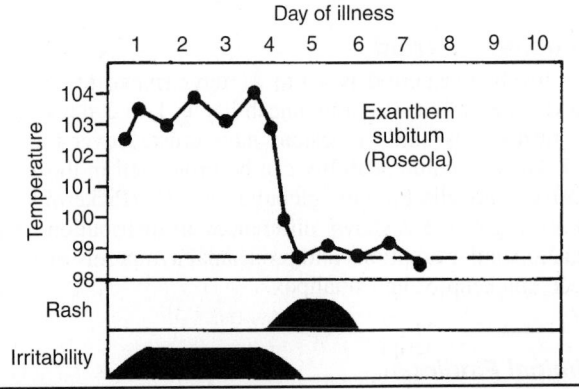

FIGURE 23-1 Schematic diagram illustrating the symptoms of roseola. (Adapted from Katz S, Gershon A, Hotez P: *Krugman's infectious diseases of children,* ed 10, Philadelphia, 1998, Mosby.)

illness is also associated with parvovirus B19, echovirus 16, other enteroviruses, measles, and adenoviruses. Until the rash develops, fever without focus and bacterial sepsis are in the differential diagnosis. If a febrile seizure occurs, meningitis is usually added to the differential diagnosis.

Management
Management is supportive.

Complications
Rare complications include febrile convulsions, meningoencephalitis, encephalitis, and hemiplegia. Associated diseases include ITP, drug sensitivity syndromes, pityriasis rosea, multiple sclerosis (MS), and hepatitis.

VARICELLA
Epidemiology
VZV infection is a common highly contagious virus belonging to the herpesvirus family. Chickenpox is the primary illness. It derives its name not from chickens but from the propensity of the lesions to resemble chickpeas. Shingles (herpes zoster) is the reactivation infection of latent VZV acquired during varicella infection (see Chapter 36).

Humans are the only reservoir of infection; illness is spread by direct contact, droplets, and airborne transmission. Victims of shingles are also infectious and can cause primary varicella illness. Immunity is usually lifelong. Symptomatic reinfection is rare, but asymptomatic reinfection occurs and symptoms are usually mild. Immunocompromised patients are at risk of developing generalized zoster. The disease tends to peak in those ages 10 to 14 years, although the overall incidence has decreased in all age groups from prior prevaccine levels (Pickering et al, 2009). Distribution is worldwide and endemic in most large cities. Epidemics occur but at irregular intervals; the greatest incidence is in late winter and spring in temperate climates. Since the advent of the varicella vaccine in 1995, varicella disease has decreased approximately 85%, and hospitalizations have decreased by about 75% (Myers et al, 2007; Pickering et al, 2009). Mild varicella breakthrough infection occurs in approximately one out of every five of those previously vaccinated, due to the efficacy of the vaccine against mild disease (70% to 90%) versus severe disease (95% to 100%) (Myers et al, 2007).

Incubation Period
The incubation period is 10 to 21 days (mean of 14 to 16 days). The period of communicability is 1 to 2 days before the rash erupts until all lesions have crusted over (about 3 to 7 days). Communicability can be prolonged in those who received varicella immune globulin or IGIV (Pickering et al, 2009). Figure 23-2 shows differences in distribution of the maculopapular eruptions and prodromal symptoms of scarlet fever, chickenpox, and smallpox.

Clinical Findings
The following two phases are seen in varicella:
1. *Prodrome:* Not always present. It is composed of low-grade fever, listlessness, headache, backache, anorexia,

mild abdominal pain, and occasionally URI symptoms. These symptoms may occur 1 to 2 days before onset of the second phase.
2. *Rash:* Classic appearance. It is centripetal, beginning on the scalp, face, or trunk. Crops of generally highly pruritic lesions progress from spots to "teardrop vesicles" that cloud over and umbilicate in 24 to 48 hours. After a few days all morphologic forms can be seen simultaneously. Scabs last from 5 to 20 days, depending on the depth of the lesions. There can be high fever, to 105° F (40.6° C). The more severe the rash, the higher the fever. Lesions can develop on all mucosal tissues, mouth, pharynx, larynx, trachea, vagina, and anus. Vaccinees that exhibit mild varicella infection rarely have more than 50 lesions (Myers et al, 2007).

Diagnostic Studies. These are of little importance because the clinical picture is easily recognized, except in the case of exposure of pregnant women. The preferred method specific for VZV is the PCR or direct fluorescent antibody done from scrapings of a vesicle base during the first 3 to 4 days posteruption. Tzanck smears of lesions demonstrate multinucleated giant cells containing intranuclear inclusion bodies, but are not specific for VZV. Serial IgG antibody titers from acute and convalescent samples can also be compared for diagnosis confirmation. The virus can be cultured from vesicular fluid, CSF, and biopsy of tissue but is less sensitive than the PCR. The WBC count is usually within normal limits.

Differential Diagnosis
The rash is classic; therefore, the diagnosis is usually not a problem (see discussion later in this chapter on differentiating varicella from smallpox). Occasionally, impetigo, cigarette burns, and insect bites can cause some confusion in children with a mild rash. Other infections that can be confused with varicella include eczema herpeticum, HSV, and Stevens-Johnson syndrome.

Management
Chickenpox is usually a benign infection in normal children. Treatment is supportive and includes management of itching with antihistamines or oatmeal baths, acetaminophen for fever, and antistaphylococcal penicillin or cephalosporins for bacterial superinfections until the bacterial agent has been identified. Children with fever for more than several days, or increasing temperatures 4 or more days after the appearance of the rash, should be evaluated closely for invasive disease. Aspirin is contraindicated because of the possibility of Reye syndrome. The use of ibuprofen for fever has been questioned because of a possible causal relationship with bacterial superinfections (Leroy et al, 2007).

Intravenous acyclovir is efficacious for immunocompromised individuals and for those with severe disease. See Table 23-3 regarding use of varicella immune globulin; it is not effective after the disease has progressed. Oral acyclovir is expensive and is not routinely recommended for most children (Pickering et al, 2009). When given to otherwise healthy children within 24 hours after eruption of the rash, there is a modest decrease in the symptoms and duration of the illness. Indications for the use of oral acyclovir is available from the CDC and AAP *Red Book* (CDC, 2009d; Pickering et al,

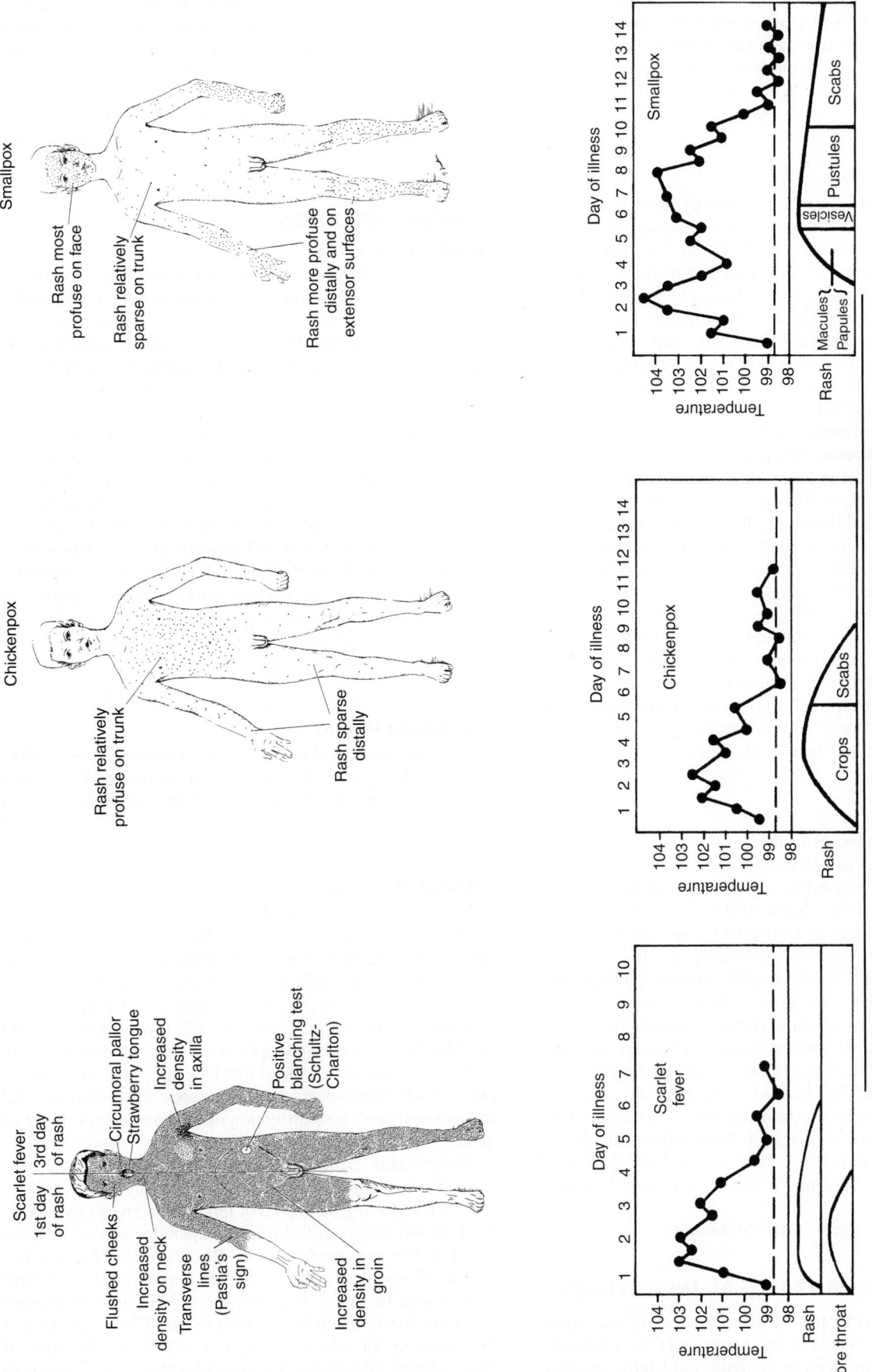

FIGURE 23-2 Differences in distribution of the maculopapular eruptions of scarlet fever, chickenpox, and smallpox. (Adapted from Katz S, Gershon A, Hotez P: *Krugman's infectious diseases of children*, ed 10, Philadelphia, 1998, Mosby.)

2009). It can also be considered for use in pregnant women with varicella, especially in their second or third trimester. For pregnant women exposed to varicella, VariZIG or IGIV can be considered. The safety to the fetus of acyclovir in the first trimester is uncertain given the low numbers thus far studied (Myers et al, 2007).

Complications
The following complications can occur: pyodermas (about a 5% incidence, causing serious invasive disease with *Streptococcus* and *Staphylococcus*); ITP (1% to 2%); pneumonia (smoking is a risk factor); CNS complications (e.g., encephalitis and Reye syndrome); and, rarely, glomerulonephritis, orchitis, hepatitis, toxic shock, osteomyelitis, necrotizing fasciitis, myositis, myocarditis, arthritis, and appendicitis. Primary varicella is associated with mortality rates of fewer than 2 to 3 per 100,000 cases with the lowest mortality rates in children 1 to 9 years old. The highest rates occur in infants, adults, and those immunocompromised.

Congenital Varicella. Neonatal involvement is directly tied to the timing of the maternal infection. Infection early in pregnancy (between 7 and 20 weeks of gestation) can result in 1% to 2% of infants exhibiting significant physical anomalies, CNS complications, and scarring (referred to as congenital varicella syndrome). Those exposed in utero after 20 weeks of gestation may have unapparent varicella and zoster early in life (Pickering et al, 2009). Because there is no time for maternal antibodies to develop and cross the placenta, newborns should be given IGIV (or VZIG if available) as soon as possible if their mothers develop varicella 5 days or less before the delivery or within 2 days postpartum. Despite having received VZIG, about 50% of infants may still develop mild varicella infection (Myers et al, 2007).

Prevention
The following are recommended:
- Children exposed to chickenpox can attend school for about 1 week. If they begin to show signs of illness, they must be kept home for 1 week. If they do not break out in a rash they may return to school. Children with active disease are to be kept home until all lesions are dry.
- Exposed patients: Use of varicella immune globulin has been discussed and can cause asymptomatic infection. Those who received immune globulin should obtain age-appropriate varicella immunization (unless contraindicated) within 5 months. In the immunocompromised, varicella titer may be obtained 2 months after varicella immune globulin to assess immune status. However, these results are not always reliable in these individuals; as an alternative, these individuals can be considered for future varicella immune globulin if exposed again (Pickering et al, 2009).
- Varicella vaccine as previously discussed.

PANDEMIC INFLUENZA VIRAL INFECTIONS
Influenza virus is an orthomyxovirus of three antigenic types, A, B, and C. Types A and B are responsible for epidemic disease; type C is attributed to sporadic mild influenza-like illness in children. Type A is further classified into two surface proteins—hemagglutinin and neuraminidase. Three hemagglutinin subtypes and two neuraminidase types are known to cause disease in humans (e.g., H1N1, HIN2, H3N2). Influenza A viruses can originate from swine and domestic or wild avian sources. Influenza is a highly contagious disease and is spread person to person by direct contact, droplet contamination, and fomites recently contaminated with infected nasopharyngeal secretions.

TYPICAL INFLUENZA
Epidemiology
In temperate climates, typical influenza epidemics always occur in the winter months, last approximately 4 to 8 weeks, and peak 2 weeks after the index case. In recent years some epidemics have lasted 3 months as a result of more than one strain of virus circulating within a community. Children shed the virus longer than adults and, therefore, are particularly prolific transmitters within a community.

After the emergence of a newly shifted subtype, the highest incidence of the illness occurs in healthy infants and children 5 to 14 years old, with an incidence of 10% to 40%. Children younger than 2 years old (especially infants less than 6 months old), those 65 years and older, and those with chronic diseases have excessively high rates of hospitalization. Though mortality figures are high for children with predisposing conditions, most fatalities occur among previously healthy children with no known risk factors; one study showed that 94% of known deaths occurred in children who had not been immunized against influenza (Pickering et al, 2009).

Incubation Period
The incubation period is 1 to 4 days. Patients become infectious 24 hours before the onset of symptoms. Viral shedding usually peaks by day 3 and ceases 7 days after the onset of illness.

Clinical Findings
Influenza patients are sick! Sudden onset of high fever (102° to 106° F [38.8° to 41° C]), headache, chills, coryza, vertigo, sore throat, pain in the back and extremities, and dry hacking cough that can resemble pertussis occur. Vomiting, diarrhea, and croup occur in young children. Infants can appear septic. Conjunctival infection, epistaxis, and myocarditis (evident by weak heart sounds and rapid, weak pulse) are common. In severe infection, there can be involvement of the lower respiratory tract with atelectasis or infiltrates. Severe myocardial involvement can cause distention of the right side of the heart and CHF.

Diagnostic Studies. Rapid influenza diagnostic test (RIDT) results are variable, ranging from sensitivities of 44% to 97% (depending on degree of influenza activity) and specificities from 76% to 100% when compared with viral cultures based on test and specimen type. Results of RIDTs are available in 15 minutes or less; some are approved for outpatient clinical use. However, their use should be based on whether the result would result in a change in the clinical care of that individual or for others at high risk (CDC, 2010h). Special viral cultures taken from the nasopharyngeal cavity by swab or aspiration within 72 hours of the onset of illness can isolate the virus in 2 to 6 days to confirm the diagnosis. Direct fluorescent antibody (DFA) and indirect immunofluorescent antibody (IFA) test results can be obtained within 3 or 4 hours and are available from hospital-based laboratories (Pickering et al, 2009). There are numerous serologic tests: viral agglutination, complement fixation, neutralization, or enzyme immunoassay (EIA). RT-PCR is both sensitive and specific. A CBC shows leukopenia.

Differential Diagnosis

The differential diagnosis includes other viral respiratory infections (common cold, parainfluenza, RSV, avian flu based on risk factors), allergic croup, epiglottitis, and bacterial URIs.

Management

Treatment is supportive (bed rest, fluids, antipyretics). Given its expense, treatment or prophylaxis with antiviral therapy (amantidine, rimantadine, zanamivir, oseltamivir) should be reserved for the following (Pickering et al, 2009):

- Children at risk of severe or complicated influenza infection (e.g., immunocompromised)
- Healthy children with moderate or severe illness
- Individuals within environments or family or social situations for which an illness would prove detrimental

When antivirals are indicated, treatment should be started within 48 hours of symptom onset and continued until the patient is asymptomatic for 24 to 48 hours. There is no approved antiretroviral for infants younger than 12 months of age. The effectiveness of the antivirals can vary from year to year based on the virus and strains in play for that season. Providers should search the CDC website for the antiviral treatment recommendations each influenza season.

Complications

Complications include Reye syndrome, respiratory infections (acute otitis media [AOM], pneumonia), acute myositis, toxic shock, myocarditis, and cystic fibrosis (CF) and asthma exacerbations followed by bacterial superinfection, usually with *H. influenzae*. Do not give aspirin to influenza sufferers!

Prevention

Influenza vaccine should be widely promoted. Antiviral prophylaxis against specific types of influenza infections may be indicated. The prophylactic doses are the same as for active influenza treatment. Though not mandatory by any professional organization, the Society for Healthcare Epidemiology of America recommends that all health care providers receive yearly influenza vaccine to protect themselves and prevent the spread of this disease to their patients and families. This action is viewed as an ethical obligation of all health care providers and personnel (Clinician Reviews, 2010).

AVIAN INFLUENZA

The avian influenza A viral strain of H5N1 has the potential to acquire genes from the influenza virus that affects other species. It is spread quickly and has morphed into a more pathogenic virus than when it first emerged in 1996. There is little natural immunity in humans; fortunately the disease in humans is still restricted and uncommon, and the virus has not yet mutated to be efficiently transmitted from person to person. To date, only humans who have had known direct contact with sick or dead poultry or wild birds or who have visited live poultry markets are most at risk for acquiring the virus. The outbreak is not expected to diminish significantly in the near future (CDC, 2008b). Human cases have been reported in Asia, Africa, the Pacific, Europe, and Near East. Indonesia and Vietnam have had the highest number of cases.

Humans who acquire the disease are severely ill, in contrast to those who experience mild symptoms with the typical "flu." Fever, malaise, myalgias, and respiratory symptoms progress to pneumonia, then to respiratory and multiorgan system failure, and then to death. Diarrhea can occur. To date the mortality rate in humans has been approximately 60%, with fatalities highest in those 10 to 19 years old (CDC, 2008b). The development of a vaccine to fight H5N1 is ongoing. If avian influenza is suspected, search the CDC website for guidance in obtaining specimens, monitoring suspected cases, and precautions by those traveling to endemic locales. The U.S. has banned importation of birds (dead or alive) and bird products (including hatching eggs) from H5N1-affected countries (list of countries available from the CDC).

OTHER VIRAL DISEASES

HUMAN IMMUNODEFICIENCY VIRUS
Pathophysiology and Epidemiology

HIV-1 and HIV-2 are retroviruses that cause disease in humans. Both serotypes cause clinically indistinguishable disease; most of the infections in the U.S. are attributed to HIV-1, less commonly to HIV-2. Retroviruses are RNA viruses that must make a DNA copy of their RNA in order to replicate. They do this by integrating into a target CD4+ T cell and then using the reverse transcriptase enzyme to convert their RNA into DNA within the cell nucleus. With transcription and translation, the HIV genes convert into messenger RNA, which can leave the nucleus with the viral genome code inside. Eventually new virions bud from the CD4+ T cells, infect other cells, and the cycle is repeated. HIV persists in infected individuals for life; latent virus protein remains in cells of the blood, brain, bone marrow, and genital tract even when the plasma viral load cannot be detected.

Although there are AIDS-like syndromes in other primates and felines, infection cannot be obtained from pets, animals, or insects. Humans are the only known reservoir for HIV-1 and HIV-2. The mode of transmission is intimate sexual contact, sharing of contaminated needles for injection, transfusion of contaminated blood or blood products, perinatal exposure, and breastfeeding. HIV has been isolated from blood (lymphocytes, macrophages, and plasma), CSF, pleural fluid, cervical secretions, human milk, feces, saliva, and urine. However, only blood, semen, cervical secretions, and human milk are implicated in transmission.

From 2006 through 2009, the annual estimated number and rate of diagnoses of HIV infection in the United States remained stable in the 40 states with confidential named-based reporting systems; approximately 79% of those infected are aware of their HIV status (CDC, 2010i, 2011). The risk of sexual transmission from just one episode of intercourse with an infected person is low. The highest per-act risk for transmission is from blood transfusion, needle sharing between drug users, receptive anal intercourse, and percutaneous needle injuries (CDC, 2006b). Accidental needlesticks in occupational settings rarely account for seroconversion and have a low infectivity rate. Less than 1% of the documented cases occurred this way. Transmission from accidental needlesticks from nonoccupational sources has not been documented. Transmission of HIV from a human bite (even when saliva is contaminated with blood) is extremely rare (CDC, 2010i). Transmission from antibody-screened blood transfusions in the U.S. is about 1 per 60,000 units (Yogev and Chadwick, 2007).

In the U.S., one of the expanding HIV-positive groups is adolescents 15 to 19 years old; rates are stable for those younger than 15 years. Racial and ethnic disparities of infection are present, with African Americans, Native Americans/Alaska Natives, Asians, and Hispanic males having higher rates, as well as men who have sex with men and those who live in urban areas (CDC, 2010i). Adolescent males are more likely to acquire the virus from male-to-male transmission; female adolescents acquire it via heterosexual transmission (72%) and IV drug use (26%) (Luzuriaga and Sullivan, 2008). Because of the long incubation period (8 to 12 years), these adolescents may not experience symptoms until they are in their 20s or 30s. A small number of children have been reported to have acquired HIV from sexual abuse (Yogev and Chadwick, 2007).

The transmission of HIV to infants can occur in several ways: in utero (5% of cases), intrapartum (13% to 18%; from infected blood and cervicovaginal secretions in the birth canal), or postpartum via breast milk (33% to 50%) (Shetty and Maldonado, 2008). If the mother has been infected with HIV during pregnancy, transmission is rare if she has low or undetectable serum levels of HIV around the time of labor and delivery. The transmission rate is higher if her initial HIV-1 infection occurs during the third trimester, when her viral load may be high but her immune activation has not fully responded (Pickering et al, 2009).

Risk of an untreated HIV-infected woman giving birth to an infected infant is 15% to 30% (Luzuriaga and Sullivan, 2008). In vaginal twin deliveries, the firstborn twin has a greater risk of developing HIV than the second. Elective cesarean delivery appears to reduce the risk of fetal infection by 87% in conjunction with zidovudine for both the mother and infant. The mother's age, advanced infection, low CD4+ T-lymphocyte count, maternal drug use, premature rupture of membranes greater than 4 hours, low birthweight, premature birth before 34 weeks, and viral load are other risk factors for increased transmission of the virus (Yogev and Chadwick, 2007).

Infection through postpartum human milk transmission can be as high as 33% and 50% in some undeveloped countries; rates can depend on the maternal state of infection, length of time she has been breastfeeding, and the presence of breast abscesses, mastitis, or nipple sores. Most HIV-1 transmission is found to occur in the initial few months of breastfeeding; the risk decreases thereafter (Luzuriaga and Sullivan, 2008). Transmission has not been reported in an infant after a single exposure to HIV-infected human milk (Havens, 2003). Transmission has been reported, however, in infants who were fed premasticated food by HIV-1 infected caregivers with bleeding gums or oral sores (Pickering et al, 2009). In developing countries where pediatric AIDS is pandemic, treatment

regimens—out of nutritional necessity—have traditionally included breastfeeding plus short-term antiretroviral drug treatment for women and infants.

Incubation Period

The incubation period is variable. The onset of symptoms of HIV infection in infants untreated perinatally is approximately 12 to 18 months; some appear within the first few months of life. Seroconversion occurs within 5 weeks in 50% of those exposed to HIV; 95% will seroconvert within 5 months (Sykes and Truax, 2010).

HIV infection can have a long latency period (longer than 5 years). Intrauterine transmission usually occurs by 10 weeks of gestation and is associated with early, severe disease in the newborn. Fifteen percent to 20% of HIV-infected children die before 4 years old (median age 11 months), whereas 80% to 85% of untreated children will experience delayed symptoms and can survive beyond 5 years of age (Pickering et al, 2009; Yogev and Chadwick, 2007).

Clinical Findings

HIV infection is often experienced as an influenza-like illness (fever, rash, sore throat, lymphadenopathy, and myalgias) for 2 to 4 weeks. These symptoms can suggest a nonspecific viral process, and a provider may not consider HIV in the differential diagnosis. At this point, the asymptomatic infection may continue for a few months to up to 15 years, depending on the viral load. The CD4+ T cells start declining at an average rate of about 50 cells/μL/year.

There are four HIV infection clinical categories for children with HIV infection, ranging from "no signs or symptoms" to "severe signs and symptoms." These categories are paired with the degree of age-specific CD4+ T-lymphocyte count and total percentage of lymphocytes to determine the stage of disease and management strategies. Newborn examinations are usually normal. Lymphadenopathy is often the first symptom, then hepatosplenomegaly. Some have failure to thrive, chronic or recurrent diarrhea, pneumonia (*Pneumocystis jiroveci* peaks at 3 to 6 months of age), oral candidiasis (in 15% to 40%), recurrent bacterial infections, chronic parotid swelling, and progressive neurologic deterioration. Those with high HIV loads develop symptoms earlier, including failure to thrive and encephalopathy. Other opportunistic diseases are *Mycobacterium avium* infection, severe CMV after 6 months old, EBV, VZV, disseminated histoplasmosis, RSV, *Mycobacterium tuberculosis*, and measles (despite vaccination).

Children—other than infants—generally have more recurrent bacterial infections, parotid gland swelling, lymphoid interstitial pneumonitis, or neurologic deficiencies that can progress to encephalopathy. *Streptococcus pneumoniae*, HIB, *Staphylococcus aureus*, and *Salmonella* organisms are common infections in pediatric AIDS patients. Sinusitis, cellulitis, glomerulopathy (especially in those of African descent), cardiac hypertrophy, anemia, CHF, and purulent middle ear infections are common. Malignancies are uncommon in pediatric AIDS.

Diagnostic Studies. Babies who are considered to have been exposed to HIV in utero demonstrate a positive virologic assay test (HIV-1 DNA PCR is the preferred assay)

| TABLE 23-6 | Testing Schedule for Human Immunodeficiency Virus in the Exposed, Non-breastfeeding Infant in the U.S. |

Test*	Time After Birth
First HIV-1 DNA PCR assay from peripheral blood (not cord blood); confirm if positive using the same test on another blood sample	Within 48 hours
Optional, HIV-1 DNA PCR assay; confirm if positive	14-21 days (some clinicians prefer this optional testing date)
Second HIV-1 DNA PCR assay; confirm if positive	1-3 months
Third HIV-1 DNA PCR assay; confirm if positive	4-6 months
Fourth HIV-1 DNA PCR assay; confirm if positive (may use RNA PCR if child older than 18 months)	12 and 24 months
Infant is considered infected if two separate samples test positive by HIV-1 DNA PCR. Infant <18 months and non-breasting is considered *definitely negative:* 2 negative tests obtained at ≥1 month and ≥4 months; two negative tests obtained at ≥6 months; and no other laboratory or clinical evidence that suggests HIV/AIDs.	

AIDS, Acquired immunodeficiency syndrome; *DNA,* deoxyribonucleic acid; *ICD,* immune complex dissociated; *HIV,* human immunodeficiency virus; *PCR,* polymerase chain reaction; *RNA,* ribonucleic acid.

*The following tests for HIV-1 are not recommended for use in those younger than 1 month of age: HIV culture; HIV p24 antigen assay; ICD p24 antigen assay; HIV-1 RNA PCR (the best option to use for children >18 months).

Hints for interpretation of results:
- Positive DNA PCR at 48 hours implies in utero transmission.
- About 93% of infected infants have a positive DNA PCR at 2 weeks of age.
- About 95% of infected infants will have a positive DNA PCR at 1 month of age.

Data from Pickering LK, Baker CJ, Kimberlin DW, et al: Children in out-of-home child care. In *Red Book 2009: Report of the Committee on Infectious Diseases* ed 28, Elk Grove Village, IL, 2009, American Academy of Pediatrics, pp 380-400.

within 48 hours of birth; those who acquire the infection in the intrapartum period test negative on this test in the first week but positive before 90 days of life. Maternal HIV IgG can persist for as long as 15 to 18 months. The HIV-1 proviral DNA assay (HIV-1 DNA PCR) identifies HIV-infected newborns early in the neonatal period, is one of the most sensitive tests, and is the only one recommended for infants less than 1 month. All the other assays have problems with false-positives, sensitivity, variable results, excessive length of time for results to be reported, or expense (Pickering et al, 2009). Table 23-6 lists recommended testing times and tests available.

Lymphopenia occurs as the disease progresses. There are decreased circulating CD4+ cells (T-suppressor, T-helper cells), and the helper-suppressor ratio is less than 1. The CDC defines an individual as suffering from autoimmune deficiency disease (e.g., AIDS) when their CD4+ T cell count is less than 200/mm^3. Some AIDS patients become seronegative late in the disease because the weakened immune system cannot manufacture antibodies.

Differential Diagnosis

The differential diagnosis includes other causes of immunologic deficiency, such as recent therapy with an immunosuppressive agent, lymphoproliferative disease, congenital immunologic states, inflammatory bowel disease, DiGeorge syndrome, ITP, chronic allergies, CF, graft-versus-host reaction, congenital CMV, toxoplasmosis, ataxia, or telangiectasia.

Management

Any information about HIV is subject to change, and the provider is cautioned to check with the CDC regarding any changes in HIV or AIDS diagnosis, treatment, and specific immunization precautions and regimens (Sherman, 2010). Treatment goals include suppressing viral replication to undetectable levels; restoring/preserving immune function; reducing HIV-associated sequelae; minimizing drug toxicity; promoting normal growth and development; and promoting quality of life (Pickering et al, 2009; Yogev and Chadwick, 2007). Initiation of antiretroviral treatment depends on the age, immune status, viral load, and clinical categories previously mentioned. Current drug regimens include combination therapy with at least three oral ARV drugs. The mainstays of therapy are the reverse transcriptase inhibitors (RTIs), nucleoside reverse transcriptase inhibitors (NRTIs) or non-NRTIs (NNRTIs), and the protease inhibitors. An injectable fusion inhibitor is also available for use in children. Treatment regimens require frequent laboratory studies and possible ARV changes throughout the life of the individual.

Primary care providers can manage infants born to HIV-infected women in consultation with an HIV or infectious disease specialist. Established protocols for the HIV-infected mother and her newborn are available. Box 23-2 outlines the protocol for the HIV-exposed newborn. The infant should be discharged from the hospital with the full 6-week course of antibiotics in hand, not just a prescription, with complete instructions for administration. This helps ensure greater compliance and continuity of prophylaxis because some insurance companies do not start paying for outpatient treatment of an infant for several weeks after birth (AAP, 2008). Treatment of a child (versus newborn) infected with HIV should only be undertaken in concert with pediatric HIV specialists because drug regimens are constantly being revised. Treatment of associated conditions with appropriate medical therapy is indicated using IGIV, antifungals, antivirals, antimycobacterials, and nutritional counseling. The CDC, AAP, and/or AIDS Treatment Information Service are excellent sources for the latest information regarding treatment. Many centers have ongoing clinical trials for which patients may be eligible.

An important role of the primary care provider in HIV treatment is helping to boost adherence rates. In addition, side effects must be monitored closely because many of the ARV drugs can interact with other commonly prescribed medications. The treatment regimens are highly challenging for parents because of complex dosing schedules and unwillingness of children to take the required medications. Many preparations are not offered in liquid form or the taste is not attractive to children. To enhance compliance, some clinicians use tools such as computer-assisted age-dependent programs; electronic pillboxes; routinely measuring drug levels; developing simpler drug protocols; studying possible social and economic factors that predict compliance and individualize

BOX 23-2 Zidovudine Regimen to Decrease Risk of Perinatal HIV Transmission to Full-Term Newborns Within 8 to 12 Hours of Birth if 35 Weeks or More

- Zidovudine (ZDV) syrup, 2 mg/kg/dose PO every 6 hours daily* within 6-12 hours of birth[†] and continuing for the first 6 weeks of life*
- Rapid HIV-1 DNA PCR testing should be performed on all infants born to a mother whose HIV-1 serostatus is unknown (and also performed on the mother) within 8-12 hours of birth so that appropriate antiretroviral prophylaxis can be started. Some states require such testing on all newborns if mother has refused testing.
- Two alternative dosing regimens can be found at www.aidsinfo. nih.gov/ContentFiles/PerinatalGL.pdf.

*For full-term infants unable to tolerate oral intake, intravenous (IV) dosage of ZDV is 1.5 mg/kg every 6 hours. For infants <35 weeks of gestation dosage is 1.5 mg/kg/dose IV, or 2 mg/kg/dose PO, every 12 hours, advancing to every 8 hours at 2 weeks of age if >30 weeks of gestation at birth or at 4 weeks of age if <30 weeks of gestation at birth.

[†]Prophylaxis starting after 48 hours of birth is not likely to prevent the transmission of HIV.

DNA, Deoxyribonucleic acid; HIV, human immunodeficiency virus; PCR, polymerase chain reaction.

Data from Panel on Treatment of HIV-infected Pregnant Women and Prevention of Perinatal Transmission: Recommendations for use of antiretroviral drugs in pregnant HIV-1-infected women for maternal health and interventions to reduce perinatal HIV-1 transmission in the United States, 2010, p 88. Available at www.aidsinfo.nih.gov/ContentFiles/PerinatalGL.pdf (accessed Nov 12, 2010); Pickering LK, Baker CJ, Kimberlin DW, et al: Red Book: 2009 report of the committee on infectious diseases, ed 28, Elk Grove Village, IL, 2009, American Academy of Pediatrics, pp 380-400.

patient care accordingly; and referring families to support networks. (See Appendix A for some helpful information about increasing medication adherence rates.)

Adolescents can present a particular noncompliance risk because of denial and fear of their infection, substance abuse and addiction, misinformation, distrust of and inexperience with the medical system, self-esteem issues, unstable living situations, and lack of familial and social support systems. It is important for the provider to be nonconfrontational yet discuss risk factors and advocate for family planning services and needle exchange programs, postexposure prophylaxis (PEP) regimens, and prompt involvement in new treatments as they become available.

Complications

HIV becomes a multisystemic illness with multiorgan complications.

Prevention and Reduction of Perinatal Transmission of HIV. The use of combination ARV therapy to reduce perinatal transmission of HIV is the norm in the U.S. The CDC, WHO, and United Nations AIDS agencies are useful resources for current treatment regimens; recommendations may vary by country.

Research efforts in underdeveloped countries have focused on different ways to prevent transmission via breastfeeding. Strategies studied have included evaluating the acceptance of formula feeding by HIV-infected women, pasteurizing breast milk, avoiding mixed breastfeeding between women, treating

breast conditions (mastitis, etc.), restricting breastfeeding to the first 6 months, and the long-term use of antiretroviral therapy in both the breastfeeding woman and her infant (Read and Committee on Pediatric AIDS, 2007; Yogev and Chadwick, 2007). One study showed that if women were treated with prophylactic medications during the first trimester, and the infant for 6 weeks antepartum with zidovudine, the transmission rate decreased to less than 8%. Another study showed a rate of less than 2% (Yogev and Chadwick, 2007).

Various studies have also demonstrated that transmission rates to infants from mothers not given zidovudine during their pregnancy can be lowered when mothers are given zidovudine at the time of labor and their infants within 24 hours of delivery for 6 weeks (Luzuriaga and Sullivan, 2008). As a result of these antiretroviral efforts, in 2010, the CDC reported a 90% decrease in reported prenatally acquired HIV and AIDS in children as compared with 1992 rates (Lampe et al, 2010). A standard antiretroviral regimen is now standard treatment for HIV-infected pregnant women and their infants. Providers need to be vigilant regarding maternal adherence with the recommended postnatal HIV prophylaxis for her infant and herself. Such adherence has been shown to be lower in women with asymptomatic HIV, who have poor social networks, who feel guilt or stigma, or who adhere poorly to their own ARV regimens (Demas et al, 2002; Wrubel et al, 2005).

- HIV-infected pregnant women and HIV-infected mothers should be counseled about the following (Pickering et al, 2009):
  - Women and their health care providers need to be aware of the potential risk of transmission of HIV infection to infants in utero and in the postpartum period and through human milk.
  - Documented, routine HIV education, and routine testing with consent of all women seeking prenatal care are strongly recommended so that each woman knows her HIV status and the methods available to prevent the acquisition and transmission of HIV to her newborn and to document whether breastfeeding is appropriate.
  - At the time of delivery, provision of education about HIV and testing with consent of all women whose HIV status is unknown are strongly recommended. Knowledge of the woman's HIV status assists in counseling on breastfeeding and helps each woman understand the benefits to herself and her infant of knowing her serostatus and the behaviors that decrease the likelihood of acquisition and transmission of HIV.
  - In general, women who are known to be HIV seronegative should be encouraged to breastfeed. However, women who are HIV seronegative but at particular high risk of seroconversion (e.g., injection drug users) should be educated about HIV with an individualized recommendation concerning the appropriateness of breastfeeding. In addition, during the perinatal period, information should be provided on the potential risk of transmitting HIV through human milk and about methods to reduce the risk of acquiring HIV infection.
- NICUs should develop policies that are consistent with these recommendations for the use of expressed human milk for neonates. Gloves should be worn by health care workers in situations in which exposure to breast milk might be frequent or prolonged, such as in milk banking. Human milk banks should follow the guidelines developed

by the FDA, CDC, and AAP. The nonprofit Human Milk Banking Association of North America sets standards of testing for all their members' milk banks.

- Adolescents must be counseled about the risk of HIV transmission (e.g., sexual transmission, sharing of needles or syringes) and the use of condoms. Condom use has been reported by 61.1% of adolescents, whereas only 12.7% report ever having had an HIV test (female rates are higher than for males) (Eaton et al, 2010).

- School attendance: Factors that must be taken into account include the risk to the immunosuppressed child of "normal germs" from healthy kids and school personnel. The benefit from attendance far outweighs the risks. Because casual transmission is unknown, there is no real risk to other children as long as the infected child can control body secretions. Children who display biting behavior or have oozing wounds should be cared for in a setting that minimizes risk to others. The child's primary care provider is the only person with an absolute need to know the child's primary diagnosis. If the family decides to inform the school, those informed should maintain confidentiality. If the family chooses not to inform the school, parents should get assurance that the school will notify them of any communicable disease outbreaks (e.g., varicella, measles) or physical altercations with others.

- Routine screening of school-age children for HIV antibodies is not indicated.

Postexposure Prophylaxis After Nonoccupational Exposure. The primary care provider may be faced with having to assess and counsel parents after their child has had an accidental puncture wound from a discarded needle found on a street, public transportation, or playground; from a wound obtained from a bite, a fight, or during a sports activity; from sexual abuse; or from exposure to breast milk from an HIV-infected woman. Though transmission is extremely rare, the provider needs to be able to address the situation with a level of understanding of the risks and current recommendations of the CDC (Fig. 23-3).

The body fluids of an HIV-infected person do not all carry the same amount of viral load or risk. For example, exposure to blood of a known HIV-infected person carries the highest risk, whereas blood-free saliva, semen or vaginal secretions, and human milk carry a low risk; urine, feces, and vomitus are unlikely to transmit the virus (CDC, 2005). Syringes that might have been used and discarded by an HIV-infected, injection-drug user generate the most concern by parents. The following information is useful when counseling parents:

- HIV viability is vulnerable to drying.
- The smaller the needle bore, the more limited the amount of blood present.
- Health care professionals stuck with a needle after withdrawing blood from an individual with full-blown clinical AIDS have a 0.3% HIV transmission risk (Levine, 2008). Most syringes (approximately 96%) used for IM or subcutaneous injection by an HIV-infected individual will not have discernible HIV RNA (CDC, 2005). There has been no documented transmission of HIV from an accidentally found, discarded needle.
- One is more likely to face greater risk from biting an individual who is HIV positive (saliva contaminated with HIV-infected blood) than from having been bitten by one infected with HIV (saliva not contaminated by infected blood).

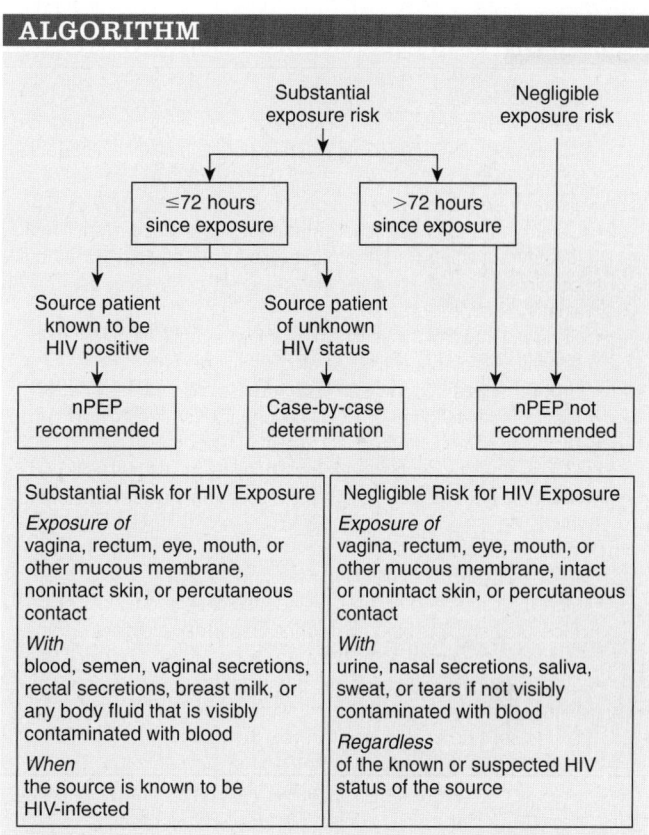

ALGORITHM

FIGURE 23-3 Algorithm for evaluation and treatment of possible nonoccupational human immunodeficiency virus (HIV) exposures. *nPEP,* nonoccupational postexposure prophylaxis. (From Smith DK, Grohskopf LA, Black RJ: Antiretroviral postexposure prophylaxis after sexual, injection drug use, or other nonoccupational exposure to HIV in the U.S.: recommendations from the U.S. Department of Health and Human Services, *MMWR Morb Mortal Wkly Rep* 54 [RR-2]:1-20, 2005. Available at www.cdc.gov/mmwr/PDF/rr/rr5402.pdf [accessed Dec 14, 2010].)

The provider and parent must weigh the unproven safety and benefits of participating in the PEP regimen against the significant toxicity of the drugs themselves. If instituted, PEP therapy needs to start within 72 hours after exposure and continue for 28 days. Close follow-up for support, medication monitoring (adherence and toxicity), and serial HIV antibody screening are needed (Box 23-3 provides some management strategies). Consult the CDC concerning the current PEP prophylaxis antiretroviral drug therapy recommended.

MEASLES (RUBEOLA)

Epidemiology

Measles (rubeola) is a *Morbillivirus* in the Paramyxoviridae family and is similar to mumps and influenza. There is only one antigenic type. Measles is typified by a rash, indicating viremia. It is a serious illness in children! The disease is associated with high mortality and morbidity rates worldwide. Humans and primates are the only known reservoir of infection. The sources of the infection include respiratory secretions, blood, and urine of infected persons. Virus is transmitted through droplet contact, fomites, and, less likely, aerosol transmission. Peak incidence of infection in susceptible persons occurs during the winter and spring months. The failure rate after the first

BOX 23-3 Management of Patients With Possible Exposure to HIV

1. Treat the exposure site.
   - Wash wounds with soap and water; flush mucous membranes with water. Give Td or Tdap booster if appropriate (see also Table 23-3).
2. Evaluate the exposure source if possible.
   - Determine the HIV infection status of the exposure source. If unknown, testing with appropriate consent should be offered if possible.
3. Evaluate the exposed person.
   - Perform HIV serologic testing to identify current HIV infection and hepatitis B and hepatitis C serologic testing as appropriate.
   - Provide or refer for counseling to address stress and anxiety.
   - Discuss prevention of potential secondary HIV transmission.
   - Discuss prevention of repeat exposure, if appropriate.
   - Report the incident to legal or administrative authorities as appropriate to the setting of the exposure and the severity of the incident.
4. Consider PEP.
   - Explain potential benefits and risks.
   - Discuss issues of drug toxicity and medication compliance.
   - Measure complete blood cell count, creatinine, and alanine transaminase concentration as baseline for possible drug toxicity.
   - Begin prophylaxis as soon as possible after exposure, preferably within 1 to 4 hours; prophylaxis begun more than 72 hours after exposure is unlikely to be effective.

   - Arrange for follow-up with HIV specialist and psychologist, if appropriate.
   - Educate about prevention of secondary transmission (sexually active adolescent should avoid sex, or use condoms, until all follow-up test results are negative).
   - Report to PEP registry at CDC.
5. Choose therapy.
   - Consider drug potency and toxicity, regimen complexity and effects on compliance, and possibility of drug resistance in the exposure source.
   - Supply 3 to 5 days of medication immediately, instructing patients to obtain remainder of medication at follow-up visit.
6. Follow up.
   - Perform initial follow-up within 2-3 days to review drug regimen and adherence, evaluate for symptoms of drug toxicity, assess psychosocial status, and arrange appropriate referrals, if needed.
   - Continue therapy for 28 days.
   - Monitor for drug adverse effects at 4 weeks with complete blood cell count and alanine transaminase concentration.
   - Evaluate for psychological stress and medication compliance with weekly office visits or telephone calls.
   - Consider referral for counseling if needed.
   - Repeat HIV serologic testing at 6 weeks, 12 weeks, and 6 months after exposure.

CDC, Centers for Disease Control and Prevention; *PEP,* postexposure prophylaxis.
From Havens PL, Committee on Pediatric AIDS: Postexposure prophylaxis in children and adolescents for nonoccupational exposure to human immunodeficiency virus, *Pediatrics* 111(6):1475-1489, 2003. Reaffirmed 2009.

vaccine at 12 months old is approximately 5%; after the second vaccine the failure rate is about 2% (Pickering et al, 2009). Modified measles can manifest in children who have been passively immunized with IG after exposure to the disease. It can also occur in infants with partial maternal immunity. The illness is an abbreviated version of typical disease.

Incubation Period

The incubation period is 8 to 12 days. A person is contagious 1 to 2 days before the onset of symptoms or 3 to 5 days before the rash, and 4 days after the appearance of the rash, or roughly 14 days (Pickering et al, 2009). The incubation period of modified measles can persist as long as 20 days. There is no carrier state; disease or two vaccinations usually confer lifelong immunity.

Clinical Findings

The clinical manifestations are divided into three stages:
1. *Incubation period:* There are no specific symptoms.
2. *Prodromal period:* This is the first sign of the illness and lasts 4 to 5 days. This stage consists of URI symptoms, low to moderate fever (greater than 101° F [38.3° C]), and cough, coryza, and conjunctivitis (the "three C's" of measles). An enanthem can be found on the oral mucosa opposite the lower molars. These Koplik spots last 12 to 15 hours. They are small, irregular, bluish white granules on an erythematous background and are pathognomonic of measles infection.
3. *Rash stage:* The rash of unmodified measles usually appears on the third or fourth day of the illness. As the rash appears, temperature rises, often to 105° F (40.5° C). The rash first appears behind the ears and on the forehead. It is

maculopapular. Papules enlarge, coalesce, and move progressively downward, engulfing the face, neck, and arms over the next 24 hours. By the end of the second 24 hours, the rash has spread to the back, abdomen, and thighs. As the legs become more involved, the face begins to clear. The entire process takes approximately 3 days. Respiratory symptoms are most severe on day 3 of the rash. The more severe the rash, the more severe the illness. It can become hemorrhagic. This type of measles can be fatal because of disseminated intravascular coagulation (DIC). After the fourth day of the rash stage, the rash begins to fade. The disease peaks; defervescence occurs. After the rash clears a residual light pigmentation occurs, lasting approximately 1 week, that desquamates. Maternal antibody level and improperly given vaccine can alter the presentation and clinical course.

With modified measles, the prodrome period can be as early as 1 to 2 days with normal to low-grade fever. URI symptoms are minimal to absent. Koplik spots usually do not appear. The rash is so mild that it is often missed.

Diagnostic Studies. A single measles IgM antibody level is useful if drawn when symptoms suggest this disease; the reactivity is low after more than 30 days. Confirmation of disease can also be made by viral isolation from urine, blood, throat or nasopharyngeal secretions or from serial IgG antibody titers that compare acute and convalescent serum specimens. Measles is a reportable disease in the U.S.

Differential Diagnosis

Any viral rash (e.g., roseola, rubella, echovirus, coxsackievirus, IM, adenovirus, and EBV), toxoplasmosis, scarlet fever, Kawasaki syndrome, meningococcemia, Rocky Mountain spotted fever, drug rashes, and serum sickness are included in the differential diagnosis.

Management

Treatment is supportive (antipyretics, bed rest, adequate fluids, air humidification, warm room, darkened room if photophobia is present). Bacterial superinfections (e.g., ear infections, bronchopneumonia, encephalitis) are treated with appropriate antibiotics. All children with encephalitis, severe pneumonia, or compromised immune systems should be managed in consultation with an infectious disease expert.

Children in the U.S. and in countries where malnutrition is an issue are at greater risk for death or morbidity with measles infection. These children, and those with severe measles, have lower vitamin A levels. Use of vitamin A is now recommended for all children despite their country of residence. Dose once daily for 2 days: less than 6 months of age, 50,000 international units; 6 through 11 months of age, 100,000 international units; 12 or more months of age, 200,000 international units (Pickering et al, 2009).

Complications

Bacterial superinfection and viral complications can manifest as a URI, obstructive laryngitis, otitis, mastoiditis, cervical adenitis, bronchitis, transient hepatitis, and pneumonia (the largest cause of fatalities in infants). The causative organism can be the measles virus itself or group A beta-hemolytic streptococci (GABHS), pneumococci, *H. influenzae,* or *S. aureus.* Infection can exacerbate underlying TB. Other complications include myocarditis, purpura fulminans ("black measles," characterized by multiorgan bleeding), encephalitis (one in 1000 cases) and other neurologic sequelae, and subacute sclerosing panencephalitis (fatal complication of wild-type measles; the disease is more prevalent in males, in rural and poorer areas, and in Hispanic children) (Mason, 2007a). There are usually no complications with modified measles.

Care of Exposed Individuals

This is done with active and passive immunization.

MUMPS

Epidemiology

Mumps is an acute generalized viral disease with painful enlargement of one or more salivary glands (usually parotid glands). Mumps is in the Paramyxoviridae family. Only one serotype is known, and humans are the only natural reservoir. The source of infection is the saliva of infected persons. The virus is spread by direct contact, aerosol transmission, fomites, and possibly, urine from infected individuals. Viremia exists, and the virus is found in blood, urine, CSF, saliva, and upper respiratory secretions. Infection is more often an outcome of undervaccination of susceptible individuals. Incidence of this illness has decreased by more than 99% in the U.S. since the advent of the mumps vaccine (Litman and Baum, 2009). Infection occurs during all seasons but is most common during late winter and spring; it affects both sexes equally. Mumps virus crosses the placenta, and infection during the first trimester increases the risk of spontaneous abortion. Fetal malformations after prenatal mumps infection have not been demonstrated (Mason, 2007b).

Incubation Period

The incubation period ranges from 12 to 25 days (usually 16 to 18 days). The period of communicability is about 1 to 2 days before glandular swelling up to 5 days after the onset of swelling. One third of patients are asymptomatic but infectious. One attack usually confers lifelong immunity. Transplacental antibodies to mumps are protective for 6 months.

Clinical Findings

There are two clinical stages:
1. *Prodromal stage:* Rare in children but can cause fever, headache, anorexia, neck or other muscular pain, and malaise.
2. *Swelling stage:* Approximately 24 hours after the prodromal stage, one (in 25% of patients) or both of the parotid glands begin to painfully swell in a characteristic manner. If both glands are affected, one generally swells before the other. The gland fills the space between the posterior border of the mandible and mastoid, pushing downward and forward to the zygoma. The ear is pushed forward and upward. This can take a few hours to a few days. The enlarged glands usually return to normal size in 3 to 7 days; 10% to 15% of cases involve only submandibular gland swelling. Rarely a maculopapular, pink discrete rash is seen on the trunk. Pain on the affected side can be elicited by having the patient eat something sour. This is known as the "pickle sign." The Stensen duct is red and swollen. Fever is usually moderate and rarely high; 20% are afebrile. Little pain is associated with submandibular infection. However, the redness subsides more slowly. The Wharton duct is frequently swollen. If sublingual salivary glands are involved, there is bilateral swelling in the submental region in the floor of the mouth. Edema caused by lymphatic obstruction of the manubrium and upper chest is reported.

Diagnostic Studies. These include viral isolation and culture, and serologic tests (enzyme immunoassay for IgG and IgM antibodies and specific mumps antibody). Leukopenia with relative lymphocytosis and an elevated amylase are typical.

Differential Diagnosis

Cervical or preauricular lymphadenitis, CMV, HIV, enteroviruses, tumor, suppurative parotitis by either bacterial or viral (coxsackievirus, parainfluenza 1 and 3) infection, idiopathic recurrent parotitis, parotid ductal obstruction, Mikulicz syndrome, uveoparotid fever, and cancer (especially lymphosarcoma) are included in the differential diagnosis.

Management

Treatment is supportive (antipyretics, bed rest as needed, diet appropriate for chewing discomfort). Corticosteroids or nonsteroidal antiinflammatory drugs (NSAIDs) are given to manage arthritic complications. Manage orchitis with bed rest and scrotal elevation.

Complications

Complications include meningoencephalitis (mostly males older than 20 years); orchitis and/or epididymitis (14% to 35% incidence in adolescents and adults); oophoritis (7% incidence in postpubertal women; fertility is not affected); severe pancreatitis (rare); thyroiditis (uncommon in children); myocarditis; deafness (1 in 15,000 cases—transient or permanent); ocular complications (swelling of the lacrimal glands or optic neuritis); arthritis (rare in children); thrombocytopenia and hemolytic anemia (usually self-limited); mastitis (rare); and glomerulonephritis (rare).

Prevention

School and daycare students should be kept home until 9 days after the onset of parotid swelling. Active and passive immunization have been discussed.

ERYTHEMA INFECTIOSUM

Epidemiology

Erythema infectiosum, or fifth disease, is caused by parvovirus B19. The virus is a member of the Parvoviridae family and a single-stranded DNA virus that replicates in erythrocyte precursors. It is called *fifth disease* because it was the fifth eruptive rash described. These rashes include scarlet fever, measles, rubella, erythema subitum (roseola infantum; sixth disease), and erythema infectiosum. Humans are the only reservoir. Erythema infectiosum is spread via vertical transmission from mother to fetus, by respiratory tract secretions, and percutaneous exposure to blood or blood products. Distribution is worldwide. It is a disease of childhood, highest in 5- to 15-year-olds, but infants and adults are not immune. Secondary spread to household contacts is up to 50% (Pickering et al, 2009). The disease occurs most commonly in late winter and early spring.

Incubation Period

The incubation period is approximately 4 to 21 days; the rash and symptoms occur between 2 and 3 weeks after exposure. The period of communicability lasts until the rash appears. Chronic infection can occur in those immunocompromised or with most types of hemolytic anemias.

Clinical Findings

The following two phases are seen in erythema infectiosum:
1. *Prodrome:* Consists of mild fever (15% to 30% of cases), myalgias, headache, malaise, URI symptoms
2. *Rash:* Appears 7 to 10 days after the prodromal stage and occurs in three stages: It first appears on the face as an intense red eruption on the cheeks (slapped cheek) with circumoral pallor that lasts 1 to 4 days. Next a lacy maculopapular eruption appears on the trunk, then moves peripherally to the arms, thighs, and buttocks. Palms and soles are generally spared. This phase can last a month. Finally, the rash subsides. Older children may have pruritus. There may be periodic recurrences precipitated by trauma, heat, exercise, stress, sunlight, or cold (see Color Plate). Children experience arthralgia less than 10% of the time; knees are more commonly involved. Adult females are more likely to complain

of polyarthropathy (Pickering et al, 2009). Arthralgia most commonly resolves in 2 to 4 weeks. Those with hemolytic anemias or who are immunocompromised may have fever, pallor, tachycardia, and symptoms of heart failure.

Diagnostic Studies. Laboratory testing is not generally indicated because the diagnosis can be made clinically. Serum B19-specific IgM confirms the presence of infection and persists for 6 to 8 weeks. Anti-B19 IgG confirms past infection. For immunocompromised individuals, viral DNA testing methods are required. There are PCR or nucleic acid hybridization tests for B19. The virus is difficult to grow in culture.

Differential Diagnosis

This is not a difficult disease to diagnose. The differential diagnoses include rubella, enterovirus disease, lupus, atypical measles, and drug rashes.

Management

There is no specific antiviral treatment. Those with hemolytic anemia or who are immunocompromised should be considered for hospitalization. IGIV offers some help for those with immunocompromised conditions.

Complications

These are few and typically not significant. All previously healthy patients usually recover without sequelae. The most frequently reported complications include arthritis (hands, wrists, knees, ankles occurring 2 to 3 weeks after onset of initial symptoms); chronic infection in those immunodeficient; aplastic crisis (more common in those with chronic hemolytic anemias, including sickle cell anemia, thalassemia, hereditary spherocytosis, or other types of chronic hemolysis); fetal hydrops and death or intrauterine growth retardation if exposed in utero (no reports of congenital anomalies) (Koch, 2007); thrombocytopenic purpura or neutropenia; myocarditis (rare); papular-purpuric "gloves and socks" syndrome (fever, pruritus, purpura, painful edema, and redness in a glove-and-sock distribution pattern) followed by petechiae and oral lesions.

Prevention

Because there is widespread unapparent infection in children and adults avoidance of known exposure can reduce but not eliminate the risk of infection. An exposed pregnant woman should consult with her health care provider. Children in the rash stage may attend school.

PARAINFLUENZA VIRUS

Epidemiology

Parainfluenza virus, a paramyxovirus, is similar to the influenza and mumps viruses and is an important cause of croup, bronchitis, bronchiolitis, and pneumonia. There are four antigenic types. Most children have been exposed to types 1, 2, and 3 by the time they are 3 years old. Type 3 is endemic, associated more with illnesses in those less than 6 months old, results in shorter immunity (a particular problem for immunocompromised patients), and outbreaks tend to peak in the spring. Types 1 and 2 usually strike children 2 to 6 years old, and outbreaks are seen more in summer and fall and in odd-numbered years; reinfections occur at any age. Type 1 is most frequently associated with croup. Type 4 infections are less well pathologically and clinically understood but are not believed to cause severe illness (Wright, 2007).

This virus is spread by direct person-to-person contact through infected nasopharyngeal secretions or from fomite contamination; it replicates only in respiratory epithelium of the upper large airways and eustachian tube environs. Infection occurs throughout the year depending on the type. By the time most children are 5 years old, they have been exposed to all of the types (Pickering et al, 2009).

Incubation Period

The incubation period is 2 to 6 days. Depending on the serotype, healthy children can shed virus for 4 to 7 days before symptom onset and up to 7 to 21 days after resolution of symptoms.

Clinical Findings

Eighty percent of parainfluenza infections affect the upper airways. This virus accounts for 50% of hospital admissions for croup and 15% of admissions for bronchiolitis and pneumonia (Wright, 2007). Sore throat is a common complaint in older children. Fever is found in only 20% of cases and is inversely proportional to the age of the child. Discrete maculopapular rashes of short duration can be found if the patient is carefully examined.

Diagnostic Studies. Routine testing is not needed. The virus can be isolated from nasopharyngeal secretions; results are usually available within 4 to 7 days (or earlier) depending on the testing technique available. Confirmation is by rapid antigen detection. Sensitivities vary when rapid antigen identification is done by immunofluorescent assays, enzyme immunoassays, and fluoroimmunoassays. Multiplex RT-PCR may also be available.

Differential Diagnosis

The differential diagnosis includes other viral URIs, allergic croup, bacterial URIs, laryngotracheitis, and other acute upper airway obstructive diseases (e.g., acute angioneurotic edema, epiglottitis, and foreign body aspiration).

Management

The treatment is supportive. Antiviral therapy is not available (Pickering et al, 2009). Oxygen saturation and hypercapnia monitoring in more severely affected children are appropriate. Antibiotics are reasonable in cases of severe infection when secondary bacterial invasion is suspected (e.g., otitis media, pneumonia). See Chapter 31 for more specific treatment recommendations based on the diagnosis. No vaccine is available. Good hand hygiene is important.

Complications

Complications are infrequent. Secondary bacterial infections, including otitis media, bronchitis, tracheitis, and pneumonia may occur, especially in those who are immunocompromised.

RUBELLA (GERMAN OR 3-DAY MEASLES)
Epidemiology

Rubella is an acute disease of childhood that occurs in two forms: postnatal and congenital. Rubella is an RNA virus of the genus *Rubivirus*, in the Togaviridae family. Humans are the only reservoir. Infection is spread through nasopharyngeal secretions or transplacentally during either apparent or silent infection. It is worldwide in distribution. The virus has been isolated in blood, stool, and urine of infected individuals. It also has been isolated on fomites for as long as 24 hours.

With the arrival of immunization, the number of epidemics declined. Most cases now occur in those unvaccinated, foreign-born, or from areas with poor vaccination coverage. Serologic studies have determined that approximately 10% of individuals born in the U.S. older than age 5 years are susceptible (Pickering et al, 2009). Males and females are equally affected. Primary maternal infection during the first trimester to the sixteenth week is most associated with congenital defects. Approximately 25% to 50% of infections are subclinical. There is transplacental immunity for approximately 5 to 6 months if the mother is immune. There is probable lifelong immunity for naturally occurring disease. Verified second attacks are rare.

Incubation Period

The incubation period is 14 to 21 days (mean 18). The period of infectivity is 3 to 8 days after exposure and for 11 to 14 days thereafter. Those who develop rashes are infectious approximately 5 days before the rash to 6 days beyond its appearance (Maldonado, 2008).

Clinical Findings

Postnatal disease is marked by three stages, and splenomegaly may be present:

1. *Prodrome:* There are mild catarrhal symptoms (fever, GI upset, sore throat, eye pain, arthralgia). This stage is occasionally missed and occurs about 1 to 5 days prior to onset of stage 3.
2. *Lymphadenopathy:* Usually begins within 24 hours, but can begin as early as 7 days before the rash appears, and can last for more than 1 week. The postauricular, posterior cervical, and posterior occipital are the primary lymph nodes involved. There is generalized lymph node involvement, and at times splenomegaly is noted.
3. *Rash:* An enanthem can appear in 20% of cases just before the general rash. The enanthem, Forchheimer spots, consists of small rose-colored to reddish spots located on the soft palate. They are not considered pathognomonic for rubella and are noted in scarlet fever and other URIs. The rubella rash can be the first obvious sign of illness. It begins on the face and can fade before it spreads to the chest during the next 24 hours. The rash is composed of discrete maculopapules that occasionally coalesce. It spreads caudally, lasting a mean of 3 days. There can be itching without a rash or a fine, branlike desquamation. A low-grade fever can occur during the eruptive phase and continue for up to 3 days. There is no photophobia; anorexia, headache, and malaise are rare.

Diagnostic Studies. Diagnosis is usually made by clinical symptoms; however, the only reliable means to check infection is by antibody testing. Serologic testing of acute and convalescent titers at least 2 weeks apart or a single elevated IgM titer is diagnostic of recent infection. However, timing is everything for the interpretation of results, for the IgM remains detectable only for about 1 to 3 weeks after onset of the rash. Immunity is now more commonly tested using latex agglutination enzyme or fluorescent immunoassay, among others. Rubella-specific IgM is an important test in the newborn. Suspected rubella can be confirmed using throat, nasal, or urine specimens by inoculation of appropriate cell media; the laboratory should be notified so that specific testing on the culture can be done.

Differential Diagnosis

The disease can be difficult to diagnose unless there is an epidemic. The rash can be confused with scarlet fever, mononucleosis, enterovirus, roseola, rubeola, erythema infectiosum, EBV, and drug eruptions.

Management

Treatment is supportive (e.g., antipyretics for fever control) unless complications (e.g., encephalitis) occur; severe thrombocytopenic purpura can be managed with corticosteroid therapy and platelet transfusions.

Complications

Complications in postnatal rubella are rare. These include arthritis (most common complication, affecting 20% of children; females are afflicted more often; onset is about 1 week after appearance of rash), ITP, and encephalitis (within 4 days of onset of rash). Myocarditis, pericarditis, follicular conjunctivitis, hemolytic anemia, and hepatitis are rare complications (Maldonado, 2008).

Prevention

Children with postnatal rubella should be kept home from school or daycare for approximately 1 week after the rash erupts. Active and passive immunization have been discussed.

Reinfection

There are conflicting studies. Because illness without rash exists, the actual numbers of reinfections are unknown. Reinfection is known to occur from wild-type virus and in those previously immunized; in pregnant women reinfection can result in congenital rubella syndrome (Mason, 2007c). Accidental revaccination of a pregnant woman should not be considered a reason for pregnancy termination alone; surveillance has demonstrated signs of infection in the infant but not congenital rubella syndrome (Pickering et al, 2009).

WEST NILE VIRUS
Epidemiology

WNV is an arbovirus (family Flaviviridae) and is related to St. Louis and Japanese encephalitis viruses. The virus was previously known to mostly inhabit Africa, West Asia, and the Middle East. Since 1999 it has spread rapidly across the U.S. It recurs yearly during warmer weather, when mosquitoes begin breeding. Temperate weather and drought conditions are also believed to encourage mosquito-borne illnesses. It is mainly spread to people by bites from infected mosquitoes. The species of mosquito mostly commonly associated with WNV feeds at dawn and dusk and breeds in standing water. Evidence points to uncommon human-to-human spread via organ transplantation, blood transfusions, placenta, through breast milk, and possible aerosol transmission. The blood supply has been screened for WNV in the United States since 2003 (Ferri, 2010).

Mosquitoes become infected by feeding on the blood of previously mosquito-infected birds and then transferring the virus via saliva to other birds, horses, humans, and other animals. A hallmark of the presence of WNV in communities has been the discovery of dead birds (notably crows, jays, and magpies). Bird-to-human transmission is not believed to occur.

Symptoms in immunocompetent humans develop 2 to 14 days after being bitten by an infected mosquito. The disease causes the highest morbidity and mortality rates in older adults, those with preexisting chronic diseases, those immunosuppressed, and in those having had organ transplants. Neuroinvasive disease affects about 1 in 150, mostly older adults (Ferri, 2010) with a mortality rate of approximately under 1% in children (Pickering et al, 2009).

Clinical Findings

Only about one quarter of individuals exhibit signs and symptoms (Zou et al, 2010), which are nonspecific and typically include fever (102° to 104° F [38.8° to 40° C]); headache; muscle aches; eye pain; rash on neck, body, arms, or legs; lymphadenopathy; weakness; anorexia; nausea; and vomiting. Myocarditis, hepatitis, or pancreatitis occur occasionally. Those with mild disease experience symptomatic relief within a week, with fatigue lingering longer. Most pregnant women who contract WNV deliver infants who show no signs of congenital WNV involvement. Those with severe infection may experience typical symptoms plus neuroinvasive involvement. CNS symptoms (severe headache, change in mental status [disorientation], awkward gait or paralysis, optic neuritis, myelitis, polyradiculitis, stiff neck and nerve abnormalities, tremors or seizures, stupor or coma), and both encephalitis and meningoencephalitis can result.

Laboratory Studies. Consider testing children with a febrile or acute neurologic illness whose history includes exposure to mosquitoes, prenatal exposure with or without breastfeeding, recent blood transfusion or organ transplant. The test of choice is IgM for WNV-specific antibody done by EIA or IFA of serum or CFS collected after 8 days (more likely detectable) of clinical symptom onset. Serial titers are then collected 2 to 3 weeks apart to compare acute and convalescent samples. Viral cultures and nucleic acid amplification are not always positive during the acute phase (Pickering et al, 2009). A CBC may be normal or show elevated WBCs, low lymphocytes, anemia; MRI or CT scan (or both) are indicated if the individual has neurologic findings. A newborn exposed in utero to WNV should have either cord or infant serum tested for IgM after delivery; the placenta and umbilical cord should be sent to a histopathologist.

Management

For asymptomatic or mild cases, no treatment is necessary. Hospitalization is indicated for those with symptoms of meningitis or encephalitis. WNV-infected pregnant women should have an ultrasound of the fetus at least 2 to 4 weeks following maternal infection to assess for structural abnormalities (CDC, 2004). A newborn whose mother was infected with WNV during her pregnancy should be examined for congenital anomalies, neurologic and hearing deficits, and signs of viral infection.

Complications

With severe infection, complications include encephalitis, meningoencephalitis, meningitis, cardiac dysrhythmias, optic neuritis, uveitis, chorioretinitis, orchitis, myocarditis, pancreatitis, GBS, respiratory muscle paralysis, and hepatitis.

Prevention

The goal of prevention is to avoid mosquito bites. Mosquito abatement programs have been instituted in communities to reduce mosquito breeding grounds. Counseling should include the following:

- Stay indoors during the mosquitoes' most active times—dawn and dusk; if must be outdoors during these times, wear light-colored, long-sleeved shirts and long pants.
- Apply insect repellent with either N,N-diethyl-3-methylbenzamide (DEET; formerly N,N-diethyl-meta-toluamide), picaridin 5% to 10%, or oil of lemon eucalyptus to exposed skin and clothing (no DEET for children less than 2 months old).
- Concentration of DEET depends on length of time of expected exposure to mosquitoes or ticks: 10% DEET confers approximately 2 hours of protection; 30% about 5 hours. Apply according to length of protection needed for children 2 months and older. Do not apply to face or hands; use sparingly. Wash DEET off with soap and water when the child is inside (AAP, 2010b).
- Do not use combination sunscreen and DEET products because sunscreen needs to be reapplied more frequently; the DEET component applied too frequently can be toxic.
- Inventory outdoor areas for standing water that serves as breeding areas for mosquitoes (e.g., old tires, pots or containers, birdbath [change once a week], pool or spa covers). Keep pools and spas clean and chlorinated.
- Use tight-fitting screens on all doors and windows.
- Report any dead birds, especially crows, jays, hawks, magpies, and owls, to local health department or pest control agency.

No vaccine is yet available for humans; equine vaccines are available and strongly recommended for horses (Pickering et al, 2009).

HANTAVIRUS PULMONARY SYNDROME
Epidemiology

Hantavirus pulmonary syndrome (HPS) was formerly referred to as hantavirus. The causative agent is Sin Nombre virus (SNV), one of 23 hantaviruses. The virus is carried by deer mice (prominent reservoir), white-footed mice, cotton rats, and rice rats. It is spread by aerosolization of the rodent's saliva, urine, and feces excretions. These rodents are distributed equally throughout the U.S.; eradication of rodents is neither feasible nor desirable given their role in biodiversity. Most cases occur in the spring and summer months but can vary depending on location and rodent population. HPS carries a mortality rate of about 30% to 40% (Pickering et al, 2009).

Incubation Period

Typically, 1 to 6 weeks after exposure to infected rodent body excreta

Clinical Findings

The illness typically involves a prodromal phase of fever, chills, headache, nausea, vomiting, diarrhea, and myalgia (notably of shoulders, lower back, upper legs) prodrome for 3 to 7 days followed by abrupt onset of pulmonary edema, cardiac decompensation, and hypotension.

Diagnostic Studies. There is early thrombocytopenia and leukocytosis with a shift to the left. The diagnosis is confirmed by detecting hanta-specific IgG and IgM antibodies to SNV using ELISA; a rapid diagnostic test is available.

Management

Treatment is supportive.

Prevention

Human avoidance of rodent waste and nests is the goal in dealing with this disease. Before people work around mouse-infested basements or outbuildings they should read the guideline about cleaning up after rodents, which is available on the CDC website.

OTHER NOTABLE VIRUSES IN CIRCULATION

As technology has become more sophisticated, researchers have been able to identify previously unidentified causative agents of infectious diseases.

Human Pneumovirus (Metapneumovirus)

Metapneumovirus (human pneumovirus; hMPV) is a respiratory pathogen of the Paramyxoviridae family. Its antigenicity is closely related to RSV, as is its symptomatology and epidemiology, including a simultaneous (and expanded) seasonal pattern. This agent should be considered as a causative agent of acute respiratory infection among hospitalized children, especially in the spring months. In the U.S. it is estimated that 5% to 10% of infant lower tract infections can be attributed to this virus. Approximately 90% of all 5-year-olds are seropositive for this agent; the peak age range is between 5 and 22 months old (Hermos et al, 2010). Symptoms of hMPV may include rhinitis, wheezing/stridor, tachypnea, abnormal tympanic membranes, pharyngitis, rhonchi, rales, and hypoxia. Those with asthma may experience an exacerbation of their illness. Chest x-rays may demonstrate diffuse perihilar infiltrates, peribronchial cuffing, lobar infiltrates, or hyperaeration. Immunoassays, PCR, and serology tests are diagnostic tests. The role of antiviral agents in treating this virus is unknown.

Human Calicivirus Infections (Norovirus and Sapovirus)

Norovirus (also called Hunter virus and Norwalk-like virus) and sapovirus belong to the calicivirus family. Transmission is person to person by the fecal-oral route, through contaminated water, or food contaminated by infected food handlers. These viruses are highly contagious and occur in closed populations, such as in daycare centers, cruise ships, or facilities for older adults. Norovirus accounts for about 90% of the sporadic epidemics of gastroenteritis in children less than 4 years old. Children often acquire the norovirus from contaminated water in public swimming pools, wading pools, and water parks despite these venues having been chlorine-treated (Pickering et al, 2009), because it is not rapidly inactivated by chlorine. The incubation period is 12 to 48 hours; the duration of illness is 12 to 60 hours; the virus can be excreted for 5 to 7 days (50% of cases), but up to 3 weeks (25% of cases) after onset of symptoms (Pickering et al, 2009). Symptoms of infection include nausea, vomiting, diarrhea, and abdominal cramps; some individuals may experience a low-grade fever, chills, headache, muscle aches, and fatigue. Vomiting may be more pronounced in children (Bhutta, 2007). Dehydration is a serious complication of this infection. This illness can recur. Diagnosis can be made with RT-PCR assay. Treatment is supportive, including rehydration. There is no antiviral treatment or vaccine. Preventive measures include good handwashing and other hygienic measures. Precautions when in public recreational water facilities include not swimming with diarrhea; not swallowing the water; washing children's perianal area with soap and water before going into the water; and taking children for frequent bathroom breaks and diaper checks. Individuals known to have been infected should not be in public water facilities for 1 week after the illness (Pickering et al, 2009).

Severe Acute Respiratory Syndrome

SARS is attributed to a coronavirus and is a frequent cause of URIs. It is spread by secretions from the respiratory tract or fomites, but the virus has been detected in stool, urine, and blood. The incubation period ranges from 2 to 10 days, after which typical clinical symptoms appear within 3 to 5 days (Pickering et al, 2009). Transmission of the virus seems most intense during the second week of one's illness. Outbreaks occur during the winter in temperate climates; young children seem particularly vulnerable. Symptoms can include fever (>100.4° F [38° C]), cough, malaise, myalgias, wheezing (rare), headaches, diarrhea, and nausea or vomiting. Severity of disease is age dependent; children younger than 12 years are less likely to transmit the infection and experience a nonspecific mild illness that lasts less than 5 days (Bitnum and Read, 2007). Teenagers may experience a more intermediate (in severity) illness with increased respiratory distress and hypoxemia (10% to 20% of cases) and require mechanical ventilation (Bitnum and Read, 2007). The fatality rate is estimated to be less than 1% in those younger than 20 years of age (Bitnum and Read, 2007; Poutanen, 2008).

Diagnostic testing should not proceed unless clinical and epidemiologic factors are suggestive of SARS. Testing initially involves antibody assays to rule out RSV and influenza A and B. The standard test for direct detection is the RT-PCR. If SARS is suggested, the provider should consult the CDC website (www.cdc.gov/ncidod/sars/clinicians.htm) for specimen collection and laboratory guidance.

Radiologic findings frequently show focal interstitial infiltrates that progress to generalized, patchy infiltrates and later consolidation. Children generally have less prominent radiographic findings. Blood tests have demonstrated leukopenia, thrombocytopenia, a platelet count in the low-normal range in about half of infected individuals, and sometimes elevated creatine phosphokinase levels and hepatic transaminases. Young children seem to resolve their abnormal laboratory findings more rapidly than do teenagers (Bitnum and Read, 2007).

Management involves strict isolation of the index case, respiratory precautions (hand hygiene, gloves, masks); CDC has infection control guidelines for the home isolation of index cases and their caregivers. Once diagnosed, the patient may need monitoring of pulse oximetry levels and be prescribed antibiotics for both typical and atypical respiratory pathogens. There has been evidence of clinical improvement with ribavirin, corticosteroids, type 1 interferons, convalescent plasma, lopinavir/ritonavir, or inhibitors of viral entry (Poutanen, 2008). Travelers should check the CDC traveler's website regarding the location of endemic SARS before embarking in order to take precautions.

POTENTIAL EMERGING VIRUSES ON THE HORIZON

Kaye and colleagues (2010) have reviewed "candidate diseases" to speculate on what might appear within the next 5 to 10 years, taking into consideration global climate changes, increasing international travel, known vectors, drug resistance, importation of wild animals (that serve as vectors), and bioterrorism. They speculate that among others, the flaviviruses dengue fever, Japanese encephalitis, and yellow fever (all with mosquito vectors), chikungunya (an alphavirus, also with a mosquito as vector), and a new pandemic of influenza (other than H5N1) are more likely to emerge in the U.S. The Global Viral Forecasting (GVF) organization monitors the emergence of deadly viruses spread from animals to humans in order to detect pandemics as they begin. The goal is to ultimately increase the "bank of genetic information" from known viruses in order to develop vaccines to stop the spread of disease. The GVF and global partners have numerous "viral listening posts" in central Africa, China, Malaysia, Madagascar, and Laos, where pandemics often start. Air travel and road development increase the transmission of these potentially dangerous viruses throughout the world.

■ Tick-Borne Diseases

Lyme disease, ehrlichiosis, Rocky Mountain spotted fever (RMSF), tick-borne relapsing fever, babesiosis, tularemia, and African tick bite fever are common tick-borne diseases in the U.S. It is important for providers to be aware of the specific tick vectors and epidemic geographic areas of the vectors. Only the first two diseases are discussed here (tularemia is discussed in the section on bioterrorism agents). A key to including tick-borne diseases in the differential diagnosis is being suspicious when an individual complains of influenza-like symptoms (fever, headache, myalgia) during summer (an unusual time for such symptoms, especially if they live and recreate outdoors in endemic areas).

LYME DISEASE
Epidemiology

Borrelia burgdorferi (Bb), a spirochete, is the causative agent that is carried and transmitted to humans by ticks. Lyme disease is the most commonly reported vector-borne infection in the U.S. and one complicated by differing standards of diagnosis and treatment. The Infectious Diseases Society of America (IDSA) and the International Lyme and Associated Diseases Society (ILADS) have widely divergent views about the nature of transmission, the properties of the spirochete, whether a chronic form of the disease exists, and approaches to treatment.

In the U.S., coastal New England, the mid-Atlantic states, Wisconsin and Minnesota, and Northern California have reported 98% of the cases (IDSA, 2010). European nations reporting the disease include Scandinavian countries and central Europe (Germany, Austria, Switzerland). When eastern blacked-legged deer tick *(Ixodes scapularis)* or western black-legged deer tick *(Ixodes pacificus)* larvae hatch in early summer, they are usually not infected. During their life cycle (nymphal and adult molt stages), the tick can feed on an infected host, and become infected with *Bb*. In the East, the natural host for *Bb* is the white-footed mouse; in the West it is mostly lizards (these are relatively poor reservoirs because only about 1% to 8% of the ticks are infected with *Bb*). The infected tick then transmits the organism to humans. The infection is more likely to be transmitted during the nymphal stage (Shapiro, 2007). The size of the tick in the nymphal stage is about 1 mm; in the adult stages from 2.5 to 4 mm. Lyme disease has been reported in habitats that are inhospitable to the tick; the vector in these cases has not been identified.

There is varied risk of transmission, depending on the percentage of ticks actually infected with *Bb*. In endemic locations annual incidence rates range from 20 to 100 per 100,000 cases; Lyme, Connecticut (a hyperendemic location) has been reported to have cases as high as 1000 per 100,000. Children 5 to 10 years of age have higher incidence rates than those who are older (Shapiro, 2007). Individual overall risk is only about 1% to 3% for developing disease after a tick bite, even in endemic areas (8% to 10% risk if bitten by a nymph) (Shapiro, 2007); coinfection with other tick-borne pathogens must be considered in endemic regions. The risk of human infection after a tick bite is related to how long the tick has fed. It takes hours for the tick to fully implant its mouth into the host's skin and days to become fully engorged. Nymphal ticks must feed for 36 to 48 hours or more and adult ticks for 48 to 72 hours before the risk of transmission of *Bb* is significant; many human victims have removed the tick before this time. However, because of the small size of the tick and possible location on the body where it is lodged (e.g., scalp), an engorged tick may not be noticed before it drops off. The disease is not regarded as being teratogenic to fetal development.

IDSA and ILADS differ on the existence of "chronic," "persistent," or "recurrent" Lyme disease. Some researchers and providers believe that patients attribute medically unexplained symptoms to chronic Lyme disease (Shapiro, 2010). On the other side, the ILADS cites the ability of *Bb* to live intracellularly and avoid antibiotics. They encourage the use of long-term combination drug treatment using other drugs not specifically used for Lyme disease to treat chronic infection (Burrascano, 2008). Additionally the ILADS views chronic infection as: (1) the result of not just infection by *Bb*, but as a result of many coinfections due to other pathogens known to be also transmitted by tick bites (*Babesia* species, *Bartonella*-like organisms, *Ehrlichia, Anaplasma, Mycoplasma,* and viruses); and (2) a result of improper treatment in the early stage of the disease that causes immune dysfunction, opportunistic infections, biologic toxins, metabolic and hormonal imbalances, and deconditioning among others. ILADS also regards *Bb* as transmittable by other routes (sexually, in utero, in breast milk from an infected mother, and by other insect vectors).

IDSA and ILADS offer current treatment guidelines on their websites (www.idsociety.org and www.ilads.org, respectively). Both organizations agree that children rarely progress to stage 2 or 3 when treated in the erythema migrans phase; those with arthritic symptoms recover completely. Parental concerns about chronic symptoms after adequate treatment need to be addressed carefully, and other behavioral or organic causes may need to be explored. A Lyme disease infectious disease specialist can help decide if further treatment is warranted.

Incubation Period

The incubation period from the bite to the rash stage is approximately 1 to 32 days (median 11 days) (Pickering et al, 2009). Late manifestation of the disease may appear months to years later. In the presence of antibiotics, *Bb* has been experimentally shown to be able to "hide" intracellularly and change form (Savely, 2006).

Clinical Findings

Lyme disease is hard to diagnosis because the symptoms can be so variable. Classic Lyme disease can be divided into three stages:

1. *Stage 1 (early localized disease):* Generally within 1 to 2 weeks after the bite, a typical rash may appear at the inoculation site (this time frame can range from 3 to 32 days); less than half of all individuals demonstrate a rash (Burrascano, 2008). Erythema migrans rash begins as a red, annular macule or papule at the site of the tick bite and progresses into large annular erythematous lesions 5 to 15 cm in diameter. Multiple lesions occur less than 10% of the time (Burrascano, 2008). The center of the lesion of erythema migrans may be clear, vesicular, or necrotic; it may be pruritic or painful. It typically is located in the axillary, periumbilical, thigh, or groin areas. The rash remains for a few weeks and fades even if untreated. In many cases the rash does not follow this classic pattern but instead may resemble nummular eczema, tinea, granuloma annulare, an insect bite, or cellulitis; the rapid enlargement of erythema migrans helps distinguish it.
2. The patient may experience fever, malaise, headache, arthralgia, and stiff neck during this phase. Without treatment, these symptoms, including the rash, may become intermittent, lasting for weeks to months.
3. *Stage 2 (early disseminated disease):* Through spirochetemia, the organism disseminates through the skin causing

multiple skin lesions (1 to 3 cm). These are morphologically similar to, but smaller than, the local lesion. They develop several days to several weeks after the primary lesions. Symptoms in children with disseminated disease include frequent headaches or stomachaches, urinary symptoms, migratory musculoskeletal pains, mood swings, irritability, obsessive-compulsive behavior, and new-onset ADHD (Savely, 2006). Infections of the eye, bone, heart, synovium, muscle, liver, spleen, and CNS can occur because of the hematogenous and lymphatic spread of the organism. The patient may experience iritis, optic neuritis, conjunctivitis, osteomyelitis, pericarditis, and myocarditis (although rare this may be manifested by varying degrees of heart block), mild arthritis, hepatitis, lymphadenitis, aseptic meningitis, and cranial neuropathies (especially seventh nerve palsy in children that lasts 2 to 8 weeks). Stage 2 can last from weeks to 2 years without treatment. Most of the symptoms (including the rash) wax and wane during this time.

4. *Stage 3 (late disease)*: Stage 3 usually begins with pauciarticular or monarticular arthritis that occurs weeks to months after the initial tick bite. The knees are most commonly affected. The joints are red, hot, and swollen, but not as painful as with other types of bacterial arthritis. Untreated, the arthritis initially resolves in a few weeks but becomes recurrent, migratory (but rarely to small joints), and chronic.

Diagnostic Studies

Lyme disease is best diagnosed by clinical and epidemiologic history (to give a probability that the patient actually has Lyme disease) and typical physical findings; only if all three exist should one proceed with serologic testing as an adjunct (Pickering et al, 2009; Shapiro, 2007). Objective signs for acute Lyme disease (per IDSA)—and the three main indicators for deciding when to perform serologic testing—are erythema migrans, facial nerve palsy, and arthritis; these three symptoms are more synonymous with actual disease versus the other nonspecific symptoms previously described (Pickering et al, 2009). Serologic tests do not become positive for weeks after a bite; delaying treatment until results are back decreases the chances of successfully treating this disease in the early stages.

Serologically positive results may also indicate prior infection rather than present acute infection because antibodies can remain elevated for years. One medical approach recommends IgM- and IgG-specific antibodies done via ELISA or IFA assay. Any positive result needs to be followed up with the Western blot test for *Bb* antibodies. IgM antibodies appear in the early stage at 3 to 4 weeks, peak at 6 to 8 weeks, then decline or persist for years. IgG-specific antibodies appear 6 to 8 weeks after inoculation and peak at 4 to 6 months; they can remain elevated indefinitely. Early antimicrobial intervention may prevent the production of Lyme antibodies. There are many false-positive cross-reactions with other spirochetes, lupus, and varicella organisms.

Another medical approach recommends using the IgM and IgG Western blot as the initial screening tool, using only a reference laboratory that reports all of the bands (e.g., IGeneX, Inc.), and that providers in endemic Lyme disease areas learn to interpret the Western blot bands. Each band differs as to specificity. By being able to read the 14 to 16 bands, suspicions of *Bb* exposure can be more finely honed and lead to better diagnosis and timely treatment (CDC epidemiologic criteria for Lyme disease considers 5 out of 10 bands as diagnostic; ILADS regards this epidemiologic criteria as a surveillance tool only and one that is inappropriately being applied for clinical diagnosis).

Borrelia burgdorferi can be cultured from a leading-edge skin biopsy of the erythema migrans lesion, as well as from blood, CSF, myocardium and synovium; however, culture is costly, takes 4 to 6 weeks, and success of isolation is low (Shapiro, 2007). Sensitivity is low with PCR; the patient should be off antibiotics for a minimum of 6 weeks prior to testing; and a positive result is significant (Burrascano, 2008). If chronic disease with *Bb* is present, a suppression in the immune system occurs which decreases the CD-57 count. This count can be used to determine how active the disease is and if relapse is likely following treatment. An increase indicates coinfection with another pathogen because it is believed that only *Borrelia* depresses the CD-57 (Burrascano, 2008).

Differential Diagnosis

The rash, if present, may suggest eczema, tinea, granuloma annulare, cellulitis, or an insect bite. Also considered in the differential diagnoses are osteomyelitis, WNV, parvovirus B19, relapsing fever, syphilis, leptospirosis, mycoplasma, septic arthritis, infectious hepatitis, nonresponsive lymphadenopathy, meningitis, MS, amyotrophic lateral sclerosis, juvenile arthritis, Bell palsy, other spirochete-caused diseases, thyroid disease, heavy metal toxicity, and vasculitis. Primary psychiatric disorders, in recalcitrant cases after appropriate treatment for Lyme disease, should also be considered.

Management

The abilities of *Bb* to hide intracellularly, to change form, and to grow slowly are reasons that the disease is more difficult to diagnose and treat (Savely, 2006). Clinical judgment is crucial in determining whether to treat a patient. The earlier in the migrans stage that treatment is started the better the long-term outcome. The primary care provider is best advised to study the literature from the Lyme Disease Association, IDSA, and ILADS, and consult with infectious disease specialists if uncertain how to proceed. The provider can feel confident about using doxycycline or amoxicillin in children when the history includes the following (Wormser et al, 2006):

- Tick is reliably identified as a nymph or adult *Ixodes scapularis* species (providers in endemic areas should have this expertise of identification, including the stages and determining degree of engorgement for criterion number 2 below).
- Tick was attached for at least 36 hours (as indicated by size of engorgement or known time of exposure). Prophylaxis can be given (see Prevention section) if started within 72 hours of tick removal for individuals 8 years or older.
- Local rate of infection with *Bb* is greater than 20% in the region where the tick was acquired (only includes parts of New England, mid-Atlantic states, Minnesota and Wisconsin).
- Clinical symptoms fit early stage symptomatology for Lyme disease.

The dosage for treatment of early localized disease (stage 1) or erythema migrans includes (Review Panel, 2010; Wormser et al, 2006):

- Less than 8 years old: Amoxicillin 50 mg/kg/day orally (PO) divided into three doses a day (maximum 500 mg/dose) for 14 to 21 days. ILADS advocates 6 weeks of treatment as long as there are no other constitutional symptoms.
- 8 years or older: Doxycycline 100 mg PO twice daily for 14 to 21 days or 4 mg/kg PO twice daily for 14 days (maximum 200 mg/day). Give a small snack with doxycycline to reduce nausea (6 weeks of treatment per ILADS).
- For individuals unable to take amoxicillin or doxycycline, use any of these: Cefuroxime 30 mg/kg/day divided twice daily PO (maximum 500 mg/dose) for 14 to 21 days; azithromycin 10 mg/kg once daily (maximum 500 mg/day) for 7 to 10 days; clarithromycin 7.5 mg/kg twice daily PO (maximum 500 mg/dose) for 13 to 21 days; or erythromycin, 12.5 mg/kg/day PO four times daily (maximum 500 mg/dose for 14 to 21 days (6 weeks per ILADS). Do not use the macrolides or first-generation cephalosporins as first-line drugs.

If an individual has removed a tick, he or she should be given guidance about the signs and symptoms of erythema migrans (see Prevention prophylaxis guidelines). Should the individual develop these within 30 days, he or she should be considered for treatment of the disease (Review Panel, 2010).

Prevention

Avoid tick-infested areas whenever possible. If in such areas, use tick skin repellent with DEET (see recommended DEET percentages under the prevention section for WNV). Inspect skin carefully every day during the tick season. Spray permethrin on clothing and wear light-colored long pants (tucked into shoes), long sleeves, and a hat. Chronic absorption of insecticides, however, can produce toxicity, especially in children; however, when used according to directions children older than 2 months can safely use DEET (Wormser et al, 2006). Alternative repellents include permethrin for clothing, Picaridin, and IR 3535.

Post–tick bite prophylaxis with doxycycline (single 200 mg dose, or children >8 years 4 mg/kg PO up to 200 mg dose per IDSA; 28 days per ILADS) can be effective in preventing the disease. However, this prophylaxis should be given only to those who live in highly endemic areas (see criteria numbers 1 and 3 under Management section) and when the tick is at least minimally engorged with blood. The IDSA postulates that chemoprophylaxis is unwarranted otherwise, because most ticks are removed before engorgement has occurred and overall risk for disease is low (Shapiro, 2007).

EHRLICHIOSIS AND ANAPLASMA INFECTIONS

Both infections are caused by distinct species of obligate intracellular bacteria carried by the lone star tick (*Amblyomma americanum,* for ehrlichial infections of which there are two species) and the black-legged or deer tick (*I. scapularis)* for anaplasmosis. The southeast, south-central, mid-Atlantic states, and the same regions in which Lyme disease occur are common endemic areas for ehrlichiosis in the United States. *Anaplasma* infections are reported more commonly in the north-central states, northeastern states (especially Connecticut and New York), and in Wisconsin and Minnesota, with a sprinkling reported from other states. Any individual who has a history of tick exposure in an endemic area, a non-specific rapid onset febrile illness during the spring or summer, and some of the following symptoms should be considered at risk for ehrlichiosis or anaplasmosis. Children are increasingly acquiring this disease, and the diseases are most likely underreported. The incubation period for both diseases ranges from 5 to 10 days after a tick bite (Pickering et al, 2009).

Both infections produce acute, systemic symptoms with fever, headache, myalgia, malaise, chills, nausea, and anorexia in about half of those infected. Less common symptoms include diarrhea and vomiting, weight loss, arthralgia, cough, and change in mental status (20% to 50% of cases). With ehrlichiosis, a rash may occur after onset of symptoms and is seen in about 60% of infected children; less than 10% of *Anaplasma* cases exhibit a rash (Pickering et al, 2009). The rash is variable in appearance, generally involves the trunk with sparing of the hands and feet, and appears about a week after the onset of other symptoms. Leukopenia, neutropenia, anemia, or thrombocytopenia with elevated hepatic transaminases can be seen on blood tests depending on the pathogen. Pleocytosis with predominance of lymphocytes and increased total protein is commonly seen in CSF samples.

Diagnosis can be made using several techniques: isolating the pathogen from blood or CSF by IgG-specific titer using an IFA assay and comparing titers between the acute and convalescent periods (2 to 4 weeks apart); detection of the pathogen from a PCR assay titer; isolating bacterial antigen from a biopsy/autopsy sample; or isolating *Ehrlichia* or *Anaplasma* organisms from a specimen grown in cell culture. The CDC can aid in advising the appropriate test. The differential diagnosis includes RMSF and Lyme disease.

Treatment of choice is doxycycline (4 mg/kg/day divided twice daily for at least 3 days after defervescence for a minimum total course of at least 7 days; maximum dose 100 mg/dose, PO or IV). Use of doxycycline is advised even in young children given the potential for life-threatening illness. Data suggest that discoloration of permanent teeth is not significant if doxycycline is taken for 14 days or less (Pickering et al, 2009). A response to treatment should occur within 1 week. Systemic complications include pulmonary infiltrates, bone marrow hypoplasia, respiratory failure, encephalopathy, meningitis, DIC, spontaneous hemorrhage, and renal failure. The mortality rate for ehrlichiosis is about 3%, and about 1% for anaplasmosis (Pickering et al, 2009). Recovery is usually complete after 1 to 2 weeks; some neurologic difficulties can remain in children who have had systemic disease. Prevention is the same for Lyme disease. Prophylaxis is not recommended due to the low risk of infection (Pickering et al, 2009).

▮ Bacterial Infections

Although less common overall than viral diseases, bacterial infections allow for interventions (including antibiotics) that can decrease the course of an illness and prevent subsequent complications. Many bacterial infections may be diagnosed clinically and treated empirically. A good understanding of the pathophysiology of common bacterial infections, and knowledge of the most likely organisms involved, allows for efficient and effective implementation of treatment. Bacterial infections of the skin and soft-tissue infections (SSTIs), lymphadenitis, osteomyelitis, fasciitis, pneumonia, meningitis, infectious diarrhea, and UTI are discussed in other chapters relevant to the system affected; fungal infections and parasitic infections are likewise found elsewhere.

TACKLING POTENTIAL METHICILLIN-RESISTANT *STAPHYLOCOCCUS AUREUS*

It is increasingly important to recognize a clinical situation in which diagnosis and management of bacterial infections requires consideration of the involvement of community-associated methicillin-resistant *S. aureus* (CA-MRSA). Knowing the prevalence in one's community of CA-MRSA is crucial for how a provider should treat severe pneumonia, cellulitis, osteomyelitis, myositis, bacteremia, endocarditis, empyema, meningitis, scalded skin syndrome, toxic shock syndrome (TSS), deep tissue abscesses (especially those that come on quickly), reported spider bites, skin and soft tissue infections, and necrotizing fasciitis. About 59% of all skin and soft-tissue infections are attributed to CA-MRSA (Davis, 2008). It is also increasingly being implicated as the causative agent in pneumonia in the younger age groups and in those without risk factors. CA-MRSA has gone from "simply" a resistant *S. aureus* to an entirely new clone that has an altered penicillin-binding protein with decreased sensitivity to most beta-lactam antibiotics. With a combination of this protein and specific genetic encoding for cytotoxicity (affects the degree of virulence) the *S. aureus* strains are able to evade neutrophils and cause leukocyte, monocyte, and macrophage destruction and tissue necrosis (Norrby-Teglund and Low, 2008).

There are some clinical clues that MRSA may be involved in the presenting symptomatology or history of an otherwise healthy individual. Miller and Kaplan (2009) summarize these as the "six C's of CA-MRSA transmission" (contact, cleanliness, compromised skin integrity, contaminated/shared objects, crowded living situation, and capsules [recent treatment with beta-lactam antibiotics]). The following illustrate these six points in more detail (Lewis, 2006; Rosenthal, 2005, 2006; Tufts and Connor Hardman, 2006):

- Individual has a boil, furuncle, or abscess without draining pus that is erythematous, warm, painful; onset may have been rapid (key finding) (Hasty et al, 2007)
- Individual fails treatment with a beta-lactam product. If individual has been in contact with a cat, consider cat-scratch disease (CSD) as a differential diagnosis (it would have been unresponsive to beta-lactam treatment)
- Other family members have similar skin infections.
- Individual has a recent history of skin infection, even if it was responsive to a beta-lactam agent
- Neonate with skin or soft tissue infection
- Skin lesion looks like a spider bite; larger lesions are more suspicious for MRSA.
- Pus is present.
- History of recurrent small, nontender, nonpruritic maculopapular lesions that become pruritic or painful; multiple lesions present
- Individual participates in contact sports (wrestling, football) where turf burns and abrasions are common, and athletes share lockers, bars of soap, towels, other equipment

- Individual may be of an ethnic minority; of lower socio-economic status; in the military; homeless; recently incarcerated; lives in a crowded environment; uses illicit drugs; participates in high-risk sexual behaviors
- Nonpregnant or pregnant woman has a breast abscess.
- Individual has no history in the past year of having been hospitalized, of having had surgery, and has no permanent indwelling medical devices passing through the skin.
- Individual attends daycare; is less than 2 years of age (Miller and Kaplan, 2009)
- Individual has CF or progressive respiratory tract infection
- Individual has a head or neck infection (retropharyngeal abscess, mastoiditis, AOM, sinusitis, periorbital and orbital infections); osteomyelitis; myositis; pneumonias with empyema; sepsis; pustulosis in neonates—these are found to be due to CA-MRSA with increasing frequency [Miller and Kaplan, 2009]).

The provider can safely treat many superficial skin lesions (e.g., impetigo, localized pustulosis in an asymptomatic neonate) without a culture using the conventional management strategies of the past. In minor infections most cases resolve whether or not the antibiotic matched the susceptibility of the organism (Norrby-Teglund and Low, 2008). In all cases, providers need to assess each case carefully and diligently and provide instructions to parents to return if the child is unresponsive to treatment. Anticipate complications and consider the clinical clues previously mentioned for skin and soft-tissue infection. The selection of a drug that covers MRSA should be made on the basis of the prevalence of MRSA within one's community, if infection was nosocomial, and the severity of the infection. See Chapters 36 and 39 for other discussions about MRSA.

Recommended management strategies (Fig. 23-4) include:
- Culture any lesion with purulent exudate or abscesses (even if treated empirically with antibiotics); for those with severe local infection; for those with signs of systemic toxicity; those who failed to respond to prior treatment (Liu et al, 2011).
- Incision and drainage (I&D) is the treatment of choice for any nondraining, but fluctuant abscess; antibiotics alone are ineffective (performing I&D prior to localization of pus is not effective and may promote more serious infection). Antibiotics are not needed after draining the abscess in most cases (consider in those that are immunocompromised or have a risk of endocarditis) (Butler, 2009).
- Send specimens to the laboratory for a Gram stain, culture and sensitivity, and "d-test" (indicates any possible inducible resistance to clindamycin). Cultures should not be taken from superficial open surface wounds due to contaminating bacteria other than the causative pathogen (Illinois Department of Public Health, 2008).
- For *deep-seated* infections without fluid fluctuation and without signs of bacteremia (fever, chills, malaise), warm compresses to localize pus are appropriate and oral antibiotics can be considered. The individual should be instructed to return for further evaluation in 24 to 36 hours for I&D (providers need to have a way to contact patient regarding status).
- For *uncomplicated soft-tissue* infection (e.g., impetigo; secondarily infected eczema, ulcers, or lacerations) and without fluid fluctuation, empiric topical mupirocin 2% is probably sufficient. Using moist heat on small furuncles to promote draining may also be sufficient (Liu et al, 2011).

ALGORITHM

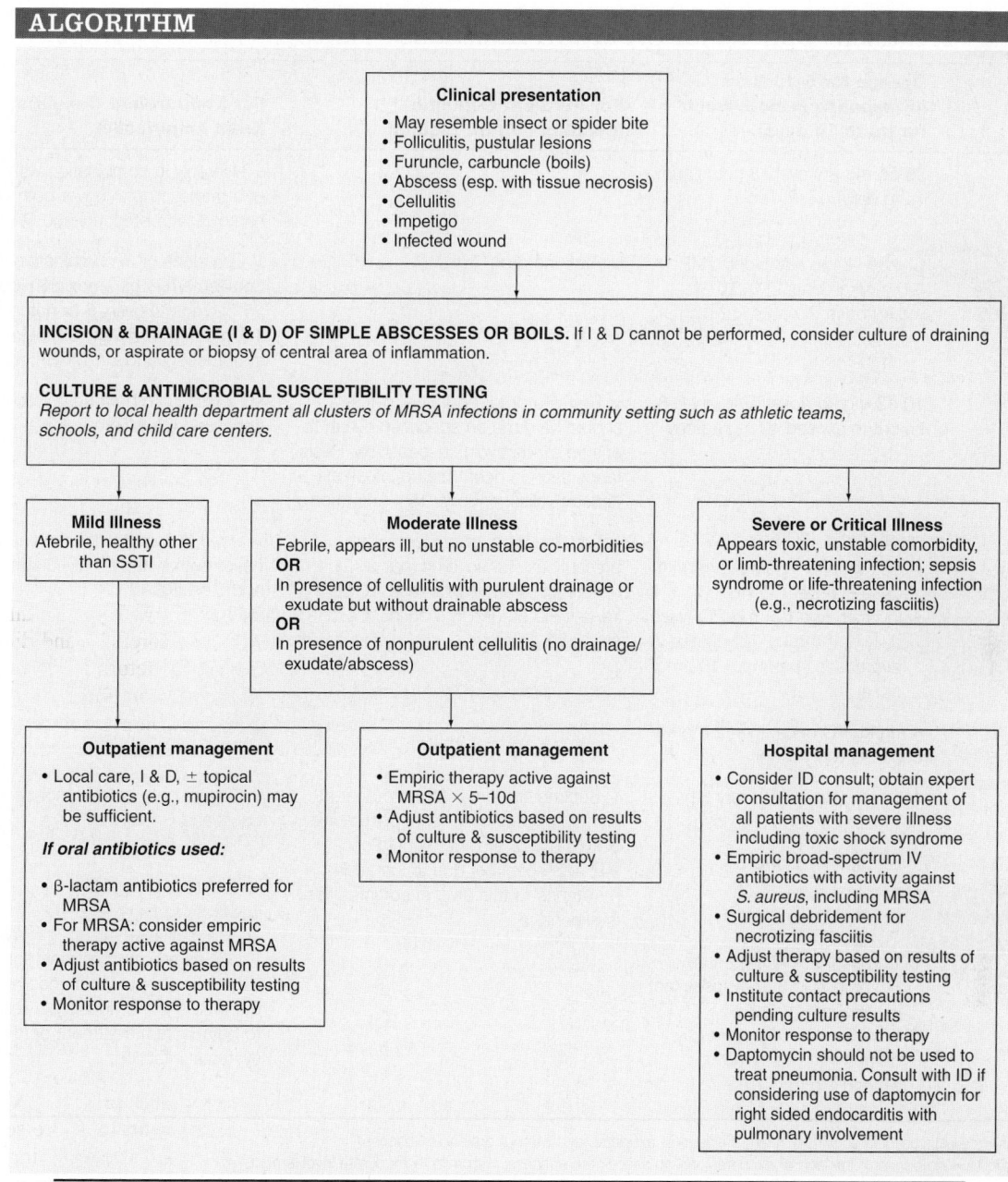

Clinical presentation
- May resemble insect or spider bite
- Folliculitis, pustular lesions
- Furuncle, carbuncle (boils)
- Abscess (esp. with tissue necrosis)
- Cellulitis
- Impetigo
- Infected wound

INCISION & DRAINAGE (I & D) OF SIMPLE ABSCESSES OR BOILS. If I & D cannot be performed, consider culture of draining wounds, or aspirate or biopsy of central area of inflammation.

CULTURE & ANTIMICROBIAL SUSCEPTIBILITY TESTING
Report to local health department all clusters of MRSA infections in community setting such as athletic teams, schools, and child care centers.

Mild Illness
Afebrile, healthy other than SSTI

Moderate Illness
Febrile, appears ill, but no unstable co-morbidities
OR
In presence of cellulitis with purulent drainage or exudate but without drainable abscess
OR
In presence of nonpurulent cellulitis (no drainage/exudate/abscess)

Severe or Critical Illness
Appears toxic, unstable comorbidity, or limb-threatening infection; sepsis syndrome or life-threatening infection (e.g., necrotizing fasciitis)

Outpatient management
- Local care, I & D, ± topical antibiotics (e.g., mupirocin) may be sufficient.

If oral antibiotics used:

- β-lactam antibiotics preferred for MRSA
- For MRSA: consider empiric therapy active against MRSA
- Adjust antibiotics based on results of culture & susceptibility testing
- Monitor response to therapy

Outpatient management
- Empiric therapy active against MRSA × 5–10d
- Adjust antibiotics based on results of culture & susceptibility testing
- Monitor response to therapy

Hospital management
- Consider ID consult; obtain expert consultation for management of all patients with severe illness including toxic shock syndrome
- Empiric broad-spectrum IV antibiotics with activity against *S. aureus*, including MRSA
- Surgical debridement for necrotizing fasciitis
- Adjust therapy based on results of culture & susceptibility testing
- Institute contact precautions pending culture results
- Monitor response to therapy
- Daptomycin should not be used to treat pneumonia. Consult with ID if considering use of daptomycin for right sided endocarditis with pulmonary involvement

FIGURE 23-4 Algorithm for management of suspected *S. aureus* skin and soft tissue infection. (Data from Illinois Department of Public Health: Methicillin-resistant *Staphylococcus aureus* in Illinois: guidelines for the primary care provider, 2008, Figure 1. Available at www.isph.state.ilus/health/infect/MRSAProvider.htm (accessed November 18, 2010). *ID*, Infection disease; *I&D*, incision and drainage; *IV*, intravenous; *MRSA, methicillin-resistant staphylococcus aureus; MSSA, methicillin-sensitive staphylococcus aureus; SSTI*, skin and soft tissue infections.

- The use of oral antibiotic treatment for any suspected methicillin-sensitive *S. aureus* is appropriate under the following circumstances and providers should contact child/family within 2 to 3 days to determine response to treatment (Table 23-7 lists antibiotic treatment options):
  - Presence of severe or extensive abscesses (e.g., involving multiple sites); or rapidly progressing infection with signs of cellulitis, systemic illness; comorbidities or immunosuppression; extreme age; abscess is in an area difficult to incise/drain (e.g., face, hand, genitalia); septic phlebitis; and/or lack of response to incision/drainage (Liu et al, 2011).

- Prevention measures for athletes and return to play guidelines are included in Box 13-6 and Table 13-8.
- For recurrent MRSA soft-tissue infections (Liu et al, 2011):
  - Review hygiene and wound care (see first two bullet points under recommended management strategies).
  - Institute environmental hygiene measures (clean surfaces in contact with skin [e.g., doorknobs, bathtubs, counters, toilet seats]).
  - Decolonization techniques (consider where ongoing transmission is occurring within a household despite adherence to hygiene and wound care strategies). May include nasal decolonization with mupirocin 2% twice

| TABLE 23-7 | Treatment Options for CA-MRSA Infections |

Antibiotic	Dosage for 5-10 Days (if response is slow, treat for up to 14 days)	For Purulent Cellulitis* (pending culture results)	For Nonpurulent Cellulitis† (treat empirically)
Amoxicillin	25-50 mg PO every 8 hours (max 1.2 g daily)		√ Use only in combination with TMP-SMX or a tetracycline to cover both beta-hemolytic streptococci and CA-MRSA.
Trimethoprim-sulfamethoxazole (TMP-SMX) (98% efficacy*)	Children 2 mo and older: TMP 4-6 mg/kg/dose; SMX 20-30 mg/kg/dose PO every 12 hr	√ First-line drug	√ Use alone or in combination with a beta-lactam (e.g., amoxicillin [dosed at 25-50 mg PO every 8 hr not to exceed 1.2 g daily]) to cover both beta-hemolytic streptococci and CA-MRSA.
Clindamycin	10-13 mg/kg/dose PO every 6-8 hr, not to exceed 40 mg/kg/day	√ First-line drug; additional d-test should be done on specimen by lab to ensure clindamycin susceptibility. Resistance seen in deep-seated infections (osteomyelitis, endocarditis, pneumonia)	√ Covers both beta-hemolytic streptococci and CA-MRSA
Doxycycline	Children 8 yr and over: • 45 kg and under: 2 mg/kg/dose PO every 12 hr • Over 45 kg: 100 mg PO twice daily or 4 mg/kg/day divided in two doses (maximum 100 mg/dose)	√ First-line drug; photosensitivity precautions. Tetracycline may also be used in children >8 yr of age (20-50 mg/kg/day PO divided in 4 doses not to exceed 2 g daily).	√ Used in combination with amoxicillin to cover both beta-hemolytic streptococci and CA-MRSA.
Minocycline	4 mg/kg PO once, then 2 mg/kg/dose PO every 12 hr	√	√
Linezolid	10 mg/kg/dose PO every 8 hr, not to exceed 600 mg/dose	√ Second-line drug; for complicated skin/soft-tissue infections, pneumonia. Before using, provider should consult with specialist due to increasing resistance to this drug in communities; is expensive	√ Covers both beta-hemolytic streptococci and CA-MRSA
Beta-lactam (e.g., cephalexin, dicloxacillin)	Cephalexin: 25-50 mg/kg/day PO divided in 3 or 4 doses (not to exceed 4 g/day) Dicloxacillin: 25-50 mg/kg/day divided in 4 doses (not to exceed 2 g/day)		√ Use as empiric treatment for beta-hemolytic streptococci; recommended for CA-MRSA in individuals not responsive to beta-lactam treatment or in those with systemic infection.

*Purulent cellulitis = cellulitis associated with purulent drainage or exudates and without drainable abscess.
†Nonpurulent cellulitis = no purulent drainage or exudates and no associated abscess; with mild to moderate involvement.
Macrolides, fluoroquinolones, second-generation cephalosporins, and rifampin (as a single agent or in combination with other drugs) are not indicated for known CA-MRSA.
CA-MRSA, Community-acquired methicillin-resistant *Staphylococcus aureus; PO,* orally (per os [mouth]).
Data from Liu C, Bayer A, Cosgrove SE, et al: *Clinical practice guidelines by the Infectious Diseases Society of America for the treatment of methicillin-resistant* Staphylococcus aureus *infections in adults and children,* 2011. Available at www.cid.oxfordjournals.org/content/early/2011/01/04/cid.ciq146.full.pdf+html (accessed Jan 8, 2011); Pickering LK, Baker CJ, Kimberlin DW, et al: *Red Book: 2009 Report of the Committee on Infectious Diseases,* ed 28, Elk Grove Village, IL, 2009, American Academy of Pediatrics, pp 610-611.

daily for 5 to 10 days; antiseptic body wash with a skin antiseptic solution (e.g., chlorhexidine) for 5 to 14 days or diluted bleach baths (¼ cup bleach for ¼ tub of water) for 15 minutes twice weekly for about 3 months. Oral antibiotics are not recommended for decolonization.

OTHER EMERGING DRUG-RESISTANT BACTERIAL INFECTIONS

Multiple drug resistant gram-negative bacteria are a major concern. Of note are *Klebsiella pneumoniae* and *Acinetobacter baumannii*, which have already gained resistance to virtually all antibiotics in hospital settings. Although the figures are not known for the U.S., in Europe two thirds of the 25,000 reported deaths in hospitals were due to gram-negative nosocomial infection. The concern of infectious disease specialists is that the resistant strains could spread outside the hospital settings (similar to CA-MRSA) if in-hospital hygienic measures are not successful (Kaye et al, 2010; Pollack, 2010).

CAT-SCRATCH DISEASE

Epidemiology

B. henselae is the causative organism for CSD. It is the most common cause of chronic persistent (greater than 3 weeks) lymphadenopathy and is a slow-growing, gram-negative bacillus. Cats are the only natural reservoir; the organism is spread between cats via the cat flea and spread to humans via skin inoculation. CSD is believed to be a common infection, with most cases occurring in patients less than 20 years old. In 90% of cases, a cat (usually a kitten) is involved (Pickering et al, 2009). Other sources of inoculation have reportedly been attributed to dog scratches, wood splinters, fish hooks, cactus spines, and porcupine quills. The disease is most prevalent in fall and winter except in tropical areas, where it shows no seasonal predilection. The incidence is greater than 24,000 cases annually in the U.S. (Stechenberg, 2007).

Incubation Period

The incubation period between injury and primary skin lesion is 7 to 12 days. The lymphadenopathy may take 5 to 50 days to develop, but averages 12 days.

Clinical Findings

In approximately one third of cases, patients manifest systemic illness; the rest are not very sick. Greater than 50% have a history of a cat scratch (Stechenberg, 2007). The illness typically presents with cutaneous findings and other key characteristics that include:

- Lesions 3 to 5 mm that arise approximately 1 week after inoculation and can persist for months; lesions occur in up to two thirds of individuals. The nonpruritic lesions initially begin as vesicles or pustules and evolve into papules. They may follow a linear pattern that follows the cat scratch. They may be misdiagnosed as impetigo secondary to an insect bite. The cutaneous lesions heal completely without scarring. From 2% to 17% of individuals may present with nonsuppurative conjunctivitis or ocular granuloma (the affected eye is not painful, with little or no discharge, but may be markedly red and swollen) with preauricular lymphadenopathy. Inoculation is surmised to be from rubbing the eye(s) following handling a cat (Stechenberg, 2007).
- One to 4 weeks after the inoculation the axillary, cervical, submandibular, preauricular, epitrochlear, inguinal, and femoral nodes closest to the lesion begin to swell (in that general order). There can be single or multiple nodes involved. The node may swell to 1 to 5 cm. The area around the infected node is usually warm, tender, indurated, and erythematous during the first few weeks. Cellulitis is uncommon, but large nodes may suppurate up to 25% of the time (Pickering et al, 2009). The lymphadenopathy usually lasts approximately 1 to 2 months and up to 1 year in some cases. Mucous membrane ulcers may occur.
- A fever of 100.4° to 102.2° F (38° to 39° C), malaise, anorexia, fatigue, and headache also accompany the lymphadenopathy in one third of patients.

Diagnostic Studies. An IFA for serum antibodies is available from commercial labs, state health departments, or the CDC. Culturing the skin lesions for *B. henselae* is unproductive. CT or ultrasonography may identify hepatic or splenic abscesses and granulomas. The CBC may be normal or show mild leukocytosis. The ESR may be elevated early in the disease process; hepatic transaminases may increase with systemic disease. Lymph node biopsy may show nonspecific bacilli.

Differential Diagnosis

The differential diagnosis includes any cause of lymphadenopathy. The most common of these are bacterial and viral infections (e.g., streptococci [especially group A beta-hemolytic], staphylococci, anaerobic bacteria, atypical mycobacteria, tularemia, brucellosis, CMV, HIV, EBV, systemic fungal infections, toxoplasmosis, malignancy). Neck masses from other sources (e.g., cystic hygromas, bronchogenic cysts, tumors) are in the differential.

Management

Symptomatic treatment is usually sufficient in most cases because CSD usually spontaneously resolves within 2 to 4 months. Antipyretics can be used for a moderate fever. Painful nodes can be treated with moist wraps or needle aspiration. Incision and drainage of nonsuppurative lesions should be avoided because of the high risk of chronic draining sinuses. Needle aspiration can yield material for diagnostic testing. Antibiotics are not generally used unless there is concern for systemic CSD or bacterial involvement of lesions. Azithromycin, clarithromycin, TMP-SMX, rifampin, ciprofloxacin, and gentamicin are commonly used. Oral azithromycin has shown some clinical success in reducing the initial lymph node volume in half the infected patients (500 mg in one dose the first day; 250 mg days 2 through 5; smaller children: 10 mg/kg/24 hours on day 1; 5 mg/kg/24 hours days 2 through 5) (Stechenberg, 2007).

Complications

A small percentage of patients manifest systemic illness. This can be associated with fever up to 106° F (41.2° C), malaise, fatigue, anorexia, weight loss, emesis, headache, hepatosplenomegaly, sore throat, exanthema, blindness secondary to stellate macular retinopathy, neurologic changes (bizarre behavior), seizures, and arthralgia. Enlarged mediastinal or pancreatic nodes can cause pleurisy, obstructive phenomena, and splenic and hepatic abscesses. Other complications include Parinaud oculoglandular syndrome (from inoculation of the palpebral conjunctivitis from rubbing the eye after touching the cat scratch), encephalopathy (5% incidence after 1 to 3 weeks of lymphadenopathy), aseptic meningitis, severe chronic systemic disease, erythema nodosa, neuroretinitis, thrombocytopenic purpura, primary atypical pneumonia, relapsing bacteremia, breast mass, endocarditis, angiomatoid papules, and osteomyelitis. Almost all of these problems generally resolve completely over several months, rarely a year (Stechenberg, 2007).

Prevention

Children should be discouraged from playing roughly with cats. Cat scratches should be washed thoroughly with soap and water. Immunocompromised individuals should stay away from cats that scratch or bite and avoid stray cats and cats younger than 1 year of age (Pickering et al, 2009).

KINGELLA KINGAE INFECTION

This organism has recently emerged from obscurity and is an important cause of invasive infections in children younger than age 5 years. The organism is part of the normal flora of the pharynx in children more than in adults; it can easily be transmitted among children in childcare settings. The incubation period is variable. Suspect in culture-negative skeletal infections of young children. History often includes recent or concomitant gingivostomatitis or upper respiratory infection. Pyogenic arthritis (most often affecting the knee, hip, ankle), osteomyelitis (distal femur), diskitis, endocarditis in children with underlying cardiac disease (it is among the HACEK group of pathogens [*Haemophilus* spp., *Actinobacillus actinomycetemcomitans, Cardiobacterium hominis, Eikenella corrodens,* and *Kingella kingae*]), meningitis, occult bacteremia, and pneumonia indicate invasive infection. It is difficult to isolate on routinely used solid culture media. The organism is susceptible to many antibiotics (penicillins, aminoglycosides, ciprofloxacin, erythromycin). Standard hygienic preventive measures should be in place in childcare settings (Pickering et al, 2009).

MENINGOCOCCAL DISEASE

Many organisms can cause meningitis (group B streptococcus, *Escherichia coli, Listeria monocytogenes,* enterococci, *S. pneumoniae, N. meningitidis, H. influenzae*). The causative organism varies with age. Only *N. meningitidis* is discussed here. (Chapter 27 also provides a general discussion of CNS infections.)

Epidemiology

N. meningitidis is a gram-negative diplococcus. It is a common commensal organism in the human nasopharynx. Groups A, B, C, W-135, and Y are largely the causes of invasive disease. Groups B, C, and Y account for 90% of invasive meningococcal disease in the U.S. and share equal incidence (Marrazzo and Hofman, 2010). Group B is a greater threat to younger children (Woods, 2007). The organism is spread from person to person via respiratory tract secretions and in most cases causes asymptomatic colonization. This can persist for weeks to months. The asymptomatic carriage rate is approximately 25% in nonepidemic periods. Disease occurs most often during winter and early spring in children, but sporadically (97% of cases) in the U.S. Children 2 years or younger have the greatest incidence with a peak occurring in children less than 1 year old. Epidemics occur in semiclosed communities (e.g., daycare centers, schools, college dormitories, and military barracks). The risk increases in environments where there is active or secondhand smoke exposure; in African-Americans, and in those from lower socioeconomic levels (Marrazzo and Hofman, 2010). Patients with functional or anatomic asplenia, sickle cell disease, agammaglobulinemia, AIDS, and complement deficiency or properdin deficiency are at increased risk for invasive or recurring meningococcal disease (Pickering et al, 2009; Woods, 2007). Adolescents from 15 to 19 years experience another peak in incidence, and college freshmen living in dormitories have slightly less than a fourfold increase in risk than their peers who are not in college (Woods, 2007). Those 15 to 24 years old have the highest mortality rate as a result of septic complications despite the fact that younger children have more meningitis (Marrazzo and Hofman, 2010).

N. meningitidis has also been found causative in other infections including conjunctivitis, otitis media, epiglottitis, arthritis, and pericarditis, urethritis in men (uncommon), and pelvic inflammatory disease in women (uncommon).

Incubation Period

The incubation period is 1 to 14 days. Patients are contagious until 24 hours after initiation of treatment.

Clinical Findings

Colonization can lead to invasive disease. Bacteremia and sepsis result and, depending on hematogenous spread, multiple patterns of illness can occur. These include bacteremia without sepsis, meningococcemic sepsis without meningitis, meningitis with or without meningococcemia, meningoencephalitis, and specific organ infection.

Presenting symptoms of meningitis can include:
- *Occult bacteremia:* This appears in a febrile child with URI or gastrointestinal-like symptoms. There may be a maculopapular rash. Often these children are treated as having a viral illness. Some have recovered without antimicrobial intervention, whereas others have developed meningococcal meningitis (58% of cases) (Woods, 2007).
- *Meningococcemia:* Symptoms may include fever (characteristic), chills, cold hands and feet, pharyngitis, headache, anorexia, purulent conjunctivitis, photophobia, myalgias/limb pain/refusal to walk (7%), myocarditis, malaise, stiff neck (less in infants), seizures, prostration, irritability, emesis, and a maculopapular or petechial rash (characteristic, follows other symptoms within 5 to 20 hours and occurs in about 7% of cases) (see Color Plate) that may quickly progress to purpura and septic shock manifested by hypertension, DIC, acidosis, adrenal hemorrhage, renal failure, myocardial failure, and coma (Woods, 2007). Fever and irritability may be the only initial symptoms in young children, whereas fever and headache are more typical in older children and adolescents (Marrazzo and Hofman, 2010).

Diagnostic Studies. The diagnosis is confirmed with a positive culture or Gram stain from blood, CSF, synovial fluid, sputum, or petechial or purpura lesion scraping. Latex agglutination testing is not recommended. PCR testing is used widely in the United Kingdom and is useful when antibiotics are given before testing, and organism growth has been suppressed. Some research and public health laboratories may offer PCR assays in the U.S. A CBC shows leukopenia or leukocytosis with increased bands and neutrophil percentages, hypoalbuminemia, hypocalcemia, metabolic acidosis with increased lactate levels, decreased platelets, and elevated ESR and CRP.

Differential Diagnosis

The list of differential diagnoses is long and includes septicemia caused by other invasive bacteria (e.g., pneumococcus or *H. influenzae,* viral meningitis, TB brain abscess, chronic otitis media, and sinusitis). Collagen-vascular diseases, primary hematologic and oncologic disease, erythema nodosa, erythema multiforme, RMSF, mycoplasma, lead encephalopathy, coxsackievirus, echovirus, rubella and rubeola infections, Henoch-Schönlein purpura, ITP, viral exanthems, typhus, typhoid, TSS, rat bite fever, gonococcemia, *S. aureus* endocarditis, and Kawasaki syndrome are also in the differential diagnosis.

Management

If the child is suspected of having meningococcemia, IV antibiotics are started pending culture results; cefotaxime or ceftriaxone are drugs of choice. If susceptibility is confirmed, aqueous penicillin G (250,000 to 300,000 units/ kg/day IV divided every 4 hours for 5 to 7 days) has been the drug of choice for infants and children. Alternative drugs (and for those with penicillin allergies) include cefotaxime, ceftriaxone, chloramphenicol (hematologic concerns with this drug), or ciprofloxacin. The patient is kept in respiratory isolation until 24 hours after the induction of treatment. Some *N. meningitidis* strains in the U.S. are partially resistant to penicillin, but no treatment failures have been reported. Penicillin resistance is reportedly high in some European countries. Early dexamethasone given within minutes before antimicrobials may reduce the incidence of residual neurologic and audiologic complications, but its use in children remains controversial. Activated protein C for meningococcal sepsis in children and adults has been studied but also remains controversial (Marrazzo and Hofman, 2010).

Control Measures

Exposed contacts must be carefully monitored. Household, school, or child contacts who develop a febrile illness must be evaluated for invasive disease promptly. High-risk household contacts have 500 to 800 times the risk as do those in the general community (Pickering et al, 2009).

- **Chemoprophylaxis** should be given within 24 hours of identification of the index case. At-risk individuals include close contacts (household, daycare, nursery school, those who shared oral secretions [kissing, shared utensils or toothbrushes]) of the index case 7 days before the onset of symptoms are at increased risk of invasive disease. Airline travel of greater than 8 hours while sitting next to an infected individual qualifies an individual for prophylaxis (Pickering et al, 2009). Casual contact with the index case, casual contact with a high-risk contact, or medical personnel (unless they performed mouth-to-mouth resuscitation, intubation, or suctioning before antibiotic therapy was instituted) are usually not considered high risk. Oral rifampin, 10 mg/kg/dose PO (maximum dose 600 mg) twice daily for a total of four doses is the prophylactic treatment of choice for those older than 1 month. Infants younger than 1 month old should be given 5 mg/kg/dose PO twice daily for a total of four doses. Ceftriaxone (125 mg IM for those less than 15 years old; 250 mg IM for those older than 15 years) in a single dose is as effective as oral rifampin; it can be given to pregnant women. Ciprofloxacin (500 mg PO in a single dose) can be given to nonpregnant adults 18 years and older (it can be given for those 1 month old or older but this is not routinely recommended; dose 20 mg/kg PO [maximum 500 mg]). Azithromycin (500 mg single dose) is effective but not recommended for routine use (Pickering et al, 2009).
- **Prophylaxis during outbreak:** Vaccine with serogroups A, C, Y, and W-135, in conjunction with chemoprophylaxis, is advisable to prevent extended outbreaks only if the identified strain is contained in the vaccine (see the discussion under Meningococcal Vaccine for guidance). No vaccine covers serogroup B infection.

Complications

Complications are caused by inflammation, intravascular hemorrhage, necrosis in multiple organ systems, and shock. Skeletal deformities and limb amputations are not infrequent.

Meningitis can lead to ataxia, seizures, pneumonia, deafness (5% to 10%), arthritis and pericarditis, visual field defects, palsies and paralysis, developmental delays, and hydrocephalus. The fatality rate from meningococcemia is approximately 40% in the U.S. (Marrazzo and Hofman, 2010) and about 10% from invasive meningococcal disease (Woods, 2007).

STREPTOCOCCAL DISEASE

Streptococci are gram-positive spherical cocci that are classified based on their ability to hemolyze RBCs. Complete hemolysis is known as beta-hemolytic. Partial hemolysis is alpha-hemolytic; nonhemolysis is gamma-hemolytic. Cell wall carbohydrate differences further subdivide the streptococci. These differences are identified as Lancefield antigen subgroups A-H and K-V. Subgroups A-H and K-O are associated with human disease. GABHS is the most virulent, though group B beta-hemolytic streptococcus can cause bacteremia and meningitis in infants younger than 3 months (rarely older) (Pickering et al, 2009). Group A beta-hemolytic and nongroup A and B streptococcus infection are discussed in this chapter; group B beta-hemolytic streptococcus is discussed in Chapter 38. (Also see discussion about rheumatic heart disease caused by group A streptococcal infection in Chapter 30.)

Group A Beta-Hemolytic Streptococcus

Epidemiology. Transmission is primarily through infected upper respiratory tract secretions or, secondarily, through skin invasion. Fomites and household pets are not vectors. Food-borne outbreaks from contamination by food handlers are reported. Streptococcus microbes most commonly invade the respiratory tract, skin, soft tissues, and blood. Both streptococcus pharyngitis and impetigo are associated with crowding, whether at home, school, or other institution. Pharyngitis is rare in infants and children less than 3 years old, but the incidence rises with age (predominantly from 3 to 15 years old) (Gerber, 2007). It is not common in adults unless there is an epidemic.

Streptococcal pharyngitis more typically occurs during late fall, winter, and spring in temperate climates. Carrier rates can be high during epidemics (20% to 50% depending on age) (Pickering et al, 2009). By contrast, streptococcus skin infection (impetigo, pyoderma) is more common in toddlers and preschool-age children and occurs more often during summer, early fall in tropical areas, or in warmer weather in temperate climates. Those at increased risk for invasive GABHS are those with varicella infection, IV drug use, HIV, diabetes, chronic heart or lung disease, infants, and older adults.

Incubation Period. The incubation period is 2 to 5 days for pharyngitis and 7 to 10 days from skin acquisition to development of impetigenous lesions. The period of communicability is from the onset of symptoms up to a few months in untreated individuals. More than 50% of individuals who acquire the organism will become ill (Pickering et al, 2009).

Clinical Findings. The following may be seen in GABHS:

- *Respiratory tract infection.* Streptococcal tonsillopharyngitis and pneumonia are described in Chapter 31. Peritonsillar abscess, cervical lymphadenitis, retropharyngeal abscess, otitis media, mastoiditis, and sinusitis symptoms may be clinical features.
- *Scarlet fever.* This is caused by erythrogenic toxin. It is uncommon in children younger than 3 years of age. The

incubation period is approximately 3 days (the range is 1 to 7 days). There is abrupt illness with sore throat, vomiting, headache, chills, and malaise. Fever can reach 104° F (40° C). Tonsils are erythematous, swollen, and usually covered in exudate. The pharynx also is inflamed and can be covered with a gray-white exudate. The palate and uvula are erythematous and reddened, and petechiae are present. The tongue is usually coated red. Desquamation of the coating leaves prominent papillae (strawberry tongue). The typical scarletina rash appears 1 to 5 days following onset of symptoms (Stevens, 2010). The exanthema is red and finely papular and makes the skin feel coarse, akin to sandpaper. The rash begins in the axilla, groin, and neck, spreads centripetally, is generalized within 24 hours, and blanches on pressure (Schultz-Charlton sign). There is circumoral pallor and the cheeks are flushed. There is increased rash density on the neck, axilla, and groin. Pastia lines, transverse linear hyperpigmented areas with tiny petechiae, are seen in the folds of the joints (see Fig. 23-2). In severe disease, small vesicles (miliary sudamina) can be found on the hands, feet, and abdomen. Rash, sore throat, and constitutional symptoms resolve in approximately 5 to 7 days (average 3 to 4 days). The rash begins to desquamate shortly thereafter. Fine branlike flakes begin on the face and slowly spread to the trunk and extremities (including fingernail margins, palms, and soles). This process may take up to 6 weeks.

- *Skin infections.* See discussion of impetigo in Chapter 36.
- *Bacteremia.* This can occur after respiratory (pharyngitis, tonsillitis, AOM) and localized skin infections. Some children have no obvious source of infection. Meningitis, osteomyelitis, septic arthritis, pyelonephritis, pneumonia, peritonitis, and bacterial endocarditis (acute rheumatic fever caused by a certain "rheumatogenic" strain) are rare but are associated with GABHS bacteremia.
- *Vaginitis.* See discussion of vulvovaginitis in Chapter 35.
- *Perianal streptococcal cellulitis.* This is uncommon and occurs in either sex. Manifestations include local itching, pain, blood-streaked stools, erythema, and proctitis. Although infection is usually the result of autoinoculation, it can be a symptom of sexual molestation if infected saliva is used as a sexual lubricant.
- *Rheumatic heart disease.* See Chapter 30.
- *Necrotizing fasciitis.* See Chapter 36.
- *Streptococcal TSS.* See Chapter 36.

Diagnostic Studies. Cultures or serologic testing differentiate the offending organism. Review diagnostic studies in the appropriate chapters previously mentioned. Anti-deoxyribonuclease (anti-DNase) is another way to measure streptococcal antibodies for the diagnosis of post-streptococcal glomerulonephritis and serious streptococcal skin infections (e.g., necrotising fasciitis).

Differential Diagnosis. A differential diagnosis is acute pharyngitis caused by viruses, especially adenoviruses or EBV (infectious mononucleosis syndrome). Other bacterial upper respiratory diseases in the differential diagnosis, though rare, include diphtheria, tularemia, toxoplasmosis, mycoplasma, tonsillar TB, salmonellosis, and brucellosis. Staphylococcal impetigo must be differentiated from GABHS pyoderma. Septicemia, meningitis, osteomyelitis, septic arthritis, pyelonephritis, and bacterial endocarditis can result from other bacteria causing similar infections.

Management. Antimicrobial therapy is the treatment of choice. See appropriate site-specific chapters for managing infections.

Complications. These are usually caused by the spread of the disease from the localized infection; many have already been discussed. Research is underway to determine whether prior infection with GABHS can produce autoimmune antibodies that cross-react with brain tissue. This occurrence is being referred to as pediatric autoimmune neuropsychiatric disorders associated with streptococcus pyogenes (PANDAS). An array of neuropsychiatric disorders is thought to result from the production of autoimmune antibodies, including obsessive-compulsive disorders, tic disorders, and Tourette syndrome. Treating with immunoregulatory therapy is investigational only (Gerber, 2007). Surgical scarlet fever can occur after wound infection, burns, or streptococcus skin infection.

Non–Group A or B Streptococci

These streptococci or Lancefield groups (principally groups C, F, and G) are associated with invasive disease in all age groups. They may cause septicemia, UTIs, endocarditis, respiratory disease (upper and lower), skin soft-tissue infection, pharyngitis, brain abscesses, and meningitis in newborns, children, adolescents, and adults. The incubation period and communicability times are unknown. Culture and antimicrobial susceptibility are essential. The habitats in humans differ as a result of resistance issues. Generally penicillin G is adequate, pending sensitivity determination (Pickering et al, 2009).

TUBERCULOSIS

TB is caused by *Mycobacterium tuberculosis* and is a very slow-growing organism, taking up to 10 weeks to grow on solid media and 1 to 6 weeks in liquid media. The degree of infectivity depends on the intensity and length of exposure to and the burden of bacilli carried by the index case. For this reason, TB is regarded as moderately infectious under most situations (Fitzgerald et al, 2009). The bacilli are spread primarily by droplet contamination from coughing, sneezing, laughing, or singing. Droplets can stay suspended in the air for hours. Fomite transmission is uncommon. The mycobacteria are isolated in less than 75% of infants and 50% of children with pulmonary TB (Pickering et al, 2009). The clinical signs and symptoms of infection depend on the child's immune response. The more effective the immune response in clearing the *M. tuberculosis* bacilli, the less destructive the disease.

Epidemiology

Individuals in the U.S. with the highest incidence of TB primarily live in urban, low-income areas and are non-Caucasian or ethnic. Foreign-born children 14 years and younger account for more than one quarter of children newly diagnosed (Pickering et al, 2009); in the non-Caucasian population TB is higher in young adults and children younger than 5 years of age (Starke and Munoz, 2007). High-risk groups for latent TB infection (LTBI) and active disease include immigrants, international adoptees, those from or travelers to high-prevalence regions (Asia, Africa, Middle East, Latin American, former Soviet Union countries), the homeless, and individuals in correctional facilities (Pickering et al, 2009). In more than 98% of cases, the portal of entry is the lung (Starke and Munoz, 2007).

Ninety-five percent of cases of TB occur in Third World countries where HIV/AIDS infection has been epidemic and health care is poor or inaccessible. Globally, one third of the world's population is infected with the mycobacteria (Starke and Munoz, 2007).

The age at the time of infection is predictive of the extent an infection will evolve into disease. Infected infants and pre-pubertal adolescents are more likely to progress to TB disease, as are those 15 to 25 years old and older adults. Generally about 3% to 4% of those infected with the bacilli progress to active disease during the first year after tuberculin conversion; thereafter, an additional 5% do so (Fitzgerald et al, 2009). These estimates are based on heavy exposures during disease-prone periods of life. Other factors that make an individual more prone to active infection include TB infection within the prior 2 years; immunocompromise (from a disease [e.g., HIV] or immunosuppressive drugs); IV drug use; those with certain diseases (e.g., Hodgkin disease, lymphoma, diabetes mellitus, chronic renal failure, malnutrition), and possibly those taking tumor necrosis factor-alpha antagonists to treat arthritis, inflammatory bowel disease, or other diseases (Pickering et al, 2009).

Congenital TB is extremely rare. An infant would most likely become infected after delivery from contact with an infected mother or other person. Exposure in utero could occur from exposure to maternal bacteremia at different stages in the course of maternal *M. tuberculosis* infection; seeding of the placenta by disseminated (miliary) TB from the mother that gained access to the fetal circulation; fetal aspiration of amniotic fluid at delivery if their mother had tuberculous endometritis; or in utero ingestion of infected amniotic fluid (Starke and Jacobs, 2008).

Incubation Period

Infection is defined as converting from a negative to a positive tuberculin skin test. The skin test is reactive within 2 to 10 weeks after initial infection. Risk of disease is highest in the first 6 months after infection. The risk continues to remain high for the subsequent 2 years after infection, but it can take years before progressing to disease. After treatment is started, infectivity may cease within days or take several weeks depending on the drugs prescribed and response of the organisms and other characteristics of the disease (e.g., for cavitary disease, response can take longer). In children less than 10 years of age, there is usually minimal cough and little expulsion of bacilli and, therefore, less contagion (Pickering et al, 2009).

Clinical Findings

Table 23-8 describes the stages of TB in children and requisite management strategies.

Primary Pulmonary Tuberculosis. Most children ages 3 to 15 years with primary pulmonary TB are asymptomatic when first noted to have a positive TB skin test. Most children with disease first develop hilar lymphadenopathy then focal hyperinflation and atelectasis (Starke and Munoz, 2007). An effective immune response eliminates most of the bacilli

TABLE 23-8	Characteristics of Tuberculosis in Children		
	STAGE		
	Exposure	**Infection (LTBI)**	**Disease**
Skin test	Negative	Positive (60%-90%)	Positive (60%-90%)
Physical examination	Normal	Normal	Usually abnormal*
Chest radiograph	Normal	Usually normal†	Usually abnormal‡
Treatment	If <4 years old or with impaired immunity (e.g., HIV)	Always	Always
Number of drugs	One	One	Three or four

*More than 50% of infants and children with pulmonary tuberculosis have a normal physical examination.
†Calcification in the lungs, hila, lymph nodes, or a small granuloma is considered infection, not disease.
‡Some children with extrapulmonary tuberculosis have a normal chest radiograph.
HIV, Human immunodeficiency virus; *LTBI,* latent tuberculosis infection.
Data from Pickering LK, Baker CJ, Kimberlin KW, et al: Tuberculosis. In *Red Book: 2009 Report of the Committee on Infectious Diseases,* ed 28, Elk Grove Village, IL, 2009, American Academy of Pediatrics; Starke JR, Munoz FM: Tuberculosis *(Mycobacterium tuberculosis).* In Kliegman RM, Behrman RE, Jenson HB, et al, editors: *Nelson textbook of pediatrics,* ed 18, Philadelphia, 2007, Saunders, pp 1240-1254.

although small numbers of bacilli can be spread throughout the body during the bacteremic phase.

Rarely, enlarging lymph nodes can encroach on the regional bronchus, causing compression and obstruction; this is more commonly seen with infants. Compression can also occur of the esophagus (causing dysphagia or aspiration) and major arteries and veins (causing edema). Inflamed nodes can erode through the endobronchial wall; fistulas can occur between the lymph node and the bronchial lumen and cause fibrosis, bronchiectasis, and pneumonia. Recurrent cough, stridor, and wheezing are signs of increasing pulmonary infection.

Symptoms in children are generally minor and slightly more evident in infants. These signs and symptoms typically occur 1 to 6 months after infection and may range from low-grade fever, and nonproductive cough and dyspnea (more common in infants) to malaise, decreased appetite, weight loss (failure to thrive in infants), night sweats, chills, erythema nodosum, and phlyctenular keratoconjunctivitis (a hypersensitivity reaction marked by elevated clear nodules with surrounding hyperemia near the limbus). Approximately 2% to 30% of children present with extrapulmonary TB symptoms (meningitis and/or granulomatous inflammation of the lymph nodes, bones, joints, skin, and middle ear and mastoid) (Pickering et al, 2009; Starke and Munoz, 2007).

Most children do not suffer significant pulmonary disease, and resolution occurs with or without appropriate treatment (Starke and Jacobs, 2008). Residual calcification of the primary focus or regional lymph nodes may be evident on x-ray.

Diagnostic Studies. The initial parenchymal inflammatory response generally does not show up on the chest radiograph; there are usually some visible localized, nonspecific infiltrates. Over time the hypersensitivity of the lung tissue and hilar lymph node inflammatory response continue. Most children generally quickly resolve the infiltrates and adenopathy, whereas the hilar adenopathy continues to enlarge in infants. The hallmark is disproportionately enlarged regional lymph nodes as compared with a relatively small pleural focus (Starke and Jacobs, 2008).

Radiography in childhood shows inconspicuous pneumonitis in the lower and middle lung fields. In adolescents, apical or subapical infiltrates are seen, often with cavitations, and no hilar adenopathy (Fitzgerald et al, 2009). Extensive pulmonary infiltrates and cavitation can be seen if there was erosion and necrosis from disseminated bacilli. Lesions may be the size of millet seeds; hence the name "miliary" TB.

Hilar adenopathy suggests TB, but culture of the organism is essential to establish the diagnosis. Specimens for culture may be obtained from gastric aspirates, sputum, bronchial washings, pleural fluid, CSF, urine or other body fluids or biopsies. Children older than 5 years and adolescents can be induced to cough to produce sputum with aerosolized hypertonic saline. When age or ability to produce sputum is a factor, an early morning gastric aspirate analyzed by fluorescent staining is an effective and sensitive testing method. These aspirates are collected on 3 separate days. However, the positive diagnostic yield from aspirates is less than 50% (Pickering et al, 2009). Histologic examination for acid-fast bacilli from biopsies can be helpful. In any case, all specimens need to be cultured.

A new system, the Cepheid GeneXpert System, is a single-use sample-processing system using a special machine. The system simplifies nucleic acid amplification (a PCR assay) directly from sputum. It not only approaches 100% sensitivity and specificity but also detects rifampin resistance and gives results in less than 2 hours. It avoids the current nucleic acid amplification methods in use to detect *M. tuberculosis* that are more complex, labor intensive, and technically difficult. Its potential use in the U.S. and globally to rapidly identify and quickly start individuals on appropriate treatment cannot be underestimated (Helb et al, 2010). Other testing of cultured organisms can be done and may use DNA probes or high-pressure liquid chromatography.

If isolate from the index case is confirmed as TB, culture material does not need to be obtained from the child. However, a culture is necessary in the following circumstances: the index case is unavailable; the child has HIV infection or immunocompromised; drug-resistant TB is suspected; or the child has extrapulmonary symptoms (Pickering et al, 2009).

The Tuberculin Skin Test. Tuberculin skin testing is based on the delayed hypersensitivity to *M. tuberculosis* antigens. The test usually becomes positive 3 weeks to 3 months (usually 4 to 8 weeks) after inhalation of the bacilli (Starke and Munoz, 2007). The preparation for skin testing is purified protein derivative (PPD). This Mantoux test uses 0.1 mL of 5 tuberculin units (TU) PPD. It is injected intradermally into the volar surface of the forearm, producing a wheal with 6 to 10 mm of induration (crucial for accurate testing). A multipuncture skin test should not be used (Pickering et al, 2009; Starke and Munoz, 2007). The Mantoux test is read 48 to 72 hours later by an experienced health care professional. The induration, not the erythema, is measured. For those having had BCG, interpretation of the skin test is the same as for nonrecipients (see prior discussion under BCG vaccine). High-risk groups (including children with HIV, beginning at 3 to 12 months of age) and patients living in areas where TB is endemic or on the rise should be skin tested yearly. Low-risk groups do not need to be routinely tested.

Pediatric patients are considered at high risk for TB if they meet any of the following medical risk criteria (Pickering et al, 2009):

- Have close contact with others who have suspected or confirmed TB
- Are immigrants or have traveled to TB-prevalent parts of the world (Asia, Middle East, Africa, Latin America, countries formerly part of the Soviet Union) (wait 10 weeks after return for screening with the tuberculin skin test) (Pickering et al, 2009)
- Have clinical signs suggestive of TB on chest radiograph or other clinical evidence suggestive of TB infection
- Are HIV positive, have an immunosuppressive disorder, or are being treated with immunosuppressive drugs
- Are exposed to individuals with HIV who are using illicit drugs
- Have other risk factors, including Hodgkin disease, lymphoma, diabetes mellitus, chronic renal failure, or malnutrition
- Are exposed to individuals residing in homeless shelters, nursing homes, correctional institutions, other residential institutions, migrant farm workers

All individuals with positive PPDs need quick clinical and radiographic evaluation. A Mantoux skin test is defined as positive for LTBI or tuberculosis disease if the following reactions occur (Pickering et al, 2009):

- Induration (5 mm or greater) in children who are in close contact with an individual with active or previously active TB cases; themselves suspected of having TB because their chest radiograph is consistent with active or previously active TB or they have clinical findings of TB; or diagnosed with immunosuppressive disorders or HIV infection, or who are receiving immunosuppressive drugs
- Induration (10 mm or greater) in children younger than 4 years of age with any of the high-risk factors listed above
- Induration (15 mm or greater) in children 4 years of age or older without any risk factors
- If the skin test shows onset of induration after 72 hours, it should be interpreted as positive.

Skin testing is not always valid: 10% to 40% of children with positive cultures can have a negative skin test. This decreased reactivity can also occur in immunocompromised patients (e.g., HIV); infants younger than 3 months of age; those with poor nutrition; those with other viral infections (notably measles, varicella and influenza); and in those with progressive TB (up to 50% with disseminated [miliary] TB or meningitis will not react until several months after receiving drug treatment) or recent TB infection (Pickering et al, 2009; Starke and Munoz, 2007). Additionally, a poor response to the skin test can occur due to inadequate handling of the Mantoux solution, improper injection technique, or interpretation error. Patients sensitized to nontuberculous mycobacteria can cross-react and have a less than 10- to 12-mm reaction to TB skin testing.

Interferon-Gamma Release Assays. Interferon-gamma release assays (IGRA) are newer screening tests approved by the FDA for detecting T-cell response to specific *M. tuberculosis* antigens. They do not distinguish between LTBI or acute disease but have the advantage of not being affected by prior BCG vaccination. The IGRA is not to be used routinely for screening in children younger than 5 years or for those immunocompromised of any age. IGRA is recommended in the following circumstances (Pickering et al, 2009):

- Immunocompetent children 5 or more years of age in place of the Mantoux to confirm suspected LTBI or active disease. A positive result is indicative of TB infection; a negative IGRA is not to be interpreted as absence of infection or disease if clinical signs and symptoms suggest otherwise.
- Can be considered in children who have received BCG and have a positive Mantoux to better determine infection when a false-positive skin sensitivity could be the result of BCG

Differential Diagnosis

The provider should consider TB in patients with symptoms of basilar meningitis, hydrocephalus, cranial nerve palsy, or stroke. Permanent neurologic dysfunction can result and has a worse prognosis in infants than in toddlers and older children. The differential diagnosis includes mycotic infections, staphylococcal pneumonia, sarcoidosis, chronic pneumonia, and Hodgkin lymphoma. Differential diagnosis in lymph node disease includes cat-scratch disease, tularemia, toxoplasmosis, tumor, brachial cysts, cystic hygroma, and pyogenic infection.

Management

A tuberculosis specialist should be consulted. After case-finding of index and contact cases and diagnostic studies, the state and/or local health department may initiate treatment and follow-up. Antitubercular drug treatment is focused on eradicating the bacilli and inhibiting their multiplication in LTBI and early pulmonary disease as quickly as possible. Rapid resolution of caseous or granulomatous lesions will not occur. It is imperative that strict adherence to drug combination regimens be followed to minimize drug resistance. Tables 23-9 and 23-10 show the recommended drugs and treatment regimens based on the disease state.

Infants of mothers diagnosed with TB disease in pregnancy should be started on treatment for LTBI after birth for 3 or 4 months (at which time a Mantoux skin test should be given), even if breastfeeding and the mother is on concurrent therapy. Treatment should start in a pregnant woman with signs and symptoms or abnormal findings on chest x-ray consistent with TB disease after the first trimester. If the pregnant woman was found to have LTBI, she should be started on LTBI treatment for 9 months after the postpartum period, and the newborn would need no further evaluation or therapy (Pickering et al, 2009).

The exclusively breastfed infant receiving isoniazid should be given pyridoxine, although it is not routinely recommended for children and adolescents (Pickering et al, 2009; Starke and Jacobs, 2008). It is also recommended for use in those individuals whose diets are either deficient in meat or milk, in those with HIV, and for pregnant adolescents; the tablets can be pulverized for easier administration. For children with meningeal, endobronchial, pericardial effusion, and miliary

TABLE 23-9 Most Commonly Used Drugs for Tuberculosis in Children

Drug	Daily Dose	Twice-Weekly Dose
Isoniazid (I)	LTBI: 10 mg/kg (max: 300 mg) Disease: 10-15 mg/kg (max: 300 mg); available as syrup or tablets; crushed tablets are more palatable than the syrup	20-30 mg/kg/dose (max: 900 mg/dose)
Rifampin (R)	10-20 mg/kg (maximum, 600 mg); available as syrup or tablets	10-20 mg/kg/dose (max: 600 mg/dose)
Pyrazinamide (Z)	30-40 mg/kg (max: 2000 mg); tablets only	50 mg/kg/dose (max: 2000 mg/dose)
Etham-butol (E) ethionamide	20-25 mg/kg (max: 2500 mg); tablets only	50 mg/kg/dose (max: 2500 mg/dose)

Note: Isoniazid and rifampin are available in a combination preparation: isoniazid 150 mg/rifampin 300 mg. Another preparation combines isoniazid 50 mg/rifampin 120 mg/pyrazinamide 300 mg. These combinations have not been studied for use in children (Starke and Jacobs, 2008).
LTBI, Latent tuberculosis infection; *max,* maximum.
Data from Pickering LK, Baker CJ, Kimberlin DW et al: *Red Book: 2009 Report of the Committee on Infectious Diseases,* ed 28, Elk Grove Village, IL, 2009, American Academy of Pediatrics, p 689.

TB, corticosteroids may be used to decrease the inflammation that is detrimental to organ function; its use also decreases mortality rates and neurologic disability.

Monitoring Response to Treatment. Tracking of index and contact cases is under the jurisdiction of state and local health departments. Initial evaluation, drug management, and follow-up may also take place in these centers. However, the primary care provider may also play a crucial role in monitoring response to treatment. The following are general monitoring guidelines (Blumberg and Leonard, 2010; Pickering et al, 2009):

- See all individuals monthly who are being treated for any stage of tuberculosis. Evaluate for antitubercular drug side effects and adherence monthly, notably for symptoms of hepatitis if on isoniazid (a rare finding in healthy infants, children, and adolescents). Educate patients to call immediately if experiencing signs of hepatoxicity (vomiting, abdominal pain, jaundice), peripheral neuritis, diarrhea, or gastrointestinal irritation. Those on pyrazinamide may experience hepatoxicity, arthralgia, or gastrointestinal disturbances. Rifampin may cause orange secretions in urine, vomiting, hepatitis, flulike symptoms, thrombocytopenia, and pruritus; those on oral contraceptives need to use a back-up method.
- Baseline liver function tests, creatinine level, and platelet count should be obtained on all individuals (this may have been at the initial evaluation by the health department); it is not necessary to monitor these unless the baseline results were abnormal or clinical assessment suggests an indication.

TABLE 23-10 Drug Treatment Regimens for Tuberculosis in Infants, Children, and Adolescents[d]

Type of Tubercular Illness	Isoniazid (I)	Rifampin (R)[a]	Pyrazinamide (Z)	Ethambutol (E)
Prophylaxis				
• Isoniazid susceptible	Daily for 9 months[b]			
• Isoniazid resistant		Daily for 6 months[c]		
• If resistant to both I and R, consult tuberculosis (TB) specialist				
Pulmonary[f] and extrapulmonary disease (miliary, lymph node, bone, joint infection)[d]	Daily for 2 months, then 2 or 3 times weekly for 4 months[e]	Daily for 2 months, then 2 or 3 times weekly for 4 months[e]	Daily for 2 months	Daily for 2 months if drug resistance is of concern and/or until drug resistance is known. Directly observed therapy (DOT) is recommended.
		OR		
	2 or 3 times/week for 2 months under DOT then 2 or 3 times weekly for 4 months under DOT[e]	2 or 3 times/week for 2 months under DOT then 2 or 3 times weekly for 4 months under DOT[e]	2 or 3 times/week for 2 months under DOT	2 or 3 times/week for 2 months under DOT until drug resistance known
• Hilar adenopathy only	Daily for 6 months	Daily for 6 months		
Meningitis[d] (treat for a total of 9-12 months)	Daily for 2 months, then once daily or twice weekly for 7-10 months	Daily for 2 months, then once daily or twice weekly for 7-10 months	Daily for 2 months	Daily for 4-8 weeks until drug susceptibility is determined. Can also use ethionamide, streptomycin, or another aminoglycoside. If suspect drug resistance to streptomycin, substitute with kanamycin, amikacin, or capreomycin.

Boxes indicate that these drug regimens are given concurrently.
[a]Rifampin resistance is more likely to occur in those with HIV infection.
[b]DOT twice a week can be used for 9 months if daily therapy cannot be achieved.
[c]DOT twice a week can be used for 6 months if daily therapy cannot be achieved.
[d]Treatment recommendations are in constant flux; it is advised that providers consult a pediatric TB specialist before initiating treatment for any type of TB infection to ensure that the most current treatment is prescribed; different regimens will be used if child also has concurrent human immunodeficiency virus (HIV) infection.
[e]DOT is desirable.
[f]For pulmonary TB, if isoniazid resistant but rifampin- and pyrazinamide-susceptible, treat with R, Z, and E for 6 months; other drug-resistance situations and drug regimens should be discussed with a TB specialist. Children with drug-resistant TB disease should be on DOT.
Data from Pickering LK, Baker CJ, Kimberlin DW, et al: Children in out-of-home child care. In *Red Book 2009 Report of the Committee on Infectious Diseases,* ed 28, Elk Grove Village, IL, 2009, American Academy of Pediatrics, p 688; Starke JR, Munoz FM: Mycobacterial infections: tuberculosis *(Mycobacterium tuberculosis).* In Kliegman RM, Behrman RD, Jenson HB, et al, editors: *Nelson textbook of pediatrics,* ed 18, Philadelphia, 2007, Saunders; Starke JR, Jacobs RF: *Mycobacterium tuberculosis.* In Long SS, Pickering LK, Prober CG, editors: *Principles and practice of pediatric infectious disease,* ed 3, Philadelphia, 2008, Churchill Livingstone.

- A sputum specimen for acid-fast bacilli smear and culture is collected monthly until two consecutive specimens are negative; a sputum specimen should be collected after 2 months of drug therapy to evaluate for relapse (check to see if done by the health department).
- If sputum culture is positive after 3 months of therapy, the bacilli need to be rechecked for drug susceptibility.
- Repeat chest radiograph after 2 months; it is good practice to take one after therapy has been completed as a baseline for comparison against any subsequent films.
- Extrapulmonary disease: Follow clinical symptoms because sputum cultures are more difficult to monitor progress.
- For those taking ethambutol, ask about presence of any visual disturbances (screen visual acuity and red-green color vision if dosages exceed 20 mg/kg/day or if on more than 2 months of treatment with this drug); if unable to test visual acuity, consider an alternate drug.
- Children can be given measles and other attenuated live-virus vaccines at age-appropriate times, unless on high-dose corticosteroids, are severely ill, or have another contraindication.

Complications

The following complications can occur with TB:
- *Progressive Primary Pulmonary Disease.* Rarely, primary TB can progress and disseminate. This occurs more frequently in infants and children younger than the age of

5 years, a result of their immune systems being immature or inadequate to the task of eliminating bacilli. The primary pleural focus enlarges and develops a large caseous center, and liquefaction forms a cavity that contains large numbers of bacilli. Symptoms in children with progressive disease are more acute and include high intermittent fevers, night sweats, severe cough, and weight loss. Pleural effusion, peritonitis, or meningitis can occur in as many as two thirds of individuals (Fitzgerald et al, 2009). In young adults the infection is usually more chronic and onset is subtle. Nonspecific symptoms include fever, anorexia, weakness, and weight loss. The physical examination should include a careful skin examination, looking for cutaneous eruptions, sinus tracts, scrotal masses, and lymphadenopathy; hepatomegaly, splenomegaly, tachypnea, dyspnea, rales, wheezes, and stridor are often found.

- *Reactivation of Pulmonary Tuberculosis.* There is potential for infection after reactivation of pulmonary TB in those who acquired their initial infection when they were older than the age of 7 years; they are highly contagious until effective treatment is started. Reactivation is more likely to occur after the child reaches adolescence and can present with either few symptoms or fever, anorexia, malaise, weight loss, night sweats, productive cough, hemoptysis, and chest pain. Full recovery is excellent with appropriate treatment (Starke and Munoz, 2007).
- *Miliary Disease.* During the early stages of the primary disease, bacilli disseminate and reach the bloodstream directly from the initial focus or by way of the regional lymph nodes. This complication of primary pulmonary disease occurs more commonly in infants, children, and adolescents, but is seen less frequently since the advent of effective drug therapy. It appears more often now in racial minorities, in those with underlying conditions that may compromise the immune system, and in older adults (Fitzgerald et al, 2009). Systemic signs such as anorexia, weight loss, and low-grade fever progress over weeks to lymphadenopathy, hepatosplenomegaly, higher fever, dyspnea, cough, rales, wheezing, frank respiratory distress, and pneumothorax or pneumomediastinum. Headache suggests meningitis; abdominal pain suggests tuberculous peritonitis (Starke and Munoz, 2007).
- *Lymph Node Disease.* This is an extrapulmonary form of TB affecting the superficial lymph nodes; it is known as *scofula.* It can be caused by drinking raw milk contaminated with *M. bovis* or after initial infection with *M. tuberculosis.* The head, trunk, neck, and inguinal and lower extremity nodes are firm (but not hard), fixed to underlying tissue, and nontender. The lymphadenopathy is usually unilateral at first and can progress to multinode involvement. Tuberculin skin testing is usually positive; a chest x-ray is normal 70% of the time. The diagnosis can be made by culturing node tissue biopsies, but the organism is found in only about 50% of cases (Starke and Munoz, 2007).
- *Pleural Effusions.* This frequently occurs in primary disease. It is caused by an extension of the bacillus into the pleural space by subpleural foci or hematogenous spread, or both. It usually occurs 6 months to years after the primary infection. Symptoms include abrupt onset of low to high fever, shortness of breath, chest pain on deep inspiration, and decreased breath sounds. Response to treatment takes several weeks; radiographic changes can continue to

be evident for months following treatment. Scoliosis can be a complication (rare).
- *Tuberculous Meningitis.* This is the most serious complication of TB. It generally follows primary pulmonary disease in 0.3% of untreated infants and young children 6 months to 4 years of age. Meningeal infection is also common in miliary TB. Bacilli migrate to the subarachnoid space. Caseous lesions can enlarge, encapsulate, and form a tuberculoma that can act just like any other CNS mass lesion. Symptoms can evolve slowly or rapidly; infants and children generally experience rapid onset. Tuberculin skin testing is negative in 50% of cases, with 20% to 50% of cases also having negative chest x-rays (Starke and Munoz, 2007). Diagnosis is via CSF culture. Symptoms include fever, malaise, irritability, drowsiness, decreased developmental milestones, nuchal rigidity, positive Kernig or Brudzinski signs, hypertonia, vomiting, seizures, and other neurologic symptoms. The provider should consider TB in the differential diagnosis for any child who presents with basilar meningitis and hydrocephaly, cranial nerve palsy, or stroke without other apparent cause. Tuberculoma (brain tumor presenting as headache, fever, seizure) is also possible in children.
- *Cutaneous Tuberculosis.* This variant is rare in the U.S., occurring in 1% to 2% of all TB cases (Starke and Munoz, 2007). It occurs in two forms: (1) the TB chancre, and (2) multiple skin lesions resulting from hematogenous spread. Those at high risk include those with HIV, those with poor hygiene, and those who are malnourished.
- *Hematogenous Spread of Tuberculosis to Other Organs or Body Systems.* Spread can be to endocrine and exocrine glands, urogenital tract, heart and pericardium, skeleton, eyes, abdomen, tonsils, adenoids, larynx, middle ear, and mastoids.
- *Multiple Drug Resistant Tuberculosis* (MDR-TB). Not only is *M. tuberculosis* gaining resistance to isoniazid and rifampin, resistance to a fluoroquinolone is also seen in a subgroup (referred to as XDR-TB) and at least one of the second-line injectable medications (capreomycin, amikacin, or kanamycin). Immigrants from countries with high rates of MDR-TB who have had prolonged exposure to ineffective drugs are influencing resistance patterns and providing a treatment challenge (Kaye et al, 2010).

■ Helminthic Zoonoses

Approximately 71% of U.S. households with children own a pet(s), so close contact is inevitable (American Veterinary Medical Association, 2007). About 75% of emerging infectious diseases are diseases of animal origin, and approximately 60% of all human pathogens are zoonotic (transmitted from an animal to a human host) in origin (CDC, 2010j). Transmission of zoonotic infections can occur by several routes:
- Direct infection by ingestion of eggs or the penetration of larvae into the body (infections such as tapeworms and roundworms are acquired from their eggs; hookworms penetrate the skin)
- Indirect infection by ingestion of larvae in food (e.g., fish, meat, snails, freshwater shrimp, land crabs)
- Exposure to an intermediary vector (e.g., mosquitoes, flies, fleas, ticks)

Domesticated dogs, cats, and wild animals (e.g., raccoons) kept as pets can be infected with intestinal helminth parasites. Mild to severe illness can result when a helminth is transmitted to children, most often by fecal contamination. Only toxocariasis larva migrans, which may be encountered in primary care, is discussed here. (See Chapter 32 for a further discussion on intestinal parasites.)

TOXOCARIASIS

Description and Epidemiology

Parasitic helminth larvae can live for extended periods in human and animal organs and tissues causing an inflammatory condition, such as toxocariasis or larva migrans (LM), which can affect many organs and tissues within the body. When LM has been identified, the most common clinical syndromes are visceral (VLM) and ocular (OLM), less typically neural (NLM), covert, and cutaneous (caused by a dog or cat hookworm, *Ancylostoma braziliense*). They can be further classified as *asymptomatic* or *clinically unapparent*.

The *Toxocara* species of roundworms found in dogs *(canis)* and cats *(catis)* commonly cause LM in humans. The raccoon ascarid, *Baylisascaris procyonis,* causes less VLM but can lead to neural LM and resultant eosinophilic meningitis. Puppies (more commonly than kittens worldwide) and kittens carry the *Toxocara* roundworm. Puppies are infected prior to birth (not true for kittens) or from their mother's milk. Dogs or cats of any age can harbor the parasite, but dogs are a more common vector. Infection with *T. canis* can cause VLM, OLM, and, in severe cases, neural LM. *T. cati* causes less VLM than *T. canis*.

Ingestion of these hardy eggs (they can remain viable for months and in inclement weather conditions) occurs from contact with excreta in contaminated soil (in sandboxes, parks, playgrounds, schoolyards, public places where dogs/cats have visited), hands, toys, or in food. Once the eggs are ingested and hatched, the larvae can penetrate the intestines and migrate to the liver, lungs, heart, brain, and muscles. With initial or mild infestations, the larvae seem to be able to reach other locations, such as the brain and eye, more easily. In humans, the larvae cannot complete their maturation into adult worms so infected individuals do not pass eggs or larvae in their excreta.

The most recent study within the U.S. showed a prevalence rate of 14% for toxocariasis; prior studies showed a rate as high as 54% in a selected kindergarten population (Nash, 2009). Young children and those less than 20 years of age are most commonly infected (Won et al, 2007). Preschool children are most commonly affected by VLM, whereas OLM occurs more often in older children and young adults.

Clinical Findings

Symptoms result from the migrating larvae and from the induced eosinophilic granulomatous inflammation. Diagnosis is based on clinical features, exposure to the feces of puppies or kittens (simply touching an infected animal is not a risk factor), and diagnostic studies.

History. Assess for history of pica or geophagia; exposure to dogs, cats, or environments where animals are known to frequent; and recent travel, fever, abdominal pain, hepatomegaly, or respiratory symptoms (cough, wheezing, asthma,

pneumonia). In the case of OLM, there may be no history of pica or previous VLM.

Physical Examination

- OLM: Posterior or peripheral subretinal mass, decreased vision, strabismus, or leukokoria
- VLM: Abdominal pain, hepatomegaly, anorexia, nausea, vomiting, lethargy, irritability, coughing, wheezing, fever, cervical adenitis, limb pain, urticaria, pruritic skin lesions or nodules. Seizures and behavioral changes are uncommon.
- NLM: The presenting symptoms may be mild (subtle neurologic or behavior changes) to severe (CNS involvement, seizures).
- Covert LM: Chronic weakness, abdominal pain, allergic signs

Diagnostic Studies

- VLM: CBC reveals leukocytosis, marked eosinophilia (>500/μL), hypergammaglobulinemia (IgG, IgM, IgE), elevated A and B blood group isohemagglutinin titers. With migration of the helminth via the portal system to the intestinal lumen, eosinophil counts are normal or slightly raised. Migration through internal or visceral organs causes the count to be more markedly elevated; the degree of eosinophilia wanes if the helminth completes its migration cycle or is able to wall itself off and avoid provoking a host eosinophilic response. ELISA is confirmatory.
- OLM: None of the above. From a specimen of vitreous-aqueous fluid, elevated *T. canis* antibody titers (ELISA with confirmatory Western blot test is less sensitive for diagnosis) are seen when compared with serum titers. CT and MRI may be used to detect granulomatous lesions in OLM.
- Overt LM: Eosinophilia, increased IgE. Covert toxocariasis may demonstrate asymptomatic eosinophilia only.
- Chest x-ray: Transient infiltrates in about 50% of cases with pulmonary symptoms (Van Voorhis and Weller, 2010).

Differential Diagnosis

Ascaris lumbricoides, B. procyonis, Fasciola hepatica, schistosomiasis, and retinoblastoma are included in the differential diagnoses.

Management

Toxocariasis should be considered in any child with nonspecific symptoms, notably recurrent abdominal pain, reactive airway disease, allergies of unknown cause, and elevated eosinophilia. A normal eosinophilia count should not predispose the provider from ruling out this infection, if suspected.

Most individuals do not require treatment because there is usually spontaneous recovery over a period of weeks to months (Dent and Kazura, 2007). A pediatric infectious disease expert should be consulted for treatment recommendations. Management is based on controlling inflammatory reactions (corticosteroids and antihistamines) and use of appropriate anthelmintic therapy (rates of successful treatment with anthelmintics are mixed) (Nash, 2009). Anthelmintic medications include albendazole (drug of choice; not FDA approved for this use; 400 mg bid PO for 5 days, all ages) and mebendazole (100 to 200 mg bid PO for 5 days, all ages). Family pets need evaluation by a veterinarian.

Education

Prevention of zoonotic infestations includes identifying possible sources of exposure, referral of pets to veterinarians for testing, decontamination of soiled environments, and prevention of further exposure. The last intervention includes education about safe pet fecal cleanup, the regular deworming of pets, good handwashing, behavioral modification in cases of pica and geophagia, and covering sandboxes when not in use. Information should be provided to families with pets, especially puppies, kittens, and raccoons, about having them tested for helminth infestations. Communities should be encouraged to promote leash laws and responsible pet ownership (cleaning up pet fecal waste), to disallow dogs from playgrounds and parks where children play, and to restrict open access to sandboxes.

The Child Presenting With Fever

Fever is defined as an abnormally elevated body temperature with a temperature of 100.4° F (38° C) per rectum or higher. (See Chapter 21 for a more complete description of the physiologic processes involved in fever mechanisms.)

The normal physiologic hypothalamic set-point is altered by many different agents. Febrile illnesses in neonates are usually the result of congenital infections, those acquired at delivery (late-onset group B streptococcal infection), those acquired in the nursery (especially in premature infants), those acquired at home (pneumococcal or meningococcal infection), or those acquired as a result of anatomic or physiologic dysfunction (e.g., renal). Other causes for fever in children are related to bacterial and viral infections, vaccines, biologic agents, tissue damage, malignancy, drugs, collagen-vascular disorders, endocrine disorders, inflammatory disorders, and other disease states. Temperatures higher than 105.8° F (41° C) are rarely of infectious origin but are due to CNS dysfunction (e.g., malignant hyperthermia, drug fever, heat stroke).

The fever-causing agents produce endogenous pyrogens that reset the hypothalamic center. This process takes approximately 90 minutes. Clinically, this means that blood cultures should be obtained before the fever spikes because there would be a greater bacterial or fungal yield.

There are two situations of invasive bacterial or viral infections that are a particular challenge for any provider dealing with neonates, infants, and young children 36 months or younger: fever without a source or focus and fever of unknown origin. Each of these situations is discussed separately, and guidelines for their management are given. A fairly objective diagnosis can be reached by completing a careful history, physical examination, and following diagnostic, assessment, and management guidelines based on age, symptoms, estimated risks, associated diseases, and immune status. A few general epidemiologic points are helpful for this discussion (Powell, 2007):

- In infants younger than 3 months, with fever, 70% of causative agents can be identified, the majority being viral (40% to 60%); a workup for bacterial disease is still necessary.
- Viruses have a seasonal pattern: RSV and influenza A in winter; enterovirus in summer and fall.

- Bacteremia occurs in approximately 5% of previously well infants younger than 3 months.
- Prior to the conjugated pneumococcal vaccine, occult bacteremia (due to *S. pneumoniae, N. meningitidis,* and *Salmonella*) was diagnosed in about 1.5% of nontoxic-appearing children between 3 and 36 months of age who had fever of 102.2° F (>39° C) rectally. More commonly infections in this age group can be attributed to otitis media, pneumonia, URIs, enteritis, UTIs, osteomyelitis, and meningitis.
- Bacteremia can be an occult infection in young infants and children (i.e., nontoxic-appearing patient whose blood culture is positive for a pathogenic organism).
- The younger the infant, the greater the uncertainty about the possibility of a serious bacterial infection, and the greater the need to rule out this possibility.

FEVER WITHOUT FOCUS IN INFANTS AND YOUNG CHILDREN

Description

The assessment of the child who has an acute fever involves a careful investigation for a source of infection. Children between birth and 24 months are at greatest risk for unsuspected occult bacteremia; it is less common in those older than 36 months. *Fever without focus* is an acute febrile illness in which the etiology of the fever is not apparent after careful history and physical examination. For the purposes of this discussion, *fever* is defined as a rectal temperature of 100.4° F (38° C) or greater in infants 0 to 90 days old; or greater than 102.2° F (39° C) in infants and children 3 to 36 months old.

Epidemiology

Table 23-11 provides a list of the most common pathogens causing bacteremia in infants less than 3 months of age. Since the advent of the *H. influenzae* type b conjugate vaccine this agent has been virtually eliminated as a cause of bacteremia in children 3 to 36 months; the *S. pneumoniae* conjugate vaccine (started routinely in 2000) is expected to follow a similar trend (Powell, 2007; Shapiro, 2008).

Clinical Findings

History. The following should be included in the history of the illness:

- Duration and degree of fever (fever documented at home by reliable caregiver should be considered accurate)
- Possible associated symptoms: Vomiting, diarrhea, respiratory symptoms, rash (especially petechiae or purpura), irritability, inconsolability, change in play activities, lethargy (level of consciousness characterized by poor or absent eye contact or failure to recognize parents or interact with persons or objects in the environment)
- Review of known exposures (family illness, contacts with other ill children, daycare contacts)
- Recent vaccination
- Recent travel history
- Past medical history of malignancy, splenectomy, shunt, indwelling catheter, immunologic disorders, recurrent bacterial infections, serious bacterial infection
- Neonatal history of complications, prior antibiotics, prior surgeries, hyperbilirubinemia
- Chronic illness

TABLE 23-11	Age-Related Causes of Serious Bacterial and Viral Infections in Very Young Infants*

Bacteremia/Meningitis

<1 mo	Group B streptococcus
	Escherichia coli (and other enteric gram-negative bacilli)
	Listeria monocytogenes
	Streptococcus pneumoniae
	Haemophilus influenzae
	Staphylococcus aureus
	Neisseria meningitidis
	Salmonella spp.
	Herpes simplex
	Enteroviruses
1-3 mo	*S. pneumoniae*
	Group B streptococcus
	N. meningitidis
	Salmonella spp.
	H. influenzae
	L. monocytogenes
	S. aureus

Osteoarticular Infections

<1 mo	Group B streptococcus
	S. aureus
1-3 mo	*S. aureus*
	Group B streptococcus
	S. pneumoniae

Urinary Tract Infection

0-3 mo	*E. coli*
	Other enteric gram-negative bacilli
	Group D streptococcus (including *Enterococcus* spp.)

*In decreasing order of frequency.

From Shapiro ED: Fever without localizing signs. In Long SS, Pickering LK, Prober CG, editors: *Principles and practice of pediatric infectious diseases,* ed 3, Philadelphia, 2008, Churchill Livingstone.

- Current medications, including antipyretics and antibiotics
- Immunization history with *H. influenzae* type b conjugate and pneumococcal conjugate vaccines

Assessment

Risk Criteria. *High risk* is regarded as:
- Any febrile infant younger than 1 month of age
- Any toxic-appearing neonate, infant, or child regardless of age, risk factors, or degree of fever
- An infant 1 to 3 months of age with a rectal fever of 100.4° F (38° C) or greater
- An infant 1 to 3 months of age with a chronic illness or underlying condition with unreliable caretakers, who was premature, has a WBC count equal to or greater than 15,000 or absolute WBC band count of greater than 1500, or greater than 5 WBCs per high-power field (hpf) in stool specimen, or catheterized spun urine sediment with greater than 10 WBC/hpf
- Continue with the workup even if an infant less than 3 months of age has otitis media.

Low risk is regarded as:
- An infant or child 3 to 36 months of age with a fever greater than 102.2° F (39° C), who is nontoxic appearing with a history of previously being healthy, has nonfocal bacterial infection, and a positive rapid influenza A test.
- An infant 3 to 6 months of age with rectal temperature greater than 100.4° F (38° C) but less than 102.2° F (39° C) who is not ill appearing
- Infant or child 3 to 36 months of age who is mildly ill appearing with rectal temperature greater than 102.2° F (39° C) but <104° F (40° C) and fewer than 15,000 WBCs; stool fewer than 5 WBCs/hpf if diarrhea present; catheterized urinalysis spun sediment of less than 10 WBC/hpf; negative chest x-ray if cough present
- Documented immunizations (or lack of) to at least two doses of both *H. influenzae* conjugate vaccine and pneumococcal conjugate vaccine (HPV7 or HPV13)

Diagnostic Studies. A negative, low-risk ambulatory workup is characterized by the following laboratory results:
- CBC: WBC count less than 15,000/mm³, absolute band count of fewer than 1500 bands/mm³
- Blood culture: No growth in 48 hours (72 hours for those immunocompromised or if fungal infection suspected in the neonate)
- Catheterized urinalysis: Fewer than 10 WBCs/hpf spun sediment, negative leukocytes and nitrites
- Catheterized urine culture: More than 100,000 single pathogen (see also Chapter 34 for diagnostic criteria for UTIs)
- When diarrhea is present: Fewer than 5 WBCs/hpf in stool
- If cough is present: Negative chest x-ray
- If petechiae are present: Normal platelet count; still need to monitor clinically

Differential Diagnosis

The differential diagnoses includes upper respiratory tract disease (e.g., viral URI, otitis media, and sinusitis); lower respiratory tract disease (e.g., bronchiolitis, pneumonia); gastrointestinal disease; musculoskeletal infections (e.g., cellulitis, septic arthritis, osteomyelitis); urinary tract infection (especially due to *E. coli*); occult bacteremia due to other pathogens in children 3 to 36 months of age (in those immunized with both Hib and pneumococcal conjugate vaccine rate is less than 0.5% of children) (Powell, 2007).

Serious bacterial agents are identified in approximately 10% to 15% in previously well neonates with fever and diagnoses such as sepsis, meningitis, UTI, enteritis, osteomyelitis, and suppurative arthritis. Other possible illnesses to consider in this age group include pyelonephritis (more often occurring in uncircumcised boys, neonates, those with urinary tract anomalies, and females), otitis media, omphalitis, mastitis, and other skin or soft-tissue infections (Powell, 2007).

Management

Research studies and analysis of data have established practice guidelines for the outpatient management of infants and children from 0 to 36 months of age presenting with fever without focus. A management algorithm for specific

ALGORITHM

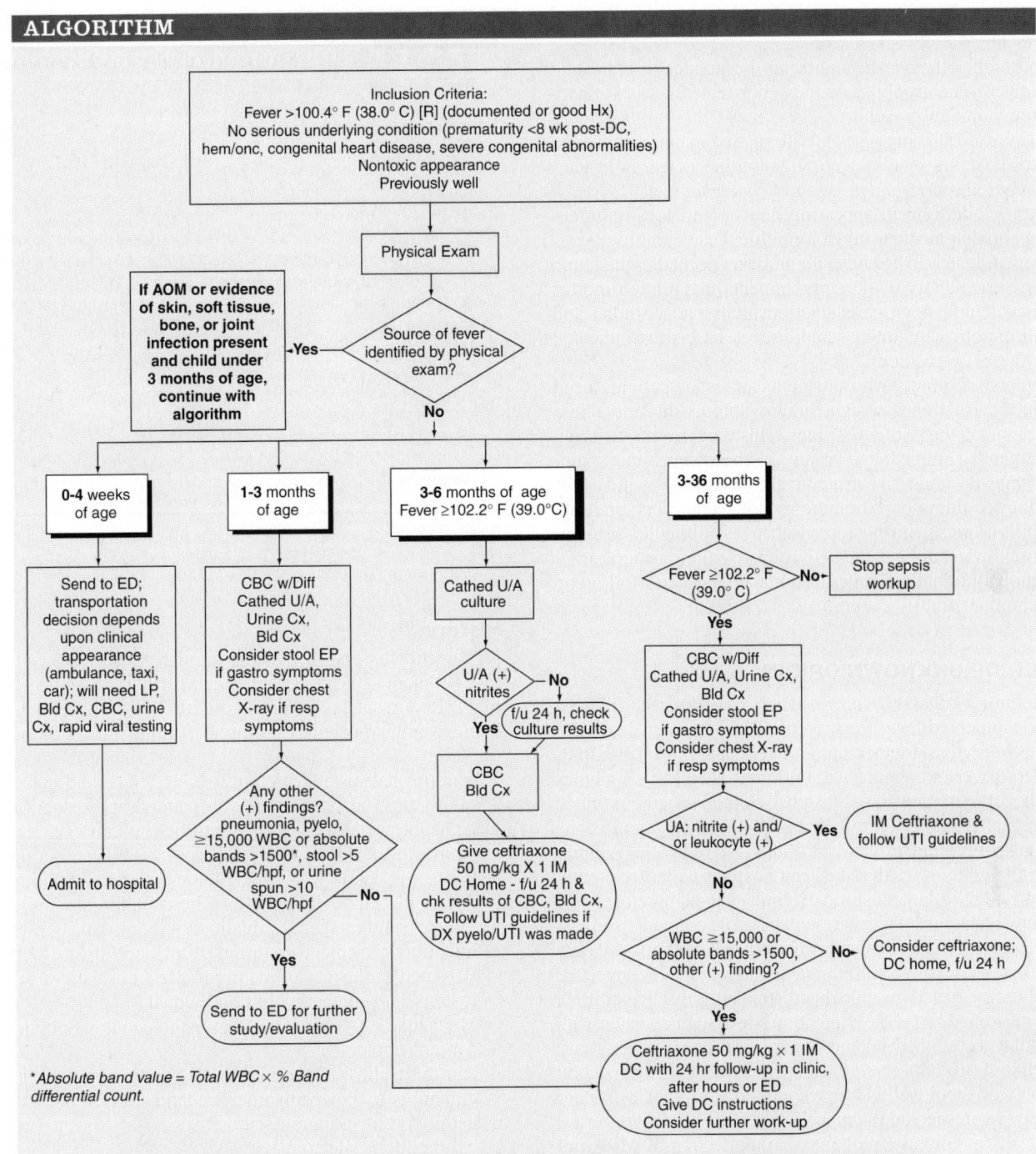

FIGURE 23-5 Fever without focus algorithm. *AOM,* acute otitis media; *Bld Cx,* blood culture; *Cathed,* catheterized; *CBC,* complete blood count; *chk,* check; *Cx,* culture; *DC,* discharge; *Dx,* diagnosis; *ED,* emergency department; *EP,* enteric pathogens (culture); *f/u,* follow-up; *h,* hours; *hem/onc,* hematologic/oncology issue; *hpf,* high power field; *Hx,* History; *IM,* intramuscularly; *LP,* lumbar puncture; *pyelo,* pyelonephritis; *R,* rectal; *resp,* respiratory; *R/O,* rule out; *U/A,* urinalysis; *UTI,* urinary tract infection; *WBC,* white blood cell count; *w/Diff,* with differential. (Modified from Children's Hospital and Health Center: *R/O sepsis algorithm,* San Diego, 1998, Children's Hospital and Health Center; Ishimine P: The evolving approach to the young child who has fever and no obvious source, *Emerg Med Clin N Am* 23:1087-1115, 2007; Powell KR: Fever without a focus. In Kliegman RM, Behrman RE, Jenson HB et al, editors: *Nelson textbook of pediatrics,* ed 18, Philadelphia, 2007, Saunders, pp 1087-1093.)

age groups based upon risk factors is found in Figure 23-5. Additionally:

- Fever with petechiae in any-age child who is *ill-appearing* is high risk for a life-threatening bacterial infection; immediate hospitalization and workup are indicated.

- Fever with petechiae but in a child who is *well-appearing*: draw a CBC, platelet count, and blood culture; observe for further petechial development (unless attributed to coughing/sneezing/emesis); if child continues to be well-appearing and has no further petechiae, manage on an outpatient basis as determined by most probable diagnosis and reason for petechiae.

- The higher the WBC count and the greater the absolute number of neutrophils or bands, the greater the risk of bacteremia in a febrile child.

Shapiro (2008) proposes an alternative management plan for those 3 months and older, in light of the decrease in bacteremia caused by *H. influenzae* and *S. pneumoniae*:

- If the child is well-appearing and has no foci of infection, no diagnostic testing or empirical use of antibiotics is needed. Instead, the child should be rechecked in the clinic in a series of follow-up appointments that allow time for clinical and laboratory evaluations. Laboratory studies and antimicrobial treatment would be prescribed as indicated by these observations.

Parents of infants who are managed as outpatients need detailed instructions on signs and symptoms that indicate a worsening of their infant's illness. Instruct parents to bring their infant in immediately if any of these signs and symptoms appear: change in or new rash; duskiness, cyanosis, or mottling; coolness of extremities; poor feeding or vomiting; irritability; cries with positional changes; difficulty in comforting or arousing; seizure activity (eye rolling or jerking of extremities); or bulging anterior fontanelle. Careful follow-up of such infants must be a priority.

FEVER OF UNKNOWN ORIGIN

The definition of *fever of unknown origin* (FUO) in children is: (1) a documented fever (rectal temperature greater than 101° F [38.3° C] or oral temperature greater than 100° F [37.8° C]) for 2 to 3 weeks or more without an etiology, that includes 3 weeks of outpatient visits, extensive studies, and continued fevers, and (2) no etiology after 1 week of evaluation in the hospital (Long and Edwards, 2008; Powell, 2007). A child with an FUO requires that the health care provider frequently rethink and reevaluate historical, clinical, and laboratory data.

Many FUOs are atypical presentations of common disorders, notably infections (account for more than one third of cases) (Long and Edwards, 2008), or rheumatologic and connective tissue diseases (e.g., juvenile rheumatoid arthritis [JRA], SLE). Few are exotic. In the U.S., infectious diseases associated with most diagnoses of FUO include mononucleosis, EBV, cat-scratch disease *(B. henselae)*, complicated UTIs, and vertebral and pelvic osteomyelitis (Long and Edwards, 2008). Other causative agents include salmonellosis, TB, rickettsial diseases, syphilis, Lyme disease, prolonged viral infections, CMV, viral hepatitis, coccidioidomycosis, histoplasmosis, malaria, and toxoplasmosis. Less common are tularemia, brucellosis, rat-bite fever, leptospirosis, drug fever, Kawasaki disease, inflammatory bowel disease, and rheumatic fever. Neoplastic conditions and AIDS have symptoms other than just fever. Fevers lasting more than 6 months have been reported in those with granulomatosis or autoimmune disease (Powell, 2007).

In children less than 6 years of age, the most common causes of FUO are UTI/pyelonephritis, respiratory illnesses, localized infections (abscess, osteomyelitis), juvenile arthritis (JA), and, rarely, leukemia. In adolescents the most common causes include TB, inflammatory bowel disease, autoimmune disorders, lymphoma, as well as the causes listed for children less than 6 years of age (Powell, 2007). Also see the differential diagnosis list that follows.

| **BOX 23-4** | Typical Findings in Patients With Fatigue of Deconditioning |

- Age >12 years
- Preillness achievement high (academic and social)
- Family expectations high (performance)
- Acute febrile illness with onset easily dated
- Family and outside attention high
- Multiple but vague complaints
- Odd complaints (e.g., 10-second "shooting" pains at multiple sites; 30-second "blindness"; stereotypic, sporadic, brief unilateral tremors, jerks, or "paralysis" lasting <1 minute)
- Tiredness, but no daytime sleep (or reversal of daytime and nighttime sleep)
- Model of chronic illness in family, recent loss of important person, change in family dynamics
- Unusual cooperation and interest during interview and examination (or unusual fearfulness and dependency on parent)
- Preserved or increased weight
- Normal physical and neurologic examination
- Normal results of screening laboratory tests

From Long SS, Edwards KM: Prolonged, recurrent, and periodic fever syndromes. In Long SS, Pickering LK, Prober CG, editors: *Principles and practice of pediatric infectious diseases*, ed 3, Philadelphia, 2008, Churchill Livingstone.

History

A careful history helps distinguish between recurrent fever episodes and those that need further evaluation as an FUO. Recurrent fevers resolve with well periods between them, suggesting an etiology of multiple self-limiting infections.

- Careful analysis of symptoms or signs, a meticulous review of systems, history of the fever pattern, and patient's age. An adolescent with complaints of low-grade fevers, or whose fever has resolved but who feels ill and is unable to attend school or social activities may have "fatigue of deconditioning" (Box 23-4). These children require the same careful medical evaluation, but rarely have a serious infection or medical condition (Long and Edwards, 2008).
- Past medical history of recurrent infections, surgery, transfusions, and contact with ill individuals
- Medication use, including over-the-counter and herbal/natural supplements
- Family medical history, including autoimmune disease or inflammatory bowel disorder; genetic background
- Family pets, pet immunization history, or exposure to wild or other domestic animals
- Unusual dietary habits (eating squirrel, rabbit, or other unusual animal meat)
- History of pica; history of travel (location; travel immunizations; water/food ingested; if returned home with travel souvenirs containing dirt, rocks, or earth-contaminated artifacts)

Clinical Findings

Physical Examination. Special attention needs to be paid to these areas:

- Skin: Presence of rashes, lesions, nailfold capillary abnormalities; presence or absence of sweating
- Mouth: Note a smooth tongue with absence of fungiform papillae; presence of candidiasis
- Throat: Exudate, erythema

- Local or generalized lymphadenopathy or hepatospleno-megaly
- Joint examination, and palpation of bones for tenderness, swelling
- Palpation/percussion of sinus and mastoid areas for tenderness; tap upper teeth
- Eye examination noting exudate, palpebral or bulbar conjunctivitis, conjunctival hemorrhages, papillary reaction; a complete ophthalmologic examination is indicated to fully evaluate for uveitis, chorioretinitis, proptosis
- Pelvic examination in adolescent females
- Rectal examination and guaiac test
- Deep tendon reflexes

Laboratory Studies. Laboratory studies are dependent on a history and physical examination that point to a specific infection or area of suspicion. Studies might include (Powell, 2007):

- CBC with differential, ESR (>30 mm/hr needs further evaluation) or CRP (no need to do both tests)
- Serologic tests for specific diseases as suggested by history and examination
- Blood cultures obtained aerobically (may require serial specimens to rule out different diseases)
- Urinalysis plus blood and urine cultures
- Mantoux skin test
- Chest, sinus, mastoid, and gastrointestinal tract radiographs may be indicated.
- Liver chemistries
- Serum protein analysis
- Heterophil antibody and antinuclear antibody titer in older children

Other tests may involve bone marrow, radionuclide scans, total body CT, MRI, echograms, ultrasounds, or biopsies.

Differential Diagnosis

Infectious diseases, collagen-vascular disease (JA, SLE), malignancies, drug fever (typically secondary to ingestion of phenothiazines, antidepressants, atropine, amphetamine, and other anticholinergic medications), nosocomial, HIV-associated illnesses, diabetes insipidus, hyperthyroidism, inflammatory bowel disease, hematoma in a confined space, anhidrotic ectodermal dysplasia, and Münchausen syndrome by proxy are included in the differential diagnosis of an FUO.

Management

Consider hospitalizing the child if there is evidence of systemic illness or failure to thrive, if the child is very young, or if the parent(s) anxiety is extreme. Otherwise the child should be followed up with frequent visits, with documented fever pattern, and other specialized tests if screening tests indicate the need or if other physical findings develop. Empiric use of antibiotics should be avoided unless the child has possible disseminated TB (Powell, 2007).

■ Infectious Agents Used in Bioterrorism

Since September 11, 2001, the U.S. has become more aware of a potential threat of infectious diseases acquired through biologic warfare. Most of these diseases have not been seen in clinical practice settings. Children are at particular risk for exposure to and absorption of biologic agents (e.g., anthrax and botulinum toxin). Factors that predispose them to such risk include being within closer proximity to the ground, having faster ventilation rates and thinner skins, having an increased risk of dehydration, and having greater undeveloped cognition.

Agents of biologic warfare are categorized by the CDC according to their potential for aerosol transmission, susceptibility of the population, degree of person-to-person transmission, expected high morbidity and mortality rates, the likelihood for delayed diagnosis, and the lack of effective and efficacious treatments. Agents at highest risk to the populace are known as category A weapons of bioterrorism. These include specific bacteria, viruses, botulinum toxin, *Bacillus anthracis* (anthrax), *Francisella tularensis* (tularemia), variola virus (smallpox), *Yersinia pestis*, and viruses of hemorrhagic fever (Ebola, Marburg, Lassa fever). Table 23-12 details each agent.

A national Laboratory Response Network has been established in the U.S. to provide standardized diagnostic testing for selected agents. This network links state and local public health laboratories with other advanced-capacity laboratories, including those at CDC.

Providers can help their communities in the early detection and prompt large-scale medical response by developing an awareness of syndromes and symptoms that might suggest a biologic warfare agent exposure. They can also join other health care providers in developing pediatric readiness plans. These readiness plans should include triage, isolation and treatment/care facilities, transportation, communication, housing, and the establishment of vaccination clinics on a massive scale for children, especially in communities where health departments and/or emergency departments may not have the procedural skills to address a severely ill pediatric population. Health alerts can be requested by e-mail from the CDC.

TABLE 23-12 Agents of Bioterrorism

Disease	Signs and Symptoms	Incubation Time (Range)	Person-to-Person Transmission	Isolation	Diagnosis	Postexposure Prophylaxis for Children and Adolescents*	Treatment in Children and Adolescents*
Anthrax (*Bacillus anthracis*) • Inhalation	Flulike symptoms (fever, fatigue, muscle aches, dyspnea, nonproductive cough, headache), chest pain; possible 1-2 days of improvement then rapid respiratory failure and shock. Meningitis may develop.	1-6 days (up to 6 weeks)	None	Standard precautions	Chest x-ray evidence of widening mediastinum; obtain sputum and blood culture. Sensitivity and specificity of nasal swabs unknown—do not rely on for diagnosis	Prophylaxis for 60 days started as soon as possible after exposure: amoxicillin†,doxycycline, ciprofloxacin Alternative: ofloxacin or levofloxacin or gatifloxacin PLUS 3 doses of Biotrax vaccine (not for children or pregnant women); other vaccines are in development	Start within 48 hours after onset of symptoms: penicillin G†,amoxicillin†,ciprofloxacin Alternative: ofloxacin or levofloxacin or gatifloxacin Do not use: cephalosporins, trimethoprim-sulfa
• Cutaneous	Intense itching followed by painless papular lesions, then vesicular lesions, developing into eschar surrounded by edema.	1-12 days	Direct contact with skin lesions may result in cutaneous infection	Contact precautions	Peripheral blood smear may demonstrate gram-positive bacilli on unspun smear with sepsis		
• Gastrointestinal (GI)	Abdominal pain, nausea and vomiting, severe diarrhea, GI bleeding, and fever.	1-7 days	None	Standard precautions	Culture blood and stool		
Botulism (*Clostridium botulinum*)	Afebrile, excess mucus in throat, dysphagia, dry mouth and throat, dizziness, then difficulty moving eyes, mild pupillary dilation and nystagmus, intermittent ptosis, indistinct speech, unsteady gait; extreme symmetric descending weakness, flaccid paralysis; generally normal mental status.	Inhalation: 12-80 hours Food-borne: 12-72 hours (2-8 days) (the consumed food probably will not be one usually associated with botulism)	None	Standard precautions	Laboratory tests available from CDC or public health department; obtain serum, stool, gastric aspirate, and suspect foods before administering antitoxin. Differential diagnosis includes polio, GBS, myasthenia, tick paralysis, stroke, meningococcal meningitis	Pentavalent toxoid (types A, B, C, D, E) may be available in the future. One 10-mL vial trivalent botulism antitoxin IV; equine antitoxin for adults after skin testing. For aerosolized exposure, immediately clean or dispose of clothes, clean/rinse hair, and use 0.1% hypochlorite bleach on contaminated surfaces.	Botulism antitoxins Supportive care Ventilation Avoid clindamycin and aminoglycosides. Infant botulism (due to C. *botulinum* type A or B): treat with botulism immune globulin (BabyBIG).

Pneumonic plague (*Yersinia Pestis*) • Pneumatic form	High fever, cough, hemoptysis, chest pain, nausea and vomiting, headache. Advanced disease: purpuric skin lesions, copious watery or purulent sputum production; respiratory failure in 1-6 days.	2-3 days (2-6 days)	Yes, droplet aerosols	Droplet precautions until 72 hours of effective antibiotic therapy	A presumptive diagnosis may be made by Gram, Wayson, or Wright stain of lymph node aspirates, sputum, or cerebrospinal fluid with gram-negative bacilli with bipolar (safety pin) staining	Start within 7 days of exposure for 1 week: Doxycycline, ciprofloxacin. A vaccine is under development	Start within 24 hours of symptom onset: Streptomycin, gentamicin. Alternatives: doxycycline or ciprofloxacin
Smallpox (variola virus)	Prodromal period: malaise, fever, rigors, vomiting, headache, and backache. After 2-4 days, skin lesions appear and progress uniformly from macules to papules to vesicles and pustules, mostly on face, neck, palms, soles, and subsequently progress to trunk. Any case of suspected smallpox should alert the provider to a possible intentional exposure. (see Fig. 23-2)	12-14 days (7-17 days)	Yes, airborne droplet nuclei or direct contact with skin lesions or secretions (e.g., saliva) until all scabs separate and fall off (3-4 weeks). Highest risk is to those within 6 feet of infected person	Airborne (includes N95 mask) and contact precautions	Swab culture of vesicular fluid or scab, send to biosafety level 4 laboratory. All lesions are similar in appearance and develop synchronously, as opposed to chickenpox. Electron microscopy can differentiate variola virus from varicella. Assistance for assessing and testing specimens available from the national Laboratory Response Network (LRN)	Ideally, early vaccine within 3 to 4 days after exposure (ideally within 72 hours); the vaccine can prevent or lessen symptoms of the disease or prevent death. Vaccinia immune globulin (VIG) can be useful for some of the complications.	Supportive care, vaccinations within 72 hours of rash; possible use of cidofovir
Tularemia	Fever, headache, acute inflammation, pharyngitis, chills, fatigue, myalgias. Any suspicious atypical pharyngitis, ulcer at the site of a tick bite, atypical pneumonia, pleuritis, and hilar lymphadenopathy are signs of this disease.	2-10 days (average 2-6 days)	No	Standard precautions blood: antibody	Respiratory secretions and blood titers (>fourfold increase). Light microscopy and fluorescent-labeled antibody, PCR	May be considered: doxycycline, ciprofloxacin, chloramphenicol. No vaccine available	Treat for 7-10 days: streptomycin, gentamicin, amikacin, doxycycline, ciprofloxacin, imipenemcilastin, chloramphenicol

Continued

TABLE 23-12 Agents of Bioterrorism—cont'd

Disease	Signs and Symptoms	Incubation Time (Range)	Person-to-Person Transmission	Isolation	Diagnosis	Postexposure Prophylaxis for Children and Adolescents*	Treatment in Children and Adolescents*
• Ulceroglandular	Skin papules, granu-lomatous lesions with necrotic, case-ous areas						
• Oculoglandular	Edematous/inflamed conjunctiva with yellow nodules, ulcers or palpebral conjunctiva/sclera. Cervical/submaxil-lary/preauricular lymphadenopathy.						
• Typhoidal	Fever >102° F (39.4° C), chills, headache, aches, vomit-ing, photophobia, hepatosplenomegaly, exanthems on upper extremities (± face and neck), diarrhea.						
• Pneumonic	Respiratory symp-toms of pneumo-nia or pleuritis. Differential diagnosis includes psittacosis, legionellosis, Q fever, mycoplasma and C. pneumoniae infec-tions, anthrax, and plague.				Pneumonic: x-ray findings of lobar/sub-segmental infiltrates, hilar adenopathy, pleural effusion, atypi-cal infiltrates		

| Hemorrhagic fevers
• Crimean-Congo
• Dengue
• Ebola and Marburg
• Hanta pulmonary syndrome
• Lassa fever | Generally: fever, muscle aches, dizziness, malaise, weakness, exhaustion, ± rash, ± headache. With disease progression: ecchymosis, bleeding from orifices with GI symptoms, can lead to shock, delirium, seizures, renal failure. | Depends on agent
Crimean: 2-10 days
Ebola/Marburg: 3-9 days
Dengue: 2-7 days
Lassa: 6-17 days | Ebola and Lassa only via blood or body fluids | Mask, contact, and standard precautions depending on agent; isolation of infected persons; DEET for mosquito-bite resistance | Virus-specific serum IgM or viral antigen, RNA, ELISA analysis of viral proteins, or virus isolation; handle in a biosafety level 4 laboratory. | No vaccines available | Hospitalization (typically ICU) for supportive care: ribavirin therapy may be useful for some agents in certain cases. For exposed persons, monitoring their temperature twice daily for 21 days is recommended; fever warrants further consideration of treatment options. |

*Contact local health department for any suspected cases and prior to starting prophylaxis or treatment; alert laboratory personnel handling specimens so they can take precautions.

†If strains are sensitive.

CDC, Centers for Disease Control and Prevention; ELISA, enzyme-linked immunosorbent assay; GBS, Guillain-Barré syndrome; ICU, intensive dare unit; IgM, immunoglobulin M; RNA, ribonucleic acid.

Modified from Centers for Disease Control and Prevention (CDC): General fact sheets on specific bioterrorism agents. Available at www.bt.cdc.gov/bioterrorism/factsheets (accessed Dec 15, 2010); North Carolina Statewide Program for Infection Control and Epidemiology (SPICE): Bioterrorist agents, 2002. Available at www.unc.edu/depts/spice/chart.pdf (accessed Dec 15, 2010). Other data from: Dennis DT, Mead PS: Yersinia species, including plague. In Mandell GL, Bennett JE, Dolin R, editors: Mandel, Douglas, and Bennett's principles and practice of infectious diseases, ed 7, Philadelphia, 2009, Churchill Livingstone; Duchin J, Malone JD: Bioterrorism. In Dale DC, editor: Infectious diseases: the clinician's guide to diagnosis, treatment, and prevention, New York, 2010, WebMD; Hodges LS, Penn RL: Francisella tularensis (tularemia) as an agent of bioterrorism. In Mandell GL, Bennett JE, Dolin R, editors: Mandel, Douglas, and Bennett's principles and practice of infectious diseases, ed 7, Philadelphia, 2009, Churchill Livingstone; Peters CJ: Viral hemorrhagic fevers as agents of bioterrorism. In Mandell GL, Bennett JE, Dolin R, et al, editors: Mandel, Douglas, and Bennett's principles and practice of infectious diseases, ed 7, Philadelphia, 2009, Elsevier; Pickering LK, Baker CJ, Kimberlin DW et al: Red Book: 2009 Report of the Committee on Infectious Diseases, ed 28, Elk Grove Village, IL, 2009, American Academy of Pediatrics; Reddy P, Bleck TP: Botulism toxin as a biological weapon. In Mandell GL, Bennett JE, Dolin R, editors: Mandel, Douglas, and Bennett's principles and practice of infectious diseases, ed 7, Philadelphia, 2009, Churchill Livingstone.

Atopic and Rheumatic Disorders

RITA MARIE JOHN AND MARGARET A. BRADY

Atopic disorders and rheumatic diseases (collagen vascular or connective tissue diseases) of childhood share certain characteristics that lend to their combined discussion in this chapter. Inflammation, chronicity, and genetic predisposition are common to both groups of disorders. The triad of atopic disorders that may or may not coexist consists of atopic dermatitis (AD), allergic rhinitis (AR) (or "hay fever"), and asthma. The two most common childhood rheumatic diseases that primary care providers are likely to encounter are juvenile idiopathic arthritis and systemic lupus erythematosus (SLE). Juvenile dermatomyositis is also a classic rheumatic disease but is less frequent in occurrence. These are collagen-vascular disorders that have localized or generalized findings marked by inflammation and an autoimmune response. Vasculitis, an inflammation of the blood vessels, is characteristic of many of the rheumatic diseases.

Fibromyalgia is a rheumatic disease that causes widespread musculoskeletal pain with generalized tender points associated with fatigue (Buskila, 2009). Brief discussions of this disease, in addition to chronic fatigue syndrome (CFS), are presented. Although the incidence of rheumatic fever has diminished significantly in the U.S., it is still a disease that merits attention by providers. Therefore, a review of its clinical presentation and treatment also is included. The immunopathogenesis and management of Henoch-Schönlein purpura (HSP), the most common systemic vasculitis syndrome of childhood, also are discussed.

Pathophysiology and Defense Mechanisms

ATOPIC OR ALLERGIC DISORDERS

Allergy involves a specific acquired alteration in the body that has an immunologic basis. An allergen acts as an antigen that then triggers an immunoglobulin E (IgE) response in genetically predisposed individuals. The union of antigen and antibody creates a cascade of events that culminates in biochemical reactions. There are four types of allergic reactions: I (manifested as typical allergic symptoms to the extreme of anaphylactic reactions), II (antibody cytotoxicity reactions), III (immune complex reactions with Arthusreactions and serum sickness as examples), and IV (cellular immune-mediated or delayed-type hypersensitivity). All four types of allergic or hypersensitivity reactions are mediated by circulating or cellular antibodies and generally can occur in any individual (Lasley and Hetherington, 2011). Type I involves local and systemic manifestations resulting from an interaction between antigen and tissue cells that have been sensitized with reaginic antibody, generally IgE (e.g., urticaria and angioedema). Type II involves reactions from antibody interacting with antigenic components on cell surfaces (e.g., hemolytic anemia and transfusion reactions). Type III is characterized by deposition of immune microprecipitates in or around blood vessels. Complement or toxic products are released. Henoch-Schönlein purpura is one example of type III-mediated reactions. A type IV allergic reaction is a delayed-type hypersensitivity interaction involving sensitized lymphocytic cells that results in the release of toxic lymphoid cell products. Cytokines are released which stimulate bone marrow precursors to produce more leukocytes that become macrophages. Examples of type IV reactions are tuberculin skin test reactions and contact dermatitis (Lasley and Hetherington, 2011).

Atopy represents a complex interaction between multiple genes and environmental exposures. Atopic disorders are forms of allergic reactivity that occur only in certain susceptible individuals with an unknown and probably genetic predisposition. Environmental factors also play a role in atopy of these individuals who exhibit a hyperresponsiveness in target organs (lungs, skin, or nose). Certain antigens (e.g., cat dander, ragweed) are problematic for atopic individuals but not for others. These atopic individuals become sensitized to the offending allergen, resulting in an atopic disorder.

The development of an atopic disorder or allergic response involves a susceptible individual who is both exposed to an offending antigen and has a predisposition to selective synthesis of IgE when in contact with common environmental antigens. If these conditions are in place and contact with an offending antigen occurs, the following biochemical chain of cascading events unfolds:

- There is a brisk proliferation of T-helper type 2 (Th2) cells that secrete cytokines: interleukin (IL)-3, IL-4, IL-5, IL-9, and IL-13.
- Cytokines are involved in IgE synthesis and activation of eosinophils.
- IgE binds to receptors on mast cells, basophils, and Langerhans cells.
- Chemical mediators that cause biochemical reactions and allergic-related injury to target organs (skin and respiratory tract) are released. Examples of chemical mediators include but are not limited to:
  - Histamine
  - Tryptase
  - Prostaglandins
  - Leukotrienes
  - Eosinophil chemotactic factor of anaphylaxis
  - Platelet-activating factor

The end result of this biochemical process is tissue injury of a target organ. Examples of tissue injury include inflammation and hyperresponsiveness, resulting in such symptoms as obstruction, increased mucus discharge, and pruritus.

Immediate allergic reactions can involve sneezing, hives, wheezing, vomiting, or anaphylaxis. Acute reactions (<30 minutes) can be followed by a late-phase response several hours (2 to 12) after the initial response. This late-phase response is due to the influx of other inflammatory cells such as basophils, eosinophils, monocytes, lymphocytes, and neutrophils and their inflammatory mediators that are recruited to the site of the acute allergic reaction (Lasley and Hetherington, 2011).

The pathogenesis of atopic diseases involves a complex interrelationship of genetic, environmental, and immunologic factors. The main defense mechanism to protect against atopic disorders is the elimination of the offending substance to prevent IgE development and antigen-antibody interaction. For example, if there is a family history of atopic disorders, breastfeeding offers the protection of limited exposure to cow's milk protein and the benefit of maternal IgA and IgG antibodies. Once chemical mediators are released, the body's protective responses reduce inflammation and repair tissue damage. Pharmacologic therapy cannot cure atopic disorders, but reduces symptoms and checks the allergic process. For example, drugs may be used to control inflammation (corticosteroids), compete with histamine for receptor sites on target tissues (antihistamines), act as a selective leukotriene receptor antagonist (e.g., montelukast), and prevent mast cell degranulation and mediator release (cromolyn sodium).

RHEUMATIC DISORDERS

Juvenile idiopathic arthritis (JIA) is the term increasingly being used as the nomenclature for what was formerly called *juvenile rheumatoid arthritis (JRA)*. JRA was used to describe a group of conditions involving chronic inflammation of synovial joints in children younger than 16 years old. Its newer nomenclature is juvenile idiopathic arthritis which includes enthesitis-related, undifferentiated, and psoriatic arthritis that had not been included in the American College of Rheumatolgy classification for chronic childhood arthritis. JIA now encompasses additional types of juvenile arthritis (e.g.,

enthesitis-related arthritis and psoriatic arthritis) beyond what had been identified under the nomenclature of JRA (Haftel, 2011; Rabinovich, 2010). Both JIA and SLE are connective tissue disorders marked by inflammatory changes in connective tissues throughout the body. The exact cause of these collagen diseases is not completely understood; however, an autoimmune basis is postulated as a key factor in rheumatic disease.

There are no natural defense mechanisms identified to prevent either of these diseases; however, periods of remission do occur in some children with SLE for unknown reasons, and many children with JIA achieve complete remission with puberty (approximately 85% complete remission rate) (Haftel, 2011). Because inflammation is a significant factor in these two rheumatic diseases of childhood, administration of corticosteroid preparations is a key therapy to control inflammation responsible for tissue injury and possible permanent tissue changes.

Juvenile Idiopathic Arthritis

The exact etiology of most forms of JIA is unknown; however, there are two theories about its causation. Genetics is believed to be a predisposing factor. Some genetic factors, such as human leukocyte antigen (HLA) alleles, appear to play a role in influencing the susceptibility to develop disease, and others influence disease severity. An external trigger such as infection or trauma seems to initiate the autoimmune reaction and cause an exaggerated immune response (Rabinovich, 2010).

The pathogenesis of JIA involves a combination of humoral and cell-mediated immunity responses with proliferation of macrophage-like and fibroblastoid synoviocytes. There is subsequent infiltration of neutrophils and lymphocytes, which is evidence of an autoimmune response. The humoral response is responsible for the release of autoantibodies (especially antinuclear antibodies), an increase in serum immunoglobulins, the formation of circulating immune complexes and complement activation. The cell-mediated reaction is associated with a T-lymphocyte response that plays a key role in cytokine production resulting in the release of tumor necrosis factor α (TNF-α), IL-1, and IL-6. B lymphocytes are activated by T-helper cells and produce autoantibodies that link to self-antigens. The B lymphocytes infiltrate the synovium with the end result of nonsuppurative chronic inflammation of the synovium that can lead to articular cartilage and joint structure erosion. Children with JIA have no demonstrable immunodeficiency (Rabinovich, 2010).

Systemic Lupus Erythematosus

Children with SLE exhibit a marked increase in the production of autoantibodies that attack the body's deoxyribonucleic acid (DNA). This leads to immune complex formation and tissue damage from either direct bonding in tissues, immune complex deposition, or a combination of both (Klein-Gitelman, 2010). Various immune phenomena are associated with SLE, including altered immunologic reactions in the T- and B-lymphocyte function. There is a loss of T-lymphocyte control and hyperactivity of B lymphocytes resulting in nonspecific and specific antibody and autoantibody production. There is a strong link between a faulty immune mechanism and SLE because this disease is characterized by inflammatory damage to target organs brought on by autoantibodies attacking self-antigens. The exact etiology of SLE is unknown, but many factors including genetics, hormones, and environment are linked to the immune dysregulation that characterizes this rheumatic disease. Environmental factors that are thought to play a role in its pathogenesis are oral contraceptive use, pregnancy, microbials (viral agents mostly), temperate climates, exposure to ultraviolet light, and certain drugs (e.g., hydralazine and procainamide).

There is an association between HLA type and complement deficiency. Characteristic pathologic findings include the production of numerous autoantibodies and impairment in the normal suppression of autoreactive B-cell clones. Immune complexes are abundant, and their clearance may be impaired. In addition, fibrinoid deposits collect in blood vessel walls in many organs that result in ischemic damage (Haftel, 2011).

■ Assessment

HISTORY

Key factors to consider in the history of a child who has an atopic disorder include the following:
- A family history or personal history of allergies, asthma, AD (eczema), or AR is frequently found; similar allergic diseases tend to be found in families.
- Pruritus is a significant finding in AD and AR.
- The rash of AD is characteristically found in certain locations of the body.
- Coughing or shortness of breath with exercise or exertion and nighttime coughing and wheezing are characteristic of asthma.
- Signs and symptoms of AR and asthma may be associated with certain allergens or key triggering agents and may be seasonal.

Key factors to consider in the history of a child who has a rheumatic disease include the following:
- History of a characteristic rash or joint involvement (arthritis), or both (common findings). May have symptoms of serositis, enthesitis, myositis, and vasculitis, which are other inflammatory markers
- Other systemic manifestations of disease such as fever and hematologic, renal, and/or pulmonary abnormalities

PHYSICAL EXAMINATION

A detailed physical examination of the cardiovascular, respiratory, integumentary, and musculoskeletal systems may reveal characteristic signs (see Chapters 30, 31, 36, and 37).

DIAGNOSTIC STUDIES

Various diagnostic studies or procedures can be used in the outpatient evaluation and management of children with either atopic disorders or rheumatic diseases. Indications for specific tests are discussed under the specific atopic or rheumatic problem.

Atopic Disorders

Routine chest radiographs are not indicated in most children with asthma because most often they are normal or only show hyperinflation. However, chest radiographs can be useful in selected cases of asthma or suspected asthma. These should

be performed with the first episode of asthma or with recurrent attacks; in a child with atypical signs or symptoms; if a secondary infection does not clear with standard therapy; or if there are signs and symptoms of significant pulmonary involvement (Lasley and Hetherington, 2011).

Pulmonary function tests, such as forced vital capacity, forced expiratory volume in 1 second, and forced expiratory flow, are important diagnostic tests to establish the diagnosis of asthma, especially in young children. Children older than 5 years can typically perform spirometry testing. Peak expiratory flow (PEF) rate and pulse oximetry measurements can be easily and quickly done in most pediatric settings and provide additional information useful to monitor and manage asthma.

Eosinophil count, determination of serum IgE concentration, in vitro serum testing (fluorescent enzyme immunoassay) (CAP-RAST, ImmunoCAP or CAP-FEIA), and in vivo skin testing (prick test) are not needed to confirm the diagnosis or to monitor treatment of the majority of children with an atopic disorder. Children with significant dermatitis or who are highly allergic may need additional or extensive diagnostic testing.

Rheumatic Diseases

Laboratory blood studies, including antinuclear antibodies (ANAs), anti–double-stranded DNA, anti-Smith (Sm) antibody, and determination of serum complement levels, are common tests ordered in children with SLE. Other related blood, serologic, and urine laboratory studies are indicated depending on organ involvement (e.g., renal involvement is a frequent complication). While there is no laboratory test that has 100% sensitivity and specificity, doing an ANA, rheumatoid factor (RF), and an anti-cyclic citrullinated peptide (anti-CCP) is recommended (Stanley and Ward-Smith, 2011). The anti-CCP is helpful for diagnosing JIA in the early stages of disease (Waits, 2010), Guidelines for the laboratory workup of SLE and JIA are discussed later in this chapter.

Imaging studies (MRI and radiographs) are done to assess and manage joint abnormalities.

■ Management

The atopic and rheumatoid disorders tend to be chronic conditions with exacerbation and remission of symptoms. Individual management strategies are based on the specific disease process and are discussed in each of their respective sections. However, certain key concepts apply to these conditions.

GENERAL MEASURES

The following general measures should be part of the management of atopic and rheumatoid disorders:
- Encourage self-care and learning about one's disease.
- Address issues of burdens associated with living with a chronic disease, such as:
  - School, peer, and family dynamics
  - Body image
  - Adolescent adjustment
  - Pain management
  - Patient-parent role in management of a long-term illness or chronic condition
- Nutrition and the avoidance of obesity, if activity is limited, or foods if they are triggers

MEDICATIONS

The control of inflammation associated with atopic disorders and rheumatoid diseases is a key principle in the management of these illnesses. Corticosteroids, whether used topically on the skin, inhaled via the nostrils or throat, taken orally for systemic effect, or taken intramuscularly or intravenously for rapid systemic absorption are a mainstay of treatment. Other pharmacologic agents commonly used are as follows:

- For atopic conditions:
  - Antipruritic agents—to control itching
  - Antihistamines—to control symptoms associated with the release of chemical mediators
  - Anticholinergics—to reduce vagal tone in the airways (may also decrease mucus gland secretion)
  - Bronchodilators—to control bronchospasm
  - Cromolyn sodium and nedocromil—to inhibit mast cell release of histamine
  - Leukotriene modifiers—to disrupt the synthesis or function of leukotrienes
  - Antibiotics—to treat secondary infections
  - Immunomodulators—to inhibit the inflammatory response. They include topical preparations and subcutaneous agents.
- Omalizumab is a recombinant DNA-derived, humanized IgG monoclonal antibody that binds to human IgE on the surface of mast cells and basophils. This anti-IgE monoclonal antibody is used as a second-line treatment for children older than 12 years who have moderate to severe allergy-related asthma and react to perennial allergens. It is used when symptoms are not controlled by inhaled corticosteroids (ICSs).
- For rheumatic diseases:
  - Analgesics (salicylates or nonsteroidal antiinflammatory drugs [NSAIDs])—to relieve arthritis or joint pain; to relieve pain in general
  - Other therapeutic agents, such as corticosteroids and/or biologic drugs to block tumor necrosis factor—to relieve signs and symptoms specific to the disease process and organ system involvement

PARENT AND PATIENT EDUCATION

Patients and parents need to be instructed about the following:

- Signs and symptoms necessitating immediate reevaluation.
- Medications—clear instructions are needed on how to administer, how much and when to give, monitoring side effects, and how long medication should be taken. A written plan is highly recommended based on either symptoms or, in the example of asthma, peak expiratory flow rate (PEFR).
- Correct administration of inhaled medications—for example, when two puffs or sprays are ordered, the child should activate one puff or spray and then inhale, followed in 1 to 2 minutes by a second puff or spray and second inhalation. A parent or child may think incorrectly that being told to take two puffs or two sprays means to activate two puffs or sprays and then inhale.
- Any other measures relevant to the treatment plan (e.g., bathing instructions, monitoring peak flow rate, avoiding allergens, and environmental control)
- Parent support groups and professional organizations and resource groups

■ Specific Immunologic Problems of Children: Common Atopic Disorders

ASTHMA

Description

Asthma is a chronic respiratory disease characterized by the following features (National Heart, Lung, and Blood Institute [NHLBI], 2007).

- Immunohistopathologic responses that produce:
  - Shedding of airway epithelium and collagen deposition beneath the basement membrane
  - Edema
  - Mast cell activation
  - Inflammatory infiltration by eosinophils, lymphocytes (Th2-like cells), and neutrophils (especially in fatal asthma)
- Airway inflammation contributes to airflow limitations, including:
  - Acute bronchoconstriction
  - Airway edema
  - Mucous plug formation
- Airflow obstruction is often reversible, either spontaneously or with treatment.
- Persistent inflammation can result in airway wall remodeling and irreversible changes.
- Airway inflammation also triggers hyperresponsiveness (to any of a variety of stimuli, such as physical, chemical, or pharmacologic agents; allergens; exercise; and cold air) and is a factor in disease chronicity. Inflammation causes bronchospasms with resultant characteristic symptomatology of wheezing, breathlessness, chest tightness, or cough typically worse at night or after exercise (Sharma and Gupta, 2010).

Asthma in children is classified as intermittent, mild persistent, moderate persistent, or severe persistent depending on symptoms, recurrences, need for specific medications, and pulmonary function measurements (Table 24-1). Children classified at any level of asthma can have episodes involving mild, moderate, or severe exacerbations. Exacerbations involve progressive worsening of shortness of breath, cough, wheezing, chest tightness, or any combination of these symptoms. The degree of airway hyperresponsiveness is usually related to the severity of asthma. Children younger than 5 years of age experience greater airway hyperresponsiveness than older children. Airway remodeling can result from chronic inflammation caused by asthma. Irreversible structural changes take place and result in decreased pulmonary function (Lasley, 2006). A child's classification can change over time.

Many children experience early- and late-phase responses to their asthma episode. The early asthmatic response (EAR) phase is characterized by activation of mast cells and their mediators, with bronchoconstriction being the key feature. EAR starts within 15 to 30 minutes of mast cell activation and resolves within approximately 1 hour if the individual is removed from the offending allergen. The late-phase asthmatic response is a prolonged inflammatory state that usually follows the EAR within 4 to 12 hours after exposure to the allergen, is often associated with airway hyperresponsiveness more severe than the EAR presentation, and can last from hours to several weeks (Liu et al, 2004).

TABLE 24-1 Classification of Asthma Severity in Children: Clinical Features Before Treatment

Classification and Step	Symptoms*	Nighttime Symptoms	Lung Function
Step 1: Intermittent	Symptoms ≤2 times per wk Asymptomatic and normal PEF between exacerbations Requires SABA 2 days/wk Exacerbations brief (few hr or days); varying intensity No interference with normal activity	≤2 times per mo	FEV_1 >80% predicted Normal FEV_1 between exacerbations
Step 2: Mild persistent	Symptoms >2 times per wk but <1 time per day Requires SABA >2 days/wk but not >1/day Exacerbations may affect activity (minor)	3-4 times per mo	FEV_1 >80% predicted
Step 3: Moderate persistent	Daily symptoms Daily use of inhaled SABA Some limitations Exacerbations affect activity, ≥2 times per wk; may last days	>1 time per wk but not nightly	FEV_1 >60% but <80% predicted
Step 4: Severe persistent	Continual symptoms Requires SABA several times/day Extremely limited physical activity Frequent exacerbations	Often 7 times per wk	FEV_1 <60% predicted

*Having at least one symptom in a particular step places the child in that particular classification.

FEV_1, Forced expiratory volume in 1 second; *PEF,* peak expiratory flow; *SABA,* short-acting β_2-agonist.

Adapted from National Heart, Lung, and Blood Institute (NHLBI): *Full report of the expert panel: guidelines for the diagnosis and management of asthma,* (EPR-3), National Institutes of Health, 2007, Bethesda, Md.

Exercise-induced bronchospasm describes the phenomenon of airway narrowing during or minutes after the onset of vigorous activity. Most asthmatics exhibit airway hyperirritability after rigorous activity and display exercise-induced bronchospasm. However, for some children, exercise is the only stimulus that triggers their asthma. Although asthma is not always associated with an allergic disorder in children, many pediatric patients with chronic asthma have an allergic component.

Epidemiology

It is not known for certain whether hyperresponsiveness of the airways is present at birth in genetically predisposed children or acquired. However, the genetic predisposition for the development of an IgE-mediated response to common aeroallergens, known as atopy, remains the strongest identifiable predisposing risk factor for asthma. A combination of genetic predisposition and exposure to certain environmental factors are the necessary components responsible for the pathophysiologic response associated with asthma.

The morbidity and mortality statistics of asthma in childhood demonstrate an alarming increase in the prevalence of asthma and its complications. In 2008, 8.7 million 5- to 17-year-olds had been diagnosed with asthma (American Lung Association [ALA], 2010). The prevalence rate for asthma is highest among children 5 to 17 years with the highest rate among African-American children (ALA, 2010). Occupational or environmental exposure can cause airway inflammation associated with asthma. Factors known to precipitate or aggravate asthma in children include the following:

- Atopic individual response to allergens—inhaled, topical, ingested
- Viral infections

- Exposure to known irritants (paint fumes, smoke, air pollutants) and occupational chemicals
- Gastroesophageal reflux
- Exposure to tobacco smoke (for infants, especially smoking by mother)
- Environmental changes—rapid changes in barometric pressure, temperature, especially cold air
- Exercise
- Psychological factors or emotional stresses (e.g., crying, laughter, anxiety attack, or panic disorder)
- AR and sinusitis
- Drugs (e.g., acetaminophen, aspirin, beta-blockers)
- Food additives (sulfites)
- Endocrine factors (e.g., obesity)

Allergen-induced asthma results in hyperresponsive airways. The majority of children with asthma show evidence of sensitization to any of the following inhalant allergens:

- House dust mites, cockroaches, indoor molds
- Saliva and dander of cats and dogs
- Outdoor seasonal molds
- Airborne pollens—trees, grasses, and weeds

There is a high prevalence of asthma in food-allergic children; egg and tree nut allergy is significantly associated with asthma (Gaffin et al, 2011).

Clinical Findings

History. In order to assess the degree of asthma severity and impairment of function, a standardized instrument can be used. Tests for this purpose are available in the guidelines summary (NHLBI, 2007, p 17). Other instruments such as the Asthma Control Questionnaire, Asthma Therapy Assessment Questionnaire, Asthma Control Test, and the Asthma Control Score are available via the Internet. The advantages of a standardized questionnaire are that it allows the health care provider to assess changes in the patient's asthma, then alter the management plan as needed. The history of a patient being seen for asthma can include the following:

- Family history of asthma or other related allergic disorders (e.g., eczema or AR)
- Conditions associated with asthma (e.g., chronic sinusitis, nasal polyposis, gastroesophageal reflux, and chronic otitis media)
- Complaints of chest tightness or dyspnea
- Cough, particularly at night and in the early morning
- Cough or shortness of breath with exercise or exertion
- Seasonal, continuous, or episodic pattern of symptoms
- Episodes of recurrent "bronchitis" or pneumonia
- Precipitation of symptoms by known aggravating factors (upper respiratory infections [URIs], acetaminophen, aspirin)

Physical Examination. The following may be seen on physical examination:

- Wheezing (may be absent if severe obstruction) or coughing
- Prolonged expiratory phase, high-pitched rhonchi
- Diminished breath sounds
- Signs of respiratory distress, including tachypnea, retractions, nasal flaring, use of accessory muscles, increasing restlessness, apprehension, agitation, drowsiness to coma
- Tachycardia, hypertension or hypotension, pulsus paradoxus
- Cyanosis of lips and nailbeds if underlying hypoxemia
- Other possible associated findings include sinusitis, atopic dermatitis, and rhinitis.

Diagnostic Studies. Laboratory and radiographic tests should be individualized to the child and based on symptoms, severity or chronology of the disease, response to therapy, and age. Tests to consider include the following:

- Oxygen saturation by pulse oximetry to assess severity of acute exacerbation. This should be a routine part of every assessment on a patient with asthma. Pulse oximetry measures the oxygen saturation (SaO_2) of hemoglobin—the percent of total hemoglobin that is oxygenated—as follows:
  - Greater than 95%, mild
  - 90% to 95%, moderate
  - Less than 90%, severe lack of oxygen
- A complete blood count (CBC) if secondary infection or anemia is suspected (also check for elevated numbers of eosinophils)
- Chest radiograph for the first episode, and then only if secondary respiratory infection or other pulmonary disorders are suspected or if child is less than 1 year old with persistent wheezing
- Sinusitis should be considered as a cause of an asthma exacerbation. However, imaging of the sinus is not routinely needed to make the diagnosis of sinusitis. (See Chapter 31 for a discussion on sinusitis and the criteria needed for ordering computed tomography [CT] scans, which are more sensitive and specific than sinus radiographs.)
- Allergic workup, including skin testing, IgE, or Immuno-CAP (refer child to pediatric allergist)
- Sweat test if cystic fibrosis is a possibility
- Pulmonary function tests:
  - Formal spirometry testing is the gold standard in children older than 4 years for diagnosing asthma.
  - Start with PEF assessment in children 4 to 5 years or older to monitor the effectiveness of β-agonist treatment (measurements before and after treatments) and assess the severity of airflow obstruction.
  - Consider the use of more sophisticated pulmonary laboratory studies for the child with severe asthma.

TABLE 24-2	Predicted Average Peak Expiratory Flow for Normal Children and Adolescents
Height (Inches)	**Males and Females (L/Minute)**
43	147
44	160
45	173
46	187
47	200
48	214
49	227
50	240
51	254
52	267
53	280
54	293
55	307
56	320
57	334
58	347
59	360
60	373
61	387
62	400
63	413
64	427
65	440
66	454
67	467

NOTE: It is recommended that peak expiratory flow (PEF) rate objectives for therapy be based on each individual's "personal best," which is established after a period of PEF rate monitoring while the individual is under effective treatment.

From National Heart, Lung, and Blood Institute (NHLBI): *Executive summary: guidelines for the diagnosis and management of asthma*, NIH Pub No 94-3042A, National Institutes of Health, 1994, Bethesda, Md; adapted from Polger G, Promedhar V: *Pulmonary function testing in children: techniques and standards*, Philadelphia, 1971, Saunders.

Pulmonary monitoring and typical findings include the following:

- PEF can be used in some children as young as 4 to 5 years. Noteworthy is the fact that values are instrument specific. Use child's personal best value as a guideline to help detect possible changes in airway obstruction; can use predicted range for height and age if personal best rate is not available (Table 24-2).

Use of the Peak Flowmeter and Its Interpretation

Steps to follow in using a peak flow meter:
1. Have child stand up.
2. Make sure that indicator is at the base of the numbered scale.
3. Ask child to take a deep breath.
4. Have the child place the peak flow meter in the mouth with the lips sealing the mouthpiece. Tell the child not to put his or her tongue in the hole of the mouthpiece.
5. Tell the child to blow out as hard and fast as possible.
6. Record the rate, but if the child coughs, do not write down that number.
7. Repeat steps 2 through 6, two more times.
8. Record the highest of the three values.

Peak Expiratory Flow Rate

The maximum flow rate that is produced during forced expiration with fully inflated lungs

Personal Best Value

The highest value that an individual achieves in measuring PEF rate over a 2-week period when his or her asthma is under good control is known as one's "personal best" value or rate. Good control is defined as when one feels well without asthma symptoms. To determine personal best, take readings twice daily, in the morning and late afternoon or evening, and 15 to 20 minutes after taking an inhaled short-acting β_2-agonist. Using the personal best value is the most accurate gauge to use to interpret changes in peak flow measurements because the child's own scores are used as the standard for comparison.

• Interpretation of PEF reading (Box 24-1 describes use of peak flowmeter and interpretation of results)—if PEF is in the:
  ○ Green zone: More than 80% to 100% of personal best signals good control
  ○ Yellow zone: Between 50% and 79% of personal best signals a caution
  ○ Red zone: Between 0% and 50% of personal best signals major airflow obstruction
• Chest radiograph findings: Typically normal and may show hyperinflation of the lungs with flattening of the diaphragm and peribronchial thickening on radiograph with or without atelectasis (Liu et al, 2007)

Differential Diagnosis

Numerous conditions can cause airway obstruction and be incorrectly confused with asthma, especially in young children and infants. Examples include the following:
• Acute bronchiolitis, laryngotracheobronchitis, bronchopneumonia
• Bronchial foreign body aspiration
• Congenital malformations of the respiratory, cardiovascular, or gastrointestinal (GI) systems
• Bronchopulmonary dysplasia
• Cystic fibrosis (CF)
• Tracheal or foreign body compression (e.g., vascular aortic ring, enlarged lymph nodes or tumors)
• Chronic lower respiratory tract infections caused by immunodeficiency disorders

• Recurrent aspirations
• Vocal cord dysfunction
• Gastroesophageal reflux disease
• Heart disease

Management

The *Full Report of the Expert Panel: Guidelines for the Diagnosis and Management of Asthma* (ERP-3) (NHLBI, 2007) provides the most recent standards for the treatment of asthma in children. Management strategies are based on whether the child has intermittent, mild persistent, moderate persistent, or severe persistent asthma (see Table 24-1). A stepwise approach is recommended. If control of symptoms is not maintained at a particular step of classification and management, the health care provider first should reevaluate for compliance and administration factors. If these factors do not appear to be responsible for the lack of symptom control, the health care provider should go to the next step. Likewise, gradual step-downs in pharmacologic therapy may be considered when the child is well controlled for 3 months. ICS may be reduced about 25% to 50% every 3 months to the lowest possible dose needed to control the child's asthma (NHLBI, 2007).

In this chapter the outpatient management of intermittent, mild persistent, moderate persistent, and severe persistent asthma is discussed, as is the outpatient management of acute exacerbations. The practitioner should refer to other textbooks for management of severe asthma requiring hospitalization.

Chronic Asthma. Treatment of chronic asthma in children is based on general control measures and pharmacotherapy. General control measures include the following:
• Avoid exposure to known allergens or irritants.
• Avoid use of acetaminophen in children at risk for asthma (McBride, 2011).
• Administer yearly influenza vaccine.
• Control environment to eliminate or reduce offending allergen.
• Provide allergen immunotherapy.
• Treat rhinitis, sinusitis, or gastroesophageal reflux.
• See section on patient education for other measures.

The pharmacologic management of asthma in children is based on the severity of asthma and the child's age. The stepwise approach to treatment (Figs. 24-1 and 24-2) is based on severity of symptoms and the use of pharmacotherapy to control chronic symptoms, maintain normal activity, prevent recurrent exacerbations, and minimize adverse side effects, and nearly "normal" pulmonary function. Within any classification, a child may experience mild, moderate, or severe exacerbations. NHLBI guidelines for assessing asthma control and initiating and adjusting asthma therapy for the various pediatric age groups are found in Figs. 24-3 and 24-4.

Important considerations to note in the pharmacologic treatment of asthma include the following:
• Control of asthma should be gained as quickly as possible by starting at the classification step most appropriate to the initial severity of the child's symptoms or at a higher level (e.g., a course of systemic corticosteroids or higher dose of inhaled corticosteroid). After control of symptoms, decrease treatment to the least amount of medication needed to maintain control.
• Systemic corticosteroids may be needed at any time and step if there is a major flare-up of symptoms.

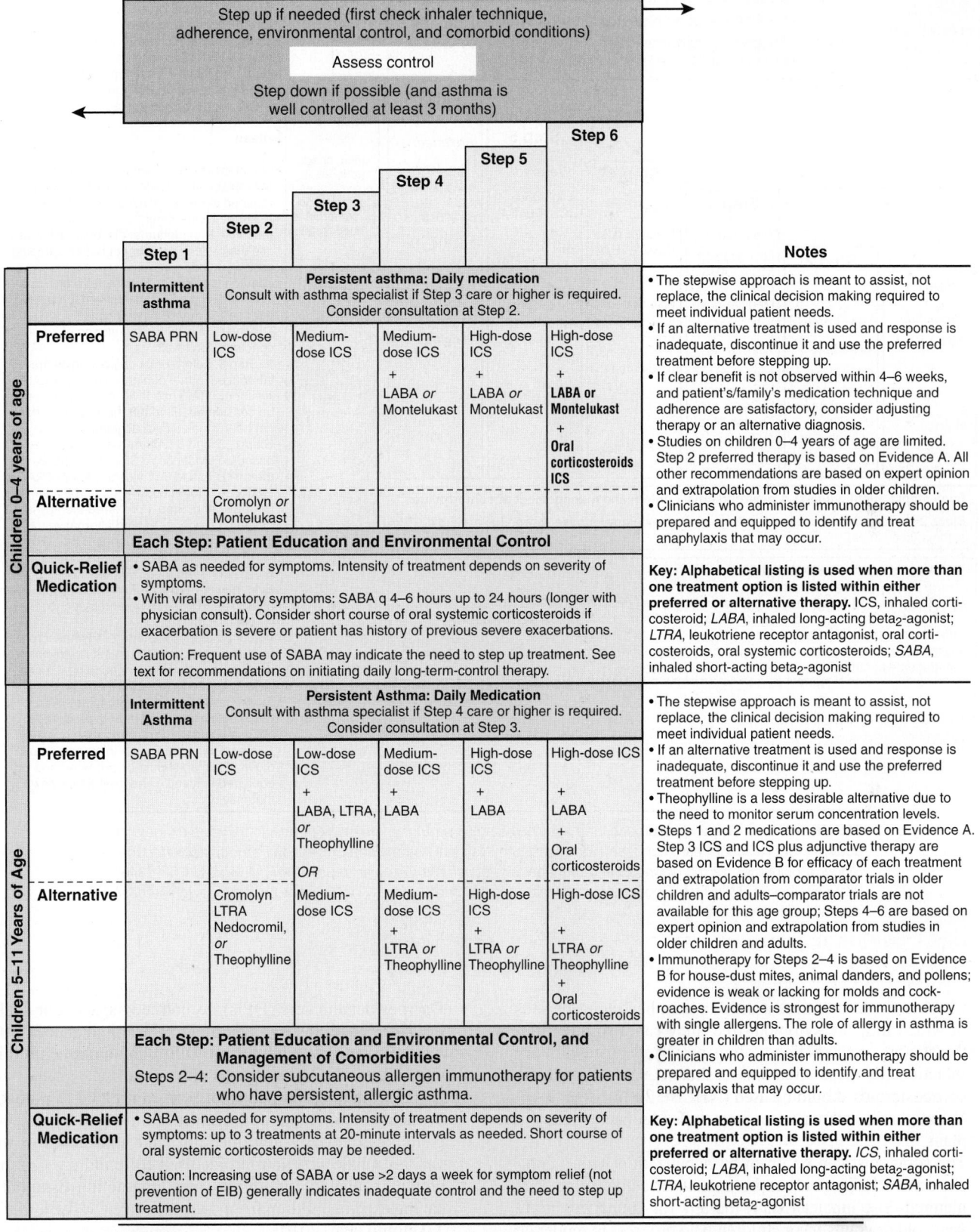

FIGURE 24-1 Stepwise approach for managing asthma in children 0 to 4 years of age and 5 to 11 years of age. (From National Heart, Lung, and Blood Institute, National Asthma and Prevention Program: *Expert panel report 3: guidelines for the diagnosis and management of asthma.* Summary report 2007, NIH Pub No. 08-5846, 2007, Bethesda, MD, U.S. Department of Health and Human Services, p 42, www.nhlbi.nih.gov/guidelines/asthma/asthsumm.pdf.)

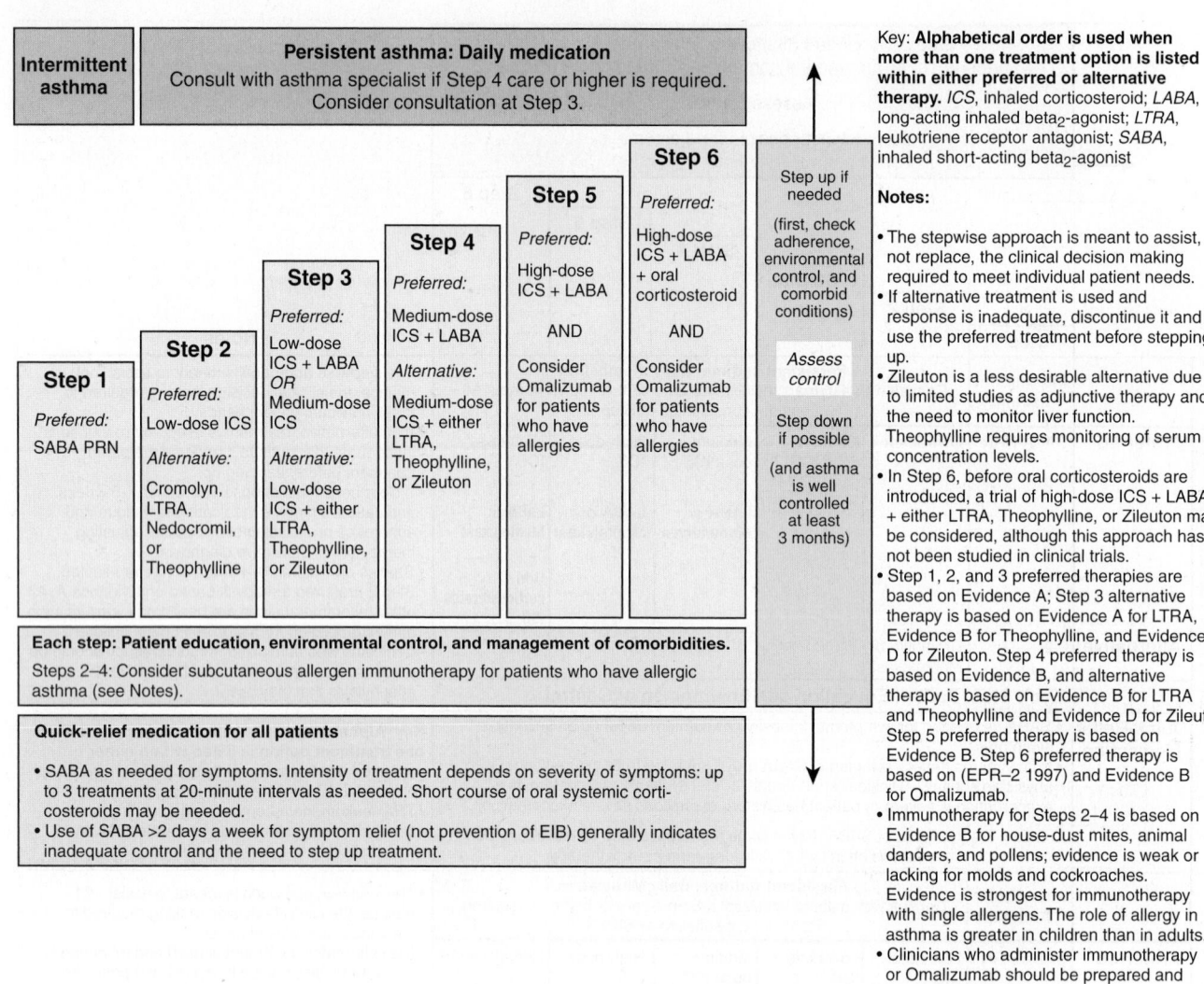

Intermittent asthma	Persistent asthma: Daily medication Consult with asthma specialist if Step 4 care or higher is required. Consider consultation at Step 3.

Step 1

Preferred:
SABA PRN

Step 2

Preferred:
Low-dose ICS

Alternative:
Cromolyn, LTRA, Nedocromil, or Theophylline

Step 3

Preferred:
Low-dose ICS + LABA OR Medium-dose ICS

Alternative:
Low-dose ICS + either LTRA, Theophylline, or Zileuton

Step 4

Preferred:
Medium-dose ICS + LABA

Alternative:
Medium-dose ICS + either LTRA, Theophylline, or Zileuton

Step 5

Preferred:
High-dose ICS + LABA

AND

Consider Omalizumab for patients who have allergies

Step 6

Preferred:
High-dose ICS + LABA + oral corticosteroid

AND

Consider Omalizumab for patients who have allergies

Step up if needed
(first, check adherence, environmental control, and comorbid conditions)

Assess control

Step down if possible
(and asthma is well controlled at least 3 months)

Each step: Patient education, environmental control, and management of comorbidities.

Steps 2–4: Consider subcutaneous allergen immunotherapy for patients who have allergic asthma (see Notes).

Quick-relief medication for all patients

• SABA as needed for symptoms. Intensity of treatment depends on severity of symptoms: up to 3 treatments at 20-minute intervals as needed. Short course of oral systemic corticosteroids may be needed.
• Use of SABA >2 days a week for symptom relief (not prevention of EIB) generally indicates inadequate control and the need to step up treatment.

Key: **Alphabetical order is used when more than one treatment option is listed within either preferred or alternative therapy.** *ICS*, inhaled corticosteroid; *LABA*, long-acting inhaled beta$_2$-agonist; *LTRA*, leukotriene receptor antagonist; *SABA*, inhaled short-acting beta$_2$-agonist

Notes:

• The stepwise approach is meant to assist, not replace, the clinical decision making required to meet individual patient needs.
• If alternative treatment is used and response is inadequate, discontinue it and use the preferred treatment before stepping up.
• Zileuton is a less desirable alternative due to limited studies as adjunctive therapy and the need to monitor liver function. Theophylline requires monitoring of serum concentration levels.
• In Step 6, before oral corticosteroids are introduced, a trial of high-dose ICS + LABA + either LTRA, Theophylline, or Zileuton may be considered, although this approach has not been studied in clinical trials.
• Step 1, 2, and 3 preferred therapies are based on Evidence A; Step 3 alternative therapy is based on Evidence A for LTRA, Evidence B for Theophylline, and Evidence D for Zileuton. Step 4 preferred therapy is based on Evidence B, and alternative therapy is based on Evidence B for LTRA and Theophylline and Evidence D for Zileuton. Step 5 preferred therapy is based on Evidence B. Step 6 preferred therapy is based on (EPR–2 1997) and Evidence B for Omalizumab.
• Immunotherapy for Steps 2–4 is based on Evidence B for house-dust mites, animal danders, and pollens; evidence is weak or lacking for molds and cockroaches. Evidence is strongest for immunotherapy with single allergens. The role of allergy in asthma is greater in children than in adults.
• Clinicians who administer immunotherapy or Omalizumab should be prepared and equipped to identify and treat anaphylaxis that may occur.

FIGURE 24-2 Stepwise approach for managing asthma in youths more than or equal to 12 years of age and adults. (From National Heart, Lung, and Blood Institute, National Asthma and Prevention Program: *Expert panel report 3: guidelines for the diagnosis and management of asthma.* Summary report 2007, NIH Pub No. 08-5846, 2007, Bethesda, MD, U.S. Department of Health and Human Services, p 45, www.nhlbi.nih.gov/guidelines/asthma/asthsumm.pdf.)

• Children with intermittent asthma may have long periods in which they are symptom-free; they can also have life-threatening exacerbations, often provoked by respiratory infection. In these situations a short course of systemic corticosteroids should be used (NHLBI, 2007).
• Variations in asthma necessitate individualized treatment plans.
• The β$_2$-agonist can be given by nebulization with a compressor. Nebulization can be a more effective route than metered-dose inhaler (MDI) therapy for young infants (2 years old or younger) or children who progress to moderate or severe airway obstruction.
• A spacer or holding chamber with an attached mask enhances the delivery of MDI medications to the lower airways of a child. Spacers eliminate the need to synchronize inhalation with activation of MDI. Older children can use the spacer without the mask.

• Dry powder inhalers (DPIs) do not need spacers or shaking before use. Instruct children to rinse their mouth with water and spit after inhalation. DPIs should not be used in children younger than 4 years old.
• Different inhaled corticosteroids are not equal in potency to each other on a per puff or microgram basis. Table 24-3 compares the daily low, medium, and high doses of the various inhaled corticosteroids used for children. Combination inhaled corticosteroid and long-acting β$_2$-agonist can be used in children from 4 years of age (NHLBI, 2007; Taketomo et al, 2010).
• For treatment of exercise-induced bronchospasm:
  ○ Warm up before exercise for 5 to 10 minutes.
  ○ Use either an inhaled short-acting β$_2$-agonist or a mast cell stabilizer (cromolyn or nedocromil) or both. Combination of both types of drugs is the more effective therapy. A long-acting β$_2$-agonist can be used in older children.

Children 0-4 years of age

Assessing severity and initiating therapy in children who are not currently taking long-term control medication

Classification of Asthma Severity

Components of Severity		Intermittent	Persistent		
			Mild	**Moderate**	**Severe**
Impairment	Symptoms	≤2 days/week	>2 days/week but not daily	Daily	Throughout the day
	Nighttime awakenings	0	1-2x/month	3-4x/month	>1x/week
	Short-acting beta₂-agonist use for symptom control (not prevention of EIB)	≤2 days/week	>2 days/week but not daily	Daily	Several times per day
	Interference with normal activity	None	Minor limitation	Some limitation	Extremely limited
Risk	Exacerbations requiring oral systemic corticosteroids	0-1/year	≥2 exacerbations in 6 months requiring oral systemic corticosteroids, or ≥4 wheezing episodes/1 year lasting >1 day AND risk factors for persistent asthma		

←——— Consider severity and interval since last exacerbation. Frequency and severity may fluctuate over time. ———→

Exacerbations of any severity may occur in patients in any severity category

Recommended Step for Initiating Therapy (See Fig. 24-1 for treatment steps.)	Step 1	Step 2	Step 3 and consider short course of oral systemic corticosteroids	

In 2-6 weeks, depending on severity, evaluate level of asthma control that is achieved. If no clear benefit is observed in 4-6 weeks, consider adjusting therapy or alternative diagnoses.

Notes

- The stepwise approach is meant to assist, not replace, the clinical decision making required to meet individual patient needs.

- Level of severity is determined by both impairment and risk. Assess impairment domain by patient's/caregiver's recall of previous 2-4 weeks. Symptom assessment for longer periods should reflect a global assessment such as inquiring whether the patient's asthma is better or worse since the last visit. Assign severity to the most severe category in which any feature occurs.

- At present, there are inadequate data to correspond frequencies of exacerbations with different levels of asthma severity. For treatment purposes, patients who had ≥2 exacerbations requiring oral systemic corticosteroids in the past 6 months, or ≥4 wheezing episodes in the past year, and who have risk factors for persistent asthma may be considered the same as patients who have persistent asthma, even in the absence of impairment levels consistent with persistent asthma.

Key: *EIB*, Exercise-induced bronchospasm.

Children 5-11 years of age

Assessing severity and initiating therapy in children who are not currently taking long-term control medication

Classification of Asthma Severity

Components of Severity		Intermittent	Persistent		
			Mild	**Moderate**	**Severe**
Impairment	Symptoms	≤2 days/week	>2 days/week but not daily	Daily	Throughout the day
	Nighttime awakenings	≤2x/month	3-4x/month	>1x/week but not nightly	Often 7x/week
	Short-acting beta₂-agonist use for symptom control (not prevention of EIB)	≤2 days/week	>2 days/week but not daily	Daily	Several times per day
	Interference with normal activity	None	Minor limitation	Some limitation	Extremely limited
	Lung function	• Normal FEV_1 between exacerbations • FEV_1 >80% predicted • FEV_1/FVC >85%	• FEV_1 >80% predicted • FEV_1/FVC >80%	• FEV_1 = 60-80% predicted • FEV_1/FVC = 75-80%	• FEV_1 < 60% predicted • FEV_1/FVC < 75%
Risk	Exacerbations requiring oral systemic corticosteroids	0-1/year (see note)	≥2/year (see note) ——————————————→		

←——— Consider severity and interval since last exacerbation. ———→
Frequency and severity may fluctuate over time for patients in any severity category.

Relative annual risk of exacerbations may be related to FEV_1.

Recommended Step for Initiating Therapy (See Fig. 24-1 for treatment steps.)	Step 1	Step 2	Step 3, medium-dose ICS option	Step 3, medium-dose ICS option, or step 4

and consider short course of oral systemic corticosteroids

In 2-6 weeks, evaluate level of asthma control that is achieved, and adjust therapy accordingly.

Notes

- The stepwise approach is meant to assist, not replace, the clinical decision making required to meet individual patient needs.

- Level of severity is determined by both impairment and risk. Assess impairment domain by patient's/caregiver's recall of previous 2-4 weeks and spirometry. Assign severity to the most severe category in which any feature occurs.

- At present, there are inadequate data to correspond frequencies of exacerbations with different levels of asthma severity. In general, more frequent and intense exacerbations (e.g., requiring urgent, unscheduled care, hospitalization, or ICU admission) indicate greater underlying disease severity. For treatment purposes, patients who had ≥2 exacerbations requiring oral systemic corticosteroids in the past year may be considered the same as patients who have persistent asthma, even in the absence of impairment levels consistent with persistent asthma.

Key: *EIB*, Exercise-induced bronchospasm; *FEV₁*, forced expiratory volume in 1 second; *FVC*, forced vital capacity; *ICS*, inhaled corticosteroids.

FIGURE 24-3 Classifying asthma severity and initiating treatment in children 0 to 4 years of age and 5 to 11 years of age. (From National Heart, Lung, Blood Institute, National Asthma Prevention Program: *Expert panel report 3: guidelines for the diagnosis and management of asthma.* Summary report 2007, NIH Pub No. 08-6846, Bethesda, MD, 2007, U.S. Department of Health and Human Services, pp 40-41. www.nhlbi.nih.gov/guidelines/asthma/asthsumm.pdf.)

		Assessing severity and initiating therapy in children ≥ 12 yr who are not currently taking long-term control medication					Notes

Components of Severity		Classification of Asthma Severity				Notes
			Persistent			
		Intermittent	Mild	Moderate	Severe	
Impairment Normal FEV₁/FVC: 08-19 yr 85% 20-39 yr 80% 40-59 yr 75% 60-80 yr 70%	Symptoms	≤2 days/week	>2 days/week but not daily	Daily	Throughout the day	•The stepwise approach is meant to assist, not replace, the clinical decision making required to meet individual patient needs.
	Nighttime awakenings	≤2x/month	3-4x/month	>1x/week but not nightly	Often 7x/week	•Level of severity is determined by both impairment and risk. Assess impairment domain by patient's/caregiver's recall of previous 2-4 weeks and spirometry. Assign severity to the most severe category in which any feature occurs.
	Short-acting beta₂-agonist use for symptom control (not prevention of EIB)	≤2 days/week	>2 days/week but not daily, and not more than 1x on any day	Daily	Several times per day	
	Interference with normal activity	None	Minor limitation	Some limitation	Extremely limited	•At present, there are inadequate data to correspond frequencies of exacerbations with different levels of asthma severity. In general, more frequent and intense exacerbations (e.g., requiring urgent, unscheduled care, hospitalization, or ICU admission) indicate greater underlying disease severity. For treatment purposes, patients who had ≥2 exacerbations requiring oral systemic corticosteroids in the past year may be considered the same as patients who have persistent asthma, even in the absence of impairment levels consistent with persistent asthma.
	Lung function	• Normal FEV₁ between exacerbations • FEV₁ >80% predicted • FEV₁/FVC normal	• FEV₁ >80% predicted • FEV₁/FVC normal	• FEV₁ >60 but <80% predicted • FEV₁/FVC reduced 5%	• FEV₁ < 60% predicted • FEV₁/FVC reduced >5%	
Risk	Exacerbations requiring oral systemic corticosteroids	0-1/year (see note)	≥2/year (see note) ⟶			Key: *FEV₁*, forced expiratory volume in 1 second; *FVC*, forced vital capacity; *ICU*, intensive care unit; *x*, times; *yr*, years.
		⟵ Consider severity and interval since last exacerbation. ⟶ Frequency and severity may fluctuate over time for patients in any severity category.				
		Relative annual risk of exacerbations may be related to FEV₁.				
Recommended Step for Initiating Therapy (See Fig. 24-2 for treatment steps.)		Step 1	Step 2	Step 3	Step 4 or 5 and consider short course of oral systemic corticosteroids	
		In 2-6 weeks, evaluate level of asthma control that is achieved and adjust therpay accordingly.				

(Left side vertical label: Children ≥12 years of age)

FIGURE 24-4 Classifying asthma severity and initiating treatment in children more than or equal to 12 years of age and adults. (From National Heart, Lung, Blood Institute, National Asthma Prevention Program: Expert panel report 3: guidelines for the diagnosis and management of asthma. Summary report 2007, NIH Pub No. 08-6846, Bethesda, Md, 2007, U.S. Department of Health and Human Services, p. 43.)

○ Use two puffs of a β₂-agonist and/or cromolyn MDI 15 to 30 minutes before exercise (Kelly and Oppenheimer, 2010). Tolerance may develop if a β₂-agonist is used more than a few times a week; it should not be used as a controller monotherapy. Those who exercise regularly should use controller medication, preferably an inhaled corticosteroid. Oral montelukast can also be used on a daily schedule at least 2 hours prior to exercise (Storms, 2010).

○ Using a scarf or mask around the mouth may decrease exercise-induced asthma (EIA) induced by cold.

Table 24-4 identifies the usual dosages for long-term control medications (exclusive of inhaled corticosteroids) used to treat asthma in children. Quick-relief medications are listed in Table 24-5.

Practice parameters are guides and should not replace individualized treatment based on clinical judgment and unique differences among patients.

Acute Exacerbations of Asthma. The treatment of acute episodes of asthma is also based on classification of the severity of the episode. Acute episodes are classified as mild, moderate, and severe. Signs and symptoms are summarized in Table 24-6. Early recognition of warning signs and treatment should be stressed in both patient or parent education, or both.

Characteristics of a *mild acute episode* are:
• Wheezing, usually at the end of expiration
• Increased respiratory rate
• No signs of respiratory distress, cyanosis, or activity restriction

• PEF or forced expiratory volume (FEV₁) greater than 70% of expected value
• Ability to speak in normal sentences between breaths

Children with a *moderate acute episode* of asthma manifest the following:
• Audible wheeze
• Use of accessory muscles
• Increase in respiratory rate
• Unable to walk or utter more than three to five words between breaths

Manifestations of a *severe acute episode* of asthma in children include the following signs of severe respiratory distress:
• Cyanosis
• Use of accessory muscles plus lower rib and suprasternal retractions; nasal flaring
• Agitation and the ability to say only single words between breaths
• Loud wheezing on inhalation and expiration (NHLBI, 2007)

The *initial pharmacologic treatment* for acute asthma exacerbations is shown in Fig. 24-5. It consists of inhaled short-acting β₂-agonists, two to six puffs every 20 minutes for three treatments by way of MDI with or without a spacer, or a single nebulizer treatment (0.15 mg/kg; minimum 1.25 to 2.5 mg of 0.5% solution of albuterol in 2 to 3 mL of normal saline).

If the initial treatment results in a good response (PEF/FEV₁ greater than 70% of the patient's best), the inhaled short-acting

TABLE 24-3 Estimated Comparative Daily Dosages for Inhaled Corticosteroids

Drug	LOW DAILY DOSE		MEDIUM DAILY DOSE		HIGH DAILY DOSE	
	Child*	Adult†	Child*	Adult†	Child*	Adult†
Beclomethasone HFA (40 or 80 mcg/puff)	80-160 mcg	80-240 mcg	>160-320 mcg	>240-480 mcg	>320 mcg	>480 mcg
Budesonide DPI (90, 180, or 200 mcg/inhalation)	180-400 mcg	180-600 mcg	>400-800 mcg	>600-1200 mcg	>800 mcg	>1200 mcg
Budesonide inhaled suspension for nebulization (child dose) (0.25 mg/2 mL, 0.5 mg/2 mL)	0.5 mg		1 mg		2 mg	N/A
Flunisolide (250 mcg/puff)	500-750 mcg	500-1000 mcg	1000-1250 mcg	>1000-2000 mcg	>1250 mcg	>2000 mcg
Flunisolide HFA (80 mcg/puff)	160 mcg	320 mcg	320 mcg	>320-640 mcg	>640 mcg	>640 mcg
Fluticasone HFA/MDI						
• MDI: 44, 110, or 220 mcg/puff	88-176 mcg	88-264 mcg	>176-352 mcg	>264-440 mcg	>352 mcg	>440 mcg
• DPI: 50, 100, or 250 mcg/inhalation	100-200 mcg	100-300 mcg	>200-400 mcg	>300-500 mcg	>400 mcg	>500 mcg
Mometasone DPI (200 mcg/inhalation)	N/A	200 mcg	N/A	400 mcg	N/A	>400 mcg
Triamcinolone acetonide (75 mcg/puff)	300-600 mcg	300-750 mcg	>600-900 mcg	>750-1500 mcg	>900 mcg	>1500 mcg

Inhaled Corticosteroids in Children 0-4 Years

	Low Daily Dose	Medium Daily Dose	High Daily Dose
Budesonide inhaled suspension for nebulization (0.25 mg/2 mL, 0.5 mg/2 mL)	0.25-0.5 mg	>0.5-1 mg	>1 mg
Fluticasone HFA: 44, 110, or 220 mcg/puff	176 mcg	>176-352 mcg	>352 mcg

*Child 5 to 11 years old.
†Adult ≥12 years old.
DPI, Dry powder inhaler; *HFA,* hydrofluoroalkane; *MDI,* metered-dose inhaler; *N/A,* not approved and no data available for this age group.

β_2-agonists can be continued every 3 to 4 hours for 24 to 48 hours. Consider a 7- to 10-day burst of oral corticosteroids.

An incomplete response (PEF or FEV_1 between 40% and 69% of personal best or symptoms recur within 4 hours of therapy) is treated by continuing β_2-agonists and adding an oral corticosteroid. The β_2-agonist can be given by nebulizer. Parents should contact their child's health care provider for additional instructions. If there is marked distress (severe acute symptoms) or a poor response (PEF or FEV_1 <40%) to treatment, the child should have the β_2-agonist repeated immediately and should be taken to the emergency department. Emergency medical rescue (911) transportation should be used if the distress is severe and nonresponsive.

If children experience acute asthma exacerbations more than once every 4 to 6 weeks, their treatment plan should be reevaluated (NHLBI, 2007).

Complications

Complications from asthma can range from mild secondary respiratory infections to respiratory arrest. Unresponsiveness to pharmacologic agents can lead to status asthmaticus and ultimately to death. Chronic high-dose steroid use leads to growth retardation and other related side effects.

Patient and Parent Education and Prevention

The practitioner needs to remember that day-to-day management of asthma is the responsibility of the child or parent. Education should be tailored to meet the patient's individual and family needs. Therefore the primary care provider should provide instruction on the following:
• Factors responsible for asthma symptoms (i.e., inflammation, airway hyperresponsiveness, and obstruction)
• Environmental control of allergens or triggers, such as smoking and dust
• Medication use (when to take, how often to take, side effects)
• Home PEF monitoring
• How to use inhalers, spacer devices, or aerosol equipment (Box 24-2)
• Proper cleaning of aerosol equipment
• What to do if symptoms worsen (what medications to add or increase; how frequently to use inhaled medication;

TABLE 24-4	Long-Term Control Medications for the Treatment of Asthma			
Medication	**Dosage Form**	**Child Dose‡**	**Adult Dose§**	**Comments**
Inhaled Corticosteroids (See Table 24-5)				
Systemic Corticosteroids (Applies to All Three Corticosteroids)				
Methylprednisolone	2-, 4-, 8-, 16-, 32-mg tabs	0.25-2 mg/kg daily in a single dose in AM or every other day as needed for control; 60 mg max dose	7.5-60 mg daily in a single dose in AM or every other day as needed for control	For long-term treatment of severe persistent asthma, administer single dose in AM either daily or on alternate days (alternate-day therapy may produce less adrenal suppression). If daily doses are required, one study suggests improved efficacy and no increase in adrenal suppression when administered at 3 PM.
Prednisolone	5-mg tabs, 5 mg/5 mL, 1 mg/mL	Same as above	Same as above	
Prednisone	1-, 2-, 5-, 10-, 20-, 50-mg tabs; 5 mg/mL, 1 mg/mL	Short-course "burst": 1-2 mg/kg/day in a single or 2 divided doses a day, max 60 mg/day for 3-10 days	Short-course "burst" to achieve control: 40-60 mg/day as single or 2 divided doses for 3-10 days	Short courses or "bursts" are effective for establishing control when initiating therapy or during a period of gradual deterioration. The bursts should be continued until patient achieves 80% PEF rate personal best or symptoms resolve. This usually requires 3-10 days, but may require longer. There is no evidence that tapering the dose following improvement prevents relapse.
Cromolyn and Nedocromil				
Cromolyn	MDI: 800 mcg/puff nebulizer; 20 mg/ampule	5-11 yr: 1 or 2 puffs 3 or 4 times a day;1 ampule 3 or 4 times a day	2-4 puffs 3 or 4 times a day; 1 ampule 3 or 4 times a day	One dose 10-15 minutes before exercise or allergen exposure provides effective prophylaxis for 1-2 hr.
Nedocromil	MDI: 1.75 mg/puff	>6-11 yr: 2 puffs 4 times a day	2 puffs 4 times a day	May decrease dose to 2 or 3 times a day when desired response achieved.
Inhaled Long-Acting β₂-Agonists (Should Not Be Used for Symptom Relief or for Exacerbations; Use With Inhaled Corticosteroids)				
Salmeterol	DPI: 50 mcg/inhalation	>4 yr: 1 activation/puff every 12 hr	1 activation/puff every 12 hr	Use with inhaled corticosteroid only. Do not use as a rescue inhaler for symptom relief or for exacerbations.
Formoterol	DPI: 12 mcg/single-use capsule	>5 yr: 1 capsule every 12 hr apart	1 capsule every 12 hr	Do not take orally; must be used with aerolizer.
Sustained-release albuterol	4-mg tab* 8-mg tab†	0.3-0.6 mg/kg/day in 2 divided doses; not to exceed 8 mg/day ≥6 yr	4-8 mg twice a day	For children 6 yr and older
Methylxanthines				
Theophylline (numerous manufacturers)	Liquids Sustained-release tabs and capsules	Maintenance oral doses for acute symptoms: 1-9 yr: 20-24 mg/kg/day 9-12 yr: 16 mg/kg/day 12-16 yr: 13 mg/kg/day (in children doses divided every 8-12 hr)	Maintenance dose for acute symptoms: 10 mg/kg/day divided every 8-12 hr; up to 900 mg max/day	Routine serum theophylline level monitoring is required (serum concentration 5-15 mcg/mL); not commonly used with pediatric patients. Smoking alters dosage requirements.
Leukotriene Modifiers				
Montelukast	4- or 5-mg chewable tab, 10-mg tab; granules 4 mg/packet	6 mo-5 yr: 4 mg a day; 6-14 yr: 5 mg a day	>14 yr: 10 mg a day >15 yr prevention of EIB: 10 mg at least 2 hr before exercise (no other doses should be given in 24 hr)	

TABLE 24-4	Long-Term Control Medications for the Treatment of Asthma—cont'd			
Medication	**Dosage Form**	**Child Dose‡**	**Adult Dose§**	**Comments**
Zafirlukast	10- or 20-mg tab	5-11 yr: 10-mg tab twice a day	>12 yr: 40 mg daily (20-mg tab twice a day)	Take zafirlukast at least 1 hr before or 2 hr after meals.
Zileuton	300- or 600-mg tab		2400 mg daily (give tabs 4 times a day)	Less desirable because of the need to monitor hepatic enzymes (ALT); used in children older than age 12 years
Combined Medication				
Fluticasone/ salmeterol	HFA: 45, 115, fluticasone 230 mcg/21 mcg salmeterol		HFA: >12 yr: 2 inhalations twice a day of 45 mcg fluticasone /21 mcg salmeterol or 115 mcg fluticasone /21 mcg salmeterol	HFA adult dose not to exceed 2 inhalations of 230 mcg fluticasone/21 mcg salmeterol twice daily
	Diskus: 100, 250, or 500 mcg fluticasone/50 mcg salmeterol	Diskus: >4-11 yr: 1 inhalation twice a day of 100 mcg fluticasone/50 mcg salmeterol; dose depends on severity of asthma	Diskus: 1 inhalation twice a day of 100 mcg fluticasone/50 mcg salmeterol; dose depends on severity of asthma	
Budesonide/ Formoterol Aerosol or powder MDI	Aerosol: 80 mcg, 160 mcg budesonide/4.5 mcg formoterol Powder: 100 mcg budesonide/6 mcg formoterol	5-11 yr: 2 puffs twice a day of aerosol 80 mcg/4.5 mcg, not to exceed 4 inhalations/ day	2 puffs twice a day — depends on severity; not to exceed 4 inhalations/ day of 160 mcg/4.5 formoterol	

*Proventil and Repetabs come in 4 mg only.
†Volmax comes in 4 mg and 8 mg.
‡≤12 yr old.
§Adult ≥12 years old.
ALT, Alanine aminotransferase; DPI, dry powder inhaler; max, maximum; EIB, exercise induced bronchospasm; MDI, metered-dose inhaler; PEF, peak expiratory flow; tab(s), tablet(s).
Adapted from the National Heart, Lung, and Blood Institute (NHLBI): Full report of the expert panel: guidelines for the diagnosis and management of asthma (EPR-3), National Institutes of Health, 2007, Bethesda, Md; Taketomo CK, Hodding JH, Kraus DM: Pediatric dosage handbook, ed 17, Hudson, OH, 2011, Lexi-Comp.

specific indications about when to seek additional medical treatment for worsening of symptoms); development of a written action/treatment plan with the child or parent to cover these issues (Fig. 24-6 shows a sample home treatment plan)

- Need to have an adequate supply of all medications (including oral corticosteroids) at home and medications readily accessible to the child at school or other settings where the child frequents
- Management of the child at school, camp, or other places away from home
- The need for regular follow-up every 1 to 6 months and as needed with exacerbations

The primary care provider should stress that asthma is a chronic disease that can be controlled—the goal of therapy is to maintain normal activity. The absence of symptoms does not mean the disease has disappeared, but that it is well-controlled. The child should wear a medical alert bracelet. Patients and parents should be acquainted with local asthma education programs and activities, such as asthma camp. Also written instructions and handouts should be provided for parents, children, and other significant individuals (e.g., school personnel).

Prognosis

Asthma is a chronic disease that for most children can be successfully managed with proper pharmacologic therapy, allergen and environmental control, and patient education. Mild asthma is more likely to disappear with increasing age than is moderate or severe asthma.

ALLERGIC RHINITIS

Description

AR is a disorder that results in inflammation of the nasal epithelium and other related local manifestations caused by the release of chemical mediators, from an antigen-antibody reaction. AR represents a type I IgE-mediated allergic response. It is a clinical diagnosis that is based on the presence of rhinorrhea, nasal pruritus and congestion, and sneezing. Manifestations can be seasonal or perennial depending on exposure to the offending agent and subsequent sensitization to the offending allergen (Lasley and Hetherington, 2011). There may be a related family or medical history of atopic dermatitis or asthma. A history of AD is associated with a 70% chance of having AR, asthma, or both—the dreaded atopic triangle (Becker, 2009).

TABLE 24-5 Quick-Relief Medications for the Treatment of Asthma

Medication	Dosage Form	Child Dose*	Adult Dose	Comments
Short-Acting Inhaled β₂-Agonists				
Metered-Dose Inhalers				
Albuterol HFA	90 mcg/puff, 200 puffs	Acute exacerbation: 4-8 puffs every 20 min for 3 doses then every 1-4 hr as needed Maintenance: 0-4 yr old, 1-2 inhalations every 4-6 hr >5 yr old, 2 puffs every 4-6 hr prn	Acute exacerbation: 4-8 puffs every 20 min for 4 hr then every 1-4 hr as needed Maintenance: 2 puffs every 4-6 hr prn	Not generally recommended for long-term treatment. Regular use on a daily basis indicates the need for additional long-term control therapy.
Pirbuterol	200 mcg/puff, 400 puffs	Acute exacerbation: 4-8 inhalations every 20 min for 3 doses then every 1-4 hr as needed Maintenance: 2 inhalations 3 or 4 times/day	Acute exacerbation: 4-8 inhalations every 20 min for up to 4 hr then every 1-4 hr as needed Maintenance: 2 inhalations 3 or 4 times/day	
Levalbuterol HFA	45 mcg/puff	Acute exacerbation: 4-8 puffs every 20 min for 3 doses then every 1-4 hr Maintenance: >5 yr: 2 inhalations every 4-6 hr	Acute exacerbation: 4-8 puffs every 20 min for up to 4 hr then every 1-4 hr as needed Maintenance: 2 inhalations every 4-6 hr	Not FDA approved for long term, daily maintenance use. Use more than 2 days/wk indicates need for long-term control therapy
				Nonselective agents (e.g., epinephrine, isoproterenol, metaproterenol) are not recommended because of their potential for excessive cardiac stimulation, especially at high doses.
Nebulizer Solution				
Albuterol	5 mg/mL (0.5%) 0.63 mg/3 mL 1.25 mg/3 mL 2.5 mg/3 mL	<5 yr: 0.63-2.5 mg in 3 mL NS every 4-6 hr prn >5 yr: 1.25-2.5 mg in 3 mL of NS every 4-8 hr prn	Adults: 1.25-5 mg in 3 mL of NS every 4-8 hr prn	May mix with cromolyn or ipratropium nebulizer solutions; may double dose for mild exacerbations.
Levalbuterol	0.31 mg/3 mL 0.63 mg/3 mL 1.25 mg/3 mL	Acute exacerbation: 0.075 mg/kg (minimum dose 1.25 mg) every 20 min for 3 doses then 0.075-0.15 mg/kg (not to exceed 5 mg) every 1-4 hr as needed Maintenance: 0-4 yr: 0.31-1.25 mg every 4-6 hr prn; >5 yr and adults: 0.31-0.63 mg every 8 hr prn	Acute exacerbation: 1.25-2.5 mg every 20 min for 3 doses then 1.25-5 mg every 1-4 hr as needed Maintenance: 0.31-0.63 mg every 8 hr as needed	Use more than 2 days/wk indicates need for long-term control therapy
Anticholinergics				
Metered-Dose Inhalers				
Ipratropium-HFA	17 mcg/puff, 200-puff canister	Maintenance: 1-2 inhalations every 6 hr (max 12 inhalations/day)	Maintenance: 2-3 puffs every 6 hr (max 12 inhalations/day)	Evidence is lacking that these drugs produce added benefit to β₂-agonists in long-term asthma therapy.
Nebulizer Solution				
Ipratropium	0.02% (2.5 mL)	Maintenance therapy: 250-500 mcg every 6 hr	250 mcg every 6 hr	Lacks evidence that ipratropium provides added benefit to β₂-agonists in long-term control

TABLE 24-5 Quick-Relief Medications for the Treatment of Asthma—cont'd

Medication	Dosage Form	Child Dose*	Adult Dose	Comments
Systemic Corticosteroids (Dosage Applies to All Three Corticosteroids Listed Below)				
Methylpred-nisolone	2-, 4-, 8-, 16-, 32-mg tabs	Short-course "burst": 1-2 mg/kg/day, max 30-60 mg/day, for 3-10 days	Short-course "burst" to achieve control: 40-60 mg/day as single or 2 divided doses for 3-10 days	Short courses or "bursts" are effective for establishing control when initiating therapy or during a period of gradual deterioration.
Prednisolone	5-mg tabs, 5 mg/5 mL, 15 mg/5 mL			
Prednisone	1-, 2.5-, 5-, 10-, 20-, 50-mg tabs: 5 mg/mL, 5 mg/5 mL			The burst should be continued until patient achieves 80% PEF rate personal best or symptoms resolve; this usually requires 3-10 days but may require longer; there is no evidence that tapering the dose following improvement prevents relapse.

*<12 yr old.
FDA, U.S. Food and Drug Administration; *max*, maximum; *NS*, normal saline; *PEF*, peak expiratory flow; *tabs*, tablets.
Adapted from the National Heart, Lung, and Blood Institute (NHLBI): *Full report of the expert panel: guidelines for the diagnosis and management of asthma* (EPR-3), National Institutes of Health, 2007, Bethesda, Md; Taketomo CK, Hodding JH, Kraus DM: *Pediatric dosage handbook,* ed 17, Hudson, OH, 2011, Lexi-Comp.

TABLE 24-6 Classifying Severity of Asthma Exacerbations*

	Mild	Moderate	Severe	Respiratory Arrest Imminent
Symptoms				
Breathless	While walking

Can lie down | While at rest (infant—softer, shorter cry; difficulty feeding)

Prefers sitting | While at rest (infant—stops feeding)

Sits upright | |
Talks in	Sentences	Phrases	Words	
Alertness	May be agitated	Usually agitated	Usually agitated	Drowsy or confused
Signs				
Respiratory rate	Increased

Guide to rates of breathing in awake children:

Age
<2 mo
2-12 mo
1-5 yr
6-8 yr | Increased

Normal rate
<60/min
<50/min
<40/min
<30/min | Often >30/min | |
| Use of accessory muscles; suprasternal retractions | Usually not | Commonly | Usually | Paradoxical thoracoabdominal movement |
| Wheeze | Moderate, often only end expiratory | Loud; throughout exhalation | Usually loud; throughout inhalation and exhalation | Absence of wheeze |
| Pulse/min | <100

Guide to normal pulse rates in children:

Age
2-12 mo
1-2 yr
2-8 yr | 100-120

Normal rate
<160/min
<120/min
<110/min | >120 | Bradycardia |
| Pulsus paradoxus | Absent <10 mm Hg | May be present 10-25 mm Hg | Often present >25 mm Hg (adult), 20-40 mm Hg (child) | Absence suggests respiratory muscle fatigue |

Continued

TABLE 24-6	Classifying Severity of Asthma Exacerbations*—cont'd			
	Mild	**Moderate**	**Severe**	**Respiratory Arrest Imminent**
Functional Assessment				
PEF percent predicted or percent personal best	≥70%	Approximately 40%-69%	<40% predicted or personal best, or response lasts <2 hr	<25%
Pao_2 (on room air) and/or	Normal (test not usually necessary)	>60 mm Hg (test not usually necessary)	<60 mm Hg: possible cyanosis	
Pco_2	<42 mm Hg (test not usually necessary)	<42 mm Hg (test not usually necessary)	≥42 mm Hg: possible respiratory failure	
Sao_2% (on room air) at sea level	>95% (test not usually necessary)	90%-95%	<90%	

*The presence of several parameters, but not necessarily all, indicates the general classification of the exacerbation. Many of these parameters have not been systematically studied, so they serve only as general guides.
Pao_2, Partial pressure of oxygen in arterial blood; Pco_2, partial pressure of carbon dioxide; *PEF,* peak expiratory flow; Sao_2, oxygen saturation in arterial blood.
From National Heart, Lung, and Blood Institute: *Full report of the expert panel: guidelines for the diagnosis and management of asthma* (EPR-3), National Institutes of Health, 2007, Bethesda, Md.

Epidemiology

AR is second only to asthma as the most common atopic disorder. There is an increased incidence in families with an atopic history. Genetic (the presence of an abnormal sensitivity that is associated with IgE production) and environmental factors are linked to its cause. Repeated exposure to the offending allergen for a period of time is an important contributing factor necessary for sensitizing the immune system to produce an allergic IgE response. Many of the allergens that cause asthma produce AR in the same child; AR is postulated to be a distinct feature of the same inflammatory process that results in asthma. Thus to effectively treat asthma, AR must also be effectively managed.

AR is rare in children less than 6 months old and, if present in infancy, is due to foods or household inhalants, not seasonal pollens. Food allergens can occasionally cause rhinitis.

In AR the mucous membranes of the nose, eyes, eustachian tubes, middle ear, sinuses, and pharynx become inflamed. The nasal mucosa is particularly vulnerable to inhaled allergens with a resulting type I, IgE-mediated allergic response. The nasal mucosa of a susceptible individual comes into contact with an allergen that binds to a specific IgE antibody. Superficial mucosal mast cells and basophils then degranulate and release chemical mediators, such as histamine and tryptase, chymase, kinins, heparin, and newly generated mediators including leukotrienes, prostaglandins, and platelet-activating factors (Sheikh and Najib, 2010). This causes an early-phase reaction of edema, cellular recruitment, and increased vascular permeability with hyperemia and increased serous and mucoid secretions. A late-phase response can occur about 4 to 8 hours later that results in additional release of chemical mediators from eosinophils, basophils, CD4 T cells, monocytes and neutrophils that cause chronic nasal inflammation (Lasley and Hetherington, 2011).

AR tends to be seasonal, perennial, or episodic. Seasonal AR (hay fever or seasonal pollenosis) typically occurs after 3 years old. Seasonal AR results from sensitization to airborne allergens such as tree, grass, and weed pollen (ragweed and other weeds) and outdoor molds. Sensitization from outdoor allergies typically occurs after the age of 3 years. In contrast, indoor allergens' effect can occur in children younger than 2 years (Becker, 2009). There can be geographic variations in seasonal AR depending on climate and when the allergens are released into the environment.

Perennial AR has year-round signs and symptoms that may be more severe in the winter. Onset of manifestations can occur before the second year of life, and offending substances tend to be indoor allergens, including the following:
- House dust mites
- Cockroaches
- Feathers
- Allergens or danders of household pets
- Indoor mold spores and seasonal pollens

Episodic AR occurs with intermittent exposure to an allergen. Thus the rhinitis is related to a distinct event, such as visiting a house where a cat dwells.

Clinical Findings

Common nasal symptoms and findings on physical examination include the following:
- Reduced patency from chronic or recurrent bilateral nasal obstruction as a result of congestion and inflammation
- Mouth breathing, snoring, nasal speech
- Pale to purplish and edema (bogginess) of nasal mucous membranes
- Clear, thin, watery to seromucoid rhinorrhea
- Nasal crease—horizontal crease across the lower third of nose
- Itching, rubbing of nose or "allergic salute"
- Nasal stuffiness, postnasal drip, paroxysms of sneezing, congested cough, or night cough
- Dennie lines, Morgan fold or atopic pleats—extra groove in lower eyelid (Fig. 24-7)

Associated manifestations include the following:
- Itching of palate, pharynx, nose, or eyes
- High arched palate

Assess Severity

- **Patients at high risk for a fatal attack require immediate medical attention after initial treatment.**

- Symptoms and signs suggestive of a more serious exacerbation such as marked breathlessness, inability to speak more than short phrases, use of accessory muscles, or drowsiness should result in initial treatment while immediately consulting with a clinician.

- Less severe signs and symptoms can be treated initially with assessment of response to therapy and further steps as listed below.

- If available, measure PEF—values of 50-79% predicted or personal best indicate the need for quick-relief medication. Depending on the response to treatment, contact with a clinician may also be indicated. Values below 50% indicate the need for immediate medical care.

Initial Treatment

- Inhaled SABA: up to two treatments 20 minutes apart of 2-6 puffs by metered-dose inhaler (MDI) or nebulizer treatments.

- Note: Medication delivery is highly variable. Children and individuals who have exacerbations of lesser severity may need fewer puffs than suggested above.

Good Response

No wheezing or dyspnea (assess tachypnea in young children).

PEF $\geq$ 80% predicted or personal best.

- Contact clinician for followup instructions and further management.

- May continue inhaled SABA every 3-4 hours for 24-48 hours.

- Consider short course of oral systemic corticosteroids.

Incomplete Response

Persistent wheezing and dyspnea (tachypnea).

PEF 50-79% predicted or personal best.

- Add oral systemic corticosteroid.

- Continue inhaled SABA.

- Contact clinician urgently (this day) for further instruction.

Poor Response

Marked wheezing and dyspnea.

PEF < 50% predicted or personal best.

- Add oral systemic corticosteroid.

- Repeat inhaled SABA immediately.

- If distress is severe and nonresponsive to initial treatment:
  —Call your doctor AND
  —**PROCEED TO ED;**
  —Consider calling 911 (ambulance transport).

- To ED.

Key: *ED*, Emergency department; *MDI*, metered-dose inhaler; *PEF*, peak expiratory flow; *SABA*, short-acting beta$_2$-agonist (quick-relief inhaler).

FIGURE 24-5 Management of asthma exacerbations: home treatment.

- Hoarseness and frequent attempts to clear the throat
- Redness of the conjunctiva, tearing, lid and periorbital edema, infraorbital cyanosis or allergic shiners (dark periorbital swelling)
- Enlarged tonsillar and adenoidal tissue
- "Cobblestone" appearance of the pharynx or palpebral conjunctivae (or both) as a result of increased lymphoid tissue
- Malocclusion if problem is chronic
- May have related sleep disturbances and performance problems at school related to lack of adequate sleep

BOX 24-2 How to Use a Metered-Dose Inhaler

Using an inhaler seems simple, but most patients do not use it correctly.

Steps for Using an Inhaler for Children Younger Than 5 Years of Age
1. The use of a mask chamber with a metered-dose inhaler (MDI) allows the delivery of inhaled medications even in an uncooperative child.
2. The child should be placed in the parent's lap, and the mask placed around the child's mouth.
3. Press down on the MDI while firmly holding the mask around the child's mouth. The child will eventually take a deep breath and inhale the medication.

Steps for Using an Inhaler for Children 5 Years or Older
Getting Ready
1. Take off the cap and shake the inhaler.
2. Breathe out all the way.
3. Hold the inhaler as shown in A, B, or C below.

Breathe in Slowly
1. Start breathing in slowly through the mouth, and then press down on the inhaler one time. (If a holding chamber is used, first press down on the inhaler.) Within 5 seconds, begin to breathe in slowly.
2. Keep breathing in slowly, as deeply as possible.

Hold Your Breath
1. Hold breath for a slow count to 10 if possible.
2. For inhaled quick-relief medicine (β_2-agonists), wait about 1 minute between puffs. There is no need to wait between puffs for other medicines.

A. Hold inhaler 1 to 2 inches in front of mouth (about the width of two fingers).

B. Use a spacer/holding chamber. These come in many shapes and can be useful to any patient.

C. Put inhaler in mouth. Do not use for steroids.

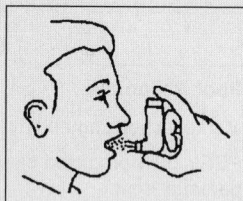
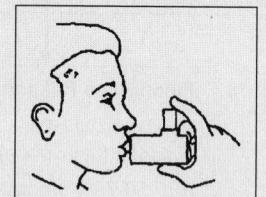
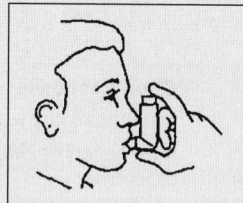

Step A or B is best, but step C can be used if patient has trouble with step A or B.

Clean Inhaler As Needed
Look at the hole where the medicine sprays out from your inhaler. If "powder" can be seen in or around the hole, clean the inhaler. Remove the metal canister from the L-shaped plastic mouthpiece. Rinse only the mouthpiece and cap in warm water. Let them dry overnight. In the morning, put the canister back inside. Put the cap on.

Know When to Replace Inhaler
For medicines taken each day: as an example, a new canister has 200 puffs (number of puffs is listed on canister), and child is told to take 8 puffs per day: 8 puffs per day for 25 days equals 200 puffs in canister. So this canister will last 25 days. If child started using this inhaler on May 1, replace it on or before May 25. Write the date on your canister. For quick-relief medicine, take as needed and count each puff. Do not put canisters in water to see if they are empty.

Adapted from National Asthma Education and Prevention Program: *Facts about controlling asthma,* NIH Pub No 97-2339. National Heart, Lung, and Blood Institute (NHLBI). Bethesda, Md. A reproducible handout.

Diagnostic Studies. Characteristic symptoms and clinical findings are the key to diagnosis. A history of atopy in the child or family member is helpful in making the diagnosis of AR. The presence of eosinophils on nasal smear can help substantiate the diagnosis, but is a nonspecific, nonuniversal finding. The presence of nasal eosinophilia often predicts a positive response to nasal corticosteroid sprays. Referrals for skin or serologic testing for IgE antibody to specific allergens should be reserved for the child with significant symptoms who does not respond to traditional management. The ImmunoCAP, in vitro serum tests, can be done to identify suspected allergens (Lasley and Hetherington, 2011).

Differential Diagnosis

Conditions to include as differential diagnoses are the common cold, purulent rhinitis, sinusitis, adenoidal hypertrophy, foreign body obstruction, nasal polyposis of cystic fibrosis, nasopharyngeal tumors, choanal atresia or stenosis, and vasomotor rhinitis. Overuse of prescription or over-the-counter (OTC) topical nasal decongestants can cause drug-induced rhinitis (rhinitis medicamentosa) as can the use of cocaine. Some individuals experience idiopathic rhinitis marked by nasal hyperresponsiveness to nonspecific triggers, such as strong smells (e.g., perfumes, bleach), tobacco smoke, or changes in environmental temperature and humidity. Hormonal rhinitis occurs during pregnancy, puberty, and in hypothyroidism,

Asthma Treatment Plan

(This asthma action plan meets NJ Law N.J.S.A. 18A:40-12.8) (Physician's Orders)

The Pediatric/Adult Asthma Coalition of New Jersey
"Your Pathway to Asthma Control"
PACNJ approved Plan available at www.pacnj.org

Sponsored by
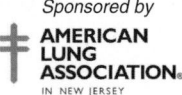
AMERICAN LUNG ASSOCIATION® IN NEW JERSEY

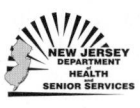

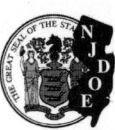

(Please Print)

Name	Date of Birth	Effective Date
Doctor	Parent/Guardian (if applicable)	Emergency Contact
Phone	Phone	Phone

HEALTHY ▐▐▐▶

You have _all_ of these:
- Breathing is good
- No cough or wheeze
- Sleep through the night
- Can work, exercise, and play

And/or Peak flow above _____

Take daily medicine(s). Some metered dose inhalers may be more effective with a "spacer" – use if directed.

MEDICINE	HOW MUCH to take and HOW OFTEN to take it
☐ Advair® ☐ 100, ☐ 250, ☐ 500 _____	1 inhalation twice a day
☐ Advair® HFA ☐ 45, ☐ 115, ☐ 230 _____	2 puffs MDI twice a day
☐ Alvesco® ☐ 80, ☐ 160 _____	☐ 1, ☐ 2 puffs MDI twice a day
☐ Asmanex® Twisthaler® ☐ 110, ☐ 220 _____	☐ 1, ☐ 2 inhalations ☐ once or ☐ twice a day
☐ Flovent® ☐ 44, ☐ 110, ☐ 220 _____	2 puffs MDI twice a day
☐ Flovent® Diskus® ☐ 50 ☐ 100 ☐ 250 ____	1 inhalation twice a day
☐ Pulmicort Flexhaler® ☐ 90, ☐ 180 _____	☐ 1, ☐ 2 inhalations ☐ once or ☐ twice a day
☐ Pulmicort Respules® ☐ 0.25, ☐ 0.5, ☐ 1.0 __	1 unit nebulized ☐ once or ☐ twice a day
☐ Qvar® ☐ 40, ☐ 80 _____	☐ 1, ☐ 2 puffs MDI twice a day
☐ Singulair ☐ 4, ☐ 5, ☐ 10 mg _____	1 tablet daily
☐ Symbicort® ☐ 80, ☐ 160 _____	☐ 1, ☐ 2 puffs MDI twice a day
☐ Other	
☐ None	

Remember to rinse your mouth after taking inhaled medicine.

If exercise triggers your asthma, take this medicine_____ _____ minutes before exercise.

CAUTION ▐▐▐▶

You have _any_ of these:
- Exposure to known trigger
- Cough
- Mild wheeze
- Tight chest
- Coughing at night
- Other:_____

And/or Peak flow from_____ to_____

Continue daily medicine(s) and add fast-acting medicine(s).

MEDICINE	HOW MUCH to take and HOW OFTEN to take it
☐ Accuneb® ☐ 0.63, ☐ 1.25 mg _____	1 unit nebulized every 4 hours as needed
☐ Albuterol ☐ 1.25, ☐ 2.5 mg _____	1 unit nebulized every 4 hours as needed
☐ Albuterol ☐ Pro-Air ☐ Proventil® _____	2 puffs MDI every 4 hours as needed
☐ Ventolin® ☐ Maxair ☐ Xopenex® _____	2 puffs MDI every 4 hours as needed
☐ Xopenex® ☐ 0.31, ☐ 0.63, ☐ 1.25 mg __	1 unit nebulized every 4 hours as needed
☐ Increase the dose of, or add:	
☐ Other	

➡ **If fast-acting medicine is needed more than 2 times a week, except before exercise, then call your doctor.**

EMERGENCY ▐▐▐▶

Your asthma is getting worse fast:
- Fast-acting medicine did not help within 15-20 minutes
- Breathing is hard and fast
- Nose opens wide
- Ribs show
- Trouble walking and talking
- Lips blue • Fingernails blue

And/or Peak flow below _____

Take these medicines NOW and call 911.
Asthma can be a life-threatening illness. Do not wait!

☐ Accuneb® ☐ 0.63, ☐ 1.25 mg _____	1 unit nebulized every 20 minutes
☐ Albuterol ☐ 1.25, ☐ 2.5 mg _____	1 unit nebulized every 20 minutes
☐ Albuterol ☐ Pro-Air ☐ Proventil® _____	2 puffs MDI every 20 minutes
☐ Ventolin® ☐ Maxair ☐ Xopenex® _____	2 puffs MDI every 20 minutes
☐ Xopenex® ☐ 0.31, ☐ 0.63, ☐ 1.25 mg __	1 unit nebulized every 20 minutes
☐ Other	

Triggers
Check all items that trigger patient's asthma:
- ☐ Chalk dust
- ☐ Cigarette Smoke & second hand smoke
- ☐ Colds/Flu
- ☐ Dust mites, dust, stuffed animals, carpet
- ☐ Exercise
- ☐ Mold
- ☐ Ozone alert days
- ☐ Pests - rodents & cockroaches
- ☐ Pets - animal dander
- ☐ Plants, flowers, cut grass, pollen
- ☐ Strong odors, perfumes, cleaning products, scented products
- ☐ Sudden temperature change
- ☐ Wood Smoke
- ☐ Foods: _____

_____
_____
_____

☐ Other: _____
_____
_____
_____

This asthma treatment plan is meant to assist, not replace, the clinical decision-making required to meet individual patient needs.

FOR MINORS ONLY:

☐ This student is capable and has been instructed in the proper method of self-administering of the non-nebulized inhaled medications named above in accordance with NJ Law.

☐ This student is _not_ approved to self-medicate.

Make a copy for patient and for physician file. For children under 18, send original to school nurse or child care provider.

PHYSICIAN/APN/PA SIGNATURE_____ DATE_____

PARENT/GUARDIAN SIGNATURE_____

PHYSICIAN STAMP

FIGURE 24-6 Sample asthma treatment plan. (From the Pediatric Asthma Coalition of New Jersey: *Asthma action plan.* Available at www.pacnj.org/pdfs/asthmatreatmentenglish2010.pdf [accessed Dec 22, 2010]).

and food-induced rhinitis is associated with consumption of hot and spicy foods.

Management

There are four strategies for the management of AR: avoidance, pharmacology, immunotherapy, and education.

Avoidance Strategies. Determining triggering factors if possible and avoiding exposure to the offending allergen or irritant as much as possible are essential. Allergens causing seasonal rhinitis are more difficult to avoid than are the indoor allergens, such as molds, because pollens are smaller and lighter and thus remain in the air longer.

Determine triggering factors if possible. Key avoidance measures for indoor allergens and irritants include the following:

- Control house dust, paying special attention to the child's bedroom.
  - Use dust mite–proof mattress and pillow covers (allergen-impermeable encasement).
  - Wash bed linens in hot water (greater than 130° F [54.4° C]) weekly.
  - Minimize (if possible, eliminate) stuffed toys in child's bedroom
  - Use vertical blinds instead of horizontal blinds or curtains.
  - Remove carpeting from bedroom.
  - Use plastic or wood furniture instead of cloth or upholstered furniture.
- Eliminate smoking from the child's environment; if household members still smoke despite education, stress that they should smoke outside the house.
- Keep pets outdoors; consider not having pets.
- Reduce mold; avoid damp basements and other sources of moisture from the home environment (see Chapter 41 for further discussion of molds).
- Indoor humidity should be less than 50%; avoid vaporizers.
- Use dehumidifiers, air conditioners with efficient filters, and air-cleaning devices with an electronic precipitator or with a high-efficiency particulate air (HEPA) filter.
- Eliminate milk, egg, or wheat for infants with perennial AR, if these prove to be offending substances.
- Vector control for cockroach elimination

Pharmacologic Therapy. Treatment depends on the severity of the symptoms and the ability of the parent or child to comply with recommendations. Intranasal corticosteroids reduce inflammation, edema, and mucus production and are typically a key component in long-term therapy to manage the symptoms associated with AR. Antihistamines are frequently used to treat the symptoms of rhinorrhea, sneezing, and nasal and eye pruritus. Pharmacologic agents should be started 1 to 2 weeks before pollen season for children with seasonal AR. For perennial AR, start with the maximum recommended dose, then taper to the minimum dose needed to control symptoms. Often children with AR benefit from a combination approach; some require only single-line therapy. Antibiotics need to be prescribed for secondary infections (sinusitis).

Oral Antihistamines

- Oral antihistamines are especially helpful in seasonal AR. The second-generation antihistamines are particularly effective in controlling symptoms of AR and are often used to manage this problem.

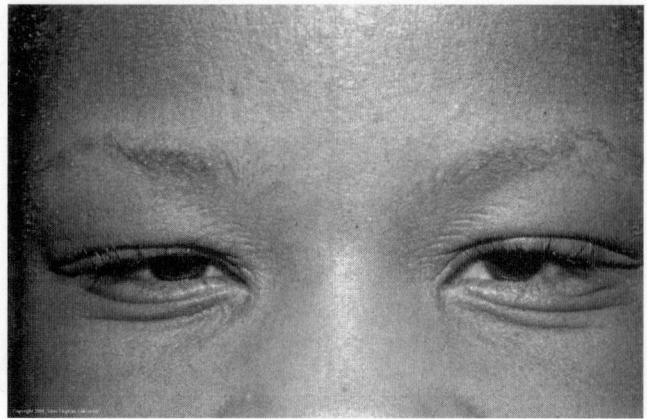

FIGURE 24-7 Dennie line or Morgan line. (From Cohen B: *Pediatric dermatology,* ed 3, Pshiladelphia, 2005, Mosby.)

- Oral antihistamines relieve symptoms of nasal itching, sneezing, and rhinorrhea, but do little to relieve nasal obstruction.
- Oral antihistamines are divided into different classes; different classes of drugs may be more effective for different children (Table 24-7).
- Dosage of drug may need to be increased until relief of symptoms is obtained or side effects are experienced.
- Patients can develop a tolerance to a particular antihistamine and may need to rotate drugs if tolerance develops.
- If side effects with one antihistamine are experienced, another antihistamine in a different class or one in the same class but with different actions should be prescribed.
- Sedating antihistamines may interfere with daytime activities and negatively affect school performance; second-generation antihistamines (e.g., cetirizine, loratadine, and fexofenadine) are associated with less sedation effect.

Topical Nasal Antihistamine

- Azelastine is a nasal antihistamine spray approved for use in seasonal AR in children 5 years and older.
- Azelastine acts by competing with histamine for histamine 1 (H_1)-receptor sites; it has a bitter taste and is associated with sedation.
- Olopatadine is a nasal spray approved for use in children older than 6 years.
- Like nasal azelastine, it is effective in reducing itching, sneezing, rhinorrhea, and congestion (Sheikh and Najib, 2010).

Decongestants

- Decongestants may help relieve nasal congestion; however, they have limited long-term benefit because of adverse effects associated with their use (Lasley and Hetherington, 2011).
- Decongestants may be used alone or in combination with an antihistamine.
- Topical decongestants can cause rebound rhinorrhea (rhinitis medicamentosa) if used for more than 3 to 5 days; errors in administration can cause systemic absorption and side effects of irritability, nervousness, and insomnia among others.
- Children less than 4 years old should not be given decongestants.

Nasal Cromolyn

- Cromolyn is an intranasal mast cell stabilizer used for seasonal or perennial AR.

TABLE 24-7	Antihistamine Classes*	
Class	**Name**	**Comments**
Ethanolamines	Diphenhydramine	Sedation, dizziness, thickening of bronchial secretions
	Clemastine	Dry mouth, fatigue, headache, somnolence, bradycardia
	Carbinoxamine	Drowsiness, CNS excitation and difficulty sleeping
Ethylenediamine	Pyrilamine	Not used in children
	Tripelennamine	Not used in children
Alkylamines	Chlorpheniramine	Drowsiness, sedation, dry mouth, GI symptoms
	Brompheniramine	Palpitations, weight gain, drowsiness, dizziness, headache
Piperazines	Hydroxyzines	Sedation, dizziness, dry mouth
Piperidines	Cyproheptadine	CNS depression or stimulation, weight gain, dry mouth
Nonsedating antihistamines	Loratadine	Dry mouth, fatigue, headache, somnolence. Approved for children ≥2 years old
	Cetirizine	Dry mouth, fatigue, headache, somnolence. Approved for children ≥2 years old
	Fexofenadine	Dry mouth, fatigue, headache, somnolence, dysmenorrhea, flulike signs. Approved for children ≥6 years old

*The CDC released a report warning about the use of cough and cold medications in children <4 years old. Products containing nasal decongestants (e.g., pseudoephedrine), antihistamines (e.g., carbinoxamine), cough suppressants (e.g., dextromethorphan), and expectorants are often used by parents of children in this age group; however, their use is associated with adverse side effects that may lead to death in children <2 yr old. This warning now applies to children less than 4 yr old.
CNS, Central nervous system; GI, gastrointestinal.
Data from CDC: Infant deaths associated with cough and cold medications—two states, 2005, *MMWR Morb Mortal Wkly Rep* 56(01):1-4, 2007. Available at www.cdc.gov/mmwr/preview/mmwrhtml/mm5601a1.htm; U.S. Food and Drug Administration: Using Over-the-Counter Cough and Cold Products in Children (www.fda.gov/ForConsumers/ConsumerUpdates/ucm048515.htm). Accessed April 26, 2011.

- It is less effective than intranasal corticosteroids, and frequent dosing is needed (Becker, 2009).

Intranasal Corticosteroids
- Corticosteroids are effective in reducing inflammation and subsequent nasal obstruction. The child should clear the nasal passages of mucus before use.
- Corticosteroids are considered one of the most effective treatments to manage AR and have been safely used in long-term management of this condition.
- Corticosteroids can be effective for relieving symptoms of nasal congestion, rhinorrhea, itching, and sneezing.
- Corticosteroids can take 1 week or more before clinical benefit is observed.
- Side effects can include local burning, irritation, sneezing, or soreness (<10% experience these symptoms). Epistaxis is related to improper technique—spraying the nasal septum (Lasley and Hetherington, 2011).
- Table 24-8 lists usual dosages per nostril for intranasal corticosteroid preparations (Taketomo et al, 2011).

Leukotriene Modifiers
- Montelukast is approved for use in seasonal and perennial AR.
- It has a moderate effect when used alone (Sheikh and Najib, 2010).

Antibiotics
- Treat secondary infections (e.g., sinusitis and otitis media) with appropriate antibiotics.

Immunotherapy. Allergen immunotherapy is indicated when symptoms are severe and have not improved with avoidance measures and pharmacologic therapy or when complications of chronic or recurrent sinusitis or otitis media and hearing loss are problematic. It should only be performed in a facility that has both the necessary equipment and health care professionals who are prepared to treat anaphylaxis.

Complications
Sinusitis may complicate AR owing to associated swelling of the mucosal lining of the sinuses with secondary infection. Likewise eustachian tube dysfunction and its sequela, serous otitis media, are common complications. Malocclusion, the development of a high-arched palate, and the typical allergic facies can result from long-standing AR. Sleep disturbances, irritability, and poor performance in school are associated with AR. In addition, chronic AR may lead to chronic cough and postnasal drip.

If a child has both AR and asthma, treatment of the child's AR is essential if the child's asthma is to be effectively managed.

Patient and Parent Education and Prevention
Because AR is often a chronic problem, parents and children need to have specific information about controlling this disorder.
- Instruct on environmental control. Handouts and a review of ways to individualize this information are essential.
- Review pharmacologic therapy, including the following:
  - Indications for and changes in medications
  - Frequency of use
  - Common side effects and contraindications
  - How to use intranasal sprays or inhalers if prescribed

Prognosis
Perennial AR can be a chronic problem unless offending allergens are identified and eliminated from the environment. If this is not possible, pharmacologic therapy is usually helpful in reducing symptoms. As the child grows and the nasal

TABLE 24-8	Intranasal Corticosteroid Preparations Used for Allergic Rhinitis: Usual Doses		
Drug	**Dose**	**Number of Inhalations or Sprays and Daily Frequency**	**Age**
Beclomethasone	42 mcg/inhalation	1 or 2 sprays twice a day (decrease to 1 spray when symptoms controlled)	6-12 yr
		1 twice to four times a day or 2 twice a day	≥12 yr
Beclomethasone—aqueous inhalation	42 mcg/inhalation 84 mcg/spray	1-2 twice a day 1-2 once daily	≥6 yr ≥6 yr
Budesonide*	32 mcg/spray	Initial: 1 spray/nostril once daily; <12 yr 2 sprays/nostril daily max; > 12 yr 4 sprays/nostril daily max	≥6 yr
Flunisolide	25 and 29 mcg/spray	1 spray/nostril three times a day or 2 sprays twice daily to a max of 4 sprays each nostril daily; maintenance dose is 1 spray daily	6-14 yr
		2 sprays/nostril twice a day to 2 sprays/nostril three times/day; maintenance 1 spray daily	≥14 yr
Fluticasone	50 mcg/spray	1 spray/nostril daily; 2 sprays daily if severe or poor response; reduce to 1 spray/nostril/day once symptoms controlled	≥4 yr
		2 sprays/nostril daily or 1 spray/nostril twice daily; may reduce to 1 spray/nostril daily once symptoms controlled	>12 yr
Mometasone	50 mcg/spray	1 spray daily 2 sprays daily	2-11 yr >12 yr
Triamcinolone AQ	55 mcg/spray	1 spray/nostrol daily; max dose 2 sprays/nostril daily	2-11yr
		2 sprays/nostril daily; may increase to 2 sprays/nostril daily; maintenance dose 1 spray/nostril daily	>12 yr
Tri-Nasal ® (Triamcinolone)	50 mcg/inhalation	2 sprays daily; may increase to 4 sprays daily or 2 sprays twice a day; titrate when symptoms controlled	>12 yr

*Reduce slowly every 2 to 4 weeks to smallest effective dose.
Data from Taketomo CK, Hodding JH, Kraus DM: *Pediatric dosage handbook,* ed 17, Hudson, OH, 2011, Lexi-Comp.

passages increase in size, symptoms may also lessen. Symptoms from seasonal AR often worsen from the adolescent years to mid-adulthood. Moving to a new environment often results in a short respite (1 to 3 years) from symptoms. However, the child frequently becomes sensitized to new airborne pollens and symptoms of seasonal AR return.

ATOPIC DERMATITIS

Description

AD is a common skin disorder of childhood that is characterized by acute and chronic skin eruptions. The term *eczema* is sometimes used interchangeably with *atopic dermatitis.* Eczema means flaring up, which describes the acute symptom complex (erythema, scaling, vesicles, inflamed papules and plaques, and crusts) seen with AD, but does not adequately describe the chronic skin changes that can result from this disorder. AD manifests a typical morphology and distribution of flexural lichenification or linearity in adults and facial and extensor involvement in infants and children. AD is frequently referred to as the "itch that rashes." With AD, the skin's ability to act as a protective barrier is impaired, resulting in xerosis (dry skin), cracking, an increase in skin markings, lichenification, and susceptibility to bacterial, viral, and fungal infections (see the Color Plate).

Epidemiology

AD affects approximately 10% to 12% of the childhood population in the U.S. with higher incidence in other countries and African-Americans and Asian children having a higher frequency in health care visits for AD (Krafchik, 2010). AD develops in 85% of children within the first 12 months of life, and in 95% of children before age 5 years. Approximately 0.9% of adults have AD; some of whom had an adult onset but the majority had AD as a child. AD is often the first manifestation of the "atopic march" with asthma and AR following. Asthma also develops in approximately 30% and AR develops in 35% of those with AD. The incidence of AD is increasing in the U.S. (Krafchik, 2010).

The exact etiology is unknown and may vary from individual to individual. Although many children have high IgE levels, an exact immune mechanism for this disorder is not evident The identification of the filaggrin (FLG) mutation has been identified as a risk factor for AD. The FLG is produced in the stratum granulosum and contributes to the natural moisture in the stratum corneum. Therefore, a lack of stratum corneum hydration and an increase in the pH caused by a defect in the FLG cause an impaired barrier function (Wollenberg and Schnopp, 2010). Immune dysregulation involving IgE sensitization resulting in a malfunction of the epithelial-barrier, epidermal barrier dysfunction, and pharmacophysiologic abnormalities

TABLE 24-9	Assessment of Atopic Dermatitis	
Onset	**Signs and Symptoms**	**Comment/Prognosis**
Initial presentation • <3 months old • 2-3 months old	Dry skin first sign Itch-scratch-itch cycle starts	Often not noticed
Infantile phase	Acute presentation—common in infants: intense itching; redness, papules, vesicles, edema; serous discharge and crusts; xerosis, dry hair, scalp; diaper area sparing; cheeks, forehead, scalp, extremities	Two thirds of cases resolve by 2-3 years
Childhood phase (starts 2 years old to puberty)	Involves wrists, hands, popliteal and antecubital fossa; eyebrows thin and broken off (Hertog sign); some only have feet involved; may have allergic-atopic facies and white dermatographism	One third continue into teenage years
Adolescent phase	Common in children and teenagers; thickened, leathery, hyperpigmented skin; scratch marks	New or recurrent problem

are implicated in its pathogenesis. A defect in the epithelial barrier integrity is a contributing factor to the onset of AD. If the epithelial barrier is impaired, transepidermal water loss in normal as well as lesioned skin increases. When the barrier's integrity is impaired due to allergy and irritants, there is cytokine production, inflammation, and the development of lesions (Spergel, 2010). Abnormalities in histamine production (increased in the skin), chemotaxis, monocytes, and cytokines are associated with AD. T-lymphocyte activation and hyperresponsiveness of Langerhans cells are also thought to be implicated in its expression. Th2 lymphocytes infiltrate the dermis in the acute stage; Th1 cells predominate in the chronic phase. A positive family history of AD is common as is a family history of atopic disease. Sweating increases itching in atopic skin, and transepidermal water loss is increased. A predisposition to development of pruritus is believed to be a key factor with variability in the extent of the skin involvement and severity of presentation (Krafchik, 2010; Laskey and Hetherington, 2011).

Clinical Findings

The following are seen in AD (Krafchik, 2010; Paller and Mancini, 2011) (Table 24-9):

- Essential diagnostic features include pruritus and eczematous changes that reflect typical age-specific morphologic patterns and a chronic or relapsing skin condition.
- More than one third of cases begin before 3 months old. Dry skin is the only initial sign. These infants are generally not brought in for health care until pruritus and the itch-scratch-itch cycle develops, generally around 2 to 3 months old.
- Acute manifestations (more common in infants) include the following:
  - Intense itching
  - Redness
  - Papules, vesicles, and edema
  - Serous discharge and crusts
  - Generalized dry skin (xerosis) with dry hair and scalp; diaper area usually spared
  - Lichenification is typically not seen

- Chronic manifestations (more common in children and adolescents) include the following:
  - Lichenification—thickened, leathery, hyperpigmented skin
  - Scratch marks
  - Generalized xerosis with flaky and rough skin
- Characteristics of infantile phase:
  - Begins from birth to 6 months old; may resolve but can continue into the childhood phase
  - Cheeks, forehead, scalp, extending to trunk as symmetric patches or to the extremities; lateral extensor surface of arms and legs
  - Tends to be acute with intense itching, erythema, papules, vesicles, oozing crusting, and generalized xerosis; the diaper area and groin are usually spared of lesions
- Characteristics of childhood phase:
  - Beginning around 2 years old and lasting to puberty or may continue from the infantile phase
  - Classic areas of involvement include the wrists (hands), neck, ankles (feet), popliteal and antecubital fossae, commonly of flexural areas; periorbital and perioral areas may also be involved.
  - Eyebrows can be thin and broken off (loss of the lateral half of the eyebrow is called Hertog sign).
  - Tends to be chronic; possible lichenification
  - Pruritus is often severe.
  - Lesions tend to be dry and papular with circumscribed scaly patches.
- Characteristics of adolescent/adult phase:
  - Begins at puberty and can commonly continue into adulthood; often involves the flexural folds (popliteal and antecubital fossae), face, neck, upper arms and back, dorsa of hands, fingers, feet, and toes
  - May be new occurrence or recurrence of a chronic condition
  - Dry skin and lichenification are prominent findings.
  - Erythematous, dry-scaling papules and plaques with fewer exudates
  - Postinflammatory hypopigmentation or hyperpigmentation that disappears

- Other key features of AD:
  - Tendency toward dry skin and a lowered threshold for itching (itch-scratch-itch cycle)
  - Tendency to worsen during dry winter months or with heat in the summer
  - Chronic AD often secondarily infected with *Staphylococcus aureus* (most commonly) or *Streptococcus pyogenes* (occasionally)
  - Hyperpigmentation may be noted especially in areas of lichenification
- Possible associated features:
  - Atopic pleats—extra groove in lower eyelid called Dennie lines or Morgan fold (see Fig. 24-7), crease across upper bulb of nose
  - Accentuated palmar and flexural creases
  - Allergic shiners, mild facial pallor, or dry hair
  - Keratosis pilaris—follicular papules occurring on the extensor aspect of the arms, anterior thighs, and lateral aspects of the cheeks
  - Nummular eczema, dyshidrotic eczema, juvenile plantar dermatitis, nipple eczema, or ichthyosis vulgaris
  - White dermatographism—a red line first appears with firm stroking of the skin, but is replaced by a white line in approximately 10 seconds but without an associated wheal; the normal reaction of skin is to develop a red line at the site of stroking, followed by a red flare, and then later a wheal in 1 to 3 minutes
  - Some with AD have an associated circumoral pallor (thought to be related to local edema and vasoconstriction)

Diagnostic Studies. Diagnosis of AD is based on characteristic historical and physical findings. A chronic or recurring rash that is pruritic and has a characteristic distribution and appearance, together with a family or personal history of atopy, are key in leading to the diagnosis of AD. Histologic examination of the skin is rarely needed and is reserved only for cases that are difficult to diagnose and to exclude other diseases. There is a more severe subtype associated with IgE responses to allergens and a higher rate of secondary infection and a milder form lacking these features (Wollenberg and Schnopp, 2010). Immunologic testing (e.g., IgE, CAP-RAST, or prick test) is not needed to confirm the diagnosis or to monitor treatment. Skin testing and desensitization are not routinely recommended for children with AD only. If secondary fungal infection is suspected, collect scrapings and use potassium hydroxide (KOH) to look for fungal hyphae.

Differential Diagnosis

Other types of dermatitis, including seborrheic dermatitis, contact dermatitis, allergic contact dermatitis, nummular dermatitis, psoriasis, and scabies, are included in the differential diagnosis. A few genetic conditions are associated with similar skin eruptions (e.g., phenylketonuria, Wiskott-Aldrich syndrome, histiocytosis X, and acrodermatitis enteropathica). Pityriasis alba can also be a differential diagnosis.

Management

Treatment strategy is based on the following key concepts:
- The itch-scratch-itch cycle must be interrupted.
- Dryness of the skin must be corrected by rehydrating the stratum corneum; good moisturization is critical.

- If there are known offending agents (irritants and allergic triggers), they must be eliminated.
- Secondary bacterial or viral infections must be treated.

Acute versus chronic care management is also a consideration. The following therapies are key factors in the control of AD.

Pharmacotherapy
- Antihistamine agents have little direct effect on pruritus, but sedating doses at night help children with pruritus—which is worse at night—fall asleep. They have limited effectiveness as monotherapy in AD. The following agents are often used (Taketomo et al, 2011):
  - Hydroxyzine has excellent antihistaminic qualities, but can cause drowsiness and behavioral changes. If an antihistamine is needed throughout the day, the usual oral dose of hydroxyzine in children is 2 mg/kg/day divided every 6 to 8 hours (Taketomo et al, 2011). This dose may need to be increased.
  - Diphenhydramine hydrochloride is also a useful antihistamine, especially if sedation is also needed. The usual oral dose of diphenhydramine hydrochloride in children is as follows: 2 to 6 years old, 6.25 mg every 4 to 6 hours with 37.5 mg/day maximum; 6 to 12 years old, 12.5 to 25 mg every 4 to 6 hours with 150 mg/day maximum; children older than 12 years, 25 to 50 mg every 4 to 6 hours with 300 mg/day maximum (Taketomo et al, 2011).
  - Doxepin is a tricyclic antidepressant with strong antihistamine activity used by dermatologists for the treatment of itch. It is not approved for use in children and the risk of suicidal ideation should be assessed if a patient is on this drug. It is also available as doxepin 5% cream but due to potential for sedation and overdosage, this formulation is not used in children.
- Nonsedating or low-sedating antihistamines may be considered (see Table 24-7).
- Topical corticosteroid preparations (TCPs) are a mainstay of therapy because they reduce inflammation and pruritus. Do not apply topical steroids containing propylene glycol because it irritates the skin (Krafchik, 2010). The classification of the TCP should be known because potent and very potent TCPs are associated with more side effects such as thinning of the skin or adrenal axis suppression than milder preparations (Wollenberg and Schnopp, 2010). A proactive approach to the treatment of AD includes twice weekly application of TCP for up to 4 months once the lesions are quiet. The rationale for this approach is that the skin is actually not normal and has a defect in hydration, which can be treated using an intermittent approach (Wollenberg and Schnopp, 2010).
  - Gels penetrate well, are somewhat more drying, and are effective in the management of acute weeping or vesicular lesions.
  - Ointments penetrate more effectively than creams or lotions and provide occlusion. They are beneficial in the management of dry, lichenified, or plaquelike areas; however, they may occlude eccrine ducts and lead to sweating.
  - When applied over large areas of dermatitis or if occlusion (covering with plastic wrap) is used, the possibility of significant systemic absorption is greatly increased, especially in infants and young children.

○ Apply a thin layer of TCP cream (acute stage) or ointment (chronic stage) to affected areas marked with acute exacerbations three or four times a day.

○ Use of fluorinated, TCP in children should only be done in consultation with a physician or a dermatology specialist. Never use fluorinated, topical corticosteroid preparations on the face; instead use 1% hydrocortisone ointment sparingly two or three times a day until symptoms improve and then withdraw. Tapering of steroids begins as the erythema and itch subsides (Wollenberg and Schnopp, 2010). Combine the baseline moisturizing skin care with an antiinflammatory. Do not use for an extended period because corticosteroids cause thinning of the skin (see Table 36-1 for a listing of topical corticosteroids by potency rating).

○ Decisions about which topical steroid and the potency to be prescribed should be based on the extent and severity of the AD. Taper to a less potent topical steroid once the AD is controlled or use it intermittently to control flares. If such steroids are rapidly discontinued, a rebound phenomenon can occur. If possible, apply topical corticosteroids within the first 3 minutes after a bath or shower because their absorption is improved when the skin is hydrated.

• Immunomodulators (tacrolimus 0.03% ointment and pimecrolimus 1% cream) can be used in nonimmunosuppressed children 2 years and older and are reserved for moderate to severe AD for those who did not respond to conventional therapy. They are approved as second-line agents for short-term and intermittent therapy but do have black box warnings. These NSAIDs block calcineurin, which is a protein phosphatase that causes T-cell activation. The most common side effect is stinging or burning, which starts 5 minutes after the application and can last for an hour but usually decreases after 1 week (Wollenberg and Schnopp, 2010), usually during the first several days of administration and in severe cases of AD. They are safe steroid-sparing agents and work well on thinner skin of the face, neck, groin, and axillae. Sun protection is needed with their use (Lasley and Hetherington, 2011).

• Skin barrier repair and treatment: Drugs (EpiCeram and Eletone) that improve the skin hydration barrier are available by prescription. These drugs are used twice a day. They are expensive and not covered by all insurance plans.

• Treatment of colonization and infection: The immune dysregulation in AD causes a tendency to colonize with *S. aureus* as well as viral infection including herpes simplex. The reduction of colonization with staphylococcus as well as treatment of infection may be equally as important (Wollenberg and Schnopp, 2010). The literature suggests that prophylactic baths with sodium hypochlorite (bleach) twice a week can decrease *S. aureus* colonization (Huang et al, 2009).

Skin Care. Hydration is a key element in the treatment of AD (Krafchik, 2010; Paller and Mancini, 2011).

• Use open wet compresses if there are weeping, oozing lesions and signs of acute skin inflammation. They also help rehydrate the skin.

○ Aluminum acetate (Burow solution in a 1:20 or 1:40 preparation). Solution should be lukewarm or body temperature.

○ Use a soft cloth that is moderately wet and not dripping; remoisten as needed. Corticosteroid topical preparations can be applied after application of compresses.

○ Apply two or three times a day to the affected skin; can use up to 5 days; effective during the acute stage of AD.

○ Aveeno or oatmeal baths help soothe acute episodes of pruritus, followed by application of a heavy cream emollient (the thicker and greasier the emollient the more effective).

• Lukewarm soaking baths for 10 minutes to reduce skin dryness. Excessive soaking in the bathtub depletes the skin of natural moisturizers. Use lukewarm, not hot, water, which can trigger itching. Use mild, unscented soap with a neutral pH, such as Dove, Oil of Olay, Aveeno, and Purpose, for the axilla and groin. Do not use drying or deodorant soaps, bubble-bath products, and oils in bath water. Immediately after bathing gently pat the child with a towel (do not completely dry the skin) and quickly apply the emollient. Some recommend two baths daily, each less than 5 minutes, immediately followed by lubricating oils or ointments as a way to restore water to the skin.

• Cetaphil, Diprobase, and Unguentum (Merck) are nondrying soap-free cleansing agents and can be substituted for bathing. Instruct parents to leave these agents on the skin; they should not be wiped off after applying. Patients with wool or lanolin sensitivity should use glycerin moisturizers, such as Cetaphil.

• Immediately after bath or shower, gently pat dry within 3 minutes; no rubbing or scrubbing. Emolliate with a moisturizer. Lubricants maintain the skin's hydration, and emollients are the treatment of choice for dry skin.

○ An ointment-based emollient (e.g., Vaseline, petrolatum jelly, Crisco, vegetable oil, whipped petrolatum, Aquaphor, and Elta) can be applied just before getting out of the bath water or just after getting out of the bath while still damp. If patients do not like the greasy feel of an ointment, other topical creams (e.g., Vanicream, Cereve, Cetaphil) can be used. This is also a good time to apply TCPs because absorption of the agent is more effective if the skin is hydrated.

• Emollients can be applied three or four times a day as needed, such as fragrance-free Eucerin cream, Crisco (plain, not butter flavored), Aveeno, Moisturel, Neutrogena, Dermasil, Curel, or petroleum jelly (an occlusive agent). If a child is sensitive to fragrances, scented creams, such as Nivea and Vaseline Intensive Care, should be avoided. TriCeram is a moisturizer that repairs the stratum corneum barrier function. It is a ceramide-dominant, lipid-based emollient. Urea-containing products, such as Aquacare cream or lotion and Ureacin Crème, soften and moisturize dry skin. Stinging is a side effect when used on fissured or flaring skin.

• Children with severe AD may need additional soaking after baths to maintain skin hydration. This should be done at bedtime. Wet gauze and bandage wraps, wrung out to dampness, can be placed on the extremities with a dry dressing over them. Cotton pajamas or soaks can also be used with a wet, wrung-dry pajama or soak next to the skin and then covered with a corresponding dry pajama or sock. For some children with AD (xerotic individuals), frequent bathing may exacerbate their pruritus and thus aggravate their skin problems. Bathing must be limited in these patients and emollients used. If a child experiences stinging when bathing during acute exacerbations, adding 1 cup of table salt into the bath may reduce the stinging sensation.

- Keep fingernails short to decrease additional skin trauma from scratching.
- Consider stopping the use of fabric softeners and using a sensitive skin detergent (e.g., All Free Clear).

Secondary Infection Management

- Systemic antibiotic agents are essential if secondary skin infection with *S. aureus* or *S. pyogenes* is suspected.
  - First-generation cephalosporins are most commonly used.
  - Be cognizant that community-based methicillin-resistant *Staphylococcus aureus* (MRSA) has been rapidly increasing (see discussion in Chapter 23 on how to identify and manage).
  - Topical antibiotic preparations are contraindicated, although the use of mupirocin has been demonstrated to reduce colony counts of *S. aureus*. Intermittent application of mupirocin to the nares and hands of patients and their caregivers twice daily for 3 weeks may decrease colonization.
  - Topical antibacterial scrubs are contraindicated because they dry out the skin and cause irritation.
- The addition of ⅛ to ¼ cup of chlorine bleach in a full tub of bath water has been shown to transiently decrease *S. aureus* colonization of the skin.
- Topical antifungal medication is recommended if KOH positive for hyphae.

Other Therapies

- Tar preparations may be added to help manage chronic and lichenified forms of dermatitis.
  - These are topical agents that have limited use.
  - Patients should be cautioned about photosensitivity.
- Systemic corticosteroid agents are rarely needed.
- Ultraviolet (UV) light treatment may benefit some; however, it is rarely used because of the risk of skin cancer.

Environmental Management

- A decrease in environmental humidity and an increase in antigen presentation are key causative factors. Therefore, increase environmental humidity and decrease exposure to antigens. Cool temperatures (e.g., through the use of air conditioning) help.
- Eliminate or avoid known or suspected offending agents. These include:
  - Nonbreathable fabrics—nylon or wool; wool is irritating, whereas soft cotton clothing is not. Clothes should be loose fitting.
  - Overheating and overdressing (heat and perspiration are irritant triggers that increase pruritus).
  - Chlorine, turpentine, harsh soaps, fabric softeners, products with fragrances, and bleach.
  - Allergenic agents, such as feather pillows, fuzzy toys, stuffed animals, pets.
  - House dust mites—careful attention to the child's bedroom is important (e.g., encasing mattresses and pillows, washing bedding in hot water weekly, frequent vacuuming, removing carpets or at least frequent cleaning are recommended).

Dietary Management

- Dietary restrictions may include eliminating cow's milk from the diet of infants predisposed to atopy. Eggs, fish, chocolate, nuts, and citrus fruits are generally not allowed until 12 months old. In some infants and young children, a food allergen may contribute to their AD; elimination of the food may reduce symptoms. However, food allergens in older children and adults are not a common trigger.
- A study on supplementing the early diet of infants with probiotics demonstrated a reduction in the occurrence of AD in the first year of life (Grüber et al, 2010).

Referral. Refer to a dermatologist if a child is unresponsive to traditional therapy or has an unusual manifestation.

Complications

Secondary skin infections are a frequent complication of AD. *S. aureus* is the most frequent bacterial organism associated with skin infection. Treatment of secondary skin infection is imperative in the management of AD. Kaposi varicelliform eruption (eczema herpeticum) is a significant complication that can result in severe illness in children. Lichenification, a secondary skin change marked by thickening of the skin, is associated with chronic itching. Keratoconus is occasionally seen and is associated with chronic rubbing of the eyelids. Individuals with AD may be prone to molluscum contagiosum, tinea, and warts. The risk of developing lymphoma is dramatically increased in individuals with AD, especially with the use of potent topical steroids and their long-term use (Krafchik, 2010).

Patient and Parent Education and Prevention for Outpatient Management

The provider should stress that AD is often a recurrent disease that can be controlled. The goal of therapy is to prevent the itch-scratch-itch cycle and hydrate the skin. Specific written instructions and handouts should be provided because management is complex.

Parents need to understand:

- The use of medications (when, how much, and how often to use; side effects; and proper application of topical preparations)
- Care of the skin
- The risks for secondary infection
- The role of environmental controls of allergens or triggers
- Possible dietary management as outlined previously
- What to do if symptoms worsen or signs of secondary skin infection appear and when to seek additional medical treatment
- Precipitating factors
  - Extreme temperatures or humidity
  - Excess sweat
  - Emotional stress
  - New clothes—wash with mild detergent (with no dyes or perfumes) before wearing them to remove formaldehyde and other chemicals
  - Harsh washing detergents—add second rinse cycle when washing clothes
  - Wearing coarse clothes
  - Excess soap and water
  - Cutaneous or systemic infection

Prognosis

With appropriate treatment, AD can generally be controlled. In two thirds of children, the symptoms of AD become less severe, with complete remission in 20%. However, there is an adolescent and adult stage of the disease. Risk factors for adult AD include widespread dermatitis as a child, family history of AD, early initial childhood age of onset, high serum IgE levels, and a history of asthma or AR (Lasley and Hetherington, 2011). Self-image problems may result if AD is severe.

■ Diseases With an Autoimmune Basis

JUVENILE IDIOPATHIC ARTHRITIS (JUVENILE RHEUMATOID ARTHRITIS)

Description

The chronic arthritides of childhood present unique challenges to the child, family, and the pediatric provider. JIA is a disease with an autoimmune basis and represents a group of conditions with onset of symptoms in children at or younger than 16 years old that causes chronic inflammation of at least one synovial joint for 6 weeks or more. As noted in the beginning of this chapter, JIA is a newer term used by the International League of Associations for Rheumatology. There are various subtypes of the chronic arthritides in children that are categorized based on differences in their disease onset, severity, duration, and pattern of complications. The three principal types of arthritis are polyarticular (five or more joints involved), pauciarticular or oligoarticular (inflammation of one to four joints), or systemic onset with fever, characteristic rash, and serositis. Some health care providers (generally outside the U.S.) prefer to call this syndrome juvenile idiopathic arthritis instead of JRA; the term JIA will likely replace the JRA classification (Haftel, 2011; Rabinovich, 2010).

Epidemiology

The exact cause of JIA is unknown. Approximately 1 in 1000 children are affected with oligoarticular, the most common arthritic subtype. Certain histocompatibility complex antigens are more prevalent in the JIA population. Cytokine production, proliferation of macrophage-like synoviocytes, infiltration with neutrophils and T-lymphocytes, and autoimmunity are thought to be the major pathologic processes causing chronic joint inflammation (Haftel, 2011; Rabinovich, 2010).

The rate of JIA is significantly higher in girls than in boys typically in oligoarticular and pauciarticular JIA. The female to male ratio in systemic onset is equal. The approximate percentage of occurrence and age breakdown for each of the subtypes follows: systemic—10% and occurs at any age; polyarticular—40% and has a late (6 to 12 years old) or early childhood onset (1 to 4 years); and oligoarticular—50% with a late or early onset. Adolescents tend to have more rheumatoid factor–positive disease (Haftel, 2011; Rabinovich, 2010).

Clinical Findings

History. The major complaints of the child with JIA are:
- Pain—generally a mild to moderate aching
- Joint stiffness—worse in the morning and after rest; arthralgia may occur during the day

Physical Examination. Associated features are:
- Nonmigratory monoarticular or polyarticular involvement of large or proximal interphalangeal joints for more than 3 months
- Systemic manifestations—fever, erythematous rashes, leukocytosis, serositis, lymphadenopathy, and rheumatoid nodules

Less commonly seen are ocular disease (e.g., iridocyclitis, iritis, or uveitis), pleuritis, pericarditis, anemia of chronic disease, fatigue, and growth failure, or leg lengths discrepancy if the arthritis is unilateral.

Key physical findings are:
- Swelling of the joint with effusion or thickening of synovial membrane, or both, noted on palpation
- Heat over inflamed joint and tenderness along joint line
- Loss of joint range of motion and function; child typically holds the affected joints in slight flexion and may walk with limp

There are three major patterns of presentation (Haftel, 2011):

1. *Systemic-onset pattern* with spiking fevers once or twice a day at approximately the same time of day that can last for months, an evanescent (lasting a few hours) pale or salmon-pink macular rash (occurs with fever), hepatosplenomegaly, leukocytosis, and polyserositis; the arthritis is typically polyarticular and follows the systemic manifestations in 6 weeks to 6 months. This group does not develop iridocyclitis.

2. *Polyarticular pattern (five or more synovial joints involved within the first 6 months of diagnosis)* of chronic pain and symmetric joint swelling; low-grade fever, fatigue, nodules, and anemia of chronic disease may be present, but are not as prominent as in acute form; uveitis occurs in this subtype; typically involves the small joints of the hands, feet, ankles, wrists, and knees and can also involve the cervical spine. Adolescents who develop this type differ from those with early onset in that they exhibit a positive RF. Adolescents who develop late-onset polyarticular JIA have a course similar to the adult entity.

3. *Oligoarticular pattern* with involvement of few joints, typically the weight-bearing joints within the first 6 months of diagnosis; synovitis may be mild and painless; joint involvement is asymmetric and involves medium-sized joints (commonly the knees) followed by the ankle and wrist; often the laboratory values do not demonstrate evidence of inflammation; and patients do not tend to have signs of systemic inflammation.

Each of the three principal types of JIA has a typical pattern of presentation. For more information on the specific presentation of the other subtypes of JIA, the primary care provider should consult other texts on this subject.

Diagnostic Studies. Diagnosis is based on physical findings and history of arthritis lasting for 6 weeks or longer and having excluded all other possible differential diagnoses; there is no diagnostic laboratory test for JIA. Most children with oligoarticular arthritis have negative laboratory markers. Those with polyarticular and systemic-onset typically have elevated acute-phase reactants and anemia of chronic disease. A positive result for RF by latex fixation may be present but occurs in less than 10% of children and rarely in those with systemic JIA. ANA may be present in up to 50% of children with oligoarticular disease. A positive ANA helps identify children at higher risk for uveitis. The anti-CCP test has been added to the initial workup of JIA as citrullinated residues are part of the essential antigenic components that are recognized by autoantibodies in rheumatoid arthritis (von Venrooij & Pruijin, 2000). This test has a specificity of 99% and a sensitivity of 70% to 75%. The use of both FR and anti-CCP improves sensitivity (Waits). Other laboratory tests that may be useful include a CBC (to exclude leukemia); ESR, and C-reactive protein (CRP) nonspecific markers of inflammation. Other findings may include lymphopenia, anemia, and hypoalbuminemia. However, laboratory studies may be normal in these children. Imaging studies (magnetic resonance imaging [MRI]) can help in managing joint pathologic conditions. Analysis of synovial fluid is not helpful in the diagnosis of JIA.

Differential Diagnosis

The various causes of monoarticular arthritis should be considered in the differential diagnosis. These include tumors, leukemia, cancer, bacterial infections, toxic synovitis, rheumatic fever, SLE, Lyme disease, spondyloarthropathies, inflammatory bowel disease, septic arthritis, and chondromalacia patellae.

Management

Children with severe involvement should be followed by a specialist in pediatric rheumatology. Other pediatric subspecialists, such as orthopedists, ophthalmologists, and cardiologists may be consulted as needed. Therapy depends on the degree of local or systemic involvement.

The main treatment goals are to suppress inflammation, preserve and maximize joint function and prevent joint deformities, and prevent blindness. Aspirin therapy has largely been replaced with the use of NSAIDs. Pharmacologic agents commonly used in the management of JIA include the following (Haftel, 2011):
- NSAIDs: Children with oligoarthritis generally respond well to NSAIDs.
  - Ibuprofen: 10 mg/kg/dose qid (maximum 1000 mg/day)
  - Tolmetin: 20 to 30 mg/kg/day divided tid (maximum 2000 mg/day)
  - Naproxen: 10 mg/kg bid (maximum 1000 mg/day)
  - Indomethacin, older than 2 years: 1 to 2 mg/kg/day divided in two to four doses (maximum 4 mg/kg/day); adults 25 to 50 mg/dose two or three times/day (maximum 200 mg/day) (Taketomo et al, 2010)
  - Celecoxib (older than 17 years) 100 to 200 mg every day to bid (maximum 400 mg/day)
- Oral or parenteral corticosteroids used as bridging therapy until other medications take effect
- Second-line medication such as hydroxychloroquine, sulfasalazine, the TNF-α agents (e.g., etanercept, infliximab, and adalimumab—drugs that soak up tumor necrosis factor, an immune-system protein, and block the inflammatory cascade), methotrexate, or anakinra are used in severe forms of JIA.
- Intraarticular corticosteroid injections are used if there is severe joint involvement.
- Pharmacologic therapy for uveitis is given as indicated by an ophthalmologist. Females with ANA-positive oligoarticular JIA are at high risk and require slit-lamp examination every 3 to 4 months. The uveitis often does not correspond to the severity of the arthritis (i.e., uveitis may be present despite quiescent arthritis).
- Physical therapy—range of motion muscle-strengthening exercises and heat treatments—is used for joint involvement, and occupational therapy is beneficial. Rest and splinting are used if indicated.
- Ophthamologic follow-up every 3 months for 4 years (even if the arthritis has resolved) for all ANA-positive JIA patients. They have a greater risk of uveitis that may not be clinically apparent but can lead to blindness if not detected and treated.

Complications

Systemic involvement can include iridocyclitis, uveitis, pleuritis, pericarditis, anemia, fatigue, and hepatitis. Residual joint damage caused by granulation of tissue in the joint space can be a problem. Children most likely to develop permanent crippling disability are those with hip involvement, unremitting synovitis, or positive RF test.

Patient and Parent Education and Prevention

The following education and preventive measures are taken:
- For children on aspirin therapy (not typically given)— educate parents about the risk of Reye syndrome and its signs and symptoms.
- Recommend yearly influenza vaccine.
- Offer chronic disease counseling as indicated in Chapter 21.
- Encourage normal play and recreation.
- Educate about side effects of medications, in addition to splinting, orthotics, and bracing requirements.
- Instruct about need to follow up with an ophthalmologist. Frequency of follow-up for uveitis screening is based on subtype of JIA and is determined by the ophthalmologist.
- Ensure that parent and child understand that physical therapy is a mainstay of treatment for chronic childhood arthritis and should be part of the child's daily routine. A daily plan that includes passive, active, and resistive exercises is important.
- Water therapy and the use of heat or cold reduce pain and stiffness. Swimming is an excellent activity for these children except those with severe anemia and cardiac disease.
- Tricycle or bike riding and low-impact dance are other beneficial activities.
- Refer to the American Arthritis Foundation, which has excellent resources for family members and children.
- Instruct on the need to involve school personnel in the identification of required school-related services through an individualized education plan (IEP) or a 504.
- Discuss the challenge of pain management and its assessment in children with chronic arthritis and encourage parents to advocate for effective pain control on behalf of their child.

Prognosis

The course of the disease is variable, and there is no curative treatment. After an initial episode, the child may never have another episode, or the disease may go into remission and recur months or years later. The disease process of JIA wanes with age and completely subsides in 85% of children. However, systemic onset, a positive RF, poor response to therapy, and the radiologic evidence of erosion are associated with a poor prognosis. Onset of disease in the teenage years is related to progression to adult rheumatoid disease.

SYSTEMIC LUPUS ERYTHEMATOSUS

Description

SLE is a chronic, systemic rheumatic disease that can involve many organ systems including the kidneys, skin, blood cells, and nervous system. Autoantibody formation resulting from hyperactive B-lymphocytes due to a loss of T-lymphocyte control on B-lymphocyte activity is a key characteristic of this immune complex disease. Cell-mediated autoimmune responses are also part of the pathogenesis of SLE (Klein-Gitelman, 2010). It is more acute and severe in children than in adults.

Epidemiology

The exact cause is unknown; however, genetics and environment are involved in its pathogenesis marked by the production of significantly increased circulating autoantibodies. Altered cellular immunity in genetically predisposed individuals is postulated as a key factor in this disease. SLE is an autoimmune disease that is characterized by ANA production. There is widespread multiorgan system inflammation as a result of altered immune regulation. In SLE, immune complexes are deposited in various tissues of the body, and their clearance is impaired. Deposits of immune complexes trigger a generalized inflammatory response that can lead to tissue damage, such as vasculitis and ischemia and numerous organ system abnormalities (commonly the heart and renal system). There is variety in both the presentation—acute life-threatening episodes or in an indolent manner—and how it is manifested over time in an individual.

The mechanism triggering immune complex formation is unknown. Onset before 8 to 9 years old is rare. SLE peaks between 11 and 15 years of age (Pongmarutani et al, 2006). Females are preponderantly affected more than males with a 4:1 ratio before puberty and an 8:1 ratio after puberty (Haftel, 2011; Klein-Gitelman, 2010).

Clinical Findings

Clinical findings depend on organ involvement. Its presentation may be abrupt or have a gradual, nonspecific onset. Fever, rash, fatigue, and joint pain are the most typical presentation in children.

History. The history may include the following:
- Joint involvement
  - Most common initial finding
  - Nondeforming arthritis with effusion and tenderness
  - Often symmetric joint involvement
- Arthralgia
- Systemic manifestations
- Low-grade fever—intermittent or sustained
- Fatigue and malaise
- Anorexia and loss of weight

Physical Examination. The following may be seen on physical examination (Haftel, 2011):
- Malar or "butterfly" rash—scaly erythematous maculopapular rash covering malar areas extending over the bridge of the nose and cheeks; may spread down the face to the chest and extremities; "butterfly" rash and other lesions can be photosensitive; seen in approximately 95% of those with SLE.
- Discoid rash with plugging of the follicles, hypopigmentation and hyperpigmentation, and scarring; discoid rash is less common in children.
- Lesions may also include small ulcerations in the skin and mucous membranes, indurations, purpura, and erythema nodosum.
- Alopecia (as a result of loss of hair follicles from discoid lupus)
- Mucous membrane manifestations (ulceration) of the mouth and nasal septum
- Gingivitis, mucosal hemorrhage, erosions, ulcerations
- Silvery whitening of the vermilion border of the lips or thickening, redness, ulceration, or crusting of the lips
- Raynaud phenomenon is present in some children
- Polyserositis—pleurisy, pericarditis, and peritonitis
- Hepatosplenomegaly and lymphadenopathy
- Signs and symptoms of central nervous system (CNS) involvement (seizures or psychosis) and cardiac (pleuritis or pericarditis) and renal involvement (e.g., cardiac failure or renal failure), which is common in children

Diagnostic Studies. Initial laboratory testing includes CBC, ANA, ESR, CRP, serum chemical analysis (metabolic and protein screen), and urinalysis. The ANA test is positive in more than 97% of children who have active, untreated SLE; the titers are usually high (Haftel, 2011). A negative ANA excludes SLE from the diagnosis except for the rare false-negative test. A positive ANA test should be followed up with testing for disease-specific types of ANA (e.g., antibodies to Sm, Ro, or La). The ANA autoantibody profile screens for anti-Sm, anti-Ro, anti-La, anti-double strand DNA, and anti-ribonucleoprotein (antiRNP) antibodies (Gamboa and Sugarman, 2008; Pongmarutani et al, 2006). Antibodies to double-stranded DNA are present in most patients with SLE and are generally exclusively seen in cases of SLE and not other disease states; antibodies directed against Sm are diagnostic of SLE but are only found in 30% of patients with SLE. Antiphospholipid antibodies may also accompany SLE and predisposes the patient to stroke (Klein-Gitelman and Miller, 2007). Leukopenia or lymphopenia, hemolytic anemia, and thrombocytopenia are frequent laboratory findings. Other laboratory and radiographic studies depend on organ involvement (e.g., chest x-ray, electrocardiogram [ECG], renal ultrasound, histopathologic studies, urine testing, and serologic testing). Proteinuria and hematuria are a hallmark of lupus nephritis.

Differential Diagnosis

Diseases that resemble SLE include rheumatic fever, malignancy, serum sickness, and viral infections. A temporary, drug-induced SLE can be caused by several pharmacologic agents, including hydantoin compounds, hydralazine, isoniazid (INH), procainamide, and sulfonamides.

Management

Children with SLE need to be followed by a specialist in collagen-vascular disorders. Other pediatric subspecialists may be consulted. Therapy depends on the degree of local or systemic involvement. Sunlight is a known trigger of SLE. Therefore, general measures include avoiding sun exposure and daylight fluorescent light, in addition to applying sunscreen for UVA and UVB protection. Prompt recognition and treatment of disease flares are essential to prevent systemic complications, so frequent clinical and laboratory monitoring is important. The following measures also may be helpful (Klein-Gitelman, 2010):

- NSAIDs are used for relief of arthritis, arthralgias, serositis, or pain (if nephritis is present, use with caution).
- Oral steroids are prescribed if renal, cardiac, pulmonary, or CNS involvement is present. They have been the mainstay of SLE for decades. The dose is adjusted depending on clinical and laboratory findings. Cautious tapering of steroids is often needed.
- Antimalarial drugs (e.g., hydroxychloroquine) may be used to treat cutaneous and musculoskeletal manifestations; it is often used as a maintenance therapy.
- Immunosuppressant agents may be added if the response to steroids is inadequate; cyclophosphamide may be added with corticosteroid therapy if the child has active nephritis or CNS lupus.
- Use of other pharmacologic agents or therapies depends on the type and level of organ system involvement; monoclonal antibody agents are being used in investigational studies.
- Vitamin D and calcium supplements are used to reduce the risk of osteoporosis related to chronic corticosteroid use.

Complications

For the most part, SLE is considered a controllable disease in children. The severity of the illness is variable. A diagnosis of SLE in childhood does not always mean a poor prognosis, especially if renal involvement or cerebritis is not present. Renal failure, CNS lupus, myocardial infarction, cardiac failure, and infection are the leading causes of death in children. Exposure to ultraviolet light may bring out or worsen skin lesions and can result in exacerbation of systemic problems that can cause death. Side effects resulting from chronic use of high-dose corticosteroids (e.g., osteoporosis, avascular necrosis) can be a problem.

Patient and Parent Education

The provider should educate patients and parents about:
- The effect of sun exposure and the need for sunscreen protection
- The need to rest between activities because fatigue is a frequent problem for children with SLE
- The fact that SLE is a chronic disease that can have periods of remission followed by exacerbations

Prognosis

SLE is a chronic disease with periods of exacerbations with waxing and waning of symptoms; however, complete remission can occur. Children with mild disease do well; those with severe major organ involvement have a poor prognosis.

FIBROMYALGIA SYNDROME

Description

Fibromyalgia (FM) is the term used to describe a chronic, idiopathic pain syndrome characterized by widespread, diffuse, nonarticular musculoskeletal pain and fatigue with multiple trigger points that are discrete painful sites. It is a benign, intermittent, noninflammatory musculoskeletal pain syndrome that is also referred to as myofascial pain syndrome, generalized pain syndrome, fibrositis, and pain amplification syndrome. It is a complex syndrome that involves fatigue, poor sleep patterns with nonrefreshing sleep, and generalized pain involving muscles, ligaments, and tendons. Symptoms are often vague and variable, with no major organ system abnormalities found. Its presentation can range from a generalized increased sensitivity to pain to a more classic pattern of specific symptoms. Fibromyalgia can occur as a primary condition or in conjunction with other rheumatologic disorders (secondary fibromyalgia) (Buskila, 2009; Haftel, 2011).

Epidemiology

The cause and pathogenesis of fibromyalgia are uncertain but thought to involve CNS malfunction with amplification of pain transmission and interpretation. Genetic predisposition is also implicated because a familial prevalence has been reported (Buskila, 2009). It is considered a subset of musculoskeletal pain syndromes. Females are affected more often than males, who tend to report lower levels of pain at specific points sites than their female counterparts (Buskila, 2009). Fibromyalgia is more common in adults, but can occur in children, generally in those older than 12 years. The prevalence of fibromyalgia in children is estimated at 6% (Haftel, 2011).

Clinical Findings

History. The history may include the following long-standing common symptoms:
- Pain at multiple sites including muscles and in the soft tissues around joints
- Pain may awaken from sleep and interfere with routine activities.
- Fatigue and malaise
- Paresthesias and complaints of headache
- Insomnia or prolonged night awakenings
- Depression (a significant number exhibit depressive symptoms) and anxiety
- School absence due to pain is not uncommon but keeps up with school work

Physical Examination. Local areas of painful (not just tender) trigger points in muscles (usually at areas of tendon insertion) with digital pressure are characteristic physical findings. Pressure causes pain at the site and in a circumferential or linear pattern surrounding the site. Common trigger points include the neck, back, lateral epicondyles, greater trochanter, and knees. Typically there is no evidence of arthritis or muscular weakness.

Diagnostic Criteria. The criteria for the diagnosis of fibromyalgia are as follows:
- A 3-month or longer history of diffuse pain associated with multiple trigger points
- Pain in 11 of 18 specific tender point sites on digital palpation (using approximately 4 kg of pressure)

Other underlying illness must have been excluded including inflammatory diseases (e.g., SLE, postinfectious fatigue that can follow Epstein-Barr [EBV] or influenzavirus infections, or mood and conversion disorders). Approximately 30% of children diagnosed as having chronic fatigue syndrome were also diagnosed with FM (Buskila, 2009; Haftel, 2011).

Diagnostic Studies. Laboratory studies are of little benefit. Blood count, liver functions, and muscle enzymes are normal. If secondary fibromyalgia is present, order appropriate tests to diagnose rheumatoid disorder. However, children with fibromyalgia can have a false-positive ANA as do 20% of normal children (without rheumatoid disorders).

Differential Diagnosis

In CFS, tiredness lasting longer than 6 months rather than pain is the major complaint (Scheffer, 2011). Fibromyalgia initially may be mistaken for other rheumatoid diseases, but does not have the associated rashes, weight loss, fever (greater than 101° F [38.3° C]), or joint swelling. Lyme disease is also in the differential.

Management

Children and their parents need reassurance that they do not have a life-threatening disease, but have a chronic condition that can be a lifelong problem. Treatment focuses on relieving symptoms and can include the following:

- Physical therapy for range-of-motion exercises, mild low-impact aerobic exercises (e.g., swimming, bicycling, and walking), and muscle strengthening
- Amitriptyline (low doses) taken before bedtime has been helpful in stabilizing abnormal sleep patterns and in reducing pain.
- Psychotherapy and relaxation techniques to help cope with this condition and deal with stress
- NSAIDs can be prescribed for pain control.
- Gabapentin can be prescribed to reduce pain sensitivity.
- Complementary therapy involves acupuncture.

Patient and Parent Education

The provider should educate patients and parents about:

- Fibromyalgia and that it is not a psychosomatic disorder
- Education about sleep hygiene
- The possibility that this could be a chronic problem, and there can be periods of remissions followed by exacerbations

Prognosis

The outcome of fibromyalgia in children varies; however, fibromyalgia in children generally has a better prognosis than it does in adults (Buskila, 2009; Haftel, 2011).

CHRONIC FATIGUE SYNDROME

Fatigue is a common complaint in adolescence. However, only a small number of children go on to have chronic issues of severe debilitating and overwhelming fatigue that presents the provider with the diagnostic challenge as to its etiology as does CFS. Children can develop idiopathic pain syndromes, which are characterized by the presence of severe disability despite the lack of physical or laboratory findings. CFS is one of the subsets of idiopathic pain syndromes as is fibromyalgia. The onset is rare in childhood but does occur in adolescence with an overall 1% prevalence rate (Scheffer, 2011). The key patient complaint is fatigue that must have a new onset, is unexplained, is not linked to ongoing exertion, and

is persistent. This fatigue is not substantially relieved by rest or sleep and results in substantial reduction in activity much lower than before the onset of their fatigue illness. About two thirds of pediatric cases have a reported onset of CFS after a preceding viral illness with pharyngitis and fever.

There are two criteria necessary for a diagnosis of CFS (Centers for Disease Control and Prevention [CDC], 2010). The first is severe chronic and debilitating fatigue present for at least 6 months or longer that is not relieved by rest and another medical or psychiatric diagnosis does not explain this physical symptom. In addition to fatigue symptoms as just described, the child needs to have at least four of the following eight symptoms to meet CFS criteria:

- Self-reported impaired short-term memory or limitations in concentration (cognitive dysfunction) that results in impaired social, academic, occupational, or personal activities
- Sore throat that is recurrent
- Painful cervical or axillary lymph nodes
- Muscle pain (myalgia)
- Multiple joint arthralgia with no swelling or redness noted
- Headaches of a new pattern or severity
- Unrefreshing sleep
- Postexertional malaise lasting for more than 24 hours

Other secondary complaints may include but are not limited to chills, night sweats, visual disturbances, dizziness, or fainting (CDC, 2010). Complaints of low-grade fever may be reported, but are generally not documented on examination. There may be a history of neuropsychiatric problems; however, in these cases, a psychiatric illness must first be excluded before a diagnosis of CFS can be made. EBV infection has been implicated in the cause of CFS. However, EBV does not explain all the symptoms. No single immunologic abnormality has been consistently identified as the causative factor. The cause of CFS remains undetermined and may possibly represent the culminating effect of multiple factors such as infectious disease, immunologic dysfunction, stress, and/or neutrally mediated hypotension (CDC, 2010). Its treatment is based on symptoms. Care must be taken in diagnosing this disorder in children, and other conditions (e.g., hypothyroidism, sleep apnea, hepatitis B or C, SLE, cancer, alcohol or drug abuse, Lyme disease, and major depressive and other psychiatric disorders) must first be ruled out. One study found that self-reported childhood trauma (particularly emotional and sexual abuse) by adults was associated with a sixfold increase in risk for the development of CFS (Heim et al, 2009).

For a definitive diagnosis of CFS once other conditions are ruled out, the child is best referred to a specialist in this area. Pharmacologic intervention generally is not effective. Psychological support (stressing that this disease is not made up) and exercise are associated with reduced disability. Children and adolescents with chronic fatigue reporting illness may have symptoms that wax and wane over time. The majority typically have substantial improvement in their symptoms or complete recovery 1 to 4 years after diagnosis (Jenson and Jones, 2007).

ACUTE RHEUMATIC FEVER
Description

Acute rheumatic fever (ARF) is a nonsuppurative complication following a Lancefield group A streptococcus (GAS) pharyngeal infection that results in an autoimmune inflammatory process involving the joints (polyarthritis), heart (rheumatic heart disease), CNS (Sydenham chorea), and subcutaneous tissue (subcutaneous nodules and erythema marginatum). Recurrent ARF with its multisystem responses can follow with subsequent GAS pharyngeal infections. Long-term effects on tissues are generally minimal except for the damage done to cardiac valves that leaves fibrosis and scarring and results in rheumatic heart disease (Lee, 2009). ARF is diagnosed based on a set of criteria called the revised Jones criteria. These criteria are used for the initial attack of ARF. Further modifications of the Jones criteria are used for recurrent ARF (see Box 30-7).

Epidemiology

The exact pathologic mechanism that is responsible for the inflammatory changes in various organs and tissues and the abnormal immune response that follows GAS is unknown. Abnormalities in the host immune response to streptococcal cell wall proteins are believed to be involved. Greater organism virulence is associated with specific M protein types and a more "mucoid" capsule. There appears to be a strong genetic influence on susceptibility to GAS infection, with a family history of rheumatic fever and a lower socioeconomic status as known risk factors. More than 80% of the worldwide cases of ARF and rheumatic heart disease occur in developing countries (Schneider, 2011; Steer and Carapetis, 2009). The latency period from infection with GAS until symptom onset of ARF is usually 2 to 6 weeks. Skin infections with GAS rarely result in ARF. Recurrence of ARF following subsequent episodes of GAS pharyngitis (symptomatic or asymptomatic infection) is high. The most commonly affected age group is children 5 to 6 years old to 15 years old (Schneider, 2011). See Chapter 30 for further discussion of ARF and cardiac involvement.

Clinical Findings and History

The diagnosis of an initial attack of ARF is based on the revised Jones criteria (see Box 30-7) and is as follows:
- Evidence of documented (culture, rapid streptococcal antigen test, or antistreptolysin O [ASO] titer) GAS pharyngeal infection
- Findings of two major manifestations or one major and two minor manifestations of ARF (Schneider, 2011; Steer and Carapetis, 2009)

Major Manifestations
- Carditis is common (pancarditis, valves, pericardium, myocardium) and can cause chronic, life-threatening disease (i.e., congestive heart failure [CHF]) with estimates of 30% to 80% of patients with ARF experiencing carditis; it is also more common in younger children than adolescents.
- Polyarthritis (migratory and painful) involving large joints and rarely small or unusual joints (e.g., vertebrae); it is the most common manifestation of ARF
- Sydenham chorea (uncommon)
- Erythema marginatum manifested as pink macules on the trunk and extremities; nonpruritic; this sign is uncommon
- Subcutaneous nodules associated with repeated episodes and severe carditis; this sign is uncommon

Minor Manifestations
- Fever (101° to 102° F [38.2° to 38.9° C]), arthralgia, history of ARF

Diagnostic Studies
- Elevated acute-phase reactants (ESR, white blood cells [WBCs], CRP)
- Leukocytosis
- Prolonged PR interval on electrocardiogram

Children may be diagnosed with ARF without evidence of a preceding streptococcal infection in the following two situations: a child with Sydenham chorea or with acquired heart disease (commonly mitral valve regurgitation without a congenitally abnormal or prolapsed valve) that can only be linked to ARF. Approximately 80% of children with ARF have an elevated ASO titer. In situations in which the ASO titer is normal and ARF is still suspected, titers for anti-DNase B or other GAS-specific antibodies should be obtained with repeat testing in 2 weeks to look for a fourfold rise in titers (Young and Strong, 2006).

Differential Diagnosis

No single diagnostic test exists for ARF, and many diseases are included in the differential diagnosis (e.g., JIA, connective tissue diseases, infective endocarditis, and Lyme disease).

Management

The treatment of ARF includes the following:
- Antibiotic therapy to eradicate GAS infection. Primary prevention requires that a GAS infection be treated within 10 days of onset. Benzathine penicillin G is the drug of choice unless there is an allergic history; erythromycin is then the drug of choice. Azithromycin and some oral cephalosporins are also sometimes used (Schneider, 2011). A patient with a history of ARF who has an upper respiratory infection should be treated for GAS whether or not GAS is recovered because asymptomatic infection can trigger a recurrence.
- Antiinflammatory therapy. Aspirin (ASA) can be used for arthritis after the diagnosis is established; it is usually given only for 2 weeks and then tapered. ASA is also used in the treatment of mild to moderate carditis. ASA and steroids provide symptomatic relief, but do not prevent the incidence of chronic heart disease. However, the use of steroids has been beneficial in the management of severe carditis, reducing its morbidity and mortality. The association of Reye syndrome with aspirin use is always a concern and must be addressed with parents. Yearly influenza immunization is critical for children on aspirin therapy.
- Chest radiographs, ECG, and echocardiography are indicated; carditis usually develops within the first 3 weeks of symptoms.
- Referral for treatment of CHF if needed. Medical management or valve replacement may be necessary.
- Bed rest is generally indicated only for children with CHF. Children with Sydenham chorea may need to be kept in bed to protect them until their choreiform movements are controlled. Steroids in the absence of other symptoms are not useful in the treatment of chorea.
- Children with severe chorea may benefit from the use of such pharmacologic agents as sodium valproate or carbamazepine (Steer and Carapetis, 2009).

The prevention of ARF includes the following:
- Treat GAS pharyngeal infections with the appropriate antibiotics. Antibacterial prophylaxis for those with a prior history of ARF is required because of their greatly increased

risk of recurrent ARF with subsequent inadequately treated GAS infections. Intramuscular penicillin G (1.2 million units every 28 days) is more effective than daily penicillin V (Schneider, 2011).

- Antibacterial secondary prophylaxis is continued for 5 years after the last ARF episode in children without carditis or until 21 years old (whichever is longer). For those with carditis and persistent myocardial or valvular disease, treatment is 10 or more years and may be lifelong (Steer and Carapetis, 2009).
- Children with a history of ARF need bacterial endocarditis prophylaxis treatment for dental or surgical procedures in addition to their regular antibiotic prophylaxis (see Chapter 30).

Complications

Chronic CHF can occur after an initial episode of ARF or follow recurrent episodes of ARF. Residual valvular damage is responsible for CHF. The risk of significant cardiac disease increases dramatically with each subsequent episode of ARF; thus prevention of subsequent GAS infections is critical. Intramuscular benzathine penicillin must be given every 4 weeks and not monthly and can be given every 3 weeks in high-risk children. The need for adherence must be stressed to parents.

■ Vasculitis Syndrome

HENOCH-SCHÖNLEIN PURPURA

Description

HSP is an overwhelming disease of childhood that is marked by acute vasculitis with associated inflammatory change of small blood vessels in various organ systems. The key feature is a palpable petechial or purpuric rash.

Epidemiology

HSP is the most common systemic vasculitis syndrome seen in children whose cause remains unknown. It often is preceded by an upper respiratory infection and can occur anytime from infancy (as early as 6 months old) to adulthood. However, it is primarily a disease of childhood that typically occurs in children 3 to 15 years old. HSP is seen slightly more frequently in males than females and occurs more frequently in winter months than other times of the year. This condition often follows a respiratory infection.

Leukocytic infiltration of tissue, hemorrhage, and ischemia are associated findings. IgA is involved in the immunopathogenesis of HSP. There is widespread leukocytoclastic vasculitis with IgA deposition in vessel walls noted as a common finding. With inflammation of the small blood vessels extravasation of blood occurs into local tissue. Patients with depositions of IgA in their renal mesangium have an associated nephritis. Although unproven, there is some conjecture that HSP may be allergy mediated (Haftel, 2011).

Clinical Findings

Clinical findings are typically characterized by a rash (palpable purpura) symmetrically distributed over the buttocks and extensor areas of the legs with arthritis. Signs and symptoms of GI and renal vasculitis are a less frequent occurrence. Arthritis occurs in approximately 80% of patients, is very painful, and has an acute onset. The lower extremities, typically the ankles and knees, are the most common arthritic sites. Approximately one half of children develop GI involvement, and one third develop renal involvement. Symptoms of renal involvement can occur as an acute or chronic problem; renal involvement tends to be mild in most cases (Haftel, 2011).

The diagnosis of HSP is based on the presence of two or more of the following four findings:
- Palpable purpura
- Bowel angina
- Diagnostic biopsy (granulocytes found in the walls of arterioles or venules on histologic examination)
- Pediatric age group (less than 20 years old at onset of symptoms)

History. A history of palpable cutaneous purpura is a hallmark of HSP. The classic presentation is purpura concentrated on the dependent areas of the body below the waist. Palpable purpura on the legs and buttocks is a key historical feature; however, the rash may occur anywhere on the body. In addition, the history may include the following:
- Urticarial or small maculopapular rash may precede purpuric lesions, but rapidly progress to purpura with areas of ecchymoses.
- Arthritis
  ○ Typically involves knees and ankles and is migratory, but can occur in any joint
  ○ May precede the appearance of purpuric lesions
- Colicky abdominal pain
  ○ Pain typically mild to moderate and may precede the onset of the rash
- Vomiting
- Hematuria (a hallmark of HSP nephritis)
- Gross or occult GI bleeding (bloody diarrhea) or significant abdominal distention—a less common finding

Physical Examination. The two most common manifestations of HSP are (Miller and Pachman, 2007):
- Skin vasculitis: cutaneous purpura—sine qua non for the diagnosis
  ○ Diameter: 0 to 2 mm
  ○ Concentrated on the legs and buttocks
  ○ Can involve trunk, face, and upper extremities
  ○ Typically lasts 3 days to 3 to 4 months
  ○ May be accompanied by edema typically involving the calves, dorsum of feet, scalp, scrotum, or labia
  ○ Starts as a pinkish maculopapular rash and progresses from red to purple to brown palpable purpura
- Arthritis
  ○ Initially incapacitates, but is self-limited and nondeforming
  ○ Commonly is periarthritis and involves the knees and ankles
  ○ Warmth, swelling, and erythema over the joints

Other common features that may be found include the following:
- Signs of GI obstruction (partial obstruction to intussusception) or bleeding
- Signs of glomerulonephritis (can occur within first few months of disease onset, but rarely presents as late renal disease)
  ○ Hypertension or azotemia
  ○ Hematuria and proteinuria (classic findings of nephritis)

Other, less common, physical findings are related to complications caused by vasculitis in other body organs (e.g., respiratory, cardiac, and CNS).

Diagnostic Studies. The diagnosis of HSP is based on clinical findings. A urinalysis must be done to check for hematuria and proteinuria. Blood urea nitrogen (BUN) and creatinine are useful to evaluate renal function. Renal biopsy may be warranted if renal involvement is severe. Checking stools for blood is important in children complaining of abdominal pain. If GI obstruction is a consideration, abdominal radiographs should be ordered. Other diagnostic studies (e.g., chest radiographs, CT scans, or electroencephalographs) are ordered based on the signs and symptoms of complications, such as shortness of breath, seizures, mental status changes, or hypertension. Such studies are useful to identify specific organ system involvement and the severity of the complication.

In HSP, the ESR, CRP, and WBC (nonspecific indicators of systemic inflammation) are elevated. Because this condition is associated with a nonthrombocytopenic purpura, the platelet count is normal or even high.

Differential Diagnosis

Diseases that cause a similar rash with renal abnormalities are part of the differential diagnosis and include poststreptococcal glomerulonephritis, hemolytic uremic syndrome, serum sickness (drug related), and SLE. Other forms of vasculitides, such as Wegener granulomatosis and polyarteritis nodosa, are considerations (Haftel, 2011).

Management

Children with HSP need to be referred to a pediatrician and subspecialists depending on organ system involvement. Hospitalization is necessary with moderate to severe GI and renal system involvement or if pulmonary, cardiac, or CNS manifestations are present. Treatment is generally supportive, and careful attention is given to maintaining hydration and electrolyte balance. In addition, the following are key components of the management plan:

- Monitor for GI blood loss.
- Monitor for hematuria and proteinuria.
- Monitor and treat hypertension.
- Prescribe analgesics and NSAIDs for arthritis.

- Prescribe systemic corticosteroids for GI disease (provides significant relief of abdominal pain).
- Acute nephritis typically responds to corticosteroids, but immunosuppressive therapy (cytotoxic drugs) may be needed in resistant cases.
- Treat complications.

The skin lesions do not require special care and resolve without treatment. Use of other pharmacologic agents or therapies depends on the type and level of organ system involvement.

Complications

Infrequent complications of HSP seen in children include myositis, orchitis, hemorrhagic cystitis, pancreatitis, cholecystitis, bowel infarction, perforation or stricture, intussusception, acute renal failure, seizures, ataxia, pulmonary hemorrhage, carditis, anterior uveitis, and episcleritis. Ileoileal intussusception is a complication marked by severe colicky abdominal pain. The arthritis associated with HSP does not leave joint damage and typically does not recur (Haftel, 2011).

Patient and Parent Education

The provider should educate patients and parents about:
- The illness, its complications, and the risk of recurrence
- The need to closely monitor for nephritis for 1 year following the initial presentation and after resolution, including blood pressure and urinalysis testing (Dedeoglu et al, 2010)

Prognosis

HSP tends to last 3 to 4 weeks and then completely resolves in most cases without significant sequelae. However, the rash can wax and wane for 1 year, and some children have recurrent disease. The presence of significant nephritis in the initial course of the disease (elevated BUN and persistent high-grade proteinuria) is a potentially serious complication with risk for long-term sequelae, such as hypertension or renal insufficiency. Less than 1% of children with HSP progress to end-stage renal disease (Haftel, 2010).

Endocrine and Metabolic Disorders

BECKY J. WHITTEMORE, ARLENE SMALDONE, AND ROBERT D. STEINER

Endocrine and metabolic disorders affect a large number of children and may be rare (e.g., nephropathic cystinosis) or relatively common (e.g., type 1 and type 2 diabetes mellitus). This chapter begins with an overview of anatomy, physiology, and pathophysiology of the endocrine and metabolic systems and general issues related to assessment and management of these disorders. Following are two sections covering endocrine and metabolic disorders as they are managed by primary care providers in collaboration with specialists. Although there is a great degree of overlap in these disorders, distinctive processes occur in each, and as such, specific conditions may involve different approaches to assessment and management.

■ Anatomy and Physiology

The endocrine system regulates growth, pubertal development and reproduction; homeostasis of the individual; and the production, storage, and use of energy. Classically the endocrine system was understood to function via hormones produced in glands with action at a distant site. Now the understanding is that hormones may also act in a paracrine fashion affecting cells adjacent to the hormone-secreting cell or in an autocrine fashion in which the hormone affects the secreting cell by diffusion. Many endocrine glands are controlled by the hypothalamic-pituitary axis. Many of the hormones of the hypothalamic-pituitary axis (or molecules that are structurally similar to such hormones) are also made in the gut and other tissues.

Hormones are often activated by a feedback loop; for example, thyrotropin-releasing hormone (TRH) from the hypothalamus stimulates pituitary thyrotropin (TSH) secretion, which in turn stimulates thyroid hormone production (T_3 [triiodothyronine] and T_4 [thyroxine]). Thyroid hormone levels provide feedback to the hypothalamus and pituitary thereby suppressing TRH and TSH secretion so that a balance is reached. In similar fashion, the adrenal glands secrete corticosteroids and the gonads produce progesterone, androgens, and estradiol, all of which influence hypothalamic and pituitary hormone production. For some systems, the setpoint changes as individuals develop. Hormone secretion can be regulated by nerve cells and by factors important in the immune system (e.g., cytokines interact with hormones that influence weight homeostasis).

Metabolic function in the body involves complex biochemical processes to transform essential amino acids, carbohydrates, and lipids to substances or energy that can be used at the cellular level; to produce molecules; and to perform cell functions. These biochemical processes or metabolic pathways are driven by enzyme activity.

■ Pathophysiology

Endocrine abnormalities occur when an alteration in regulation of the normal feedback system results in hyposecretion or hypersecretion of one or more hormones. Multiple factors cause alterations in hormone production. These factors include tumors, trauma, infection, systemic disease, genetic disorders, congenital malformation or agenesis of an endocrine gland, idiopathic causes, and iatrogenic causes (e.g., medications). The defect or problem can originate at the pituitary-hypothalamic level, in organ abnormalities, or for unknown reasons that lead to unresponsiveness to endogenous hormone. Hypothyroidism and hyperthyroidism are examples of disease entities in which the interrelationships of the hypothalamic-pituitary-thyroid axis may be altered at any one of these sites.

Many metabolic diseases are caused by inborn errors of metabolism. An alteration in genetic constitution results in disrupted biochemical functioning. For example, in children with phenylketonuria (PKU, a deficiency of the enzyme phenylalanine hydroxylase), the essential amino acid phenylalanine accumulates, resulting in mental retardation if not treated within the first weeks of life. Type 1 diabetes mellitus is an example of an acquired immune-mediated metabolic disease. In diabetes, a reduction in insulin production or deficiency of its action results in abnormal metabolism of carbohydrate, protein, and fat.

■ Assessment

Endocrine and metabolic disorders disrupt organs throughout the body and can alter various body functions. Assessment requires a thorough family history, physical examination, and specific diagnostic testing for the suspected disorder.

HISTORY

- What is the child's growth pattern since birth?
- Has there been a recent alteration in growth pattern?
- Is the child taking any medications that could affect endocrine or metabolic function?
- Have there been signs or symptoms of endocrine or metabolic dysfunction?
- Was there maternal exposure to radioiodine, goitrogens, or iodine medication during pregnancy?
- When did the child first show signs of sexual development?
- What is the child's diet and exercise history?
- Is there a family history of endocrine, autoimmune, or metabolic disorders?
- Does the child have unusual odors, recurrent vomiting, or unexplained lethargy?

PHYSICAL EXAMINATION

A detailed examination should include the following:
- Measure stature. Supine length is preferred for children younger than 2 years old. Use a stadiometer for children older than 2 or 3 years. Plot height, weight, and head circumference on a standardized growth chart appropriate to the child's age and gender. In addition, growth charts are available for children with certain genetic conditions, such as Down and Turner syndromes, and should be used to assess growth patterns of children with these conditions (see Appendix B). Serial measurements are critical to assess growth patterns over time.
- Check for proportionate appearance. Measure sitting and standing heights for upper to lower segment ratio (see Chapter 32).
- Assess height age (the age corresponding to the child's height when plotted at the 50th percentile on a growth chart) and growth velocity (linear growth in centimeters or inches over the past year).
- Inspect the child's genitalia for signs of either normal or ambiguous genitalia.
- Identify the stage of sexual development using Tanner staging (see Chapter 8).
- Note facial, axillary, and pubic hair for presence, distribution, and texture.
- Examine the skin for presence of striae and acanthosis nigricans (see Color Plate) of the neck, axilla, breast, knuckles, and skinfolds.
- Palpate the neck for thyroid gland symmetry and size, noting enlargement or presence of nodules.
- Examine for presence of dysmorphic features.
- Examine the abdomen noting any organomegaly.
- Complete general neurologic examination.

Acquired endocrine disorders are often due to either hyposecretion or hypersecretion of a specific hormone or combination of hormones, and the child may or may not appear ill. Signs of dehydration, exophthalmos, and tachycardia are

physical findings associated with endocrine pathology. Newborns with metabolic disorders may initially appear well, but physical signs develop with metabolic activity. Characteristic physical findings associated with specific disease entities are presented later in this chapter.

DIAGNOSTIC TESTS

Measurement of hormone levels is a key tool in the diagnosis of endocrine disorders. Specific blood and urine studies that identify end products of abnormal metabolism or elevated or diminished levels of various substances such as glucose, galactose, or amino acids are important in the diagnosis of metabolic disorders. Accurate interpretation of data requires strict adherence to laboratory protocol for collecting and managing specimens. Additionally, not all laboratories have the ability to conduct tests that are sensitive to the hormone or substance being measured (e.g., measurement of hormones in precocious puberty requires high sensitivity; measurement of ammonia levels requires strict procedures when obtaining the sample).

Radiographic and imaging studies (e.g., bone age, ultrasonography, computed tomography [CT], and magnetic resonance imaging [MRI]) are also important diagnostic tools in evaluating certain endocrine and metabolic disorders.

Many of these studies are expensive and can put additional emotional stress on a family that is already uncertain about their child's condition.

■ Management Strategies

GENERAL MEASURES

Clinical consequences for the child affected by an endocrine or metabolic disorder vary from mild to severe. Undiagnosed and untreated, these disorders may lead to irreversible mental retardation, physical disability, neurologic damage, or death. Early detection, accurate diagnosis, and timely intervention are necessary to achieve favorable outcomes. Chronic disease issues and the effects of these diseases on lifestyle must also be addressed:

- Family, school, peer, and emotional adjustment
- Body image, self-esteem, and social competence
- Disease understanding, acceptance, and self-care
- Regimen adherence

A successful outcome depends on the patient and family receiving support and encouragement in self-care, learning about the disease, and understanding the patient-parent role in managing a long-term illness or chronic condition.

GENETIC COUNSELING

Genetic counseling is often necessary. Implications are significant for the family of a child with endocrine or metabolic disorders that are genetically linked (see Chapter 40).

MEDICATIONS

Pharmacologic therapy, including hormone replacement, whether temporary or lifelong is often essential for management of these disorders. Medications may be administered via injection, creating distress in both the child and caregiver. Short, clear instructions about medications are important; how much to give, when and how to administer, possible side effects, and when to make adjustments in medication are key messages to convey.

DIETARY CONSIDERATIONS

Metabolic diseases often require strict adherence to dietary plans and restrictions. Parents, patients, other caregivers, and school personnel must be aware of the dietary needs and restrictions and the effect of diet on the disease process. They must also be given support in order to adjust to the economic, social, and psychological demands created by such restrictions.

PATIENT AND PARENT EDUCATION

Close supervision and frequent follow-up are necessary for children with metabolic and endocrine disorders. These children are best evaluated initially and periodically by a multidisciplinary team with expertise in pediatric endocrinology and/or clinical genetics (metabolic diseases). Parent and patient education should include:
* Nature of the disorder
* Treatment plan
* Possible complications
* Plan for long-term follow-up including the timing and process of transition to adult care services

The multidisciplinary team can provide the education and support needed. The primary care provider, as a part of this team, is in an ideal position to reinforce the plan of care. Additionally, essential primary health care needs and anticipatory guidance cannot be overlooked.

Disorders of Endocrine Function

Endocrine pathologies most commonly seen in children can be assessed by considering the following seven areas:
* Disturbance of growth
* Abnormalities of pubertal development
* Adrenal conditions
* Disorders of sexual maturation
* Thyroid conditions
* Diabetes mellitus, types 1 and 2
* Posterior pituitary gland dysfunction

■ Growth Disorders

Children grow in a predictable way, and deviation from a normal growth pattern can be the first sign of an endocrine disorder. Every effort should be made to collect serial growth data so that a pattern of growth can be assessed and current growth velocity determined. Care must be taken to obtain accurate supine (for children under 2 or 3 years old) or standing measurements and to plot the child's length or height on the appropriate growth chart (see Appendix B). A child's predicted growth potential is based in large part on genetic potential and may change with altered nutritional status and illness patterns. An estimate of the expected stature (±2 standard

---

BOX 25-1 | Classification of Growth Retardation

Primary growth abnormalities
* Osteochondrodysplasia
* Chromosome abnormalities
* Intrauterine growth restriction
* Dysmorphic syndromes
Genetic short stature
* SHOX gene haploinsufficiency
Secondary growth failure
* Malnutrition
* Chronic illness
* Endocrine disorders
  ○ Hypothyroidism
  ○ Cushing syndrome
  ○ Pseudohypoparathyroidism
  ○ Rickets
  ○ IGF-1 deficiency
    * Growth hormone deficiency
    * Growth hormone insensitivity
    * Defects in IGF-1 synthesis
Variants of normal growth
* Constitutional delay of growth
* Puberty

IGF-1, Insulin-like growth factor 1; *SHOX*, short stature homeobox.

deviations where 1 standard deviation equals 2 inches [4.5 cm]) for a particular child can be made by calculating a midparental target height:

Target height for boys : (mother's height + 5 inches [13 cm]) + (father's height)/2

Target height for girls : (father's height − 5 inches [13 cm]) + (mother's height)/2

Growth disorders may be classified as primary or secondary. Primary growth disorders include skeletal dysplasias, chromosomal abnormalities (e.g., Turner syndrome), and genetic short stature. Secondary growth disorders may result from undernutrition, chronic disease, endocrine disorder, and idiopathic (constitutional) growth delay [CGD]) (Box 25-1). The following discussion focuses on growth hormone deficiency (GHD) and CGD (Table 25-1).

GROWTH HORMONE DEFICIENCY
Description
Growth hormone (GH) is an anterior pituitary hormone released in response to sleep, exercise, and hypoglycemia. Secretion of GH occurs in a series of irregular and pulsatile bursts throughout the day and night, with most GH activity occurring during sleep. GH deficiency (GHD) may be either congenital or acquired. Individuals may also be resistant to GH, and GHD increases with age and immunodeficiency.

Epidemiology
Estimates of the incidence of idiopathic GHD vary; an epidemiologic study conducted in Denmark reported an incidence of child-onset GHD of 2.58/100,000 for boys and 1.7/100,000 for girls (Stochholm et al, 2006).

TABLE 25-1 Short Stature: Characteristics of Growth Hormone Deficiency and Constitutional Growth Delay in Children

Condition	Etiology	Onset	Presentation	Endocrine/Metabolic Disturbance
Growth hormone deficiency (GHD)	Idiopathic (most common) Pituitary or hypothalamic disease Trauma Minor organic hypothalamic lesion Infection Radiation	Congenital or acquired	Slow growth rate with normal birthweight Signs and symptoms of increased intracranial pressure Microphallus Proportional short stature Delayed bone age	Deficiency or impairment in secretion of growth hormone-releasing hormone
Constitutional growth delay (CGD)	Variation of normal growth Not a disease	First years of life with impaired growth	Growth velocity is normal after 3 years of age Delayed puberty with pubertal growth spurt Delayed bone age Positive family history	None—final height is appropriate for parents' height

Clinical Findings

Findings that suggest a GHD include hypoglycemia, deficiencies of other pituitary hormones, presence of midline defects, history of treatment with cranial radiation, and low serum levels of insulin-like growth factor 1 (IGF-1) or insulin-like growth factor binding protein 3 (IGFBP-3).

History. A history obtained to evaluate the short or slowly growing child should include:
- Details of pregnancy, delivery, and newborn period
  - Mother's health during pregnancy
  - Birthing process, type, and presence of complications
  - Birth length and weight
  - Neonatal course, including history of prolonged jaundice, hypoglycemia, microphallus (often diagnostic of congenital GHD)
  - Dysmorphia, especially midline facial defects or eye abnormalities
- Parents' and siblings' height, weight, and growth pattern
- Age at which growth decelerates
- Chronic illness(es)
- Symptoms of hypothyroidism or other known pituitary hormone deficiency
- Trauma or insult to the central nervous system (CNS)
- Signs of an intracranial lesion

Physical Examination. Physical examination of the short or slow-growing child should include:
- Identification of clinical clues to chronic illness or dysmorphic syndrome (e.g., childlike facies with large, prominent forehead)
- Evaluation of the fundi for signs of increased intracranial pressure
- Palpation of the thyroid gland for the presence of a goiter
- Evaluation of the stage of puberty
- Measurement of body proportions including arm span, height and upper-to-lower (U/L) body segment ratio to exclude a skeletal dysplasia (dwarfing condition). Interpretation of the U/L body segment ratio is dependent on the age of the child. At birth the U/L ratio is approximately 1.7:1; at 3 years of age it is approximately 1.3:1; and at 7 years and older approximately 1:1 (Keane, 2007).

Diagnostic Tests. If growth velocity is subnormal (including when prior heights are not available), initial evaluation should include:
- Complete blood count (CBC) and erythrocyte sedimentation rate (ESR)
- Urinalysis
- Screening for gastrointestinal (GI) illness when appropriate (e.g., celiac disease screening [serum immunoglobulin A (IgA) and transglutaminase], irritable bowel disease, stool for ova and parasites)
- Chemistry panel
- Growth factors (IGF-1 and IGFBP-3)
- Thyroid function tests: Free T_4 and TSH should be obtained to exclude both pituitary TSH deficiency and primary hypothyroidism
- Bone age x-ray of left wrist and hand
- Karyotype to rule out Turner syndrome in girls. Turner syndrome occurs in approximately 1:1500 to 1:2500 girls. Girls with Turner mosaicism may not manifest the typical clinical findings of Turner syndrome (e.g., cubitus valgus, webbing of the neck) thus highlighting the importance of karyotyping all females presenting with short stature (Loscalzo, 2008) (see Chapter 40).
- Measurement of GH production may be necessary. Because secretion of GH is pulsatile, random serum measurement of the hormone is inadequate; stimulation testing using agents such as arginine, levodopa (L-dopa), clonidine, and/or glucagon is needed to accurately assess GH production.

Differential Diagnosis

Individual children with short stature may not fit nicely into a single category, but may have multiple factors contributing to their stature. Many chronic illnesses can slow linear growth, likely through a variety of mechanisms including malnutrition, acidosis, anorexia, and deficiencies of minerals (e.g., zinc and iron) and vitamins necessary for growth (Box 25-2). Typically children with poor growth as a result of chronic illness are underweight for height; their weight gain slows prior to growth deceleration. Thyroid hormones are essential to growth during childhood; sex steroids are important for

<table>
<tr><td>

BOX 25-2 Chronic Illness Contributing to Growth Failure

- Gastrointestinal disease
  - Celiac disease
  - Inflammatory bowel disease
  - Cystic fibrosis
- Cardiovascular disease
  - Cyanotic heart disease
  - Congestive heart failure
- Renal disease
  - Uremia
  - Renal tubular acidosis
- Hematologic disorders
  - Chronic anemia
- Inborn errors of metabolism
- Pulmonary disease
- Chronic infection
- Anorexia nervosa

</td><td>

BOX 25-3 FDA-Approved Indications for Growth Hormone Therapy

- Growth hormone deficiency
- Growth failure caused by chronic renal failure
- Turner syndrome
- Prader-Willi syndrome
- Intrauterine growth restriction with failure to catch up by 2 years old
- Idiopathic short stature
  - Height more than 2.25 standard deviations below the mean for age and gender
  - Unexplained short stature with poor height prognosis

FDA, U.S. Food and Drug Administration.

</td></tr>
</table>

normal growth during the pubertal growth spurt. Deficiency of these hormones is characterized by subnormal growth velocity, normal to increased weight for height, and delay in bone age.

Management

Children should be referred to a pediatric endocrinologist if hypothyroidism, low IGF-1 and IGFBP-3 or other hormone deficiency is confirmed, or for unexplained persistent slow growth without evidence of chronic illness. The U.S. Food and Drug Administration (FDA) has approved a number of indications for GH therapy (Box 25-3) (Schwenk, 2006). GH dosing is based on a child's body weight with doses ranging from 0.15 to 0.30 mg/kg/wk. Response to GH therapy is greater for children receiving daily injections compared with those receiving three injections per week. During the first year of therapy, growth velocity may exceed normal growth rates as much as fourfold. Reported side effects of GH include glucose intolerance, pseudotumor cerebri, edema, growth of nevi, slipped capital femoral epiphyses, and scoliosis (Schwenk, 2006). The cost of GH therapy may present an economic burden to the family and referral to a social worker to assist in finding financial support may be appropriate.

CONSTITUTIONAL GROWTH DELAY
Description

CGD is a common growth pattern variation and should not be considered a disease entity. When the child has no evidence of chronic illness, has a delay in bone age, and is growing at a normal rate for bone age, the likely diagnosis is CGD. These children generally reach normal adult height, although they may be slightly short compared with other family members.

Clinical Findings

History. The history may include the following:
- Normal length and weight at birth
- Slowed linear growth between 1 to 3 years of age and then normal growth velocity; normal height velocity is the most critical factor in diagnosing CGD

- Height at or slightly below the third percentile on standardized growth charts
- Delayed pubertal development
- History of similar growth patterns in other family members

Physical Examination. Findings on physical examination include:
- Delayed bone age with growth velocity normal for bone age
- Final height prediction based on bone age within range of calculated target height
- Neurologic examination within normal limits

Diagnostic Tests. The same screening tests used to evaluate GHD are performed to rule out pathologic conditions.

Management

Reassurance and support should be provided to the child and family regarding ultimate height and development. An endocrine referral may be necessary to differentiate CGD from GHD and for possible hormone replacement therapy.

GROWTH EXCESS

Some children, in contrast to those with CGD, are tall for their family as young children, enter puberty early, yet ultimately reach a height within the normal range for their family. Rarely will this accelerated growth require referral to a pediatric endocrinologist. Tall stature in comparison with parents' height or rapid growth velocity in childhood can represent an underlying abnormality, however, including:
- Primary skeletal abnormalities such as Marfan syndrome, Klinefelter syndrome, and other overgrowth syndromes
- Overnutrition that advances the bone age and the timing of puberty. In these children, weight gain occurs first, and weight percentile is farther above the growth curve than height percentile.
- Excess adrenal androgens or gonadal steroids. These children have physical examination findings of early puberty.

Pubertal Disorders

The physical changes of puberty occur in response to production of sex steroids by the ovaries or testes (see Chapter 8). Hypothalamic gonadotropin-releasing hormone

(GnRH) regulates the release of luteinizing hormone (LH) and follicle-stimulating hormone (FSH) from the pituitary gland, which in turn stimulates gonadal hormone secretion.

By midgestation the fetal hypothalamic-pituitary-gonadal axis is intact; at term, the production of GnRH, LH, and FSH in this system is low. When placental and maternal hormones are removed at delivery, unrestrained production of these hormones occurs in the newborn, and the infant experiences a "mini puberty" between 2 weeks and 3 months of postnatal life. After infancy the hypothalamic GnRH pulse generator is more sensitive to feedback inhibition from the brain, and by 1 year of age, LH and FSH decrease to the prepubertal range, and the child enters a "latency" period that continues until puberty. Puberty occurs when the feedback inhibition is released and GnRH is again produced (Greiner and Kerrigan, 2006; Nathan and Palmert, 2005). The timing of the release correlates better with bone age than chronologic age.

The initiation of puberty in girls is earlier now compared with past decades and varies by race and ethnicity. A large epidemiologic study using data from 1300 girls who participated in the third National Health and Nutrition Examination Survey (NHANES) demonstrated that Tanner stage 2 breast development was present in less than 5% of non-Hispanic Caucasian girls with normal body mass index (BMI) by the age of 8 years; however, thelarche (breast bud development) is a normal finding in non-Hispanic black and Mexican-American girls before 8 years of age. Although girls are starting puberty at a younger age than in past generations, the timing of menarche and reaching Tanner stage 5 have not changed dramatically (Rosenfield et al, 2009). Menarche typically occurs within 3 years from the start of breast development; 95% of girls will have signs of puberty by the age of 12 years and achieve menarche by the age of 14 years. Boys normally begin puberty from age 9 to 14 years. The first sign of puberty is increased testicular volume in 85% of boys. Clinicians should be concerned when puberty presents early or is delayed.

EARLY PUBERTY

Early puberty is divided into four categories: premature thelarche, premature adrenarche, isolated menarche, and true precocious puberty. Premature thelarche, isolated breast development without any other features of puberty, occurs in infant and toddler girls and is sometimes present at birth. This breast development, likely due to estrogens produced during the mini puberty of infancy or increased responsiveness of the breast primordia, can take months or years to resolve and rarely progresses to true precocious puberty.

Premature adrenarche is the early onset of pubic hair in either boys (prior to 10 years of age) or girls (prior to 8 years of age) not associated with other features of true puberty. Premature adrenarche may be caused by a mild form of congenital adrenal hyperplasia (CAH), exposure to topical testosterone, or rarely, adrenal tumor. Most often the condition is idiopathic. Children with idiopathic premature adrenarche are at increased risk for polycystic ovary syndrome and metabolic syndrome (Ibáñez et al, 2009).

Isolated menarche is an uncommon condition in which girls have one to a few episodes of vaginal bleeding without breast development. In this condition, sexual abuse, vaginal tumor, a functional estrogen-producing ovarian cyst, and primary hypothyroidism all need to be excluded.

BOX 25-4 | Disorders of Puberty

Central Precocious Puberty
- Idiopathic
- CNS disorder
  - Hamartoma
  - Tumor
  - CNS radiation
  - Infection
  - Trauma
- Hypothyroidism
- hCG-secreting tumor

Peripheral Precocious Puberty
Girls
- McCune-Albright syndrome
- Ovarian cyst
- Estrogen-secreting ovarian or adrenal tumor

Boys
- Severe, non–salt wasting, congenital adrenal hyperplasia
- Testotoxicosis (activating mutation of the LH receptor)
- Testicular tumor

CNS, Central nervous system; *hCG*, human chorionic gonadotropin; *LH*, luteinizing hormone.

PRECOCIOUS PUBERTY

Description

True precocious puberty refers to the onset of multiple features of puberty earlier than the normal range. Features may include accelerated linear growth, breast development or penile enlargement, and pubic hair development. Depending on the duration of symptoms, the bone age may be advanced. Precocious puberty can be divided into two broad categories: central, gonadotropin dependent; or peripheral, gonadotropin independent (Box 25-4). Prolonged exposure to exogenous sex hormones (mother's birth control pills or father's topical testosterone) (Aksglaede et al, 2006) and exposure to chemicals that disrupt endocrine function (see Chapter 41) can cause precocious puberty (Cesario and Hughes, 2007).

Epidemiology

In the U.S. the incidence of precocious puberty is 0.01% to 0.05% per year. Precocious puberty is more common in females compared with males and in African-American children compared with Caucasian children (Muir, 2006). Any lesion that disrupts the normal connections between the brain and the hypothalamus can cause central precocious puberty. This condition is most often idiopathic in girls. Boys have a 30% incidence of CNS tumors in situations of central precocious puberty.

Clinical Findings

Children who present with features of puberty at a younger age than normal should have an evaluation as to the etiology. Children who start to develop signs of puberty at the early end of the normal range should be evaluated if they have rapid progression of pubertal signs resulting in a bone age more than 2 years ahead of chronologic age, or new CNS-related findings (e.g., headaches, seizures, focal neurologic defects) (Kaplowitz, 2009).

History. The history should include details (age of onset, progression, duration) of pubertal symptoms (breast tissue, pubic hair, phallic enlargement, acne, body odor, oily scalp), pattern of growth, any symptoms suggestive of a CNS lesion, and pattern of puberty in family members. Any exposure to topical estrogens or testosterone, oral estrogens, or environmental estrogen disruptors should be determined.

Physical Examination. Physical examination should include:

- Assessment of stature and growth velocity
- Description of the child's Tanner stage
- Breast development should be evaluated by palpation rather than inspection to differentiate between the presence of true breast tissue versus fat deposition (Rosenfeld et al, 2009)
- Pubic and axillary hair (girls)
- Penile length, testicular volume, and pubic and axillary hair (boys) (see Chapter 8)

Diagnostic Tests

- Premature thelarche: No laboratory studies are necessary in the infant or toddler girl unless she has other features of true puberty or continued increase in breast size
- Premature adrenarche: Serum 17-hydroxyprogesterone (17-OHP) to exclude CAH and a 24-hour urine collection for 17-ketosteroids or imaging of the adrenal glands to exclude an adrenal tumor
- Isolated menarche: Thyroid function tests to exclude primary hypothyroidism, and pelvic ultrasound to rule out the presence of an ovarian cyst or pelvic tumor

Diagnostic tests for children with true precocious puberty include:

- Bone age x-ray
- LH, FSH, and estradiol or testosterone (use a laboratory with a sensitive assay that will detect early pubertal values at the lower end of the range)
- If LH and FSH are high (in pubertal range: indication of central etiology), an MRI is indicated to exclude CNS tumor.
- If LH and FSH are low (in prepubertal range: indication of peripheral puberty), complete a GnRH stimulation test to distinguish central from peripheral puberty.
- If etiology is peripheral:
  - Pelvic ultrasonography of girls
  - Testicular ultrasonography of boys
  - Serum 17-OHP to rule out a severe form of CAH

Management

Treatment of precocious puberty should be done with the guidance of a pediatric endocrinologist. Management will depend on the underlying disorder, age of the child, degree of advancement of the bone age, and the child and family's emotional response to the condition. Radiation, surgery, or chemotherapy is indicated in the case of CNS tumors. A long-acting GnRH agonist may be used to bring serum sex steroids to prepubertal levels. Treatment of precocious puberty is important to increase final adult height.

DELAYED PUBERTY

Description

Puberty is considered delayed when a boy 14 years or older or a girl 13 years or older has no clinical features of puberty on physical examination.

BOX 25-5 Etiology of Delayed Puberty

Chronic Illness
- GI with poor weight gain
- Chronic renal failure
- Anorexia nervosa or bulimia
- Chronic anemia
- Respiratory or cardiac disease
- Medication-induced poor weight gain

CGD
- Endocrine diseases associated with delayed bone age
- Hypothyroidism

GHD
- Failure of the hypothalamic-pituitary-gonadal axis

CGD, Constitutional delay of growth; *GHD,* growth hormone deficiency; *GI,* gastrointestinal.

BOX 25-6 Failure of the Hypothalamic-Pituitary-Gonadal Axis

Hypothalamic Pituitary Dysfunction (LH/FSH Deficiency)
- Multiple pituitary hormone deficiency
- Isolated gonadotropin deficiency
  - Kallmann syndrome (anosmia and gonadotropin deficiency)
- Hyperprolactinemia
- Functional deficiency associated with decrease in calories or extreme exercise

Gonadal Failure
Girls
- Turner syndrome
- Oophoritis
- Galactosemia
- Chemotherapy induced

Boys
- Vanishing testes syndrome (in utero testicular torsion)
- Chemotherapy or radiation

FSH, Follicle-stimulating hormone; *LH,* luteinizing hormone.

Epidemiology

Any chronic condition that delays the bone age may cause delayed puberty because the timing of puberty correlates better with bone age than chronologic age (Box 25-5). In addition, failure of any part of the hypothalamic-pituitary-gonadal axis may also delay puberty (Box 25-6). The most common cause of delayed puberty is CGD (Louis et al, 2008).

Clinical Findings

History and Physical Examination. History and physical examination should focus on clinical clues indicating a chronic illness, symptoms or signs of hypothyroidism, prior history of CNS insult, or new CNS symptoms suggesting hypopituitarism. Review of systems should include questions about pattern of growth, especially growth velocity, sense of smell, and galactorrhea.

Diagnostic Tests. Laboratory investigation should include:

- Focused screening for acute or chronic illness (CBC, sedimentation rate, urinalysis, liver enzymes, electrolytes [renal function])
- Bone age x-ray
- Free T$_4$ and TSH
- IGF-1 and IGFBP-3, if GHD is suspected
- Serum prolactin
- LH and FSH (when gonadal failure is present, LH and FSH are abnormally elevated)

Management

A referral to a pediatric endocrinologist is necessary to determine the etiology and necessary treatment. Hormonal replacement is the treatment of choice for hypogonadism.

■ Adrenal Disorders

ANATOMY AND PHYSIOLOGY

Adrenal gland steroid production is under the control of the hypothalamic-pituitary axis. The hypothalamus secretes corticotropin-releasing hormone (CRH) in a pulsatile fashion, which stimulates production and secretion of adrenocorticotropic hormone (ACTH) by the pituitary gland. ACTH regulates adrenal glucocorticoid (cortisol) and androgen production. Cortisol is produced in a series of enzymatic steps (Fig. 25-1) and is highest in the morning, low in the afternoon and evening, and lowest at midnight. Secreted in response to hypoglycemia, hypotension, pain, or other stressful events,

cortisol has negative feedback on the synthesis and secretion of CRH, vasopressin, and ACTH.

The adrenal gland also produces mineralocorticoid hormones (aldosterone), regulated by renal production of renin interacting with angiotensinogen to create angiotensin. The renin-angiotensin system is involved in regulation of salts, especially sodium; blood pressure; and renal blood flow. Aldosterone production also occurs in enzymatic steps, many of which are common to the cortisol production pathway.

ADRENAL INSUFFICIENCY
Description

Adrenal insufficiency is characterized by a deficiency of hormones produced by the adrenal cortex; deficits of cortisol and aldosterone are perhaps the most important to body function. In primary adrenal insufficiency (hypofunctioning adrenal gland), glucocorticoid (cortisol) and mineralocorticoid (aldosterone) hormones are deficient, whereas in secondary adrenal insufficiency (hypothalamic or pituitary defect), only a glucocorticoid deficit is found. Thus, children with both forms of adrenal insufficiency have hypoglycemia and hypotension caused by cortisol deficiency. Only those with a primary adrenal insufficiency are at risk for salt-wasting crisis (hyponatremia, hyperkalemia, acidosis, and dehydration) caused by aldosterone deficiency.

Epidemiology

Primary adrenal insufficiency may be due to an inability to produce cortisol secondary to an enzyme defect in the adrenal steroid pathway (CAH), hypoplasia of the adrenal gland, or

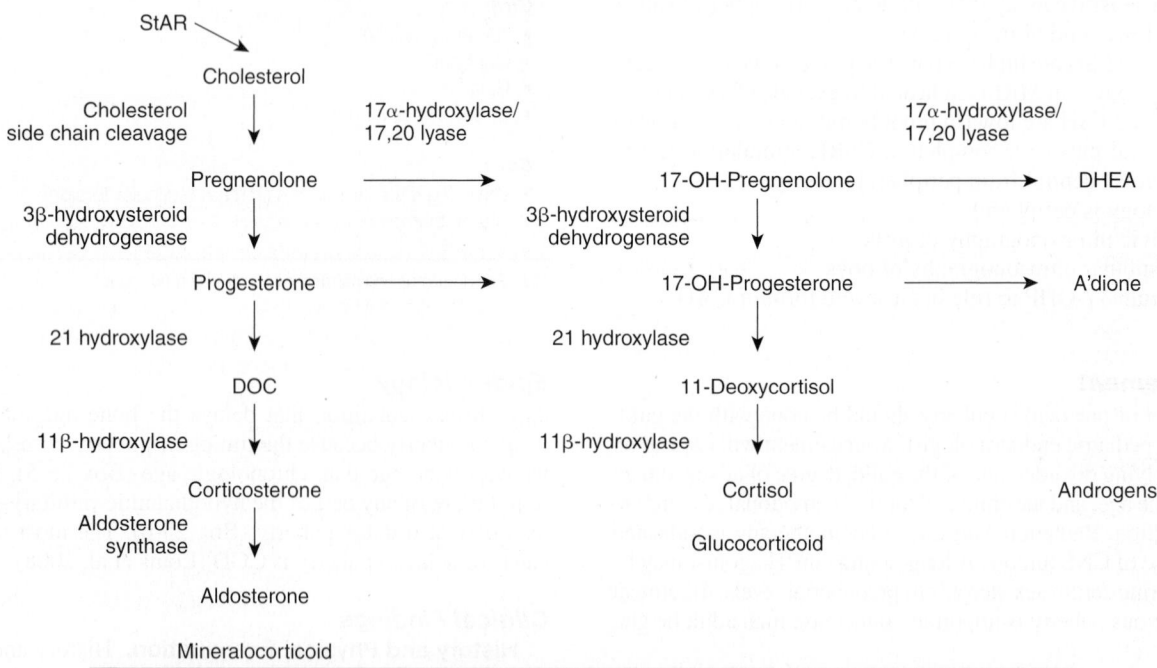

FIG. 25-1 Adrenal steroidogenesis. After the steroidogenic acute regulatory (StAR) protein–mediated uptake of cholesterol into mitochondria within adrenocortical cells, aldosterone, cortisol, and adrenal androgens are synthesized through the coordinated action of a series of steroidogenic enzymes in a zone-specific fashion. *A'dione,* Androstenedione; *DHEA,* dehydroepiandrosterone; *DOC,* deoxycorticosterone. (From Stewart PM: The adrenal cortex. In Larsen PR, Kronenberg HM, Melmed S, et al, editors: *Williams textbook of endocrinology,* ed 10, Philadelphia, 2003, Saunders, p 495.)

an acquired defect (Box 25-7). Lesions of the hypothalamus or pituitary lead to secondary adrenal insufficiency. Suppression of the hypothalamic-pituitary-adrenal axis secondary to steroid use can also lead to adrenal insufficiency. Infants born extremely prematurely (24 to 28 weeks' gestation) sometimes demonstrate symptoms of adrenal insufficiency because of immaturity of the hypothalamic-pituitary-adrenal axis.

Secondary adrenal insufficiency can occur as a result of ACTH deficiency, as one of multiple hypothalamic-pituitary deficiencies, or rarely as an isolated problem. Most often the infant or child has a syndrome known to be associated with hypopituitarism (for example septo-optic dysplasia), has also been discovered to have GHD, or has a destructive lesion (e.g., tumor or radiation to the brain) or prior CNS trauma.

CAH is caused by a deficiency of any of the enzymes in the cortisol pathway. In addition to interrupting normal cortisol production, the most common enzymatic abnormality, 21-hydroxylase (21-OH) deficiency, causes shunting of cortisol precursors to the androgen pathway resulting in production of elevated levels of adrenal androgens in utero. Female infants born with classic CAH typically have ambiguous genitalia (e.g., enlarged clitoris and/or posterior fusion of the labia) from this excessive androgen exposure in utero. However, male infants have no signs of CAH at birth with the exception of subtle hyperpigmentation and possible mild enlargement of the penis (Antal and Zhou, 2009). About 75% of children with CAH caused by 21-OH deficiency also have aldosterone deficiency. Newborn screening programs now routinely test for the presence of CAH caused by 21-OH deficiency to detect CAH early to avoid a potentially life-threatening salt-wasting crisis in affected infants.

Clinical Findings

History. Symptoms of cortisol deficiency include a history of:
- Poor appetite
- Failure to thrive or weight loss
- Weakness
- Vomiting

BOX 25-7 Adrenal Insufficiency

Deficiency of CRH or ACTH
- Isolated deficiency
  - Congenital
  - Acquired as a result of hypophysitis
- Multiple pituitary hormone deficiencies
  - Congenital (septo-optic dysplasia, midline defects)
  - Acquired (CNS trauma, infection, tumor, radiation)

Primary Adrenal
- Congenital
  - Congenital adrenal hyperplasia (most common 21-OH deficiency)
  - Adrenal hypoplasia (X-linked, autosomal recessive, ACTH receptor defect)
- Acquired
  - X-linked, adrenoleukodystrophy
  - Autoimmune (Addison disease)
  - Infection

21-OH, 21-Hydroxylase; *ACTH,* adrenocorticotropic hormone; *CNS,* central nervous system; *CRH,* corticotropin-releasing hormone.

Symptoms of aldosterone deficiency include:
- Vomiting
- Poor feeding
- Lethargy
- Dehydration

Physical Examination. On physical examination the infant or child often shows the following signs:
- Dehydration
- Hypotension
- Excessive pigmentation of the skin and mucous membranes (present only with primary adrenal insufficiency)

Diagnostic Tests. Laboratory tests include:
- Serum glucose (hypoglycemia)
- Blood gases and bicarbonate (for metabolic acidosis)
- Electrolytes (low sodium, elevated potassium with aldosterone deficiency)
- Serum cortisol (a cortisol value greater than 20 mcg/dL indicates adrenal sufficiency. A value lower than that must be interpreted in the clinical context in which the sample was drawn. Often an ACTH stimulation test, performed in collaboration with a pediatric endocrinologist, is needed to conclusively diagnose both primary and secondary adrenal insufficiency).
- Serum ACTH (elevated in primary adrenal insufficiency)
- Serum 17-OHP (diagnostic in children with suspected CAH caused by 21-OH deficiency)
- Serum renin level (elevated with aldosterone deficiency)
- Aldosterone level (low with aldosterone deficiency)

Plasma renin and aldosterone levels are interpreted best if they are drawn when serum sodium levels are low.

Management

Treatment of adrenal insufficiency includes hormone replacement and is best managed by a pediatric endocrinologist. An adrenal crisis is a medical emergency requiring immediate and vigorous administration of intravenous dextrose, normal saline, and stress doses of hydrocortisone. Intravenous stress doses of hydrocortisone succinate vary with age: 25 mg in children younger than 3 years; 50 mg in children ages 3 to 12 years; and 100 mg in children older than age 12, administered every 6 hours. Parents should be instructed regarding the need for stress doses of hydrocortisone when their child has a febrile illness, surgery, or trauma; they should also be taught how to administer hydrocortisone via intramuscular injection in case the child is vomiting or otherwise unable to swallow or retain oral medication. This injection allows parents extended time to seek further medical advice or intervention.

Long-term therapy of CAH includes oral hydrocortisone in replacement doses of 8 to 10 mg/m^2 (8 to 10 mg per square meter of body surface) in children with ACTH deficiency or primary adrenal insufficiency. Children with CAH tend to have higher hydrocortisone needs. If present, aldosterone deficiency must be treated with fludrocortisone acetate. Treatment of CAH requires a fine balancing act to replace steroids, thereby preventing androgen overproduction. Excess steroid intake can lead to delayed growth; not enough steroids contribute to rapid bone age growth and ultimate short stature. Individual treatment plans are essential to meet the specific needs of individual children. The primary care provider should be familiar with the medical endocrinology treatment plan and reinforce it at routine well- and sick-child visits.

HYPERADRENAL STATES

Epidemiology

Cortisol excess is most commonly caused by exogenous glucocorticoid treatment of an illness (e.g., serious asthma, to prevent rejection after a transplant, or as part of chemotherapy protocols). Endogenous cortisol excess may be due to a pituitary tumor producing ACTH, adrenal tumor, or to ectopic production of ACTH from a nonpituitary tumor (rare in children).

Clinical Findings

Clinical features of cortisol excess include:
- Weight gain
- Growth failure
- Osteopenia
- Hypertension
- Delayed puberty
- Plethora (hypervolemia)
- Skin: Acne, purple striae, hirsutism
- Compulsive behavior

Almost all children with simple obesity are of normal height or are tall for their age, and cortisol excess can be excluded on physical examination alone. When growth is slow or growth data are missing and cortisol excess needs to be excluded by laboratory evaluation, a 24-hour urine collection for free cortisol or a late evening serum or salivary cortisol is the best screening test.

Management

When children receive glucocorticoids for underlying illness for longer than 7 to 10 days, the steroid dose should be weaned rather than abruptly discontinued to allow the hypothalamic-pituitary-adrenal axis to recover normal function and sometimes to prevent a flare-up of the underlying disease. Procedures for tapering the dose are empiric, but in general, the longer the patient has been on glucocorticoids, the longer the taper. Withdrawal plans are based on the goal of treating the patient with the least amount of glucocorticoids in order to avoid long-term adverse effects while avoiding potential adrenal insufficiency during withdrawal. Decreasing the dose to a physiologic dose while monitoring the cortisol level is one method to wean. A morning cortisol value of 20 mcg/dL suggests it is safe to wean further or, if the patient is already on half maintenance dose, discontinue the medication (Carroll and Findling, 2009; Hopkins and Leinung, 2005). Even after the steroid has been safely discontinued, the patient may not be able to respond adequately to severe stress for as long as 6 to 12 months.

■ Disorders of Sex Development

DESCRIPTION

Abnormalities of sexual differentiation usually present in infancy with ambiguous genitalia. The spectrum of physical examination findings ranges from the appearance of a normal male penis and normal scrotum but without palpable gonads, to an infant who looks mostly female with mild enlargement of the clitoris. True hermaphroditism, in which the infant has both male and female gonadal structures, is rare.

Infants with 46 XY chromosomes who have complete androgen insensitivity (androgen receptor defect) have genitalia that appear female; these children are not detected in the newborn period unless a karyotype is performed for some other reason. Children with complete androgen insensitivity may not be identified until the time of an inguinal hernia repair when a testis is discovered or during the teen years when they fail to develop pubic hair or menstruate.

EPIDEMIOLOGY

Disorders of sex development occur when the XX fetus is exposed to excess androgen in utero, the XY fetus is unable to produce or respond to androgens, or, rarely, true hermaphroditism. The most common cause of disordered sex development is CAH that exposes an XX fetus to excess androgens during fetal life (see Fig. 25-1). Other much less common virilizing conditions include aromatase deficiency or virilizing tumor in the mother. In an XY fetus, disordered sex development can result from inadequate androgen production or partial androgen insensitivity (Kolon, 2008).

CLINICAL FINDINGS

All infants should receive a complete genital examination before discharge from the nursery. The initial laboratory evaluation of an infant with ambiguous genitalia should be directed by a pediatric endocrinologist and includes:
- Karyotype. This test can be done quickly (within 48 to 72 hours) if the cytogenetics laboratory is alerted to the urgency. Subsequent laboratory evaluation is based on karyotype results.
- In XY infants, measurement of the precursors of testosterone, testosterone, and dihydrotestosterone
- In XX infants, serum 17-OHP to establish a diagnosis of 21-OH deficiency
- Serum müllerian inhibitory substance can also be measured or can be assessed indirectly by obtaining an ultrasound or genitogram

MANAGEMENT

The family needs to be counseled immediately. The primary health care provider has a responsibility to document the abnormality and refer to a specialist team that includes a pediatric endocrinologist, medical geneticist, and pediatric urologist. The initial studies should be sent with the referral. The specialist team should meet with families and educate them about the normal process of genital development, the cause of their child's abnormality, the evaluation process, and the determination of gender for childrearing. Female is the appropriate sex of rearing for XX infants with CAH and for infants with complete androgen insensitivity. Sex of rearing in incompletely masculinized XY infants is complicated, and waiting to assign the sex of rearing until the evaluation is complete is imperative (Kolon, 2008). Treatment of the underlying cause, if known (e.g., CAH), is essential.

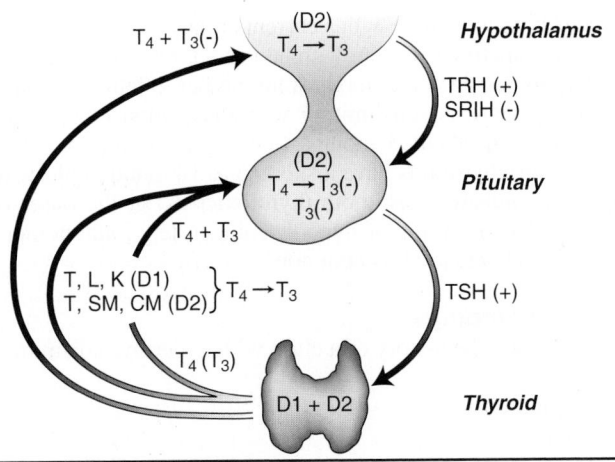

FIG. 25-2 Interrelationships of the hypothalamic-pituitary-thyroid (HPT) axis. Secreted thyroxine (T₄) must be converted to triiodothyronine (T₃) to produce its effects. This conversion may take place in tissues such as the liver (L), kidney (K), and thyroid (T) catalyzed by the type 1 iodothyronine deiodinase, D1. Type 2 (D2) is present in human thyroid (T), skeletal muscle (SM), possibly cardiac muscle (CM), and the pituitary and hypothalamus. *SRIH,* somatotropin release-inhibiting factor (somatostatin hormone); *TRH,* thyrotropin-releasing hormone; *TSH,* thyroid-stimulating hormone. (From Melmed S, Polonsky KS, Larsen PR, editors: *Williams textbook of endocrinology,* ed 12, Philadelphia, 2011, Saunders.)

■ Thyroid Disorders

ANATOMY AND PHYSIOLOGY

The hypothalamic-pituitary-thyroid axis begins functioning in utero (Fig. 25-2). The hypothalamus produces TRH, which in turn stimulates pituitary production of TSH. TSH stimulates the thyroid gland to secrete primarily T₄, which is converted in peripheral tissues to T₃. Both T₃ and T₄ bind to thyroid-binding proteins, primarily thyroid-binding globulin (TBG). The free, unbound form of T₃ and T₄ is biologically active. T₄ inhibits hypothalamic TRH and pituitary TSH secretion. Thyroid hormone has an important role in growth and development, basal metabolic activity, oxygen consumption, brain development, and metabolism of lipids, carbohydrates, and proteins.

HYPOTHYROIDISM

Description and Epidemiology

Primary hypothyroidism (hypothyroidism caused by a problem in the thyroid gland itself) may be either congenital or acquired. Congenital hypothyroidism (CH) affects 1 in 3000 to 4000 infants (Schulze et al, 2009) with female infants more commonly affected. Congenital hypothyroidism results from an abnormality in development of the thyroid gland during fetal life (dysgenesis or agenesis) or a problem with the ability of the thyroid to make thyroid hormone. Less frequently, CH may result from an abnormality at the level of the pituitary or hypothalamus (affecting 1 in 100,000 infants). CH is the most common cause of preventable mental retardation. Untreated congenital hypothyroidism leads to irreversible brain damage and variable degrees of growth failure, deafness, and neurologic abnormalities. Earlier detection of CH through improvements in newborn screening combined with more aggressive

thyroid hormone replacement regimens (10 to 15 mcg/kg/day) at diagnosis, has led to improved developmental outcomes for newborns with CH.

The most common cause of acquired hypothyroidism in children in the Western world is Hashimoto thyroiditis, an autoimmune condition leading to destruction of the thyroid gland (Counts and Varma, 2009). Worldwide, iodine deficiency is the main cause of acquired primary hypothyroidism and has led to salt iodination as a public health measure in many countries. Hypothyroidism can also be due to a TSH deficiency that is secondary to pituitary disease or dysfunction of the hypothalamus (central hypothyroidism). Other causes of acquired hypothyroidism are listed in Box 25-8.

Clinical Findings

History. Growth failure, goiter, delayed or arrested puberty, delayed dentition, weight gain, fatigue, dry skin, hyperlipidemia, decline in school performance, and menorrhagia can be present in the child with hypothyroidism. A family history of thyroid disease or other autoimmune conditions is frequently present. A history of risk factors for hypopituitarism (e.g., CNS insult, frequent headaches, midline defects) is useful information when assessing the risk for TSH deficiency.

Physical Examination. The clinical manifestations of primary hypothyroidism vary with the age of the child. At birth the newborn may appear completely normal, thus the importance of newborn screening programs for early identification of hypothyroidism. The most common neonatal signs are prolonged jaundice, constipation, and umbilical hernia. Infants with CH may also have a large anterior and posterior fontanelle, macroglossia, and decreased muscle tone, and may be poor feeders. They may have respiratory distress and poor peripheral circulation with cool, cyanotic skin in the extremities.

Physical examination findings of older children who present with acquired hypothyroidism include delayed growth or subnormal growth velocity, goiter, weight gain, and delayed return of the deep tendon reflexes. Children with central hypothyroidism (thyroid deficiency secondary to pituitary or hypothalamus dysfunction) may show poor growth, increased weight for height, and features suggestive of hypopituitarism such as midline facial or eye abnormalities.

Diagnostic Tests. For primary hypothyroidism:
- The diagnosis of CH is usually made in infancy, detected by newborn screening tests. Newborn screening programs test filter paper blood spots using one of two screening strategies: a primary TSH/backup T₄ method or a primary T₄/backup TSH method to identify newborns with either

TABLE 25-2	Thyroid Hormone Dosing
Age	**L-Thyroxine (mcg/kg/day)**
0-6 months	10-15
6-12 months	6-8
1-5 years	5-6
6-12 years	4-5
>12 years	2-3

Adapted from Lee C, Custer JW, Rau RE: Drug doses. In Custer JW, Rau RE, editors: *The Harriet Lane handbook: a manual for pediatric house officers*, ed 18, Philadelphia, 2009, Mosby; Polak, M, Van Vliet G: Disorders of the thyroid gland. In Sarafoglou K, Hoffmann GR, Roth KS, editors: *Pediatric endocrinology and inborn errors of metabolism*, New York, 2009, McGraw-Hill Medical.

primary or central hypothyroidism. When a result is abnormal, the primary care provider or hospital of record and regional center is contacted to obtain a confirmatory free T_4 and TSH serum sample. A serum sample is also indicated if clinical features of CH are detected. Retesting may be necessary.

- For children with Down syndrome retesting is recommended at 6 and 12 months old and then annually (Carroll et al, 2008).
- In older children TSH is abnormally elevated and the free serum T_4 is either within the normal range or low.

For central hypothyroidism:
- Free serum T_4 is low with a normal TSH.

For children with TBG deficiency:
- Total T_4 is low, but free T_4 and TSH are normal. TBG level should then be measured to confirm TBG deficiency.

Management

TBG does not require treatment. Hypothyroidism is treated with replacement doses of levothyroxine sodium. The dose varies by age and weight (Table 25-2). Ongoing laboratory monitoring and follow-up are age-dependent. Because normal thyroid function in the first 3 years of life is critical for normal cognitive development, more frequent monitoring is necessary for infants and young children. In general, an elevated TSH (in primary hypothyroidism) or depression of the free T_4 (in central hypothyroidism) indicates the need to increase the dose of medication. Following an adjustment in thyroid hormone replacement, thyroid function testing should be repeated in 4 to 6 weeks to be sure the new dose is adequate.

HYPERTHYROIDISM

Description

Hyperthyroidism occurs in childhood when the thyroid gland overproduces thyroid hormone or when a child is given too large a dose of thyroid hormone replacement.

Epidemiology

Graves disease, an autoimmune condition, is the most common cause of hyperthyroidism (LaFranchi, 2007). In this condition thyroid-stimulating immunoglobulin binds to the TSH receptor resulting in excessive thyroid hormone production.

Infants born to women with a current or past history of Graves disease sometimes present with neonatal Graves disease, secondary to passage of antibody from mother to fetus. Neonatal Graves disease is self-limiting with dissipation of maternal antibodies by about 3 months of age. Some children with Hashimoto thyroiditis have a short (6 to 18 months) phase of hyperthyroidism (Hashimoto thyrotoxicosis) at the onset of disease. Other causes of hyperthyroidism (e.g., autonomous thyroid nodules) are less common.

Clinical Findings

History. The history of a child with hyperthyroidism may include:
- Palpitations
- Tremor
- Increased appetite often accompanied by weight loss
- Fatigue
- Muscle weakness
- Emotional lability
- Poor concentration with decreased school performance
- Hyperdefecation
- Poor sleep

Physical Examination. Often observed findings in hyperthyroidism include:
- Goiter (almost 100%)
- An audible thyroid bruit may be present
- Tachycardia
- Wide pulse pressure
- Underweight for height
- Eyelid lag or exophthalmos (approximately 50% of children with Graves disease have exophthalmos)
- A hyperfunctioning nodule in the thyroid may be present
- Warm, moist skin
- Tremor or hyperreflexia

Diagnostic Tests. The free T_4 and total T_4 levels will be elevated and the TSH suppressed below the sensitivity of the assay. Measuring a T_3 level is helpful in hyperthyroidism because it may be more dramatically elevated than the T_4 and be a better marker to monitor.

Management

Children with hyperthyroidism should be referred to a pediatric endocrinologist for discussion of treatment options (i.e., medical therapy using antithyroid drugs, subtotal thyroidectomy, or radioiodine ablation) and ongoing management (LaFranchi, 2007).

■ Diabetes Mellitus

Diabetes mellitus is a group of conditions characterized by inadequate insulin secretion, insulin resistance, or both. These dynamics lead to defective metabolism of carbohydrate, protein, and fat and subsequent hyperglycemia (Alemzadeh and Wyatt, 2007). Diabetes affects approximately 186,300 individuals 20 years old or younger in the U.S. (National Diabetes Information Clearinghouse, 2007). New cases are more frequently diagnosed during the autumn and winter months (Cooke and Plotnick, 2008). In addition to the most familiar forms—type 1 (formerly called insulin-dependent diabetes mellitus [IDDM] or juvenile-onset diabetes) and type 2

BOX 25-9 Types of Diabetes Other than Type 1 and Type 2

Genetic Defects in Beta-Cell Function
- Maturity-onset diabetes of youth (MODY) syndrome
- Mitochondrial DNA mutations
- Wolfram syndrome (diabetes insipidus, diabetes mellitus, optic atrophy, deafness)
- Thiamine responsive

Drug or Chemical Induced
- Glucocorticoids
- L-Asparaginase
- Antirejection medications

Conditions Affecting Function of the Exocrine Pancreas
- Cystic fibrosis
- Pancreatitis
- Trauma
- Hemolytic uremic syndrome (HUS)

Infections
- Congenital rubella
- Cytomegalovirus (CMV)

Genetic Syndromes With Diabetes
- Prader-Willi
- Turner
- Alström
- Down
- Neonatal diabetes

TABLE 25-3 Comparison of Type 1 and Type 2 Diabetes

	Type 1	Type 2
Age at onset	All ages	≥10 years
Gender	Equal distribution by gender	More frequent in females
Race/ethnicity	May occur in all racial and ethnic groups Most frequent in Non-Hispanic Caucasians	More frequent in African-Americans, Asians, Native Americans, Hispanics
Obesity	Obesity not related to type 1 diabetes	>90%
Family history of diabetes	Uncommon	Common
Hypertension	Uncommon	Common
Acanthosis nigricans	Rare	Common
Polycystic ovary syndrome	Rare	Common
Ketosis, diabetic ketoacidosis	Occurs in approximately one third of new cases of diabetes	Uncommon
Islet autoimmunity	Present	Uncommon

(formerly called non–insulin-dependent diabetes mellitus [NIDDM] or adult-onset diabetes)—there are others (Box 25-9). The incidence of type 1 and type 2 diabetes is increasing dramatically in children in the U.S. and other countries throughout the world (Ma and Chan, 2009; Patterson et al, 2009). Table 25-3 shows the distinguishing features of type 1 and type 2 diabetes.

TYPE 1 DIABETES

Epidemiology

Type 1 diabetes is caused by autoimmune destruction of pancreatic beta cells in the islets of Langerhans thought to be triggered by a preceding environmental event in genetically susceptible individuals. This destruction of beta cells results in an absolute deficiency in insulin secretion, reduced biologic effectiveness, or both. High blood glucose levels are a result of the defective metabolism of carbohydrate, protein, and fats; normal metabolic function depends on sufficient amounts of circulating insulin. Insulin deficiency results in uninhibited gluconeogenesis and a blockage in the use and storage of circulating glucose. Based on 2002-2003 data from the SEARCH for Diabetes in Youth study, 15,000 new cases of type 1 diabetes and 3700 new cases of type 2 diabetes occur per year among children (birth to 19 years old) in the U.S. (SEARCH for Diabetes in Youth, 2010). Type 1 diabetes is much more common among children than is type 2, representing 80% of all diabetes in children 9 years old and younger (0.76 cases per 1000 children), and 91% of all

diabetes in non-Hispanic Caucasian youth 10 to 19 years old (2.8 cases per 1000 children). Among Hispanic youth 10 to 19 years old, 78% of diabetes is type 1; among African-Americans, 69%; among Asian or Pacific Islanders, 60%; but for American Indians, only 34% of diabetes is type 1 (Liese et al, 2006; Mayer-Davis et al, 2009). The process of developing the disease can be gradual, but children may become ill quite suddenly once symptoms manifest. Onset of symptoms can present at any age. Although children are most often diagnosed during the time of puberty, the highest age-specific increase has occurred in young children with approximately 20% of new cases diagnosed in children 5 years old or younger (Roche et al, 2005). Females and males are affected in equal numbers (Alemzadeh and Wyatt, 2007).

Clinical Findings

History. As diabetes develops, the symptomatology reflects the decreasing degree of beta cell mass, increasing insulinopenia and hyperglycemia, and increasing ketoacids. A provider's level of suspicion should rise when any child has inappropriate polyuria, dehydration, poor weight gain, and flulike symptoms. With type 1 diabetes the child may have had a viral infection, cold, or flu; parents may notice increased urination and thirst during the recovery period, with additional signs and symptoms appearing over a period of days or weeks. Children may exhibit significant weight loss, fatigue, and lethargy. Twenty percent to 40% of children do not seek treatment

until they develop ketoacidosis (Alemzadeh and Wyatt, 2007). The following early symptoms are often reported:
- Polydipsia
- Polyphagia
- Polyuria
- Nocturia
- Blurred vision
- Weight loss
- Fatigue
- Vaginal moniliasis

As ketoacid accumulates, the following history is reported:
- Abdominal pain
- Nausea, vomiting
- Fruity-smelling breath
- Weakness (caused by dehydration)
- Mental confusion
- Coma

Physical Examination. Although children typically have polyuria, polydipsia, and weight loss, the physical examination of children with new-onset type 1 diabetes may be remarkably benign. Findings can range from benign to severe. Look for:
- Dehydration (child may not look clinically dehydrated unless actively vomiting)
- Weight loss or slow weight gain; assess height and weight over time
- Muscle wasting
- Tachycardia
- Slow, labored breathing (Kussmaul) (if ketotic)
- Flushed cheeks and face (if ketotic)
- Fruity-smelling breath (if ketotic)
- Vaginal yeast, thrush, or other infection

Diagnostic Tests. Urine testing and blood glucose measurements are generally all that are required to make the diagnosis.
- Urine for glucose and ketones
- Metabolic screen for acid-base status to exclude diabetic ketoacidosis
- Hemoglobin A_{1c} (HbA$_{1c}$) equal to or greater than 6.5% (American Diabetes Association [ADA], 2010). In their study, Ehehalt and colleagues (2010) found that all children with HbA$_{1c}$ greater than 6.35% were subsequently diagnosed with type 1 diabetes, despite lack of other symptoms.
- Blood sugar
  - Fasting plasma glucose equal to or greater than 126 mg/dL
  - Random plasma glucose equal to or greater than 200 mg/dL
  - Postprandial (2 hours after eating) plasma glucose equal to or greater than 200 mg/dL
- Screen for concomitant associated autoimmune conditions (primary hypothyroidism and celiac disease affect approximately 5% of children with type 1 diabetes) (ADA, 2010).
- Capillary blood samples, reagent sticks, and glucose meters should only be used for monitoring diabetes control and not for diagnosing diabetes mellitus.

Differential Diagnosis

Type 1 diabetes must be distinguished from stress-induced hyperglycemia, which in some studies occurs in up to 4% of normal children during a serious illness. Thyroiditis and/or celiac disease may be present at initial diagnosis of type 1 diabetes.

Management

The treatment goals for children with type 1 diabetes are to achieve normal growth and development, optimal glycemic control, and positive psychosocial adjustment to diabetes while minimizing acute or chronic complications. Each child is different, and treatment of new-onset type 1 diabetes must be individualized to determine target blood glucose levels, diet, and insulin regimen best suited to the individual child. The ADA publishes and makes available on their website standards of care each year for the management of diabetes in children.

Diabetes treatment and education approaches for children and adolescents with type 1 diabetes are well-defined and supported by strong evidence from multicenter randomized controlled trials; these trials demonstrate that glycemic control through use of intensive insulin management prevents and/or delays development of microvascular complications of diabetes (Diabetes Control and Complications Trial Research Group, 1993, 1994). Management of new-onset type 1 diabetes involves determining the insulin regimen and dose best suited to the individual child, target range for blood glucose levels, and best methods to manage the child's diet. Children and families must learn how to inject insulin, monitor blood glucose levels, quantify the amount of carbohydrate in food, prevent hypoglycemia, manage diabetes during illness, and adjust insulin dose or carbohydrate intake for strenuous activities. These children and families need ongoing access to certified pediatric diabetes educators, pediatric dietitians, and psychologists or social workers when necessary.

Each component of the treatment regimen is discussed in the following text.

Initial Management. All children with type 1 diabetes should be started on insulin at diagnosis. Children with ketoacidosis should be admitted to the hospital for intravenous insulin treatment, fluid replacement, and careful monitoring to prevent cerebral edema that, although rare, can cause significant morbidity or mortality.

Whenever possible, children should be referred immediately to a children's diabetes center for initiation of insulin therapy and diabetes education. Traditionally most children with new-onset type 1 diabetes were hospitalized to initiate insulin therapy. However, current practice in many diabetes centers is to routinely manage these children as outpatients unless diabetic ketoacidosis is present. A systematic review of studies suggests that outpatient management at initial diagnosis of type 1 diabetes has no disadvantages regarding glycemic control, complications, psychosocial factors, or total costs (Clar et al, 2007).

Insulin. Insulin therapy choices are many. The selection of an insulin regimen depends on the age of the child, family preferences and lifestyle, the family's social and educational resources, and the clinician's comfort level. All children require medical nutrition therapy that must match the insulin schedule. The most frequently used insulin preparations are listed in Table 25-4. For general guidelines regarding insulin dosing, goals for glycemic control, and blood glucose target ranges by age group, see Table 25-5.

TABLE 25-4 Types of Insulin

Insulin	Onset (minutes)	Peak (hours)	Duration (hours)
Short Acting			
Regular	30 to 60	2 to 3	4 to 6
Rapid Acting			
Aspart	10 to 15	1/2 to 1	3 to 4
Lispro	10 to 15	1/2 to 1	3 to 4
Glulisine	10 to 15	1/2 to 1	3 to 4
Intermediate Acting			
NPH	120 to 240	6 to 10	14 to 16
Long Acting			
Detemir	Slowly	6 to 8	6 to 24
Glargine	120 to 180	No peak	20 to 24

TABLE 25-5 Insulin Dosing (Units/kg/Day), Blood Glucose Target Levels, and HbA_{1C} Goals by Age

Age (years)	Blood Glucose Targets (mg/dL)	Total Daily Insulin (Units/kg/Day)	% of Total Dose as Basal Insulin	HbA_{1C} Goal
0 to 5 years	100 to 200	0.6 to 0.7	25 to 30	<8.5%
6 to 12 years	90 to 180	0.7 to 1.0	40 to 50	<8%
13 to 19 years	90 to 150	1.0 to 1.2	40 to 50	<7.5%

Adapted from Alemzadeh R, Wyatt DT: Diabetes mellitus in children. In Kliegman RM, Behrman RE, Jenson HB, et al, editors: *Nelson textbook of pediatrics,* ed 18, Philadelphia, 2007, Saunders; American Diabetes Association (ADA): Standards of medical care in diabetes-2011, *Diabetes Care* 34(Suppl 1):S11-S61, 2011.

Two starting insulin strategies exist with some variations. A traditional regimen would include short-acting insulin (lispro or aspart) combined with intermediate-acting NPH insulin at breakfast, short-acting insulin at dinner, and NPH insulin at bedtime. This plan has the advantage that a school-age child will not require an injection at school, but the disadvantage that the timing of meals must remain consistent each day with the child eating a set amount of carbohydrate at meals and snacks. With this type of regimen, most young children require three meals and three snacks, whereas teens require three meals and two snacks daily.

The other regimen is a basal bolus routine using a long-acting insulin analogue administered at breakfast (infants and toddlers) or bedtime (teens) to provide a steady background amount of insulin with boluses of short-acting insulin at meals and with snacks. This regimen allows unreliable eaters to match their carbohydrate intake with insulin; children may be flexible with the timing of meals and snacks. However, this regimen requires more injections. Families learn to use a carbohydrate-to-insulin ratio (to cover the carbohydrate content of the meal/snack) and a blood sugar correction formula (if the blood glucose is above the target range) to determine each quick-acting insulin dose.

The usual sites for insulin injection are the legs, arms, abdomen, hips, and buttocks. School-age children and adolescents can be encouraged to use their abdomen as a regular injection site. However, young children with minimal subcutaneous abdominal fat may have difficulty with this site. Rotation of injection sites is necessary to prevent lipohypertrophy and poor absorption of insulin.

Insulin may be injected using a syringe, an insulin pen, or continuous subcutaneous insulin infusion (CSII) via an insulin pump. The insulin pump is particularly useful for delivering a basal bolus of insulin. It infuses short-acting insulin into the subcutaneous tissue through a small flexible, soft cannula. The cannula is replaced in a new site by the wearer or the family every 2 or 3 days. The pump is programmed to deliver small amounts of insulin on a continuous basis (basal insulin) and bolus insulin at the time of meals and snacks to cover the amount of carbohydrate eaten. The amount of insulin delivered in a bolus is determined by the user and may be adjusted for level of activity. Insulin pumps are not "automatic," require more work and deeper understanding of diabetes than subcutaneous injections, and put the child at risk for ketosis if the catheter kinks or becomes obstructed or if the pump malfunctions. Several deaths have been reported among adolescents using insulin pumps, and this group may need special consideration when deciding to use an insulin pump (Cope et al, 2008). Nonetheless, use of insulin pumps is considered safe and efficacious even with young children (Churchill et al, 2009) and is becoming an increasingly popular way to deliver insulin in children with type 1 diabetes.

After insulin treatment has been started, children may enter a "honeymoon period" during which insulin doses decrease. Close follow-up—often daily phone calls—after beginning insulin therapy is necessary to prevent hypoglycemic episodes. Generally, insulin dose adjustments are based on the blood glucose patterns over several days. In general, the insulin dose is decreased if any unexplained severe hypoglycemic events occur.

Monitoring Blood Sugar Levels. Children and families are taught to self-monitor blood glucose (SMBG) before meals, at bedtime, and sometimes in the middle of the night. Blood glucose meters have benefited from continued advances in technology; many provide results within 5 seconds, and store blood glucose values. In addition, the continuous glucose monitor (CGM) has been approved for use in children. Different from the traditional glucose meter, the CGM requires placement of a catheter in subcutaneous tissue where a sensor, transmitter, and receiver measure and report both real-time interstitial glucose levels and directional trending graphs every few minutes. Alarms warn of low and high blood glucose levels using individually determined preset blood glucose ranges. Research suggests that use of the CGM could be effective in lowering HbA_{1c} and decreasing hypoglycemic episodes, but that children and adolescents are less likely than adults to continue its use (Juvenile Diabetes Research Foundation Continuous Glucose Monitoring Study Group, 2010).

Adjusting Insulin Dosages. Parents and teens are taught to make adjustments in insulin based on blood sugar patterns. They analyze what time of day the blood glucose is consistently outside of the target range (either too low or too high) and adjust the insulin dose that caused the problem. Usually parents can safely make up to a 10% adjustment in the problematic insulin dose. With practice and guidance, many families eventually feel comfortable adjusting the insulin dose independently; others may feel more comfortable conferring with their diabetes care provider.

Initial management of new-onset diabetes also includes:

- At diagnosis, screening for hypothyroidism by thyroid peroxidase and thyroglobulin antibodies testing; annual screening thereafter
- At diagnosis, screening for celiac disease by measuring tissue transglutaminase or antiendomysial antibodies; screening thereafter if growth failure, abdominal symptoms or failure to gain weight/weight loss is present.

Ongoing Management. Children with type 1 diabetes should be seen every 3 to 4 months with careful attention paid to diabetes management including:

- Home glucose monitoring results. Age-related targets for fasting and before-meal glucose are:
  - Children 5 years or less: 100 to 180 mg/dL
  - 6 to 12 years: 90 to 180 mg/dL
  - 13 to 19 years: 90 to 130 mg/dL
- Frequency of hypoglycemia
- HbA_{1c} (HbA_{1c} closely correlates with average blood glucose concentrations over the past 3 months.). Age-related targets are:
  - Children 5 years or less: less than 8.5%
  - 6 to 12 years: less than 8%
  - 13 to 19 years: less than 7.5%
- Physical activities
- Emotional adjustment to the disease
- Social issues, such as peer pressure
- Eating issues (young women with diabetes have an increased incidence of eating disorders, such as "diabulemia" in which insulin dosage is decreased in order to lose weight) (Alemzadeh and Wyatt, 2007)
- A physical examination that focuses on:
  - Growth and weight gain
  - BP
  - Stage of puberty
  - Examination of the injection sites looking for lipodystrophy
  - Clues for other autoimmune disease (thyroiditis and celiac disease)

Ongoing management of type 1 diabetes also includes the following referrals and monitoring:

- Referral for a dilated and comprehensive eye examination 3 to 5 years after diabetes onset in children 10 years of age and older. The examination should then be repeated annually.
- Annual screening for microalbuminuria with random spot urine sample for microalbumin-to-creatinine ratio in children who have had diabetes for more than 5 years and are 10 years of age or older (ADA, 2011)
- Annual screening for hypothyroidism
- Appropriate referrals for psychological counseling and nutritional review
- Collaboration with school nurses, teachers, and administrators to ensure that treatment regimens are followed in the school or daycare setting

Medical Nutrition Therapy. Nutrition is an essential component of diabetes management. Diets should be healthy and calories spread over three meals and two or three snacks daily when the child is using NPH insulin. Caloric requirements are based on the child's age, body weight, and activity level. Calories are distributed among protein (15%), carbohydrates (55%), and fat (less than 30% of caloric intake with less than 7% in the form of saturated fats) and account for food preferences including those pertinent to culture and ethnicity. The meal plan for a child with diabetes should include the same healthy foods that clinicians recommend to all their pediatric patients. The goal is to balance food intake with insulin dose and activity to maintain blood glucose levels within the target range and to prevent hyperglycemic and hypoglycemic episodes.

A pediatric dietitian is essential to provide ongoing guidance to the child and family. Various approaches to nutrition therapy are being used. Carbohydrate counting is an approach that allows greater flexibility for children using basal bolus insulin regimens. A meal plan based on food exchanges is also commonly used, particularly for children using an insulin regimen with NPH. Children with diabetes can safely eat sugary treats on occasion by including those treats within their prescribed carbohydrate allotment. Low-calorie (e.g., saccharin, aspartame, sucralose, acesulfame potassium) and reduced-calorie (e.g., sorbitol and xylitol) sweeteners are safe in moderation. Fad diets are discouraged (ADA, 2011).

Exercise. Exercise is encouraged in all children, including children with diabetes, to promote cardiovascular fitness, control weight, and enhance social interaction and self-esteem. Exercise lowers blood glucose levels by increasing uptake of glucose into the tissues. Therefore, children and families are taught to either decrease the insulin dose or take extra carbohydrates prior to exercise to compensate for this effect. Because exercise may affect blood glucose levels for several hours after exercise has occurred, parents need to be aware of the risk of nocturnal hypoglycemia on active days and monitor blood glucose levels more frequently. Children and adolescents with type 1 diabetes should not be excluded from participation in sports activities, including competitive sports.

Complications

Morbidity and mortality in type 1 diabetes come from metabolic derangements and from long-term complications that affect the small and large blood vessels. Chronic high blood sugar has been shown to cause the long-term complications of microvascular disease (retinopathy, nephropathy, neuropathy, depression, cognitive defects) and macrovascular disease (arterial obstruction with gangrene of extremities and ischemic heart disease). These complications can be prevented or their rate of progression slowed by improving glycemic control through use of intensive insulin regimens consisting of multiple daily injections or CSII. After 15 years of having diabetes, an individual has a 98% risk of developing diabetic retinopathy; lens opacities occur in 5% of individuals younger than 19 years old (Alemzadeh and Wyatt, 2007). Treatment success may be hampered by ongoing psychosocial issues and neuropsychiatric problems.

Patient and Parent Education

Providing families and children with information that helps them gain control of a very difficult disease is crucial. The National Diabetes Education Program offers education materials specifically targeted to both type 1 and type 2 diabetes (http://ndep.nih.gov). Education of the child, family, and caregivers should include insulin therapy, SMBG, nutrition and meal planning, exercise, managing sick days, school issues, coping skills, and prevention of complications. Those with diabetes should always wear a form of medical identification. School personnel must be informed of the plan of care and must implement an individualized care plan for the child.

TYPE 2 DIABETES
Description and Epidemiology
Type 2 diabetes begins with increased tissue resistance to insulin, resulting in hyperinsulinemia and hyperglycemia. Although pancreatic beta cells initially produce insulin, hyperglycemia creates an increased insulin demand; with increasing demand for insulin over time, the pancreas loses its ability to effectively secrete insulin. Autoimmune destruction of pancreatic beta cells does not typically occur. During puberty growth hormone secretion as part of the pubertal growth spurt further increases resistance to insulin action for those predisposed to type 2 diabetes. Adolescents with normally functioning pancreatic beta cells secrete additional insulin to compensate for this puberty-related effect. However, when beta cells do not function properly, metabolic decompensation begins and leads to a state of pre-diabetes (impaired fasting glucose and/or impaired glucose tolerance) with eventual progression to type 2 diabetes (ADA, 2000).

Type 2 diabetes is strongly associated with environmental factors such as obesity, sedentary lifestyles, and high-caloric lipid-rich foods. Children who are born to a mother with gestational diabetes, who are small for gestational age at birth (sign of intrauterine undernutrition), who are overweight or obese, and who have a family history of type 2 diabetes are at increased risk for type 2 diabetes (Cowell, 2008). Research is ongoing to identify more clear connections between the environment and diabetes in children (The Environmental Determinants of Diabetes in the Young [TEDDY] Study Group, 2008).

Type 2 diabetes accounts for up to 45% of all new total diabetes cases in the U.S. and has a stronger genetic predisposition than type 1 diabetes (Mohamadi and Cooke, 2010). Among Native Americans 10 to 19 years old, 76% of all cases of diabetes are type 2 with 51 per 1000 cases in Pima Indians. Type 2 diabetes is least common among non-Hispanic Caucasians (6% of all diabetes cases) (Liese et al, 2006). The prevalence of type 2 diabetes may be underreported, especially because children may have no symptoms or mild symptoms for a long period. Children usually are diagnosed during the teenage years, between 10 and 19 years old, and some centers have seen a greater than 10-fold incidence in this age group.

Clinical Findings
The symptoms of type 2 diabetes may be absent or subtle, so children at risk should be screened. The ADA provides guidelines for screening children at risk:
- Screen if overweight (BMI of greater than 85th percentile for age and gender or weight greater than 120% of ideal weight), plus any two of following risk factors:
  - Family history of type 2 diabetes in first- or second-degree relative

- Race/ethnicity (Native American, African-American, Latino, Asian-American, Pacific Islander)
  - Signs of insulin resistance or conditions associated with insulin resistance (e.g., acanthosis nigricans, polycystic ovary syndrome, hypertension, dyslipidemia)
  - Maternal history of diabetes or gestational diabetes mellitus (GDM) during child's gestation
- Screen every 3 years.
- Use fasting plasma glucose test following diagnostic criteria for diabetes discussed earlier.
- Use clinical judgment to screen for type 2 diabetes in high-risk patients who do not meet these guidelines.

History. The history of patients with type 2 diabetes may include:
- Polydipsia
- Polyphagia
- Polyuria
- Nocturia or bedwetting
- Blurred vision
- Obesity, especially central
- Report of a hyperpigmented velvet-like rash in skinfolds
- Frequent or slow-healing infections
- Fatigue
- History of premature adrenarche
- Symptoms of sleep apnea
- Family history of type 2 diabetes

Physical Examination. The physical examination should include assessment of height, weight, stage of pubertal development, and blood pressure. The following findings may be present:
- Dehydration
- Overweight (BMI greater than 85th percentile for age and gender) or obesity
- Weight loss (less common)
- Acanthosis nigricans noted in the axilla, base of the neck, groin, knuckles, and other skinfolds (see Color Plate)
- Vaginal yeast, thrush, other infection
- Polycystic ovary syndrome symptoms (e.g., acne, hirsutism)
- Hypertension

Diagnostic Tests. Screening should be conducted in high-risk children without symptoms (see earlier guidelines) and should include:
- Urine for glucose and albumin (can be performed in the office)
- Children can have ketoacidosis if they have gone undiagnosed for a long time.
- Fasting blood sample for blood glucose, HbA_{1c}, lipid panel, TSH and free T_4, and insulin level

In symptomatic children, diagnosis is made if the following exist:
- Random plasma glucose concentration equal to or greater than 200 mg/dL (11.1 mmol/L)
- Fasting plasma glucose equal to or greater than 126 mg/dL (7 mmol/L)
- Postprandial (2 hours after eating) plasma glucose equal to or greater than 200 mg/dL (11.1 mmol/L)
- HbA_{1c} equal to or greater than 6.5% (ADA, 2010)

Differential Diagnosis
Some obese children have type 1 diabetes and may be misdiagnosed as type 2. The presentation of type 1 diabetes can be of slower onset in older children and adults. Maturity-onset

diabetes of youth (MODY) is a group of autosomal dominant, single-gene disorders that may clinically look like type 2 diabetes. Children with MODY, on average, are younger (mean age 10.8 versus 12.8 years), less likely to be overweight or obese (50% versus 92%), and less likely to be from an ethnic minority group (0% versus 56%) compared with children presenting with new-onset type 2 diabetes (Ehtisham et al, 2004). Depending on the diagnostic results, further laboratory studies to evaluate female hyperandrogenism (serum free testosterone, 17-OHP) and sleep apnea may be indicated.

Management

Treatment of type 2 diabetes in youth remains in its infancy and lacks the strong evidence base of type 1 diabetes. The Treatment Options for Type 2 Diabetes in Adolescents and Youth (TODAY) study, a 15-center randomized controlled trial sponsored by the National Institute of Diabetes and Digestive and Kidney Diseases (NIDDKD), begun in 2003 and projected to end in 2012, is studying the best treatment options for type 2 diabetes in individuals 10 to 17 years old. The study compares the effectiveness of three treatment options for type 2 diabetes in youth: (1) metformin (currently the only oral diabetes agent approved for use in children); (2) metformin plus rosiglitazone; and (3) metformin plus an intensive behavioral intervention (TODAY Study Group, 2010). Pharmacotherapy is discussed more fully below.

As with type 1 diabetes, the treatment plan for children with type 2 diabetes must be individualized. The treatment goal is the normalization of blood glucose values:

- HbA_{1c} less than or equal to 7%
- Low-density lipoprotein (LDL) less than 110 mg/dL
- High-density lipoprotein (HDL) greater than 45 mg/dL
- Triglycerides less than 125 mg/dL

Successful control of the associated complications such as hypertension and hyperlipidemia is important. Ongoing management strategies include the following:

- Annual dilated and comprehensive eye examination to monitor for microvascular changes (e.g., retinopathy, nephropathy)
- Annual urine test for microalbumin
- HbA_{1c} and plasma glucose levels monitored every 3 to 4 months for those whose therapy has changed or who are not meeting glycemic goals. Children who are meeting goals and have stable glycemic control can be monitored every 6 months.
- Follow-up every 3 to 4 months on lifestyle, nutrition, and other complications of obesity discussed in more detail in the following text.

Lifestyle Changes: Nutrition and Exercise. When discovered early, type 2 diabetes may respond to lifestyle changes such as alterations in diet and exercise. The TODAY Lifestyle Program (LSP) is an intensive long-term family-based intervention to change eating and exercise behaviors in children with type 2 diabetes who are severely overweight (TODAY, 2010). These changes must be comprehensive. Medical nutrition therapy (MNT) is an important part of the treatment plan. Referral to a registered pediatric dietitian is essential, with the goals of weight loss and regulating nutritional intake. A low-fat diet, self-monitoring of weight, and being physically active are important components of MNT. Successful weight management may consist of weight maintenance rather than

weight loss depending on the child's age and BMI. Changes in family eating patterns can contribute to weight maintenance or loss that may normalize insulin levels.

Sports and regular exercise are strongly encouraged in children and adolescents with diabetes. Regular vigorous exercise (a minimum of 30 to 60 minutes a day) helps control weight and even modest weight loss has been shown to reduce insulin resistance (ADA, 2010). Overweight or obese adolescents may lack self-esteem or motivation to participate in school sports activities but may be willing to walk as a form of exercise. Use of pedometers has been effective in improving physical activity levels in adolescents particularly when individualized behavioral goals are set (Adams et al, 2009; Butcher et al, 2007).

Additional lifestyle changes include tobacco cessation and breastfeeding of infants by adolescent mothers with type 2 diabetes or those who had GDM.

Pharmacotherapy. The primary treatment for children and adolescents with type 2 diabetes is education and lifestyle modification, particularly improvement of nutritional and physical activity behaviors leading to weight loss. In the U.S., however, less than 10% of children with type 2 diabetes are successful in achieving glycemic control with diet and exercise alone (ADA, 2000). If lifestyle changes are not successful in normalizing blood glucose levels, pharmacologic agents should be added to the treatment regimen. Metformin is the only oral agent approved for use in children with type 2 diabetes and is the drug of choice. Little research has been done on the use of other hypoglycemic agents in children. Most children are begun on metformin in doses up to 1000 mg twice a day. Metformin rarely causes hypoglycemia, so blood glucose need only be checked before breakfast and 2 hours after dinner. Mild gastrointestinal side effects may occur with metformin use and are usually self-limiting. Metformin users can experience vitamin B_{12} deficiency probably secondary to malabsorption, especially with higher doses and longer use. Providers should counsel patients taking metformin to increase foods high in vitamin B_{12}; they should also have a high suspicion of vitamin B_{12} deficiency if clinical signs appear. Although there is no consensus on requiring laboratory testing, patients taking metformin, especially long-term users, should probably be assessed regularly for vitamin B_{12} deficits and high homocysteine levels (de Jager et al, 2010). Should the patient fail to respond to metformin, a combination of two oral agents may be used (Table 25-6).

When a patient with type 2 diabetes has ketonuria or is in diabetic ketoacidosis, insulin therapy is needed initially. These patients are started on the same insulin regimen with home glucose monitoring and a precise food plan as patients with type 1 diabetes. Typically the insulin needs are higher than in patients with type 1 diabetes because of insulin resistance. Following stabilization of blood glucose levels, it may be possible to gradually wean the insulin and begin metformin. Over time the natural course of type 2 diabetes can result in the body's inability to produce sufficient endogenous insulin, making treatment with oral agents ineffective. If this occurs, insulin replacement using a long- and/or short-acting insulin is necessary.

Medication may also be needed to control hypertension (Tan, 2009) and dyslipidemia, two frequent comorbidities of type 2 diabetes in youth. Guidelines for treatment of dyslipidemia in pediatric patients focus on children 8 years of age or older, particularly when dyslipidemia is accompanied by other cardiovascular risk factors such as obesity or diabetes (Daniels et al, 2008).

TABLE 25-6 Oral Medications for Type 2 Diabetes Mellitus

Drug	Action/Comments
Biguanides (metformin HCl)*	Decreases the amount of sugar produced by the liver; increases insulin sensitivity of the liver and muscles. No direct effect on beta-cells in pancreas. Used as first-line monotherapy.
Sulfonylureas (glimepiride, glyburide)	Stimulates beta-cells to make more insulin; may make body tissue more sensitive to insulin. Side effects include weight gain, hypoglycemia; no effect on lipids; possible liver toxicity. Not approved for use in children. Used as second-line therapy in combination with thiazolidinediones
Thiazolidinediones† (pioglitazone)	Increases insulin sensitivity at the cellular level; improves glucose usage. Side effects include weight gain; unknown if may cause edema and congestive heart failure in children.
Meglitinides (repaglinide)	Stimulates beta-cells; no known effect on insulin sensitivity.
Glucosidase inhibitors (acarbose, miglitol)	Slows down the conversion of ingested carbohydrates to sugar in the intestine. Side effects primarily gastrointestinal distress.

*Approved by the U.S. Food and Drug Administration (FDA) for use in children.
†FDA has restricted access to rosiglitazone maleate, only available to participants in Avandia-Rosiglitazone Medicines Access Program.

Complications

Complications of type 2 diabetes are similar to those of type 1 diabetes (microvascular and macrovascular diseases). Nephropathy is a more common complication in those with type 2 than type 1 diabetes. Nonalcoholic fatty liver disease and eventual dependence on insulin for control can occur.

Patient and Parent Education

The same education needs apply to children with type 1 and type 2 diabetes: information about the nature of the disease; strategies and techniques to manage the physical disease (e.g., medication, insulin, nutrition, exercise); networks, support, and skills to cope with emotional and psychological issues; collaboration with school personnel and wearing a form of medical identification. The National Diabetes Education Program is an invaluable resource for providers and children and their families.

■ Obesity

EPIDEMIOLOGY

The prevalence of obesity has increased in children and adults around the world. A more detailed discussion of obesity is found in Chapter 10.

In most children, overweight and obesity are due to an imbalance between calories consumed and calories burned.

Almost all children with excess caloric intake will be tall for their age and/or have a normal to rapid growth velocity. Therefore, every child should have a BMI calculated and compared with normative data at each clinic visit.

From an endocrine perspective, the mechanisms of weight homeostasis are complex and involve hypothalamic hormones, hormones produced by adipocytes (e.g., leptin), and the gut (e.g., gherlin) (Chia and Boston, 2006). In most children, no single hormone deficiency or excess explains obesity. The presence of a recognizable genetic or endocrine dysfunction accounts for, at most, 5% of children who are overweight (Sondike and Jeffrey, 2009).

Several "classic" hormone situations may cause obesity, including hypothyroidism, cortisol excess, and GHD. In these conditions, the child is likely to be short or growing at a subnormal growth velocity. Several genetic conditions predispose children to being overweight (e.g., Prader-Willi syndrome). Developmental delay and dysmorphic features are key to identifying these conditions.

DIAGNOSTIC TESTS

Children with a BMI greater than the 85th percentile for age and gender should be screened for a number of conditions:
- Abnormalities in glucose tolerance with a fasting glucose or an oral glucose tolerance test
- Nonalcoholic steatohepatitis with liver function tests of aspartate aminotransferase (AST), alanine aminotransferase (ALT)
- Dyslipidemia with a fasting lipid panel
- Thyroid function with a thyroid panel
- Sleep apnea by history of snoring, daytime somnolence
- Polycystic ovary syndrome with a free and total testosterone level (if symptomatic with irregular menses, acne, or hirsutism)
- Hypertension with a BP measurement
- Orthopedic issues by history (e.g., slipped capital femoral epiphysis)
- Psychological issues by history (some children with obesity suffer from low self-esteem, behavior problems, or depression)

MANAGEMENT

Children with type 2 diabetes, polycystic ovary syndrome, or other metabolic or endocrine disorders associated with obesity should be followed in concert with a pediatric endocrinologist. Those with obesity alone are more effectively treated in the primary care office with nutritional counseling and ongoing support to achieve a more active lifestyle (Nieman and McKnight, 2010). In general, the goal is weight maintenance, not loss, in the overweight child without any of the previously mentioned complications; it is expected that these children will eventually grow into their weight and achieve a BMI less than the 85th percentile. For children with an overweight-related complication, weight loss of 1 pound per month would be an appropriate goal; more rapid weight loss in children who have not yet reached their growth potential may be associated with slowing in linear growth.

Consensus is lacking as to the most effective way to manage obesity. Goals for reducing calories consumed and increasing daily exercise must be made within the context of each family; success is more likely to be achieved if the entire family participates in lifestyle changes. Providers must work closely with families to ensure consistent follow-up, to assess the effectiveness of interventions, and to modify the treatment strategy if necessary (see Chapter 10).

◼ Posterior Pituitary Gland Disorders

Abnormal posterior pituitary function is uncommon in pediatrics. Children with inappropriately dilute urine for the clinical situation may only be identified when they develop hypernatremic dehydration, secondary enuresis, or polyuria. They may also be discovered in an evaluation of a child at risk for hypopituitarism. If a screening of first morning urine shows low specific gravity in the absence of urinary glucose, a pediatric endocrinologist should be consulted.

Introduction to Inborn Errors of Metabolism

Inborn errors of metabolism (IEM) encompass a wide range of inherited disorders with alterations of specific biochemical reactions. The term "inborn error of metabolism" was coined by Garrod in 1908 to describe the hereditary alteration in enzyme reactions he observed in the first identified "inborn error," alkaptonuria, and use of the term has persisted (Lanpher et al, 2006).

Although individually rare, IEM have a collective incidence of approximately 1 in 1500 live births (Raghuveer et al, 2006), and all health care providers will likely encounter a child with an IEM at some point in their career. Clinical consequences for the affected individual vary from mild to severe. Early detection, accurate diagnosis, and rapid intervention are necessary to achieve favorable outcomes; prevent irreversible mental retardation, physical disability, neurologic damage, or death; and reduce long-term financial burden and human suffering. This section discusses the classification and pathophysiology of IEM; overviews newborn screening, including common clinical presentations and emergency management of conditions found in the newborn period; and presents a brief overview of the diagnosis and treatment of a few more common disorders.

◼ Classification of Inborn Errors of Metabolism

Classification of IEM presents a challenge because of the number and diversity of disorders. Proposed classification systems have suggested categorizing based on affected organ (e.g., neurologic or hepatic diseases), organelle (e.g., mitochondrial or lysosomal disorders), age of presentation (e.g., neonatal or adult onset), large- or small-molecule diseases, or affected metabolic pathway (e.g., urea cycle defect [UCD] or defects of amino acid metabolism) (see Table 25-7).

TABLE 25-7	Classification of Inborn Errors of Metabolism With Partial List of Disorders
Classification	**Disorders**
Amino acid disorders	Maple syrup urine disease Phenylketonuria Tyrosinemia Homocystinuria
Organic acidemias	Propionic acidemia Methylmalonic acidemia
Urea cycle disorders	Ornithine transcarbamylase deficiency Citrullinemia
Carbohydrate disorders	Galactosemia Glycogen storage disease Hereditary fructose intolerance
Fatty acid oxidation disorders	MCAD VLCAD LCHAD
Mitochondrial disorders	Leigh disease MNGIE syndrome Pearson syndrome
Peroxisomal disorders	Zellweger syndrome Adrenoleukodystrophy Infantile Refsum disease
Lysosomal storage disorders	Hurler syndrome Fabry disease Gaucher disease Niemann-Pick disease
Purine and pyrimidine disorders	Lesch-Nyhan disease Hereditary orotic aciduria
Metal metabolism disorders	Wilson disease

LCHAD, Long-chain 3-hydroxyacyl-CoA dehydrogenase deficiency; *MCAD*, medium-chain acyl CoA dehydrogenase deficiency; *MNGIE*, mitochondrial neurogastrointestinal encephalopathy; *VLCAD*, very long-chain acyl CoA dehydrogenase deficiency.

◼ Pathophysiology

Most metabolic disorders are caused by an inherited defect, generally of a single enzyme or its cofactor, resulting in altered function of a metabolic pathway. Autosomal recessive inheritance patterns are most common.

Figure 25-3 provides an overview of the major metabolic pathways. The majority of defects are caused by a single gene mutation encoding a specific enzyme whose function is to facilitate the conversion of various substances (substrates, [e.g., foodstuffs]) into others (metabolic products, [e.g., urea]). The block in the pathway variably leads to accumulation of substrate proximal to the block (e.g., lysosomal storage disorders); accumulation of toxic metabolites (e.g., galactose by-products in galactosemia); deficiency of a product distal to the block (e.g., tyrosine in PKU); feedback inhibition or activation by the metabolite; or some combination thereof. Loss of enzyme function varies by degree, altering the clinical phenotype, the clinical course,

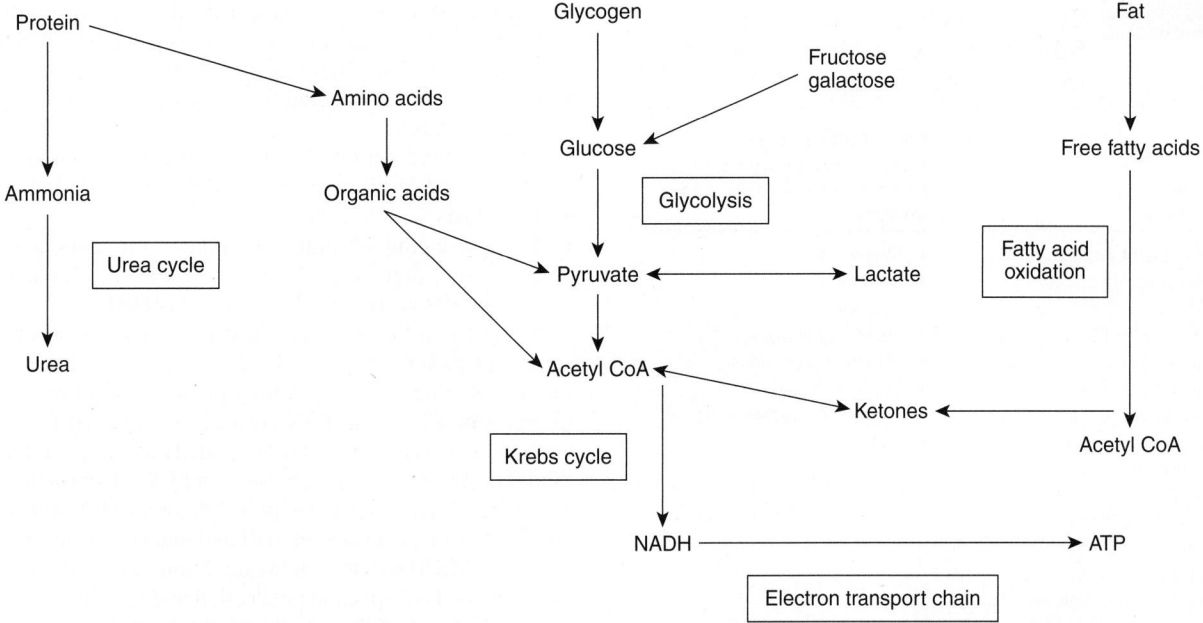

FIG. 25-3 Overview of major metabolic pathways. *Acetyl CoA*, Acetyl coenzyme A; *ATP*, adenosine triphosphate; *NADH*, nicotinamide adenine dinucleotide. (From Logan A: Metabolic disease. In Cheng A, Williams BA, Sivarajan VB, editors: *The hospital for sick children handbook of pediatrics*, ed 10, Toronto, 2004, Saunders, p 474.)

and the response to treatment among individuals with the same diagnosis.

Assessment of Inborn Errors of Metabolism

DESCRIPTION

IEM are rare but should be included in the differential diagnosis of any critically ill neonate, as well as infants, children, adolescents, and young adults presenting with symptoms that are progressive or otherwise unexplained. The timing of symptom onset in relation to initiation of feedings can be an important clue. Infants with IEM almost always appear normal at birth with effects of the disease becoming apparent over the course of days to months. As substrates or toxic metabolites accumulate, such as in organic acidemias, nonspecific symptoms that may be indistinguishable from sepsis typically appear. Finding a cause of symptoms, however, does not necessarily rule out the possibility of IEM (Thomas and Van Hove, 2009) (e.g., electrolyte abnormalities diagnosed as renal Fanconi syndrome may be caused by underlying cystinosis).

CLINICAL FINDINGS

History

A thorough family and individual history is important to identify possibilities of IEM. Details in a family and patient history that should raise suspicion include:

- Consanguinity
- Decompensation when ill greater than anticipated for the nature of the illness (commonly seen in acidosis)
- Developmental delay, psychomotor retardation, or loss of milestones

- Failure to thrive
- Frequent infections
- Family history of IEM
- Siblings with unexplained infant or neonatal death
- Symptoms seen with a change in diet
- Unusual odor (sweat, urine, or cerumen)

Physical Examination

A complete examination is essential, with attention to dysmorphia, muscle tone, ocular symptoms, organomegaly, and respiratory function. Box 25-10 provides an overview of symptoms suspicious for an inborn error at various ages.

Diagnostic Tests

Effective intervention for IEM depends on the ability to identify the disorder before the onset of symptoms. Screening for the presence of IEM allows the provider to identify the condition before damage has occurred. The capability to screen for IEM dates to the early 1960s when an inexpensive test for PKU using a small blood sample collected on a filter paper was developed (Guthrie and Susi, 1963); 400,000 newborns in 29 states were part of a pilot study that confirmed the effectiveness of this test to detect PKU. As a result, states instituted screening programs for newborn infants, and today, virtually all of the millions of infants born each year in the U.S. are screened (see Chapter 38).

Technologic advances have allowed for screening a wide array of disorders, and the newborn screening test encompasses much more than screening for PKU. Although every state mandates newborn screening, each state, using a developed set of criteria, independently determines which conditions will be screened. This practice leads to some discrepancies among states (National Newborn Screening & Genetics Resource Center, 2011).

BOX 25-10 Symptoms Suggesting an Inborn Error of Metabolism in Children by Age

Neonates and Infants	Older Children and Adolescents (in Addition to Those of Neonates and Infants)
• Abnormal neurologic examination	• Ataxia
• Acidosis	• Dementia
• Cardiomyopathy	• Dystonia or chorea
• Coagulopathy	• Mental retardation
• Coarse facial features	• Muscular weakness
• Dysmorphic features	• Ophthalmoplegia
• Hyperammonemia	• Progressive deterioration
• Hypotonia or hypertonia	• Skeletal changes
• Jaundice	
• Metabolic acidosis	
• Neutropenia and/or thrombocytopenia	
• Ocular findings (retinitis pigmentosa, cherry red spots, cataracts or corneal clouding)	
• Organomegaly	
• Respiratory distress (apnea or tachypnea)	
• Seizures	
• Unexplained hypoglycemia	
• Vomiting	

Laboratory studies are generally necessary in the diagnosis of IEM; however, determining what studies to perform is not straightforward. Consider performing a newborn screening test on any significantly ill neonate, unless proof of prior collection is obtained. If the ill neonate was discharged early (before 48 hours postpartum), a second screen should be done at 10 to 14 days of age (see Chapter 38). Testing for common (i.e., nonmetabolic) causes of presenting symptoms should not be sacrificed for metabolic testing, but it is not always wise to wait until all routine tests have been performed and the results known before submitting samples for metabolic disease testing. This additional step facilitates workup should the patient be referred to a metabolic specialist. When the ill child has signs and symptoms of what could be an IEM, the primary care provider should consult early with a metabolic specialist rather than wait for results of tests. For chronic presentations, after common etiologies are ruled out, refer to a metabolic specialist for testing beyond routine analysis.

Initial laboratory studies for the neonate with a suspected IEM include:
- CBC with differential
- Blood glucose
- Blood urea nitrogen (BUN) and creatinine
- ALT, AST, bilirubin
- Coagulation studies
- Blood gases
- Serum electrolytes with special attention to anion gap = $Na^+-(Cl^- + HCO^-_3)$ (normal anion gap is between 8 and 12 mEq/L)
- Plasma ammonia (collected free flowing [no tourniquet, no heelstick, preferably no capillary tubes] immediately placed on ice and analyzed within 45 to 60 minutes)
- Plasma lactate (collected free flowing)
- Creatine kinase
- Plasma (and variably urine) quantitative amino acids; plasma acylcarnitine profile, and plasma carnitine
- Urinalysis
- Urine-reducing substances, ketones (if acidotic and hypoglycemic), organic acids, mucopolysaccharides and oligosaccharides if storage disease is suspected

Many labs offer a metabolic panel, typically on urine, but some labs prefer urine and blood. This test varies among laboratories. Testing may also consist of biochemical or molecular (deoxyribonucleic acid [DNA]) analysis obtained from blood. Other more invasive tests may be needed including cerebrospinal fluid (lactate, amino acids, glucose), or biopsy from skin, liver, or muscle (enzyme assays). Additionally, for the child with chronic encephalopathy, consider an MRI and magnetic resonance spectroscopy (MRS) for brain imaging. Familiarity with the appropriate methods of specimen collection and handling (before and during shipment of the samples to the laboratory) is important because inappropriate practices alter the quality of the sample, potentially leading to unreliable results and missed cases.

MANAGEMENT

Management of metabolic disorders varies depending on the specific condition, its severity, and whether it is an acute or chronic presentation. Caregivers of children with a known diagnosis of inborn errors (e.g., those that cause hyperammonemia) become very astute at early recognition of symptoms in their child and should be viewed as crucial partners in the health care team.

Metabolic Emergencies

Emergency management of metabolic disorders requires hospital admission and specialist care. The goal of emergency management is twofold: prevent catabolism and remove toxic substrates or metabolites. Aggressive management is necessary to avert or reduce neurologic sequelae. This acute care management may require intravenous medications (including glucose to halt catabolism), diet restriction (e.g., no protein for 24 to 48 hours or until mental status is back to baseline), hemodialysis, or life support.

Stable Metabolic Disorders

The variability of IEM requires individual management tailored to the patient's specific diagnosis and phenotype. However, the following strategies provide several broad categories from which treatments are drawn.
- Control substrate accumulation:
  ○ Restrict dietary intake (e.g., restricting phenylalanine intake in PKU).
  ○ Control endogenous production of the substrate (e.g., give high-calorie, no-protein feeds during illness to prevent catabolism, which would release amino acids).
  ○ Accelerate removal of the substrate (e.g., administer sodium benzoate/phenylacetate in UCDs to increase elimination of waste nitrogen through an alternate pathway).

- Dietary supplementation
  - Replace or supplement the diet with products that become deficient distal to the metabolic block or if the diet is medically restricted (e.g., arginine or citrulline in UCDs).
- Vitamin and cofactor replacement
  - Increase the supply of certain vitamins that act as cofactors to metabolic reactions to improve function of the residual enzyme activity. Vitamin replacement is also important with severely restricted diets.
- Enzyme replacement therapy (ERT)
  - ERT (an intravenous infusion of enzyme replacement given every 1 to 4 weeks) is becoming more widely available in the clinical setting for lysosomal storage diseases.
- Bone marrow or organ transplant
  - Stem cell transplantation using exogenous bone marrow or cord blood as a donor site is clinically available for some disorders, but is in early stages of widespread clinical use (Prasad and Kurtzberg, 2010).
  - Organ transplant can essentially "cure" some metabolic diseases by transplanting an organ in which the mutant genes are expressed. Liver transplantation has shown success in some cases of IEM.

COMPLICATIONS

Multiple complications such as renal failure, hypertension, spinal cord compression, and carpal tunnel syndrome may be seen with IEM, often necessitating a multidisciplinary management team.

■ Specific Metabolic Disorders of Children

DISORDERS OF CARBOHYDRATE METABOLISM

This group of disorders is caused by the inability to metabolize the monosaccharides glucose, galactose, and fructose; and the polysaccharide glycogen. Aberrant glycogen synthesis or disorders of gluconeogenesis also contribute to faulty carbohydrate metabolism.

GLYCOGEN STORAGE DISEASES
Description and Epidemiology
Glycogen is a glucose polymer stored in muscle and the liver, and deficiency of any enzyme involved in the metabolic pathway of glycogen can affect biosynthesis or degradation of glycogen in the organ in which the enzyme is expressed. This deficiency results in a variety of presentations of disease. Glucose-6-phosphatase deficiency (type 1), lysosomal acid α-glucosidase deficiency (type 2, Pompe disease), debrancher deficiency (type 3), and liver phosphorylase kinase deficiency (type 9) are the most common early childhood presentations. Overall frequency of all forms is 1:20,000 live births (Raghuveer et al, 2006).

Clinical Findings
Signs and symptoms may include cardiomegaly, hepatosplenomegaly, hypoglycemic seizures, lactic acidosis, ketosis, hyperlipidemia, elevated transaminases, easy fatigability, hypotonia, and muscle weakness.

Diagnostic Tests. Enzyme assays and mutation analysis are available for essentially all identified forms of glycogen storage disease.

Management
Treatment varies depending on the specific defect. Types 1, 3, 4, and 9 all affect enzyme activity in the liver, which is responsible for homeostasis of plasma glucose. Treatment is aimed at maintaining normal blood glucose levels and may require continuous feedings through a gastrostomy tube, frequent feedings throughout the day, and ingestion of uncooked cornstarch slurry at bedtime. Parents and children must be aware of symptoms of low blood sugar, and home glucose monitoring is recommended. Enzyme replacement therapy for Pompe disease is available.

GALACTOSEMIA
Description
Galactosemia results from a disorder of galactose metabolism. The classic form of galactosemia is caused by deficient galactose-1-phosphate-uridyltransferase (GALT) activity. Dietary galactose is most commonly ingested as lactose, the principal carbohydrate in human milk and commercial non-soy formulas. The metabolism of galactose undergoes many enzymatic reactions. A block at the level of the GALT enzyme results in accumulation of galactose-1-phosphate (gal-1-P) and other galactose derivatives, leading to the clinical symptoms.

Epidemiology
Incidence of the classic autosomal recessive form is estimated at 1 in 40,000 live births (Schulze et al, 2009).

Clinical Findings
Infants with classic galactosemia appear normal at birth, but demonstrate clinical manifestations after milk feeding. Although galactosemia is typically discovered on newborn screening, neonates may show clinical signs before results of the screening are known. Therefore, galactosemia should remain in the differential diagnosis of any ill neonate. Clinical manifestations of severe, untreated galactosemia include poor weight gain, lethargy, jaundice, vomiting, coagulopathies, and *Escherichia coli* sepsis. Vitreous hemorrhage has been reported.

Diagnostic Tests. Urine-reducing substances are positive in recently fed (lactose-containing formulas or breast milk) infants. Serum glucose may be decreased. GALT activity in red cells is deficient, and liver enzymes and gal-1-P levels are elevated.

Management
Treatment of classic galactosemia consists of eliminating dietary galactose. Ensure that the child is receiving appropriate calcium supplementation.

Controversy surrounding appropriate treatment of variants (e.g., Duarte galactosemia) continues with some centers recommending dietary restriction, some recommending no therapy, and others using soy formula during the first year.

Complications

Long-term complications of untreated galactosemia include cirrhosis, cataracts, and irreversible brain damage; death can occur. Despite treatment, most children with classic galactosemia develop speech impairment, and some develop impaired motor function. Premature ovarian failure is also common.

UREA CYCLE DISORDERS

Description and Epidemiology

A defect in any enzyme of the urea cycle results in hyperammonemia secondary to the body's inability to detoxify waste nitrogen through its normal conversion to urea. Ammonia is an end product of amino acid catabolism and is highly toxic to the CNS. Five enzymes are required for the conversion of ammonia to urea, and deficiency in any of these enzymes results in disease. Incidence of the disorder is approximately 1:30,000 births (Rezvani, 2007).

Clinical Findings

In infants, symptoms are related to the effects of hyperammonemia, start after protein ingestion, and include vomiting, lethargy, irritability, malaise, and potential seizures and coma. Older children may exhibit ataxia, confusion, agitation, irritability, and combativeness.

Diagnostic Tests. No specific findings are typically found with initial laboratory testing.

- BUN may be low.
- Ammonia level greater than 100 mmol/L (or lower in older children) evokes concern (normal values are typically less than 35 mmol/L).
- Enzyme assays are available for diagnosis of most of the disorders.
- Genetic mutation analysis may confirm diagnosis of some of the disorders.

Management

Treatment of acute hyperammonemia is completed by acute care staff with the goal being to establish a source of glucose and rapidly decreasing ammonia levels. Principles of treatment of chronic UCDs are very similar, but also include limiting endogenous protein catabolism and dietary protein consumption under the supervision of a metabolic dietitian.

Complications

Despite appropriate treatment, children with UCDs are vulnerable to metabolic decompensation, mild to moderate mental retardation, and premature death.

AMINO ACID METABOLISM DISORDERS: AMINOACIDOPATHIES AND ORGANIC ACIDURIAS AND ACIDEMIAS

More than 30 defects of amino acid metabolism are attributed to enzyme or cofactor defects. Although all of these disorders result from defects in amino acid metabolism, they are generally classified as aminoacidopathies or organic acidurias or acidemias, depending on whether amino acids or organic acids are detected in urine or plasma. The more common aminoacidopathies include PKU, maple syrup disease (MSD), tyrosinemia types 1 and 2, and homocystinuria.

PHENYLKETONURIA

Description and Epidemiology

Classic PKU is the most common form of PKU and results from deficiency of the enzyme phenylalanine hydroxylase, which converts phenylalanine to tyrosine. Untreated PKU leads to elevated phenylalanine concentrations in the blood and brain and results in CNS damage with profound mental retardation. More prevalent in Caucasians, PKU is an autosomal recessive trait with an incidence of approximately 1:10,000 (Schulze et al, 2009).

Clinical Findings

No clinical manifestations are noted at birth, and the effects of high phenylalanine levels may not be apparent in the first few months, by which time, if untreated, irreversible brain damage has occurred. Children with more advanced, untreated disease tend to have lighter skin and hair than typical for their race and develop an eczematous rash and a musty or mousy odor related to buildup of phenylacetic acid.

PKU should be detected on newborn screening. Infants with classic PKU ingesting a normal diet will have serum phenylalanine levels greater than 1200 mmol/L on confirmatory testing for PKU, whereas others with milder hyperphenylalaninemia will have intermediate levels.

Differential Diagnosis

Biopterin is a cofactor for phenylalanine, tyrosine, and tryptophan hydroxylases. Children with biopterin defects may be detected on newborn screening, but will continue to deteriorate despite usual dietary intervention for PKU. Testing blood and urine pterins and biopterin enzymes is recommended in any child with high phenylalanine levels because treatment for biopterin defects is different than PKU treatment.

Management

Treatment for PKU involves limiting the dietary intake of phenylalanine, with a goal of serum phenylalanine levels between 120 and 360 mmol/L in infants and young children. Phenylalanine is an essential amino acid and cannot be eliminated entirely, thus patients need to receive enough to meet growth needs. To obtain the essential amino acids and to meet energy and other nutritional needs, the diet is supplemented with a medically modified formula, free of phenylalanine. Over the child's first year or two of life, parents are educated on the phenylalanine content of foods; the child's phenylalanine level is frequently monitored; and a phenylalanine "allowance" is established based on the child's dietary tolerance. The current recommendation is "diet for life" to prevent long-term cognitive and neurologic sequelae. Medically modified low-phenylalanine food products are available online and directly, with insurance reimbursement in some states. Pregnant teenagers with PKU must maintain very strict dietary restrictions to protect the fetus. Consultation with or referral to a dietitian is essential.

CLASSIC HOMOCYSTINURIA

Description and Epidemiology

Homocystinuria due to cystathionine synthase deficiency is the most common form of these disorders, with a prevalence of approximately 1:200,000 (Schulze et al, 2009). Discussion of homocystinuria caused by defects in vitamin metabolism and deficiency of methylenetetrahydrofolate reductase (MTHFR) is beyond the scope of this chapter.

Clinical Findings

Clinical manifestations are nonspecific and include failure to thrive and developmental delay.

Diagnostic Tests. Plasma and urine amino acid testing is completed to evaluate concentrations of:
- Methionine (elevated levels may be found on the newborn screening, but values rise slowly, and high methionine levels may not be detected on specimens obtained from affected infants in the first few days after birth; a second newborn screening is necessary)
- Homocystine
- Total homocysteine

Management

Some children respond to vitamin B_6 therapy; and plasma homocystine and methionine concentrations are monitored. If the child responds, treatment with vitamin B_6 is continued. Children who do not respond to vitamin B_6 are placed on a methionine-restricted diet with frequent monitoring of plasma amino acids and total plasma homocystine. Betaine is administered. Folate and vitamin B_{12} optimize conversion of homocystine to methionine.

Complications

Treatment outcomes are variable, and these children are at high risk for metabolic stroke, though prognosis is good for those with the classic form of homocystinuria identified on newborn screening. Untreated patients develop ocular lens dislocation, progressive mental retardation, thromboembolic events, convulsions, and skeletal abnormalities resembling Marfan syndrome.

DISORDERS OF FATTY ACID OXIDATION

MEDIUM-CHAIN ACYL-CoA DEHYDROGENASE DEFICIENCY

Description and Epidemiology

Fatty acids are an important energy resource for the body, used during times of fasting and stress when glycogen stores become depleted. Defects can occur at any point in fatty acid transport or the mitochondrial beta-oxidation pathway, yielding more than 20 disorders in which individuals are unable to metabolize fatty acids. The more common fatty acid oxidation disorders are: medium-chain acyl-coenzyme A (acyl-CoA) dehydrogenase deficiency (MCAD), very long-chain acyl-CoA dehydrogenase deficiency (VLCAD), and long-chain 3-hydroxyacyl-CoA dehydrogenase deficiency (LCHAD). The incidence of all disorders ranges from 1:15,000 to 1:200,000. MCAD is quickly becoming one of the most common IEM identified in infants by newborn screening with an estimated incidence of 1:15,000 live births (Schulze et al, 2009).

Clinical Findings

Common manifestations include hypoglycemia during fasting; cardiomyopathy; muscle weakness; and inappropriately low or absent ketone production during times of stress, fasting, and illness. Individuals with MCAD may be asymptomatic for a lifetime or have premature death. Fasting may lead to complications including hypoketotic hypoglycemia, hypotonia, lethargy and vomiting progressing to seizures, coma, encephalopathy, and death. Up to 25% of patients die during their first episode, 50% may never be symptomatic, and the overall prognosis for survivors is excellent because fasting tolerance improves with age (Stanley and Bennett, 2007). Any increase in energy demand may tip the balance and result in a metabolic crisis as vital organs are deprived of fuel. Fatty acid oxidation disorders have been implicated as the cause of death in 5% of sudden unexpected death in infancy (Schulze et al, 2009).

Diagnostic Tests. Expanded newborn screening will identify the majority of fatty acid oxidation defects. Confirmatory tests for MCAD include:
- Plasma acylcarnitine profile
- Enzyme assay
- Mutation analysis

Hypoglycemia or normoglycemia may be present during times of illness, and blood glucose monitoring is not a reliable measure of metabolic status in these children.

Management

Treatment varies and may include fasting avoidance, dietary restriction of long-chain fats, supplementing the diet with medium-chain fats, and carnitine supplementation to prevent secondary deficiency.

For individuals with MCAD, avoidance of fasting is the mainstay of treatment. Infants should not fast for longer than 4 hours for the first 4 months. For each month of age, 1 hour of fasting can be added up to a maximum of 10 to 12 hours. These guidelines do not apply during times of higher energy demand (Walter, 2009). If the child awakens during the night, this could indicate hypoglycemia and the need for a snack. Providers should maintain a low threshold for recommending intravenous glucose infusions during times of illness and fever when energy requirements increase. Monitor carnitine level and supplement with oral carnitine 50 to 100 mg/kg/day in divided doses if free carnitine level is below the reference range.

Complications

The most serious consequence of this group of disorders is the inability to use fatty acids for energy production and lack of ketone production (burned for energy) during times of fasting, which may result in death.

LYSOSOMAL DISORDERS

Lysosomal storage disorders (LSDs) are caused by an accumulation (storage) of glycoproteins, glycolipids, or glycosaminoglycans (as in mucopolysaccharidosis [MPS]) within lysosomes and various tissues, which leads to the various clinical presentations and symptoms. Incidence for all LSDs is 1:7700 live births (Raghuveer et al, 2006); the condition typically presents in later infancy to adulthood (Hoffmann and Mayatepek, 2005). Symptoms vary depending on the site of storage and the specific disorder and may include hepato-splenomegaly, coarse facies, corneal clouding, mental retardation, thrombocytopenia, bone pain, neuralgia, abnormal liver function studies, respiratory problems, hydrocephalus, and cardiomyopathy. Enzymatic assay and mutation analysis are available for most disorders. Initial diagnostic testing for MPS consists of screening urinary glycosaminoglycans (urine MPS screen). Treatment varies from symptom management to ERT with varying degrees of success.

DYSLIPIDEMIA: HYPERCHOLESTEROLEMIA AND HYPERLIPIDEMIA

Description and Epidemiology

Dyslipidemias are disorders of lipoprotein metabolism, some of which lead to increased levels of total cholesterol (TC) and LDL cholesterol, a varied presentation of triglycerides (TG), and/or decreased levels of HDL cholesterol.

Dyslipidemias can be acquired (secondary) or genetic (primary). Secondary hyperlipidemias result from exogenous factors such as obesity, drugs (e.g., isotretinoin, oral contraceptives, antipsychotics), and alcohol; endocrine or metabolic disorders (e.g., hypothyroidism, diabetes); storage disease

(e.g., glycogen storage disease); obstructive liver disease (e.g., biliary atresia); and other causes, such as anorexia nervosa.

Among primary dyslipidemia, familial hypercholesterolemia is most common. Familial hypercholesterolemia results from pathogenic mutation in the LDLR gene (most common) or the apoB/E protein. These mutations compromise the receptor cells' ability to facilitate clearance of LDL cholesterol through the liver; as a result, LDL accumulates in the body. Triglycerides are usually normal. The two types of familial hypercholesterolemia are heterozygous, which is common (1:300 to 500), and homozygous, which is exceedingly rare (1:1,000,000). Homozygous hypercholesterolemia is characterized by extremely high LDL levels (e.g., 600 mg/dL or more) and a poor outcome if the patient does not have very aggressive early treatment; treatment may include LDL apheresis and possible liver transplant. Even with treatment, atherosclerotic vascular disease is common by 30 years old (Shankarappa et al, 2009).

Clinical Findings

Hyperlipidemia does not typically present as a clinical illness in children. Although not all children with dyslipidemia will have cardiovascular problems as adults, screening of children

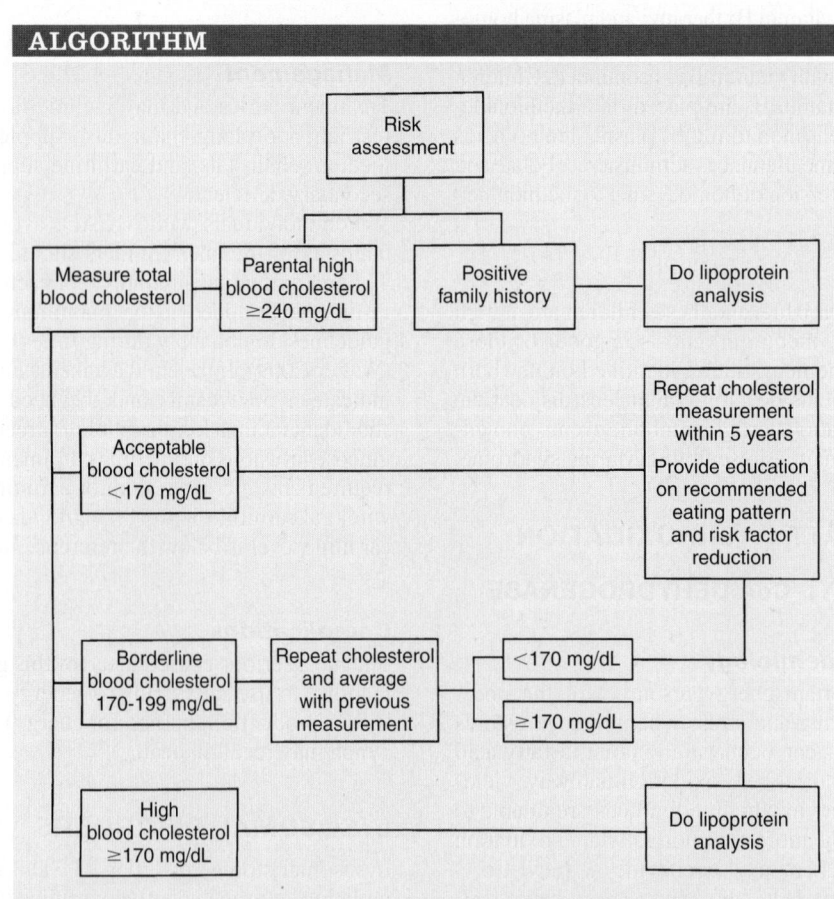

FIG. 25-4 Risk assessment of children based on high parental blood cholesterol or a positive family history of premature atherosclerotic disease. (Reprinted from National Cholesterol Education Program: *Report of the Expert Panel on Blood Cholesterol Levels in Children and Adolescents,* National Heart, Lung, and Blood Institute, PHS NIH Pub No. 91-2732, U.S. Department of Health and Human Services, Washington, DC, 1991, U.S. Government Printing Office.)

at risk is important to identify those with hyperlipidemia and hypercholesterolemia and intervene in an effort to prevent problems from occurring. The current recommendation is to screen children and adolescents with a positive family history of dyslipidemia (TC level of greater than 240 mg/dL) or premature (55 years or older for men and 65 years or older for women) cardiovascular disease (CVD). Screening is recommended for children with incomplete or absent family history data and those with other risk factors related to cardiac disease (e.g., overweight, obesity, hypertension, cigarette smoking, or diabetes mellitus) (Daniels et al, 2008).

History. Risk factors for hypercholesterolemia and hyperlipidemia found in the history include:
- Overweight or obesity (most predictive of dyslipidemia)
- Family history of hypercholesterolemia (e.g., parent with TC greater than 240 mg/dL)
- Family history of premature atherosclerotic disease
- Diabetes mellitus
- Hypertension
- Cigarette smoking
- Use of atypical antipsychotic drugs (e.g., risperidone, olanzapine, clozapine, ziprasidone)

Physical Examination. The child may have no clinical signs or symptoms or may have:
- Overweight or obesity (BMI more than the 85th percentile)
- Hypertension
- Xanthomas (may be seen with familial hypercholesterolemia; tendon xanthomas in adolescents)

Diagnostic Tests. The clinical conditions of dyslipidemia can be determined by lipoprotein analysis (Figs. 25-4 and 25-5). Precise genetic etiology is not needed for therapeutic decisions.

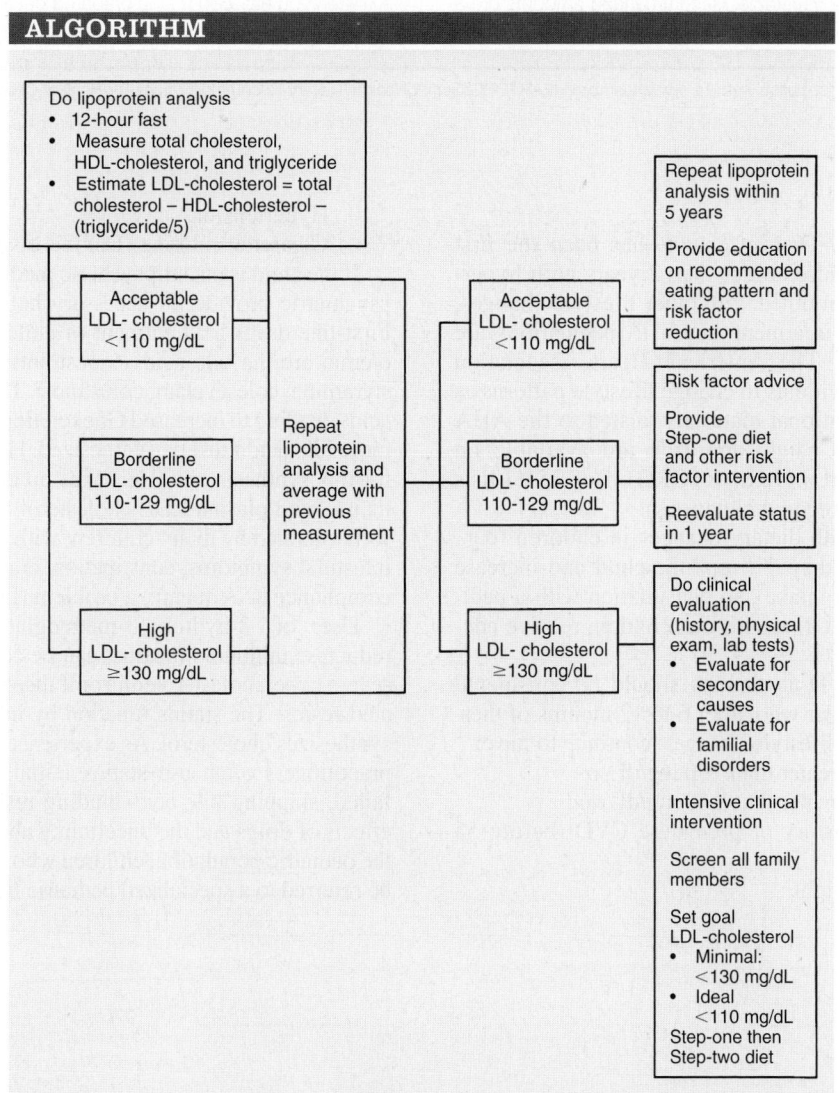

ALGORITHM

Do lipoprotein analysis
- 12-hour fast
- Measure total cholesterol, HDL-cholesterol, and triglyceride
- Estimate LDL-cholesterol = total cholesterol − HDL-cholesterol − (triglyceride/5)

Acceptable LDL-cholesterol <110 mg/dL

Borderline LDL-cholesterol 110-129 mg/dL

High LDL-cholesterol ≥130 mg/dL

Repeat lipoprotein analysis and average with previous measurement

Acceptable LDL-cholesterol <110 mg/dL

Borderline LDL-cholesterol 110-129 mg/dL

High LDL-cholesterol ≥130 mg/dL

Repeat lipoprotein analysis within 5 years

Provide education on recommended eating pattern and risk factor reduction

Risk factor advice

Provide Step-one diet and other risk factor intervention

Reevaluate status in 1 year

Do clinical evaluation (history, physical exam, lab tests)
- Evaluate for secondary causes
- Evaluate for familial disorders

Intensive clinical intervention

Screen all family members

Set goal LDL-cholesterol
- Minimal: <130 mg/dL
- Ideal <110 mg/dL
Step-one then Step-two diet

FIG. 25-5 Classification, education, and follow-up of patients based on low-density lipoprotein (LDL) cholesterol level. *HDL,* High-density lipoprotein. (Reprinted from National Cholesterol Education Program: *Report of the Expert Panel on Blood Cholesterol Levels in Children and Adolescents,* National Heart, Lung, and Blood Institute, PHS NIH Pub No. 91-2732, U.S. Department of Health and Human Services, Washington, DC, 1991, U.S. Government Printing Office.)

BOX 25-11   American Heart Association Diet and Lifestyle Recommendations for Infants, Children, and Families to Reduce Cardiovascular Disease

- Balance calorie intake and physical activity to achieve or maintain a healthy body weight; incorporate enough moderate physical activity to use at least 200 kcal/day.
  - All children ages 2 and older should engage in a minimum of 60 minutes of moderate-intensity, age-appropriate physical activities each day; these may be done in blocks of time: one 60-minute, two 30-minute, or four 15-minute periods.
- Try to exclusively breastfeed for the first 4 to 6 months after birth.
- Try to maintain breastfeeding for 12 months.
- Introduce other sources of nutrients at about 4 to 6 months.
- Limit juice to 4 to 6 oz per day; feed juice from a cup only; use only 100% juice.
- Minimize intake of beverages and foods with added sugars (e.g., soda, candy).
- Do not overfeed children; they can usually self-regulate the number of calories they need.
- Consume a diet rich in vegetables and fruits; each meal should include at least 1 fruit or vegetable. Recommended amounts are a range of:
  - 1 cup of fruit *and* ¾ to 1 cup of vegetables per day for children 1 to 3 years old (the larger amount for 2- to 3-year-olds)
  - 2 cups of fruit *and* 3 cups of vegetables per day for a 14- to 18-year-old boy.
- Choose whole-grain, high-fiber foods; limit refined grain products. At least half of all grains should be whole grain. Recommended total grain intake ranges from 2 oz per day for a 1-year-old to 7 oz per day for a 14- to 18-year-old boy.
- Serve fat-free and low-fat dairy foods. A recommended range of intake includes:
  - 2 cups of milk (or equivalent) for children 1 to 8 years old
  - 3 cups of milk (or equivalent) for children 9 to 18 years old
- Serve fish regularly; avoid commercially prepared fried fish.
- Limit intake of total fat to 30% to 35% for children 2 to 3 years old; 25% to 35% total calories for children 4 to 18 years old. Limit saturated fat, trans fat, and cholesterol.
- Choose and prepare foods with little or no salt.
- When you eat food that is prepared outside of the home, follow the AHA diet and lifestyle recommendations.

Adapted from American Heart Association website: www.heart.org/HEARTORG/GettingHealthy/Dietary-Recommendations-for-Healthy-Children_UCM_303886_Article.jsp.

Management

Lifestyle Changes. Dietary change has been the first step in treatment of children older than 2 years with hypercholesterolemia and, combined with other lifestyle changes, remains a mainstay of treatment—even if medications are added to the regimen. The American Heart Association (AHA) encourages individuals to change lifestyle patterns as well as alter diet; educational materials related to the AHA Therapeutic Lifestyle Change approach are available on their website (www.heart.org/HEARTORG) (Box 25-11 lists AHA diet and exercise recommendations).

Many issues arise with dietary changes in children (e.g., increasing dietary fiber may "fill up" the child and increase the risk of poor nutrient intake), so consultation with a pediatric dietitian is essential to ensure that children receive adequate nutrition.

Pharmacotherapy. Drug therapy should be considered in children 8 years or older who, after 6 to 12 months of therapy focused on diet and lifestyle changes, continue to have:

- LDL concentration greater than 190 mg/dL, *or*
- LDL concentration greater than 160 mg/dL *and*
  - Positive family history of premature CVD (before 55 years old) *or*
  - Obesity or overweight

- Hypertension
- Cigarette smoking (Daniels et al, 2008)

If the child is on antipsychotic medication, a consult with the psychiatric provider is necessary before beginning treatment. First-line drugs for treatment of children with hypercholesterolemia are the bile acid sequestrants or "resins" (e.g., cholestyramine, colesevelam, colestipol). These drugs bind with bile acids, leading to increased GI excretion of bile acids. As a result, more bile acid must be synthesized. Hepatic cholesterol is used for this synthesis; the liver takes up circulating cholesterol for its use, and plasma LDL cholesterol decreases. Resins are not well tolerated by many children, with adverse effects of gastrointestinal symptoms, constipation, cramping, and bloating, and compliance is frequently a problem (Daniels et al, 2008).

Use of 3-hydroxy-3-methylglutaryl-CoA (HMG-CoA) reductase inhibitors (statins) can be considered if the child has severe hypercholesterolemia or if there is a poor response to bile acid resins. The statins function by inhibiting the enzyme that synthesizes cholesterol. As experience in children accumulates, practitioners often use statins initially after diet therapy has failed, skipping bile acid–binding resins. Because of the side effects of drugs and the uncertainty about their long-term use in the pediatric population, children who need drug therapy should be referred to a specialized pediatric lipid center for treatment.

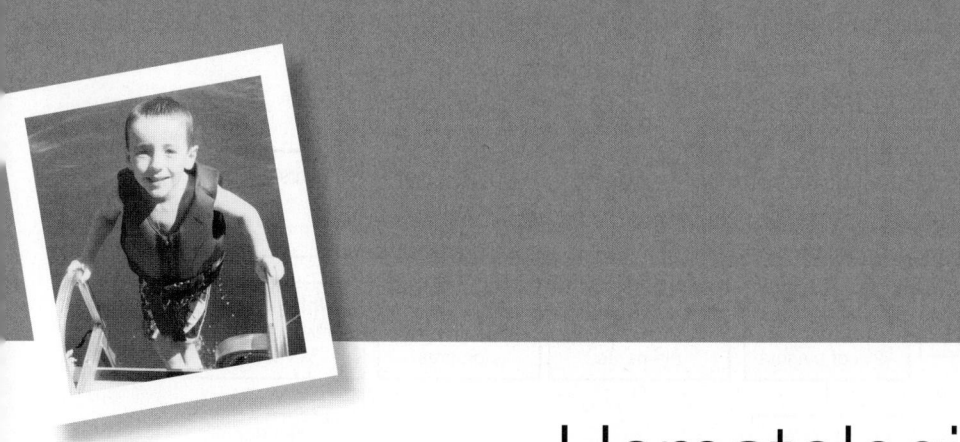

Hematologic Disorders

VERONICA KANE AND MARTHA K. SWARTZ

The hematologic system is a massive fluid organ that permeates the entire body, delivering nutrients and other vital elements throughout. Essential body functions carried out by blood include the transfer of respiratory gases, hemostasis, phagocytosis, and the provision of cellular and humoral agents to fight infection. Abnormalities of blood cells are seen in various disease states and alterations in nutrition, necessitating the use of diagnostic hematologic studies to differentiate common nutritional deficiencies with straightforward treatments from rare diseases with a genetic or chronic component for which extensive referral and a multidisciplinary approach are needed. Because of the effect of impaired cellular nutrition on normal growth and development of sensitive systems in pediatrics, early diagnosis of blood disorders is vital to ensure the best possible prognosis.

■ Anatomy and Physiology

Blood is made of cellular components, each with specialized functions, and a fluid component called plasma, which serves as the transport medium. The cells that comprise whole blood are categorized as erythrocytes (red blood cells [RBCs]); leukocytes (white blood cells [WBCs]); and thrombocytes (platelets). Leukocytes are further differentiated into subtypes (lymphocytes, granulocytes, and monocytes). Abnormally high or low counts of any of the cell categories may indicate the presence of a large variety and many forms of diseases. Due to its sensitivity in screening for a variety of disorders, the complete blood count (CBC) is among the most performed studies and is commonly used in routine health screening. Plasma is the clear yellow fluid in which proteins (primarily albumins, globulins, and fibrinogen) are the major solutes. These plasma proteins maintain intravascular volume, contribute to the coagulation of blood, and are important in acid-base balance. Figure 26-1 shows the breakdown of all components of whole blood.

Blood formation in the human embryo begins in the yolk sac during the first several weeks of gestation. During the second trimester blood is formed primarily in the fetus's liver, spleen, and lymph nodes. In the last half of gestation, hematopoiesis shifts from the fetal liver and spleen to the bone marrow, where, by birth, most blood formation takes place. Most erythropoiesis occurs in the last month of gestation. The bone marrow produces erythrocytes, granulocytes, monocytes, and platelets and provides lymphocytes and lymphocytic precursors to the spleen, lymph nodes, and other lymphatic tissues.

ERYTHROCYTES

Erythropoietin, produced primarily by renal glomerular epithelial cells, regulates erythrocyte (RBC) production. In response to a decrease in the number of circulating RBCs or a decrease in the oxygen pressure (Pao_2) of arterial blood, erythropoietin stimulates the bone marrow to convert certain stem cells to proerythroblasts. Substances essential for RBC formation include iron, vitamin B_{12}, folic acid, amino acids, and other nutrients.

The RBC matures through the following stages: proerythroblast, erythroblast, normoblast, reticulocyte, and erythrocyte. As cellular differentiation occurs, the nucleus present in the early forms of the cell is extruded and replaced by hemoglobin (Hgb). The RBC assumes its characteristic anucleated biconcave disk shape, which is easily distorted, thereby enabling it to pass through small capillaries and sinuses without being destroyed. The large surface-to-volume ratio of the semipermeable membrane facilitates rapid gas exchange.

The youngest RBCs are the reticulocytes. After release from the bone marrow, reticulocytes stay in circulation for about 1 day before becoming mature RBCs. The *reticulocyte count* is about 4% to 6% for the first 3 days of life, which reflects the relatively greater amount of erythropoiesis that occurs in the fetus. This increased reticulocyte count is followed by a sudden drop around 1 year of age to 0.5% to 1.5%, which remains the norm for the rest of life (Table 26-1). In cases of low RBC levels, such as anemia or sudden blood loss, the effectiveness of the body's early response to treatment or progress of healing can be measured via the reticulocyte count. A mature RBC survives about 120 days before it is destroyed through phagocytosis in the spleen, liver, or bone marrow.

In the presence of anemia the reticulocyte count needs to be corrected to account for the decrease in circulating RBCs and the shift of immature reticulocytes prematurely from

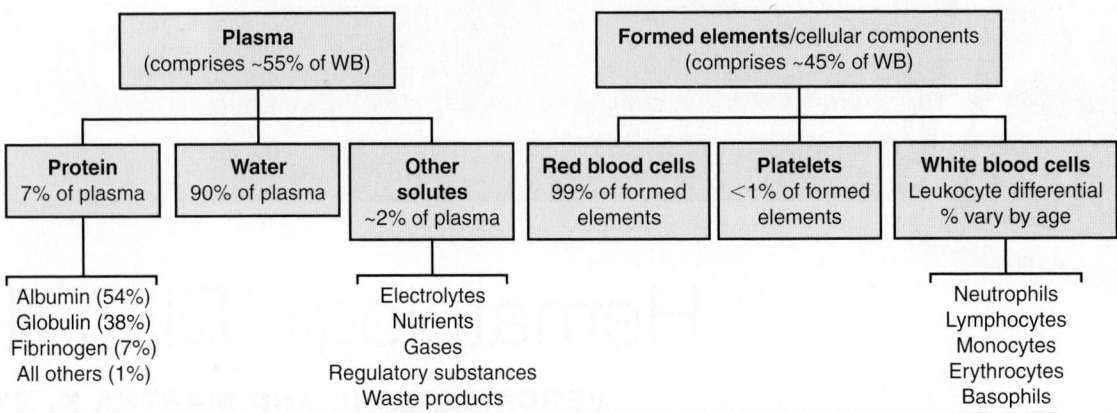

FIGURE 26-1 Composition of whole blood.

marrow into blood. This correction is the *reticulocyte production index.*

Table 26-2 presents an overview of the common clinical diagnostic blood tests including those used to assess red blood cell functioning.

Hemoglobin

Hgb is the oxygen-carrying protein molecule in the RBC. Production of Hgb requires circulating iron, the synthesis of a protoporphyrin ring, and the production of globin. Each Hgb molecule is comprised of two pairs of polypeptide chains. The globin portion contains protein in a precise sequence of amino acids that is coded by genes located on chromosome 16 and chromosome 11. Normal hemoglobin contains two alpha- and two beta-chains. These chains then attach to heme groups, large iron-containing disks, and porphyrin, a nitrogen-containing organic compound.

Each of the four iron atoms in the Hgb molecule combines reversibly with an atom of oxygen to form oxyhemoglobin. This reaction occurs when the oxygen concentration is relatively high, as in the lungs, where oxygen crosses the alveolo-capillary membrane and saturates about 96% of the Hgb. The percentage of oxyhemoglobin is the arterial oxygen saturation (SaO_2), and it is measured through pulse oximetry or arterial blood gas determination. When the oxygen concentration is lower, as in the tissues, oxygen is released from Hgb to meet cellular demands.

Erythrocyte Development

Many dietary elements are essential to the developmental process of mature RBCs, including amino acids, carbohydrates, lipids, vitamin B_{12}, folate, vitamin C, and iron. Free Hgb, which is released during red blood cell lysis, is transported to the reticuloendothelial system by haptoglobin. The reticuloendothelial system is located in the spleen, liver, and bone marrow and is where the lysis substrates, iron, amino acids, carbohydrate, and lipids are reclaimed. Transferrin transports iron to the bone marrow and into the maturing RBC, where it is incorporated into the new heme molecule. As this new cell matures, the nucleus eventually is extruded and the RBC is released into circulation as a reticulocyte. Within 1 to 2 days the reticulocyte becomes a mature RBC. The average life span of the RBC is 120 days.

Structural Variations

Hgb molecules normally represent the majority of the body's Hgb and, in adult Hgb, are composed of two fundamental subunit chains, alpha (α) and beta (β). Equal numbers of each chain are essential for normal cell function. An imbalance of the chains damages and destroys RBCs thereby producing anemia.

Various forms of Hgb are found in the embryo, fetus, and adult, depending on changes in globin chain synthesis. At birth, approximately 70% of Hgb is made up of fetal hemoglobin (Hgb F), which is composed of two α-chains and two gamma-chains (γ). By 12 months of age, 95% of a person's Hgb typically consists of adult Hgb molecules (Hgb A), which are composed of two α- and two β-polypeptide chains attached to four heme groups. In the majority of individuals, Hgb F remains present at levels of less than 2%. Hgb A_2 is another type of adult Hgb but consists of two α- and two delta (δ)-chains. Hbg A_2 normally makes up about 2.5% of the total Hgb and may be increased in beta-thalassemia. Mutations occur whenever there are gene defects in either of the subunit chains resulting in Hgb variants. Any alteration of the amino acid sequencing on the chromosomes (11, 16) that code production of the beta globin chain results in one of over 600 identified variants of Hgb. Some abnormal hemoglobins are the result of amino acid substitutions. While many mutations are innocuous, with indiscernible physiological impact, other structural defects are devastating.

Among the most commonly occurring Hgb variants are Hgb S (sickle), Hgb C, Hgb E, persistence of Hgb F, and Hgb H. The incidence of these hemoglobins tends to peak within certain regional or racial populations. Atypical combinations of Hgb variants can occur, each with its own resulting condition or problems. *Hemoglobin electrophoresis,* which separates each hemoglobin out on a gel medium, is used to differentiate the Hgb variants from Hgb A thus aiding in the diagnosis of specific hemoglobinopathies (Ohls and Christensen, 2007; Wu, 2006).

Diminished production of one of the two subunit chains results in disorders referred to as "thalassemias." Thalassemias are categorized into two types: alpha and beta, and are named based on the affected chain. In the carrier state for alpha-thalassemia, there is one α-chain present enabling the production of adequate amounts of hemoglobin with no symptoms in the carrier. In alpha-thalassemia the beta-globulin subunits cluster into groups of four in the absence of any

TABLE 26-1 Hematologic Values and Normal Leukocyte Differential Count During Infancy and Childhood

Hematologic Values

Age	HEMOGLOBIN (g/dL) Mean	Range	HEMATOCRIT (%) Mean	Range	RETICULOCYTES (%) Mean	MCV (fL) Lowest	LEUKOCYTES (WBC/mm³) Mean	Range	NEUTROPHILS (%) Mean	Range	LYMPHOCYTES (%) Mean*	EOSINOPHILS (%) Mean
Cord blood	16.8	13.7-20.1	55	45-65	5	110	18,000	(9000-30,000)	61	(40-80)	31	2
2 weeks	16.5	13-20	50	42-66	1		12,000	(5000-21,000)	40		63	3
3 months	12	9.5-14.5	36	31-41	1		12,000	(6000-18,000)	30		48	2
6 months-6 years	12	10.5-14	37	33-42	1	70-74	10,000	(6000-18,000)	45		48	2
7-12 years	13	11-16	38	34-40	1	76-80	8000	(4500-13,500)	55		38	2
Adult												
Female	14	12-16	42	37-47	1.6	80	7500	(5000-10,000)	55	(35-70)	35	
Male	16	14-18	47	42-52		80						3

Other Red Cell Indices

RDW: 0-3 d, <18; 1-6 mo, <16.5; 7 mo-2 yr, <16; 2-8 yr, <15; 13-18 yr, <14.5
MCHC: 1-2 wk, 28-38%; 1-6 mo, 30-36%; 7 mo-adults, 31-37%

Normal Leukocyte Differential Count

Age	GRANULOCYTES Segmented Neutrophils (%)	Band Neutrophils (%)	Eosinophils (%)	Basophils (%)	AGRANULOCYTES Lymphocytes (%)	Monocytes (%)
Birth	47 ± 15	14.1 ± 4	2.2	0.6	31 ± 5	5.8
6 months	23	8.8	2.5	0.4	61	4.8
12 months	23	8.1	2.6	0.4	61	4.8
2 years	25	8	2.6	0.5	59	5
4 years	34 ± 11	8 ± 3	2.8	0.6	50 ± 15	5
6 years	43	8	2.7	0.6	42	4.7
8 years	45	8	2.4	0.6	39	4.2
10 years	46 ± 15	8 ± 3	2.4	0.5	38 ± 10	4.3
12 years	47	8	2.5	0.5	38	4.4

Absolute neutrophil count (ANC) = WBC × (% seg + band).
*Relatively wide range.
FL, Femtoliters; MCHC, mean corpuscular hemoglobin concentration; MCV, mean corpuscular volume; RDW, red cell distribution width; WBC, white blood cell.
Data from Kliegman RM, Behrman RE, Jenson HB, et al, editors: Nelson textbook of pediatrics, ed 18, Philadelphia, 2007, Saunders; Taketomo CK, Hodding JH, Kraus: Pediatric dosage handbook, ed 17, Hudson, OH, 2011, Lexi-Comp, p 1676; Wallach J: Interpretation of diagnostic tests, ed 8, Philadelphia, 2006, Lippincott Williams & Wilkins.

TABLE 26-2	Clinical Diagnostic Interpretation
Test	**Description**
Complete blood count (CBC)	Broad screening test for illnesses that cause alteration in red blood cell indices and white blood cell count
CBC with differential	Additionally assesses the amounts of the white cell subtypes present in a given sample of whole blood
CBC with peripheral smear	Additionally assesses the size and shapes of a sample of RBC
Red blood cell (RBC)	Increased with polycythemia vera and fluid loss—diarrhea, burns, dehydration. Decreased with anemia.
Hemoglobin (Hgb)	Iron-binding portion of RBC
Hematocrit (Hct)	Calculation of the percentage of RBC in a given volume of whole blood
Mean corpuscular volume (MCV)	Determines the volume of the average RBC in femtoliters; increased (macro) with B_{12}, folic acid deficiency, hypothyroid; decreased (micro) with iron deficiency, thalassemia, lead poisoning, anemia of chronic disease
Mean corpuscular hemoglobin (MCH)	Average amount of Hgb in red cells. Used in determining type and severity of anemia. Mirrors MCV
Mentzer Index = MCV/RBC	Differentiates between iron deficiency and thalassemia. Ratio <13: Thalassemia Ratio >13: Iron deficiency, hemoglobinopathy
RBC distribution width (RDW)	Increased RDW indicates mixed population of RBCs; immature RBCs are larger than mature, so increase is associated with anemias
Reticulocyte count (Retic)	A percentage of the circulating erythrocytes; this reflects the bone marrow production of new RBCs, reticulocytes, and their subsequent release into the bloodstream. Important in assessing the body's response to an anemic state.
Reticulocyte production index (RPI)	A calculation to more accurately reflect the reticulocyte production in the diagnosis of anemia because the absolute RBC count decreases in anemia; it indicates whether the bone marrow is responding and corrects for the degree of anemia $$RPI = ReticCount \times \frac{Hemoglobin\ (observed)}{Normal\ hemoglobin} \times 0.5$$ RPI >3 associated with hemolysis or blood loss; <2 reflects decreased or ineffective production for the degree of anemia
Absolute neutrophil count (ANC)	Refers to the total number of neutrophil granulocytes present in the blood. Normal value: ≥1500 cells/mm³ Mild neutropenia: ≥1000 to <1500 cells/mm³ Moderate neutropenia: ≥500 to <1000 cells/mm³ Severe neutropenia: ≤500 cells/mm³
Poikilocytosis	Refers to an increase in abnormal RBCs of any shape where they make up 10% or more of the total population
White blood cell (WBC)	May be increased with infections, inflammation, cancer, leukemia; decreased with some medications, some severe infections; bone marrow failure

α-chains with which to partner. These beta-tetramers are incapable of carrying oxygen, and the affected fetuses die in utero *(hydrops fetalis)*. In beta-thalassemia major, the α-chains do not bind with each other but rather degrade in the absence of β-chains. Conversely, in beta-thalassemia minor, there are sufficient β-chains present to bind with the abundant α-chains to create functional Hgb molecules and a resultant asymptomatic mild microcytic anemia.

There are also altered states of Hgb, such as occurs with methemoglobin. In this condition, the ferrous form of iron oxidizes to the ferric state causing the *heme* moiety to be incapable of carrying oxygen. If reduced Hgb levels exceed 5 g/dL serious tissue hypoxia and cyanosis can occur.

Methemoglobinemia can be congenital or caused by exposure to certain drugs and chemicals.

Normal Values

Hgb levels in a newborn range from 12.5 to 20.5 g/dL and then drop to its lowest point around 2 to 4 months of age (Wu, 2006). This drop represents a physiologic anemia caused by the shortened survival of fetal RBCs and the rapid expansion of blood volume during this period. A decrease in Hgb can also develop secondary to a decrease in RBC production, blood loss, or increased RBC destruction. Due to the effect of these processes, oxygen transport to the tissues is adversely

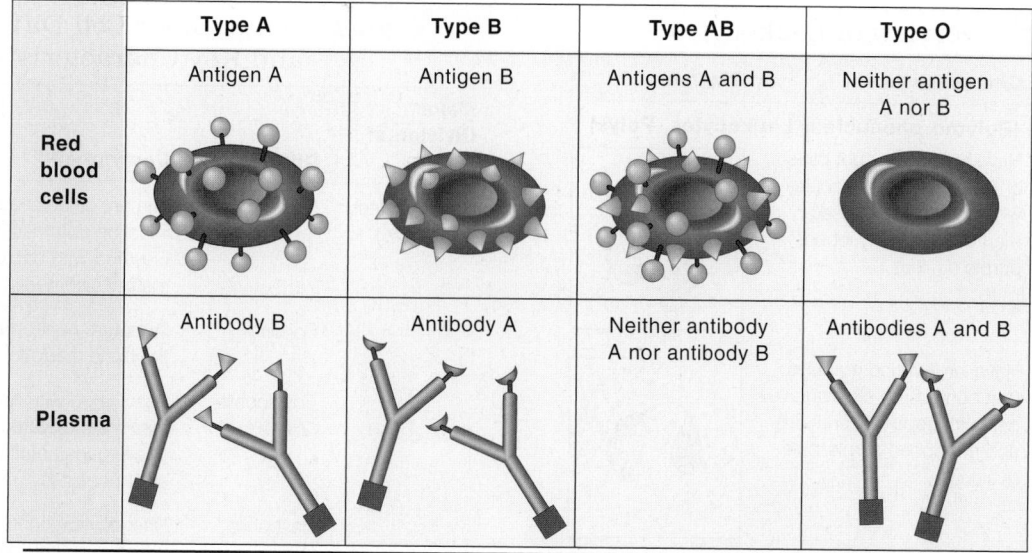

	Type A	Type B	Type AB	Type O
Red blood cells	Antigen A	Antigen B	Antigens A and B	Neither antigen A nor B
Plasma	Antibody B	Antibody A	Neither antibody A nor antibody B	Antibodies A and B

FIGURE 26-2 Red cell antigenicity. (From Patton K: *Anatomy & physiology,* ed 7, St. Louis, 2010, Mosby.)

affected and the individual can become clinically anemic. Table 26-1 summarizes the RBC indices.

Antigenic Properties of Red Blood Cells

Red cells are classified into different types according to the presence of antigens on the cell membrane. The antigenicity is genetically determined and represents contributions from both parents. The most common antigens are designated A, B, and Rh. A person inherits either A or B antigen (type A or B blood), both antigens (type AB blood, which is the universal recipient), or neither antigen (type O blood, which is the universal donor) (Fig. 26-2). In the U.S., 85% of Caucasians and 95% of African-Americans are Rh-positive (Guyton and Hall, 2010). Clinically these distinctions become important when blood transfusions are necessary or in the assessment for maternal-fetal blood incompatibilities. The International Society for Blood Transfusion recognizes more than 20 blood group systems (including Rh and ABO).

LEUKOCYTES

Leukocytes, or WBCs, are larger and fewer in number than erythrocytes. Normally about 5000 to 10,000 leukocytes are contained in a microliter of blood. The primary function of WBCs is protection of the body from invasion by foreign organisms and distribution of antibodies and other immune response components. When levels reach critical low and high values for leukocytes there are great risks to the child. A WBC count of less than 500/mm^3 places the patient at risk for a fatal infection. However, a WBC count greater than 30,000/mm^3 indicates massive infection or a serious disease such as leukemia.

Five distinct types of WBCs can be grouped into two broad classifications: granulocytes (also known as polymorphonuclear leukocytes [PMNs], or "polys") and agranulocytes. Granulocytes contain large granules and horseshoe-shaped nuclei that become segmented and are connected by thin strands (Table 26-3). With Wright stain the cytoplasm stains blue or pink. Granulocytes are further divided into neutrophils;

eosinophils, which absorb the acid dye eosin; and basophils, which absorb a basic dye. The agranulocytes include lymphocytes (also known as immunocytes) and monocytes.

Granular Leukocytes (Polymorphonuclear Leukocytes, Polys)

Neutrophils, Basophils, Eosinophils. In children, granulocytes comprise 40% to 70% of all WBCs. They mature in the bone marrow through the following stages: stem cells, myeloblasts, promyelocytes, myelocytes, metamyelocytes, band forms, and, finally, mature segmented neutrophils. This maturational process takes approximately 6 to 11 days. Once a neutrophil is released into the bloodstream it circulates for about 6 to 9 hours before entering the tissues, where the major function of PMNs is phagocytosis of harmful particles and cells, particularly bacterial organisms. Thus neutrophils are the primary WBC involved in fighting bacterial infections.

A frequency distribution of the types of WBCs is obtained by the differential count, and quantitative alterations within the categories are important diagnostically (Table 26-4). A relative increase in the number of circulating immature neutrophils (band forms, metamyelocytes, and myelocytes) is referred to as a "shift to the left," a term derived from how the differential count used to be tabulated on written forms. This phenomenon is indicative of an inflammatory process or the body's immunologic response to an acute bacterial infection. The phrase "shift to the right" indicates an increase in the total lymphocyte count.

Basophils, which account for less than 1% of circulating leukocytes, are closely related to tissue mast cells. Both cells react immediately in the face of a hypersensitivity reaction by granules releasing heparin and histamine into the bloodstream during systemic allergic reactions. Renal disease, rare carcinomas, and medications such as estrogen and antithyroid agents are among the reasons for increased basophils.

Eosinophils (1% to 2% WBCs) have two main functions: to immediately release histamine in hypersensitivity reactions and to destroy parasites. Other causes of eosinophilia include connective tissue and collagen vascular diseases, immunodeficiencies, and neoplasms, such as carcinoma, lymphoma, and Hodgkin disease. Eosinophils contain receptor sites for

TABLE 26-3	Overview of Leukocytes	
Cell Type	**Characteristics**	**Diagram**
Granulocytes (Polymorphonuclear Leukocytes, Polys)		
Neutrophils	Have small, fine, light pink or lilac acidophilic granules when stained and a segmented, irregularly lobed, purple nucleus	
Eosinophils	Have large round granules that contain red-staining basic mucopolysaccharides and multilobed purple-blue nuclei	
Basophils	Coarse blue granules conceal the segmented nucleus. Granules contain histamine, heparin, and acid mucopolysaccharides.	
Agranulocytes		
Lymphocytes	Small cells with a large, round, deep-staining, single-lobed nucleus and very little cytoplasm. The cytoplasm is slightly basophilic and stains pale blue.	
Monocytes	Large cells with a prominent, multishaped nucleus that sometimes is kidney shaped. Chromatin in the nucleus looks like lace, with small particles linked together like strands. The gray-blue cytoplasm is filled with many fine lysozymes that stain pink with Wright stain.	

Data from Bullock B, Henze R: Hematology: adaptations and alterations in function. In Bullock B, editor: *Focus on pathophysiology*, Philadelphia, 2000, Lippincott Williams & Wilkins, p 359; McCance K, Huether S: *Pathophysiology: the biologic basis for disease in adults and children*, ed 5, St Louis, 2006, Mosby.

TABLE 26-4	White Blood Cell Differential and Key Characteristics	
Major Division of WBCs	**Differential**	**Description**
Granulocytes (50%-75%)	Neutrophils	Primary defense against bacterial infection and mediating stress. Elevated with bacterial or inflammatory disorders
	Bands (<1%)	Immature neutrophils put out by the bone marrow
	Eosinophils (2%-4%)	Associated with antigen-antibody response; elevated with exposure to allergens or inflammation of skin, parasites
	Basophils (1%-2%)	Phagocytes: contain heparin, histamines, and serotonin. Increased in leukemia, chronic inflammation, hypersensitivity to food, radiation therapy. Mast cells
Nongranu-locytes (30%-40%)	Lympho-cytes (25%-35%)	Primary components of the immune system. Elevated with viral infections, leukemia, radiation exposure; decreased with diseases affecting the immune system
	Monocytes (<2%)	Elevated in infections and inflammation, leukemia; decreased with some bone marrow injury, leukemias

WBCs, White blood cells.
Data from Wu AHB: *Tietz clinical guide to laboratory tests*, ed 4, Philadelphia, 2006, Saunders; and Gilbert-Barness E, Barness LA: *Clinical use of pediatric diagnostic tests*, Philadelphia, 2006, Lippincott Williams & Wilkins.

immunoglobulin E (IgE), levels of which are elevated in people with allergies; they also prevent clot formation in the microcirculation. Eosinophils are found in the mucosa of the gastrointestinal (GI) tract and in the lungs and are weakly phagocytic.

Agranulocytes-Leukocytes

Lymphocytes. Lymphocytes (or immunocytes) comprise 25% to 35% of WBCs. Although not phagocytic, they protect the body against specific antigens. They originate in the bone marrow, but differentiate in lymphoid tissues, such as the spleen, liver, thymus, lymph nodes, and intestines. Thymus-dependent lymphocytes, or T cells, are part of the cell-mediated immune response in which cytotoxic agents and macrophages are synthesized. B-cell lymphocytes are precursors of the humoral immune response whereby the cells are transformed into plasma cells that release immunoglobulins or antibodies into the bloodstream. Lymphocytes are an important defense component.

Monocytes. Monocytes, which contain a large lobulated nucleus, are relatively immature cells that circulate for about 8 hours before migrating to tissues where they assume their mature form as macrophages. They constitute 4% to 6% of WBCs with the absolute monocyte count of 0.1 to 0.9 × 10^9/L. After briefly circulating in the peripheral vascular system, monocytes migrate to the tissue to mature and become part of the monocyte/histiocyte/immune cell system. Fixed and mobile macrophages are located primarily in the liver, spleen, lymph nodes, and GI tract and make up the mononuclear phagocyte system. Like granulocytes, which are the first line of defense against microbe invasion, their primary function is phagocytosis of bacteria and cellular debris. Monocyte elevation occurs in collagen vascular disease, Hodgkin disease, non-Hodgkin lymphoma, and chronic infections such as tuberculosis, and syphilis.

TABLE 26-5	Blood Coagulation Factors
Factor (International Nomenclature)	**Common Synonyms**
I	Fibrinogen
II	Prothrombin*
III	Tissue thromboplastin, thrombokinase
V	Proaccelerin, labile factor, accelerator globulin
VII	Proconvertin,* stable factor
VIII	Antihemophilic globulin (AHG), antihemophilic factor (AHF),antihemophilic factor A
IX	Plasma thromboplastin component (PTC), Christmas factor,* antihemophilic factor B
X	Stuart-Prower factor, Stuart factor*
XI	Plasma thromboplastin antecedent (PTA), antihemophilic factor C
XII	Hageman factor, contact factor, antihemophilic factor
XIII	Fibrin-stabilizing factor (FSF), plasma transglutaminase
Kininogen	Fitzgerald factor
Prekallikrein	Fletcher factor

*Vitamin K dependent.

PLATELET CELLS AND COAGULATION FACTORS

The smallest cellular components in blood are the platelets, or thrombocytes, which are essential to hemostasis and clot formation. Circulating platelets are fragments of megakaryocytes, which are precursor cells that form in the bone marrow. The normal platelet count ranges from 150,000 to 300,000 cells/mm^3.

When a blood vessel is injured (or in the presence of intrinsic damage to the blood), platelets adhere to the inner surface of the vessel and form a hemostatic plug. As platelets degrade, a series of at least 13 clotting factors or proteolytic enzymes are released that bring about the clotting process in a cascading sequence of successive reactions. These clotting factors are listed in Table 26-5.

The basic reactions that occur in the sequential process of blood coagulation are as follows: factor X activates and prothrombin (factor II) converts to thrombin, which then catalyzes the conversion of fibrinogen (factor I) to fibrin. Fibrin provides the matrix in which blood cells aggregate to form a clot. A deficiency of any of the proteins in the pathway leads to a clotting disorder. In particular, if factor VIII is deficient (as in classic hemophilia A) or the number of platelets is inadequate (thrombocytopenia), activation of factor X is impaired. Figure 26-3 illustrates the entire coagulation cascade. Age-specific coagulation values exist for each aspect of the coagulation process and should be referenced for proper assessment and treatment management.

Pathophysiology

Hematologic problems are generally classified as disorders of RBC function, WBC function, and platelet and coagulation function. These three broad categories are further divided into disorders of blood cell production, maturation, or destruction. Although most RBC disorders result in a decrease quantity of cells or cell abnormalities, it is important not to forget the congenital, though rare, proliferative disorder, primary *polycythemia (polycythemia rubra vera)*. This entity is a panmyeloproliferative disorder. Children usually have hepatosplenomegaly, neurologic and cardiovascular symptoms caused by erythrocytosis, diarrhea and pruritus due to histamine release related to granulocytosis, and thrombosis or hemorrhage from thrombocytosis (Burns and Camitta, 2007). Knowledge of these pathophysiologic classifications gives the pediatric provider a rationale for routine screening and useful algorithms to guide further clinical investigation.

Assessment of Disorders of Erythrocytes

HISTORY

A comprehensive history and physical examination are essential to unravel the mystery behind suspected hematologic disorders. Many hematologic processes have genetic bases. In order to discern inheritable disorders, it is necessary to identify the child's ethnicity and race(s), plus obtain a detailed family medical history. Certain disorders occur with greater frequency in individuals of certain races or ancestrally from specific geographic regions. One example of this phenomenon is *sickle cell anemia* (SCA) which primarily affects those of African ancestry. Recording all family health data in a genogram provides visual clues to patterns of heritability and assists with narrowing the diagnostic possibilities.

The provider should obtain information about *family members* with a history of any of following:
- Genetically based disorders (include, but are not exclusive to, sickle cell or thalassemia disease or trait)
- Anemia
- Jaundice
- Splenomegaly
- Gallbladder disease
- Lead exposure
- Bleeding tendencies
- Drug and toxin exposure
- Bone marrow failure
- Chronic illnesses

Maternal history is significant in young children and should include:
- Pregnancy and delivery
- Gestational drug ingestion
- Anemia during pregnancy
- Transfusion
- Pica, eating nonfood product

A comprehensive review of a *child's medical history* and *a review of systems* are fundamental. Particular attention should focus on the following:
- Prematurity (especially if anemia detected in infancy)
- Environmental exposures (lead, cadmium, pesticides, toxic waste, etc.)
- Any chronic illnesses

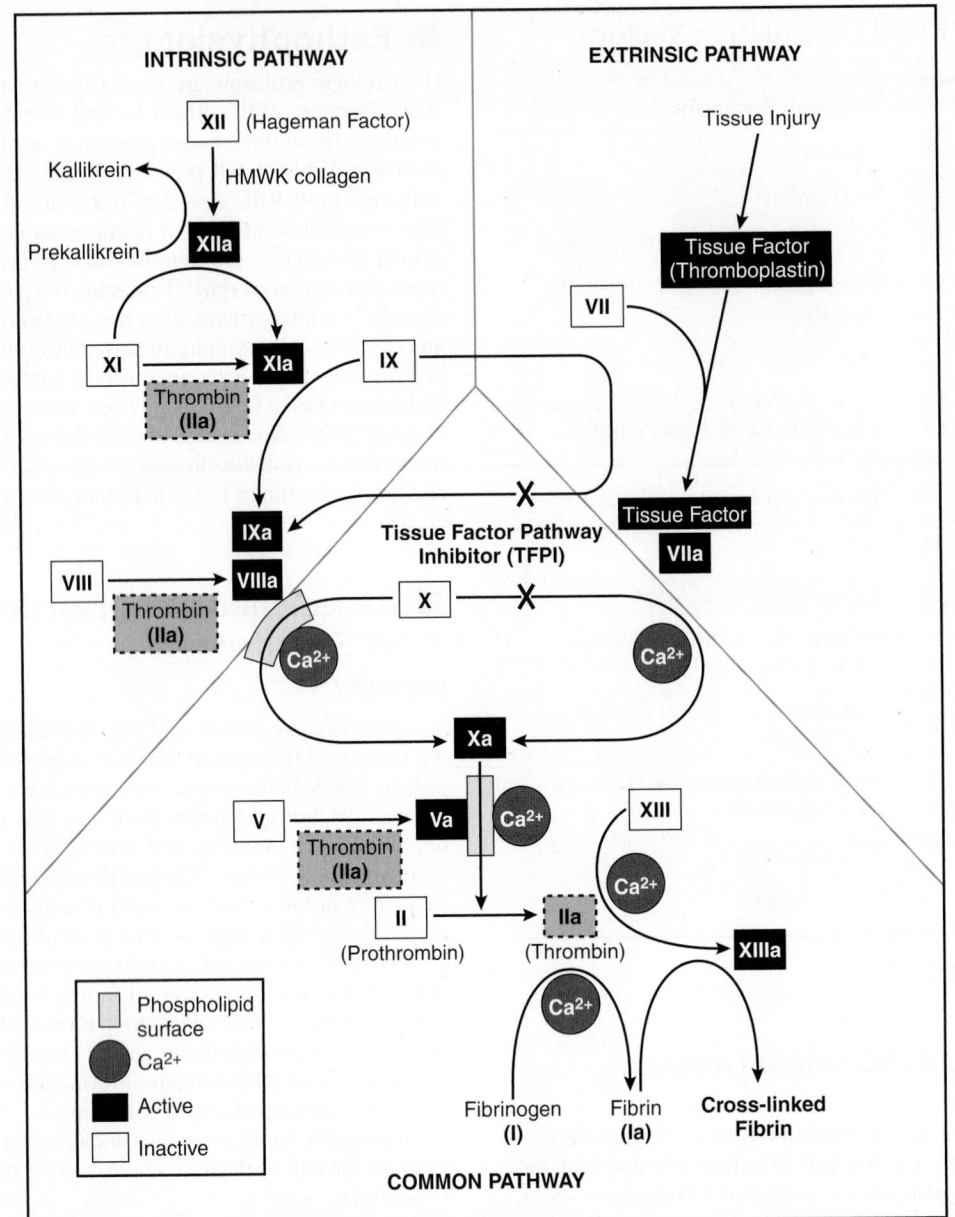

FIGURE 26-3 The classical coagulation cascade. Note the common link between the intrinsic and extrinsic pathways at the level of factor IX activation. Factors in white boxes represent inactive molecules; activated factors are indicated with a lowercase *a* and a black box. *HMWK,* High-molecular-weight kininogen. Not shown are the inhibitory anticoagulant pathways. (From Kumar V, Abbas A, Fausto N, et al: *Robbins basic pathology,* ed 8, Philadelphia, 2007, Elsevier.)

- Growth changes or weight loss, unexplained
- Persistent pallor, *ashiness*
- Adenopathy
- Evidence of endocrinopathy
- Jaundice episodes (including in the newborn period)
- Extremity pain, with or without swelling
- Prolonged or usual blood loss (particularly from mucous membranes)
- Unexplained petechiae, easy bruising
- Behavioral changes: Irritable, quiet, restless, subdued
- GI disorders: Liver disease, abdominal pain, changes in stool patterns
- Bone fractures
- Changes in stool characteristics indicating GI bleeding

- Lack of energy, fatigue
- Recent acute infections or drug exposure
- International travel and immunization history

The *nutritional history* of the child (and of the breastfeeding mother) should include the following:

- Dietary intake of iron sources, quantities and types of milk, and meat
- Type and dosing of vitamin supplements, include possibility of excessive ingestion
- A 24-hour dietary recall
- Any history of pica, protracted mouthing behaviors (particularly when iron deficiency or plumbism is suspected)

Newborn screening panel results need to be reviewed. In most states routine screening of newborn cord blood is done to detect genetic and metabolic disorders, such as sickle cell disease, sickle cell trait, and other hemoglobinopathies. The primary care provider needs to verify and document the infant's results in the medical record.

PHYSICAL EXAMINATION

The physical examination of the child should be comprehensive and include vital signs and growth documentation. The following positive signs are particularly important to identify due to their association with specific problems:

- Pallor (especially of the conjunctivae, buccal mucosa, and palmar creases)
- Jaundice (indicates a hemolytic process)
- Petechiae (indicates multiple cell involvement)
- Retinal hemorrhages (hemolytic disorders)
- Excessive bruising, multiple stages (coagulopathy)
- Bleeding from mucous membranes (coagulopathy)
- Lymphadenopathy (infection, malignancy)
- Frontal bossing and/or prominent maxilla (secondary to bone marrow expansion in thalassemia major)
- Joint or extremity pain (sickle cell, leukemia)
- Heart murmurs (may be heard with anemias), signs of congestive heart failure, or tachycardia (acute process with poor compensation)
- Hepatomegaly or splenomegaly (splenomegaly—associated with hemolytic processes, malignancy, acute infection; hypersplenism due to portal hypertension)
- Congenital anomalies that are associated with hematologic disorders

▇ Pancytopenia

Pancytopenia is marked by a decrease in all three formed elements of the blood—erythrocytes, leukocytes, and platelets. A child usually presents with clinical findings of infection or bleeding rather than anemia because of the longer life span of RBCs compared with platelets and WBCs. As such it is not a single disease, but results from a combination of disease processes. Pancytopenia is caused by one of three processes:

- Production failure (intrinsic bone marrow disease as occurs in aplastic anemia)
- Sequestration (as occurs with hypersplenism)
- Increased peripheral destruction of mature cells (Panepinto and Scott, 2011; Zitelli and Davis, 2007)

The child should be referred to a pediatric hematologist for treatment focused at correcting the underlying mechanism, such as hematopoietic stem cell transplantation (failure of production), splenectomy, or other treatments aimed at reducing peripheral destruction of cells or sequestration.

Erythrocyte Disorders

▇ Anemia

CLASSIFICATION OF THE ANEMIAS

Anemia is a reduction in circulating red blood cells and results from a reduction in RBC production, abnormalities of the RBC itself, shortened RBC life span or RBC destruction, or an acute or chronic loss of circulating RBCs. Various anemias are more common in specific races and geographic populations, such as SCA and glucose-6-phosphate dehydrogenase (G6PD) deficiency in people of African and Mediterranean decent. Nutritional deficiencies and toxic ingestions play integral roles in the incidence of anemias (i.e., folic acid deficiency, B_{12} deficiency, iron deficiency anemia [IDA], lead poisoning). Anemia affects many systems because it causes stress on the cardiovascular and respiratory systems. This may manifest as decreased exercise tolerance, fatigue, shortness of breath, or congestive heart failure. However, the majority of children and adolescents with anemia are asymptomatic.

RBCs may be described by the cell size, shape, or color (e.g., hypochromic, microcytic; macrocytic; normochromic, normocytic). The use of this standardized nomenclature facilitates the diagnostic process by distinguishing the various anemias (Table 26-6). For instance, IDA is microcytic (small cell) and hypochromic (pale), whereas aplastic anemia is macrocytic (large), and anemia from malignancies and chronic illness tends to be normocytic (Fig. 26-4).

In toddlers and young children, approximately 90% of anemias are caused by either IDA, lead poisoning (also called *plumbism*), infection, or hemoglobinopathy. The first two of these problems result from a reduction in available Hgb for nutrient transport within the RBC. This reduction of circulating Hgb results in small, pale RBCs (microcytic, hypochromic) with decreased oxygen-carrying potential. Inadequate RBC production can be either acquired or constitutional resulting is such anemias as aplastic anemia, red cell aplasia, and transient erythroblastosis of childhood (TEC). Table 26-7 outlines the history, physical findings, and laboratory diagnosis and treatment of the common RBC anemias in infants and children.

Another classification system defines anemias by the type of problem with RBC production (Fig. 26-5). Hypoproliferative anemias result from a failure in erythrocyte marrow production. These anemias tend to be normocytic-normochromic with a reticulocyte count less than 2, giving the semblance of the body not responding to the anemia. Among the causes for the hypoproliferative anemias are iron deficiency, marrow damage, decreased stimulation of the marrow (as in renal disease), inflammation, and metabolic disorders. Maturational anemias, in which there is a defect in nuclear maturation, are caused by nutritional disturbances, such as deficiencies in folic acid and vitamin B_{12} and exposure to chemotherapeutic agents. In chronic illnesses there may be a decrease in red cell survival time, the bone marrow response or impaired iron transport. Such an effect is often seen in chronic inflammatory illnesses, chronic infections, renal and liver disease, endocrine disorders, and malignant neoplastic diseases. In the last category increased cell destruction produces hemolytic anemias. The hemolysis may be caused by defects in the red cell membrane, hereditary hemoglobinopathies (as in SCA), or congenital enzyme defects. Among these syndromes are hereditary spherocytosis (HS) and G6PD deficiency.

EPIDEMIOLOGY

Despite steady declines in the U.S., anemia continues to be a major health problem here and to an even greater extent internationally. Iron deficiency is the most common cause of anemia, even as cases steadily decline when nutritional practices improve.

TABLE 26-6	Acute Anemia in Childhood and Adolescence				
Classification	**History**	**Physical Findings**	**Screening Tests**	**Diagnostic Tests**	**Treatment**
I. Microcytic					
Iron deficiency anemia	Infant and toddler Excessive cow's milk ingestion Poor solid food intake	Waxy, sallow appearance of skin	Hgb: 8-11 g/dL (moderate); <7 g/dL (severe) MCV: <60 fL Retic: ↓ to sl ↑	Serum Fe: ↓ TIBC: ↑ % Saturation: ↓	Ferrous sulfate, 4-6 mg/kg/day of elemental iron Discontinue cow's milk Limit formula to <24 oz/day and encourage solid food
Homozygous thalassemia (Cooley anemia)	Infant and toddler Growth failure Ethnic background consistent	Hepatospleno-megaly Frontal bossing	MCV: 50-60 fL	Hgb: var ↓	Hypertransfusion program; chelation therapy if iron overload, hematopoietic stem cell transplantation
II. Macrocytic					
Diamond-Black-fan anemia Megaloblastic anemia	(See III) Normocytic Variable, depending on etiology	Variable, depending on etiology	Hgb: var ↓ MCV: ↑ Retic: ↓ Platelets and WBC: ↓ Hypersegmented polys	Bone marrow: megaloblastic Vitamin B_{12} level: nl to ↓ Folate Others	Variable, depending on etiology (e.g., folic acid, vitamin B_{12} transfusion)
III. Normocytic **A. Production Defect**					
Diamond-Black-fan anemia	Age of onset: 65% <6 mo old 90% <1 yr old Insidious onset	25% with physical abnormalities	Hgb: <8 g/dL MCV: ↑ in 30% (100% after treatment) Retic: <1%	Bone marrow: erythroid hypoplasia and lymphocytosis Hgb F: ↑ RBCi antigen: ↑	Prednisone: 2-5 mg/kg/day
Transient erythroblastopenia of childhood	1 to 3 yr old Viral illness in preceding 3 mo	None	Hgb: 3-9 g/dL MCV: normal Retic: <1%	Bone marrow: erythroid hypoplasia	Supportive
Aplastic anemia	Bleeding Infection	Petechiae, purpura Infection Multiple anomalies possible with Fanconi anemia	Hgb: var ↓ MCV: ↑ in Fanconi anemia Retic: ↓ Platelets and WBC: ↓	Bone marrow: hypoplasia of all hematopoietic elements	Variable
B. Hemolytic					
Autoimmune hemolytic anemia	Jaundice Gastrointestinal symptoms Dark, red urine	Icterus Hepatospleno-megaly	Hgb: var ↓ Retic: ↑ (occ ↓) Smear: microspherocytes	Direct Coombs' test: positive	Corticosteroids: prednisone or intravenous equivalent: 2-6 mg/kg/day Transfusion indicated
Hemolytic-uremic syndrome	Infant and toddler Viral prodrome Gastrointestinal bleeding in 20% Sudden pallor, purpura CNS symptoms	Purpura Hypotension CNS abnormalities	Hgb: 7-8 g/dL Retic: ↑ Platelets: ↓ Smear: microangiopathy	None Renal tests: failure	Supportive: early dialysis ? Plasma infusion/exchange ? Antiplatelet drugs
C. Blood loss					
Splenic sequestration crisis of sickle cell (SS) disease (internal blood loss)	SS disease: 5 mo to 2 yr old Hgb SC or S-thalassemia: all ages Sudden weakness, dyspnea, abdominal distention Shock	Hypotension Massive splenomegaly	Hgb: <4 g/dL Retic: ↑ Smear: sickle cells	None	Plasma expanders: whole or reconstituted blood

?, Questionable use; *CNS,* central nervous system; *Fe,* iron; *Hgb,* hemoglobin; *MCV,* mean corpuscular volume; *mo,* months; *nl,* normal; *occ,* occasionally; *polys,* polymorphonuclear leukocytes; *RBCi,* red blood cell i antigen; *Retic,* reticulocyte; *sl,* slightly; *TIBC,* total iron-binding capacity; *var,* variably; *WBC,* white blood cell count.

Adapted from Burg F, Ingelfinger J, Polin, R, Gershon A, editors: *Current pediatric therapy,* ed 18, Philadelphia, 2006, Saunders.

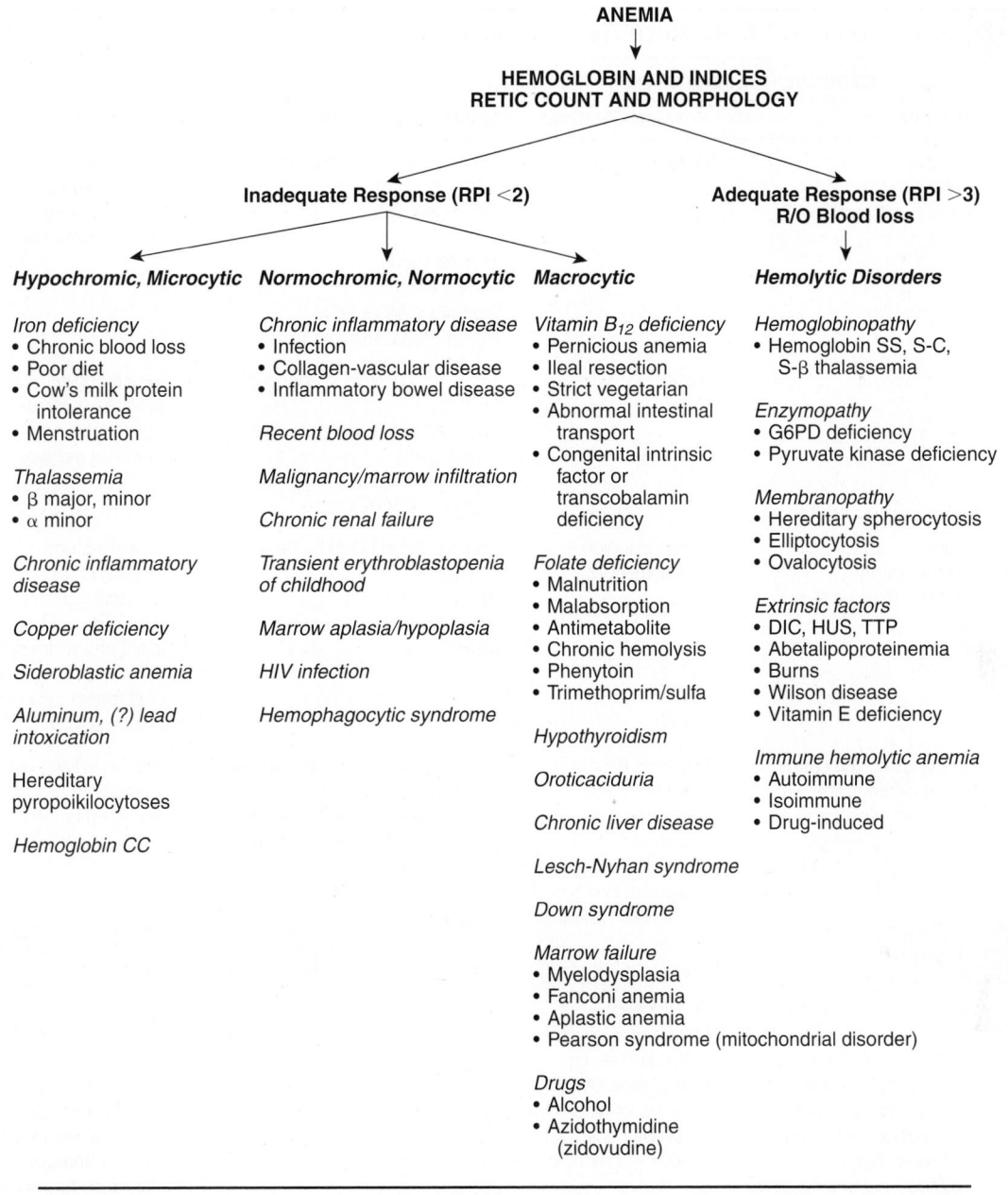

ANEMIA

**HEMOGLOBIN AND INDICES
RETIC COUNT AND MORPHOLOGY**

Inadequate Response (RPI <2)

**Adequate Response (RPI >3)
R/O Blood loss**

Hypochromic, Microcytic

Iron deficiency
• Chronic blood loss
• Poor diet
• Cow's milk protein
  intolerance
• Menstruation

Thalassemia
• β major, minor
• α minor

*Chronic inflammatory
disease*

Copper deficiency

Sideroblastic anemia

*Aluminum, (?) lead
intoxication*

*Hereditary
pyropoikilocytoses*

Hemoglobin CC

Normochromic, Normocytic

Chronic inflammatory disease
• Infection
• Collagen-vascular disease
• Inflammatory bowel disease

Recent blood loss

Malignancy/marrow infiltration

Chronic renal failure

*Transient erythroblastopenia
of childhood*

Marrow aplasia/hypoplasia

HIV infection

Hemophagocytic syndrome

Macrocytic

Vitamin B$_{12}$ deficiency
• Pernicious anemia
• Ileal resection
• Strict vegetarian
• Abnormal intestinal
  transport
• Congenital intrinsic
  factor or
  transcobalamin
  deficiency

Folate deficiency
• Malnutrition
• Malabsorption
• Antimetabolite
• Chronic hemolysis
• Phenytoin
• Trimethoprim/sulfa

Hypothyroidism

Oroticaciduria

Chronic liver disease

Lesch-Nyhan syndrome

Down syndrome

Marrow failure
• Myelodysplasia
• Fanconi anemia
• Aplastic anemia
• Pearson syndrome (mitochondrial disorder)

Drugs
• Alcohol
• Azidothymidine
  (zidovudine)

Hemolytic Disorders

Hemoglobinopathy
• Hemoglobin SS, S-C,
  S-β thalassemia

Enzymopathy
• G6PD deficiency
• Pyruvate kinase deficiency

Membranopathy
• Hereditary spherocytosis
• Elliptocytosis
• Ovalocytosis

Extrinsic factors
• DIC, HUS, TTP
• Abetalipoproteinemia
• Burns
• Wilson disease
• Vitamin E deficiency

Immune hemolytic anemia
• Autoimmune
• Isoimmune
• Drug-induced

FIGURE 26-4 Use of the complete blood count, reticulocyte count, and blood smear in the diagnosis of anemia. *DIC,* Disseminated intravascular coagulation; *G6PD,* glucose-6-phosphate dehydrogenase; *HIV,* human immunodeficiency virus; *HUS,* hemolytic-uremic syndrome; *R/O,* rule out; *RPI,* reticulocyte production index; *TTP,* thrombotic thrombocytopenic purpura. (From Scott J: Hematology. In Kliegman R, Marcdante K, Jenson H, Behrman R, editors: *Nelson essentials of pediatrics,* ed 5, Philadelphia, 2006, Saunders.)

The thalassemias are a group of inherited disorders that cause a significant number of pediatric anemias. One of the most common single gene disorders in the world is alpha-thalassemia. This genetic disorder affects more than half of the population in the southwest Pacific, one fourth in western Africa, and 5% to 10% in the Mediterranean region. Historically the disease was rare in the U.S., although approximately 30% of African-Americans are genetic carriers for this disease. However, the incidence is increasing with the recent surge in Asian immigration. Beta-thalassemia manifests with greater numbers in Mediterranean, northern African, and Indian peoples, whereas SCA is highest among African populations, and all are rare in persons of northern European ancestry.

WORKUP FOR ANEMIA

Anemia may be suspected on the basis of clinical judgment, but is often detected though hematocrit (Hct) and Hgb screening. Understanding which tests to order and how to interpret laboratory data are integral to analyzing the information communicated by the hematopoietic system (see Tables 26-1 and 26-2). Laboratory norms vary slightly with the individual lab so evaluate the child's results in accordance with local lab

| **TABLE 26-7** | Red Blood Cell Disorders Associated With Anemia in Infants and Children |

Disease	CLINICAL PRESENTATION		Laboratory Diagnosis	Treatment
	History	Physical Findings		
Iron deficiency	Fatigue Irritability Excess milk intake	Pallor or none	RBC hypochromic, microcytic MCV ↓ Serum iron ↓ TIBC ↑ % Saturation ↓ Ferritin ↓ Blood in stool or urine Ratio of MCV/RBC >13	Correct diet Eliminate source of bleeding Ferrous SO_4 up to 6 mg/kg/day of elemental iron
Alpha- and beta-thalassemia trait	None Pallor Family history	None Pallor	RBC hypochromic, microcytic MCV ↓↓ Basophilic stippling (beta-thalassemia trait) ↑ Hgb A_2 (beta-thalassemia trait) Ratio of MCV/RBC <13	None for child Test both parents Genetic counseling Avoid iron therapy
Hereditary spherocytosis	None Family history History of neonatal jaundice	Pallor, jaundice Splenomegaly	Spherocytosis Coombs' test negative Reticulocyte % ↑ Osmotic fragility increased MCHC ↑	No splenectomy if Hgb >10 g/dL (100 g/L) and reticulocyte <10% Folic acid (0.5 mg daily <5 yr old; 1 mg daily >5 yr old) Splenectomy; immunizations for pneumococcus, *Haemophilus influenzae,* and meningococcus; penicillin prophylaxis
Chronic inflammation	Depends on the cause of the inflammation and the severity of anemia (fatigue to symptoms of congestive heart failure)	Depends on the cause of the inflammation and the severity of anemia (pallor to signs of congestive heart failure)	Nonspecific tests: erythrocyte sedimentation rate Acute-phase reactants: C-reactive protein, fibrinogen, haptoglobin Serum ferritin Serum iron and TIBC % iron saturation Bone marrow iron stores Bone marrow sideroblasts	Treat underlying disease or condition Treat anemia
Lead intoxication	Pica—ingestion of nonfood substances, especially those containing lead Neurobehavioral problems (e.g., irritability, poor appetite, inattention, hyperactivity) Neurodevelopmental delay (e.g., learning problems to severe cognitive dysfunction)	Poor speech Visuomotor integration problems Encephalopathy, neuropathy, cerebral edema if severe poisoning	Basophilic stippling Erythrocyte protoporphyrin blood lead	Eliminate source of lead in the child's environment Diet rich in iron and calcium Iron supplementation, 4-6 mg/kg/day to reduce further absorption of lead Chelation therapy based on lead levels and symptoms (use Centers for Disease Control and Prevention guidelines)

MCHC, Mean corpuscular hemoglobin concentration; *MCV,* mean corpuscular volume; *RBC,* red blood cell; *TIBC,* total iron-binding capacity.
Adapted from Segel G, Hirsh M, Feig S: Managing anemia in a pediatric office practice: part 1, *Pediatr Rev* 23:75-83, 2002.

norms. The initial laboratory evaluation of suspected anemia includes the following:

- CBC
- Reticulocyte count
- Peripheral smear to examine the morphologic characteristics and staining properties of the RBC

A standardized vocabulary is used to describe the characteristics of erythrocytes that enable the provider to differentiate and categorize the disorders. The language of morphology is summarized in Box 26-1 with examples of associated disorders.

Following an abnormal screening for Hgb or Hct, further diagnostic studies may be indicated to delineate the type of acute anemia. The provider may wish to consider ordering serum iron (Fe), free erythrocyte protoporphyrin (FEP), total iron-binding capacity (TIBC), serum ferritin, and the red (cell) distribution width (RDW) if that was not included in the CBC. Table 26-8 presents a summary of how these laboratory findings relate in differentiating the microcytic anemias.

MICROCYTIC ANEMIA

By far the most common of the anemias in children, microcytic anemia often results from a defect in hemoglobin (from inadequate availability or usage of a substrate) or globin synthesis (as in inherited hemoglobinopathy). Chronic inflammation,

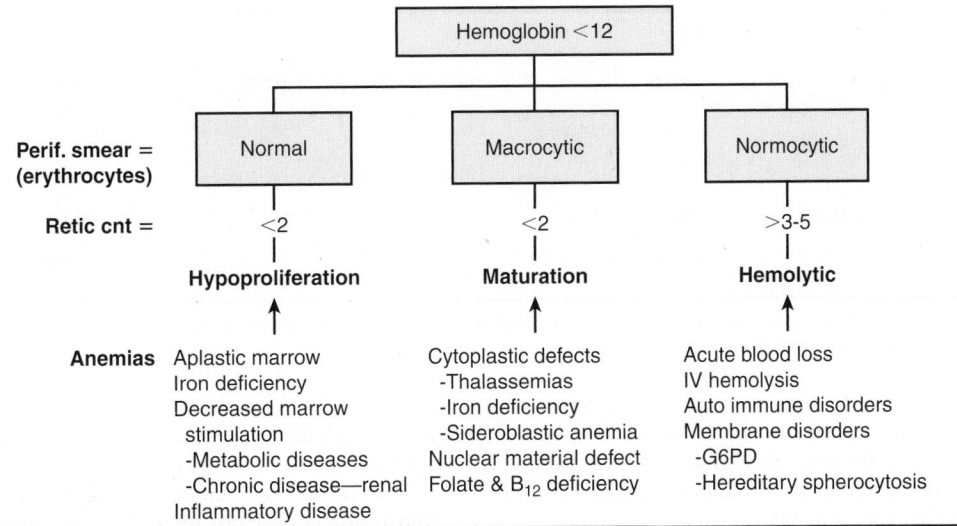

FIGURE 26-5 Classification of anemia by underlying erythrocyte disorder. (Adapted from Hillman RS, Ault KA, Rinder HM: *Hematology in clinical practice,* ed 4, New York, 2005, McGraw-Hill.)

BOX 26-1 Erythrocyte Morphology

Macrocytic Erythrocyte/Megalocyte (Abnormally Large Red Blood Cells)
- Pernicious anemia
- Lack of vitamin B_{12} and folic acid
- Megaloblastic anemia and liver disease

Schistocyte (Fragmented Cell, Helmet Cell)
- Microangiopathic hemolytic anemia
- Disseminated intravascular coagulation
- Thrombotic microangiopathies
- Thrombocytopenic purpura
- Glomerulonephritis
- Hemolytic-uremic syndrome
- Giant hemangioma

Anisocytosis (Unequally Sized RBC)
- Iron deficiency
- Sideroblastic anemia
- Vitamin A deficiency
- Kwashiorkor
- Hemoglobin H disease
- Barts hemoglobin
- Folate and vitamin B_{12} deficiency

Sideroblasts (Erythroid Precursor, Ringed RBC Body Has Iron Available but Cannot Incorporate It into Hemoglobin)
- Myelodysplastic syndrome
- Acute myelogenous leukemia
- Sideroblastic anemia

Membrane Abnormalities
- Acanthocytes or spur/spike cells
- Codocytes or target cells
- Echinocytes and burr cells
- Elliptocytes and ovalocytes
- Spherocytes

Target Cells (Abnormal Hypochromic RBCs That Have a Bull's-eye Appearance)
- Thalassemia
- Hemoglobin C
- Hemoglobin S (sickle cell anemia)
- Iron deficiency
- Postsplenectomy
- Liver disease (obstructive)

Elliptocyte-Ovalocyte
- Hereditary spherocytosis
- Thalassemia
- Iron deficiency
- Myelophthisic anemia
- Megaloblastic anemias
- Posttransfusion

Sickle Cells
- Sickle cell disease
- Hgb SC
- Hgb S thalassemia
- Parasites
- Malaria, babesiosis

Acanthocytes (Spur Cell)
- Postsplenectomy
- Cirrhosis
- Pyruvate kinase deficiency
- Uremia
- Infantile pyknocytosis

Dacryocytes—Teardrop
- Extramedullary hematopoiesis
- Myelophthisic anemia
- Severe hemolytic anemia
- Erythroleukemia

Data from Rodak BF, Fritsma GA, Doig K: *Hematology: clinical principles applications*, ed 3, St Louis, 2007, Saunders.

TABLE 26-8	Microcytic Anemias					
Diagnosis	**MCV**	**RBC Number**	**RDW**	**Ferritin**	**TIBC**
Iron deficiency anemia	Low or normal	Low	High (>14%)	Low	High
Thalassemia trait	Low	Normal to high	Normal (<14%)	Normal	Normal
Viral suppression or chronic depression	Normal or low	Low	Normal	High	Low
Lead poisoning	Low or normal	Low	Normal to high	Normal to high	Normal

MCV, Mean corpuscular volume; *RBC*, red blood cell; *RDW*, red (blood cell) distribution width; *TIBC*, total iron-binding capacity.
From Burg F, Ingelfinger J, Polin R, Gershon A, editors: *Current pediatric therapy*, ed 18, Philadelphia, 2006, Saunders.

plumbism, and iron deficiency result in decreased iron delivery to the marrow. In the thalassemias, globin chain synthesis is defective and, though rare in children, in sideroblastic anemias the heme synthesis malfunctions.

In addition to obtaining a CBC, key laboratory tests for the microcytic anemais include TIBC and Fe to differentiate IDA from the rest of the possible disorders. If the anemias of chronic illness and iron deficiency are ruled out, or if there is treatment failure, a hemoglobin electrophoresis with a quantitative Hgb A$_2$ and F can diagnosis hemoglobinopathy, such as thalassemia. Bone marrow aspiration with iron staining is used to diagnose sideroblastic anemia, but this disorder is rare in children. Table 26-8 compares the microcytic anemias laboratory findings.

IRON DEFICIENCY ANEMIA

Epidemiology

In children ages 1 through 3 years of age, IDA affects approximately 6% of Caucasians, 8% of African-Americans, and 17% of Mexican-Americans. Eleven percent of adolescent girls develop IDA primarily due to rapid growth, heavy menses, and nutritionally inadequate diets. Most infants between 9 and 24 months old, earlier in preemies, have IDA secondary to inadequate dietary iron intake (Brotanek et al, 2005). Approximately 30% of the global population suffers from iron deficiency (Ohls and Christensen, 2007). Because of iron supplementation, the incidence of IDA among children in the U.S. has been declining (Recht, 2009). Iron deficiency correlates with rapid increases in body size and blood volume during the first 2 years, along with diets low in iron, such as occurs with an overuse of goat's or cow's milk. The deficient iron intake is also associated with prolonged bottle-feeding. Brotanek and colleagues (2005) reported increasing incidence of IDA with increasing duration of bottle-feeding. IDA occurred in 3.8% of bottle-fed infants younger than 12 months, 11.5% of bottle-fed infants between 13 and 23 months, and 12.4% of bottle-fed infants between 24 and 48 months The higher incidence of IDA in Mexican-Americans is thought to be due to approximately one third (36.8%) of Mexican-American children still being bottle-fed at 24 to 48 months.

Celiac disease commonly contributes to the development of iron deficiency in affected persons by decreasing absorption of up to 46% of ingested iron. Small bowel resection is the only other condition that produces this degree of iron malabsorption. Disorders and treatments that decrease gastric acidity also impede iron absorption. Disorders causing insensitive blood loss (polyps, ulcers, hemorrhagic telangiectasia,

and diverticulitis) also deplete iron stores, as do parasitic infestations (Andrews et al, 2008).

The American Academy of Pediatrics (AAP) Committee on Nutrition recommends universal Hgb screening for anemia at 12 month of age (Baker, 2010). This screening should include an assessment of risk factors for iron deficiency and IDA. Risk factors include: (1) history of prematurity or low birthweight; (2) exposure to lead; (3) exclusive breastfeeding beyond 4 months without iron supplementation; (4) weaning to whole cow's milk without iron sources; (5) feeding problems; (6) special health care needs; (7) low socioeconomic status; and (8) Mexican-American descent. If children are at risk for IDA, a repeat Hgb/Hct should be performed as often as indicated. Screening Hgb can be performed on children younger than 1 year of age when risk factors warrant it. Menstruating females may also require screening for IDA due to the monthly blood loss, rapid growth, and potentially inadequate diet. When screening for IDA or any other routine health screening recommendation, remember that screening is not just a one-time test—the effectiveness of treatment must be determined through follow-up testing. Thus after the routine 12-month Hgb/Hct testing, risk assessment for anemia should be performed at all preventive pediatric health care visits with follow-up blood testing if positive (Levine, 2011).

Effects of Iron Deficiency

Many studies demonstrate that iron deficient states in the first few years of life are associated with subsequent cognitive deficits well into adulthood, though direct causality is difficult to prove. Further complicating the picture of causality is that lead poisoning is often a comorbid condition to IDA. The presence of low levels of iron facilitates intestinal absorption of lead. Lead poisoning and iron deficiency have significant effects on the developing brain. Due to these factors lead screening is an integral part of pediatric primary care. Early in the child's life there is critical and rapid brain development—the brain grows to 95% of its adult size by age 2 years. Nutritional deficits that result in IDA or plumbism can cause lasting damage, perhaps manifesting as diminished reading and math computational ability. A child at risk for lead exposure should typically have blood drawn to determine the level of lead at 9 to 12 months old and again at 24 months old. Local health departments determine the prevalence of lead poisoning in their area and issue guidelines related to blood lead screenings for targeted children in their catchment areas (AAP Committee on Practice and Ambulatory Medicine, 2000; Markowitz, 2007; Woolf et al, 2007). If the initial blood lead level is 20 mcg/dL or greater on a single visit or persistent levels of 15 mcg/dL occur over a 3-month period, environmental investigation and individual case management are necessary. Levels of 5 to 10 mcg/dL may also cause learning problems (Levine, 2011), but substantive data to confirm this supposition are pending.

Clinical Findings

History. Conduct a detailed history for hematologic disorders mentioned at the beginning of this chapter, but keep in mind that even children with moderate to severe anemia may be asymptomatic. Some key elements to remember are:
- Infants and toddlers may be irritable and restless but this only occurs with Hgb less than 8 g/dL and is often noticed in retrospect, after treatment. Pica may be present in unusual circumstances.
- Anorexia has been reported with Hgb levels less than 8 g/dL.
- Developmental delays (mental and motor areas) and behavioral disturbances that may be irreversible have been reported in infants and young children; adolescents may experience cognitive impairment (Recht, 2009).

Physical Examination. In mild to moderate iron deficiency, few symptoms are seen, but all systems must be methodically assessed. The child may appear normal, or pallor may be present. Rarely, in anemias that develop slowly, the physical examination may reveal tachycardia or systolic murmurs and signs of congestive heart failure. If symptoms of severe anemia exist, the examination should include stool guaiac testing.

Diagnostic Tests. The two most commonly used screening tests for IDA are Hgb and Hct, with Hgb being the more direct and sensitive marker of anemia compared with hematocrit measurements (Wu, 2006). IDA is frequently identified in routine screenings of Hgb level via capillary sampling. Excessive squeezing of the finger for capillary sample may produce inaccurate results (lower Hct), so proper technique is essential. Venous sampling is the most reliable indicator. IDA is likely if there is a low Hgb level for age (in the range of 8 to 11 g/dL), a history of low iron intake, and no concern about other possible causes for the anemia or the possibility of another hemoglobinopathy. Table 26-9 provides laboratory cut off values for anemia. If the age of the child and the dietary patterns are consistent with IDA, many clinicians begin a trial of iron supplementation without further diagnostic testing and then follow the child's Hgb and reticulocyte counts. The red blood cell distribution width is the earliest marker of iron deficiency. Serum ferritin is low with iron deficiency. Other tests that should be considered if a child is unresponsive to iron supplementation are serum iron, TIBC and transferrin saturation (Recht, 2009), and C-reactive protein (Baker et al, 2010).

Mild to moderate IDA is characterized by Hgb levels of 7 to 10 g/dL. Levels less than 4 g/dL necessitate consultation with a hematologist; and levels of 7 or less should be carefully evaluated as to whether the child needs referral to hematology. If treatment is effective, follow-up Hgb in 1 month should reveal a 1 g/dL improvement.

There is a high comorbidity between IDA and lead poisoning (Pb >10 mcg/dL) because lead molecules block iron from binding to protoporphyrin by inhibiting essential mitochondrial membrane function and interfering with enzymes. In low iron states the lack of iron results in an accumulation of erythrocyte protoporphyrin in blood.

TABLE 26-9 Age- and Gender-Specific Laboratory Cutoff Values for Anemia

Age (years)	Hemoglobin Concentration (g/dL)	Hematocrit (%)	MCV(fL)
1 to <2	<11	32.9	<77
2 to <5	<11.1	33	<79
5 to <8	<11.5	33.5	<80
8 to <12	<11.9	35.4	<80
12 to <15, male	<12.5	37.3	<85
15 to <18, male	<13.3	39.7	<85
12 to <15, female	<11.8	35.7	<85
15 to <18, female	<12	35.9	<85

MCV, Mean corpuscular volume.
From Burg F, Ingelfinger J, Polin R, Gershon A, editors: *Gellis and Kagan's current pediatric therapy,* ed 17, Philadelphia, 2002, Saunders.

The typical profile for IDA is:
- Microcytic, hypochromic RBCs on CBC
- Low or normal mean corpuscular volume (MCV); low RBC number
- High RDW (greater than 14%)
- Low ferritin
- High TIBC
- Mentzer Index greater than 14 (IDA more likely)

Differential Diagnosis

Iron deficiency should be differentiated from other microcytic, hypochromic anemias, such as lead poisoning, thalassemia minor, anemia of chronic disease, and hereditary sideroblastic anemia (see Fig. 26-4). In lead poisoning the FEP may be more than 200 mcg/dL, and basophilic stippling may be seen on the RBCs in the peripheral smear. Beta-thalassemia is indicated by elevations in Hgb A_2 on electrophoresis and Mentzer Index less than 13.

If there is no response to iron therapy, a more extensive workup should include a CBC with differential, platelet count, RBC indices, and reticulocyte count. A peripheral blood smear should also be examined to assess the number and morphology of RBCs, WBCs, and platelets. The differential diagnosis for anemia can then be determined on the basis of whether RBC production is adequate or inadequate, and whether the cells are microcytic, normocytic, or macrocytic (see Fig. 26-4). The reticulocyte production index (RPI) corrects the reticulocyte count for the degree of anemia present and indicates whether the bone marrow is responding appropriately to the anemia. The formula for calculating the RPI is:

$$RPI = \text{Reticulocyte count} \times \frac{\text{Hemoglobin}_{\text{(observed)}}}{\text{Hemoglobin}_{\text{(normal)}}} \times 0.5$$

An RPI greater than 3 indicates increased production of reticulocytes, which suggests either hemolysis or blood loss. An RPI less than 2 suggests decreased or ineffective production of reticulocytes in the marrow for the degree of anemia. Other causes of anemia, such as blood loss with occult rectal bleeding, should be considered in children with a low Hgb level on screening who eat a normal diet with adequate servings of iron-rich foods. Additional investigation is warranted in children less than 6 months or greater than 18 months or who demonstrate no response to treatment after 2 to 4 weeks. For those children with low Hgb/Hct who do not have a history suspicious for IDA, the investigation must expand to include less common sources for the anemia. Findings of severe anemia or atypical hematologic results require consultation and further investigation. Pairing the classification of the cells with the clinical findings, red cell indices, and additional diagnostic tests enables the provider to determine the appropriate treatment plan.

Management

Treatment for IDA consists of iron supplementation, typically as ferrous sulfate (4 to 6 mg/kg/day of elemental iron in three divided doses or 3 mg/kg/day in one or two divided doses for mild or moderate IDA) (McPherson and Tender, 2006). The child's Hgb/Hct and reticulocyte count should be reassessed in 4 weeks following initiation of treatment. If there is an adequate response to treatment with supplemental iron, a diagnosis of IDA is confirmed (Recht, 2009). Responses to treatment with iron supplementation are important diagnostically and therapeutically. Peripheral reticulocytosis may be seen after the first 4 days of treatment, and Hgb should return to a normal level within 4 to 6 weeks. If a therapeutic response is observed (Hgb increase of greater than 1 g/dL or greater than 3% increase in hematocrit), iron supplementation should continue for 2 to 3 months to replace depleted iron stores. Hematologic and iron status should be rechecked 6 months after iron supplements are stopped to determine resolution of the anemia and adequacy of iron stores (McPherson and Tender, 2006).

Iron Requirements. Full-term infants accumulate almost 80% of their iron stores during the last trimester of pregnancy. Maternal conditions can contribute to less iron being transferred to the fetus, such as anemia, maternal hypertension with intrauterine growth retardation, or even gestational diabetes. In the case of preterm births, the decreased amount of iron stores is depleted rapidly as the infants experience rapid postnatal growth. Preterm infants require an iron intake of at least 2 mg/kg/day through 12 months of age. If breastfed, the supplementation should begin by 1 month of age (Baker et al, 2010).

Breast milk provides an average iron content of 0.35 mg/L with the average volume consumed of 0.78 L/day (Institute of Medicine [IOM], 2003). An adequate intake of 0.27 mg/day was calculated and the IOM further determined that no correction of this recommended intake was needed during the first 6 months. However there is large variation in the iron content in human milk so the content of maternal milk may not always provide for the needs of the growing infant. Formula-fed infants receive sufficient iron intake of 12 mg/dL in standard infant formulas. Whole milk should be avoided until after 12 months of age.

The IOM calculated that the iron recommendations increase dramatically to 11 mg/day between 7 and 12 months based on cells sloughing and demands of increasing body mass. As the rate of growth decreases in toddlerhood, so does the nutritional requirements of iron, down to 7 mg/day between the ages of 1 and 3 years. Iron deficiency becomes more prevalent during this age as well, reaching 6.6% to 15.2% depending on ethnicity and socioeconomic status, although the occurrence of IDA is 0.9% to 4.4%. Despite these seemingly low levels of incidence, IDA accounts for more than 40% of the anemias of toddlerhood. Supplementation for this age group is through liquid supplement until 36 months of age. Chewable multivitamins can be used for children older than 3 years of age (Baker et al, 2010).

Complications

Adherence issues and alternative diagnoses should be explored if there is no response to iron supplementation. Dietary counseling is critical and families may need support with making necessary changes. Iron deficient states can exist in the absence of anemia as a precursor to IDA and require intervention. A more extensive determination of the child's iron status is obtained by measuring serum iron, iron-binding capacity, and the venous lead level. Stool guaiac should be checked for occult blood loss.

Children with extremely low Hgb, hypotension, or signs of congestive heart failure should be referred to a pediatric hematologist and may need hospitalization. Laboratory results that also indicate referral are neutropenia, thrombocytopenia, nucleated RBCs, or immature myeloid elements. When disorders of erythrocytes, platelets, and leukocytes are found, a bone marrow disorder is probable.

Education and Prevention

Parents or caretakers should be counseled to increase iron-rich food sources in their child's diet. Whole cow's milk should be avoided in infants younger than 12 months old due to the low iron content and possibility of insensible GI blood loss. After 12 months of age, cow's milk ingestion should be limited to 24 ounces per day. Goat's milk should not be the sole diet for the child due not only to lack of iron, but also its lack of folic acid. For full-term infants, dietary iron supplementation (as in iron-enriched infant cereal) should begin at 4 to 6 months of age. For preterm infants, supplementation with oral iron drops should begin as early as 2 months of age. Education for children taking iron supplements include advising parents to avoid giving the iron with meals or milk, that vitamin C juice enhances absorption, and that the child's stools will probably turn black. Foods containing soy can inhibit the absorption of iron. Any dental staining associated with taking iron can be cleaned. Parents should also be cautioned to keep the medication safely out of reach to prevent accidental ingestion.

THALASSEMIAS

The thalassemias are a group of hereditary, hypochromic anemias that are associated with the absence or decreased synthesis of the normal Hgb polypeptide chains—usually the α- and ß-globin chains—and a relative excess of the other chains. The protein abnormality results in hemoglobinopathies whose names are based on the altered globulin chain (Cunningham, 2010; DeBaun and Vichinsky, 2007). The possibility of thalassemia increases if the onset of anemia and symptoms is prior to 3 to 6 months of age and there is a family history of anemia, miscarriage, jaundice, gallstones, anemia, or splenomegaly.

Categorizing the thalassemias is less straightforward than with many anemias because although the heterozygous disease is hypochromic and microcytic, the homozygous diseases are also hemolytic. There is anemia and increased erythropoiesis. The erythropoiesis results in bone marrow expansion but the pathogenesis of this is not fully understood. Focal osteomalacia and delayed bone maturation are at least partially explained by suboptimal blood transfusions and iron overload (Mahachoklertwattana et al, 2003). The effect on long-bone architecture makes the child more susceptible to fractures. Furthermore, the marrow expansion results in frontal bossing and hyperplasia of the maxillary bones leading to typical facies.

Alpha-Thalassemias

The alpha-thalassemias are composed of several variant hemoglobins that are responsible for the various presentations as discussed earlier. Current nomenclature often refers to the subtypes by including indication of the number of gene deletions of α-globin, with severity of symptoms increasing with more deletions. Three gene deletions result in severe, even fatal manifestation of disease. Two gene deletions present with hypochromia; the absence of gene deletions causes mild anemia and often erythrocytosis. A single globin gene deletion is clinically insignificant (Segel, 2007).

There are two manifestations of the disease expression of alpha-thalassemia. The homozygous Hgb type, Barts hemoglobin with four γ-chains, results in *hydrops fetalis* and is incompatible with life because of severe anemia. However, homozygous Hgb H disease is a microcytic, hypochromic anemia that most often manifests as a hemolytic anemia, hepatosplenomegaly, and mild jaundice, and sometimes includes thalassemia-like bone changes. During times of physiologic stress the child may require RBC transfusion.

There are two different carrier states of alpha-thalassemia. In alpha-thalassemia trait the child exhibits microcytosis and hypochromia, but has normal percentages of Hgb A_2 and Hgb F. The other trait state is referred to as a *silent carrier* state, but can have either a silent hematologic phenotype or present with microcytic hypochromia and some erythropoiesis.

Management. Hgb H disease exacerbations may necessitate occasional transfusion during hemolytic or aplastic crises. No treatment is indicated for the carrier trait expressions of disease.

Beta-Thalassemia Minor/Minima

Description. Beta-thalassemia minor and minima disease, also known as trait, is associated with a mild, hypochromic, microcytic anemia in which Hgb levels are 2 to 3 g/dL below normal, and the MCV averages 65 fL. These children need to be monitored for iron accumulation but are otherwise asymptomatic (Segel, 2007). The disease may be confused with iron deficiency or lead poisoning and can be differentiated by measuring serum iron or lead levels, transferrin saturation, or serum ferritin levels (see Table 26-6). It is particularly important to correctly diagnose this condition in order to avoid unnecessary administration of iron supplements that could result in iron overload. The primary diagnostic feature is increased Hgb A_2 (greater than 3.5%) on electrophoresis.

Clinical Findings. Clinically most individuals with thalassemia trait are asymptomatic, although mild pallor and splenomegaly may be found. An Hgb of 9.5 to 11 g/dL and an MCV of less than 80 fL/cell is commonly seen in prepubertal children. The MCV/RBC count per milliliter is less than 13 (the Mentzer Index). In contrast, the Mentzer Index of iron deficiency is usually greater than 13; however, some sources use 13.5 as the indicator for IDA (Segel et al, 2002a; Ziteli and Davis, 2007). The degree of anemia may be exacerbated in concurrent illness or pregnancy.

Management. No specific treatment is known for beta-thalassemia minor. Primary emphasis should be on education of all family members and genetic testing, and counseling should be offered.

Beta-Thalassemia, Intermedia

This variant of thalassemia is the result of various mutations that cause a disorder with a clinical severity that spans from the mild symptoms of the beta-thalassemia trait to the severe manifestations of beta-thalassemia major. Classification is typically based on the severity of the symptoms and the types of treatments necessary rather than by the specific genotype. Diagnosis and management are clinically based with a goal toward maintaining a satisfactory Hgb of at least 6 to 7 g/dL without the regular need for RBC transfusions.

Beta-Thalassemia Major

Description. Homozygous forms are thalassemia intermedia and thalassemia major. Homozygous beta-thalassemia major (or Cooley anemia) is associated with severe anemia resulting from decreased or absent production of Hgb A and hemolysis caused by the precipitation of excess α-chains in the RBCs.

Clinical Findings. Affected infants usually become symptomatic in the first year of life and have pallor, failure to thrive, hepatosplenomegaly, and a severe anemia with an average Hgb of 6 g/dL and low MCV (60 to 70 fL). RBC morphology reveals significant microcytosis, poikilocytosis, hypochromia, target cells, and nucleated RBCs. Hgb A_2 and Hgb F levels are elevated.

Management. Proper management of the child requires collaboration with a pediatric hematologist. Red blood cell transfusions are usually necessary every 2 to 4 weeks to maintain a hemoglobin level between 9 and 10 g/dL as the goal. To help with future crossmatching, the provider should obtain a complete typing of the patient's erythrocyte profile before the first transfusion. This helps decrease difficulties with subsequent transfusions. Splenectomy may be indicated as well. Stem cell transplantation is effective for the small percentage of young children with a human leukocyte antigen (HLA) match and no organ dysfunction. Allogeneic hematopoietic transplantation has been documented to produce approximately an 85% to 87% long-term survival rate in children (Gaziev et al, 2008). Gene therapy is being investigated and holds promise for those with this major disorder.

Iron chelation is necessary to treat the hyperferric state produced by repeated transfusions and prevent complications primarily of the heart, liver, and endocrine system (Takeshita, 2010). Chronic iron chelation therapy is necessary in order to remove the excess iron that results from the frequent transfusions. Deferoxamine is administered parenterally usually via a pump overnight. It is time consuming and is associated with abdominal pain. Deferasirox is an oral agent, taken once daily, at a dose of 20 mg/kg/day; it stabilizes the ferritin levels, thus achieving a negative iron balance. Iron excretion through chelation is further aided by the ingestion of vitamin C. The iron is excreted through the kidneys, so hydration and monitoring of renal status is vital.

Complications. If the condition is left untreated, bone marrow expansion causes the characteristic facies with frontal bossing and maxillary overgrowth. Other complications of disease and treatment include osteopenia, thrombolytic symptoms, cardiopulmonary problems, asplenia secondary to splenectomy, cholelithiasis, and extramedullary hematopoiesis.

The medications used to chelate the iron have additional side effects. Deferasirox, the daily oral agent, commonly produces headache, nausea, vomiting, joint pain and fatigue. It has a black box warning of GI hemorrhage, as well as kidney and liver failure.

Deferoxamine has risks associated with intravenous medication administration (infection), and vision and hearing loss. Additionally there are the inherent risks and complications of transfusion including transfusion reaction, fever and, though rare, hepatitis, or human immunodeficiency virus (HIV) infection.

The disease, its complications, and treatments are painful for the child and monopolize a large portion of the children's and families' lives. Families need not only professional support and education, but also interaction with other families affected by this disorder, such as through the Thalassemia Support Foundation or Cooley's Anemia Foundation.

MACROCYTIC ANEMIA

MEGALOBLASTIC ANEMIAS

Description
Megaloblastic anemias are characterized by oval macrocytes and hypersegmented PMNs in the peripheral blood and megaloblasts in the bone marrow.

Epidemiology
Relatively rare megaloblastic anemias are due primarily to a lack of folic acid, vitamin B_{12}, or both. These two substances function as coenzymes in nuclear protein synthesis. Megaloblastic anemias may develop if the diet lacks these two substances or if the gastric intrinsic factor necessary for the absorption of vitamin B_{12} is absent. Peak incidence is between 4 and 7 months of age.

Clinical Findings
History. Suspicion of megaloblastic anemia should be high if there is any history of young infants who are being fed a diet of powdered cow's milk products or goat's milk. These are deficient in folic acid and vitamin B_{12}. Of equal concern are older children who have strict vegetarian diets and any child with signs of severe nutritional deficiencies, absorption

problems, or who have tapeworm infestations. Children with folic acid deficiency tend to have irritability, inadequate weight gain, and chronic diarrhea.

Physical Examination. Physical findings relate to the severity of the anemia but commonly include:
- Weakness, pallor
- Beefy-red, smooth, sore tongue

Diagnostic Tests. The following results may be seen:
- Elevated MCV (greater than 100 fL) and decreased reticulocyte count
- Blood smear showing nucleated RBCs and macroovalocytes with anisocytosis and poikilocytosis
- Normal white cell count and platelet count, but possibly decreased in more severe cases
- Large and hypersegmented neutrophils; possible large platelets
- In suspected folic acid deficiency—RBC folate level is decreased, iron and B_{12} levels tend to be normal or elevated.

Management
Management of folic acid deficiency and juvenile pernicious anemia (caused by a lack of vitamin B_{12}) is typically best done in consultation with a pediatric hematologist. Treatment is dietary supplementation and correction of the underlying disorder (e.g., infection) if possible.

In folic acid deficiency confirmed by measurement of the RBC folate level, folic acid may be administered in a dose of 0.5 to 1 mg/day and continued for 3 to 4 weeks until a hematologic response has occurred. This is followed by maintenance therapy with a multivitamin containing 0.2 mg of folate. Prolonged use of high-dose folic acid should be avoided (Glader, 2007; Ohls and Christensen, 2007). In vitamin B_{12} deficiency, a prompt hematologic response is usually seen after parenteral administration of vitamin B_{12}. If neurologic involvement is present, 1 mg of vitamin B_{12} should be given intramuscularly daily for at least 2 weeks. A maintenance dose of a 1 mg intramuscular injection of vitamin B_{12} is administered monthly throughout the patient's life (Glader, 2007; Ohls and Christensen, 2007).

NORMOCYTIC ANEMIAS

Anemias that have an RBC size within the normal value range are termed normocytic. Normocytic anemias tend to coincide with chronic illness, B_{12} deficiency, traumatic blood loss, or pregnancy. They are not common in children. Final determination of the etiology extends beyond blood cell indices and includes further chemistry laboratory tests, such a blood urea nitrogen (BUN), creatinine, serum glutamic-oxaloacetic transaminase (SGOT), alkaline phosphatase, bilirubin, erythrocyte sedimentation rate, urinalysis, and thyroid profile.

TRANSIENT ERYTHROBLASTOPENIA OF CHILDHOOD

Description
Idiopathic erythroblastopenia of childhood, or TEC, is a benign disorder of unknown cause that occurs in children during the first few years of life, usually after 1 year old. It is characterized by anemia, reticulocytopenia, and erythroid hypoplasia of the bone marrow.

Etiology

The cause of this transient suppression of erythropoiesis with resultant decreased red cell production is not clear, although it frequently follows a viral infection. Thus viral and immunologic mechanisms are suspected (Glader, 2007; Recht, 2009). TEC is associated with temporary failure of erythropoiesis caused by probable viral suppression or as a result of an IgG-mediated autoimmune response.

Clinical Findings

History. TEC occurs mainly in previously healthy children between 6 months and 3 years old. The child may have a history of a preceding infection.

Physical Examination. Patients have symptoms of anemia, typically a gradually increasing pallor. Parents may report noticing decreased energy levels or fatigue in their child. Pallor and fatigue develop over a course of days and are often associated with viral symptoms, such as fever, malaise, lethargy, abdominal pain, or upper respiratory symptoms. Jaundice may be noted, especially if the child has a preexisting hemoglobinopathy (Huang and Portwine, 2009).

Diagnostic Tests. The following are seen in TEC:
- Anemia (in which the Hgb content may be as low as 2.5 g/dL or only slightly decreased but is generally around 6 to 8 g/dL)
- Markedly low reticulocyte count
- WBC count usually normal
- Platelets normal or elevated
- High serum iron level reflecting decreased utilization
- Bone marrow aspiration results indicating erythroid hypoplasia

Differential Diagnosis

The syndrome can be differentiated from congenital hypoplastic anemia (Diamond-Blackfan syndrome) by the normal size of the RBCs (MCV less than 80 fL). Approximately 25% of children with Diamond-Blackfan syndrome have dysmorphic features (e.g., short stature, congenital heart disease, and mental retardation), whereas children with TEC have a normal physical examination (Recht, 2009).

Management

TEC is self-limited, with recovery taking place 1 to 2 months after diagnosis. No specific treatment is indicated, although transfusions may be required for severe anemia. A referral to a hematologist may be needed.

HEMOLYTIC ANEMIA

Hemolytic anemias are caused by premature destruction of RBCs and increase marrow production of reticulocytes. They can be classified as either hereditary or acquired and should be suspected in cases of an elevated reticulocyte count in the absence of bleeding or heparin therapy. In particular, the hereditary and congenital anemias manifest in infancy and early childhood. They may be due to a variety of hemoglobinopathies or to defects in the red cell membrane. Determining the etiology of hemolysis necessitates careful history taking, including family medical history, child's medical history, diet, medication intake, and environmental exposures. Confirmation of the diagnosis comes from Hgb electrophoresis, Heinz body stain, and osmotic fragility test.

SICKLE CELL ANEMIA AND TRAIT

Etiology

Sickle cell disease describes a group of complex, chronic disorders that are characterized by hemolysis, unpredictable acute complications that may become life threatening, and the possible development of chronic organ damage. Children who have homozygous inheritance have SCA or disease (Hgb SS). Their bodies do not form the normal Hgb A molecule, but rather synthesize hemoglobin S (Hgb S), which carries the amino acid valine instead of glutamic acid. Because of this change, Hgb S tends to polymerize or come out of solution at low PaO_2, low pH, low temperature, and low osmolality. This process collapses the RBC giving it a "sickled" shape and produces a chronic hemolytic anemia. The new shape is rigid and clogs small blood vessels producing ischemia, pain, and other vaso-occlusive problems.

Epidemiology

Sickle cell disease has an autosomal recessive inheritance pattern. It is found most often in people of African descent, but is also detected among ethnic groups from the Mediterranean, the Caribbean, Central and South America, and India. Due to migration it now occurs worldwide. In the U.S., sickle cell disease occurs in about 1:400 African-American infants and 1:36,000 Hispanics (DeBaun and Vichinsky 2007). Sickle trait occurs in 8% of African-Americans. This incidence exceeds that of most other serious genetic disorders in children, including cystic fibrosis and hemophilia; only alpha-thalassemia is more common (Modell and Darlison, 2008). Routine neonatal screening identifies most infants with sickle cell disease born in the U.S. because it is mandated in all states and the District of Columbia. It is still important to do a careful family medical history because many adults do not realize they are carriers.

Clinical Findings

Children with sickle cell trait who are heterozygous (Hgb A + Hgb S) for the gene essentially have a benign clinical course. Their RBCs contain only 30% to 40% Hgb S, and sickling does not occur under most conditions. It is only in rare instances of hypoxia, such as in shock, while flying in unpressurized aircraft, or traveling to high elevations, that signs of vaso-occlusion can occur. However, the presence of sickle cell trait has been implicated as a causative factor in the sudden deaths of young military recruits, college football players, and some teens. Extreme exercise, typically to exhaustion, dehydration, and relative hypoxia (altitude) are major confounding factors (Mitchell, 2007).

The symptoms of sickle cell disease are multisystem, necessitating vigilant care to minimize occurrence of crises and complications. Common symptoms include:
- Fatigue and anemia
- Pain crises
- Dactylitis (swelling and inflammation of the hands and/or feet) and arthritis
- Bacterial infections
- Lung and heart injury

- Leg ulcers
- Priapism
- Splenic sequestration (sudden pooling of blood in the spleen) and liver congestion
- Aseptic necrosis and bone infarcts (death of portions of bone)
- Eye damage
- Abdominal pain

Physical Examination. Symptoms typically begin to emerge in the second 6 months of life as the amount of Hgb S increases and Hgb F declines. Subsequently, painful, vaso-occlusive crises occur. Due to the multisystem nature of complications these children need prompt, detailed evaluation and intervention. After 5 years old, splenomegaly usually disappears because of autoinfarction of the organ. Rates of height and weight gain usually slow after 7 years old, and puberty may be delayed 3 to 4 years.

Diagnostic Tests. The following laboratory results are seen in sickle cell disease (Panepinto and Scott, 2011; Segel et al, 2002b).

- Hematocrit of 20% to 29%
- Hgb 6 to 10 g/dL (severe)
- Reticulocyte count elevated: 5% to 15%
- Normal to increased WBC and platelet count
- MCV greater than 80 fL; mean corpuscular hemoglobin concentration (MCHC) greater than 37 mg/dL
- Hgb electrophoresis (after infancy), isoelectric focusing or high performance of liquid chromatography showing a predominance of Hgb S and no Hgb A.
- Morphology: Irreversibly sickled cells or chronic elliptocytes, Howell-Jolly bodies, nucleated RBCs

Hgb electrophoresis results in a newborn with sickle cell trait will be Hgb FAS, and Hgb FS for a child with either SCA or sickle beta-zero thalassemia (SBO). Normal results of Hgb electrophoresis are Hgb FA.

Differential Diagnosis

Chronic hemolytic anemia should be included in the differential diagnosis. Other syndromes characterized by hemolytic anemia and vaso-occlusion are Hgb SC disease and a combination of Hgb S with alpha- or beta-thalassemia. These diseases may be differentiated through electrophoresis and family testing if necessary. Prenatal genetic testing is available in instances of high suspicion; otherwise mandated newborn screening will render the diagnosis in most cases before symptoms present.

Management

Management of the child with SCA is complicated and should be done in consultation with a pediatric hematologist. Individuals with sickle cell disease still need regular primary care services and coordination of consultative services and information. Growth is closely monitored, immunizations need to be done on time, parents require support, and communication with specialty services should be coordinated, such as an annual ophthalmologic examination by a retinal specialist. Care is comprehensive, spanning normal well-child issues through acute crises and hospitalization. Some of the key aspects of care for the child with SCA are as follows:

- Hydration, illness prevention, and pain management are fundamental aspects of disease management. Nonsteroidal antiinflammatory drugs (NSAIDs) or acetaminophen may be adequate for mild to moderate pain, but narcotics should be used when these are not adequate for management (as with anyone taking narcotics, abuse and addiction issues must be considered).
- CBC and reticulocyte count are monitored every few months.
- All the usual immunizations of childhood are to be administered on time including 13-valent pneumococcal conjugate and 23-valent pneumococcal polysaccharide vaccines. Meningococcal vaccine is administered for children older than 2 years (Orkin et al, 2008); however, under special circumstances MPSV4 may be given to children as young as 3 months. An annual flu vaccination is essential.
- Invasive bacterial infection is the leading cause of death in young children with SCA. Penicillin V prophylaxis (125 mg orally, twice daily) is initiated by 2 months old. At 3 years old, increase the dose to 250 mg orally twice a day, and continue at least until the fifth birthday (AAP, 2002; DeBaun and Vichinsky, 2007; Orkin et al, 2008; Taketomo et al, 2011).
- Folic acid supplementation at 1 mg/day is typically given to adults to prevent folate deficiency due to hemolysis. It is not standard therapy for children unless a folic acid deficiency is suspected (Ashok and Bertolone, 2010).
- Aggressive treatment of infections and maintenance of hydration and body temperature are used to prevent hypoxia and acidosis; volume replacement may be necessary to prevent circulatory collapse.
- Treatment of coexisting medical problems associated with lower O_2 saturations, such as asthma and obstructive sleep apnea.
- In children with severe SCA, hydroxyurea is used to reduce the number of painful crises and incidences of acute chest syndrome (a leading cause of death in adolescents with SCA). It is a preventive medication and not effective during the acute crisis. Hydroxyurea use is associated with a lower need of blood transfusions and fewer hospital visits. There is some early evidence suggesting it helps improve growth and preserves organ function. Despite these benefits, side effects do occur including increased risk for serious infection. As always, the practitioner must carefully weigh all risks and benefits before integrating this medication into the treatment plan.
- Annual stroke prevention screening of major intracranial vessels with transcranial Doppler ultrasound evaluation is planned for 2- to 16-year-old children. A reading of greater than 200 cm/sec time-averaged mean maximal velocity indicates high risk for stroke (Orkin et al, 2008; Panepinto and Scott, 2011).

Children with sickle cell disease are usually co-managed by specialists in hematology and their primary care provider. Emergency admission or referral is necessary in the presence of the following:

- Fever (to rule out sepsis) greater than 101° F (38.3° C)
- Pneumonia, chest pain, or other pulmonary symptoms (acute chest syndrome)
- Sequestration crisis (splenomegaly with decreased Hgb or Hct)
- Aplastic crisis (decreased Hct and reticulocyte count)
- Severe painful crisis
- Unusual headache, visual disturbances

- Priapism
- Consultation is also necessary for the chronic sequelae of persistent bone pain or leg ulcers, pregnancy, and contraception. Stem cell transplantation may be a consideration in children with significant disease and is curative in some persons. Gene therapy is under investigation and may be available in the future. New medications are under investigation as well.

Complications

Because of functional asplenia, the greatest concern is febrile illness indicating infection and possible sepsis. In view of the serious threat of pneumococcal sepsis in children younger than 5 years old, all complaints of fever, poor feeding, lethargy, and irritability should be clinically evaluated. The consequences of hemolysis may include chronic anemia, jaundice, cholelithiasis, and delayed growth and sexual maturation. Vaso-occlusion and tissue ischemia may result in acute and chronic injury to virtually every organ system, with stroke being a major concern.

Patient and Family Education

The parents of children with sickle cell anemia need a great deal of support in raising a child with a genetically transmitted chronic disease. Clear patterns of communication should be established between the family and the provider using a partnership model. Initial education includes the genetics and pathophysiology of the disease and the importance of regular health maintenance visits. Discussion should emphasize the need for early evaluation and treatment of febrile illness, acute splenic sequestration, aplastic crisis, and acute chest syndrome. Parents can be taught to palpate their child's spleen. Any downward displacement or enlargement of the spleen below the left costal margin can be marked off and serially measured at specified periods of time (Pitts and Record, 2010). As the child grows the family should be educated about other potential clinical complications, such as stroke, enuresis, priapism, cholelithiasis, delayed puberty, retinopathy, avascular necrosis of the hip and shoulder, and leg ulcers.

Preventive Care

Preventive measures include the following:
- Timely administration of routine immunizations, including pneumococcal and meningococcal vaccines, and yearly influenza vaccine
- Prophylactic antibiotics
- Genetic counseling for those with sickle cell trait
- Support groups
- Educating adolescents with the trait about their status and the risk of disease transmission
- Hematopoietic stem cell transplant (the only intervention that can cure sickle cell disease with strict inclusion criteria identified for transplant eligibility)
- Gene therapy (under investigation)

HEREDITARY SPHEROCYTOSIS

Description

HS is a hemolytic anemia characterized by a deficiency or abnormality of the RBC membrane protein spectrin, which reduces the RBC surface area. The RBC membranes assume a more spherical shape. Hence RBCs are more likely to be sequestered and prematurely destroyed in the spleen (Recht, 2009). HS causes mild chronic hemolysis to severe transfusion-dependent anemia (Berkow and Schwartz, 2006).

Incidence

HS occurs in 1 in 5000 persons of preponderantly northern European ancestry.

Clinical Findings

Physical Examination. Jaundice usually appears in the newborn period, and it may be difficult to differentiate HS from hyperbilirubinemia caused by ABO incompatibility. After 2 years of age splenomegaly is usually present. Chronic fatigue, malaise, and abdominal pain may also be noted.

Diagnostic Tests. Laboratory findings in HS include the following:
- Chronic anemia (Hgb is 6 to 10 g/dL)
- Reticulocyte count ranges from 5% to 20%.
- On peripheral smear, a small proportion of the RBCs is spherocytic and smaller than normal and lacks the central pallor of the usual biconcave disk-shaped cell.
- Osmotic fragility of the cells is increased, as is the rate of autohemolysis of incubated blood.

Management

The treatment of choice for children with severe HS requiring multiple transfusions is splenectomy, which usually produces a clinical cure. It should be deferred until 5 or 6 years of age because of the increased risk of encapsulated bacterial infection before that age. Risks associated with splenectomy are postsplenectomy sepsis, penicillin-resistant pneumococci infection, pulmonary hypertension, and ischemic heart disease and stroke seen in HS patients (Berkow and Schwartz, 2006; Recht, 2009). Pneumococcal and meningococcal vaccines should be given before splenectomy.

After splenectomy, prophylactic penicillin therapy (less than 5 years old: 125 mg orally twice a day; greater than 5 years old: 250 mg orally twice a day) through adulthood is recommended. Because of increased hemolysis, children with HS and active hemolysis should receive 1 mg of folic acid daily until splenectomy. Splenectomy is an effective strategy to eliminate most of the hemolysis associated with HS (Segel, 2007).

Complications

Aplastic crises (often indicated by fever, fatigue, abdominal pain, and jaundice) associated with parvovirus and other viral infections are the most serious complications during childhood. Febrile illnesses should be vigorously treated. A child who is post splenectomy and has a temperature greater than 101.5° F (greater than 38.5° C) without an obvious source of infection should be hospitalized and treated with intravenous antibiotics until blood cultures prove to be negative (Panepinto and Scott, 2011). Gallstone formation can occur as a result of chronic hemolysis, and ultrasounds should be performed every 5 years and before splenectomy (Berkow and Schwartz, 2006).

GLUCOSE-6-PHOSPHATE DEHYDROGENASE DEFICIENCY

Description

A drug-induced hemolytic anemia can be caused by genetic deficiency of the G6PD enzyme in the RBC. Symptoms are generally associated with infections or exposure to oxidant metabolites of certain drugs that cause precipitation of Hgb, injury to the red cells, and rapid hemolysis.

Epidemiology

The G6PD gene is found on the X chromosome. G6PD deficiency is transmitted as an X-linked recessive trait. In the U.S., about 10% of African-American males and 1% to 2% of African-American females are affected. It may also occur in a more severe form in Greeks, Italians, Arabs, Southeast Asians, and Chinese.

Clinical Findings

History. Patients generally have a history of recent infection (particularly hepatitis) or oxidant drug ingestion—specifically, aspirin-containing antipyretics, sulfonamides, antimalarials, antihelmintics, naphthaquinolones, and fava beans. The degree of hemolysis is dependent on the amount of the drug ingested and the extent of enzyme deficiency.

Physical Examination. The patient may have pallor and jaundice if there is chronic hemolysis, or have jaundice, pallor, lethargy, irritability, headache, and red or dark clear urine after drug ingestion.

Diagnostic Tests. Several dye reduction tests provide the diagnosis. Screening tests available to measure a deficiency of G6PD should be used in high-risk groups. Only a few states include G6PD in their routine newborn screening panel. These tests measure G6PD enzyme activity in the RBC. After a hemolytic crisis, however, screening may produce a false-negative result because the younger blood cells that remain after hemolysis may show normal enzymatic activity. This is thought to be associated with higher G6PD activity taking place in reticulocytes. The enzyme assay should be obtained 2 to 3 months after an episode (Recht, 2009; Segel et al, 2002b).

Management

No specific treatment is available. Red cell transfusion and supportive therapy may be indicated in cases of severe anemia. Keeping the child well hydrated and monitoring for renal failure are important during hemolytic crisis.

Patient and Family Education

Patients should avoid the offending drugs—the most common being aspirin, sulfonamide antibiotics, and antimalarials—and foods.

Platelets and Coagulation Disorders

Platelet disorders should be ruled out in children before undergoing extensive surgery, and in children with petechiae, frequent nosebleeds, mucous membrane bleeding, or excessive bleeding from minor trauma. Evaluation of these complaints includes a family history of bleeding or platelet disorders and a history of drug or toxin exposure. Initial laboratory studies should include a CBC, platelet count, prothrombin time (PT), and activated partial thromboplastin time (aPTT). The diagnoses that may be differentiated with these tests are idiopathic thrombocytopenic purpura (ITP), hemophilia, von Willebrand disease, and leukemia. The coagulation cascade (see Fig. 26-3) provides a mechanism for understanding the interconnectedness of all the factors involved in coagulation.

DIAGNOSTIC TESTS

- Platelet count (normal range is 150,000 to 300,000/mm^3)
- Platelet function tests, such as platelet function analyzer (PFA).
- PT (normal range is 11.5 to 14 seconds).
- aPTT is the method used to determine partial thromboplastin time (PTT) and is commonly still referred to as the PTT (normal range is 25 to 40 seconds).
- Specific coagulation factor assays determine which clotting factors are absent.

The PT and aPTT measure all of the clotting factors except factor XIII. If the platelet count is normal, the aPTT or PT is prolonged, or both, a coagulation factor deficiency is possible. The typical laboratory findings of hemophilia are normal PT and PFA and an abnormal aPTT (Scott and Montgomery, 2007).

If the PT and aPTT are elevated in association with thrombocytopenia, the probable diagnosis is disseminated intravascular coagulopathy (DIC), which is a syndrome secondary to an underlying disorder, such as sepsis, malignancy, toxins, or liver failure. In DIC there is a systemic activation of the coagulation process. Extensive, ongoing activation of coagulation results in the depletion of platelets and coagulation factors, which then leads to bleeding and thrombosis (Briones and Abshire, 2006).

IMMUNE OR IDIOPATHIC THROMBOCYTOPENIC PURPURA

Description

Immune or idiopathic thrombocytopenic purpura (ITP) is the most common of the thrombocytopenic purpuras in childhood and is believed to be an autoimmune response in which circulating platelets are destroyed. It usually occurs after viral illnesses (Panepinto and Scott, 2011; Recht, 2009). In many cases the cause is autoimmune.

Epidemiology

Most cases occur between 2 and 4 years of age, and the incidence is increased in fair-skinned children. Approximately 80% of cases resolve within 6 months, even without treatment. If ITP lasts longer than 6 months, it is termed chronic ITP (Recht, 2009). Secondary causes include leukemia, medications (e.g., quinine, heparin), lupus erythematosus, cirrhosis, HIV, hepatitis C, congenital causes, and von Willebrand factor deficiency. These causes must be excluded.

Clinical Findings

ITP is essentially a clinical diagnosis and not established by a single diagnostic test though most symptoms do not develop until the platelet count is less than 20,000/mm^3. It is characterized by the following:

- Acute onset of petechiae, purpura, and bleeding in an otherwise healthy child; the bruising or bleeding may be most prominent over the legs.
- A viral illness 1 to 4 weeks before onset in 70% of cases.
- Hemorrhage of the mucous membranes, particularly the gums and lips.
- Nosebleeds that can be severe and difficult to control.
- Menorrhagia in an adolescent female.
- Liver, spleen, and lymph nodes are not generally enlarged.

Diagnostic Tests. Laboratory findings in ITP include:
- Low platelet count (less than 150,000/mm^3) with an otherwise normal CBC
- Normal PT and aPTT
- Megathrombocytes on the peripheral smear
- Normal WBC and RBC counts

Differential Diagnosis

If the smear shows fragmented RBCs, BUN and creatinine levels should be measured to rule out hemolytic-uremic syndrome. If the PT and aPTT are elevated with thrombocytopenia, DIC is a possibility, and cultures should be taken to identify sources of infection. A prolonged PT and aPTT with a normal platelet count suggest a coagulation factor deficiency. If the syndrome is complicated by prolonged thrombocytopenia, neutropenia, anemia, bone pain, or congenital anomalies, the child should be referred to a hematologist for possible bone marrow aspiration to rule out acute lymphocytic leukemia (ALL) and other disorders. In a sick, febrile child with isolated thrombocytopenia, petechiae, or purpura, the major diagnosis to consider first is meningococcemia. These children should also be referred, hospitalized, and treated for presumed sepsis.

Management

The prognosis with ITP is excellent, with spontaneous recovery in 75% of pediatric cases in the first 3 months (Scott, 2007). Most cases can be managed on an outpatient basis without any specific therapy. If the platelet count is greater than 50,000/mm^3 and no bleeding is observed, children and parents should be advised to avoid contact sports, aspirin ingestion, and any other herbal or pharmacologic agents that interfere with platelet function and to notify the practitioner of any excessive bleeding. Epistaxis can be treated with local measures. In severe cases (platelets less than 50,000/mm^3) after diagnosis of leukemia is ruled out, a short course of corticosteroid therapy may reduce severity in the initial phases. Intravenous immunoglobulin (IVIG) is also given to children with active severe bleeding and who have contraindications for steroid use; WinRho (Anti-D) is given intravenously with the dose depending on Hgb level; Rh(D) immune globulin is useful only in Rh-positive individuals. Splenectomy, immunosuppressives, and anti-CD20 antibody are options for those children with refractory or chronic ITP (Briones and Abshire, 2006; Recht, 2009).

Complications

The most serious complication is intracranial hemorrhage, which occurs in less than 0.5% of cases. Complaints of significant headache necessitate a careful neurologic evaluation (Recht 2009).

HEMOPHILIA A AND B AND VON WILLEBRAND DISEASE

Description

Inherited coagulation deficiencies are described according to the absent coagulation factor. Most result in abnormal bleeding. Hemophilia results from a deficiency of factor VIII (hemophilia A) or factor IX (hemophilia B). In hemophilia A and B, absence or deficiency of the coagulation factor results in prolonged bleeding either spontaneously from small vessels or as a result of trauma.

A rough guide to gauge the severity of hemophilia is the percentage of function of the factor levels with 100% (100 units/dL) equal to the function of factor found in 1 mL of normal plasma. The clotting factor levels associated with severity of bleeding are as follows: less than 1 unit/dL (<1%), severe; between 1 and 5 units/dL, moderate; and more than 5 units/dL, mild (Orkin et al, 2008).

In plasma, factor VIII binds with von Willebrand factor (vWF), which is a specific circulatory protein and acts as a carrier protein. von Willebrand disease (also known as vascular hemophilia) is a heterogeneous group of hereditary bleeding disorders caused by a quantitative or qualitative abnormality of vWF protein (Table 26-10). In type I the protein is quantitatively reduced; in type II it is qualitatively abnormal; and it is absent in type III.

Epidemiology

Because the genes for the coagulation factors are sex linked (carried on the X chromosome) and recessive, the disease affects primarily males. Females are generally only carriers of the disorder. About 1 in 5000 males is affected with hemophilia; and approximately 80% to 85% have hemophilia A and 10% to 15% have hemophilia B (Orkin et al, 2008). von Willebrand disease occurs in both sexes with an incidence of 1 in 100 individuals. It is the most common inherited bleeding disorder and is associated with either a qualitative or quantitative defect in vWF (Briones and Abshire, 2006; Orkin et al, 2008). The primary sites of bleeding differ depending on whether the problem is hemophilia A or B or von Willebrand disease. The fibrin/clotting cascade is available in Figure 26-3 for review.

Clinical Findings

The following are seen in hemophilia:
- A positive family history in the vast majority of cases
- Excessive bruising
- Prolonged bleeding from mucous membranes after minor lacerations, immunizations, circumcision, or during menstruation (menorrhagia)
- Hemarthrosis characterized by pain and swelling in the elbows, knees, and ankles
- A greatly prolonged aPTT
- A specific assay for factor VIII or IX activity confirms the diagnosis.

Clinical findings associated with von Willebrand disease include the following:
- Mucous membrane bleeding (epistaxis, menorrhagia), easy bruising, and excessive posttraumatic or postsurgical bleeding

TABLE 26-10	Comparisons of Hemophilia A, Hemophilia B, and von Willebrand Disease		
	Hemophilia A	**Hemophilia B**	**von Willebrand Disease**
Inheritance factor deficiency	X-linked factor VIII	X-linked factor IX	Autosomal dominant vWF and VIIIC
Bleeding site(s)	Muscle, joint, surgical	Muscle, joint, surgical	Mucous membranes, skin, surgical, menstrual
PT	Normal	Normal	Normal
aPTT	Prolonged	Prolonged	Prolonged or normal
Bleeding time	Normal	Normal	Prolonged or normal
Factor VIII coagulant activity (VIIIC)	Low	Normal	Low or normal
von Willebrand factor antigen (vWF: Ag)	Normal	Normal	Low
von Willebrand factor activity (vWF: Act)	Normal	Normal	Low
Factor IX	Normal	Low	Normal
Ristocetin-induced	Normal	Normal	Normal, low, or increased at low-dose ristocetin
Platelet aggregation	Normal	Normal	Normal
Treatment	DDAVP* or recombinant VIII	Recombinant IX	DDAVP* or vWF concentrate

aPTT, Activated partial thromboplastin time; *PT,* prothrombin time; *vWF,* von Willebrand factor.
*Desmopressin (DDAVP) for mild to moderate hemophilia A or type I von Willebrand disease.
From Scott J: Hematology. In Kliegman R, Marcdante K, Jenson H, Behrman R, editors: *Nelson essentials of pediatrics,* ed 5, Philadelphia, 2006, Saunders, p 718.

- History of ecchymosis of trunk, upper arms, and thighs
- Factor VIII clotting activity usually decreased
- vWF antigen usually decreased
- Decreased vWF
- Normal platelet count but isolated decreased platelet count associated with type 2B (Briones and Abshire, 2006; Scott and Montgomery, 2007)
- Bleeding time and aPTT generally prolonged, but may be normal (Orkin et al, 2008)

Management

Treatment of hemophilia consists of prevention of trauma and replacement therapy to increase factor VIII or factor IX activity in plasma. Plasma-derived and recombinant factor concentrates are available for replacement with recombinant factor preferred.

Hemarthrosis is the leading type of significant local bleeding. Local measures include the application of cold and pressure to affected, painful joints. As with all bleeding disorders, aspirin and nonsteroidal antiinflammatory medications should be avoided. Anticipatory guidance should be directed at avoiding high-risk behaviors and contact sports and wearing a bike helmet. Physical therapy may be needed to assist with decreased mobility caused by hemarthrosis and joint scarring. Psychosocial intervention may be needed to help families avoid overprotectiveness or permissiveness (Scott and Montgomery, 2007).

Ideally most children with hemophilia should be enrolled in a local hemophilia treatment center to facilitate a collaborative, interdisciplinary approach to management. The primary provider should remain central to the care of the child. All immunizations should be given subcutaneously with a 26-gauge needle, followed by firm pressure at the site for several minutes. Iron replacement may also be necessary in children with severe bleeding disorders.

von Willebrand disease is treated depending on the type and severity of the bleeding. The treatment of von Willebrand disease is desmopressin (DDAVP) and factor VIII-vWF concentrates. Local measures to control bleeding may also be part of the treatment plan (Briones and Abshire, 2006; Scott and Montgomery, 2007). Adjunctive therapy (e.g., estrogen and/or aminocaproic acid) depends on the type of von Willebrand disease (type 1, 2A, 2B, 2M, 2N, or 3) which is determined by the level of qualitative or quantitative factor deficiency. The use of aminocaproic acid, an antifibrinolytic agent, is sometimes recommended for dental extraction and nosebleeds (Scott and Montgomery, 2007)

A written treatment plan tailoring replacement product dosage based on the location of the bleed should be in the chart and given to the parents to carry with them. The child should wear a Medic-Alert bracelet or necklace.

Complications

In patients with hemophilia A and B, bleeding occurs when coagulation factor levels decrease particularly in closed areas, such as the joints. Brain hemorrhage can be a serious consequence of head trauma. Continued hemorrhage results in anemia and eventually hypovolemic shock.

The use of therapeutic replacement materials derived from blood carries inherent risk, especially infections. Hepatitis infection was a problem in the past. Infection with HIV unfortunately was frequently seen in patients who were exposed to multiple donors before the revision of blood donor screening tests and the use of heat-treated concentrates.

White Blood Cell Disorders

White Blood Cell Count

The WBC count is used as an indicator of infection or illness; the percentages of the different types of cells also provide useful diagnostic information. The WBC count is automated and is a routine part of the CBC. The WBC differential is obtained on a smear of blood one cell layer thick, usually with a Wright stain procedure that contains both basic and acidic dyes. The absolute neutrophil count (ANC) is calculated from the results of the differential: if WBCs = 3600/mm^3, percentage of segmented neutrophils = 20, percentage of band neutrophils = 5, lymphocytes = 60, monocytes = 10, and eosinophils = 5, then

$$ANC = WBC \times (\% \text{ Seg} + \text{Band})$$
$$= 3600 / mm^3 \times 0.25 = 900 / mm^3$$

White Blood Cell Dysfunction

The WBC count and differential are useful diagnostic guides in the management of a variety of childhood illnesses. The normal range of granulocyte and lymphocyte counts varies throughout childhood. Leukocytosis is an increase in the number of circulating leukocytes, primarily with a neutrophilic response parcticularly to bacterial infections (Box 26-2). A relative increase in the number of circulating immature neutrophils ("left shift") is a defensive mechanism in response to an inflammatory process or acute bacterial infection. Multiple WBC indices abnormalities should raise suspicion of a malignant disorder.

Alterations of Granulocytes

Neutropenia (measured as the ANC) is defined as a decrease in the number of circulating neutrophils and bands (ANC) in the peripheral blood to fewer than 1500 cells/mm^3 for children older than 1 year and to fewer than 1000 cells/mm^3 in infants between 2 weeks and 1 year of age (Orkin et al, 2008). There are some racial differences in neutrophil counts with some African-American children having slightly lower counts than Caucasian children. Neutropenia is classified as mild (ANC of 1000 to 1500 cells/mm^3), moderate (ANC of 500 to 1000 cells/mm^3), or severe (ANC <500 cells/mm^3).

Neutropenia results from decreased cellular production (as in various hematologic diseases, infections, drug-induced states, and nutritional deficiencies), increased peripheral destruction (as in autoimmune disorders), or peripheral pooling (as in bacterial infections, hemodialysis, and cardiopulmonary bypass). Most cases of neutropenia are discovered during evaluation of the WBC count in a child with an acute febrile illness, and the most common infectious causes are hepatitis A and B, respiratory syncytial virus, influenza A and B, Epstein-Barr virus, and cytomegalovirus. General management of neutropenic patients includes careful identification and prompt treatment of any suspected or proven infections.

Neutropenia is frequently seen in preterm infants and those with intrauterine growth retardation. Because the neutrophil storage pool in newborn infants is only 20% to 30% of that of adults, it is easily depleted under stressful conditions, such as

BOX 26-2 Key Characteristics of Leukocytosis

- Definition: Elevated total WBCs due to an increase in one of five types of WBCs:
  ○ Neutrophilic leukocytosis
  ○ Lymphocytic leukocytosis
  ○ Eosinophilic leukocytosis
  ○ Monocytic leukocytosis
  ○ Basophilic leukocytosis
- Differential count
  ○ Percentages: always add up to 100%
  ○ Left-sided shift: granulocytes >75% of WBC
  ○ Right-sided shift: nongranulocytes >40% of WBC

WBC, White blood cell.

infection with resultant sepsis (Stoll, 2007). Isoimmune neonatal neutropenia is a transient process resulting from transplacental transfer of maternal antibodies to fetal neutrophil antigens. Antineutrophil antibodies can be detected in maternal and infant serum (Fuleihan, 2011; Orkin et al, 2008).

The largest group of neutropenic patients includes children who are receiving chemotherapy. They are at risk for developing severe life-threatening bacterial infections depending on the degree and duration of neutropenia. Despite improvements in supportive care and treatment with granulocyte colony–stimulating factor (G-CSF), bacterial and fungal infections remain a major cause for morbidity and mortality in these patients (Sulis et al, 2006).

Qualitative abnormalities of granulocytes are usually related to defects of phagocytosis. Although individually rare, these defects may be genetic or acquired. Malnutrition, sepsis, diabetes, and leukemia are acquired disorders related to defects in leukocyte function, particularly phagocytosis and microbicidal activity (Mitchel, 2007; Orkin et al, 2008). Granulomatous diseases are relatively rare disorders of granulocytes, particularly neutrophils, in which the enzymes necessary for bactericidal activity are lacking. Such diseases result in severe, recurrent infections of the skin, lymph nodes, lungs, liver, and bone.

Lymphocytic Disorders

Lymphocytosis is produced by viral illnesses, including mumps, measles, rubella, rubeola, varicella, mononucleosis, and hepatitis. Pertussis and chronic lymphocytic leukemia also elevate the lymphocyte count. An increase in the number of atypical lymphocytes is evident in infectious mononucleosis, cytomegalic inclusion disease, and toxoplasmosis.

Cancer

Leukemia refers to a group of malignant diseases with qualitative and quantitative changes in circulating leukocytes. It is characterized by diffuse, abnormal growth of leukocytic precursors in the bone marrow. This uncontrolled increase in immature WBCs suppresses normal hematopoietic stem cells and leads to anemia and thrombocytopenia. Life-threatening infections occur because of a decrease in the function of circulating WBCs. Leukemias are further classified according to the course of the illness and the types of cells and tissues involved.

Malignant lymphomas, as in Hodgkin disease, are solid neoplasms that are lymphocytic in origin. Lymphocytes are the only WBCs involved—the malignant process occurs during their maturation or storage in bone marrow. They are associated with lymphadenopathy and tumor development in the liver, spleen, thymus, bone marrow, and submucosa of the GI and respiratory tracts. As in leukemia, immune deficiencies develop and are followed by infection. Most lymphoid neoplasms are of B-cell origin, with T-cell tumors making up the remainder. Hodgkin lymphoma is set apart from non-Hodgkin lymphomas by the presence of the malignant Hodgkin and Reed-Sternberg (HRS) giant cells in the neoplastic tissue. Also, in Hodgkin disease, within the involved nodes the HRS cells account for less than 1% of affected tissue, thus the nonneoplastic inflammatory cells usually greatly outnumber the tumor cells (Schnitzer, 2009).

LEUKEMIAS

Description

The leukemias represent a group of malignant hematologic diseases in which normal bone marrow elements are replaced by abnormal, poorly differentiated lymphocytes known as blast cells. Genetic abnormalities in the hematopoietic cells take over and result in unregulated clonal proliferation of malignant cells (Tubergen and Bleyer, 2007). Leukemias are classified according to cell type involvement (i.e., lymphocytic or nonlymphocytic) and by cellular differentiation. ALL is characterized by preponderantly undifferentiated WBCs.

Epidemiology

The leukemias are the most common form of childhood cancer. They account for approximately 41% of pediatric malignancies in children less than 15 years of age. ALL accounts for about 80% of childhood leukemia cases, with a peak incidence between 2 and 6 years old. ALL represents 23% of cancer diagnoses among children younger than 15 years of age, occurring in about 1 of every 29,000 children in the U.S. each year (National Cancer Institute, 2010). Acute myeloid leukemia (AML) accounts for about 18% of all cases. Most of the other leukemias are of the chronic myeloid form (Kupfer, 2009; Tubergen and Bleyer, 2007).

As with all types of malignancy, the exact cause of leukemia is unknown. Several factors associated with increased risk have been identified, including infection, radiation, chemical and drug exposure, and genetic factors (e.g., Down syndrome).

Clinical Findings

Most of the clinical signs and symptoms of leukemia are related to leukemic replacement of the bone marrow and the absence of blood cell precursors. The child may be anemic, pale, listless, irritable, or chronically tired and have the following:

- A history of repeated infections, fever, weight loss
- Bleeding episodes characterized by epistaxis, petechiae, and hematomas

- Lymphadenopathy and hepatosplenomegaly
- Bone and joint pain

Central nervous system (CNS) symptoms are rare at the time of diagnosis but can present due to an intracranial or spinal mass (Satake and Yoon, 2010). All these symptoms may be vague or nonspecific, in which case it is important for the provider to have a high index of suspicion for cancer.

Diagnostic Tests. The following are used to diagnose leukemia:

- CBC with differential WBC, platelet, and reticulocyte counts. Thrombocytopenia is present in up to 85% of cases, and anemia is also usually present. WBC count may be elevated, normal, or low with varying levels of neutropenia.
- Peripheral smear may demonstrate malignant cells.
- Bone marrow examination shows an infiltration of blast cells replacing normal elements of the marrow.

Approximately 90% of children with ALL have genetic alterations in their leukemic blast cells including changes in the number of chromosomes and their structure with recurrent translocations noted in about half of the cases (Satake and Yoon, 2010). Further classification regarding cell type, morphologic characteristics, and cell surface markers is generally made at the cancer treatment center to which the child is referred.

Management

Approximately 75% to 80% of children diagnosed with ALL are thought to be curable. Key genetic features are critical factors in the management plan. The treatment program for most types of acute leukemia involves a 28-day induction phase (usually with vincristine, prednisone, and L-asparaginase), with the goal of inducing a complete remission and restoring normal hematopoiesis. This is followed by a consolidation phase of therapy and then a maintenance phase of therapy. Chemotherapy, CNS therapy (cranial irradiation, which is now reserved only for a high-risk child—those with CNS disease or high WBC counts at diagnosis, or intrathecal administration of chemotherapy), and systemic administration of corticosteroids are the key interventions. The use of cranial irradiation as part of therapy is decreasing. For children with ALL who relapse, the need for allogeneic stem cell transplantation is not considered until the second complete remission. However, children with the Philadelphia chromosome or those who are not in remission by the end of the first induction phases are considered high risk for relapse and need to consider transplantation sooner. Minimal residual disease measurement is part of current protocol treatment to determine the end-of-leukemic induction burden and ALL outcome (Satake and Yoon, 2010).

For those with AML, allogeneic stem cell transplantation from an HLA-matched sibling or parent is considered in the first complete remission (Weinblatt, 2010).

Long-term sequelae of cancer therapy for ALL have been identified in research studies and include effects on cognition and neuropsychological functioning. CNS irradiation has been linked to learning disabilities and impaired IQ, especially in children younger than 5 years of age who also received intrathecal therapy. As a result, cranial radiation dosages have been reduced, and earlier neuropsychological testing is recommended. Other documented potential late effects of ALL treatment include congestive heart failure, avascular necrosis, and osteoporosis (Meck et al, 2006; Monteleone and Meadows, 2009). Late effects associated with common childhood cancers are further discussed at the end of this chapter.

Risk-directed treatment based on high-risk features at diagnosis (i.e., WBC count, age, cytogenetics, response to therapy, minimal residual disease, immunophenotype, CNS status, ethnic background, and gender) and transplantation options has drastically improved cure rates. TEL/AML1 is present in about 20% of children with ALL and is considered the most favorable prognostic marker; in contrast to the presence of the Philadelphia chromosome, which is associated with a poor prognosis. AML also has genetic markers that are associated with a more or less favorable prognosis (Silverman, 2009). It is hoped that the incidence and severity of late-term effects will likewise diminish.

The role of the primary care provider is crucial to facilitate proper referrals and effective interdisciplinary communication and to assist the family in their coping and adaptation processes. Regular child health supervision visits are also important and should not be overlooked. The provider should ensure that immunizations are given as appropriate and that the child is monitored for failed remission or metastasis (CNS and testicles are common sites) and late effects.

LYMPHOMAS

NON-HODGKIN LYMPHOMA

Description

The non-Hodgkin lymphomas (NHLs) are a diverse group of solid tumors of the lymphatic tissues that form from malignant proliferation of T cells, B cells, or indeterminate lymphocyte cells. Different classification systems have been used to categorize these tumors. In pediatrics the common types of NHL are small noncleaved cell lymphoma (Burkitt and non-Burkitt subtypes, B-cell origin), lymphoblastic lymphoma, and large cell lymphoma (Johnston, 2010). NHLs account for 6% of all pediatric cancers (Kupfer, 2009).

Epidemiology

The incidence rate in children younger than 19 years old from 2003 to 2007 was 11.8 per 1 million children (National Cancer Institute, 2010). NHL occurs most frequently in children during the second decade of life and infrequently in children less than 3 years old. It is the most frequent malignancy in children with acquired immunodeficiency syndrome and is also associated with Epstein-Barr and cytomegalovirus infections.

Clinical Findings

The most common site of origin is in the lymphoid structures of the intestinal tract. The most common manifestations in children are (1) acute abdomen, including abdominal pain, distention, fullness, and constipation and (2) nontender lymph node enlargement. Histologic differences account for varying disease sites; lymphoblastic NHLs often present as intrathoracic tumors; in contrast, small noncleaved cell lymphomas commonly present as abdominal tumors. Other sites include the CNS and the bone marrow. Initial presentation is often with advanced disease of stages III or IV (Cairo and Bradley,

2007). Duration of symptoms before a diagnosis is made is typically 1 month or less (Johnston, 2010).

Diagnostic Tests. Diagnostic studies are ordered depending on the location of the lymphoma and symptoms. They include CBC with differential, chest radiograph, ultrasound, computed tomography (CT) or magnetic resonance imaging (MRI) scan or positron emission tomography (PET) of the area in question, gallium and/or bone scan, bone marrow aspirates and biopsies, lumbar puncture with CNS fluid analysis, CBC, liver function tests, lactate dehydrogenase, uric acid and electrolyte levels, and 8-hour creatinine clearance if indicated (Johnston, 2010).

Management

The diagnosis is confirmed by surgical biopsy, and the extent of the disease process and staging can be determined by scans, bone marrow aspiration, and lumbar puncture. Because of rapid developments in treatment and the importance of careful histologic evaluation, these children should be referred to a major pediatric cancer center for care.

Lymphomas are sensitive to chemotherapy. Cranial irradiation or intrathecal chemotherapy is part of the treatment plan if CNS involvement is present. Maintenance therapy may be continued for 6 months to 2 years. The prognosis has improved dramatically. The 5-year relative survival rate is 81.7% based on 2003-2007 statistics for children 0 to 19 years (National Cancer Institute, 2010).

HODGKIN DISEASE

Description

Like the NHLs, Hodgkin disease is a malignancy of the reticuloendothelial and lymphatic systems and involves B cells. It usually originates in a cervical lymph node and spreads to other lymph node regions and, if left untreated, to organ systems, including liver, spleen, bone, bone marrow, and brain. Unlike the NHL, involvement of the bone marrow and CNS is rare (de Alarcon and Metzger, 2008). Clinical and pathologic staging of the disease is usually done by specialists according to the Ann Arbor staging criteria.

Epidemiology

Hodgkin disease represents 50% of the lymphomas of childhood. It is rare in children younger than 5 years old. The frequency of Hodgkin disease in children between the ages of 15 and 20 years old is 12.1 cases per 1 million (de Alarcon and Metzger, 2008). Clusters of cases in families suggest a genetic predisposition. Hodgkin disease is associated with immunodeficiencies and infection with Epstein-Barr virus (EBV) and cytomegalovirus virus as is NHL (deAlarcon and Metzger, 2008).

Clinical Findings

The most common manifestations of Hodgkin disease include the following:
- Painless enlargement of the lymph nodes, usually in the cervical area; the nodes may feel firm, are often matted together, and are nontender to palpation
- Chronic cough if the trachea is compressed by a large mediastinal mass

- Fever, decreased appetite, weight loss, and night sweats
  Diagnostic Tests. Hematologic findings are often normal, but may include the following:
- Anemia
- Elevated or depressed leukocytes or platelets
- Elevated sedimentation rate and C-reactive protein; serum copper and ferritin level
- Abnormal liver function test results
- Urinalysis may have proteinuria
- Imaging studies: chest radiography, ultrasound, CT, MRI, and PET

Management

The diagnosis is confirmed by histologic examination of an excised lymph node, followed by bone marrow studies to determine the extent of the disease. The child should receive treatment at a pediatric oncology center in collaboration with the primary provider. Optimal results are obtained through irradiation, chemotherapy with numerous agents or a combination of both. Data from 2003 to 2007 indicate a 95.1% relative survival rate for children 0 to 19 years (NCI, 2010). Infertility is problematic for those receiving high doses of alkylators; sperm banking is discussed as an option for males before starting therapy. Approximately 30% of children who survive Hodgkin disease develop secondary malignancy 30 years later, typically thyroid, breast, nonmelanoma skin cancers and non-Hodgkin lymphoma and acute leukemia. Therefore, lifelong monitoring is necessary (de Alarcon and Metzger, 2008).

LATE EFFECTS OF CHILDHOOD CANCERS

Estimates are given that 1 in 450 adolescents and young adults is a long-term cancer survivor (Monteleone and Meadows, 2009). Any adverse effect that does not resolve after completion of therapy or a problem that develops after completion of therapy is labeled as a late effect of childhood cancer. Late effects can be attributed to radiation therapy, chemotherapy, or a combination of both and can occur later during puberty or with aging. Common problems have been identified, and pediatric survivors of cancer need to be monitored for these issues. Problems need to be identified early and promptly addressed. They can include the following (Meck et al, 2006; Monteleone and Meadows, 2009):

- Short stature from cranial irradiation and intensive chemotherapy
- Precocious puberty after cranial irradiation and hypothyroidism with neck or mantle radiation therapy (RT)
- Avascular necrosis of the bone caused by high-dose steroid therapy—more pronounced in young children—and with local irradiation
- Osteoporosis from cranial irradiation, glucocorticoids, and antimetabolites
- Leukoencephalopathy resulting from cranial irradiation, methotrexate, glucocorticoids

- Peripheral neuropathy and hearing loss from cisplatin
- Cognitive dysfunction, stroke, and seizures from intrathecal chemotherapy, certain systemic chemotherapy agents, and radiation. Cranial radiation effects are dose dependent and more deleterious on young developing brains
- Vision, auditory, and skeletal changes from head and neck radiation
- Obesity and gonadal dysfunction resulting from a neuroendocrine effect
- Potential alterations in pubertal development and gonadal function if given high-dose alkylating agents, especially in puberty and to girls
- Cardiomyopathy and arrhythmias if given anthracyclines. Children given these drugs need to be educated just before their teen years about avoiding alcohol, which increases the likelihood of cardiotoxicity, and cautioned about cigarette smoking
- Pericardial effusion, constrictive pericarditis, or late coronary artery disease from radiation therapy that includes all or part of the heart (e.g., Hodgkin disease)
- Pneumonitis and pulmonary fibrosis from chest and thorax radiation and with such chemotherapy agents as bleomycin and carmustine
- Malignant glioma associated with cranial irradiation and sarcomas associated with musculoskeletal radiation
- Secondary leukemias (usually AML) associated with therapy with alkylating agents and epipodophyllotoxins. Secondary solid tumors are associated with RT.
- Glomerular or tubular injury, renal insufficiency with heavy metals (e.g., cisplatin)
- Infertility and early menopause with alkylator therapy
- Cystitis or bladder dysfunction with cyclophosphamide
- Delayed recovery of normal immune function (may need readministration of immunization)
- Psychosocial effects associated with chronic illness (e.g., less likely to go to college, marry, and be employed).
- Cancer relapse
- Peripheral neuropathies
- Possibility of hepatitis C virus infection if the child had a blood transfusion before 1992
- Bone marrow transplant recipients can also experience unique late effects associated with this treatment and require monitoring. Medical insurance coverage may also be problematic in later years

Monitoring programs for childhood cancer survivors provides a rich source of data to guide cancer treatment and its follow-up. All survivors of childhood cancers need regular health care supervision from a provider who is aware of their prior treatment modalities and knowledgeable of late effects, aware of their risk of occurrence, and comfortable with risk-based monitoring for such problems. Healthy lifestyles and dietary practices, and avoidance of sun, alcohol, recreational drug use, and tobacco should be stressed (Meck et al, 2006; Monteleone and Meadows, 2009).

Neurologic Disorders

CATHERINE G. BLOSSER, ANNE C. ALBERS, AND MELISSA REIDER-DEMER

Central nervous system (CNS) problems can affect many systems and present in a variety of ways and degrees. No other body system has as much influence on a child's development. The challenge for health care providers is to be able to screen and identify neurologic problems; know when to appropriately refer to specialists; be able to monitor the general health of the patient and provide routine preventive care; serve as a case manager based on school and health care issues; help coordinate resources; and support families as they deal with the challenges of grief and long-term care.

◼ Anatomy and Physiology

ANATOMY

Briefly, the nervous system is divided into two parts: the CNS and the peripheral nervous system (PNS). The CNS consists of the brain and spinal cord. The PNS is made up of a network of afferent nerves and sense organs, which send information to the brain, and the efferent nerves, which send information out to the body for responses. Descending tracts from the brain to the gray matter of the spinal cord include the extrapyramidal tract, which conveys information from the cerebellum to the motor cells of the anterior column, and the pyramidal tract, which is the main motor pathway from the cerebral cortex to the spinal nerves and carries messages for voluntary movement. Most pyramidal tract fibers cross in the medulla, so the left half of the brain controls the right side of the body and vice versa. The anatomic units of the brain and their functions are listed in Table 27-1 and shown in Figures 27-1 and 27-2.

AUTONOMIC NERVOUS SYSTEM

The visceral activities of the body (i.e., blood vessels, glandular secretions, gastrointestinal tract, cardiac muscle) are controlled by the autonomic nervous system (ANS). The ANS is comprised of the sympathetic system and the parasympathetic system, which are principally under the control of the hypothalamus. When the hypothalamus receives information from the cortical centers (e.g., visual, auditory, olfactory) and sensory stimuli from the various parts of the body (e.g., organs, glands), it functions as a "switchboard" between the two systems. Generally, both systems supply the same organs, glands, and smooth muscles. The sympathetic system begins in the thoracolumbar area of the spinal cord and extends distally; its function is often

referred to as the "fight or flight" reaction. It is most active when an individual is physically or mentally stressed. The parasympathetic system begins in the medulla and midbrain with relays to the thalamus and higher centers. Enervation results in slowed activity, a decreased metabolic rate, and the conservation of energy; this system is active when an individual is mentally or physically relaxed. The principal sympathetic system neurotransmitters are epinephrine and norepinephrine. The parasympathetic fibers produce acetylcholine. The two systems function in balance—one excites and the other inhibits (Box 27-1). The enteric system is a component of the ANS, but does not play a role specifically in neurology. This system consists of a meshwork of nerve fibers that innervate the digestive system.

PHYSIOLOGY

Nerve impulses are transmitted along a nerve fiber through changes in polarization of the membrane, during which electrical activity is produced. Certain chemicals diffuse across the synapses between nerves and end organs. There are approximately fifty substances that act as neurotransmitters in the brain. The main categories of neurotransmitters are acetylcholine (a primary transmitter released by neurons projecting through the cerebral cortex and limbic system), amino acids (e.g., glutamate, aspartate, glycine, gamma aminobutyric acid [GABA]), biogenic amines (e.g., norepinephrine, dopamine, serotonin, histamine), and the largest family, neuropeptides (e.g., endorphins, angiotension II, melatonin, oxytocin, and many others). All of the neurotransmitters play an important role in either excitation or inhibition of neurons.

◼ Pathophysiology and Defense Mechanisms

The nervous system is intimately related to functioning of the entire body; problems in any part of the system can have neurologic implications. Examples include uncontrolled firing of cerebral neurons (seizures); the inability of cerebral neurons to fire or the inability of the CNS to process stimuli and respond accordingly (coma); or the inability of peripheral nerves to respond to or receive signals through the pyramidal system of afferent and efferent nerves (paralysis). Other problems occur when special areas of the nervous system or individual nerves are damaged. Broad incapacity occurs with neurotransmitter problems. Many

TABLE 27-1	Anatomic Units of the Nervous System and Functions

Anatomic Unit	Functions
I. Central nervous system	
A. Brain	
1. Forebrain—cerebrum	
a. Cortex (gray matter)	Posterior—motor skills
(1) Frontal area	Anterior—decision-making, emotions, memory, judgment, ethics, abstract thinking Broca's area—speech
(2) Parietal area	Sensory integration, language, reading, writing, pattern recognition
(3) Temporal area	Memory storage, auditory processing, olfaction, limbic system in deep temporal lobe—arousal
(4) Occipital area	Visual processing
b. Diencephalon	
(1) Thalamus	Receives and sorts sensory input, modulates motor impulses from cortex
(2) Hypothalamus	Integrates autonomic functions
2. Midbrain	Connects brain with cerebellum, pons, medulla
3. Hindbrain	
a. Pons	Bridges cerebellum, medulla, midbrain; cranial nerves (CN) V, VI, VIII arise here
b. Medulla	Proximal end of spinal cord; contains reticular system—arousal; CN IX to XII arise here
c. Cerebellum	Coordination and movement; balance; smooth movements
B. Cranial nerves	Sensory and motor components; olfaction; vision; hearing; facial, tongue, pharyngeal, eye, shoulder movements
II. Spinal cord	
A. Dorsal roots	Afferent sensory fibers
B. Ventral roots	Efferent motor fibers
III. Protective layers	
A. Meninges	Protection of delicate nervous tissues
B. Ventricles	
C. Cerebrospinal fluid	

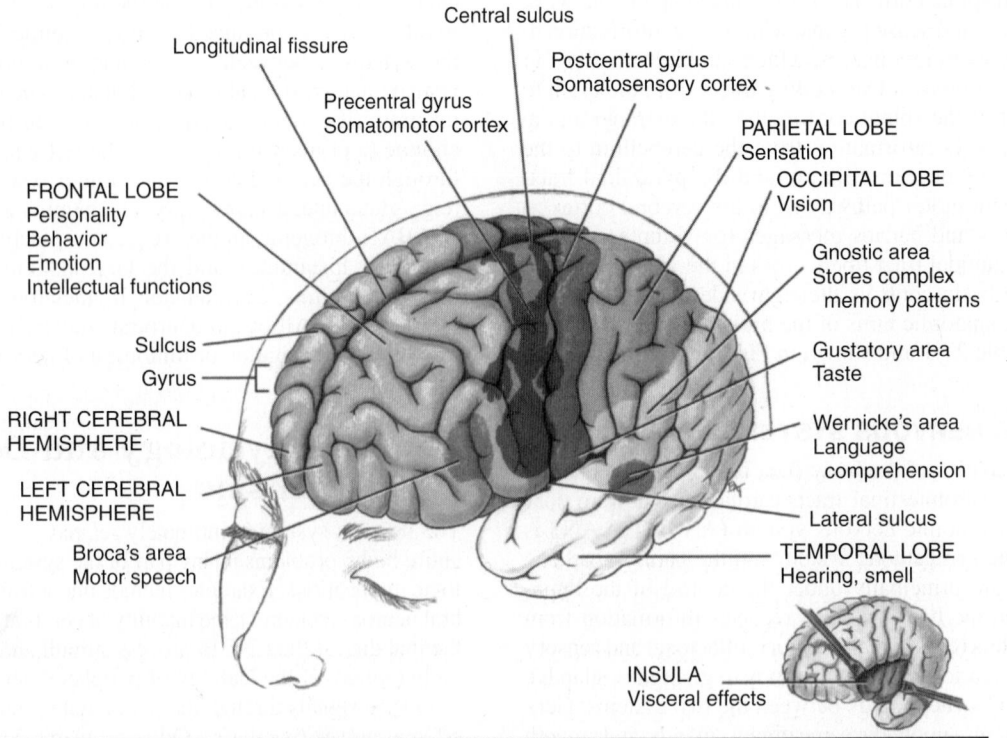

FIGURE 27-1 Lobes and functional areas of the cerebrum. (From Polaski AL: *Luckmann's core principles and practice of medical-surgical nursing,* Philadelphia, 1996, Saunders.)

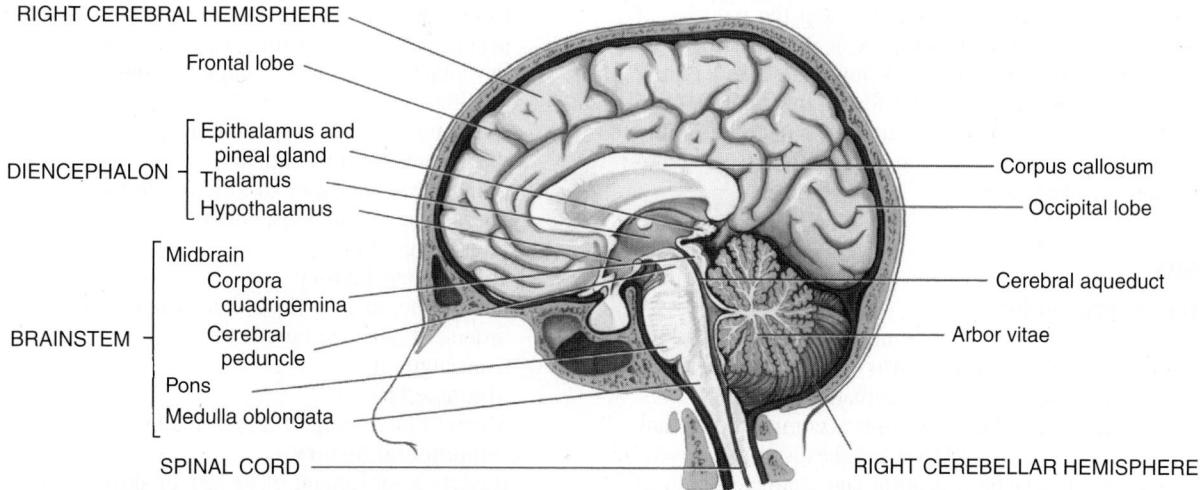

RIGHT CEREBRAL HEMISPHERE
Frontal lobe
DIENCEPHALON
- Epithalamus and pineal gland
- Thalamus
- Hypothalamus

Corpus callosum
Occipital lobe

BRAINSTEM
- Midbrain
  - Corpora quadrigemina
  - Cerebral peduncle
- Pons
- Medulla oblongata

Cerebral aqueduct
Arbor vitae

SPINAL CORD
RIGHT CEREBELLAR HEMISPHERE

FIGURE 27-2 Midsagittal section of the brain showing the major portions of the diencephalon, brainstem, and cerebellum. (From Polaski AL: *Luckmann's core principles and practice of medical-surgical nursing*, Philadelphia, 1996, Saunders.)

BOX 27-1	Autonomic Nervous System: Parasympathetic and Sympathetic Functions

Parasympathetic System

Pupil constriction
Increased watery saliva
Lacrimal gland vasodilation
Coronary vessel vasoconstriction
Bronchial muscle constriction
Stomach peristalsis
Colon peristalsis
Genitalia vasodilation
Urinary bladder constriction
Skin vessel dilation

Sympathetic System

Pupil dilation
Increased viscous/thick saliva
Coronary vessel vasodilation
Bronchial muscle relaxation
Stomach constriction
Adrenaline secretion
Colon relaxation
Sphincter relaxation
Sphincter constriction
Genitalia vasoconstriction
Urinary bladder relaxation
Skin vessel constriction

CNS disorders have interactive genetic, immunologic, and infectious factors that are probably causative (e.g., multiple sclerosis, cerebral palsy). Other causative factors include:

- *Systemic Problems.* The brain is extremely sensitive to changes in physiology anywhere in the body. Thus, any metabolic change, whether from external or internal factors (autoimmune, inflammatory, infectious causes), affects the CNS. Examples include delirium from toxins, diabetic coma, meningitis, epilepsy, ataxias, and chorea.

- *Neurodegenerative Disorders.* Neurodegenerative disorders result from a loss of structure or function of neurons in the brain or spine, including death of neurons. Many neurodegenerative diseases are caused by genetic mutations (e.g., multiple sclerosis, Rett syndrome).

- *Genetic Problems.* Many medical disorders have a genetic component that directly affects the nervous system. Some of the single-gene defects may have direct neurologic effects (such as neurofibromatosis), whereas others, typically inborn errors of metabolism, can have indirect effects via the abnormal metabolites released (e.g., phenylketonuria). Other examples of disorders with a genetic component include Tourette and Rett syndromes.

- *Structural Defects.* Because the CNS is structurally complex, there are many opportunities for defects to occur in utero. Examples of such defects include hydrocephaly, anencephaly, and spina bifida.

- *Trauma.* Head and spinal cord injuries are common and can have long-term, serious consequences for the child. Such complex neurologic tissue does not always heal in a way that results in full recovery of function(s).

- *Tumors and Cancer.* Benign or cancerous tumors evolve when there is a problem with cellular division. Problems with the body's immune system can also lead to such tumors. Peripheral nerves can regenerate somewhat if conditions are optimal. In the spinal cord the axons of injured neurons cannot regrow within the cord, but they can grow in peripheral nerves outside the cord. In this case, if the cut ends are reconnected with special attention to the myelin sheath, regeneration of the injured nerve begins at the proximal end of the neuron soon after injury. The growth rate is approximately 2.5 to 3 mm per day (Menkes and Moser, 2006).

Assessment of the Nervous System

Assessment of the nervous system requires a careful history of the patient and family, and a detailed physical examination. The examiner needs to determine if a neurologic disorder exists and, if so, the disorder's location and the patterns of impairment. For children with complex or severe neurologic problems, social, environmental, developmental, and family issues need thorough exploration. Historical information from patients more than 3 years old and from one or more family members provides the most accurate picture. Imaging or laboratory studies may be required.

HISTORY

- **History of present illness**
  - Onset: When did the first symptoms appear? Was the onset insidious or sudden? Was it associated with an injury, insult, or recent exacerbating event? If yes, describe the event. Was the onset accompanied by any constitutional symptoms? How has the disorder evolved?
  - Pain and/or headache: Location and character, path of radiation, severity, extent of disability produced, effect of various activities or stimuli (including light sensitivity), relief measures, changes from day to night, effects of previous treatment, presence of pain or discomfort in other parts of the body
  - Sensory deficits: Changes in hearing, vision, taste, loss of pain sensation, vertigo, dizziness, numbness, tingling
  - Injury: How, when (time and date), why, where, mechanism or manner in which the injury was produced: accidental or nonaccidental? Immediate treatment provided? If past injury, at what age did the injury occur?
  - Reflexive responses: Vomiting, coughing, primitive reflexes, tics, clonus
  - Behavioral changes: Irritability, stupor, changes in appetite, lack of attention, random activity, emotional lability, changes in school performance
  - Motor and balance changes: Ataxia, spasticity, increased or decreased tone
- **Medical history**
  - Prenatal history: Maternal and paternal ages, alcohol, drug ingestion (including environmental toxins, such as fish contaminated with mercury), radiation exposure, nutrition, prenatal care, injuries, hyperthermia, smoking, human immunodeficiency virus (HIV) or other infectious disease exposure, maternal illness, bleeding, toxemia, diabetes, previous abortions and stillbirths
  - Birth history and neonatal course: Place of birth, complications, labor and delivery, resuscitation, trauma, congenital anomalies, feeding history (reflux, colic, frequent formula changes), jaundice, convulsions, infection, gestational age, sleep disturbances, multiple birth. Low birthweight and failure to thrive have a strong effect on child development (Msall, 2009).
  - Injuries or infections: Meningitis, encephalitis, head injuries, seizures—types, frequency, medications; frequent musculoskeletal injuries (can suggest coordination or impulsive behavior).
  - Cardiovascular or respiratory disorders
  - Environmental exposure to toxins (e.g., lead exposure)
  - Metabolic disorders: Diabetes mellitus, thyroid disease. Hypoglycemia causes confusion, convulsion, loss of consciousness. Hyperglycemia causes lethargy, coma. Hyperthyroidism causes tremor. Hypothyroidism causes weakness, coma.
  - Past neurologic disease and tests: Tics, hydrocephaly, genetic screening, or imaging studies done
  - Psychiatric disorders: Hallucinations, delusions, and illusions
  - Drug ingestion: Lead poisoning, dietary/herbal supplements, and pharmaceuticals
  - Urinary tract disease: Uremic syndrome manifests with confusion, convulsions, coma
  - Physical growth
- **Family disease history**
  - Family members with similar symptoms or genetic disorders; obtain a pedigree
  - Consanguinity
  - Migraine history
  - Mental functioning of family members
- **Developmental history**
  - Review achievement of or loss of skills in all developmental milestone categories—language, gross motor, fine motor, social, and cognitive—and school performance. The Ages & Stages, Denver Developmental Screening Test II, and the World-class Instructional Design and Assessment (WIDA-ACCESS Placement Test [W-APT]) are useful.
- **Functional health**
  - Inquire about the effects of symptoms on all areas of health promotion and safety, nutrition, elimination, activity, communication, role relationships, values and beliefs, sexuality, sleep, coping (management style) and stress tolerance, temperament, and self-concept. The "management style" of family members is crucial to assess because it suggests how different family members may react over time to any chronic illness of their child (Shevell, 2009).
- **Social context**
  - Inquire about the family composition (including critical family events such as additions or losses of family members); home, neighborhood, and school environment; culture and ethnicity; other stressors; strengths; resources; childcare; financial issues (socioeconomic status, poverty); identified social supports (e.g., family, friends, health professionals); and community agencies involved with the family and child.
- **Review all systems plus**
  - Allergies, immunizations, hearing, vision, dental, skin integrity, behavior, nutritional status, and eating disorders

PHYSICAL EXAMINATION

The following should be noted:
- Growth pattern, including height, weight, body mass index (BMI), and head circumference
- Abnormalities of the skin (café au lait macules, angiomas, other pigmentation changes)
- Anomalies (for example, unusual facies, shape and number of digits, low-set ears)
- Cardiovascular system (including blood pressure)
- Musculoskeletal system: Gower's sign, calf muscle hypertrophy, and muscular function
- Hearing
- Vision: eye problems, including cataract, corneal clouding, cherry-red spot, change of visual function

- Tanner stage
- Hepatomegaly/splenomegaly

Specifics of the Neurologic Examination

The neurologic examination moves from the highest level of functioning to the lowest. Cerebral function is tested first; then cranial nerves, motor function, and sensory function; and finally reflexes. The neonate's neurologic functioning is largely subcortical. Therefore, the examination is more limited than in an older infant or child. In infants and children, watching them carefully while collecting the history and actively playing with them in an age-appropriate manner provides a great deal of neurologic information. A tennis ball, some small toys (e.g., a small car), a bell, and something that attracts attention (e.g., a pinwheel) are useful throughout the examination.

Behavior and Mental Status. Test the following cortical functions:
- Responsiveness
- Judgment
- Language and speech (receptive, expressive, written); speech flow, voice quality, organization of thoughts
- Memory
- General knowledge
- Ability to relate to others: parents versus strangers
- Mood and affect

Cranial Nerve Function. The majority of neurological examinations assess cranial nerves (CN) II through XII because CN I (the olfactory) is difficult to assess in children and is not functional until 5 to 7 months old. Vision (CN II) is indicated by blinking in response to a bright light. In the neonate, CN III, IV, and VI can be tested by assessing the ability to track through the visual fields. Facial grimaces test for CN V and VII. Hearing (CN VIII) can be tested with a small bell, finger rub, or snap. The gag reflex tests CN IX and X.

Motor Examination. Gait, posture, coordination, balance, strength, symmetry, quality of movement, and tone are aspects of the motor examination. Information can be gained from questioning the parent because it is often difficult to elicit the needed skills in the time and environment given.
- *Muscle strength and size.* Look at muscle size, contour, and symmetry. Have the child stand from a lying position. Look for Gower's sign (i.e., a child using the arms to push off from bent knees and gradually climbing the body and straightening up, which is common in children with muscular dystrophy). Ask the child to move extremities against resistance and to grip your fingers hard. The presence of muscular hypertrophy or hypotrophy should be noted.
- *Muscle tone.* Muscle tone might be considered the resting strength of the muscle. Is the trunk control and/or extremities floppy, rigid, or somewhat stiff when the child is resting or active? How difficult is it to move body parts passively? Tone may be increased or decreased all over or differ between the legs and the trunk and arms.
- *Fine motor coordination.* Fine motor coordination is tested by having the child pick up small pieces, write, stack blocks, copy pictures, turn book pages, put puzzles together, or do other hand activities.
- *Involuntary movements.* Tremors are fine involuntary movements. Chorea or choreiform movements are large,

irregular jerking and writhing movements. Athetoid movements are slow writhing movements, especially of the hands and feet. Dystonia is an uncontrolled change in tone with movement and a tendency to hyperextend the joints.
- *Reflexes.* When a reflex is abnormal, the question is, why? Did the impulse not go through, or did the child have a problem in the ability to move responsively because of problems in efferent signals or muscle tissue contractility? (See section on reflexes that follows.)
- *In an infant, assessing posture and muscle tone is fundamental.* Motor testing should include observation for symmetry of movements, consistent fisting of the hands, opisthotonos, scissoring, abnormal tone, and tremors. The infant's cry can be an indicator of several diseases (e.g., it is high pitched with increased intracranial pressure, resembles mewing in cri du chat syndrome, and is hoarse with hypothyroidism).

Sensory Examination. Examine for pain sensation and stereognosis. The accuracy of interpretation of this part of the examination is always limited in infants and young children. Use a light pinprick to check for mild pain sensation.

Reflexes
- Deep tendon reflexes include the biceps, brachioradialis, triceps, patellar, and Achilles.
- Superficial reflexes include the upper abdominal, lower abdominal, cremasteric, gluteal, and plantar.
- Primitive reflexes include sucking, rooting, asymmetric tonic neck, grasp, trunk incurvation, stepping, and others found in Table 27-2. These primitive reflexes can be absent or decreased in a satiated or sleepy infant. Tendon reflexes can be tested in an older child. In older children and adults, a Babinski sign is an important sign of upper motor neuron disease.

Cranium Examination. The neurologic examination should always include measurement of head circumference until the child is 2 years of age and if it appears abnormally large or small in an older child. Inspect the skull for symmetry and shape. Auscultation over the skull or above the eyes may reveal a cranial bruit. Percussion of the skull can give a sound resembling a cracked pot when the sutures are separated, as with increased intracranial pressure. The anterior fontanelle should normally be slightly depressed with very faintly perceived pulsations.

Autonomic Nervous System. Alterations in blood pressure, sweating, or body temperature can be indicators of ANS problems.

Meningeal Signs. Evidence of meningeal irritation, such as with meningitis, include positive Kernig and Brudzinski signs. A Kernig sign is positive if resistance and head or neck pain are elicited when the patient bends over from the waist and touches fingers to toes. In an infant, the Kernig sign can be tested by extending the leg at the knee with the infant lying supine. A positive sign can be as subtle as facial grimacing. A positive Brudzinski sign is evidenced by the patient spontaneously flexing the hip and knees after the examiner passively flexes the neck.

DIAGNOSTIC STUDIES

- Radiographs have relatively little diagnostic value for the neurologic system since the advent of computed tomography (CT) and magnetic resonance imaging (MRI). CT scans

TABLE 27-2	Primitive Reflexes				
Reflex	**Age Appears**	**Age Disappears**	**How to Elicit**	**Response**	**Notes**
Newborn Reflexes					
Rooting	Birth	3-4 mo	Head midline, stroke perioral area	Infant opens mouth and turns head to stimulated side	Absence indicates CNS disease or depressed severe infant; sleeping infant may not respond
Sucking	Birth	3-4 mo	Place nipple or finger 3-4 cm into mouth	Suck should be strong: push finger up and back; note rate	Absence indicates CNS depression; satiated or sleeping baby may not respond well
Asymmetric tonic neck reflex (ATNR)	Birth	4-6 mo	With baby supine, side; hold 15 sec	Arm and leg extend on facial side; arm and leg on other side flex	Obligatory response when child cannot get out of position is abnormal; persistence beyond 4-6 mo indicates CNS lesion (e.g., CP)
Palmar grasp	Birth	3-6 mo	Place finger into infant's palm and press against palm	Infant flexes all fingers around examiner's finger	Grasp should be strong and symmetric
Trunk incurvation (Galant)	Birth	2 mo	Suspend baby prone; stroke 2-3 cm from spine with fingernail	Baby flexes toward stimulus	Asymmetry is significant; tests for spinal cord lesions; should not persist after 6 mo
Stepping	Birth	6-8 wk	Infant is held as though weight bearing with feet on surface	Infant steps along, raising one foot at a time	Tests brainstem, spinal column; absence indicates paralysis or depressed baby
Moro	Birth	4 mo	Present loud noise or allow infant's head to drop slightly	Arms spread and fingers extend and then flex; then arms come toward each other; cry is possible	Asymmetry indicates paralysis or fractured clavicle, absence indicates brainstem problem, usually severe; persistence also abnormal
Crossed extension	0-4 mo	Passively extend one leg and press knee to table; prick sole of that foot with pin	Other leg should slightly extend and adduct	
Plantar grasp	Birth	8-10 mo	Place finger firmly against base of toes	Toes should curl down	Tests S1-S2 spinal nerves; lessens by 8 mo, suspect any asymmetry
Later Reflexes					
Landau	3 mo	15 mo-2 yr	Suspend infant prone by supporting abdomen	Infant should lift both head and legs	Abnormal if arm tone increased with internal rotation, arm held at side, or arm does not lift as noted
Neck righting	6 mo	2 yr	With infant supine, turn head to one side	Infant's trunk rotates in direction of head	Absent or decreased can indicate spasticity; can also rotate trunk and then look for head to follow; tests midbrain
Parachute	6-8 mo	Never	Suspend infant prone and lower quickly toward table	Infant should extend arms, hands, fingers	Response should be symmetric and "protective"

CNS, Central nervous system; *CP*, cerebral palsy.

display differences in density of the intracranial tissues and structures. MRI provides additional information related to aneurysms (e.g., hemorrhages, calcifications, abscesses), brain structure, and the cellular activity of various parts of the neurologic system (e.g., tumors, CNS, spinal cord, and malformations). There may be a medical need to order more specific tests, such as a magnetic resonance angiogram (used to detect blood vessel stenosis and aneurysms) or functional magnetic resonance imaging (fMRI—used to detect subtle metabolic changes in the brain that indicate how certain parts of the brain are working). A neurologic consultant can advise when these would be necessary.

- Laboratory studies provide indicators of systemic disease, infection, or inflammation. They are especially important for children receiving medication for seizures. Drug levels, liver function, and blood studies may need to be monitored routinely.
- Lumbar puncture provides information about metabolism, infections, and trauma.
- The electroencephalogram (EEG) provides information about the electrical activity of the CNS, which is important in assessing function rather than structure.
- Ultrasonography can be useful in infants to evaluate brain tissue.
- Other studies can include polysomnography (helps assess narcolepsy, apnea of infancy, certain movement disorders, and nocturnal seizures); electromyography (tests muscle activity); nerve conduction studies; evoked responses (brainstem—auditory, somatosensory, and visual); electronystagmography (measures eye movements to assess vertigo and postconcussion syndrome); and cerebral arteriography (visualizes cerebral blood vessels to evaluate vascular anomalies and tumors).

■ Management Strategies

COUNSELING

Counseling for neurologic problems involves several components. The family should understand the pathologic condition, including possible etiologies, and the treatment plan; be provided with information about the prognosis with and without treatment and any genetic implications of the diagnosis; and have sufficient time to ask questions about all these issues. Counseling also involves helping families cope with the diagnosis and its short- and long-term implications for the child and family. A plan of care needs to be mutually agreed on and fluid enough to adapt to changes in the child's condition.

Information about a diagnosis needs to be delivered truthfully, compassionately, and promptly using appropriate terminology. Correct language not only influences how parents relate to their child's condition but also communicates to others a more accurate reflection of the child's abilities (e.g., schools, employers). Examples of appropriate terminology include:

- *Impairment:* Existence of a deviation from normal activity or an inability to control an involuntary movement (one can be impaired without being disabled)
- *Disability:* A restriction in an ability to execute a normal activity of daily living that someone of similar age could execute (all people with disabilities are impaired)

- *Handicap:* Existence of a disability that prevents the person from achieving a normal role in society that someone of a similar age is expected to achieve (all people with handicaps have disabilities)
- *"Extra needs"* versus *"special needs"* is a more socially acceptable and easily understood term to use when referring to a person.

ANTICIPATORY GUIDANCE
Neurologic Development

Families are sometimes concerned about problems that providers believe are within normal limits. No neurology referral is necessary in these situations. The family needs to understand the anticipated pattern of neurologic development including timelines and markers that they can use to monitor their child's development. Misperceptions about the implications of minor variations must be dealt with, and the family should always be given the opportunity to return for further assessment or discussion if concerns remain. The temperament of the child and the child's learned social behavior versus pathologic symptoms may need to be addressed (e.g., breath holding vs. seizures).

Educational Needs

Many neurologic problems in children affect learning, although neurologic problems are not synonymous with mental retardation. Sensory problems affect the child's ability to receive the input necessary for learning. Motor problems affect both the child's ability to interact with the environment and the ability to communicate or indicate understanding. Management should always consider the educational needs of the child. Special infant or preschool early intervention educational programs can assist the child to learn by using the most appropriate learning modalities. Teachers often need assistance in understanding the limitations and strengths of the child. Parents need to be encouraged to develop close communication with the educational staff because this relationship is mutually beneficial for optimizing the learning experience of the child.

Genetics Counseling

Many neurologic conditions are genetic in origin. Genetic implications are best communicated through formal genetics counseling; feelings of parental guilt need to be addressed. See Chapter 40 for guidance.

PHYSICAL, OCCUPATIONAL, AND SPEECH THERAPY

Physical therapy (PT) can be useful to help restore or maintain function or to teach new motor skills. The physical therapist should be accustomed to dealing with children. PT services are often combined with occupational and speech therapy to promote maximal development. Early intervention programs offer such assistance in many states and are generally free to qualifying patients. Should any services be denied, families should be advised to inquire about the appeal process in their state. Federal funding is available in most states for therapy programs for children from birth through 2 years of age.

SOCIAL SERVICES

Children and families with children that experience multiple handicapping conditions frequently have ongoing issues of coping, monitoring, and management of medical and financial resources. Medical social workers, public health nurses, and case managers can provide invaluable assistance for these families for continuity and coordination of care.

MEDICATIONS

A variety of medications are used to control the effects of neurologic problems. These may include antiepileptic drugs (AEDs), mood stabilizers, and antidepressants. Most require time for the effects to become apparent, need dosage adjustments, and are affected by the metabolism of the individual child. Periodic measurement of blood levels is often needed. Side effects of medications need to be weighed against their beneficial effects. Many require tapering of dosages when treatment with the medication is to be discontinued.

Specific Neurologic Problems of Children

■ Degenerative Disorders

Degenerative disorders consist of a group of neurodegenerative disorders whose etiologies affect either the gray matter or white matter of the brain. Degenerative disorders are believed to be the result of biochemical or metabolic dysfunctions (in turn caused by genetic, immune-mediated demyelination, or by unknown etiologies) that lead to anatomic or functional insults to major portions of the brain. These insults can affect the basal ganglia, cerebellum, brainstem, spinal cord, peripheral and cranial nerves, or cerebrum. Such insults can also follow infections or an altered immune state.

Gray matter diseases involve neurons, and their onset is heralded by seizures, a decrease in cognitive functioning, and visual changes. Gray matter disorders include Menkes syndrome (also called kinky-hair syndrome), progressive infantile poliodystrophy, neuronal ceroid-lipofuscinoses, and Rett syndrome, which is discussed later in the chapter. White matter diseases usually lead to demyelination and are evidenced by decreasing motor skills, ataxia, and spasticity. Such disorders include Schilder disease, acute disseminating encephalomyelitis, acute hemorrhagic leukoencephalitis, and multiple sclerosis (MS) (discussed later). The diagnosis is based on age of onset, clinical features (signs and symptoms), genetic transmission, and chemical and chromosomal studies. It also must be determined if the episodes of disability are single (monophasic) or polyphasic (relapses close to initial onset of symptoms with similar areas of involvement).

In the case of inflammatory demyelination, separate events are determined by whether or not they occur more than 30 days apart and involve separate white matter pathways. In an initial acute demyelinating event it may be difficult to determine a diagnosis; the extent of motor, visual, and neurologic involvement needs to be determined in all events. If a demyelinating event is suspected, the child should be referred to a neurologist (preferably pediatric) for a comprehensive evaluation and diagnosis.

RETT SYNDROME

A mutation in the X-linked, methyl-CpG-binding protein 2 gene (MECP2) occurs in 80% of females with classic Rett syndrome features (Percy and Lane, 2009). This gene contains instructions for protein synthesis of methyl cytosine–binding protein. MECP2 is abundant in the brain. When not disabled by mutation, it silences certain genes that control motion and emotion. This neurodevelopmental disorder was previously thought to affect only females and to be lethal to males. However, there has been some reported variation to this X-linked Rett syndrome gene occurring in males that is not lethal and results in mental retardation and neurologic impairment; some have Klinefelter syndrome (XXY) (Percy and Lane, 2009). Defects in MECP2 also occur in patients with autism, schizophrenia, learning disabilities, and neonatal encephalopathy (National Institute of Neurology Disorders and Stroke [NINDS], 2010a). Most females with Rett syndrome represent de novo mutations (Percy and Lane, 2009).

Rather than cause brain degeneration, Rett syndrome arrests maturation of certain areas of the brain. The patient is typically female with an onset of symptoms at 5 to 18 months of age. Those affected cease to gain developmental milestones. CNS irritability and withdrawal develop, and then these girls begin to lose skills, including speech and hand skills. Stereotypic hand movements, slowed head growth leading to microcephaly, autistic-like behavior, dementia, and disorganized breathing and apnea followed by hyperpnea occur. Seizures, scoliosis, and spastic paraparesis and quadriparesis are late developments in the syndrome.

Deoxyribonucleic acid (DNA) tests for the presence of mutations in MECP2 and are typically found to be about 80% accurate in diagnosing children with Rett syndrome (Proud and Elias, 2009). This is likely attributed to the possibility that 20% to 30% of the affected patients inherit only a part of the gene that is affected, and it remains undetected with current laboratory testing.

Physical, occupational, and speech therapies and seizure management are important to preserve functional abilities. As with all neurodevelopmental problems, families need significant support and social services. Life expectancy varies depending on complicating factors, but many live well into middle age (Percy and Lane, 2009). Differential diagnoses include cerebral palsy (CP), autism, psychosis, and other neurodegenerative diseases.

MULTIPLE SCLEROSIS
Description and Epidemiology

MS occurs in 5% of children before the age of 16 (Banwell, 2009). It is exceptional to have symptoms occur before a child is 10 years old (0.2% to 2% of all cases). Two to three times as many females as males are affected. It is widely believed that MS is an autoimmune inflammatory neurodegenerative disorder of the CNS. Macrophages, activated T-lymphocytes, and other destructive molecules are stimulated by yet not fully understood events. These inflammatory cells cause both CNS demyelination and axon damage within the white brain matter, including the optic nerve. Research is focused on environmental (including geography and living north of 40 degrees latitude), infectious, toxic, immunologic, hormonal, or genetic causes. No specific virus has been isolated, although the most promising agent seems to be the Epstein-Barr virus. Some scientists propose that it is multifactorial (National MS Society, 2010).

Overall the clinical course is variable. The disease is typified by two phases: initial relapse and remittance and secondary progression. The episodes of focal neurologic dysfunction can last weeks or months, followed by partial or complete recovery. The more relapses occur earlier in the disease, the more quickly the progression to irreversible disability. It is recognized that focal inflammation of the brain is active, even during the remission phase, and there seems to be a point of no return for the brain's coping mechanism. This coping mechanism appears to allow for a degree of adaptation for different types of mechanisms of inflammation that originate from outside the CNS, from target-determined changes in immune cells and microglial activation, and from the accumulation of cortical gray matter lesions. Immunoglobulin G (IgG) antibodies have been found in several acute demyelinating presentations and may be the future characterization of phenotypes (Banwell, 2009). However, once irreversible disability begins, the rate of progression is independent of the frequency of relapses.

Clinical Findings

Symptoms are the same for children as for all other ages. These include (Banwell, 2009):

- Unilateral weakness or ataxia (frequent presenting symptom).
- Symptoms that last more than 24 hours.
- Headache (may be severe, prolonged, generalized).
- Vague paresthesias of lower extremities, distal portions of hands and feet, and face.
- Visual disturbance (diplopia, blurred vision, or sudden loss of vision as a result of optic neuritis).
- Concurrent optic neuritis and transverse myelitis (referred to as neuromyelitis optica or Devic disease).
- Vertigo, dysarthria, and sphincter disturbances are uncommon. Neurogenic bladder may present in acute transverse myelitis.
- Repeated episodes are frequently preceded by fever, nausea and vomiting, and lethargy may occur within months or years of each other.

Diagnostic Studies

- Neuroimaging. An MRI (gadolinium enhanced) early in the course of the disease can be important in predicting the clinical future. In children demyelination of white matter presents as well defined and perpendicular to the corpus callosum. Evidence of disturbance of the blood-brain barrier is thought to be a better predictor than the number of T2 white matter lesions for developing inflammatory MS lesions and atrophy. Gray matter lesions are believed to play a role but are undetectable using current imaging.
- Later in the course of the disease, nonconventional neuroimaging techniques (magnetization transfer imaging and imaging for whole brain atrophy) are more useful than the gadolinium-enhanced MRI for tracking the progression of disability.
- Other studies may include a lumbar puncture (may show oligoclonal bands) and visual-evoked responses.

Differential Diagnosis

A diagnosis of MS can be considered during the initial episode of a neurologic dysfunction that affects a certain region of the body and occurs over a limited period of time. Brain tumor, focal encephalitis, nonviral infections with focal cerebritis or abscess formation, cerebrovascular diseases, leukodystrophies, and systemic vasculitis, mitochondrial, vitamin B_{12} deficiency (with macrocytic anemia), and spinal cord symptoms should be considered after initial presentation. After a remission and exacerbation pattern is established, consider multiple cerebral emboli, systemic vasculitis, or recurrent infections in a susceptible host (Banwell, 2009).

Management

There are no therapies to slow the disease once the progressive phase has started. Therefore, research is focused on finding therapies to slow the early progression of the disease. Treatment involves exercises—resistance, aerobic, and stretching—and routines that promote agility and speed. The use of corticosteroids during exacerbations is traditional therapy. Intravenous methylprednisone results in a faster resolution of visual disturbances and is a widely used treatment for the pediatric population. Other treatments used in adolescents and adults are immunomodulatory therapies (high-dose, high-frequency interferon or low-frequency interferon and glatiramer acetate, cyclophosphamide, natalizumab, and mitoxantrone); these treatments reduce the frequency of contrast-enhancing lesions (Banwell, 2009). Another treatment under study is the use of intravenous immunoglobulin (IVIG), which is postulated to work by binding to circulating antibodies and preventing them from entering the CNS. Adult data show a favorable response, but the studies in young children are limited (Banwell, 2009). Treatment decisions are not dependent on MRI imaging alone. Tools to monitor subtle changes in abilities are often used, such as the McDonald criteria for multiple sclerosis (Hawkes and Giovannoni, 2010). Continuing research is targeting a variety of the mechanisms and processes of the disease to prevent and treat relapses, alter disease progression, and discover neuroprotective factors.

■ Nondegenerative Disorders

BENIGN PAROXYSMAL VERTIGO

Benign paroxysmal vertigo (BPV) may be incorrectly diagnosed as epilepsy. It typically develops in toddlers (median age 18 months) but rarely occurs after 5 years old. BPV is also a known precursor to the development of migraines later in life (Wilkinson, 2009). The history may include rapid onset of an attack that lasts seconds to minutes; daily attacks that occur in clusters over several days and then may not recur for weeks or months; and a possible history of motion sickness. Symptoms are likely to have resolved by the time the child is examined. The physical examination findings consist of:

- Acute unsteadiness; the child may fall or refuse to walk or sit; may grab on to a parent or object for steadiness.
- Nystagmus may be present; no loss of consciousness with events.
- Vomiting and nausea may be present and be quite prominent.

TABLE 27-3	Terms Used to Describe Cerebral Palsy	
Movement Type	**Description**	**Associated Impairments**
Spastic	Inability of a muscle to relax	Often evident after 4-6 months; retarded speech; convergent strabismus; toe-walking; flexed elbows; delayed walking until 18-24 months; one third have seizures
Athetoid	Inability to control muscle movement (continuous, writhing movements)	Infant has difficult feeding as a result of tongue thrust, is initially hypotonic with head lag; increasing tone with rigidity over time; speech delay
Ataxic	Problems with balance and coordination	Tremors
Body Part Involved		
Diplegic	Affects both legs more than both arms	Most have limited use of legs; can walk often with aids; walk typically "scissor-like" with knees bent in and crisscross over each other
Hemiplegic	Affects one side of the body (upper extremity is usually affected more than the lower extremity)	Often not detected at birth; right side often more affected than left; 50% develop seizures; growth arrest of affected limb(s); individuals usually able to walk
Tetraplegic/Quadriplegic	Affects all four extremities, trunk and head	Affects upper extremities more than lower; 50% with grand mal seizures; IQ impairment can be severe; most unable to walk or stand
Specific Problems With Movement or Function		
Dystonia	Involuntary, slow, sustained muscle contraction	Abnormal posture, writhing motion of arms, legs, trunk
Choreic	Disorganized tone	Uncontrollable jerky movements of toes and fingers
Tremor	Involuntary, rhythmic movements of opposing muscles; can affect extremities, head, face, vocal cords, trunk	
Ballismus	Violent, jerky movements; may affect only one side of body	
Rigidity	Stiffness	

- Appearance of child is frightened and/or pale.
- Child may be lethargic or drowsy; some children may sleep and return to normal activities on awakening (Martin Sanz and Barona de Guzman, 2007).
- Neurologic examination is essentially negative except for abnormal vestibular function.

One possible diagnostic study involves ice water caloric testing to detect abnormal vestibular function. The clusters of attacks may be managed with diphenhydramine, 5 mg/kg/24 hr (maximum 300 mg/24 hr) PO, IM, IV, or per rectum. Once diagnosis is made, parental reassurance is key. Children may be inappropriately diagnosed as having epilepsy and started on anticonvulsants; attacks will not respond to such drugs.

CEREBRAL PALSY

Description

The term *cerebral palsy* is used to designate a mixed group of motor disorders that affect motor function and are caused by static injury to developing brains (Brunstrom and Tilton, 2009). This is a chronic, nonprogressive disorder that impairs control of movement by damaging motor areas in the brain. Symptoms appear within the first few years of life. Depending on the area affected and the extent of damage, children with CP can also have mental impairment (up to 66%); seizures (up to 50%); a lag in growth and development; neurosensory disorders affecting touch, pain, and continence; perceptual disorders; impaired vision and hearing; speech, swallowing, or chewing difficulties; and other learning or emotional difficulties. The degree of brain injury can vary from person to person, and the degree of impairment is not necessarily profound but can vary as well (Brunstrom and Tilton, 2009).

There are three major types of CP: spastic, athetoid (or dyskinetic), and ataxic. Spastic is when the muscles stiffen, causing muscle tightness. Athetoid affects the muscles that enable smooth, coordinated movement and maintain body posture; without this control movement becomes involuntary and purposeless. The ataxic type affects balance and coordination. Children may exhibit varying degrees of involvement and severity; capabilities may improve over time depending on the degree of involvement and treatment. Table 27-3 lists more terms that describe CP.

Epidemiology

CP was once believed to be caused only by birth complications (neonatal or perinatal asphyxia or trauma), but the Collaborative Perinatal Project demonstrated that most children with CP were born at term without complicated labors and deliveries (Johnston, 2007). The etiology is unknown in a large percentage of cases. Small-for-gestational-age, low birth-weight (less than 1000 g), or preterm babies (less than 37 weeks of gestation), and multiple births are at greater risk for CP. Complicated labor and delivery, breech presentation, Apgar score of less than 3 at 10 minutes or more; traumatic delivery; microcephaly; exposure to maternal infection (evidenced by chorioamnionitis, inflamed placental membranes, umbilical cord inflammation, foul-smelling amniotic fluid, maternal temperature greater than 100.4° F [38° C] during labor, or urinary tract infection [UTI]); maternal vaginal bleeding (between the sixth and ninth month of pregnancy); severe proteinuria late in pregnancy; maternal hyperthyroidism, mental retardation, and seizures; intracranial hemorrhage; toxemia; preeclampsia; antepartal hemorrhage; postmaturity; fetal distress; maternal stroke; coagulation in the fetus or newborn; and neonatal seizures are considered risk factors (Menkes and Moser, 2006). Other etiologies may include intrauterine drug exposure (e.g., alcohol, cocaine, tobacco, crack cocaine), intrauterine infections (e.g., cytomegalovirus, toxoplasmosis, rubella), and congenital brain malformations. In the U.S. it is estimated that children who acquire CP postnatally account for 10% to 20% of those with the disorder. In such cases, the cause can be attributed to meningitis, encephalitis, head trauma (e.g., secondary to shaken baby syndrome or other abuse, car accidents, falls), and kernicterus (Brunstrom and Tilton, 2009).

The prevalence is 1 to 3 per 1000 live births across many studies. Wilson-Costello and colleagues' study (2007) showed that the use of antenatal steroids and cesarean deliveries decreased neurodevelopmental impairment, sepsis, severe cranial ultrasound abnormalities, and postnatal steroid use in extremely low-birth-weight infants. This resulted in a decrease in the rate of cerebral palsy from 13% to 5% and a decrease in neurodevelopmental impairment from 35% to 23%.

Clinical Findings

History. The history should include pathologic, developmental, and functional health patterns.

Pathology
- Prenatal/natal history of risk factors as listed previously
- Seizures
- Hearing and vision or ocular problems, such as strabismus, nystagmus, optic atrophy
- Change in growth parameters, especially decreased head circumference
- Early head injury or meningitis
- Muscle tone (can be hypotonic before 6 months old then become hypertonic, as evidenced by unusual posture or favoring one side). Preterm infants with generalized, prolonged, and cramped synchronized movements are more often diagnosed with CP at a later time (Brunstrom and Tilton, 2009).

Development. Milestones may be delayed but should still be attained; persistent primitive reflexes are common (e.g., Moro and tonic neck). Hand preference before 1 year old is highly suspect.

Functional Health Patterns. Assess the following:
- Feeding history of regurgitating through the nose, inability to coordinate suck and swallow, inability to advance the diet to textured foods—in short, oral-motor coordination problems
- Irritability or depressed affect (including unusual sleepiness) as a neonate
- Difficulty with movement, cuddliness, grasp and release, self-feeding, and head control to look around; inability to change position per developmental level

- Persistent primitive reflexes
- Communication problems, either in language or speech proficiency

Physical Examination
- Skin: Dermatologic signs of syndromes, such as neurofibromatosis, may be present.
- Orthopedic examination: Scoliosis, contractures, and dislocated hip may be present.
- Neurologic examination: The following may be seen:
  - Deep tendon reflexes increased
  - Tone increased, although occasionally decreased; hypotonia before 6 months old is common. Tone may also be mixed.
  - Minimal muscle atrophy
  - No fasciculations
  - Persistent primitive reflexes (e.g., tonic neck and Moro after 6 months old)
  - Delayed reflexes (e.g., parachute reflex remains absent after 9 to 10 months old; side-protective reflexes remain absent after 5 months old)
  - Asymmetric movements
  - Preferred handedness before 1 to 2 years old
  - Structural defects, such as hydrocephaly or microcephaly
- Vision and hearing: Visual refractive errors occur in 50% of children; strabismus is found in 33%. Hearing problems may have resulted from the initial brain insult.
- Development: Assess gross motor, fine motor, language, and personal social skills. The Denver Developmental Screening Test II (Denver II) can be used for initial screening. Motor milestones are commonly delayed. Note quality of movements (e.g., smoothness of gait, grasping, clarity of speech).
- Feeding: Note a reversed swallow wave; uncoordinated suck and swallow; decreased tone of the lips, tongue, and cheeks; increased gag reflex; involuntary tongue and lip movements; increased sensitivity to food stimuli; poor occlusion; and delayed inhibition of the suck reflex.
- Evaluate the diet, height, weight, and BMI for adequate nutrition.

Diagnostic Studies
- Imaging studies. A CT scan can be obtained to identify brain malformations. An MRI will aid the visualization of structures and abnormalities that are nearer to bony structures.
- Chromosomal and metabolic studies. These studies can be done to identify genetic disorders, especially single-gene defects.
- Lumbar puncture if sepsis is suspected.

Differential Diagnosis

The first and main requirement is to differentiate central from peripheral disorders. CP is always central and is characterized by brisk deep tendon reflexes. Many other conditions can have CP motor involvement features. These conditions include sepsis from intrauterine infections, fetal alcohol syndrome, hydrocephalus, tumors, agenesis of the corpus callosum or other brain malformations, Tay-Sachs disease, phenylketonuria, Lesch-Nyhan syndrome, spinal cord injury, hypothyroidism, muscle diseases, seizures, and many genetic and metabolic disorders (e.g., cerebral folate deficiency) (Djukic, 2007; Steinfeld et al, 2009). Mental retardation results in delayed milestones but should not result in increased reflexes. Neuromuscular disorders are associated with signs of weakness, muscle atrophy, and decreased deep tendon reflexes. These disorders typically present with a missed milestone.

Management

The management of children with CP described here can serve as a model for the management of children with a variety of neurologic problems.

- *Referral of suspected cases.* Children with CP should be evaluated and cared for at centers that provide interdisciplinary caregivers, including a developmental pediatrician, gastroenterologist, orthopedist, neurologist, nurse, speech pathologist, physical and occupational therapists, education consultant and psychologist, and social worker. Care may also involve an ophthalmologist, feeding clinic and nutritionist services, and genetics counseling.
- *Family education about the diagnosis.* Families need to understand the diagnosis and its nonprogressive but incurable characteristics. They need to understand that the extent of brain damage is not always related to the extent of disability; no one can predict what the future for a given child will be. Children who receive special services—physical therapy, speech therapy, and other interventions—have better outcomes than children who are left to develop on their own. United Cerebral Palsy has educational materials and a variety of services available.
- *Family support.* Generally, families grieve when given the diagnosis of CP and need support during this time. Support groups or opportunities to meet other families with affected children are often helpful. The emotional needs of siblings must not be overlooked. The social worker can be very helpful to families trying to cope with complex health problems.
- *Financial resources.* CP services are long term and expensive. Many children will be eligible for Supplemental Security Income or state program benefits for the severely handicapped. Respite care may be available. The Individuals with Disabilities Education Act of 1997 (IDEA) requires children with disabilities to be assessed for and instructed in the use of assistive devices along with appropriate referrals to regional centers. Some insurance companies try to avoid the costs of long-term care and therapy. Medical social workers and public health nurses can be very helpful in connecting families to appropriate services.
- *Nutrition.* Children with CP often have inadequate nutrition because of their problems with biting, sucking, chewing, swallowing, and self-feeding. Additionally, children with athetosis may need as much as 50% to 100% more calories to support their increased caloric needs because of their constant writhing movements. Children with spasticity, on the other hand, may need fewer calories because of their decreased movements. Occasionally, the problems are so severe that a gastrostomy is needed, sometimes with fundoplication to prevent reflux and aspiration. Special positioning, feeding therapy, and special feeding devices can help. High nutrient density is a key to providing a nutritious diet (i.e., getting more nutrients into the same volume of food) (also see Chapter 10). Feeding clinics are often helpful.

- *Elimination.* Constipation is common because of lack of exercise, inadequate fluid and fiber intake, medications, poor positioning, low abdominal muscle tone, and other factors. Stool softeners, such as docusate sodium, may help. Laxatives, such as senna concentrate or Milk of Magnesia, may be useful but should not be used long term. Osmotic agents may also be used (e.g., polyethylene glycol). Bladder control and urinary retention are also problems in CP; these children are three times more likely to suffer UTIs (Richardson and Palmer, 2009).
- Most children achieve bladder control between 3 and 10 years old. For some, toilet training may be difficult, especially for those with mental retardation.
- *Dentistry.* Orofacial muscle tone can contribute to malocclusion. Problems with oral mobility make daily dental hygiene difficult, leading to more gum disease. The side effects of some seizure medications can include swollen gums and tooth decay. A careful dental care program is necessary (see Chapter 33: Dental Care of Children with Extra Needs).
- *Drooling.* Inability to manage oral secretions results in drooling. Social isolation, wet clothing, skin excoriation, malodorous breath, discomfort, choking, gagging, and aspiration can make these oral secretions a serious problem. The anticholinergic, glycopyrrolate, is approved for use in those 3 to 16 years old with chronic excessive drooling from neurologic conditions. This cherry-flavored oral solution (1 mg/5 mL) is dosed at 0.05 to 1 mg by mouth two or three times daily. Side effects may be problematic (e.g., dry mouth, vomiting, constipation, flushing, urinary retention, and nasal congestion). Clinical improvement in drooling has been demonstrated in up to 78% of children and adolescents who used this drug (Waknine, 2010). Surgical intervention is a last resort and commonly involves removing the submandibular gland or nerves, or cutting or rerouting the salivary duct.
- *Respiratory.* Positioning problems, an increase in gastroesophageal reflux disorder, and difficulty in clearing secretions place children with CP at higher risk for respiratory problems, notably pneumonias (especially from aspiration). The duration of respiratory symptoms with upper respiratory infections (URIs) is increased in these children because they may have congenital paralysis or sleep-related obstruction (Daniel, 2006; Hill et al, 2009). A tracheotomy may be necessary in severe cases of upper airway obstruction or difficulty.
- *Skin.* The skin in sedentary children is more likely to break down and cause decubitus. There is an increased incidence of skin latex allergies with CP (Behrman and Adler, 2008).
- *Movement and mobility.* Positioning and seating, standing, transportation, bathing, dressing, mobility for play and getting to school are important to assess and manage. Occupational and physical therapists are essential to these aspects of care, and families need their help incorporating various strategies into their homes and lifestyles. The goals of therapy are to improve physical conditioning and gain maximal independence in mobility, fine motor activities, self-care, and communication by promoting efficient movement patterns, inhibiting primitive reflexes, and achieving isolated extremity movements. Bracing, postural support and seating systems, adaptive devices, and early intervention programs beginning in infancy are important. Open-front

walkers, quadrupedal canes, gait poles, wheelchairs, and motorized wheelchairs are beneficial in helping children explore their environment more efficiently. Although the condition is not progressive in terms of the brain lesion, contractures, scoliosis, dislocated hips, and other deformities can develop if the child is allowed to maintain abnormal positions for long periods; range-of-motion exercises are a long-term need. Orthopedic care may be necessary. Constraint-induced therapy (the use of the more functional side is restricted) can both improve mobility function and sustain function longer than conventional physical therapy in children with CP (Taub et al, 2004).

- *Medications.* Antispasmodic medications (baclofen, tizanidine, diazepam, and dantrolene) may be used to minimize contractures and spasticity. They are appropriate for children needing only a mild decrease in their muscle tone or in those with widespread spasticity. For results, dosages often need to be high, and side effects can result (drowsiness, upset stomach, high blood pressure, and possible liver damage with chronic use).

- Botulinum toxin A injections are used to eliminate pain, minimize contractures, delay or prevent surgery, and maximize function (Quality Standards Subcommittee of the American Academy of Neurology and the Practice Committee of the Child Neurology Society et al, 2010). Although botulinum toxin A has become standard treatment in pediatrics, it is used off-label (NINDS, 2010b). Its use is dependent on the recommendation of—and after a thorough evaluation by—a pediatric physiatrist, pediatric neurologist, or pediatric orthopedic surgeon, and after input of therapists and family. It is injected directly into muscles (sometimes guided by an electromyogram or electrical stimulation). The child may experience mild flu-like symptoms and transient worsening of spasticity; for this reason, injections are best followed by physical and occupational therapies that help strengthen the antagonist and agonist muscles (NINDS, 2010b). The dosage administered depends on which muscles are being selected and muscle size. Results are generally seen within 5 to 7 days and last 3 to 4 months. The toxin has been safely used in infants older than 1 month. Resistance can occur because neutralizing antibodies can develop. Therefore, only the smallest possible effective dose must be used, and at least 3 months must lapse between injections. Contraindications include diffuse hypertonia, myasthenia gravis (MG), motor neuron disease, injection into an infected muscle, caution in pregnancy (fetal complications have been seen in animal studies), and caution when it is coadministered with an aminoglycoside or another agent that interferes with neuromuscular transmission (toxin effect can be increased) (Quality Standards Subcommittee of the American Academy of Neurology and the Practice Committee of the Child Neurology Society et al, 2010). The numerous side effects should be thoroughly understood by care providers.

- *Communication.* With the combined problems of lack of oral-motor control and the high incidence of mental retardation, communication can be a problem. Speech therapy may be of assistance; augmentative devices, such as computers with voices, can allow for language development and communication of needs even without oral speech. Hearing deficits need to be identified and managed by an audiologist.

- *Vision.* Visual acuity, eye tracking, and binocularity are key factors to be assessed by a pediatric ophthalmologist (Brunstrom and Tilton, 2009).

- *Osteopenia.* Individuals with CP are at risk of bone density loss secondary to their inability to ambulate and place weight on their bones. Some medical providers prescribe bisphosphonates off-label to children (NINDS, 2010b).

- *Pain.* Spastic muscles, strain on compensatory muscles, and frequent or irregularly occurring muscle spasms can cause chronic and acute pain. Diazepam, gabapentin, and complementary therapies (distraction, biofeedback, relaxation, therapeutic massage) can help (NINDS, 2010b).

- *Special Education.* Early intervention programs and specialized educational programs through school systems are often beneficial.

- *Other Treatments.* Surgery is used to release contractures or to sever overactivated nerves (called a selective dorsal root rhizotomy). Selective dorsal root rhizotomy (of spinal nerves) plus intrathecal baclofen decrease spasticity and increase range of motion of affected limbs. Intrathecal baclofen uses an implantable pump to deliver the drug, a muscle relaxant. The pump is programmable with an electronic telemetry wand. Pumps have been successfully implanted in children as young as 3 years of age; this treatment has small but significant risks of complications. It is most efficacious in children who have some motor movement control and who have few muscles to treat that are not fixed or rigid (NINDS, 2010b). Intense physical therapy is an instrumental adjunct treatment.

- Strength training can help with balance and weakness. Functional electrical stimulation (involves insertion of a microscopic wireless device into specific muscles or nerves) has been used to activate and strengthen muscles in the hand, shoulder, and ankle. It should be regarded as experimental in CP and is used only as an alternative treatment if other treatments fail to relax muscles or relieve pain (NINDS, 2010b).

- Alcohol "washes" (injections of alcohol into targeted nerves) are sometimes used. Benefits can last from months to 2 years or more; side effects include significant risk of pain or numbness. Research is moving in the direction of developing chemodenervation techniques that deliver injected antispasmodic medications more precisely to target and relax muscles (NINDS, 2010b).

- "Patterning" is a controversial physical therapy (child is taught elementary movements, such as crawling, before advancing to walking skills). The American Academy of Pediatrics and other organizations do not endorse this technique because of the lack of evidence-based studies. Likewise, the Bobath technique (involves inhibiting abnormal movement patterns in favor of more normal ones) has provoked strong reservations about efficacy. Conduction education (use of rhythmic activities combined with physical maneuvers on special equipment) has failed to consistently produce improvement (NINDS, 2010b).

Complications

Approximately one half of children with CP develop seizures within the first year or two (Dodson, 2008). Children who receive no intervention have poorer functional abilities; they make less progress developmentally and are at risk for

BOX 27-2	Problems Associated With Cerebral Palsy

Cognitive
Learning disabilities
Mental retardation

Seizure Disorders
Language and Speech Disorders
Articulation
Vocal strength and quality
Language processing

Vision
Refractive errors
Strabismus
Amblyopia
Cataracts
Retinopathy of prematurity
Cortical blindness
Homonymous hemianopsia (hemiplegia)

Hearing
Conductive
Sensorineural

Other Sensory
Tactile hypersensitivity or hyposensitivity
Dyspraxia
Balance and movement problems
Proprioception difficulties
Stereognosis

Motor
Prolonged primitive reflexes
Absence of protective reflexes
Delayed motor milestones
Hip subluxation and dislocation
Scoliosis
Contractures

Feeding and Eating Problems
Chewing, sucking, and swallowing deficits
Drooling
Hypoxemia
Fatigue
Underweight and overweight
Gastroesophageal reflux
Aspiration

Bowel
Constipation
Encopresis

Urinary
Bladder control
Urinary retention
Urinary tract infections

Dental
Malocclusions
Enamel deficits and caries
Gum hyperplasia (with phenytoin)

Pulmonary
Respiratory infections
Pneumonia

Skin
Decubitus
Latex allergy

Behavioral and Emotional
Behavioral disorders
Attention-deficit disorder, with and without hyperactivity
Self-injurious behaviors
Depression
Autism
Growth failure
Other

Data from Jackson Allen P, Vessey J: *Primary care of the child with a chronic condition*, ed 5, St Louis, 2010, Mosby.

unnecessary contractures and deformities. Box 27-2 lists associated problems seen in CP. Children who are immobile, who are profoundly retarded, or who need special feeding have a decreased life expectancy (Katz, 2003).

Prevention and Screening
The incidence of CP can be decreased to some extent through good prenatal care. Recent research is centered on several processes believed to play a causative role in CP. These research endeavors include identifying genes that may be associated with abnormal neuronal migration; evaluating the role that excessive amounts of glutamate in the brain play in overexcitation and death of neurons; investigating whether synthetic neuroprotective substances can be developed (neurotrophins) and given to an infant after stroke or hypoxia; and continuing to evaluate the relationship between elevations in interferons or other inflammatory cytokines that result from maternal infection and interrupt normal fetal brain development. Also, RH incompatibility during pregnancy may cause CP in the

child if not treated (NINDS, 2010b). During the 28th week of pregnancy, immunoglobulin (RhoGAM) can be administered to the mother to prevent CP in this situation.

BELL PALSY
Description
Bell palsy is sudden, acute unilateral paralysis or weakening of any facet of the facial nerve without sensory loss. There is edema of CN VII and venous congestion in areas of the nerve canal. It is conjectured that the disease stems more from a postinfectious (especially herpetic) allergic response or immune demyelinating facial neuritis rather than from viral invasion. Implicated infectious agents include Epstein-Barr (20% of cases), mumps, herpes simplex and herpes zoster, and Lyme disease (Williams and Maria, 2009). There may be a genetic predisposition that involves trigeminal and auditory nerve pathways. Onset is rapid and can progress to maximal intensity within hours. Symptoms may last for 1 to 9 weeks (average 2 to 4 weeks) with spontaneous remission and recovery.

Clinical Findings

History. The patient may initially experience localized pain or tingling in one ear and then experience sagging on one side of the face with the eyelid completely or partially closed. The history usually reveals a URI within the previous 2 weeks or exposure to cold temperature.

Physical Examination. A neurologic assessment of all facial nerve functions may be difficult in children and is not critical to make an accurate diagnosis. The clinician should note the following:

- Unilateral motor changes in the forehead, cheek, and perioral area; face muscles pull to the normal side when the child makes facial expressions
- Normal blood pressure
- Dribbling liquids from the weak side; eating and drinking are more difficult.
- Hypersensitivity to loud noises
- Eyelid fails to close on the affected side, and complete blinking may be absent; exposure keratitis may be present.
- Taste (50% of patients; anterior two thirds of tongue), lacrimation, and salivation may be impaired.
- No limb weakness
- Any skin lesions to suggest herpes on the affected side of the face (would indicate active viral infection of the nerve or its motor neurons)

Diagnostic Studies. It is widely accepted that diagnostic testing is not indicated unless the patient fails to improve over a 6-week period or other neurologic symptoms occur.

Differential Diagnosis

Included in the differential diagnosis are Guillain-Barré syndrome (usually includes an additional symptom of absent tendon reflexes of limbs), hypertension, congenital absence of the depressor angularis oris muscle, infection, trauma (the use of forceps during delivery can cause a facial nerve compression neuropathy that spontaneously resolves within a few days to weeks), Melkersson syndrome (involves recurrent facial palsies with swollen lips, tongue, cheeks, or eyelids), Möbius syndrome, acute otitis media, poliomyelitis, histiocytosis X, varicella, post-DTP (diphtheria-tetanus-pertussis) vaccine reaction, facial nerve tumors, neurofibroma, infiltration of facial nerves with leukemic cells, rhabdomyosarcoma of the middle ear, and brainstem infarcts.

Management

If lid closure is incomplete, prescribe methylcellulose eyedrops or ocular lubricant to the affected eye several times daily and patch the eye if the child plays outdoors, during active play, and when sleeping. Steroid use is still somewhat controversial but its use has demonstrated improvement in outcome (oral prednisone is dosed at 1 mg/kg/day for 1 week, then tapered for 1 week; start within the first 3-5 days) (Sarnat, 2007). Because of a possible etiology of herpes, some practitioners administer acyclovir within 72 hours of symptom onset and in conjunction with the steroid therapy, dosing at 40 mg/kg/day (Williams and Maria, 2009). Its use remains controversial in pediatrics (Sarnat, 2007). Worster and colleagues' (2010) research failed to demonstrate any significant benefit when acyclovir was added to a steroid-only regimen.

Complications

The younger the child, the more complete the remission, usually 100% (Williams and Maria, 2009). If recovery is incomplete, lack of salivation in response to food, lack of lacrimation, facial contractures, and tics may occur.

EPILEPSY AND SEIZURE DISORDERS

Description and Epidemiology

Seizures are due to the misfiring of the cortical neurons of the brain. Convulsive seizures occur when misfiring causes episodes of involuntary contraction of voluntary muscles. Table 27-4 summarizes the types of seizures. When seizures are recurrent and unrelated to fever, the disorder is called *epilepsy*. Seizures represent either brain dysfunction or significant underlying disorders. A patient may demonstrate characteristics of more than one type of seizure. Epilepsy most often has two characteristics: the seizures recur, and the seizure events are unprovoked.

Different kinds of seizures arise from disorders in diverse parts of the brain. Seizures can result from a variety of genetic, symptomatic, or idiopathic conditions. More than 30,000 genes are expressed in the brain, and approximately 20% of individuals with epilepsy have a genetic etiology. Several familial epilepsies have been identified. These include benign neonatal convulsions, juvenile myoclonic epilepsy, and progressive myoclonic epilepsy (Camfield and Camfield, 2009).

Clinical Findings

History. Historical questioning should include the following:

- Description of the seizure: Focal or generalized, loss of consciousness, aura, length of postictal sleep or confusion, duration of the episode, and associated illness
- Any underlying medical diagnosis (e.g., diabetes, renal disease, cardiovascular disorder)
- Previous CNS infection or birth trauma
- Intrauterine infection, trauma, bleeding
- Toxic exposure or drug use
- Anticonvulsant medication stopped abruptly
- Recent head injury
- Family history of seizures
- Any noted missed milestones

Physical Examination. The following should be determined on physical examination:

- Focal abnormalities, weakness
- Presence of seizure activity during the examination
- Hypertension (for renal disease)
- Systemic disease
- Cardiovascular disorder
- Neurocutaneous disease, café au lait spots of neurofibromatosis, ash leaf spots or adenoma sebaceum of tuberous sclerosis, facial hemangioma of Sturge-Weber syndrome
- Signs of head trauma
- Transillumination of the skull in infants

Diagnostic Studies. These are typical diagnostic test recommendations:

- Complete blood count (CBC) (including platelets, liver function tests [LFTs])—useful for diagnostic purposes or as a baseline before anticonvulsant therapy is started
- Metabolic screen

TABLE 27-4 Classification of Seizures

Seizure Type	Age	Pattern	Comments
I. Partial or focal seizure			
A. Focal simple		Begins locally; Consciousness not impaired; lasts 10-20 seconds	Affects one hemisphere
1. With motor symptom	Any age	Any part of body: includes Jacksonian seizure	From birth trauma, inflammation, idiopathic, stroke, tumors (individual shows progressive neurologic symptoms)
2. With sensory or somatosensory symptom	Any age	"Pins and needles," numb; auras include lights, tastes, sound	
3. With autonomic symptom	Any age	Recurrent abdominal pain, headache, sweat, laugh, cry, tachycardia, dilated pupil	May have migraine quality; family history of migraine or seizures
4. Compound form	Any age		
B. Complex focal	Any age; may be hard to recognize in young child	Consciousness impaired; clonic activity, forced head/eye deviation, focal tonic posturing, automatisms—purposeless motor activities (e.g., lip smacking, repetitious swallowing/chewing, finger/hand fidgeting, tics); lasts 1-2 minutes	
1. Impaired consciousness only		Staring spell	
2. With cognitive symptom		May have confusion	
3. With affective symptom		Aura of fear	
4. With "psychosensory" symptom		May have odd smell/taste; visual or auditory hallucination	
5. With "psychomotor" symptom		Automatism	
6. Compound form			
C. Focal seizures, secondary generalized		Seizure begins in one part of body but then generalizes	Aura can let person seek safe position
II. Idiopathic localization-related seizures			
A. Benign focal (or rolandic)	4-13 years		Resolves by adolescence; treatment may not be needed
1. Diurnal		Alert; unilateral twitching, drooling, paresthesia of face, gums, tongue, buccal mucosa; may progress into hemiclonic or hemitonic movements; Advances to generalization	
2. Nocturnal			With or without postictal weakness of affected side
III. Generalized seizure			
A. Absence (Petit mal)	4-12 years	Lasts 5-30 seconds; lapses of consciousness (short staring "spells"); can have associated movements; no falling; no aura	Usually no aura; Hyperventilation for 3-4 minutes can trigger seizure; blinking lights can also trigger
B. Myoclonic (infantile spasms)	Infancy	Head drops or sudden flexing; may suddenly cry out; older children exhibit trunk or extremity flexion	Hypsarrhythmia on EEG with no normal background activity; difficult to treat
C. Clonic		Rhythmic jerking	
D. Tonic		Intense muscle contraction	
E. Tonic-clonic	Any age; most common type of seizure	Grand mal; begins with loss of consciousness; stiffening, violent jerking; postictal phase of sleep and confusion; 15% incontinent	Aura in some; may have abdominal pain or headache; life threatening if continues, producing hypercarbia, respiratory acidosis, lactic acidosis; some occur in sleep
F. Atonic	Childhood	Similar to myoclonic; aka "drop attacks;" duration <15 minutes	Child often falls; injury protection important

aka, Also known as; EEG, electroencephalogram.

- Blood glucose—standard in all patients
- Urine and serum toxicology—only if illicit drug exposure is suspected
- Lumbar puncture—only if child is younger than 6 months; any aged patient with persistent changes in mental status or failure to return to baseline functioning; patients with meningeal signs
- EEG—standard in all children after first nonfebrile seizure. An abnormal EEG supports the seizure diagnosis. However, a normal EEG when the child is not seizing does not rule out a seizure disorder. Video EEG (VEEG) over 1 to 6 days is another option to identify seizure activity.
- MRI—imaging studies are not routinely indicated if the initial seizure is followed by a normal neurologic examination and return to baseline mental status. Imaging is recommended: (1) if the patient demonstrates cognitive changes after several hours and postictal focal dysfunction (signs of increased intracranial pressure, such as found with tumors, abscesses, strokes, or vascular malformations); (2) if the seizure lasted more than 15 minutes; (3) in infants younger than 6 months old; and (4) if any new onset of focal neurologic deficit has occurred. An MRI is now the preferred imaging study over CT scans because of its increased sensitivity.
- CT scan—used only in cases of marked cognitive, motor, or neurologic dysfunction of unknown etiology (e.g., head injury, brain infection or tumor, abscesses); abnormal EEGs; or focal seizure symptoms that may or may not evolve into a generalized seizure.
- Polysomnography (simultaneous EEG, electromyogram, electrocardiogram [ECG], and electrooculogram) can be useful to assess nocturnal seizures.

Differential Diagnosis

Consider breath-holding, inattentive staring, benign shudders, self-gratification behavior, tantrums, cyclic vomiting, benign paroxysmal vertigo, syncope, migraine headaches, gastroesophageal reflux, night terrors, conversion disorder, metabolic problems, tumors or other CNS problems, or a cardiovascular problem. Vertigo has been confused with epilepsy. Tics (involuntary, spasmodic, nonrhythmic, repetitive movements) are stereotypic but not associated with impaired consciousness and at times can be suppressed by the patient.

Pseudoseizures. A pseudoseizure may be difficult to distinguish from true seizures, even after direct observation. It is the most common manifestation of a conversion disorder in children (Kronenberger and Dunn, 2009). Suspect pseudoseizures in a patient with a documented underlying seizure disorder who has gained more recent control; 15% to 30% of children have coexisting epilepsy (Kronenberger and Dunn, 2009). In such cases the pseudoseizures serve as attention-getting behaviors for the child who misses the attention gained before control. Pseudoseizures also may be seen in adolescents; more often in girls than in boys (3:1). Stress and anxiety, especially within the family, are found in 50% of cases. Abuse and/or traumatic injury can be seen in as many as 30% to 50% of these children (Kronenberger and Dunn, 2009). Distinguishing characteristics of pseudoseizures include the following:

- Unilaterally or bilaterally coordinated motor activity more like thrashing and jerking (scissor-like movements) rather than characteristic tonic-clonic movements; no aura or complaints of malaise; heart palpitations; feeling like choking before seizure onset
- Occur only before a witness; occur at home; do not interrupt play
- Normally reactive pupils to light
- Are situation specific and have a gradual onset
- No associated tongue biting or injury
- Have an abrupt recovery—no postictal state
- Discomfort, distress expressed; sometimes ataxia, fumbling; consciousness may be impaired, but the patient is not unconscious
- No incontinence
- No EEG changes, even during episodes

Treatment for pseudoseizures involves developing alternative gains to seizure behavior. Most children stop after the diagnosis is made and interventions are in place. A referral for counseling may be indicated in a multifaceted approach of therapy and drugs for psychological illness, depending on the etiology. Assess previous somatic complaints, stress factors, peers, family, illness modeled in the home. If suspected, but the history is unclear, a VEEG should be considered. No anticonvulsants are used in the case of children who do not have an underlying seizure disorder. Comorbidities of major mood disorders have been seen in up to 30% of cases (Kronenberger and Dunn, 2009).

Management

Referral. If a seizure disorder is suspected, refer to a neurologist for diagnosis and initiation of treatment. Antiepileptic drugs (AEDs) are usually prescribed, especially after a second seizure. Delaying treatment does not affect ultimate control, but early diagnosis and intervention can often reduce the disabilities and risks associated with the condition.

Management of Stable Patients With Diagnosed Seizure Disorders. The primary care provider (PCP) can monitor stable children with seizures, including continuing the prescription for their anticonvulsant(s), monitoring drug levels, and performing case management. Approximately one third of children who have a history of cognitive or motor impairments will have a recurrent unprovoked seizure within 1 year.

Drug Monitoring. All providers working with patients receiving anticonvulsants should be familiar with the common drugs (Table 27-5) and their major side effects. Helping with compliance issues is also a component of the monitoring role (also see discussion in Appendix A regarding methods to increase compliance). If possible, start with one drug with the fewest side effects and describe how the drug works with the child and parent, with an explanation of side effects. Key points for drug monitoring include:

- Patients can be controlled with subtherapeutic blood levels.
- Patients can be free of side effects at levels beyond the therapeutic range.
- Phenytoin saturates the enzyme system; therefore, even a small increase in dosage can cause a marked increase in blood levels.
- Half-lives and steady state concentrations vary by patient and when new AEDs are introduced or when other non-AEDs being taken (e.g., antibiotics, antipyretics). Half-lives are longer with the introduction to a new drug; steady concentrations (and elimination) of the drug are achieved at five half-lives.
- If gastrointestinal side effects occur, decreasing the dosage and increasing the frequency of administration may help;

TABLE 27-5	Antiepileptic Drug Therapy for Children*		
Seizure Type	**Drug**	**Therapeutic Blood Levels (g/mL)**	**Laboratory Monitoring**
Partial, generalized tonic-clonic in children >2 years old; contraindicated for absence and myoclonic	Carbamazepine	4-12	Baseline CBC at 6-12 weeks, then annually; drug blood levels
Partial, generalized, status epilepticus	Phenytoin	10-20	Drug blood levels
Simple partial, tonic-clonic	Phenobarbital	15-40	None
Absence	Ethosuximide	40-100	None
First-line generalized seizures if >10 years old, myoclonic, absence	Valproic acid	50-120	Baseline CBC with differential, LFTs; CBC with differential, SGOT, and drug levels especially in the first 6 months
Partial, tonic-clonic, myoclonic	Primidone	5-12	None
Partial, myoclonic, infantile spasm	Vigabatrin	1.4-14	Visual fields every 3-6 months
Partial, generalized, Lennox-Gastaut syndrome	Felbamate[†]	Not monitored	LFTs, CBC with differential, platelets, reticulocyte count monthly (requires close monitoring)
Refractory partial-onset, rolandic	Gabapentin—usually an adjunct drug with other AEDs used for partial seizures	5-15	Depends on other AED used
Partial, Lennox-Gastaut syndrome, absence, atonic, juvenile myoclonic	Lamotrigine	2-20	
Partial, generalized and Lennox-Gastaut (adjunct drug); partial, tonic-clonic	Topiramate	2-25	None
Partial	Oxcarbazepine Lacosamide	5-50	None
Partial, generalized	Zonisamide	10-40	None
Partial	Levetiracetam	20-60	None
Partial, generalized	Tiagabine—adjunct drug only	5-70	None
Partial, absence, myoclonic, infantile spasms, Lennox-Gastaut syndrome, akinetic	Clonazepam	>0.013	LFTs, CBC with differential

*See an appropriate pharmacology reference for dosing.
[†]Drug used only for refractory epilepsy; now approved for use in children ≥2 years old with Lennox-Gastaut syndrome; otherwise for use in children ≥14 years old.
AEDs, Antiepileptic drugs; *CBC,* complete blood count; *LFTs,* liver function tests; *SGOT,* serum glutamic-oxaloacetic transaminase or AST.
Data from Fenichel G: *Clinical pediatric neurology: a signs and symptoms approach,* ed 4, Philadelphia, 2001, Saunders; Johnston MV: Seizures in childhood. In Kliegman RM, Behrman RE, Jenson HB et al, editors: *Nelson textbook of pediatrics,* ed 18, Philadelphia, 2007, Saunders, pp 2457-2475; Riviello JJ: General concepts in seizure management. In Burg FD, Ingelfinger JR, Polin RA et al, editors: *Current pediatric therapy,* ed 18, Philadelphia, 2006, Saunders; White HS, Wilcox, KS: Comparative anticonvulsants profile and proposed mechanism of action of antiepileptic drugs. In Pellock JM, Bourgeois BFD, Dodson WE, editors: *Pediatric epilepsy diagnosis and therapy,* ed 3, New York, 2008, Demos.

try changing to an enteric-coated pill or taking the drug after eating.
- Administer drug twice daily or daily for better compliance.
- The first signs of toxicity usually include sedation, changes in behavior, and changes in cognition; other drug toxicities may cause decreases in memory and attention span or interpersonal relationship difficulties. It is important to note that some patients may exhibit these changes and have drug levels within the normal range.
- Metabolites of the drugs can cause hypersensitivity side effects.
- Monitor routine drug levels based on the clinical picture with trough levels (random drug levels are rarely helpful).

- Some herbal products interfere with seizure control (e.g., ginkgo and kava) (Fu et al, 2008). Also see Table 42-2 in Chapter 42.

Antiepileptic Drug Withdrawal. After 2 years or longer without seizures, most pediatric neurologists will consider gradually withdrawing anticonvulsant therapy after obtaining an EEG. Patients with histories of benign epilepsy with rolandic spikes or with idiopathic generalized seizures are more likely to be successfully withdrawn. Those with complex partial seizures and juvenile myoclonic seizures are more likely to have a recurrence once medication has been withdrawn. Drug withdrawal should occur over a span of several months because abrupt weaning might cause status epilepticus (SE) (Shih and Ochoa, 2009).

Children with mental retardation, CP, focal motor deficits, age of onset younger than 2 years, symptomatic seizures, and abnormal EEGs are not appropriate candidates for weaning. Weaning is supervised closely, with one drug removed at a time. Of children who have been seizure-free for 2 years and have low risk factors, 70% to 75% remain seizure-free without drugs. If seizures do recur, 50% do so within the first 6 months of weaning and 60% to 75% within 2 years. Three fourths of recurrences occur during weaning or within the first year (Shinnar and O'Dell, 2008). If the onset of seizures occurred during a time of anoxia, head injury, meningitis, or encephalitis, the AED treatment can be stopped after recovery from the condition is complete. The child can always be restarted should there be a recurrence.

Ketogenic Diet. The ketogenic diet is useful in young children with all types of seizures, particularly in those with myoclonic forms, infantile spasms, atonic-kinetic types, and with the mixed seizures of Lennox-Gastaut syndrome (Kossoff et al, 2009). The diet is considered when the side effects of AEDs are intolerable or when allergies to AEDs preclude administration. The ideal child is between 2 and 5 years old because the desired steady state of ketosis is easier to maintain. The diet is stringent and requires utmost vigilance to the ratios of calories, protein, fat, carbohydrates, vitamins, and minerals. It is best managed under very tight control with medical and dietetic leadership. Side effects usually involve abdominal pain and diarrhea. A prescreening process, including psychological testing to determine the child's and family's emotional functioning, coping, and problem-solving abilities, is recommended. A dietitian should screen the child for nutrition and growth status. A nurse should interview the family for understanding of and education about the protocol. The diet is started while the child is admitted to the hospital, where metabolic and neurologic states can be monitored. A follow-up study of children who had remained on a ketogenic diet for 3 to 6 years demonstrated that 34% had a greater than 90% reduction in their seizures (Nordli and DeVivo, 2008).

Surgery. Surgical interventions have been successful in helping some children with complex partial seizures; however selection of appropriate children must be done with great care. *Focal resection* surgery is used only in children whose epileptic focus is localized, who have failed to respond to AEDs, and whose development has been assessed over time. Seizure-free rates after resection have been documented to reach 60% to 80%, with minimal loss of neurologic function depending on the type of surgery (Duchowny, 2008). *Hemispherectomy or interhemispherectomy* can be curative. Side effects of the surgery include hemiparesis, incontinence, stuttering, and poor hand coordination. *Temporal lobotomies* are an option for treating intractable partial complex seizures localized to the temporal area; side effects are aphasia and superior quadrant visual loss. Slightly more than 50% of candidates achieve freedom from seizures. *Callosotomy and vagus nerve stimulation*, as palliative surgeries, are options for children with multiple regions of hemispheric involvement that result in intractable seizures. In *vagus nerve stimulation* (VNS), a programmed device—"pacemaker of the brain"—is implanted in the anterior chest wall. A wire wraps around the left vagus nerve and sends regular, mild pulses of electrical energy to the brain via the nerve. A patient with an aura can stimulate the device to prevent a seizure. For those without an aura, the device is set on specific parameters given the patient's seizure pattern. With VNS, seizures and side effects can be better controlled. Children as well as adults are good candidates.

Counseling. Older children and parents need to understand the diagnosis, treatment (including specifics of the prescribed AED), necessary follow-up, and long-term prognoses. Myths (e.g., epilepsy is synonymous with mental retardation) and negative attitudes continue to surround epilepsy and may need to be addressed. Laws vary from state to state regarding driving, but generally a teenager who has been seizure-free for 2 years and has demonstrated good drug compliance should be allowed to drive. One study revealed that fatal car crashes attributed to seizures were rare versus those caused by other medical conditions (Tiamkao et al, 2009). Many antiseizure medications are teratogenic; therefore, contraception is essential for sexually active females.

Children with epilepsy may experience social stigmas and problems with self-esteem. Other mental health problems may also occur in these children as they try to cope with a chronic disease. Parents are encouraged to treat children as normally as possible and seek appropriate support groups.

Safety. Uncontrolled seizures can present safety hazards for an unsupervised child. The child and family need to consider the situations that the child will be in and be sure that someone knows what to do if a seizure occurs, including school personnel. Safety helmets worn at all times are sometimes warranted if falls and head injury occur frequently. Swimming alone is never recommended, but swimming, contact sports, and climbing are to be allowed if the child is well controlled and there is constant supervision during these activities. Refer to Chapter 13 for a further discussion of sports and activities for those with seizure disorders.

Immunizations. The decision to give pertussis vaccine to children with neurologic seizures or other neurologic conditions needs to be made on an individual basis. Children who will be in childcare centers, special clinics, or residential care centers should be immunized if possible. Progressive neurologic conditions with developmental delays or nonfebrile seizures are reasons for deferral of pertussis vaccine until the underlying cause has been determined. Infants and children with a personal history of seizures have been noted to have an increased risk of post-DPT immunization seizures, less so with the acellular pertussis form of DPT (DTaP). These seizures generally have been found to be febrile, self-limited, brief, and generalized. There has been no evidence that such febrile seizures lead to brain damage, predispose one to epilepsy, or aggravate neurologic disorders. Other neurologic conditions that predispose one to seizures or neurologic deterioration or a seizure history in an infant younger than 1 year old should result in consideration of deferral of pertussis immunization until the child is near or at 1 year of age (AAP, 2009). DTaP and acetaminophen at the time of administration and every 4 hours for the first 24 hours may be given to allay concerns of fever or other adverse effects. The efficacy of using acetaminophen prior to and following immunizations is discussed in Chapter 23.

Complications

Status epilepticus (SE) are seizures that may be continuous, or frequent, without recovery between episodes. *Nonconvulsive SE* is characterized by continuous abnormal EEG activity without tonic-clonic activity. *Convulsive SE* typically involves tonic-clonic activity in two or more seizures between which there is no recovery of consciousness or a prolonged single seizure lasting more than 30 minutes (it has been suggested that the seizure duration criteria be shortened to 5 minutes) (Mahajan, 2009). A child who has generalized tonic-clonic seizures and who is in SE is at risk for brain damage and intellectual deficits (Leszczyszyn and Pellock, 2008; Prasad, 2009). Lack of oxygenation, decreased cerebral perfusion, metabolic acidosis, hypoglycemia, hyperkalemia, lactic acidosis, increased temperature, and increased intracranial pressure can all result in significant risk of morbidity and mortality. Such an occurrence needs to be handled as a medical emergency. SE can be triggered by an acute brain infection, progressive neurologic disease, AED failure, or, rarely, a febrile seizure in an otherwise healthy child without other risk factors. However, most cases of SE occur in children with underlying neurologic deficits. It is difficult to diagnose SE in children with absence or complex partial seizures because the children may just appear confused (Leszczyszyn and Pellock, 2008). Adverse outcomes can include behavioral problems, mental retardation, and focal motor deficits. Diazepam rectal gel is recommended for use by health care providers, parents, and caregivers (including school personnel) in children more than 2 years old who have a seizure lasting more than 5 minutes. It is administered once and takes effect in 5 to 15 minutes. Its use has decreased emergency department visits by 67%; it is safe at higher than recommended doses; and it has less than a 1% incidence of respiratory depression. The most common side effect is somnolence. It is available in a premeasured portable syringe and dosed according to age and weight (Leszczyszyn and Pellock, 2008).

FEBRILE SEIZURES

Description and Epidemiology

Febrile seizures are the most common type of seizures in children. They are brief, generalized, clonic or tonic-clonic in nature, and can be either simple or complex. A concurrent illness is present with rapid fever rise to at least more than 102.2° F (39° C), but the fever is not necessarily that high at the time of the seizure. Little postictal confusion is associated with febrile seizures. Simple febrile seizures last less than 15 minutes and do not recur during the same febrile illness period. Complex febrile seizures last longer than 15 minutes, can recur on the same day, and can have focal attributes (even during the postictal phase). Most (57%) febrile seizures occur 1 to 24 hours after fever onset (Wolf and Shinnar, 2009).

The etiology of febrile seizures is unclear and by definition excludes seizures that are caused by intracranial illness or are related to an underlying CNS problem. The risk is higher in children with a family medical history for febrile seizures or in those with predisposing factors (e.g., neonatal intensive care unit [NICU] stay more than 30 days, developmental delay, daycare attendance). Additionally, it is conjectured that these seizures may be disease-specific or related to peak temperature reached during the febrile episode (Wolf and Shinnar, 2009).

Two percent to 4% of all children have febrile seizures, depending on ethnicity (e.g., Japanese children have a 9% to 10% risk factor). Febrile seizures generally occur in children between 1 month and 5 years of age with 93% occurring between 6 months and 3 years old. Fifty percent will recur in the first 6 months and 90% within 2 years; the overall risk

of recurrence is between 30% and 50% (Wolf and Shinnar, 2009).

Clinical Findings

History. Include the following:

- Description of seizure duration, type (generalized or focal), frequency in 24 hours
- Relationship of the seizure to a febrile episode and level of temperature
- Any abnormal neurologic findings noted before the seizure (is not consistent with a febrile seizure)
- Family history of afebrile or febrile seizures
- Maternal smoking in the perinatal period
- Prematurity or neonatal hospitalizations for more than 28 days
- Parents' perception of development of child

Physical Examination. The physical examination is the same as that described earlier for seizures.

Diagnostic Studies. Diagnostic studies include the following (Wolf and Shinnar, 2009):

- Lumbar puncture in infants younger than 12 months old and who may also have used an antibiotic prior to seizure onset, and/or who have signs of meningeal irritation (Baren, 2009; Ghotbi and Shiva, 2009).
- Blood glucose in all children
- CBC, calcium, electrolytes, urinalysis are optional but frequently included
- EEG if neurologic signs are present or seizure was atypical
- MRI for complex febrile seizure features or if any doubt exists about the diagnosis

Differential Diagnosis

Consider sepsis, meningitis, metabolic or toxic encephalopathies, hypoglycemia, anoxia, trauma, tumor, and hemorrhage. Febrile delirium and febrile shivering can be confused with seizures. Breath-holding spells can mimic febrile seizures; however, the former are always related to crying or tantrums. Febrile seizures come at unpredictable times during sleep, eating, play, or other generally calm times and are related to the onset of an illness. Epileptic seizures occur without concurrent illness and at unpredictable times.

Management

- Protect the airway, breathing, and circulation if the seizure is still occurring. Place the child in a side-lying position to prevent aspiration or airway obstruction.
- Do not put anything into the child's mouth during the seizure.
- Time the duration of the seizure and observe whether it is focal or generalized.
- Reduce the fever with acetaminophen or ibuprofen (oral or suppository) after the seizure has stopped, although the use of antipyretics will not necessarily prevent another febrile seizure.
- The child should be seen shortly after the seizure. Advise transport to an emergency center if the seizure lasts more than 10 minutes.
- Most medical providers agree that anticonvulsants are not recommended for febrile seizures, but they may be considered if the child has abnormal neurologic findings

or developmental delays; the initial seizure was complex febrile, *and* there is a family history of afebrile seizures; or if the child has recurrent, prolonged simple febrile seizures.

Prophylaxis for Those With Recurrent Febrile Seizures

Prolonged anticonvulsant prophylaxis is not recommended. Phenytoin and carbamazepine antiepileptics are not useful; sodium valproic acid can be effective but the side effects do not justify its use (Wolf and Shinnar, 2009). If prophylaxis is indicated, diazepam by mouth 0.3 mg/kg every 8 hours (1 mg/kg/24 hr) can be given over the course of the febrile illness (usually for 2 to 3 days). Another approach is to use rectal diazepam in a gel form (dosed at 0.5 mg/kg for children 2 to 5 years of age) at the time of a seizure; this will prevent recurrence for approximately 12 hours. Side effects of diazepam include transient ataxia, lethargy, and irritability that can be decreased by adjusting the dosage (Johnston, 2007). An alternative to diazepam, if transient ataxia or lethargy exists, is daily phenobarbital to achieve a blood level of 15 mcg/mL. Phenobarbital, however, has behavioral side effects that are often intolerable to the family.

Education

The family should receive information about febrile seizures, their risks, and their management. Education should include information explaining the febrile seizure; reassurance that no long-term consequences are associated with febrile seizures; information that febrile seizures recur in some children and that nothing can be done to prevent the seizures; and first-aid information in case another seizure occurs at some time. The decision to use prophylaxis is up to the parents and the PCP on a case-by-case basis. A follow-up phone call after the event is useful.

Complications

SE can result (Mahajan, 2009). Death or persisting motor deficits do not occur in patients with febrile seizures. No indication has been found that intellect or learning is impaired. An affected child has an increased risk for the development of epilepsy (less than 5%) if the seizure is prolonged and focal; if the child has repeated seizures with the same febrile episode; or if the child has had a prior neurologic deficit, a family history of epilepsy, or both. Two thirds of children who have had one simple febrile seizure will have no more. The younger the age at onset (less than 18 months old) of the first febrile seizure, the lower the temperature threshold is needed to cause the child to seize and the more likely the child is to have a recurrence.

BRACHIAL PLEXUS

Description and Epidemiology

A stretch injury of the brachial plexus in neonates can occur during a difficult vaginal delivery; such injury has also been reported following cesarean births. Injury involves the upper cervical nerve roots C5 and C6 (Erb-Duchenne palsy) and the lower cervical nerve roots C7, C8, and T1 (Klumpke palsy). The injuries are attributed to traction of the involved nerves (with mild affect) to more serious complete nerve root avulsion from the spinal cord. Partial diaphragmatic paralysis can result because innervation comes from C3, C4, and C5.

Neonatal risk factors for plexus injuries include high birthweight, shoulder dystocia, a lengthy labor, breech delivery, maternal gestational diabetes, and forceps or vacuum extraction. The incidence is approximately 3 per 1000 live births for Erb palsy. Klumpke palsy is rare (about 0.5% of plexus palsies) and is believed to be caused by delivering the head before the upper arm in a breech baby whose arms are extended. Up to 81% of infants may have nerve root avulsions of the upper roots following breech delivery (Nelson, 2009). Brachial plexus injuries can also occur to children restrained with a seatbelt during an automobile accident.

Clinical Findings

Physical Examination. Typically, soon after birth, the infant is found to have asymmetric active range of motion of the arms. On further evaluation the following may be determined:
- Erb palsy: "Waiter's tip" positioning of the arm (shoulder adduction and internal rotation with wrist flexion); there may be some sensory impairment; ability to fist is a favorable sign for a good outcome.
- Klumpke palsy: Paralyzed hand and forearm with good shoulder and elbow function.
- Total plexus avulsion: Completely flaccid upper extremity.
- The neonatal physical examination should include a careful evaluation of the Moro reflex (for symmetry), respiratory effort, evidence of Horner syndrome (ptosis, myosis [pupillary contraction], anhidrosis [absence of sweat]), and the neuromuscular function of the involved extremity. After the neonatal period, examine for posterior shoulder dislocation (would present as markedly limited external rotation) or bony deformity of the glenoid.

Diagnostic Studies. If nerve root avulsion is suspected, high-resolution CT myelography, fast spin-echo MRI, and electromyography and nerve conduction studies can be used to evaluate the injury.

Differential Diagnosis

Consider ipsilateral clavicle fracture (with resultant pain that can explain the immobility of the extremity) and Horner syndrome (also presents with ptosis, myosis, and anhidrosis in addition to avulsion of the T1 nerve root).

Management

Gentle range-of-motion exercises by parents and scheduled follow-up appointments to note progress by the PCP are routine. Surgical exploration and repair of neurolysis and nerve grafting may be undertaken in those with nerve root avulsion. However, there are no standardized outcome measurements, and comparison between studies has been inconclusive (Nelson, 2009; Terzis and Kokkalis, 2009). Older children with permanent functional limitations may be candidates for corrective shoulder surgery.

Prognosis

The majority of brachial plexus palsies (80% to 95%) spontaneously resolve over several weeks to several months. By the third month, recovery of biceps function (active motion against gravity) is evidenced. Should wrist, thumb, and finger extension occur by this time, a complete recovery can be expected. In those with nerve root avulsions, early intervention is crucial to achieve some functional recovery.

GUILLAIN-BARRÉ SYNDROME

Description

Guillain-Barré syndrome is an immune-mediated polyneuropathy that mainly affects peripheral nerves. The paralysis follows a respiratory (notably *Mycoplasma pneumoniae*) or gastrointestinal (notably *Campylobacter jejuni* or *Helicobacter pylori*) viral infection by approximately 10 days. Infection with West Nile virus has also been implicated, as well as cases that have followed immunization with rabies, influenza, polio (oral), and possibly conjugated meningococcal vaccines (Sarnat, 2007). Most patients have acute demyelinating neuropathy. Known variants include acute motor axonal degeneration (as evidenced by ophthalmoparesis, ataxia, and areflexia) and acute sensory neuropathy. New descriptions of the syndrome include reference to cranial nerve involvement and myelopathy (Morrison, 2009).

Clinical Findings

History. The following are reported:
- Nonspecific viral infection (gastrointestinal or respiratory) occurring within recent past
- Weakness or neurologic changes in sensory, motor, or visual systems. Onset is gradual, progressing in an ascending order (known as Landry ascending paralysis), starting in the lower extremities and progressing to the bulbar muscles over days or weeks; maximum weakness reached within 2 to 3 weeks.
- Fever

Physical Examination
- Tenderness and pain in muscles with palpation
- Irritability
- Inability or refusal to walk due to flaccid tetraplegia or quadriplegia
- Paresthesia may or may not be present.
- Respiratory insufficiency
- Dysphagia, facial weakness
- Extraocular muscle involvement rare; papilledema and visual acuity changes may be seen.
- Miller-Fisher syndrome may be seen (acute external ophthalmoplegia, ataxia, areflexia [often early in disease]).
- Signs of viral meningitis or meningoencephalitis
- Urinary retention or incontinence (20% of cases and is usually transient in nature)
- Blood pressure and cardiac rate changes, including bradycardia, postural hypotension, asystole

Diagnostic Studies
- CSF studies: Elevated CSF protein (usually greater than twice upper limit of normal); normal glucose, no pleocytosis (fewer than 10 white blood cells [WBCs]/mm^3)
- Negative blood cultures; viral cultures rarely conclusive
- Normal or mildly elevated creatine kinase (CK) level; antiganglioside antibodies (against GM1, GD1) may be elevated in axonal neuropathy form of the disease
- Decreased motor nerve conduction velocities; slowed sensory nerve conduction
- EMG: Shows acute denervation of muscle

Differential Diagnosis

Bickerstaff brainstem encephalitis, meningitis, meningoencephalitis, spinal muscle atrophy, HIV, metabolic diseases, and West Nile virus are included in the differential diagnoses.

Management

Hospitalization is paramount for observation and for handling complications of respiratory muscle paralysis. IVIG for 5 days is standard protocol. Plasmapheresis, and/or immunosuppressive drugs may be used in cases unresponsive to IVIG. Care is supportive (respiratory, prevention of decubitus, treatment of secondary bacterial infection). Rehabilitative therapy should begin early. Pain management should be aggressive during treatment and rehabilitation therapy (Morrison, 2009).

Complications

Chronic varieties of Guillain-Barré can occur, as evidenced by recurrence or lack of improvement of symptoms over months or years. Children may have relapses. Unresolved weakness, flaccid tetraplegia or quadriplegia, and bulbar and respiratory muscle compromise may linger or remain and last longer than 2 months. This is then considered chronic inflammatory demyelinating radiculopathy.

HEADACHES

Description and Epidemiology

Headaches of all types are one of the most common reasons parents seek medical care for their children (Raieli, 2010). They are common during childhood, increasing in frequency and incidence during adolescence. Headaches fall into two classifications—acute and chronic. Table 27-6 lists the more common types found in these classifications. A person may experience different types of headaches, and migraines may be particularly difficult to diagnose because they can be expressed differently and incompletely during childhood.

The exact physiologic mechanism and etiology for many headaches have not been conclusively determined. Headache pain occurs when pain-sensitive intracranial structures are activated. Such structures include the arteries of the circle of Willis and some of their branches, meningeal arteries, large veins and dural venous sinuses, and part of the dura near blood vessels. Muscles around the head, neck, scalp, eyes, jaw teeth, sinuses and the external carotid artery and its branches, are pain sensitive structures external to the skull. Stimulation of these structures results in more localized pain that is carried by cranial nerves V, VII, IX, and X. In contrast, intracranial stimulation refers pain imprecisely (e.g., occipital lobe tumor). The pain-sensitive blood vessels can be stimulated by inflammation, trauma, traction, compression, malignant infiltration, and other disturbances (Boes et al, 2008). Hershey and colleagues' study found that a coenzyme Q10 (CoQ10) deficiency may be present in children with frequent migraines (Hershey et al, 2007).

Studies indicate that 40% of children will experience a headache by the age of 7 years and 75% by 15 years of age (Rubin et al, 2010). In particular, migraine headaches are common in children and may go unrecognized by a health care provider (Bigal et al, 2008). Prevalence rates for migraine headaches are reported to be: age 3 (3% to 8%); age 5 (19.5%); age 7

TABLE 27-6	Most Common Types of Headaches			
Characteristic	**Vascular (Migraine)**	**Cluster**	**Chronic, Daily, Low Grade**	**Tension**
Prevalence	1.2%-3.2% occurrence in children 3-7 years old (greater incidence in males); 4%-11% occurrence prepuberty (no gender difference in incidence); 8%-23% postpuberty (female:male = 3:2)	Uncommon in children before 20 years; male predominance (Majumdar, 2009)	All ages, increased incidence in midteen females	All ages; commonly starts during adolescence; both sexes affected
History	Positive family history (90%, particularly on maternal side of family) (Haslam, 2007); can have history of motion sickness	Family history is rare Rarely begins in childhood; headaches generally recur on the same side History of cigarette smoking or second hand cigarette smoke exposure during childhood (Rozen, 2010)	May have had episodic symptoms suggestive of migraine with or without aura that evolved into daily chronic headache (70% in one study [Moore and Shevell, 2005]) Family history of migraine Chronic use of nonprescription analgesics or caffeine (including caffeinated drinks); social, psychological, emotional factors, posttrauma	Positive family history with childhood onset; fatigue, stress, depression, exertion
Pattern	Recurrent pattern May have aura; most commonly without aura Bilateral in young children changing to unilateral in adolescence Transitory neurologic changes (nausea and vomiting, malaise, personality changes, photophobia, phonophobia) Appears sick; incapacitates Periodic "ice-pick" pain on top of head described by adolescents Resolves after sleeping Pain typically lasts 1-3 hours but up to 72 hours in some cases	Unilateral headache recurring daily over 2-12 weeks with 6 months to 2 years between occurrences; clusters can occur several times in a year Pain occurs in bursts lasting 30-90 minutes and repeated several times a day Hurts to lie down, pain intense (constant, throbbing, stabbing, burning, squeezing), scalp tender, conjunctiva injected, tearing, nasal congestion, ptosis, eyelid edema, agitation; retro-orbital, periorbital, occipito-nuchal regions Often occurs within 60 to 90 minutes after falling asleep Can be associated with nausea, vomiting, photophobia, aura (Rozen, 2011), phonophobia	Throbbing pain, anxiety, malaise if does not take the above listed analgesia Occurs at least 15 days/month for 3 months Pain generally bilateral (bifrontal or bitemporal), low intensity, dull ache, may interfere with activities and school attendance Occurs at variable times of day	Bilateral, diffuse (site may shift), dull, usually mild-moderate intensity; aching pain ("tight band around head"), located in neck and back of head; rarely incapacitating May appear on awakening and continue all day; does not increase with activity *Episodic:* No nausea or vomiting, photophobia, phonophobia, or neurologic changes; negative neurologic examination *Chronic:* may have nausea Lasts 30 minutes, all day, or for up to 7 days Can occur at same time as more classic migraine headache
Trigger	Stress, tension, anxiety, perimenstrual or periovulation timing, fatigue, sustained exercise, head trauma, menstrual cycle, sexual activity, hunger, bright lights, odors, alcohol, certain foods (cheese, chocolates, citrus fruits particularly in children [Lewis, 2009]), noise, travel, cold weather	None	Withdrawal from analgesics or caffeine; stress or emotional upsets; postconcussion syndrome	Stress, depression, musculoskeletal dysfunction

Continued

| TABLE 27-6 | Most Common Types of Headaches—cont'd | | | |

Characteristic	Vascular (Migraine)	Cluster	Chronic, Daily, Low Grade	Tension
Differential diagnosis	Benign occipital epilepsy of childhood (same visual changes as migraine, but are followed by either unilateral or tonic-clonic, complex partial seizure pattern, then headache and nausea—occurs usually as child falls asleep); hemiplegic or basilar-type migraine; benign paroxysmal torticollis or vertigo; abdominal migraine; cyclic (or cyclical) vomiting syndrome	Chronic paroxysmal one-sided head pain (hemicrania), migraines, temporal arteritis, sinusitis, glaucoma	Tension headaches, migraine with or without aura	Migraine, brain tumor, cervical, ocular, and temporomandibular disorders, chronic sphenoid sinusitis
Diagnostic tests	None (EEG if suspected benign occipital epilepsy; neurologic examination is abnormal; atypical history and pattern)	None	None	None
Treatment (see a pediatric pharmacology reference for dosing)	*Acute:* See Table 27-9 *Prophylaxis:* See Table 27-9* *Others:* Biofeedback and relaxation (see also Chapter 42, Table 42-5)	*Prevention:* Lithium, verapamil, valproic acid, topiramate, melatonin *Suppression:* prednisone 1 mg/kg/day for 5 days, then taper for 2 weeks *Acute attack:* Sumatriptan (injection or nasal), oxygen, lithium. Oxygen is treatment of choice (inhale 100% oxygen for 20 min at 8-15 L/min following onset [70% effective]); zolmitriptan	*Acute only:* Ibuprofen, naproxen, acetaminophen, or other nonsteroidal antiinflammatory drug (with clear limits to their use); antidepressants; amitriptyline (>12 yrs); antihistamine cyproheptadine (3-12 yrs)	*Acute:* Analgesics, nonsteroidal antiinflammatory drugs, amitriptyline, tizanidine *Chronic:* Antidepressants (treatment of choice; start with low dose and increase every 3-7 days; try for at least 1-2 months), beta-blockers, anticonvulsants *Other:* Massage; relaxation techniques; cold; alternating warm compresses to occipital area

*Prophylaxis is indicated if the child has two to four severe episodes a month or cannot attend school regularly.
Data from Haslam RHA: Headaches. In Kliegman RM, Behrman RE, Jenson HB et al: *Nelson textbook of pediatrics,* ed 18, Philadelphia, 2007, Saunders, pp 2479-2483; Lewis DW, Bigal ME, Winner PL: Migraine and the childhood periodic syndromes. In Winner P, Lewis DW, Rothner AD, editors: *Headache in children and adolescents,* ed 2, Hamilton, Ontario, 2008a, BC Decker; Lewis DW, Bigal ME, Winner P: "Other" primary headaches in children and adolescents. In Winner P, Lewis DW, Rothner AD, editors: *Headache in children and adolescents,* ed 2, Hamilton, Ontario, 2008c, BC Decker; Lewis DW: Pediatric migraine, *Neurol Clin* 27(2):481-501, 2009; Majumdar A: Cluster headache in children—experience from a specialist headache clinic, *Eur J Paediatr Neurol* 13(6):524-529, 2009; Moore AJ, Shevell M: *Chronic daily headaches in pediatric neurology practice,* 2005. Available at www.medscape.com/viewarticle/501997 (accessed March 28, 2011); Rozen TD: Trigeminal autonomic cephalalgias, *Neurol Clin* 27(2):537-556, 2009; Rozen TD: Cluster headache as the result of secondhand cigarette smoke exposure during childhood, *Headache* 50(1):130-132, 2010; Rozen TD: Cluster headache with aura, *Curr Pain Headache Rep* 15(2):98-100, 2011; Unger J: Pediatric migraines: clinical pearls in diagnosis and therapy, *Consult Pediatricians* 5(9):545-551, 2006.

(37% to 51%); and 7 to 15 years of age (57% to 82%). Before 10 years of age, the incidence is higher in males than females. After age 11 the prevalence is higher in females (Bigal et al, 2008). The mean age at onset of migraine is at age 7.2 years for males and 10.9 years for females (Lewis et al, 2004).

It is the clinician's job to discern between symptoms that suggest that a headache is primary (e.g., tension-type, cluster, migraine type) or due to a secondary cause (e.g., tumor, hydrocephaly, infection, intoxication [lead, carbon monoxide], idiopathic intracranical hypertension, increased intracranial pressure). Key historical questions and a thorough workup are mandatory in order to exclude secondary headache etiology. In the absence of findings suggestive of a secondary headache, a more certain diagnosis of a primary headache disorder can be made. The International Headache Society provides succinct clinical criteria (available at www.ihs-classification.org) to help the provider evaluate, delineate between, and classify primary headaches (e.g., including migraines with or without aura and migraine subtypes) and secondary headaches.

Clinical Findings

History. Children less than 12 years of age often have a poor sense of time and may not serve as the best historians (Bigal et al, 2008). Important questions to ask the child and parent(s) include:

- *Duration.* Recent severe onset is worrisome.
- *Frequency and triggers.* Children with recurrent, low-intensity headaches, with no neurologic changes, and who recover completely between episodes are unlikely to have serious intracranial etiology. Triggers can include ovulation

---

BOX 27-3 Classification of Pediatric and Adolescent Migraine

With Aura*

Individual experiences >2 attacks
Meets all the criteria for migraine without aura
Individual has at least three of the following symptoms:
- ≥ one reversible aura symptom*
- At least one aura develops slowly over >5 minutes, or two or more aura symptoms occur in succession
- Aura does not last >1 hour
- Headache begins during or follows the aura in <1 hour
- Headache cannot be attributed to another disorder

Without Aura

Individual experiences ≥ five attacks
Headache episode lasts 1 to 72 hours
Headache has two or more of the following characteristics:
- Located bilaterally or unilaterally in frontotemporal region (not occipital)
- Pulsation present
- Intensity is moderate to severe
- Is aggravated by routine physical activity
Headache has one or both of the following and is not attributable to another disorder:
- Nausea and/or vomiting
- Photophobia and/or phonophobia

---

*Aura symptoms: *typical aura* includes visual (flickering lights, spots, lines, blurred vision, scotoma), sensory (pins, needles, numbness of hands and feet), or speech (aphasia) symptoms (or any combination) without motor weakness; *hemiplegic aura* includes unilateral sensory (numbness face, arm, leg) and motor signs (unilateral weakness), and aura can last for days; *basilar-type aura* includes vertigo, tinnitus, diplopia, blurred vision, scotoma, ataxia, occipital headache, possibly dilated pupils, ptosis, and alterations in consciousness that may precede a generalized seizure.
Data from Lewis DW, Bigal ME, Winner PL: Migraine and the childhood periodic syndromes. In Winner P, Lewis DW, Rothner AD, editors: *Headache in children and adolescents,* ed 2, Hamilton, Ontario, 2008a, BC Decker.

---

or menstruation, exercise, food or odors, and stress. Other triggers can include chocolate, processed meats, aged cheeses, nuts, altered amounts of caffeine intake, dairy products, shellfish, and some dried fruits. Such findings as perimenstrual exacerbation, food triggers, and a stable pattern to the headache with intervals of wellness over a long time period are reassuring symptoms that suggest primary headache (Bigal et al, 2008).

- *Location.* Occipital or consistently localized headaches can indicate underlying pathology. Facial pain might be sinusitis. Ocular motor imbalance can produce a dull periorbital discomfort, whereas temporomandibular joint pain tends to localize around the periauricular or temporal areas.
- *Quality and severity of pain.* Sharp, throbbing, or pounding pain is probably vascular (migraine). Dull and constant pain may be tension or organic. Severity can be assessed by asking about limitations to activities and missed school days. How many "different kinds of headaches" are experienced?
- *Age of onset.* Progression of the headaches over time, and longest period of time without symptoms.
- *Home management* and medications including dosage and self-coping activities.
- *Associated symptoms* can include nausea, vomiting, visual changes, dizziness, paresthesia, neck/shoulder pain, back pain, otalgia, abdominal pain, hypersomnia, food cravings, confusion, ataxia, pallor, photophobia, and phonophobia. Changes in gait, personality, mentation, or behavior that do not occur at the same time as the headache are worrisome and merit further evaluation with medical referral. There are some precursor symptoms and conditions that can indicate a predisposition to migraines. These include cyclic vomiting (see Chapter 32), abdominal migraine (see Chapter 32), and benign paroxysmal vertigo. Alone, they do not warrant extensive or expensive workups unless the diagnosis is unclear. These conditions may evolve into migraine without aura in later childhood (Lewis et al, 2008a).
- *Head trauma.* If associated with headache, a subdural hematoma or postconcussive syndrome must be considered.

- *Psychologic symptoms.* Evaluate for the presence of depression, school stressors, or concerns about family functioning.
- *Family history.* Most children with headache, especially migraine, have a family history of headaches.

Distinguishing Features of Headache Types
- *Migraine and migraine with aura* can be differentiated by the presence or absence of aura symptoms (Box 27-3). Characteristics of migraines include nausea; abdominal pain; vomiting; unilateral pain; pulsating pain; relief with sleep; an aura; visual changes such as dark or blind spots; and a history of a family member (usually on the maternal side) with migraine without aura in 90% of cases (Haslam, 2007). Dizziness and motion sickness may be described. Infants and toddlers may present with irritability, sleepiness, and pallor. In preadolescents, common migraine symptoms are more likely. Nausea and vomiting might not occur, and the pain can be more frontal. Lethargy and sleep can follow. Visual changes are rare, and the pain quality is variable. Times between headaches are pain free.
- *Abdominal migraine* is rare; symptoms include midline pain, nausea, and vomiting with minimal or no headache. Such symptoms can also be suggestive of complex partial seizures (see Chapter 33).
- *Muscle contraction or tension headaches.* The pain is dull and bifrontal or occipital, with nausea and vomiting occurring only rarely; there is no prodrome. Tension headaches can last for days or weeks but generally do not interfere with activities. In children it can be difficult to differentiate migraine and tension-type headaches. Psychosocial stress seems to be a major factor in tension and chronic daily headaches in both children and adolescents.
- *Secondary headaches* (or those headaches that have a pathologic process) (Box 27-4). Key historical markers are sudden onset of hyperacute or increasing pain severity or accompanying neurologic signs. These require prompt referral. Presenting symptoms of these headaches include (Bigal et al, 2008; Lewis et al, 2008b):
  - Headache pain that is worse in the morning on awakening and standing up, then fades

BOX 27-4 Signs and Symptoms Suggestive of Intracranial Structural Pathology

Infants
Full anterior fontanelle
Open metopic and coronal sutures
Poor growth
Impaired upward gaze
Abnormal head growth
Shrill cry
Lethargy
Vomiting

Children
Persistent unilateral headache
Papilledema
Abnormal eye movements (or one or both eyes suddenly turn in)
Ataxia
Hemiparesis
Abnormal deep tendon reflexes
Severe, excruciating headache of recent onset, unlike any previously experienced; no normal period of functioning between episodes of headache
Cranial bruits
Personality changes

Data from Chutorian AM: Headaches. In Burg FD, Ingelfinger JR, Polin RA et al, editors: *Current pediatric therapy*, ed 18, Philadelphia, 2006, Saunders.

○ Headache increases in frequency and severity over a period of only a few weeks
○ Pain that wakens the child from sleep
○ Vomiting but not nausea; vomiting may relieve the headache
○ Visual disturbances, diplopia, edema of the optic disc
○ Increased pain with straining, sneezing, coughing, defecation, or changes in position
○ Occipital region and neck pain (brain tumors tend to originate in the posterior fossa area in children [Lewis et al, 2008b])
○ Educational, mental, personality or behavioral alterations, irritability
○ Seizures
○ Unsteadiness
○ Fever
○ Family history of neurological disorders (e.g., brain tumors, neurofibromatosis, vascular malformations)
○ Child has a history of a ventriculoperitoneal shunt, meningitis, hydrocephaly, or tumor.

Physical Examination. A complete physical and neurological examination is in order. Particular areas to assess include (Lewis et al, 2008b):
• Blood pressure, supine and standing with 2-minute interval between them
• Height and weight
• Head circumference (all children)
• Eyes: Palpate for tenderness; check disks, movements
• Ears: Patency of canals, normal tympanic membranes, absence of tumors
• Neck: Palpate muscles; check range of motion for nuchal rigidity

TABLE 27-7 How to Proceed When the Complaint Is Dizziness

Complaint of Dizziness	Studies Indicated
Lightheaded	None
Double vision (posterior fossa location)	MRI
Sensation of whirling motion of oneself or of room or objects (vertigo)	MRI
Confusion	MRI, EEG, comprehensive metabolic screen

EEG, Electroencephalogram; *MRI,* magnetic resonance imaging.

• Sinuses (frontal and maxillary)
• Teeth (percuss, inspect)
• Temporomandibular joints (mouth and jaw): Palpate and check range of motion
• Thyroid gland
• Bones and muscles of skull: Palpate for tenderness; listen for cranial bruits; check range of motion of cervical spine
• Extremities: Tandem gait
• Nerves: Palpate supraorbital, trochlear, occipital nerves; assess CN IX-XII
• Reflexes: Pronator drift test
Diagnostic Studies. Imaging studies are rarely indicated unless the history suggests intracranial pressure (see Box 27-4); there is a sudden onset, increased severity, or change in headache pattern; the neurological examination is abnormal; or when a complaint of "dizziness" fits the criteria listed in Table 27-7. A CT scan without contrast is usually adequate to determine the presence of a brain tumor. If abnormal, an MRI should be done. An EEG should be obtained if the history and physical examination suggest a seizure process. If there is a history of external trauma, such as from a motor vehicle accident, cervical and spinal x-rays should be ordered.

Differential Diagnosis

The differential diagnosis consists of sinusitis, an intracranial mass, pseudotumor cerebri, sleep disorder, hyperthyroidism, hypertension, cyclic vomiting, abdominal migraine, BPV, and temporomandibular joint dysfunction. Visual acuity is rarely a cause of headaches. These and other causes of headaches in children are outlined in Table 27-8.

Management

Refer all patients with organic (structural) headaches. Parents seek medical attention for pain relief for their child, in addition to reassurance that there are no intracranial processes occurring (brain tumors). Each child with headaches requires an individually tailored strategy that may include pharmacologic and nonpharmacologic modalities.

For nonorganic headaches (e.g., no tumor, aneurysm, or metabolic or structural cause), the patient should be taught pain and stress management techniques; nonsteroidal antiinflammatory drugs (NSAIDs) are the first-line pharmaceutical

TABLE 27-8	Additional Causes of Headaches in Children
Cause	**Characteristics**
Drugs	
Cocaine	Migraine-like pain in patient with no history of migraine headaches
Marijuana	Frontal, mild
Analgesics, methylphenidate, oral contraceptives, steroids, and cardiovascular agents	Pain follows administration (of drug) or withdrawal (typical of analgesics)
Food additives (nitrites, monosodium glutamate common)	Pain occurs only in individual genetically sensitive; pain is diffuse, throbbing after ingestion
Physiologic	
Vasculitis	Uncommon in children; can occur as part of a collagen-vascular disease, such as systemic lupus erythematosus
Chronic hypertension	Low-grade occipital pain on awakening or frontal during day
Eyestrain	Dull, aching pain behind eyes relieved when eyes are closed; caused by muscular fatigue during prolonged ocular convergence; not a refractive error
Temporomandibular joint (TMJ) syndrome	>8 years old; pain on one side of face and vertex of TMJ; may be a history of jaw injury
Whiplash and neck injury	Pain dull, aching in neck, shoulders, upper arms with poor neck rotation; no nausea or vomiting; caused by muscles contracted to "splint" area of dysfunction in cervical joint areas or soft tissue
Following partial or generalized seizure	Diffuse pain
Infectious illness (viral or bacterial): meningitis, sinusitis, pharyngitis, upper respiratory infection; fever (Lewis et al, 2008b)	Pain may be nonspecific
Dental disease	Uncommon
Malfunctioning shunt or hydrocephalus	History of ventriculoperitoneal, ventriculopleural, or ventriculoatrial shunt
Toxins—Carbon monoxide, lead	Dull, aching pain
Tumor, brain abscess, subarachnoid or intracranial hemorrhage	Progressive worsening; can be severe; worst in early morning and with lying down (brain tumors)
Exertional	Sharp and occurs after exercise
Posttraumatic head injury	Pain can be severe when associated with epidural hematoma; if not associated with epidural hematoma, can start within hours up to weeks following injury (Lewis et al, 2008b).

for acute treatment. There can be significant loss of school attendance as a result of headaches, but attendance should be mandatory. A quiet rest period may be allowed at school if needed, and school nurses can be helpful in developing a plan for this. If the child remains home, activities should be restricted to bed and all homework completed. The child should be returned to school if the pain improves during the school day. Minimize attention to the headache. Relaxation exercises or biofeedback training can be helpful. Trigger factors should be avoided. Refer to Chapter 42 for complementary and alternative therapies.

The goals of treating acute-onset migraines include abortive therapy; reducing frequency, severity, and length of treatment; reducing loss of impairment; improving overall quality of life; avoiding escalation of medications; optimizing self-care abilities of the patient and family; using beneficial and cost-effective treatment; and minimizing medication side effects. Many of the newer medications for migraines (e.g., triptans) have not been adequately tested for safety and efficacy in children and adolescents, with the exception of sumatriptan and zolmitriptan (refer to Table 27-9 for treatment options). An 8- to 12-week course of preventive treatment is necessary to determine efficacy, and daily regimens should be used only for a set period of time. Lewis (2009) recommends treating throughout the school year and then gradually curtailing daily agents during the summer months. An alternative for younger children is to use shorter courses of preventive medications (6-8 weeks) followed by gradual weaning. All individuals with migraines benefit from regular sleep, exercise, moderate caffeine intake, and adequate hydration. Medications should be taken as soon as possible after the onset of the headache; should be taken in the prescribed dosage; should be available

TABLE 27-9 Therapies for Pediatric Migraine

Drug	Dosage	Notes from Studies (Lewis, 2004, 2010; Unger, 2006)
Acute Treatment of Nonspecific Acute Migraine *Medications (these should be tried first in acute management)*		
• Acetaminophen (gel capsule)*	• 10-15 mg/kg PO every 4 hr up to 500 mg every 4 hr	• Acetaminophen has faster onset of action than ibuprofen
• Ibuprofen* (gel capsule)	• 7.5-10 mg/kg PO every 4 hr up to 800 mg every 8 hr	• Ibuprofen showed greater headache resolution than acetaminophen (rebound headache can occur)
• Naproxen sodium	• Children: 5-7 mg/kg PO every 8-12 hr • Adolescents: 250-325 mg PO every 8-12 hr (max 1250 mg/24 hr)	• Safe and effective
• Dimenhydrinate	• 2-5 yr: 12.5-25 mg PO every 6-8 hr (max 75 mg/24 hr) • 6-12 yr: 25-50 mg PO every 6-8 hr (max 150 mg/24 hr) • >12 yrs: 50-100 mg PO every 4-6 hr (max 400 mg/24 hr)	• Use when vomiting is a major symptom
Migraine-Specific Acute Medications* *5-HT$_1$-receptor agonists (triptans)*		

• Sumatriptan*	• Consider for children >12 yr old when there is no response to analgesics
	  ○ Nasal spray*: 5 mg/spray; 5-20 mg each nostril once (may repeat every 2 hr if headache unresolved; max dosage 40 mg/24 hrs)
	  ○ Subcutaneous (self-administered): 3 or 6 mg once (may repeat in 1 hr; max dosage 12 mg/24 hrs)
	  ○ Oral: 25-100 mg once (may be repeated every 2 hr; max 200 mg/24 hr); available in tablets: 25, 50, or 100 mg
		• Triptans are all FDA approved for those ≥18 yr old; they are regarded safe, and well tolerated in children ≥12 yr old; efficacy rates for the triptans (*except for sumatriptan nasal spray and oral zolmitriptan*) are essentially the same as for placebos; they may prolong an aura.
		• If the first dose is given in the outpatient setting, the patient should be monitored for 1 hr.
		  ○ Side effects: Hot flushes; nausea and vomiting, chest/neck/head pressure, tingling, bad taste (nasal agents)
		  ○ DBCT: When compared with placebo, nasal sumatriptan significantly reduces headache; side effects present with sumatriptan vs placebo.
		  ○ Inadequate data to support use of subcutaneous sumatriptan use in children; do not use in basilar-type and hemiplegic migraine or in those with cardiovascular disease, uncontrolled hypertension, or who have used MAO inhibitor in prior 2 weeks. Has been used off-label in children <12 yrs who have not responded to typical analgesic regimens.

• Zolmitriptan	• ≥18 yr: 2.5-5 mg PO repeated every 2 hr prn (max 10 mg/24/hr)	Limited studies in children <18 yrs: no significant benefit seen in one study in children 12-17 yrs.
• Rizatriptan	• ≥18 yr: 5-10 mg PO repeated every 2 hr prn (max 30 mg/24/hr) (ODT available)	Studies limited in children; one study found no difference in symptom relief between drug and placebo; side effects well tolerated.
• Naratriptan	• ≥18 yr: 2.5 mg PO once, repeated once in 4 hr, prn	Do not use concurrently with an SSRI or SNRI because serotonin syndrome can occur.
• Almotriptan	• ≥12 yr: 6.25 mg PO once, repeat once in 2 hr prn (max 2 doses/24 hr)	
• Frovatriptan	• ≥18 yr: 2.5 mg PO at onset; repeat every 2 hr, prn (max 7.5 mg/24 hr)	
• Eletriptan	• ≥18 yr: 20-40 mg PO, repeated every 2 hr prn (max 80 mg/24 hr)	
Prophylaxis Treatment (Maintain Use for at Least 1 Year) *Antidepressants*		
• Amitriptyline (nortriptyline and desipramine have not been studied)	• Starting dosage 5-10 mg PO at bedtime, increasing every 2 wk towards maximum of 1 mg/kg/day	• Not assessed in controlled studies but is one of the most widely used agents • Efficacy in 50%-80% of children • Adverse effects: somnolence, dry mouth, dysrhythmia (order an ECG if dose exceeds 25 mg/day) • Use with caution in children ages <12 yr
• Trazodone	• 7-18 yr: 1 mg/kg/day PO divided tid	• Mixed results; no appreciable side effects

TABLE 27-9	Therapies for Pediatric Migraine—cont'd	
Drug	**Dosage**	**Notes from Studies (Lewis, 2004, 2010; Unger, 2006)**
Anticonvulsants		
• Divalproex sodium	• 10-30 mg/kg/day PO bid in divided doses up to 40 mg/kg/day	• Open-label trials only done: Showed 50% reduction in headache frequency in children ages 7-16 yr • Adverse effects: Weight gain, heartburn, hair loss, dizziness • Not for use in children ages <2 yr
• Topiramate	• 5-10 mg/kg/day PO divided bid up to maximum dose 100 mg/day • Adolescents: Start with 15-25 mg PO dose at bedtime; gradually increase to 50 mg bid on a weekly or every-other-week basis; benefit may be seen at 25 mg at bedtime	• Gaining wide acceptance for efficacy; well-designed study showed benefit at 50 mg bid dosing with more than 80% of patients showing >50% improvement after 8 weeks of treatment • Adverse effects: Weight loss, episodes of paresthesia, cognitive slowing, loss of appetite, dizziness, irritability; monitor any change in school/cognitive performance • Indicated in epilepsy for children as young as 2 yr
• Levetiracetam		• Open label studies done in children (no well-controlled studies) showed promising results of >50% reduction in migraine frequency.
• Zonisamide		• Small open label study of children 10-17 yrs showed ⅔ of children had >50% reduction in mixed refractory headaches.
Antiserotonergic agents		
• Cyproheptadine	• Age <2 yr: Not recommended • 2-6 yr: 0.25 mg/kg/day PO (tablet or syrup) • Age ≥7 yr: 2 mg PO daily; then titrate to 3-4 mg PO daily OR • < 10 yrs without overweight problems: 2-4 mg PO at bedtime; may be gradually increased to bid-tid use if side effects not problematic	• Used more in toddlers because weight gain (due to appetite stimulation) and somnolence are primary adverse effects in older children; sedation more problematic at doses higher than 4-8 mg/24 hr • In children ages 3-12 yr, drug was effective in up to 83% of patients, per retrospective study. • Do not use methysergide in children <10 yr and do not use for more than 3 mo (prolonged use can cause retroperitoneal or pulmonary fibrosis).
Antihypertensives		
• Beta-blocker: propranolol (timolol, atenolol, metoprolol, nadolol have not proven effective [Lewis, 2009])	• ≥7-8 yr: 10-20 mg PO tid; start with 10 mg/24 hr and increase by 10 mg/week	• May take up to several weeks to a month to be effective • May lower blood pressure or cause depressive adverse effects or exercise-induced asthma • 71% of children 7-16 yr had complete remission using 60-120 mg/day in a DBCT; other trials failed to show any improvement in headache frequency. • Do not use in children with history of asthma; use with caution in children with depression (Gunner et al, 2008)
• Alpha-agonist (clonidine)		• No significant difference in headaches between clonidine and placebo groups
• Calcium channel blocker (Flunarizine)	• 5-13 yr: 5 mg PO at bedtime (may be increased to 10 mg at bedtime)	• Probably effective for reducing frequency • Not available in the U.S.

*Recommended as most effective treatment for acute migraine in children and adolescents (Maria, 2009).

bid, twice daily; *DBCT,* double-blind controlled trial; *ECG,* electrocardiogram; *FDA,* U.S. Food and Drug Administration; *MAO,* monoamine oxidase; *max,* maximum; *ODT,* orally disintegrating tablet; *PO,* by mouth; *SNRI,* serotonin-norepinephrine reuptake inhibitor; *SSRI,* selective serotonin reuptake inhibitor; *tid,* three times daily; $5-HT_1$, 5-hydroxytryptamine receptor agonists.

Data from Edmunds MW, Mayhew MS: *Pharmacology for the primary care provider,* ed 3, St Louis, 2009, Mosby; Gunner KB, Smith HD, Ferguson LE: Practice guideline for diagnosis and management of migraine headaches in children and adolescents: part two, *J Pediatr Health Care* 22(1):52-59, 2008; Haslam RHA: Headaches. In Kliegman RM, Behrman RE, Jenson HB et al, editors: *Nelson textbook of pediatrics,* ed 18, Philadelphia, 2007, Saunders, pp 2479-2483; Lewis D, Ashwal S, Hershey A et al: Practice parameter: pharmacological treatment of migraine headache in children and adolescents, *Neurology* 63(12):2215-2224, 2004, reviewed as current information in 2010; Lewis DW: Pediatric migraine, *Neurol Clin* 27(2):481-501, 2009; Lewis DW: Almotriptan for the acute treatment of adolescent migraine, *Expert Opin Pharmacother* 11(14):2431-2436, 2010; Maria BL: Current pharmacotherapy for pediatric migraine: In Maria BL, editor: *Current management in child neurology,* ed 4, Hamilton, Ontario, 2009, BC Decker, p 87; Unger J: Pediatric migraines: clinical pearls in diagnosis and therapy, *Consult Pediatr* 5(9):541-551, 2006.

at home, school, or work; and the overuse of analgesics is to be avoided (more than three doses per week) (Lewis, 2009).

Prophylactic therapy is considered when migraines cause a child to miss school regularly and when the child suffers severe headaches two to four times a month with a clear sense of functional disability (Haslam, 2007). Anticonvulsants are also used, especially if the child has a seizure disorder. Other medications to consider might include beta-blockers, antidepressants, NSAIDs, or calcium channel blockers.

Complications

Brain tumors, abscesses, hematomas, and arteriovenous malformations in children are generally associated with ataxia, papilledema, intellectual changes, or behavioral changes. These processes crowd out other intracranial structures, precipitating edema and interfering with the normal actions of CSF and vessels. Infants may initially accommodate well to the increase in intracranial pressure because of the ability of their cranial sutures to expand.

HEAD INJURY

Description

Traumatic brain injury (TBI) involves tissue damage to the brain and its surrounding structures, and injury can range from mild to severe. Head injuries can be either open or closed. Open head trauma produces more focal injuries. Closed head trauma causes more multifocal or diffuse damage. Primary effects are from the initial injury and are related to mechanical forces that tear connections within the brain and cause contusions where the brain hits the skull surfaces (e.g., shaken baby syndrome). Axons to distant areas, fibers in the corpus callosum connecting the two hemispheres, or both

can be torn. Contusions and hemorrhage can occur. Secondary effects of the trauma, such as hypoxia, ischemia, hypotension, brain swelling, hemorrhage, contusion, and status epilepticus, can affect recovery.

The most common causes of head trauma differ according to age. Infants and toddlers are more likely to obtain head trauma from falls and physical abuse. Children 0 to 4 years and 15 to 24 years old have the highest risk of traumatic brain injury. Young children receive their head injuries from falls and pedestrian and bicycle accidents, whereas adolescents receive their TBI from motor vehicle accidents (Centers for Disease Control and Prevention [CDC], 2010a; Dawodu, 2009). Concussions are commonly related to sports injuries. See Chapter 13 for information on posttrauma management of head injuries related to sports.

Clinical Findings and Management

Chapter 39 discusses assessment, diagnostic studies, and management of a head-injured patient including the Glasgow Coma Scale (GCS), which has been traditionally used to measure the severity of head injury. Modification to the GCS for pediatrics has resulted in the implementation of the Pediatric GCS scoring system (Menkes and Ellenbogen, 2009). However, such predictive scales of outcome should not be the sole determinant of patient management. See Table 27-10 for a useful head injury acuity assessment guideline. Guidelines for sports-related injuries and when children might resume sports activities are found in Chapter 13.

Posttrauma Sequelae. The PCP is likely to encounter posttrauma patients. The duration of coma is predictive of subsequent neurologic function, and prognosis is good if mortality does not occur in the first 48 hours (Menkes and Ellenbogen, 2009). Minor head injury without neurologic

TABLE 27-10	Head Injury Acuity		
Characteristic	**Mild/Low Risk**	**Moderate/Moderate Risk**	**Major/High Risk**
Length of time patient was unconscious or had posttraumatic amnesia	<1 hour	1-24 hour	>24 hours
Glasgow Coma Scale score	13-15	9-12	3-8
Symptom	Usually alert in the emergency department with headache, dizziness, lethargy, irritability; withdrawn, may or may not be labile	Occasional brain swelling and hematomas Brief LOC, seizure, vomiting Headache, concentration, problem-solving and memory problems; symptoms can last for several months	Impaired LOC, focal neurologic findings, skull injuries Approximately 50% mortality rate
Sequelae	Repeated "minor" damage (e.g., head trauma with sports) can result in change in neuropsychology (attention, arousal, and information processing). ADHD, decreased attention span, emotional changes, sleep disturbances, memory problems, headache, language deficits can result	Same as for "mild" with concentration, problem-solving and memory problems; symptoms can last for several months	Seizures, hemiparesis, aphasia, cognitive problems, behavior changes Anxiety, attention problems (concentration, problem-solving and memory problems); symptom can last for several months (e.g., ADHD)

ADHD, Attention-deficit/hyperactivity disorder; *LOC,* loss of consciousness.
Data from Menkes JH, Ellenbogen MD: Traumatic brain and spinal injuries in children. In Maria BL, editor: *Current management in child neurology,* ed 4, Hamilton, Ontario, 2009, BC Decker, pp 624-637.

changes generally has no resulting deficit. In major head injuries, correlation between the extent of the injury to the extent of the dysfunction is predictive of outcome in 70% of cases. After severe injury, cognitive function changes generally will not improve after 12 months, but speech and motor difficulties may continue to see improvement for up to several years. A neuropsychological evaluation may be helpful to plan appropriate educational and behavioral management.

Children (2 to 6 years old) are usually more impaired than adolescents, secondary to immature brain development and general vulnerability. However, children and adolescents are more likely to show improvement in cognitive and social skills than adults who suffered the same degree of head trauma. Such improvement may evolve steadily over several years. Approximately 5% of hospitalized children with a head injury suffer a seizure within the first week; another 5% experience a seizure after this time (Rosman, 2006).

Prevention

- Wear helmets when using bicycles, skateboards, scooters, motorcycles, inline skates, snowboarding, ski racing, and when appropriate for sports participation. The proper fitting of helmets can be found in Chapter 13.
- Protect children from falls in the home or from playground equipment. Discourage the purchase of residential trampolines (see Chapter 13 for information on trampoline injuries and prevention strategies).
- Use appropriate seat restraints when riding in motor vehicles.

DISTURBANCES OF HEAD GROWTH

Macrocephaly

Macrocephaly is defined as a head circumference more than 2 standard deviations (SD) above the mean for age and sex or one that increases too rapidly. "Large" heads may be genetic and only of statistical significance; the provider's initial evaluation should be to measure both parents' head circumferences (see Appendix B for charts). Macrocephaly can also be attributed to hydrocephaly, megalencephaly (enlarged brain), subdural hematoma, tumor, thickening of the skull, or other problems. Benign familial macrocephaly may occur as a part of, or be related to, a genetic syndrome (anatomic or metabolic) such as Sotos syndrome (cerebral gigantism) and neurofibromatosis type 1. Infants with anatomic megalencephaly have macrocephaly at birth, but those with a metabolic etiology are normocephalic at birth. In cases of excessive volumes of CSF, the fluid may be located within the brain (in the ventricular cavities) or outside the brain, in the subarachnoid spaces.

A CT scan can be diagnostic with consultation or referral if abnormal. A CT interpretation of "benign enlargement of the subarachnoid spaces" (BESS) generally requires no further treatment. The subarachnoid enlargement resolves by school age, although the macrocephaly remains. This finding is found more often in boys, and there is a family history of macrocephaly in most cases (Di Muzio, 2011).

Hydrocephaly

See Chapter 38 for the discussion on congenital hydrocephalus.

Microcephaly

Microcephaly is defined as a head circumference 2 SD below the mean for age and sex or a head in which the growth is increasingly slower than normal. On examination the skull appears to be normally shaped; palpation may reveal some overlapping bones along the suture lines. This disorder can result from conditions in which the brain never formed correctly because of genetic or chromosomal abnormalities. Disease processes that interfere with normal brain growth can also be causative (these infants have normal head circumferences at birth). Brain damage that occurs prenatally may or may not always be evident initially in the newborn; a decreasing head circumference curve may start to occur after the infant reaches 3 to 6 months of age.

Commonly, microcephalic children have delayed developmental milestones and neurologic problems. Management of microcephaly is supportive, may involve an interdisciplinary team, and is directed toward management of the resulting deficits. Protein-calorie malnutrition, craniosynostosis, and hypopituitarism are treatable causes of microcephaly. Referral to a neurologist should be made for diagnostic purposes.

Craniosynostosis

Skull malformations may be due to primary or secondary causes. Congenital (or "true" or "primary") craniosynostosis involves early closure or absence of one or more cranial sutures. When more than one suture is involved, there is more likely to be an associated genetic disorder; craniosynostosis can be found in more than 60 genetic syndromes (e.g., Crouzon, Apert, Carpenter, Chotzen, Pfeiffer), but all of these syndromes also have extracranial features (DeMyer, 2009). Growth along the remaining open suture lines produces progressive skull deformity in one or more directions. The skull is flat over the closed suture(s). Increased intracranial pressure may result as the brain tries to grow within the confined space, but this does not always occur. Primary craniosynostosis occurs in 1 per 2000 to 2500 births (DiRocco et al, 2009), is ethnically neutral, and can vary in type and prominence between genders. The sagittal suture is most commonly fused (referred to as scaphocephaly or dolichocephaly) and accounts for 60% of all cases. Figure 27-3 illustrates the different descriptions for skull deformities seen.

Secondary synostosis results when outside forces put pressure on the growing cranium, causing the skull to become misshapen (referred to as *deformational plagiocephaly*). Secondary synostosis is most commonly seen with premature infants (termed *deformational scaphocephaly*), after shunting an infant with hydrocephaly, in children who have microcephaly and aberrant positioning in utero, during birth, or perinatally because of torticollis or positioning traditions. The success of the Back to Sleep campaign has resulted in an increase of infants with secondary (or pressure-related) occipital flattening. Such occipital deformity is not accompanied by compensatory suture line growth that would be seen with a primary lambdoidal synostosis. This type tends to correct when the child attains vertical posture (DeMyer, 2009).

Clinical Findings

Physical Examination. Monitor cranial symmetry for the first year. This is best done by looking down at the top of the head, noting the position of the ears and cheekbones. Typically, a deformational plagiocephaly will form a parallelogram

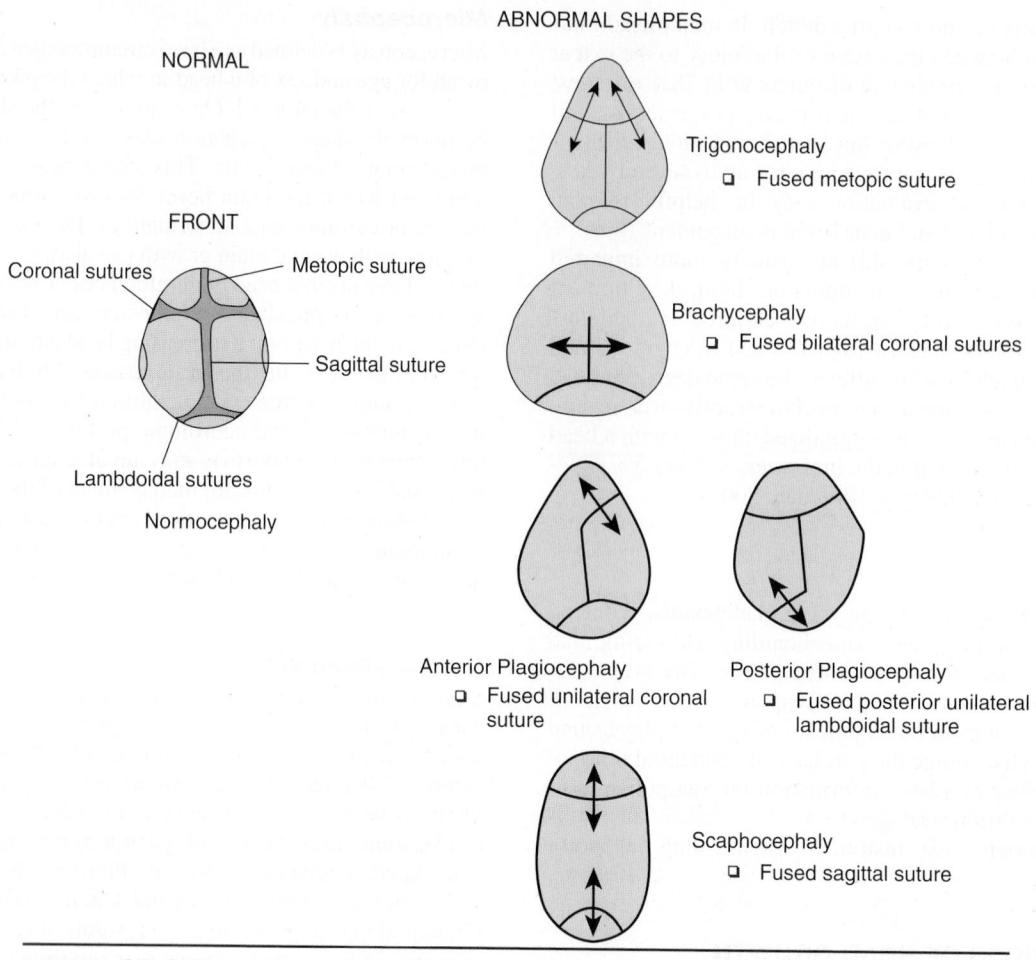

FIGURE 27-3 Characteristics of skull deformities seen with craniosynostosis. (Adapted from Cohen MM: *Craniosynostosis update 1987, Am J Med Genet Suppl* 4:99-148, 1988.)

characterized by unilateral occipital flattening and contralateral occipital bossing, ipsilateral ear displacement anteriorly, and associated parietal bossing and cheekbone prominence on the side of the occipital flattening. In contrast, the deformity of lambdoidal craniosynostosis does not assume a parallelogram shape, may be present at birth, has less frontal asymmetry than positional plagiocephaly, the ear ipsilateral to the occipital flattening is posterior and displaced inferiorly to the contralateral ear; the deformity may become more severe over time. Figure 27-4 compares these two deformities (DeMyer, 2009).

Symmetry of neck rotation should also be included in the examination to rule out torticollis. Infants with torticollis typically have some limitation of neck rotation away from the side of their occipital flattening.

Diagnostic Studies. A CT scan is standard for a skull shape deformity. Deformational plagiocephaly does not require imaging studies in most situations when the history and physical examination are diagnostic. If the child has neurologic findings, an MRI is also indicated (DeMyer, 2009).

Differential Diagnosis

In about 5% of young infants, the frontal metopic suture may normally be prominent. This prominence is not clinically significant, does not signify craniosynostosis, and does not require intervention.

Management

If craniosynostosis is suspected, refer the child to an experienced pediatric neurosurgeon or craniofacial plastic surgeon. Treatment is often surgical, but in some cases reassurance, repositioning, exercises for any associated torticollis, and clinical follow-up are sufficient. If the condition is genetic, management needs to be planned according to the problems associated with the syndrome. Genetic counseling is important.

PCPs can anticipate concern about deformational plagiocephaly by counseling parents at the newborn visit to: (1) lay infant down in the Back to Sleep position for sleep, alternating positions (i.e., left and right occiputs); (2) when awake and observed, place infants prone; (3) during feedings have parents avoid holding an infant in a manner that avoids putting pressure on the flattened part of the skull; and (4) have infants spend minimal time in car seats or other upright devices that maintain supine positioning. Improvement should occur over a 2- to 3-month period if interventions are instituted early. Throughout the first year, emphasize tummy time. Monitor head shape during all well-child visits. The majority of positional plagiocephalies are self-limited; sometimes physical therapy is indicated in recalcitrant cases (e.g., with torticollis).

For positional plagiocephaly, orthotic cranial molding helmet therapy may be prescribed when repositioning and exercises are not successful. The helmet is individually engineered to allow growth where needed and restrict it where the

Positional molding

Unilateral lambdoid synostosis

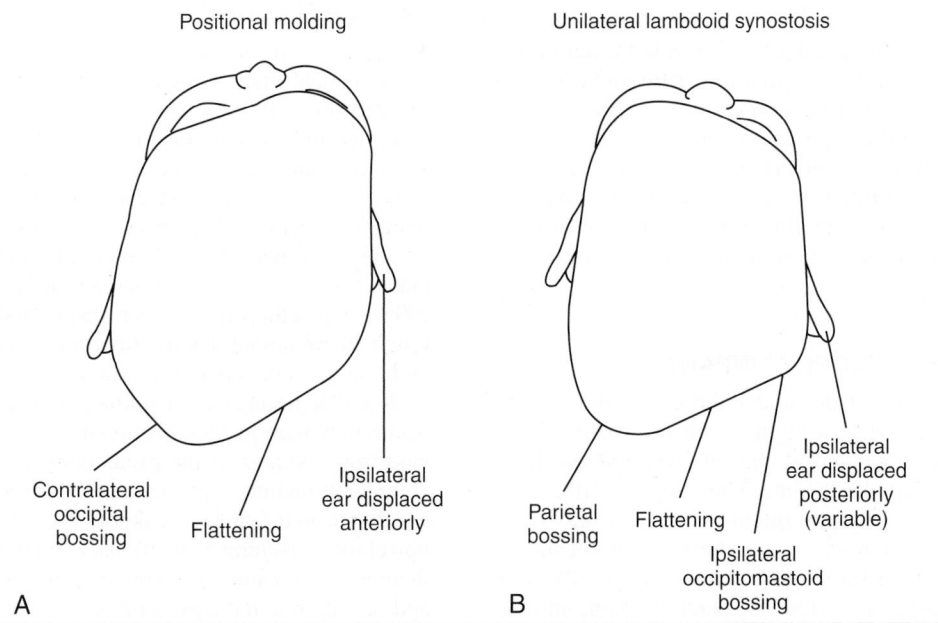

Contralateral occipital bossing

Flattening

Ipsilateral ear displaced anteriorly

Parietal bossing

Flattening

Ipsilateral occipitomastoid bossing

Ipsilateral ear displaced posteriorly (variable)

A

B

FIGURE 27-4 Differences between positional molding **(A)** and unilambdoid synostosis **(B)**. (From Gruss JS, Ellenbogen RG, Whelan MF: Lambdoid synostosis and posterior plagiocephaly. In Lin KY, Ogle RC, Jane JA, editors: *Craniofacial surgery: science and surgical technique,* Philadelphia, 2002, Saunders.)

head is prominent; it needs to be worn for 23 hours a day for 4 to 6 months, can lead to odor and skin breakdown, is costly, and may not be covered by health insurance (Taub and Pierce, 2011). One study showed 36% to 54% improvement in asymmetry in those infants whose parents were most compliant in using the helmet over the 6-month study period (Robinson and Proctor, 2009).

CENTRAL NERVOUS SYSTEM INFECTIONS
Description and Epidemiology
All the infections of the CNS have similar symptoms. These infections can be manifested acutely (over 1 to 24 hours) or chronically (over 1 to 7 days or more). Bacteria, viruses, fungi, spirochetes, protozoa, and parasites can all cause CNS infection. The meninges, superficial cortical structures, blood vessels, and brain parenchyma can be involved. The most common microbes are (Bale, 2009):
- Newborn to 2 months old: Group B and D streptococci, *Escherichia coli* and other gram-negative enterobacteria, *Listeria monocytogenes,* and occasionally *Haemophilus influenzae.*
- Two months to 12 years old: Bacterial infections—*H. influenzae* type B, *Neisseria meningitidis,* and *Streptococcus pneumoniae* are the most common. In those with immune deficiencies *Pseudomonas aeruginosa, Staphylococcus aureus,* coagulase-negative staphylococci, *Salmonella* spp. and *L. monocytogenes* can be implicated.

Clinical Findings
History. The following may be reported:
- Upper respiratory tract or gastrointestinal symptoms accompanied by fever
- Increasing lethargy and irritability
- Recent head injury or neurosurgical procedure
- Immunodeficiency diseases

Physical Examination. Findings on physical examination include the following:
- Systemic signs, including fever; malaise; impaired heart, lung, or kidney function
- CNS signs, including headache; stiff neck and spine; nausea and vomiting; fever or hypothermia; changes in mental status, ranging from irritability to lethargy or coma; seizures; and focal or sensory deficits in cranial nerves, notably III, IV, and VI
- Presence of Kernig or Brudzinski signs of meningeal irritation (may be absent in a young infant)
- Bulging fontanelle and increasing head circumference in a young infant
- Papilledema—a late finding in older children or adolescents
- Cranial nerve palsies
  By age, the most common findings are as follows:
- From 0 to 3 months old: Fever, hypothermia, lethargy, irritability, poor feeding, apnea, focal seizures, enteric or respiratory symptoms, nuchal rigidity, and a bulging fontanelle (infrequent)
- From 3 months to 5 years old: Petechial rash, localized CNS signs as described earlier
- From 6 to 18 years old: Petechial rash, CN VII palsy (Lyme disease), sinusitis symptoms, localized CNS signs

Diagnostic Studies. Blood cultures, CBC with differential, urinalysis, chemistry panel, and lumbar puncture for CSF studies are done. Enterovirus meningitis and herpes simplex virus rapid tests are available. EEGs, CT or MRI scan, and brain biopsy may be needed.

Management and Complications
The PCP needs to refer all children with potential CNS infection as rapidly as possible. Hypovolemia, hypoglycemia, hyponatremia, acidosis, septic shock, increased intracranial pressure, and other complications can occur quickly

and need aggressive management. Hearing loss can occur in all forms of meningitis, and all children with meningitis merit postinfection auditory evaluation. Blindness, hydrocephaly, CP, seizures, and developmental delays can also occur depending on the type of organism involved. Outcomes are typically based on the type of infectious agent and severity of initial infection; age of patient (the younger, the worse the outcome); length of symptoms before the diagnosis and initiation of treatment; and antibiotic and dosage.

THE HYPOTONIC "FLOPPY" INFANT

When supported with a hand under the chest, the normal infant will hold the back straight or nearly so, the arms flexed and slightly abducted at the elbows, and the head slightly up at less than 45 degrees. The "floppy" infant will droop over the hand. A floppy infant is alert but has hypotonia and depressed spontaneous movements, which should arouse suspicion. Other symptoms seen in a range of known causes include seizures, failure to react to pain, muscle wasting, absent reflexes, tongue fasciculation, and unilateral muscular movement defects (Ryan, 2009). Etiologies usually focus on a metabolic or CNS dysfunction or a systemic illness. Most conditions involving the CNS are serious and lasting; others may be transitory, such as brachial plexus nerve palsy after birth or congenital myasthenia gravis. Hypotonic infants can increase their tone over the first year of life and then demonstrate spastic CP. A baby can have low tone but still not lack strength when actively moving. The infant may also be weak, which means that its maximal effort lacks strength. Floppy infants with brisk reflexes almost certainly have a CNS disorder. Prenatal substance abuse has resulted in neonatal hypotonia (Ryan, 2009). All floppy babies need to be referred to specialists, including a geneticist. The diagnostic tool of choice is the MRI; sometimes muscle biopsies or various neurophysiologic studies are used. Many conditions of floppy infant syndrome do not respond well to treatment; rehabilitation can help maximize function. The key is to discern central from peripheral neuropathy, as well as assessing the fatigability of the muscle (Ryan, 2009).

REYE SYNDROME

Reye syndrome is an encephalopathy process often associated with influenza A and B. It is a systemic disorder of mitochondrial function occurring during or after a viral infection and, more often, with the use of salicylates during such viral illnesses (Beutler et al, 2009). Infrequent cases are seen with varicella or nonspecific respiratory infections, notably *H. influenzae* type B. A decline in incidence has been associated with the decreased use of salicylates.

Unless treated, the clinical course in Reye syndrome proceeds in predictable stages after the initial prodromal symptoms of the illness: severe vomiting progresses to irrational behavior; to stupor and coma; to apnea, fixed pupils, and decorticate posturing with increasing brain edema; and then to death. Management involves immediate referral with admission to a hospital for supportive care. About 70% of patients survive, some with severe neurologic sequelae. Infants are more severely affected than older children.

TETHERED CORD

The spinal cord is attached to the base of the brain and free at the caudal end, allowing for freedom of movement during growth, activities, and skeletal changes (including such abnormalities as scoliotic curves). With a tethered cord, however, the caudal end is fixed by a ropelike filum terminale at or below the L2 level. This can cause abnormal stretching and damage to nerve cells, fibers, and blood vessels. Eventually, symptoms of neurologic deterioration occur. It is often associated with a congenital spinal anomaly, such as spina bifida (90%), but tethering can also result from bony protrusions, tough membranous bands, lipomas, tumors, cysts, scarring, and trauma in the area of the cauda equina.

Not all tethering leads to clinical symptoms. If symptoms do occur, they manifest as functional deficits to nerves that emanate from the area of the cauda equina. Common findings or complaints include asymmetry of leg or foot growth and muscle wasting in an infant, leg weakness, incontinence of bladder and bowel (or worsening of such), back or leg pain (especially with flexion or extension), groin or genitorectal pain, loss of reflexes and sensation in the legs, scoliosis, or deformity of the legs or hips (NINDS, 2010c). Symptoms are not necessarily evident in infancy but can be manifested in early childhood to adulthood. The following skin changes are often seen in individuals later diagnosed with tethered cord or other spinal abnormalities: dimples above the gluteal cleft or within the cleft (dimples at the coccyx are generally benign), spinal hair tufts, a deviated gluteal fold, spinal fatty deposits, midline birthmarks, and sacral sinuses or tracts (see Color Plate).

If a provider is suspicious of a tethered cord, an MRI of the spine is the gold standard for viewing the parenchymal anatomy. A referral to a pediatric neurosurgeon is also indicated. Surgery is usually the treatment of choice and can halt and prevent further neurologic dysfunction. If a child has reached full skeletal height with minimal symptoms, monitoring is all that is often done. Be watchful for retethering in children who have had surgery for tethered cord; this can occur as the child gets older. A child with a history of repaired spina bifida needs to be closely monitored for early symptoms of tethered cord.

ARNOLD-CHIARI MALFORMATION

Arnold-Chiari malformations consist of two types of uncommon congenital spinal cord anomalies whose sequelae are usually not evident until late childhood or into adulthood. Type I malformation involves the downward elongation (herniation) of the caudal end of the cerebellar vermis through the foramen magnum. Type II malformation is present in 0.5 to 1 per 1000 of children with spina bifida myelomeningocele. The herniation can lead to brainstem and upper cervical cord compression that may ultimately cause necrosis of both structures. The etiology is believed to be secondary to embryonic segmentation disorders of the neural tube (Salman and Maria, 2009).

The symptoms of a malformation may not be readily apparent. Type I malformation can cause headache, neck pain, atrophy and decreased reflexes in the lower extremities, sensory losses, and scoliosis. Any child with myelomeningocele should be suspected of having type II malformation. Type II malformation involves the same herniation as type I plus an alteration in the shape and development of the medulla. Further symptoms of type II may include hydrocephaly, respiratory distress, syncope, poor feeding, vomiting, dysphagia, tongue paralysis, and cardiopulmonary failure. Epilepsy is not related. Diagnosis is made by MRI and the condition may inadvertently be found at the time of an MRI for a possibly unrelated reason (e.g., headache). Management strategies are not always successful; surgery to relieve the compression or a ventriculoperitoneal shunt may be tried in symptomatic cases. Older children may benefit from a cervical laminectomy to relieve compression as the child grows.

MYELOMENINGOCELE

Description

Failure during embryogenesis of the vertebrae, skull, meninges, brain, or spinal cord to be encapsulated by the lamina of the vertebrae along the dorsal midline of the body is referred to as a dysraphic defect. Myelomeningocele refers to the protrusion of both the spinal cord nerve roots (myelo) and the three layers of membranes (meninges) that cover the spinal cord and brain through this spinal defect. The protruding dural sac may contain only the meninges (10% to 20% of cases) or both meninges and nerve roots (the remaining cases). The term *spina bifida cystica* is often used interchangeably with myelomeningocele. When the vertebral arches fail to close, but there is no subsequent herniation of cord or meninges, the term *spina bifida occulta* is used. Most cases of spina bifida cystica occur in the thoracolumbar area (90%). Meningoceles may also protrude through the skull and may or may not be covered with skin. Such a cranial meningocele consists only of a CSF-filled meningeal sac; no nerve roots are involved, and therefore no neurologic deficits exist. However, there may be brain malformation under the mass that does have neurologic consequences. Encephaloceles or cephaloceles refer to cranial lesions that contain a meningocele sac plus cerebral cortex, cerebellum, or portions of brainstem that protrude from fissures in the occipital (most common), frontal, or nasal cavity areas of the skull.

Epidemiology

Closure of the neural tube usually occurs during the third and fourth weeks of gestation. Genetic and environmental factors are believed to play a causative role in the failure of the closure to occur. A woman who has had a previous child born with dysraphia has about a 3% to 4% recurrence rate with future pregnancies (Kinsman and Johnston, 2007) and Hispanic women are at higher risk (CDC, 2010b). A lack of sufficient levels of folic acid and vitamin A increases the incidence of neural tube defects (NTDs). All women of childbearing age are encouraged to take 0.4 mg/day of folic acid. A woman wishing to conceive, or who has had a prior pregnancy that resulted in a neural tube defect, should take 4 mg/day for 4 weeks before conception and through the first trimester (CDC, 2009). Intake of certain drugs and toxins is associated with neural tube defects; they include folic acid antagonists (trimethoprim, carbamazepine, phenytoin, phenobarbital, primidone), retinoic acid derivatives (e.g., vitamin A, a paradox given that insufficient levels also cause the defect), valproic acid, and alcohol. Diabetes mellitus (including gestational diabetes), maternal hyperthermia during the first month of pregnancy, trisomy 13 and 18, and Meckel syndrome are also risk factors (Kinsman, 2009).

The rate of affected pregnancies with neural tube defects dramatically dropped after the mandatory fortification of cereal grains with folic acid. Since 2004, the incidence has leveled off to about 3000 affected pregnancies in the U.S. rather than continue to decline. The incidence worldwide is approximately 300,000 births (CDC, 2010b). There is speculation that this leveling may be due to overall decreases in serum folate, red blood cell (RBC) folate concentrations in nonpregnant women, and to some nonfolate risk factors yet to be identified (CDC, 2007; 2010b). Proposed explanations for the decline in serum folate include increasing obesity rates (obese individuals metabolize folate differently), low-carbohydrate diet trends (which requires the elimination of breads, cereals, and other products that contain the mandatory fortified folic acid-enriched flour), the popularity of whole-grain breads (which have lower natural folate levels), the reduction in the mean folate content of certain enriched breads, and maternal diabetes (CDC, 2007).

A maternal serum test showing an increase in the concentration of alpha-fetoprotein is diagnostic; if elevated, an ultrasound and amniocentesis are performed (alpha-fetoprotein is the primary plasma protein within the fetus, and amniotic fluid and is elevated if there is a defect in the skin of the fetus). Cranial ultrasounds should be done to look for hydrocephaly and cephaloceles (and in turn the Arnold-Chiari type II malformation). It is preferable that these infants be delivered by cesarean section.

Clinical Findings

See Chapter 38 for the history and physical examination. Other physical anomalies can accompany myelomeningocele including cleft lip and palate, omphalocele, diaphragmatic hernia, tracheoesophageal fistula, congenital heart disease, bladder exstrophy, and imperforate anus.

Management and Complications

In the neonatal period, serial cranial ultrasounds are conducted to watch for the development of hydrocephaly, if this condition has not shown up prenatally. Surgical resection and closure of the involved neural tube structures are done within a week after birth; often shunting for hydrocephaly is also required. If surgery is not done during that time, death may result in the first year from meningitis or sepsis. Intrauterine surgery has also been successful in closing the defect and preventing exposure of the neural tube to amniotic fluid and possible postnatal infection. If the defect occurs in a high spinal region or there is clinical hydrocephalus at birth, survival is also compromised.

The PCP's role includes delivering well-child care, assessing and treating acute illnesses (especially UTIs and constipation), monitoring shunt function, checking for skin breakdown, and communicating with and often coordinating services between a myriad of specialists that will be involved (e.g., orthopedists, ophthalmologists [strabismus is common], neurologists, nephrologists, physical therapists, social workers, geneticists).

Genitourinary management entails teaching parents (and eventually the child) how to regularly catheterize a neurogenic bladder. Periodic urine cultures, assessing renal function (with serum electrolytes, creatinine), and, depending on the child's course, ordering appropriate imaging studies (renal scans, intravenous pyelograms [IVPs], ultrasounds) fit within the PCP's role. In addition, the PCP needs to be alert to the onset of symptoms indicative of Arnold-Chiari type II malformation and tethered cord, and watch for seizures (15% incidence), learning difficulties, and attention-deficit/hyperactivity disorder (ADHD). Bowel training can help control stool incontinence.

Prognosis

With aggressive early treatment, survival rates can be as high as 85% to 90%; deaths more commonly occur before 4 years of age. Normal intelligence is seen in 70% of survivors, but they experience more learning and seizure problems. Continence can sometimes be achieved with an artificial urinary sphincter or bladder augmentation when the child is older. Functional mobility depends on the level and degree of the defect and on the intact function of the iliopsoas muscle. A child with a defect in the sacral and lumbosacral area almost certainly will be able to achieve functional ambulation. Of those with a higher defect, about half will achieve mobility using braces and canes (Kinsman, 2009).

MYASTHENIA GRAVIS
Description and Epidemiology

Myasthenia gravis (MG) is an autoimmune disorder that produces an immune-mediated neuromuscular blockade or neuromuscular junction disorder. It originates when circulating receptor-binding antibodies decrease the number of available acetylcholine receptors (AChRs) on the postsynaptic muscle membrane or motor endplate. This leaves the motor endplate less responsive than normal (Vajsar, 2009).

MG is nonhereditary in most cases; however, three rare presynaptic congenital forms exist. Symptoms of congenital MG start at or close after birth and persist. Myasthenic mothers may have infants with a transient neonatal myasthenic syndrome as a result of the transfer of placental anti-AChR antibodies. Once the infant's own receptors regenerate and reinsert into synaptic membranes, the symptoms resolve. Children with MG can also experience other autoimmune diseases (e.g., systemic lupus erythematosus, thyroiditis, rheumatoid arthritis, diabetes mellitus).

MG affects approximately 40 per 1 million population; about one fifth of these develop symptoms before 20 years of age. The nonhereditary form of MG can occur any time after birth, although onset before 1 year old is rare (Vajsar, 2009). There is no racial or geographic predilection.

Clinical Findings

Physical Examination. The key findings of this disorder include:

- Ptosis and some degree of extraocular muscle weakness (usually the first symptom). Older children may complain of double vision; younger children may endeavor to hold their eyelids open with their fingers. The ocular signs may be asymmetric.
- Dysphagia. Infants commonly have feeding problems; older children fatigue when chewing. There may be slurred speech and a snarling appearance when trying to smile.
- Muscular weakness of neck flexor muscles (infants), limb-girdle and distal muscles of the hands. Symptoms do not include muscle fasciculations, myalgias, or sensory symptoms. Ten percent of patients have limb weakness as the initial symptom (Vajsar, 2009). Other times, the weakness may be so mild as to only occur after exercise.
- Rapid muscular fatigue as evidenced by inability to:
  - Hold an upward gaze for 30 to 90 seconds
  - Sustain a chin to chest position, while supine
  - Maintain arm abduction for more than 1 to 2 minutes
  - Sustain rapid hand-fisting movements for long periods of time

Twelve percent of infants born to mothers with MG develop symptoms within 72 hours of birth—respiratory insufficiency, dysphagia, hypotonia, weakness, poor spontaneous motor activity, weak cry, poor sucking, choking, expressionless face, and absent Moro reflex. Symptoms generally resolve within 12 weeks. With congenital MG, symptoms are permanent, there is no remission, and these children do not experience myasthenic crises.

Diagnostic Studies

- A short-acting cholinesterase inhibitor (edrophonium chloride) is given as a clinical test; it should cause spontaneous improvement in the ptosis and ophthalmoplegia within seconds; other muscles should fatigue less rapidly.
- An EMG is more diagnostic than a muscle biopsy.
- Estimation of the number of AChRs per endplate and in vitro endplate function studies are also possible. An assay of plasma antibodies to AChRs is often inconclusive; only one third of adolescents and an occasional prepubertal child show these antibodies present.
- Other tests can include serologic antinuclear antibodies and immune complexes; thyroid profile; CK level (normal with MG); chest x-ray (any enlarged thymus needs to be followed up with a tomography or CT scan of the anterior mediastinum); ECG (should be normal); muscle biopsy may be considered.

Differential Diagnosis

Hypothyroidism (caused by Hashimoto thyroiditis), polymyalgia rheumatica, MS, progressive external ophthalmoplegia, Guillain-Barré syndrome, Möbius syndrome, congenital ptosis, congenital myopathies, myotonic dystrophy, and glycogen-storage disease are in the differential.

Management

MG (including neonatal MG) is treated with anticholinesterase therapy (pyridostigmine) because it is longer acting and produces less severe side effects than neostigmine. The initial dosage is age and weight dependent and is then titrated upward until the patient responds, side effects are controlled, or until increases are no longer effective. Corticosteroids, cytotoxic agents (azathioprine and cyclosporine), or thymectomy may also be considered, especially if symptoms are severely debilitating (bulbar or respiratory involvement). Corticosteroids should be administered on an alternate-day regimen. Plasmapheresis and IVIG are alternative treatments and limited in scope. There is some controversy regarding their use; they are only used for short-term management since they produce only temporary remission (Sarnat, 2007; Vajsar, 2009).

Complications

Complications include growth retardation from steroids and possible immunodeficiency in adulthood after thymectomy. Long-term therapy with anticholinergics may lead to cholinergic crises that present similarly to myasthenic crises (Vajsar, 2009).

TIC DISORDERS

Tics, or habit spasms, are found in children and adults. Boys are two to three times more likely to be affected than girls. The most common time for onset is 6 to 8 years old (range is from 2 to 15 years of age) with maximum severity between 8 and 12 years of age (Singer, 2009). Types of tic disorders are simple and complex; motor, verbal, or both; and acute or chronic (lasting longer than 1 year). Some tics can be suppressed with effort and are not a part of voluntary movements. Other forms of tics wax and wane and tend to decrease when the child is out of school. Duration of affliction can be lifelong; half of the children with tics outgrow them in late adolescence. Others may experience this resolution only to see them recur in middle age. Tics are not associated with degenerative diseases.

Simple motor tics usually affect the head, eyes, or face (eye blinks, eyebrow raising, nose flaring, grimacing, lip smacking); head or arm jerking, kicking, toe curling, and shoulder shrugging can also occur. More complex motor tics include head shaking; touching; hitting; jumping; smelling objects; repeating movements; self-mutilating activities such as lip biting; and other behavior. Initial vocal tics include sniffing, grunting or snorting, throat clearing, and coughing. Hissing and barking can occur, but swearing is rare in children. If swearing (or coprolalia) is repressed by the patient, it usually results in barking or coughing noises; this occurs in about 10% of patients (Singer, 2009).

Tourette syndrome is the most complex of the tic disorders. It is believed to be caused by a combination of neurobiologic, psychological, hereditary (autosomal dominant with varying levels of penetrance, which is gender related), and environmental factors. Imaging studies have demonstrated the lack of normal striatum asymmetry. The tics can vary in severity over time. Boys with Tourette syndrome frequently have concomitant ADHD, whereas girls are more likely to experience obsessive-compulsive disorder (OCD). Another potentially associated precursor is beta-hemolytic streptococcus infection (pediatric autoimmune neurophysiologic disorder associated with strep infections [PANDAS]) especially if the child presents with sudden onset of symptoms (Singer, 2009). To meet the diagnostic criteria for Tourette syndrome, the tics must:

- Be a combination of motor and verbal tics, not necessarily concurrent
- Be repeated many times every day for more than 1 year with a waxing and waning course but demonstrate a progressive pattern overall
- Begin before 21 years old
- Not be related to some other medical condition (e.g., seizures, Huntington disease, or postviral encephalitis), medications, or other substances (Singer, 2009)

Differential Diagnosis

Consider hyperkinesis; choreiform (harder to suppress and occurs during voluntary movements) or dystonic movements; genetic disorder, such as Huntington or Wilson disease; OCD; structural lesion in the brain; and pharmacologic side effect.

Management

Tics should be ignored, given their tendency to wax and wane. The decision to treat with medicine depends on how much the tics bother the child rather than the parents as well as psychosocial, functional, impairment with tics, or classroom disruption (Singer, 2009). Treatment should include a combination of behavioral therapy and medication. Pharmacologic management of motor or vocal tics includes first- and second-tier medications. First-line drugs include clonidine or guanfacine along with baclofen, clonazepam, topiramate, or levetiracetam. Second-tier drugs include haloperidol, pimozide, and risperidone (Singer, 2009). Drugs may need to be rotated to maintain effectiveness over time. Because of the comorbidity with ADHD and OCD, management strategies must also involve the family, educational systems, and other supportive measures, including medication.

Eye Disorders

CATHERINE G. BLOSSER AND TERI MOSER WOO

Ophthalmic diseases occur most often in the very young or elderly, with the exception of eye trauma, refractive errors, and some other disorders (e.g., retinoblastoma [RB]). Infants and children are particularly susceptible to permanent central visual loss (amblyopia), opacities (congenital cataracts), refractive errors not associated with amblyopia, strabismus (ocular misalignment), and other conditions that interfere with visual acuity (ptosis, anisometropia). With early detection and correction these conditions do not lead to permanent loss in the mature central visual system of the older child or adult (American Association for Pediatric Ophthalmology and Strabismus [AAPOS] and American Academy of Ophthalmology [AAO], 2007). When caring for children with eye problems, priorities include promoting optimal growth and development of the ocular structures and maximizing visual acuity. To this end, primary care providers (PCPs) seek to promote good vision and health, detect abnormalities, treat those conditions that fall within their scope of practice, refer patients with conditions requiring an ophthalmologist's expertise, and provide education and reassurance to parents and children. Care of blind or visually impaired children is discussed in Chapter 15.

■ Standards for Visual Screening and Care

Standards and guidelines for visual screening and eye care in children are set by a number of agencies and professional groups. Pediatric-focused objectives related to vision in the proposed U.S. Department of Health and Human Services (USDHHS) *Healthy People 2020* draft (2009) propose to:
- Increase the proportion of preschool children ages 5 years and younger who receive vision screening.
- Reduce blindness and visual impairment in children and adolescents ages 17 years and younger.
- Reduce uncorrected visual impairment due to refractive errors.
- Increase the use of personal protective eyewear in recreational activities and hazardous situations around the home.

The U.S. Preventive Services Task Force (USPSTF) *Guide to Clinical Preventive Services* (2004) notes that:
- Screening tests have reasonable accuracy in identifying strabismus, amblyopia, and refractive errors in children

younger than 5 years. Providers should be alert for signs of ocular misalignment when examining infants and children. Treating strabismus and amblyopia early greatly reduces long-term amblyopia and improves visual acuity.

The joint recommendation of the American Academy of Pediatrics (AAP), American Association of Certified Orthoptists, AAPOS, and the AAO includes the following (AAP et al, 2007):
- Well-child examinations should include ocular history, vision assessment, external inspection of the eyes (including pupils and red light reflex), lids, and ocular mobility. This also includes an evaluation of fixation and following (binocularly and monocularly) starting at birth, with patched visual acuity screening starting at 3 years old (Tables 28-1, 28-2, and 28-3). If the child is uncooperative, retesting should occur 6 months later. Inability to fix and follow after 3 months of age warrants a referral to a pediatric ophthalmologist or an eye specialist trained to treat pediatric patients. Subsequent testing should occur at 4, 5, 10, 12, 15, and 18 years old. A subjective historical assessment should occur during visits at all other ages. Children who are difficult to screen after two attempts or who demonstrate any other eye abnormality should undergo photoscreening techniques to detect amblyopia, media opacities, and treatable ocular disease processes.

For high-risk children, the AAO (2009) recommends that asymptomatic children have a comprehensive examination by an ophthalmologist if they have any of the following:
- Health and developmental problems that make screening by the primary care clinician difficult or inaccurate (e.g., retinopathy of prematurity [ROP], or diagnostic evaluation of a complex disease with ophthalmologic manifestations)
- A family history of conditions that cause or are associated with eye or vision problems (e.g., RB, significant hyperopia, strabismus [particularly accommodative esotropia], amblyopia, congenital cataract, or glaucoma)
- Multiple health problems, systemic disease, or the use of medications that are known to be associated with eye disease and vision abnormalities (e.g., neurodegenerative disease, juvenile rheumatoid arthritis, systemic steroid therapy, systemic syndromes with ocular manifestations, or developmental delay with visual system manifestations).

TABLE 28-1	Normal Visual Developmental Milestones
Birth-2 weeks	Infant sees and responds to change in illumination; refuses to reopen eyes after exposure to bright light; increasing alertness to objects; fixes on contrasts (e.g., black and white); jerky movements; pupillary reaction present.
2-4 weeks	Infant fixes and follows on an object, though sporadically.
By 3-4 months	Infant recognizes parent's smile; looks from near to far and focuses close again; beginning development of depth perception; follows 180-degree arc; reaches toward toy; few exodeviations; esotropia abnormal.
By 4 months	Color vision near that of an adult; tears are present.
By 6-10 months	Infant fixes on and follows toy in all directions; movements smooth.
By 12 months	Vision is close to fully developed.

TABLE 28-2	Visual Acuity Norms (Snellen Equivalents)	
	Forced Choice Preferential Looking (FPL)	**Age Visual-Evoked Potential (VEP)**
Birth	20/400	20/800
2 months	20/400	
4 months	20/200	20/600
6 months	20/150	20/400
12 months	20/50	20/20
18-24 months	20/25 or 20/20	
5 years	20/25 or 20/20	

VEP does not require a motor response of the primary visual cortex. FPL may involve more cortical processing, which matures more slowly than the visual cortex. Adapted from Eustis HS, Guthrie ME: Postnatal development. In Wright KW, Spiegel PH, editors: *Pediatric ophthalmology and strabismus,* New York, 2003, Springer; Stout A: Pediatric eye examination. In Wright KW, Spiegel PH, editors: *Pediatric ophthalmology and strabismus,* New York, 2003, Springer.

■ Development, Physiology, and Pathophysiology of the Eye

DEVELOPMENT OF THE OCULAR STRUCTURES

At 21 days of gestation, the human embryo is one fifth of an inch long, and the first recognizable ocular tissue is visible on each side of the head. By the end of the eighth week the eyes have moved medially toward the front of the face. The eyelids are completely formed, and the edges of the upper and lower lids fuse to seal the eye while it develops. At 16 weeks of gestation the eyes are fully anterior, and over the ensuing weeks they continue to move closer to the bridge of the nose. By the seventh month of pregnancy, the fetus can open its eyes.

Development of the eye as a visual organ is not complete at birth, yet newborns have the ability to fix their gaze, follow an object to midline, and react to a change in the intensity of light. Over the first 2 to 3 months of extrauterine life, the ability to focus at any range develops as the eyes become coordinated horizontally and vertically. By 3 months old infants can follow moving objects, and by 4 months they can indicate visual recognition of familiar objects. The shape and contour of the eyeball changes, and visual acuity and binocularity gradually increase with age. The volume of the orbits doubles by the time the child is 1 year old and almost doubles again by 6 to 8 years old. Eye growth is completed at 10 to 13 years. The corneal dimension, however, changes minimally from full-term newborn to adulthood.

During early childhood the visual pathways that ensure central vision are developing. The brain must receive equally clear, bilaterally focused images at the same time for this development to occur. The adult visual field is obtained by 10 years old. The visual pathways are amenable to the greatest corrective influences (e.g., adequate treatment of amblyopia) until 7 to 8 years old. Research has demonstrated that the visual system of teens and adults with amblyopia might still retain substantial plasticity (Scheiman et al, 2005; Zhou et al, 2006).

ANATOMY AND PHYSIOLOGY OF THE EYE

The eyeball consists of three layers of tissue: the fibrous tunic, the vascular tunic, and the inner tunic or retina. The fibrous tunic consists of the sclera and the cornea. The vascular tunic, the middle layer, is composed of the choroid, the ciliary body, and the iris (Fig. 28-1). All the structures of the eye are dedicated to accurate and efficient functioning of the innermost layer of the eyeball, the retina. The optic disc consists only of nerve fibers (no rods or cones), so no visual images are formed here. Thus, it is referred to as the blind spot.

The inside of the eyeball consists of the anterior and posterior cavities (see Fig. 28-1). The anterior cavity is divided into anterior and posterior chambers. The anterior chamber lies between the cornea and the iris. The posterior chamber lies between the iris and the suspensory ligament. Aqueous humor circulates throughout these chambers to maintain intraocular pressure (IOP) and link the circulatory system with the avascular lens and cornea. The other cavity within the eyeball, the posterior cavity, lies between the lens and the retina. The gelatinous vitreous humor found in this cavity contributes to the maintenance of IOP and holds the retina in place. The lens, which separates the cavities, hangs by the suspensory ligament. Six muscles guide movement of the globe. Four rectus muscles (superior, inferior, lateral, and medial) move the eyeball up, down, in, and out, respectively. Two oblique muscles (superior and inferior) rotate the eyeball on its axis. Cranial nerve (CN) III (oculomotor), CN IV (trochlear), and CN VI (abducens) innervate these muscles.

The focusing of light rays involves four basic processes: refraction of light rays, accommodation of the lens, constriction of the pupil, and convergence of the eyes. *Refraction* is the bending of light rays as they pass from one transparent medium (air) to another (cornea or lens). The lens modifies the degree of refraction to create the sharpest image on the retina. *Accommodation* is the ability of the lens to focus on close objects by increasing its curvature. The normal eye refracts light rays from an object 20 feet away to focus a clear image

TABLE 28-3 Recommended Ages and Methods for Pediatric Eye Evaluation Screening

Recommended Age	Method	Indications for Referral to an Ophthalmologist
Newborn-3 months	Red reflex Ocular history Inspection	Abnormal or asymmetric Structural abnormality
3-6 months (approximately)	Fix and follow Ocular history Red reflex Inspection	Failure to fix and follow in a cooperative infant Abnormal or asymmetric Structural abnormality
6-12 months and until child is able to cooperate for verbal visual acuity	Fix and follow with each eye Alternate occlusion Ocular history Corneal light reflex Red reflex Inspection	Failure to fix and follow Failure to object equally to covering each eye Asymmetric Abnormal or asymmetric Structural abnormality
≥3 years and every 1-2 years after 5 years	Visual acuity* (monocular) Ocular history Corneal light reflex/cover-uncover reflex Red reflex Inspection Attempt ophthalmoscopy	3 years: 20/50 or worse; 5 years: 20/40 or worse >5 years: 20/30 or worse, or two lines of difference between the eyes Asymmetric/ocular refixation movements Abnormal or asymmetric Structural abnormality

*Pictures (Lea Hyvärinen [LH/LEA] symbols or Allen cards for 2- to 4-year-olds); "tumbling E" or HOTV for ≥4-year-olds; or vision-testing machines.
NOTE: These recommendations are based on panel consensus. Although the child may be retested if screening is inconclusive or unsatisfactory, undue delays should be avoided; if inconclusive on retesting, referral for comprehensive pediatric medical eye evaluation is indicated. Use of medication for pupillary dilation facilitates evaluation of the red reflex. See text for recommended medication.
Data from American Academy of Pediatrics (AAP) Committee on Practice and Ambulatory Medicine and Section on Ophthalmology, American Association of Certified Orthoptists, American Association of Pediatric Ophthalmology and Strabismus, American Academy of Ophthalmology (AAO): Eye examination in infants, children, and young adults by pediatricians: policy statement, *Pediatrics* 111(4):902-907, 2003, reaffirmed 2007.

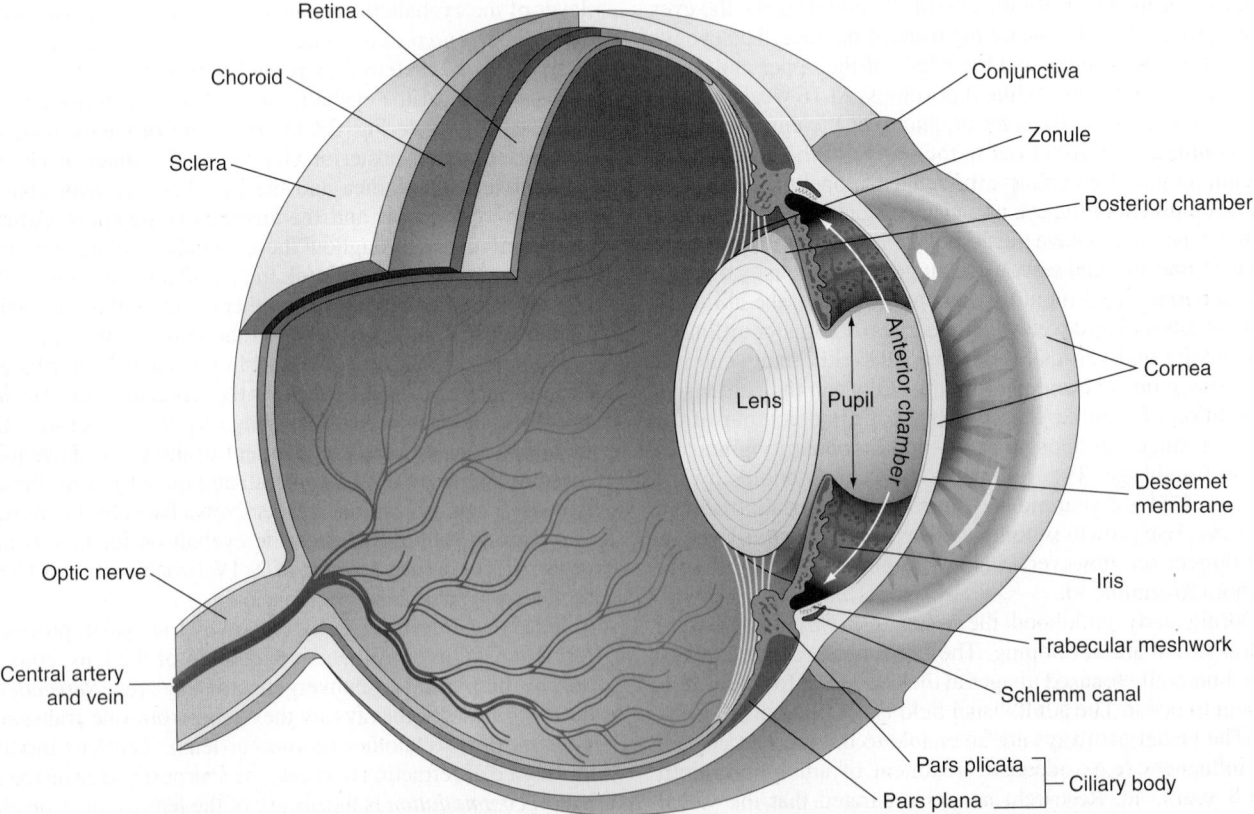

FIGURE 28-1 Anatomy of the eye. (From Kumar V, Abbas AK, Fausto N, et al: *Robbins and Cotran pathologic basis of disease,* professional edition, ed 8, Philadelphia, 2010, Saunders.)

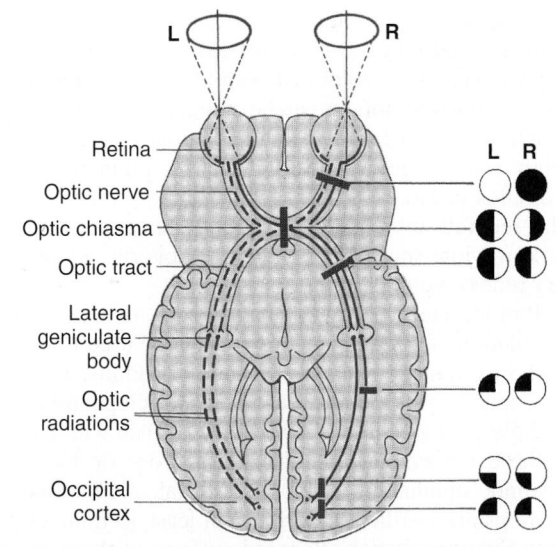

FIGURE 28-2 Visual pathway. On the right are diagrams of the visual fields with areas of blindness darkened to show the effects of injuries in various locations. (From Anderson PD: *Basic human anatomy and physiology: clinical implications for the health professions,* Sudbury, MA, 1984, Jones and Bartlett. Copyright ©1984, Jones and Bartlett Publishers, www.jbpub.com. Reprinted with permission.)

onto the retina; hence the fraction 20/20 is used to denote the accepted standard of normal vision. The circular muscle fibers of the iris, which contract in response to light, cause constriction of the pupil. Regulating the light entering the eye can also facilitate production of a precise image. To maintain single binocular vision, close objects require the eyes to rotate medially so that the light rays from the object hit the same points on both retinas. This rotation is called *convergence.* A normal neonate demonstrates disconjugate fixation, but convergence and accommodation normally develop by 3 to 4 months, with parallel alignment by 5 to 6 months without nystagmus or strabismus. Jerky eye movements can be seen until 2 months, after which time smooth tracking movements are expected.

After an image is formed on the retina, light impulses are converted into nerve impulses and transmitted to the visual centers located in the occipital lobes of the cerebral cortex. Lesions in various places along the neural tracts from the eye to the cortex cause different types of loss of visual fields (Fig. 28-2).

PATHOPHYSIOLOGY OF THE EYES

Potential problems with the eyes or visual system can take the form of specific disorders, infections, or injuries to the eye. The most common disorders of the eye interfering with vision are refractive errors (myopia, hyperopia, astigmatism, and anisometropia). Less common disorders include strabismus, amblyopia, ptosis, nystagmus, cataracts, glaucoma, ROP, and RB. Infections and injuries may be relatively minor and superficial or critical and involve deep tissues of the eye. Certain systemic diseases (e.g., juvenile rheumatoid arthritis) and medications (e.g., steroids) can also affect the eyes and warrant extra assessment measures.

■ Assessment

Assessment of the eye, as with all body systems, requires a thoughtful history, careful physical examination, and certain specialized screening tests.

HISTORY

- General medical history including birthweight; pertinent prenatal, perinatal, postnatal factors (e.g., prematurity, infections); past hospitalizations and surgery; general health and development
- Family medical history of ocular problems (including eye surgeries), such as glaucoma, blindness, poor vision, difficulty walking in dim light, photophobia, use of thick glasses, lazy eye, strabismus, nystagmus, leukokoria, RB, congenital cataracts
- History of chronic systemic disease in patient or family (e.g., inflammatory bowel disease; connective tissue disorders; cardiac defects of Marfan syndrome; midfacial hypoplasia; abnormalities of teeth, umbilical cord, or urinary tract; neurologic or skin anomalies; developmental delay; mental retardation; diabetes; sickle cell hemoglobinopathies; Tay-Sachs disease; tuberculosis)
- Presence of allergies and specific allergens
- Current medications (e.g., steroids); past or present substance abuse
- Child's ocular history, which includes:
  - Date (and results) of the last vision screening and prior eye problems or diseases, including diagnoses and treatments
  - If history of eye injury: unilateral or bilateral injury? Were there visual changes or photophobia? What treatment was received?
  - Prescription and use of eyeglasses or contact lenses. Does the child have glasses that were prescribed? Are they used? If not, why?; use of sunglasses with ultraviolet (UV) protection or protective eyewear for sports activities
- Symptoms or indications of eye dysfunction or disease:
  - Older children may report visual loss or change in vision, such as blurring, diplopia, spots, and halos. Younger children may be observed to have problems with fixing or focusing (holding objects up close to see), tracking, squinting, head tilt, eye-hand coordination, grasp, gait, balance, behavior, and changes in the ability to maintain eye contact; eyelid droop
  - Photophobia may present as irritability, shielding, or rubbing of the eyes
  - Swollen eyelids, pruritus, excessive tearing or discharge, erythema, burning, eye fatigue, strabismus
  - Constant blinking, chronic bulbar conjunctival injection

PHYSICAL EXAMINATION

The physical examination can be challenging, depending on the child's age. The components need to be done quickly to accommodate the child's short attention span. Knowledge of visual developmental milestones is essential in assessing a child's visual capabilities (see Table 28-1).

- Gross inspection should be made of the external structures with a penlight (lids, bulbar and palpebral conjunctiva, cornea, lacrimal structures, and the size, symmetry, and reactivity of the pupils), orbits, eye muscle balance, and mobility.

- The red reflex is tested in all ages. It needs to be assessed for color, intensity, and clarity (opacities or white spots). A rule of thumb is that if the examiner cannot see into the eye (e.g., absent red light reflex), the patient cannot see out.
- In children more than 5 years old, funduscopic examination allows for visualization of the retina, choroid, fovea, macula, optic disc and cup, and entry and exit of the vessels and nerves.
- Examination of the eye is sometimes facilitated by using a cotton-tipped applicator to evert the eyelid. Eyelid eversion is accomplished by having the patient look down while the examiner grasps the lashes with the thumb and index finger, places the applicator in the middle of the lid, pulls the eyelid down and out, and everts it over the applicator.
- Growth parameters (especially head growth and shape) and the head and neck or other structures should be examined if a systemic condition is suspected.

SCREENING TESTS
Conducting Screening Tests

Fatigue, hunger, anxiety, and environmental distractions can interfere with vision testing. Testing should always precede the administration of immunizations or any procedure that might cause discomfort. While testing, observe children for behavior indicating that they are having difficulty, such as straining, squinting, excessive blinking, head tilting or shaking, or thrusting the trunk or head forward. The tendency to peek out from behind the eye shield may or may not reflect difficulty; the child may do so out of a desire to be successful and please the tester. The examiner should resist the tendency to correct a mistake or give the child nonverbal clues that can influence the results. Three-year-old children who have difficulty performing any of the vision tests in the PCP's office should be tested again within 6 months; those unable to perform when older than 4 years of age should be retested in 1 month (AAP et al, 2007). A child who is uncooperative on the second attempt should be referred for a formal examination (AAPOS and AAO, 2007).

Red Light Reflex

The red light reflex should be tested at every well examination, including the initial newborn examination. Performing an adequate red light reflex test (Bruchner test) allows the clinician to detect the presence of asymmetric refractive errors, strabismic deviations, and abnormalities in the ocular media (e.g., cataracts, corneal abnormalities, RB). Disease processes involving the cornea, lens, vitreous, or retina block the light from entering or exiting the pupil and result in an abnormal red light reflex. The recommended technique follows:

- Darken the examination room (a lighted room causes the pupils to constrict, resulting in a poor red reflex). The darker the room, the easier it is to detect more subtle asymmetries between the red reflexes.
- Stand an arm-length away from the infant or child and use the ophthalmoscope light set at 0 or +1 to illuminate the face.

- Look at both pupils simultaneously and separately. Examining the red reflex slightly off axis to the center of the pupil enhances the color (ask a child to look to one side or use a distraction; infants can be approached from the side). In children with fair skin pigmentation, the red reflex is bright red-orange; in those with darker pigmentation, the red reflex is dark red-brown.
- The red reflexes should be symmetric; any asymmetry, dark or white spots, opacities, or leukokoria (white pupillary reflex) requires either:
  ○ Prompt referral to an ophthalmologist, or
  ○ Dilation of the pupils. Dilation may be used to enhance the examination in questionable situations. In infants younger than 9 months, use 0.25% cyclopentolate with 2.5% phenylephrine. In infants older than 9 months, use the cyclopentolate/phenylephrine drops or 1% tropicamide ophthalmic drops (AAP et al, 2008). One or 2 drops are instilled in each eye at least 15 minutes prior to the examination. Rare side effects to these medications include tachycardia, hypertension, urticaria, cardiac arrhythmias, or contact dermatitis.

Photoscreening, in which a calibrated camera takes a photograph under prescribed lighting conditions, may be used to assess the red light reflex and screen for ambylopia, although more research is indicated before this technique is a consistently reliable method of screening children because results vary among photoscreening apparatus and operators (AAP, 2008a). Medial opacities and refractive errors can also be discerned using this technique, particularly in preverbal or developmentally delayed children.

Infants with a positive family history of RB should be referred to an ophthalmologist familiar with the disease for examinations under anesthesia or dilation starting at 1 to 6 weeks old. Infants with a history of or with a relative having congenital cataracts, congenital retinal dystrophies (e.g., Leber congenital amaurosis, retinitis pigmentosa), malformation of the eye and related brain structures (e.g., coloboma, microphthalmia, anophthalmia, optic nerve hypoplasia), metabolic disorders (e.g., albinism, Hurler syndrome, Tay-Sachs disease), or other retinal or lenticular problems should also be referred to an ophthalmologist for a dilated examination (AAP, 2008b; Teplin et al, 2009).

Some pediatric ophthalmologists recommend routine dilation at the 2-month well-child examination, instilling the drops as the infant is weighed. Adequate dilation is achieved within 15 to 30 minutes, in time for the physical examination. Such dilation also enhances the detection of infantile cataracts (Murphee and Christensen, 2003).

Visual Acuity Testing

Visual acuity screening (see Tables 28-2 and 28-3), for both near and distance vision, should be performed on all children during routine physical examinations, when problems with visual acuity are suspected, and/or when eye trauma occurs. The American Optometric Association recommends comprehensive examinations at 6 months, 2 and 4 years, and every 2 years afterward (AOA, 2002). The AAO recommends a formal screening by the age of 5 years and sees no added benefit in having comprehensive examinations for asymptomatic children (AAPOS and AAO, 2007). If the child wears eyeglasses or contact lenses, visual acuity measurement must be obtained with correction.

Color Vision Testing

The human retina contains 6 million red and green cones and approximately 1 million blue cones. Alterations in color vision occur when the normal photopigments in the photoreceptor cones are replaced with different ones. Color ranges are then interpreted or perceived differently.

Red-green color deficiency is an X-linked inherited disorder or may indicate optic nerve disease. Inherited color deficiencies are more common in males and affect up to 8% of males and 5% of females (Tomsak, 2008). Color vision deficiency may also be acquired. A patient with acquired deficiency may have had normal color vision and then experienced color changes and losses. Diabetes, infections, optic neuritis, and toxins are systemic conditions that can lead to such losses. Blue-yellow deficiency is the most common type of acquired color deficiency.

Significant color blindness can affect school performance; can have safety implications, in that the child may be unable to distinguish traffic or vehicle brake lights; and can affect career choices. Color vision is tested by using the Richmond pseudoisochromatic plates (formerly Hardy-Rand-Rittler plates) or Ishihara plates. Children 3 to 4 years old are usually able to comply with testing directions, but the test does not routinely need to be administered (parents may request testing when their child is young and makes errors when asked to identify colors). In a child who is truly color deficient, the colors are not misnamed.

Peripheral Vision Testing

Examination of peripheral visual fields provides information about retinal function, the neuronal visual pathway to the brain, and the function of CN II (optic nerve). In an infant, assessment is limited to a rough estimate of peripheral visual fields by watching the child's response to a familiar object (e.g., bottle, toy) or a threatening gesture as it is brought into each of the four quadrants. In children mature enough to cooperate, peripheral visual fields can be measured by confrontation or by finger counting. Peripheral visual fields should be approximately 50 degrees upward, 70 degrees downward, 60 degrees medially (toward the nose), and 90 degrees laterally.

Testing for Ocular Mobility and Alignment

The Hirschberg test (also called the *corneal light reflex*) evaluates extraocular muscle function by projecting a small light source onto the cornea of the eye with the child looking straight ahead. A normal test reveals the reflected light as a small white dot symmetrically located in the same position of each eye (often slightly nasal of center). The cover-uncover test and the alternating cover test should be performed with the child fixating straight ahead, first on a near point object and then on a far point object about 20 feet away (Fig. 28-3). The process is sometimes aided by asking the child questions about the object (e.g., "How many cows do you see?" in a picture that has been placed for this purpose on the wall). During the alternating cover test, the examiner rapidly covers and uncovers the eye while shifting between the two eyes. Any orbital movement is an indication of misalignment.

Assessment of Visual Loss

If significant visual disturbance is suspected, the following functional vision assessments should be performed, the results documented, and the child referred immediately to an ophthalmologist:

- Shine a penlight into the eye from a lateral position and turn the light off and on several times to assess light perception. If the child can identify when the light is on or off, vision is described as "LP" (light perception).

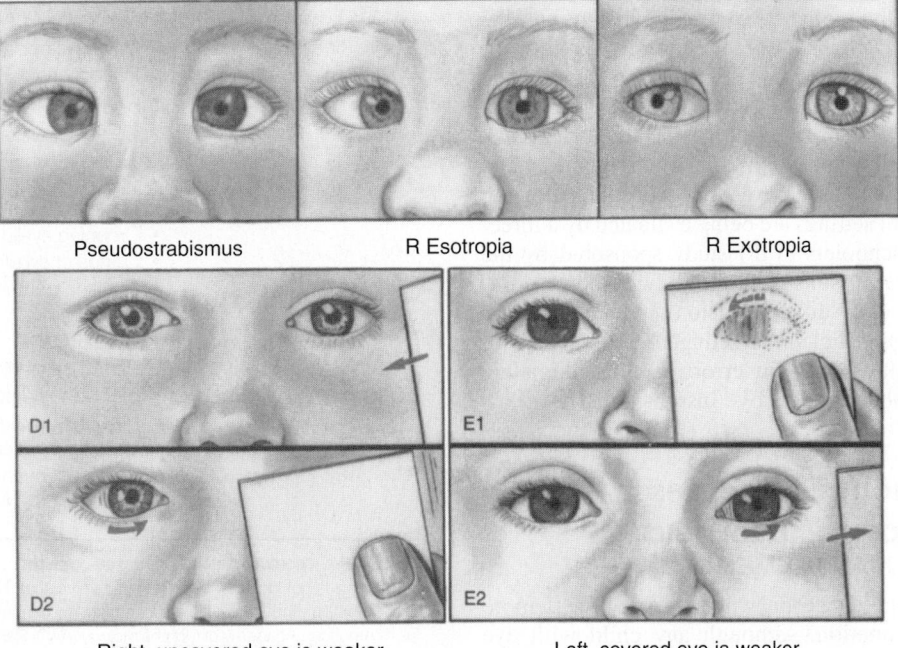

Pseudostrabismus R Esotropia R Exotropia

Right, uncovered eye is weaker   Left, covered eye is weaker

FIGURE 28-3 Extraocular muscle function testing (corneal light reflex and cover test). (From Jarvis C: *Physical examination and health assessment,* ed 2, Philadelphia, 1996, Saunders.)

- If hand movement (H/M) can be seen 12 inches from the child's face, it is documented as "H/M at 1 ft." Indication of search and recognition should be seen as the hand is slowly moved back and forth with periodic cessation.
- Ask the child to count the number of fingers (C/F) seen when one, two, or three fingers are held up 12 inches from the child's face. If the child is correct, document the vision as "C/F at 1 ft."

DIAGNOSTIC STUDIES

Laboratory and Imaging Studies

Cultures and Gram stain of eye discharge are done if identification of infection or particular organisms would be helpful in guiding management. Ultrasound (not to be used in cases of a suspected ruptured globe), computed tomography (CT), or magnetic resonance imaging (MRI) are sometimes useful in determining a diagnosis of orbital cellulitis, trauma, or tumor, or in substantiating a concern about the central nervous system (CNS). An MRI should not be used in the case of a suspected intraocular metal foreign body.

Fluorescein Staining

Fluorescein staining may be used to determine the extent of damage to the corneal or conjunctival epithelium as a result of trauma, infection, or exposure to a foreign body. Moisten a small strip of fluorescein tape with sterile water and place it in the lower conjunctival cul-de-sac. Allow the fluorescein to mix with tears. Examine the cornea with a cobalt blue filter light; any injury will take up the fluorescein stain and appear as a greenish area. Too much of the stain will cloud the entire cornea.

Other Visual Testing Tools

Three primary visual electrodiagnostic or electrophysiologic tests are used by ophthalmologists to provide insight into the functioning of the visual pathway. Preferential looking, or forced choice preferential looking (FPL), testing can be done in the PCP's office (requires use of special black-and-white and gray-striped cards to provide the spatial frequencies). A digital camera can be used to take images of the pupillary and red reflexes. The various visual screening procedures done in ambulatory and school settings are being evaluated by a three-phase Vision in Preschoolers (VIP) study sponsored by the National Eye Institute. Results of the study will more definitively indicate which of 11 different vision screening tests are more sensitive and specific for targeting preschoolers with amblyopia, strabismus, refractive errors, and/or idiopathic decreased visual acuity (National Eye Institute, 2010).

■ Management Strategies

REFERRAL FOR OPHTHALMOLOGIC AND SPECIALTY MANAGEMENT

See Table 28-4 for guidance on when to refer for a more comprehensive examination. Although any child with eye pathologic conditions should be referred to an ophthalmologist, optometrists can be a valuable resource in caring for children with refractive errors or certain common eye conditions

---

TABLE 28-4 Indications for a Comprehensive Pediatric Medical Eye Evaluation

Indication	Specific Examples
Risk factors (general health problems, systemic disease, or use of medications that are known to be associated with eye disease and visual abnormalities)	• Prematurity (birthweight less than 1500 g or gestational age 30 weeks or less) • Retinopathy of prematurity • Intrauterine growth retardation • Perinatal complications (evaluation at birth and at 6 months) • Neurologic disorders or neurodevelopmental delay (at diagnosis) • Juvenile idiopathic arthritis (at diagnosis) • Thyroid disease • Cleft palate or other craniofacial abnormalities • Diabetes mellitus (5 years after onset) • Systemic syndromes with known ocular manifestations (at 6 months or at diagnosis) • Chronic systemic corticosteroid therapy or other medications known to cause eye disease • Suspected child abuse
A family history of conditions that cause or are associated with eye or vision problems	• Retinoblastoma • Childhood cataract • Childhood glaucoma • Retinal dystrophy/degeneration • Strabismus • Amblyopia • Eyeglasses in early childhood • Sickle cell anemia • Systemic syndromes with known ocular manifestations • Any history of childhood blindness not due to trauma in a parent or sibling
Signs or symptoms of eye problems by history or observations by family members*	• Defective ocular fixation or visual interactions • Abnormal light reflex (including both the corneal light reflections and the red fundus reflection) • Abnormal or irregular pupils • Large and/or cloudy eyes • Drooping eyelid • Lumps or swelling around the eyes • Ocular alignment or movement abnormality • Nystagmus • Persistent tearing, ocular discharge • Persistent or recurrent redness • Persistent light sensitivity • Squinting/eye closure • Persistent head tilt • Learning disabilities or dyslexia

NOTE: These recommendations are based on panel consensus.
*Headache is not included because it is rarely caused by eye problems in children. This complaint should first be evaluated by the primary care physician.
From American Academy of Ophthalmology (AAO) Pediatric Ophthalmology Panel: *Pediatric eye evaluations: screening and comprehensive ophthalmic evaluation PPP*, 2007. Available at www.one.aao.org/ce/practiceguidelines/ppp_content.aspx?cid=761ac199-5cfe-42f4-b40b-33f9d5f0d364 (accessed Nov 8, 2010).

(e.g., corneal abrasions, foreign bodies). PCPs should acquaint themselves with the statutory guidelines for scope of practice and prescription privileges as designated by the state boards of optometry within their state to optimize referral possibilities.

Ophthalmologic or optometric management of potential or present central vision deficiencies may include the following strategies:

Occlusion. Various techniques may be used to treat strabismus and improve or prevent amblyopia by blocking vision in the sound eye. These include occlusion (patching), occlusive contact lens (a last resort method), optical penalization (over-plusses the lens on the sound eye), or pharmacologic penalization with 0.5% or 1% atropine (not used in infants).

Corrective lenses. In children, eyeglasses are used to correct refractive errors. Gas-permeable or soft contact lenses can be successfully worn by children as young as 8 years (Jones et al, 2009). Keratorefractive (laser-assisted in situ keratomileusis [LASIK]) surgery is undergoing worldwide research for its applicability in children with low to moderate myopia, severe anisometropia, bilateral high ametropia, and refractive amblyopia; however, its use remains controversial (Daoud et al, 2009; Fecarotta et al, 2010). The AAO discourages LASIK surgery in individuals younger than 18 years old and provides guidelines regarding suitable candidates for the procedure (AAO, 2007a, 2008a).

General guidelines for glasses and contact lenses can be found in Box 28-1. Glasses must be changed frequently in children because of head growth. Because the child may be reluctant to wear eyeglasses that hurt or pinch, parents should assess the fit of the eyeglasses on a monthly basis and watch for behavior that indicates discomfort in a preverbal child (e.g., constantly removing glasses, rubbing at the frames or face).

Contact lenses (includes daily wear [hard lenses] and soft, extended and/or disposable wear lenses), in addition to the cosmetic benefit, can provide better refractive error correction than eyeglasses, thereby enhancing visual acuity and the total corrected field of vision. Studies have also shown that their use improves how children feel about their appearance, athletic abilities, and what friends think of them (Jones-Jordan et al, 2010). Eye health can be promoted by reinforcing instructions regarding proper contact lens care and reminding the patient that contact lenses should not be worn when the eye is inflamed or topical ophthalmic medications are being used.

Until recently "plano" (noncorrective, decorative, or theatrical contact lenses used for cosmetic purposes) have been available for purchase from non-vision care resources. Severe eye injuries (including blindness) resulted when people bypassed the usual regulatory safeguards (proper fit, adequate instruction on use, and hygiene). Such cases prompted the AAO to sponsor legislation that required the U.S. Food and Drug Administration (FDA) to regulate the lenses as medical devices (AAO, 2005). The law requires that these types of lenses be properly fitted and dispensed by prescription only from a qualified eye care professional. Another type of plano lens includes those with light-filtering tints. These block or enhance certain colors and are designed for sports use by tennis players, golfers, baseball players, spectators, trapshooters, and skiers.

OPHTHALMIC MEDICATIONS

Caution and precision must be exercised when administering ocular medications to children because their smaller body mass and faster metabolism may potentiate the action of the drugs and result in adverse ocular and systemic side effects. Topical ophthalmic medications, such as antibiotics, mydriatics, and corticosteroids, are frequently found in ointment or solution vehicles. These topical agents are primarily used for treating disorders affecting the anterior segment of the eye. Solubility is one of several factors that influence the absorption of topical ophthalmic medications. Those that are water soluble (e.g., anesthetics, steroids, and alkaloids) penetrate the corneal epithelium easily. Fat-soluble preparations (e.g.,

---

BOX 28-1 Recommendations for Use of Corrective Lenses

Eyeglasses
- Polycarbonate lenses are lightweight, strong, and shatterproof; scratch-resistant coating is recommended.
- Silicone nose pads with nonskid surfaces prevent glasses from slipping.
- Comfort cables secure frames by wrapping around the child's ears and are available for children 1 to 4 years old. Straps are recommended for infants less than 1 year old and allow them to roll and lie down.
- Flexible hinges allow outward bending for easy removal by the child.
- Match the frame to the child's facial shape and features to encourage compliance; if old enough, allow the child to choose the frames.
- To encourage compliance with infants and children, do not fight them when they remove glasses; be persistent, replace the glasses, and provide distraction. Parents may need to set the glasses aside for a few hours before trying again. Seek counsel from the prescribing provider for further help.
- Tinted lenses can be used for photosensitivity; ultraviolet (UV) light filters are helpful with aphakia (absence of lens), congenital absence of iris, and albinism.

- Do not place the glasses down with lenses in contact with hard surfaces.
- Clean glasses daily with liquid soap and a soft cloth (do not use paper products).

Contact Lenses
- Contact lenses are appropriate for children 8 years and older; children need to be able to demonstrate ability to manage lens hygiene, including insertion and removal.
- Contact lenses are helpful for an aphakic child who would otherwise need very thick glasses that distort images.
- Wear protective outer eyewear for sports.
- Do not wear contact lenses if one or both eyes are inflamed or when using topical ophthalmic medications. Children with recurrent conjunctival or corneal infections, inadequate tears, severe allergies, or excessive exposure to dust or smoke should not wear contact lenses.
- Omit wearing extended-wear contact lenses (usually worn overnight) for 1 night a week in order to perform lens hygiene procedures.

most antibiotics) do not penetrate the epithelium of the cornea unless it is inflamed.

Topical Antibiotics

Prescription of topical antibiotics is ideally based on empirical evidence of infection. The best choice of a topical antibiotic is one that is not often prescribed for problems in other body systems. Topical ophthalmologic preparations, such as fluoroquinolones, sulfacetamide, and trimethoprim/polymyxin B, are effective and rarely produce a hypersensitivity reaction. Topical penicillins, on the other hand, are to be avoided. The pros and cons of these antibiotics are addressed in later sections of this chapter. Ophthalmic ointments are generally preferred over solutions for use in children, especially infants, because they last longer, do not sting, do not need to be given as often, and are less likely to be absorbed into the lacrimal passage. However, they do temporarily interfere with vision because they coat the eye, and they can cause contact dermatitis. Special care must be taken to ensure that the tip of the tube or dropper is not contaminated. Ophthalmic ointment should be transferred from the tube to moistened cotton swabs (one for each eye) and then rolled into the lower portion of each conjunctival sac.

Ophthalmic Corticosteroids

Although ophthalmic corticosteroids are effective in the treatment of ocular inflammation and traumatic iritis (excluding ocular allergy), a patient with a condition severe enough to warrant consideration of corticosteroid use should be referred to an ophthalmologist. Steroids are associated with numerous complications, such as an increased incidence of herpes simplex keratitis and corneal ulcers, fungal keratitis, corneal perforation and intraocular sepsis, glaucoma, slowed healing of corneal abrasions and wounds, increased IOP, cataract formation, and permanent loss of sight. They should be used only for significant ocular allergy, anterior uveitis, external eye inflammatory diseases associated with some infections, ocular cicatricial pemphigoid, and following some types of eye surgery. They should never be used for suspected eye infections, for red eye of unknown origin, or in immunocompromised children. A child receiving long-term ophthalmologic steroids should be assessed frequently for signs of adrenal suppression or other side effects. Encourage parents to keep scheduled tonometry appointments at 2- to 3-month intervals.

Other Topical Preparations

Topical decongestants or antihistamines or a combination of the two, mast cell stabilizers, and nonsteroidal antiinflammatory drugs (NSAIDs) are used in treating various ophthalmologic conditions such as allergic conjunctivitis. Over-the-counter vasoconstrictors or vasoconstrictor-antihistamine preparations can be tried first for mild allergic conjunctivitis. Cycloplegic agents are used for iritis.

Systemic Medications

In ocular infections involving the posterior segment and the orbit, systemic antibiotic preparations are necessary. A combination of topical and systemic antibiotics can also be used.

In general, these conditions warrant referral to an ophthalmologist. Systemic drugs may also cause damage to the eyes (Table 28-5).

EYE INJURY PREVENTION

Ocular trauma accounts for one third of all cases of acquired blindness in children. Male-to-female trauma incidence ratio is 4:1, with males 11 to 15 years old outnumbering all other age groups. Ninety percent of the injuries could be prevented by using protective eyewear (AAO, 2008b). The majority of the injuries are the result of sports-related accidents (50% of all eye injuries), toy darts, sticks, stones, fireworks, BB shot, paintball sports, other projectiles, and alpine skiing (AAO, 2008b; Olitsky et al, 2007). Other causes include battered child syndrome (40% have ocular findings), birth trauma, fingers/fists/other body parts in the eye, fireworks (firecrackers, sparklers, rockets), and airbags (though the injury is less than that suffered in cars without airbags or when the airbags failed to deploy). Slightly more than 44% of eye injuries occur in the home (AAO, 2008b).

The areas most affected by superficial trauma include the cornea (50%), conjunctiva (49%), and sclera; the most serious eye injuries involve the cornea, iris, lens, and optic nerve and may result from anterior chamber hyphema, vitreous hemorrhage, or retinal tear or detachment (AAO, 2008b). Listman (2004) reported that 43% had best vision of 20/200 at follow up after injury.

Prevent Blindness America's 2020 goal is to reduce injury-related vision loss by 50% by emphasizing eye safety measures (Prevent Blindness America, 2008). Parental supervision and education of children regarding prevention of eye injury are essential to minimize these injuries. Prevention includes such fundamental concepts as the following:

- Children need to be instructed to:
  - Not run with or throw sharp objects
  - Use protective eyewear when hammering, using power tools or lawnmowers, or participating in a sport where there is a higher risk of ocular injury (see list under Sports Protection)
  - Use orthodontic headwear that breaks away if force is applied
  - Not shine laser pointers in eyes
  - Use eye wash fountains when indicated
- Parents further need to be instructed to:
  - Store harmful chemicals and sharp objects out of the reach of small children
  - Limit and supervise the use of BB guns, air rifles, paintball devices, darts, and fireworks. The Prevent Blindness America (2008) organization does not support playing paintball games. At the very least, games should be supervised by a responsible adult and protective eyewear should be worn by participants.

Sunglasses

Ultraviolet (UV) A and UVB radiation from the sun can damage the lens and retina of the eye and cause cataracts and other conditions harmful to vision later in life (e.g., macular degeneration). Sunlight has more UVA than UVB, but UVB is more damaging. Sunglasses should be used to minimize such damage by absorbing these light wavelengths, even if wearing

TABLE 28-5 Systemic Drugs, Herbs, and Nutritional Supplements That Can Cause Ocular Side Effects

Drug	Ocular Side Effects	Intervention
Corticosteroids (prednisone at dosage of 15 mg/day for ≥1 year)	Cataracts, increased IOP	Monitor with ophthalmologic examinations.
Digoxin at moderately toxic ranges	Snowy, flickering, yellow vision	Resolves when drug is administered in correct range.
Isoniazid in greater than recommended dosages	Loss in color vision, decreased visual acuity, and visual field changes	Effects are reversible only if discovered early. Ophthalmologic examination is indicated before treatment and every 6 months; any changes warrant stopping isoniazid and referring to an ophthalmologist.
Isotretinoin	Pseudotumor cerebri (after initiating treatment) with resultant blurred vision, visual field loss, and varying visual acuity changes including optic neuritis, dry eye, decreased night vision, and transitory myopia	Monitor for symptoms. Annual eye exam recommended while on isotretinoin.
Minocycline hydrochloride	Pseudotumor cerebri and orthostatic blackouts, evidenced by blurred vision, visual field loss, varying visual acuity changes, diplopia; scleral pigmentation	Monitor for symptoms; scleral pigmentation may not resolve.
Phenytoin and carbamazepine	Blood levels in moderately toxic ranges can produce diplopia, blurred vision, nystagmus; sensitivity to glare	Resolve when therapeutic doses are within normal ranges.
Topiramate	Acute angle closure glaucoma; mydriasis; ocular pain; decreased visual acuity (myopia)	Onset of symptoms within 3-14 days after medication started. Stop medication. Treatment may include cycloplegics, hyperosmotic therapy, topical antiglaucoma medications.
Quetiapine	Cataracts	Monitor with ophthalmologic examinations.
Oral contraceptives (estrogen and/or progesterone)	Optic neuritis, pseudotumor cerebri, dry eyes	Monitor
Fluoxetine/SSRIs	Dry eye, blurred vision, mydriasis, photophobia, diplopia, conjunctivitis, and ptosis	Monitor
Herbs		
Canthaxanthin (taken to produce artificial suntan; food coloring)	Decreased visual acuity; retinopathy	
Cassava with prolonged usage	Decreased visual acuity; retinopathy	Contains natural cyanide so it is important that this plant is processed correctly.
Datura (may be used by those with asthma, influenza, coughs)	Mydriasis	
Ginkgo biloba	Retrobulbar and retinal hemorrhage; hyphema	
Licorice	Decreased visual acuity	
Vitamin A	Intracranial hypertension	

IOP, Intraocular pressure; *SSRIs,* selective serotonin reuptake inhibitors.

Data from Anderson AC: Ocular toxicology. In Shannon MW, Borron SW, Burns MJ, editors: *Haddad and Winchester's clinical management of poisoning and drug overdose,* ed 4, Philadelphia, 2007, Saunders; National Registry of Drug-Induced Ocular Side-Effects: *2006 AAO syllabus.* Available at www.piodr.sterling.net (accessed Jan 6, 2007); Reed Brandon, Hua Len: *Potential ocular side effects of select systemic drugs.* Faculty Scholarship, paper 3, 2010. Available at www.commons.pacificu.edu/cgi/viewcontent.cgi?article=1002&context=coofac (accessed Nov 14, 2010); Trobe J: *The physician's guide to eye care,* San Francisco, 2001, The Foundation of the American Academy of Ophthalmology.

UV-treated contact lenses. It is never too early to start wearing sunglasses. Wearing a hat with a wide (3-inch) brim only cuts the radiation exposure in half.

Sunglasses that have large-framed wraparound lenses with side shields provide the best protection. They should provide 99% to 100% protection from the UVA and UVB short waves, which range from 280 nanometers (nm) to 380 nm or more (Prevent Blindness America, 2008). The lens and frame should be constructed of nonbreakable plastic or polycarbonate. The protection comes from the chemical coating on top of, or incorporated into, the lenses. Gray, brown, and green colors are sufficient for general purposes and lead to minimal color distortion. Darker colors or polarized lenses alone do not offer the protection that is needed unless they specifically state otherwise. Sunglasses that are for fashion purposes or that do not list the UV protective wave spectrum should be avoided. Lenses should only be purchased if they carry the American National Standards Institute (ANSI) label or American Optometry Association (AOA) notation. ANSI communicates their standards by labeling their lenses Z80.3 and "general purpose," "special purpose" (for snow and water sports), and "cosmetic use" (lowest protection) (Bishop et al, 2009). In addition to the requisite UVA and UVB protection, the AOA recommends purchasing only lenses that state that they screen out 75% to 90% of visible light, are gray (for best color perception), and cause no distortion in vision (AOA, 2008).

Sports Protection

Eye protection is recommended for any child or adolescent participating in sports that have a high eye injury rate. Protective glasses or goggles are mandatory for all functionally one-eyed individuals (with best corrected vision worse than 20/40 in the poorer-seeing eye) or for any athlete who has had eye surgery or trauma or whose ophthalmologist recommends eye protection (AAO, 2003; Prevent Blindness American, 2008). Additionally, these children or adolescents should not participate in boxing or full-contact martial arts. Caution is also recommended in these individuals if they choose to wrestle, even though there is a low rate of reported injury. Specific protective eyewear is available; however, there are no standards for eyewear in this sport. Eye protection is also recommended for hockey, fencing, boxing, full-contact martial arts, racquetball, lacrosse, squash, basketball, baseball, tennis, badminton, soccer, volleyball, water polo, fishing, golf, field hockey, paintball games, pool activities, and football.

Protective eyewear should be properly fitted and selected specifically for the sport. A complete list of recommended eyewear for each sport is available online from the AAO website (www.aao.org). The list serves as a useful handout for parents. A headband or wraparound earpieces should be used to secure the glasses. Parents should only buy the protective eyewear certified by American Society for Testing and Materials (ASTM), the Hockey Equipment Certification Council (HECC), Canadian Standards Association (CSA), Protective Eyewear Certification Council (PECC), or National Operating Committee on Standards for Athletic Equipment (NOCSAE) for use in the particular sport. Fashion or street-wear glasses are inadequate, as is safety eyewear that carries an ANSI Z87.1 rating. Sports eye guards should have protective lenses designed to stay in place or pop outward in case of a blow to the eye (Prevent Blindness America, 2008).

Athletes who need prescription eyewear can either choose polycarbonate lenses in a sports frame that is ASTM F803 rated for the specific sport, wear polycarbonate contact lenses plus the appropriate protective eyewear, or wear an attached over-the-glasses eye guard that also meets specifications of ASTM F803. Younger children who do not fit into manufactured protective eyewear may be fitted with 3-mm polycarbonate lenses with ANSI Z87.1 rating. However, adequate protection cannot be guaranteed and perhaps another choice of sport should be discussed.

Laser Pointers

Lasers are rated on a scale of I to IV, with class I lasers used in laser printers and class IV used in research lasers. The FDA strengthened its message to manufacturers regarding the labeling and safety of laser pointers in 2009, stating class IIIa lasers may be used as pointers, but class IIIb (laser light shows, industrial lasers) and class IV lasers should not be used (FDA, 2009). Lasers traditionally available to the public had a maximum output of from 1 to 5 milliwatts (mW). Although harmless when used as intended by lecturers, potential injury from direct, intentional, prolonged exposure to the retina is of concern if the pointers are used as toys. A literature review found that these types of retinal injuries are not common and that exposure from a brief sweep across the eye by a class II or IIIa laser causes no injury (Ajudua and Mello, 2007). However, there are case reports of children and adolescents buying high-powered lasers from the Internet (with outputs ranging from 150 to 700 mW) and suffering permanent retinal injury and vision loss after playing with them (Wyrsch et al, 2010). It is recommended that laser devices not be made available as toys to children and adolescents.

VISION THERAPY, LENSES, AND PRISMS

Vision therapy, lenses, and prisms are controversial methods of treatment claimed by some to be effective therapy for learning disabilities and dyslexia (AAP, 2008c). These interventions consist of (1) visual training, including muscle exercises, ocular pursuit, tracking exercises, or "training" glasses (with or without bifocals or prisms); (2) neurologic organizational training (laterality training, crawling, balance board, perceptual training); and (3) wearing of colored lenses.

In a joint statement, the AAP and other organizations (AAP et al, 2009) state there is insufficient evidence to support the contention that vision abnormalities cause disabilities, including dyslexia. Therefore, vision therapy "to improve visual function by training is misdirected" (AAP et al, 2009, p 8). The joint statement further notes that the literature supporting vision therapy is "poorly validated," anecdotal, and consists of poorly controlled studies. Recommendations regarding vision care for children with learning disabilities include (AAP et al, 2009) the following:

- PCPs should perform periodic eye and vision screening for all children according to national standards and refer those who do not pass screening to ophthalmologists.
- Children with a suspected or diagnosed learning disability in which vision is felt to play a role by parents, educators, or physicians should be referred to an ophthalmologist.
- Ophthalmologists should identify and treat any significant ocular or visual disorder present.

- PCPs should recommend only evidence-based treatments and educational accommodations to school districts.
- Diagnostic and treatment approaches for dyslexia that lack scientific evidence of efficacy such as behavioral vision therapy, eye muscle exercises, or colored filters and lenses are not endorsed or recommended.

When counseling parents who inquire about vision therapy, the clinician should be aware of the pressure that parents may be under from optometrists who may be advocating vision therapy for learning disabilities and the divergent opinions held by educators and the ophthalmologic community about this modality of treatment. Managing a child with academic difficulties requires a multidisciplinary approach involving education and psychological and other medical specialists. Screening for ocular defects early is a routine part of primary care practice, and defects should be referred to the appropriate specialist.

Common Eye Disorders

VISUAL DISORDERS

REFRACTIVE ERRORS AND AMBLYOPIA

Description

Alterations in the refractive power of the eye include myopia, hyperopia, astigmatism, accommodation, and anisometropia. In a normal eye, light from a distant object focuses directly on the retina. When variations in axial length of the eyeball or curvature of the cornea or lens exist, light focuses in front of or behind the retina. This abnormal focusing produces an alteration in the refractive power of the eye that results in a visual acuity deficit (Box 28-2 provides more complete definitions).

Etiology

Genetic and heritable conditions account for approximately half of the children with visual impairment in the U.S. Cortical visual impairment, ROP, and optic nerve hypoplasia are the most prevalent conditions in preschool children (Teplin et al, 2009). Amblyopia is usually a unilateral deficit in which there is defective development of the visual pathways needed to attain central vision. Clear focused images fail to reach the brain and result in reduced or permanent loss of vision. The condition is labeled (or typed) according to the structural or refractive problem that is causing the poor visual image to reach the brain: *deprivational,* or obstruction of vision (e.g., caused by ptosis, cataract, nystagmus); *strabismic* (caused by strabismus or lazy eye); or *refractive* (myopia, hyperopia, astigmatism, anisometropia).

Refractive errors are the most common visual disorders seen in children. Approximately 20% of children have significant refractive errors by their teen years. Myopia may be present at birth, but it is more likely to develop between the ages of 6 and 9 years and continue to increase throughout adolescence; 10% of individuals before the ages of 7 or 8 years have refractive errors (Frederick, 2008). Mild hyperopia is normal in a young child but should decrease rapidly between 7 and 14 years old. Amblyopia affects approximately 2% to 3% of children in the general population (Braverman, 2009).

BOX 28-2	Descriptive Terms for Refractive Errors

Myopia, or nearsightedness, exists when the axial length of the eye is increased in relation to the eye's optical power. As a result, light from a distant object is focused in front of the retina rather than directly on it. A myopic child sees close objects clearly, but distant objects are blurry.

Hyperopia, or farsightedness, exists when the visual image is focused behind the retina. As a result, distant objects are seen clearly, but close objects are blurry.

Astigmatism exists when the curvature of the cornea or the lens is uneven; thus the retina cannot appropriately focus light from an object regardless of the distance, which makes vision blurry close up and far away. Rarely, astigmatism can be caused by an alteration in the corneal sphere caused by a soft tissue mass on the inner aspect of the eyelid, such as a chalazion or hemangioma.

Anisometropia is a different refractive error in each eye. It may consist of any combination of refractive errors discussed above, or it may occur with aphakia.

Definitions of varying degrees of visual impairment include:
- Legal blindness: Best corrected distance acuity in the better eye is less than 20/200, a visual field restriction in the better eye of less than 20 degrees, or both.
- Low vision: Corrected acuity is in the 20/70 to 20/200 range; these individuals generally meet requirements for special education.

Clinical Findings
- Squinting
- Fatigue
- Headaches (rare)
- Pain in or around eyes
- Dizziness
- Mild nausea
- Developmental delay
- Tendency to cover or close one eye when concentrating
- Family history of refractive errors, strabismus, or amblyopia

Management
- Refer to an ophthalmologist or optometrist for prescription corrective lenses. School-age children and teenagers should participate in the selection of frames; contact lenses may be considered. Extended-wear contact lenses may be prescribed in unilateral aphakia, severe anisometropia, corneal scarring with irregular astigmatism, and keratoconus.
- Older children should have an annual refraction and eyeglass evaluation.
- Unilateral visual occlusion may be necessary, and occasionally surgery may be necessary.
- Support and reassurance according to the child's developmental level are needed during the period of adjustment to contact lenses or eyeglasses.
  - Infants and toddlers need distraction, with consistent replacement of glasses once removed.
  - Verbal children may be aided by the use of positive reinforcement, such as sticker charts.

BOX 28-3 Descriptive Terms for Strabismus

A **phoria** is an intermittent deviation in ocular alignment that is held latent by sensory fusion. The child can maintain alignment on an object.

A **tropia** is a consistent or intermittent deviation in ocular alignment. A child with a tropia is unable to maintain alignment on an object of fixation.

Phorias and tropias are classified according to the pattern of deviation seen:

• Hyper- (up) and hypo- (down) are used to classify vertical strabismus.
• Exo- (away from the nose) and eso- (toward the nose) describe horizontal deviations.
• Cyclo- describes a rotational or torsional deviation.

Complications

Untreated or insufficiently treated amblyopia in young childhood results in irreversible and lifelong visual loss.

STRABISMUS
Description

Strabismus is a defect in ocular alignment, or the position of the eyes in relation to each other; it is commonly called "lazy eye." In strabismus, the visual axes are not parallel because the muscles of the eyes are not coordinated; when one eye is directed straight ahead, the other deviates. As a result, one or both eyes appear crossed. In children, strabismus may be manifested as a phoria or a tropia (Box 28-3). Pseudostrabismus is present when the sclera between the cornea and the inner canthus is obscured by closely placed eyes, a flat nasal bridge, or prominent epicanthal folds (see Fig. 28-3). In children older than 7 to 9 years who have acquired tropia, double vision occurs. In those less than 6 to 7 years old, cortical suppression of vision in the deviated eye results, which stops the diplopia, but leads to amblyopia. Exo-deviations may be constant or intermittent—the intermittent type occurs more often (Olitsky et al, 2007). Both types of strabismus may be hereditary or the result of various eye diseases (e.g., neuroblastoma), trauma, systemic or neurologic dysfunction that paralyzes the extraocular muscles, uncorrected hyperopia, craniofacial abnormalities, accommodation and accommodative convergence. Esotropia can also been seen in those with a history of prematurity, low birthweight, cerebral palsy, hydrocephalus, and maternal substance abuse or tobacco use (AAO, 2007c; Olitsky et al, 2007).

Epidemiology

The incidence of ocular misalignments is approximately 1% to 6% and each type varies by population (e.g., there are more exo-deviations in Japan; more eso-deviations in Ireland). Accommodative esotropia is most visible when the child is looking at a near object, occurs between 1 and 8 years of age (average between 2 and 3 years), and is seen in children with a history of acquired intermittent or constant crossing (AAO, 2007b).

Variable alignment is common in the newborn. Most have straight eyes; up to 70% can exhibit transient exotropia, which should resolve by 6 months of age, and 0.5% to 2% have esotropia. Up to 25% of esotropia that occurs between age 3 and

6 months resolves over time (AAO, 2007b). Congenital esotropia is ascribed to an infant with an onset less than 6 months of age who did not have a deviation as a newborn. Accommodative esotropia is an inward deviation caused by high hyperopia (AAO, 2007b; Diamond, 2008).

Clinical Findings

• Intermittent exotropia in normal children 6 months to 4 years old who are ill or tired or when they are exposed to bright light or with sudden changes from close to distant vision. It is more often seen when the child is looking with distant fixation.
• When only one eye is affected, the child always fixates with the unaffected eye.
• When both eyes are affected, the eye that looks straight at any given time is the fixating eye.
• The angle of deviation may be inconsistent in all fields of gaze, actually changing in some forms of strabismus.
• Persistent squinting, head tilting, face turning, overpointing, awkwardness, marked decreased visual acuity in one eye, or nystagmus may be seen.
• Cataracts, RB, anisometropia, and severe refractive errors are found infrequently.

Diagnostic Techniques. The corneal light reflection technique and the cover-uncover and alternating cover tests are used to screen for strabismus. Asymmetry of light reflection on the cornea is indicative of a deviation in ocular alignment. The cover-uncover test is used to detect tropias, whereas the alternating cover test detects phorias (see Fig. 28-3). The photoscreener can also be used to detect strabismus.

Management

• Any ocular misalignment seen after 4 months old is considered suspicious, and the child should be referred. Hypertropia or hypotropia, exotropia, acquired esotropia or exotropia, cyclovertical deviation, or any fixed deviation is an indication for referral as soon as it is first observed.
• The unaffected ("good") eye is occluded (using an adhesive bandage eyepatch, an occlusive contact lens, or an overplussed lens), which forces the child to use the deviating eye. Pharmacologic penalization with the daily instillation of 0.5% to 1% atropine sulfate is also used and studies show that it is as effective as conventional occlusion (Li and Shotton, 2009).
• Surgical alignment of the eyes may be necessary, but this does not preclude additional amblyopia therapy.
• Orthoptic exercises as a treatment modality are indicated only in certain forms of intermittent strabismus or when the visual axes are nearly aligned.
• Corrective lenses may or may not be indicated, depending on the presence of refractive errors.
• Assessment for amblyopia should be done at every visit, even after straightening the eyes, because changes in alignment can occur through the fifth year.
• The ocular status of an affected child's siblings is monitored.
• Local botulinum toxin injection may also be used with certain deviations.

Although response to treatment is more rapid in younger children, age should not be used as the deciding factor for referring a child with amblyopia. Although change is minimal in children over age 12 years, there have been reports of improvement with treatment even into adulthood (AAO, 2007b).

Complications
Amblyopia (secondary visual loss) occurs in 30% to 50% of children with strabismus (AAO, 2007c; Olitsky et al, 2007). Uncorrected strabismus can have a negative effect on self-esteem.

BLEPHAROPTOSIS
Description and Etiology
Blepharoptosis or ptosis is drooping of the upper eyelids affecting one or both eyes. It can be congenital or acquired, secondary to trauma or inflammation. Congenital ptosis is caused by striated muscle fibers of the levator muscle being replaced by fibrous tissue. It can be transmitted as an autosomal dominant trait. Other possible etiologies include trauma to CN III during the birthing process, trauma to the eyelid or neck, chronic inflammation (particularly of the anterior segment of the eye), or a neurologic disorder (myasthenia gravis, botulism, muscular dystrophy). Parents may remark that one eye appears smaller. In severe cases, children may have a chin-up head position or adapt by raising their brow.

Management
- Refer to an ophthalmologist. If vision is compromised, surgery is performed in an effort to prevent amblyopia and developmental delay. The amblyopia should be under treatment prior to surgical correction for the ptosis (Olitsky et al, 2007). Surgical correction depends on the degree of levator muscle compromise (Custer, 2008).
- Correct any underlying systemic disease.
- Evaluate for anisometropia (unequal refractive errors in each eye), anisocoria, and decrease in pupillary light reflex.

NYSTAGMUS
Description and Epidemiology
Nystagmus is the presence of involuntary, rhythmic movements that may be pendular oscillations or jerky drifts of one or both eyes. Movement is horizontal, vertical, rotary, or mixed.

Nystagmus can occur in association with albinism, high refractive errors, CNS abnormalities, tumors, post-infection (e.g., coxsackievirus B, cytomegalovirus [CMV], *Haemophilus influenzae* meningitis), various diseases of the inner ear and the retina, middle ear trauma, visual loss before 2 years old, and pharmacologic toxicity. Congenital nystagmus accounts for 80% of all nystagmus (Quiros and Yee, 2008). The child may have a birth history of prematurity, intraventricular hemorrhage, intrauterine psychogenic drug exposure, developmental delays, hydrocephaly, or be an infant of a mother with gestational diabetes.

Clinical Findings
The clinician should closely observe the nystagmus and note as much as possible about the type of movement (up, down, sideways), frequency (number of oscillations per a time unit),

distance of movement, field(s) of gaze within which the nystagmus is evident (e.g., field of gaze straight ahead, left, or up), and any compensatory head or neck postures of the child. The movements may be constant or varied, depending on the direction of gaze and head position. Oscillation of the newborn's eyes is common and exists for a short time during the neonatal period (Haslam, 2007). Involuntary oscillation (opsoclonus) that persists or occurs beyond the initial weeks of life indicates a pathologic condition (Olitsky et al, 2007; Quiros and Yee, 2008).

Management
Management consists of treating any underlying systemic disorder and referring the patient to an ophthalmologist. Any acquired nystagmus is most worrisome and requires prompt evaluation.

CATARACTS
Description and Epidemiology
Cataract, a partial or complete opacity of the lens affecting one or both eyes, is the most common cause of an abnormal pupillary reflex. Some cataracts are considered clinically significant, others insignificant. They are categorized as congenital or acquired.

Cataracts may be the result of infection (e.g., congenital rubella, CMV, toxoplasmosis), trauma to the eye (including physical abuse, airbag deployment), metabolic disease (e.g., galactosemia, hypocalcemia), long-term use of systemic corticosteroids or ocular corticosteroid drops, prematurity, CNS anomalies (e.g., craniosynostosis, cranial defects), genetic defects (e.g., Down syndrome, albinism), and demyelinating sclerosis and ataxia-telangiectasia. They may also be seen in children who have other ocular abnormalities, such as strabismus or pendular nystagmus, and in children with diabetes mellitus, atopic dermatitis, or Marfan syndrome. There may be a family history of cataracts; if present in multiple family members, a referral to a geneticist is indicated (Dahan, 2008).

Worldwide, cataracts are responsible for visual loss in up to 10% of children (Tesser et al, 2005). Approximately 1.2 to 6/10,000 births demonstrate infantile cataracts in the U.S.; most are isolated defects. Incidence rates vary between industrialized nations (lower) and undeveloped countries (believed to be higher) (Bashour et al, 2009).

Clinical Findings
- A history of maternal prenatal infection, drug exposure, or hypocalcemia may be elicited.
- Cataract appears as an opacity on the lens, unilateral or bilateral.
- Visual acuity deficits may vary.
- A pale red reflex in people of color should not be confused with a cataract.

Management
Management depends on the size, density, and location of the cataract. Often congenital or infantile cataracts can be monitored over several years for a progression that could produce amblyopia; some types of cataracts do not progress (Dahan, 2008; Tesser et al, 2005). Surgical removal of the lens optically

clears the visual axis. The resultant aphakic refractive error is most often corrected with contact lenses. Ophthalmic surgeons may insert an intraocular lens into the posterior chamber to partially correct aphakia, with residual refractive error corrected with spectacles. Any sensory deprivation amblyopia is treated aggressively and spectacles are prescribed beginning at age 4 months (Dahan, 2008).

Complications

Complications include amblyopia, which can be a particular challenge to treat; residual anisometropia; aniseikonia (unequal ocular image between eyes); or intraocular competition.

Prognosis

The ultimate degree of visual function depends on the cataract type, age at time of surgery, underlying disease(s), age of onset and duration, and presence of amblyopia or other ocular abnormalities. If the cataract is dense and present at birth, outcomes are better if removed within the first few weeks of life or before the age of 2 months (Teplin et al, 2009). Visual outcomes are variable, with poorer results seen with congenital unilateral cataracts than with congenital incomplete bilateral cataracts (Harper and Shock, 2008). Children with histories of cataract surgery may exhibit later inflammatory sequelae, glaucoma, retinal detachment, secondary membranes, and orbital architectural distortions (Olitsky et al, 2007).

GLAUCOMA

Description and Epidemiology

Glaucoma is a disturbance in the circulation of aqueous fluid that results in an increase in IOP and subsequent damage to the optic nerve. It is classified according to age at the time of its appearance and other associated conditions. Congenital glaucoma occurs in the first 2 to 3 years of life; it occurs because of a congenital abnormality of the structures that drain the aqueous humor. Fortunately, it is rare and generally caught early. The incidence is approximately 1 in 10,000 live births in the U.S. and rates vary among countries worldwide (Brandt, 2008).

Twenty-five percent of cases are diagnosed as newborns, 60% before 6 months old, and 80% by 12 months old; 65% to 80% occur bilaterally (Brandt, 2008). It is also seen in association with other developmental anomalies, such as neurofibromatosis; diffuse facial nevus flammeus (port-wine stain); Sturge-Weber, Marfan, Hurler, or Pierre Robin syndromes; intraocular hemorrhage; or intraocular tumor. There is a higher incidence in children with a history of congenital cataracts (up to 25% of children who have glaucoma have had prior cataract surgery) (Olitsky et al, 2007).

Secondary or juvenile glaucoma (a term used when glaucoma occurs in those between 3 and 30 years of age) occurs when the drainage network for aqueous humor becomes obstructed after ocular infection, trauma, systemic disease, or long-term corticosteroid use.

Clinical Findings

Parents may report that something is unusual about their child's eyes. This occurs more often in unilateral glaucoma when the orbital size discrepancy is more noticeable.

The clinician should then note the following symptoms of infantile glaucoma:

- "Classic triad" of tearing, photophobia, and excessive blinking or blepharospasm caused by irritation (only 30% of patients manifest this triad). Infants may turn away from light (Olitsky et al, 2007).
- Hazy corneas
- Corneal edema. Corneal and ocular enlargements are common in infants and young children (Brandt, 2008). Bulbar conjunctival erythema, and visual impairment may occur. If the condition is bilateral, parents may not notice any difference in the size of the corneas.

Symptoms of secondary glaucoma include the following:
- Extreme pain, vomiting
- Blurred or lost vision
- Tunnel vision
- Pupillary dilation
- Erythema (often in only one eye)
- Change in configuration of optic nerve cupping, with asymmetry between the eyes and loss of vision over time

Management

Early diagnosis is important. The goal is normalization of IOP and prevention of optic nerve damage along with correction of associated refractive errors and prevention of amblyopia.

- Refer to an ophthalmologist. Primary treatment is surgery as early as possible (often multiple surgeries are required). Medications may be used as part of the medical management; drug therapy may be difficult as a result of its prolonged nature, drug side effects, and adverse system effects.
- Parent and patient education must emphasize the importance of medication compliance and discourage excessive physical or emotional stress and straining during defecation.
- A medical identification tag is worn at all times.
- Follow-up is for life, often every 3 to 6 months.
- Ophthalmoscopic examination (including tonometry) is needed for every member of the family.

Complications

The following may occur over time despite treatment: permanent vision loss secondary to stretching of the cornea and sclera with resultant scarring, glaucomatous optic nerve damage, or amblyopia.

RETINOPATHY OF PREMATURITY

Description and Epidemiology

ROP is a multifactorial retinal vasculopathologic disease primarily caused by early gestational age with low birth weight. It involves the abnormal growth of the retinal vessels in incompletely vascularized retinas of premature infants. Previously ROP was called *retrolental fibroplasia*. An international classification system provides guidance for understanding this disease and for predicting outcome. ROP is classified according to the distance to which the vascularization has progressed away from the optic nerve (zone I, II, or III), severity of inflammatory changes (stage), duration (clock hours), extent of disease, presence of plus disease (degree of large vessel engorgement and tortuosity), scarring patterns, prethreshold and threshold ROP (a clinical subclassification system), and presence of Rush disease (rapidly progressing ROP, especially posterior retina) (Reynolds, 2005).

Developing retinal vessels grow outward from the optic nerve. The immature and incompletely vascularized retina is in a state of hypoxia, which stimulates the production of vascular endothelial growth factor (VEGF). Requisite levels of VEGF are needed to maintain the integrity of and stimulate retinal vessel growth. Exposure to supplemental oxygen presents an additional risk factor, although it is not totally clear what durations and concentrations of oxygen are detrimental when survival of the very smallest babies depends on prolonged oxygen and ventilation. Higher oxygen concentrations produce lower VEGF levels and result in slowed vessel growth. Over several weeks, an avascular retina becomes ischemic, and, in turn, stimulates renewed VEGF production. The increase in VEGF stimulates vessel growth but not necessarily in an ordered manner. Other factors may increase the risk of ROP and include history of maternal third-trimester bleeding, preeclampsia, diabetes, heavy smoking; in utero ischemia, hypercarbia, and hypocarbia; neonatal patent ductus arteriosus, sepsis, exchange and replacement transfusions, use of prostaglandins, lactic acidosis, congenital anomalies (e.g., anencephaly and trisomy 18), multiple birth, and being of a racial or ethnic group other than Black (Neal and Engmann, 2003; Phelps, 2010).

ROP occurs primarily in premature infants born at or less than 28 weeks of gestation or weighing less than 1500 g. The risk is higher with lower birth weights; infants between 1000 and 1251 g have a 47% incidence, and infants smaller than 1000 g a 80.6% incidence (Drenser and Capone, 2008). Infants demonstrating an unstable clinical course, despite a birth weight more than 1500 g, also are at higher risk (Olitsky et al, 2007).

Clinical Findings

ROP is initially diagnosed by a pediatric ophthalmologist while the infant is in the nursery (at 32 to 44 weeks postconception). Once the baby is discharged, the following may be seen:

- Leukokoria (white fibrovascular tissue in the retrolental space), glaucoma, cataracts
- Pupillary rigidity
- Vitreous haziness, hemorrhage
- Retinal and iris changes
- Pallor of optic nerve
- Strabismus
- Cataracts
- Detached retinas (often with secondary glaucoma, entropion, and eye infections)

An infant (especially if full or near term) not previously diagnosed with ROP with detached retinas or leukokoria needs an ophthalmologic evaluation to rule out genetic disorders (e.g., Norrie syndrome, familial exudative vitreoretinopathy [X-linked recessive]).

Management

ROP progresses at variable rates. Initial ophthalmologic examinations should be done on all infants born at less than 28 weeks' gestation or weighing 1500 g or less or those born at more than 1500 g or 29 to 34 weeks with an unstable course during hospitalization. Examinations should occur at 31 to 32 weeks of postconceptual or postmenstrual age or 4 to 6 weeks of chronologic age; any vitreoretinal sequelae need to be followed throughout life (Drenser and Capone, 2008; Olitsky et al, 2007). The PCP's role in managing ROP is to ensure that all infants fitting these criteria (even in those whose ROP resolved or who did not have ROP) receive the initial and follow-up ophthalmologic examinations (within 2 weeks or less after discharge) by a specialist experienced in examining preterm infants. The PCP further needs to:

- Discuss with parents the implications of their child's disease.
- Monitor for late sequelae or ROP progression (e.g., strabismus, pseudostrabismus, amblyopia, myopia, anisometropia, leukokoria, and cataracts).
- Assist children who have sequelae to maximize their potential by referring to early intervention services for low-vision children, to low-vision community support services, and to family support groups.
- Refer all children for yearly ophthalmologic follow-up if ROP required any treatment (even if ROP has resolved completely); less frequent follow-up is needed if no treatment was needed.

Cryosurgery or laser photocoagulation is used to arrest the progression of abnormally growing blood vessels (laser is treatment of choice) (Olitsky et al, 2007). Surgical reattachment of detached retinas has had disappointing results.

Complications

Complications can arise secondary to ROP or the treatment. Retinal detachment, strabismus, amblyopia, cataracts, serious myopia, nystagmus, astigmatism, anisometropia, uveitis, hyphema, macular burns, occlusion of the central retinal artery, glaucoma, and cicatrix (residual retinal scars) leading to later vision loss are possible. Any cicatricial formation is complete at about 8 months old. Less than 2% to 3% of infants have any visually threatening complications (Reynolds, 2005).

Prevention

Minimizing or preventing ROP can be accomplished by decreasing the occurrence of premature births and minimizing the oxygen needed. The efficacy of preventive vitamin E for high-risk infants has not been proven (Olitsky et al, 2007).

RETINOBLASTOMA
Description and Epidemiology

RB is one type of intraocular tumor. It is a rare malignant tumor of the retina but is the most common tumor in childhood. Incidence is highest in infants and young children and extremely low in children 6 years and older (Augsburger et al, 2008). A single or multiple tumors may be found in one or both eyes.

Hereditary and nonhereditary forms may occur; carrier and prenatal diagnosis is now possible. Bilateral disease and multifocal tumors are usually found in hereditary forms, whereas the nonhereditary forms are unilateral and unifocal (30% to 40% of cases). Unilateral disease occurs 60% to 70% of the time, is due to genetic mutation, and is commonly recognized by 25 months of age. The median age of diagnosis in children with bilateral disease is 12 months and 24 months in children with unilateral disease (Augsburger et al, 2008). The overall incidence is under study, but is estimated to occur once in 12,000 to 18,000 live births. Alaska Native children and New Mexico American Indians have a higher incidence than Caucasian children in the U.S. (Lanier et al, 2003).

The diagnosis of RB in developing countries can be delayed and the care suboptimal due to poor education, lower socio-economic conditions, and inadequate access to health care (Rodriguez-Galindo et al, 2008). The extraocular spread of retinoblastoma due to delayed diagnosis makes the possibility of death a real concern in developing countries.

Clinical Findings

- Positive family history
- Strabismus is often the most common finding.
- Unilateral or bilateral white pupil (leukokoria), described often as an intermittent "glow, glint, gleam, or glare" by parents, usually in low-light settings (Augsburger et al, 2008)
- Decreased visual acuity
- Possible orbital cellulitis and photophobia (causes pain), hyphema, abnormal red reflex, nystagmus, glaucoma, hypopyon (pus in anterior chamber of eye), or signs of global rupture

Diagnosis is made via CT scan with contrast and/or echography and/or MRI. Other tests may include fundus photography, fluorescein angiography, ocular ultrasonography, or fine-needle aspiration.

Management

Refer the patient to an ophthalmologist for diagnosis and management by a multidisciplinary team. An international classification system for intraocular RB lists the criteria of tumors based on their size, location, number, and degree of invasiveness or seeding. Depending on the diagnosis, treatment may involve external beam radiation, cryotherapy, laser photocoagulation, episcleral plaque brachytherapy, or systemic chemotherapy. Early detection and advances in treatment have led to less enucleation and less use of external beam radiation, preserving sight. In those with advanced tumors requiring enucleation, the hydroxyapatite implant provides excellent cosmetic appearance and acceptable motility of the implant (Shields and Shields, 2005). Siblings and parents should receive a referral for fundi examinations.

Frequent follow-up (every 3 months until 6 or 7 years old) to assess treatment and monitor for recurrence is important. Up to 45% of children treated with eye-preserving therapy will develop new or recurrent ocular tumors that require further treatment (Augsburger et al, 2008).

Complications

Metastasis (most commonly to bone or bone marrow) is possible if the diagnosis is delayed. Those who survive are at high risk for a secondary nonocular malignancy, cataracts, vitreous hemorrhage, neovascular glaucoma, lacrimal duct or gland injury, impaired orbit bone growth, radiation retinopathy,

optic neuropathy, or extraocular tumor with CNS or bone marrow suppression (Grabowski, 2006). Untreated children with RB usually die from intracranial metastasis (Augsburger et al, 2008).

Prognosis

The size and extent of the tumor determine the prognosis. Children who survive RB have an increased risk of death from nonretinoblastoma over their lifetime. The current evidence indicates there is a 20% risk of survivors developing a malignancy within 25 years of treatment. From the time of diagnosis until about 2 years after, the most common malignancies are pineoblastoma and intracranial retinoblastoma; therefore, these children should be monitored closely after RB treatment (Augsburger et al, 2008).

INFECTIONS

CONJUNCTIVITIS

An estimated 4 million cases of bacterial conjunctivitis occur in the United States annually (Smith and Waycaster, 2009). Conjunctivitis is an inflammation of the palpebral and occasionally the bulbar conjunctiva. It is the most frequently seen ocular disorder in pediatric practice. Approximately 78% of the time, bacteria are the cause of the infection (Patel et al, 2007). A 2010 study showed the causative bacteria to be most commonly *H. influenzae* (68%), *Streptococcus pneumoniae* (20%), and *Staphylococcus aureus* (up to 8%) (Meltzer et al, 2010); both gram-negative and gram-positive organisms are implicated. Conjunctivitis also occurs as a viral or fungal infection or as a response to allergens or chemical irritants. Bacterial conjunctivitis is often unilateral, whereas viral conjunctivitis is most often bilateral. Unilateral disease can also suggest a toxic, chemical, mechanical, or lacrimal cause. Blockage of the tear drainage system (e.g., from meibomianitis or blepharitis), injury, foreign body, abrasion or ulcers, keratitis, iritis, herpes simplex virus (HSV), and infantile glaucoma are other known causes. A major indicator of etiology is also age of the patient (Table 28-6).

Conjunctivitis in the Newborn (Ophthalmia Neonatorum)

Description and Epidemiology. Conjunctivitis in the newborn, also known as ophthalmia neonatorum or neonatal blennorrhea, is a form of conjunctivitis that occurs in the first month of life. In most states, conjunctivitis of the newborn is a reportable infectious disease. It occurs in 0.3% to 11% of newborns. A common cause is chemical conjunctivitis from the prophylactic instillation of silver nitrate at birth, which is one reason the product is no longer recommended. *Chlamydia trachomatis* is the cause of 2% to 50% of cases of ophthalmia neonatorum, and 50% of newborns with a mother positive for *C. trachomatis* at the time of delivery will contract the disease. Various bacteria account for 30% to 50% of cases (*Staphylococcus, Streptococcus, Pseudomonas, H. influenzae, Escherichia coli, Corynebacterium species, Moraxella catarrhalis, Klebsiella pneumoniae, Pseudomonas aeruginosa*). *Neisseria gonorrhoeae* and HSV are also implicated (AAP, 2009a).

TABLE 28-6 Types of Conjunctivitis

Type	Incidence/Etiology	Clinical Findings	Diagnosis	Management (see text for dosages)
Ophthalmia neonatorum	Neonates: *Chlamydia trachomatis, Staphylococcus aureus, Neisseria gonorrhoeae* (GC), herpes simplex virus (HSV). Silver nitrate reaction occurs in 10% of neonates	Erythema, chemosis, purulent exudate with GC; clear to mucoid exudate with chlamydia	Culture (ELISA, PCR), Gram stain, R/O GC, chlamydia	Saline irrigation to eyes until exudate gone; follow with erythromycin ointment • For GC: ceftriaxone or cefotaxime IM or IV • For chlamydia: EES PO • For HSV: antivirals IV or PO
Bacterial conjunctivitis	In neonates 5-14 days old, preschoolers, and sexually active teens: *Haemophilus influenzae* (nontypeable), *Streptococcus pneumoniae, S. aureus,* GC	Erythema, chemosis, itching, burning, mucopurulent exudate, matter in eyelashes; ↑ in winter	Cultures (optional); Gram stain (optional); chocolate agar (for GC) R/O pharyngitis, GC, AOM, URI, seborrhea	• Neonates: Erythromycin 0.5% ophthalmic ointment • ≥1 year old: fourth-generation fluoroquinolone • For concurrent AOM: treat accordingly for AOM. • Warm soaks to eyes three times a day until clear • No sharing towels, pillows • No school until treatment begins
Chronic bacterial conjunctivitis (unresponsive conjunctivitis previously treated as bacterial in etiology)	School-age children and teens: bacteria, viruses, *C. trachomatis,*	Same as above; foreign body sensation	Cultures, Gram stain; R/O dacryostenosis, blepharitis, corneal ulcers, trachoma	• Depends on prior treatment, laboratory results, and differential diagnoses • Review compliance and prior drug choices of conjunctivitis treatment • Consult with ophthalmologist
Inclusion conjunctivitis	Neonates 5-14 days old, and sexually active teens: *C. trachomatis*	Erythema, chemosis, clear or mucoid exudate, palpebral follicles	Cultures (ELISA, PCR), R/O sexual activity	• Neonates: erythromycin PO • Adolescents: doxycycline, azithromycin, EES, erythromycin base, levofloxacin PO
Viral conjunctivitis	Adenovirus 3, 4, 7; HSV, herpes zoster, varicella	Erythema, chemosis, tearing (bilateral); HSV and herpes zoster: unilateral with photophobia, fever; zoster: nose lesion; spring and fall	Cultures, R/O corneal infiltration	• Refer to ophthalmologist if HSV or photophobia present • Cool compresses three or four times a day
Allergic and vernal conjunctivitis	Atopy sufferers, seasonal	Stringy, mucoid exudate, swollen eyelids and conjunctivae, itching (key finding), tearing, palpebral follicles, headache, rhinitis	Eosinophils in conjunctival scrapings	• Naphazoline/pheniramine, naphazoline/antazoline ophthalmic solution (see text) • Mast cell stabilizer (see text) • Refer to allergist if needed

AOM, Acute otitis media; *ELISA,* enzyme-linked immunosorbent assay; *EES,* erythromycin ethylsuccinate; *IM,* intramuscular; *IV,* intravenous; *PCR,* polymerase chain reaction; *PO,* oral; *R/O,* rule out; *URI,* upper respiratory infection.

Clinical Findings
History and Physical Examination
- Chemical conjunctivitis usually occurs in the first 24 to 72 hours of life.
- Septic conjunctivitis caused by:
  - Bacteria usually occur from 5 to 14 days of life.
  - *C. trachomatis* usually begins between 5 to 14 days of life; it can also occur in newborns born via cesarean section with intact membranes.
  - *N. gonorrhoeae* usually appears in the first 3 to 5 days of life (up to 28 days).
  - HSV presents at birth or in the first 4 weeks of life.

Symptoms most commonly seen include the following:
- Chemical-induced conjunctivitis frequently manifests as nonpurulent discharge and edematous bulbar and palpebral conjunctiva.
- *C. trachomatis* specifically causes moderate eyelid swelling and palpebral or bulbar conjunctival injection and moderate thick, purulent discharge.
- *N. gonorrhoeae* specifically causes acute conjunctival inflammation, lid edema, erythema, and excessive, purulent discharge.
- Bacteria present with conjunctival erythema, purulent discharge.

- HSV specifically causes mild conjunctivitis, erythema, corneal opacity, serosanguineous discharge, and vesicular rash on eyelids and is often unilateral.

There may be a maternal history of vaginal infection during pregnancy or current sexually transmitted infection (STI).

Laboratory Studies. Swabs and scrapings must be done. Gram and Giemsa staining, direct immunofluorescent monoclonal antibody staining, cultures, enzyme-linked immunosorbent assay (ELISA), or polymerase chain reaction (PCR) testing can be used. Any infant younger than 2 weeks of age should be tested for gonorrhea. A culture for gonorrhea (on chocolate agar or Thayer-Martin medium) or aggressive scraping for a Gram stain is used for diagnosis (do not just sample the purulent discharge). If gonorrhea is suspected, also check for *C. trachomatis*.

Management

- Irrigate the eyes with sterile normal saline until clear of exudate.
- *Gonococcal conjunctivitis:* Infants should receive a 10- to 14-day course of intravenous or intramuscular cefotaxime. Ceftriaxone is another option, but should be avoided in neonates with hyperbilirubinemia. Ocular morbidity (corneal infection with possible scarring or perforation) can result in missed infections. Infants born by cesarean delivery need to receive prophylaxis against this agent.
- *Nongonococcal conjunctivitis:* A topical ophthalmic antibiotic preparation, such as erythromycin 0.5% ointment (0.25- to 0.5-inch strip to each eye), is applied three or four times a day, or moxifloxacin (four times a day for at least 5 days) (AAP, 2009b). The eyes should be cleansed with water or saline applied to cotton balls before instilling the ointment into the lower conjunctival sac.
- *Herpes simplex conjunctivitis:* Hospitalization and topical and systemic antivirals are needed. Two thirds of infectious cases can spread to the CNS, mouth, and eyes; one third to the skin (Mills and Khazaeni, 2006).
- *Chlamydia:* Assess for systemic infection (pharyngitis, ear infection, pneumonia). Treatment is with oral erythromycin base or ethylsuccinate (50 mg/kg/day in four divided doses) for 14 days. Topical treatment is not indicated because it does not lower the risk for a subsequent pneumonia caused by *Chlamydia* (see Inclusion Conjunctivitis in the next section).
- Chemical-induced conjunctivitis resolves spontaneously within 3 to 4 days without specific treatment.
- Mothers and their sexual partners should receive treatment if gonococcal and/or chlamydial infections occur in their newborns.

Prevention. The Centers for Disease Control and Prevention (CDC) recommends prophylactic administration of antibiotic eye medication within 1 hour of delivery to prevent ophthalmia neonatorum. The eyelids should be wiped gently with sterile cotton prior to application. Erythromycin ointment 0.5% (0.25 to 0.5 inch to each eye) is the recommended prophylaxis agent and the only one now marketed for this purpose in the U.S. The previously designated alternative, tetracycline ophthalmic ointment 1%, is no longer marketed in the U.S., nor is silver nitrate 1% (CDC, 2009a). Should a shortage of erythromycin occur, as happened in 2009, PCPs can find recommended alternative medications on the CDC website (CDC, 2009b). Povidone-iodine in a 2.5% solution is in use outside the U.S. Prophylaxis is required by law in most states and territories to prevent gonococcal conjunctivitis in the newborn. However, prophylaxis does not prevent neonatal chlamydial conjunctivitis or extraocular infection. It should be determined at the time of the first visit whether infants born at home have received this prophylaxis.

Inclusion Conjunctivitis (Chlamydia)

Epidemiology. Inclusion conjunctivitis is usually caused by one of eight known strains of *C. trachomatis* and is most often seen in a neonate or sexually active adolescent. Neonates usually demonstrate symptoms within the first 5 to 14 days of life (to 6 weeks), whereas *N. gonorrhoeae* symptoms are usually detected earlier. Nasopharyngeal infection with *C. trachomatis* is found in 50% of those with inclusion conjunctivitis.

Clinical Findings
History and Physical Examination

- Maternal history of an STI or a history of a sexual partner with an STI
- Conjunctival erythema and mild to severe mucopurulent to bloody discharge, usually bilateral
- Follicular reaction (large, round elevations) in the conjunctiva of the lower eyelids; conjunctiva may bleed if stroked
- Associated cervicitis, urethritis, or rectal infection
- Infants may have symptoms suggestive of chlamydial pneumonia at 1 to 3 months old.

Laboratory Studies. Definitive diagnosis of *Chlamydia* can be made by isolating the organism by tissue culture and by nucleic acid amplification (NAA) testing (AAP, 2009c). Conjunctival scrapings for Giemsa staining are indicated. Scrapings must contain epithelial cells because *Chlamydia* is an obligate intracellular organism (AAP, 2009c). Other nonculture tests for *Chlamydia* include direct fluorescent antibody (DFA) and enzyme immunoassay (EIA). A specimen should also be gathered appropriately to test for gonorrhea because of the comorbidity of these two organisms. Ocular morbidity can result if gonorrhea is missed (refer to Chapter 31 for guidance on pneumonia caused by *C. trachomatis*).

Management. Treatment options have expanded from the traditional use of oral erythromycin ethylsuccinate (EES) to other macrolides, azithromycin, and clarithromycin. There is an increased incidence of idiopathic hypertrophic pyloric stenosis (IHPS) in infants less than 6 weeks old following systemic EES. However, this has not altered the recommendation of EES as the preferred treatment. The risk of using azithromycin and clarithromycin has not been fully established, although there have been reports of IHPS after the use of azithromycin (AAP, 2009c). Medical providers who treat newborns with EES should discuss the signs and potential risks of developing IHPS with parents.

Treatment recommendations include:
- A 14-day course of oral EES (50 mg/kg/day in four divided doses or 500 mg twice a day for 14 days). A second 14-day course is sometimes required because the failure rate with EES is 10% to 20%. Either EES is repeated, or oral azithromycin (20 mg/kg/24 hours daily for 3 days) has been found effective (AAP, 2009c). Providers are encouraged to use systemic EES with caution; if no other alternatives are viable, they need to have a high index of suspicion for the development of IHPS.
- Trimethoprim-sulfamethoxazole (0.5 mL/kg/day in two divided doses for 14 days) is an alternative systemic

treatment after the neonatal period (AAP, 2009c), and azithromycin and clarithromycin have been used, although they are not FDA approved in this age group.

- Doxycycline (200 mg twice a day for 7 days), erythromycin base (2.5 g, divided four times daily for 7 days), EES (3.2 g, divided four times daily for 7 days), azithromycin (1 g orally in a single dose), ofloxacin (600 mg divided twice daily for 7 days), or levofloxacin (500 mg daily for 7 days) can be used in young adults.
- Topical ointment (erythromycin, moxifloxacin) is sometimes recommended despite systemic drug treatment; the AAP notes that such concurrent treatment is unnecessary and ineffective (AAP, 2009c).
- Mothers of infants with *C. trachomatis* conjunctivitis, partners of such mothers, and partners of sexually active adolescents also need examinations and treatment for 2 weeks with tetracycline or erythromycin.

Complications. Complications include chlamydial pneumonia (5% to 20% of infants will develop pneumonia if their mother has a chlamydial infection at delivery), nasopharyngeal colonization (in up to 50% of infants treated for inclusion conjunctivitis), or gastroenteritis in infants (AAP, 2009c). Complications may occur 6 to 8 weeks following the conjunctivitis.

Bacterial Conjunctivitis

Description and Epidemiology. Acute bacterial conjunctivitis (commonly called *pinkeye*) is a contagious and easily spread disease. *H. influenzae* is the most common organism isolated in children who are younger than 7 years (Hautala et al, 2008; Smith and Waycaster, 2009). *S. pneumoniae, M. catarrhalis,* and adenovirus are also common pathogens. It is most common in the winter and in toddlers and preschoolers. Since the introduction of the *S. pneumoniae* vaccine in 2000, the incidence of vaccine-type invasive pneumococcal infections has decreased by 99%; the incidence of invasive pneumococcal disease has decreased by 77% in children younger than 5 years (AAP, 2009d).

Clinical Findings

- Erythema of one or both eyes, usually starting unilaterally and becoming bilateral (*key* finding) (see Color Plate)
- Yellow-green purulent discharge (*key* finding) (see Color Plate)
- Encrusted and matted eyelids on awakening (*key* finding) (see Color Plate)
- Burning, stinging, or itching of the eyes and a feeling of a foreign body
- Photophobia
- Petechiae on bulbar conjunctiva
- Symptoms of upper respiratory infection, otitis media, or acute pharyngitis
- Vision screen should be normal and documented in the patient's record

Laboratory Studies. Routine culture testing is *not necessary*. Gram stain and culture can be done if the conjunctivitis is chronic, recurrent, or difficult to treat.

Differential Diagnosis. Bacterial conjunctivitis requires consideration of nasolacrimal duct obstruction in infants, ear infection, Kawasaki syndrome, foreign body, corneal abrasion, uveitis, herpetic conjunctivitis, poor compliance, or wrong choice of drug. Cultures or scrapings are appropriate for unresolved infection.

Management. Bacterial conjunctivitis is considered a self-limited disease (unless caused by gonorrhea or *Chlamydia*) that usually resolves within 8 to 10 days. However, because both gram-negative and gram-positive organisms have been implicated, children who receive topical antibiotics demonstrate faster clinical improvement, can return to daycare or school faster, and cause less parental work loss. The common practice of prescribing antibiotics for conjunctivitis, however, has led to an increasing rate of drug resistance. It is imperative that providers make their diagnosis judiciously and then treat with an effective drug that is more likely to be tolerated and taken as directed. For this reason, older children and teens may be treated conservatively without using antibiotics. This prevents the overuse of antibiotics and takes into consideration the self-limited nature of this disease.

Choose broad-spectrum coverage that has the lowest resistance rate, greatest compliance, and best penetration of tissues. The cost of ophthalmic antibiotics varies significantly. If patients have a large copay for brand-name drugs or if they lack paid drug coverage, cost should be factored in when prescribing for this self-limited disease.

Parents can be instructed to put pressure over the lacrimal duct when instilling the medication to prevent drainage into the nasolacrimal system. If improvement is not seen in 3 days after treatment is initiated, refer to or consult as appropriate with an ophthalmologist. Contacts should not be worn during conjunctivitis treatment. Disposable lenses should be discarded and permanent contacts sterilized before reinserting (Jacobs, 2009).

For uncomplicated bacterial conjunctivitis, treatment includes (Jacobs, 2009; Rubenstein and Virasch, 2008):

- Sodium sulfacetamide 10% ophthalmic solution or ointment; not effective against *H. influenzae;* stings; can cause allergic reactions (including Stevens-Johnson syndrome). Dosage: 1 or 2 drops four times a day for 5 to 7 days.
- Trimethoprim sulfate plus polymyxin B sulfate ophthalmic solution. Dosage: 1 or 2 drops four times a day for 5 to 7 days.
- Erythromycin 0.5% ophthalmic ointment is recommended for patients with sulfa allergy and for infants. Dosage: ½-inch ribbon four times a day for 7 days.
- Azithromycin drops for children older than 12 months. Dosage: 1 drop twice a day for 2 days, then 1 drop daily for 5 days.
- Fluoroquinolone ophthalmic drops including besifloxacin, ciprofloxacin, gatifloxacin, levofloxacin, moxifloxacin, ofloxacin may be prescribed for children older than 12 months. Dosage: 1 or 2 drops four times a day for 5 to 7 days (regimens vary by medication).

The aminoglycosides (neomycin, tobramycin, gentamicin) are to be avoided because of possible hypersensitization, severe allergic reactions, and increasing resistance (Wagner et al, 2010).

Conjunctivitis-Otitis Syndrome

This syndrome is usually caused by *H. influenzae.* Treat for the otitis media (see Chapter 29). Concurrent use of a topical antibiotic is not necessary.

Patient Education. If only one eye is involved, it is likely that the infection will spread within a day or two to involve both eyes. The patient (or parent) is instructed to do the following:

- Cleanse the eyelashes several times a day with a weak solution of no-tears shampoo and warm water. The importance of wiping from the inner canthus outward and using a different cloth or cotton ball for each eye should be emphasized.

- Use warm soaks three or four times a day to relieve itching and burning.
- Instill the prescribed ophthalmic solution or ointment into the lower conjunctival sac. A moistened cotton swab may be used to facilitate instillation of ointments. Dosing while the child is sleeping greatly increases compliance and, therefore, effectiveness.
- Wash hands frequently and avoid shared linens to limit spread of the infection.

Also treat seborrheic dermatitis on the scalp and face if present (refer to Chapter 36 for treatment recommendations). Daycare center exclusion policies vary (some allow return once the treatment is started, while others only after completing 1 to 2 days of treatment). Improvement in the child's condition should be seen within 48 hours. If medication compliance is not in question and improvement is not seen within 72 hours of administration, the parent should be instructed to return so that a smear of the exudate can be taken for culture and sensitivity testing.

Complications. If the infection proves recalcitrant to treatment, eye pain is present, vision is blurred, or ophthalmoscopic examination reveals a bulging iris and a contracted, fixed pupil, suspect more serious inflammation of the uveal tract (iritis, cyclitis, or choroiditis). Refer immediately to an ophthalmologist to avoid ocular morbidity.

Viral Conjunctivitis
Epidemiology. Viral conjunctivitis is usually caused by an adenovirus but can also be caused by herpes simplex, herpes zoster, enterovirus, molluscum contagiosum, or varicella virus. It is more common in children older than 6 years and in the spring and fall (see Table 28-6).

Clinical Findings
- Tearing and profuse clear, watery discharge (*key* findings)
- Fever, headache, anorexia, malaise, upper respiratory symptoms (pharyngitis-conjunctivitis-fever triad with adenovirus [*key* findings])
- Pharyngitis with enlarged preauricular nodes (*key* findings)
- Itchy, red, and swollen conjunctiva
- Hyperemia and swollen eyelids
- Photophobia with measles or varicella rashes
- Herpetic vesicles on the eyelid margins and eyelashes (marginal blepharitis) or on the conjunctiva and cornea (keratoconjunctivitis)

Management
- Good hygiene is essential. Viral conjunctivitis is self-limited and should resolve in 7 to 14 days. Conjunctivitis is often difficult to distinguish from keratitis. If there is any question about diagnosis, refer for ophthalmologic assessment.
- Warm or cold compresses and artificial tears can be used.
- Prophylaxis with antibiotics is not recommended (Wagner et al, 2010).
- Antihistamine or vasoconstrictive ophthalmic solutions may be used for symptomatic relief.
- If HSV infection is suspected, immediate referral to an ophthalmologist is indicated. Topical corticosteroids should be avoided because they may worsen the course.
- Molluscum on the eyelid margins requires referral for excision.

Conjunctivitis-Pharyngitis Syndrome
This syndrome is more likely to be caused by adenovirus than by a bacterium. Treat accordingly.

Complications. Involvement of deeper layers of the cornea (keratitis) can occur and must be differentiated from conjunctivitis. Scarring of the cornea resulting in blindness is a significant complication of HSV infection. If in any doubt, refer to an ophthalmologist for a slit-lamp examination.

Allergic Conjunctivitis
Description and Epidemiology. Allergic conjunctivitis usually occurs in childhood but can occur after adolescence. Four types of allergic conjunctivitis have been identified: (1) hay fever–associated conjunctivitis is characterized by mild injection and swelling and is associated with exposing the eyes to environmental allergens (dust, grass, molds, animal dander) and may be associated with generalized allergic reaction including nasal congestion; (2) vernal conjunctivitis is more severe, with peak incidence in 10- to 12-year-olds, occurs in boys at twice the rate of girls, and has an increased prevalence in warm weather; (3) atopic keratoconjunctivitis occurs in those with atopic dermatitis and/or asthma (Rubenstein and Virasch, 2008). It affects the lower tarsal conjunctiva, usually occurs in late adolescence, is notable for significant (beyond that seen in allergic conjunctivitis) itching, burning, and tearing that are often chronic. Giant papillary conjunctivitis is a fourth type and occurs most often in contact lens wearers; it occurs 10 times more frequently in those wearing soft contacts than hard contacts (Rubenstein and Virasch, 2008).

Seasonal allergens (notably grass pollens and ragweed) cause allergic conjunctivitis. Rhinitis, eczema, and asthma may be associated conditions. The incidence is up to 40% of the general population and is experienced by approximately 32% of atopic children (Bielory and Friedlaender, 2008).

Clinical Findings
- Severe itching and tearing (*key* findings)
- Family history of atopy or seasonal allergies
- Rhinitis, eczema, asthma
- Acute attacks precipitated by allergens (e.g., pollen, animals, molds, dust, dust mites, occasionally food)
- Redness and swelling of the conjunctiva or eyelid (or both) (see Color Plate)
- Follicular reaction of the conjunctiva
- Stringy, mucoid discharge
- Bilateral involvement most common
- Cobblestone papillary hypertrophy in the tarsal conjunctiva
- Vision screening should be normal; document in patient's record

Laboratory Studies. Conjunctival or nasal smears (using Wright stain) reveal numerous eosinophils.

Management
- Prevention is best; avoid allergens.
- For mild cases, saline solution or artificial tears are administered along with cool compresses. Refrigerated eyedrops are more soothing.
- The next step is topical decongestants, oral or topical antihistamines, topical mast cell stabilizers, or topical NSAIDs (Rubenstein and Virasch, 2008). The decongestants do not decrease the allergic response, but do relieve erythema, injection, and lid edema. Prescribed agents can provide quicker, more long-term relief with fewer side effects than over-the-counter agents. Vasoconstrictors should be avoided because

of rebound hyperemia (Rubenstein and Virasch, 2008). Patients may be treated with systemic antihistamines (fexofenadine, loratadine, or cetirizine) if systemic symptoms are present (see Chapter 31 for management of allergies).

- ○ Topical decongestants include naphazoline hydrochloride ophthalmic solution (1 or 2 drops every 3 to 4 hours).
- ○ A combination antihistamine-decongestant is more effective than either agent alone: naphazoline hydrochloride plus antazoline ophthalmic solution (1 or 2 drops four times a day) can be used sparingly to reduce ocular congestion, irritation, and itching.
- Topical mast cell stabilizers may be helpful for maintenance therapy, chronic allergies, or vernal conjunctivitis.
  - ○ Cromolyn sodium 4%: 1 or 2 drops every 4 to 6 hours for children older than 4 years on a regular basis
  - ○ Nedocromil sodium 2%: 1 or 2 drops two times a day
  - ○ Pemirolast potassium: 0.1% or lodoxamide tromethamine 0.1% 1 or 2 drops four times a day for children older than 2 years
- Topical olopatadine hydrochloride 0.1% is a mast cell stabilizer combined with an antihistamine for children older than 3 years (1 drop 8 hours apart).
- Topical NSAIDs can be used for late-phase treatment of itching and burning.
  - ○ Ketorolac tromethamine 0.5%, 1 drop four times a day up to 1 week in children older than 12 years; it often stings when applied.
- Topical steroids must be used with caution because of possible side effects (increased IOP, potential for viral infection, contraindication with herpes, potential to cause cataracts, and poor corneal healing). An ophthalmologist should be consulted before using. At maximum, they should be used for 1 week.
- Refer to an allergist for allergen immunotherapy when rhinitis is present because therapy can lead to better control without the need for medication.
- Refer to an ophthalmologist if unresponsive to treatment or if the following is present: corneal abrasions, impaired vision, need for corticosteroids, severe keratoconjunctivitis, or atypical manifestations.
- Maintain a high threshold of suspicion for herpes-induced blepharitis or atopic keratoconjunctivitis if pain is present.

Complications. Some forms of allergic conjunctivitis (e.g., vernal conjunctivitis) can lead to corneal ulceration, scarring and vision loss, corneal degeneration, and changes in the corneal curvature (Jun et al, 2008).

BLEPHARITIS

Description and Etiology

Blepharitis is an acute or chronic inflammation of the eyelash follicles or meibomian sebaceous glands of the eyelids (or both). It is usually bilateral. There may be a history of contact lens wear or physical contact with another symptomatic person. It is commonly caused by contaminated makeup or contact lens solution. Poor hygiene, tear deficiency, rosacea, and seborrheic dermatitis of the scalp and face are also possible etiologic factors. The ulcerative form of blepharitis is usually caused by S. aureus. Nonulcerative blepharitis is occasionally seen in children with psoriasis, seborrhea, eczema, allergies, lice infestation, or in children with trisomy 21.

Clinical Findings

- Swelling and erythema of the eyelid margins and palpebral conjunctiva
- Flaky, scaly debris over eyelid margins on awakening; presence of lice
- Gritty, burning feeling in eyes
- Mild bulbar conjunctival injection
- Ulcerative form: Hard scales at the base of the lashes (if the crust is removed, ulceration is seen at the hair follicles, the lashes fall out, and an associated conjunctivitis is present)

Differential Diagnosis

Pediculosis of the eyelashes.

Management

Explain to the patient that this may be chronic or relapsing. Instructions for the patient include:

- Scrub the eyelashes and eyelids with a cotton-tipped applicator containing a weak (50%) solution of no-tears shampoo to maintain proper hygiene and debride the scales.
- Use warm compresses twice daily for 5 to 10 minutes and wipe away lid debris.
- Apply antistaphylococcal antibiotic (e.g., erythromycin 0.5% ophthalmic ointment, 0.25 to 0.5 inch into each eye three or four times daily) until symptoms subside and for at least 1 week thereafter. Ointment is preferable to eyedrops because of increased duration of contact with the ocular tissue.
- Treat associated seborrhea, psoriasis, eczema, or allergies as indicated.
- Remove contact lenses and wear eyeglasses for the duration of the treatment period. Sterilize or clean lenses before reinserting.
- Purchase new eye makeup; minimize use of mascara and eyeliner.
- Use artificial tears for patients with inadequate tear pools.

Chronic staphylococcal blepharitis and meibomian keratoconjunctivitis respond to oral erythromycin (250 mg daily for maintenance). Doxycycline (50 to 100 mg twice daily), tetracycline, or minocycline can be used chronically in children older than 8 years (Ganatra and Goldstein, 2008).

HORDEOLUM

Description

Commonly called a stye, hordeolum is an infection of either the sebaceous glands (Zeis or Molls glands), the eyelids (external hordeolum), or the meibomian glands of the eyelid (internal hordeolum). The causative organism is S. aureus or, rarely, P. aeruginosa.

Clinical Findings

A tender, swollen red furuncle is seen. In an external hordeolum, the swelling is generally smaller, superficial, and located along the lid margin. An internal hordeolum is larger and may point through the skin or conjunctival surface (Neff and Carter, 2008). The patient complains of a foreign body sensation. An internal hordeolum on the palpebral conjunctiva can be inspected by rolling back the eyelid. (See Color Plate)

Differential Diagnosis

If the hordeolum does not resolve, consider cellulitis of the lid or orbit, sebaceous cell cancer, or pyogenic granuloma.

Management

- Rupture often occurs spontaneously when the furuncle becomes large and a point develops. Removal of an eyelash near the furuncle frequently promotes rupture.
- Warm, moist compresses three or four times daily, 10 to 15 minutes each time, facilitate the process of rupturing. Hygiene for the eye can be maintained by scrubbing the eyelashes and eyelids with a cotton-tipped applicator containing a weak (50%) solution of no-tears shampoo once or twice a day.
- Antistaphylococcal ointment (e.g., 0.5% erythromycin, 0.25 to 0.5 inch into each eye 3 or 4 times a day) until 2 to 3 days after resolution is effective treatment.
- Steroids are not indicated.
- Refer to an ophthalmologist for incision and drainage if the hordeolum does not rupture on its own after coming to a point or for multiple or recurrent hordeolum.

CHALAZION

Description

Chalazion is a chronic sterile inflammation of the eyelid resulting from a lipogranuloma of the meibomian glands that line the posterior margins of the eyelids. It is deeper in the eyelid tissue than a hordeolum and may result from an internal hordeolum or retained lipid granular secretions.

Clinical Findings

Initially, mild erythema and slight swelling of the involved eyelid are seen. After a few days the inflammation resolves, and a slow growing, round, nonpigmented, painless (*key* finding) mass remains. It may persist for a long time and is a commonly acquired lid lesion seen in children. (See Color Plate)

Management

- Acute lesions are treated with hot compresses.
- Refer to an ophthalmologist for surgical incision or topical intralesional corticosteroid injections if the condition is unresolved or if the lesion causes cosmetic concerns. A chalazion can distort vision by causing astigmatism as a result of pressure on the orbit.

Complications

Recurrence is common. Fragile, vascular granulation tissue called pyogenic granuloma that enlarges and bleeds rapidly can occur if a chalazion breaks through the conjunctival surface.

NASOLACRIMAL DUCT CONDITIONS: DACRYOSTENOSIS AND DACRYOCYSTITIS

Description and Epidemiology

Nasolacrimal duct obstruction, or dacryostenosis, is an abnormal obstruction (imperforate valve of Hasner) of the nasolacrimal duct that prevents tears from flowing into an opening in the nasal mucosa. Dacryocystitis is an inflammation of the involved nasolacrimal duct; infection can result. Nasolacrimal duct obstruction is fairly common in neonates (up to 6% of live births [Olitsky et al, 2007]). It is thought to be due to a membrane at birth that covers the nasolacrimal duct, which then fails to break down quickly. It may also occur at any age secondary to trauma to the duct or to a chronic duct obstruction complicated by an upper respiratory infection. The condition is also found more frequently in those with craniofacial disorders and Down syndrome. Congenital failure of the duct to canalize may be unilateral or bilateral, and clinical signs appear 2 to 6 weeks after birth when tear production develops. Duct blockage usually resolves spontaneously in 96% of infants by 12 months of age (Olitsky et al, 2007). When infection is present it is most commonly caused by *S. aureus* and is often unilateral (other isolates include streptococci and *E. coli*).

Clinical Findings

- Continuous or intermittent tearing, stickiness, and mucoid discharge at the inner canthus that can become purulent
- Blepharitis in lids and lashes
- Occasional nasal obstruction and drainage
- Expression of thin mucopurulent exudate from the punctum lacrimale
- Fluorescein dye, instilled bilaterally in the inferior conjunctival sac and checked in 2 and 5 minutes with a cobalt blue light source, will disappear if duct is patent.

The following additional symptoms may be noted if bacterial superinfection is present:

- Tenderness and swelling over the lacrimal duct (can be exquisite) (see Color Plate)
- Eyelids stuck shut on awakening
- Edema and erythema of the tear sac (most prominent in the triangular area just below the medial canthus)
- Excoriation and thickening of the periorbital skin
- Conjunctival injection
- Fever
- Expression of purulent material
- Mucocele of inner canthal tendon (unusual; presents as a bluish mass)
    Laboratory Studies. A white blood cell (WBC) count (elevated) and cultures are obtained from the expressed exudate if the inflammation is severe.

Differential Diagnosis

Punctual or canalicular atresia, conjunctivitis, foreign body, congenital glaucoma, dacryocele, intraocular inflammation, and nasal mucosal edema are differential diagnoses.

Management

Treatment goals are to minimize stagnation in the tear duct and prevent infection.

- Daily massage of the lacrimal sac may be performed to facilitate canalization of the duct. The technique involves placing a clean finger over the medial canthus and pressing in a posterior direction until the fingertip enters the space behind the inferior bony orbital ridge. Gentle pressure applied in a downward and medial direction transmits

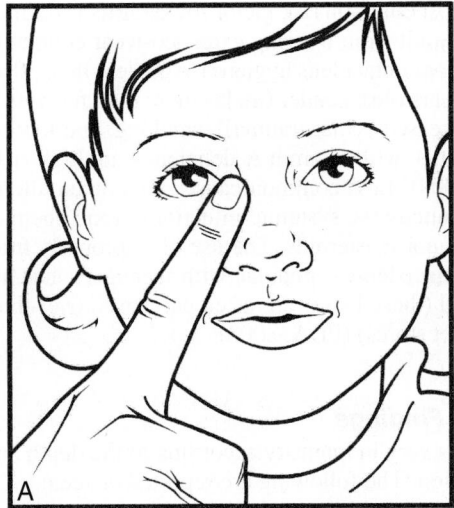

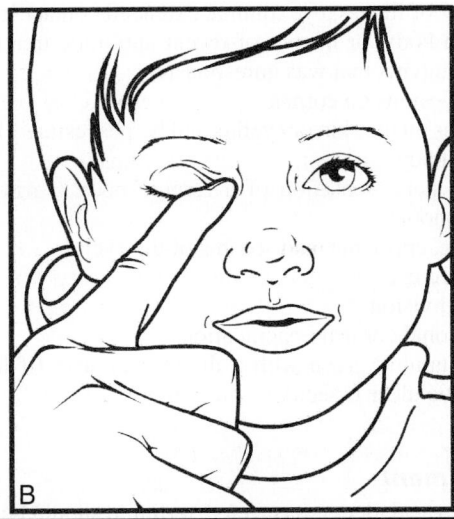

FIGURE 28-4 Technique to clear nasolacrimal duct obstruction. **A,** Incorrect technique. **B,** Correct technique. The finger is pushing behind the bone, "in and up." Note that the fingertip is not visible in the proper technique.

hydrostatic force through the nasolacrimal duct to the obstruction (Fig. 28-4). This technique should be performed about 10 times, two or three times a day. The eyelid should be cleaned with plain water after massage (Olitsky et al, 2007).

- For excessive mucopurulent exudates the following choices may be administered: topical ophthalmic ointment or ophthalmic drops (drops may penetrate more quickly), such as 0.5% erythromycin (0.25 to 0.5 inch into each eye three or four times a day) for 5 days or polymyxin B/trimethoprim (1 drop three or four times a day) for 1 to 3 weeks with massage and frequent cleansing of secretions. The duct may open spontaneously with resolution of the bacterial infection.
- Saline drops into the nose, followed by aspiration before feeding and at bedtime, help relieve any concurrent nasal congestion.

If the mucopurulent exudate persists for 1 to 2 weeks despite the above interventions, the infant or child needs a referral to an ophthalmologist regardless of age. Some ophthalmologists may probe the duct in an infant as early as 4 months old, whereas others wait until 9 to 12 months old. If probing fails to alleviate the problem (which is unusual), surgery may be required for placement of a tube stent or for a dacryocystorhinostomy (DCR). Chronic obstructions usually indicate bacterial colonization, which generally will persist without probing (Palay and Krachmer, 2005). When fever, marked erythema, swelling, tenderness, and toxic appearance occur, hospitalization is indicated for parenteral antibiotics (Wald, 2007).

Complications

Periorbital or orbital cellulitis is a complication of chronic dacryocystitis.

PERIORBITAL CELLULITIS

Description and Epidemiology

Periorbital cellulitis, or inflammation of the tissues surrounding the involved eye, is often associated with trauma or focal infection near the eye, eyelid abscess, bacteremia, or sinusitis. It is predominantly an infection in children, spread from the upper respiratory tract or middle ear.

It is most commonly seen in children up to 6 years old. It can also occur with infected lacerations, abrasions, insect stings or bites, impetigo, or a foreign body where the infection is spread via venous or lymphatic channels. It may also be secondary to paranasal sinusitis (Nageswaran et al, 2006). The etiology is often unknown, but the bacteria most commonly responsible for periorbital cellulitis are streptococcal organisms (these are nonvaccine streptococcal strains in children who have received both *H. influenzae* type B [HIB] and heptavalent pneumococcal conjugate vaccine), *S. aureus*, and, until the introduction of the HIB vaccine, HIB (Olitsky et al, 2007; Wald, 2007). *M. catarrhalis* can also be a causative agent in children younger than 4 years of age.

Clinical Findings

- Acute febrile illness (temperature higher than 102.2° F [39° C] if associated with bacteremia)
- Swelling and erythema of tissues surrounding the eye; upper lid affected more often than the lower lid.
- Deep red eyelid (color is purple-blue with *H. influenzae* infection)
- Symptoms of bacteremia or sinusitis (headache, decreased vision)
- Orbital discomfort or pain, proptosis, or paralysis of extraocular muscles

Laboratory Studies. Depending on the severity and speed of progression of the cellulitis, the following are useful:

- Complete blood count (CBC) with differential (WBC count usually greater than 15,000 if bacteremic)
- Blood cultures and culture of purulent wounds near the eye
- Lumbar puncture (infants younger than 1 year old)
- CT scan to rule out sinusitis, orbital cellulitis, or subperiosteal abscess
- Visual acuity, extraocular movement, and pupillary reaction testing

Differential Diagnosis

Conjunctivitis (bilateral conjunctival inflammation), cavernous sinus thrombosis, and orbital cellulitis (proptosis, limited extraocular movement, and reduced visual acuity) are the differential diagnoses in children; in neonates consider conjunctivitis, dacryocystitis, and ruptured dacryocystocele.

Management

The child may be managed as an outpatient if:

- The cellulitis is mild.
- The orbit is not involved (full eye movements are present, no pain with eye movement, visual changes, or ptosis).
- The child exhibits no symptoms of systemic bacterial sepsis.
- The child is older than 1 year.

Management must be made on a case-by-case basis. Consultation is needed when proptosis, ophthalmoplegia, or changes in visual acuity occur; these conditions are suggestive of orbital cellulitis.

Outpatient management consists of:

- Ceftriaxone (50 to 75 mg/kg [up to a maximum of 1 g] intramuscularly divided every 12 hours). The child is monitored daily until blood cultures are negative for 48 hours or clinical improvement is seen. Oral antibiotics may then be used to complete a 7- to 14-day course. Amoxicillin (high-dose), amoxicillin with clavulanic acid, and cefixime are first-line choices for treatment. If a rapid clinical response is not seen, further evaluation and treatment should be done. Warm soaks to the periorbital area every 2 to 4 hours for 15 minutes may provide comfort and speed healing. The parent is advised to call immediately if there is any change in condition.

Hospitalization and intravenous administration of antibiotics followed by a 10-day course of oral antibiotics are required for any of the following (Olitsky et al, 2007; Wald, 2008):

- Moderate to severe cases of cellulitis
- A poor response to outpatient management
- A purulent wound near the eyelid
- Children younger than 1 year old
- Children with suspected sepsis

Complications

Complications include orbital cellulitis or extension of the infection into the orbit, subperiosteal or orbital abscess, optic neuritis, retinal vein thrombosis, panophthalmitis, meningitis, epidural and subdural abscesses, and cavernous sinus thrombosis.

KERATITIS AND CORNEAL ULCERS

Description and Epidemiology

Inflammation of the cornea (keratitis) can cause a dramatic alteration in visual acuity and can progress to corneal ulceration and blindness. It is a medical emergency and requires prompt referral to an ophthalmologist (Mills, 2009). A corneal ulcer begins as a well-defined infiltration at the center or edge of the cornea and subsequently suppurates and forms an ulcer that may penetrate deep into the corneal tissue or spread to involve the width of the cornea. Involvement is usually unilateral. The causative agents include viruses (HSV-1, varicella-zoster, hepatitis C), bacteria (*H. influenzae, Moraxella, S. aureus, S. pneumoniae, Pseudomonas, N. gonorrhoeae,* Enterobacteriaceae [including *Klebsiella, Enterobacter, Serratia,* and *Proteus*]), fungi (rare), and protozoa.

The most common risk factor for keratitis is trauma (which can also result from wearing extended-wear contact lenses or having poor contact lens hygiene). Age (less than 30 and more than 50 years old), gender (males more than females [secondary to increased ocular trauma]), smoking, and low socioeconomic status, with vitamin A deficiency are high risk factors (Mills, 2009). Less common causes include an allergic reaction, conjunctivitis, systemic infections, toxic chemicals, and the use of corticosteroids. The use of improperly fitted decorative contact lenses, popular with teenagers, has also been implicated (these lenses are often purchased over-the-counter from outlet stores) (FDA, 2008).

Clinical Findings

Symptoms vary in intensity according to the depth and extent of ulceration. The following are reported or seen:

- Exposure to an infected individual
- History of illness, eye trauma, extended contact lens wear, foreign body, or history of recent antibiotic treatment for conjunctivitis that was unresponsive
- White lesions on cornea
- Vesicles on the skin or eyelids and herpes lesions elsewhere on the body
- Severe pain, sensation of a foreign body ("gritty"), and photophobia
- Tearing, erythema, and spasms of the eyelid
- Inflamed eye
- Blurred vision
- Occasional corneal opacification
- Area staining green with a fluorescein strip (if herpes, a dendritic ulcer is seen)

Management

When a corneal ulcer is suspected, the child should be referred immediately for a slit-lamp examination. Delay can result in loss of vision in the eye. Do not attempt to treat. Visual acuity outcome is good when these ulcers are treated aggressively with the appropriate agent (Mills, 2009).

- Steroids should never be used.
- Treatment with antivirals, such as trifluridine or vidarabine, may be used to speed healing in herpes simplex infections.

Complications

Corneal opacification, scarring, and loss of vision can occur if treatment is delayed.

INFLAMMATION OF THE UVEAL TRACT

Description and Epidemiology

Inflammation of the uveal tract (iris, ciliary body, choroids) and other ocular structures is often called *uveitis*. The inflammation may be anterior (affecting the iris, ciliary body, or both) or posterior (affecting the choroid). Adjacent ocular structures can also be involved, including the retina, vitreous, sclera, lens, and optic nerve. The inflammation may be acute or chronic. In the U.S., the incidence is about 6% in children; those with juvenile idiopathic arthritis (JIA) and a spondyloarthropathy account for most of those cases. Globally, rates in children range from 2.2% to 33.1% of all cases (Walton, 2010). Many processes have been implicated, broadly divided into infectious and noninfectious. Known etiologies include viral or bacterial infections, ocular trauma, and infection elsewhere in the eye. Other causes include allergy, malignancy, and systemic diseases, such as JIA, inflammatory bowel, Kawasaki syndrome, herpes simplex, tuberculosis, Lyme disease, cytomegalovirus (CMV), toxoplasmosis, syphilis, acquired immunodeficiency syndrome (AIDS), ulcerative colitis, rubella retinitis, and Stevens-Johnson syndrome (Olitsky et al, 2007; Walton, 2010; Weiss, 2008).

Clinical Findings

- Acute onset of pain (*key* finding)
- Red eye, photophobia, and blurred or decreased vision (*key* findings)
- Excessive tearing and eyelid edema
- Conjunctival erythema
- Circumcorneal injection
- Hypopyon (pus layer in the bottom of the anterior chamber) (see Color Plate)
- Cloudy appearance of the eye with a bulging iris and a contracted, irregular, or fixed pupil (see Color Plate)
- If chronic, there may be no ocular pain, photophobia, redness, or tearing.
- There may be a history of prior viral infection, joint pain, trauma, gastrointestinal problems.

Differential Diagnosis

Conjunctivitis is the differential diagnosis.

Management

Evaluate and treat any underlying systemic disease. Refer the patient to an ophthalmologist; definitive diagnosis is made by slit-lamp examination. The prognosis is improved with early treatment. Cycloplegics and topical or systemic corticosteroids (depending on the cause of the inflammation) are often used in treatment. Cycloplegic-mydriatics are used regularly to prevent posterior synechiae (adhesions of iris to lens and cornea); NSAIDs may be used as adjunct treatment.

Complications

Anterior and posterior synechiae, changes in IOP, corneal edema, various degrees of visual impairment, papillary scarring, retinal detachment, glaucoma, enucleation, and cataracts are possible complications.

TRACHOMA

Description and Epidemiology

Trachoma is a chronic infectious disease of the eye characterized by follicular keratoconjunctivitis with neovascularization of the cornea. It is the second leading cause of blindness in the world. It is caused by one of the two *C. trachomatis* bivars that exist in the world. It is endemic in the Middle East and Southeast Asia. It is rare in the U.S. but is endemic among Navajo Indians in the southwestern U.S. (Hammerschlag, 2007). It is contagious, often spread from eye to eye by flies.

Clinical Findings

- Inflammation
- Pain
- Photophobia
- Excessive tearing
- Granulation follicles on the upper tarsal conjunctiva, eventual inversion (entropion) of the eyelid leading to corneal trauma, scarring, and blindness
  Laboratory Studies. Cultures and staining are done.

Management

Consult with an ophthalmologist because treatment is difficult and recommendations vary. The World Health Organization (WHO) recommends treating with azithromycin (single dose of 20 mg/kg, maximum 1 g) (AAP, 2009c; Hammerschlag, 2007). Other drugs used include oral doxycycline (for children older than 8 years) or erythromycin for 40 days; or a topical antibiotic ointment (erythromycin, tetracycline, sulfacetamide [twice daily for 2 months or intermittently over 6 months]) to rapidly reduce inflammation to prevent scar formation (AAP, 2009c). Steroids are contraindicated. Reinforce the need for frequent handwashing and careful cleansing of the eyes. Discourage sharing of towels and handkerchiefs.

◼ The Injured Eye

CORNEAL ABRASION

Description

Damage to or loss of the epithelial cells of the cornea in the form of a corneal abrasion or tear is relatively common. Scratches from forceps delivery, paper, brushes, fingernails, contact lens overuse, improperly fitted cosmetic contact lenses, airbag deployment, plants, or foreign body in the conjunctival sac are often responsible.

Clinical Findings

- Evidence and sensation of a foreign body
- Severe pain and photophobia
- Tearing and blepharospasm
- Decreased vision
- Conjunctival erythema
- On examination, disrupted tear film over the corneal epithelium is seen with a penlight.
- Fluorescein staining with superficial uptake is indicative of a minor corneal abrasion. If the fluorescein staining goes deeply into the cornea, subepithelial corneal damage (e.g., corneal ulceration or corneal tear) is possible. Vertical striations on the cornea suggest a foreign body embedded under the eyelid.

Management

- Refer severe corneal injuries or possible subepithelial damage to an ophthalmologist. Refer those who wear contact lenses with an abrasion to an ophthalmologist to rule out bacterial corneal infection (a prophylactic topical antibiotic [e.g., gentamicin or ciprofloxacin] may be prescribed in these circumstances to cover *Pseudomonas*).

- If no symptoms of corneal infection, use topical antibiotics (0.5% erythromycin or polysporin drops or ointment [preferred as more lubricating]) four times daily. The use of a patch does not improve healing or decrease pain and a poorly applied patch may cause a corneal abrasion (Olitsky et al, 2007). An abrasion generally heals in 24 to 48 hours. Some specialists apply a soft contact lens as a protective barrier.
- Advise the patient to return daily for follow-up evaluation or refer for slit-lamp examination within 24 to 36 hours. If responding, continue the ointment for 2 to 3 days. If no improvement is seen after 24 to 48 hours or if symptoms worsen, refer to an ophthalmologist.
- Use elbow restraints for the infant to ensure that the eye is not rubbed or further irritated.
- Oral analgesics or ophthalmologic NSAIDs (e.g., ketorolac 0.5%) may be used to ease the discomfort. Do not use topical anesthetics because they are toxic to the epithelium.

FOREIGN BODY
Description and Epidemiology
A superficial foreign body (FB) in the eye is usually lodged on the surface of the eye or superficially in the cornea. It rarely results in serious trauma, but they may penetrate the globe (intraocular) with more serious consequences. Foreign bodies commonly occur in younger children during play and in older children during sports; they can include dirt, dust, metallic particles, or alkaline products from the deployment of an airbag.

Clinical Findings
Be sure to include in the history if the individual was working on a metal-on-metal activity. The following may be noted:
- Pain and foreign body sensation
- Foreign body visible in the conjunctival sac
- Tearing
- Inflammation
- Irregular or peaked pupil
- Photophobia
- Opaque lens
- Perforating wound to the cornea or iris
- Fluorescein staining may be useful if no foreign body is visualized.
  Diagnostic Studies. Ultrasonography or CT scan may be needed, depending on the foreign body and its location. An MRI is contraindicated.

Management
- Never remove an intraocular foreign body (including a metal object or fragment) and never remove a foreign body if the history indicates that a projectile object was possibly involved in the injury or patient has had LASIK procedure. Refer immediately to an ophthalmologist.
- View the upper bulbar conjunctiva by having the patient look down while the upper lid is pulled away from the globe and the upper recess illuminated. Evert the eyelid to visualize the superior tarsal conjunctiva.
- Use of a topical anesthetic (proparacaine 0.5% or tetracaine 0.5%, 1 drop—may repeat at 3- to 5-minute intervals) facilitates patient cooperation

- If not visualized but suspected, remove an extraocular foreign body via irrigation with sterile saline or sterile eye irrigant.
- If the object is visualized, either irrigate or gently lift object away with a moistened cotton-tipped swab (after instillation of topical anesthetic). The latter technique should be used only for cooperative individuals and for small FBs in order to avoid further trauma to the epithelial surface.
- If any difficulty is encountered, stop all efforts, patch the eye, and refer the patient immediately to an ophthalmologist.
- After removing any extraocular object, instill fluorescein stain and inspect the cornea with cobalt-blue light to look for green staining or lines; check visual acuity. Follow guidelines for managing a corneal abrasion.
- Reschedule the patient in 24 hours or refer to an ophthalmologist for follow-up.
- In the case of an airbag deployment (talc, cornstarch, and/or baking soda are released), irrigate the eyes with sterile saline or sterile eye irrigant and carefully examine the eye(s) for further evidence of trauma.

Complications
Sympathetic ophthalmia, chronic siderosis, or a uveitis of the injured eye can occur any time from 10 days to many years after a penetrating injury of the globe.

BURNS
Etiology
Burns to the eyes and surrounding tissues can be thermal (caused by exposure to steam, flame, intense heat [e.g., touching cornea with a curling iron], cinders, or cigarettes), chemical (e.g., cleaning agents, fertilizers, pesticides, battery fluid, or laboratory products), or induced by UV light (e.g., from bright snow, laser pointers, or a sunlamp). The amount of damage to the eye is directly related to the length of exposure and the nature of the source of the burn. Chemical burns are true emergencies because of the progressive damage that can occur. Alkaline solutions are especially damaging. Burns on the eyelids are classified and treated the same as burns elsewhere on the body.

Clinical Findings
- Pale or necrosed appearance of the surrounding skin and eyelids
- Opacity of corneal tissue
- Visual impairment (decreased acuity)
- Initial exquisite pain or delayed complaints of pain (e.g., in UV burns, pain emerges about 6 hours after exposure)
- Photophobia
- Tearing within 12 hours of exposure
- Swollen corneas
- Fluorescein stain revealing pinpoint uptake

Management
- Instill a topical anesthetic if available.
- Chemical burns require immediate, ongoing, copious irrigation. With the eyelids held apart, instill a steady, gentle

solution of tepid water, saline, or Ringer irrigation for 20 to 30 minutes or until the pH of the tear film is 7.3 to 7.7. The pH should be rechecked after 30 minutes to ensure it maintains this level. Refer to an ophthalmologist after irrigation to determine the extent of the damage. Do not patch the eye; allow tearing to continue to cleanse the eye. Cool compresses applied to the surrounding skin may be comforting. Hospitalization may be needed for sedation and analgesia.

- Thermal burns may be treated the same way as corneal abrasions (Weaver and Rosen, 2010).
- UV burns are treated by using topical antibiotic prophylaxis, patches, and analgesics. Healing should occur in 1 to 2 days.

LACERATIONS OF THE ORBIT
Description
Lacerations from injuries cause perforation of the cornea and lead to uveal prolapse. They are described as to whether they are of the anterior segment (cornea, anterior chamber, iris, lens) or posterior segment (sclera, retina, vitreous).

Clinical Findings
The clinical findings (only a few of the more obvious are mentioned here) depend on which segment is involved.
- Anterior segment
  - Irregular pupil (retracted or peaked)
  - Iris prolapse
- Posterior segment
  - Poor red light reflex
  - Decreased vision
  - Black tissue or fluid seen under the conjunctiva

Management
Apply an eye shield (can be made from a cup) to protect the eye. Refer the patient immediately to an ophthalmologist to rule out damage to the globe and surrounding structures.

TRAUMATIC HYPHEMA
Description and Epidemiology
A hyphema is an accumulation of visible blood or blood products in the anterior chamber of the eye and is the result of blunt trauma to the globe without penetration or perforation. This condition is most often caused by balls, fists or fingers, elbows, rocks, exploding airbags, and sticks. It may also occur in infants with birth trauma or in patients with RB, abnormal iris vessels (rubeosis), leukemia, juvenile xanthogranuloma of the iris, or abnormal hematologic profiles, such as sickle cell trait or disease, or secondary to child abuse. Seventy-five percent of these injuries occur in males (Crouch et al, 2007).

Clinical Findings
Vision, pupil motility, the lids and adnexa, the cornea and anterior segment, and the red light reflex should be assessed. The following may be noted (Olitsky et al, 2007):
- History of traumatic eye injury
- Somnolence (often associated with intracranial trauma)

- Blood appearing as a dark red fluid level between the cornea and iris on gross examination or as a hazy-appearing iris
- Inability to detect a bilateral red light reflex
- Pain, photophobia, and tearing
- Visual acuity changes and impaired vision (light perception and hand motion perception)
- Abnormal pupillary reflex

Management
The goals of treatment include resolving the hyphema, making the patient comfortable, and preventing complications. No consensus has been reached on how to best accomplish such treatment (e.g., whether or not to hospitalize, use systemic medications, or which medications to use). There is a risk of recurrent bleeding. However, the following steps should be taken:
- Refer the patient immediately to an ophthalmologist. A slit-lamp examination is indicated.
- Restrict oral intake until the child has been seen by an ophthalmologist.
- Place a perforated eye shield (not a patch) over the eye—avoid pressure to prevent reinjury.
- If a hematologic disorder is detected, ensure quick intervention and close follow-up.

The following steps are commonly recognized for treatment of traumatic hyphemas:
- Outpatient management is acceptable for those with small hyphemas (grade I): Elevate the head of the bed to 30 degrees. Child should wear a Fox shield; maintain bed rest with bathroom privileges for 5 days; participate in no strenuous activities for 10 days; have daily eye examinations to check for blood staining and IOP. Cycloplegic agents may be used (Olitsky et al, 2007).
- Children should be hospitalized with a hyphema of grade II or III, those with sickle cell, if there is an increase in IOP, or if there is a question about compliance with outpatient treatment.
- Acetaminophen is the analgesic of choice; avoid aspirin and NSAIDs because they may add to the risk of a rebleed. Sedatives may be necessary in pediatric patients.
- Surgery may be necessary to remove the trapped blood from the chamber if (1) it is causing an increase in IOP; (2) in sickle cell patients; to prevent corneal blood staining; (3) if the hyphema remains without some clearing in the first 4 days; or (4) a clot is pressing against the corneal epithelium (Olitsky et al, 2007).
- After hospital discharge, the child should be followed closely by an ophthalmologist because long-term monitoring is necessary to detect possible traumatic cataract, retinal detachment, or glaucoma.

Complications
A second hemorrhage can occur within 3 to 5 days of the first, increasing the risk of glaucoma, amblyopia, or corneal blood staining that can result in permanent visual loss. This rebleed occurs in approximately 7% to 38% of all cases. The larger the hyphema, the more likely the child is to rebleed. Patients with abnormal hematologic profiles (e.g., sickle cell hemoglobinopathies) are more likely to have visual loss because of optic atrophy (Crouch et al, 2007).

Prognosis

Success in treatment is determined by the recovery of visual acuity. When less than a third of the anterior chamber is filled with blood, approximately 80% regain acuity of 20/40 or better. When more than half (but less than total) of the chamber is filled, this same visual acuity is regained in about 60%. However, only 35% of those with total hyphema will have this return in acuity. In children younger than 6 years of age, about 60% have good visual return (Crouch et al, 2007).

RETINAL DETACHMENT

Description and Epidemiology

Retinal detachment is detachment of the neurosensory retina from its retinal pigment epithelium base within the globe. It is rare in children, so suspicion should be high for traumatic causes (e.g., child abuse), a congenital abnormality or syndrome (aphakia, cataracts, Ehlers-Danlos, Stickler, Marfan, Norrie syndromes), or specific disease (ROP, viral retinitis, RB, or various retinopathies) (Olitsky et al, 2007). Some detachments may not be diagnosed for months or years after a blunt trauma injury (Weichel et al, 2005). There may be concurrent ocular disease or a family history of retinal detachment.

Clinical Findings

- Blurry vision that becomes progressively worse
- Dark cloud in one visual field, flashing lights, or a "shower of floaters"
- Darkening of retinal vessels on funduscopic examination
- Gray elevation at the site of detachment

Management

Instruct the patient not to eat and refer to an ophthalmologist for evaluation.

ORBITAL HEMATOMA AND CONTUSION OF THE GLOBE

Description and Etiology

This condition is usually the result of a blow to the globe. The degree of damage depends on the energy of the object hitting the globe. Such injuries commonly occur as a result of sports activities, motor vehicle accidents, assault, BB gun accidents, or airbag deployment.

Clinical Findings

- Milky white appearance of the retina
- Visual acuity changes
- Severe bruising of the eyelids and periorbital tissues
- Lens dislocation
- Retinal detachment or edema
- Vitreous, retinal, or choroid hemorrhage
- Rupture of the eyeball

Management

Refer the patient immediately to an ophthalmologist. A closed head injury, damage to the skull, and facial bone fractures need to be ruled out via CT scan, MRI, or ultrasound radiography.

Occasionally cryopexy or laser photocoagulation surgery is needed for contusions of the globe.

Complications

Possible complications include permanent visual loss, retinal necrosis, subretinal hemorrhage, and retinal or macular holes.

ORBITAL FRACTURES

Description and Etiology

An orbital fracture is a fracture of the walls of the orbit secondary to blunt trauma to the orbital rim or eye(s). The orbital floor is thin and subject to fracture. The inferior rectus muscle may become caught in the fracture site. The usual cause of an orbital fracture is a blow or blunt trauma to the orbit (e.g., ball, fist, motor vehicle accident [hitting the dashboard], fall).

Clinical Findings

- Pain, diplopia
- Numbness below orbit
- Ecchymosis of the lids, nosebleed, trouble chewing
- Limited ocular movement (especially upward) and weakness in downward movement
- Globe displacement with a sunken-eye appearance or a protruding eye
- Bony discontinuity or "step-off"
- Subcutaneous emphysema in surrounding tissues and edema
- Enophthalmos
- Corneal laceration
- Irregular pupil
- Hyphema or absent red light reflex

Diagnostic Studies. Plain film radiography and CT scan are the best imaging modalities (Olitsky et al, 2007).

Management

- An orbital fracture is an ophthalmologic emergency requiring immediate intervention and referral. Diagnostic studies are performed to rule out injury to the skull and cranial contents. Open reduction may be necessary if any of the orbital bones are displaced or to rule out displacement of the globe or enophthalmos.
- Icing the injury for 24 hours, followed by heat for 2 to 3 days, allows the swelling to subside before surgical repair. Surgery is often best done within 2 to 7 days up to 2 to 4 weeks, depending on the injury (Wright, 2003).
- Antibiotic prophylaxis is administered. Nasal decongestants may also be used.

PTERYGIUM

A pterygium is a fibrovascular mass of thickened bulbar conjunctiva that extends beyond the limbus onto the cornea. Elastic and hyaline degenerative changes occur. The lesion is usually triangular and more commonly found on the nasal side of the orbit. It is caused by irritation of the bulbar conjunctiva from sunlight, wind, dust, fumes, or airborne allergens; it can also be hereditary. Growth rates of the lesions vary. A pinguecula may precede the pterygium, which occurs as a yellow-white, slightly raised mass on the bulbar conjunctiva. The lesion is usually painless, may itch, and may be accompanied by occasional complaints of blurred vision if the lesion enlarges.

Because a pterygium is uncommon in children, the clinician needs to consider other causes: papillomas, dermoids, keratoacanthomas, an epithelial inclusion or a dermoid cyst, or a rare malignancy (Wilson et al, 2003). Treatment involves protecting against irritants (use of goggles or sunglasses, or topical lubricants, such as artificial tears) and using mild vasoconstrictors or short-term steroids for inflammation. Surgical removal may be needed if the pterygium impedes vision. Recurrence after surgical removal, restricted ocular mobility (especially with abduction), and diplopia may be complications.

SUBCONJUNCTIVAL HEMORRHAGE

Subconjunctival hemorrhage is splotchy bulbar conjunctival redness that spontaneously occurs or is secondary to increased intrathoracic pressure (from coughing, sneezing, straining, or trauma) that results in the bursting of conjunctival vessels. It is commonly found in neonates as a benign occurrence to a vaginal delivery. The hemorrhages are painless and usually spontaneously resolve within 2 to 3 weeks. No treatment is indicated unless there is pain, vision loss, or photophobia, which indicate a referral to an ophthalmologist. Spontaneous hemorrhages can (rarely) occur with hypertension, diabetes mellitus, and blood dyscrasias, or can be a sign of a ruptured globe if there is a history of trauma (Sharma and Brunette, 2010; Wright, 2003).

EYELID CONTUSION ("BLACK EYE")

An eyelid contusion is usually a result of blunt injury to the eye and surrounding tissues. The result is bruising, swelling, and often an impressive appearance ("black eye"). If the child complains of increased pain or swelling, decrease in visual acuity, double vision, flashing lights or "floaters" or develops a bilateral "raccoon eyes" appearance, an ophthalmologic evaluation is needed to rule out a more serious eye injury (e.g., ruptured globe, basilar skull fracture, detached retina, hyphema). Examine all eye structures before excessive swelling sets in. Treatment consists of elevating the head and intermittent ice compresses for 48 hours. A CT scan may be warranted (Sharma and Brunette, 2010).

■ Deformities of the Eyelids

ENTROPION

Entropion is a condition in which the eyelids invert so that the cilia or epithelium rubs against the corneal surface, causing abrasion or irritation. The upper and lower eyelids may be involved. There is a rare congenital form. Examination reveals evidence of lid laxity. Pain or irritation and photophobia are typical symptoms. Complications include corneal scarring and corneal infections. Management involves surgical intervention.

ECTROPION

Ectropion is a rare condition in which the eyelid margins evert. The condition may be congenital, seen after infection, or secondary to scarring after trauma, radiation, or prior surgery. It can be confused with euryblepharon. Management involves lubrication for mild cases; surgery is indicated for chronic or symptomatic cases.

EURYBLEPHARON

Euryblepharon appears as a wide palpebral fissure with the appearance of a sagging half of the lower eyelid (temporal side) or a pulling away of the lid from the orbit. It can have a genetic etiology (e.g., Down syndrome), be associated with other ocular anomalies (e.g., congenital cleft lip, strabismus, congenital ptosis), or be seen in association with nonocular anomalies (e.g., hypospadias, inguinal hernias, dental anomalies). It is often confused with ectropion. It is usually a mild cosmetic condition that the child may outgrow. No treatment is indicated unless chronic tearing or exposure keratitis occurs; in such cases, reconstruction can be done.

Ear Disorders

ANN M. PETERSEN-SMITH AND SHIRLEY BECTON McKENZIE

The ear serves two functions—hearing and equilibrium. The ear includes both external and inner ear structures. Malfunctions of any of the ear structures can have impact on the ear itself as well as surrounding tissues. Additionally, ear dysfunction can cause systemic problems that have a lifelong impact. Adequate hearing is important for speech and language acquisition, academic performance, and socialization. Pediatric primary care providers must have an understanding of normal ear anatomy and physiology and be able to confidently identify, assess, and diagnose ear disorders in children. Deafness is discussed in Chapter 15.

■ Standards for Hearing Screening

The Joint Committee on Infant Hearing (JCIH) (2007), the U.S. Preventive Services Task Force (USPSTF) (2008), and the National Institute on Deafness and Other Communication Disorders (NIDCDH) (2004) advocate for universal detection of hearing loss before a child is 1 month of age. These organizations also recommend follow-up of abnormal newborn hearing screening by 3 months of age and appropriate family-centered intervention by 6 months of age. A USPSTF review cited that children identified by universal newborn hearing screening had better language outcomes at school age than those not screened and had earlier referral, diagnosis, and management than those identified by other means (Nelson et al, 2008). According to the 2007 Executive Summary of the Joint Commission on Infant Hearing, infants who pass newborn screening but have other risk factors for hearing loss should have at least one diagnostic audiologic assessment by 24 to 30 months of age. Screening of newborns or infants can be done by using evoked otoacoustic emission testing or automated auditory brainstem response. All U.S. states and territories and the District of Columbia have established Early Hearing Detection and Intervention (EHDI) programs. In addition, various locations in Canada and Europe offer newborn hearing screening programs (Centers for Disease Control and Prevention [CDC], 2010).

The American Academy of Pediatrics (AAP) *Bright Futures* guidelines (Hagan et al, 2008) recommends puretone audiometry at 3, 4, 5, 6, 8, 10, 12, 15, and 18 years of age, with subjective assessment at other ages. More frequent hearing, speech-language, and communication screening are indicated for children at high risk for hearing loss including those with persistent or recurrent acute otitis media (AOM), middle ear effusion (MEE), and those with chronic exposure to loud noises.

■ Development, Anatomy, and Physiology

DEVELOPMENT

Development of the ear begins during the third week of gestation and is complete by the third month of embryonic life. Insult to the fetus during this time can cause irreparable damage to the ear and negatively affect hearing. Ear development occurs at the same time as kidney development, so malformation or dysfunction in one system should alert the health care provider to problems in the other.

ANATOMY AND PHYSIOLOGY

The external ear is responsible for transmission of sound waves from outside the ear to the middle ear and for clearance of debris. The canal contains glands that secrete sweat, sebum, and cerumen that help lubricate the hair follicles and aid in the removal of debris. Patency of the ear canal is imperative for proper functioning.

The tympanic cavity constitutes the middle ear. The tympanic membrane (TM) is at the proximal end of the external auditory canal (EAC) and separates the external ear from the middle ear. The middle ear is a small chamber in the temporal bone that contains the ossicles—the malleus, incus, and stapes—which function to transmit sound waves from the EAC to the inner ear. The malleus lies against the TM, which vibrates when sound waves hit it. The stapes rests against the oval window, and its vibration causes the oval window to stimulate the fluids of the inner ear.

The eustachian tube has three physiological functions with respect to the middle ear: (1) ventilation of the middle ear to equalize air pressure in the middle ear with atmospheric pressure and to replace oxygen that has been absorbed; (2) protection from nasopharyngeal sound, pressure, and secretions; and (3) drainage of secretions from the middle ear into the nasopharynx.

The inner ear functions to transmit sound and aid in balance. Vibrations of the TM, ossicles, and oval window set the inner ear fluids in motion. The fluid sound waves reach the cochlea, wherein lies the organ of Corti, which contains the hearing receptor hair cells. The hair cells transmit impulses to the auditory nerve (cranial nerve VIII), which transmits stimuli to the auditory cortex of the temporal lobe in the brain. The equilibrium receptors lie in the semicircular canals and vestibule of the inner ear. The semicircular canals respond to changes in direction of movement. The vestibule contains receptors essential to the maintenance of equilibrium.

Pathophysiology and Defense Mechanisms

PATHOPHYSIOLOGY

The processes that negatively affect the ear are usually localized; however, pathological ear conditions can be related to systemic dysfunction or disorders. Common localized pathological conditions include viral, bacterial, or fungal infections in the inner, middle, and outer ear; foreign bodies in the ear; and trauma. Neurological dysfunction, poor immunological competence, and congenital anomalies are common disorders that can affect the ear and its functions. External influences, such as excessive noise in the environment, can cause irreparable damage to the ear's hearing function.

DEFENSE MECHANISMS

Debris formed by keratinizing cells in the ear is lubricated and extruded by the cilia in the EAC. Maintenance of an acidic pH in the ear canal prevents the growth of pathogenic bacteria. Additionally the surface lining of the external ear is water resistant and has ample blood and lymph supplies. These characteristics and the antibacterial properties of cerumen help protect against invading microorganisms. In comparison with the distal end of the EAC, the proximal end has fewer hair fibers, a thinner epithelial layer, and more nerve fibers that cause great discomfort when touched. This sensitivity to pain serves a protective function by deterring the insertion of foreign bodies into the ear, thus preventing damage to the middle ear.

The inner ear is also well protected inasmuch as the structures for both hearing and equilibrium are set deep within the skull.

Assessment

HISTORY

The history of a patient with an ear disorder should include the following:
- Medical history significant for craniofacial abnormalities (e.g., cleft lip or palate) or syndromes associated with craniofacial anomalies (Down syndrome, Treacher Collins syndrome)
- Prematurity

- Medical history pertinent to ear conditions (e.g., central nervous system infections, otitis media, trauma)
- Pain (onset, location, quality, duration, alleviating or aggravating factors)
- Associated symptoms, such as fever, vomiting and diarrhea, nasal congestion, or other symptoms of upper respiratory infection
- Itching or discharge
- Tinnitus or hearing loss
- Exposure to risk factors: Environmental tobacco smoke (ETS), bottle propping, pacifier use, childcare, noise, swimming
- Diabetes mellitus
- Family history of ear dysfunction
- Family history of/or presence of kidney malformation

PHYSICAL EXAMINATION

The physical examination includes the following:
- Inspection of the external structures of the ear for symmetry, skin abnormalities, discharge, or lesions.
  - The inner and outer canthi of the eye should form a straight line with the superior portion of the pinna. If the pinna inserts below this line, the ear is considered low-set, which can be associated with a number of genetic and congenital syndromes and renal issues.
- Assessment of developmental milestones related to hearing and speech development (Box 29-1)

BOX 29-1 Developmental Milestones Used to Assess Hearing

Birth to 3 Months
Startles (Moro reflex) to loud noise
Awakens to sounds
Blinks or widens eyes to noises

3 to 6 Months
Quiets to parent's voice
Stops activity to listen to new sound
Looks for source of sound
Reciprocates vocally and initiates sounds

6 to 12 Months
Coos and gurgles with inflection
Responds to simple phrases
Turns to localize sound in any plane
Responds to own name

12 to 18 Months
Points to unexpected sound or familiar objects when asked
Follows simple direction without cues
Imitates some sounds, first words by 12 to 15 months old

18 to 24 Months
Points to body parts when asked
Has expressive vocabulary of 20 to 50 words
50% of speech intelligible to strangers

Data from Northern J, Downs M: *Hearing in children*, ed 4, Baltimore, 1991, Williams & Wilkins.

- Palpation and rotation of the external ear for tenderness and inflammation; push on the tragus and apply pressure to the mastoid process.
- Otoscopic examination, which is best accomplished in a young child at the end of the physical examination with the child on an examining table or seated on the parent's lap. Pulling the ear downward, outward, and backward can enhance visualization of the EAC in infants and small children. In older children and adolescents, the EAC is lifted upward and backward, slightly away from the head.
- Decreased TM mobility secondary to effusion is noted through pneumatic otoscopy, tympanometry, or acoustic reflectometry.
- Examine the canal for redness, edema, or discharge. Assess all 360 degrees of the TM, the bony processes, and the cone of light (see Color Plate). Look for air-fluid level or bubbles behind the TM. Note any retraction, perforation, redness or other alteration in color, fibrosis, bulging, or retraction.

COMMON DIAGNOSTIC STUDIES

- *Evoked otoacoustic emission (EOAE) testing* is the method of hearing screening used for universal newborn screening. Dr. David Kemp first described the phenomenon of otoacoustic emissions in 1978. He found that the normal-hearing ear has the ability to emit detectable sounds called spontaneous otoacoustic emissions. The normal ear also emits these sounds when given a stimulus (EOAE) and

provides evidence that the outer hair cells of the cochlea are functioning appropriately and hearing is likely to be intact. EOAE is efficient, highly sensitive, and easy to perform in a quiet, cooperative child, which makes it conducive for use in newborns. However, the EOAE does not quantify hearing deficit and may not identify auditory nerve dysfunction; ambient room noise and an uncooperative child may interfere with the test and provide unreliable results. Improvements in EOAE and auditory brainstem response technology have resulted in highly acceptable levels of hearing sensitivity and specificity at relatively low cost (Nelson et al, 2008).

- *Auditory brainstem response (ABR)* measures the initiation of sound-induced electrical signals in the cochlea. The ABR measures the functioning of the peripheral auditory system and neurological pathways related to hearing. Although it is not a direct measure of hearing, ABR allows for inferences to be made about hearing thresholds. The ABR is useful in identifying hearing loss in a young infant or in children unable to cooperate with EOAE or audiometry. Occasionally sedation is required. Neurological abnormalities may make interpretation of an ABR impossible. Automated ABR is available as a screening device.
- *Audiometry,* useful in assessing hearing loss in older children, measures hearing threshold via bone or air conduction, or both, in decibels at varying frequencies (Tables 29-1 and 29-2). Twenty dB is about as loud as a whisper, 40 dB is normal speaking loudness, and 90 dB produces pain. The frequencies of normal speaking range from

TABLE 29-1	Audiologic Tests for Infants and Young Children				
Test	**Characteristics**	**Age Range**	**Advantages**	**Disadvantages**
Behavioral observation audiometry (BOA)	Behavioral test: responses to noisemakers or calibrated sounds are observed	0 to 5 months	Low cost	Insensitive to unilateral or less than severe hearing loss; highly subject to observer bias; child tires rapidly when subjected to repeated stimuli
Visual reinforced audiometry (VRA)	Behavioral test: child is given an animated toy for turning to sounds	5 to 24 months	Low cost; child responds at softer levels and for longer periods compared with BOA	Insensitive to unilateral loss (unless earphones used); need two examiners to reduce bias
Play audiometry	Behavioral test: child is trained to respond to tones by playing game	2 to 5 years	Low cost; can detect unilateral and mild hearing loss	Requires cooperation of child
Screening audiometry	Behavioral test: child raises hand or responds verbally to tones at fixed levels (20 to 25 dB)	4 years and older	Can be performed by trained paraprofessional in most children 4 years and older; can detect unilateral and mild hearing loss	Further tests required if failed
Otoacoustic emission (OAE)	Physiological test: response of inner ear to brief clicks or tones is measured with specialized instrument	Any	Child's response not needed; takes less than 2 minutes if child is quiet; can be performed by a trained paraprofessional; low cost; can detect unilateral and mild hearing loss	Cannot tell type or degree of loss; further tests required if failed
Auditory brainstem response (ABR) audiometry	Physiological test: averaged number of responses of brainstem to brief tones or clicks	Any	Child's response not needed; can detect unilateral and mild loss; can determine degree and slope of loss (with tone bursts and bone conduction testing)	Requires audiologist and equipment to administer and interpret; expensive; requires sedation beyond about 6 months old

dB, Decibels.

in place. In a systematic review of the effectiveness of different cerumen removal methods, Clegg and colleagues (2010) found that sodium bicarbonate, olive oil, and water are more effective than no treatment. They also found that the effectiveness of irrigation versus mechanical cerumen removal was equivocal.

Mechanical cerumen removal (curettage) requires skill and the use of a cerumen spoon. This method is not as messy and may be as effective as irrigation. Blunt plastic ear curettes may be less traumatic than the metal variety. Always carefully explain the procedure to parents and inform them that the ear canal is extremely sensitive and fragile and bleeds easily when touched. This may prevent an adverse parent reaction when there is blood on the curette or in the ear canal.

FOLLOW-UP AND REFERRAL

The need for follow-up for ear disorders depends on the age of the child, the diagnosis, the treatment plan, and the response to treatment. Kershner (2007) suggests that follow-up for OM should be individualized. Young infants with a severe infection, children with continuing fever or pain, and those given a safety-net antibiotic prescription (SNAP) should have phone follow-up within a few days. Infants and children with recurrent ear infections should be seen for follow-up within 2 weeks and those with only sporadic ear disease within a month. Kershner (2007) suggests that older children need no follow-up after an ear infection if there was complete resolution of symptoms.

An otolaryngology referral is indicated for unusual ear conditions, congenital malformation of the head and neck structures, craniofacial anomalies, sensory dysfunction involving hearing or speech, when appropriate therapy for OM has failed, or if ongoing effusion or infection persists. Myringotomy (and/or PET insertion) is indicated when there is severe, refractory pain; hyperpyrexia; facial paralysis, mastoiditis, labyrinthitis; or central nervous system infection; immunological compromise; and an ear infection that has failed two courses of antibiotics (Kershner, 2007). Referral to an audiologist is necessary if the ear pathology is prolonged or when the child's ability to hear is questioned. Speech and language evaluations are imperative to resolve questions about whether the child's verbal development is delayed because of persistent or recurring ear problems. Chapter 31 addresses criteria for tonsillectomy and adenoidectomy.

Pressure-Equalizing Tubes

Recommendations for the use of PETs in children with persistent MEE, who are otherwise well, are being reconsidered. Paradise and colleagues (2007) found that the placement of PETs in children less than 3 years of age with persistent OME did not result in significant improvement in developmental outcomes, including speech and language acquisition. The authors concluded that waiting to insert PETs (6 months for bilateral effusion and 9 months for unilateral effusion) had no detrimental effect on development and resulted in fewer procedures with equivocal outcomes. Browning and associates (2010) found that PETs placed for persistent MEE in otherwise healthy children provided only a short-term improvement in hearing and that PETs have no effect on speech and language development. The analysis also found that in children who had a persistent MEE for more than 12 weeks and documented hearing loss had some benefit from PETs for up to 6 months but then the effect diminished. By then the tubes had likely fallen out or the condition had resolved.

Placing PETs takes less than 15 minutes and is usually done using general anesthesia. The child is usually discharged after about an hour and is treated with antibiotic otic drops for several days. Children with persistent hearing loss after PET placement should be further evaluated (Spielmann et al, 2008). The examiner can establish that the tube is functioning properly if the tube spans the eardrum, the lumen is unobstructed, and no MEE is present. If appropriate functioning of the tube cannot be established, pneumatic otoscopy or tympanometry may be useful. A flat (type B) tympanogram with large-volume measurements confirms appropriate function of the PET. A normal (type A) tympanogram suggests a clogged or extruded tube. The use of ototopical drops for 5 to 7 days can occasionally clear a clogged PET. Otic suspensions that are mildly acidic should be used because they are less irritating to middle ear mucosa. If the child can taste the drops or complains of stinging, the drops are most likely reaching the middle ear space, which indicates a functioning tube.

Generalized water precautions for children with PETs are controversial. A child with PETs does not need to take precautions during bathing, showering, or surface swimming because water does not enter the middle ear space (Wang et al, 2009). Diving and head dunking may allow water into the middle ear space. Chlorinated pools have few bacteria, and earplugs are probably unnecessary. However, lakes, ponds, rivers, and bath water may have high bacterial counts, so earplugs are recommended if head dunking may occur.

Viral myringitis or early AOM without otorrhea in a child with PETs will most likely resolve spontaneously because of increased middle ear ventilation. Tympanostomy tube otorrhea (TTO) occurs usually when a child with PETs has an upper respiratory infection and has drainage coming from the tubes. TTO usually involves the same bacterial pathogens seen in AOM. Ototopical antibiotics are recommended because of their ability to concentrate the medication in the middle ear space; however, it is imperative that purulent material be removed from the canal prior to instilling the drops. Eardrops containing fluoroquinolone, with or without a corticosteroid, are the preferred treatment for TTO even in recurrent AOM (Granath et al, 2008; Schmelzle et al, 2008; Wall et al, 2009). Ototopical medications are listed in Table 29-3.

If the otorrhea has not improved after 5 to 7 days of topical therapy, treatment with oral antibiotics is appropriate. If the otorrhea is resistant to both treatments, referral to an otolaryngologist is recommended.

Many PETs fall out well before their usefulness has been expended. Once the PET has been extruded from the TM, follow-up every 6 to 12 months is suggested until the tube falls out of the external canal. For the rare set of PETs that remains in situ, surgical removal is suggested after 2 years. Complications of PETs include otorrhea, otitis externa (OE), granuloma, cholesteatoma, PET obstruction, persistent TM perforation, and tympanosclerosis. Bacterial biofilms can form on implanted prostheses, including PETs, and tend to be resistant to systemic antibiotics (Bakaletz, 2007).

TABLE 29-3 Commonly Used Topical Preparations for Otitis Externa and Analgesia

Product Name (Manufacturer)	Antibiotic	Antiinflammatory	Acid	Comments
Analgesic				
Auralgan AB Otic Allergen Aurodex (available in generic formulation)	None	None	None	Benzocaine in a glycerin and propylene base Used for anesthesia for ear pain Should not be used if integrity of TM in question
Antibiotics (Not Ototoxic)				
CiproDex (Alcon)	Ciprofloxacin	Dexamethasone		Use ≥6 months old Contains steroid
Floxin Otic (Daiichi Pharmaceutical)	Ofloxacin	None	Acetic and boric	Does not contain steroid
Vasocidin Ophthalmic (Ciba Vision Ophthalmics)	Sulfacetamide	Prednisolone		No documented ototoxicity with either agent Excellent broad-spectrum coverage Contains steroid
Antibiotics (Ototoxic)				
Cortisporin Otic Suspension Pediotic (King Pharmaceutical)	Polymyxin B and neomycin	Hydrocortisone	Hydrochloric	May be painful on instillation Neomycin may cause cutaneous irritation Should not be used if integrity of TM in question Can be ototoxic
Cipro HC Otic (Alcon Labs)	Ciprofloxacin	Hydrocortisone	Glacial acetic acid	Use ≥1 year old Contraindicated with TM perforation
Cleansing and Antipruritic Agent (Ototoxic)				
Domeboro Otic (Bayer Pharmaceutical Division)	None	None	Acetic	Excellent choice for cleansing of the EAC Aluminum acetate helps to prevent itching Do not use if integrity of TM in question

EAC, External auditory canal; *TM,* tympanic membrane.

PREVENTION OF NOISE-INDUCED HEARING LOSS

Noise is a common cause of sensorineural hearing loss (SNHL) in children, and the pattern of damage depends on the frequency, intensity, and duration of the noise (Gifford et al, 2009). Any structure in the ear can be permanently damaged by noise greater than or equal to 140 dB. (See Chapter 41 for discussion of this environmental hazard and a list of risky noise sources.)

■ Specific Ear Problems in Children

OTITIS EXTERNA

Description

OE, commonly called "swimmer's ear," is an inflammatory reaction of the EAC, which may also involve the pinna or TM. Inflammation is evidenced as (1) simple infection with edema, discharge, and erythema; (2) furuncles or small abscesses that form in hair follicles; or (3) impetigo or infection of the superficial layers of the epidermis. OE can also be classified as mycotic OE, caused by fungus, or as chronic external otitis, a diffuse low-grade infection of the EAC. Severe infection or

systemic infection can be seen in children who have diabetes, who are immunocompromised, or who have received head and neck irradiation.

Epidemiology

OE results when the protective barriers in the EAC are damaged by mechanical or chemical mechanisms. OE is most frequently caused by retained moisture in the external ear canal, which changes the acidic environment of the external ear canal to a neutral or basic environment, thereby promoting bacterial or fungal growth. Chlorine in swimming pools adds to the problem because it kills the normal ear flora and allows the growth of pathogens. Excessive cleaning or scratching of the ear canal can remove some of the protective cerumen, creating abrasions in the thin ear canal skin that will allow organisms to enter the deeper tissue. *Pseudomonas* is also associated with the use of hearing aids or protectors, drainage from AOM, and ear trauma. Otitis externa is most often caused by *Pseudomonas aeruginosa* and *Staphylococcus aureus* but it is not uncommon for the infection to be polymicrobial.

Furunculosis of the external canal is generally caused by *S. aureus* and *Streptococcus pyogenes*. Otomycosis is usually caused by *Aspergillus* or *Candida* and is caused by recent use of systemic or topical antibiotics or steroids. Otomycosis is also more common in children with diabetes or immune dysfunction, accounts for 10% of OE, and is most commonly caused by *A. niger, Escherichia coli, Klebsiella pneumoniae,* and group B streptococci are more common in neonates.

Long-standing ear drainage may suggest a foreign body, chronic middle ear problem, such as a cholesteatoma, or granulomatous tissue. Bloody drainage may indicate trauma, severe OM, or granulation tissue. Chronic or recurrent OE may result from eczema, seborrhea, or psoriasis. Eczematous dermatitis, moist vesicles, and pustules are seen in acute infection, and crusting is more consistent with chronic infection.

Clinical Findings

History. The following can be found:
- Itching and irritation progressing to severe pain
- Pressure and fullness in ear and occasionally hearing loss that can be conductive or sensorineural
- Rare systemic complaints and symptoms
- Rare hearing loss and otorrhea
- Sagging of the superior canal, periauricular edema, and preauricular and postauricular lymphadenopathy with more severe disease. Extension to the surrounding soft tissue results in the obstruction of the canal with or without cellulitis.

Physical Examination. Findings on physical examination can include the following:
- Pain, often quite severe, with movement of the tragus or on attempts to examine the ear with an otoscope
- Swollen EAC with debris, making visualization of the TM difficult or impossible
- Rare otorrhea
- Occasional regional lymphadenopathy
- Tragal tenderness with a red, raised area of induration that can be deep and diffuse or superficial and pointing, which is characteristic of furunculosis
- Red, crusty or pustular spreading lesions
- Black spots over the TM, indicative of mycotic infection
- Dry-appearing canal with some atrophy or thinning of the canal and virtually no cerumen visible with chronic OE
- Presence of PET or perforation of TM (avoid use of ototoxic drops)

Diagnostic Studies. Culturing the discharge from the ear is not customary, but may be indicated if clinical improvement is not seen during or after treatment, there is severe pain, the child is a neonate, or immunocompromised or chronic or recurrent OE is suspected. Culturing requires a swab premoistened with sterile nonbacteriostatic saline or water.

Differential Diagnosis

AOM with perforation, TTO, chronic suppurative otitis media (CSOM), necrotizing OE, cholesteatoma, mastoiditis, posterior auricular lymphadenopathy, dental infection, and eczema are all possible differential diagnoses.

Management

The following steps outline the management of OE:
- Eardrops are the mainstay of therapy for OE (see Table 29-3). Acetic acid drops can be effective in mild episodes of OE but resolution of symptoms may be delayed (Kaushik et al, 2010). In moderate to severe cases, antibiotics with steroid otic drops are the treatment of choice. Symptoms should be markedly improved within 7 days but resolution of the infection may take up to 2 weeks (Kaushik et al, 2010). Drops should be used until all symptoms have resolved. Ototoxic drugs should not be used if there is a risk of perforation rather than OE.
  - Antibiotic agents should be chosen based on efficacy, low incidence of adverse effects, cost, and likelihood of compliance. Neomycin, polymyxin, or hydrocortisone drops should not be used if there is a nonintact TM because this drug is known to cause allergic reaction manifested by redness, irritation, itching, and drainage (Younis, 2010).
  - The quinolone products are effective against *Pseudomonas, S. aureus,* and *Streptococcus pneumoniae,* which may be a factor if the OE is a complication of AOM.
  - Neomycin is effective against *S. aureus,* but has no activity against *Pseudomonas.* Polymyxin, which is often found in combination with neomycin and hydrocortisone, has good *S. aureus* and *Pseudomonas* coverage.

It is important to apply tragal pressure after each drop of medication to ensure that the medication gets to the middle ear space.
- If significant swelling is present, insert a wick into the EAC (Haddad, 2007). A foam (Pope), cotton, hydrogel polymer (Merocel XL) or gauze (0.25 inch) wick usually works well. The tip of the wick is lubricated with water-based lubricant just before insertion into the ear. Once in place the wick should be impregnated with antibiotics for as long as it remains in the auditory canal (this may require reapplication of drops every 2 to 3 hours). Wicks are usually removed after several days. The wick will fall out when the swelling has subsided, and treatment with direct application of drops to the ear canal should continue for the entire course.
- Oral or parenteral antibiotics are generally not needed except for severe OE, systemic illness (fever, lymphadenitis), or failed topical treatment.
- Avoid cleaning, manipulating, and getting water into the ear. Swimming is prohibited during acute infection.
- Administer analgesics for pain. Narcotic analgesics may be necessary for severe pain and are indicated for short-term use.
- Debridement with a cotton-tipped applicator, self-made cotton wick, or calcium alginate swabs is indicated once the inflammatory process has subsided and can enhance the effectiveness of the ototopical antibiotic drops (Haddad, 2007).
- Lance a furuncle that is superficial and pointed with a 14-gauge needle. If it is deep and diffuse, a heating pad or warm oil-based drops can speed resolution.
- If impetigo is present, clear the canal by using half-strength hydrogen peroxide or other antiseptic solutions, followed by a warm-water rinse. Apply an antibiotic ointment (mupirocin) once or twice a day for 5 to 7 days. The child should avoid touching the ear. Fingernails should be short and hands cleansed with antibacterial soap. Systemic antibiotics are generally unnecessary.
- Mycotic OE is treated with antifungal solutions such as clotrimazole-miconazole, nystatin, or other antifungal agents including *m*-cresyl acetate 2.5%, gentian violet, and thimerosal 1:1000 (Haddad, 2007). The canal may be

cleansed with a 5% boric acid in ethanol solution followed by antifungal solution.

If the child is not improved within 72 hours (relief of otalgia, itching, and fullness), recheck to confirm diagnosis. Lack of improvement may be due to obstructed ear canal, foreign body, poor adherence, or contact sensitivity among other things. A follow-up visit may be necessary after 1 to 2 weeks for reevaluation of the OE and removal of debris. If symptoms are worsening or there is no improvement in a week, a referral to an ear, nose, and throat (ENT) specialist or dermatologist is indicated.

Complications

Infection of surrounding tissues with impetigo, irritated furunculosis, and malignant OE with progression and necrosis caused by *Pseudomonas* are possible complications. Involvement of the parotid gland, mastoid bone, and infratemporal fossa is rare (Haddad, 2007).

Prevention

The patient should be instructed to do the following:
- Avoid water in the ear canals.
- Use well-fitting earplugs for swimming especially in "dirty water."
- Use acidic drops (diluted vinegar or diluted alcohol) three to five drops daily, especially after swimming or bathing, to prevent the recurrence of OE (Haddad, 2007; Spektor, 2010).
- Use a blow dryer on warm setting to dry the EAC (Younis, 2010).
- Avoid persistent scratching or cleaning of the external canal.
- Avoid prolonged use of ceruminolytic agents.

FOREIGN BODY IN THE EAR CANAL

Description

A foreign body in the external ear canal is a problem frequently seen by pediatric health care providers, in emergency departments, and by otolaryngologists worldwide (Ologe et al, 2007).

Epidemiology

Foreign bodies are usually placed or thrown into the ear canal by the child or other children. Insects can also be found in the canal. Leaves and other plant materials can be intentionally inserted into the EAC as a form of native remedy (Shafi et al, 2010).

Clinical Findings

History. The history can include the following:
- Child reports putting something into the ear or having something thrown at him or her
- Complaints of itching, buzzing, fullness, or an object in the ear
- Persistent cough or hiccups
- Unilateral otalgia and otorrhea
- Asymptomatic

Physical Examination. A foreign body is visible with the naked eye or by otoscopic examination.

Management

Adequate visualization in a cooperative patient and a skilled provider with the appropriate equipment are the keys to successfully removing a foreign body in the EAC. It is critical that the object be removed on the first attempt because the success rate is markedly decreased after the first attempt (Dwivedi et al, 2009). A provider has one attempt to remove the object and if the object is not successfully removed, then a referral to an ENT specialist is recommended (Heim and Maughan, 2007).

Foreign bodies in the lateral one third of the ear canal are the easiest to remove. Foreign bodies in the medial two thirds of the ear canal are more difficult to remove because the canal is narrower, is lined with bone, is quite vascular, and is exquisitely sensitive. The TM lies at the most medial part of the EAC. Straighten the ear canal by pulling on the pinna, and gently shake the patient's head; occasionally the foreign body will fall out.
- Disk batteries must be removed emergently.
- Spherical objects are the most difficult to remove and should be referred to an otolaryngologist.
- Soft, irregularly shaped objects are generally graspable with a bayonet forceps, alligator forceps, or curved hook.
- Round or breakable objects can be removed using a wire loop, a curette, or right-angle hook that is slowly advanced beyond the object and withdrawn carefully.
- If the object is made of iron, nickel, or cobalt, try using a magnet to retrieve it.
- Insects in the ear canal should be killed with mineral oil or lidocaine and the child should be referred for otomicroscopic removal (Haddad, 2007).
- Irrigation can only be done if the tympanic membrane is intact and should be done using fluid at body temperature and a commercial irrigator or 60-mL syringe with an angiocatheter on the end (Haddad, 2007).
  - ○ Irrigation may only serve to push the object farther into the ear canal.
  - ○ Do not irrigate if the object is a disk battery or vegetable matter or if the TM is not intact.
- If available, suctioning with a Schuknecht foreign body catheter with umbrella may work.
- Refer the patient to an otolaryngologist if the object cannot be extracted on the first attempt, the object cannot be removed without causing further damage or worse pain, the child is unable to cooperate, or the foreign body has a higher likelihood of failure (in the medial third of the ear canal, spherical shape, etc.) (Dwivedi et al, 2009; Haddad, 2007; Heim and Maughan, 2007).
- Ear blocks (regional anesthesia) are not recommended.
- Consider conscious sedation if the clinical setting is appropriate.
- Once the object is removed, topical antibiotic drops with steroid are recommended for any drainage and to decrease inflammation.

Complications

Infection, perforation of the TM, and damage to the ossicles are possible if the object is not removed.

Prevention

Educate children and their parents not to put objects into the ear.

TABLE 29-4	Types of Acute Otitis Media
Type	**Characteristics**
AOM	Suppurative effusion of the middle ear
Bullous myringitis	AOM in which bullae form between the inner and middle layers of the TM and bulge outward
Persistent AOM	AOM that has not resolved when antibiotic therapy has been completed or AOM recurs within days of treatment
Recurrent AOM	Three separate bouts of AOM within a 6-month period or four within a 12-month period; often a positive family history of OM and other ENT disease

AOM, Acute otitis media; *ENT,* ear, nose, and throat; *OM,* otitis media; *TM,* tympanic membrane.

ACUTE OTITIS MEDIA

Description

AOM is an acute infection of the middle ear (see Color Plate). The AAP and AAFP *Clinical Practice Guidelines* (2004a) require the presence of the following three components to diagnose AOM:
- Recent, abrupt onset of signs and symptoms of middle ear inflammation and effusion (ear pain, irritability, otorrhea and/or fever)
- MEE as confirmed by bulging TM; limited or absent mobility by pneumatic otoscopy; air-fluid level behind TM; otorrhea
- Signs and symptoms of middle ear inflammation as confirmed by distinct erythema of the TM or distinct otalgia interfering with normal sleep or activity

Characteristics of different types of AOM are defined in Table 29-4.

Epidemiology

AOM often follows eustachian tube dysfunction (ETD). Common causes of ETD include upper respiratory infections, allergies, and environmental tobacco smoke (ETS). ETD leads to functional eustachian tube obstruction and decreases the protective ciliary action in the eustachian tube. When the eustachian tube is obstructed, negative pressure develops as air is absorbed in the middle ear (see Color Plate). The negative pressure pulls fluid from the mucosal lining and causes an accumulation of sterile fluid. Bacteria pulled in from the eustachian tube lead to the accumulation of purulent fluid. Young children have shorter, more horizontal, and more flaccid eustachian tubes that are easily disrupted by viruses, which predisposes them to AOM. Respiratory syncytial virus and influenza are two of the viruses most responsible for the increase in the incidence of AOM seen from January to April. Other risk factors associated with AOM are listed in Box 29-2.

S. pneumoniae, nontypeable *Haemophilus influenzae, Moraxella catarrhalis,* and *S. pyogenes* (group A streptococci) are the most common infecting organisms in AOM (Gould and Matz, 2010). In the past, *S. pneumoniae* was responsible for the majority of AOM with *H. influenzae* and *M. catarrhalis* only responsible for up to 40%. With the introduction of the heptavalent pneumococcal conjugate vaccine

BOX 29-2	Risk Factors for Otitis Media, Chronic Otitis Media, or Otitis Media With Effusion

- Genetic susceptibility/sibling with history of OM
- Non-Hispanic Caucasian children
- Prematurity
- Younger than 2 years of age
- Unimmunized
- Daycare attendance
- Sharing a bedroom
- Breastfeeding for less than 6 months
- Parental smoking and other environmental tobacco smoke exposure
- Environmental pollution exposure
- Overweight or obese
- Feeding in supine position
- Autumn season
- Male gender
- Early onset OM
- Bilateral OME
- Lower socioeconomic status

(PCV7) in 2000, the incidence of AOM caused by *S. pneumoniae* decreased and for the first time *H. influenzae* became the most common bacteria causing AOM (Coker et al, 2010; Casey and Pichichero, 2004). However, there had been an increase in AOM caused by *S. pneumoniae* type 19A, which was not included in the PCV7 vaccine. The 19A strain is now responsible for more than 50% of pneumococcal infections in the U.S. (Casey et al, 2010). The PCV13 vaccine, which was introduced in 2010, contains the 19A strain and should further decrease the incidence of pneumococcal infection in children. Additional vaccines purported to be more effective in preventing otitis media are in development (O'Brien et al, 2009; Vergison et al, 2010).

Most episodes of AOM occur in the first 24 months of life, with 39% of infants in the U.S. having their first AOM before 9 months of age and 62% by 2 years of age (Daly et al, 2010). Children with bilateral AOM tend to be younger and are more likely to have *H. influenzae* and severe inflammation of the tympanic membrane, which may explain why children with bilateral disease are more likely to have persistent symptoms (McCormick et al, 2007).

Clinical Findings

History. Rapid onset of signs and symptoms:
- Ear pain with possible ear pulling in the infant; may interfere with activity and/or sleep
- Irritability in an infant or toddler
- Otorrhea
- Fever

Other key factors or symptoms:
- Prematurity
- Craniofacial anomalies or congenital syndromes associated with craniofacial anomalies
- Exposure to risk factors
- Disrupted sleep or inability to sleep
- Lethargy, dizziness, tinnitus, and unsteady gait
- Diarrhea and vomiting
- Sudden hearing loss

- Stuffy nose, rhinorrhea, and sneezing
- Rare facial palsy and ataxia
  Physical Examination
- Presence of MEE, confirmed by pneumatic otoscopy, tympanometry, or acoustic reflectometry, as evidenced by:
  ○ Bulging TM (see Color Plate)
  ○ Decreased translucency of TM (Shaikh et al, 2010)
  ○ Absent or decreased mobility of the TM (see Color Plate)
  ○ Air-fluid level behind the TM
  ○ Otorrhea
- Signs and symptoms of middle ear inflammation indicated by either:
  ○ Erythema of the TM. (Amber is usually seen in OME; white or yellow may be seen in either AOM or OME [Shaikh et al, 2010].)
- Distinct otalgia that interferes with normal activity or sleep
- In addition, the following TM findings may be present:
  ○ Increased vascularity and obscured or absent landmarks (see Color Plate).
  ○ Red, yellow, or purple TM (redness alone should not be used to diagnose AOM, especially in a crying child)
  ○ Thin-walled, sagging bullae filled with straw-colored fluid seen with bullous myringitis

Diagnostic Studies. Pneumatic otoscopy is the simplest and most efficient way to diagnose AOM. Tympanometry reflects effusion (type B pattern). Tympanocentesis to identify the infecting organism is helpful in the treatment of infants younger than 2 months old. In older infants and children, tympanocentesis is rarely done and is useful only if the patient is toxic or immunocompromised or in the presence of resistant infection or acute pain from bullous myringitis. If a tympanocentesis is warranted, refer the patient to an otolaryngologist for this procedure.

Differential Diagnosis

OME, mastoiditis, dental abscess, sinusitis, lymphadenitis, parotitis, peritonsillar abscess, trauma, ETD, impacted teeth, temporomandibular joint dysfunction, and immune deficiency are differential diagnoses. Any infant 2 months old or younger with AOM should be evaluated for fever without focus and not just treated for an ear infection.

Management

Many changes have been made in the treatment of AOM because of the increasing rate of antibiotic-resistant bacteria related to the injudicious use of antibiotics. Ample evidence has been presented that symptom management may be all that is required. Sixty-one percent of children with AOM will have symptom resolution within 24 hours and nearly 75% by 1 week whether they received antibiotics or placebo (Gould and Matz, 2010).

Whether to treat AOM remains controversial (Coker, 2010; Shaikh et al, 2009). Treatment options are decided based on the child's age, the illness severity, and the certainty of diagnosis.

1. Pain management is the first principle of treatment.
   - Weight-appropriate doses of ibuprofen or acetaminophen should be encouraged to decrease discomfort and fever.
   - Topical analgesics such as benzocaine or antipyrine/benzocaine otic preparations can be added to systemic

TABLE 29-5 Criteria for Treatment or Observation in Children With Acute Otitis Media

Age	Certain Diagnosis	Uncertain Diagnosis
<6 months of age	Antibacterial therapy, analgesics	Antibacterial therapy; analgesics
6 months to 2 years of age	Antibacterial therapy	Antibacterial therapy if severe illness; observation option* if nonsevere illness; analgesics
≥2 years of age	Antibacterial therapy if severe illness. Observation option if nonsevere illness*	Observation option*; analgesics

*Observation option discussed in text.
Data from Marchisio P, Bellussi L, DiMauro G, et al: Acute otitis media: from diagnosis to prevention: summary of the Italian guideline, *Int J Pediatr Otolaryngol* 74:1209-1216, 2010; Shaikh N, Havey K, Paradise JL, et al: The Cochrane library and acute otitis media in children: an overview of reviews, evidence-based child health, *Cochrane Rev J* 4(2):390-399, 2009.

pain management if the tympanic membrane is known to be intact. Topical analgesics should not be used alone (Marchisio et al, 2010).
   - Distraction, oil application, or external use of heat or cold may be of some use.
2. Observation or "watchful waiting" for 48 to 72 hours (Table 29-5) allows the patient to improve without antibacterial treatment. Pain relief should be provided, and a means of follow-up must be in place; options for follow-up include:
   - Parent-initiated visit or phone call for worsening or no improvement
   - Scheduled follow-up appointment
   - Routine follow-up phone call
   - SNAP to be started if the child's symptoms do not improve or if they worsen in 48 to 72 hours (Table 29-6).
   - Communication with the parent, reevaluation, and the ability to obtain medication must be in place.
   - Watchful waiting studies in children 6 months to 12 years old with nonsevere AOM have demonstrated the safety, effectiveness, and decreased antibiotic use when parents share in the decision-making and there is close follow-up (Siegel, 2010). Of 100 average-risk children, amoxicillin treatment has a modest effect; 80% of children would get better within 3 days without antibiotic, an additional 12 improve with antibiotic, but 3 to 10 children would develop rash and 5 to 10 would develop diarrhea (Coker, 2010).
3. Antibacterial therapy should be instituted for all children younger than 6 months of age with a diagnosis of AOM; for those ages 6 months to 2 years with a definitive diagnosis; and for children older than 2 years of age with severe illness (see Tables 29-6 and 29-7). Treatment with antibiotics should be for 10 days for children younger than 2 years of age or when there is a risk of treatment failure. A 5-day therapy regimen may be appropriate in well children older than 2 years (Marchisio et al, 2010).
   - Amoxicillin (40 to 90 mg/kg/day) divided twice a day remains the first-line antibiotic for AOM.

TABLE 29-6   Recommended Antibiotics for Patients Treated Initially With Observation or With Antibiotic Treatment

Illness severity	INITIAL ANTIBIOTIC TREATMENT AT DIAGNOSIS		CLINICALLY DEFINED TREATMENT FAILURE AFTER 48-72 HOURS OF OBSERVATION		CLINICALLY DEFINED TREATMENT FAILURE AFTER INITIAL TREATMENT WITH ANTIBIOTIC	
	Recommended	Alternate for Penicillin Allergy	Recommended	Alternate for Penicillin Allergy	Recommended	Alternate for Penicillin Allergy
Temperature <102.2° F (39° C), mild symptoms	Amoxicillin, 80-90 mg/kg/day	Non-Type 1: cefdinir Type 1: azithromycin	Amoxicillin, 80-90 mg/kg/day	Non-Type 1: cefdinir Type 1: azithromycin	Amoxicillin-clavulanate, 90 mg/kg/day of amoxicillin, with 6.4 mg/kg/day of clavulanate	Non-Type 1: ceftriaxone, 3 days; Type 1: clindamycin
Temperature >102.2° F (39° C) and/or severe otalgia	Amoxicillin-clavulanate, 90 mg/kg/day of amoxicillin, with 6.4 mg/kg/day of clavulanate	Ceftriaxone IM, 1 or 3 consecutive daily doses	Amoxicillin-clavulanate, 90 mg/kg/day of amoxicillin, with 6.4 mg/kg/day of clavulanate	Ceftriaxone IM, 3 consecutive daily doses	Ceftriaxone, 3 days	Tympanocentesis, clindamycin

Adapted from American Academy of Pediatrics and American Academy of Family Physicians: Clinical practice guideline: diagnosis and management of acute otitis media, *Pediatrics* 113(5):1454, 2004; University of Michigan Health System: *Otitis media guideline,* 2007. Available at www.guideline.gov/content.aspx?id=11685&search=otitis+media (accessed on March 17, 2011).

- With resistant infection or severe illness (fever greater than 102.2° F [39° C] or moderate to severe otalgia) or suspected beta-lactamase bacteria, amoxicillin-clavulanate should be started at 80 to 90 mg/kg/day of the amoxicillin component divided twice a day.

If there is a documented hypersensitivity reaction to amoxicillin, the following antibiotics are acceptable:
- Non-Type I hypersensitivity reaction
  - Cefdinir 14 mg/kg/day in one or two doses
  - Cefpodoxime 10 mg/kg/day once daily
  - Cefuroxime 30 mg/kg/day in two divided doses
- Type 1 hypersensitivity reaction, macrolides can be used, though they provide poor coverage for *H. influenzae:*
  - Azithromycin (10 mg/kg on day 1 and 5 mg/kg on days 2 to 5)

Other possibilities include:
- Ceftriaxone 50 mg/kg given parenterally daily in one to three doses over a 5-day period may be effective for the vomiting child, the child unable to tolerate oral medications, or the child who has failed amoxicillin-clavulanate.
- Clindamycin 30 to 40 mg/kg/day in three divided doses (may be considered for ceftriaxone failure but should only be used if susceptibilities known)

A listing of medications that are acceptable to treat OM is found in Table 29-7.
4. Recommendations for follow-up include:
   - After 48 to 72 hours if a child has not showed improvement in ear symptomatology, the child should be seen to confirm or exclude the presence of AOM. If the initial management option was an antibacterial agent, the agent should be changed.
5. Persistent and recurrent AOM
   - Persistent AOM occurs when antibiotic therapy has been completed and evidence of AOM is still present, or

AOM recurs within days of treatment. Retreatment with a broader-spectrum antibiotic is suggested.
- Persistent MEE is common after resolution of acute symptoms and should not be seen as a need for continuing antibiotics (see section on OME).
- Recurrent AOM is present when more than three distinct and well-documented bouts of AOM have occurred in 6 months or four or more episodes in 12 months.
6. An otolaryngology referral is indicated when appropriate therapy for OM has failed. Myringotomy or placement of PETs can help relieve discomfort and decrease the likelihood of further infection. Indications for tympanostomy and the insertion of PETs were discussed in an earlier section.
7. The pediatric provider is encouraged to keep current on updated recommendations for the treatment of AOM because of the rapid changes in resistance patterns and newly developed treatments.
8. Other issues in treating AOM
   - Decongestants and antihistamines are not helpful in the treatment of AOM.
   - Antimicrobial ototopical drops (ofloxacin or ciprofloxacin) or ophthalmic drops (tobramycin or gentamicin) are indicated if the TM is perforated, the child has otorrhea, or has patent, draining PETs.
   - Xylitol, a sugar found in fruits and the bark of birch trees, has bacteriostatic effects against *S. pneumoniae* and interferes with bacterial adhesion to mucous membranes. It appears to have some suppressive effects in preventing ear infections. Having the child drink an oral solution of xylitol or chew a stick of sugar-free gum at least three times a day may reduce the recurrence rate. Recent studies suggest that the liquid form seems to cause fewer gastrointestinal symptoms (Vergison et al, 2010; Vernacchio et al, 2007).
   - There is no safe or effective herbal treatment for the treatment of AOM or OME.

TABLE 29-7	Medications Used to Treat Acute Otitis Media	
Drug	**Dose**	**Comments**
Amoxicillin	80-90 mg/kg/day every 12 hr	First choice unless contraindicated
Amoxicillin-clavulanate	80-90 mg/kg/day every 12 hr with clavulanate <10 mg/kg/day	Good beta-lactamase coverage; costly and more likely to cause diarrhea
Azithromycin	10 mg/kg/day on day 1 (max dose 500 mg/day) then 5 mg/kg/day on days 2-5 given daily (max dose 250 mg/day)	Children older than 6 mo, 5-day treatment course Macrolide Primarily used with penicillin allergy Should not be used as first-line
Cefdinir	14 mg/kg/day every 12 hr or daily	Broad-spectrum third-generation cephalosporin
Cefixime	8 mg/kg every 12 hr or daily	Broad-spectrum third-generation cephalosporin; reduced efficacy against *S. pneumoniae*
Cefpodoxime	10 mg/kg/day daily	Broad spectrum of coverage, costly; third-generation cephalosporin
Cefprozil	30 mg/kg/day every 12 hr	Broad spectrum of coverage, cost similar to other cephalosporins; intermediate potency second-generation cephalosporin; moderate taste
Ceftibuten	9 mg/kg/day given daily	Children older than 6 mo; third-generation cephalosporin; active against beta-lactamase; reduced efficacy against *S. pneumoniae*
Ceftriaxone	50 mg/kg/day IM in 1-3 doses over 3 days	Costly; third-generation cephalosporin
Cefuroxime	30 mg/kg/day every 12 hr 125 mg every 12 hr if younger than 2 yr old 250 mg every 12 hr if 2-12 yr old 250-500 mg every 12 hr if older than 12 yr	Broad spectrum of coverage, costly; most potent second-generation cephalosporin; poor taste
Clarithromycin	15 mg/kg/day every 12 hr	Children older than 6 mo, 5-day treatment course Macrolide Primarily used with penicillin allergy Should not be used as first-line
Clindamycin	30-40 mg/kg/day given every 8 hr	Should not be used unless culture and sensitivities are done

Data from Taketomo CK, Hodding JH, Kraus DM: *Pediatric dosage handbook*, ed 16, Hudson, OH, 2009, Lexi-Comp.

Complications

Persistent AOM, persistent OME, TM perforation (see Color Plate), OE, mastoiditis, cholesteatoma, tympanosclerosis (see Color Plate), hearing loss of 25 to 30 dB for several months, ossicle necrosis, pseudotumor cerebri, cerebral thrombophlebitis, and facial paralysis are possible complications.

Prevention and Education

The following interventions, shown to be helpful in preventing AOM, should be encouraged:
- Pneumococcal vaccine; specifically PCV13, which contains subtype 19A (Pelton and Leibovitz, 2009)
- Annual influenza vaccine may help prevent OM, especially in high-risk children who attend daycare centers (Marchisio et al, 2009).
- *H. influenzae* type b vaccine, although recommended, is not helpful in preventing AOM because the *H. influenzae* responsible for AOM is usually nontypeable.
- Xylitol chewing gum or liquid as tolerated (Vernacchio et al, 2006).
- Exclusive breastfeeding until at least 6 months old is protective against single and recurrent episodes of AOM, although the mechanism of protection is not completely understood (Sabirov et al, 2009).

- Choose licensed daycare facilities with fewer children.
- Avoid bottle propping, feeding infants lying down, and passive smoke exposure.
- Avoid the use of pacifiers. Although the relationship cannot be fully explained, multiple studies have shown that pacifier use increases the incidence of AOM (Vergison et al, 2010).
- Educate regarding the problem of drug-resistant bacteria and the need to avoid the use of antibiotics unless absolutely necessary; if antibiotics are used, the child needs to complete the entire course of the prescription and follow up if symptoms do not resolve.

OTITIS MEDIA WITH EFFUSION

Description

The diagnosis of OME is made when there is evidence of MEE without signs or symptoms of acute ear infection (see Color Plate). MEE decreases the mobility of the TM and interferes with sound conduction.

Epidemiology

OME can occur spontaneously with ETD caused by an inflammatory process after AOM, viral illness, anatomic abnormalities, barotrauma, allergies, or a combination of these conditions.

ETD changes the middle ear mucosa in the following sequence: (1) the mucosa becomes secretory with increased mucus production; (2) the mucus becomes viscous as the mucosa absorbs water; and (3) fluid becomes stuck behind the TM. Bacterial biofilms may explain the persistence of OME. Biofilms are mixed microorganisms enclosed in a polymeric matrix that adhere to surfaces, such as the middle ear mucosa (Bakaletz, 2007; Hall-Stoodley et al, 2006; Tonnaer et al, 2006).

ETD can cause OME, which then can become AOM. OME is a natural consequence of both treated and untreated AOM. Approximately 90% of all children will have OME at some time before school age, with an increased frequency between 6 months and 4 years old; 75% of OME episodes resolve within 3 months (Gould and Matz, 2010).

Risk factors for chronic OME are listed in Box 29-2.

Clinical Findings

History. The following features may be noted in the affected child:

- Often asymptomatic and afebrile
- Intermittent complaints of mild ear pain
- Fullness in the ear ("popping" or the feeling of "talking in a barrel")
- Complaint of hearing loss in older children
- Dizziness or impaired balance
- Chronic vomiting with failure to thrive, which can be related to chronic OME

Physical Examination. Pneumatic otoscopy reveals decreased TM mobility. An abnormal-appearing TM, often described as dull, varying from bulging and opaque with no visible landmarks to retracted and translucent with visible landmarks and an air-fluid level or bubble, may be seen (see Color Plate). Head and neck structures should be examined for abnormalities.

Diagnostic Studies. The tympanogram is flat-type B. The audiogram can show hearing loss of 15 to 31 dB.

Differential Diagnosis

Differential diagnoses include AOM; all causes of hearing loss and anatomic abnormalities; persistent unilateral OME can indicate nasopharyngeal carcinoma.

Management

Recommendations in the 2004 OME guidelines (AAP, 2004b) pertaining to children 2 months to 12 years old include:

- Documenting in the medical record at each visit the presence and duration of effusion, whether it is unilateral or bilateral, and any associated symptoms
- Identifying children at risk for speech, language, or learning problems
- Using watchful waiting in those children who are not at risk because of the likelihood of spontaneous resolution of OME
- At-risk children are defined as having developmental delays because of sensory, physical, cognitive, or behavioral factors (e.g., hearing loss independent of OME, speech or language delays, pervasive or other developmental disorders, syndromes or craniofacial disorders, blindness, cleft palate). These children should be promptly referred for hearing, speech, and language evaluation.

| **BOX 29-3** | Risk Factors for Hearing Loss Caused by Otitis Media With Effusion[*] |

- Bilateral OME for 4 months or longer
- If two or more present:
  - OME present for longer than 8 weeks
  - Speech development slower than peers
  - Speech less clear than previously
  - Child decreases amount of talking
  - Child less responsive to name and other familiar sounds
  - Child says "Huh?" or "What?" frequently
  - Child sits close to TV or wants volume louder
  - Child has difficulty learning (reading, spelling)
  - Child is hyperactive or overly inattentive

[*]Child should be tested audiologically if one or two of the above is present.
OME, Otitis media with effusion.
Modified from Daly KA, Hunter LL, Giebink GS: Chronic otitis media with effusion, *Pediatr Rev* 20(3):89, 1999.

- Children considered not at risk should be watched for 3 months from the onset of effusion or diagnosis because 75% effusion resulting from AOM resolves within 3 months.
  - Follow-up during the 3 months with pneumatic otoscopy and/or tympanogram is at the clinician's discretion.
  - Reexamination is recommended at 3- to 6-month intervals until the effusion dissipates, significant hearing loss is identified, or structural abnormalities of the TM or middle ear are suspected (retraction pockets, ossicular erosion, areas of atelectasis or atrophy).
  - Hearing and language testing is recommended if OME lasts for 3 months or longer or at any point if language delay, learning problems, or significant hearing loss is suspected. Box 29-3 lists risk factors for hearing loss.
- Referral rationale, expectations, and decision-making process should be communicated to the parent when referral to an otolaryngologist is made. Duration of effusion, reason for referral, and any relevant information should be communicated to the otolaryngologist.
  - Bilateral myringotomy with insertion of tympanostomy tubes as discussed earlier in the chapter
- Other recommendations:
  - There is no evidence that decongestants, antibiotics, and nasal steroids are of any benefit in the management of OME (Williamson et al, 2009).
  - Limited studies suggest that second-generation antihistamines might be of some benefit if the OME is associated with allergies (Goodrich et al, 2009).
  - Tonsillectomy or adenoidectomy alone should not be used to treat OME.
  - The use of complementary and alternative medicine as a treatment for OME lacks scientific evidence documenting efficacy and the uncertain balance of harm and benefit.

Complications

Complications include recurrent AOM and hearing loss that may be temporary conductive or, over time, permanent high-frequency SNHL.

Prevention and Education

- Stress the importance of follow-up until the TM and hearing are normal. Advise parents of the length of time (weeks to months) required for resolution of OME.
- Remind parents of their important role in language development of their child. Conversation and parent interaction through reading and play, along with affirmative sounds and gestures, are the most important factors in language development and school readiness.
- Strategies for maximizing hearing for the child:
  - Face the child and get within 3 feet before speaking.
  - Enunciate clearly; speak slower and louder.
  - Use visual clues and repeat as necessary.
  - Turn off competing background noise (music, radio, television).
  - Request preferential seating in the classroom.

CHOLESTEATOMA
Description

Cholesteatoma is usually the result of a chronic ear infection and involves the formation of an epidermal inclusion cyst of the middle ear or mastoid consisting of desquamated debris from the keratinizing, squamous epithelial lining of the middle ear (see Color Plate). As the cholesteatoma grows in size, it can destroy the surrounding structures. Hearing loss, dizziness, and facial muscle paralysis are rare complications.

Epidemiology

Cholesteatomas can be congenital, primary acquired, or secondary acquired (Spilsbury et al, 2010). Varied theories explaining their formation include an inflammatory process, perforation of the TM, and failure of desquamated tissue to clear from the middle ear. The incidence rate is unknown.

Clinical Findings

History. The history may be negative with congenital cholesteatomas. The history with an acquired cholesteatoma might include:
- Chronic OM with malodorous purulent otorrhea
- Vertigo and hearing loss
- History or presence of PET

Physical Examination. A pearly white lesion is present on or behind the TM. Aural polyps are considered cholesteatomas unless proven otherwise. Congenital cholesteatomas are often in the most anteroinferior position of the TM.

Differential Diagnosis

Tympanosclerosis, debris from chronic OME, malignant rhabdomyosarcoma, and aural polyps are some of the differential diagnoses.

Management

Accurate diagnosis and immediate otolaryngological referral for surgical excision are needed.

Complications

Complications include irreversible structural damage, permanent bone damage, facial nerve palsy, hearing loss, and intracranial infection, especially in untreated cases.

MASTOIDITIS
Description

Mastoiditis is a suppurative infection of the mastoid cells.

Epidemiology

Mastoiditis may accompany AOM. The mucoperiosteal lining of the mastoid air cells becomes inflamed, with subsequent progressive swelling and obstruction of drainage from the mastoid. Common organisms identified include *S. pneumoniae*, *H. influenzae*, *M. catarrhalis*, *S. aureus*, *S. pyogenes*, and *Mycobacterium tuberculosis* (rare). Gram-negative *E. coli*, *Proteus*, and *Pseudomonas* are more common in chronic mastoiditis, more virulent infections, and young infants. Antibiotic treatment for AOM does not safeguard against and may actually mask mastoiditis with a normal TM. Intracranial complications of mastoiditis are common and may develop despite treatment.

The exact incidence of mastoiditis is unknown but has been described as low since the introduction of antibiotics. It is most common in children from infancy to adolescence with a peak between 6 and 13 months of age; gender distribution is equal. Although uncommon, it is potentially life threatening. It is important to note that the watchful waiting and SNAP approaches to AOM and OME have not increased the incidence of acute mastoiditis (Ho et al, 2008).

Clinical Findings
History and Physical Examination
- Concurrent or recurrent AOM
- Fever and otalgia
- Persistent OM unresponsive to antibiotic therapy
- Postauricular swelling. Infants may have swelling above the ear, displacing the pinna inferiorly or laterally. Older children have swelling that pushes the earlobe superiorly and laterally.

Diagnostic Studies
- CT can provide definitive anatomical information.
- Tympanocentesis with culture and Gram stain help identify offending organism.

Differential Diagnosis

Include other causes of postauricular inflammation or swelling such as lymphadenopathy, periauricular cellulitis, perichondritis of auricle, mumps, or tumors of the mastoid bone.

Management

Urgent ENT referral is imperative. Hospitalization, intravenous antibiotics, and mastoidectomy are usually required.

Prevention

The pneumococcal conjugate vaccine has reduced the incidence of mastoiditis caused by *S. pneumoniae*.

SENSORINEURAL AND CONDUCTIVE HEARING LOSS

Description

Hearing loss is defined as bilateral pure-tone hearing loss of 40 dB or more at frequencies of 500, 1000, and 2000 Hz in the better ear. Three types of hearing loss are recognized: sensorineural, conductive, or mixed. Either or both ears may be involved.

SNHL is most commonly associated with dysfunction of or damage to the cochlea (inner ear) and less often associated with damage to the auditory nerve (cranial nerve VIII). SNHL that is related to the auditory nerve is usually labeled auditory neuropathy or auditory dyssynchrony, neither of which is amenable to treatment with hearing aids, but may respond to cochlear implants. SNHL can be congenital or acquired, mild or severe, and is permanent.

Conductive hearing loss (CHL), either congenital or acquired, implies a problem in the outer or middle ear, and results from blocked transmission of sound waves from the EAC to the inner ear (e.g., AOM, OME). The cochlea functions normally. Bone conduction is usually normal with decreased air conduction. Conductive hearing loss is usually in the range of 20 to 60 dB (Gregg et al, 2004). MEEs result in an average hearing loss of 27 to 31 dB.

Mixed hearing loss involves a combination of SNHL and CHL. Abnormalities are identified in outer, middle, and inner ear spaces. Central hearing loss occurs when the nerves or nuclei of the central nervous system, either in the pathways to the brain or the brain itself, are damaged or impaired (Gifford et al, 2009).

Epidemiology

SNHL and CHL can be associated with craniofacial anomalies (e.g., aural atresia, cleft lip or cleft palate, external ear deformity without atresia, dysmorphic facies without external ear deformity), genetic aberrations or congenital deformities (e.g., white forelock, café au lait spots, family history of SNHL, metabolic abnormalities), or environmental exposure (e.g., ototoxic drugs, bacterial or viral meningitis, other infectious diseases, loud noises, head trauma).

SNHL can occur when hair cells in the cochlea are injured by exposure to excessive noise over a variable period. SNHL can also come from prenatal and perinatal exposure (e.g., intrauterine infections, toxic chemicals, erythroblastosis fetalis). It is estimated that 80% of congenital SNHL is due to recessive inheritance (Mehra et al, 2009). Multiple genes associated with various types of SNHL have been identified.

CHL can also be congenital or acquired. Congenital causes include aural stenosis or atresia and ossicle malformations. Acquired conductive hearing loss can be caused by AOM, OME, foreign bodies in the ear canal, cerumen impaction, TM perforation, cholesteatoma, ossicular discontinuity, collapsing ear canals, otosclerosis, and tympanosclerosis (Gifford et al, 2009).

The overall prevalence of congenital deafness is estimated to be 1 in 1000 births. The incidence for varying degrees of hearing loss in healthy infants is 3 in 1000 and increases to 6 in 1000 when well and at-risk infants are pooled together (Laury et al, 2009). Unilateral hearing loss affects 0.4 to 34 per 1000 newborns and 1 to 50 per 1000 school-age children (Lieu et al, 2010).

Clinical Findings

History. Hearing loss is often a "silent disease." Careful consideration and attention to identified risk factors are essential in identifying hearing loss in children.

The risk factors for SNHL in newborns include the following (Gifford et al, 2009; Joint Committee on Infant Hearing, 2007):

- Birthweight less than 1500 g
- Severe depression at birth (e.g., Apgar score of 0 to 3 at 5 minutes, failure to initiate a response by 10 minutes, or hypotonia at up to 2 hours old)
- Neonatal intensive care unit admission for 2 days or longer
- Prolonged mechanical ventilation for greater than 10 days
- Persistent pulmonary hypertension
- Long QT syndrome (usually profound hearing loss)
- Congenital infections, such as toxoplasmosis, bacterial meningitis, syphilis, rubella, cytomegalovirus, and herpes
- Metabolic disorders, such as phenylketonuria (PKU) and galactosemia
- Endocrine disorders, such as adrenal hyperplasia and hypothyroidism
- Craniofacial anomalies, including morphological abnormalities of the pinna and ear canal
- Genetic syndromes, such as sickle cell disease, Usher syndrome, neurofibromatosis, Waardenburg syndrome, osteopetrosis, or findings associated with other genetic syndromes known to include hearing loss
- Hyperbilirubinemia requiring exchange transfusion or causing kernicterus
- Family history of hereditary childhood SNHL
- Ototoxic drug exposure

The risk factors for hearing loss in children 1 month to 3 years old include (Joint Committee on Infant Hearing, 2007):

- Parental or caregiver concern regarding hearing, speech, language, or developmental delay; parents tend to be about 12 months ahead of care providers in identifying hearing loss in children (Harlor and Bower, 2009)
- Kidney malformation
- Family history of permanent childhood hearing loss
- Stigmata or other findings associated with a syndrome known to include SNHL, conductive hearing loss, or ETD
- Syndromes associated with progressive hearing loss, such as neurofibromatosis and osteopetrosis
- Neurodegenerative disorders, such as Hunter syndrome, or sensorimotor neuropathies, such as Friedreich ataxia and Charcot-Marie-Tooth disease
- Head trauma with loss of consciousness or skull fracture
- Bacterial meningitis
- Ototoxic medication exposure
- Diabetes mellitus
- Recurrent or persistent OME for at least 3 months

Other risk factors or indicators for hearing loss include the following:

- Failure to learn to speak at the appropriate age or failure to respond to auditory stimuli; speech that sounds like baby talk or is monotone and difficult to understand; avoidance of speaking

- Failed school screening audiogram; decreased note taking; seeming to misunderstand, ignore, confuse, or miss what is being said
- Aggression, increased physical complaints, difficulty in school and social situations
- Environmental exposure to firecrackers, toy cap pistols, firearms, loud music, loud television, squeaking toys, and machines (e.g., snowmobiles, farm equipment, lawn mowers)
- History of head or neck irradiation

Physical Examination. The following may be found in children with SNHL and conductive hearing loss:

- Abnormal hearing screening during routine newborn or well-child care visits or other office visits. For children younger than 6 months old, an ABR test is recommended. Behavioral testing using a conditioned response or an ABR is appropriate for children older than 6 months.
- A complete physical examination with special attention to the eyes, skin, and skeletal and nervous systems is needed.
- Ears—preauricular pits, auricular malformation or appendage, abnormal TM integrity, or impaired mobility with pneumatic otoscopy.
- Eyes—cataracts, corneal opacities, coloboma, blindness, nystagmus, exophthalmos, night blindness, heterochromia iridis, or blue sclerae (associated with genetic disorders that can cause SNHL)
- Craniofacial anomalies or genetic stigmata associated with SNHL (see Epidemiology)

Diagnostic Studies. EOAE and ABR are the diagnostic tests used for newborn hearing screening. After that period of time, audiometry is the preferred hearing testing of choice. If the cause of the hearing impairment is evident (cholesteatoma, ossicle malformation, OM), the diagnostic workup is limited. If the cause of the hearing loss is not readily apparent, consider the following diagnostic tests:

- Urinalysis, serum blood urea nitrogen, and creatinine to rule out renal disease
- Complete blood count, thyroid function tests, sickle cell screen
- TORCH (toxoplasmosis, other agents, rubella, cytomegalovirus, herpes simplex) screen in newborns
- Genetic testing
- Electrocardiogram (ECG) (long QT syndrome)
- Ophthalmological examination
- Computed tomography (CT) as indicated to rule out inner ear malformation

Differential Diagnosis

Mixed SNHL with conductive hearing loss and central hearing loss are included in the differential diagnosis.

Management

The following should occur for any child with suspected hearing loss:

- Refer if suspected hearing loss to an audiologist and otolaryngologist for full evaluation as soon as possible. In the referral include information about the patient's symptoms, history or physical findings, and any known diagnosis associated with hearing loss.
- Refer for surgical intervention as indicated.
- Treat known medically related conditions (diabetes, hypothyroidism).
- Genetic counseling
- Encourage the use of amplification devices as appropriate. They may be personal (e.g., hearing aids) or group (e.g., teacher microphone).
- Cochlear implants with an external speech processor are sometimes used for profound SNHL. If implants are in place, it is imperative that the child's immunizations are up to date, specifically pneumococcal conjugate vaccine.
- Recommend special school and teaching strategies, such as front-of-room placement and facing the child when speaking.
- Evaluate and treat AOM and OME if present (see the AOM and OME sections).
- Screen for hearing loss if bilateral MEE is present for 3 months or longer.
- Ensure a family-centered approach in making decisions regarding interventions for the child (e.g., Individuals with Disabilities Education Act [IDEA]).
- Refer to Chapter 15 for discussion of children who are hearing impaired.

Complications

Significant hearing loss impedes speech, language, cognitive development, and social interaction skills.

Prevention

- Good prenatal care
- Provide Rho(D) immune globulin to prevent erythroblastosis fetalis in susceptible women.
- Treat prenatal and perinatal infections promptly.
- Avoid ototoxic drug use.
- Immunize against mumps, rubella, varicella, *H. influenzae* type b, *S. pneumoniae*, influenza, and other diseases that can cause SNHL through central nervous system damage.
- Recommend avoidance of environmental factors associated with hearing loss.

Cardiovascular Disorders

JULIE MARTCHENKE AND CATHERINE G. BLOSSER

Most cardiovascular problems in the pediatric population are due to congenital heart disease (CHD), which occurs in 0.4% to 5% of all live births, 3% to 4% of stillborns, 10% to 25% of abortuses, and 2% of premature infants (patent ductus arteriosus [PDA] excluded) (Botto et al, 2008). Incidence rates vary depending on diagnostic techniques used and the inclusion and exclusion criteria of studies. By 1 week of age, 40% to 50% of infants with CHD have been detected. Some defects, such as small ventricular septal defects (VSDs) or bicuspid aortic valves, may cause no disability to a child; however, they pose a risk for bacterial endocarditis and may cause great concern for parents and caregivers.

The primary care provider (PCP) must maintain a high index of suspicion regarding any signs or symptoms of cardiovascular disease. This facilitates early identification and referral of infants and children with potential cardiovascular problems. PCPs also assist in the management of patients with CHD before and after heart surgery or procedures. Providers need to be attentive to the needs of the whole child because the focus of subspecialists and the family is on the heart disease. They also support families and children once a diagnosis is made and educate families about prevention of acquired heart disease.

■ Anatomy and Physiology

FETAL CIRCULATION

Knowledge of the fetal circulation is essential for understanding the circulatory changes that occur in the newborn at delivery (Fig. 30-1). Fetal circulation has four unique features that differ from postnatal circulation:
- Oxygenation of the blood occurs in the placenta, not the lungs.
- Fetal pulmonary vascular resistance is high, and systemic vascular resistance is low (high pressure on the right side of the heart, low pressure on the left side).
- The foramen ovale, the opening in the septum between the two atria, permits a portion of the blood to flow from the right atrium directly to the left atrium.
- A PDA provides a connection between the pulmonary artery and the aorta that allows blood to flow from the pulmonary artery to the aorta and bypass the fetal lungs.

Oxygen is diffused into the fetal circulation from the maternal uterine arteries in the placenta. From the placenta oxygenated blood flows through the umbilical vein and is diverted through the liver to the inferior vena cava (IVC) by the ductus venosus. When this well-oxygenated blood reaches the right atrium, it flows preferentially toward the atrial septum, through the foramen ovale, and into the left atrium. Oxygenated blood then flows into the left ventricle and out the aorta. Approximately two thirds of the blood from the aorta flows toward the head and neck to ensure that the fetal brain constantly receives well-oxygenated blood.

Venous blood returns from the head and upper extremities through the superior vena cava (SVC) to the right atrium. This blood preferentially flows toward the tricuspid valve into the right ventricle. From the right ventricle the blood enters the pulmonary artery. Because pulmonary vascular resistance is high and systemic resistance is low, most blood in the pulmonary artery flows through the ductus arteriosus into the descending aorta to supply oxygen and nutrients to the trunk and lower extremities. Only a small amount of blood flows into the pulmonary circuit to perfuse the lungs.

The fetal circulation is best described as two parallel circuits, with the left ventricle supplying blood to the upper extremities and the right ventricle serving the lower extremities and the placenta. At the time of transition to extrauterine life, these separate blood flows become a serial circuit.

NEONATAL CIRCULATION

A number of complex events occur at birth that rapidly shift the fetal circulation toward a neonatal circulation pattern. Clamping the umbilical cord, with subsequent removal of the placenta as the oxygenating organ, causes an immediate circulatory change in which the lungs become the new source of oxygenation. This change causes an increase in systemic vascular resistance (systemic blood pressure [BP]). With the first breath, mechanical inflation of the lungs and an increase in oxygen saturation bring about a dramatic fall in pulmonary vascular resistance and, consequently, increased pulmonary blood flow. This begins constricting the ductus arteriosus. As the pressures within the heart become relatively higher on the left side and lower on the right, the foramen ovale closes. Functional closure

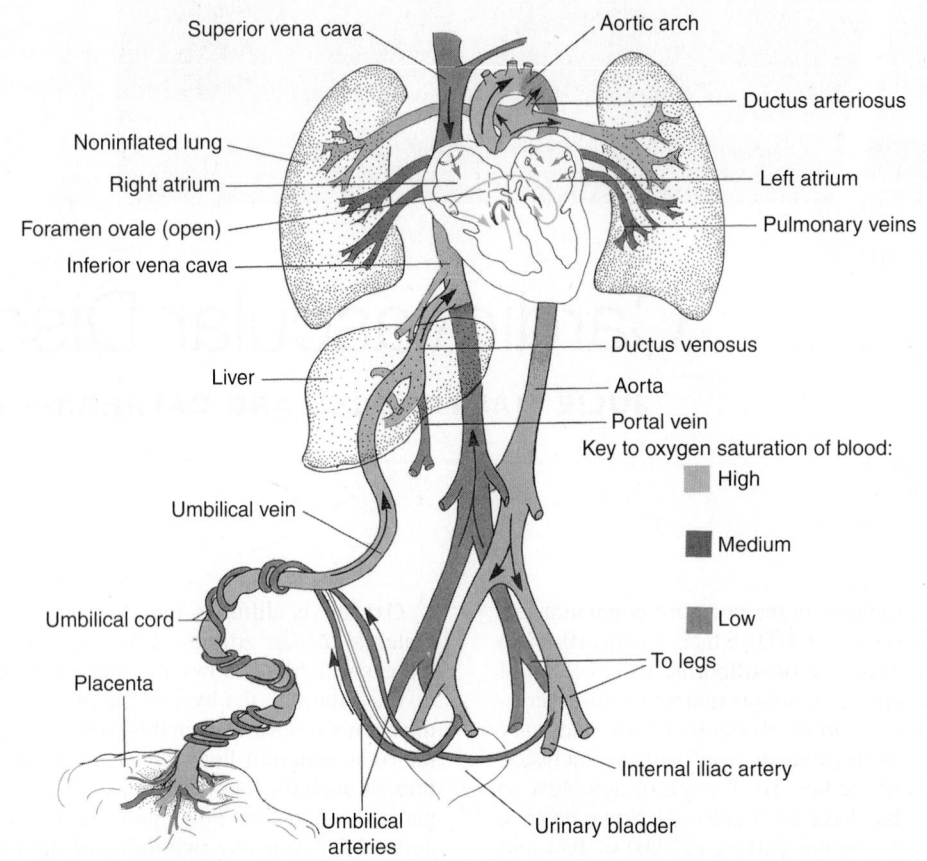

Superior vena cava
Aortic arch
Ductus arteriosus
Noninflated lung
Right atrium
Left atrium
Foramen ovale (open)
Pulmonary veins
Inferior vena cava
Ductus venosus
Liver
Aorta
Portal vein
Key to oxygen saturation of blood:
High
Umbilical vein
Medium
Umbilical cord
Low
Placenta
To legs
Internal iliac artery
Umbilical arteries
Urinary bladder

FIGURE 30-1 Fetal circulation. (From Gorrie TM, McKinney ES, Murray SS: *Foundations of maternal-newborn nursing,* Philadelphia, 1994, Saunders.)

of the ductus arteriosus and foramen ovale usually occurs within the first hours to days of life, and a serial circuit forms out of the once-parallel pulmonary and systemic circulation.

The transition toward complete anatomic closure, or obliteration of fetal structures by tissue growth or constriction, is more gradual. Pulmonary vascular resistance drops gradually over the first 6 to 8 weeks of life, which may protect the pulmonary circulation against volume overload in some congenital heart anomalies. If not noted earlier, shunt murmurs or symptoms of congestive heart failure (CHF) gradually become apparent as the infant approaches 8 weeks of age. At this time, resistance to flow is less, and shunting to the pulmonary bed increases.

Conditions that cause persistence of fetal shunts allow unoxygenated blood to flow from the right side of the heart to the left. Any murmur or cyanosis in a newborn should be carefully monitored and evaluated to detect cardiac abnormalities.

NORMAL CARDIAC STRUCTURE AND FUNCTION

The heart is a muscular four-chambered organ located in the mediastinum, the space in the chest between the lungs. The four chambers are divided into two larger muscular pumping chambers, the ventricles, and two smaller receiving chambers, the atria. Desaturated systemic blood returns to the right atrium by way of the inferior and superior venae cavae. The blood passes from the right atrium through the tricuspid valve to the right ventricle. The right ventricle pumps the blood through the pulmonic valve into the pulmonary artery and the lungs,

where it is oxygenated. Blood returning from the lungs enters the left atrium by way of the pulmonary veins and then passes through the mitral valve into the left ventricle. The left ventricle pumps the blood through the aortic valve into the aorta to provide oxygenated blood for the systemic circulation.

The heart valves are one-way valves that open and close because of pressure changes within the heart, controlling the flow of blood from chamber to chamber. The tricuspid valve has three cusps held in place by the chordae tendineae. The pulmonary valve directs blood flow from the right ventricle into the pulmonary artery, which bifurcates into right and left arteries to allow flow into both lungs. The pulmonary veins entering the left atrium contain no valves, so blood can flow freely from the lungs into the atrium. The mitral valve controls flow from the left atrium into the left ventricle. The aortic valve controls flow from the high-pressure left ventricle out to the body.

CONDUCTION SYSTEM

Myocardial contraction is stimulated by electrical depolarization along the conduction tract within the heart. Depolarization begins at the sinoatrial node, which is high in the wall of the atrium. This node acts as the pacemaker of the heart by regularly beginning the depolarizing impulses of each heartbeat. The wave of depolarization travels from the sinoatrial node throughout the atria and produces contraction of the atrial muscle. The impulses reach the atrioventricular (AV) node, which is located in the lower portion of the right atrium at the junction of the atrium and ventricle. From the AV node, the depolarization wave passes through the bundle of His, the fibers extending from the AV node along the intraventricular septum. Depolarization spreads through the left and right branches of the bundle of His and through the Purkinje fibers extending into the ventricular muscle. Impulses then spread throughout the ventricles and cause contraction. The electrocardiogram (ECG) demonstrates this pattern of changing electrical impulses.

HEART SOUNDS

At the time of ventricular contraction, the beginning of systole, the mitral and tricuspid valves close and produce the first heart sound (S_1). S_1 is the "lubb" of lubb-dupp. Although the left side of the heart reacts slightly before the right side, closure of the mitral and tricuspid valves occurs so closely together that S_1 usually appears as a single sound. S_1 is best heard at the left lower sternal border and is synchronous with the apical and carotid pulses.

After the blood has been ejected, the heart relaxes, the mitral and tricuspid valves open, and the aortic and pulmonary valves close to keep the blood from rushing back into the ventricles. This closure results in the second heart sound (S_2). S_2 is normally split with inspiration in children. S_2 reflects the onset of diastole and is the "dupp" of lubb-dupp. The intensity and splitting of S_2 is one of the most important parts of the pediatric cardiac examination. S_2 is best heard at the upper left sternal border in the pulmonic area.

Pathophysiology

The term *congenital heart disease* implies only that a cardiovascular malformation is present at birth. It does not indicate the etiology or the cause of the malformation. When CHD is diagnosed in an infant or child, parents may incorrectly assume that they are somehow responsible for the child's defect. Health care professionals must be clear about what is and what is not known about CHD to spare parents needless worry and guilt.

It is assumed most CHD is due to a complex interaction of genetic (including gender) and environmental or intrauterine factors, although currently about 75% of CHDs have no identified cause. However, as more genetic testing becomes available and further research is done, it is becoming clearer that the genetic contribution to CHD is greater than previously thought (Pierpont et al, 2007).

The heart is essentially formed by 6 weeks of fetal life, a time when the fetus is most susceptible to infectious or teratogenic exposure or to predisposing genetic or chromosomal factors. Up to 25% of children with CHD also have noncardiac abnormalities (Goldmuntz and Lin, 2008).

Table 30-1 lists the most common known chromosomal abnormalities associated with heart disease. Information about ordering genetic tests and resources for families is available from the National Institutes of Health (NIH) website (http://www.nih.gov/) and in-depth information about specific genetic defects or syndromes is available from Online Mendelian Inheritance in Man (OMIM) website (http://www.ncbi.nlm.nih.gov/omim). Genetic testing should also be done in children who have, in addition to CHD, other congenital anomalies, dysmorphic features, neurocognitive deficits, growth

retardation, mothers with multiple miscarriages, or siblings with congenital defects (Goldmuntz and Lin, 2008).

Two percent to 4% of CHD is caused by well-documented teratogens and maternal conditions or environmental influences. Teratogens known to affect the heart include maternal use of thalidomide, cocaine, lithium, fluconazole, phenothiazine, alcohol, anticonvulsants, and retinoic acid. Maternal exposure to pesticides and solvents has also been associated with CHD. Infection, especially cytomegalovirus, mumps, or rubella, contracted in the first 8 weeks of gestation can cause CHD. Infants born to mothers with insulin-dependent diabetes, systemic lupus erythematosus (SLE), and phenylketonuria also have increased risk for various cardiac defects (Goldmuntz and Lin, 2008) (Box 30-1 and Table 30-1).

Assessment of the Cardiovascular System

Cardiac assessment includes a comprehensive history, a thorough physical assessment, and a variety of diagnostic tests.

HISTORY

Cardiac evaluation includes review of the family, maternal, fetal, neonatal, and infant medical history, in addition to growth and development (see Box 30-1 for risk factors).

PHYSICAL EXAMINATION

Physical assessment in a child with suspected CHD should be adapted to the age of the child (Box 30-2). Be flexible, yet thorough, in any evaluation and include all aspects of the physical examination in an order that best suits the comfort and needs of the infant, child, or adolescent.

Vital Signs

Heart rate, respiratory rate, and BP vary considerably throughout childhood. Measurements of vital signs must be obtained on each visit with the child at rest because crying and exercise affect results. Refer to charts for normal ranges for various age groups, gender, and height for comparison.

- *Heart rate* (Table 30-2). Heart rates should always be obtained by auscultation of the heart in children younger than 10 years old. Assessment should include rate and rhythm variations. An increased heart rate can be caused by excitement, anxiety, hyperthyroidism, heart disease, anemia, or fever. Assess the rhythm for regularity.
- *Pulses.* Pulses should be checked in the upper and lower extremities and evaluated for character (strength) and variation between the different sites. A bounding pulse may indicate a PDA or aortic insufficiency. Weak or "thready" pulses may indicate CHF or an obstructive lesion, such as severe AS. Good brachial pulses in conjunction with weak or absent femoral pulses may indicate coarctation of the aorta (COA).
- *BP.* The National Institutes of Health National High Blood Pressure Education Program (NIH-NHBPEP) (2004) on BP control in children and adolescents recommends measuring BP annually beginning at 3 years of age. Providers should auscultate BP on children 3 years or older. In

| TABLE 30-1 | Congenital Malformation Syndromes Associated With Selected Congenital Heart Disease |

Disorders	Resultant Heart Defect(s)/Occurrence
Syndromes With Chromosomal/Gene Disorders	
Trisomy 21 (Down syndrome)	Atrioventricular septal defect, VSD, ASD, PDA, TOF (50%)
Trisomy 18 (Edwards syndrome)	VSD, ASD, PDA, COA, bicuspid aortic or pulmonary valve (99%)
Trisomy 13 (Patau syndrome)	VSD, PDA, dextrocardia (90%)
Turner syndrome (XO)	Bicuspid aortic valve, COA (35%), pulmonic stenosis
Marfan syndrome (FBN1 gene)	Mitral valve prolapse, aortic root dilation
22q11.2 deletion syndrome	Interrupted aortic arch, truncus arteriosus, TOF, perimembranous VSD, aortic arch anomalies
Klinefelter variant (XXXXY)	PDA, ASD (15%)
Williams syndrome	PS, supravalvular AS
Noonan syndrome (PTPN11)	Valvular pulmonic stenosis, hypertrophic cardiomyopathy
CHARGE (gene CHD7)	Truncus arteriosus, interrupted aortic arch type B
Jacobsen (11q23 deletion)	Hypoplastic left heart syndrome, COA
Long QT syndrome	Palpitations, syncope, sudden death
Holt-Oram syndrome (TBX5)	ASD, VSD
Cri du chat syndrome (5p)	VSD, PDA, ASD (25%)
Neurofibromatosis	PS, COA
Nonhereditary Syndromes	
Fetal alcohol syndrome	VSD, PDA, ASD, TOF (25%-30%)
Fetal hydantoin syndrome	PS, AS, COA, PDA, VSD, ASD (<5%)
Fetal trimethadione syndrome	TGA, VSD, TOF (15%-30%)
Infant of diabetic mother	TGA, VSD, COA (3%-5%); cardiomyopathy (10%-20%)
Pierre Robin syndrome	VSD, PDA (29%); ASD, COA, TOF (less commonly)
VATERL association	VSD, other defects (>50%)
Congenital diaphragmatic hernia	VSD, TOF (25%)
Cornelia de Lange (de Lange) syndrome	VSD (30%)
Other System Malformations	
Hydrocephalus	VSD, ECD, TOF (6%)
Dandy-Walker syndrome	VSD (3%)
Tracheoesophageal fistula and/or esophageal atresia	VSD, ASD, TOF (21%)
Imperforate anus	TOF, VSD (12%)

AS, Aortic stenosis; *ASD,* atrial septal defect; *COA,* coarctation of the aorta; *ECD,* endocardial cushion defect; *PDA,* patent ductus arteriosus; *PS,* pulmonary stenosis; *TGA,* transposition of the great arteries; *TOF,* tetralogy of Fallot; *VATERL,* vertebral anomalies, anal atresia, cardiovascular anomalies, tracheoesophageal fistula, esophageal atresia, renal and/or radial anomalies, limb defects; *VSD,* ventricular septal defect.

Data from Goldmuntz E: The genetic contribution to congenital heart disease, *Pediatr Clin North Am* 51:1721-1737, 2004; Lin A, Belmont J, Malik S: Heart. In Stevenson R, Hall J, editors: *Human malformations and related anomalies,* ed 2, Oxford, 2006, Oxford University Press; Park MK, Troxler RG: *Pediatric cardiology for practitioners,* ed 4, St Louis, 2002, Mosby.

selected cases, in which the index of suspicion of heart disease is high, providers should check BPs in younger children. It is important to always use a BP cuff that is appropriate for the child's size. For arm pressure, the width of the cuff should be two thirds the length of the upper arm measured from the axilla to the antecubital space. A cuff that is too narrow or does not fit around a chubby arm may cause an erroneously high reading. Cuff sizes of 3, 5, 7, 12, and 18 cm should be on hand in order to accommodate the array of pediatric patient sizes. Initial evaluation should compare the pressure in all four extremities. Pressure in all extremities should be equal, with pressure in the legs being

---

BOX 30-1 Risk Factors Suggestive of Congenital Heart Disease

Perinatal Risk Factors

Maternal infections and exposures (CMV, rubella, other viral syndromes)

Maternal use of tobacco, alcohol, street drugs, retinoic acid, hydantoins, lithium, valproates

Maternal chronic disease (CHD, lupus, insulin-dependent diabetes, phenylketonuria)

Maternal age at child's birth (increase in chromosomal abnormalities after 40 years old)

Maternal pregnancy history (excessive weight gain, gestational diabetes)

Neonatal Risk Factors

Fetal or newborn distress (aspiration, hypoxia, cyanosis)

Prematurity (increased incidence of CHD in premature infants)

Presence of associated anomalies (genetic or chromosomal abnormalities or syndromes)

Neonatal infections (GBS)

Birthweight (term infants, <2500 g; SGA, <2 standard deviations from the mean for gestational age)

Newborn Risk Factors

Murmur at birth or early infancy

Hypertension (at birth or beyond)

Feeding difficulty (SOB, easily fatigued, diaphoresis, poor intake)

Cyanosis (increase with crying, feeding, exertion)

Tachypnea (persistent, with crying, feeding)

Toddler, School-Age, and Teenage Risk Factors

Deviation from normal growth and development (normal milestone development, following own growth curve)

Deviation from activity level appropriate for chronologic age (unable to keep up with peers; unable to run or ride bike)

Frequent respiratory tract infections (pneumonia, URIs that last longer than normal)

Prior murmurs, blue spells

Documented GABHS infection

Hypertension (documented on a minimum of three separate visits)

Chest pain with exertion

SOB with exertion (beyond normal peers)

Syncope or dizziness (especially associated with noted heart rate change)

Tachycardia or bradycardia (fluttering in chest, racing heart)

Family History Risk Factors

CHD (especially siblings, parents, first-degree relatives)

Sudden death or premature myocardial infarction (before 50 years old)

Hypertension

Rheumatic fever

Genetic syndromes

Hypercholesterolemia

CHD, Congenital heart disease; *CMV,* cytomegalovirus; *GABHS,* group A beta-hemolytic streptococcus; *GBS,* group B streptococcus; *SGA,* small for gestational age; *SOB,* shortness of breath; *URIs,* upper respiratory infections.

BOX 30-2 Developmental Approach to Cardiac Assessment

Infants

Complete the assessment with the infant in the parent's arms to keep the infant quiet and cooperative.

Perform uncomfortable aspects of the examination after auscultation to ensure a quiet listen.

Keep the infant covered and warm to minimize discomfort and physiologic changes associated with chilling.

Observe color, respiratory effort, and general effort level while the baby is quiet.

Toddlers

Approach the child quietly, calmly, and slowly. A loud, boisterous greeting may frighten the toddler.

Complete the assessment wherever the child is most comfortable—sitting on the floor, in the parent's lap, on the examination table.

Allow the child to handle a stethoscope while the history is being taken.

Have a toy or distraction item available during the examination.

Consider "listening" to the parent's heart first to improve comfort with the examination.

School Age

Clearly explain the plan and expectations before the examination.

Answer the child's questions honestly.

Talk about topics of interest (school, sports) during the examination.

School-age children may be modest and prefer to keep a gown on during most of the examination.

School-age children may be helpful in discussion of symptoms and events surrounding current concerns.

Adolescents

Questions should be directed at the adolescent and parent.

Communicate in a manner that conveys honesty, professionalism, and interest in their concerns.

Ensure privacy related to both the physical examination and information sharing.

Provide a choice of having a parent present for any or all aspects of the history and examination.

Adolescents are very "body aware" and need reassurance that their concerns are valid, even when the symptom is within normal limits.

---

slightly higher (10 to 20 mm Hg) in a child who walks. Lower extremity pressure is measured with the stethoscope placed over the popliteal artery. The NIH periodically publishes norms for BP by gender, age, and height; they are found in Tables 30-3 and 30-4 (NIH-NHBPEP, 2004).

- *The pulse pressure* (difference between systolic and diastolic pressure) is normally 20 to 50 mm Hg throughout childhood. A wide pulse pressure caused by an abnormally

low diastolic pressure may be an indication of PDA, aortic regurgitation, or other cardiac pathologic conditions.

- *Respiratory rate.* Evaluation of the respiratory system includes the respiratory rate, assessment of effort, and breath sounds in all five lobes of the lungs. It is important to evaluate the respiratory rate in a quiet infant or child. A respiratory rate greater than 40 in a young child or 60 in a newborn who is quiet, resting, and afebrile warrants

TABLE 30-2	Normal Heart Rates (Beats per Minute) in Infants and Children		
Age	Resting (Awake)	Resting (Asleep)	Exercise/ Fever
Newborn	100-180	80-160	Up to 220
1 week-3 months	100-220	80-200	Up to 220
3 months-2 years	80-150	70-120	Up to 220
2-10 years	70-100	60-90	195-215
10-20 years	55-90	50-90	195-215

further evaluation. An infant with CHD may be happily tachypneic and not show significant signs of grunting, intercostal retractions, nasal flaring, or tracheal tug (up and down movement of the trachea with each inspiration).

- *Oxygen saturation.* Oxygen saturation is considered to be an essential vital sign in many settings. It is important to obtain oxygen saturations in new babies or new patients because cyanosis is often subtle and not always readily perceptible to all examiners. Pulse oximetry alone may detect cyanotic heart disease in asymptomatic newborns, preventing possible mortality and morbidity from delayed diagnosis (Mahle et al, 2009).

General Appearance

The provider should observe an infant while obtaining a history and before performing any other part of the physical examination. General nutritional state, respiratory effort, color, physical abnormalities, and distress or discomfort level should be observed.

- During this observation period note the presence of unusual facial characteristics (e.g., malformed ears, wide-spaced eyes, noticeable anomalies) or extracardiac anomalies (e.g., cleft lip or palate, polydactyly, microcephaly) that may be associated with a syndrome or chromosomal abnormalities. Children may have obvious stigmata, such as those seen with Down syndrome, Marfan syndrome (unusually tall with an arm span wider than the head-to-toe height), Turner syndrome (webbed neck, prominent ears), or fetal alcohol syndrome (microcephaly and pinched facies), all of which are associated with CHD.
- Overall skin color should be assessed for signs of mottling or central cyanosis while the infant is at rest. Cyanosis caused by heart disease is recognized as a pale blue or ruddy red color of the mucous membranes (lips, tongue, nailbeds). The tongue is the best indicator because it lacks pigmentation and is abundantly served by the vascular system. Peripheral cyanosis or acrocyanosis, a blueness or pallor noted around the mouth and on the hands or feet, can be a normal variant, especially if it intensifies when the infant is cold. Clubbing of the fingers and toes may be seen in children with long-standing cyanosis.
- Note any wheezing, nasal flaring, retractions, prominent neck veins, or head bobbing with respirations.
- Note also signs of peripheral or periorbital edema. Edema or puffiness around the eyes may be evident in an infant with CHF even in the absence of peripheral edema of the

hands or feet. True pitting edema of the feet is an unusual finding in an infant with CHF.
- Measure and plot height and weight on standardized charts, including Down and Turner syndrome charts, at each assessment. Although many children with CHD fall within the normal ranges of height, weight, and development, a large number of infants and children with heart disease experience poor weight gain, less than normal linear growth, and delays in achieving developmental milestones.

Palpation

Palpate all five areas of the chest: the aortic, pulmonic, tricuspid, and mitral areas, and Erb's point (Fig. 30-2). Chest palpation is best accomplished by using the open palm of the hand near the base of the fingers. The hand should be gently moved across the chest to assess abnormal precordial activity, including pulsations, lifts, heaves, or thrills, and to determine the location of the apical impulse. The apical impulse is used to determine the size of the heart and is the most lateral point at which cardiac activity can be palpated. In infants and children, the impulse is normally palpated at the apex of the heart in the fourth intercostal space just to the left of the midclavicular line. At approximately 7 years old, the point shifts to the fifth intercostal space. In the presence of cardiomegaly, the apical impulse is shifted laterally or downward.

- Thrills are a palpable vibration caused by turbulent blood flow through abnormal structures or defects in the heart. The turbulent flow may be due to valvular narrowing or stenosis or defects, such as VSD.
- Assess peripheral pulses (radial, brachial, carotid, dorsalis pedis, and posterior tibial) for amplitude and intensity. In COA, the examiner will note decreased or absent femoral pulses and impulse lag if the radial pulse is palpated simultaneously. A fast pulse rate may indicate arrhythmia or CHF.
- The liver and spleen should be assessed for enlargement. A liver more than 1 cm below the right costal margin in an older infant or child may indicate hepatomegaly and is an important finding. Infants may have a palpable liver edge as a normal finding.
- The back should be examined for scoliosis, a finding associated with enlarged hearts.

Auscultation of Heart Sounds

- The examiner should approach auscultation of the heart in the same manner for every child either beginning at the base or apex of the heart. Ideally, assess heart sounds in a quiet environment when the child is cooperative.
- Four individual heart sounds can be heard: S_1, S_2, S_3, and S_4. S_1 and S_2 represent normal heart sounds, whereas the presence of S_3 or S_4 may indicate cardiac enlargement or volume overload.
- At each area of examination, the provider should accurately identify the first (S_1) and second (S_2) heart sounds.
- S_1 has the following characteristics:
  - It is heard in the beginning of systole and indicates closure of AV valves (mitral and tricuspid).
  - It may be differentiated from early systolic clicks by the low frequency of the sound (clicks have a higher frequency). It is best heard with the diaphragm of the stethoscope.
  - It is usually loudest at the apex.

TABLE 30-3 Blood Pressure Levels in the 90th and 95th Percentiles for Girls 1 to 17 Years Old by Percentiles of Height

Age	Height Percentiles* BP†	SYSTOLIC BP (mm Hg)							DIASTOLIC BP (mm Hg)						
		5%	10%	25%	50%	75%	90%	95%	5%	10%	25%	50%	75%	90%	95%
	↓														
1	90th	97	97	98	100	101	102	103	52	53	53	54	55	55	56
	95th	100	101	103	104	105	106	107	56	57	57	58	59	59	60
2	90th	98	99	100	101	103	104	105	57	58	58	59	60	61	61
	95th	102	103	104	105	107	108	109	61	62	62	63	63	65	65
3	90th	100	100	102	103	104	106	106	61	62	62	63	64	64	65
	95th	104	104	105	107	108	109	110	65	66	66	67	68	68	69
4	90th	101	102	103	104	106	107	108	64	64	65	66	67	67	68
	95th	105	106	107	108	110	111	112	68	68	69	70	71	71	72
5	90th	103	103	105	106	107	109	109	66	67	67	68	69	69	70
	95th	107	107	108	110	111	112	113	70	71	71	72	73	73	74
6	90th	104	105	106	108	109	110	111	68	68	69	70	70	71	72
	95th	108	109	110	111	113	114	115	72	72	73	74	74	75	76
7	90th	106	107	108	109	111	112	113	69	70	70	71	72	72	73
	95th	110	111	112	113	115	116	116	73	74	74	75	76	76	77
8	90th	108	109	110	111	113	114	114	71	71	71	72	73	74	74
	95th	112	112	114	115	116	118	118	75	75	75	76	77	78	78
9	90th	110	110	112	113	114	116	116	71	72	72	73	74	75	75
	95th	114	114	115	117	118	119	120	76	76	76	77	78	79	79
10	90th	112	112	114	115	116	118	118	73	73	73	74	75	76	76
	95th	116	116	117	119	120	121	122	77	77	77	78	79	80	80
11	90th	114	114	116	117	118	119	120	74	74	74	75	76	77	77
	95th	118	118	119	121	122	123	124	78	78	78	79	80	81	81
12	90th	116	116	117	119	120	121	122	75	75	75	76	77	78	78
	95th	119	120	121	123	124	125	126	79	79	79	80	81	82	82
13	90th	117	118	119	121	122	123	124	76	76	76	77	78	79	79
	95th	121	122	123	124	126	127	128	80	80	80	81	82	83	83
14	90th	119	120	121	122	124	125	125	77	77	77	78	79	80	80
	95th	123	123	125	126	127	129	129	81	81	81	82	83	84	84
15	90th	120	121	122	123	125	126	127	78	78	79	79	80	81	81
	95th	124	125	126	127	129	130	131	82	82	82	83	84	85	85
16	90th	121	122	123	124	126	127	128	78	78	79	80	81	81	82
	95th	125	126	127	128	130	131	132	82	82	83	84	85	85	86
17	90th	122	122	123	125	126	127	128	78	79	79	80	81	81	82
	95th	125	126	127	129	130	131	132	82	83	83	84	85	85	86

*Height percentile determined by standard growth curves.
†BP (blood pressure) percentile determined by a single measurement.
From National Institutes of Health, National High Blood Pressure Education Program Working Group on High Blood Pressure in Children and Adolescents (NIH-NHBPEP): The fourth report on the diagnosis, evaluation, and treatment of high blood pressure in children and adolescents (1996, revised 2005). Available at www.nhlbi.nih.gov/guidelines/hypertension/child_tbl.pdf (accessed Oct 2, 2010).

TABLE 30-4 Blood Pressure Levels in the 90th and 95th Percentiles for Boys 1 to 17 Years Old by Percentiles of Height

Age	Height Percentiles* BP†	SYSTOLIC BP (mm Hg)							DIASTOLIC BP (mm Hg)						
		→ 5%	10%	25%	50%	75%	90%	95%	5%	10%	25%	50%	75%	90%	95%
1	90th	94	95	97	99	100	102	103	49	50	51	52	53	53	54
	95th	98	99	101	103	104	106	106	54	54	55	56	57	58	58
2	90th	97	99	100	102	104	105	106	54	55	56	57	58	58	59
	95th	101	102	104	106	108	109	110	59	59	60	61	62	63	63
3	90th	100	101	103	105	107	108	109	59	59	60	61	62	63	63
	95th	104	105	107	109	110	112	113	63	63	64	65	66	67	67
4	90th	102	103	105	107	109	110	111	62	63	64	65	66	66	67
	95th	106	107	109	111	112	114	115	66	67	68	69	70	71	71
5	90th	104	105	106	108	110	111	112	65	66	67	68	69	69	70
	95th	108	109	110	112	114	115	116	69	70	71	72	73	74	74
6	90th	105	106	108	110	111	113	113	68	68	69	70	71	72	72
	95th	109	110	112	114	115	117	117	72	72	73	74	75	76	76
7	90th	106	107	109	111	113	114	115	70	70	71	72	73	74	74
	95th	110	111	113	115	117	118	119	74	74	75	76	77	78	78
8	90th	107	109	110	112	114	115	116	71	72	72	73	74	75	76
	95th	111	112	114	116	118	119	120	75	76	77	78	79	79	80
9	90th	109	110	112	114	115	117	118	72	73	74	75	76	76	77
	95th	113	114	116	118	119	121	121	76	77	78	79	80	81	81
10	90th	111	112	114	115	117	119	119	73	73	74	75	76	77	78
	95th	115	116	117	119	121	122	123	77	78	79	80	81	81	82
11	90th	113	114	115	117	119	120	121	74	74	75	76	77	78	78
	95th	117	118	119	121	123	124	125	78	78	79	80	81	82	82
12	90th	115	116	118	120	121	123	123	74	75	75	76	77	78	79
	95th	119	120	122	123	125	127	127	78	79	80	81	82	82	83
13	90th	117	118	120	122	124	125	126	75	75	76	77	78	79	79
	95th	121	122	124	126	128	129	130	79	79	80	81	82	83	83
14	90th	120	121	123	125	126	128	128	75	76	77	78	79	79	80
	95th	124	125	127	128	130	132	132	80	80	81	82	83	84	84
15	90th	122	124	125	127	129	130	131	76	77	78	79	80	80	81
	95th	126	128	129	131	133	134	135	81	81	82	83	84	85	85
16	90th	125	126	128	130	131	133	134	78	78	79	80	81	82	82
	95th	129	130	132	134	135	137	137	82	83	83	84	85	86	87
17	90th	127	128	130	132	134	135	136	80	80	81	82	83	84	84
	95th	131	132	134	136	138	139	140	84	85	86	87	87	88	89

*Height percentile determined by standard growth curves.

†BP (blood pressure) percentile determined by a single measurement.

From National Institutes of Health, National High Blood Pressure Education Program Working Group on High Blood Pressure in Children and Adolescents (NIH-NHBPEP): The fourth report on the diagnosis, evaluation, and treatment of high blood pressure in children and adolescents (1996, revised 2005). Available at www.nhlbi.nih.gov/guidelines/hypertension/child_tbl.pdf (accessed Oct 2, 2010).

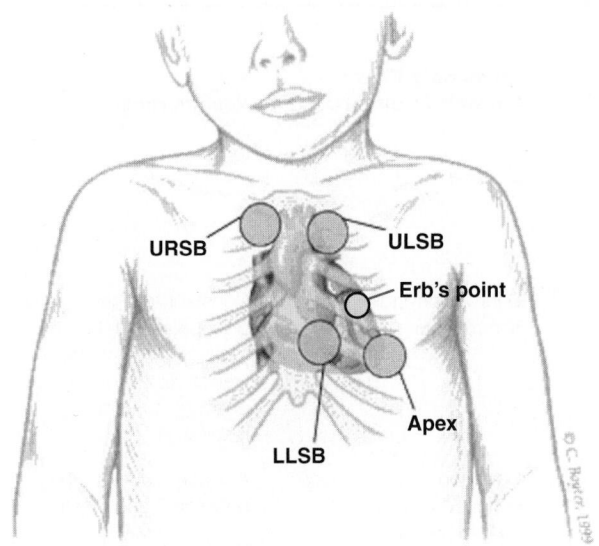

Upper right sternal border (URSB; aortic listening area)
- Aortic valve clicks of aortic stenosis, venous hum

Upper left sternal border (ULSB; pulmonic listening area)
- Pulmonary valve clicks of pulmonary stenosis, pulmonary flow murmurs, atrial septal defect, PDA, venous hum

Lower left sternal border (LLSB; tricuspid area)
- Ventricular septal defects, Still's murmur, tricuspid value regurgitation, hypertrophic cardiomyopathy, subaortic stenosis

Apex (mitral area)
- Aortic or mitral valve clicks, mitral valve regurgitation

Erb's point
- Aortic ejection click of aortic stenosis, or dilated aortic root

FIGURE 30-2 Traditional auscultatory areas for clicks and murmurs. (Adapted from McConnell M, Adkins S, Hannon D: Heart murmurs in pediatric patients: when do you refer? *Am Fam Pract* 60[2]:558-565, 1999. © C Boyter, 1999.)

- S_2 has the following characteristics:
  - It is composed of the aortic (A_2) and pulmonic (P_2) components and marks the end of systole.
  - S_2 is normally split with inspiration because pulmonic valve closure lags behind aortic valve closure. S_2 becomes single with expiration.
  - S_2 is best assessed at the upper left sternal border in the pulmonic area.
  - Pulmonary hypertension causes early closure of P_2 and accentuation of S_2, which may sound like a loud, single second heart sound.
  - Absence of one of the semilunar valves (as in pulmonary atresia) causes single S_2.
  - Wide splitting of S_2 without becoming a single sound on expiration may indicate increased pulmonary flow (typical of ASD).
- S_3 and S_4 have the following characteristics:
  - S_3 is associated with rapid ventricular filling; it may be heard in a quiet infant or child with a rapid heart rate.
  - S_3 "gallop" is best heard at the apex with the bell of the stethoscope during early diastole. When combined with S_1 and S_2, it gives an impression of the word

"Kentucky." S_3 is easier to appreciate when the child is in the left lateral decubitus position.
  - S_4 is always pathologic; it represents increased force of atrial contraction and ventricular distention.
  - S_4 "gallop" sounds like the word "Tennessee." It is best heard in late diastole just before S_1.
  - S_4 is low-pitched and is best heard at the apex with the bell of the stethoscope.
- Clicks: Ejection clicks are heard early in systole, immediately after S_1, and may sound like a split first heart sound. Pulmonic ejection clicks are high in frequency, vary with respiration, and disappear with inspiration. An aortic ejection click, heard best at Erb's point, is constant in intensity with a sound of a "snap" or a "click." Nonejection clicks are heard best in midsystole, or midway between S_1 and S_2 in the cardiac cycle at the apex. These clicks are best heard in patients who are leaning forward or standing, may disappear with inspiration, and are due to mitral valve prolapse (Park, 2008). Figure 30-2 describes cardiac conditions associated with each of these clicks.

Murmurs

Up to 80% of children may have a murmur, especially beginning at 3 to 4 years old (Park, 2008). It may be caused by normal blood flow through normal cardiac structures (innocent or physiologic murmur) or by turbulent blood flow caused by a defect or abnormal cardiac structures. Murmurs may be intensified by anything that increases cardiac output (e.g., anemia, fever, exercise).

Innocent or Functional Murmurs. Functional or innocent cardiac murmurs are common in children and can be evident in newborns. Table 30-5 describes common types of innocent murmurs; Box 30-3 describes the characteristics of an innocent murmur. Families and older children with innocent murmurs should be reassured that there is no cardiac pathology. They should be informed that this murmur may come and go and may be louder at times of fever, anxiety, pain, or exercise, and that activities do not need to be limited or any special precautions taken.

Criteria for Describing a Heart Murmur. Every murmur is assessed according to the criteria listed in Table 30-6. These are further illustrated and discussed in Figure 30-3. Characteristics of pathologic murmurs needing referral are listed in Box 30-3. The presence of a murmur causes great anxiety for a family awaiting a diagnosis. All murmurs should have a second opinion from a pediatric colleague or pediatric cardiologist if the diagnosis is uncertain or there is a suspicion of heart disease (Allen et al, 2008).

Common Diagnostic Studies. If the provider intends to refer for a cardiology consult, performing any of the following routine diagnostic studies is not cost-effective. The cardiology consultant will be able to determine with greater discrimination which, if any, tests should be ordered (Allen et al, 2008).

- *Chest radiograph.* Radiography provides the following information: cardiac size and size of specific chambers and great vessels, cardiac contour, status of pulmonary blood flow, and status of the lungs and other surrounding tissue (Fig. 30-4).
- *ECG.* ECG monitors the electrical activity of the heart from different locations and in different planes of the body. The ECG gives information about forces of ventricular contraction, hypertrophy, chamber dilation, and rhythm.

TABLE 30-5	Common Innocent Murmurs			
	Stills	**Pulmonary Flow Murmur of Childhood**	**Pulmonary Flow Murmur of Infancy**	**Venous Hum**
Other names	Innocent Vibratory Functional Physiologic "Head start" murmur	Flow murmur	Peripheral pulmonary stenosis	
Description	Midsystolic, louder in supine position or with inspiration	Early systolic to midsystolic; decreases or disappears with standing; increases with cardiac output or in supine position	Short, midsystolic ejection murmur	Constant swishing sound, disappears with head turning, compression of jugular vein(s), or supine position; varies with respirations
Age	Any age, but most common between 2 and 6 years	Any age, but more commonly heard in thin-chested adolescents between 8 and 14 years	Common during newborn period, especially in preterm infants	Any age, but commonly between 2 and 8 years
Best heard	Midpoint, left lower/apex and midsternal border; does not radiate	Pulmonary outflow area; radiates to lung fields	Murmur radiates from left upper sternal border to both axilla and back, usually gone by 6 months	In upright position, left and right upper chest below clavicles
Quality	Short, vibratory, musical, "twangy string," medium-pitched	Soft, blowing with normally split S_2; no click or thrill	Soft with middle to high pitch	Soft, high pitch; does not radiate
Intensity	Grades II (rarely III)	Grades I-II	Grades I-II	Grades II-III
Differential diagnosis	Small VSD, IHSS	ASD, PS	Supravalvular PS or AS	PDA

NOTE: Innocent murmurs typically increase with cardiac output (excitement, fever, anemia).

AS, Aortic stenosis; *ASD,* atrial septal defect; *IHSS,* idiopathic hypertrophic subaortic stenosis; *PDA,* patent ductus arteriosus; *PS,* pulmonic stenosis; *VSD,* ventricular septal defect.

Adapted from Allen H, Phillips J, Chan D: History and physical examination. In Allen HD, Driscoll DJ, Shaddy RE et al: *Moss and Adams' heart disease in infants, children, and adolescents: including the fetus and young adult,* ed 6, Philadelphia, 2001, Lippincott Williams & Wilkins; Bernstein D: Evaluation of the cardiovascular system. In Kliegman RM, Behrman RE, Jenson HB et al: *Nelson textbook of pediatrics,* ed 18, Philadelphia, 2007, Saunders.

BOX 30-3	Auscultatory Findings—The Innocent Versus Pathologic Murmur

The Innocent Murmur
- Usually grade I-II/VI in intensity and localized
- Changes with position (sitting to lying)
- May vary in loudness or presence from visit to visit
- May increase in loudness (intensity) with fever, anemia, exercise, or anxiety
- Musical or vibratory in quality
- Systolic in timing except for venous hum, which is continuous
- Duration is short
- Best heard in LLSB or pulmonic area (except for venous hum)
- Rarely transmitted
- May disappear with Valsalva maneuver, position, or gentle jugular pressure
- Vital signs: normal
- ECG: normal
- General health status: good

Possible Pathologic Murmur: *Refer these to a pediatric cardiologist*
- A murmur in a patient with a syndrome known to have a high incidence of CHD (e.g., trisomy 21)
- Any diastolic murmur
- Any systolic murmur that is associated with a thrill
- Pansystolic murmurs
- Continuous murmurs that cannot be suppressed
- Systolic clicks
- Opening snaps
- Fixed splitting of the second heart sound not associated with bundle branch block
- An accentuated S_2
- S_4 gallops
- Not positional
- Grade ≥III/VI
- Harsh quality

CHD, Congenital heart disease; *ECG,* electrocardiogram; *LLSB,* left lower sternal border.

Data from Lucas JF, Saul JP: Innocent murmurs. In Burg FD, Ingelfinger JF, Polin RA et al, editors: *Current pediatric therapy,* ed 18, Philadelphia, 2006, Saunders.

TABLE 30-6	Describing a Heart Murmur	
Grade or intensity: • Does not necessarily indicate severity of the problem • May be altered with positional change from supine to sitting	Grade I: Barely audible; heard faintly after a period of attentive listening Grade II: Soft but easily audible Grade III: Moderately loud, no thrill Grade IV: Loud, present Grade V: Loud, audible with stethoscope barely on the chest Grade VI: Heard without stethoscope (rare)
Timing with cardiac cycle	Systolic Diastolic Continuous
Location on chest where murmur is loudest	Aortic or pulmonic listening areas, URSB, ULSB, Erbs point, LLSB, apex
Radiations or transmission to other locations	To back To apex To carotids
Quality	Musical Harsh blowing
Duration	Point of onset and length of time systole and diastole murmurs last (e.g., "early systole, heard throughout cardiac cycle")
Pitch	Low Middle High

LLSB, Left lower sternal border; *ULSB,* upper left sternal border; *URSB,* upper right sternal border.

• *Echocardiogram.* Echocardiography uses reflected sound waves to identify intracardiac structures and their motion. The types of recordings include two-dimensional, M-mode, contrast, Doppler, and tissue Doppler studies (Fig. 30-5). Fetal echocardiography can diagnose CHD as early as 16 to 18 weeks' gestation (high-frequency transvaginal echocardiography as early as 10 weeks' gestation), as well as dysrhythmias and hemodynamic changes (Kleinman et al, 2008).

• *Complete blood count (CBC).* CBC rules out severe anemia or polycythemia as a cause of a murmur.

Other diagnostic tests may include the following:

• *Cardiac catheterization.* An opaque catheter is introduced into the heart chambers via a large peripheral vessel. The cardiologist measures pressures and saturation in chambers and vessels and uses dye to outline anatomy. This provides information about cardiac output, vascular resistance, and the response of the heart to exercise and medications.

• *Hyperoxia test.* Supplementation of 100% oxygen results in "pinking" and increased arterial oxygen saturation when the disease is primarily pulmonary; minimal or no color improvement indicates that the disease is cardiac. More commonly, simple pulse oximetry saturations are used to evaluate for cyanosis.

• *Magnetic resonance imaging (MRI).* This technique uses a strong magnetic field to cause movement of nuclei to yield an image of the heart structures and information about chamber volumes and function.

• *Exercise testing.* A graded treadmill or bicycle ergometer is used to determine cardiac output (myocardial blood flow and rhythm) response to exercise for endurance and capacity measurement.

SYSTOLIC MURMURS

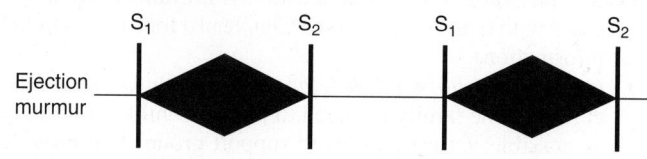

• Comprise most murmurs heard and occur between S_1 and S_2.
• Are either regurgitation murmurs (e.g., the holosystolic murmur of a VSD that begins with S_1 and continues throughout systole) or ejection murmur caused by flow of blood through narrowed or stenotic areas (e.g., AS).
• Best heard at second left or right intercostal space (ICS)
• Begin with or after S_1 and end with or before S_2.
• Include all innocent and physiologic murmurs.

DIASTOLIC MURMURS

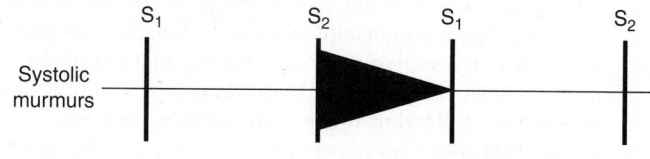

• Typically occur between S_2 and before or at S_1.
• Always indicate cardiac pathology.
• Murmur that starts with S_2 and has a decrescendo quality is most commonly due to aortic or pulmonic regurgitation.
• Mid-diastolic "rumble," a short low-pitched rumble heard best at the apex, is commonly due to atrioventricular valve stenosis or increased flow across a nonstenotic valve, such as seen with a large VSD or PDA.

CONTINUOUS MURMURS

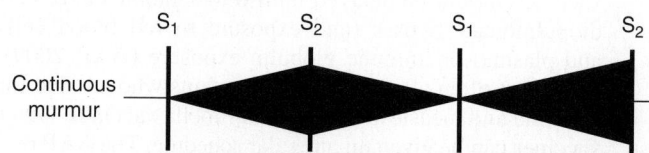

• Start at S_1 and go completely through systole and diastole.
• Most common cause is PDA.
• These murmurs need to be differentiated from the coexistence of separate systolic and diastolic murmurs and venous hums.

FIGURE 30-3 Types of heart murmurs. (Adapted from Allen HD, Gutgesell HP, Clark EB et al, editors: *Moss and Adams' heart disease in infants, children, and adolescents, including the fetus and young adult,* ed 6, Philadelphia, 2001, Lippincott Williams & Wilkins, p 150.)

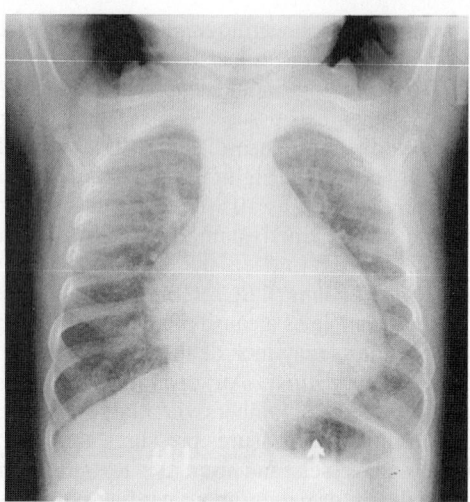

FIGURE 30-4 Chest radiogram of a 3-month-old with ventricular septal defect (VSD) and congestive heart failure (CHF). Cardiomegaly with increased pulmonary vascular markings from pulmonary venous congestion is visible.

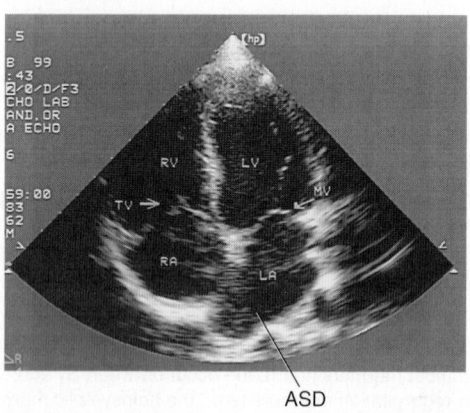

ASD

FIGURE 30-5 Echocardiogram of a 2-year-old with an atrial septal defect (ASD).

■ Management Strategies

REFERRAL

If a provider suspects cardiac disease or is unsure about findings, it is best to refer the patient to a pediatric cardiologist if available. Findings suggestive of cardiac disease are the presence of cyanosis, symptoms of CHF, a pathologic murmur, or a murmur that is difficult to differentiate in the presence of poor growth and development. A murmur alone in a child who is otherwise doing well should be referred to a pediatric cardiologist for further evaluation in a timely but not urgent time frame (2 to 4 weeks). Newborns should be evaluated within 1 or 2 days of noticeable signs or immediately depending on the severity of their symptoms. An infant with suspected disease who has a murmur, symptoms of CHF, cyanosis, or poor feeding should be evaluated as soon as possible by a pediatric cardiologist. An older child with dizziness, chest pain with exertion, dysrhythmia, dyspnea, syncope, signs of CHF, or abnormal vital signs should also be referred as soon as possible.

FAMILY SUPPORT

Families need the support of their PCP to help them understand the diagnosis, to cope with the short- and long-term consequences, and to advocate for them within the referral system, which may be an overwhelming experience. Because of the stress involved in initial diagnosis, many parents do not absorb all information presented and may need multiple opportunities to ask questions and learn about the diagnosis.

Parents and their designated support people should clearly understand the diagnosis and have diagrams of the defect and general information to take away with them for future reference. Should medication be necessary, parents should understand the reason for the drug and the regimen for administration and side effects. They should have a good understanding of the signs and symptoms of deterioration (e.g., CHF) and clear information regarding how to proceed should symptoms develop. Infant and child cardiopulmonary resuscitation certification is critical for anyone caring for a child with a heart condition.

PRIMARY HEALTH CARE FOR CHILDREN WITH CARDIOVASCULAR DISEASES

The goals of primary health care for a child with cardiovascular disease include the following:

- *Adequate nutritional intake and optimal growth.* Depending on the child's condition, the family may need help in modifying the diet to provide maximum calories or limit various types of foods. The young infant with CHF may need 24, 27, or 30 kilocalories per ounce of formula or fortified breast milk. The child may also need a nasogastric or gastric tube to obtain adequate calories because he or she may be unable to suck adequately. Children with cyanotic conditions may initially have adequate weight gain. The provider should refer to a nutritionist if available for assistance with complex diets (see Chapter 10 for more detailed information).
- *Optimal psychosocial development and functioning.* Discuss with the family the need to treat the child as normally as possible. Direct parents to support groups that provide informational and emotional support for families. Provide support to siblings of the affected child as well. Poor sibling bonding and unexpressed fears and anger in young siblings toward an infant with a severe or chronic disease can affect their relationships and family dynamics for many years. A retrospective review of studies that pertained to the long-term psychological adjustment of children and adolescents following open heart surgery for CHD concluded that these survivors are at risk for psychological maladjustment and impaired health-related quality of life (Latal et al, 2009).
- *Optimal preventive and primary health care.* Live virus vaccines should be delayed until 6 to 7 months after cardiopulmonary bypass (and exposure to red blood cells and plasma) or immune globulin exposure (AAP, 2009). This most often affects 1-year-old infants who are due for varicella and measles, mumps, and rubella vaccines. Other vaccines can be given on a regular schedule. The AAP recommends provision of respiratory syncytial virus (RSV) prophylaxis for infants less than 2 years old who have cyanotic or complicated CHD. (Refer to the current AAP

Red Book or Centers for Disease Control and Prevention [CDC] website for immunization schedule.)

- *Prevention of avoidable complications.* Prevention of respiratory infections through good handwashing and avoiding contact (if possible) with others with upper respiratory infection (URI) symptoms, should be emphasized. Vaccination against seasonal influenza is prudent.

- *Prevention of infective endocarditis* (IE). Although uncommon in children, IE (also called subacute bacterial endocarditis [SBE]) is associated with a high morbidity and mortality rate (discussed later in this chapter) and warrants primary prevention whenever indicated. Standards for prophylaxis against SBE are available in Box 30-4, and Tables 30-7 and 30-8. A high index of suspicion for IE should be maintained if any unusual clinical findings (e.g., petechiae, fever) are present after any procedure. Children with CHD appear to have more severe gingival inflammatory conditions, with a concomitant increase in *Haemophilus* species, *Actinobacillus actinomycetemcomitans, Cardiobacterium hominis, Eikenella corrodens,* and *Kingella* species (HACEK) and other microbes known to cause endocarditis compared with other children (Steelman et al, 2003). The reason for this is not clear. Good dental hygiene is extremely important for these patients.

- *Optimal fitness.* Reassure the parents that the child generally "self-limits" activity according to ability. The cardiology provider should be consulted regarding exercise limitations before entrance into sports or any activities that require strenuous physical exertion. Parameters for sports participation for children with various forms of cardiac diseases or conditions can be found in Chapter 13, Table 13-5.

- *Optimal neurodevelopmental adaptation to school and life tasks.* Several studies have shown relatively high

incidences (up to 50%) of neurodevelopmental impairments in school-age children who had open heart surgery in infancy (Majnemer et al, 2008). Although mean intelligence scores are generally within the average range, many of these children have difficulties with visuospatial tasks, fine motor functions, higher order language skills, memory and attention. They may be impaired in their ability to coordinate lower-order skills to perform higher-order tasks. In one study, 25% of children who had neonatal heart surgery had developmental disabilities. A few studies show that there is brain injury and immature brain development in infants with CHD prior to heart surgery, presumably due to disordered fetal circulation (Miller el al, 2007).

◼ Congenital Heart Diseases

CONGESTIVE HEART FAILURE

CHF refers to a progressive clinical and pathophysiologic syndrome found in many children with heart problems. The symptoms vary with age of the child and the root cardiac problem. Box 30-5 provides information on age specific signs and symptoms of CHF. Besides functional changes, CHF is marked by changes in neurohormonal and molecular changes within the heart (Hsu and Pearson, 2009a).

CHF in children can be caused by congenital malformations leading to volume overload (such as a large VSD) or pressure overload (such as AS) or more complex heart disease. CHF can also occur in children with structurally normal hearts due to cardiomyopathy or secondary to dysrhythmias, ischemia, toxins, or infections (Table 30-9). These conditions are discussed in more detail later in this chapter. One set of authors estimate CHF affects 12,000 to 35,000 children each year (Hsu and Pearson, 2009a).

The largest group of infants and children with CHF are those with excessive left to right shunting through unrepaired congenital defects. CHF is somewhat of a misnomer in these cases, as the myocardium generally responds quite well to the challenge of excessive blood volume for a long time and cardiac output remains adequate. However, the compensatory response to this excessive workload does provoke electrolyte and fluid imbalances as well as a host of other neurohormonal changes. Children with heart failure from systolic or diastolic cardiac dysfunction from infections, obstruction, or dysrhythmia need treatment to ameliorate fluid and electrolyte imbalances, increase contractility, and decrease cardiac afterload.

A greater understanding of the underlying neurohormonal mechanisms of CHF has been detailed and aided by therapies in the adult population. Depending on the underlying pathophysiology, the same patterns of elevated neurohormonal and inflammatory mediators (aldosterone, norepinephrine, natriuretic peptides, tumor necrosis factor, and renin) occur in children. In adult populations large-scale studies have shown the value of blocking some of the chronic neurohormonal changes to CHF with agents such as aldosterone inhibitors, angiotensin inhibitors, and sympathetic inhibitors (beta-blockers). To date, however, no large-scale pediatric study has been able to show positive effects with this change in CHF therapeutic focus. However, based on adult evidence and some small pediatric studies, the International Society of Heart and Lung Transplantation recommended angiotensin-converting enzyme

---

BOX 30-4 Cardiac Conditions Associated With the Highest Risk of Endocarditis: Prophylaxis Recommended

Prophylaxis is recommended for individuals who have had:
- Procedures that involved the application of prosthetic valves
- Procedures that involved the use of prosthetic material to repair cardiac valves
- A history of infective endocarditis
- Unrepaired cyanotic congenital heart disease, including palliative shunts and conduits
- Completely repaired congenital heart defect with prosthetic material or device(s) whether via surgery or catheterization for the first 6 months after the procedure due to the endothelialization of prosthetic material within that period
- Repaired congenital heart disease with residual defects (e.g., residual ventricular septal defect) at the site of or adjacent to an area of a prosthetic patch or prosthetic device
- A cardiac transplant and then develop cardiac valvulopathy

Data from Nishimura RA, Carabello BA, Faxon DP et al: ACC/AHA 2008 guideline update on valvular heart disease: focused update on infective endocarditis. A report of the American College of Cardiology/American Heart Association Task Force on Practice Guidelines: endorsed by the Society of Cardiovascular Anesthesiologists, Society for Cardiovascular Angiography and Interventions, and Society of Thoracic Surgeons, *Circulation* 118:887-896, 2008.

TABLE 30-7	Procedures for Which Endocarditis Prophylaxis Is or Is Not Recommended in High-Risk Individuals	
	Prophylaxis Recommended	**Prophylaxis *Not* Recommended**
Dental	Dental extractions Periodontal procedures Dental implant placement and reimplantation of avulsed teeth Root canal instrumentation Initial placement of orthodontic braces but not brackets Teeth or implant cleaning where bleeding is expected Postoperative suture removal	Restorative dentistry Routine anesthetic injections through noninfected tissue Intracanal endodontic treatment; postplacement and buildup Rubber dam placement Placement of removable prosthodontic or orthodontic appliances Bleeding from trauma of lips or oral mucosa Taking oral impressions Fluoride treatments Taking oral radiographs Orthodontic appliance adjustment or placement of brackets Shedding of primary teeth
Respiratory tract	Tonsillectomy or adenoidectomy Surgery involving respiratory mucosa	Endotracheal intubation Flexible bronchoscopy without biopsy Pressure tympanostomy tube insertion/removal Rigid bronchoscopy
Skin	Procedures involving infected skin or skin structures	Uncomplicated skin biopsy Tattooing (but this is highly discouraged in high-risk individuals)
Musculoskeletal tissue	Procedures involving infected musculoskeletal tissue	
Genitourinary tract	Cystoscopy or urinary tract manipulation in patients with enterococcal infection	Vaginal delivery Cesarean section Urethral catheterization without infection Therapeutic abortion Circumcision Hysterectomy
Gastrointestinal tract		GI tract procedures including esophagogastroduodenoscopy or colonoscopy
Other procedures		Cardiac catheterization, including device placement and pacemakers

Data from Nishimura RA, Carabello BA, Faxon DP et al: ACC/AHA 2008 guideline update on valvular heart disease: focused update on infective endocarditis. A report of the American College of Cardiology/American Heart Association Task Force on Practice Guidelines: endorsed by the Society of Cardiovascular Anesthesiologists, Society for Cardiovascular Angiography and Interventions, and Society of Thoracic Surgeons, *Circulation* 118:887-896, 2008.

(ACE) inhibitors for moderate to severe left ventricular dysfunction (Hsu and Pearson, 2009b). The traditional armamentarium of heart failure therapies (i.e., diuretics, inotropes, and afterload reducers) is likely to be added in the future after further elucidation of the neurohormonal responses in children with the different conditions listed in Table 30-9. The role of monitoring B natriuretic peptides (amino acid polypeptides secreted by the *ventricles* in response to stretching) in managing CHF is also evolving.

LEFT-TO-RIGHT SHUNTING CONGENITAL HEART DISEASE (ACYANOTIC)

Pulmonary overflow lesions have a communication between the two sides of the heart through which extra blood shunts from the high-pressure, oxygenated left side of the heart to the low-pressure, deoxygenated right side of the heart. The result is an increase in pulmonary blood flow (Fig. 30-6). These lesions are acyanotic in nature. Table 30-10 illustrates the distinguishing features of left-to-right versus right-to-left shunting disorders.

ATRIAL SEPTAL DEFECT
Description and Epidemiology

An ASD is a defect or hole in the atrial septum. Of the four types of ASD, the most common involves the midseptum in the area of the foramen ovale and is called an ostium secundum–type defect (Fig. 30-7). Defects of the sinus venosus type are high in the atrial septum, near the entry of the SVC, and are frequently associated with anomalous pulmonary venous return. A primum ASD is in the lower portion of the septum and is most often seen in children with Down syndrome. The rarest form of ASD is an unroofed coronary sinus (see Table 30-10 for incidence figures). Usually ASDs occur spontaneously; however, there are a few identified genetic mutations which cause familial ASDs (Porter and Edwards, 2008).

Clinical Findings
History
- Often completely asymptomatic
- May fatigue easily or have exertional dyspnea
- May be somewhat thin

TABLE 30-8 Prophylactic Regimens for Dental Procedures*

Route	Agent	Regimen†
Able to take oral medication	Amoxicillin	Adults: 2 g PO; children: 50 mg/kg PO (max 2 g)
Unable to take oral medication	Ampicillin or‡	Adults: 2 g IM or IV; children: 50 mg/kg IM or IV (max 2 g)
	Cefazolin or ceftriaxone	Adults: 1 g IM or IV; children: 50 mg/kg IM or IV (max 1 g)
If penicillin allergic, oral	Clindamycin or‡	Adults: 600 mg PO; children: 20 mg/kg PO (max 600 mg)
	Cephalexin or cefadroxil or	Adults: 2 g PO; children: 50 mg/kg PO (max 2 g)
	Azithromycin or clarithromycin	Adults: 500 mg PO; children: 15 mg/kg PO (max 500 mg)
Penicillin allergic and unable to take oral medication	Clindamycin or‡	Adults: 600 mg IM or IV; children: 20 mg/kg IM or IV (max 600 mg)
	Cefazolin or ceftriaxone	Adults: 1 g IM or IV; children: 50 mg/kg IM or IV (max 1 g)

IM, Intramuscular; *IV,* intravenous; *max,* maximum, *PO,* orally.
*Antibiotic regimens are procedure specific; refer to the American Heart Association reference for nondental prophylaxis recommendations.
†Take 30-60 minutes prior to the procedure.
‡Or other first- or second-generation oral cephalosporin in equivalent adult or pediatric dosage. Cephalosporins should not be used if there is a history of anaphylaxis, angioedema, or urticaria with penicillins.
Data from Nishimura RA, Carabello BA, Faxon DP et al: ACC 2008 guideline update on valvular heart disease: focused update on infective endocarditis. A report of the American College of Cardiology/American Heart Association Task Force on Practice Guidelines: endorsed by the Society of Cardiovascular Anesthesiologists, Society for Cardiovascular Angiography and Interventions, and Society of Thoracic Surgeons, *Circulation* 118:887-896, 2008.

BOX 30-5 Signs and Symptoms of Congestive Heart Failure

Infants
Tachypnea
Tachycardia
Rales or wheezing
Cardiomegaly and hepatomegaly
Periorbital edema
Poor feeding
Poor weight gain
Diaphoresis

Children-Teens
Tachypnea
Tachycardia
Rales or wheezing
Cardiomegaly and hepatomegaly
Orthopnea
Shortness of breath or dyspnea with exertion
Peripheral edema
Poor growth and development

TABLE 30-9 Conditions That Can Lead to Congestive Heart Failure in Children

Age	Condition
Premature infant	Patent ductus arteriosus
Birth to 1 week	Hypoplastic left heart syndrome Coarctation of the aorta Critical aortic stenosis Interrupted aortic arch Arteriovenous malformations Tachycardia Cardiomyopathy
1 week to 3 months	Ventricular septal defect Truncus arteriosus Atrioventricular canal (endocardial cushion defect) Total anomalous pulmonary venous return Coarctation Tachycardia Patent ductus arteriosus Aortic stenosis Tricuspid atresia
Older than 1 year	Bacterial endocarditis Rheumatic fever Myocarditis

- May have a history of frequent upper respiratory tract infections or pneumonia

Physical Examination
- Typically a murmur may not be noticed until the child is 2 to 3 years old, when examination of a quiet child can be performed.
- Mild left precordial bulge or palpable lift at the left sternal border may be seen.
- S_1 is normal or split, with accentuation of the tricuspid valve closure sound.
- S_2 is often split widely and is relatively fixed in relation to respiration in patients with normal pulmonary pressure.

- A grade I to III/VI, widely radiating, medium-pitched, not harsh systolic crescendo-decrescendo murmur is heard best at the pulmonic area. If the shunt is large, increased blood flow across the tricuspid valve is responsible for a mid-diastolic, rumbling murmur at the left lower sternal border (LLSB).

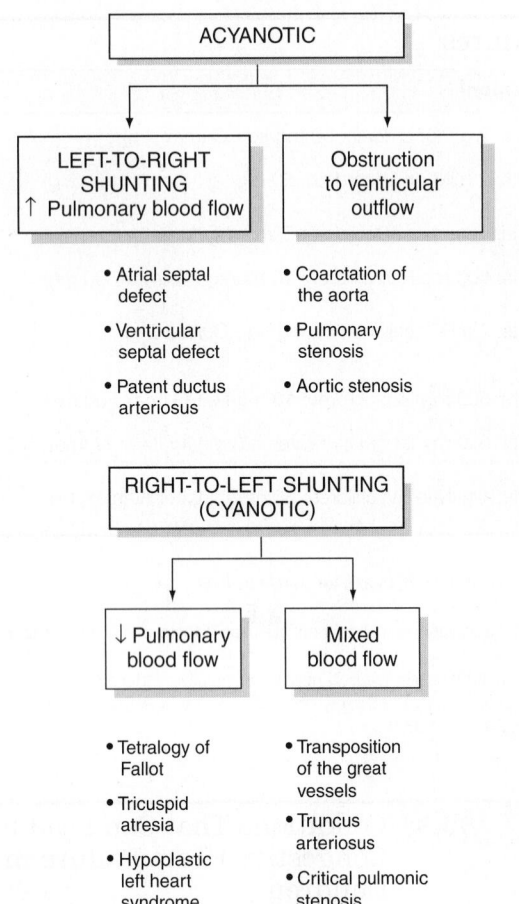

FIGURE 30-6 Classification of congenital heart disease (CHD).

- In older patients (teenage or older), pulmonic and tricuspid murmurs decrease in intensity, and the second heart sound may be single and accentuated. A diastolic murmur of pulmonic incompetence can appear.

Diagnostic Studies
- Chest radiography may reveal cardiac enlargement. The main pulmonary artery may be dilated and the pulmonary vascular markings increased.
- The ECG shows right axis deviation with right atrial enlargement. Lead V1 usually shows a right bundle branch block with a rSR′ pattern. P wave may be tall showing right atrial enlargement. The PR interval may be prolonged. However, the ECG can be normal in small left-to-right defects. The ECG should be assessed for AV prolongation.
- The echocardiogram identifies the specific location of the defect in the atrial septum and shows right-sided chamber enlargement.
- Cardiac catheterization is rarely necessary unless the diagnosis is in doubt, shunt size is indeterminable, or pulmonary vascular disease is suspected (Porter and Edwards, 2008).

Management

Management of ASD includes the following:
- Small defects found in infancy may close on their own.
- Larger defects require intervention, usually after 1 year and before school entry or when the defect is identified in

an older child. Interventional cardiologists can now close most ASDs in the cardiac catheterization lab with a closure device. If the defect is large or unfavorable to device closure, cardiac surgeons can patch it. Surgical mortality rate is less than 1%.
- SBE prophylaxis precautions are necessary only in the first 6 months after cardiac surgery (see Table 30-7).
- Long-term outcome is excellent for patients after ASD repair.
- Five to 10% of adults with uncorrected ASDs develop severe irreversible pulmonary hypertension that is disabling and life-shortening.

VENTRICULAR SEPTAL DEFECT

Description and Epidemiology

A VSD is a hole or defect in one of the areas of the ventricular septum. There are four types of VSDs: perimembranous, supracristal (type of VSD occurring in the outflow part of the right ventricle [RV] above crista supraventricularis), inlet, and muscular. The most common type is the perimembranous VSD (Fig. 30-8). VSDs are associated with many congenital defects, but 95% demonstrate no chromosomal anomaly (see Table 30-1). Approximately 30% to 50% of these defects are small; the vast majority of these close by 4 years old (McDaniel and Gutgesell, 2008).

Clinical Findings
History
- A murmur is often not heard immediately after birth. When pulmonary vascular resistance falls (normally at 2 to 8 weeks old), more blood is shunted across the VSD from left ventricle to right ventricle and hence to the pulmonary circulation. This causes a classic loud murmur and possibly heralds the beginning of CHF symptoms.
- Parents may note signs and symptoms of CHF (see Box 30-5).
- Small defects may be completely asymptomatic.

Physical Examination
- Small VSD
  - Harsh, high-pitched, grade II to IV/VI holosystolic murmur at LLSB
  - All other findings within normal limits
- Large VSD
  - Low-pitched, grade II to V/VI holosystolic murmur at LLSB
  - VSD murmur that becomes higher pitched over time indicates that the defect is becoming smaller
  - Diastolic rumble at the apex
  - Thrill along the left sternal border
  - Signs of progressing CHF after the first weeks of life (see Box 30-5).
  - S_3 or S_4 gallop if CHF is present (McDaniel and Gutgesell, 2008)

Diagnostic Studies
- Chest radiography findings vary depending on the size of the shunt. Children with small shunts have a normal heart size and pulmonary vascular markings that are just beyond the upper limits of normal. Patients with large shunts have cardiac enlargement involving both the left and right ventricles and left atrium, as well as pulmonary vascular markings that are significantly increased (see Fig. 30-4).

TABLE 30-10   Congenital Heart Disease: Differential Diagnosis of Cardiac Defects

Feature	Atrial Septal Defect	Ventricular Septal Defect	Patent Ductus Arteriosus	Transposition of the Great Vessels	Tetralogy of Fallot	Tricuspid Atresia	Aortic Stenosis	Pulmonic Stenosis	Coarctation of the Aorta
Incidence of total CHD	7%-10%, 2:1 female to male	25%; > females	10%; 2:1 females	2%-5%, 3:1 male	3.5%-9%; > males	<3%	5%, 4:1 male	8%-10%	5%
Age at initial presentation	Variable; may be asymptomatic into adulthood	Variable depending on size; large by 4-8 wk old; small by 6 mo old	Neonate to 3 mo old	Newborn	Usually by 6 mo old	Newborn	Depends upon severity; critical in newborn	Depends on severity; newborn to school-age	First week of life or 3-5 yr old
Clinical findings	Murmur, typically on preschool examination	CHF or murmur	CHF or murmur	Cyanosis	Cyanosis	Cyanosis	Murmur, CHF; older child, chest pain	± Cyanosis; murmur	CHF in newborn; hypertension in preschooler
Auscultation	Midsystolic murmur at ULSB with wide-split second heart sound	Holosystolic murmur at LLSB	Continuous murmur under left clavicle, referred to back	Usually no murmur	Early SEM at second left ICS; holosystolic murmur at LLSB	ASD murmur, may be associated with PDA	SEM at URSB; systolic click at apex with bicuspid valve	Late SEM ULSB, intermittent systolic to back ejection click	SEM in left intraclavicular region with transmission
Radiologic findings	May have mild cardiomegaly	Normal or cardiomegaly	Cardiomegaly	Egg-shaped heart	Boot-shaped heart	Cardiomegaly	Normal	Normal	Rib notching
Pulmonary vasculature	Normal to slightly increased	Normal or increased	Increased markings	May have increased markings or be normal	Decreased pulmonary vascularity	Decreased pulmonary markings	Normal	Decreased in severity	Normal
ECG	May have rSR pattern in V1, right atrial enlargement	Combined ventricular hypertrophy	Combined ventricular hypertrophy	RV hypertrophy	RV hypertrophy	Right atrial enlargement, absent RV voltage	LVH	RV hypertrophy	RV hypertrophy

ASD, Atrial septal defect; *CHF*, congenital heart failure; *ECG*, electrocardiogram; *ICS*, intercostal space; *LLSB*, left lower sternal border; *LVH*, left ventricular hypertrophy; *PDA*, patent ductus arteriosus; *RV*, right ventricular; *SEM*, systolic ejection murmur; *ULSB*, upper left sternal border; *URSB*, upper right sternal border.

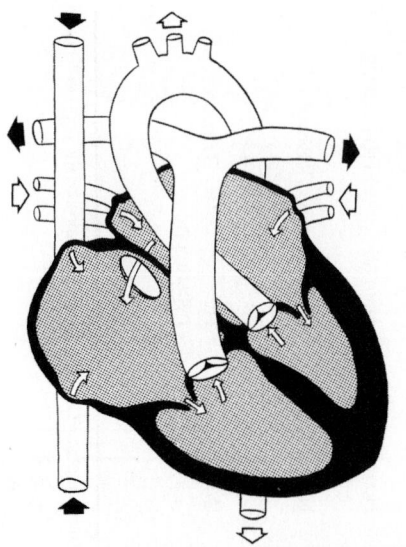

FIGURE 30-7 Atrial septal defect (ASD). (Used with permission of Ross Products Division, Abbott Laboratories, Columbus, OH 43216. From *Clinical education aid no 7*. Copyright 1970 Ross Products Division, Abbott Laboratories.)

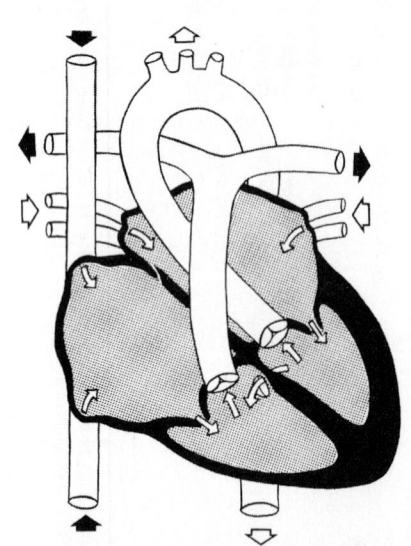

FIGURE 30-8 Ventricular septal defect (VSD). (Used with permission of Ross Products Division, Abbott Laboratories, Columbus, OH 43216. From *Clinical education aid no 7*. Copyright 1970 Ross Products Division, Abbott Laboratories.)

- The ECG is normal for patients with small defects and may show left ventricular hypertrophy (LVH) or biventricular hypertrophy (BVH) with large shunts.
- Echocardiography provides visualization of defects and pinpoints the exact anatomic location. In "pinhole" VSDs, a murmur may be present; however, a defect may not be visualized on the echocardiogram.
- Cardiac catheterization is rarely necessary except when there is a question of elevated pulmonary vascular resistance or when the VSD can be closed in the catheterization laboratory (McDaniel and Gutgesell, 2008).

Management
- Infants with small defects and no symptoms of CHF are monitored every 3 to 6 months throughout the first year of life and then biannually to assess for closure of the defect. Some defects may never close and cause no difficulty. SBE prophylaxis is not recommended.
- Larger defects with signs of CHF are managed as follows:
  ○ Lanoxin, diuretics, ACE inhibitors, and beta-blocker dosages are prescribed, as needed, by a cardiologist.
  ○ The provider must monitor nutritional intake and weight gain in these infants and children. It is also important to teach families to fortify an infant's calories to 24, 27, or even 30 kcal/oz, as needed. Arrange for enteric nutritional support via nasogastric tube for young infants struggling to meet their caloric needs.
- Families must be taught the signs and symptoms of developing or progressing CHF (see Box 30-5).
- Surgery or device closure will be done if no improvement is seen over weeks or months.
  ○ SBE prophylaxis precautions are necessary for 6 months after surgery (see Tables 30-7 and 30-8).
  The long-term outcome is excellent after VSD repair (McDaniel and Gutgesell, 2008).

ATRIOVENTRICULAR SEPTAL DEFECT (ATRIOVENTRICULAR CANAL DEFECT OR ENDOCARDIAL CUSHION DEFECT)
Description and Epidemiology
The endocardial cushion is a central cardiac structure that includes the septal portions of the mitral and tricuspid valves and lower portion of the atrial septum and upper portion of the ventricular septum. In AV septal defects, variable portions of the endocardial cushion are absent. Complete AV septal defect implies the absence of this cushion, leading to a primum ASD, a single AV valve (composed of leaflets of the intended mitral and tricuspid valves), and an inlet VSD. There may also be partial, transitional, and intermediate defects with less profound abnormalities and usually less severe symptoms (Fig. 30-9). Four to 5% of congenital heart defects are complete or partial AV canal defects; 75% of patients with complete AV canal defect have Down syndrome (Cetta et al, 2008).

Clinical Findings
History
- Children with only a primum ASD (partial AV canal) may not manifest symptoms.
- In infants with complete AV canal defects, parents may note signs and symptoms of CHF (see Box 30-5).
Physical Examination
- Partial AV canal (primum ASD) findings are the same as those with secundum ASD. There may also be a soft blowing murmur of mitral regurgitation in the apex and or infrascapular area.
- Complete AV canal defect
  ○ Low-pitched, grade II to V/VI holosystolic murmur at LLSB. A murmur may not be evident at birth but increases in loudness at 2 to 8 weeks after pulmonary vascular resistance falls.
  ○ Diastolic rumble at the apex; thrill along the left sternal border.

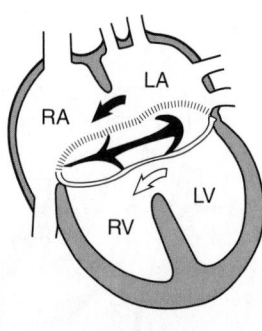

FIGURE 30-9 Complete atrioventricular canal defect (also known as a complete endocardial cushion defect). An ostium primum atrial septal defect *(solid arrow)* and an inlet ventricular septal defect (VSD) *(open arrow)* are present. *LA,* Left atrium; *LV,* left ventricle; *RA,* right atrium; *RV,* right ventricle. (Used with permission of Park MK, Troxler RG: *Pediatric cardiology for practitioners,* ed 4, St Louis, 2002, Mosby.)

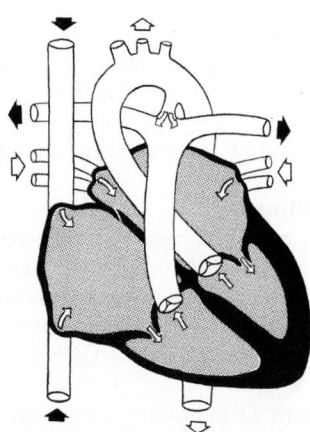

FIGURE 30-10 Patent ductus arteriosus. (Used with permission of Ross Products Division, Abbott Laboratories, Columbus, OH 43216. From *Clinical education aid no 7.* Copyright 1970 Ross Products Division, Abbott Laboratories.)

- ○ Signs of progressing CHF after the first weeks of life; S_3 or S_4 gallop if CHF is present
- ○ Some infants maintain neonatal high pulmonary vascular resistance and do not show signs of CHF. Instead they may manifest signs of pulmonary hypertension with loud single S_2, precordial heave, minimal murmur, and perhaps desaturation with agitation or effort (Cetta et al, 2008).

Diagnostic Studies
- Chest radiography findings vary depending on the size of the shunt. Children with small shunts have a normal heart size and pulmonary vascular markings that are just beyond the upper limits of normal. Patients with large shunts (complete AV canal defect) have cardiac enlargement involving both the left and right ventricles and left atrium, as well as increased pulmonary vascular markings (see Fig. 30-4).
- The ECG usually shows superior axis between −40 and −160 degrees. Right ventricular hypertrophy (RVH) is usually present, and LVH or BVH in large shunts may be present. In 50% of children, the PR interval is prolonged.
- Echocardiography (two-dimensional, Doppler, or transesophageal) provides visualization of the size of ASD and VSD defects, size and other characteristics of the AV valve(s), and relative sizes of the RV and LV.
- Cardiac catheterization if there is a question of elevated pulmonary vascular resistance.

Management
- Children with a partial AV canal defect that consists of a primum ASD and possibly a cleft mitral valve are monitored every 3 to 6 months throughout the first year of life and then biannually until the defect is closed surgically during toddler or preschool years. These children usually do not have signs of CHF, though they may gain weight slowly. They rarely manifest difficulty with pulmonary hypertension after surgery.
- Infants with a complete AV canal defect usually need surgical correction in the first 6 months of life. Some infants develop pulmonary hypertension and become increasingly desaturated before surgery. Most infants need CHF medical management before surgery that includes:
  - ○ Digoxin, diuretics, ACE inhibitors, and beta-blockers
  - ○ Monitoring nutritional intake and weight and fortifying infant formula or breast milk as previously discussed; enteric nutritional support via nasogastric tube may be needed.
  - ○ Educating families on the signs and symptoms of developing or progressing CHF.
  - ○ Surgical repair consists of closure of the defect and reconstruction of the common AV valve into separate tricuspid and mitral valves. Residual mitral and/or tricuspid insufficiency is common after surgery. Surgical mortality is less than 2%; SBE prophylaxis precautions are necessary for only 6 months.

PATENT DUCTUS ARTERIOSUS
Description and Epidemiology
In the normal newborn functional closure of the ductus arteriosus occurs in the first 12 to 72 hours. Permanent sealing of the ductus arteriosus occurs in 2 to 3 weeks (Moore et al, 2008). The ductus arteriosus may remain patent in some infants and leave a connection between the aorta and the pulmonary artery. As pulmonary vascular resistance falls, aortic blood is shunted into the pulmonary artery and recirculates through the lungs (Fig. 30-10) (see Table 30-10 for incidence figures). The frequency of PDAs increases with decreasing gestational age in premature infants; it is as high as 45% to 80% in very young infants less than 1750 g (Moore et al, 2008). PDA occurs with many congenital malformation syndromes (see Table 30-1).

Clinical Findings
History
- The infant or child may be asymptomatic if the PDA is small.
- Increasing signs of CHF may appear in the first weeks of life in larger PDAs.
Physical Examination
- In the immediate postnatal period, the murmur is soft, systolic, and heard along the left sternal border, under the left clavicle, and in the back.

- After the first weeks of life, a typical grade II to V/VI, harsh, rumbling, continuous "machinery murmur" is heard in the left infraclavicular fossa and pulmonic area with a thrill at the base.
- Physical findings of CHF may be present with a large shunt (see Box 30-5).
Diagnostic Studies
- Chest radiographic findings: With a small to moderate shunt, the heart is not enlarged; with larger shunts, enlargement of both left atrial and ventricular is apparent. Pulmonary vascular markings may be increased.
- ECG: LVH with large shunts; QRS axis is normal or rightward.
- Echocardiogram: Demonstrates the patent ductus and usually enlargement of the left atrium (Moore et al, 2008).

Management
- Indomethacin or ibuprofen may be given to preterm infants to effect closure when there is significant left-to-right shunt.
- An asymptomatic infant with a small left-to-right shunt from a PDA is followed for spontaneous closure for approximately 2 years. Patients with large shunts or infants with pulmonary hypertension should have their PDA surgically closed within the first few months of life to prevent the development of progressive pulmonary vascular obstruction. Surgical ligation of the ductus is a low-risk procedure because cardiopulmonary bypass is not necessary.
- Interventional cardiologists now close many PDAs in children older than 8 months by inserting coils into the shunt in the cardiac catheterization laboratory.
- Families should be reassured that their child will live an active, normal life.
- SBE prophylaxis precautions are recommended for the 6-month period after the surgical or device closure.

RIGHT-TO-LEFT SHUNTING CONGENITAL HEART DISEASE (CYANOTIC)

Cyanotic CHD represents 10% to 18% of all congenital heart lesions (Goldmuntz and Lin, 2008). Cardiac cyanosis is due to obstruction of pulmonary blood flow or mixing of oxygenated and unoxygenated blood. Visible cyanosis occurs when oxygen saturation in blood reaches around 85%. Cyanosis is more readily apparent with polycythemia and less readily apparent with anemia or the presence of fetal hemoglobin. Polycythemia is a compensatory mechanism to increase the oxygen-carrying capacity in cyanotic patients; however, it increases the risk for cerebral thromboses (Park, 2008). The most common heart conditions causing cyanosis in the immediate newborn period are listed in Figure 30-6. Table 30-10 illustrates the different presentations and management of conditions when comparing left-to-right and right-to-left shunting CHDs.

TRANSPOSITION OF THE GREAT ARTERIES
Description and Epidemiology
TGA results from incomplete septation and migration of the truncus arteriosus during fetal development. In TGA the aorta arises from the right ventricle and the pulmonary

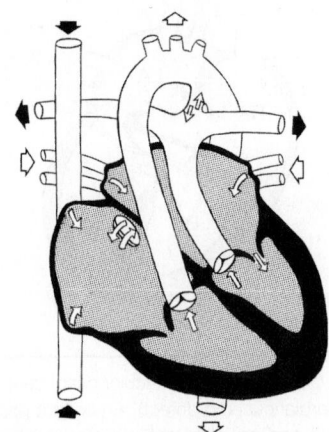

FIGURE 30-11 Complete transposition of the great vessels. (Used with permission of Ross Products Division, Abbott Laboratories, Columbus, OH 43216. From *Clinical education aid no 7*. Copyright 1970 Ross Products Division, Abbott Laboratories.)

artery arises from the left ventricle. The aorta receives the deoxygenated systemic venous blood and returns it to the systemic arteries. The pulmonary artery receives oxygenated pulmonary venous blood and returns it to the pulmonary circulation (Fig. 30-11). With TGA there may be a number of other heart malformations, most commonly VSD, PDA, and coronary artery defects (see Table 30-10 for incidence figures).

Clinical Findings
History
- Cyanosis is immediately evident by 1 hour of birth (52%) or within the first day after birth (92%). Because TGA and VSD allow mixing of oxygenated and unoxygenated blood, occasionally children with these defects who are less cyanotic present as late as 3 months old.
- CHF symptoms may be present.
- Affected infants are often large for gestational age with retardation of growth and development after the neonatal period.
Physical Examination
- Infants may have no murmur at birth or may have a murmur characteristic of associated lesions, such as VSD, ASD, or PDA.
- S_2 is loud and single because of the anatomic placement of the great arteries in TGA.
Diagnostic Studies
- Chest radiography and ECG findings may be normal in the early newborn period, or the heart may appear egg shaped.
- ECG findings show right axis deviation and RVH.
- Echocardiography shows the pulmonary artery arising from the left ventricle and the aorta arising from the right (Wernovsky, 2008).

Management
- Immediate referral to a pediatric cardiac center is necessary. Correction of electrolyte and acid-base imbalance may be necessary.
- Give intravenous prostaglandin E_1 (PGE$_1$) to delay closure or reopen the ductus arteriosus.

- A balloon atrial septostomy may be performed in the catheterization laboratory to promote mixing of oxygenated and unoxygenated blood in the atria.
- The arterial switch (Jatene procedure) is usually performed in the first few days of life.
- These patients are monitored closely throughout life with annual echocardiogram follow-up.
- SBE prophylaxis precautions are indicated for life.

Prognosis

Without treatment there is a 50% mortality rate in the first month of life and 90% by the first year. Operative mortality is from 5% to 17%; there are excellent long-term results after surgery (Wernovsky, 2008). However, long-term patency and growth of the coronary arteries warrant close monitoring. Neopulmonic stenosis and neoaortic regurgitation may occur after the arterial switch. Refer any patient with a history of arterial or atrial switch to a pediatric cardiologist, especially with a history of palpitations, syncope, and/or shortness of breath with exertion.

TETRALOGY OF FALLOT
Description and Epidemiology

TOF (also referred to as TET) is a combination of four anatomic cardiac defects resulting in right ventricular outflow tract obstruction: (1) pulmonary valve stenosis, (2) RVH, (3) VSD, and (4) an aorta that overrides the ventricular septum (Fig. 30-12). There is a spectrum of severity in TOF, and it is the most common cyanotic lesion. In the most severe forms the pulmonary valve and artery are atretic (not patent). This is referred to as TOF pulmonary atresia, and these infants are quite cyanotic as newborns. In the mildest form, "pink TETs," the infant may not display signs of cyanosis because the valvular stenosis is mild, and their symptoms may be similar to a large VSD. In most cases of TOF, however, right-to-left shunting across the VSD and cyanosis increase over the first months of life as a result of increasing obstruction in the right ventricular outflow tract (Siwek et al, 2008) (see Table 30-10 for incidence figures). Children with chromosome 22q11.2 deletion syndrome or Down syndrome may have this defect (see Table 30-1).

Clinical Findings
History
- Cyanosis
  - In cases with mild right ventricular outflow obstruction, cyanosis may be so slight that it is not initially evident, or it may be present at birth (with severe obstruction).
  - Dyspnea and cyanosis (including hypercyanotic episodes, or "TET spells") increase by 2 to 4 months old, especially with crying, feeding, and/or defecation. The infant may have a history of poor weight gain.

Physical Examination. The severity of symptoms depends on the degree of right ventricular outflow obstruction. The following examination findings may be evident:
- Cyanosis of the mucous membranes and dyspnea
- A grade III to V/VI, harsh systolic ejection murmur at the left mid- to upper sternal border (VSD murmur and symptoms of a large VSD). There may be palpable thrill and a holosystolic murmur at the LLSB.
- A sternal lift secondary to right ventricular hypertrophy

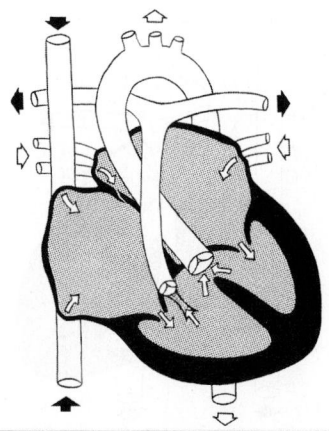

FIGURE 30-12 Tetralogy of Fallot (TOF). (Used with permission of Ross Products Division, Abbott Laboratories, Columbus, OH 43216. From *Clinical education aid no 7.* Copyright 1970 Ross Products Division, Abbott Laboratories.)

Diagnostic Studies
- Chest radiography may show a boot-shaped heart with decreased pulmonary vascular markings.
- ECG shows RVH and right axis deviation and may show a conduction delay in V1.
- An echocardiogram shows the extent of the pulmonary obstruction and demonstrates the anatomy of the overriding aorta and VSD.
- Pulse oximetry values decrease over time, with resultant increase in hemoglobin and hematocrit values.
- Cardiac catheterization, in the most severe forms, to delineate pulmonary artery anatomy.

Management
- In neonates with severe pulmonary obstruction, the ductus arteriosus is maintained or reopened with PGE$_1$ until more definitive repair or palliation is possible.
- For hypercyanotic episodes, the child should be cradled in a knee-chest position, soothed, and given oxygen and perhaps morphine sulfate subcutaneously until the spell subsides. The knee-chest maneuver increases systemic resistance, decreases right-to-left shunting, and increases pulmonary blood flow, perhaps alleviating symptoms. Immediate intervention is required for infants who are "spelling," especially if the previously mentioned maneuvers do not end the spell. (Children have died when such episodes have not been adequately addressed.) Most children are surgically repaired before hypercyanotic spells begin (Siwek et al, 2008).
- Complete repair with open-heart surgery is usually performed in infancy.
- Lifelong cardiology follow-up for pulmonic regurgitation or late arrhythmias. Recent studies indicate that progressive right ventricular dilation leads to increasing QRS duration on ECG. QRS duration of 180 ms significantly increases the risk of ventricular tachycardia and sudden death (Aboulhosn and Child, 2008). A cardiology consult is indicated before clearing for sports participation (Maron et al, 2005).
- SBE prophylaxis precautions are indicated before surgery and generally 6 months after repair.

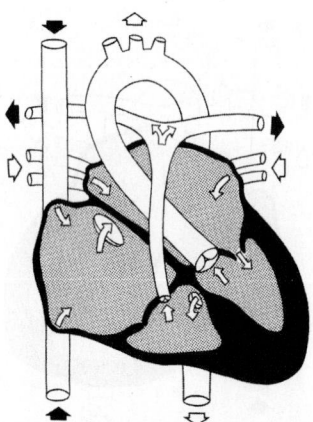

FIGURE 30-13 Tricuspid atresia. (Used with permission of Ross Products Division, Abbott Laboratories, Columbus, OH 43216. From *Clinical education aid no 7.* Copyright 1970 Ross Products Division, Abbott Laboratories.)

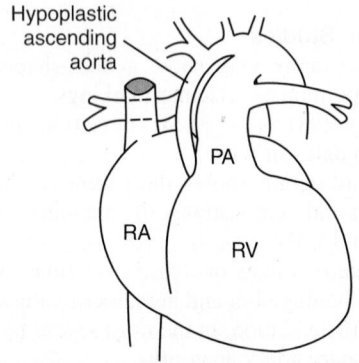

FIGURE 30-14 Hypoplastic left heart syndrome. (Adapted from Park MK, Troxler RG: *Pediatric cardiology for practitioners,* ed 4, St Louis, 2002, Mosby.)

TRICUSPID ATRESIA, HYPOPLASTIC LEFT HEART SYNDROME, AND OTHER SINGLE VENTRICLE DEFECTS

Description and Epidemiology

Hypoplastic left and right heart and single ventricle defects are a heterogeneous group of heart problems that together comprise perhaps 5% to 6% of congenital defects. In most cases there is functionally only one ventricle involving either right or left morphology that must do the work of pumping blood to both the systemic and pulmonary circulations (Figs. 30-13, 30-14, and 30-15). Oxygenated and deoxygenated blood mix in this ventricle, and the child is cyanotic. Most of these children require palliative cardiac procedures.

Tricuspid atresia results in the absence of communication between the right atrium and the right ventricle (see Fig. 30-13). TGA also occurs in 50% of these patients. The right ventricle is usually hypoplastic. Less than 3% of all children with CHD have tricuspid atresia. Up to 20% have multiple cardiac abnormalities (VSD, PDA, ASD). The etiology of this condition is unknown (Epstein, 2008).

Hypoplastic left heart syndrome occurs in 2.5% of heart defects. Intrauterine stenosis of either the mitral or aortic valves or both, results in a small left ventricle and hypoplasia of the ascending aorta and arch (see Fig. 30-14). The cause

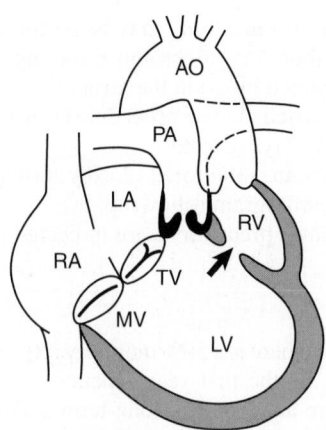

FIGURE 30-15 Single ventricle defect. (Used with permission of Park MK, Troxler RG: *Pediatric cardiology for practitioners,* ed 4, St Louis, 2002, Mosby.)

is unknown although it is linked to some genetic syndromes, such as Jacobsen syndrome (Tweddell et al, 2008).

Clinical Findings

History

- Cyanosis in the first week of life with dyspnea on exertion; fatigue with the effort of crying or feeding with subsequent poor weight gain

Physical Examination

- A murmur may be present; usually a single S_1 and/or S_2 is heard.
- Cyanosis is generally evident as soon as the ductus arteriosus closes.
- Hepatomegaly (may or may not be present)

Diagnostic Studies

- Chest radiography is generally normal initially, with changes occurring as the degree of cardiomegaly and obstruction of the pulmonary blood flow progresses.
- ECG findings depend on the type of single ventricle disease, but are always abnormal for age. Right ventricular forces are diminished in tricuspid atresia.
- Two-dimensional echocardiography is diagnostic and shows the specifics of the anatomy (Tweddell et al, 2008).

Management

- Intravenous PGE_1 may be indicated in newborns. Most children are initially palliated with aortopulmonary shunts or Norwood, Sano, or hybrid procedures depending on their anatomy. At 4 to 6 months of age, palliation is continued with a Glenn anastomosis of the SVC to the pulmonary artery. The third stage of palliation is the Fontan procedure, which occurs at 2 to 4 years old; the IVC is connected to the pulmonary artery. Some children are considered for cardiac transplantation early in life if their anatomy is not amenable to the Fontan pathway (Twedell et al, 2008).
- Families require support throughout the child's life. Frequent surgeries and hospitalizations can interfere with normal social development. Early recognition and intervention for developmental delays are important to the child's future.
- SBE prophylaxis is recommended while the child remains cyanotic (see Box 30-4; see Tables 30-7 and 30-8).

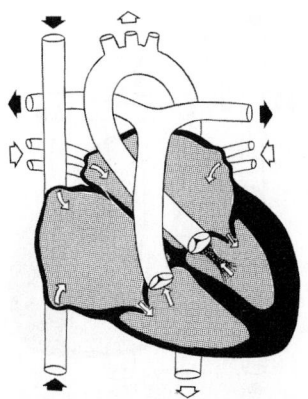

FIGURE 30-16 Subaortic stenosis. (Used with permission of Ross Products Division, Abbott Laboratories, Columbus, OH 43216. From *Clinical education aid no 7.* Copyright 1970 Ross Products Division, Abbott Laboratories.)

Complications

Complications include development of collateral arterial and venous vessels, protein-losing enteropathy, dysrhythmias and many others. A decrease in exercise tolerance throughout life can be expected, in addition to left or right ventricular dysfunction. There may be fewer complications with surgical palliation at earlier ages. For those with severe long-term complications, heart transplantation can be an option (Tweddell et al, 2008).

OBSTRUCTIVE CARDIAC LESIONS

AORTIC STENOSIS AND INSUFFICIENCY
Description and Epidemiology

AS or narrowing may occur at the aortic valvular, subvalvular, or supravalvular level. Valvular stenosis is the most common form (Fig. 30-16). The stenotic aortic valve is usually bicuspid rather than tricuspid. Stenosis causes increased pressure load on the left ventricle leading to LVH and, ultimately, ventricular failure. The imbalance between increased myocardial oxygen demand of hypertrophied myocardium and coronary blood supply may lead to ischemia and the risk of fatal ventricular arrhythmias. The bicuspid AV generally becomes more stenotic and often regurgitant (insufficient) over time. However, some infants are born with critical AS and require urgent intervention. Children with only a congenital bicuspid aortic valve and no stenosis or regurgitation have a 2% risk of developing symptoms by adolescence (Schneider and Moore, 2008) (see Table 30-10 for incidence figures).

Twenty percent of patients with AS have associated cardiac abnormalities, such as COA and VSDs (Schneider and Moore, 2008) (see also Table 30-1). Females with Turner syndrome have increased incidence of obstruction at all levels of left heart outflow tract (Goldmuntz and Lin, 2008).

Clinical Findings
History
- Growth and development may be normal.
- Activity intolerance, fatigue, chest pain (angina pectoris), or syncope can develop or increase with age.
- CHF, low cardiac output, and shock may be evident in newborns with severe AS.

- Sudden death, presumably due to dysrhythmias, can occur with increasing severity of stenosis and exertion.
Physical Examination
- BP may reveal a narrow pulse pressure. The apical impulse may be pronounced with moderate to severe stenosis.
- A grade III to IV/VI, loud, harsh systolic crescendo-decrescendo murmur is best heard at the upper right sternal border with radiation to the neck, LLSB, and apex.
- With a valvular lesion, a faint, early systolic click at the LLSB may be heard.
- With aortic insufficiency, an early diastolic blowing murmur is heard at the LLSB to apex.
- In the most severe lesions, S_2 is single or closely split; S_3 or S_4 heart sounds may also be heard.
- A thrill may be present at the suprasternal notch (Schneider and Moore, 2008).
Diagnostic Studies
- Chest radiographs are usually normal or may show LVH. Adults frequently develop radiographic evidence of calcification over time on the aortic valve.
- ECG can be normal or reveal LVH and inverted T-waves.
- 24-hour Holter monitors may demonstrate ventricular dysrhythmia.
- Echocardiograms are the diagnostic examinations of choice (Schneider and Moore, 2008).

Management
- The type and timing of treatment depends on the severity of the obstruction.
- Balloon valvuloplasty of the stenotic valve is the initial palliative treatment of AS in the newborn. However, the AV generally has to be surgically addressed later (Schneider and Moore, 2008).
- In older children, AV replacement is necessary for severe AS and/or insufficiency; unfortunately, none of the current replacement options are ideal or enduring for children. Mechanical valves are prothrombotic and require anticoagulation with warfarin. Heterograph and homograft valves have limited durability in the aortic position, and the Ross procedure requires placement of the homograft in the pulmonic position, leading to future replacements of that valve as it stenoses (Schneider and Moore, 2008).
- Patients with mild AS can participate in all sports, but should have annual cardiac examinations. Patients with moderate AS should chose low-intensity sports, such as golf, bowling, table tennis, or softball, as guided by their cardiologist. Patients with severe AS or moderate AS with symptoms should avoid competitive or intensive sports because there is a risk of sudden death from ventricular dysrhythmias (Maron et al, 2005) (see also Chapter 13, Table 13-5).
- Any aortic root dilation (commonly seen with bicuspid or stenotic aortic valves) may require intervention to prevent aortic dissection.
- SBE prophylaxis is necessary for 6 months after surgery.

PULMONIC STENOSIS
Description and Epidemiology

Normally the pulmonary valve opens to allow the flow of blood from the right ventricle into the pulmonary artery. In pulmonic stenosis, there is narrowing at the subpulmonic, valvular, or supravalvular area. Right-sided pressure is increased as the ventricle pumps against the obstruction. RVH occurs as a result of this increased load. Pulmonary stenosis can also occur in the main and/or branch pulmonary arterial system. Mild pulmonic stenosis is usually identified on routine examination. Many patients also develop poststenotic dilation of the pulmonary artery (see Table 30-1 for associated congenital malformation syndromes and Table 30-10 for incidence figures).

Clinical Findings
History
- The patient is usually asymptomatic, with a murmur noted on routine physical examination.
- Exertional dyspnea and fatigue are noticeable as stenosis progresses.
- Cyanosis from right-to-left shunting over the foramen ovale may be evident with critical pulmonic stenosis in the newborn.
- Growth and development are usually normal except in cases of Turner or Noonan syndrome in which short stature is common.

Physical Examination
- A grade II to IV/VI, harsh, mid- to late systolic ejection murmur is heard at the upper left sternal border over the pulmonic region with transmission along the left sternal border, neck and back, and into both lung fields.
- An intermittent systolic ejection click may be evident in the pulmonic area that decreases with inspiration and increases with expiration.
- Cyanosis and symptoms of right-sided CHF can occur in severe pulmonic stenosis in the newborn.

Diagnostic Studies
- Chest radiographs may be within normal limits in infants or show prominent main pulmonary artery segments in 80% to 90% of cases. Right-sided cardiac enlargement and decreased peripheral pulmonary vascular markings may be evident if heart failure develops.
- ECG may be normal with mild stenosis; with moderate to severe pulmonic stenosis, right axis deviation and RVH occur.
- Echocardiograms confirm the diagnosis, identifying the gradient and monitoring progression of the stenosis.
- Cardiac catheterization may be used to delineate location of the main and branch pulmonary artery stenoses.

Management
- Interventional cardiologists perform balloon valvuloplasty in neonates and older children with stenosis greater than 50 mm Hg. If unsuccessful, surgical valvuloplasty or replacement may be indicated. Interventional catheterization with stents and balloons is also used for branch stenosis.
- With mild stenosis, families must be encouraged to treat their children normally and not limit their activity. Moderate stenosis can progress to severe narrowing during periods of rapid growth, such as during infancy or adolescence (Prieto and Latson, 2008).
- SBE prophylaxis is not considered necessary except in the 6-month postoperative period or if prosthetic material is used (see Box 30-4).

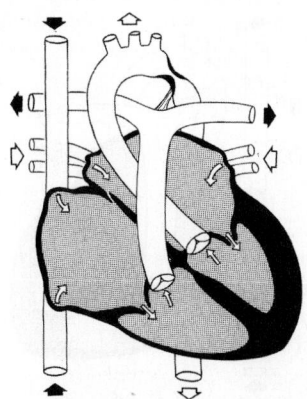

FIGURE 30-17 Coarctation of the aorta (COA). (Used with permission of Ross Products Division, Abbott Laboratories, Columbus, OH 43216. From *Clinical education aid no 7*. Copyright 1970 Ross Products Division, Abbott Laboratories.)

COARCTATION OF THE AORTA
Description and Epidemiology
COA is a narrowing of a small or long segment of the aorta (Fig. 30-17). Coarctation may occur as a single defect caused by a disturbance in the development of the aorta or may be secondary to constriction of the ductus arteriosus. The severity of the coarctation, its location, and the degree of obstruction determine the effect of the coarctation. Systolic and diastolic hypertension exists in vessels proximal to the narrowing. Hypotension is present in vessels below the area of narrowing (Beekman, 2008). Patients with Turner syndrome have close to a 10% incidence of coarctation (Goldmuntz and Lin, 2008) (see Table 30-10 for other incidence figures).

Clinical Findings
History. In older children, coarctation may go unnoticed until hypertension or a murmur are detected. Retrospectively, children with coarctation may have had complaints of leg pain with exercise or headaches. Severe neonatal coarctation presents early in life with tachypnea, poor feeding, and possibly cool lower extremities. COA in newborns is not always apparent until the ductus closes and decreases blood flow to the lower body.

Physical Examination
- Upper extremity hypertension with lower extremity hypotension are present, although milder cases may cause only a minimal discrepancy between upper and lower extremity BPs. In severe cases, poor lower extremity perfusion may be noticed with lower body mottling or pallor.
- Delayed timing and absent or weak arterial femoral and other distal pulses may occur.
- Bounding brachial, radial, and carotid pulses may occur.
- Signs of CHF may be evident.
- A systolic ejection murmur may be detected in the left infraclavicular region with transmission to the back.
- A ventricular heave at the apex can be palpated.
- A gallop rhythm may occur in infants with CHF.

Diagnostic Studies
- Chest radiography may reveal a normal or slightly enlarged heart and increased pulmonary vascular markings.
- ECG findings depend on the severity of the lesion and the age of the patient. In infants, RVH may be seen; in older children, LVH develops secondary to hypertension.

- Echocardiography is helpful in confirming the diagnosis and locating the constricted aortic segment. It may also show associated cardiac abnormalities.
- MRI can define the location, severity, and anatomy of the aortic arch.

Management

- In critical neonatal coarctation, PGE_1 is used to maintain or reopen the ductus.
- If possible, surgical resection of the constricted area and anastomosis of the upper and lower portions of the aorta is performed. Restenosis is more likely to occur if repair was before 1 year of age (Beekman, 2008). Cardiologists may dilate or stent the coarcted area in recoarctation or mild coarctation. Other procedures, including bypass grafting, may be necessary with unusually long coarcted segments. Surgical mortality is rare (Beekman, 2008).
- In older children with long-standing hypertension, antihypertensive medication may be required for several months after repair. Long-term prognosis is excellent unless there are associated intracardiac defects. BP should be monitored postoperatively for recoarctation.
- Patients with previous coarctation repairs may participate in any competitive sport if residual BP gradient between arm and legs is less than 20 mm Hg and peak systolic BP is normal at rest and with exercise. However, during the first year after surgery, high-intensity static exercises, such as weight lifting and wrestling, should be avoided (Maron et al, 2005).
- SBE prophylaxis is no longer considered necessary except in the 6-month postoperative period or if prosthetic material is used (see Box 30-4).

LONG-TERM ISSUES FOR CHILDREN AND YOUNG ADULTS WITH CONGENITAL HEART DISEASE

Description

Because of the success of pediatric cardiac surgery, 85% of children born with CHD live to adulthood; however, they require close supervision to assess their cardiac function and need for further interventions. Some studies estimate there are now more adults with CHD than children with the same problems. Surgeries performed on these adults during their childhood were not corrective, but palliative to different degrees. The severity of residual problems varies depending on the defect, type of surgical correction, and individual patient. However, very few of these individuals born with CHD would have made it to adulthood without some residual cardiac problem. To assist these patients, regional centers for the care of adults with CHD are developing (Pierpont et al, 2007).

Management

Late adolescent patients should be referred to adult congenital heart specialists for follow-up of moderate to complex lesions, for determining when future surgeries (cardiac and noncardiac) may be best performed, and for risk assessment for pregnancy. Details about residual problems for each cardiac defect are beyond the scope of this text. However, key points

in the evaluation of an older child or young adult with CHD are presented.

Chronic Cyanosis. Chronic cyanosis leads to difficulty with homeostasis and polycythemia. Clotting properties of platelets are often adversely affected, and friable collateral vessels develop in the pulmonary circulation. Conversely, polycythemia and dehydration can predispose these patients to thromboemboli (Aboulhosn and Child, 2008). Cyanotic older children and young adults often have limited cardiac reserve and a tendency for renal dysfunction associated with surgery, anesthesia, or physiologically stressful events.

Cardiac Chamber Dilation (Atrial or Ventricular). Many older CHD patients have insufficiency in one or more valves, often as a residual effect of previous surgery. Over long periods this leads to chamber dilation in the chamber receiving backflow. This dilation is well tolerated for many years but eventually affects function and leads to dysrhythmias initiated in the dilated tissues and dilation of other valves. Because the process is gradual, patients are often not cognizant of a change in function and may wait until the process is advanced before seeking care.

Dysrhythmias and Heart Blocks. Rhythm disturbances can occur as a result of long-standing cyanosis, the aforementioned chamber dilation, and fibrotic suture lines. Often episodes of palpitations bring older congenital heart patients to care (Aboulhosn and Child, 2008).

Ventricular Hypertrophy. Ventricular hypertrophy caused by stenotic outflow vessels or valves can, over time, predispose patients to myocardial ischemia, poor ventricular compliance, and serious ventricular dysrhythmias (Aboulhosn and Child, 2008).

■ Preventing Sudden Cardiac Death

The PCP has a responsibility to screen for causes of sudden cardiac death whenever performing a sports physical examination or assessing a complaint of chest pain, syncope, or palpitations. This can be a daunting challenge because none of the most common causes of sudden cardiac death are easily diagnosed by history or examination. The incidence of sudden cardiac death (non–sudden infant death syndrome [SIDS]) in children is 8 to 62 per 1,000,000 (McCormack, 2009). In the U.S. the most frequent causes of sudden death identified at autopsy are (in order of frequency) hypertrophic cardiomyopathy (HCM) (also called idiopathic hypertrophic subaortic stenosis and hypertrophic obstructive cardiomyopathy); coronary artery anomalies; myocarditis; arrhythmogenic right ventricular dysplasia; and aortic rupture and stenosis (Maron et al, 2009). Some portion of sudden death is caused by fatal dysrhythmias induced by congenital causes, such as long QT syndrome, Wolff-Parkinson-White and Brugada syndromes. These are not found on physical autopsy but are identified by genetic autopsy (testing for genetic abnormalities known to cause sudden death). Some of these conditions are discussed later in this chapter.

A full discussion of this topic is beyond the scope of this chapter; however, a few general guidelines can be offered. The PCP needs to do a full history including family history as well as a cardiac examination. Refer to a pediatric cardiologist if syncope, chest tightness, seizures, hypertension, or palpitations occur with exercise. Refer also if child has a history of heart disease, rheumatic fever, myocarditis, Kawasaki disease, or if there is a family history of sudden death, congenital coronary heart disease, long QT, hypertrophic cardiomyopathy, or Marfan syndrome. Also refer if there is evidence of stigmata of Marfan syndrome, murmurs, clicks, or elevated BP. Also see Chapter 13 for a discussion about sudden death in terms of assessing risk factors during the preparticipation physical examination for sports.

■ Acquired Heart Disease

CHEST PAIN

Description and Epidemiology

Chest pain in the pediatric population is a common complaint and does not usually represent a serious cardiovascular problem. However, chest pain of any kind can cause great anxiety for children, adolescents, and their parents. It is important to thoroughly evaluate this complaint with a careful history (especially note a family history of sudden death or early cardiac disease) and a thorough physical examination. ECG and other laboratory tests may be indicated if findings are present. Reassurance is of utmost importance, as most pediatric patients with chest pain do not have cardiac pathologic conditions (Driscoll, 2008).

The most frequent cause of chest pain is musculoskeletal, originating in the chest wall or chest cage. Costochondritis, Tietze syndrome, idiopathic chest pain, precordial catch syndrome, slipping-rib syndrome, hypersensitive xiphoid syndrome, trauma, and muscle strain are diagnoses assigned to specific types of chest pain; all are of musculoskeletal origin, are benign, and rarely require any treatment. The pain is often related to sports or casual athletic activity. Chest wall pain, particularly with exercise, may indicate exercise-induced asthma, but rarely indicates cardiac disease. Chronic chest pain that is vague and occurs over many months in a variety of circumstances, particularly around stressful events, may be psychogenic (anxiety or hyperventilation). Pain associated with syncope, exertional dyspnea, or irregularities in heart rhythm needs careful evaluation for a cardiac cause. Usually children or adolescents who have pain of cardiac origin describe a specific history with details that are consistent from event to event.

The incidence of chest pain in children seen emergency departments (EDs) is approximately 0.288%; it occurs slightly more often in males. The mean age at initial evaluation is 12 to 14 years. Most cases resolve spontaneously (Driscoll, 2008).

Clinical Findings

History. To determine the etiology of the chest pain, the provider should inquire about the following:
- Past medical history or family history for sudden death, heart disease or condition, asthma, eczema, Marfan syndrome, sickle cell disease
- Past sports activities, including friendly wrestling at home
- Previous trauma or muscle strains
- Characteristics of the chest pain
  - Relationship of pain to exercise; any syncope or exertional dyspnea
  - Any burning, substernal pain that worsens with reclining or with spicy foods (gastrointestinal etiology)
  - Pain that is sharp or stabbing, lasting several seconds to minutes, located over the midsternum or infranipple area, and occurring with nonexertion or deep inspirations (more likely musculoskeletal in origin)
  - Pain that awakens the patient (more likely organic)
- Any other associated symptoms, such as fever, nausea, vomiting, headaches, or choking episodes
- Any recent, major stressful events
- Medication, tobacco, or other drug use, including oral contraceptives (embolism)

Physical Examination. A complete chest (lungs and heart) and abdominal examination should be performed. Key findings to focus on include the presence of the following:
- Cardiac murmur, rubs, or clicks
- Point tenderness of one or more costochondral joints exaggerated with physical activity or deep inspirations (costochondritis or Tietze syndrome [if associated with warmth, swelling, or tenderness over costochondral junction])
- Irregular heart rhythm (cardiac disease)
- Shortness of breath, coughing, wheezing, chest pain with exercise
- Rales, wheezing, tachypnea, decreased breath sounds (pulmonary disease)

Diagnostic Studies. In most cases only the history and physical are necessary to make the diagnosis; other tests are not indicated unless the following problems are suspected:
- Febrile, cardiac, or pulmonary condition: Obtain a chest radiograph.
- Exercise-induced asthma: Perform a pulmonary function test with exercise.
- Rhythm disturbance: Order a 24-hour Holter monitor or stress test (or both).
- Signs of CHD, pericarditis, or myocarditis: Order an ECG.

Differential Diagnosis

The differential diagnosis includes disorders that can present with chest pain, such as musculoskeletal, respiratory (asthma, pneumonia, embolism, pneumothorax), psychogenic, and gastrointestinal disorders (reflux esophagitis, esophageal foreign body). Other miscellaneous entities, such as sickle cell crisis, aortic abdominal aneurysm (Marfan syndrome), pleural effusion (collagen-vascular disorders), herpes zoster, and shingles need to be considered.

Management

- When chest pain has no clear-cut etiology, the child appears well, and all aspects of the evaluation are normal, reassurance may be the most important treatment. Frequently, when reassured that the pain has no organic cause, the pain subsides or becomes less of an issue for the child.
  - Costochondritis and Tietze syndrome are usually responsive to nonsteroidal antiinflammatory treatment and rest.
  - Antacids may be tried if esophagitis is suspected; see Chapter 32.
  - See management of esophageal foreign body ingestion in Chapter 32.
  - See Chapters 13 and 31 for management of exercise-induced asthma and respiratory diseases.
- If pulmonary, gastrointestinal, or cardiac disease is a concern, treatment, referral, or evaluation is necessary. Chest pain associated with exercise should be referred to a cardiologist.

- Follow-up is indicated to ensure that no new findings have emerged, to ensure that the child is participating in normal activities, and to monitor for potential psychoemotional problems. (Driscoll, 2008)

HYPERTENSION

Definition and Epidemiology

Hypertension is defined as a systolic or diastolic (or both) BP in the 95th or higher percentile for age, sex, and height on at least three separate occasions. High-normal or prehypertensive BP is defined as average systolic or diastolic BP in the 90th percentile or higher, but less than the 95th percentile. Normal BP is defined as systolic and diastolic BP below the 90th percentile for age, sex, and height. Stage 1 hypertension is BP that ranges from the 95th percentile for age, sex, and height or above 120/80 to 5 mm Hg above the 99th percentile. Stage 2 hypertension is BP greater than 5 mm Hg above the 99th percentile (NIH-NHBPEP, 2004).

Hypertension is a significant problem affecting 2% to 5% of children and adolescents. Increasingly, children are found to have high BP associated with obesity, sedentary lifestyles, and stress. Secondary hypertension is more commonly seen in children less than 6 years old (at significant or severe hypertension levels) (NIH-NHBPEP, 2004). The primary cause of secondary, severe hypertension is renovascular or parenchymal renal diseases. Other causes include coarctation of aorta, endocrine disorders, genetic disorders such as Williams syndrome, neurofibromatosis and tuberous sclerosis, drugs, and central nervous system (CNS) tumors (Grinsell and Norwood, 2009). The onset of primary hypertension is more likely to occur after 10 years old. Neonates with hypertension are severely ill with neurologic, cardiac and renal symptoms. One large study of 14,000 children at a large academic health center found considerable underdiagnosis of pediatric hypertension. Electronic records of 507 children showed elevated BPs on three separate primary care visits; however, only 26% were diagnosed with hypertension (Hansen et al, 2007).

Clinical Findings

The goal of the clinical history and physical examination is to look for causes of secondary hypertension, comorbidities of primary hypertension, and signs of end-organ damage of prolonged hypertension of either type.

History

- Neonatal history of prolonged mechanical ventilation and umbilical catheterization
- Diet, activities, and other habits (e.g., smoking, drinking)
- Sleep history, particularly symptoms of sleep apnea (Enright et al, 2003)
- Medications taken, including oral contraceptives, cold medications, steroids, and diet aids
- Chronic illness, especially renal disease, past history of urinary tract infections, diabetes, or seizures
- Headache, chest pain, dyspnea, muscle weakness, palpitations, abdominal pain, facial palsy, decreased vision, excessive sweating
- Family history of a first-degree relative with myocardial infarction (especially before 50 years old), stroke, hypertension, diabetes, hyperlipidemia, sudden cardiac death, polycystic kidney disease, neurofibromatosis, pheochromocytoma, or obesity

Physical Examination

- Body habitus, especially overweight (per body mass index [BMI]); poor growth (height, weight); signs of metabolic syndrome
- Dysmorphic features
- Edema, pallor, flushing, skin lesions (suggestive of tuberous sclerosis or SLE)
- Absent, diminished, or pounding pulses in all extremities
- Fundi abnormalities, enlarged thyroid gland, abdominal mass, flank bruit; decreased visual acuity, facial palsy
- Elevated BP

Accurate BP measurement is essential using an appropriate-size cuff with the cubital fossa supported at the heart level. The right arm is preferred for comparison with normative charts; right thigh measurement is also recommended if elevated pressure is suspected. The individual should be seated and have been resting in that position for 3 to 5 minutes. Deflation should be controlled at 2 to 3 mm Hg per second. Systolic pressure is recorded at the onset of tapping sounds; diastolic pressure is recorded at the disappearance (not the muffling) of sounds. Some authorities recommend recording the pressure twice on each occasion and using an average of each to record. BP elevation must be confirmed on three separate occasions.

Diagnostic Studies. Laboratory evaluation of stage 1 or 2 HTN should focus on searching for causes of secondary hypertension, comorbidities of primary hypertension, and target organ damage of either primary or secondary hypertension. The search for secondary causes of hypertension needs to be individualized.

- One study suggests that in children with mild to moderate hypertension and positive family history or elevated BMI, workup should be limited to serum cholesterol, echocardiogram, and renal ultrasound. These researchers also suggest ambulatory BP monitoring (Wiesen et al, 2008).
- Children less than 10 years of age with stage 2 hypertension require more aggressive laboratory evaluation compared with older children with stage 1 hypertension and obesity. CBC, erythrocyte sedimentation rate (ESR), C-reactive protein (CRP), urinalysis and culture, electrolytes, blood urea nitrogen, creatinine, and plasma renin levels, renal nuclear medicine scans, and renal ultrasound are screening studies for the most common secondary causes of hypertension.
- If renal vascular disease is suspected, the workup is best managed by a nephrologist because newer technologies, such as MRI and spiral computed tomography (CT), are replacing angiography.
- Additional organ assessments include echocardiography for LVH and COA and a thorough ophthalmologic examination (NIH-NHBPEP, 2004).

Management

Figure 30-18 shows an algorithm to manage children with high BP.

- BP measurements should be done annually on all children 3 years and older, with baseline and serial measurements documented carefully in the child's record. Standardized BP norms are available (see Tables 30-3 and 30-4).
- Prehypertension: At least two follow-up BP measurements should be taken within 1 to 2 months of the initial reading to determine whether this high reading is a single, isolated

ALGORITHM

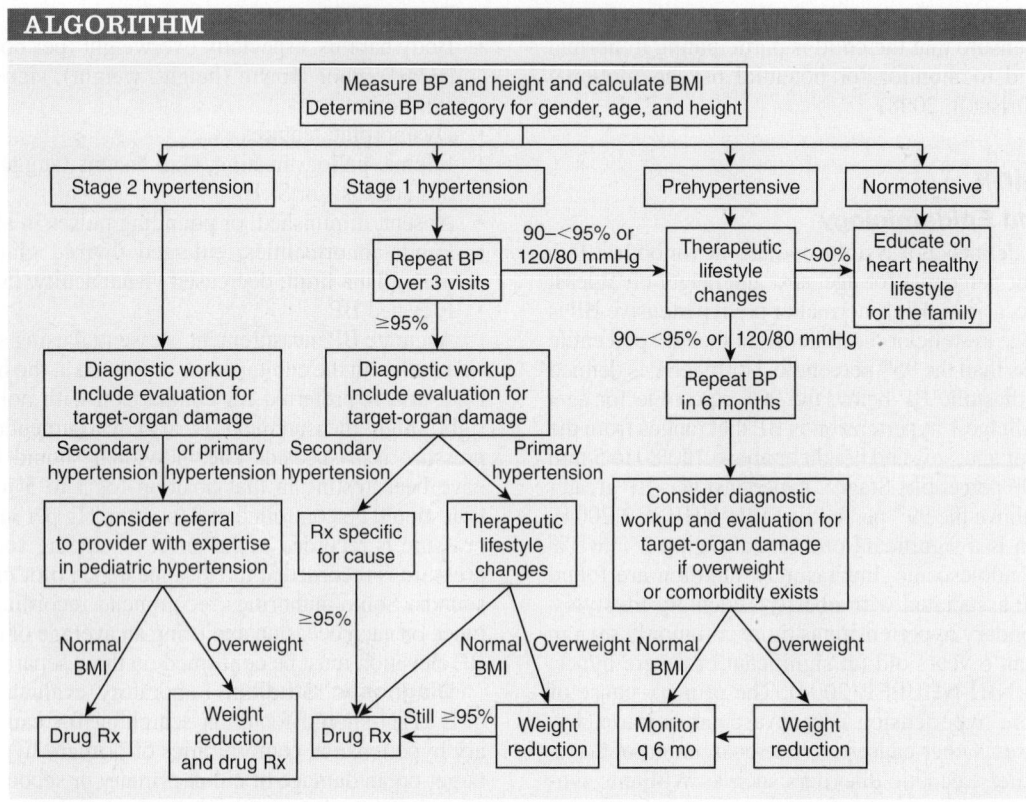

FIGURE 30-18 Hypertension management algorithm. *BMI,* Body mass index; *BP,* blood pressure; *Rx,* prescription. (Used with permission of the National Institutes of Health, National High Blood Pressure Education Program Working Group on High Blood Pressure in Children and Adolescents [NIH-NHBPEP]: The Fourth Report on the Diagnosis, Evaluation, and Treatment of High Blood Pressure in Children and Adolescents, *Pediatrics* 114[Suppl]: 555-576, 2004, p 571.)

event. If subsequent readings fall below the 95th percentile, the child should continue with routine BP checks during annual visits.

- Hypertension, secondary to overweight, can be as serious as hypertension secondary to other organic disease and should be treated as such. For those with high-normal BP without any indication of organic disease, treatment should consist of nonpharmacologic intervention: diet, exercise, and weight management. Caloric restriction with exercise is more effective than caloric restriction alone (NIH-NHBPEP, 2004). Recommendations should include the following:
  - ○ Dietary intervention to control or reduce overweight is covered in Chapter 10. High sodium foods and sodium supplements should be eliminated.
  - ○ Increase physical exercise and sports participation to 30 to 60 minutes a day balanced with relaxation techniques. Aerobic, not static or isometric exercise, is recommended. See Chapter 13 for information on sports activities, readiness, and conditioning strategies; Table 13-7 discusses management for sports participation for those with hypertension.
  - ○ Avoid smoking, caffeine, alcoholic beverages, and illicit drug consumption.
- Patients with secondary hypertension, primary hypertension with symptoms, LVH, or insufficient change in hypertensive status after 6 to 12 months of diet and exercise therapy should start medications (NIH-NHBPEP,

2004). The provider should refer the patient to a specialist who has experience using antihypertensive agents in children. The goal is to reduce systolic or diastolic BP below the 95th percentile. If a concurrent condition exists, the goal becomes reducing BP to the 90th percentile (medication recommendations are in Table 30-11). A single drug, usually an ACE inhibitor, angiotensin-receptor blocker (ARB), beta-blocker, calcium channel blocker, or diuretic should be started at the lowest recommended dose and advanced until the desired BP is reached. If maximum dose or adverse side effects are reached, a second medication should be added. Step-down therapy may be possible for overweight children who lose weight and achieve BP goals. Studies of antihypertensives in children indicate racial differences may exist in the medication effect of ACE inhibitors; ARBs or beta-blockers were not studied. Side effect profiles are similar to those found in adults (Flynn, 2008).

Complications

Long-term BP elevation leads to an increase in left ventricular mass, increased carotid intimal medial thickness, and coronary artery calcification, especially if combined with overweight, lipid and lipoprotein abnormalities, and tobacco use. There are some indications of cognitive impairments in children with hypertension as well (Flynn, 2008). Yearly echocardiograms are recommended to evaluate LVH.

TABLE 30-11	Antihypertensive Medications for Children		
Class	**Drugs**	**Dose and Dosing Interval**	**Comments**
Angiotensin-converting enzyme (ACE) inhibitors	Captopril	Initial dose: 0.3-0.5 mg/kg/dose; max dose: 6 mg/kg/day; tid dosing	ACE inhibitors are contraindicated in pregnancy. Check serum potassium and creatinine periodically. All can be compounded into a suspension.
	Enalapril	Initial dose: 0.08 mg/kg/day up to 5 mg/day; max dose: 0.6 mg/kg/day up to 40 mg; daily to bid dosing	
	Lisinopril	Initial dose: 0.07 mg/kg/day up to 5 mg/day; max dose: 0.6 mg/kg/day up to 40 mg/day; daily dosing	
Alpha- and beta-blocker	Labetalol	Initial dose: 1-3 mg/kg/day; max dose: 10-12 mg/kg/day up to 1200 mg/day; bid dosing	
Beta-adrenergic antagonist	Propranolol	Initial dose: 1 mg/kg/day divided bid; usual dose 2-4 mg/kg/day; max dose: 16 mg/kg/day	Asthma, heart failure, and insulin-dependent diabetes are contraindications. Monitor heart rate for excessive bradycardia. Athletic performance may be impaired.
	Metoprolol	Initial dose: 1-2 mg/kg/day: max dose: 6 mg/kg/day up to 200 mg/day; bid dosing	
	Atenolol	Initial dose: 0.5-1 mg/kg/day; max dose: 2 mg/kg/day up to 100 mg/day; daily to bid dosing	
Angiotensin-receptor blocker (ARB)	Irbesartan	Children 6-12 yr: 75-150 mg/day	ARB inhibitors are contraindicated in pregnancy. Check serum potassium and creatinine periodically.
	Losartan	Initial dose: 0.7 mg/kg/day up to 50 mg/day; max dose: 1.4 mg/kg/day up to 100 mg/day; single daily dose	
Calcium channel blocker	Amlodipine	Children 6-17 yr: 2.5-5 mg once daily	Amlodipine and isradipine can be compounded into a suspension. May cause tachycardia.
	Isradipine	Initial dose: 0.15-2 mg/kg/day; max dose: 0.8 mg/kg/day up to 20 mg/day; tid-qid dosing	
	Extended-release nifedipine	Initial dose: 0.25-0.5 mg/kg/day up to 5 mg/day; max dose: 3 mg/kg/day up to 120 mg/day; daily to bid dosing	
Central-adrenergic agonists	Clonidine	Children 12 yr: initial dose: 0.2 mg/day, divided bid; max dose: 2.4 mg/day	May cause dry mouth or sedation. Sudden cessation can cause rebound.
Peripheral alpha agonist	Prazosin	Initial dose: 0.05-0.1 mg/kg/day; max dose: 0.5 mg/kg/day up to 50 mg/day once; tid dosing	
Direct vasodilators	Hydralazine	Initial dose: 0.75 mg/kg/day; max dose: 7.5 mg/kg/day up to 200 mg/day divided; dosed qid	Fluid retention and tachycardia commonly occur. Hydralazine can cause lupus-like syndrome in some patients.
	Minoxidil	Initial dose: 0.2 mg/kg/day; max dose: up to 50 mg/day; daily to tid dosing	Minoxidil can cause hypertrichosis.
Diuretics	Chlorthalidone	Initial dose: 0.3 mg/kg/day; max dose: 2 mg/kg/day up to 50 mg/day	Patients on diuretics should have electrolytes monitored. Potassium-sparing diuretics (spironolactone, triamterene, amiloride) can cause hyperkalemia, especially when given with ACE inhibitor or ARB. Chlorthalidone may cause azotemia in patients with renal disease.
	Furosemide	Initial dose: 0.5-2 mg/kg/day per dose; max dose: 6 mg/kg/day; dosed daily to bid	
	Hydrochlorothiazide	Initial dose: 1 mg/kg/day; max dose: 3 mg/kg/day up to 50 mg/day; dosed daily	
	Spironolactone	Initial dose: 1.5 mg/kg/day, max dose: 3.3 mg/kg/day; dosed daily or bid	

bid, Twice daily; *max*, maximum; *kg*, kilogram; *qid*, four times daily; *tid*, three times daily; *yr*, year.

Prevention

- Because much of hypertension is related to lifestyle, prevention through optimal health promotion and maintenance is essential. Regular health maintenance, including evaluation of BP and health education regarding risk factors, is critical. Counseling should emphasize both behavioral modification and parental involvement. Decreasing body mass index and increasing aerobic fitness have been shown to reduce elevations in age-related BP. Specific preventive measures include the following:
  - ○ Good nutrition
  - ○ Prevention of overweight
  - ○ Decrease in dietary fat and sodium
  - ○ Aerobic exercise daily for at least 30 minutes
  - ○ Stress management
  - ○ Avoidance of caffeine, tobacco use, and prescription or over-the-counter medications that can exacerbate high BP (e.g., cold medications with ephedrine or phenylephrine, steroids)
  - ○ Monitoring of BP if oral contraceptives are used

KAWASAKI DISEASE

Description and Epidemiology

Kawasaki disease (KD) (also known as mucocutaneous lymph node syndrome or infantile polyarteritis) is characterized by an acute generalized systemic vasculitis occurring throughout the body. Although the etiology of KD remains unknown, clinical evidence supports an infectious cause. It exhibits geographic and seasonal outbreaks, in the late winter and early spring. Person-to-person spread is low, but it occurs with greater frequency in siblings (1%).

Between 9.1 and 32.5 per 100,000 children (depending on race) contract KD each year in the U.S. (Wood and Tulloh, 2009). Genetic susceptibility is probably an important contributor, as evidenced by the differential racial incidence and higher rates of occurrence among siblings. Although all racial groups are susceptible, the incidence is highest in Asian-American children, followed by African-Americans and Hispanics; rates are lowest in Caucasian children. There is a 1.5:1 male-to-female ratio. More than 85% of cases occur in children younger than 5 years of age (Wood and Tulloh, 2009). KD is self-limited and is the most common cause of acquired heart disease in children in Japan and the U.S. (Wood and Tulloh, 2009).

Clinical Findings

The classic diagnostic criteria are listed in Box 30-6. However, children can have atypical or incomplete KD with coronary anomalies shown by echocardiogram. Children younger than 6 to 12 months of age may have more atypical findings. Figure 30-19 shows a decision-making algorithm for suspected atypical or incomplete KD. There are four stages in which changes in cardiovascular pathology occur, depending on the length of time since the onset of symptoms.

Stage 1. The acute phase (days 0 to 14) begins with an abrupt onset of high fever (greater than 102.2° F [39° C]) that is unresponsive to antipyretics or antibiotics. Typically significant irritability, bilateral nonpurulent conjunctival injection, erythema of the oropharynx, dryness and fissuring of the lips, "strawberry tongue," cervical lymphadenopathy,

---

BOX 30-6 Diagnostic Criteria for Kawasaki Disease

The child must exhibit fever for 5 days plus four of the other five criteria or, if fewer than four criteria, coronary vessel involvement:
1. Bilateral conjunctival injection without exudate
2. Polymorphous rash that may be urticarial or pruritic
3. Inflammatory changes in the lips and oral cavity
4. Changes in the extremities, such as peripheral edema, erythema of the palms and soles, or desquamation of the hands and feet (convalescent period)
5. Cervical lymphadenopathy that is often unilateral, anterior cervical

Data from Newburger J, Takahasi M, Gerber M et al: Diagnosis, treatment and long-term management of Kawasaki disease: a statement for health professionals from the Committee on Rheumatic Fever, Endocarditis, and Kawasaki Disease, Council on Cardiovascular Disease in the Young, American Heart Association, *Pediatrics* 114(6):1708-1733, 2004.

---

a polymorphous rash, erythema of the urethral meatus, tachycardia, and edema of the extremities are noted. During the acute phase, there may be pericardial, myocardial, endocardial, and coronary artery inflammation. The child typically is tachycardic and has a hyperdynamic precordium with a gallop rhythm and a flow murmur. Rarely, children have low cardiac output syndrome from poor myocardial function.

Stage 2. The subacute phase (2 to 4 weeks after illness onset) begins with resolution of the fever and lasts until all other clinical signs have disappeared. Irritability may be prolonged throughout this phase.

Desquamation of the fingers (at the junction of nail tip and digit) occurs first, followed by desquamation of the toes. Transient jaundice, abnormal liver function tests, arthralgia or arthritis, transient diarrhea, orchitis, facial palsy, and sensorineural hearing loss may occur. Coronary artery aneurysms appear during this period, more so in untreated children. Common sites for aneurysm, in order of frequency, are the proximal left anterior descending coronary, proximal right coronary, left main coronary, left circumflex, and distal right coronary artery.

Stage 3. During the convalescent phase, all clinical signs of KD have resolved, but laboratory values may not have returned to normal. This phase is complete when all blood values are normal (6 to 8 weeks from onset).

Stage 4. The chronic phase is from 40 days to years after illness onset. Coronary complications, if present, can persist into adulthood.

Diagnostic Studies

- CBC with differential, ESR, platelet count, CRP, liver transaminases, gamma-glutamyltransferase (GGT), and urinalysis. Occasionally the ESR is normal but CRP is elevated. Stage 1 is typified by an elevated ESR and platelet count (as high as 700,000/mm³); elevated CRP; leukocytosis with left shift; slight decreases in red blood cells and hemoglobin; hypoalbuminemia; increased α_2-globulin; and sterile pyuria. It is important to note that the platelet count may be initially normal, with gradual increase after the seventh day of fever.
- Blood, urine, cerebrospinal fluid, and group A beta-hemolytic streptococcus (GABHS) pharyngeal cultures may be indicated given the patient's symptomatology (to rule out other sources of fever).

ALGORITHM

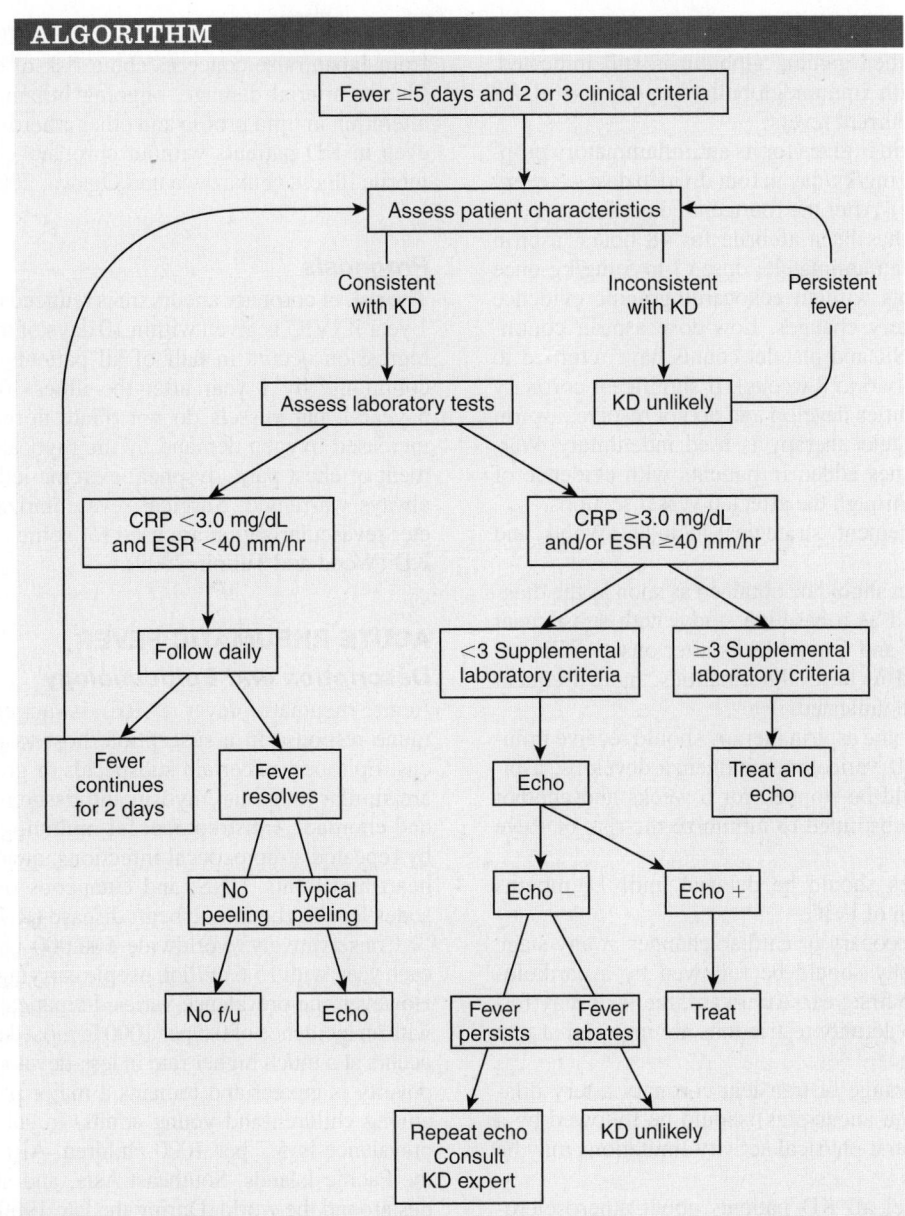

FIGURE 30-19 Algorithm for evaluation of suspected incomplete Kawasaki disease (KD). (Redrawn from Newburger J, Takahashi M, Gerber M et al: Diagnosis, treatment and long-term management of Kawasaki disease: a statement for health professionals from the Committee on Rheumatic Fever, Endocarditis, and Kawasaki Disease, Council on Cardiovascular Disease in the Young, American Heart Association, *Pediatrics* 114[6]:1708-1733, 2004, p 1709.)

- Echocardiograms at acute illness, 2 weeks and 6 to 8 weeks after onset of fever are performed to evaluate for coronary, myocardial, and pericardial inflammation. Angiography, MRI, and cardiac stress testing may be considered.

Differential Diagnosis

The differential diagnosis includes measles, adenovirus, scarlet fever, drug reactions, Stevens-Johnson syndrome, erythema multiforme, mononucleosis, juvenile arthritis, leptospirosis, inflammatory bowel disease, sarcoidosis, SLE, rickettsial infection, and toxic shock for the triad of red eyes, prolonged fever, and rash (Wood and Tulloh, 2009).

Management

Early diagnosis is essential to prevent aneurysms in the coronary arteries and extraparenchymal muscular arteries. Goals of treatment include: (1) evoking a rapid antiinflammatory response, (2) preventing coronary thrombosis by inhibiting platelet aggregation, and (3) minimizing long-term coronary risk factors by exercise, diet, and smoking prevention.

- Treatment includes the following (Wood and Tulloh, 2009):
  - Intravenous gamma globulin (IVIG) therapy (a single dose of 2 g/kg over 10 to 12 hours, ideally in the first 10 days of the illness) to reduce the incidence of coronary artery abnormalities. The use of immunoglobulin after the tenth day must be individualized. If a patient is found to have an abnormal echocardiogram, fever,

tachycardia, or other signs of inflammation beyond the tenth day, then gamma globulin is still indicated. Retreatment with immunoglobulin may be useful for persistent or recurrent fevers

○ High-dose aspirin is given for its antiinflammatory properties (80 to 100 mg/kg/day in four divided doses—every 6 hours initially). After the fourteenth day of illness and once the child has been afebrile for 48 hours, aspirin is continued at an antiplatelet dose (3 to 5 mg/kg once daily) in patients without echocardiographic evidence of coronary artery changes. Low-dose aspirin continues until the ESR and platelet counts have returned to normal (typically 6 to 8 weeks). If significant coronary artery abnormalities develop and do not resolve, aspirin or other antiplatelet therapy is used indefinitely. Warfarin is sometimes added in patients with evidence of turbulent flow through the affected vessel sections.

Additional management strategies include (Wood and Tulloh, 2009):

- An echocardiogram should be obtained as soon as the diagnosis is established as a baseline study, with subsequent studies at 2 weeks and 6 to 8 weeks after onset of illness. If a child is found to have abnormalities, more frequent evaluations may be indicated.
- All patients on chronic aspirin therapy should receive influenza vaccination. If varicella or influenza develops, aspirin treatment should be stopped for 6 weeks and another antiplatelet drug substituted to minimize the risk of Reye syndrome.
- Live-virus vaccines should be delayed until 11 months after administration of IVIG.
- Patients without coronary or cardiac changes at any stage on echocardiography should be followed by a cardiologist throughout the first year. Afterward, the PCP may follow the patient; no activity restrictions are imposed at that point.
- Patients with any range of transient coronary artery dilation (including giant aneurysms) should be followed by a cardiologist for years; physical activity limitations may be imposed.
- Follow and counsel all KD patients about atherosclerosis risk factors (Fukazawa and Ogawa, 2009; Tierney and Newberger, 2007) (see Complications discussion).

Complications

The acute disease is self-limited; however, during the initial stage (acute phase), inflammation of the arterioles, venules, and capillaries of the heart occurs and can later progress to coronary artery aneurysm in 15% to 25% of untreated children (less than 5% when treated appropriately) (Wood and Tulloh, 2009). The process of aneurysm formation and subsequent thrombosis or scarring of the coronary artery may occur as late as 6 months after the initial illness. Other possible complications include recurrence of KD (less than 2%); CHF or massive myocardial infarction; myocarditis or pericarditis, or both (30%); pericardial effusion; and mitral valve insufficiency. Mortality (1.25%) from KD occurs from cardiac sequelae 15 to 45 days after onset of fever (Wood and Tulloh, 2009). Children with coronary dilation or aneurysms (especially those greater than 4 mm) may have long-term coronary endothelial changes that place the child at risk for early ischemic disease; they may

also develop dyslipidemias (Wood and Tulloh, 2009). Studies from Japan raise concerns about risk of early atherosclerosis (due to arterial damage, ongoing inflammatory process, and alteration in lipid profile and other atherosclerosis risk factors) even in KD patients without coronary changes during acute febrile illness (Fukazawa and Ogawa, 2009).

Prognosis

The risk of coronary aneurysm is reduced in patients older than 1 year if IVIG is given within 10 days of the illness. Aneurysm regression occurs in half of all patients who develop them, commonly by 1 year after the illness (80% resolve within 5 years), but vessels do not dilate normally in response to increased oxygen demand by the myocardium. Prompt treatment of chest pain, dyspnea, extreme lethargy, or syncope is always warranted. Surgical revascularization and transcatheter revascularization are used for some coronary sequelae of KD (Wood and Tulloh, 2009).

ACUTE RHEUMATIC FEVER
Description and Epidemiology

Acute rheumatic fever (ARF) is an exaggerated autoimmune response in a susceptible host to group A streptococcus. Epitopes on certain subspecies of group A streptococcus are similar to human myosin and tissue of the mitral annulus and chordae. Antistreptococcal immunoglobulins, stimulated by repeated streptococcal infections, attack the patient's own heart and joints, CNS, and cutaneous tissue. Repeated episodes lead to rheumatic heart disease (RHD) (Yani, 2008).

Conservatively, worldwide 500,000 children acquire ARF each year, with 15.6 million people carrying the burden of RHD. However, the prevalence varies dramatically around the world with an incidence of 0.5 per 1000 in most developed countries; it occurs at a much higher rate in less-developed countries, where poverty is greater and remains a major public health problem among children and young adults. In sub-Saharan Africa the prevalence is 5.7 per 1000 children. ARF is also endemic in the Pacific Islands, Southeast Asia, and aboriginal communities around the world. During the late 1960s and 1970s the disease almost disappeared in the U.S. and Western Europe only to resurge in the mid-1980s in the intermountain states. It is the leading cause of acquired heart disease in children worldwide, occurring most commonly in school-age children 5 to 15 years old (Yani, 2008). Resultant RHD has severe economic ramifications in developing countries due to resulting disability and premature death (World Health Organization [WHO], 2004).

Figure 30-20 shows the pathogenic pathway of ARF and RHD. In developed countries the strains of streptococci that induce ARF are rare and usually cause throat infection; they do not cause skin infections, such as impetigo. However, this is not always true in developing countries or subpopulations with high ARF prevalence (such as Australian Aborigines). In these populations, impetigo streptococcal infections do precede ARF (Yani, 2008). Some children are also more susceptible to the ARF immune response based on their human leukocyte antigen (HLA) class.

Repeated streptococcal infections appear to prime the immune response in the child before the first episode of ARF. Once the immune system is primed to the pathogen and triggered by repeated exposures, CD4 cells attack cardiac myosin

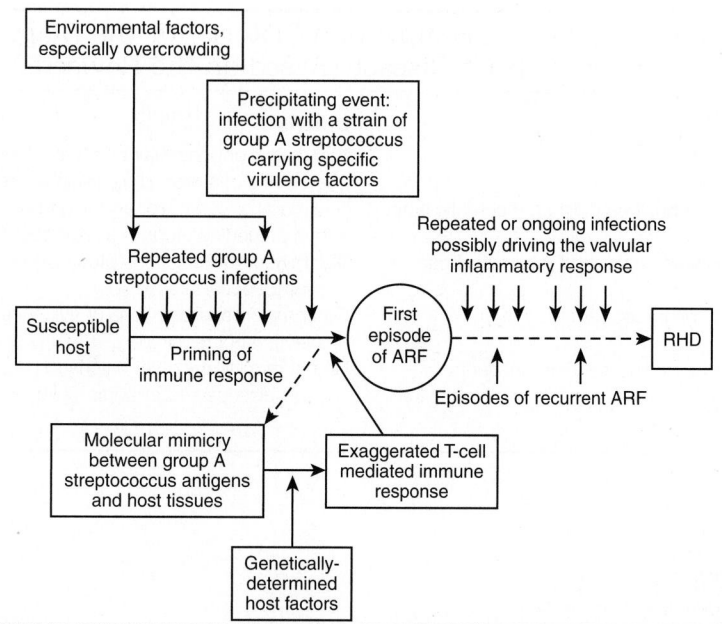

FIGURE 30-20 Pathogenetic pathway for acute rheumatic fever (ARF) and rheumatic heart disease (RHD). (Used with permission of Carapetis J, McDonald M, Wilson N: Acute rheumatic fever, *Lancet* 366:155-168, 2005, p 157.)

BOX 30-7 | **Jones Criteria for Rheumatic Fever***

Evidence of Preceding GABHS Infection
- Positive throat culture or rapid streptococcal antigen test result
- Elevated or rising streptococcal antibody titer

Minor Manifestations
- Arthralgia
- Fever
- Elevated acute-phase reactants
- Elevated erythrocyte sedimentation rate
- Elevated C-reactive protein

Major Manifestations
- Carditis
  - Tachycardia out of proportion to degree of fever
  - Cardiomegaly
  - New murmurs or change in preexisting murmurs
  - Muffled heart sounds
  - Precordial friction rub
  - Precordial pain
  - Changes in electrocardiogram (especially prolonged PR interval)

- Polyarthritis
  - Swollen, hot, red, painful joint(s)
  - After 1 to 2 days, affects different joints (migratory)
  - Favors large joints—knees, elbows, hips, shoulders, wrists
- Erythema marginatum
  - Erythematous macules with clear center and wavy, well-demarcated border
  - Transitory
  - Nonpruritic
  - Primarily affects trunk and extremities (inner surfaces)
- Chorea
  - Sudden, aimless, irregular movements of extremities
  - Involuntary facial grimaces
  - Speech disturbances or emotional lability
  - Muscle weakness (can be profound)
  - Muscle movements exaggerated by anxiety and attempt at fine motor activity; relieved by rest
- Subcutaneous nodes
  - Nontender swelling
  - Located over bony prominence
  - May persist for some time and then gradually resolve

*The presence of two major or one major and two or more minor criteria with evidence of preceding GABHS infection indicates a high probability of rheumatic fever.
GABHS, Group A beta-hemolytic streptococcus.
From Dajani AS, Ayoub E, Bierman FZ et al: Guidelines for the diagnosis of rheumatic fever: Jones criteria, updated 1992, *Circulation* 87:302-307, 1993; Ferrieri P, for the Jones Criteria Working Group: Proceedings of the Jones criteria workshop, *Circulation* 106(19):2521, 2002. Reviewed and reaffirmed the prior updated 1992 Jones criteria.

---

and laminin (in valve membranes) because these proteins appear similar to the M-protein on the streptococci. This classically occurs during a latent period of 10 to 20 days following streptococcal infection. First episodes of ARF usually occur before adolescence, and any cardiac damage may resolve if no further episodes occur (through prevention by antibiotic prophylaxis). However, in the developing world or in high prevalence communities, reexposure without prophylaxis is common, inducing worsening RHD with each new episode.

Clinical Findings

The diagnosis of ARF has traditionally been based on a set of guidelines known as the Jones criteria (Yani, 2008) (Box 30-7). The presence of two major or one major and two minor criteria with evidence of a preceding GABHS infection indicates a high probability of ARF. Children with fewer manifestations can also have ARF. Arthritis of large joints occurs in 65% of cases, carditis in 50%, chorea in 15% to 30%, cutaneous nodules in 5%, and subcutaneous nodules in less than 7%.

BOX 30-8 **2002-2003 World Health Organization Criteria for the Diagnosis of Rheumatic Fever and Rheumatic Heart Disease (Based on the Revised Jones Criteria)**

Diagnostic Categories	**Criteria**
Primary episode of rheumatic fever (RF)[1]	Two major* or one major and two minor** manifestations **plus** evidence of a preceding group A streptococcal infection***
Recurrent attack of RF in a patient **without** established rheumatic heart disease[2]	Two major or one major and two minor manifestations **plus** evidence of a preceding group A streptococcal infection
Recurrent attack of RF in a patient **with** established rheumatic heart disease	Two minor manifestations **plus** evidence of a preceding group A streptococcal infection[3]
Rheumatic chorea. Insidious onset rheumatic carditis[2]	Other major manifestations or evidence of group A streptococcal infection not required
Chronic valve lesions of rheumatic heart disease (RHD) (patients presenting for the first time with pure mitral stenosis or mixed mitral valve disease)[4]	Do not require any other criteria to be diagnosed as having rheumatic heart disease and/or aortic valve disease

* Major manifestations	• Carditis • Polyarthritis • Chorea • Erythema marginatum • Subcutaneous nodules
** Minor manifestations	• Clinical: fever, polyarthralgia • Laboratory: elevated acute phase reactants (erythrocyte sedimentation rate or leukocyte count)
*** Supporting evidence of a preceding streptococcal infection within the last 45 days	• Electrocardiogram: prolonged PR interval • Elevated or rising antistreptolysin-O or other streptococcal antibody, or • A positive throat culture, or • Rapid antigen test for group A streptococci, or • Recent scarlet fever

1. Patients may present with polyarthritis (or with only polyarthralgia or monoarthritis) and with several (three or more) other minor manifestations, together with evidence of recent group A streptococcal infection. Some of these cases may later turn out to be rheumatic fever. It is prudent to consider them as cases of "probable rheumatic fever" (once other diagnoses are excluded) and advise regular secondary prophylaxis. Such patients require close follow-up and regular examination of the heart. This cautious approach is particularly suitable for patients in vulnerable age groups in high-incidence settings.
2. Infective endocarditis should be excluded.
3. Some patients with recurrent attacks may not fulfill these criteria.
4. Congenital heart disease should be excluded.
From World Health Organization: *Rheumatic fever and rheumatic heart disease: report of a WHO expert consultation.* 2001, Table 4.1, p 23. Available at www.who.int/cardiovascular_diseases/resources/trs923/en (accessed July 22, 2010).

The symptoms of carditis may be vague and insidious with decreased appetite, fatigue, and pains. A high-pitched holosystolic murmur is heard at apex with radiation to the infrascapular area as well as tachycardia and often a gallop rhythm.

There is some growing concern that strict adherence to the Jones criteria could lead to underdiagnosis of ARF. This criticism is specifically based on the criterion of having a compulsory documentation of previous GABHS infection, which may not have been an available or affordable test in developing countries (Pereira et al, 2007; WHO, 2004). WHO criteria are offered in Box 30-8.

Diagnostic Studies
- Rapid streptococcal antigen screening or streptococcal culture is done during the acute illness in children older than 2 years. However, up to two thirds of children with ARF may have negative streptococcal results when tested in the latency period after acute pharyngitis.
- Other tests include antistreptolysin-O titer (ASO), CBC, ESR, and CRP.
- Echocardiograms evaluate valve damage and function.

Management
- Treatment and prevention of GABHS infection are essential.

- Antiinflammatory agents are used to control clinical manifestations of the disease although there is no clear proven benefit. Children with more severe carditis often are given steroids; the lesser cases are given salicylates for 4 to 6 weeks (Yani, 2008).
- Supportive therapy as appropriate is given including surgical valve replacement if necessary.
- Prevention of recurrence can be achieved with prompt identification and treatment of future GABHS infections. In approximately 70% to 80% of patients, valvular disease will resolve if they are compliant in taking antibiotic prophylaxis after the first episode of RHD. This requires penicillin injections every 3 to 4 weeks or daily oral penicillin VK or erythromycin until at least age 40 for those who have had RHD. For patients who have had RF but no carditis, antibiotics are given for 5 years or until age 21, whichever is longer (Yani, 2008).
- See Chapters 23 and 31 for further discussion of treating group A streptococcal infections.

Complications
Carditis presents with mitral and possibly aortic regurgitation in 95% of cases, usually within 2 weeks of RF illness. The mitral valve becomes leaky due to annular dilation and

elongation of the chordate that attach leaflets to the left ventricle. With moderate to severe mitral regurgitation CHF develops; recurrent episodes of RF lead to worsening valve disease.

INFECTIVE ENDOCARDITIS

Description and Epidemiology

IE (formerly SBE) is a condition in which a bacterial or fungal infection invades traumatized endocardial surfaces of the heart, most commonly the cardiac valves. IE usually occurs in children or adults with underlying structural cardiac abnormalities (CHD, ARF) (rarely in those without structural heart disease) and in those with indwelling catheters and devices that are commonly used in oncology or neonatal patients. The incidence of IE has increased as more children with CHD are surviving because of aggressive treatments. Half of cases occur in children older than 10 years, but infection can occur in any age group.

Turbulence caused by stenotic valves, previous surgical repairs, or high-velocity jets (from blood flowing under force through a structural heart defect) traumatizes cardiac endothelium and leads to thrombogenesis. Clumps of platelets and fibrin provide a nidus for circulating bacteria or rarely fungi. The bacteria or fungi multiply, shielded from circulating white cells by the platelet-fibrin matrix. These vegetations cause further damage by destroying nearby valve tissue and extending to surrounding endothelium.

Gram-positive cocci cause 80% of cases of IE in children. *Streptococcus viridans* is the most common causative organism, followed by *Staphylococcus aureus*. HACEK (HACEK refers to a grouping of gram-negative bacilli: *Haemophilus* species) *(H. parainfluenzae, H. aphrophilus, H. paraphrophilus), Actinobacillus actinomycetemcomitans, Cardiobacterium hominis, Eikenella corrodens,* and *Kingella* species organisms are less commonly implicated (Taubert and Gewetz, 2008). Children with CHD appear to have more severe gingival inflammatory conditions, increased plaque accumulation, and more HACEK microbes, which leads to endocarditis (Steelman et al, 2003). Fungal endocarditis is the most severe form with alarming mortality especially in immunocompromised patients and neonates (Taubert and Gewetz, 2008).

Endocarditis is relatively rare in the U.S., accounting for 1 in 1280 pediatric admissions per year (92% of these admissions have CHD or an indwelling catheter). Patients who have had palliative surgery for cyanotic heart disease and those with prosthetic aortic valve replacements are at highest risk for IE (Taubert and Gewetz, 2008). In developing countries where there is a high prevalence of RHD, there is a concurrent increase in IE because RHD-damaged valves are vulnerable to IE.

Clinical Findings

History and Physical Examination

- Acute manifestations: Short duration of illness, high fever (greater than 102.2° F [39° C]), myalgias, night sweats, arthralgias, headache, general malaise, decreased appetite, increase in intensity of preexisting murmur or new onset of murmur
- Embolization symptoms: Hematuria, acute onset of respiratory distress, splenomegaly, neurologic changes (stroke, brain abscesses, hemorrhage, meningitis), petechiae (in

conjunctiva, buccal mucosa, palatal area, nailbeds, palms, and soles). The classical findings— Janeway lesions (flat, nontender lesions on palms and soles), Osler nodes (small raised lesions on pad of fingers and toes), Roth spots (retinal hemorrhages with a central white spot) and splinter hemorrhages—occur rarely in children (Taubert and Gewetz, 2008).

Diagnostic Studies

- The diagnosis is based on clinical findings and results of blood cultures. A persistent low-grade fever in a patient with known cardiac abnormalities should be evaluated immediately with three sets of blood cultures over 24 hours from different sites before the administration of empirical antibiotic therapy. This detects 97% of cases of IE. When three cultures are positive for the same organism, IE must be considered and treatment instituted. The modified Duke criteria for diagnosis can be a useful guideline and are based on clinical, microbiologic, echo, and pathologic data (the Duke criteria are available at www.wikipedia.org/wiki/infectious_endocarditis) (Taubert and Gewetz, 2008).
- The ESR, CRP, and WBC count are elevated in the acute stage; anemia may be evidenced.
- Two-dimensional echocardiography

Management

Treatment should begin as soon as IE is suspected in order to decrease the subsequent morbidity and mortality associated with untreated bacteremia. High doses of appropriate antibiotics are given intravenously for 4 to 6 weeks, although some adults are successfully treated for 2 weeks (Taubert and Gewetz, 2008).

Complications

Infection carries high morbidity and mortality rates and can lead to destruction of heart valves or disseminated sepsis. Septic and thrombotic emboli from bacterial or fungal vegetations can cause abscesses and ischemic damage to distant areas, such as the brain, abdominal viscera, and extremities (Taubert and Gewetz, 2008).

Prevention

For children with high-risk cardiac conditions (previous endocarditis; unrepaired or palliated cyanotic CHD; prosthetic or bioprosthetic valve, shunt, or conduit; repaired CHD with residual defects adjacent to the site of the prosthetic patch or device; and heart transplant recipients) prophylactic antibiotic therapy is given before all dental procedures involving manipulation of gingival tissue. Endocarditis prophylaxis is also recommended for 6 months after heart surgery for all congenital heart patients (Nishimura et al, 2008) (see Tables 30-7 and 30-8).

MYOCARDITIS AND CARDIOMYOPATHY

Myocarditis is a rare inflammatory illness of the muscular walls of the heart. It may go unrecognized in children whose inflammatory process resolved spontaneously, or it may progress to fulminant disease resulting in chronic cardiomyopathy or even death. Myocarditis is often caused by viral infections, most commonly adenoviruses, coxsackievirus A and B, parvovirus B19, echoviruses, and poliovirus. Influenza, cytomegalovirus (CMV), varicella, mumps, human immunodeficiency virus (HIV), RSV, and rubella are other viral causes. Nonviral infections (fungal, bacterial, protozoal, rickettsial), various medications, autoimmune or inflammatory disorders (e.g., ARF, SLE), toxic reactions to infectious agents, or other disorders (e.g., KD) may also be etiologic agents; however, the etiology is often unknown. Myocarditis may occur in epidemics, usually in infants in association with coxsackievirus B (Towbin, 2008).

The inflammatory process in the myocardium leads to dilation of all cardiac chambers, especially the left ventricle. This leads to poor function and stretching of mitral annulus with regurgitation. Eventually the healing process begins (hopefully) but this may lead to replacement of myofibers with fibroblasts and scar formation. This leads to decreased elasticity and performance and creates the substrate for ventricular dysrhythmias (Towbin, 2008).

Clinical Findings

History. As the interstitial inflammation process progresses, cardiac function decreases and symptoms of CHF become evident. The following history is characteristic:

- Infants (may be manifesting intrauterine exposure): Fever, irritability or listlessness, episodes of pallor, diaphoresis; tachypnea or respiratory distress; poor appetite and vomiting
- Children and adolescents: Recent flulike or gastrointestinal viral illness (10 to 14 days previously); lethargy, low-grade fever, pallor; decreased appetite and abdominal pain; exercise intolerance, rashes, palpitations, respiratory distress (late finding)

Physical Examination

- Pallor, mild cyanosis, skin cool and mottled with poor perfusion (in infants)
- Rapid laborious respirations, grunting, decreased pulse oximetry reading
- Tachycardia, gallop rhythm, muffled heart sounds, apical systolic murmur, weak pulses
- Hepatomegaly, jugular venous distention (older children and adolescents)

Diagnostic Studies. Refer patients with symptoms suggestive of myocarditis to a pediatric cardiologist. Diagnostic testing usually involves chest radiography, ECG, two-dimensional echocardiography, CBC, ESR, CRP, cardiac and liver enzymes, viral titers, blood cultures, metabolic studies (e.g., thyroid and carnitine), and viral cultures or PCR from the myocardial tissue.

Differential Diagnosis

Sepsis, asthma, recurrent vomiting, and chronic viral illness are in the differential diagnosis.

Management

- Treatment is supportive with bed rest and medications, such as digitalis, diuretics, ACE inhibitors, and beta-blockers. Occasionally, anticoagulation and antidysrhythmia medications may be used. Many experimental therapies appear promising, including the use of IVIG and

interferon-β (Towbin, 2008). Severe cases may require hospitalization for mechanical ventilation and inotropic support. Recovery often takes 2 to 3 months; follow-up is indefinite. Pericardial effusion and pericarditis can occur concurrently. Long-term ACE inhibitor therapy is recommended for nearly all children with asymptomatic left ventricular dysfunction and with symptomatic HF (Harmon et al, 2009).

Complications and Prognosis

- Scarring of the myocardium may occur and cause persistent heart failure and ventricular dysrhythmias. Cardiac transplantation may be necessary in some patients with myocarditis or cardiomyopathy. However, approximately 50% of children go on to complete recovery (Towbin, 2008).

PERICARDITIS

Pericarditis refers to an inflammation or other abnormality of the pericardium, the sac that surrounds the heart. Excess fluid accumulates in the pericardial space and causes the normally compliant pericardium to distend. As intrapericardial pressure increases, the heart becomes compressed and its ability to fill is limited. Pericarditis may be seen in individuals without a history of cardiac disease. Viral infection (usually coxsackievirus or adenovirus) is the most common cause of pericarditis in children (40% to 75% of cases). Other etiologic agents include infections (tuberculosis, other bacteria), trauma, hypersensitivity to medication (isoniazid [INH], hydralazine), collagen-vascular and connective tissue diseases (ARF, juvenile rheumatoid arthritis, SLE), KD, postsurgical complications, and complications of systemic infection. Pericarditis is most common in children younger than 2 years of age and demonstrates equal sex distribution (Rheuban, 2008). It is a serious illness that may have rapidly fatal consequences if not diagnosed and treated in a timely manner. The following findings should alert the provider to refer the patient to a pediatric cardiologist:

- History of precordial or substernal chest pain altered by respiration, coughing, or position (may not be found in small children); lethargy, loss of appetite, abdominal pain; fever, irritability; tachycardia; viral illness 10 to 14 days before onset of symptoms
- Physical examination findings: Distended neck veins; tachycardia, pericardial friction rub (an early sign heard best along the left sternal border with the patient leaning forward) or muffled heart sounds (if the effusion is large); Kussmaul sign (slow, deep respirations); pulsus paradoxus, a decrease in BP of greater than 10 mm Hg during inspiration with patient in a supine position; hepatomegaly
- ECG can show diffuse ST segment elevation (80%), PR depression, and T-wave inversion.
- Chest x-ray may show enlargement of cardiac silhouette.
- Echocardiogram will show relative quantities of pericardial fluid and compression of cavities if large effusion is seen (Rheuban, 2008).

Myocarditis is the main differential diagnosis. Management consists of pericardiocentesis if tamponade becomes evident, nonsteroidal antiinflammatory drugs (NSAIDs) and analgesics, or, rarely, sternotomy or thoracotomy to control any intrapericardial bleeding. Cardiac tamponade can occur with large or rapid effusions. There is a relapse rate of 15% if the causative agent was viral. Most children recover fully within 3 to 4 weeks (Rheuban, 2008).

Heart Conduction Disturbances

CARDIAC DYSRHYTHMIAS

Epidemiology

Approximately 14 per 100,000 pediatric ED visits are for cardiac dysrhythmias (or arrhythmias). The most common dysrhythmias are sinus tachycardia (most prevalent), supraventricular tachycardia (SVT), bradycardia, and atrial fibrillation (Doniger and Sharieff, 2006). Genetic defects cause some dysrhythmias, most notably long QT syndrome and familial ASD or conduction abnormality defect (Goldmuntz and Lin, 2008). Most abnormal heart rhythms in children with structurally normal hearts are benign, but a dysrhythmia in a child with a cardiac abnormality can be lethal. Any child who has a dysrhythmia or syncope with exertion requires an evaluation for underlying cardiac disease.

Dysrhythmias can manifest as a primary disorder or as a consequence of cardiac or other systemic disorders. The following dysrhythmias (see Table 30-3 for normal heart rates) may be noted:

- Sinus dysrhythmia—variable heart rate that increases with inspiration and decreases with expiration. This is a normal finding in children.
- Bradycardia or slow heart rate for age
  - Sinus bradycardia is the most common cause of bradycardia in children and may be due to hypoxia, acidosis, increased intracranial pressure, abdominal distention, hypothermia, or hypoglycemia. It may also be caused by drugs, such as beta-blockers or digoxin. Mild slowing may be due to increased vagal tone or cardiac conditioning (e.g., athletes) (Doniger and Sharieff, 2006).
  - Complete AV block can either be congenital, as seen in infants of mothers with an autoimmune disease, such as SLE, or may be acquired after cardiac surgery. Certain rare cardiac defects, such as L-transposition of the great arteries and heterotaxy, are also associated with complete heart block. The hemodynamic effect of a slow heart rate depends on how slow it is (Doniger and Sharieff, 2006).
- Tachycardias
  - Sinus tachycardia is caused by predisposing factors that increase cardiac output, including fever, anxiety, infection, drug exposure, dehydration, pain, hyperthyroidism, or anemia among many others. Treatment is directed at the underlying disorder (Doniger and Sharieff, 2006).
  - SVTs are the most common pathologic tachycardias in children:
    - AV reentrant tachycardia is the most common SVT. In AV reentrant tachycardia, there is an additional pathway for impulse transmission from atria to ventricles besides the normal AV node. AV reentrant tachycardias often first present in infants younger than 4 months of age and again in young adolescents (Doniger and Sharieff, 2006). Rarely (less than 10%), children with asymptomatic Wolff-Parkinson-White (WPW) syndrome have potentially life-threatening dysrhythmias.
    - A less common SVT is AV nodal tachycardia, which is also a reentrant tachycardia caused by dual AV node pathways.
    - The rarest type of SVT is ectopic atrial tachycardia caused by an ectopic focus in the atrium. This SVT is much more difficult to diagnose and treat.
- Long QT syndrome–induced ventricular tachycardia. The QT interval is longer than normal in some people as a result of a congenital abnormality or exposure to certain drugs and toxins (a list of such substances is available at www.qtdrugs.org). A QT interval corrected for the heart rate (QTc) of greater than 0.44 second in males and 0.46 second in females is worthy of investigation (McCormack, 2009). If a long QT syndrome is assessed on ECG and there are concerning symptoms (dizziness, palpitations, syncope) or family history, refer to a pediatric cardiologist. All family members need screening if an index case is identified.
- Premature atrial contractions. Depolarization may or may not be conducted through the AV node. Premature contractions can be seen in an infant or child with an otherwise normal heart. It is not unusual to see multiple premature atrial contractions on the ECG of a newborn.
- Premature ventricular contractions—premature QRS complex with a prolonged duration or morphologic difference from the preceding QRS. Occasional premature ventricular contractions are also seen in otherwise normal infants. Premature ventricular contractions that are uniform in appearance, which means that they have the same QRS complex appearance every time, are usually of no consequence.

Clinical Findings

History

- Bradycardia with a sudden decrease in heart rate can cause syncope or severe dizziness.
- SVT can be of sudden onset and variable duration.
  - Infants tolerate several hours of SVT with rates up to 250 beats per minute before demonstrating evidence of poor feeding, irritability, or pallor that can eventually lead to CHF if not converted.
  - Older children may feel quite ill after a few minutes and have complaints of "butterflies" in the chest, dizziness, palpitations, pain in the neck, abdominal pain with nausea and vomiting, and syncope.

Physical Examination

- Slow or fast heart rate; rhythm—regular, irregular, or regularly irregular

Diagnostic Studies. Tests include ECG (the basic screening tool) and 24-hour Holter monitoring or event monitoring if symptoms are sporadic and the ECG is normal.

Differential Diagnosis

The differential diagnosis includes any condition that may elevate or slow heart rate.

Management

A sinus dysrhythmia requires no treatment. Refer all other rhythm abnormalities to a pediatric cardiologist for evaluation. Other findings that require a referral include abnormal ECG; history of unusual heart rhythm; history of syncope or dizziness on exertion with palpitations; or history of cardiac abnormality, heart surgery, or WPW syndrome. For recurrent SVTs, the child or parent may be taught to monitor the heart rate and use vagal maneuvers to break the spell, such as bearing down (Valsalva maneuver).

Complications

Death can occur with some dysrhythmias if untreated.

■ Syncope

DESCRIPTION AND EPIDEMIOLOGY

Syncope is a transient loss of consciousness due to a decrease in cerebral flood flow; recovery is relatively prompt. In assessing a syncopal episode, the provider must distinguish between a simple fainting event versus whether the event is a symptom or a red flag for a serious cardiovascular, neurologic, or other medical condition. The focus of this section on syncope is distinguishing between normal and cardiovascular etiologies associated with syncope. It is important, and often tricky, to distinguish between the two. Symptoms such as dizziness and visual changes may suggest an impending faint or collapse (i.e., cardiac arrest). However, any syncope in a child with heart disease or that is associated with exercise requires immediate evaluation of an underlying cardiac condition.

Ineffective cerebral blood flow due to ineffective cardiac output or cardiovascular control can result in a true syncopal episode. In *cardiac* syncope, this occurs due to a combination of obstruction to left ventricular filling, left ventricular ejection, or ineffective contraction along with an underlying structural, functional, or electrical heart condition (e.g., aortic stenosis, cardiomyopathy, coronary disease) (see discussion earlier in this chapter regarding sudden cardiac death). It often comes without prodromal symptoms or may be associated with palpitation or chest pain (angina). *Simple fainting* (also called neurocardiogenic syncope [NCS]) is neurally mediated and leads to disordered cardiac and vascular regulation. In this case vasodilation, cardiac slowing, and hypotension with resultant cerebral ischemia lead to the individual passing out. NCS may also be further delineated by such specific names as vasovagal syncope, cardioinhibitory syncope, pallid breath-holding spells (or reflex anoxic seizures), vasodepressor syncope, postural orthostatic tachycardia syndrome, or others (Newburger et al, 2006). Ninety-five percent of the time, the syncope is vasodepressive or vasovagal (Sondheimer et al, 2009). Additional causes include neurologic (headache, seizure, transient ischemic attack), psychiatric (depression, panic attack, conversion reaction), and systemic or metabolic (drugs, carbon monoxide, electrolyte imbalance/problems) (Alexander, 2006).

The relatively high incidence of syncope contrasts with a low incidence of aborted and cardiac-related sudden death (1 per 100 patient years) in the pediatric and young adult population. Simple, or common, fainting occurs in approximately 20% to 50% of children from birth to 20 years of age (Sondheimer et al, 2009); 10% to 40% of adolescents have an episode of fainting or presyncopal symptoms after provocative testing (Newburger et al, 2006). Toddlers may faint with breath-holding spells, most commonly between the ages of 6 months and 3 years. More than 65% of these cases resolve

by 5 years or age and the majority by 8 years (after this time, they are usually classified as convulsive syncope). Breath-holding syncope has an incidence of approximately 5% and occurs in boys and girls with equal frequency (Newburger et al, 2006). Simple fainting in female adolescents supersedes that of males. Approximately 20% of adolescents have a history of breath-holding spells as toddlers (Sondheimer et al, 2009).

Clinical Findings

History. A thorough history that focuses on triggers and presyncopal symptoms is the most critical "test" of syncopal causation (Table 30-12). Ninety percent of the time, there is a positive family history of events similar to those the child experiences (Sondheimer et al, 2009). Important information to obtain includes the following:

- A triggering factor, such as exercise, pain, or an emotional event (e.g., anxiety, panic)
- A prior incident or incidents of syncope or fainting (e.g., venipuncture, seeing blood, experiencing an injury)
- An associated injury, clonic-tonic movements, or vertigo
- Associated chest pain, palpitations, tachycardia, or bradycardia

TABLE 30-12	Relative Frequency of Premonitory Symptoms and Residual Findings With Common Neurally Mediated Syncope Versus More Serious Cardiac Syncope

	Neurally Mediated	Cardiac Syncope
Symptoms		
Premonitory symptoms	+++	±
Lightheadedness	+++	+/±
Palpitations	+	++
Occurs while upright	+++	+
Occurs while sitting	+/±	+
Emotional trigger	++	++
Exercise trigger	+	++
Residual Findings		
Pallor	+++	+/±
Incontinence	−	+
Disorientation	−	+
Fatigue	++	±
Diaphoresis	++	±
Injury	+	++

+++, Very common (>~50%); ++ common (>~20%); + not rare (>~5%); ± uncommon (<5%); − rare (<~1%).
From Newburger JW, Alexander ME, Fulton DR: Innocent murmurs, syncope, and chest pain. In Keane JF, Lock JE, Fyler DC, editors: *Nadas' pediatric cardiology*, ed 2, Philadelphia, 2006, Saunders. Reprinted with permission.

- A family history of sudden death before age 40; congenital deafness; long QT syndrome; cardiomyopathy; recurrent adolescent or toddler syncope that was outgrown (Newburger et al, 2006)
- The possibility of pregnancy or the use of drugs; list other medications
- A history of exercise-induced asthma, respiratory distress, or other concomitant medical disorder
- A known psychological stress or stressors at home or school or in social environments
- Standing for any length of time prior to the episode indicates orthostasis; history of "head rushes" when standing up
- In a hot environment, sweating, dehydration; hunger
- Nausea, constriction of visual fields ("world going dark") prior to episode
- Any postepisode symptoms such as dizziness, pallor, clammy feeling, exhaustion, headache
- A history of otherwise being well, active, with minimal medical issues
- Arousal after fainting within 1 to 2 minutes; recovery may have taken more than 1 hour
- Stiffening, jerking motions during unconsciousness (tonic-clonic muscular contractions of face [including fixed upward deviation of eyes], trunk, and extremities mimicking epilepsy occurs in approximately 50% of individuals) (Johnston, 2007)
- Other activities prior to episode: hair grooming, coughing, micturition, neck stretching (Sondheimer et al, 2009)

Physical Examination. A detailed neurologic examination is needed if the syncopal episode suggests a seizure disorder. Careful evaluation of the head, eyes, ears, nose, and throat is done if vestibular disease is likely. A cardiovascular examination is especially important.

Diagnostic Tests. The majority of individuals with cardiac syncope are identified either by a history of associated presyncopal symptoms with exercise, abnormal ECG, family history of dysrhythmia, or abnormal physical examination (Newburger et al, 2006). The diagnosis of neurally mediated syncope can confidently be made based on history, examination, and ECG. The diagnostic workup to distinguish between the two consists of:

- Orthosatic vital signs: More than a 30 mm Hg drop in BP after standing for 5 to 10 minutes, or a baseline systolic pressure of less than 80 mm Hg in an adolescent
- Hemoglobin, if anemia is suspected. CBC, random glucose, and glucose tolerance tests have low yields and are not recommended routine tests for syncope.
- 12-lead ECG, looking for left ventricular hypertrophy, WPW syndrome, AV and interventricular conduction defects, electrical myopathies (e.g., long QT syndrome). If ECG results are borderline or family history is highly suggestive of cardiac etiology, ECGs on siblings and parents may be useful. Twenty-four hour Holter monitoring and portable event monitoring can be useful to rule out serious disease.

- Echocardiography: Can be useful when history, physical, ECG, family history suggest cardiac disease or cardiac syncope
- Cardiac catheterization: Can be useful in those with CHD who have symptoms of syncope, palpitations, nonsustained ventricular tachycardia, other dysrhythmias.
- Head-up tilt testing produces false-positive results. It is used more as a confirmatory test of vasodepressive syncope in individuals with frequent, recurrent syncopal episodes. In adolescence, an assessment of the level of anxiety may be a better predictor of future faints than the head-up tilt test. Studies have shown that 40% of asymptomatic adolescent volunteers experience presyncopal symptoms with a 70-degree tilt (Newburger et al, 2006).
- Treadmill exercise testing may be used in some individuals with problematic syncope.

Management

If cardiac syncope is suspected, a referral to a pediatric cardiologist for further evaluation is paramount. Restrict the child from sports participation until then.

For neurally mediated syncope, education (regarding cause, prevention, and how to abort a syncopal event) is key. Prevention involves ensuring good hydration (along with decreasing caffeine and increasing sodium intake) and initiating antigravity techniques at the onset of presyncopal sensations (isometric leg or arm contractions; positional shifts from supine to upright; squatting or lying down; possibly using compression socks). Having the individual rest for 5 to 10 minutes either supine or with legs up if prodromal symptoms occur or after a fainting episode is important (standing up too quickly after an episode may trigger repeated syncope). Tilt training and upright, weight-bearing aerobic exercises have also been used. Concomitant cognitive-behavioral therapy is indicated if the episodes are psychogenic in etiology.

In refractory cases, pharmacologic management may play a role, though this should not be first-line treatment. These therapies may involve the use of volume enhancement (using fludrocortisone; 0.1 mg/kg/day); limiting excessive catecholamine drive (using beta-blockers, such as atenolol; 0.5 to 2 mg/kg/day); vagolytic agents (disopyramide; 2.5 mg/kg four times daily), and/or selective serotonin reuptake inhibitors (SSRIs) (Sondheimer et al, 2009). If drug therapy is used, the typical duration is for 1 year followed by weaning. Pacemaker implantation has been used in rare cases.

Differential Diagnosis

Differential diagnosis includes migraine with confusion or stupor, seizures, hypoglycemia, hysteria, hyperventilation, vertigo, carbon monoxide poisoning, electrolyte imbalance, drugs, and cardiovascular disease including underlying dysrhythmia (Sondheimer et al, 2009).

Respiratory Disorders

RITA MARIE JOHN AND MARGARET A. BRADY

Respiratory problems are a leading cause of illness in children and a major reason for health care visits. Viral upper respiratory infections (URIs), pharyngitis, and otitis media are common diagnoses seen every day by practitioners. Parents seek health care to confirm the appropriate management of upper respiratory disorders for common cold, otitis media, rhinosinusitis, and tonsillopharyngitis. Parents seeking to relieve their child's upper respiratory tract symptoms may use a variety of over-the-counter medications or try to pressure the primary care provider to prescribe cold medications or antibiotics. In contrast, a child with a lower respiratory tract disorder such as asthma or bacterial pneumonia can experience a potentially life-threatening illness that demands prompt attention. Providers who ask key questions about the history of the respiratory symptoms; do a systematic and complete examination of the upper and lower airways, including the sinuses; and, if indicated, order specific laboratory tests and radiographic examinations can determine an accurate diagnosis and develop a successful treatment plan in most cases. When children have complicated problems, they can be referred with baseline information to the appropriate medical specialist for additional studies and treatment.

■ Anatomy and Physiology

UPPER RESPIRATORY TRACT

The upper respiratory tract includes the nostrils, nasopharynx, larynx, upper part of the trachea, eustachian tubes, and sinuses. Air is warmed and humidified as it travels through the nasal passages, and particles are filtered out by coarse nasal hairs. The nasal passages are lined with lysozymes, secretory immunoglobulin A (IgA) and IgG in nasal mucus to defend against microbial invasion. The nasal mucosa is continuous and similar to the sinus mucosa except that the nasal mucosa is thicker with more glands (Cherry and Shapiro, 2010). A blanket of mucus covers the surface epithelium of the nasal and sinus mucosa. The mucociliary action of the paranasal epithelium moves secretions from the sinuses to the nasal cavity. The frontal, maxillary, and anterior parts of the ethmoid sinuses drain to the middle meatus of the nose, whereas the sphenoid and posterior parts of the ethmoid sinuses drain to the superior meatus of the nose (DeMuri and Wald, 2010). Secretions need to be able to move through patent ostia into the nose. The quality of secretions and normally functioning cilia are key factors in the movement of secretions into the nose. Inflammation of nasal mucosa frequently causes edema and disruption of the sinus secretions. If there is significant swelling of the ostia due to URI or allergic inflammation, or mechanical or local obstruction, ostial obstruction results and obstruction of the sinus secretions occurs. Cilia movement and mucus flow allow the sinuses to be free of pathogens.

The maxillary sinuses are present by the second trimester of gestation but are not fully pneumatized until a child is about 4 years old. Ethmoid sinuses develop by the fourth month of gestation and form the thin lateral walls of the orbit of the eye. They are pneumatized at birth and can be visualized on plain radiographs when the child is 1 to 2 years old. The sphenoid sinuses start to form in the first 2 years of life but remain rudimentary until age 6 when they become visible on radiographs. They reach their permanent size, but not shape, by age 12 years. As a result, the nasal cavity and paranasal sinuses reach adult proportion by age 12 (Cherry and Shapiro, 2010). The sinuses become clinically significant sites of infection as follows:

- Maxillary and ethmoid sinuses as early as late infancy
- Sphenoid sinuses around the third and fourth years of life
- Frontal sinuses around the sixth to tenth years of life

The epiglottis deflects swallowed material toward the esophagus to protect the larynx. The vocal cords form a V-shaped opening known as the glottis. The subglottic space is beneath the vocal cords, and its walls converge toward the cricoid ring to form a complete ring of cartilage around the larynx. In children less than 2 to 3 years old, the cricoid ring is the narrowest part of the airway; in older children and adults, the glottis is narrowest. The rings of tracheal cartilage support the trachea and the mainstem bronchi.

The trachea and airways of the infant and young child are more compliant than those of an adult. Hyperextension of the neck can constrict the airway of infants. Consequently, changes in intrapleural pressure lead to greater changes in an infant's or young child's airways compared with the effect that such changes would exert on adult airways, thereby causing an increased risk of airway collapse. Similarly, increased chest wall compliance in young infants makes them more vulnerable to adverse events, and their respiratory muscles cannot effectively handle sustained, intense respiratory workload that occurs during severe pulmonary illnesses (Sarnaik and Heidemann, 2007).

LOWER RESPIRATORY TRACT

The right lung has three lobes, upper, middle, and lower, with the upper and middle being separated by a minor fissure. The left lung has two lobes, upper and lower, separated by a major fissure. The upper left lobe has an area called the *lingula* that corresponds to the right middle lobe. The right mainstem bronchus is shorter and wider than the left bronchus. It forms a smaller angle away from the trachea than the left bronchus does. This anatomic variation explains why foreign bodies (FBs) usually lodge in the right mainstem bronchus. Although the body surface and the number of respiratory airways and alveoli increase 10-fold from birth to adult life, the tissue available for gas exchange increases approximately 20-fold. The newborn's chest is cylindrically shaped and has relatively horizontal ribs, which limits the infant's ability to expand his or her chest. Because there is greater transverse growth in the lower part of the chest wall, the shape of the chest changes during the first few years of life. This differential growth results in the ribs being positioned lower anteriorly than posteriorly. The change in positioning of the ribs adds rigidity to the thorax of older children.

The diaphragm is the main muscle of respiration, and the intercostal, sternocleidomastoid, spinal, neck, and abdominal muscles are accessory muscles that can be used to increase effort. Normal exhalation occurs from elastic recoil of the lung.

Primitive airways appear at approximately the fourth week of gestation. At about the sixteenth week of gestation, the number of bronchial branches equals that in adults. Subsequent growth continues by increasing the length of the respiratory tract. During the sixteenth to twenty-sixth weeks of gestation, vascularization of the future respiratory portion of the lung occurs. Cartilage, glands, and muscles of the airways and type II alveolar cells are formed by week 28. Type II cells allow the fetus to produce a phospholipid called surfactant. The airways continue to grow, and terminal sac formation occurs. At approximately week 36, the terminal sacs divide, and alveoli are formed. Approximately 50 million primitive alveoli are present at birth.

After birth the alveolar ducts branch off the third respiratory bronchioles. Alveoli continue to form and number 100 to 200 million in older children and 200 to 600 million in adolescents. The alveolar sacs continue to increase in size. The adult lung contains approximately 300 million alveoli.

Other structures important for gas exchange and pulmonary function are present at birth and include cartilage, mucus glands, goblet cells, and ciliated cells of the conducting airways. The airways above the bronchioles are lined with ciliated pseudostratified columnar cells as well as goblet cells. Mucus is produced from the mucus glands that line the respiratory tract. The cilia play a critical role of sweeping mucus and debris toward the upper respiratory tract. Smooth muscle is also present; therefore, even very young infants can have bronchospasm. Beyond the bronchioles a thin layer of surfactant that reduces surface tension and prevents airway collapse.

Airway resistance is higher in newborns and young children than in adults. The airways of young infants and children are easily obstructed by inflammation, FBs, or mucous. The maximal inspiratory pressure generated by an infant is equal to that of an adult. However, the chest wall and supporting structures are softer and more flexible, so chest wall retraction is greatest in young infants. The chest wall of a newborn is highly compliant.

■ Pathophysiology Involved in Airway Disease

All lung disorders cause some form of airway obstruction. Narrowing of the airway lumen results from one or more of the following:

- Presence of intraluminal material (e.g., secretions, tumors, or foreign matter)
- Mural thickening (e.g., edema or hypertrophy of the glands or mucosa)
- Contraction of smooth muscle (e.g., spasm)
- Extrinsic compression

These factors rarely occur in isolation. They cause pulmonary malfunction by impairing tracheobronchial hygiene and impeding normal airflow. Severe airway obstruction can occur in infants or young children from very small blockages because of their airway size.

The two major types of airway obstruction are complete and partial. In complete obstruction neither airflow nor drainage of secretions occurs. Such occlusion leads to lobar atelectasis after the residual gas diffuses into the pulmonary circulation. In partial airway obstruction, airflow and secretion drainage occur but are impaired. Partial obstruction can be further divided into two separate classifications. The first consists of a bypass valve obstruction caused by narrowing of the lumen; a wheeze may be produced. Although resistance to flow is increased, air can still flow in during inspiration and out during expiration. The second is a check-valve or ball-valve obstruction; air entry is possible, but during expiration the lumen is completely occluded so that escape of air is impossible. Bronchial FBs and emphysema are associated with bypass, check-valve, or ball-valve obstructions that result in overinflation of lung airways.

Airway obstruction that occurs above the level of the secondary bronchi generally interferes more with inspiration than expiration. If the obstruction is complete and above the bifurcation of the trachea, asphyxia and death can result. Partial obstruction may result in severe dyspnea, stridor (a harsh high-pitched inspiratory sound), and subcostal retractions. Coughing removes nonfixed, high airway obstruction. Poor inspiratory airflow limits the coughing effectiveness. The sound produced by coughing may indicate the level of airway obstruction and assists in making a diagnosis. Obstructions next to the larynx produce a cough that sounds croupy or barking. Obstructions in the trachea or major bronchi produce a brassy sound.

Lower airway obstructions result from peripheral lesions that are usually diffuse in location and involve bronchioles smaller than 3 mm. The usual mechanism of narrowing is spasm, accumulation of secretions, edema of the mucous membrane, extrinsic compression, or any combination of these factors. Complete airway obstruction causes atelectasis. A large percentage of the lung volume needs to be involved before symptoms become apparent; small atelectatic changes do not produce obvious clinical manifestations.

The primary clinical manifestation of lower airway obstruction occurs during expiration. Wheezing is the principal sound patients make if the obstruction allows enough air to pass through the narrowed lumen. Chest excursion diminishes, and the expiratory phase prolongs. Increased airway resistance during exhalation results in overinflation of the lungs, which in turn eventually increases the anteroposterior diameter of the chest. Chronic overinflation results in the "barrel chest" typical of a patient with chronic lung disease such as cystic fibrosis (CF) or emphysema. The accumulation of fluids and inflammation in the lower airways usually results in a repetitive hacking, ineffectual cough. On physical examination, percussing an overinflated chest elicits hyperresonance.

Symptoms worsen as obstruction increases. The body attempts to compensate by using accessory muscles to assist in breathing. Dyspnea can result and may include orthopnea and exercise intolerance. Cyanosis appears as the oxygen saturation drops below 85% and is an ominous sign. Mild obstruction is marked by reduced respiratory rate and increased tidal volume; severe obstruction is characterized by increased respiratory rate, increased retractions with the use of accessory muscles, anxiety, and cyanosis.

Fine crackles or rales indicate respiratory pathology and are short, crackling sounds heard during inspiration. These sounds are caused by airways suddenly opening after having been previously closed. The gas pressure between the compartments equalizes and creates the crackling sound. Fluid accumulation in the airways may also result in crackles. Crackles or rales are not cleared by coughing.

Airway obstruction is the underlying etiology for the most common forms of pediatric lung diseases. Restrictive disease is less common in pediatric patients and is characterized by decreased lung compliance with relatively normal flow rates. Examples of causative factors include neuromuscular weakness, lobar pneumonia, pleural effusion or masses, severe pectus excavatum, or abdominal distention. Key findings of restrictive lung disease are rapid respiratory rate and decreased tidal volume/capacity (Carter and Marshall, 2011; Sarnaik and Heidemann, 2007).

■ Defense Systems

The respiratory defense system includes mechanical and biologic processes. Mechanical defenses include:

- Filtering of particles
- Warming and humidifying of inspired air
- Clearing of airway through mucociliary and coughing actions
- Spasm and breathing changes

Approximately 75% of inspired air is warmed as it passes through the nose, paranasal sinuses, pharynx, larynx, and upper portion of the trachea. Final warming and humidifying of the airstream take place in the trachea and large bronchi. Heat and moisture are removed during the expiratory phase of respiration. The nose has a large surface area on which particles larger than 5 mm are trapped and filtered to prevent them from entering the lower airways. The trachea and bronchioles are lined with various defensive cells and mucus glands. Goblet cells secrete the mucous layer that lies on the tip of cilia. Particles entering the conducting airway are quickly cleared by the mucociliary defenses. Coughing is a reflex mechanism that has three phases: (1) inspiratory, (2) compressive, and (3) expiratory (Chang, 2009). Through forceful expiration foreign bodies and other materials can be removed from the airways; coughing propels particles. Young infants and children cannot effectively expectorate mucus, so they swallow it. Cough reflex loss causes aspiration and pneumonia. Temporary breathing cessation, reflex shallow breathing,

laryngospasm, and even bronchospasm are compensatory efforts aimed at stopping foreign matter from further entry into the lower respiratory tract. However, these respiratory efforts offer limited protection and have significant drawbacks.

Biologic processes that protect the respiratory system include:

- Phagocytosis
- Absorption of noxious gases in the vasculature of the upper airway
- Absorption of particles by the lymph system

Phagocytosis, aided by the secretory immunoglobulin IgA plus interferon, lysozyme, and lactoferrin, is the principal antimicrobial defense. Particles reaching the alveoli can be phagocytized by alveolar macrophages and polymorphonuclear cells, cleared from the lung by the mucociliary system, or carried by lymphocytes into regional nodes or the blood. These particles can take days to months to clear.

The respiratory defense system is at risk for compromise from numerous environmental factors. Damage to epithelial cells is caused by a variety of substances and gases such as sulfur, nitrogen dioxide, ozone, chlorine, ammonia, and cigarette smoke. Hypothermia, hyperthermia, morphine, codeine, and hypothyroidism can adversely alter mucociliary defenses. Dry air from mouth breathing during periods of nasal obstruction, tracheostomy placement, or inadequately humidified oxygen therapy results in dryness of the mucous membrane and slowing of the cilia beat. Cold air is also irritating to the lower airways.

Phagocytic ability is also reduced by many substances, including ethanol ingestion and cigarette smoke. Hypoxemia, starvation, chilling, corticosteroids, increased oxygen, narcotics, and some anesthetic gases also impair phagocytosis. Recent acute viral infections can reduce antibacterial killing capacity. Damage from infection and chemical irritants may or may not be reversible.

Recurrent respiratory infections in children merit investigation for immunodeficiencies or other underlying diseases such as primary ciliary dyskinesia or cystic fibrosis. The mnemonic SPUR can help determine which children need further workup:

S = severe infection
P = persistent infection and poor recovery
U = unusual organisms
R = recurrent infection (Bush, 2009)

Immunodeficiencies should be considered if the child has eight or more new ear infections in a year, two or more serious sinus infections, persistent oral candidiasis, 2 or more months on antibiotics without improvement, and/or the need for intravenous (IV) antibiotics to clear infections. Also consider immunodeficiencies if there is recurrent pneumonia, failure to thrive, a family history of immunodeficiency, or two or more deep skin infections (Bush, 2009).

■ Assessment of the Respiratory System

The history provides valuable information about the causes, progression, and potential complications of a child's respiratory condition. The physical examination and diagnostic testing allow the provider to determine the extent of respiratory distress.

HISTORY

- History of the present illness can be assessed using the mnemonic PQRST:
  - P = Promoting, preventing, precipitating, palliating factors
    - *Contacts.* Are any family members or close contacts (e.g., daycare, school) ill with similar signs and symptoms?
    - *Prevention.* Are you using any medications to prevent colds (e.g., zinc lozenges, echinacea, and vitamin C are touted in the lay press as prevention measures, but may have negative side effects in children and adolescents)?
    - *Progression.* Are the respiratory signs or symptoms increasing in severity, lessening, or about the same? Is the child easily fatigued, less active, having trouble sleeping, or working harder to breathe?
    - *Treatment.* Have any over-the-counter or prescription drugs been used? Have any other treatment modalities been used, including folk cures, complementary therapies, or home remedies?
  - Q = Quality or quantity
    - How severe are the symptoms? Is the illness interfering with school attendance or play? Are breathing problems affecting the child's ability to sleep and eat?
  - R = Region or radiation
    - Does the child complain of chest pain?
  - S = Severity, setting, simultaneous symptoms or similar illnesses in the past
    - *Key signs and symptoms.* Has the child had symptoms or signs of a daytime or nighttime cough, fever, vomiting, malaise, rhinorrhea, sore throat, lesions in the mouth, retractions, cyanosis, dyspnea, or increased respiratory effort? Table 31-1 lists key characteristics and causes of cough.
    - *Associated symptoms.* Has there been a decrease in appetite or feeding? Any rashes, headaches, or abdominal pain?
    - *Similar illnesses in the past.* Does the child have a history of respiratory tract infections, allergies, or asthma? How many similar infections has the child had (e.g., croup, pneumonia, rhinosinusitis, streptococcal tonsillopharyngitis, frequent colds)?
  - T = Temporal factors
    - When did the illness begin?
    - Was the onset acute or insidious or proceeded by the common cold?
    - How long has it lasted? How has it changed over time?
    - Does the child have a history of respiratory tract infections, allergies, or asthma? How many similar infections has the child had (e.g., croup, pneumonia, rhinosinusitis, streptococcal tonsillopharyngitis, frequent colds)?
- Family history
  - Do others in the family have a history of allergies or asthma?
  - Is there any family history of immunodeficiency, ear-nose-throat, or respiratory problems?
  - Does anyone in the family have genetic diseases such as CF or alpha 1-antitrypsin deficiency?
- Review of systems
  - Note any infections, constitutional diseases, or congenital problems that might have a respiratory component.
- Environment
  - Does anyone in the family or in the daycare setting smoke? Does the child live or attend school in an urban or industrial area subject to air pollution (e.g., near a major highway, industrial plant, or bus terminal)?

PHYSICAL EXAMINATION

When determining respiratory distress, think about the total presentation and not just individual isolated findings. Consider the anxiety level, respiratory rate and rhythm, use of accessory muscles, color, breath sounds, grunting, and pulse oximetry results. Information pertinent to the physical examination of a child with suspected respiratory disease includes the following:

- Measurement of vital signs and observation of general appearance:
  - A normal respiratory rate is age dependent and, if elevated, is a key indicator of lower respiratory involvement.
  - The level of anxiety, nasal flaring, and position of comfort are useful indicators of respiratory distress. Changes in skin color may be subtle or obvious depending on the level of deoxygenation. Grunting is a sign of small airway disease.
- Inspection of:
  - Nose: Look for rhinorrhea—clear, mucoid, mucopurulent; FBs, erosion, polyps, lesions, bleeding; septal position; and color of the mucous membrane.
  - Throat, pharynx, and tonsils: Look for lesions, vesicles, exudate, enlargement of any structure, or other abnormalities. If epiglottitis is a consideration, do not inspect the mouth or attempt to elicit a gag reflex.
  - Chest: Look at the depth, ease, symmetry, and rhythm of respiration. These are key indicators of lower respiratory tract involvement. The use of accessory muscles and the presence of retractions should be noted. A prolonged expiratory phase is associated with respiratory obstruction in the lower airways.
- Palpation or percussion (or both) of:
  - Paranasal and frontal sinus: Palpate for signs of sinus tenderness, knowing that this is a very insensitive physical assessment finding. Note: Take child's age into consideration when determining likelihood of sinus pathology.
  - Chest: Percuss for signs of dullness or hyperresonance caused by consolidation, fluid, or air trapping.
- Auscultation of the chest:
  - Upper tract: Pathology frequently causes noisy breathing, snoring, stridor, rhonchi and can be a source of referred breath sounds (Mellis, 2009).
  - Lower tract: Pathology is suggested by fine crackles or rales, rhonchi, rattles, and polyphonic and monophonic wheezing (Mellis, 2009).

DIAGNOSTIC TESTS

Diagnostic procedures used to evaluate respiratory illness in children managed as outpatients include the following:

- Monitoring oxygenation by pulse oximetry and blood gases:
  - Pulse oximetry can be used to continuously measure pulse rate and peripheral oxygen saturation in arterial

TABLE 31-1 Key Characteristics of Cough, Common Causes, and Questions to Ask in a Pediatric History

Key Characteristics to Consider and Questions to Ask

Age factor	Infants have a weak, nonproductive cough.
Quality	Staccato-like (*Chlamydia trachomatis* in infants); barking or brassy (croup, tracheomalacia, habit cough); paroxysmal or inspiratory whoop (pertussis or parapertussis); honking (psychogenic). Is the cough wet or dry?
Duration	*Acute* (most causes are infectious and last less than 2 weeks), *subacute* cough lasts from 2-4 weeks; *recurrent* (associated with allergies and asthma), or *chronic* lasting greater than 4-8 weeks (e.g., CF, asthma). Is the cough continuous or intermittent?
Productivity	Mucus producing or nonproductive?
Timing	During the day, night (associated with asthma), or both?
Effect on parent and child	Are parents frustrated with the cough? Is it causing them to lose sleep and work time? Are they concerned that the child may have something serious?
Associated symptoms	Fever—may indicate bacterial infection (pneumonia) Rhinorrhea, sneezing, wheezing, atopic dermatitis—associated with asthma and allergic rhinitis Malaise, sneezing, watery nasal discharge, mild sore throat, no or low fever, not ill appearing—typical of URI Tachypnea—pneumonia or bronchiolitis in infants (infants may not have a cough)
Exposure to infection or travel	Has the child been out of the country (tuberculosis)? Is there a member of the household being treated for "bronchitis" or another cough illness?

Causes

Congenital anomalies	Tracheoesophageal fistula, vascular ring, laryngeal cleft, vocal cord paralysis, pulmonary malformations, tracheobronchomalacia, congenital heart disease
Infectious agent	Viral (RSV, adenovirus, parainfluenza, HIV, metapneumovirus, human bocavirus), bacterial (tuberculosis, pertussis, *Streptococcus pneumoniae*), fungal, and atypical bacteria (*Chlamydia* and *Mycoplasma*)
Allergic condition	Allergic rhinitis, asthma
Other	FB aspiration, gastroesophageal reflux, psychogenic cough, environmental triggers (air pollution, tobacco smoke, wood smoke, glue sniffing, volatile chemicals), CF, drug induced, tumor, congestive heart failure

CF, Cystic fibrosis; *FB,* foreign body; *HIV,* human immunodeficiency virus; *RSV,* respiratory syncytial virus; *URI,* upper respiratory infection.
Adapted from Chang AB: Cough, *Pediatr Clin North Am* 56:19-31, 2009; Cherry JD: Croup (laryngitis, laryngotracheitis, spasmodic croup, laryngotracheobronchitis, bacterial tracheitis, and laryngotracheobronchopneumonitis. In Cherry J, Demmler-Harrison G, Kaplan S et al, editors:. *Feigin & Cherry's textbook of pediatric infectious diseases,* ed 6, Philadelphia, 2010, Saunders, pp 254-268.

blood. The oxyhemoglobin saturation percentage (SpO_2) is digitally displayed. Results generally correlate well with simultaneous arterial saturation (SaO_2). With anoxia, there is a rise in organic phosphate content within the red blood cells that results in more O_2 available to tissues. People living at higher elevations suffer from chronic hypoxia. When first arriving at a high elevation, many individuals experience a transient mountain sickness with symptoms that include headache, insomnia, irritability, breathlessness, nausea, and vomiting. This phenomenon lasts approximately 1 week before acclimatization begins. The affected person begins to increase production of red blood cells (RBCs). Finally, a functional nonpathologic right ventricular hypertrophy takes place. These effects last as long as the person remains at high elevation. Severe altitude sickness can lead to cerebral and pulmonary edema and can be life-threatening.

○ Blood gas studies can help the provider assess possible respiratory collapse and are used in acute care settings. A rising $Paco_2$ is an ominous sign.

• Unless there is chronic or complicated rhinosinusitis, imaging in acute rhinosinusitis remains controversial because uncomplicated URIs can cause abnormalities of the paranasal sinuses (Cherry and Shapiro, 2010; DeMuri and Wald, 2010). Radiographic imaging in respiratory disease may be necessary, including radiographs, ultrasonography, magnetic resonance imaging (MRI), and computed tomography (CT) of the sinuses, soft tissues of the neck, and chest. Abnormalities of the nasal mucosa such as thickening may reflect inflammation. Chest radiographs should be done in both posteroanterior and lateral positions because lesions may only be seen in one of the two views. Fluoroscopy is useful in the evaluation of stridor and abnormal movement of the diaphragm. Several other pulmonary studies may be ordered by the medical specialists to whom the child is referred. Contrast studies (e.g., barium esophagogram) are useful for patients with recurrent pneumonia, persistent cough, tracheal ring, or suspected fistulas. Other imaging studies that might be needed to assess these children include bronchograms (useful in delineating the smaller airways), pulmonary arteriograms (evaluation of the pulmonary vasculature), and radionuclide studies (evaluation of the pulmonary capillary bed). Pulmonary function tests are discussed in Chapter 24 in the section on asthma.

- Other specialized tests, including sweat testing, cultures and blood work, are addressed under the specific illness.
- Endoscopy (bronchoscopy and laryngoscopy), bronchoalveolar lavage, percutaneous tap, lung biopsy, and microbiology studies are other helpful diagnostic procedures if used appropriately. Children who have unusual signs and symptoms that require such procedures should be referred to medical specialists.

Basic Respiratory Management Strategies

GENERAL MEASURES

Children who are significantly ill or have unusual manifestations need referral to or consultation with a pediatrician or pediatric subspecialist. General management measures include the following:

- *Fluid.* Hydration is important to keep mucous membranes and secretions moist. Intake of fluids should be encouraged and parents of young children should be given guidelines regarding the type, amount, and frequency of fluids and feedings that their child should take.
- *Oxygen administration.* The use of supplemental oxygen is important to help relieve hypoxemia in most children who have acute respiratory distress. Depression of the respiratory drive is possible with supplemental oxygen administration if the central nervous system (CNS) chemoreceptors are blunted by hypercapnia. However, children at risk for blunting are those with issues related to chronic hypercapnia and are generally easily recognized because they tend to have chronic severe respiratory diseases such as CF and bronchopulmonary dysplasia. In acute situations, administer oxygen using an appropriately sized mask or a high-flow O_2 source held near the child's face if a mask frightens the child. The safe, acceptable range of O_2 saturation is 92% to 95%; higher levels may lead to oxygen toxicity (Chin, 2010; Robinson and Van Asperen, 2009). Children seen in primary care settings who require supplemental oxygen should be transported to an acute care hospital setting via emergency medical services for evaluation and stabilization.
- *Humidification.* For a child with laryngotracheobronchitis (LTB), taking the child out into the cold night air or opening a freezer door may be beneficial. There is no evidence for the use of steam or humidification in croup (Everard, 2009). A cold-mist vaporizer helps provide moisture to the nares and oropharynx during a common cold, but the vaporizer must be cleaned daily so that it will not become a source of infection.
- *Bulb syringe.* Because infants are obligate nose breathers, parents should be instructed in use of the nasal bulb syringe to relieve obstruction of the infant's nares with mucus. Use the bulb syringe gently and intermittently because improper use can cause irritation, inflammation, and respiratory obstruction from tissue damage. Providing parents with written instruction on suctioning the infant's nose with a bulb syringe is advantageous. Cincinnati Children's

Hospital Medical Center has home instructions for this technique available on its website.
- *Normal saline nose drops, nasal rinses, or spray.* Use before feedings and when mucus is thick or crusted. Follow by suctioning the nares with a bulb syringe. Saline nasal rinses are widely available commercially and are helpful for older children and adolescents.

MEDICATIONS

The following pharmacologic agents may be needed to treat various respiratory illnesses:

- *Antibiotics.* Specific agents are discussed in the section on individual illnesses. If an antibiotic is prescribed, the drug should be taken until completed.
- *Analgesics and antipyretics.* Acetaminophen and ibuprofen may be prescribed for relief of pain or fever.
- *Decongestants and antihistamines.* The use of decongestants and antihistamines does not shorten the course of a disease, but can provide relief of nasal symptoms. However, due to the risk of overdosage and unsupervised ingestions, these agents should not be used in children younger than 4 years of age (Centers for Disease Control and Prevention [CDC], 2008). Practitioners need to use caution in prescribing these agents in children younger than 6 years.
- *Expectorants.* Water is one of the most effective expectorants. Over-the-counter agents provide some symptomatic relief, but do not shorten the course of respiratory illnesses. Do not use in children younger than 4 years (CDC, 2008).
- *Cough medication.* Cough suppressant medications should be prescribed judiciously because coughing is a protective mechanism to clear secretions. In review of evidence-based guidelines for the intervention in pediatric cough, the only cough medication that was recommended was honey, provided the child was more than 1 year old (Chang, 2009). However, the study results may be the result of a placebo effect (Paul et al, 2007).

All health care providers must be cognizant of their role in the prevention of superinfections caused by the indiscriminate use of antibiotics.

PATIENT AND PARENT EDUCATION

Frequent handwashing and avoiding touching eyes and nose can help prevent the spread of infection. Parents should be educated about assessment and management of changes in the child's condition. Significant educational issues are identified in Box 31-1.

Indications for Tonsillectomy and Adenoidectomy

Controversy remains about the need for tonsillectomy, adenoidectomy, or both, particularly for less affected children (Burton and Glasziou, 2009). Tonsillectomy has been found to be beneficial in children who are severely affected with recurrent tonsillitis (Morris, 2009). Tonsillectomy may be helpful in the syndrome of periodic fever, aphthous stomatitis, pharyngitis, and cervical adenitis (PFAPA syndrome) (Garavello et al, 2009; Licameli et al, 2008) and in obstructive sleep apnea. The provider must weigh the pros and cons of

BOX 31-1 Parental Education for At-Home Care of the Child With a Respiratory Tract Infection

Infection: Issues to Discuss

Fluid: Give guidelines on type, amount, and frequency of fluids child should take.

Humidification: For laryngotracheobronchitis, take the child out into the cold night air or open a freezer door. In dry climates, humidifiers help in common colds; instruct about cleaning of nebulizers and humidifiers (see below).

Bulb syringe: Instruct to use the bulb syringe gently and intermittently for suctioning the nares.

Normal saline nose drops or spray: Use before feedings and when mucus is thick or crusted. Follow by suctioning nares with bulb syringe.

Other educational issues to cover:

- Indications for immediate reevaluation of child:
  o Signs and symptoms of respiratory distress
  o Other indicators of worsening of illness (e.g., toxic appearance, malaise, feeding difficulty)
- Information on when to expect improvement in the child's symptoms and, if symptoms do not improve as expected, what to do next
- Clear instructions about medications—how much to give, when to give, side effects to watch for, how long to give, and the necessity of completing the course of antibiotics
- Infection control information if needed—handwashing and disposal of infected secretions; the CDC has excellent written and video education materials available on handwashing at www.cdc.gov/Features/HandWashing.
- Care of nebulizers and humidifiers—to prevent the growth of organisms, nebulizers and humidifiers should be cleaned daily with soapy water, rinsed thoroughly, soaked for one half hour in a solution of one part vinegar to two or three parts distilled water, and then air-dried. Control III® disinfectant is a commercial product that can be substituted for vinegar; however, it is expensive.
- Instructions on next return visit

recommending a tonsillectomy, adenoidectomy, or both and consider whether a wait-and-see approach is the best strategy to determine if growth and time will negate the need for surgery (Burton and Glasziou, 2009). Cold steel tonsillectomy is associated with less pain and bleeding postoperatively than the traditional method of diathermy (Morris, 2009).

Adenoidectomy can also be considered if appropriate medical treatment fails to correct obstructive adenoidal hypertrophy, recurrent or chronic otitis media (after tympanostomy tube placement has been tried), and chronic unresponsive rhinosinusitis. The treatment of choice for sleep obstructive apnea is a tonsilloadenoidectomy (Schechter and Section on Pediatric Pulmonology Subcommittee on Obstructive Sleep Apnea Syndrome, 2002). Children with behavioral problems including attention-deficit/hyperactivity disorder (ADHD) may have obstructive sleep apnea as the cause of their ADHD behaviors.

For any relative indication for tonsillectomy, the risk-benefit ratio of the procedure must be weighed. Significant morbidity and mortality rates are associated with tonsillectomy including complications such as anesthesia problems, hemorrhage, and infection (Burton and Glasziou, 2009). Approximately 6% of children who are younger than age 3 years experience respiratory complications following tonsillectomy. The morbidity and mortality rates connected with adenoidectomy are not as high as with tonsillectomy.

■ Upper Respiratory Tract Disorders

THE COMMON COLD

Description and Epidemiology

The common cold is a frequent problem seen in pediatric practice, and parents often seek information from their child's primary health care provider as to whether their child's symptoms represent a typical URI or indicate the beginning or advancing signs of a more serious illness. Young children have on average 6 to 10 URIs or colds per year. Viruses cause most common colds with 50% resulting from infection by the more than 100 serotypes of rhinoviruses. Parainfluenza viruses, respiratory syncytial virus, coronavirus, and human metapneumovirus are also common agents (Cherry and Nieves, 2010). Other agents that occasionally cause cold symptoms include adenovirus, enterovirus, influenza viruses, reoviruses, and human bocavirus. Daycare and preschool attendance are associated with an increased number of common colds in young children and their spread to school-age children in the family. The acquisition of a common cold virus occurs via inoculation of the nose and possibly the conjunctiva. Colds can be spread through direct inhalation of virus from a sneeze, nasal blowing, or inoculation via fingers from nasal secretions or fomites. Mental stress, lack of sleep, high basal levels of catecholamines, infrequent exercise, smoking, and low vitamin C intake are risk factors for colds in adults, but these have not been studied in children (Cherry and Nieves, 2010).

Pathophysiology

When a person has a common cold, there is an increase in the number of polymorphonuclear leukocytes (PMN) in the nasal submucosa and epithelium. The presence of PMN, rather than bacterial colonization, changes the color of nasal mucus, with green mucus due to PMN enzymatic activity and yellow mucus being caused by the simple presence of PMN (Winther et al, 1984). With rhinovirus there is an increase in bradykinins and albumin in the nasal secretions, but no increase in histamines. Rhinovirus and coronaviruses do not cause destruction of the nasal epithelium, but adenovirus and influenza have a significant destructive effect on the respiratory epithelium.

Clinical Findings

Symptoms of a viral cold include nasal congestion, cough, rhinorrhea, fever, and pharyngitis (Bush, 2009; Cherry and Nieves, 2010).

History. The following may be reported:

- Gradual onset
- Prominent nasal symptoms of rhinorrhea (key finding)
- Sore throat and dysphagia
- Mild cough
- Low-grade fever
- After a variable period of 1 to 3 days, nasal secretions are thicker and more purulent, leading to nasal excoriation.

Physical Examination. Virus-specific findings include:

- Conjunctiva: Mild injection
- Nose: Red nasal mucosa with secretions of varying colors depending on the degree of nasal mucosa destruction and PMN activity

- Throat: Mild erythema
- Lymph: Anterior cervical lymphadenopathy with freely movable nodes less than 2 cm
- Chest: Clear to auscultation and without adventitious sounds

Diagnostic Tests. Usually a throat culture is not done if the child has predominantly nasal symptoms but complains of throat irritation (Cherry and Nieves, 2010). However, if a diagnosis of common cold is in doubt, a rapid strep test followed by a culture if negative should be done. Cultures are useful in differentiating viral infection from group A beta-hemolytic streptococcus (GABHS) infection.

Differential Diagnosis

The most common differentials are allergic rhinitis, rhinosinusitis, and adenoiditis (Table 31-2). Colds can be associated with pharyngitis or, when tonsillar involvement is significant, tonsillopharyngitis (tonsillitis). When tonsillar involvement is minor, the term *nasopharyngitis* is used.

Management

Only supportive care is needed for a viral URI (see Basic Respiratory Management Strategies, General Measures and Patient Education, earlier). Antibiotics are not appropriate treatment. The use of decongestants, antihistamines, and cough medication is not indicated for children younger than 4 years old and should be used with caution in children younger than 6 years old. The child should receive symptomatic relief for fever, pain, and nasal congestion using normal saline and an antipyretic. Fluid intake should be encouraged. Controlled trials have not found sufficient evidence to recommend zinc lozenges, vitamin C, heated humidified air (Bukutu et al, 2008) or echinacea (Cherry and Nieves, 2010; Linde et al, 2006).

Complications

Common colds are self-limiting but can be complicated by otitis media, rhinosinusitis, or tonsillitis.

PHARYNGITIS, TONSILLITIS, AND TONSILLOPHARYNGITIS

Description

Pharyngitis is an inflammation of the mucosa lining the structures of the throat including the tonsils, pharynx, uvula, soft palate, and nasopharynx. The illness is generally acute and involves an inflammatory response including erythema, exudate, or ulceration. The etiology could include a number of viruses and bacteria. If there are nasal symptoms, it is called nasopharyngitis but if there are no nasal symptoms, the disease is called pharyngitis or tonsillopharyngitis. Most pharyngitis is caused by viruses (Cherry, 2010a; Martin, 2010). Adenovirus is the most common cause of nasopharyngitis (Cherry, 2010a). Other viruses include Epstein-Barr virus (EBV), herpes simplex virus (HSV), cytomegalovirus (CMV), enterovirus, influenza virus, parainfluenza, and human immunodeficiency virus (HIV). The viral organisms generally present with upper nasal symptoms. The common bacterial etiology includes *Streptococcus pyogenes* (group A streptococcus), *Corynebacterium diphtheriae*, *Arcanobacterium haemolyticum*, *Neisseria gonorrhoeae*, group C and group G streptococci, and *Mycoplasma pneumoniae.*

Acute Viral Pharyngitis, Tonsillitis or Tonsillopharyngitis

Epidemiology. Adenoviruses are more likely to cause pharyngitis as a prominent symptom. Other viruses (e.g., rhinovirus) are associated with pharyngitis as a minor symptom and rhinorrhea or cough as predominant features. The enterovirus (coxsackievirus, echovirus), herpesvirus, and EBV are also common. Viral infections occur year-round, but peak seasonally. Therefore, it is helpful to know what agents are currently infecting children in the community. It can be difficult to differentiate viral from bacterial infections because of overlapping symptoms (Morris, 2009). However, hoarseness, cough, coryza, conjunctivitis, diarrhea, enanthems, and exanthems are classic features of a viral infection, which is often spread to siblings and classmates via close contact (Cherry and Nieves, 2010).

Clinical Findings

History. The following may be reported:
- Pain
- Myalgia and arthralgia
- Fever
- Sore throat and dysphagia

Physical Examination. Common findings include:
- Reactive lymphadenopathy
  Virus-specific physical findings include the following:
- EBV can produce exudate on the tonsils, soft palate petechiae, and diffuse adenopathy.
- Adenovirus can cause a follicular pattern on the pharynx (Cherry, 2010a).
- Enterovirus can produce vesicles or ulcers on the tonsillar pillars and posterior fauces; coryza, vomiting, or diarrhea may be present.
- Herpesvirus produces ulcers anteriorly and marked adenopathy.
- Parainfluenza and respiratory syncytial virus (RSV) cause more lower respiratory tract disease (e.g., croup, pneumonia, and bronchiolitis) with their typical respiratory signs of stridor, rales, or wheezing.
- Influenza usually has more systemic complaints.

Diagnostic Tests. If a diagnosis of viral infection is in doubt, a rapid strep test or a culture should be done. Cultures are useful in differentiating viral infection from GABHS infection. If infectious mononucleosis is suspected in a child, a complete blood count (CBC) can identify a lymphocytosis and atypical lymphocytes. However, heterophile antibody testing can be helpful in school-age children and adolescents but may yield a false negative in preschool and younger children and during the first weeks of infection (Bell and Fortune, 2006; Smellie et al, 2007). Epstein-Barr antibody titers to early antigen, EBV IgM, EBV IgG, as well as long-term antibodies (Epstein-Barr nuclear antigen [EBNA]) need to be done to confirm the diagnosis if the results of the tests are not diagnostic.

Management. For viral infection, only supportive care is needed, including fever and sore throat pain relief with acetaminophen or ibuprofen. Fluid intake should be encouraged.

TABLE 31-2 Differentiations of Common Upper Respiratory Infections in Children

Site of Infection	Symptoms	Duration of Symptoms (Days)	Etiologic Agent	Management	Duration of Treatment	Comments
The common cold (viral URI)	Malaise, sneezing, watery nasal discharge, mild sore throat, may have a fever, not ill appearing	0-10	Adenovirus, rhinovirus, RSV, parainfluenza, enterovirus	No antibiotics; symptomatic Rx (e.g., saline nose drops, increased fluids); for infants, bulb-syringe the nose before meals and bedtime; for older children, humidifier		If lasts longer than 10-14 days, consider other diagnosis (e.g., rhinosinusitis)
Acute rhinosinusitis	Persistent nasal symptoms for more than 10 days with URI, nasal drainage—purulent or discolored, cough Acute presentation with high fever, purulent rhinitis	10-30	Streptococcus pneumoniae, Moraxella catarrhalis, nontypeable Haemophilus influenzae	Amoxicillin, erythromycin; trimethoprim-sulfamethoxazole, or amoxicillin-clavulanic acid	10 days	By 7 days should be asymptomatic; change antibiotics 48-72 hours after start of treatment if no response
Subacute rhinosinusitis	Same as above but persistent for at least 30 days	30-84	Same as above; may be beta-lactamase producing	Amoxicillin-clavulanic acid		Initial acute infection did not clear, need to switch antibiotics
Chronic/ recurrent rhinosinusitis	Malaise, easy fatigability, unilateral or bilateral nasal discharge, postnasal discharge, nasal obstruction if middle turbinate significantly obstructed	Recurrent >10 to <28 but symptom free for at least 10 days in between bouts Chronic >84	Same as above plus alpha-hemolytic streptococci and Staphylococcus aureus	Amoxicillin-clavulanic, azithromycin, staph coverage	3-6 weeks	May need endoscopic sinus surgery if chronic rhinosinusitis does not respond to prolonged medical management; investigate differential diagnoses or underlying issues (e.g., allergic rhinitis)

RSV, respiratory syncytial virus; Rx, medication; URI, upper respiratory infection.

Acute Bacterial Pharyngitis and Tonsillitis

Epidemiology. The most common bacterial cause of pharyngitis and tonsillitis in children and adolescents is GABHS, which accounts for about 15% to 30% of infections in children with acute sore throat and fever. Group C and group G streptococci can cause pharyngitis, but antibiotic treatment does not prevent its only nonsuppurative complication, glomerulonephritis (Gerber et al, 2009). *Arcanobacterium haemolyticum* is more common in adolescents but is difficult to culture because the organism grows slowly (Martin, 2010). *Neisseria gonorrhoeae* (GC) is a cause of adolescent pharyngitis if the patient engages in oral sex. *Mycoplasma pneumoniae* and *Chlamydophila pneumoniae* are associated with cough along with pharyngitis. *C. diphtheriae* is an extremely rare cause of pharyngitis in the United States. If the throat culture is positive for *Staphylococcus aureus*, *Streptococcus pneumoniae* or *Haemophilus influenzae*, treatment is not needed as these represent normal flora (Congeni, 2009).

Clinical Findings

History. The following characterize GABHS infection:
- Most commonly found in 5- to 15-year-old children; infrequent in children younger than 2 years old
- Abrupt onset without nasal symptoms
- Constitutional symptoms such as arthralgia, myalgia, headache
- Moderate to high fever, malaise, prominent sore throat, dysphagia
- Nausea, abdominal discomfort, vomiting, headache
- Presentation in late winter or early spring
- *N. gonorrhoeae* (GC) has no distinctive finding on examination from other pharyngitis.
- Lack of a cough or nasal symptoms, along with an exudative, erythematous pharyngitis with a follicular pattern and typical historical findings point to GABHS.
- *A. haemolyticum* causes an exudative pharyngitis with marked erythema and a pruritic, fine, scarlatiniform rash (Martin, 2010).

Physical Examination. The following may be seen:
- Petechiae on soft palate and pharynx, swollen beefy-red uvula, red enlarged tonsillopharyngeal tissue
- Tonsillopharyngeal exudate that is yellow, blood-tinged (frequently)
- Tender and enlarged anterior cervical lymph nodes
- Bad breath
- Stigmata of scarlet fever may be seen—scarlatiniform rash, strawberry tongue, circumoral pallor
- Variable presentation; may have mild pharyngeal erythema without tonsillar exudate or cervical adenopathy

Diagnostic Tests. A rapid strep test (rapid antigen detection test [RADT]) has a high specificity but variable sensitivity; therefore, a positive test indicates that a symptomatic person has strep infection and should be treated (Gerber et al, 2009). However, a negative test does not mean that streptococcal infection is not present (Gerber et al, 2009; Martin, 2010). Gerber and associates (2009) suggest that practices that do not perform a back-up test must show that their RADT has a sensitivity and specificity equal to culture. It is important not to do a strep test unless the patient has signs and symptoms, since a positive rapid strep test or a positive throat culture can identify a carrier state. The most common tests used to document past GABHS infection involve obtaining antibody titer to various streptococcal enzymes such as antistreptolysin O (ASO) or anti-deoxyribonuclease B tests (anti-DNase B) (Gerber et al, 2009). The ASO titer rises 1 week postinfection and peaks 3 to 6 weeks after infection. The DNase B test rises 1 to 2 weeks after infection, peaks 6 to 8 weeks following infection, and remains elevated for months even in the face of a mild infection with GABHS. As a result, these tests should not be used to diagnosis GABHS infection in a patient.

Management. The goal of antibiotic therapy is to shorten the course and severity of illness, prevent the spread of illness to others, and avoid the development of suppurative and nonsuppurative complications. Suppurative complications include otitis media, rhinosinusitis, peritonsillar abscess, mastoiditis, cervical adenoiditis, and meningitis, whereas nonsuppurative complications include acute rheumatic fever, acute glomerulonephritis, and poststreptococcal reactive arthritis. As stated, antibiotics do not prevent the development of acute glomerulonephritis. If the rapid strep test result is positive, antibiotics should be started immediately. The drug of choice for the treatment of GABHS is penicillin, for children not allergic to it, because of its cost, narrow spectrum of antimicrobial activity, and infrequent adverse reactions (Martin, 2010). The management plan includes the following:
- Antimicrobial therapy (based on clinical need)—one of the following (American Academy of Pediatrics [AAP], 2009; Gerber et al, 2009, Taketomo et al, 2011):
  - Penicillins
    - Phenoxymethyl penicillin (penicillin V potassium) orally for 10 days: for children less than 60 pounds (27 kg), 250 mg two or three times a day for 10 days; for children more than 60 pounds, adolescents, or adults, the dose is 500 mg two or three times a day for 10 days (AAP, 2009; Gerber et al, 2009).
    - Amoxicillin suspension is often used with young children because it is more palatable (efficacy seems equal to penicillin). It must be taken for 10 days. Amoxicillin at 50 mg/kg once a day to a maximum of 1 g can be used orally for 10 days (AAP, 2009; Gerber et al, 2009).
    - Benzathine penicillin G intramuscular (IM) (600,000 units as a single dose if less than 60 pounds [27 kg]; 1.2 million units as a single dose for larger children and adults).
  - If allergic to beta-lactams:
    - A 10-day course of a narrow-spectrum (first-generation), orally administered cephalosporin is acceptable, particularly if the child is allergic to penicillin. However, in up to 5% of penicillin-allergic patients, there is a crossover allergy to cephalosporin. Patients with a type I allergic reaction should not be treated with a first-generation cephalosporin (AAP, 2009).
    - Clindamycin at 20 mg/kg/day divided in three doses for children older than 3 years.
    - Azithromycin at 12 mg/kg once a day to a maximum of 500 mg. It should be noted that macrolide resistance is as high as 5% to 8% in some parts of the U.S. (Gerber et al 2009).
    - Clarithromycin at 15 mg/kg/day divided in two doses (maximum 250 mg twice a day)
  - If evidence of penicillin resistance is present, a beta-lactamase–resistant antibiotic can be used, such as amoxicillin-clavulanate or dicloxacillin.
- Supportive care—antipyretics, fluids, rest.
- Repeat culture is not generally needed except in situations in which it is necessary to ensure eradication of the organism.

- Continued symptoms of streptococcal pharyngitis and a positive culture for streptococcus may represent an actual treatment failure or a new infection with a different serologic type of streptococcus.
- Noncompliance with pharmacologic therapy can explain treatment failure, and in these instances, an injection of benzathine penicillin is recommended.
- For a compliant patient with recurrence, narrow-spectrum cephalosporins, clindamycin, or amoxicillin-clavulanic acid or a combination of penicillin with rifampin are reasonable alternatives (Gerber et al, 2009).
- If clinical relapse occurs, a second course of antibiotic is indicated, as discussed earlier. If recurrent infection is a problem, culturing of the family for the chronic carrier state is advised.
- Fomites such as bathroom cups, toothbrushes, or orthodontic devices may harbor GABHS and should be cleaned or discarded.
- Children can return to school when they are afebrile and have been taking antibiotics for at least 24 hours.

Complications. Major nonsuppurative late complications caused by GABHS are rheumatic fever, poststreptococcal reactive arthritis, and acute glomerulonephritis. Suppurative complications include cervical adenitis, rhinosinusitis, otitis media, pneumonia, mastoiditis, and retropharyngeal or peritonsillar abscess. Recurrent GABHS tonsillopharyngitis can also be a problem. Sydenham chorea is linked to GABHS infection. In addition, the onset or worsening of other neuropsychiatric disorders (e.g., obsessive-compulsive disorder, Tourette syndrome, or tic disorder) has been associated with streptococcal infection, but this association is not proven (Gerber et al, 2009). The acronym used to describe this phenomenon is PANDAS (pediatric autoimmune neuropsychiatric disorders) (Gerber et al, 2009; Morer et al, 2006).

RHINOSINUSITIS

Description

Rhinosinusitis involves inflammation and secondary infection of the paranasal sinuses and the adjacent nasal mucosa (See and Evans, 2007). The American Academy of Otolaryngology-Head and Neck Surgery developed clinical guidelines for the treatment of rhinosinusitis (Pearlman and Conley, 2008) and stressed the importance of differentiating viral URIs from acute bacterial sinusitis. Three symptoms were required for the diagnosis of acute rhinosinusitis—purulent nasal discharge, nasal obstruction, and facial pain, pressure, or fullness lasting between 10 days and 4 weeks. It is estimated that 5% to 10% of URI are complicated by rhinosinusitis (Cherry and Shapiro, 2010). Common causes of rhinosinusitis includes a viral infection; allergic and nonallergic rhinitis; anatomic problems such as abnormality of the ostiomeatal complex or septal deviation; cigarette smoking; swimming and diving; high-elevation climbing; and dental infections (See and Evans, 2007). Rhinosinusitis can have three clinical presentations (DeMuri and Wald, 2010):

- Persistence of URI symptoms for longer than 10 days and less than 30 days without improvement
- Severe symptoms with a high fever and purulent rhinitis at the onset and lasting at least 3 to 4 days
- Biphasic illness in which there is worsening on day 6 or 7 of a common cold in which the patient develops an increase in respiratory symptoms, nasal congestion, or a new onset or recurrence of a fever.

The maxillary and anterior ethmoid sinuses are most frequently involved in children because they are present at birth, but only the ethmoidal sinuses are pneumatized. The frontal sinuses begin their development at 7 years old with complete development at adolescence. The three key elements that keep the sinuses patent include ostia patency, normally functioning cilia, and quality of secretions. Inflammation and edema of the mucous membranes lining the sinuses cause obstruction and set up an ideal situation for bacteria to invade the sinus cavities. Certain conditions predispose children to chronic sinus infections, including allergies, nasal deformities, CF, nasal polyps, and HIV infection.

Rhinosinusitis can be divided into acute or chronic, in which symptoms persist for 12 weeks. Risk factors for the development of chronic rhinosinusitis include anatomic blockage; irritant and allergen exposure; defects in mucociliary function; immunodeficiency; and chronic infection with bacteria, viruses, or fungi. As a result a persistent swelling of the sinonasal mucosa impairs sinus drainage. Chronic rhinosinusitis can be divided further into three distinct syndromes—chronic rhinosinusitis without polyps, chronic rhinosinusitis with polyps, and allergic fungal rhinosinusitis (Brook, 2010). Patients with chronic rhinosinusitis who develop new symptoms of rhinosinusitis, are referred to as having acute-on-chronic rhinosinusitis. Remember that sinus inflammation is part of the natural history of a cold or allergic rhinitis. Thick, yellow discharge is a common and normal finding with a URI. Therefore, the pediatric provider must be cautious to not overdiagnose rhinosinusitis and subsequently indiscriminately use antibiotics (DeMuri and Wald, 2010).

Epidemiology

The various sinuses develop, aerate, and become clinically important at different times during childhood. Ethmoiditis can occur after 6 months old, in contrast to frontal rhinosinusitis, which is first seen around 10 years old. The common bacterial organisms responsible for superinfections are *S. pneumoniae*, nontypeable *H. influenzae*, *Moraxella catarrhalis*, and, less often, *S. aureus*, other streptococci, and anaerobes. Anaerobic bacteria are prominent in chronic rhinosinusitis and include *Prevotella* spp., *Porphyromonas* spp., *Fusobacterium nucleatum*, and *Peptostreptococcus* spp. Anaerobic and staphylococcal agents are implicated in chronic rhinosinusitis. Recent data from middle ear bacteria indicate that *H. influenzae* is slightly more prominent as a pathogen with a slight decrease in *S. pneumoniae* as the prominent pathogen (DeMuri and Wald, 2010). The presence of antibiotic-resistant organisms is associated with prior antibiotic therapy. The role of viruses in rhinosinusitis is not clear. Cases of recurrent and chronic rhinosinusitis are often caused by recurrent viral URIs associated with daycare attendance, smoking in the home, older siblings at home who reinfect the child, or certain predisposing conditions, such as allergies, nasal polyps, immunodeficiency disorders, or CF—the latter two conditions predispose to infections with *Aspergillus* and *Zygomycetes*.

Clinical Findings in Acute Rhinosinusitis

The time frame of symptoms determines the classification of rhinosinusitis as described earlier. The clinical guidelines for sinusitis propose that two cardinal symptoms be present:

- Purulent rhinorrhea
- Either facial pressure or nasal obstruction

Other suggestive signs and symptoms include:

- Headache, fever, fatigue, maxillary dental pain, cough, decreased ability to smell (hyposmia), no smell, and ear pressure or fullness (Hwang, 2009)
  Additional key issues:
- Cough worse at night because sinus drainage down the pharyngeal wall can induce cough and vomiting (Cherry and Shapiro, 2010)
- Periorbital cellulitis—a sign of ethmoid sinusitis in children (Cherry and Shapiro, 2010)
- Occasionally malodorous breath or ears feel full; more than half of all patients with sinusitis also have abnormal middle ear findings (Cherry and Shapiro, 2010)

Diagnostic Tests. If clinical findings suggest rhinosinusitis, radiographs are not needed. If there are symptoms of orbital, intracranial, or soft-tissue abscess, radiographic imaging should be done (Pearlman and Conley, 2008). Facial swelling, acute rhinosinusitis unresponsive to 48 hours of antibiotics, a child with a toxic appearance, chronic or recurrent rhinosinusitis, and chronic unresponsive asthma are also indications for imaging studies, including sinus radiographs, ultrasonograms, or CT scanning. CT is the accepted imaging study for acute or chronic rhinosinusitis (Pearlman and Conley, 2008). Coronal sections show lesions in the ostiomeatal complex and axial images can delineate orbital complications (Cherry and Shapiro, 2010); however, the AAP recommends its use only in children older than 6 years who are undergoing operative procedures (AAP Subcommittee on Management of Sinusitis, 2001). Nasal cultures are difficult to obtain because they must be taken from the middle ostium in the middle meatus (Cherry and Shapiro, 2010). Transillumination is subjective and difficult to perform in children.

Differential Diagnosis

Viral URI, allergic rhinitis, and other causes of headache are the differential diagnoses. Remember that rhinosinusitis may exacerbate asthma.

Management

Symptomatic pain relief with acetaminophen or ibuprofen has been shown to be helpful (Morris, 2009). Although 60% to 80% of acute rhinosinusitis episodes resolve without antibiotics in about 4 weeks, antimicrobial therapy increases the speed of resolution and reduces the amount of mucosal damage (Hwang, 2009). Antibiotics should be prescribed for a course of 10 days in rhinosinusitis or, if the child is responding slowly but not symptom-free, an additional 7 days. Most children show dramatic improvement in 3 to 4 days (fever and nasal discharge abating). Failure to improve in 48 hours suggests a resistant organism or complications. The course of therapy may be up to 21 days in acute rhinosinusitis and up to 6 weeks in chronic rhinosinusitis.

In uncomplicated acute rhinosinusitis in children, the first-line treatment should be amoxicillin because it is efficacious, safe, and inexpensive (Pearlman and Conley, 2008).

- Amoxicillin (80 to 90 mg/kg/day), amoxicillin-clavulanate, cefpodoxime, proxetil, or cefuroxime axetil as initial therapy if the child has *not* taken antibiotics in the past 4 to 6 weeks. The AAP has also recommended amoxicillin 40 to 45 mg/kg/day, but this treatment should not be given if there are high rates of resistance (DeMuri and Wald, 2010).

  - If allergic to amoxicillin—azithromycin, clarithromycin, erythromycin, or trimethoprim/sulfamethoxazole (TMP-SMX) (failure rates are up to 38% with TMP-SMX)
- Children at risk for resistant bacterial infections (antibiotic therapy within prior 1 to 3 months, daycare attendance, less than 2 years old, failure to respond within 72 hours) should receive high-dose amoxicillin-clavulanate (80 to 90 mg/kg/day amoxicillin and 6.4 mg/kg/day clavulanate).

The management of chronic rhinosinusitis is more complicated because bacteria are generally only one of other contributing factors. Referral to an otolaryngologist is often needed. Additional management considerations include the following:

- *Decongestants.* There is no randomized-controlled trial (RCT) to support the use of topical decongestants. However, if a decongestant is used by the patient, it should be limited to 5 days to avoid rebound edema (rhinitis medicamentosa) (Hwang, 2009). In older children moderate evidence shows that decongestants may be used if there is significant nasal obstruction (Morris, 2009).
- *Topical corticosteroids.* The use of intranasal steroids may decrease symptoms in patients with uncomplicated sinusitis (Zaimanovici and Yaphe, 2007).
- *Antihistamine.* Antihistamines and intranasal steroids may have a role in recurrent or chronic rhinosinusitis if allergic manifestations are present (see the management section for allergic rhinitis). See Chapter 24 for information on the use of decongestants and antihistamines.
- *Saline irrigation.* The use of buffered isotonic saline into the nasal cavity by squeeze bottle or neti pot (in late childhood and adolescence) may be helpful in allergic rhinitis, recurrent acute sinusitis, and chronic sinusitis. Because clinical guidelines do not support or negate the use of saline, it can be used by patients to help thin secretions (Hwang, 2009) and is recommended by some allergists.
- Children with complications or signs of invasive infection should be referred to the appropriate medical specialist. Surgical drainage by an otolaryngologist, treatment of allergies and control of allergic rhinitis by an allergist, or both may be necessary.
- Comfort measures include the use of acetaminophen, ibuprofen, or codeine for severe pain. A humidifier helps relieve the drying of mucous membranes associated with mouth breathing. Increase oral fluid intake.
- Diving is contraindicated with rhinosinusitis.
- Prevention includes good allergy management, relief of nasal airway obstruction, and attention to persistent nasal discharge (Cherry and Shapiro, 2010).

Complications

Chronic or recurrent rhinosinusitis may result in referral to an otolaryngologist or allergist. Orbital cellulitis secondary to ethmoiditis is a serious, life-threatening complication that is a medical emergency. It is manifested by swelling and erythema of the eyelids, proptosis, decreased extraocular movements, and altered vision. Intracranial complications, such as cavernous sinus thrombosis, subdural empyema, and brain abscess, can also occur. Chronic rhinosinusitis is also associated with intractable wheezing in children with asthma (Cherry and Shapiro, 2010).

DIPHTHERIA

Description

Diphtheria is a rare infection in the U.S. with only five cases reported annually. It is a dangerous disease because it causes a membranous obstruction of the upper airway, including the trachea. It also produces a toxin leading to a peripheral neuropathy, myocarditis, and acute tubular necrosis (AAP, 2009). Local infection is associated with a low-grade fever, and gradual onset of symptoms over 1 to 2 days. Diphtheria can also present as otic, conjunctival, and cutaneous infections.

Epidemiology

Humans are the only reservoir, and the organism is spread by respiratory droplets as well as contact with skin lesions. Although rare, fomites can act as a vehicle of transmission, and raw milk and milk products can transmit *C. diphtheriae*. The bacterium is a gram-positive rod with four biotypes (mitis, intermedius, belfanti, and gravis) that can be toxigenic or nontoxigenic (AAP, 2009). Diphtheria is caused by the toxigenic strain of *C. diphtheriae* or, less commonly, *C. ulcerans*. The toxigenic strains produce two exotoxins—enzymatically active A domain and binding B domain. The binding B domain promotes entry of A into the cell. Asymptomatic carriers can transmit the organism. The incubation period averages from 2 to 7 days but occasionally can be longer (AAP, 2009). The incidence of respiratory diphtheria is greater in the fall and the winter but skin infections are more common in the summer. Endemic areas include Africa, Latin America, Asia, and the Middle East. Fully immunized individuals can carry the bacteria asymptomatically and may present with a mild sore throat (AAP, 2009).

Clinical Findings

Disease may be mild or asymptomatic in partially or fully immunized individuals and severe if unimmunized. Characteristic signs and symptoms follow.

Primary Infection

- Low-grade fever
- Grayish, adherent pseudomembrane found in either the nasopharynx, pharynx, or trachea
- Sore throat, serosanguineous or seropurulent nasal discharge, hoarseness, cough
- Cutaneous lesions (nonhealing ulcers with dirty gray membrane or colonization of preexisting dermatoses) infected with diphtheria (seen less often)

Toxin Production. The ability of a strain of *C. diphtheriae* to produce toxin is related to bacteriophage infection of the bacterium, not to colony type.

- Toxin production is more lethal than the primary infection and can induce the following:
  - Myocarditis and electrocardiographic changes
  - Respiratory compromise
  - Cranial nerve and local neuropathies
  - Peripheral neuritis

Diagnostic Tests. A confirmatory diagnosis is based on a positive culture of *C. diphtheriae*. Specimens should be obtained from the nose, throat, any skin lesions, and either beneath the membrane or from a portion of the membrane.

Because a special culture medium is needed, the lab needs to be notified if *C. diphtheriae* is suspected. Toxigenicity tests are performed if *C. diphtheriae* is confirmed (AAP, 2009). Culture results take 8 to 48 hours; however, treatment begins when diphtheria is suspected. Do not wait for laboratory confirmation. Results of the CBC may be normal or show a slight leukocytosis and thrombocytopenia.

Differential Diagnosis

Acute streptococcal pharyngitis and infectious mononucleosis are included in the differential diagnosis of pharyngeal diphtheria. A nasal FB or purulent rhinosinusitis can resemble nasal diphtheria; epiglottitis, laryngeal diphtheria, and viral croup can also cause obstruction.

Management

Children with diphtheria require hospitalization. Treatment consists of the following:

- *Antitoxin administration (hyperimmune equine antiserum).* A single dose needs to be administered if there is a high index of suspicion prior to a positive culture result (AAP, 2009). Allergic reaction to the serum occurs in 5% to 20%, so a scratch test should be performed prior to administration. Intravenous immunoglobulin has not been approved for use.
- *Antimicrobial therapy.* Erythromycin given orally or parenterally for 14 days or penicillin G for 14 days either IM or IV or penicillin G procaine IM for 14 days. This is not a substitute for antitoxin administration.
- Supportive care for respiratory, cardiac, and neurologic complications as appropriate
- Standard and droplet precautions until two cultures are negative
- Immunization after recovery because disease does not necessarily confer immunity
- Monitoring and antimicrobial prophylaxis of contacts regardless of immunization status
- Care for respiratory, cardiac, and neurologic complications

Prevention

Universal immunization against diphtheria with regular booster injections is the only effective method of control. Infection can occur in immunized or partially immunized children, but in these individuals the disease severity is greatly diminished. Disease generally occurs in nonimmunized children; the frequency of severe life-threatening complications in this group is high. Care of a child exposed to diphtheria is individualized and based on immunization status, likelihood of follow-up, and compliance with antimicrobial therapy. The AAP Committee on Infectious Diseases' *Red Book* lists specific guidelines that should be followed for the care of exposed children.

PERTUSSIS

Description

Pertussis is caused by a gram-negative bacillus, *Bordetella pertussis* (AAP, 2009). *B. pertussis* produces a variety of components that are highly antigenic as well as biologically active. These include pertussis toxin, adenylate cyclase toxin, dermonecrotic toxin, fimbriae, filamentous hemagglutinin, pertactin, and autotransporters. These substances cause significant damage to host immune function and cause local tissue damage in the respiratory tract.

The classic cough of pertussis lasts 6 to 10 weeks, but in 50% of adolescents can last longer than 10 weeks (AAP, 2009). This infection is also known as whooping cough because of the high-pitched inspiratory whoop following spasms of coughing. This classic cough is not limited to the very young because it occurs in 72% to 100% of adolescent cases with post-tussive vomiting noted in 50% to 70% of adolescent cases (Powell, 2007). Table 31-3 shows the stages of pertussis with accompanying symptoms. The cough is an attempt to dislodge plugs of necrotic bronchial epithelial tissue and thick mucus. If this disease occurs in unvaccinated infants younger than 1 year old, it is often associated with pneumonia, seizures, and encephalopathy. Pertussis in older children and vaccinated children is complicated by syncope, sleep disturbances, rib fracture, incontinence, and pneumonia (AAP, 2009). Outbreaks of pertussis still occur despite the availability of an effective vaccine. Older children and adults can be the vector of pertussis because their symptoms are not severe. Transmission occurs via aerosolized droplets; children are most contagious during the catarrhal stage and the first 2 weeks after the cough onset (AAP, 2009).

Epidemiology

Classic pertussis is either a primary disease or reinfection. There are six species of *Bordetella*. The most common types are *B. pertussis* and *B. parapertussis* (*B. parapertussis* causes a mild pertussis-like illness). *B. bronchiseptica* infrequently causes respiratory infection and *B. holmesii* causes bacteremia. The last three bacteria are not affected by the vaccine. Transmission of these gram-negative pleomorphic bacilli is by aerosol droplet from coughing or from close contact with infected individuals. Contaminated droplets are inhaled and adhere to the ciliated epithelium of the nasopharynx. The incubation period is between 6 and 21 days. Cases of pertussis occur in adults, who act as a reservoir for the bacteria. Thus the usual source of *B. pertussis* infection in infants is an unrecognized infection in an adult family member with a cough. The highest incidence of mortality occurs in infants less than 1 month old (Cherry and Heininger, 2010).

Clinical Findings

Manifestations of this disease vary by age group, stage of disease, immunization status, and the presence of transplacentally acquired antibodies (Cherry and Heininger, 2010). There is the classic illness and an asymptomatic infection. The latter occurs in patients who are vaccinated or as a primary illness in those who are not vaccinated.

Characteristics of the classic disease in infants and young children are found in Table 31-3.

Specific findings in infants younger than 6 months old are generally severe, particularly in neonates, and include:
- Apnea (common) often with seizures caused by hypoxemia
- No inspiratory whoop
- Severe pneumonia and pulmonary hypertension, which are common

Findings in older children include (Smith, 2011):
- Persistent, irritating, nonproductive cough that may last for months; resembles a prolonged bronchitic illness
- May have severe paroxysms of coughing but generally no whooping sound
- Low-grade fever

Diagnostic Tests. While culturing for *B. pertussis* is considered the gold standard for pertussis (it is 100% specific), it is difficult to do because it requires collection from the nasopharynx with a calcium alginate fiber-tipped swab and immediate placement into a special transport medium (Regan-Lowe). Culture can be negative if the person has been ill for 3 weeks or more, has previously been vaccinated, or if antibiotics have been started. The organism is found most frequently during the catarrhal or early paroxysmal stage. Polymerase chain reaction (PCR) is increasingly popular due to its improved sensitivity and rapid result. PCR testing is done using a Dacron swab or nasal wash from the nasopharynx. However, the U.S. Food and Drug Administration (FDA) has not licensed any PCR tests for this purpose.

Commercial tests for elevated immunoglobulins to pertussis toxins are available; however, the FDA has not licensed any for diagnostic use. An elevated IgG to pertussis toxin 3 to 4 weeks after cough can be suggestive of a pertussis infection, but it is not definitive. IgA and IgM analyses lack sensitivity. Leukocytosis (20,000 to 50,000/mm^3) with 70% to 80% lymphocytes (lymphocytosis) is a common finding in infants and young children, but is rare in adolescents (AAP, 2009).

Differential Diagnosis

In the classic form of the disease, the diagnosis is clear due to the paroxysmal cough. However, the cause can be *B. parapertussis* as well as *B. pertussis*. The presence of a

TABLE 31-3	Stages of Pertussis	
Stage of Pertussis	**Length of Time**	**Manifestation**
Catarrhal	1-2 weeks	• Upper respiratory infection similar to common cold • Mild cough, coryza, sneezing, and low-grade fever (to 101° F [38.3° C])
Paroxysmal	2 to 4 weeks	• Fever is absent or minimal • Persistent staccato, paroxysmal cough ending with an inspiratory whoop • Vomiting at the end of paroxysmal coughing and whoop • Cyanosis, sweating, prostration, and exhaustion after coughing
Convalescent	3 weeks to 6 months	• Symptoms wane over a 6-month period • Waning of paroxysmal coughing episodes

Data from American Academy of Pediatrics: Summaries of infectious diseases. In Pickering LK, Baker CJ, Kimberlin D et al, editors: *Red Book: 2009 Report of the Committee on Infectious Diseases*, ed 28, Elk Grove Village, IL, 2009, American Academy of Pediatrics.

marked lymphocytosis in a child with a persistent cough illness points to *B. pertussis*. However, *C. pneumoniae*, adenoviruses, bocaviruses, and other viral agents can present in a similar fashion. Gastroesophageal reflux, cystic fibrosis, asthma, and foreign bodies should be included in the differential diagnosis.

Management

- Treatment with antimicrobial agents in the macrolide class is the treatment of choice.
- Due to the development of pyloric stenosis when erythromycin is used in infants younger than 1 month, azithromycin is the drug of choice.
- Antibiotic treatment choices include (Taketomo, 2011):
  - Azithromycin at 10 mg/kg in a single dose for 5 days is given to infants from 0 to 6 months of age.
  - Azithromycin in infants older than 6 months of age (5-day treatment: a single dose of 10 mg/kg/day [maximum of 500 mg] on day 1, then a single dose of 5 mg/kg/day [maximum of 250 mg] on days 2 to 5).
  - Clarithromycin for children older than 1 month (15 mg/kg/day in two divided doses for 7 days with a maximum dose of 1 g/day).
  - Erythromycin is used in all age groups except for infants younger than 1 month; for infants and children (40 to 50 mg/kg/day in four divided doses for 14 days with a maximum dose of 2 g/day) and adults (500 mg every six hours for 14 days).
- Antimicrobial therapy given in the paroxysmal stage does not alter the course of pertussis, but does limit the spreading of the organism (AAP, 2009).
- Corticosteroids should not be used.
- The use of albuterol and other beta 2-adrenergic medications is not supported by controlled, prospective studies (Guinto-Ocampo and McNeil, 2010).

Care of Exposed Children. Recommendations regarding isolation and prophylactic measures for exposed children and adults include the following (Guinto-Ocampo and McNeil, 2010):

- Immunization coverage with diphtheria-tetanus-acellular pertussis (DTaP) or Tdap depending on age group.
- Chemoprophylaxis with erythromycin (40 to 50 mg/kg/day [maximum, 2 g/day] orally in four divided doses for 14 days) is the drug of choice for all household and close contacts, including children in daycare and the staff and playmates, irrespective of their immunization status; azithromycin or clarithromycin is better tolerated by adolescents. Start as soon after exposure as possible. An alternate approach that can be used with only adults is to follow closely and treat with macrolides with the first appearance of respiratory signs or symptoms.
- The utility of chemoprophylaxis after 21 days of exposure to the index case is not clear (AAP, 2009).
- Close monitoring of respiratory symptoms for 20 days after last contact with an infected individual

Complications

Secondary bacterial pneumonia, seizures, epistaxis, subconjunctival hemorrhage, encephalopathy, and death can occur. Activation of tuberculosis is associated with pertussis infection.

Prevention

The recommended guidelines for the initial series of DTaP vaccines and booster doses should be followed. Remember that just one DTaP immunization can reduce the severity of symptoms in an infant infected with pertussis. Only children with valid contraindications to receiving pertussis vaccine, as identified in Chapter 23, should be excluded from receiving the vaccine.

Immunity following either natural pertussis infection or illness or vaccination is *not* long lasting. Immunity wanes over time, and the vaccine does not confer active immunity. Pertussis in older children, adolescents, and adults is a mild, often unrecognized disease that if transmitted to an unimmunized infant can result in life-threatening illness. Universal immunization of children younger than 7 years old and adolescents is crucial to control this disease.

RECURRENT EPISTAXIS

Epidemiology

Recurrent epistaxis is common in children, with an incidence of 30% in children from 0 to 5 years, 56% in school-age children 6 to 10 years, and 64% in adolescents (Kubba, 2006). It is even higher for families living in dry climates or during the winter months when artificial heating is used. The cause is often benign and typically related to mechanical trauma to the area (e.g., nose picking), and, thus, it is generally self-limiting. Other factors that can cause mucosal irritation that result in bleeding include coagulopathies, allergies, neoplasms (e.g., rhabdomyosarcoma), polyps, hemangiomas, chronic rhinitis, URI, FB, chronic use of topical nasal sprays containing corticosteroids or antihistamine decongestants, and viral or bacterial infections of nasal tissue. In adolescents, epistaxis may result from the use of recreational drugs such as cocaine. In more than 95% of cases the anterior portion of the nasal septum, called Kiesselbach area, is the usual site of involvement (Schlosser, 2009). The blood supply of Kiesselbach area comes from the external carotid through the external maxillary artery. Posterior nosebleeds are far more common in older adult patients. The relationship between hypertension and epistaxis is controversial because it is unclear whether blood pressure elevation is caused by anxiety due to the nosebleed (Schlosser, 2009). A coagulopathy, generally von Willebrand disease or platelet aggregation disorders, can manifest as recurrent epistaxis, but a careful history will reveal easy bruising.

Clinical Findings

History. The following may be reported:
- Recent nasal trauma including nose-picking
- Allergies or a recent URI
- Unexpected bruising or bleeding from other sites
- Frequent nosebleeds (unilateral or bilateral)
- Tarry stools (the result of swallowed blood)

The provider should always question about a family history of excessive bleeding episodes or bleeding disorders. In addition, topical nasal medication use, or in the case of the teen, cocaine or other inhaled recreational drugs should be explored.

Physical Examination. Nares visualization may include fresh clots, old clots, and/or raw, red skin. The nasal mucosa on the medial surface of the anterior septum may be dry, cracked, excoriated, or scabbed. The bilateral epistaxis, blood in the oropharynx, and difficult to control bleeding suggest posterior bleeding (Gifford and Orlandi, 2008).

Diagnostic Tests. A baseline hematocrit may be indicated in severe or chronic epistaxis. It can reveal iron deficiency anemia secondary to the bleeding. Unless the history points to a coagulopathy or the nosebleeds are recurrent and refractory to treatment, coagulation studies are not indicated (Schlosser, 2009).

Differential Diagnosis

A bleeding disorder or nasal tumor is characterized by epistaxis that is severe, prolonged, and recurrent. Red flags for other disorders include epistaxis in a child younger than 2 years old, evidence of bleeding at other sites, or bleeding that lasts longer than 20 minutes (Kubba, 2006). If these abnormalities occur and a coagulopathy is suspected, order a CBC, platelet count, prothrombin time (PT), activated partial thromboplastin time (aPTT), and ristocetin cofactor. If epistaxis is associated with a traumatic injury, evaluate for the presence of a nasal fracture and/or septal hematoma.

Management

The following steps are recommended:
- Have the child sit upright and lean forward to prevent swallowing the blood.
- Apply direct pressure at the nasal ala (pinch the nares together at the bony structure) for 5 minutes; 15 minutes if there is still bleeding. Have the parent watch the time because perceptions of time are subjective (Manes, 2010).
- Packing and topical vasoconstrictor drugs are occasionally needed.
- Use a bedside humidifier to moisten the air in dry climates or in winter with forced-air heating. Normal saline nose sprays are also effective.
- Apply topical antibiotic to the site of the septal scab for 5 to 7 days to keep moist, reduce itching, and assist healing. In one single-blind control trial, the daily use of nasal Vaseline provided no additional benefit compared to no treatment (Loughran et al, 2004).
- Topical agents such as Nosebleeds QR are hydrophilic polymers that form an artificial scab when they come into contact with blood. These can be applied via a swab to Kiesselbach plexus. Local applications of a solution of oxymetazoline or Neo-Synephrine (0.25 1%) can also be used (Haddad, 2007).
- Silver nitrate sticks can be used to cauterize exposed vessels if bleeding persists; however, the site must be easily accessible, visible, and not bleeding briskly. It has a high failure rate and is associated with nasal septum atrophy.
- Nasal packing with absorbable oxycellulose material if bleeding continues or the site cannot be localized; if packing is used, prescribe oral antibiotics to reduce the risk of secondary rhinosinusitis and toxic shock syndrome.
- Treat the underlying cause of the problem (e.g., trauma from nose-picking; dry air; topical nasal sprays).
- Teach parents to leave alone blood scabs because removal may precipitate further bleeding.

Prevention

Preventive measures include instructions on a good nasal regimen to keep the nasal mucosa moist. Such strategies include vaporizer use and normal saline nose drops or sprays or the application of petroleum jelly to the anterior nasal cavity daily (Manes, 2010). If the child uses nasal corticosteroids, make sure the child directs the spray laterally rather than toward the septum. This reduces epistaxis related to nasal spray (Schlosser, 2009).

NASAL FOREIGN BODY
Description

Young children tend to insert all types of FBs into a body orifice. Nasal FBs can be noted immediately by the parent or lie undetected until classic symptoms appear.

Clinical Findings

History. A persistent or recurrent unilateral purulent nasal discharge is reported. Foul odor, epistaxis, nasal obstruction, and mouth breathing are less commonly reported symptoms (Haddad, 2007). Young children will often deny inserting a foreign body.

Physical Examination. The classic symptom of a nasal foreign body is unilateral, purulent, foul-smelling nasal discharge. If the foreign body is embedded in granulation tissue or mucosa, it may take on the appearance of a nasal mass.

Differential Diagnosis

Nasal polyps, purulent rhinitis, adenoiditis, rhinosinusitis, and nasal tumors are conditions that cause bilateral or unilateral discharge.

Management

Management involves the following (Haddad, 2007; Tom and Shah, 2006):
- Detection of an FB in the nasal cavity, which establishes the diagnosis
- Removal of the nasal FB, depending on its location, its composition, and the skill of the practitioner. Alligator forceps, suction with narrow tips, and cotton-tipped applicators with collodion with or without topical vasoconstrictor drugs (to reduce swelling) can be used. Other techniques include using a hook or curette to roll the object out. A 5-French catheter with a balloon can be advanced past the FB; inflate the balloon before removing the catheter and (it is hoped) the object with it.
- Good lighting (use a headlight) is essential, as is immobilization of the young child via papoose board.
- Elevation of the child's head and suctioning of blood and secretions
- Otolaryngology referral is merited for young children who cannot cooperate or when the FB is extremely difficult or dangerous to remove, such as paper clips or staples. Providers must remember that the FB can be forced deeper into the nose if the practitioner is inexperienced at nasal FB removal.

▪ Extrathoracic Airway Disorders
CROUP (LARYNGOTRACHEITIS AND SPASMODIC CROUP)
Description

Croup (laryngotracheitis and spasmodic croup) causes disease in children less than 6 years old (Cherry, 2008). Croup involves swelling and erythema of the lateral walls of the trachea below the vocal cords in an area called the subglottis (Wald, 2010).

It results in rapid, acute, upper airway obstruction of varying degrees at the larynx, and is characterized by a harsh, barking cough and inspiratory stridor. Although viral agents are the cause of most croup, bacterial croup, also called bacterial tracheitis, laryngotracheobronchitis, or laryngotracheobronchopneumonitis, presents with not only inflammatory cell infiltration of the tracheal walls but also ulceration, pseudomembranes, and microabscesses (Cherry, 2008). Unlike viral croup, bacterial croup results in thick pus within the trachea and lower airways.

Epidemiology

Parainfluenza type 1 is the most common viral agent responsible for fall outbreaks. Other causative agents include other parainfluenza types, influenza, human coronavirus HL-63 (Wald, 2010), metapneumovirus, adenoviruses, and rhinovirus. Parainfluenza type 3 is associated with severe croup (Cherry, 2008). Viral croup is most common in children between 6 and 36 months old (60% are younger than 24 months) and occurs most often in the cold season of the year. The incubation period is 3 to 6 days (Cherry, 2008). Males are affected more often than females. Recurrent croup and recurrent laryngitis can develop in children until 6 years old. A positive family history has been noted in a small percentage of children in whom croup develops. Croup lasts approximately 5 days. With growth, the child's laryngeal tracheal airway is less vulnerable to the effects of viral infections and less susceptible to obstruction.

Clinical Findings

Clinical manifestations depend on the infectious agent responsible for the croup and the extent of the upper airway involvement.

History. The history typically includes the following:
- URI prodromal symptoms (rhinorrhea, conjunctivitis, or both) are sometimes present before stridor.
- Fever within the first 24 hours
- Intermittent stridor—mild to moderate. Classically, this presents as a barky cough.
- Gradual onset of symptoms (2 to 3 days)
- Symptoms worse at night (Bjornson and Johnson, 2008)
- May or may not have sore throat
- Improvement within a few days for most children with viral croup

Physical Examination. The following can be seen:
- Slight dyspnea, tachypnea, and retractions
- Mild, brassy, or barking cough (harsh sounding)
- Stridor—a high-pitched, harsh sound from turbulent airflow that is generally inspiratory, but may be biphasic
- Temperature is typically low grade, but may be elevated to 104° F (40° C).
- If visualized on examination of the mouth, the epiglottis will appear normal.
- Substernal and chest wall retraction in severe cases
- Prolonged inspiration
- Wheezing and rales may be heard if there is additional lower airway involvement.

Diagnostic Tests. Croup is a clinical diagnosis. Radiography of the soft tissues of the neck and chest displays a classic pattern of subglottic narrowing ("steeple sign") on posteroanterior views, but is usually not done unless there is a question about the diagnosis. Microbiology cultures of the pharynx can be helpful in selected cases that have atypical presentations with severe fever, toxic presentations, and severe inspiratory stridor.

Differential Diagnosis

Differential diagnoses include acute epiglottitis; acute spasmodic croup (no signs of infection); FB aspiration; retropharyngeal abscess; extrinsic compression from tumors, trauma, or congenital malformations; angioedema (anaphylaxis) or early asthmatic attack; laryngotracheobronchitis or laryngotracheobronchopneumonitis, infectious mononucleosis; and psychogenic stridor (Alberta Clinical Practice Guidelines Working Group, 2003). Table 31-4 differentiates acute laryngotracheitis from other common causes of stridor.

Management

Therapy depends on the cause, severity, and location of the disease. The aim of therapy is to provide adequate respiratory exchange. Table 31-5 shows management of the patient based on severity.

- *Humidified air.* A Cochrane review showed no evidence that inhalation of humidified air improved the outcome in croup scores in children with mild to moderate croup (Moore and Little, 2006). There is no evidence that the use of steam or cold humidification is harmful. However, cold air can be helpful. Often a ride in a car at night with the windows down accomplishes the same result. Occasionally vomiting relieves the bronchospasm.
- *Nebulized epinephrine.* This has been extensively studied in croup and can have short-term benefit of about 2 hours. The use of nebulized epinephrine can decrease the need for intubation (Cherry, 2008). This therapy requires close cardiorespiratory monitoring and should not be used in most primary care settings.
- *Corticosteroids.* Corticosteroids decrease inflammation and cell damage without prolonging the viral shedding duration. Meta-analysis of randomized trials shows corticosteroids improve the patient's condition (Russell et al, 2004). Steroids can be administered orally, intramuscularly, or by nebulizer. Recommended steroids include IM or oral dexamethasone (0.6 mg/kg orally) and nebulized budesonide with mild or moderate croup in an outpatient setting. However, dexamethasone at 0.6 mg/kg is more effective than prednisone and nebulized budesonide (Bjornson and Johnson, 2008; Cherry, 2008). IM dexamethasone can be used in a vomiting child. Otherwise, oral dexamethasone should be used because the rate of oral absorption equals that of IM therapy (Cherry, 2010b). The use of these agents should be limited to 1 to 2 days to avoid immunosuppression and the possibility of secondary bacterial tracheitis. However, one dose of dexamethasone has been shown to reduce inflammatory edema and to prevent destruction of ciliated epithelium (Cherry, 2008; 2010b). This one-time dose of dexamethasone (0.6 mg/kg) can be given as part of outpatient management. Antibiotics are not indicated.
- *Cold medications:* Cough and cold medicines are not indicated in croup, and their use has not been shown to be helpful (Cherry, 2008).

TABLE 31-4 Differentiating Common Respiratory Diseases That Can Cause Stridor or Similar Signs

Characteristic	Acute Laryngotracheitis	Epiglottitis	Laryngotracheobronchitis	Diphtheria	Foreign Body
Peak age	3-36 months old	1-5 years old	3 months to 36 months old	Any age/unimmunized	Toddlers
Onset	Gradual, acute onset at night	Rapid	Acute	Gradual onset over 1-2 days	Acute symptoms or gradual onset
Common findings	URI, seal-bark cough, mild to moderate dyspnea, symptoms worse at night	Sore throat, dysphagia, anxiety with inspiratory distress without significant stridor, drooling, muffled speech, looks toxic, tripod position	Hoarseness with barking cough, inspiratory stridor and toxic presentation with purulent sputum	Membranous nasopharyngitis, obstructive laryngotracheitis with local infection presenting as sore throat, nasal discharge, hoarseness	Coughing and/or choking episode, dyspnea, wheezing, cyanosis, signs and symptoms of secondary infection
Respiratory efforts	Rate generally <50	Marked distress	Marked distress	Minor to significant signs and symptoms of obstruction	Minor to significant distress
Fever	Common—low grade	High (ranges from 101.8° to 104° F [38.8° to 40° C])	High (102.2° F [39° C])	Low grade	Normal to low grade
CBC	Generally normal	High, left shift	High, left shift	Normal to slight leukocytosis, decreased thrombocyte count	Normal unless secondary infection
Organism(s)	Usually viral: parainfluenza, adenovirus, RSV	Usually *Haemophilus influenzae* type B (HIB)	Usually *Staphylococcus aureus*	*Corynebacterium diphtheriae*	
Specific laboratory tests	None	None	None	Positive culture	None
Radiographic view with findings	Lateral or AP of neck/subglottic narrowing	Lateral of neck/thumb sign	Lateral of neck/subglottic narrowing	Signs of obstruction in severe cases	May see localized hyperinflation, mediastinal shift, atelectasis
Treatment	Humidification, corticosteroids in selected cases	Hospitalization, cephalosporin, corticosteroids	Hospitalization, staphylococcus coverage	Hospitalization, erythromycin/penicillin, antitoxin	FB removal, treatment of secondary infection or bronchospasm
Intubation	Rare	Usually necessary	Frequently necessary	May be necessary	Endoscopy to remove FB
Prevention	None	Immunization—HIB	None	Immunization—DTaP	Education on childproofing home and monitoring child

AP, Anteroposterior; *CBC,* complete blood count; *DTaP,* diphtheria-tetanus-acellular pertussis; *FB,* foreign body; *LTB,* laryngotracheobronchitis; *RSV,* respiratory syncytial virus; *URI,* upper respiratory infection.

- *Bronchodilators:* If bronchospasm is also suspected, the use of bronchodilators in the usual doses prescribed for relief of asthma as discussed in Chapter 24 may be advantageous.
- *Oxygen*: Blow-by oxygen is used if the oxygen saturation falls below 92% (Alberta Clinical Practice Guidelines Working Group, 2003).
- *Other modalities:* In severe croup a helium-oxygen mixture known as heliox can be used.

Indications for Hospitalization

Children in distress with respiratory rates between 70 and 90 breaths per minute or exhibiting stridor at rest should be hospitalized. A child with a temperature higher than 102.2° F (39° C) should be carefully evaluated; hospitalization may be necessary if other worrisome symptoms are present. Racemic epinephrine by aerosol may help, but typically leads to rebound swelling several hours later. Corticosteroids are used

TABLE 31-5 Croup Severity and Treatment Based on Severity

	Mild	Moderate	Severe	Impending Respiratory Failure
Symptoms	Occasional croupy cough No retractions No chest wall retractions	Frequent croupy cough Audible stridor and suprasternal and sternal retractions at rest No agitation	Frequent croupy cough Tachypnea Prominent inspiratory and occasional expiratory stridor Agitation and distress	Audible stridor at rest Sternal retractions Lethargy Decreased level of consciousness with dusky color
Treatment				
Education of parent	X	X	X	X
Corticosteroid	X	X	X	X
Nebulized epinephrine			X	X
Blow-by oxygen			X	X until intubation
Intubation				X

Data from Alberta Clinical Practice Guidelines Working Group: *Guidelines for diagnosis and management of croup*, Alberta, ON, Canada, 2003. Available at www.albertadoctors.org/bcm/ama/ama-website.nsf/AllDoc/87256DB000705C3F87256E05005534E2/$File/CROUP.PDF.

(dexamethasone 0.5 to 2 mg/kg/dose every 8 hours IV), and IV hydration may be necessary (Cherry, 2008).

Complications

Increasing obstruction of the airways causes continuous stridor, nasal flaring, and suprasternal, infrasternal, and intercostal retractions. With further obstruction, air hunger and restlessness occur and are quickly followed by hypoxia, weakness, decreased air exchange, decreased stridor, increased pulse rate, and eventual death from hypoventilation. Anything that taxes the child's respiratory efforts, such as crying or feeding, causes more respiratory distress. Examination of the nasopharynx with a tongue depressor may result in sudden respiratory compromise. Severely ill children should be evaluated for acute epiglottitis. Viral pneumonia complicates about 1% to 2% of croup cases.

ACUTE SPASMODIC CROUP

Some children are prone to recurrent episodes of acute LTB. The etiologic agents are similar to those in laryngotracheitis (Cherry, 2008; Wald, 2010), but the condition occurs in families with a history of croup. Spasmodic croup presents with minimal coryza and acute onset of nighttime croup in a well child or a child with very mild cold symptoms. There is no fever, no pharyngitis, and a normal epiglottis. The episode is usually milder and of short duration, but symptoms may be recurrent. The treatment plan is the same as indicated for acute LTB. Spasmodic croup tends to respond well to exposure to cool air.

EPIGLOTTITIS

Epidemiology

Epiglottitis (supraglottitis) is characterized by inflammation of the epiglottis, the aryepiglottic folds, and the ventricular bands at the base of the epiglottis. The causative organism is *Haemophilus influenzae* type B (HIB). It occurs usually in children

between 1 and 5 years old with 25% of cases in children younger than 2 years old. The disease is 4 to 10 times higher in Navajo Native Americans and Alaskan Eskimos (Cherry, 2010c). Since the introduction of the HIB vaccine, there has been a drastic decline in the number of children with invasive infections caused by this organism; fortunately, epiglottitis is now a rare event. The following organisms have been implicated as causes of supraglottitis: *S. pneumoniae, S. aureus, H. parainfluenzae,* group A, B, C and G streptococcus, and *Bacillus* spp. (Cherry, 2010c).

Clinical Findings

History. There is an abrupt onset of fever, severe sore throat, dyspnea, inspiratory distress without stridor, and drooling. The child looks acutely ill and toxic.

Physical Examination. Findings include the following:

- Inspiratory and sometimes expiratory stridor
- Drooling, aphonia (muffled voice), and high fever
- Rapidly progressive respiratory obstruction and prostration
- Flaring of the ala nasi and retraction of the supraclavicular, intercostal, and subcostal spaces
- Child assumes a position of hyperextension of the neck

No attempt should be made to examine the posterior pharynx because stimulation of the area can induce spasm and obstruction of the epiglottis and lead to respiratory arrest.

In older children, one may find:

- Complaints of sore throat and dysphagia
- Stridor, irritability, restlessness, and brassy cough (uncommon)
- Airway obstruction follows within 2 to 24 hours. The child sits up with arms back, trunk forward, neck hyperextended, and chin thrust forward (tripod position).
- A rare, unusual finding is that of just a hoarse cough and a cherry-red epiglottis.

Diagnostic Tests. Blood cultures should be ordered. If the possibility of epiglottitis is thought to be remote in a patient with croup, a lateral neck radiograph may be obtained before the physical examination is undertaken. Absence of the "thumb" sign on the radiograph rules out the condition. A health care professional capable of supporting the airway and skilled in intubation must accompany the child to the radiology department and back.

Management

The time from the onset of symptoms until death may be only a matter of hours. Acute epiglottitis is a pediatric otolaryngologic emergency because of the risk of sudden airway obstruction. The goal of therapy is to establish an airway and appropriately start antimicrobials. If epiglottitis is suspected, do not examine the throat. Do not place the child in the supine position, and immediately transport the child to the hospital via emergency medical services. The child should be examined in the operating room by an otolaryngologist or an emergency department physician skilled in performing an emergency tracheostomy. An airway must be established, either a nasotracheal airway or a tracheostomy. The diagnosis is confirmed in the operating room by depressing the tongue to view the swollen cherry-red epiglottis. An expert in establishing an airway needs to be present because there is a risk of reflex laryngospasm, with acute and complete airway obstruction.

Begin the following treatments:
- Establish an airway, preferably by nasotracheal intubation (Cherry, 2010c).
- Administer IV broad-spectrum antibiotics to cover *H. influenzae.*
- Administer oxygen and respiratory support.

The acute infection rarely lasts more than 48 to 72 hours. However, idiopathic pulmonary edema can follow (in up to 9% of patients) after the establishment of an airway due to the changes in pulmonary microvascular pressure subsequent to relieving the obstruction. As improvement occurs, the child can be extubated, but antibiotic therapy should be continued for 10 days. Patients heal completely. Untreated or undertreated patients have a significant mortality rate. Remember that the time from the onset of symptoms to death can be a matter of hours. If *H. influenzae* is identified as the causative agent, rifampin prophylaxis (20 mg/kg in a single dose [maximum, 600 mg] for 4 days) should be given to all household contacts of the patient whose household has:
- At least one child younger than 4 years old who is unimmunized or incompletely immunized
- Children less than 12 months old who have not received the primary series of HIB vaccine
- Immunocompromised children (AAP, 2009; Cherry, 2010c)

In addition, if there are two cases of invasive HIB disease in a daycare center or nursery within 60 days, all members of the nursery need to receive prophylaxis (AAP, 2009).

Prevention

Routine immunization against HIB, the leading cause of epiglottitis, is the primary means of prevention. Handwashing is also an effective method of preventing spread of infection.

BACTERIAL TRACHEITIS (LARYNGOTRACHEOBRONCHITIS AND LARYNGOTRACHEOBRONCHOPNEUMONITIS)
Description and Epidemiology

Bacterial tracheitis, also known as laryngotracheobronchitis and laryngotracheobronchopneumonitis, is an acute potentially dangerous bacterial infection of the upper airway that does not involve the epiglottis. This condition is marked by an inflammatory process involving the larynx, trachea and bronchi with adherent or semiadherent mucopurulent membranes within the trachea. It can occur at any age, but typically is seen in the 3- to 10-year-old child. Bacterial tracheitis usually follows a viral respiratory infection (generally parainfluenza virus type 1). The child typically has had a prior croup episode or influenza virus and then becomes secondarily infected with *S. aureus,* the most common organism cultured, group A streptococci, *H. influenzae,* or *M. catarrhalis* (Bjornson and Johnson, 2008). No gender differentiation has been noted in the incidence or severity of symptoms (Cherry, 2010b).

Clinical Findings

History. The child initially starts with a URI including croup over a period of 2 to 7 days. A secondary bacterial infection occurs, and then suddenly the child becomes markedly worse.

Physical Examination. Copious purulent sputum is seen in older children. However, the extent of lower respiratory tract involvement is not realized due to the upper airway obstruction from infection. Inspiratory stridor develops, but there are rales, wheezing, an increased respiratory rate, and air trapping. The child looks toxic.

Diagnostic Tests. The diagnosis is based on confirming a bacterial upper airway infection. The white blood cell (WBC) count is elevated. Leukocytosis with a left shift is noted. Bacterial tracheitis can be differentiated from epiglottitis by its slower clinical course and a normal-appearing epiglottis on examination. The "classic" features of acute epiglottitis are absent (e.g., no thumb sign on a lateral neck film). However, pulmonary infiltrates and air trapping are seen on chest x-ray.

Management

Management includes the following:
- The usual treatments for croup are ineffective, and hospitalization is necessary.
- Intubation or tracheostomy is usually necessary to bypass the swelling that develops at the level of the cricoid cartilage and to manage the copious purulent secretions.
- Antibiotics that cover staphylococcus are administered.
- Oxygen and airway support are necessary.
- Most patients become afebrile in 48 to 72 hours if the condition is promptly recognized and treated. The child is weaned from the artificial airway and usually does well.

◼ Intrathoracic Airway Disorders
FOREIGN BODY ASPIRATION
Description

The symptoms and physical findings associated with aspiration of an FB depend on the nature of the material aspirated, plus the location and degree of the obstruction. The cough reflex protects the lower airways, and most aspirated material is immediately expelled with coughing. Onset of a sudden episode of coughing without a prodrome or signs of respiratory infection should make the provider suspicious of FB aspiration.

Epidemiology

Objects that are either too large to be eliminated by the mucociliary system or cannot be expelled by coughing eventually lead to some form of respiratory symptomatology. Obviously a large FB occluding the upper airway can cause suffocation. A small object in the lower respiratory tree may not produce symptoms for days to weeks. Obstruction results from either the FB itself or edema associated with its presence. Hot dogs are one of the most common causes of fatal aspiration. Toddlers commonly aspirate an FB; however, FB aspiration occurs in children of all ages.

Laryngeal Foreign Body

Clinical Findings

History. A rapid onset of hoarseness and the development of a chronic croupy cough with aphonia are reported. Be suspicious of a prior FB aspiration in children with cough, unilateral wheezing, and recurrent pneumonia.

Physical Examination. The child can also have hemoptysis, dyspnea, wheezing, and cyanosis.

Diagnostic Tests. In cases of suspected FB aspiration, expiratory or lateral decubitus chest radiographs should be ordered. Because most FBs are not radiopaque, radiographs may not be useful in the diagnosis. However, if a chest radiograph does not reveal an FB but shows local emphysema—an area that does not inflate or deflate—suspect FB aspiration (Carter and Marshall, 2011). If the history suggests FB aspiration, bronchoscopy must be undertaken. Direct laryngoscopy might reveal the presence of foreign matter.

Tracheal Foreign Body

Clinically the child has a history of a brassy cough, hoarseness, dyspnea, and possibly cyanosis. The most characteristic signs of tracheal FB aspiration are the homophonic wheeze and the audible slap and palpable thud sound produced by the momentary expiratory effect of the FB at the subglottic level.

Bronchial Foreign Body

The initial clinical findings are similar to those seen in either tracheal or laryngeal FB aspiration. Blood-streaked sputum may be expectorated. Children aspirating a metallic object often complain of a "metallic taste" in their mouths. If the object is nonobstructive and nonirritating, few or no initial symptoms may be seen. A small object can act as a bypass valve, and homophonic wheezes can be heard; emphysema or atelectasis can develop as the result of a large obstruction caused by a bronchial FB. The child may have limited chest expansion, decreased vocal fremitus, atelectasis, or emphysema-like changes with resulting hyporesonance or hyperresonance. Diminished breath sounds are often found. Crackles, rhonchi, and wheezes can be present if air movement is adequate. Most objects are aspirated into the right lung. A careful medical history may reveal a forgotten episode of choking.

Clinical Findings

History. An initial episode of coughing, gagging, and choking is described. Some objects are inhaled with no choking (e.g., a spear of grass). Hemoptysis rarely occurs as an early symptom, but on rare occasions does occur as an initial symptom months or years after the aspiration event took place.

Physical Examination. If the acute episode is missed or not appreciated, a latent period of mild "wheezing" or cough may be seen. Lobar pneumonia, intractable wheezing, and status asthmaticus can develop.

Diagnostic Tests. Clinical suspicion is the clue to this diagnosis. Inspiratory and forced expiratory chest radiographs and chest fluoroscopy are useful in identifying radiolucent FBs (Fig. 31-1).

Management. The patient should be referred to a pulmonary specialist for bronchoscopy. If the object is removed via bronchoscopy before permanent damage occurs, recovery is usually complete. Secondary lung infections and bronchospasms should be treated as suggested in the section on management of pneumonia and asthma.

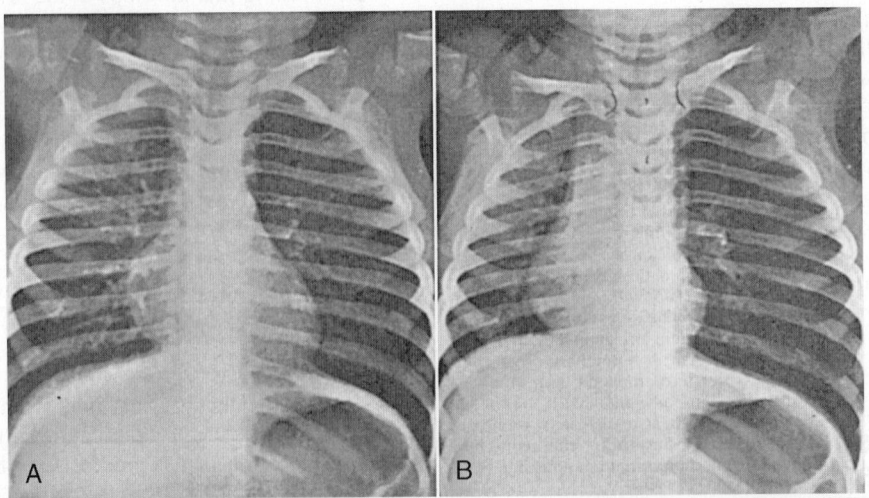

FIGURE 31-1 Obstructive overinflation caused by a peanut fragment in the left mainstem bronchus. **A,** Inspiration. **B,** Expiration. (From Ornstein D: Foreign bodies in the larynx, trachea, and bronchi. In Behrman RE, Kliegman RM, Jenson HB, editors: *Nelson textbook of pediatrics*, ed 16, Philadelphia, 2000, Saunders, p 1281.)

Complications. If the FB is vegetable matter, vegetal or arachidic bronchitis can occur. This severe condition can be characterized by sepsis-like fever, dyspnea, and cough. If the material has been there for a long time, suppuration can occur.

BRONCHITIS
Description

Bronchitis is a common diagnosis and can be classified as acute or chronic. Acute bronchitis is a febrile, cough illness lasting less than 3 weeks with rhonchi and referred breath sounds (Braman, 2006; Cherry, 2010d). It is associated with inflammation of the large airways including the trachea and the large- and medium-sized bronchi. There is associated destruction of the ciliated epithelium by the causative agent. This illness is associated with pharyngitis as well as rhinitis.

Chronic bronchitis is characterized by a productive cough lasting for more than 3 months (Hanson and Shearer, 2010). It is usually a symptom of another chronic disorder (e.g., allergies, asthma, CF, cigarette smoking). Bronchitis involves conducting airways with complete amounts of bronchial tube cartilage.

Epidemiology

This condition is usually preceded by a viral URI. Although a virus is the most common cause of acute bronchitis, weakened tissue can succumb to a secondary bacterial infection. The common viral agents implicated in bronchitis are influenzavirus, RSV, adenovirus, and parainfluenza virus. Other viral agents include rhinovirus, enterovirus, human metapneumovirus, human bocavirus, and the newer human coronavirus. *S. pneumoniae, B. pertussis,* and *H. influenzae* are the most commonly cultured bacterial organisms. *M. pneumoniae* and *C. pneumoniae* are also causative agents. *Pseudomonas aeruginosa* is the common agent in children with CF. The incidence of the disease peaks in midwinter and declines by midsummer with an increase in the fall. Male incidence predominates over females during the first 6 months of life.

Clinical Findings

The usual course of illness can be divided into three phases: a prodrome in which fever and URI symptoms predominate, a 6-day period of marked tracheobronchial symptoms with malaise and fever, and a recovery period lasting 1 to 2 weeks with cough and expectoration (Cherry, 2010d).

History. The following are reported:
- A dry, hacking, unproductive cough that begins a few days after the onset of rhinitis and fever
- Complaints of low substernal discomfort or burning chest pain aggravated by coughing
- Initially the cough is dry, harsh, and sometimes brassy in younger children. However, as it progresses, cough becomes productive, and because younger children swallow the sputum, vomiting and gagging can occur.

Physical Examination. Findings can vary and include the following:
- Variable rhinitis
- Low-grade or no fever
- Signs of nasopharyngeal infection and conjunctivitis
- Coarse breath sounds, rhonchi, and coarse, changing rales

Diagnostic Tests. Chest x-ray is not routinely done unless pneumonia is suspected. Reliance on procalcitonin levels to determine if the patient has a bacterial infection needs more research before widespread use (Christ-Crain and Opal, 2010).

Differential Diagnosis

Pertussis should be considered in patients with a cough lasting 2 to 3 weeks because it is found in 10% of patients with chronic cough. Children with recurrent acute bronchitis must be evaluated for underlying pathologic conditions. Respiratory tract anomalies, FB aspiration, bronchiectasis, immunodeficiency, allergy, rhinosinusitis, anatomic problems such as gastroesophageal reflux and tracheoesophageal fistulas, tonsillitis, exposure to air pollutants, adenoiditis, and CF must be considered in the differential diagnosis. Check for tobacco or marijuana use in teenagers. In chronic bronchitis, primary ciliary dyskinesia, cystic fibrosis, foreign body, congenital anomalies, reflux, aspiration, asthma, allergies, autoimmune diseases, immune deficiency, and bacteria pathogens such as *B. pertussis, M. pneumoniae,* and *C. pneumoniae* should be considered (Hanson and Shearer, 2010).

Management

For acute bronchitis, no specific therapy is known, and most patients require none. Care is primarily supportive.
- *Analgesia:* For pain
- *Hydration:* Intake of fluids to avoid dehydration
- *Antiviral/antibiotics:* If influenza A is the likely etiologic agent, and there is underlying pulmonary diseases, antiviral therapy should be used. Because most cases of acute bronchitis are from viral sources, antibiotics are not indicated. If *M. pneumoniae* or *C. pneumoniae* is suspected, macrolides can be used.
- *Cough suppressants:* There is no evidence to support the use of cough suppressants. Antihistamines should not be used because of their excessive drying effect; these agents tend to prolong the symptoms.
- *Bronchodilators:* There is no evidence to support the use of inhaled β-agonists unless there is obstruction and wheezing at the onset of illness (Braman, 2006). A chest x-ray should be considered if there is evidence of a complex bacterial illness. Mucus generally thins in 5 to 10 days, and the cough decreases.

For chronic bronchitis, treatment depends on whether an underlying cause is found. Bronchodilators, cromolyn sodium, corticosteroids, and anticholinergic agents are used for the treatment of chronic cough associated with asthma or underlying chronic lung disease. If reflux is the cause, underlying treatment of the reflux is indicated. Avoidance of tobacco smoke, dust exposure, and air pollution is important. Antibiotics are used for chronic bronchitis if there is a strong likelihood of developing an underlying bacterial infection (Hanson and Shearer, 2010).

Complications

In normal, healthy children, the condition is not serious; however, malaise continues for another week or so after the cough lessens. In undernourished or chronically ill children, otitis, rhinosinusitis, and pneumonia are common.

BRONCHIOLITIS

Description

Bronchiolitis is also called infectious asthma, asthmatic bronchitis, wheezy bronchitis or virus-induced asthma. It is characterized by signs of a URI. However, the predominant pathophysiology is obstruction of the lower respiratory tract as a result of acute inflammation, edema, and necrosis of the epithelial cells of the small bronchioles. This results in bronchospasm and increased mucus production. It is a communicable disease found primarily in infancy. Bronchiolitis is the term used for an infant seen with wheezing for the very first time and is the leading cause of hospitalizations for infants. It presents with cough, fever, coryza, tachypnea, expiratory wheezing, air trapping, and inspiratory crackles. In mild cases, symptoms can last for 1 to 3 days. In severe cases, cyanosis, air hunger, retractions, and nasal flaring with symptoms of severe respiratory distress within a few hours may be seen. Apnea can occur and may require mechanical ventilation (Welliver, 2010).

Epidemiology

Bronchiolitis is a viral illness predominantly caused by RSV, especially in outbreaks (Everard, 2009; Welliver, 2010). Parainfluenza virus (types 1 through 3), adenovirus, *M. pneumoniae*, influenzavirus, adenovirus, human metapneumovirus, rhinovirus, enterovirus, and herpes simplex generally cause the remainder of cases in decreasing prevalence. Adenovirus and RSV can cause long-term complications. The incubation period for RSV is 4 to 6 days and typically occurs from late fall through early spring with virtually no outbreaks in the summer (Welliver, 2010). Typically the illness begins with URI symptoms of cough, cold, coryza, and rhinorrhea and progresses over 3 to 7 days with symptoms of audible wheezing and noisy, raspy breathing (Smith, 2011). More than 80% of the cases of bronchiolitis occur in infants less than 1 year of age with a male-to-female ratio of 1.5:1 (Welliver, 2010). It is spread by close contact with infected respiratory secretions or fomites. The most frequent mode of transmission is hand carriage of contaminated secretion. The source of infection is an older family member with a "mild" URI. Older children and adults have larger airways and tolerate the swelling associated with this infection better than infants do. Most cases of bronchiolitis resolve completely, but recurrence of infection is common, and symptoms tend to be mild.

Risk factors for severe RSV disease are high levels of RSV in the nasopharynx, having genetically smaller airways, family history of asthma, airway reactivity, premature birth, chronic lung disease, and immunodeficiency. Environmental risk factors include crowding, passive smoking, and absence of breastfeeding. RSV-specific IgE, eosinophils, and chemokines may play a role in the pathogenesis of bronchiolitis (Welliver, 2010).

Clinical Findings

History. The following are reported:

- Initial presentation of URI symptoms (cough, coryza, and rhinorrhea) lasting for 3 to 7 days
- Gradual development of respiratory distress marked by noisy, raspy breathing with audible wheezing
- Low-grade to moderate fever up to 102° F (38.9° C)
- Decrease in appetite
- No prodrome in some infants; rather they have apnea as the initial symptom

Physical Examination. Findings include the following:

- Coryza
- Mild conjunctivitis in 33% (Welliver, 2010)
- Pharyngitis
- Otitis media in up to 15% (Welliver, 2010)
- Heterophonous wheezing
- Crackles may be heard throughout the breathing cycle
- High respiratory rate (approximately 40 to 80 breaths per minute)
- Varying signs of respiratory distress and pulmonary involvement (e.g., nasal flaring, grunting, retractions, cyanosis, prolonged expiration)
- Abdominal distention
- Palpable liver and spleen, pushed down by hyperinflated lungs

Diagnostic Tests. The routine use of chest radiographs in previously healthy infants with mild RSV bronchiolitis is not indicated. Evidence-based guidelines from the AAP Subcommittee on Diagnosis and Management of Bronchitis (AAPB) and the Scottish Intercollegiate Guidelines Network (SIGN) are strongly against routine chest radiography (AAPB, 2006; SIGN, 2006). In severe illness, a chest x-ray may be ordered to rule out pneumonia, but its use must be weighed against the dangers of radiation exposure. The findings of chest radiography can vary, and even with severe illness the x-ray can be clear with a flattened diaphragm and an increase in anteroposterior diameter. Areas of atelectasis can appear like a pneumonitis, but true pneumonia is uncommon. Early bacterial pneumonia can be difficult to detect and cannot be ruled out by radiographs. Virologic testing is weakly recommended in the AAPB and SIGN guidelines. Enzyme-linked immunosorbent assays or fluorescent antibody techniques to look for RSV are the diagnostic procedures of choice in most laboratories. Viral culture of nasal washings can be done in severe cases to confirm RSV, parainfluenza viruses, influenza viruses, and adenoviruses. PCR is helpful in deciding about isolation of cohorts with the same infection in the hospital setting. Hematologic testing is not recommended in the latest guidelines. If a CBC is done for another reason, a mild leukocytosis may be seen with 12,000 to 16,000/mm^3. Routine laboratory tests are usually not required to confirm the diagnosis because they lack specificity.

Differential Diagnosis

Making the diagnosis is not usually a problem. In mild afebrile cases, bronchial asthma can be confused with bronchiolitis. Other differentials include foreign body, circulatory failure, congenital heart disease irritants, gastroesophageal reflux, metabolic causes, allergic pneumonitis, vascular rings, lung cysts, and lobar emphysema (Welliver, 2010).

Management

Evidence-based guidelines were published by the AAPB as well as the SIGN and are similar (Everard, 2009). Most infants with mild signs of respiratory distress can be treated as outpatients.

- Supportive care consists of adequate hydration and use of antipyretics.
- Transcutaneous oxygen saturation monitoring is strongly recommended.

- Fluid intake is strongly recommended to prevent dehydration.
- The following are strongly not recommended:
  - β-agonist
  - Adrenaline
  - Antibiotics (unless indicated for another problem)
  - Inhaled or oral corticosteroids
  - Physiotherapy
  - Viral therapy (ribavirin)
  - Antileukotriene therapy
  - Humidification or steam

Parents need to understand:

- The management of rhinitis (use of saline drops and suctioning of nares)
- Indications for the use of antipyretics
- Signs of increasing respiratory distress or dehydration that call for hospitalization
- Guidelines for feeding an infant with signs of mild respiratory distress (amount of fluid needed per 24 hours; smaller, more frequent feedings; monitoring of the respiratory rate; and guarding against vomiting)

Infants younger than 2 months old and older infants with signs of severe respiratory distress should be hospitalized. Signs that suggest increasing respiratory distress include the following (Smith, 2011):

- Progressive stridor or stridor at rest
- Apnea
- Increasing respiratory rate (sleeping rate of greater than 50 to 60 breaths per minute)
- Restlessness, pallor, or cyanosis
- Hypoxia recorded by either blood gas (Po_2 less than 60 mm Hg) or pulse oximetry (less than 92% on room air)
- Rising Pco_2 (recorded by blood gas)
- Inability to tolerate oral feedings
- Depressed sensorium
- Presence of chronic cardiovascular or immunodeficiency disease
- Parent unable to manage at home for any reason

In-hospital management focuses on supportive care and includes suctioning of upper airways, which is critical; humidified supplemental oxygen; and elevation of the child to a sitting position at a 30- to 40-degree angle. The infant's neck should be extended to 30 to 40 degrees. IV fluids are frequently needed because respiratory distress interferes with nursing or bottle feeding. There are subsets of infants with bronchiolitis who demonstrate significant bronchodilator responsiveness. Therefore, all infants (especially those with a family history of asthma or atopy) with significant wheezing should be given a one-time trial of an aerosolized beta 2-adrenergic treatment. If after an initial one-time trial there is no improvement, additional use of bronchodilators should be abandoned (AAPB, 2006; Everard, 2009).

Occasionally a hospitalized child is not able to be quickly weaned back to room air. Home management of these patients requiring oxygen is extremely difficult and should be undertaken only by someone with excellent pulmonary skills and in consultation with a pediatrician or pediatric pulmonologist. The child should have an O_2 saturation study before discharge to help determine the O_2 requirements at rest, feeding, play, and sleep. A pneumogram to rule out apnea may also be indicated. Strict outpatient follow-up is mandatory for as long as the child is receiving home O_2.

Complications

The first 48 to 72 hours after the onset of cough are the most critical. Apneic spells are common in infants. The child is ill-appearing and toxic, but gradually improves. The fatality rate associated with bronchiolitis is about 1% to 2%. Prolonged apnea, uncompensated respiratory acidosis, and profound dehydration secondary to loss of water from tachypnea and an inability to drink are the factors leading to death in young infants with bronchiolitis. In some children, bronchiolitis can cause minor pulmonary function problems and a tendency for bronchial hyperreactivity that lasts for years. RSV bronchiolitis has been associated with the development of asthma, but its role in the causality of asthma is still debated. Recurrent episodes of wheezing can be seen during childhood in patients with a history of bronchiolitis. This persists into adolescence in 10% of the children still wheezing. However, this figure may not be different from the general population (Welliver, 2010).

Prevention

Palivizumab is an RSV-specific monoclonal antibody used to provide some protection from severe RSV infection for high-risk infants (see Chapter 23). Educate caregivers about decreasing exposure to and transmission of RSV, especially those with high-risk infants. Advice should include limiting exposure to childcare centers, if possible; handwashing; avoiding tobacco smoke exposure; and scheduling RSV prophylaxis vaccination, when indicated.

NONBACTERIAL AND BACTERIAL PNEUMONIA

Pneumonia is a lower respiratory tract infection with consolidation of the alveolar spaces involving the airways and parenchyma of the lung. It can be lobar, interstitial, or bronchopneumonial. Lobar pneumonia involves infection of the alveolar space that results in consolidation; it is described as "typical" pneumonia. Atypical pneumonia describes patterns of consolidation that are not localized. In interstitial pneumonia, cellular infiltrates attack the interstitium, which makes up the walls of the alveoli, the alveolar sacs and ducts, and the bronchioles; this type of pneumonia is typical of acute viral infections, but may also be a chronic process. Nonbacterial pneumonia is the most common pulmonary infection in children and adolescents (Boyer, 2010). Aside from viruses, this category includes atypical bacterial pneumonia caused by *M. pneumoniae*, *C. pneumoniae*, and *Chlamydia trachomatis*. Respiratory viruses account for 40% of acquired pneumonia (Ranganathan and Sonnappa, 2009). Pneumonitis is a general term used to describe lung inflammation that may or may not be associated with consolidation.

Bacterial pneumonia occurs as a primary infection caused by organisms that spread from the nasopharynx, or as a secondary complication of a viral pneumonia (Ranganthan and Sonnappa, 2009). *S. pneumoniae* is the leading cause of bacterial pneumonia in all age groups except newborns (Klein, 2010). Certain bacterial pneumonias have a specific pattern of disease: *S. pneumoniae* causes a lobar pneumonia, whereas *S. aureus* presents with empyema, abscess, and pneumatocele formation (Klein, 2010). Irritation of the pleura causes chest pain in children with pneumonia.

Lobar and interstitial pneumonia and bronchiolar and bronchial inflammation can coexist in a child (Klein, 2010). Table 31-6 differentiates the various forms of pneumonia commonly found in infants, children, and adolescents. Table 31-7 shows the most common organisms by age. Treatment is often empirical and varies with age.

Description

Primary bacterial pneumonia is less common in childhood than secondary bacterial infection after a viral infection. Viral pneumonia often involves both the conducting airways and the alveoli. This type of pneumonia is a common problem in young children and can result in serious illness in a young infant. The onset of viral pneumonia is gradual over a 1- to 2-day period of coryza, respiratory congestion, fever, cough, and increasing fretfulness (Boyer, 2010). Viral infection affects the lung defenses by altering normal secretions, inhibiting phagocytosis, modifying the normal bacterial flora, and disrupting the epithelial layer. Thus the many childhood viruses set the stage for secondary bacterial infection. Children with immunologic problems or chronic illnesses are prone to primary bacterial pneumonia and experience recurrent pneumonias or fail to clear the initial infection completely. Differentiating bacterial from viral pneumonia is particularly important in infants younger than 6 months.

Mycoplasma pneumonia, or primary atypical pneumonia, is the most common cause of pneumonia in children older than 5 years through the young adult years. This disease is usually mild and self-limited. *Chlamydia* pneumonia is a characteristic pneumonia resulting from the transmission of *C. trachomatis* from the infected genital tract of the mother to the infant. It does not become apparent until the infant is 2 to 19 weeks old.

Epidemiology

Infecting organisms associated with pneumonia vary by age (see Table 31-7). Ninety percent of childhood bacterial pneumonia is caused by *S. pneumoniae* (Klein, 2010). Pneumococcal pneumonia occurs most commonly in the late winter and early spring, after the cycle of viral URIs. Asymptomatic carriers play a more important role in dissemination of disease than do sick contacts. Children younger than 4 years old suffer the highest attack rate. Pneumonia caused by community-acquired methicillin-resistant *Staphylococcus aureus* (MRSA) has become a worrisome occurrence especially with influenza infection. *S. aureus* presents with chills, high and prolonged fever, dyspnea, and pleuritic chest pain (Klein, 2010).

Viruses that cause pneumonia in children of all ages are identified in Table 31-7. *M. pneumoniae,* an organism without a cell wall, is transmitted from one symptomatic patient to another

---

TABLE 31-6 Differentiating Various Forms of Pneumonia in Infants, Young Children, and Adolescents

Characteristic	Bacterial	Viral	*Mycoplasma pneumoniae* and *Chlamydophila pneumoniae*	*Chlamydia trachomatis*
Common age	All ages	All ages	>5 years old	2-19 weeks old (typically 1-3 months old)
Onset	Acute; gradual	Acute; gradual	Slow	Gradual
Clinical findings	Depend on age; starts with URI, cough, dyspnea, tachypnea, rales, decreased breath sounds, grunting, retractions, toxic look; potential progression to severe respiratory distress	Depend on age; cough, coryza, hoarseness, crackles, wheezing, stridor	Persistent cough, malaise, headache	Tachypnea, staccato cough, crackles, wheezing rare, 50% have signs or history of conjunctivitis
Fever	Acute onset of fever (≥102.2° F [>39° C])	Present	>102.2° F (>39° C)	Afebrile
CBC	WBCs often elevated >15,000/microliter	Normal or slight elevation of WBC	Normal	Eosinophilia in 75% of cases
Organism(s)	90% caused by *Streptococcus pneumoniae*	RSV, parainfluenza, influenza (types A and B)	*M. pneumoniae* *C. pneumoniae*	*Chlamydia trachomatis*
Radiographic findings	Lobar consolidation	Transient lobar infiltrates	Varies, interstitial infiltrates	Hyperinflation, infiltrates
Treatment	Depends on bacteria and age of child; amoxicillin, penicillin, methicillin, cefuroxime, gentamicin, vancomycin	Supportive care	Erythromycin/clarithromycin	Erythromycin

CBC, Complete blood count; *RSV,* respiratory syncytial virus; *URI,* upper respiratory infection; *WBCs,* white blood cells.

by droplet spread. The incubation period is 2 to 3 weeks, and asymptomatic carriage after infection can last for weeks. Due to prenatal screening, the incidence of *C. trachomatis* infection of the newborn has decreased but should be considered in a mother with inadequate or no prenatal care. *C. trachomatis* is an organism that has many subtypes within the species. Approximately 50% of infants born to infected mothers acquire this infection, but only 5% to 20% of these infants develop *C. trachomatis* pneumonia with a typical onset between 1 and 3 months of age.

Clinical Findings in Infants and Young Children

Age influences the clinical manifestations of pneumonia and differing infectious agents cause different presentations and symptoms. However, the difference in presentation of viral or bacterial pneumonia is not always clear or easy to differentiate. Remember that neonates may have respiratory manifestations without a fever, or fever only with subtle or no physical findings suggestive of pneumonia.

History. The following may be reported (Boyer, 2010; Klein, 2010):
- Initial history of a mild URI for a few days—similar for both bacterial and viral.

TABLE 31-7 Age Variants in Pneumonia Microorganisms

Age	Viral Organisms	Bacterial Organisms
Neonatal	Cytomegalovirus	More common • Group B streptococci • Gram-negative enteric bacteria • *Listeria* • *Chlamydia trachomatis* Uncommon organisms • *Streptococcus pneumoniae* • Group D streptococcus • Anaerobes
Infants	Most common • Respiratory syncytial virus • Parainfluenza • Influenza • Adenoviruses • Metapneumovirus	Less common • *S. pneumoniae* • *Haemophilus influenzae* • *Mycoplasma pneumoniae* • *Mycobacterium tuberculosis* • *Bordetella pertussis* • *Pneumocystis jiroveci*
Preschool children	Most common • Respiratory syncytial virus • Parainfluenza • Influenza • Adenoviruses • Metapneumovirus	Less common • *S. pneumoniae* • *H. influenzae* • *M. pneumoniae* • *M. tuberculosis* • *C. pneumoniae*
School-age children	Respiratory viruses as above	• *M. pneumoniae* • *C. pneumoniae* • *S. pneumoniae* • *M. tuberculosis*

Adapted from Ranganathan S, Sonnappa S: Pneumonia and other respiratory infections, *Pediatr Clin North Am* 56:140, 2009.

- Abrupt high fever with temperatures greater than 103.3° F (39.6° C), chills, cough, and dyspnea suggest bacterial pneumonia.
- Other manifestations include restlessness, shaking chills, apprehension, shortness of breath, malaise, and pleuritic chest pain. Irritation of the pleura causes chest pain in children with pneumonia.
- History of group B streptococcal or *C. trachomatis* infection in the mother
- Prenatal drug use or lack of prenatal care is a risk factor for serious bacterial infection (SBI) in the neonate.
- Slower onset of respiratory symptoms, cough, wheezing, or stridor with less prominent fever suggests viral pneumonia.
- Bacterial pneumonia is less likely in a wheezing child (Ranganathan and Sonnappa, 2009).
- With *C. trachomatis*, the infant is typically afebrile; prior, concurrent, or no history of inclusion conjunctivitis reported.

Physical Examination. Typical findings seen in all types of pneumonia include:
- Nasal flaring, grunting, retractions
- Tachypnea generally greater than 60 breaths per minute in infants less than 2 months old, greater than 50 breaths per minute in children 2 to 11 months old, or greater than 40 breaths per minute at rest in children 1 to 5 years old (may be the only clue), tachycardia, air hunger, cyanosis are significant findings
- Fine crackles, dullness, diminished breath sounds
In bacterial pneumonia:
- Splinting the affected side to minimize pleuritic pain or lying on the side in a fetal position helps compensate for decreased air exchange and improves ventilation.
- Tachypnea and retractions
- Progression to delirium, circumoral cyanosis, and posturing
- Other findings can include:
  - Presence of a pleural effusion and signs of congestive heart failure
  - Abdominal distention, downward displacement of the liver or spleen
- Nuchal rigidity without meningeal infection from involvement of the right upper lobe
- Decreased peripheral perfusion and capillary refill
- Lethargy
In viral pneumonia:
- Wheezing
- Downward displacement of the liver or spleen
In primary atypical bacterial pneumonia (*C. trachomatis*):
- *C. trachomatis* pneumonia characterized by repetitive, staccato cough with tachypnea, cervical adenopathy, crackles, and rarely wheezing
- Conjunctivitis is associated with *C. trachomatis* (Ranganathan and Sonnappa, 2009).

Clinical Findings in Children and Adolescents
History. The patient can have:
- Sick contacts at home
- Travel history
- Inadequate immunization coverage
- FB aspiration
- Asthma
- Environmental exposure
- Initial history of URI

- History of a sudden onset of shaking chills, followed by a high fever, cough, chest pain; these symptoms are associated with bacterial pneumonia
- A prodrome of chills, headache, sore throat, gastrointestinal symptoms, and malaise is often associated with atypical bacterial pneumonia.

Physical Examination. Symptoms vary, and there is overlap between bacterial and viral pneumonia. Typical findings seen in all types of pneumonia include:

- Elevated respiratory rate, accessory muscle use, wheezes or adventitious sounds such as crackles, retractions, tachypnea, decreased tactile and vocal fremitus, diminished breath sounds
- Dullness plus fine and crackling rales on the affected side
  In bacterial pneumonia:
- Changes in level of consciousness
- Dry, hacking, productive cough (with rust-colored or bloody sputum if expectorated)
  In primary atypical bacterial pneumonia (*M. pneumoniae* and *C. pneumoniae*):
- URI symptoms, low-grade fever (temperature less than 102.2° F [39° C])
- Dry cough with scant sputum
- Rhinorrhea is not commonly reported nor found
- Typically hear minimal changes or harsh breath sounds and rhonchi on auscultation

Diagnostic Tests. A chest x-ray should not be routinely performed in children with pneumonia (Ranganathan and Sonnappa, 2009). The British Thoracic Society (2002) guidelines recommend the use of a chest x-ray in a child younger than 5 with a fever greater than 104° F (40° C) and without features of bronchiolitis. Radiographic evidence of pneumonia includes abscesses, lobar infiltrates, effusions, or cavities. However, no other chest x-ray findings are helpful in differentiating bacterial from viral pneumonia (Kumar and McKean, 2004).

Direct fluorescent antibody (DFA) testing of nasopharyngeal washings may help determine the viral agent, but is generally reserved for children needing hospital admission. The WBC count is normal or mildly elevated with a predominance of lymphocytes in viral pneumonia. Infants and children with significant lower respiratory symptoms may require hospitalization and more extensive diagnostic testing. In such cases the usual findings in a bacterial pneumonia include the following:

- WBC count is elevated (greater than 20,000/mm^3) with predominant neutrophils.
- Arterial blood gases are consistent with hypoxia.
- The organism may be found by culture of nasopharyngeal scrapings (not always accurate), tracheal aspirates, blood (10% to 20% of cases are positive; however, if positive, this confirms the causative pathogen), or lung tap fluid.
- Radiographs are consistent with lobar or segmental consolidation or a round pneumonia with pleural effusion in up to 30% of children. Frontal and lateral films are needed for adequate visualization. Staphylococcal pneumonia involves the right lobe 65% of the time. Pneumatoceles are common in staphylococcal pneumonia (Klein, 2010).
- Blood, urine, and CSF cultures should also be obtained in infants younger than 2 months as part of a septic workup.

BOX 31-2 Criteria for Hospital Admission for Pneumonia

- Tachypnea: >60 breaths/min in infants <2 months; >50 breaths/min in children 2 to 11 months old; or >40 breaths/min at rest in children 1 to 5 years old
- Grunting, dyspnea or apnea
- Severe respiratory distress
- Oxygen saturation less than 92% with the need for supplemental oxygen (pulse oximetry reading or arterial blood gas)
- Toxic appearance
- Failure to respond to appropriate oral antibiotic
- Neonate to 3 months old
- Poor oral intake with signs of dehydration
- Pulmonary complications noted on radiographs—abscess, empyema, pneumatocele
- Social issues at home that indicate parent or caretaker cannot appropriately monitor and/or care for the child

---

Blood cultures should also be done in older children who are hospitalized and suspected to have bacterial pneumonia (Kumar and McKean, 2004).

Differential Diagnosis

The child's age and characteristic signs and symptoms as identified previously help distinguish viral from bacterial pneumonia. Other disease entities and conditions to consider in the differential diagnosis are bronchiolitis, congestive heart failure, acute bronchiectasis, FB aspiration, pulmonary abscess, parasitic pneumonia, and endotracheal tuberculosis. Also right lower lobe pneumonia can be confused with appendicitis. Right upper lobe pneumonia can often closely resemble meningitis.

Management

Most otherwise healthy older children can be managed as outpatients. Guidelines for admission are identified in Box 31-2. Neonates must always be admitted to the hospital if diagnosed with pneumonia regardless of infecting pathogen. Young infants may also need hospitalization unless *C. trachomatis* is suspected. All children with pneumonia require supportive care with antipyretics, hydration, and rest. Antibiotics should be reserved for those with suspected bacterial infection only. Serious infections may require hospitalization for respiratory therapy including humidified oxygen, pulmonary therapy, and/or intubation.

Guidelines for outpatient and inpatient treatment of pneumonia by age and certain specific pathogens are as follows (Ranganathan and Sonnappa, 2009; Taketomo et al, 2011):

- *Outpatient antibiotic treatment* (5 to 10 days' duration of therapy): Oral antibiotics are considered safe for most children with pneumonia (Ranganathan and Sonnappa, 2009).
  - *One month to 4 months old:* May need to admit unless chlamydia suspected: Treat chlamydia with oral azithromycin for 5 days or erythromycin base or ethylsuccinate for 14 days (AAP, 2009).

○ *Four months to 4 years old:* Amoxicillin 80 to 100 mg/kg/day, divided every 6 to 8 hours for 10 days

○ *Five years and older:* Azithromycin 12 mg/kg/day once a day for 5 days (maximum dose 500 mg), amoxicillin 80 to 100 mg/kg/day divided twice a day or three times a day for 10 days or amoxicillin with clavulanic acid with 80 to 90 mg amoxicillin dosage and use the 7:1 dosage form or Augmentin ES 600 mg/5 mL for 10 days. If chlamydia pneumonia or mycoplasma pneumonia is suspected, azithromycin is an appropriate choice.

○ Erythromycin, azithromycin, or clarithromycin is the recommended treatment if *M. pneumoniae* or *C. pneumoniae* is suspected.

• *Inpatient treatment:* Testing to identify the pathogen is important for selection of appropriate antimicrobial therapy.

○ *Neonate:* Ampicillin and cefotaxime, ceftriaxone, or gentamicin

○ *One month to 5 years old:* Cefuroxime and add vancomycin if rapid progression of illness

○ *Five years and older:* Cefotaxime and azithromycin and add vancomycin if rapid progression of illness

• The recommended treatment for *S. aureus* pneumonia is nafcillin, cephazolin, clindamycin (for MRSA) with vancomycin as an alternative. (Smith, 2011).

Prognosis

By the second to third day of treatment, auscultation should reveal a change in respiratory sounds as the infection begins to consolidate. Increased fremitus, tubular breath sounds, and the disappearance of crackles may be noted. Most children have an uneventful recovery, but it is important to inform parents that their child's cough can last for several weeks. Routine rechecks with chest x-rays are not recommended because radiographic findings may take 6 to 8 days to normalize. If pneumonia recurs or persists for longer than 1 month, the child needs further evaluation for underlying disease.

Complications

Empyema is common in staphylococcal and GABHS infections. Scarring of the airways and lung tissue can cause dilated bronchi, which results in bronchiectasis. Lung abscess can result if the pneumonia causes necrosis of the lung tissue. *M. pneumoniae* can spread to the blood, CNS, heart, skin, or joints. A child with sickle cell disease and pneumonia caused by *M. pneumoniae* has more severe pulmonary disease than the average child does. Children with recurrent pneumonias should be referred for further pulmonary evaluation.

Prevention

Identify and treat pregnant women with *C. trachomatis.* Universal vaccination against influenza, HIB, and pneumococcal infection is essential. For high-risk neonates monthly injections of humanized monoclonal RSV antibody are essential (Klein, 2010) (see Chapter 23).

CYSTIC FIBROSIS
Description

CF is a multisystem genetic disorder manifested by chronic obstructive pulmonary disease (COPD), gastrointestinal disturbances, and exocrine dysfunction. Over the past decade the life expectancy for individuals with CF increased to 37.4 years (O'Sullivan and Freedman, 2009).

Epidemiology

CF occurs in approximately 1 in 3000 Caucasian births. Although not common, it does occur in 1 in 15,000 to 20,000 African-American, 1 in 4000 to 10,000 Hispanic, and 1 in 350,000 Japanese births (O'Sullivan and Freedman, 2009). This autosomal recessive genetic disorder involves mutation of the CF transmembrane conductance regulator protein (CFTR), which is expressed in epithelial cells and blood cells. The gene is on chromosome 7, but more than 1500 CFTR mutations have been identified, though the functional importance of only a few of those mutations is known.

CFTR functions in sodium transport through the epithelial sodium channel, regulates the adenosine triphosphate (ATP) channels, and is involved in bicarbonate chloride exchange. The CFTR gene defect causes defective ion transport, airway surface liquid depletion, and defective mucociliary clearance (Ratjen, 2009).

The CFTR mutations can be grouped into five classes. Understanding the type of mutation helps direct the type of therapy and has taken on new importance in targeted CF treatment. The most common defect, found in 66% of cases, is a deletion of phenylalanine in position 508 (D508) (Ratjen, 2009). Polymorphism in non-CFTR genes may explain the difference in the manifestations of the genetic change within different families. Ultimately, the mucus obstruction that results causes inflammation and infection. This failure to conduct ions across the epithelial cell membranes leads to problems in the lungs, biliary tree, pancreas, intestines, vas deferens, and sweat glands. This results in mucus thickening and target organ damage in the lungs and exocrine glands.

In the lung, there is airway depletion, which leads to ciliary collapse and decreased mucociliary transport. Ultimately, the mucous obstruction causes chronic inflammation and infection, and bacterial colonization in trapped mucous secretions (O'Sullivan and Freedman, 2009; Ratjen, 2009).

Clinical Findings

CF is a multisystemic progressive illness with varying levels of severity. Table 31-8 shows age variants in clinical manifestations. Clinical manifestations may include the following (O'Sullivan and Freedman, 2009):

• *Pulmonary.* CF is a major cause of severe chronic lung disease in children. The lungs of children with CF are normal at birth but become inflamed with chronic airway infection within a short time following birth. The respiratory epithelium exhibits marked impermeability to chloride and excessive sodium reabsorption. Mucus is viscous, and dehydration of the airway secretions occurs leading to

TABLE 31-8 Clinical Manifestations of Cystic Fibrosis: From Neonatal Period to Adolescence

Stage of Childhood	Clinical Manifestations
Neonatal period	Meconium ileus Prolonged jaundice Intestinal atresia
Infancy	Cough Colonization with bacteria in mucus Bacterial pneumonia Failure to thrive Hypoproteinemia Abdominal distention Cholestasis Rectal prolapse Steatorrhea Distal intestinal obstruction syndrome (DIOS) Hemolytic anemia
Childhood	Polyps Steatorrhea Rectal prolapse DIOS Idiopathic pancreatitis Liver disease
Adolescence	Allergic bronchopulmonary aspergillosis Chronic pansinusitis Nasal polyposis Bronchiectasis Hemoptysis Idiopathic pancreatitis Osteoporosis

Adapted from O'Sullivan B, Freedman SD: Cystic fibrosis, *Lancet* 373:1891-1904, 2009.

dysfunctional mucociliary transport, airway obstruction, and chronic infections. Pulmonary system manifestations run the clinical spectrum from chronic, dry, frequent cough and sputum production to respiratory failure. Bronchitis, bronchiolitis, bronchiectasis, and pneumonia occur frequently. Bronchospasm resembling acute or chronic asthma may be present. The airways become colonized with *S. aureus, H. influenzae,* and, finally, *P. aeruginosa. Burkholderia cepacia* is a slower-growing organism found in children with CF. Infection is found in infancy. Pulmonary disease usually becomes progressive and leads to cor pulmonale, respiratory failure, and death by adulthood. Other respiratory problems associated with CF include recurrent acute rhinosinusitis, nasal polyps, and allergic bronchopulmonary aspergillosis (ABPA) which starts by childhood and continues into adulthood. Digital clubbing is common.

- *Gastrointestinal tract and nutrition.* During infancy, meconium ileus, pancreatic insufficiency, and rectal prolapse can be manifestations of CF. Meconium ileus develops in up to 15% of newborns born with CF. A meconium ileus syndrome equivalent can also develop in older patients, with desiccated fecal material

causing gastrointestinal obstruction. Eighty-five percent of affected children have failure to thrive because of pancreatic enzyme insufficiency. Edema with hypoproteinemia may also be present. These children have thick fat-laden stools (steatorrhea), poor muscle mass, and delayed maturation. Infants with CF who are fed soy-based formulas do very poorly, and severe hypoproteinemia and anasarca quickly result. During childhood, intussusception, hepatitic steatosis, biliary fibrosis, and rectal prolapse can occur. Childhood problems continue into adulthood. Clinically apparent cirrhosis occurs in 15% of patients with subsequent risk of portal hypertension. Adenocarcinoma of the digestive tract can occur. Other gastrointestinal problems associated with CF include volvulus, duodenal inflammation, gastroesophageal reflux, bile reflux, fibrosing colonopathy, and poor fat absorption that leads to vitamin A, K, E, and D deficiencies with resulting anemia, neuropathy, night blindness, osteoporosis, and bleeding disorders.

- *Hepatobiliary tract.* Biliary cirrhosis occurs in 2% to 3% of children with CF and is characterized by jaundice, ascites, hematemesis from esophageal varices, and splenomegaly. Hepatic steatosis is also a known complication of CF. Adolescent patients may experience biliary colic and cholelithiasis.
- *Endocrine.* Recurrent acute pancreatitis is not uncommon. Cystic fibrosis–related diabetes mellitus (CFRD) with relative insulin deficiency develops as the patient ages due to autolysis of the pancreas as the pancreas body becomes fatty. CF patients need annual blood glucose screening because by adulthood up to 30% of patients develop CFRD (O'Sullivan and Freedman, 2009).
- *Musculoskeletal.* Vitamin D deficiency may result in osteoporosis when bone reabsorption exceeds bone formation.
- *Reproductive.* Affected children have delayed sexual development. The vas deferens is nonfunctional and atrophied due to CFTR dysfunction, leading to azoospermia and male sterility. The incidence of inguinal hernia, hydrocele, and undescended testes is also high. Females experience secondary amenorrhea, cervicitis, and decreased fertility. A pregnancy is usually carried to term if pulmonary function is not severely compromised.
- *Sweat glands.* Excessive salt loss can lead to hypochloremic alkalosis, especially in warm weather or after gastroenteritis. Children with CF often taste salty because of elevated amounts of sodium chloride (NaCl) lost in endogenous sweat. Dehydration and heat exhaustion are concerns.

Diagnostic Tests. The diagnosis of CF is made on the basis of clinical features and laboratory findings. Patients must have one of more of the clinical features of CF, which include chronic sinopulmonary disease, gastrointestinal and nutritional abnormalities, salt loss syndrome, chronic metabolic alkalosis or male urogenital abnormalities resulting in obstructive azoospermia (Saiman and Hiatt, 2010). In addition, one or more laboratory findings that indicate a CFTR abnormality must be present. The results of the sweat test are determined differently depending on age. The diagnosis of CF can be made in patients with clinical features of the disease under the following guidelines:

- The concentration of sweat chloride is greater than 60 mmol/L.

- The concentration of sweat chloride is in the intermediate range of 30 to 59 mmol/L for infants less than 6 months or in the range of 40 to 59 mmol/L for older individuals.
- The child has two disease-causing CFTR mutations (O'Sullivan and Freedman, 2009).

Sweat tests should be done at a laboratory that regularly deals with children and routinely does these tests. Sodium chloride concentration goes up with age but a concentration greater than 66 mmol/L is still a diagnostic level. A result of greater than 60 mEq/L of chloride on two specimens is in the diagnostic range for CF. Children with hypoproteinemia may elicit false-negative sweat test results.

The second test is genetic analysis for the CFTR mutation. In general, a test that looks for the 40 most common disease-causing mutations that occur in 90% of the CF population is done first (O'Sullivan and Freedman, 2009). Full sequence analysis will detect most mutations. Prenatal diagnosis has greater than 90% sensitivity for detecting a CF gene mutation on the long arm of chromosome 7. Newborn screening looks for immunoreactive trypsin (IRT) in the blood spot taken at birth. A very high IRT needs to be repeated in 1 to 3 weeks; when there is an elevation, a DNA analysis looking for CFTR mutation is done.

If the patient does not meet the classic criteria, nasal transepithelial potential difference (NPD) can be measured. This test is not available at all centers.

Glycosylated hemoglobin levels may be elevated in older children because of impaired pancreatic functioning. Pulmonary function tests are used to follow the clinical course.

Management

Children with CF have complicated treatment regimens and should be monitored by a multidisciplinary team at a CF-accredited center. Pulmonary, nutritional, physical, and pharmacologic (antibiotic and antiinflammatory) therapy and psychological counseling must be individualized for each child at each stage of the illness. Home-based maintenance therapy for pulmonary and nutritional interventions is critical. With pulmonary exacerbations, children with CF generally have hospital stays for at least 2 weeks for aggressive pulmonary and antibiotic therapy. Oral antibiotics are used to clear colonization and infection. The Cystic Fibrosis Foundation ranked treatments for CF using the USPSTF recommendation to grade pulmonary treatments and reported that dornase alfa and inhaled tobramycin have the strongest evidence for use in patients with moderate to severe disease with *P. aeruginosa* and in mild disease. Other treatments listed below should be used in specific patient populations.

- Inhaled dornase alfa (recombinant human deoxyribonuclease): Daily dornase selectively cleaves the DNA and reduces the mucus viscosity, which improves airway clearance.
- Inhaled tobramycin: 300 mg twice a day in 28-day on-off cycles. Tobramycin is an aminoglycoside that results in bacterial death by inhibiting bacterial protein synthesis by binding to 30S and 50S ribosomal units.
- Inhaled hypertonic saline: Use at 4 mL twice a day. It works by drawing water into airways. It is a cheaper therapy; there still needs to be more research done on this modality.

- Chronic administration of azithromycin: Effective for both its antibiotic and antiinflammatory properties by lowering cytokine production
- Ibuprofen: Reduction of inflammation but should begin use before inflammation starts
- Inhaled β-agonist

Lung transplantation is a viable therapy for selected patients who have terminal lung disease (Saman and Hiatt, 2010).

■ Pectus Deformity

DESCRIPTION

Pectus excavatum, or funnel chest, is the most common congenital deformity of the anterior chest wall and results in sternal concavity (Gokhale and Selbst, 2009). Midline narrowing of the thoracic cavity and restriction in chest wall movement are characteristic with an increase in the effect during childhood and adolescence. This can lead to decreased filling of the right heart chamber, lowering cardiac output and a decreased exercise tolerance.

Pectus carinatum is much less common than pectus excavatum. It also progresses during puberty. In pectus carinatum, there is a bowing out of the sternum (also called "pigeon chest"). Although this shape may be cosmetically unattractive, there are fewer complaints about shortness of breath, chest pain, or dyspnea. Both types of deformity can lead to psychological distress for the child.

EPIDEMIOLOGY

Children with upper airway obstruction have a higher incidence of pectus excavatum, but many children with this defect are identified at birth or within the first year of life and have no underlying pulmonary problem. The cause of pectus excavatum in these instances is often unknown. Chest wall deformities are found in 66% of patients with Marfan syndrome (Gokhale and Selbst, 2009).

CLINICAL FINDINGS

History

The parent may note a depression (excavatum) or bowing out (carinatum) of the sternum. Fatigue, shortness of breath, decreased exercise tolerance, or chest pain can be reported. Depression may be a complaint due to changes in self-image.

Physical Examination

The finding in pectus deformities include:
- Posterior depression of the sternum and costal cartilage (in pectus excavatum)
- Anterior bowing of the sternum (carinatum)

Diagnostic Tests

Diagnostic tests include:
- Chest radiography
- Exercise testing if substantial pectus excavatum deformity is present

- Other cardiac (echocardiogram) and pulmonary function studies as suggested by the degree of excavatum deformity and symptomatology

MANAGEMENT

If the excavatum deformity is the result of a pulmonary disease, early treatment of the underlying pulmonary problem occasionally resolves the skeletal deformity. Surgical repair depends on the severity of the defect, demonstration of a decrease in pulmonary function, progression of the defect on serial radiographs, or sometimes the patient's and parents' wish for cosmetic repair. If the patient is male with an associated scoliosis or has a severe pectus carinatum or excavatum, evaluate for Marfan syndrome. Surgery for children with pectus carinatum, if done, is usually for cosmetic purposes.

COMPLICATIONS

Pectus excavatum can also affect cardiac and pulmonary function.

Gastrointestinal Disorders

NANCY BARBER STARR, CATHERINE G. BLOSSER, MARGARET A. BRADY, CATHERINE E. BURNS, ARDYS M. DUNN, AND ANN M. PETERSEN-SMITH

The gastrointestinal (GI) system, also known as the digestive system, is essential for lifelong health. This system provides the nutrients that give the body's cells the energy needed to function. Sustained operation and maintenance of this system are essential for normal growth and development and for the effective functioning of other organ systems.

The pediatric primary care provider plays an integral role in the care of children with GI dysfunction. A thorough understanding of the anatomy, physiology, and common disorders of the GI system is needed to appropriately assess and treat pediatric GI problems. This chapter focuses on pathologic GI disorders commonly seen in children. Other problems of the GI system, such as obesity, anorexia, bulimia, encopresis, and constipation, are discussed in Chapters 10, 12, and 19.

■ Anatomy and Physiology

The GI system begins to develop during the third week of gestation. The primitive gut is initially formed and then divides into the foregut, midgut, and hindgut. The structures further develop in an intricate and complex fashion to become the digestive tract and accessory organs.

The GI tract extends from the mouth to the anus. It includes the organs of digestion and accessory organs, such as the liver, pancreas, and gallbladder. The system provides the following functions: ingestion of food, movement of food from the mouth toward the rectum, mechanical dissolution of food, chemical dissolution of food, absorption of nutrients, and expulsion of waste products. The mouth serves as the site for ingestion, chewing, and mixing of food with saliva. The tongue senses the texture and taste of foods, which initiates salivation and the release of gastric juices in the stomach. The esophagus transports food from the mouth to the stomach by *peristalsis*, the sequential contraction and relaxation of the musculature in the esophagus. The upper esophageal sphincter prevents air from being swallowed while breathing. The lower esophageal sphincter (LES) prevents food from being regurgitated from the stomach, which is important because intraabdominal pressure exceeds intrathoracic and atmospheric pressures. The stomach serves as a reservoir for ingested foods. It secretes digestive juices, mixes food with the gastric fluids,

and propels the liquid material into the small intestine. The small intestine's primary function is absorption of nutrients (carbohydrates, fats, proteins, minerals, and vitamins) into the systemic circulation. Absorption occurs through villi, which cover the mucosal folds and serve as the functional unit of the intestine. Each villus contains an artery, a vein, and a lymph vessel that transport nutrients from the intestine into the systemic circulation. The villi are covered with enterocytes, whose major role is the digestion of carbohydrates and proteins. Enterocytes secrete proteins and enzymes known as brush border enzymes, which assist in digestion.

Carbohydrates must be converted to monosaccharides before their absorption is possible. This process begins in the mouth, where the salivary enzyme amylase breaks down complex starches into disaccharides. The brush border enzymes in the small intestine convert disaccharides into monosaccharides (sucrose to glucose and fructose, lactose to glucose and galactose, and maltose to glucose). When this process is hindered, disaccharides remain osmotically active and can cause diarrhea.

Fat absorption, which occurs mainly in the jejunum, is accomplished through the addition of lipases secreted by the pancreas. Lipases break down fats into particles that are easily absorbed by the villi. Fats then rely on the lymphatic system for absorption.

Proteins are converted to amino acids by pancreatic enzymes. The resulting amino acids are further divided into smaller amino acid particles that are absorbed via the brush border into the systemic circulation. After appropriate absorption of nutrients, the small intestine is left with the initial fecal liquid. This liquid is then propelled by peristalsis into the large intestine. The large intestine removes water from the fecal liquid and allows for short-term storage. The fecal mass, which consists of waste products, bacteria, intestinal secretions, and shed cells, is pushed into the sigmoid colon.

Entry of feces into the rectum stimulates the defecation reflex. This reflex stretches the rectal wall, relaxes the internal anal sphincter, and thereby creates the need to defecate. If this urge is ignored, further fluid resorption occurs as the stool is retained, resulting in an increase in stool mass and dryness. Excessive stretching of the colon from the hard, dry stool bolus can lead to decreased peristalsis, further complicating the retention of stool.

■ Pathophysiology

The GI tract can be affected by illness, injury, or other problems that prevent it from functioning normally. Dysfunction can be localized or systemic. Categories of dysfunction include the following: disorders of motility; infection; malabsorption syndromes; impairment of digestion, absorption, and nutrition; congenital malformations and genetic syndromes; metabolic disorders; behavioral problems; injuries and trauma; and food intolerances such as lactose and gluten intolerance.

■ Assessment

HISTORY

The history assesses the following:
- Family history of any GI disease (e.g., gallbladder disease, ulcers, or allergy to any food product)
- Past medical history related to the GI system (e.g., illnesses, surgeries, anatomic problems, such as cleft lip or palate, esophageal atresia)
- Feeding habits and nutrition history or current diet (what, when, how often, what tolerated)
- Changes in appetite
- Presence of pain (onset, location, type, quality, aggravating and alleviating factors)
  - *Epigastric* pain usually indicates pain from the liver, pancreas, biliary tree, stomach, and upper part of the small bowel (duodenum).
  - *Periumbilical* pain is generated from the distal end of the small intestine, cecum, appendix, and ascending colon.
  - *Colonic* visceral pain is lower abdominal pain that can be dull, diffuse, cramping, or burning.
  - *Suprapubic* discomfort indicates distal intestine, urinary tract, and pelvic organ dysfunction.
  - *Referred* pain is a diagnostic challenge. For example, because of convergent nerve pathways, inflammation of the diaphragm can generate pain that is perceived as shoulder or lower neck pain. When visceral pain is overwhelming, referred pain occurs.
  - *Acute* continuous pain is more indicative of an acute process.
  - *Secondary autonomic nervous system stimulation* associated with acute abdominal pain can produce symptoms of sweating, nausea, vomiting, pallor, and anxiety.
- Bowel habits (frequency, times per week, consistency, associated pain, the need for medications or enemas)
- Constipation and diarrhea (patient's definition of each, how often they occur, treatment tried)
- Thirst level (increased or decreased)
- Food intolerance or allergy (what foods, symptoms, treatment)
- Heartburn, belching and flatulence, vomiting
- Other signs or symptoms (e.g., apnea or asthma that may be caused by gastroesophageal reflux [GER])

PHYSICAL EXAMINATION

When assessing a suspected GI problem, a head-to-toe physical examination is indicated.

- Plot growth parameters, including weight for height, to establish proportionality of the patient and exclude certain growth aberrations from the diagnosis.
- Determine body mass index (BMI). The BMI is one of the first indicators used to assess body fat and is a common method of tracking weight problems and obesity in children 2 years and older (see Chapter 10 for more details).
- Determine hydration status (skin turgor, mucous membranes, peripheral pulses, tears, capillary filling).
- Inspect the abdomen for visible peristalsis, rashes, lesions, asymmetry, masses, enlarged organs, and pulsations.
- Auscultate for frequency of bowel sounds (normal is 5 to 20 per minute).
- Percuss for density and to measure organs.
- Palpate both lightly and deeply.
- Assess peritoneal irritation:
  - Have the patient walk standing straight up or cough.
  - Have the patient stand on tiptoes and fall onto the heels or jump.
  - Palpate for rebound tenderness and a positive Rovsing sign.
  - Check for the obturator sign: A supine patient flexes the right thigh at the hip with the knee bent and internally rotates the hip. The sign is positive when it induces abdominal pain.
  - Check for the psoas sign: The patient lies on the left side and extends and then flexes the right leg at the hip. A positive sign is one that induces abdominal pain.
- Perform a rectal examination when intraabdominal, pelvic, or perirectal disease is suspected (the newborn examination should always routinely assess for anal stenosis). Include external inspection and internal palpation for masses, stool, or irregularities. The index finger is typically used because of its increased sensitivity; however, in infants and young children, use the fifth finger. Insert a gloved, lubricated finger into the rectum. Place the other hand on the abdomen for a bimanual examination. Young pediatric patients should be supine with their feet held together and knees and hips flexed, putting their legs over their abdomen. Adolescent males can be lying on their side or standing with the hips flexed and the upper part of the body on the examination table. Adolescent females can be lying on their side or, if a concurrent pelvic examination is to be done, in the lithotomy position.
- Perform a gynecologic examination if a pathologic pelvic condition is suspected (see Chapter 35).

COMMON DIAGNOSTIC STUDIES

Laboratory tests are performed as indicated:
- Urinalysis (UA) and urine culture
- Complete blood count (CBC) with differential
- Serum chemistry screen, liver profile, lipid profile, erythrocyte sedimentation rate (ESR), C-reactive protein (CRP), thyroid function
- Stool examination for ova and parasites (O&P), culture, blood, white blood cells (WBCs), pH, reducing substances
- Fecal fat collection for 72 hours to rule out fat malabsorption
- Pregnancy test
- Urine tests for gonorrhea or chlamydia, Papanicolaou (Pap) smear and vaginal cultures and/or smears if pelvic or gynecologic pathologic condition is suspected

Imaging of the abdomen may include the following (Clayton, 2010):

- *Radiography*
  - ○ Abdominal x-ray, as the preliminary study; available, less expensive, with lower radiation
  - ○ Upper and lower GI series with fluoroscopy demonstrate anatomy and function
  - ○ Air contrast enema (diagnose and treat intussusceptions)
  - ○ Bone age (to assess suspected growth abnormalities)
  - ○ Chest radiographs (to rule out pneumonia)
- Ultrasound (US)—no ionizing radiation, noninvasive, relatively inexpensive (especially for pyloric stenosis, intussusceptions, appendicitis, cholelithiasis, trauma)
- Computed tomography (CT) scan—used only after other imaging studies; quick, but invasive, increased radiation, possible sedation (helpful in nephrolithiasis, appendicitis [the gold standard], intraabdominal masses, pancreatitis)
- Magnetic resonance imaging (MRI)—noninvasive and no ionizing radiation; more costly, sedation may be required (useful in a wide range of disorders)
- Nuclear medicine (scintigraphy)—provide functional and quantifiable data (especially with biliary disease, GER, and Meckel diverticulum)

Specialized tests may also be considered:
- Barium swallow
- Duodenal aspirate to identify existing infection
- Esophageal pH probe to establish gastroesophageal reflux disease (GERD), with a pH of less than 4 representing a reflux episode
- Capsule endoscopy
- Breath hydrogen test if lactose intolerance is suspected
- Sweat chloride test if cystic fibrosis (CF) is suspected (see Chapter 31)

■ Management Strategies

MEDICATIONS

Many common medications are used to treat various GI disorders:

- Antibiotics, antifungals, or anthelmintics for bacterial, fungal, or parasitic infections
- Antiemetics for nausea or vomiting
- Antidiarrheals occasionally for persistent diarrhea or diarrhea associated with chronic disease, but never for acute diarrheal diseases because toxins need to be excreted from the body
- Stool softeners, laxatives, and cathartics for acute treatment and long-term management of constipation and encopresis (see Chapter 12)
- Medications that alter GI motility or tone to treat GERD
- Oral steroids, parenteral steroids, and other immunosuppressants in the treatment of inflammatory bowel disease
- Pain medication and antispasmodics in selected acute and chronic GI conditions
- Medications that alter gastric acidity to treat GERD and ulcer disease
- Iron supplementation as supportive therapy for chronic disease

Probiotics and Prebiotics

Probiotics are foods or dietary supplements with viable microorganisms that alter the microflora of the host, stimulating favorable growth and/or activity of bacteria. Prebiotics are supplements or foods with nondigestible ingredients that benefit the host by stimulating favorable growth and/or activity of probiotic bacteria. Probiotics have been studied more extensively than prebiotics, with modest effectiveness shown in the prevention of acute infectious diarrhea as well as the treatment of acute viral gastroenteritis and in the prevention of antibiotic-associated diarrhea. There is also some evidence of effectiveness in preventing necrotizing enterocolitis in low birthweight infants, and in treating *Helicobacter pylori* gastritis, irritable bowel syndrome, chronic ulcerative colitis, and colic. Prebiotics may be of some benefit in preventing infection in healthy infants. Though these products seem to be safe in healthy infants and children, there is some concern about the safety of administering them to high-risk children including immunocompromised, ill preterm infants, and/or children with indwelling medical devices (Thomas et al, 2010; Weng and Walker, 2006). See Chapter 42 for further information about using probiotics.

NUTRITION AND ACTIVITY

A nutritional plan that meets the recommended daily needs should be encouraged to promote normal GI function, growth, and development. Intake of fluids to ensure hydration is equally important. Dysfunction of the GI tract can be either short term or long term and can require alterations in dietary intake. Consultation with a registered dietitian is important in designing an adequate nutritional plan for a child with a long-term GI problem (see Chapter 10 for more detail).

Age-appropriate activity should be encouraged on a regular basis to help maintain normal GI function. Some GI maladies require short-term rest, but generally the system functions better when activity is regular and consistent.

COUNSELING AND EDUCATION

It is important to spend time assessing and planning for the unique needs of a child with GI dysfunction. Helping the family understand the disease or disorder and its course, prognosis, and management is essential to normalize life for the child.

■ Upper Gastrointestinal Tract Disorders

DYSPHAGIA

Description

Dysphagia, or difficulty swallowing, may be caused by a variety of disorders. Younger children may be unable to swallow, and older children can have awareness that something is wrong with their swallowing ability or may complain of something being stuck in their throat (globus). The physiology of swallowing is complex with oral, pharyngeal, and esophageal phases. The *oral phase* refers to ingestion, mastication, and the propulsion of food to the back of the mouth as a bolus. The *pharyngeal phase* includes the swallowing and transfer of food from the pharynx to the esophagus. Airway closure is critical during the pharyngeal phase, and the child needs to have intact motor and sensory pharyngeal protective mechanisms to prevent aspiration. The *esophageal phase* allows food to pass into the stomach.

Epidemiology

Dysphagia may occur as a result of a structural defect, neurologic or motor disorders, or mucosal injury. Structural defects make it more difficult to swallow solids than liquids. Common structural defects include esophageal narrowing (stricture, web, or tumor) or extrinsic obstruction (vascular ring). Nonstructural causes arise from motility disorders of the oropharynx or esophagus and are uncommon in children. Prematurity and neurologic impairment from disorders such as cerebral palsy or muscular dystrophy can be causes of dysphagia. Mucosal injury most commonly occurs from GERD or gastritis, but can also be due to caustic ingestion or medication. The number of children with swallowing difficulties has escalated because the advances in technology have increased the survival of children with special health care needs.

Clinical Findings
History
- Progressive dysfunction
- Persistent drooling or cough
- Discomfort with swallowing or a sense of food getting stuck
- Picky eating (e.g., a child who prefers liquids to solids) or food refusal
- Heartburn, halitosis, chest pain
Physical Examination
- Observe the infant or child feeding, paying special attention to the adequacy of the child's oral motor skills and safety of swallowing.
- Perform a complete physical examination, paying particular attention to mouth, throat, and neck.
Diagnostic Studies. Diagnostic tests may include:
- Lateral neck films
- Barium swallow (usually the initial procedure because it is especially effective in detecting esophageal narrowing)
- Fiberoptic endoscopy evaluation of swallowing
- Videofluoroscopy swallowing study
- Manometry (gold standard for diagnosing motor disorders)
- MRI (for structural abnormalities)
- Electromyography

Differential Diagnosis

Obstructive and compressive lesions usually cause trouble only with solids. Physiologic dysfunction is usually associated with systemic disease, and the patient has trouble with both liquids and solids. A dysfunctional feeding relationship between child and feeder can manifest as dysphagia.

Management

Difficulty with swallowing requires evaluating associated cognitive, developmental, and behavioral issues. A multidisciplinary approach is recommended to provide a comprehensive, cost-effective evaluation and consistent care for the child and family. Health professionals from otolaryngology, gastroenterology, nutrition, occupational therapy, psychology, and speech-language pathology may be involved.

VOMITING AND DEHYDRATION
Description

Vomiting is the forceful emptying of gastric contents coordinated by the medullary vomiting center and/or the chemoreceptor trigger zone of the brain. It is differentiated from regurgitation, which is a passive reflux of gastric contents. It can be caused by GI or extraintestinal disorders that are either acute or chronic. Vomiting can be classified as projectile (often arising from the central nervous system [CNS]) or nonprojectile (often seen in GER), and bilious, bloody, nonbilious, or nonbloody.

The age of the child helps to formulate an appropriate list of potential diagnoses (Chandran and Chitkara, 2008).
- Newborn or young infant—infectious process, congenital gastrointestinal anomaly, CNS abnormality, or inborn errors of metabolism
- Infants and young children—gastroenteritis, GERD, milk/soy protein allergies, pyloric stenosis or obstructive lesion, inborn errors of metabolism, intussusception, child abuse, intracranial mass lesion
- Older children and adolescents—gastroenteritis, systemic illness, CNS (cyclic vomiting syndrome [CVS], abdominal migraine, meningitis, brain tumor), intussusception, rumination, superior mesenteric artery syndrome, pregnancy

Dehydration is the loss of water and extracellular fluid. Volume depletion or hypovolemia (loss of extracellular fluid) and dehydration are used interchangeably. Dehydration is classified by the Centers for Disease Control and Prevention (CDC) (2008) as minimal to none (<3%), mild to moderate (3% to 9%), or severe (>9%). It can also be differentiated between infants and older children respectively as mild (5% and 3%), moderate (10% and 6%), or severe (15% and 9%) (Mahajan, 2009).

Epidemiology

Vomiting. Vomiting is one of the most common symptoms in childhood. Nonbilious vomit is generally caused by infection, inflammation, and metabolic, neurologic, or psychological problems. An obstructive lesion generally causes bilious vomiting. Bloody vomit accompanies active bleeding in the upper GI tract (gastritis, peptic ulcer disease).

Following is a list of potential causes of vomiting by site of origin:
- Oropharynx: Cleft palate and laryngopharyngeal cleft
- Upper GI: Congenital stricture, foreign body, gastritis and/or esophagitis, gastric web, pyloric stenosis, tracheoesophageal fistula, vascular ring, peptic ulcer disease (PUD)
- Small intestine: Annular pancreas, choledochal cyst, intestinal atresias and stenosis, intestinal malrotation with volvulus, intestinal pseudo-obstruction
- Colon: Hirschsprung disease, intussusception, meconium ileus, necrotizing enterocolitis, fecal impaction
- Hepatobiliary or pancreatic dysfunction
- Infections: Bacterial enteritis, otitis media, sepsis, urinary tract infection (UTI), viral gastroenteritis (VGE), hepatitis
- Neurologic: Congenital anatomic malformation, gray and white matter degenerative disorders, hydrocephalus, kernicterus, brain tumors, migraine headache, head trauma

- Other: Cow's-milk protein allergy (CMP intolerance), inborn errors of metabolism, maternal drug exposure and/or withdrawal, toxic ingestions, appendicitis, cyclic vomiting, pneumonia, drug or alcohol ingestion, eating disorders, pregnancy

Dehydration. Dehydration is overwhelmingly the result of an infectious process, primarily viral, that often causes diarrhea. Children are at increased risk due to their higher surface area–to–volume ratios, higher rate of insensible loss, and in younger children the inability to communicate or actively replenish losses. Depending on the cause of dehydration, water and salts (primarily sodium chloride) may be lost in physiologic proportion or disparately, producing one of three types of dehydration: isonatremic (isotonic), hypernatremic (hypertonic), and hyponatremic (hypotonic). When dehydration is caused by simple diarrhea, homeostatic mechanisms can usually maintain sodium concentrations in the serum, resulting in isonatremia. When vomiting occurs with diarrhea and water intake is less, there is greater water loss than salt loss, potentially resulting in hypernatremic dehydration. When there is massive stool loss of water and salt and only water is ingested, there is a large salt loss, potentially resulting in hyponatremia.

Clinical Findings

History. The vomiting history should assess the following:
- History of illnesses, surgeries, or hospitalizations
- Medications currently being taken (including over-the-counter, herbal, cultural, and homeopathic remedies)
- Recent exposure to illness, injury, or stress; recent travel (including camping); swimming activities
- Possibility of poisoning

- Family history of GI disease or fetal or neonatal deaths (metabolic syndrome, congenital anomaly)
- Onset and duration of vomiting, quality and quantity, presence of blood or bile, odor, precipitating event
- Relationship of vomiting to meals, time of day, or activities
- Vomiting early in the morning
- Presence of associated symptoms: Diarrhea, fever, ear pain, UTI symptoms, vision changes, cough, headache, seizures, high-pitched cry, polydipsia, polyuria, polyphagia, anorexia

The dehydration history should assess the following:
- Mental status and thirst
- Parental concern regarding decreased tearing or urination, or depressed fontanelle in infants

Physical Examination
- Growth parameters and vital signs
- Neurologic examination: Nuchal rigidity, decreased level of consciousness, and behavioral changes, which can include irritability or lethargy. Sensorium remains intact until there is greater than 6% of weight loss as a result of dehydration. Hypotension is a late manifestation of dehydration.
- Abdominal examination: Inspect for distention, abdominal scars from previous surgery (may be associated with obstruction and/or adhesions), or visible peristaltic waves. Auscultate bowel sounds (i.e., increased with gastroenteritis, decreased with obstruction, absent with ileus or peritonitis). Palpate the abdomen for pain and/or rebound tenderness. Assess abdominal organs (liver and spleen size, masses). Perform a rectal examination as indicated.
- Respiratory examination: Tachypnea, decreased oxygen saturation, stridor
- Assessment of dehydration (Table 32-1)

TABLE 32-1	Assessment of Dehydration		
	DEGREE OF DEHYDRATION		
Symptoms	**Minimal or None** (<3% loss of body weight)	**Mild to Moderate** (3% to 9% loss of body weight)	**Severe** (>9% loss of body weight)
Mental status	Well; alert	Normal, fatigued or restless, irritable	Apathetic, lethargic, unconscious
Thirst	Drinks normally; might refuse liquids	Thirsty; eager to drink	Drinks poorly; unable to drink
Heart rate	Normal	Normal to increased	Tachycardic; bradycardic in severe cases
Quality of pulses	Normal	Normal to decreased	Weak, thready, or impalpable
Breathing	Normal	Normal; fast	Deep
Eyes	Normal	Slightly sunken	Deeply sunken
Tears	Present	Decreased	Absent
Mouth and tongue	Moist	Dry	Parched
Skinfold	Instant recoil	Recoil in <2 seconds	Recoil in >2 seconds
Capillary refill	Normal	Prolonged	Prolonged; minimal
Extremities	Warm	Cool	Cold; mottled; cyanotic
Urine output	Normal to decreased	Decreased	Minimal

From Centers for Disease Control and Prevention Disaster Safety: *Information for health care providers: guidelines for the management of acute diarrhea*, 2008. Available at http://emergency.cdc.gov/disasters/hurricanes/pdf/dguidelines.pdf (accessed Jan 21, 2011).

○ One of the most useful clinical signs of hydration is capillary refill time (CRT). Normal CRT is less than 2 seconds. CRT, skin turgor, and tachypnea, considered together, are most helpful in determining dehydration (Steiner et al, 2004).

○ A clinical dehydration scale (CDS) is a predictive tool regarding length of stay and need for intravenous fluids (Goldman et al, 2008). The four parameters used for assessment are general appearance, eyes (sunken or not), moistness of mucous membranes, and presence of tears.

○ Mahajan (2009) provides five points to assess the level of dehydration: volume deficit with history and physical, osmolar disturbance (serum sodium and osmolality), acid-base disturbance (blood pH, P_{CO_2}, serum bicarbonate), potassium, and renal function (blood urea nitrogen [BUN]), creatinine, urine specific gravity.

Diagnostic Studies. Diagnostic studies are performed as indicated by the probable diagnosis:

- Complete blood count (CBC) with differential, blood culture
- Electrolytes, including BUN and creatinine, glucose, and liver function tests
  ○ Serum bicarbonate less than 17 mEq/L (differentiates mild from moderate/severe hypovolemia) (Mahajan, 2009)
  ○ Serum sodium less than 130 (hyponatremic) or more than 150 (hypernatremic)
- CRP and ESR
- Serum lactate, organic acids, ammonia for metabolic disorders (may only be abnormal during episodes of vomiting)
- UA and urine culture
- Toxicology screen
- Stool for culture and occult blood, leukocytes, parasites, fat, pH, reducing substances
- Rapid strep test and/or throat culture
- Pregnancy test
- Abdominal radiographs (suspected obstruction or foreign body ingestion, organomegaly, or a palpable mass)
- Chest radiograph (suspected pneumonia)
- US (abscesses, masses, stenoses, cysts, appendicitis, pyloric stenosis)
- Barium swallow or enema (malrotation, pyloric stenosis, GER, masses)
- Endoscopy (obstruction, hemorrhage, infection; collect biopsies)
- Esophageal pH probe analysis, scintiscan
- CT scan or MRI to diagnose masses, inflammation, herniations, perforations, and obstructions
- Electroencephalogram (EEG)

Differential Diagnosis

See Table 32-2.

Management

Vomiting

- Identify and alleviate the cause as soon as possible.
- Antiemetics, though not recommended in acute gastroenteritis, or when cause is unknown, may at times be warranted. Newer medications such as 5-HT3 receptor antagonists

(ondansetron or granisetron) do not have adverse effects on the CNS and may be indicated in older children (Chandran and Chitkara, 2008; Ulshen, 2009).

- Refer to specialist for persistent vomiting, recurrent vomiting, or vomiting associated with significant underlying process.

Dehydration

- Determine the degree of dehydration.
  ○ If minimal, mild, or moderate, oral rehydration solution (ORS) with 70 to 90 mEq/L sodium, 25 g/L glucose, 20 mEq/L potassium, 30 mEq/L base (in the form of citrate, acetate, or lactate) with a defined osmolarity of 240 to 300 mOsm/L is recommended.
  ○ If severe, immediate and aggressive intervention is needed (e.g., intravenous [IV] fluids).
  ○ Pediatric subcutaneous rehydration using recombinant human hyaluronidase is an alternate method, effective when used in children with mild to moderate dehydration who require parenteral therapy (Allen et al, 2009).
- Initial rehydration, maintenance of fluids, and replacement of ongoing losses are stages of treatment (Table 32-3). Physiologically sodium and glucose are coupled in transport across the intestinal brush border into systemic circulation to maximize rehydration. Administration of fluid should be in frequent, small (5 mL or less) amounts. Larger amounts may be given as tolerated. Plain water, juices, soda, milk, and sports drinks should be avoided because these liquids are hyperosmolar and do not provide appropriate replacement of sugars and electrolytes. A pediatric emergency department using ORS in children with moderate dehydration showed not only successful rehydration, but also a decreased length of stay, less staff use, and more satisfied parents (Bell, 2010). Palatability of ORS does not affect the quantity consumed (Freedman et al, 2010). Homemade solutions can be used when premade ORS is not available (see http://rehydrate.org). Refeeding should resume as quickly as possible because the gut needs nutrition to facilitate mucosal repair following injury.
- Antiemetics. A single dose of an oral disintegrating tablet of ondansetron (2 mg for children 8 to 15 kg, 4 mg for children 15 to 30 kg, and 8 mg for more than 30 kg) reduces vomiting, decreases the chance of dehydration, and increases the success of oral hydration (Amir, 2007; Freedman et al, 2006; Roslund et al, 2006).
- Monitor urine output.
- Treat fever.
- Refer if the child has a toxic appearance, severe dehydration, projectile vomiting, abnormal examination, vomiting for greater than 12 hours, or vomiting of blood, bile, or fecal matter, or significantly decreased urine output.

Complications

Dehydration, fluid and electrolyte imbalance, aspiration pneumonia, hemorrhage, or a tear of the esophagus are possible.

Patient Education

Providing written information to the parent about care that is needed during all stages of oral rehydration therapy is helpful. Also include information about signs that indicate the child

TABLE 32-2 Differential Diagnosis of Vomiting in Infants and Children

Infant	Child	Adolescent
Common Conditions		
Gastroenteritis	Gastroenteritis	Gastroenteritis
GERD	GERD	GERD
Overfeeding	Gastritis	Gastritis
Anatomic obstruction: pyloric stenosis, malrotation with intermittent volvulus, intestinal duplication, Hirschsprung disease, antral/duodenal web, foreign body, or incarcerated hernia	Toxic ingestion: lead, iron, or vitamins A and D	Toxic ingestion
Systemic infection: UTI, pneumonia, hepatitis	Systemic infection: UTI or pyelonephritis; pneumonia; hepatitis	Systemic infection
Pertussis syndrome	Pertussis syndrome	Pertussis syndrome
Otitis media	Otitis media, sinusitis Appendicitis, small bowel obstruction Migraine Medication: ipecac, digoxin, theophylline, etc.	Sinusitis Appendicitis, small bowel obstruction, IBD Migraine Medication: ipecac abuse/bulimia Pregnancy, PID

Rare Conditions
- Other gastrointestinal disorders: achalasia, gastroparesis, peptic ulcer, food allergy or pancreatitis
- Neurologic: hydrocephalus, subdural hematoma, intracranial hemorrhage or mass, infant migraine, Chiari malformation, or meningitis
- Metabolic/endocrine: galactosemia, hereditary fructose intolerance, urea cycle defects, or amino and organic acidemias, congenital adrenal hyperplasia
- Renal: obstructive uropathy or renal insufficiency
- Cardiac: congestive heart failure or vascular ring
- Others: pediatric falsification disorder (Munchausen syndrome by proxy), child neglect or abuse, cyclic vomiting syndrome, or autonomic dysfunction

GERD, Gastroesophageal reflux disease; *IBD,* inflammatory bowel disease; *PID,* pelvic inflammatory disease; *UTI,* urinary tract infection.
Adapted from Blanchard S, Czinn S: Peptic ulcer disease in children. In Kliegman RM, Behrman RE, Jenson HB et al: *Nelson textbook of pediatrics,* ed 18, Philadelphia, 2007, Saunders, pp 1572-1574; Vandenplas Y, Rudolph C, Di Lorenzo C, et al: Pediatric gastroesophageal reflux clinical practice guidelines: joint recommendations of the North American Society for Pediatric Gastroenterology, Hepatology, and Nutrition (NASPGHAN) and the European Society for Pediatric Gastroenterology, Hepatology, and Nutrition (ESPGHAN), *J Pediatr Gastroenterol Nutr* 49(4):498-547, 2009. Used with permission of Lippincott Williams & Wilkins.

is worse or not responding to treatment in the expected time frame.

CYCLIC VOMITING SYNDROME

Description

CVS is characterized by recurrent, discrete, self-limited episodes of vomiting between which are completely symptom-free periods. CVS is often associated with abdominal migraines (discussed on p 765). During episodes there is intense nausea and unremitting vomiting (a median of six times per hour at peak) often with bilious emesis (83%) and severe abdominal pain (80%) (Li et al, 2008). Accompanying symptoms include pallor, listlessness, anorexia, nausea, retching, abdominal pain, headache, and photophobia. The periods of vomiting may last hours or even days; the symptom-free periods may last for weeks or even years. Consensus criteria for CVS have been established for diagnosis (see www.naspghan.org).

Epidemiology

Although the typical child with CVS is healthy up to 90% of the time, there are substantial morbidity and medical costs when episodes occur because of missed days of school (average 24 per child), high rate of IV rehydration, the cost of laboratory and imaging studies, endoscopic procedures, emergency department visits, and missed work by a parent (Li et al, 2008).

The etiology of CVS is unknown, but there is a link with migraines. Cyclic vomiting may occur any time between infancy and young adulthood, most commonly diagnosed between 3 and 7 years old. Girls are affected more often than boys (60:40), as are Caucasian, elementary school–age children. Affected individuals tend to have mothers and maternal grandmothers who have a higher incidence of migraine headaches, depression, anxiety, irritable bowel syndrome (IBS), and hypothyroidism (Boles et al, 2005; Li et al, 2008). CVS is often a precursor of later classic migraines.

TABLE 32-3	Treatment Based on Degree of Dehydration		
Degree of Dehydration	**Rehydration Therapy**	**Maintenance**	**Replacement of Ongoing Losses**
Minimal or none	Not applicable	0-10 kg: 100 mL/kg/24 hr 10-20 kg: 1000 mL +50 mL/kg for each kg over 10 kg >20 kg: 1500 mL + 20 mL/kg for each kg over 20 kg	<10 kg body weight: 60-120 mL oral rehydration solution (ORS) for each diarrheal stool or vomiting episode >10 kg body weight: 120-240 mL ORS for each diarrheal stool or vomiting episode
Mild to moderate	ORS: 50-100 mL/kg body weight over 3-4 hr or 10-20 mL/kg/hr	Same	Same
Severe	Lactated Ringer solution or normal saline* intravenously in boluses of 20 mL/kg body weight until perfusion and mental status improve, then administer 100 mL/kg body weight ORS over 4 hr or 5% dextrose in ½ normal saline intravenously at twice the maintenance fluid rates	Same	Same: if unable to drink, administer through nasogastric tube or administer 5% dextrose in ¼ normal saline with 20 mEq/L potassium chloride intravenously

Nutrition
- Continue breastfeeding.
- Lactose-containing formulas are usually well-tolerated. If lactose malabsorption appears clinically substantial, lactose-free formulas can be used.
- Return to regular milk in smaller amounts more often.
- Resume age-appropriate normal diet after initial rehydration, including adequate caloric intake for maintenance.
- Complex carbohydrates, fresh fruits, lean meats, yogurt, and vegetables are all recommended.
- Avoid fatty foods and foods high in simple sugars.
- Avoid carbonated drinks or commercial juices.

*In severe dehydrating diarrhea, normal saline is less effective for treatment because it contains no bicarbonate or potassium. Use normal saline only if Ringer lactate solution is not available, and supplement with ORS as soon as the patient can drink. Plain glucose in water is ineffective and should not be used.
Adapted from Centers for Disease Control and Prevention Disaster Safety: *Information for health care providers: guidelines for the management of acute diarrhea*, 2008. Available at http://emergency.cdc.gov/disasters/hurricanes/pdf/dguidelines.pdf (accessed Jan 21, 2011).

Clinical Findings
History
- Red flags have been identified (Box 32-1)
- Family history positive for migraine headache is common
- A prodromal period (some combination of pallor, anorexia, nausea, abdominal pain, or lethargy) and/or a recovery period (from ill to playing again) that is brief
- Episodes that begin and end abruptly
- Episodes more likely to occur early in the morning (3:00 to 4:00 AM) or on awakening
- An identifiable trigger is commonly seen in children—physical stress (infection, lack of sleep, menstrual periods) or psychological stress (birthdays, holidays, school-related), or food products (e.g., chocolate, cheese, monosodium glutamate)
- Intense nausea not relieved by vomiting
- Headache, motion sickness, photophobia, phonophobia, or vertigo may occur

Physical Examination. Physical examination is normal, although children with CVS appear substantially more ill than children with viral gastroenteritis. If any red flags are present, further workup is indicated.

Diagnostic Studies. *Screening labs* during a vomiting episode help exclude other diagnoses:
- Electrolytes including HCO_3
- Upper GI radiographs (to exclude malrotation)

BOX 32-1	Red Flags of Cyclic Vomiting Syndrome

- Abdominal signs (e.g., bilious vomiting, abdominal tenderness, and/or severe abdominal pain, hematemesis)
- Triggering events (e.g., fasting, high-protein meal, or intercurrent illness)
- Abnormal neurologic examination (e.g., severely altered mental status, abnormal eye movements, papilledema, motor asymmetry, and/or gait abnormality [ataxia])
- Progressively worsening episodes or conversion to a continuous or chronic pattern

- Abdominal US in refractory cases (rule out transient hydronephrosis)
- If hyponatremic or hypoglycemic, rule out Addison disease and fatty acid oxidation

Differential Diagnosis
CVS is a diagnosis of exclusion. Severe GI symptoms can indicate hydronephrosis, cholelithiasis, pancreatic disease, or ureteropelvic junction. CVS precipitated by concurrent illness, fasting, or high-protein meals can indicate a metabolic

CHAPTER 32 Gastrointestinal Disorders **747**

BOX 32-2 Lifestyle Changes for Cyclic Vomiting Syndrome

1. Keep a journal of potential precipitating factors in order to identify triggers (75% of children can be helped by this alone).
   - Recognize the role of excitement as a trigger (e.g., downplay big events)
   - Avoid trigger foods (chocolate, cheese, monosodium glutamate, hot dogs, aspartame, antigenic foods)
   - Avoid excessive energy output
2. Provide supplemental carbohydrate for fasting-induced episodes or high-energy demand times (e.g, fruit juices or other sugar-containing drinks, snacks between meals, before exertion, or at bedtime).
3. Maintain healthy lifestyle.
   - Regular aerobic exercise, avoiding overexercising
   - Regular meal schedules—don't skip meals
   - Maintain good sleep hygiene
   - Maintain good hydration
   - Avoidance or moderation in consumption of caffeine

Data from Li B, Lefevre F, Chelimsky GG et al: North American Society for Pediatric Gastroenterology, Hepatology, and Nutrition Consensus Statement on the Diagnosis and Management of Cyclic Vomiting Syndrome, *J Pediatr Gastroenterol Nutr* 47:379-393, 2008.

BOX 32-3 Prophylactic Medication for Cyclic Vomiting Syndrome

Children 5 Years or Younger
- Cyproheptadine (first choice): 0.25 to 0.5 mg/kg/day divided bid or tid
- Propranolol (second choice): 0.25 to 1 mg/kg/day, most often 10 mg bid to tid; taper when discontinuing; monitor resting heart rate

Children Older Than 5 Years
- Amitriptyline (first choice): 0.25 to 0.5 mg/kg at bedtime, increase weekly by 5 to 10 mg, until 1 to 1.5 mg/kg; monitor electrocardiogram (ECG) before starting and 10 days after peak dose
- Propranolol (second choice): see above

Data from North American Society for Pediatric Gastroenterology, Hepatology, and Nutrition Consensus Statement on the Diagnosis and Management of Cyclic Vomiting Syndrome, 2008. Available at www.naspghan.org/user-assets/Documents/pdf/PositionPapers/CVS statement.pdf. Accessed June 20, 2011.

disorder. An abnormal neurologic examination is suggestive of increased intracranial pressure. Approximately 10% of children with CVS-like history have a specific underlying disorder. Although uncommon, Munchausen by proxy syndrome has been known to mimic CVS in a child given ipecac (Li et al, 2008).

Management

If there are no findings suggestive of another disorder, a trial of therapy is targeted at prophylaxis during the well phase and at acute and supportive measures during the three phases of the episode—prodrome, vomiting, and recovery. Consideration of the child's clinical course, frequency and severity of attacks, and resultant morbidity directs the plan.

Well Phase: Prevention and Prophylaxis
- Lifestyle changes (up to 70% respond with decreased episode frequency) (Li et al, 2008) (Box 32-2).
- Daily prophylactic therapy if abortive therapy fails consistently or episodes are frequent and/or severe (Box 32-3). Doses can be titrated every 1 to 4 weeks to achieve therapeutic dose for at least two CVS cycles. Phenobarbital and supplements (L-carnitine and coenzyme Q10) have also been used.

Episode: Acute Interventions
- Supportive measures include early intervention—within 2 to 4 hours of onset of symptoms: dark, quiet environment and replacement of fluids, electrolytes, and calories. If anxiety is a trigger, relaxation exercises are reported helpful.
- Pharmacologic: Administer abortive therapy as early as possible
  - Antimigraine (triptans) in children older than 12 years of age with infrequent and/or mild episodes (fewer than one per month); sumatriptan 20 mg intranasally at onset is contraindicated if basilar artery migraine.
  - Antiemetic (5-HT3 receptor antagonist): Ondansetron 0.3 to 0.4 mg/kg/dose IV every 4 to 6 hours (up to 20 mg)
  - Sedatives for unrelenting nausea and vomiting to induce sleep: Lorazepam (with ondansetron) is considered most effective, but chlorpromazine with diphenhydramine can be used.
  - Analgesic: Ketorolac 0.4 to 1 mg/kg IV every 6 hours (max dose 30 mg, max daily dose 120 mg) with ranitidine for severe midline abdominal pain; morphine or hydromorphone can be added.
  - Treatment of specific symptoms can include histamine 2 receptor antagonists (H$_2$RAs) or proton pump inhibitors (PPIs) for epigastric/dyspeptic pain, antidiarrheals for diarrhea, short acting angiotensin-converting enzyme (ACE) inhibitors for hypertension, and/or anxiolytic medication for anxiety (panic) triggers.
- Complementary modalities (e.g., biofeedback, massage, imagery) have also been used (also see Chapter 42 under Headaches).

Referral. Referral is recommended if red flag symptoms occur or if the child fails to respond to appropriate acute treatment and/or prophylaxis. (Response is defined as at least a 50% reduction in episode frequency and/or severity of vomiting during attacks over a 2-month period of therapy).

Complications

Dehydration, electrolyte derangement, metabolic acidosis, hematemesis, and weight loss can be complications of an acute episode. Ongoing esophagitis may require acid suppression. Frequent or prolonged episodes may lead to growth failure. Abdominal epilepsy is an uncommon cause of cyclic vomiting; an EEG is useful in evaluation and anticonvulsants can be helpful in treatment (Ulshen, 2009).

Patient Education

Work with families using their knowledge of the child to determine individual triggers and develop an plan of care for all stages.

TABLE 32-4	Symptoms and Signs That May Be Associated With Gastroesophageal Reflux	
Symptoms and Signs by Age	**Symptoms and Signs for All Children**	**Signs**
Infancy: regurgitation; signs of esophagitis (irritability, arching, choking, gagging, feeding aversion); failure to thrive. Usually symptoms resolve between 12 and 24 months of age. Obstructive apnea, stridor, lower airway disease by which reflux complicates a primary airway disease (e.g., bronchopulmonary dysplasia). Otitis media, sinusitis, lymphoid hyperplasia, hoarseness, vocal cord nodules, laryngeal edema. *Older children*: regurgitation during preschool years, complaints of abdominal and chest pain, neck contortions (arching, turning of head), asthma, sinusitis, laryngitis	• Recurrent regurgitation with/without vomiting • Weight loss or poor weight gain • Ruminative behavior • Heartburn or chest pain • Hematemesis • Dysphagia, odynophagia • Respiratory disorders such as wheezing, stridor, cough, hoarseness	• Esophagitis • Esophageal stricture • Barrett esophagus • Laryngeal/pharyngeal inflammation • Recurrent pneumonia • Anemia • Dental erosion • Apnea spells • Apparent life-threatening events

Adapted from Vandenplas Y, Rudolph C, Di Lorenzo C et al: Pediatric gastroesophageal reflux clinical practice guidelines: joint recommendations of the North American Society for Pediatric Gastroenterology, Hepatology, and Nutrition (NASPGHAN) and the European Society for Pediatric Gastroenterology, Hepatology, and Nutrition (ESPGHAN), *J Pediatr Gastroenterol Nutr* 49(4):498-547, 2009 (p 519).

GASTROESOPHAGEAL REFLUX DISEASE

Description

GERD refers to the passage of gastric contents into the esophagus from the stomach through the LES. It is a normal physiologic process that occurs several times a day in healthy infants, children, and adults. "GERD is present when the reflux causes troublesome symptoms and or complications" (Vandenplas et al, 2009, p 499). GERD is the most common esophageal disorder in children (Orenstein et al, 2007).

Epidemiology

The etiology of GERD is unclear and probably multifactorial. Inappropriate relaxation of the LES with failure to prevent gastric acid reflux into the esophagus, prolonged esophageal clearance of the gastric refluxate, and impaired esophageal mucosal barrier function are the likely causes of most GERD (Suwandhi et al, 2006). LES function usually is influenced by intraabdominal pressure, hormones, neurologic control, and age. Young infants have increased intraabdominal pressure because of their inability to sit upright. They can also regurgitate when they cough, cry, or strain. In healthy infants, regurgitation is highest in the first month of life (73%) and decreases to 50% by the fifth month of life. During the first 2 months of life, 20% of infants regurgitate more than four times per day. After age 1 year, less than 4% of infants regurgitate daily. Weight gain is less in infants who regurgitate more than four times per day and breastfed babies regurgitate less than formula-fed babies (Hegar et al, 2009).

Alterations in swallowing, pharyngeal coordination, esophageal motility, and delayed gastric emptying are also potential factors related to GERD. Increased muscle tone, chronic supine positioning, and altered GI motility exacerbate GERD. *Helicobacter pylori (HP)* has been associated with GERD. Children with *HP* are about six times more likely to develop GERD than non–*HP*-positive children. *HP* has not been found in infants less than 1 year of age (Moon et al, 2009).

One study found GERD in 2% of healthy children, ages 7 to 16 years (Pashankar et al, 2009). The American Academy of Otolaryngology-Head and Neck Surgery (AAO-HNS) states that 10% of infants younger than 1 year with regurgitation develop significant complications (GERD) (AAO-HNS, 2011). Up to 70% of infants less than 1700 g may have GERD; 40% have symptomatic improvement by 4 months old, and 85% are symptom-free by 12 months old (Sondheimer, 2005). Risk factors include neurologic impairment, obesity, cystic fibrosis, hiatal hernia, and family history of GERD.

Clinical Findings

Common signs and symptoms by age that should lead the clinician to suspect GERD are found in Table 32-4, although, according to the guidelines, there is no symptom or symptom complex that is diagnostic of GERD or predicts response to therapy. In older children and adolescents, history and physical examination may be sufficient to diagnose GERD. The most common symptom is "heartburn." Recurrent regurgitation with or without vomiting, weight loss or poor weight gain, ruminative behavior, hematemesis, dysphagia, and respiratory disorders such as wheezing, stridor, cough, apnea, hoarseness, and recurrent pneumonia are also associated with GERD.

History. Box 32-4 summarizes the history for GERD that should be collected according to the national guidelines. *Warning signs* that merit urgent investigation of vomiting are found in Box 32-5.

Physical Examination
• Review of height, weight, and head circumference
• Signs of failure to thrive (FTT)
• Torticollis: Neck arching
• Hoarseness
• Anemia
• Tooth erosion resulting from destruction of enamel by gastric acids caused by frequent vomiting
• Rash, recurrent diarrhea, persistent vomiting, or early-morning vomiting (symptoms of other primary disease with GERD as a secondary problem)

Diagnostic Studies. In most infants with vomiting and in older children with regurgitation and heartburn, a history

---

BOX 32-4 History for the Child With Suspected Gastroesophageal Reflux Disease

Feeding and Dietary History
- Amount/frequency (overfeeding)
- Preparation of formula
- Recent changes in feeding type or technique
- Position during feeding, burping technique and frequency

Behavior During Feeding
- Choking, gagging, coughing, arching, discomfort, refusal

Pattern of Vomiting
- Frequency and amount, pain, forceful
- Blood or bile
- Associated fever, lethargy, diarrhea

Medical History
- Prematurity
- Growth and development, previous weight and height gain (growth charts)
- Past surgery, hospitalizations
- Newborn screen results
- Recurrent illnesses, especially croup, pneumonia, asthma
- Symptoms of hoarseness, fussiness, hiccups, apnea
- Other chronic conditions
- Medications: current, recent, prescription, nonprescription

Family Psychosocial History
- Sources of stress
- Maternal or paternal drug use
- Postpartum depression

Family Medical History
- Significant illnesses
- Family history of gastrointestinal disorders
- Family history of atopy

Adapted from Vandenplas Y, Rudolph C, Di Lorenzo C et al: Pediatric gastro-esophageal reflux clinical practice guidelines: joint recommendations of the North American Society for Pediatric Gastroenterology, Hepatology, and Nutrition (NASP-GHAN) and the European Society for Pediatric Gastroenterology, Hepatology, and Nutrition (ESPGHAN), *J Pediatr Gastroenterol Nutr* 49(4):498-547, 2009 (p 519). Used with permission of Lippincott Williams & Wilkins.

BOX 32-5 Warning Signals Requiring Urgent Investigation in Infants With Regurgitation or Vomiting

- Bilious vomiting
- Gastrointestinal bleeding, hematemesis, hematochezia
- Consistently forceful vomiting or onset of vomiting after 6 months of life
- Failure to thrive
- Diarrhea or constipation
- Fever
- Lethargy
- Hepatosplenomegaly
- Bulging fontanelles, macrocephaly, or microcephaly
- Seizures
- Abdominal tenderness or distension
- Documented or suspected genetic/metabolic syndrome

Adapted from Vandenplas Y, Rudolph C, Di Lorenzo C et al: Pediatric gastro-esophageal reflux clinical practice guidelines: joint recommendations of the North American Society for Pediatric Gastroenterology, Hepatology, and Nutrition (NASP-GHAN) and the European Society for Pediatric Gastroenterology, Hepatology, and Nutrition (ESPGHAN), *J Pediatr Gastroenterol Nutr* 49(4):498-547, 2009 (p 506). Used with permission of Lippincott Williams & Wilkins.

---

and physical examination are sufficient to reliably diagnose GERD, recognize complications, and initiate treatment. An empiric trial of acid suppression with a PPI for 4 weeks may be used as a diagnostic test in older children and adolescents but is not recommended in infants and young children.

Nonradiologic diagnostic tests as indicated:
- CBC with differential to rule out anemia and infection
- UA and urine culture
- Stool for occult blood
- Testing for *HP*

The following specialized tests may be obtained following consultation with a physician or a pediatric gastroenterologist.
- Esophageal pH monitoring has been the gold standard to diagnose reflux. However, the presence of reflux may not correlate with the severity of illness and some gastric contents may not be acidic. Transnasal pH placement may be uncomfortable, decrease appetite and activity, and thus underestimate the true incidence of reflux episodes (Dranove, 2008). Typically, patients are asked to discontinue H_2 blockers for 72 hours before the test and PPIs for 1 week before the study.
- Multichannel intraluminal esophageal impedance (MII) measures episodes of reflux independent of the pH of the fluid. It is especially useful for making a diagnosis in children with respiratory events related to reflux because it can measure multiple indices, such as heart rate, oxygenation, sleep state, and apnea episodes. It can also measure the height of refluxed material, and the content and direction of the reflux (liquid, air, or both). It is preferred by many gastroenterologists because it can measure acid and non-acid reflux (50% of reflux in infants is nonacidic). Cost, time to interpret results, and lack of consensus about norms for frequency or length of nonacidic reflux events are disadvantages to this study (Dranove, 2008; Vandenplas et al, 2009).
- Wireless pH monitoring is also available. A pH probe is placed transorally, temporarily attached to the esophageal mucosa where it is programmed to record events for 48 hours. The capsule typically sloughs in about 5 days. Failure to attach, chest pain, feeling of foreign body, and premature detachment are negative aspects of this technology.
- Endoscopy to obtain a biopsy can help determine severity of reflux esophagitis. It can rule out esophagitis and other pathologic conditions if deemed necessary. It may also be used to redilate strictures.
- Barium upper GI series should only be used if obstruction or an anatomic abnormality of the upper GI tract is suspected.
- Radionuclide scan with scintiscan and esophageal and gastric ultrasonography studies are not recommended for routine evaluation of GERD.

Differential Diagnosis

The clinician should also consider other causes of vomiting as found in Table 32-2.

Management

See Figures 32-1, 32-2, and 32-3, and Table 32-5.

Pharmacologic. Acid-suppression agents are the mainstays of treatment. These pharmacologic agents include H_2RAs, PPIs, and buffering agents:

- H_2RAs: Cimetidine, ranitidine, famotidine, nizatidine
- PPIs: Omeprazole, lansoprazole, rabeprazole, pantoprazole, esomeprazole

PPIs are superior to H_2RAs in relieving symptoms and mucosal healing and do not result in tolerance as do H_2RAs. However H_2RAs and buffering agents have a rapid onset of action and are useful in on-demand treatment (Vandenplas et al, 2009) (Table 32-6).

There is insufficient evidence to justify the routine use of prokinetic agents such as cisapride, metoclopramide, domperidone, bethanechol, erythromycin, or baclofen for GERD. Because safe and convenient alternatives are available that are more acceptable to patients, chronic antacid therapy is generally not recommended for patients with GERD (Vandenplas et al, 2009).

Nutrition. Feeding techniques, volumes, and frequency of feeding should be normalized. A trial of extensively hydrolyzed protein formula may be used for 2 to 4 weeks in formula-fed infants with vomiting. Thickening agents for formula (1 tablespoon rice cereal/ounce formula) reduce regurgitation, but not significantly (Hegar et al, 2008). In older children and adolescents there is no evidence to support specific dietary restrictions to decrease symptoms. Obesity is related to GERD (Pashankar et al, 2009), so weight management could be helpful.

Lifestyle. Because prone positioning is associated with increased risk of sudden infant death syndrome (SIDS), supine positioning during sleep in infants is recommended. Positioning infants upright may worsen reflux. There may be some benefit in older children to left-side positioning during sleep or elevation of the head of the bed (elevate the head of the bed and don't add pillows because it may increase abdominal flexion and compression).

Surgical. Antireflux surgery strategies such as fundoplication are used for management of cases that have not responded to less invasive strategies, have life-threatening complications, or will have long-term dependence on medical therapy in which compliance or patient preference precludes ongoing use. However, the surgery is not necessarily curative. For example, in one study of fundoplication in children with CF, 12% had repeat surgery, 48% had recurrent GERD symptoms, and only 28% discontinued GERD medications (Vandenplas et al, 2009). Now that PPI therapy is so successful, fundoplication may become less common (Orenstein et al, 2007).

Complications

Complications include chronic cough, FTT, irritability, and malnutrition. Esophageal injury secondary to reflux results in bleeding, stricture formation, and Barrett esophagus. GERD is circumstantially associated with significant asthma, recurrent

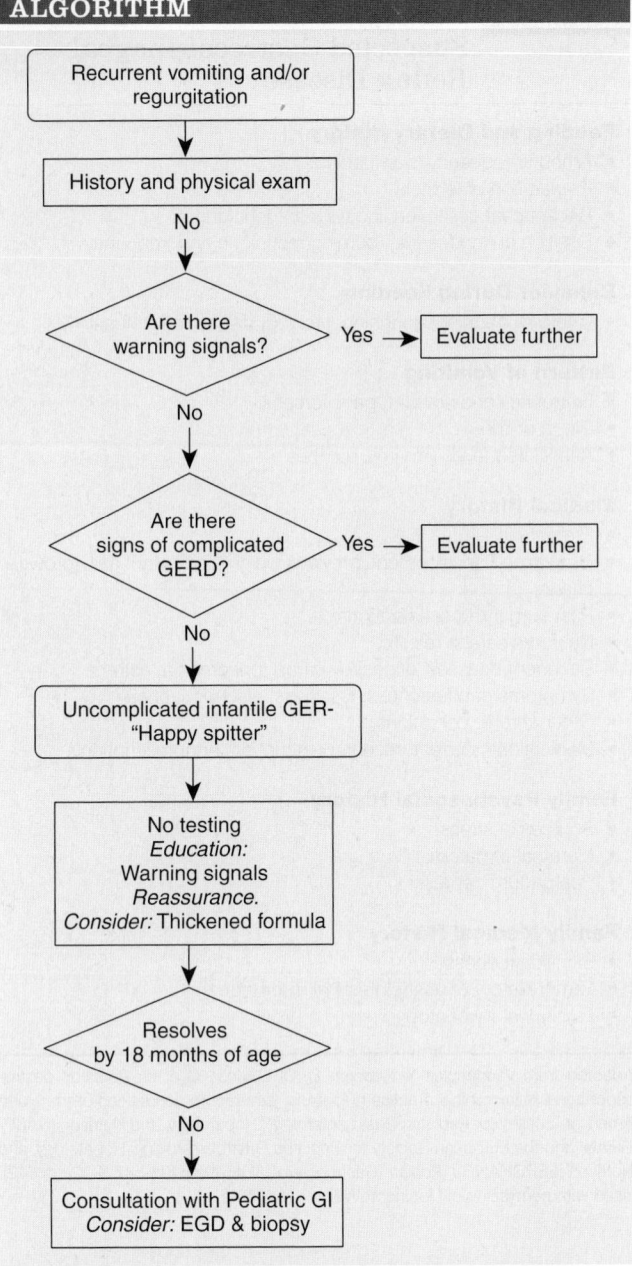

ALGORITHM

FIGURE 32-1 Approach to the infant with recurrent regurgitation and vomiting. (From Vandenplas Y, Rudolph C, Di Lorenzo C et al: Pediatric gastroesophageal reflux clinical practice guidelines: joint recommendations of the North American Society for Pediatric Gastroenterology, Hepatology, and Nutrition [NASPGHAN] and the European Society for Pediatric Gastroenterology, Hepatology, and Nutrition [ESPGHAN], *J Pediatr Gastroenterol Nutr* 49[4]:498-547, 2009.)

pneumonia, or laryngeal disorders. In the majority of infants with apnea or apparent life-threatening event, GERD is not the cause. However, in the rare case where a relationship is suspected, pH monitoring in combination with polysomnographic recording and precise, synchronous symptom recording may aid in establishing cause and effect (Vandenplas et al, 2009). Red flags in infants are bilious vomiting and/or hematemesis. See Box 32-5.

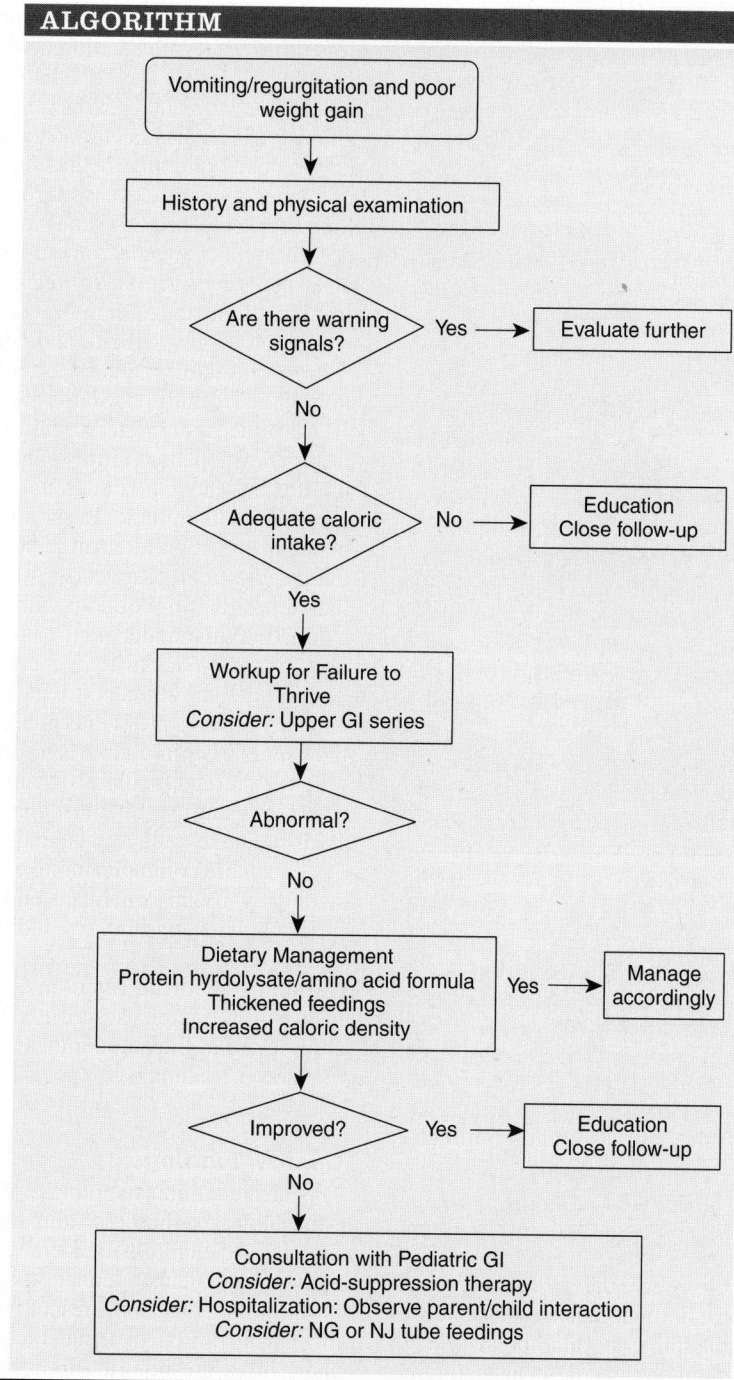

FIGURE 32-2 Approach to the infant with recurrent regurgitation and weight loss. (From Vandenplas Y, Rudolph C, Di Lorenzo C et al: Pediatric gastroesophageal reflux clinical practice guidelines: joint recommendations of the North American Society for Pediatric Gastroenterology, Hepatology, and Nutrition [NASPGHAN] and the European Society for Pediatric Gastroenterology, Hepatology, and Nutrition [ESPGHAN], *J Pediatr Gastroenterol Nutr* 49[4]:498-547, 2009.)

Patient Education

- Assure parents of infants that regurgitation is usually self-limited and symptoms improve as the child grows. Parental education and reassurance are recommended for infants with uncomplicated regurgitation.
- Remind parents that GERD may temporarily worsen during illness.
- Review medication information, including dosages and side effects.

PEPTIC ULCER DISEASE

Description

Peptic ulcer disease (PUD) consists of a group of gastric and duodenal disorders ranging from gastritis to ulceration. With duodenal ulcers (DUs), mucosal defects penetrate the duodenal mucosa and submucosa. Gastric ulcers (GUs) result from mucosal defects that penetrate the gastric mucosa and submucosa. Peptic ulcers are different in children compared to adults in clinical presentation, as well as

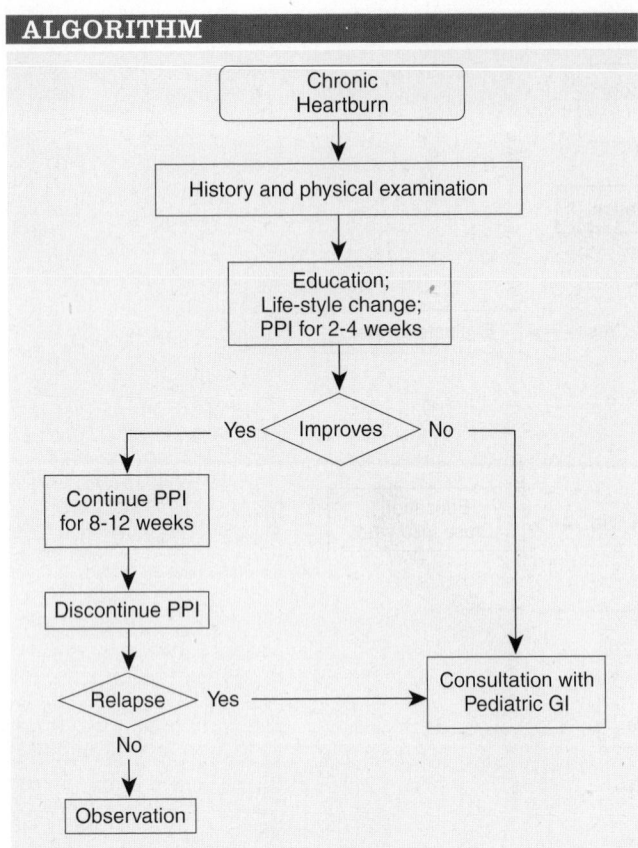

FIGURE 32-3 Approach to the older child or adolescent with heartburn. (From Vandenplas Y, Rudolph C, Di Lorenzo C et al: Pediatric gastroesophageal reflux clinical practice guidelines: joint recommendations of the North American Society for Pediatric Gastroenterology, Hepatology, and Nutrition [NASPGHAN] and the European Society for Pediatric Gastroenterology, Hepatology, and Nutrition [ESPGHAN], *J Pediatr Gastroenterol Nutr* 49[4]:498-547, 2009.)

in prevalence rates, types of ulcer disease, and complications (Sultan et al, 2009).

Epidemiology

PUD is classified as primary or secondary. Most *primary* ulcers are duodenal, have no underlying cause, and tend to be chronic with resulting granulation tissue and fibrosis. They tend to recur. They are more common in adolescents and rare in children. *Secondary* ulcers are more often gastric, generally more acute, and associated with known ulcerogenic events. Severe erosive gastropathy can result in bleeding ulcers or gastric perforations, more commonly in the stomach than duodenum. Head trauma, severe burns, use of corticosteroids, and NSAIDs are associated with secondary ulcers. Aspirin or nonsteroidal antiinflammatory drugs (NSAIDs) cause mucosal injury by direct injury or inhibiting cyclooxygenase and prostaglandin formation. Chronic therapy with these medicines causes gastric mucosal damage but is not associated with ulcer formation. Stress ulceration usually occurs within 24 hours of critical illness (e.g., may occur in 25% of critically ill children in intensive care units [ICUs]) (Blanchard and Czinn, 2007). Preterm and term infants in neonatal intensive care units (NICUs) can also develop gastric mucosal

lesions with bleeding or perforation. *Idiopathic* ulcers are found in *HP*-negative children who have no history of taking NSAIDs; 15% to 20% of pediatric duodenal ulcers are of this type (Blanchard and Czinn, 2007). A strong familial predisposition for PUD has been noted, and most children with DUs have a positive family medical history, a key finding. There is no evidence that diet plays a role in the formation of ulcers. Smoking can cause DUs and slow the rate of healing.

Peptic ulcers result from an imbalance between protective and aggressive factors. *Protective* factors include the water-insoluble mucous gel lining, local production of bicarbonate, regulation of gastric acid, and adequate mucosal blood flow. *Aggressive* factors include the acid-pepsin environment, infection with *HP*, and mucosal ischemia. Colonization rates with *HP* have been suggested to be 8% to 63%, with higher rates in less-developed countries. Colonization likely occurs early in life, but the infection often remains asymptomatic with low-grade inflammation or no mucosal changes. In any case, peptic ulcers in children are much less related to *HP* infection than they were in past years (Sultan et al, 2009). Studies show that almost half of children with ulcers are *HP* negative (Tam et al, 2009). In another study of Canadian children with upper GI symptoms *HP*-positive rates were 7% (Segal et al, 2008).

PUD has an estimated frequency of 1 case in 2500 hospital admissions and a prevalence rate of 1.7% in primary care practices and 1.8% in endoscopic procedural diagnosis. PUD is rare in children less than 10 years old and is usually related to secondary causes. It is most common among youths between 12 and 18 years of age. The male-to-female ratio is about 2 to 3:1. It is more common among children of low socioeconomic status, in African-Americans and Hispanics, and children living in crowded, unsanitary conditions who share a bed (Sultan et al, 2009).

Zollinger-Ellison syndrome (ZES) is a rare syndrome involving refractory severe PUD caused by gastric hypersecretion due to the autonomous secretion of gastrin by a neuroendocrine tumor.

Clinical Findings

The most common symptom of PUD is vague, dull abdominal pain; however, the presenting symptoms vary depending on the age of the child. Hematemesis or melena is reported in up to 50% of patients. Neonates can present with gastric perforation. Infants usually present with feeding difficulty, vomiting, crying episodes, hematemesis, or melena. Epigastric pain and nausea are reported more often by school-age children and adolescents. The classic adult symptom of PUD, pain alleviated by ingestion of food, is present in only a minority of children. More often, children present with symptoms outlined in the following text. Most children presenting with epigastric or periumbilical pain do not have PUD, but rather functional bowel disorder, IBS, or functional dyspepsia. They rarely present with acute abdominal pain with ulceration from perforation or symptoms of pancreatitis from a posterior penetrating ulcer (Blanchard and Czinn, 2007).

History

- Asymptomatic or symptoms can wax and wane. Remissions may last from weeks to months.
- Pain with eating, dyspepsia; can awaken individual from sleep.
- GI tract bleeding (may be a presenting symptom).

TABLE 32-5	Management Strategies for Infants and Children With Gastroesophageal Reflux	
Population	**Diagnostic Tests**	**Management Strategies**
Infant with uncomplicated recurrent regurgitation (GER)	None needed	Parental education and reassurance In formula-fed babies, a thickened formula may reduce over-regurgitation and vomiting but does not reduce the reflux itself.
Infants with recurrent vomiting and poor weight gain (GERD)	Diet history, urinalysis, CBC, serum electrolytes, blood urea nitrogen, serum creatinine Other tests as indicated	For breastfed infants, continue to breastfeed. For formula-fed babies, 2-week trial of extensively hydrolyzed formula or amino acid–based formula to exclude cow's-milk allergy. Increase caloric density. Thicken formula if needed. Educate regarding formula intake needed to sustain normal weight gain. Refer to pediatric gastroenterologist if management fails to improve symptoms and weight gain.
Infants with unexplained crying and/or distressed behavior	Evaluate for cow's-milk allergy, neurologic disorders, constipation, infection (especially UTIs).	Empiric trial with extensively hydrolyzed protein formula or amino acid–based formula. No evidence to support the empiric use of acid suppression for the treatment of irritable infants. However, if irritability persists and no condition other than GERD remains, then continued support of parents with the anticipation of improvement over time; workup to establish the relationship of reflux to feeding or to diagnose esophagitis; or trial of antisecretory therapy, although there is a potential risk for adverse effects. Clinical improvement following empiric therapy may result in spontaneous symptom resolution or placebo response.
Child older than 18 months with chronic regurgitation or vomiting	Consider diagnosis other than GERD. Testing may include upper GI endoscopy, esophageal pH/MII, and barium upper GI series.	Treatment depends on diagnosis.
Heartburn in older children and adolescents	No further studies needed if problem is episodic and not severe	On-demand therapy with buffering agents, sodium alginate, or H₂RA may be used for occasional symptoms. For chronic heartburn, lifestyle changes such as diet change, weight loss, smoking avoidance, sleeping position, no late-night eating, and a 2-week trial with a PPI may help. PPI can be continued for up to 3 months if symptoms resolve. Persistent heartburn after that time should be referred to a pediatric gastroenterologist.
Reflux esophagitis—endoscopically diagnosed	No further studies needed	PPI for 3 months is initial therapy. Trial of tapering the dose and then withdrawal of PPI. Chronic relapsing esophagitis may be the diagnosis if PPI cannot be withdrawn and may involve long-term therapy with PPI or antireflux surgery.

CBC, Complete blood count; *GER,* gastroesophageal reflux; *GERD,* gastroesophageal reflux disease; *GI,* gastrointestinal; *H₂RA,* histamine 2-receptor antagonist; *UTI,* urinary tract infection; *MII,* multichannel intraluminal esophageal impedance; *PPI,* proton pump inhibitor.
Adapted from Vandenplas Y, Rudolph C, Di Lorenzo C et al: Pediatric gastroesophageal reflux clinical practice guidelines: joint recommendations of the North American Society for Pediatric Gastroenterology, Hepatology, and Nutrition (NASPGHAN) and the European Society for Pediatric Gastroenterology, Hepatology, and Nutrition (ESPGHAN), *J Pediatr Gastroenterol Nutr* 49(4):498-547, 2009.

- Infants: Poor feeding, GI bleeding, vomiting, intestinal perforation, slow growth; history of prematurity or term birth spent in a NICU.
- Toddlers and preschoolers: Poorly localized abdominal pain, vomiting, GI bleeding. May worsen after eating; irritability; anorexia.
- School-age children and adolescents: Poorly localized epigastric or right lower quadrant pain. Pain is often described as dull, aching, and lasting from minutes to hours. Nocturnal pain is common in older children. Relief from antacids is reported by less than 33% of children. If the pain awakens the child, worsens with food, and is relieved by fasting, this may help distinguish GI pathology from psychogenic pathology, although these symptoms are infrequently described in children. Recurrent vomiting may occur.
- GI bleeding may lead to iron deficiency anemia with symptoms of fatigue, headache, dyspnea, and malaise.
- Family history of PUD

- Predisposing factors: Alcohol, smoking, aspirin, NSAIDs, corticosteroids, emotional stress, serious systemic disease, sepsis, hypotension, respiratory failure, multiple traumatic injuries, and extensive burns.
- ZES presents with severe peptic ulceration, kidney stones, watery diarrhea, or malabsorption (fasting serum gastrin level >200 pg/mL and baseline gastric acid hypersecretion at more than 15 mEq/hr).

Physical Examination. A careful physical examination should be performed; however, there may be no physical findings. The physical examination should include the following:
- Height, weight, head circumference, BMI, and percentiles
- Vital signs
- General observation of the appearance of the child
- Assessment of perfusion: Mental status, heart rate, pulses, capillary refill, pallor
- Assessment of hydration: Mucous membranes and skin turgor

TABLE 32-6	Medications Used for GERD and Acid Suppression in Peptic Disease

Medication	Pediatric Dose
H₂-Receptor Antagonists	
Cimetidine	20-40 mg/kg/day up to 400 mg divided 2 times/d infants 1-2 mg/kg/day every 6 hr
Famotidine	1-2 mg/kg/day up to 20 mg every 8-12 hr; 40 mg/day for young adults
Nizatidine	>6 mo old: 5-10 mg/kg/day divided 2 times/d
Ranitidine	4-6 mg/kg/day up to 150 mg divided 2 or 3 times/d
Proton Pump Inhibitors	
Lansoprazole	0.8-4 mg/kg/day; start at 1 mg/kg/day. Dose range: <30 kg: 15 mg/day, >30 kg: 30 mg/day
Omeprazole	1-3.3 mg/kg/day daily or 2 times/d; start at 1 mg/kg/day; dose range: <20 kg: 10 mg/day, >20 kg: 20 mg/day. Approved for use in those >2 yr old
Rabeprazole	Adult dose: 20 mg/day
Pantoprazole	Adult dose: 40 mg/day
Esomeprazole	Ages 1-17 yr: >8 kg but <20 kg: 5 or 10 mg daily for 8 weeks >20 kg: 10-20 mg daily for 8 weeks (Tolia et al, 2010) Contents of capsule may be mixed with 1 tablespoon of applesauce for easier swallowing, if needed.
Cytoprotective Agent	
Sucralfate	40-80 mg/kg/day

d, Day; *GERD*, Gastroesophageal reflux disease.
Adapted from Blanchard SS and Czinn SJ: Peptic ulcer disease in children. In Kliegman RM, Behrman RE, Jenson HB et al: *Nelson textbook of pediatrics*, ed 18, Philadelphia, 2007, Saunders.

- Careful mouth inspection for ulcers (associated with Crohn disease) and dental enamel erosion (associated with GERD)
- Lung examination for wheezing (associated with GERD)
- Abdominal examination for tenderness and hepatosplenomegaly
- Rectal examination (to assess perirectal disease)
- Pelvic examination in sexually active female patients with pain
- Testicles and inguinal examination in male patients

Diagnostic Studies. Endoscopy with mucosal biopsy is the diagnostic test of choice, and validates *HP* infection. However, if a child has mild PUD, minimal laboratory studies are needed. Diagnostic studies to consider include the following (Sultan et al, 2009):

Laboratory Studies
- Initially: CBC (anemia is associated with chronic infection with *HP* or acute or chronic blood loss due to ulcer perforation into the abdominal cavity), albumin (low) and ESR

(high) are red flags for systemic disease. May also consider stool for guaiac and *HP* (especially in children).
- If child is unstable, severe, or has chronic, recurrent symptoms, or serious complications consider also iron studies; *HP* serology (most useful in teenagers, only helpful in children if negative due to high false-positive rate); prothrombin time and activated partial thromboplastin time [aPTT] (useful to identify coagulopathy); electrolyte, BUN, creatinine levels (to assess volume depletion); arterial blood gases (acidosis); urinalysis (hydration, infection, or stones); serum gastrin and gastrin-releasing peptide levels (in patients with refractory ulcers to exclude ZES). NOTE: PPIs must be discontinued 2 weeks before gastrin level measurement. Type and crossmatch for blood may also be done.

Imaging Studies
- Abdominal or chest x-ray for perforation
- Upper GI series helps diagnosis in about 70% of children (sensitivity higher for duodenal ulcers). A fibrinous clot in the ulcer may lead to false-negative findings. Barium studies have false-positive rates as high as 30% to 40%. Gastric outlet obstructions often due to pyloric lesions can be identified (Sultan, 2009).
- Angiography is sometimes done if there is a massive bleed and endoscopy cannot be performed.

Procedures
- Esophagogastroduodenoscopy (EGD) is the procedure of choice in children for detecting PUD because it allows direct visualization of mucosa, localization of source of bleeding, and collection of biopsy specimens. It is also used therapeutically for acute bleeding.

Studies to Detect HP
- Histologic examination and culture of biopsies obtained via endoscopy is the gold standard; sensitivities to antibiotics should be done concurrently.
- C-urea breath test is the noninvasive diagnostic test of choice; it is sensitive in children older than 2 years, but requires special equipment.
- Stool monoclonal antibody test is an alternate, is sensitive and specific, and is especially useful to monitor after eradication.
- Serum IgG antibody titer for *HP* (level >500 units [normal 0 to 200]) in children older than 12 years; a positive result only means exposure to disease. This test should neither be the sole basis for starting therapy nor used to test for eradication.

Differential Diagnosis

All other causes of abdominal pain, especially GERD, IBS, GI bleeding, cholelithiasis, cholecystitis, pancreatitis, lactose intolerance, hyperkalemia, and hypercalcemia are in the differential.

Management

- The goals of treatment include ulcer healing, elimination of the primary cause, relief of symptoms, and prevention of complications.
- Medications
  - H₂RAs or PPIs are first-line therapy (see Table 32-6). PPIs have the best effect if given before a meal
  - Antacids: Any liquid preparation, 0.5 mL/kg, given between 1 and 3 hours after eating and before bed

○ *Eradication* therapy for *HP* is indicated for children with a duodenal or gastric ulcer identified by endoscopy and histopathology. *Empiric* therapy for suspected *HP* is not recommended. There is increasing antibiotic resistance to *HP*. Therapy is not indicated for gastritis without PUD, recurrent abdominal pain (RAP), or for children with asymptomatic PUD or with a family member with PUD. See Table 32-7 for treatment guidelines when *HP* is confirmed. Compliance with the treatment regimen is the single most important determinant of eradication. Eradication rates are more than 90%. The test of cure can either be the stool antigen test or the urea breath test (Ables et al, 2007).

- Referral to a gastroenterologist should occur if there is:
  ○ Lack of improvement or inability to wean off meds
  ○ History of hematemesis, melena, occult blood in stools, anemia, and/or weight loss
- Idiopathic ulcers: The preferred treatment is acid suppression with either H$_2$RAs or PPIs. Patients should be followed closely and, if symptoms recur, acid suppression restarted. PPIs are preferred for maintenance in children older than 1 year.
- ZES: PPIs are the mainstay of treatment and must be started promptly (Blanchard and Czinn, 2007).

Complications

Acute hemorrhage, chronic blood loss, penetration of the ulcer into the abdominal cavity, or adjacent organs may produce shock, anemia, peritonitis, or pancreatitis. Obstruction can occur if inflammation and edema are extensive. Hemorrhage occurs in 15% to 20% of patients and perforation occurs in 5% (Sultan et al, 2009). Recurrence, gastric outlet obstruction, gastric adenocarcinoma, and gastric lymphoma are other possible complications. The highest rates of mortality are found in young infants with secondary stress ulcers in which GI bleeding or hemorrhage occur, sometimes catastrophically.

Patient Education, Prevention, and Prognosis

Treatment success depends on the child completing the drug regimen. PUD in children is being actively studied, and clinicians must be aware of ongoing changes. With the introduction of H$_2$RAs and PPIs and the recognition that *HP* can be treated, the incidence of complications has decreased dramatically.

■ Lower Gastrointestinal Tract Disorders

INFANTILE COLIC

Description

Infantile colic is characterized by persistent crying in infants younger than 3 months old. The average infant cries for 2 to 3 hours per day. In contrast, an infant with colic usually cries for more than 4 hours per day. Wessel and colleagues in 1954 established the original criteria known as "the rule of threes": beginning at 1 to 2 weeks of life, periods of crying for 3 or more hours per day, 3 or more days per week, lasting for 3 or more weeks (Wessell et al, 1954). Illingsworth (1985)

TABLE 32-7	Three Regimens for Eradication of *Helicobacter pylori* Disease in Children
Medications*	**Dosage**
Option 1 (3 drugs)	
1. Amoxicillin	50 mg/kg/day divided twice daily up to max 1 g twice daily
2. Clarithromycin	15 mg/kg/day divided twice daily up to max 500 mg twice daily with food
3. Omeprazole	1 mg/kg/day divided twice daily up to max 20 mg twice daily
Option 2 (3 drugs)	
1. Clarithromycin	15 mg/kg/day divided twice daily up to max 500 mg twice daily with food
2. Metronidazole	20 mg/kg/day divided twice daily up to 500 mg twice daily
3. Omeprazole	1 mg/kg/day divided twice daily up to max 20 mg twice daily
Option 3 (4 drugs)†	
1. Bismuth subsalicylate (antimicrobial effect)	8-12 yr: ⅔ to 1 tablet/caplet four times/d chew or dissolve tablets in mouth before swallowing
	>12 yr: 2 tablets/caplets four times/d chewed or dissolved prior to swallowing
2. Tetracycline	>8 yr: 20-50 mg/kg/day divided four times/d to max 3 g daily. Take 1 hr before or 2 hr after meals.
3. Metronidazole	20 mg/kg/day divided twice daily up to max 500 mg twice daily
4. Omeprazole (or comparable acid inhibitory doses of another PPI) *or* an H$_2$ blocker (cimetidine, famotidine, nizatidine, or ranitidine)	1 mg/kg/day divided twice daily up to max 20 mg twice daily

*All regimens consist of three drugs given simultaneously and should be prescribed initially for 7 (minimum) to 14 days (higher eradication rates).

†Only for children 8 years or older. Follow-up breath or stool test can confirm eradication; some cases require additional treatment course of 14 days.

d, Day; *max,* maximum; *PPI,* proton pump inhibitor; *qid,* fours times daily.

Data from Pickering LK, Baker CJ, Kimberlin DW et al: *Red Book: 2009 Report of the Committee on Infectious Diseases,* ed 28, Elk Grove Village, IL, 2009, American Academy of Pediatrics; Sultan MI, Li B UK, Greene MT: Helicobacter pylori *infection: treatment and medications.* Updated 2010. Available at www.emedicine.medscape.com/article/929452-treatment (accessed Feb 5, 2011).

described colicky infants as having attacks of screaming in the evening with classic motor features that included flushed face, furrowed brow, and clenched fists, with legs drawn up and a piercing high-pitched scream.

Epidemiology

No specific cause of colic has been identified, and multiple independent causes are felt to contribute, with both physical and psychosocial factors playing a role. Organic causes for excessive crying account for less than 5% of infants (Freedman et al, 2009). Differences in functional biomarkers (breath hydrogen production in response to lactose-containing milk, intestinal permeability changes, circulating gut hormones, food intolerance, gut microflora and inflammatory markers) may indicate pathology (Moore, 2009). Two studies on aberrant intestinal microflora and inflammation show effects on gut motor function and gas production by coliform bacteria *Escherichia coli* (Savino et al, 2009) and *Klebsiella* (Rhoads et al, 2009). In these studies probiotic supplementation provided significant improvement in symptoms.

Psychosocial factors that may play a role in intensity of colic include the perception of a stressful pregnancy, negative childbirth experience, unsatisfying interactions among family members, and overstimulation. The parents' inability to accurately interpret and respond to the infant's cries may contribute to colic. The stress created by a crying baby contributes to ineffective parental communication and interventions, family dysfunction, parental anxiety, and fatigue. In a study by Megel and colleagues (2011) mothers with infants who cry persistently had a sense of loss, not only of her competence as a mother but also of the infant she brought home from the hospital. Until the colic resolved, the mothers went through cycles of "searching" for the feeling of being a "good" mother.

Carey's study on colic (1972) described colicky babies as having a low sensory threshold. Keefe (1988) suggested the term irritable infant syndrome "characterized by excessive crying, increased activity, and difficulty falling asleep" (p 76) and attributed symptoms to the infant's inability to regulate state. More recent studies do not support the notion that colic is a manifestation of a child with "difficult temperament," but more likely just a manifestation of the spectrum of variation of typical behavioral development and maturation (Keefe et al, 2006a,b; Moore, 2009). The fact that colic tends to go away completely by 4 months of age may support this notion.

The incidence of colic varies greatly depending on the definition used. Studies using the Wessel definition tend to cite an incidence of about 20% of infants. However, other studies range as high as 40% (Megel et al, 2011; Moore, 2009; Savino et al, 2010).

Clinical Findings
History
- Infant is younger than 3 months old and cries 3 hours or more a day for 3 days or more per week
- Demands frequent feeding and is often fussy while feeding
- Has excessive gas
- Is inconsolable or is comforted for short periods only
- Is "tense" or "tight" and keeps legs stiff and fists clenched tightly
- Red flags in the history indicating a potential organic cause for crying include apnea, cyanosis, struggling to breathe; excessive spitting or vomiting; and stool retention.

Physical Examination. If possible see the family during a crying time. A thorough examination must be completed to rule out other pathologic conditions and should include the following:
- Body temperature and evaluation of growth parameters
- Full body examination to look for signs of trauma or abuse
- Abdominal examination for distention, masses, tenderness, and bowel sounds
- Stool for blood or mucus

Diagnostic Studies. If the child is gaining weight and has a normal examination, no other laboratory tests are indicated.

Differential Diagnosis
All other causes of abdominal pain are in the differential diagnosis. Also included are UTI, other infection, corneal abrasion, or traumatic injury.

Management
- No treatment is totally effective for infantile colic. The goal of treatment is to manage the situation until the colic resolves itself. Parents and providers who are flexible, creative, and persistent in seeking solutions are most likely to be successful. Recommendations for providers include (Megel et al, 2011):
  - Rule out potential physiologic causes of crying.
  - Review strategies already used and offer other suggestions (Box 32-6).
  - Allow the mother to talk about effects on herself and other family members.
  - Acknowledge the challenges of the situation and the mother's efforts to help.
  - Follow up by phone call or visit.

Complications
Stress created by a crying baby can contribute to parental feelings of hostility, anger, and guilt, ultimately leading to poor parent-child interaction. Early termination of breastfeeding, postpartum depression, shaken baby syndrome, unnecessary treatment for GERD, postpartum resumption of cigarette smoking, and SIDS have a demonstrated relationship to an infant's excessive crying (Fireman, 2006; Karp, 2008). Parents may self-impose isolation because they do not want to burden others with the crying infant, may fear being perceived as an inadequate parent, and/or fear the infant's safety in the hands of a sitter (Megel et al, 2011). Parents may respond by unintentionally physically or emotionally abusing their infant. Rao and colleagues (2004) found that infants who had excessive uncontrolled crying that persisted beyond 3 months old, without other neurologic deficits, were more likely to have cognitive deficits in childhood. These infants should be followed closely.

Patient Education, Prevention, and Prognosis
Given the risk for child abuse, the National Center for Shaken Baby Syndrome "Period of PURPLE Crying" campaign has materials to educate parents about the characteristics of early (first 3 months of life) crying. *P* stands for peak, *U* for unpredictability of crying bouts, *R* for resistance to soothing, *P* for pain-like expression, *L* for long crying bouts, and *E* for evening clustering.

FOREIGN BODY INGESTION
Description
Most foreign body ingestions are not serious; objects pass through the gut without consequence. Most swallowed items are radiopaque; coins and small toy objects are the most

---

BOX 32-6 Management Strategies for Infantile Colic

Nutritional

- Supplementation with probiotics may be helpful (Savino, 2010; Savino et al, 2009; Thomas et al, 2010).
- Elimination of certain foods from the diet of breastfeeding mothers may prove beneficial: cow's-milk products, eggs, peanuts, tree nuts, wheat, soy, fish, cruciferous vegetables, and chocolate (Hill et al, 2006; Rosen et al, 2007).
- Hydrolyzed formula has shown some effectiveness in a small study (Rosen et al, 2007).
- Dr. Brown's Natural Flow Bottle decreased fussing and crying in babies with colic (Cirgin-Ellett et al, 2006).

Parent Education and Support

- Affirm the baby's good health and reinforce the parents' efforts to comfort their infant.
- Acknowledge the importance of the concern. Allow parents to express feelings of anger, guilt, and frustration.
- Help parents distinguish infant cries and understand typical infant crying, crying associated with illness, and infant state.
- Encourage parents to take time off by seeking help from family or friends.
- Repeat information because parents are often sleep deprived and anxious.
- Meet the infant's needs: feed, sleep, hold, suck, and stimulate.
- Reduce stimulation (quiet, dark, motionless) and avoid the overtired state (nap within 1 to 2 hour of wakefulness).
- Promote regularity and predictability of feeding and sleeping.
- Keep a diary of baby's fussing, crying, and sleeping; analyze to develop a clear daily routine and identify patterns that may be addressed by behavioral intervention (e.g., attunement, self-soothing).

Soothing Techniques

- Encourage sucking at breast, fist, fingers, or pacifier.
- Provide rhythmic activities: rock, swing, jogger, bouncing, walking, and dancing.
- Swaddling reduces crying, improves sleep, and shortens periods of distress (Evanoo, 2007; Karp, 2008; van Sleuwen, 2007).
- Provide "white" noise: lullabies, shushing, nature-recorded sounds, heartbeat or womb-recorded sounds, and hair dryer or vacuum cleaner sounds.
- Kangaroo care (skin-to-skin) contact may be beneficial.
- Car rides, crib vibrators, infant massage, and increased holding (front carrier) (Evanoo, 2007)

Complementary Therapies (see also Chapter 42)

- Probiotics have shown significant improvement in episodes and length of crying (Rosen et al, 2007; Savino, 2009, 2010).
- Herbal teas (chamomile, vervain, licorice, fennel, and lemon balm) showed a reduction in crying (57%) versus control (26%) (Rosen et al, 2007).
- Gripe water (mixture of herbs and herb oils) is touted to provide relief from flatulence and indigestion, but is not entirely without risk. Parents need to avoid products that contain alcohol or are made outside the U.S. (Roberts et al, 2004).
- Fennel seed oil: a study showed improvement of 65% over the control group (24%) (Rosen et al, 2007).
- Sucrose solutions are well proven to offer analgesic effect for single procedure in newborn infants (Harrison et al, 2010); also showed an improvement of 63% over placebo (5%) in one study but the effect was short-lived (30 minutes) (Rosen et al, 2007).
- Chiropractic, osteopathic, and massage interventions have also been used.
- Homeopathic remedies are considered benign because they are low concentration. However, one study of a homeopathic remedy, Galicol Baby, showed an association between an apparent life-threatening event and use of this remedy in infants (Aviner, 2010).

---

commonly ingested items. Food impactions are less common in children than adults. Most ingestions of foreign bodies occur in children between 6 months and 3 years of age (80%) and more than 125,000 ingestions occur annually in patients younger than 19 years (Conners, 2010). Teens may have psychiatric problems or engage in risk-taking behaviors leading to foreign body ingestion. Disk battery ingestions have increased dramatically in the past few years and are very serious (Litovitz et al, 2010).

Epidemiology

Esophageal Foreign Bodies. Esophageal foreign bodies lodge at three spots most commonly—at the thoracic inlet where skeletal muscle changes to smooth muscle (between the clavicles at about C6) (70%), at the midesophagus where the aortic arch and carina overlap the esophagus (15%), or at the LES (15%). Pointed objects or small objects such as pills or small button batteries may lodge anywhere along the slightly moist esophageal mucosa. Up to 30% of children with foreign bodies lodged in the esophagus are asymptomatic (Orenstein, 2007). Common symptoms include an initial episode of choking, gagging, and coughing. Excessive salivation; dysphagia; food refusal; emesis/hematemesis; or pain in the neck, throat, or sternal notch areas may follow. Respiratory symptoms

such as stridor, wheezing, cyanosis, or dyspnea may occur if the esophageal body impinges on the larynx or tracheal wall. Cervical swelling, erythema, or subcutaneous crepitations may indicate perforation of the oropharynx or proximal esophagus (Conners, 2010; Orenstein, 2007). Drooling or pooling of secretions may be related to an esophageal foreign body or abrasion of the esophagus as a result of swallowing the object. Disk batteries cause a liquefactive necrosis, electrical discharge leading to low-voltage burns, and pressure necrosis. Some patients have documented severe erosion or ulceration in as little as 2 hours after ingestion (Kimball et al, 2010). Emergency endoscopic removal is essential. Children who have swallowed lithium batteries greater than or equal to 20 mm diameter are at greatest risk of problems due to battery ingestion.

Abdominal Foreign Bodies. Most ingested objects that reach the stomach pass through the remainder of the GI tract without difficulty (Wyllie, 2007). Items greater than 5 cm in diameter or 2 cm in thickness tend to lodge in the stomach and need to be retrieved. Thin objects longer than 10 cm may not make the duodenal sweep turn and also need to be retrieved. In infants and toddlers, objects greater than 3 cm in length or 20 mm in diameter may not pass through the pyloric sphincter. Open safety pins or other pointed objects such as needles or thumbtacks also should be retrieved.

Perforation after ingestion occurs in only 1% of ingestions. Perforation occurs near physiologic sphincters, areas of angulation, congenital malformations of the gut, or near areas of previous bowel surgery. Coins made with nickel have been reported to interact with gastric acid to cause stomach ulceration (Conners, 2010). Abdominal distention or pain, vomiting, hematochezia, and unexplained fever are symptoms related to ingestions lodging in the stomach or intestinal areas. Items that pose a greater risk include multiple small magnets that may cling together across the bowel wall, leading to pressure necrosis; items containing lead; and batteries, which usually do not cause problems but might lead to symptoms if there is leakage of alkali or mercury from battery degradation. Lithium toxicity has been reported. Nickel in coins can lead to allergic symptoms in children with a nickel allergy.

Rectal Foreign Bodies. Children sometimes put items into their rectum. Small blunt objects usually will pass spontaneously, but large or sharp objects should be retrieved after sedation to relax the anal sphincter.

Clinical Findings
History, Physical Examination, and Laboratory Studies. Specific physical findings are unusual. Abrasions, streaks of blood, or edema of the hypopharynx may occasionally indicate a foreign body. Laboratory studies are usually not helpful, although they may be useful to identify potential infection.

Imaging Studies. Most foreign bodies are radiopaque. A single frontal radiograph that includes the neck, chest, and entire abdomen is usually sufficient to locate the object. Subsequent radiographs may be useful to more fully evaluate the patient. Esophageal objects should be precisely located with frontal and lateral chest radiographs and to make sure that there are not two objects closely aligned. Coins in the esophagus are usually seen on the frontal view, whereas tracheal coins are more often seen from the side view (Conners, 2010). Having the child ingest a small amount of dilute contrast material may help locate radiolucent objects. Endoscopy may be needed and also allows removal of the object.

Management
Most objects do not require special care. Patients who are drooling may require suction.

Esophageal Foreign Bodies. Objects in the esophagus should generally be considered impacted. Removal is mandatory except for blunt objects that have been in place less than 24 hours. Disk batteries and sharp objects should be removed without waiting. Endoscopy is the method of choice for removal except that experienced gastroenterology practitioners may use a Foley catheter to pull the object up or a bougienage method to push the object into the stomach. Only experienced clinicians working with healthy children who ingested an item less than 24 hours previously should try these methods. They are preceded by a radiograph to be sure the item has not moved in the immediate period before the procedure and followed by another radiograph to be sure there are not any retained parts or complications such as a pneumomediastinum.

Stomach/Lower Gastrointestinal Tract Foreign Bodies. Most foreign bodies that reach the stomach may be left to pass through the system, usually within 2 to 3 days. Very sharp items may perforate the bowel and should be removed endoscopically from the stomach or surgically from the intestine. Button batteries in the stomach or intestine may be left to pass but should be removed if the family has not identified the battery in the stool after 2 to 3 days. It should be removed endoscopically from the stomach at that time or watched with repeat radiographs to be sure it is progressing through the tract if it is in the intestine. Items may not pass through the gut if the child has a bowel abnormality or has had bowel surgery. Use of laxatives is not necessary. Inducing vomiting may lead to aspiration.

Complications
Systemic reactions from allergy or toxic response to massive ingestion can occur. Retained foreign bodies may cause erosion, abrasion, local scarring, obstruction, abscess, FTT, perforation, pneumomediastinum, pneumonia, or other respiratory disease. Complications from the removal process can occur. Traumatic epiglottitis can occur from trauma during swallowing or a fingersweep trying to dislodge the item.

APPENDICITIS
Description
Appendicitis is inflammation of the appendix that leads to distention and ischemia that can result in necrosis, perforation, and peritonitis or abscess formation. Although a classic presentation is easy to discern, appendicitis can mimic many other intraabdominal conditions, making diagnosis tricky.

Epidemiology
Following a closed-loop obstruction of the appendiceal lumen by a fecalith, lymphoid tissue, tumor, parasite, foreign body, or inspissated CF secretions, the appendix becomes distended, experiences increased bacterial overgrowth, and becomes subject to ischemia and necrosis. Peritoneal inflammation around the infected appendix causes the characteristic symptoms. There is about a 36- to 72-hour maximum window from the onset of pain to the rupture of the gangrenous appendix. Rupture results in the release of inflammatory fluid and bacteria into the abdominal cavity, resulting in infection of the peritoneum with resultant generalized peritonitis. The infected fluid may be walled off by the omentum and loops of small bowel with resultant abscess formation and localized pain (Katz et al, 2009).

The average age of appendicitis in children is 6 to 10 years old, with a male-to-female ratio of approximately 2:1. It is rare in infancy. The incidence is 4 cases per 1000 children. Perforation is most common in younger children (under 5 years), and is complicated by the fact that appendicitis is less common in this age group and that the ability of very young children (less than 5 years) to communicate location and type of pain is not yet well developed (Katz et al, 2009). Thus it is challenging at times to make a timely diagnosis.

Clinical Findings
History
* The most reliable information is gained from the sequence of symptoms (Katz et al, 2009).

○ Pain: Initially poorly defined periumbilical pain (earliest sign); acute onset of severe pain is not typical of acute appendicitis. A shifting of pain to the right lower quadrant may occur after a few hours and becomes more intense, continuous, and localized.

○ Nausea and vomiting: typically occurs after pain; however, in retrocecal appendicitis, this may be reversed. In gastroenteritis, vomiting precedes the pain.

○ Anorexia occurs (although up to 50% of children state that they are hungry).

○ Stool is low volume with mucus; diarrhea is atypical but can occur (gastroenteritis has high-volume, watery stools).

○ Fever is neither sensitive nor specific for appendicitis; many children present as afebrile or with low-grade fever. High fever may be associated with perforation.

• A scoring system may be helpful (Kharbanda et al, 2005). A score of 5 or less is highly sensitive in the exclusion of the diagnosis of appendicitis.

○ Nausea (2 points)
○ Focal right lower quadrant (RLQ) pain (2 points)
○ Migration of pain (1 point)
○ Difficulty walking (1 point)
○ Rebound tenderness and/or pain with percussion (2 points)
○ Absolute neutrophil count more than $6.75 \times 10^3/\mu L$ (6 points)

• The process evolves over 12 hours, with the potential for infants and young children to become sick much more quickly.

• Following perforation, symptoms lessen, with less vomiting, fever greater than 101° F (38.3° C), and the most comfortable position being on the side with the legs flexed.

• Infants demonstrate irritability, pain with movement, and flexed hips.

• The child may become quiet because crying and movement hurt.

Physical Examination. A complete physical examination is necessary. Reexamination may be needed in 4 to 6 hours.

• Presence of involuntary guarding, RLQ rebound tenderness, maximal pain over McBurney point (1.5 to 2 inches in from the right anterior superior iliac crest on a line toward the umbilicus) on abdominal examination (most reliable finding); percussion is best method for eliciting rebound tenderness.

• Heel-drop jarring test (on toes for 15 seconds, dropping down forcefully on heels); inability to stand straight or climb stairs; winces when getting off examination table or riding in a car over bumps; child most comfortable with bent knees

• Positive psoas sign or obturator sign (or both)

• Rovsing sign (pressure deep in left lower quadrant with sudden release elicits RLQ pain) strongly suggests peritoneal irritation (Katz et al, 2009; Ross and LeLeiko, 2010).

• Tenderness and possibly a mass (abscess) on the right side on rectal examination

• Scoring systems, such as those described earlier, are available and can help focus attention on signs and symptoms necessary for the diagnosis.

Diagnostic Studies. The following may be noted with appendicitis (Katz et al, 2009; Ross and LeLeiko, 2010):

• CBC with differential may show an increased WBC count (>10,000) with an increased neutrophil count. This occurs in 70% to 90% of those with acute appendicitis. However, an elevated WBC count may be neither sensitive nor specific in the clinical diagnosis of appendicitis; during the first 24 hours of symptoms it is often within a normal range.

• Amylase, lipase, and liver enzymes help to differentiate liver, gallbladder, or pancreatic issues.

• UA can show small numbers of WBCs (<20) and red blood cells (RBCs) (<20 per high-power field).

• Examination of stool may demonstrate blood and pus (rare finding).

• Abdominal radiographs can show a fecalith, especially if rupture has occurred.

• US demonstrates enlargement of the appendix and changes in its wall, increased field around the appendix, or an abscess. US has excellent specificity, but only fair sensitivity and is operator dependent.

• CT with contrast has the highest accuracy, especially in adolescents. CT compared with US has higher sensitivity and specificity, is not operator dependent, and may be more cost effective in preventing an unnecessary appendectomy. An appendiceal diameter of greater than 6 mm is considered diagnostic (in both US and CT).

• A β-human chorionic gonadotropin (β-hCG) test to rule out pregnancy or ectopic pregnancy

Differential Diagnosis

The differential diagnosis includes vomiting and gastroenteritis (fever and crampy abdominal pain with vomiting, diarrhea, or both), constipation, UTI (fever, chills, and urinary symptoms), pregnancy, PID or organ pathologic condition, pneumonia, duodenal ulcer (gnawing and burning pain), intestinal obstruction (crampy pain), peritonitis (worse pain when jumping or coughing), and intussusception (child younger than 2 years old with a right upper quadrant [RUQ] mass). (See also Fig. 32-4.)

Management

• A surgical consultation for an appendectomy is needed. Administering opioid narcotics for pain before surgical consultation effectively reduces acute abdominal pain, does not impede the diagnostic process, and does not lead to an inappropriate increased use of CT scanning preoperatively.

• Open appendectomy (OA) or laparoscopic appendectomy (LA) is indicated in nonperforated appendicitis. LA is marginally more expensive than OA; however, LA allows for earlier return to normal activities and reduced postoperative pain (Katz et al, 2009).

• The management of perforated appendicitis is controversial including whether to perform LA or OA procedures. Urgent appendectomy may not be indicated in cases of perforated appendicitis. Instead, surgeons may choose to perform appendectomy once fluid resuscitation and antibiotics have been administered. Some surgeons choose a nonoperative approach as long as the child's clinical condition improves with antibiotic treatment and may perform an appendectomy 8 to 12 weeks after recovery (Katz et al, 2009).

ALGORITHM

Differential Diagnosis

Accidental injury	Ectopic pregnancy	Pneumonia
Accidental ingestion	Food intolerance	Renal stones
Anaphylactoid purpura	Gastroenteritis	Sickle cell anemia
Appendicitis	Hemolytic uremic syndrome	Tortion of ovary or testicle
Child abuse	Mechanical obstruction	Trauma
Constipation	Mononucleosis	Urinary tract infection
		Viral syndrome

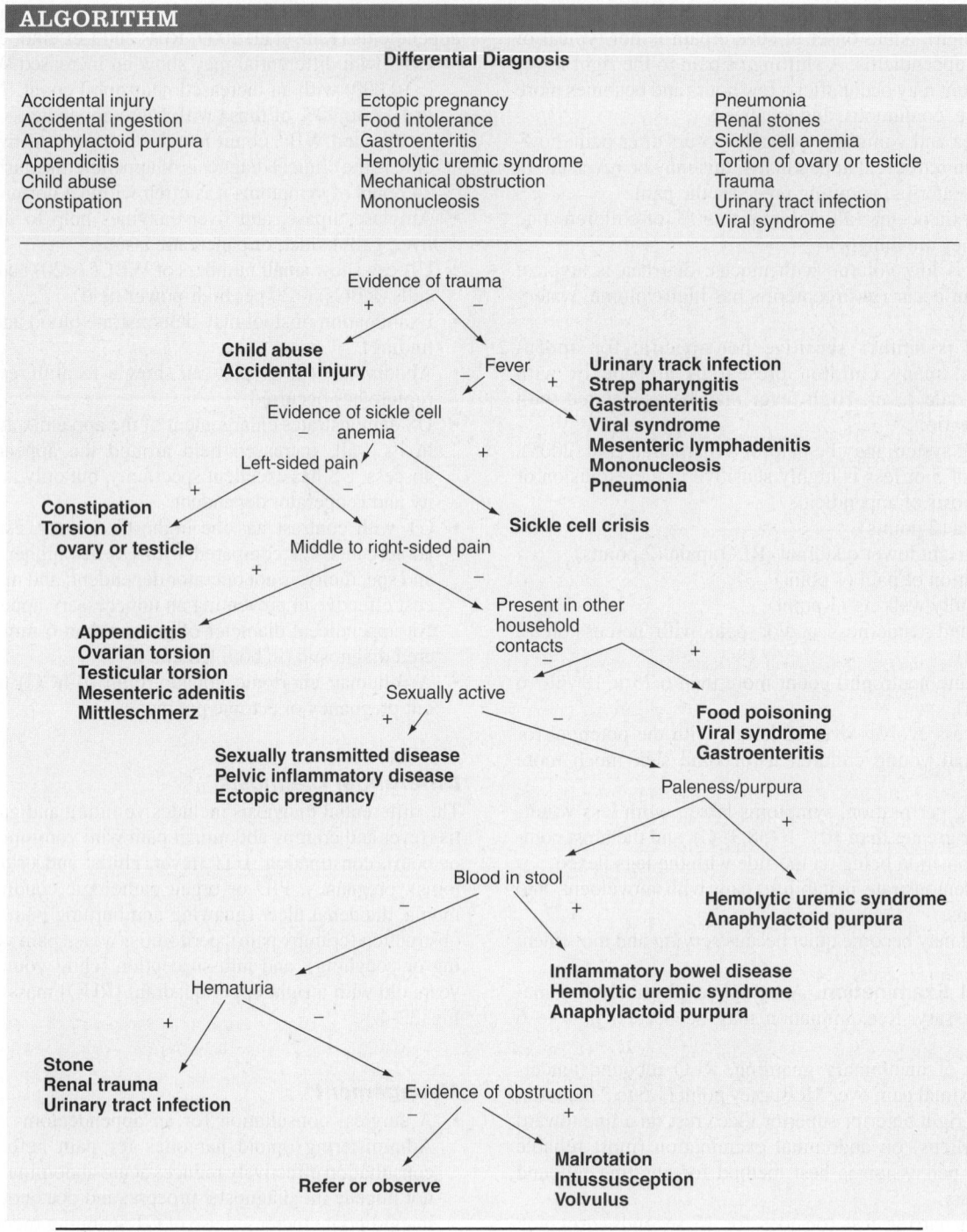

FIGURE 32-4 Decision tree for differential diagnosis of acute abdominal pain. (From Schwartz MW, Curry TA, Sargent J, editors: *Pediatric primary care: a problem-oriented approach,* ed 3, St Louis, 1997, Mosby.)

- IV and preoperative antibiotics are given if perforation is suspected.
- Patients should be seen for follow-up 2 to 4 weeks after surgery. If appetite, bowel function, energy, and activity level are normal; no pain or fever is present; findings on physical examination are normal; and the wound is well healed, the child can resume unrestricted activity. If at the 2- to 4-week follow-up the child has signs of delayed infection, abnormal bowel function, or unexplained weight loss, refer back to the surgeon.

Complications

Perforation, peritonitis, pelvic abscess, ileus, obstruction, sepsis, shock, and death can occur.

INTUSSUSCEPTION

Description

Intussusception involves a section of intestine being pulled antegrade into adjacent intestine with the proximal bowel trapped in the distal segment. The invagination of bowel

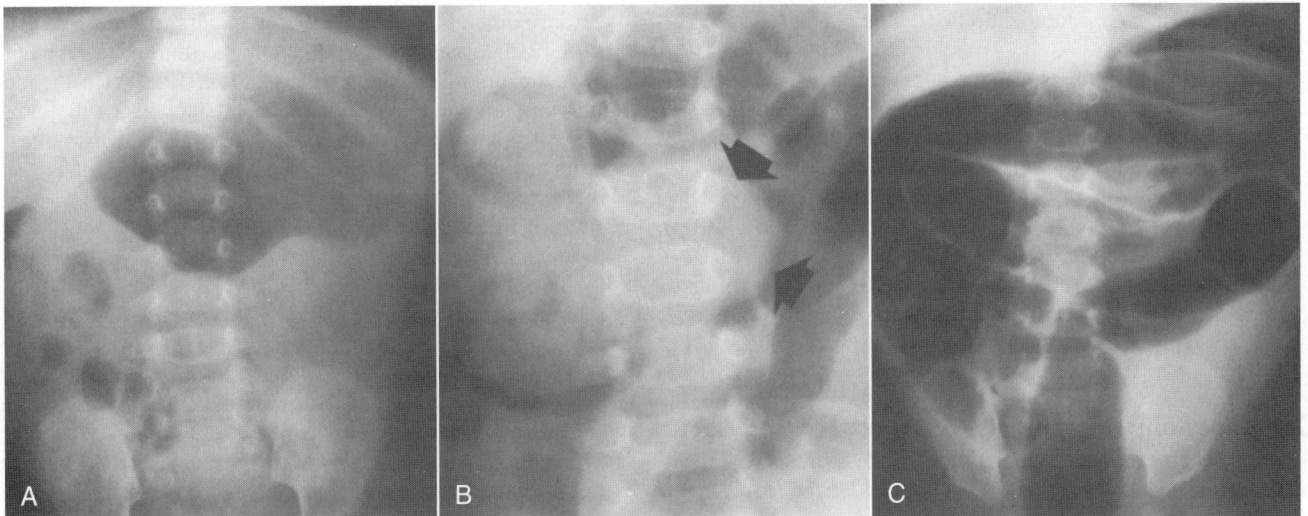

FIGURE 32-5 Intussusception. **A,** Plain abdominal radiograph demonstrating a gas-filled stomach and relatively little gas in the distal end of the bowel. This baby had typical clinical features of intussusception and a palpable upper abdominal mass. Therefore, an enema with air was performed. **B,** The intussusception *(arrows)* is outlined by air. **C,** Reduction is proved by air refluxing into loops of small bowel. (From Burg FD, Ingelfinger JR, Wald ER, editors: *Gellis and Kagan's current pediatric therapy,* ed 15, Philadelphia, 1999, Saunders.)

begins proximal to the ileocecal valve and is usually ileocolic, but it can be ileoileal or colocolic.

Epidemiology

Intussusception is thought to be the most frequent reason for intestinal obstruction in children (Ross and LeLeiko, 2010) and results from an imbalance of longitudinal forces along the intestinal wall (Blanco and Chahine, 2010). The cause is not generally apparent (idiopathic); in some children, there is a known medical predisposing factor such as polyps, Meckel diverticulum, Henoch-Schönlein purpura, constipation, lymphomas, lipomas, parasites, rotavirus, adenovirus, and foreign bodies. Intussusception may also be a complication of CF. Intussusception most commonly occurs between 5 and 10 months of age and is also the most common cause of intestinal obstruction in children 5 months to 3 years. In younger infants intussusception is generally idiopathic and responds to nonoperative approaches. Children older than 3 years are more likely to have a lead point caused by polyps, lymphoma, Meckel diverticulum, or Henoch-Schönlein purpura; therefore, a cause must be investigated (Blanco and Chahine, 2010).

Clinical Findings
History
- The classic triad for intussusception, intermittent colicky (crampy) abdominal pain, vomiting, and bloody mucous stools, are present in only one third of cases (Blanco and Chahine, 2010):
  ○ Paroxysmal, episodic abdominal pain with vomiting every 5 to 30 minutes. Vomiting is nonbilious initially. Some children do not have any pain.
  ○ Screaming with drawing up of the legs with periods of calm, sleeping, or lethargy between episodes
  ○ Stool, possibly diarrhea in nature, with blood ("currant jelly")
- A history of a URI is common.

- Lethargy is a common presenting symptom.
- Fever may or may not be present; can be a late sign of transmural gangrene and infarction.
- Severe prostration is possible.
Physical Examination
- Observe the baby's appearance and behavior over a period of time; often the child appears glassy-eyed and groggy between episodes, almost as if sedated.
- A sausage-like mass may be felt in the RUQ of the abdomen with emptiness in the RLQ (Dance sign); observe the infant when quiet between spasms.
- The abdomen is often distended and tender to palpation.
- Grossly bloody or guaiac-positive stools.
Diagnostic Studies
- An abdominal flat-plate radiograph can appear normal, especially early in the course and reveal intussusceptions in only about 60% of cases (Fig. 32-5). A plain radiograph may show sparse or no intestinal gas or stool in the ascending colon with air-fluid levels and distension in the small bowel only.
- Abdominal US is very accurate in detecting intussusception and is the test of choice (Ross and LeLeiko, 2010). It shows "target sign" and the "pseudokidney" sign and can also be used to evaluate resolution following air contrast enema.
- An air contrast enema is both diagnostic and a treatment modality.

Differential Diagnosis

The differential diagnosis includes incarcerated hernia, testicular torsion, acute gastroenteritis, appendicitis, colic, and intestinal obstruction

Management
- Emergency management and consultation with a pediatric radiologist and a pediatric surgeon

- Rehydration and stabilization of fluid status; gastric decompression
- Radiologic reduction using a therapeutic air contrast enema under fluoroscopy is the gold standard.
- Surgery if perforation, peritonitis, or hypovolemic shock is suspected or radiologic reduction fails.
- IV antibiotics are often administered to cover potential intestinal perforation.
- A period of observation following radiologic reduction is recommended (12 to 18 hours); clear discharge instructions to return with any recurrence of symptoms are required, and close phone follow-up for up to 72 hours is prudent.

Complications

Swelling, hemorrhage, incarceration, and necrosis of the bowel requiring bowel resection may occur. Perforation, sepsis, shock, and reintussusception (reported to typically be <10%, usually within 72 hours of radiologic reduction but can occur up to 36 months later) can all occur (Blanco and Chahine, 2010). Recurrence is associated with lead points.

CHILDHOOD FUNCTIONAL ABDOMINAL PAIN AND FUNCTIONAL ABDOMINAL PAIN SYNDROME

Description

Children who have recurrent abdominal pain with no specific organic etiology are said to have functional abdominal pain (FAP), also known as RAP, often a puzzling problem for providers. FAP is much more common than organic reasons for abdominal pain. The Rome III criteria are used as the diagnostic standards (Rasquin et al, 2006). These criteria include:
- FAP. The following must occur at least once per week for at least 2 months before diagnosis:
  - Episodic or continuous abdominal pain
  - Insufficient criteria for other functional GI disorders
  - No evidence of an inflammatory, anatomic, metabolic, or neoplastic process to explain symptoms
- Functional abdominal pain syndrome (FAPS): One or more of the following must occur at least once per week for at least 2 months before diagnosis and include childhood FAP criteria at least 25% of the time:
  - Some loss of daily functioning
  - Additional somatic symptoms, such as headache, limb pain, or difficulty sleeping

Epidemiology

FAP is a fairly common pediatric complaint. The cause of the pain remains unclear, but the pain is genuine. There is no evidence of visceral hypersensitivity in the rectum (Rasquin et al, 2006) as occurs with IBS. Affected children have an involuntary predisposition for the development of physiologic pain (e.g., a family history of FAP). Temperament and personality can make the child more vulnerable to environmental stressors (often minor) that precipitate the sensation of pain. Children who are perfectionists and have a tendency toward anxiety are more likely to experience FAP. Stress at school, home, with friends, or because of a novel social situation may be associated with FAP symptoms (Bishop, 2011). Positive and negative reinforcement can modify the pain.

Approximately 15% to 35% of children worldwide have recurrent abdominal pain with about one third of those having no specific organic disorder (Gottsegen, 2010). FAP is the most common pain complaint of preschoolers and accounts for 2% of pediatric visits (Scheffer, 2011). The peak incidence of FAP occurs between the ages of 7 and 12 years (Bishop, 2011).

Clinical Findings
History
- A complete review of systems
- Parental history of FAP
- A careful psychosocial history (home, school, parents, friends); secondary gains from symptoms and lack of coping skills. Endeavor to determine the degree of functional impairment.
- Existence of associated symptoms, such as headache, joint pain, anorexia, vomiting, nausea, excessive gas, and altered bowel pattern
- Comorbidity of anxiety and/or depression (in children or adults), behavioral problems, a negative life event
- Identification of alarm symptoms or red flags (Box 32-7); there is an association between these symptoms and an organic cause to the chronic pain (Bishop, 2011; Gottsegen, 2010).
- Presence of Rome criteria for FAP or FAPS (see prior description)
- Report of abdominal pain often accompanied by a dramatic reaction (clutching abdomen, doubling over, or throwing self to ground)
- Determination that symptoms may be worse in the morning, preventing the child from going to school and resulting in school avoidance
- Report that pain medications do not alleviate pain
- Illicit drug use
- Sexual activity or abuse and possibility of pregnancy

Physical Examination. Following initial examination, reexamination should be done during an acute episode and with each subsequent visit. The physical examination is usually normal, but should include:
- Weight, height, and BMI plotted on growth curves
- Vital signs (temperature, heart rate, respiratory rate, blood pressure)
- Abdominal examination: presence of pain, rebound tenderness, masses
- Perianal and rectal examination
- Complete neurologic examination
- Pelvic examination as indicated
- Examination of skin and joints
- Alarm symptoms (see Box 32-7)

Diagnostic Studies. There are two different approaches the clinician can consider.
- In their discussion of the application of the Rome III criteria, Rasquin and colleagues (2006) recommend that any testing be reserved for the presence of alarm symptoms or specific symptoms of organic disease. In these situations, testing would include:
  - CBC, ESR, CRP, UA, and urine culture if FAPS is suspected. If indicated, a biochemical profile (liver and kidney function); stool for ova, parasites, and culture; and breath hydrogen testing may be useful
  - US, endoscopy with or without biopsy, and esophageal pH monitoring as indicated by alarm symptoms

Alarm Symptoms for Functional Abdominal Pain

Red Flags on History
- Localization of the pain away from the umbilicus, especially right or left upper quadrant
- Pain associated with a change in bowel habits, particularly chronic, severe diarrhea; constipation; or nocturnal bowel movements
- Pain associated with night wakening
- Repetitive, significant emesis, especially if bilious
- Constitutional symptoms, such as recurrent fever, loss of appetite or energy
- Recurrent abdominal pain occurring in a child younger than 4 years old
- Blood in stool or emesis

Red Flags on Physical Examination
- Unexplained fever
- Unintentional loss of weight or decline in height velocity
- Organomegaly
- Localized abdominal tenderness, particularly removed from the umbilicus
- Perirectal abnormalities (e.g., fissures, ulceration, or skin tags)
- Joint swelling, redness, heat, or discoloration
- Ventral hernias of the abdominal wall

- After performing a complete history and physical examination, Bishop and associates (2011) suggest the following *initial* approach for ordering diagnostic studies to evaluate FAP:
  - CBC, ESR, amylase, lipase, UA, and abdominal ultrasound (liver, bile ducts, gallbladder, pancreas, kidneys, ureters)
  - A 3-day trial of a lactose-free diet
  - If results are negative and there are no red flags, further testing is not needed.
  - Fecal calprotectin assay can also be a good initial test in a child with recurrent abdominal pain and changes in stool habits (Diamante et al, 2010).
- *Follow-up* evaluation with additional and more invasive GI or other testing should be considered if there are positive results noted in the initial diagnostic testing, symptoms progress, or warning signs develop. These may include such testing as CT, endoscopy, celiac disease serology, and/or colonoscopy.

Differential Diagnosis

There is no evidence that the presence of the associated symptoms, a negative life event, or the presence of anxiety or depression can help distinguish between organic and FAP. Figure 32-6 outlines a decision tree for differential diagnosis of chronic abdominal pain. The following are included in the differential diagnosis: all organic causes of abdominal pain, including urinary tract, GI tract (IBS, celiac disease, intestinal malformations), and extraabdominal causes; malabsorption syndromes (usually with diarrhea, belching, flatulence, and bloating); lactose intolerance; constipation; abdominal pain associated with depression (usually includes social isolation, decreased activity and attention span, difficulty sleeping, and irritability); and school avoidance (usually associated with severe pain and anxiety on weekday mornings only).

Management
- Establish a therapeutic parent-child-practitioner relationship to improve patient satisfaction, adherence to treatment, symptom reduction, and other outcomes.
- Explain the brain-gut interaction and that biobehavioral methods are the most effective evidence-based treatments of FAP (Gottsegen, 2010).
- Use medications judiciously. H_2-blockers should not be used unless dyspepsia is present. Citalopram has been used in clinical trials with promising results in children with internalizing disorders and recurrent abdominal pain (Campo et al, 2004).
- Discuss the possibility with the child and parent that the pain can be functional (inorganic) early in the visit. Assure them that the symptoms are real and will be addressed.
- Encourage return to school and normalization of lifestyle. Limit attention given for pain episodes.
- Consider the use of complementary and alternative (CAM) medical approaches (see Chapter 42). If certain dietary practices seem to cause pain, a more bland diet may be helpful (e.g., a lactose-free diet with documented lactose intolerance). Avoiding sorbitol and fructose may be useful if malabsorption is considered a contributing factor. There is a lack of high-quality evidence that dietary intervention (fiber supplements, lactose-free diets, or lactobacillus supplementation) is an effective strategy in managing FAP in children (Huertas-Ceballos et al, 2009). A mind-body approach is often useful, combining relaxation, behavioral management, stress coping training, meditation, and biofeedback. Acupuncture, massage, and hypnosis have also been shown to help with chronic abdominal pain.
- Explore psychological triggers and use management strategies for the pain. Discuss how stressful events and emotional issues might affect the pain. Suggest distraction to shift attention from abdominal pain to other activities; attending school is a good distraction. Biofeedback provides evidence to the child that he or she can change muscle tension, skin temperature, and relaxation. Relaxation and guided imagery decrease abdominal pain.
- Identify, treat, and refer for any significant psychological issues. Psychotherapy and family therapy may be of some benefit. Cognitive behavioral therapy has also been helpful for all forms of FAP (Gottsegen, 2010). Using a biopsychosocial approach is especially helpful for FAPS. Refer for psychological dysfunction (maladaptive behavior, conversion reaction, depression, anxiety).
- Discuss alarm symptoms (see Box 32-7) so that the parents and child can identify changes in status and illness.
- Establish regular follow-up.

Prognosis and Complications

FAP can be a lifelong and chronic condition. Although one third of cases resolves within 2 months of diagnosis, one third has a long-term course with similar complaints in adulthood. The final third of cases has chronic complaints of pain (often headache) instead of abdominal pain that continue through adulthood (Kohli and Li, 2004; Walker et al, 2010). Male gender, onset of FAP before 6 years old, a delay in diagnosis greater than 6 months, and a family history of somatic pain, as first reported by Apley and Naisch (1958), are factors still predictive of a poor long-term prognosis.

ALGORITHM

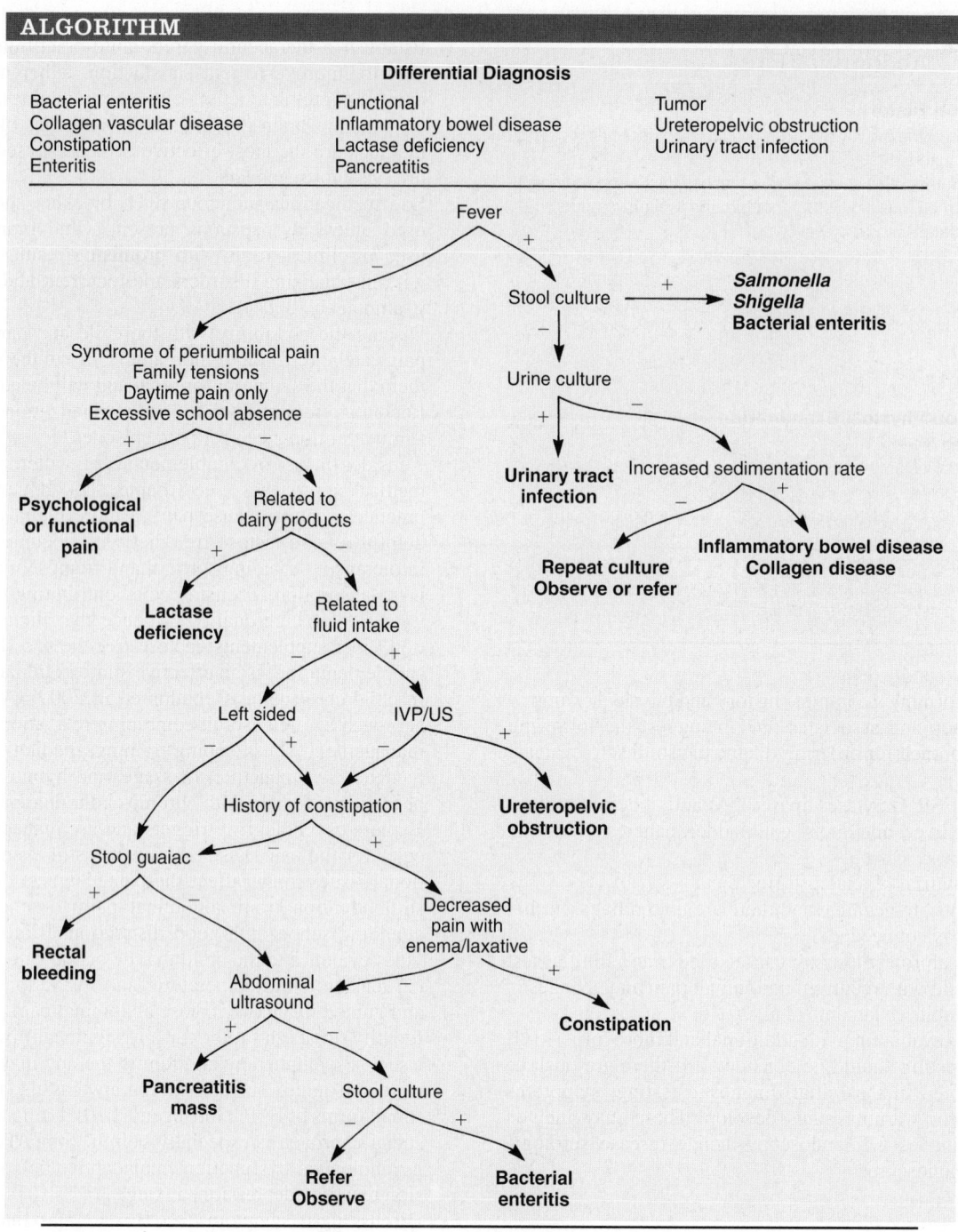

FIGURE 32-6 Decision tree for the differential diagnosis of chronic abdominal pain. (From Schwartz MW, Curry TA, Sargent J et al, editors: *Pediatric primary care: a problem-oriented approach,* ed 3, St Louis, 1997, Mosby.)

IRRITABLE BOWEL SYNDROME

Description

IBS is defined as chronic or FAP with altered bowel habits and bloating that is not explained by structural or biochemical abnormalities (El-Baba, 2010). It is considered a functional gastrointestinal disorder. The criteria for IBS (also known as IRB Rome III diagnostic criteria) must include *all* of the following at least once per week for at least 2 months before diagnosis:

- Abdominal discomfort (an uncomfortable sensation not described as pain) or pain associated with two or more of the following at least 25% of the time:
  - Improved with defecation
  - Onset associated with a change in frequency of stool
  - Onset associated with a change in form (appearance) of stool
- No evidence of an inflammatory, anatomic, metabolic, or neoplastic process that explains the child's symptoms

Epidemiology

Visceral hypersensitivity and brain-gut interaction are thought to be involved in the pathology of IBS. The hypersensitivity may be associated with infection, allergy, inflammation, or intestinal trauma. Twin studies and positive family history suggest a genetic predisposition; GI infections have also been documented. Disordered gut motility may be associated with IBS, as may be early stressful events, and ineffective coping mechanisms (Rasquin et al, 2006). Psychological comorbidity (somatic symptoms, anxiety, and depression) has also been reported. Approximately 16% of children 11 to 17 years of age report symptoms of IBS. Children with recurrent abdominal pain are at increased risk for IBS during adolescence and adulthood (El-Baba, 2010).

Clinical Findings
History
- Rome criteria symptoms for IBS (see prior description)
- Abnormal stool frequency (four or more stools per day and two or fewer stools per week)
- Abnormal stool form (lumpy/hard or loose/watery or alternating constipation and diarrhea)
- Abnormal stool passage (straining, urgency, or feeling incomplete evacuation)
- Passage of mucus
- Bloating or feeling of abdominal distention
- Dyspepsia (present in 30% of pediatric patients)
- Potential triggering events and psychosocial factors
- Family history of IBS
- Psychosocial history
- Nutrition history: Fiber and water intake, excessive sorbitol or fructose intake
Physical Examination
- Normal physical examination; normal growth curves and BMI
- Absence of alarm signals
Diagnostic Studies. There are no specific laboratory markers for IBS.

Differential Diagnosis
See FAP for differential diagnosis.

Management
- Confirm and explain diagnosis.
- The goal is to modify severity of symptoms. Identify and develop strategies to deal with triggering events and psychosocial factors.
- Antidepressants and serotonergic agents have not been widely used in children.
- Treatment options for IBS include (Bishop, 2011):
  ○ Amitriptyline or selective serotonin reuptake inhibitors in difficult or persistent cases
  ○ High-fiber diet or fiber supplements are useful to manage symptoms with constipation-predominant IBS.
- Peppermint oil (one enteric-coated capsule three times daily) and/or probiotics (try different ones and monitor response because some help more with bloating and flatulence, pain or constipation; lactobacillus and bifidobacteria are commonly used) have been found to provide excellent symptom relief (Pirotta, 2009).
- Dietary modifications may be helpful with IBS. Avoid trigger foods known to exacerbate pain episodes: caffeine, sorbitol, fatty food, large meals, gas-producing foods, such as carbonated beverages, lactose (with lactose intolerance), and cruciferous vegetables.

ABDOMINAL MIGRAINE
Description
Abdominal migraine is thought to be part of a continuum with migraine and cyclic vomiting syndrome (see earlier section). It typically occurs in children rather than adults. The diagnosis is often difficult to determine during the first episode but becomes evident with cyclic episodes. The diagnostic criteria for abdominal migraine (also known as Rome III diagnostic criteria for abdominal migraine) must include *all* of the following (Dafer, 2010; Rasquin et al, 2006):
- Paroxysmal episodes of intense, acute periumbilical (midabdominal) pain that lasts from 1 to 72 hours
- Intervening periods of usual health lasting weeks to months
- Pain that interferes with normal activities
- Pain associated with two or more of the following: Nausea, vomiting, anorexia, headache, photophobia, or pallor
- No evidence of an inflammatory, anatomic, metabolic, or neoplastic process that explains the symptoms
- These criteria need to be present two or more times in the preceding 12 months.

Epidemiology
Family migraine history is common (Dafer, 2010; Ulshen, 2009). Abnormal visual-evoked responses, hypothalamic-pituitary-adrenal axis abnormalities, and autonomic dysfunction are possible mechanisms. Abdominal migraine affects 1% to 4% of children and tends to be more common in girls than boys (3:2), with a mean onset at 7 years old and a peak at 10 to 12 years old (Chandran and Chitkara, 2008; Rasquin et al, 2006).

Clinical Findings
History
- Rome criteria for abdominal migraine (see prior description)
- Family history of migraine or motion sickness
- History of motion sickness
- Most episodes last hours to days with a 1-hour minimum.
- Aura not frequently experienced
- Headache complaints typically absent or minimal
- May have prodrome symptoms of fatigue and drowsiness
Physical Examination
- Normal physical examination; normal growth curves and BMI
- Absence of alarm signals
Diagnostic Studies. There are no laboratory markers for abdominal migraine. EEG is not necessary unless other symptoms are present such as seizure and episodes of confusion (Dafer, 2010). During the first or worst episodes appropriate laboratory and neurologic studies may be needed to exclude other serious conditions or diseases (Dafer, 2010; Mitchell, 2009).

Differential Diagnosis
The diagnosis is often difficult to determine during the first episode. Obstructive GI and renal processes, biliary tract disease, recurrent pancreatitis, familial Mediterranean fever, and metabolic disorders, such as porphyria, should be ruled out. Cyclic vomiting is thought to be a severe variant of abdominal migraine (Mitchell, 2009).

Management

- Identify and avoid triggers: Caffeine, nitrates, and amine-containing foods; excessive emotional stress; travel; prolonged fasting; altered sleep; flickering or glaring lights.
- Sleep often relieves symptoms; antiemetics may abort an attack (Dafer, 2010).
- Abdominal migraine should respond to migraine prophylactic therapy (cyproheptadine, amitriptyline, topiramate). A positive response helps confirm diagnosis.

Prognosis

The child may develop migraine headaches later in life (Dafer, 2010).

MALABSORPTION SYNDROMES: CELIAC DISEASE, LACTOSE INTOLERANCE, COW'S-MILK PROTEIN INTOLERANCE OR ALLERGY

Malabsorption syndromes can be caused by many different genetic, congenital, and acquired conditions and usually lead to an initial decrease in weight followed by a deceleration in height velocity. This chapter discusses celiac disease, lactose intolerance, and cow's-milk protein intolerance (CMPI).

Description and Epidemiology

Celiac disease is a common autoimmune disease triggered in susceptible individuals by dietary exposure to wheat gluten and related proteins in barley and rye. Celiac disease is associated with human leukocyte antigens (HLAs). Autoantibodies to the enzyme tissue transglutaminase (TTG) create an affinity to HLA-DQ2 or HLA-DQ8, activate T cells, and lead to inflammation of mucosal tissue; as a result, intestinal damage can occur (Schuppan et al, 2009). Four types of celiac disease have been noted: typical, with mostly GI symptoms; extraintestinal; silent; and latent. The last three may not have GI symptoms even though serology and/or intestinal mucosal changes occur (Setty et al, 2008). A number of conditions or variables may contribute to the development of celiac disease. It is suggested that demographic changes such as immigration from developing to developed countries increase exposure to gluten and an increased incidence of celiac disease follows (Logan and Bowlus, 2010). Celiac disease is greater among infants born by cesarean section; the development of enteric homeostasis in the newborn period may be altered, increasing susceptibility (Decker et al, 2010). Repeated rotavirus infections may increase risk of celiac disease (Stene et al, 2006), although parent-reported gastroenteritis occurring at the time gluten was introduced into the child's diet does not appear to be associated with celiac disease (Welander et al, 2010). Celiac disease can be associated with autoimmune diseases (e.g., type 1 diabetes, thyroid disease, and Sjögren syndrome) and with nonautoimmune diseases (e.g., Down syndrome, immunoglobulin A [IgA] deficiency). Celiac disease has a worldwide distribution with overall prevalence of 1% (Mustalahti et al, 2010). The most typical presentation occurs between 6 months and 2 years old.

Lactose intolerance is a clinical syndrome characterized by abdominal pain, diarrhea, nausea, flatulence, and bloating after the ingestion of lactose-containing foods. The symptoms are caused when lactose, a disaccharide (glucose and galactose) found exclusively in mammalian milk, is not absorbed in the gut. It is usually secondary to a deficiency of the lactose enzyme. Increased lactose draws fluid and electrolytes into the intestine, resulting in an osmotic diarrhea. Intestinal bacteria also metabolize excess lactose in the gut, creating methane, carbon dioxide, and hydrogen gases that lead to bloating and flatulence. Four types of lactase deficiency have been noted:

- Primary lactase deficiency, also known as lactase nonpersistence, is the most common cause of lactose intolerance. It develops in most children after weaning and at varying ages and is more common in various ethnic groups. The prevalence of primary lactase deficiency has not been established in the U.S., though it is found more often in Hispanic, African-American, Ashkenazi Jewish, Asian, and American-Indian populations than in Caucasian European-Americans.
- Secondary lactase deficiency results from small bowel injury (e.g., gastroenteritis, chemotherapy, chronic diarrhea) and is more common in infancy.
- Congenital lactase deficiency is an extremely rare congenital absence of lactase, but if left untreated, can be fatal in early infancy.
- Developmental lactase deficiency describes the lactase deficiency that occurs in preterm infants born before 34 weeks because of the immaturity of the intestinal tract (Heyman, 2008).

CMPI and *cow's-milk allergy* (CMA) can have similar clinical pictures; however, the body's immune response differs in each of these conditions. CMPI is a nonallergy hypersensitivity to cow's-milk protein (CMP), whereas CMA is antigen mediated. Most CMA is IgE mediated, an expression of atopy in which eczema, allergic rhinitis, and/or asthma may also be seen. Some cases of CMA are probably cell mediated, presenting with primarily GI symptoms (Fiocchi et al, 2010).

CMA typically develops in the neonatal period, peaks in infancy, and tends to remit during childhood. Approximately 2% to 5% of infants have CMA by food challenge and elimination diet (Fiocchi et al, 2010). IgE-mediated CMA decreased from about 4% in 2-year-olds to less than 1% in 10-year-olds (Matricardi et al, 2008). Up to 80% of children with CMA develop tolerance within 3 to 4 years of diagnosis (Fiocchi et al, 2010).

Clinical Findings

General History for Malabsorption Syndromes. Careful medical and family medical histories are very important in the evaluation of a malabsorption syndrome and are often the key to the diagnosis. In addition, a complete dietary history is needed to distinguish between undernutrition and malabsorption. Important historical findings include:

- Past surgical and trauma history
- Growth failure (a common symptom of nutritional deficiency and malabsorption)
- Delayed puberty can coexist with malabsorption.
- A voracious appetite or particular food avoidance present in small children with malabsorption syndromes
- Chronic diarrhea with frequent, large, foul-smelling, pale stools
- Excessive flatus with abdominal distention

- Pallor, fatigue, hair and dermatologic abnormalities, digital clubbing, dizziness, cheilosis, glossitis, peripheral neuropathy (symptoms of vitamin deficiency seen with malabsorption).
  Disease-Specific History. In addition to the above, the following may stand out:
  Celiac Disease
- Chronic or intermittent diarrhea, persistent or unexplained GI symptoms (e.g., nausea and vomiting), sudden or unexpected weight loss, and prolonged fatigue (National Institute for Health and Clinical Excellence [NICE], 2009)
  Lactose Intolerance
- Abdominal pain, diarrhea, nausea, flatulence, and bloating often related to the amount of lactose ingested.
  CMPI and CMA
- Family history of allergy and/or atopy
  General Physical Examination
- Growth parameters and percentiles (weight, height, BMI, head circumference)
- Skinfold thickness and lean body mass
- Tanner stage
- Examination for delayed growth and puberty
  Disease-Specific Physical Examination
  Celiac Disease
- Impaired growth, FTT, unexplained iron deficiency anemia, abdominal distention, bloating or cramping pain
- May have no symptoms at all despite evidence of small bowel changes; maintain a high suspicion for celiac disease in children with metabolic bone disease (such as rickets or osteomalacia), low-trauma fractures, or those with dental enamel defects. An estimated 85% to 90% of individuals with celiac disease are undiagnosed (NICE, 2009).
  Lactose Intolerance
- Abdominal distention
  CMPI and CMA. Symptoms may be immediate or late onset (Fiocchi et al, 2010).
- Immediate
  ○ Anaphylaxis (rare) but can be life-threatening
  ○ GI: Lip or tongue swelling, oral pruritus, nausea, vomiting
  ○ Skin: Urticaria, rash, flushing, angioedema
  ○ Respiratory: Nasal pruritus, sneezing, rhinitis, congestion, wheezing, dyspnea, chest tightness
- Late onset (1 hour to several days after ingestion of CMP)
  ○ Typically, non–IgE-mediated allergic reaction
  ○ Symptoms are mostly GI: Varied, including nausea, vomiting, abdominal pain, diarrhea, bloody stool, GERD-like symptoms, pyloric stenosis, malabsorption, FTT, IBD
  ○ Can see skin reaction (with both IgE- and non–IgE-mediated allergy); eczema
  ○ Respiratory: Heiner syndrome is very rare.
  Diagnostic Studies
- Stool assessment for occult blood, WBCs, and culture; liquid stool for pH and reducing substances; 72-hour fecal fat collection or Sudan stain for stool fat
- Spot stool testing for alpha 1-antitrypsin level to establish the diagnosis of protein-losing enteropathy
- Sweat chloride test (in the presence of steatorrhea to evaluate for CF)

- Stool for O&P. Giardiasis is a common intestinal infection causing malabsorption. See later discussion for symptoms suggestive of infestation.
- CBC with differential, mean corpuscular hemoglobin concentration (MCHC), iron, folic acid, and ferritin
- Serum calcium, phosphorus, magnesium, alkaline phosphatase, serum protein, liver function tests, vitamin D and its metabolites, vitamins A, B_{12}, E, and K
- Human immunodeficiency virus (HIV) testing (for symptoms of FTT and chronic diarrhea)
- Small bowel biopsy helps identify diseases of the small bowel mucosa and obtain material for culture and sensitivity.
- Plain abdominal radiographs and barium contrast studies as indicated
- Abdominal US can detect masses and stones in the hepatobiliary system.
- Retrograde studies of the pancreas and biliary tree if indicated
- Bone age
  Specific Tests for Celiac Disease
- Serologic testing should be done if there is clinical suspicion of celiac disease, the child has an associated disorder, or there is a first-degree relative with celiac disease. Gluten should be eaten in more than one meal every day for 6 weeks prior to testing. Recommended serologic tests include IgA tissue transglutaminase antibody (tTGA) and IgA endomysial antibody (EMA) because of their high sensitivity and specificity (NICE, 2009). EMA is more expensive and less accurate in children younger than 2 years of age (Gelfond and Fasano, 2006).
- Home blood testing is not recommended (NICE, 2009).
- If serologic testing is positive, refer for colonoscopy and biopsy for a definitive diagnosis, although colonoscopy may not be necessary if the tTGA level is greater than 100 units/mL (Mubarak et al, 2011).
- Careful follow-up of growth parameters, tTGA testing after 6 months of gluten-free diet (GFD), and then yearly (NASPGHAN, 2005).
- Bone density testing (bone problems may be first symptom of celiac disease).
  Specific Tests for Lactose Intolerance
- Lactose hydrogen breath test is the gold standard. Children should not be taking antibiotics at the time of the study because the intestinal bacteria that act on lactose may be diminished.
- Trial of a lactose-free diet for 2 weeks, being aware of hidden sources of lactose. Symptoms should disappear with the diet and reappear when lactose is reintroduced.
- Bone density if calcium deficit is suspected (lactose is necessary for calcium absorption into bone, and lactose-free diets can predispose to osteoporosis).
- If secondary cause of lactose intolerance is suspected, continue workup for all other causes of malabsorption.
  CMPI and CMA
- Elimination diet followed by a double-blind placebo-controlled oral food challenge in an allergist's office is test of choice for CMA.
- Skin patch test for allergies may be performed.
- Serum IgE antibodies testing may be performed.
- Diagnosis of CMPI is made when there is clinical improvement on CMP-free diet.

Differential Diagnosis

Organic and inorganic FTT, colic, short stature, chronic diarrhea, CF, immunodeficiency, cholestatic liver disease, GERD, and IBD are included in the differential diagnoses.

Management

Celiac Disease

- A strict GFD for life is currently the only effective treatment for celiac disease. The standard for being gluten-free is a limit of 20 ppm of gluten (NASPGHAN, 2005). Adding pure oats to a GFD can improve palatability and increase fiber and vitamin B intake (Pulido et al, 2009) without causing a systemic or autoantibody response (Koskinen et al, 2009). Unfortunately, many oat products can be contaminated with gluten during manufacturing.
- Alternative treatments are being explored, including enzyme therapy, developing genetically engineered grains, inhibiting tTGA in the intestine, and correcting intestinal barrier defects (particularly increased permeability) (Fasano et al, 2008).
- A lactose-free diet for young children may be helpful. This is generally not the case in adolescence and adults unless they are lactose intolerant (NASPGHAN, 2005).

Lactose Intolerance

- Test to ensure that the individual actually has lactose intolerance.
- Reduce exposure to lactose
  - Avoid lactose-containing milk and other dairy products, including goat's milk.
  - Use lactose-free dairy products (e.g., milk prehydrolyzed with lactase).
  - Use alternate milk sources (soy, rice, etc.).
- Use oral lactase supplements.
- Ensure adequate intake of calcium and vitamin D from other food products.
- Most individuals with primary lactase deficiency can ingest dairy products in small to moderate amounts, especially if taken with other foods (Suchy et al, 2010).

CMPI and CMA (Fiocchi et al, 2010)

- Breastfeed.
- Restrict milk and milk products from the diet of breastfeeding mothers.
- If formula fed, use extensively hydrolyzed formula initially. Partially hydrolyzed formula is *not* appropriate for infants with CMA.
- Use amino-acid formula for infants who demonstrate severe allergy (e.g., prior history of anaphylaxis) or who do not respond to extensively hydrolyzed formula.
- Extensively hydrolyzed soy formula is appropriate for infants after 6 months of age only; before 6 months, infants fed soy formula are at risk for nutritional deficit.
- Avoid use of other mammals' milk (e.g., sheep, goat, camel) due to risk of cross-allergic reaction.
- After age 2 years formula is not appropriate, but ensure daily dietary intake of 600 to 800 mg calcium.
- Probiotics may be helpful in creating tolerance, but more clinical research is needed.
- Have EpiPen if anaphylaxis is a concern.
- Monitor growth and development carefully.
- Refer to an allergist or gastroenterologist if symptoms are severe; immunotherapy is not recommended.

- Annual reevaluation of sensitivity, preferably an oral food challenge under medical supervision.

Complications and Prognosis

Celiac Disease. Growth failure is the primary complication of celiac disease. With delayed diagnosis or inadequate treatment, there is risk for fractures and osteoporosis (due to reduced bone mineral density), lymphoma, autoimmune diseases (e.g., type 1 diabetes, thyroid disorders), primary biliary cirrhosis, and primary sclerosing cholangitis. Sensory peripheral neuropathy may be related to gluten sensitivity (Hadjivassiliou et al, 2010). Celiac crisis consisting of abdominal distention, explosive watery diarrhea, dehydration with hypoproteinemia, electrolyte imbalance, hypotensive shock, and lethargy, although rare, can be the first indication of celiac disease, and can be life threatening (Mones et al, 2007). Prognosis is improved with lifelong GFD.

Lactose Intolerance. Unabsorbed lactose does not cause clinical intestinal damage despite clinical symptoms. Bone density loss may occur if there is inadequate calcium and vitamin D. Other conditions misdiagnosed as lactose intolerance may worsen.

CMPI and CMA. CMPI usually resolves by 1 to 3 years old; when there are only GI symptoms, CMPI resolves completely. CMA cannot be reversed, and there is a high likelihood of other food allergies. Complications include rickets, poor growth, and FTT.

POLYPS

Description and Epidemiology

Intestinal polyps in children may be benign or present a risk for subsequent cancer or other conditions (e.g., anemia). *Solitary polyps*, often called juvenile polyps, are the most frequently seen (90%) polyps in children (Lee et al, 2010). They are most often found in preschool-age children (4 to 5 years old), are usually located in the rectosigmoid area, have an incidence of about 2% in children less than 10 years old, and are considered to present negligible or no risk for malignancy (Manfredi, 2010). Polyps are also found in familial adenomatous polyposis (FAP), juvenile polyposis syndrome (JPS), phosphatase and tensin homolog (PTEN) hamartoma tumor syndrome, and Peutz-Jeghers syndrome (PJS), all of which are autosomal dominant conditions with variable penetrance.

Clinical Findings

History

- May be asymptomatic. A careful family history is imperative to identify children at risk for polyposis.
- Painless, bright red rectal bleeding (hematochezia). Usually the blood coats or is mixed in with the stool. Bleeding can be daily, intermittent, or infrequent. Large volume blood loss is extremely rare.
- FAP: Nonspecific complaints, diarrhea, constipation, or changes in bowel habits

Physical Examination

- Anorectal examination to find polyp or other source of rectal bleeding
- Pallor and edema caused by anemia and hypoproteinemia from GI hemorrhage and protein-losing enteropathy indicate a heavy polyp burden.

- Extraintestinal symptoms of FAP include ophthalmologic changes (may see hypertrophy of retinal pigment); dental anomalies (supernumerary or unerupted teeth); osteomas of skull, jaw or extremities; and multiple lipomas.

Diagnostic Studies
- CBC with differential and ESR, CRP, prothrombin time, and partial thromboplastin time
- Fecal occult blood test, even if blood appears to be present
- Stool culture for bacterial pathogens and O&P
- Colonoscopy to the terminal ileum with biopsy evaluation is the diagnostic test of choice.
- Upper endoscopy if there is concern for gastric or duodenal polyps. Small-bowel video capsule endoscopy may be used.
- Barium contrast of upper intestine

Management
- Refer to a pediatric gastroenterologist for management and follow-up screening.
- Treatment involves resection of the polyp(s), usually with diagnostic or surveillance screening. If multiple polyps are present, bowel resection (colectomy) is common. For FAP, colectomy is standard therapy.
- Children with one or two juvenile colonic polyps at diagnosis usually need no further follow-up.
- Follow-up is required if:
  - There is a family history of polyps (i.e., all children are at risk for polyposis).
  - The child has three or more polyps on colonoscopy.
  - Polyps are found outside the colon.
  - Extraintestinal symptoms are present.
- Follow-up varies by condition, severity, and pediatric specialist provider (Alkhouri et al, 2010; Barnard, 2009; Manfredi, 2010). Genetic testing to determine presence of gene mutation is usually done at 8 to 10 years of age.
- Ophthalmologic evaluation
- Genetic counseling

Complications

Children with polyps are at risk for colorectal, gastric, duodenal, pancreatic, and extraintestinal cancer as adults (usually appearing in the fourth decade of life or later). Psychological issues related to having a hereditary condition with uncertain long-term outcomes (i.e., high risk for malignancies) can cause family problems.

ANAL FISSURE
Description and Epidemiology

Anal fissures are small tears in the anal mucosa. The usual cause of an anal fissure is passage of frequent or hard stools. Anal stenosis and other trauma can also be causative factors. Anal fissures are the most common cause of rectal bleeding in all pediatric groups.

Clinical Findings
History
- Crying with bowel movement
- Bright red streaks of blood in the stool or diaper
- Withholding of stool

Physical Examination. With the patient in the knee-chest position and the anus slightly everted, small tears in the anal mucosa can be visible. An otoscope with a large speculum is needed if the external fissures are not readily visible. A digital anal examination with the fifth finger rules out anal stenosis.

Differential Diagnosis

Other sources of lower intestinal hemorrhage, such as infection, formula intolerance, necrotizing enterocolitis, intussusception, juvenile polyps, hemolytic-uremic syndrome, Henoch-Schönlein purpura, irritable bowel disease, and vascular lesions are included in the differential diagnosis. Sexual abuse should be considered in children with large, irregular, or multiple fissures.

Management
- Treat the cause (see Chapter 12).
- Local wound care should include sitz baths twice a day and application of 0.5% hydrocortisone cream or K-Y jelly to the anus.

Complications

Recurrence is common. Constipation causes a fissure, which leads to a stool withholding-encopresis–painful stooling cycle.

Prevention

Preventive measures include avoiding constipation, encouraging regular toileting habits, and avoiding the use of laxatives and enemas.

■ Inflammatory Bowel Disease

IBD is thought to be a dysregulated immune response of intestinal mucosa to microbes in genetically susceptible individuals. Defects may be present in both the barrier function of intestinal epithelium and the immune system (Henderson et al, 2011; Xavier and Podolsky, 2007). Three primary types of IBD are recognized: Crohn disease (CD), ulcerative colitis (UC), and unclassified IBD (IBDU). See Table 32-8 for features contrasting Crohn disease and UC. Symptoms of IBD in children can be difficult to interpret and a definitive diagnosis between CD and UC may be elusive, especially in early, active disease. Numerous contacts with health care providers may be necessary to establish a diagnosis, and the initial diagnosis may change as the disease progresses (Benchimol et al, 2009). Several indices are used to assess and classify IBD: The Crohn's Disease Activity Index (CDAI) and the Pediatric Ulcerative Colitis Activity Index (PUCAI) rate the severity of disease (Noble and Turner, 2008; Turner et al, 2007). The Paris classification, a modification of the Montreal classification, identifies the location of the disease in children (Levine et al, 2011; Satsangi et al, 2006), and the Cardiff-Hughes classification gives guidelines on diagnosis and scoring of perianal disease (Hughes, 1992).

The incidence of IBD appears to be increasing worldwide, especially the incidence of Crohn disease and pediatric-onset IBD (Benchimol et al, 2011). IBD can occur at any age, with

TABLE 32-8	Features of Crohn Disease and Ulcerative Colitis	
Feature	Crohn Disease (CD)	Ulcerative Colitis (UC)
Age at onset	10-20 years old	10-20 years old
Area of bowel affected	Can affect any part of the GI system; often in terminal ileum or colon; may be small bowel only; small bowel and cecum; small bowel and colon; or colon only; occasionally isolated perianal disease	Affects colon and rectum; entire colon may be inflamed (pancolitis); may have subtotal colitis or "ileal backwash" (i.e., superficial inflammation of ileum proximal to splenic flexure); may be left-sided (distal to splenic flexure); may have proctitis (limited to rectum or distal 15 cm)
Distribution	Segmental; disease-free "skip" areas common	Continuous distal to proximal
Endoscopic, radiographic or biopsy findings	Segmental or patchy areas of lesions; noncaseating granulomas; cobblestone appearance of bowel wall; linear/serpiginous ulcers and transverse fissures; fixation and separation of loops; small bowel strictures/stenoses; bowel or perianal fistulas; perianal abscesses or large (>5 mm) skin tags	Superficial inflammation of mucosa; friable tissue with exudates and granularity; loss of vascular pattern; small perianal skin tags (<5 mm)
Intestinal symptoms	Abdominal pain, bloody diarrhea, anorexia	Abdominal pain with or around time of stooling, bloody diarrhea, urgency, and tenesmus
Extraintestinal manifestations: Seen more often in CD than UC; similar types for both conditions	Ophthalmologic conditions (uveitis, iritis, conjunctivitis) more likely in CD	Primary sclerosing cholangitis more likely in UC

CD, Crohn disease, *GI*, gastrointestinal.
Data from Working Group of the North American Society for Pediatric Gastroenterology, Hepatology, and Nutrition and Crohn's and Colitis Foundation of America: Differentiating ulcerative colitis from Crohn disease in children and young adults: clinical report, *J Pediatr Gastroenterol Nutr* 44(5):653-674, 2007; Jose FA, Garnett EA, Vittinghoff E et al: Development of extraintestinal manifestations in pediatric patients with inflammatory bowel disease, *Inflamm Bowel Dis* 15(1):63-68, 2009.

a peak onset between 15 and 30 years. Up to 25% of cases are in children and adolescents and 4% are found in children less than 5 years of age (Mamula et al, 2008). IBD in infants is extremely rare (Kappelman and Grand, 2008), but is increasing in some areas (Benchimol et al, 2009). In contrast to adults, children diagnosed with IBD are more likely to have CD than UC, to have more severe or extensive disease (both CD and UC), more vague symptoms, more extraintestinal symptoms (e.g., arthralgia), and more relapses (Guariso et al, 2010: Kelsen and Baldassano, 2008; Turner and Griffiths, 2011).

CROHN DISEASE

Description

Crohn disease is a chronic disease with dysregulated inflammation and cytokine production in the intestinal tract. Any part of the GI tract can be involved, although the terminal ileum and colon are most commonly affected. Esophageal disease, often without upper GI symptoms, has been found in about 20% of all CD cases, and perianal disease is common (Ammoury and Pfefferkorn, 2011). Inflammation is usually transmural, affecting the entire wall of the intestine, creating fissures and fistulas. Unaffected areas of intestine are called "skip" areas.

Epidemiology

The exact cause is unknown, although it is likely due to environmental exposure that triggers an abnormal immune reaction in a genetically susceptible individual. CD peaks in late adolescence and early adulthood, then again in middle

adulthood (50 to 70 years); 25% to 40% of cases are diagnosed in childhood and adolescence. The CDC estimates the worldwide incidence rate for CD is between 0.1 and 16 per 100,000 individuals; prevalence rate is about 400 per 100,000 (CDC, 2010). It is more common in Caucasians, and males and females are affected about equally, except in esophageal disease, which is more common in boys than girls (Ammoury and Pfefferkorn, 2011). Siblings are more likely to have CD than is the general population. Approximately 10% to 15% of cases are rediagnosed as UC within the first year of illness (Bourreille et al, 2009).

Clinical Findings
History
- Fever, usually low grade, of unknown etiology
- Weight loss (average of 5 to 7 kg)
- Delayed growth velocity, short stature, delayed bone age
- Arthralgias and/or arthritis in large joints, occasional joint destruction
- Obstructive symptoms associated with meals, bloating, early satiety
- Pain in the umbilical region and RLQ; may awaken at night
- Anorexia
- Malabsorption and lactose intolerance
- Diarrhea (with or without blood or mucus) and pain with stooling
- Jaundice
- Oral aphthous ulcers, especially during exacerbations of the illness
- Use of tobacco
- Positive family history

Physical Examination

- Carefully measure growth parameters (height, weight, and BMI).
- Perform an abdominal examination while observing for RLQ tenderness and a mass.
- Perianal skin tags, deep anal fissures, and perianal fistulas strongly suggest CD.
- Clubbing of digits may be present.
- Erythema nodosum is common.

Diagnostic Studies. The following are ordered as needed:

- Inflammatory markers: ESR, CRP
- Nutritional labs: Albumin, total protein (consider iron panel, calcium, zinc, alkaline phosphatase, folate, vitamin B_{12})
- Other blood tests: CBC with differential (consider liver enzymes—aspartate aminotransferase [AST], alanine transaminase [ALT], total bilirubin, gamma-glutamyltransferase [GGT]; amylase; lipase)
- Stool: Routine culture, O&P, *C. difficile* (with recent antibiotic use), blood, WBCs, and fecal alpha 1-antitrypsin; fecal calprotectin assay (good initial test in a child with recurrent abdominal pain and changes in stool habits [Diamante et al, 2010])
- Radiologic studies: Bone age (usually delayed by 2 years), bone density, abdominal plain films, upper GI series with small bowel follow-through, abdominal CT with contrast
- Ileocolonoscopy is a first step to assess for CD. Other endoscopic studies include small bowel capsule endoscopy (SBCE), push enteroscopy, single- or double-balloon enteroscopy, interoperative enteroscopy or spiral enteroscopy (Bourreille et al, 2009). Esophageal endoscopy is recommended in children diagnosed with CD who have perianal disease (Ammoury and Pfefferkorn, 2011).
- Screen for tuberculosis (TB) if child is at risk (see Chapter 23 for risk criteria). Biologic agents used in CD therapy can activate latent TB (Chiappini et al, 2009).

Differential Diagnosis

Rheumatoid arthritis, systemic lupus erythematosus, hypopituitarism, acute appendicitis, peptic ulcer, intestinal obstruction, intestinal lymphoma, anorexia, chronic granulomatous disease, sarcoidosis, and growth failure are included in the differential diagnosis. Abdominal TB and Hermansky-Pudlak syndrome are rare conditions with Crohn-like symptoms (Chiappini et al, 2009; Damen et al, 2010).

Management

The goals of therapy are to (1) control the disease; (2) prevent relapses; and (3) achieve normal nutrition, growth, and lifestyle. Treatment is pharmacologic, nutritional, surgical, and psychosocial. The following management steps are taken:

- Refer to a pediatric gastroenterologist for colonoscopy, endoscopy, more definitive diagnosis, consultation, and follow-up care.
- In the U.S., corticosteroid management is most common. In Europe, however, exclusive enteral nutrition (EEN) is the first-line therapy (Lochs et al, 2006). EEN is given for 6 to 8 weeks as initial therapy to induce remission and control inflammation. It also fosters mucosal healing, decreases the need for medications, and enhances nutritional status (Day et al, 2007; Mallon and Suskind, 2010; Shamir 2010).
- Medications:
  - Corticosteroids (e.g., prednisone, budesonide) are used orally, rectally, or intravenously for acute inflammation of mild to moderate disease. They are not intended for use in remission.
  - 5-Aminosalicylates (balsalazide, sulfasalazine, olsalazine, and mesalamine) orally or rectally for mild disease to control inflammation
  - Immunomodulator agents are used (azathioprine, 6-mercaptopurine, methotrexate, and cyclosporine) for severe small or large bowel disease, steroid-dependent or refractory disease, severe fistula, and growth failure.
  - Biologic agents (e.g., infliximab, a chimeric, anti-tumor necrosis factor-alpha [anti-TNF-alpha] antibody) for steroid-dependent or refractory disease, perirectal fistula, and maintenance of remission, can be given alone or in combination with immunomodulators. One IV infusion of infliximab has been shown to induce remission in CD (Akobeng and Zachos, 2009). Greater mucosal healing follows treatment with immunomodulators and biologic agents than with corticosteroids (Ardizzone et al, 2010) and improved growth is seen with early anti-TNF-alpha treatment (Malik et al, 2011).
  - Antibiotics are used for acute infections (ampicillin, gentamicin, clindamycin, ciprofloxacin, or metronidazole).
  - Adjunctive therapy, including growth hormone prior to or at the time of puberty, enhances optimal growth (Heyman et al, 2008; Savage, 2010).
- Severe disease can require hospitalization, total parenteral nutrition, a nasogastric tube for decompression, or surgery. Studies indicate that 15% to 20% of children require surgery within 2 years of diagnosis and most patients eventually require surgery (Newby et al, 2008; Pacilli et al, 2011). Surgery before puberty has been shown to improve growth, though there is a high relapse rate (55%) (Pacilli et al, 2011), and surgery does not cure the disease.
- Monitor growth and pubertal changes.
- An ophthalmologic examination is needed to rule out underlying ophthalmologic manifestations of the disease.
- Refer for nutritional counseling during remission, to prevent or correct malnutrition, and to maintain and promote growth. See Chapter 10 for specific nutritional recommendations.
- Encourage participation in social activities, such as support and fitness groups (e.g., Team Challenge, a fund-raising running event for CD and colitis), and CD camps. Refer for psychosocial and family therapy as indicated.

Complications

Intestinal obstruction with scarring and strictures is the major complication of CD. Growth failure (especially linear growth) is extremely common. Fistula and abscesses can occur, but perforation and hemorrhage are rare. Primary sclerosing cholangitis, pancreatitis, pericarditis, arthritis, peripheral neuropathy, and an increased risk of lymphoma and colon cancer are other complications of CD (Benavente and Morís, 2011; Navaneethan and Shen, 2010; Peyrin-Biroulet et al, 2011; von Roon et al, 2007). Treatment with corticosteroids or immunosuppressors increases the risk for opportunistic infections and inadequate response to immunizations (Lu et al, 2009). Care must be taken with long-term use of biologics in children because of a risk of infection or malignancy (de Zoeten and Mamula, 2008). The child and family are at risk for social functioning difficulties, anxiety, depression, somatization disorders (Bryant et al, 2011), and school difficulties (Kunz et al, 2010).

Prevention and Prognosis

Follow recommended therapy to prevent sequelae. Crohn disease is progressive and without cure, although about 55% of individuals are in remission at any one time and only about 1% of individuals experience continuous active disease (Ardizonne et al, 2010). Child-onset disease tends to be more severe and require more immunosuppressive treatment than adult-onset disease (Pigneur et al, 2010).

ULCERATIVE COLITIS

Description

UC is a chronic inflammatory bowel disease largely limited to the rectum and colon. Lesions are typically continuous and involve the epithelial lining of the bowel. Up to 80% of patients with pediatric-onset UC have moderate to severe disease (Markowitz et al, 2006) and are more likely to experience inflammation above the splenic flexure. Between 4.5% and 20% have a colectomy within 5 years of diagnosis (Gower-Rousseau et al, 2009; Portela et al, 2010). Pediatric patients, especially those less than 10 years old, may appear to have no lesions in the rectum, leading to a misdiagnosis of Crohn disease (Glickman and Odze, 2008).

Epidemiology

The cause is unknown, but the disease has a multifactorial basis (i.e., heredity, diet, environment, immunologic alterations, and ineffective mucosal integrity). The annual incidence rate in the U.S. is 10 to 12 cases per 100,000, and the overall prevalence rate is 35 to 100 cases per 100,000 individuals. Peak onset occurs among 15- to 25-year-olds, and 20% of all cases are in children and adolescents (Mamula et al, 2008). Unlike CD, UC does not appear to be increasing significantly internationally (Benchimol et al, 2009, 2011).

Clinical Findings

History

- Fever
- Weight loss (average of 4 kg)
- Delayed growth and sexual maturation
- Arthritis and/or arthralgias of the large joints
- Anorexia
- Diarrhea
- Lower abdominal cramping, left lower quadrant pain
- Pain increased before stooling and passing flatus
- Stool with bright red blood and mucus
- Nocturnal stooling
- Oral aphthous ulcers
- Skin lesions (erythema nodosum, pyoderma gangrenosum, and diffuse papulonecrotic eruptions)

Physical Examination

- Carefully measure growth parameters (weight, height, and BMI) and perform a complete physical examination. Abdominal examination can reveal rebound tenderness if the disease is severe.

Diagnostic Studies

- CBC with differential, iron-binding capacity, total protein, albumin, ESR, CRP (children with low WBC counts and normal to near-normal hematocrit levels are more likely to have a mild course and are at lower risk for colectomy [Moore et al, 2011])
- Stool for WBCs, blood, and culture (bloody diarrhea with negative stool culture characteristic of UC)
- Bone age (usually delayed up to 2 years)
- Colonoscopy (diffuse mucosal inflammation)
- Perinuclear neutrophil cytoplasmic antigen (positive in 60% to 70% of cases)
- Fecal calprotectin assay (good initial test in a child with recurrent abdominal pain and changes in stool habits [Diamante et al, 2010])

Differential Diagnosis

Shigella, Salmonella, Yersinia, Campylobacter, E. coli, C. difficile, IBS, self-limited colitis, and Crohn disease are in the differential diagnosis.

Management

The goals of therapy are to (1) control the disease; (2) prevent relapses; and (3) achieve normal nutrition, growth, and lifestyle. Treatment is pharmacologic, nutritional, surgical, and psychosocial. Management involves the following:

- Refer for colonoscopy, biopsy, definitive diagnosis, consultation, and close follow-up care.
- Medications (Ng and Kamm, 2009):
  ○ 5-Aminosalicylic acid (balsalazide, sulfasalazine, osalazine, mesalamine) orally or rectally; first-line drug used to induce remission in acute disease and for long-term maintenance therapy; may be the only drug used in milder cases or in those with higher incidence of proctitis (Portela et al, 2010).
  ○ Parenteral or oral steroids for moderate to severe disease, tapered doses for remission
  ○ Hydrocortisone rectal preparation for tenesmus
  ○ Immunomodulator agents (azathioprine, 6-mercaptopurine) for persistent, active, or steroid-refractory disease or to wean off steroids. Alternative immunomodulatory drugs include tacrolimus (U.S. Food and Drug Administration [FDA]–approved calcineurin inhibitor to prevent graft rejection) as a bridge to thiopurine therapy, methotrexate, and 6-thioguanine; if first-line immunomodulator agents are ineffective, biologic agents are recommended prior to using these alternative medications.
  ○ Biologic agents (infliximab) for induction of remission and maintenance in steroid-refractory and moderate to severe disease
  ○ Cyclosporin monotherapy is as effective as or more effective than corticosteroids for initial treatment of fulminating disease.

- Probiotics (e.g., VSL#3, *Saccharomyces boulardii*) may provide benefits when used with other therapies in mild to moderately active disease.
- Curcumin (active ingredient in turmeric) may assist in maintenance of inactive disease.
- Iron supplementation to correct anemia; multivitamin
- Nutrition (see Chapter 10 for nutritional recommendations):
  - Diet: High in protein and carbohydrate, normal amount of fat, and decreased roughage. Omega-3 fatty acids (in contrast to omega-6 fatty acids) have an antiinflammatory effect on the bowel, though there is not enough evidence currently to recommend their use for treatment of UC (Turner et al, 2011).
  - Lactose is poorly tolerated.
  - Parenteral or enteral nutritional supplements (60 to 70 cal/kg/day) may be used.
  - Refer for nutritional therapy to prevent or correct malnutrition and maintain and promote growth.
- Monitor growth.
- Surgery may be indicated (complete proctocolectomy with permanent ileostomy is curative).
- Refer for ophthalmologic examination to rule out ophthalmologic manifestations of the disease.
- Refer for psychosocial therapy as indicated. Depressive disorders are common.
- Assess immunization status and ensure child is up to date; there is controversy regarding immunizing with live vaccines (e.g., varicella) (Lu et al, 2009).

Complications

Complications can include growth failure, toxic megacolon, intestinal perforation, liver disease, sepsis, cancer of the colon (a long-term sequela—1% to 2% per year after 10 years of disease), arthritis, uveitis, malnutrition, as well as behavioral and emotional problems similar to those of children with celiac disease.

Prevention and Prognosis

Follow the recommended therapy to optimize remission, maintain inactive disease state, and prevent complications. Prognosis is good for patients with mild disease and those who respond quickly to initial therapy. Those with untreated or poorly treated disease are at increased risk for colectomy and colon cancer. In one study of children who had colectomy, 73% reported pouchitis (inflammation of the ileal pouch), and 56% required a second surgery, but overall quality of life, BMI, and number of offspring were equal to that of control subjects (Pakarinen et al, 2009).

■ Failure to Thrive

Description

FTT is a broad term referring to a symptom of a lack of weight gain proportional to age as determined by standardized growth charts. The diagnosis is based on a child's weight but the definition varies in the literature. It is also called growth deficiency, growth delay, protein energy malnutrition, faltering weight, and faltering growth. FTT should be considered if any of the criteria in Box 32-8 are found. The pathway to FTT

| **BOX 32-8** | Criteria that Define Failure to Thrive |

- Weight less than 80% of median weight for length
- Weight for length less than 80% of ideal weight
- Weight for length less than the 10th percentile
- Body mass index for chronologic age less than 5th percentile
- Weight for chronologic age and sex less than 5th percentile or more than 2 standard deviations below the mean
- Length for chronologic age and sex less than 5th percentile
- Weight deceleration crossing more than two major percentile lines on age and population appropriate growth chart
- Height, head circumference, and developmental skills may be affected

---

is based on "disruptions in the complex system of biological, psychosocial, and environmental factors contributing to a child's growth and development" (Stephens et al, 2008, p 265). FTT in early childhood reflects general undernutrition (Olsen et al, 2007).

Epidemiology

FTT has three basic causes: inadequate caloric intake, inadequate caloric absorption, and excessive caloric expenditure. The most common cause is nutritional deficiency without an underlying medical condition (>80%) (Krebs and Primak, 2009; Panetta et al, 2008; Rabinowitz et al, 2010; Stephens et al, 2008). Generally the prevalence rates are thought to be around 5% to 10% in the U.S. (Casey, 2009; Daniel et al, 2008; Rabinowitz et al, 2010). Children living in poverty and/or from developing countries with higher rates of malnutrition and/or HIV infection are more likely to have FTT (Bauchner, 2007). Rates may be increasing, as more preterm infants are surviving.

Onset between 2 weeks and 4 months is more often associated with congenital disorders, serious somatic illness, and with deviant mother-infant interactions. Onset between 4 and 8 months in otherwise healthy children is more clearly associated with feeding problems (Olsen et al, 2010). In chronic cases, weight for height may appear to be normal because of concurrent reductions in velocity. The length of time over which weight loss is experienced in order to be considered FTT, has not been determined; 2 months has been suggested (Casey, 2009).

Clinical Findings and Risk Factors

Clinical findings include poor weight gain associated with poor intake, vomiting, food refusal, food fixation, abnormal feeding practices, presence of anticipatory gagging, irritability, chronic physical problems in any body system, or psychosocial problems. Inborn errors of metabolism should be suspected with history of acute, severe, and potentially life-threatening symptoms, liver dysfunction, recurrent vomiting, neurologic symptoms, cardiomyopathy, impairment of vision or hearing, renal symptoms, dysmorphic features, organomegaly, and/or high anion gap acidosis, lactic acidosis, or hypoketotic hypoglycemia (Ficicioglu and an Haack, 2009). In more severe cases, height, head circumference, and developmental progress may also be affected.

Panetta and colleagues (2008) studied the predictive value of a set of predefined symptoms and signs that might point toward "nonorganic" versus "organic" etiologies for FTT. They found that the presence of vivacity, food restriction, and/or feeding rituals and poor appetite were more predictive of nonorganic (or inadequate caloric intake) and that vomiting, diarrhea, irregular bowel movements, and abdominal distention were more typical symptoms of organic (or malabsorption/excessive expenditure of calories). Vomiting and abdominal distention were noted to be of particular significance. Panetta and associates' review also noted that infants hospitalized for FTT predictably related to social encounters and objects differently, depending on what their eventual causative deficiency proved to be. Infants with organic causes were more likely to prefer close, personal interactions (i.e., with touching/holding) than those later diagnosed as having a nonorganic deficiency due to psychosocial factors (preferred distant social encounters and relating to inanimate objects).

Therefore, a thoughtful approach to the history (medical, developmental-behavioral, nutritional, and social), physical examination, and limited laboratory evaluation of children with FTT can be more predictive than relying on a battery of laboratory tests or empiric hospitalization. The following should be included in the assessment (Bauchner, 2007; Casey, 2009; Ficicioglu and Haack, 2009; Panetta et al, 2008; Rabinowitz et al, 2010).

History. General parental concerns about the child's weight and growth need to be addressed. Look for conditions that would negatively affect the child's growth potential, increase the caloric needs, decrease the availability or use of calories, or affect the child's ability to feed or willingness to feed or factors that might affect the parent's ability or interest in feeding the child.

Prenatal
- Maternal health including chronic illness such as diabetes mellitus, HIV, CMV; habits such as nutrition, alcohol, cigarette use, infection
- Obstetric complications such as toxemia, hemorrhage, and multiple pregnancies

Perinatal
- Perinatal factors: Birthweight, Apgar scores, complications, length of stay in the hospital, congenital anomalies, neurologic insults, newborn screening results, weight for gestational age

Neonatal
- Intraventricular hemorrhage, seizures, hypoxia, extreme hyperbilirubinemia, infection

Postnatal Health
- Health: Hospitalizations, medications, surgeries, accidents, illnesses
- Serious or recurrent infections
- Recurrent symptoms such as vomiting, diarrhea, wheezing, snoring
- Chronic health condition (Table 32-9)
- Collection and interpretation of growth data, percentiles, BMI, height for weight over time
- Stooling and voiding history: Diarrhea, constipation, vomiting, poor urine stream
- Careful review of systems

Developmental Trajectory and Temperamental Style
- Developmental and behavioral history

TABLE 32-9	Major Causes of Failure to Thrive
System	**Cause**
Gastrointestinal	GER, CD, pyloric stenosis, cleft palate or cleft lip, lactose intolerance, Hirschsprung disease, milk protein intolerance, hepatitis, cirrhosis, pancreatic insufficiency, biliary disease, IBD, malabsorption, food alkalines
Cardiac	Cardiac diseases leading to congestive heart failure
Renal	UTI, renal tubular acidosis, diabetes insipidus, chronic kidney disease
Pulmonary	Asthma, bronchopulmonary dysplasia, CF, anatomic abnormalities of the upper airway; obstructive sleep apnea. Recurrently infected adenoids and tonsils.
Endocrine and metabolic	Hypothyroidism, diabetes mellitus, adrenal insufficiency or excess, parathyroid disorders, pituitary disorders, growth hormone deficiency; inborn errors of metabolism
Neurologic	Mental retardation, cerebral hemorrhage, degenerative disorders, cerebral palsy
Infectious	Parasitic or bacterial infections of the GI tract, tuberculosis, HIV
Congenital	Many genetic abnormalities
Malignancy and autoimmune disorders	Many cancers of childhood, collagenvascular disease, juvenile idiopathic rheumatoid arthritis
Nutritional	Lack of calories, lack of micronutrients including vitamin A, zinc, iron
Hematologic	Sickle cell disease and others
Prenatal	Small for gestational age, perinatal infection
Psychosocial	Depression, anorexia nervosa, bulimia, maternal depression, child abuse or neglect, ADHD, autism, chronic pain
Environmental toxins	Heavy metal poisoning; other toxins

ADHD, Attention-deficit/hyperactivity disorder; *CD,* celiac disease; *CF,* cystic fibrosis; *GER,* gastroesophageal reflux; *GI,* gastrointestinal; *HIV,* human immunodeficiency virus; *IBD,* inflammatory bowel disease; *UTI,* urinary tract infection.

Family and Psychosocial History
- Social and family factors: Family composition, caregiving environment, daycare, family support, poverty, parent-child relationship, parenting attitudes, typical day
- Family health history: Size and growth, developmental disabilities, inherited diseases that may affect growth and development

Physical Examination
- Weight, height, BMI, and head circumference (in those younger than 2 years of age) plotted on standardized growth curves and percentiles, including weight-for-height graphs (include past and present growth parameters)

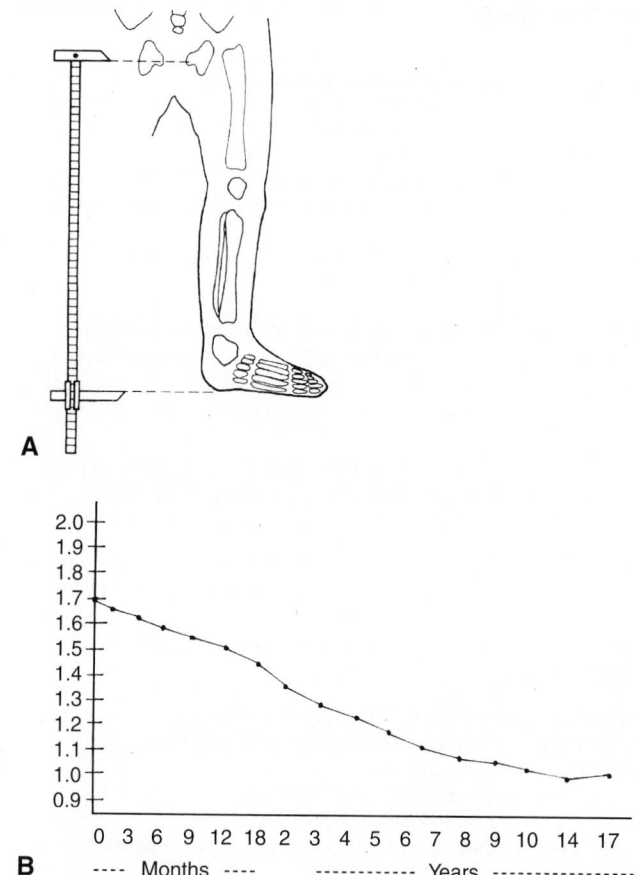

A

B

FIGURE 32-7 Upper: lower (U:L) segment ratios. **A,** To calculate U:L segment ratios use the following formula: (height – lower segment)/lower segment. **B,** Normal U:L segment ratios. 1.7 at birth, 1.3 at 3 years old, 1 at 14 years old. High U:L ratios are characteristic of short limb dwarfism or bone disorders, such as rickets. (From Siberry GK, Iannone R, editors: *The Harriet Lane handbook,* ed 15, St Louis, 2000, Mosby, p 278.)

- Skinfold measurements: Loss of subcutaneous fat; general wasting (more common in developing countries; seen with malignancy, HIV, cerebral palsy [CP], inflammatory diseases)
- Vital signs (temperature, pulse, respiratory rate, blood pressure)
- Hydration status
- Presence of dysmorphic features
- Upper and lower segment measurements (Fig. 32-7) to rule out dwarfism
- Skin, hair, nails, and mucous membranes: Scaling skin (seen with zinc deficiency); rough or hard skin (with hypothyroidism); edema (with protein deficiency); alopecia (with hypervitaminosis, kwashiorkor, or syphilis); hair color/texture changes (with zinc deficiency, Menkes kinky hair disease); spoon-shaped nails (with iron deficiency or GI diseases); cyanosis (with heart disease); and labial fissures (with vitamin deficiency)
- Evidence of abuse or neglect: Unexplained burns or skin lesions; fractures; retinal hemorrhages; unwashed skin; diaper rash; untreated impetigo; uncut and dirty fingernails; unwashed clothing
- Oral findings: Dental caries, tonsillar hypertrophy, submucous cleft palate, or tongue enlargement. May require

oral-motor function studies including lip/tongue/swallowing assessment.
- Respiratory compromise (with CF, bronchopulmonary dysplasia)
- Cardiovascular examination for congenital heart disease
- Abdominal: Lymphadenopathy, hepatosplenomegaly, masses, distention (with malignancy, inborn errors of metabolism, and immunodeficiency)
- Endocrine: Thyroid enlargement, precocious or ambiguous sexual development
- Neuromuscular tone and strength, cranial nerves for swallowing (CP)
- Hypertonicity/hyperreflexia for CP

Diagnostic Studies
- Feeding assessment: Nutritional and feeding history for calorie, protein, micronutrient intake.
  - Quality of food for age and ability to suck, chew and swallow
  - Social nature of the feeding event and family eating patterns (meals and child feeding)
  - Feeding history: Caloric intake; feeding behavior; feeding cues; cues to hunger and satiety; progression to solids; frequency of feedings; amount taken per feeding; preparation of formula (overdilution)
  - Twenty-four-hour diet recall for infants, 3-day diet history for older children eating solid foods
  - Parental understanding of nutrition and feeding of children
- Developmental assessment
- Laboratory and imaging studies as delineated in Table 32-10

Differential Diagnosis
See Tables 32-9 and 32-10.

Management
Management is often best addressed by an interdisciplinary team that includes pediatrics (with specialty consultants for specific medical conditions), nutrition (may include lactation specialist), mental health, other community resources (e.g., Women, Infants, and Children [WIC] program, food stamps, Medicaid, housing authorities), and social work personnel. Community nurse home visits can aid in observations (mealtime behaviors, such as food refusal, spitting, food throwing, oral retention), assessment, and support.
- Manage treatable causes with prompt attention to urgent, life-threatening medical conditions.
- Restore nutritional intake and appropriate intake patterns.
- Provide nutritional rehabilitation: Vitamin supplementation with iron, zinc, and minerals; calorically enriched formula and foods (up to 150 cal/kg/day for infants <6 months old). In older infants and toddlers, solids should be offered before liquids, and they should not be force fed (Bauchner, 2007). See Chapter 10 for further information related to nutrition for FTT. The expected normal weight gain by age should be (Casey, 2009):
  - Birth to 3 months old: 25 to 30 g/day
  - Three to 6 months old: 15 to 20 g/day
  - Six to 12 months old: 10 to 15 g/day
  - Twelve months and older: 5 to 10 g/day

TABLE 32-10	Evaluation Studies for Failure to Thrive		
Generic Cause	**Associated Conditions**	**Physical Findings**	**Diagnostic Evaluation**
Inadequate caloric intake	Poor food intake Chronic illness Inappropriate type/volume of feeding Anorexia, bulimia Food not available, parental withholding Poverty, neglect	Signs of neglect or abuse Minimal subcutaneous fat Protuberant abdomen	Complete dietary history Complete psychosocial evaluation Basic metabolic profile, vitamin D (calcidiol), lead, zinc, iron screening, albumin for protein status in severe FTT
Inadequate caloric absorption	Gastrointestinal causes (malabsorption, chronic vomiting, pancreatic insufficiency, celiac disease, chronic reflux, inflammatory bowel disease) Chronic renal disease, cystic fibrosis, inborn errors of metabolism, infestations	Dysmorphism suggestive of chronic disease, organomegaly, skin/mucosal changes	CBC/ESR, basic metabolic profile, serum electrolytes (include total CO_2 to rule out renal tubular acidosis), UA and urine culture, sweat test, stool studies for fat, reducing substances, O&P, and culture Review of newborn metabolic screening tests Extremity radiographs if indicated (e.g., rickets)
Excessive caloric expenditure	Hyperthyroidism, chronic disease (cardiac, renal, endocrine, hepatic), malignancy	Dysmorphisms, skin dysmorphology, cardiac findings, abdominal mass or lymphadenopathy, hepatosplenomegaly	TSH, CBC/ESR, serum protein, albumin, alkaline phosphatase, BUN, creatinine, liver function tests Chest radiograph Renal US and voiding cystourethrography
Growth failure	Genetic, familial short stature, small for gestational age, hypothyroidism	Short stature, dysmorphisms, decreasing height growth with symmetric weight to height	Thyroid studies, HIV screening Karyotype (especially in small girls for Turner syndrome) Bone age Developmental testing Growth hormone (expensive, often done later in workup)

BUN, Blood urea nitrogen, *CBC,* Complete blood count; *ESR,* erythrocyte sedimentation rate; *FTT,* failure to thrive; *HIV,* human immunodeficiency virus; *O&P,* ova and parasites; *US,* ultrasound; *TSH,* thyroid-stimulating hormone.
Data from Casey PH: Failure-to-thrive. In Carey WB, Crocker AC, Coleman WL et al, editors: *Developmental-behavioral pediatrics,* ed 4, Philadelphia, 2009, Saunders, pp 583-591; Stephens MB, Gentry BC, Michener MD et al: What is the clinical workup for failure to thrive? *J Fam Pract* 57(4):264-266, 2008.

- Provide parent education and support and improve parent-child interaction.
- Treat underlying chronic condition.
- Make referrals as needed including feeding clinics.
- Evaluate for normal weight gain by age every 1 to 3 weeks. Catch-up growth can occur rapidly but can take up to 2 weeks before growth occurs with more involved cases. One must be careful to not overshoot the mark, resulting in overweight (Casey, 2009).
- Hospitalize for evaluation and intervention to protect from abuse when intentional etiology is suspected, to avoid further starvation and sequelae, to manage extreme child-parent interaction problems, to provide care when outpatient management is not feasible or practical and to provide more intensive care after failure of outpatient management.

Prognosis

The goal of nutrition management is to achieve symmetry of weight and height and genetic growth potential. Nutritional effects of chronic conditions may persist if not treated with the primary condition. Outcomes are variable depending on the underlying condition and severity.

Most children achieve expected growth and development. However, because brain growth occurs maximally in the first 6 months of life, nutritional insufficiency in an infant can severely affect long-term development and social/emotional health. Subtle neurodevelopmental abnormalities, the home environment, and the quality of nurturing by caregivers can affect outcomes. Many studies document that FTT can result in long-term detrimental effects—short stature, lower cognitive functioning, poorer academic functioning, and increased risk for adult diseases such as cardiovascular disease, obesity, hypertension, and diabetes (Casey, 2009).

■ Lower Gastrointestinal Tract Infections and Infestations

Acute and chronic diarrhea result from alterations in the normal functioning of the intestinal system. The altered intestinal mechanisms that result in diarrhea vary; briefly, diarrhea can occur as a result of:

- Nonabsorbable solutes in the GI tract, when fluids exceed the transport capacity, or when water-soluble nutrients are not absorbed (osmotic diarrhea). Such nutrient malabsorption and/or excessive fluid intake account for most chronic diarrhea (NASPGHAN, 2005); dumping syndrome, lactase deficiency, overfeeding, and malabsorption syndromes are causative conditions.

- Invasion, inflammation, and/or release of toxins by bacteria or viruses (such as in traveler's diarrhea) that decrease absorption and increase secretion and transportation of electrolytes and water from mucosal crypt cells in the small intestine into the bowel lumen (secretory diarrhea). As an example, viruses injure the absorptive mature mucosal surface cells, thereby altering the release of disaccharides and preventing the conversion of carbohydrates to monosaccharides necessary for normal absorption. Congenital disorders, mucosal disorders, and tumors can also lead to secretory diarrhea.
- Mutations in the ion transport proteins, such as chloride-bicarbonate exchange
- Alterations in the anatomy of the intestinal surface or functional ability due to inflammation or surgical procedures (e.g., short bowel syndrome, celiac disease, IBS) with a subsequent loss of fluids, electrolytes, macro- and micronutrients, and normal peristalsis.
- A change in intestinal motility, either increased or decreased (e.g., irritable bowel, bacterial overgrowth due to stasis [pseudo obstruction], toddler's diarrhea)
- Altered immune function

ACUTE DIARRHEA

Description and Epidemiology

The term *acute gastroenteritis* was formerly used to describe acute diarrhea, but this term is technically a misnomer because the etiology of diarrhea does not technically involve the stomach (Guandalini et al, 2010). With acute diarrhea, there is a disruption of the normal intestinal net absorptive versus secretory mechanisms of fluids and electrolytes, resulting in excessive loss of fluid into the intestinal lumen. This can lead to dehydration, electrolyte imbalance, and in severe cases, death in those also malnourished (Grimwood and Forbes, 2009). In children less than 2 years of age, this translates to a daily stool volume of more than 10 mL/kg (this definition excludes the normal breastfeeding stooling of five or six stools per day). In children older than 2 years of age, diarrheal stooling is described as occurring four or more times in 24 hours. The duration can last up to 14 days.

Viruses can injure the absorptive surface of mature villous cells, which reduces the amount of fluid absorbed. Some can release a viral enterotoxin (e.g., rotavirus). A loss of water and electrolytes ensues, and there can be volumes of watery diarrhea, even if the child is not being fed. Bacterial and parasitic agents can adhere and/or translocate, causing noninflammatory diarrhea. Bacteria can also damage the anatomy and functional ability of the intestinal mucosa by direct invasion. Some bacteria release endotoxins, whereas others release cytotoxins that result in the excretion of fluid, protein, and cells into the intestinal lumen and an inflammatory response in some cases. Abnormal peristalsis for any reason can result in acute diarrhea. The enteric pathogens are spread through the fecal-oral route and by ingestion of contaminated food or water.

Worldwide, the burden of acute diarrhea is huge, resulting in 3 to 5 billion cases and nearly 2 billion deaths (20% of total child deaths) in children younger than 5 years of age (particularly vulnerable) (Bell, 2010; Grimwood and Forbes, 2009; Guandalini et al, 2010; Norman et al, 2010). Developing countries also see their share of the burden of this disease

(approximately 10%), attributable to poor water, sanitation, and hygiene (Norman et al, 2010). Globally, females have higher rates of *Campylobacter* species infections and hemolytic uremic syndrome, otherwise the incidence of cases shows no gender preference. Nontyphoidal *Salmonella, Shigella, Campylobacter, E. coli* organisms (bacteria); rotavirus, norovirus, enteric adenovirus (viruses); and *Giardia, Cryptosporidium,* and *Strongyloides* (parasites) cause most disease (Bhutta, 2007; Grimwood and Forbes, 2009). *Shigella, E. coli, Giardia lamblia, Cryptosporidium parvum,* and *Entamoeba histolytica* are particularly infectious in small amounts. The term "dysentery" is used to indicate infection with specific species of *Shigella* and *Salmonella* (e.g., *Shigella dysenteriae*).

In the U.S. those most vulnerable include Native Americans and Native Alaskans, where remote residential locations or living on reservations compromise sanitation and safe water supplies, and where severe rotavirus diarrhea occurs (Grimwood and Forbes, 2009). About 200,000 U.S. hospitalizations occur annually due to diarrheal illness, with 300 deaths (Bell, 2010). The most common viral pathogens are noroviruses and rotavirus, followed by adenoviruses and astroviruses. Food-borne bacterial or parasitic diarrheal diseases are most commonly due to *Salmonella* and *Campylobacter* species, followed by *Shigella, Cryptosporidium, E. coli* O157:H7, *Yersinia, Listeria, Vibrio* (*V. cholerae* and other species), and *Cyclospora* species. *C. difficile* has been associated with pseudomembranous colitis and diarrhea after the use of antibiotics, but is not the causative agent in most antibiotic-associated diarrhea in children in the U.S. (Bhutta, 2007).

Tables 32-11 and 32-14 discuss the characteristics of diarrheal diseases caused by bacteria, viruses, and parasites that a primary care provider is more likely to encounter and need to differentiate. Infections due to *Cryptosporidium, E. coli* O157:H7, *Giardia, Listeria, Salmonella, Shigella,* and *V. cholerae* are required to be reported to the CDC. The enteric pathogens encountered more in daycare settings include rotavirus, astrovirus, calicivirus, *Campylobacter, Shigella, Giardia,* and *Cryptosporidium* species (Guandalini et al, 2010).

Nausea and vomiting are not good indicators of the severity of a condition; however, the absence of or low-grade fever, mild to moderate periumbilical pain, and watery diarrhea are more typically associated with less serious bacterial infection and suggest small intestine involvement (Bhutta, 2007). The following are more indicative of potentially serious infection in the upper intestine:
- Food-borne illness suspected
- Bloody diarrhea, weight loss, dehydration, severe abdominal pain, and fever
- Diarrhea lasting several days with more than three stools per day
- Neurologic involvement on physical examination

Clinical Findings
History
- Pattern of diarrhea: Onset, number of stools, volume, frequency
- Appearance of stool: Odor, mucoid and/or bloody
- Associated symptoms: Abdominal pain, nausea, vomiting, or fever
- Number of wet diapers in the past 24 hours and approximate time of last void

TABLE 32-11   Diarrheal Illnesses Due to Common Bacterial or Viral Pathogens

Etiology	Incubation Period	Signs and Symptoms	Duration of Illness	Route of Transmission	Laboratory Testing	Treatment and Complications (see Table 32-12 for dosages)
Campylobacter jejuni	2-5 days	• Diarrhea (foul smelling), cramps, fever, nausea and vomiting; diarrhea may be bloody in neonates. • Occurs in warm weather months.	2-10 days	Raw and undercooked poultry, unpasteurized milk, contaminated water; low inoculum dose produces infection.	Routine stool culture; *Campylobacter* requires special media and incubation temperature; positive gross blood, leukocytes; CBC: ↑ WBCs.	• Supportive care: For severe cases, antibiotics such as erythromycin, azithromycin, and quinolones (more drug resistance) may be indicated early in the diarrheal disease for 5-7 days. Guillain-Barré syndrome can be sequelae.
Clostridium difficile	Unknown	• Variety of symptoms and severity are seen: mild to explosive diarrhea, bloody stools, abdominal pain, fever, nausea, vomiting. • Illness unusual in neonates and infants (they have asymptomatic colonization); otherwise occurs in children of all ages (Fisher, 2007).	During or after several weeks of antibiotic use; can occur without being associated with such treatment	Fecal-oral; antimicrobial therapy can increase risk of acquiring.	Stool cultures; enzyme immunoassay for toxin A, or A and B; positive gross blood, leukocytes; CBC: ↑ WBCs; ESR normal.	• Discontinue current antibiotic (any antibiotic, but notably ampicillin, clindamycin, second- and third-generation cephalosporins) (Fisher, 2007). • Fluids and electrolyte replacement are usually sufficient. If antibiotic is still needed or illness is severe, treat with oral metronidazole (drug of choice in children) or vancomycin for 7-10 days. • Supplement with probiotics. Lactobacillus GG, *Saccharomyces boulardii* are recommended (Jones, 2010; Shane, 2010). • Complications include pseudomembranous colitis, toxic megacolon, colonic perforation, relapse, intractable proctitis, death in debilitated children.
Enterohemorrhagic *Escherichia coli* (EHEC) including *E. coli* O157:H7 and other Shiga toxin–producing *E. coli* (STEC)	1-8 days	• Severe diarrhea that is often bloody, abdominal pain and vomiting. • Usually little or no fever. • More common in children <4 yr old.	5-10 days	• Undercooked, beef, especially hamburger, unpasteurized milk and juice, raw fruits, vegetables (e.g., sprouts, spinach, lettuce), salami (rarely). • Contaminated water, petting zoos.	Stool culture; *E. coli* O157:H7 requires special media to grow. If *E. coli* O157:H7 is suspected, specific testing must be requested. Shiga toxin testing may be done using commercial kits; positive isolates should be forwarded to public health laboratories for confirmation and serotyping. Stool grossly positive for blood.	• Supportive care: Monitor CBC, platelets, and kidney function closely. *E. coli* O157:H7 infection is also associated with hemolytic uremic syndrome (HUS), which can cause lifelong complications. • Studies indicate that antibiotics may promote the development of HUS.

Organism	Incubation	Signs/Symptoms	Duration	Transmission	Diagnosis	Treatment/Prevention
Enterotoxigenic E. coli (ETEC) and enteroadherent E. coli (frequent cause of traveler's diarrhea)	1-3 days	Watery diarrhea, abdominal cramps, some vomiting; often cause of mild traveler's diarrhea	3 to >7 days	Water or food contaminated with human feces	Stool culture. ETEC requires special laboratory techniques for identification. If suspected, must request specific testing.	Supportive care: Antibiotics are rarely needed except in severe cases. Recommended antibiotics include TMP-SMX and quinolones. See www.cdc.gov/travel.
Listeria monocytogenes	9-48 hours for gastrointestinal symptoms, 2-6 weeks for invasive disease	• Rare, but serious. Fever, muscle aches, and nausea or diarrhea. • Pregnant women may have mild flulike illness, and infection can lead to premature delivery or stillbirth. • Older adults or immunocompromised patients may have bacteremia or meningitis. • Infants infected from mother at risk for sepsis or meningitis	Variable	Thrives in salty and acidic conditions: fresh soft cheeses, ready-to-eat deli meats, hot dogs; also unpasteurized milk, inadequately pasteurized milk. Multiplies at low temperatures, even in properly refrigerated foods.	Blood or cerebrospinal fluid cultures. Asymptomatic fecal carriage occurs; therefore, stool culture usually not helpful. Antibody to listeriolysin O may be helpful to identify outbreak retrospectively.	Supportive care and antibiotics: IV ampicillin, penicillin, or TMP-SMX are recommended for invasive disease.
Adenovirus, enteric	3-10 days	Children >4 years	Variable	Fecal-oral, throughout year; can remain viable on inanimate objects	Stool specimen for adenovirus antigen via rapid commercial immunoassay techniques or per electron microscopy.	Supportive care Preventive care: Good handwashing and diapering precaution
Norovirus	12-48 hours	Abrupt-onset watery diarrhea, nausea, vomiting, abdominal cramps	• 24-60 hr • Often associated with closed venues (child care centers, cruise ships)	Fecal-oral; contaminated food (ice, shellfish, ready-to-eat foods [e.g., salads, bakery products], or water)	No commercial assay available; CDC can support laboratory evaluation or state and local health department laboratories can perform RT-PCR assays.	Supportive care: May need to treat dehydration and/or electrolyte imbalance Preventive care: Hand hygiene, clean surfaces and food preparation areas; no swimming in recreational venues for 2 weeks after symptoms resolve (Pickering et al, 2009)
Rotavirus	1-3 days; prevalent during cooler months in temperate climates	Acute-onset fever, vomiting, and watery diarrhea occur 2-4 days later in children <5 years, especially those between 3-24 months	3-8 days	Fecal-oral; viable on inanimate objects; rarely contaminated water or food	Enzyme immunoassay and latex agglutination assays for group A rotavirus antigen; virus can be found by electron microscopy and specific nucleic acid amplification methods.	Supportive care: May need to correct dehydration and electrolyte imbalances. Oral IG has been used in those immunocompromised. Preventive care: Rotavirus vaccine; hygiene and diapering precautions in day care facilities

Continued

TABLE 32-11 Diarrheal Illnesses Due to Common Bacterial or Viral Pathogens—cont'd

Etiology	Incubation Period	Signs and Symptoms	Duration of Illness	Route of Transmission	Laboratory Testing	Treatment and Complications (see Table 32-12 for dosages)
Salmonella spp.	1-3 days	Diarrhea, fever, abdominal cramps, rebound tenderness, vomiting. *S. typhi* and *S. paratyphi* produce typhoid with insidious onset characterized by fever, headache, constipation, malaise, chills, and myalgia; diarrhea is uncommon, and vomiting is not usually severe.	4-7 days	Contaminated eggs, poultry, unpasteurized milk or juice, cheese, contaminated raw fruits and vegetables (alfalfa sprouts, melons). *S. typhi* epidemics are often related to fecal contamination of water supplies or street-vended foods.	Routine stool cultures; positive leukocytes and gross blood. CBC: WBC can be slightly ↑ with left shift, ↓, or normal.	• Supportive care: *Only consider antibiotics* (other than for *S. typhi* or *S. paratyphi*) for infants <3 months of age, those with chronic GI disease, malignant neoplasm, hemoglobinopathies, HIV, other immunosuppressive illnesses or therapies (Pickering et al, 2009). If indicated, consider ampicillin or amoxicillin, azithromycin, or TMP-SMX; if resistance shown to any of those, use IM ceftriaxone, cefotaxime; or azithromycin or quinolones. • A vaccine exists for *S. typhi* in certain cases.
Shigella spp.	24-48 hours	• Abdominal cramps, fever, and diarrhea. Stools may contain blood and mucus. • Seen most commonly in those 6 months to 3 years	4-7 days	Food or water contaminated with human fecal material. Usually person-to-person spread, fecal-oral transmission. Ready-to-eat foods touched by infected food workers, (e.g., raw vegetables, salads, sandwiches)	Routine stool cultures; gross blood, leukocytes. CBC: normal or slightly ↑ WBCs with left shift.	Supportive care: If antibiotics indicated (severe disease, dysentery, immunocompromised), test first for susceptibility. Oral ampicillin (amoxicillin less so) or TMP-SMX recommended in the U.S.; for organism resistance, use IM ceftriaxone for 2-5 days; PO ciprofloxacin; azithromycin (oral cephalosporins not useful). If child is at risk of malnutrition, supplement with vitamin A (200,000 international units). No swimming in recreational pools/slides for 1 week after symptoms resolve (Pickering et al, 2009).
Yersinia enterocolytica and *Y. pseudotuberculosis*	24-48 hours	• Appendicitis-like symptoms (diarrhea and vomiting, fever, and RLQ pain) occur primarily in older children and young adults. May have a scarlatiniform rash or erythema nodosum with *Y. pseudotuberculosis* • Seen in all ages	1-3 weeks, usually self-limiting	Undercooked pork, unpasteurized milk, tofu, contaminated water. Infection has occurred in infants whose caregivers handled chitterlings.	Stool, vomitus, or blood culture. *Yersinia* requires special medium to grow. If suspected, must request specific testing. Serology is available in research and reference laboratories.	Supportive care: If septicemia or other invasive disease occurs, antibiotic therapy with gentamicin or cefotaxime (doxycycline and ciprofloxacin also effective) after susceptibility testing is done.

CBC, complete blood count; *CDC,* Centers for Disease Control and Prevention; *ESR,* erythrocyte sedimentation rate; *IG,* immunoglobulin; *IM,* intramuscular; *IV,* intravenous; *PO,* oral (per mouth); *RLQ,* right lower quadrant; *RT-PCR,* reverse transcriptase polymerase chain reaction assay for detection of RNA in stool; *TMP-SMX,* trimethoprim-sulfamethoxazole; *WBCs,* white blood cells; ↑, increased; ↓, decreased.
Adapted from Department of Health and Human Services, Centers for Disease Control and Prevention: Diagnosis and management of food borne illnesses: a primer for physicians and other health professionals, *MMWR Morb Mortal Wkly Rep* 53(RR04);7-9, 2004. Additional information from Fisher MC: Pseudomembranous colitis (*Clostridium difficile*). In Kligman RM, Behrman RE, Jenson HB et al: *Nelson textbook of pediatrics,* ed 18, Philadelphia, 2007, Saunders, pp 1230-1231; Pickering LK, Baker CJ, Kimberlin DW et al: *Red Book: 2009 Report of the Committee on Infectious Diseases,* ed 28, Elk Grove Village, IL, 2009, American Academy of Pediatrics.

- Dietary consumption: Changes in diet that might correlate with increased stooling; ingestion (and when) of raw or poorly cooked foods (e.g., raw or undercooked eggs, meat, shellfish, fish, poultry), unpasteurized or under-pasteurized milk or juices, home-canned foods, fresh produce (fruits/vegetables), soft cheeses, deli meats
- If given, response to oral rehydration therapy
- Food allergies
- Family members or close friends with similar illness or other GI diseases
- Daycare, school attendance, recreational swimming exposure (even if chlorinated): Illness patterns and contacts at these locations; walking in soil without shoes
- Travel history: Foreign or coastal areas; camping or travel where untreated water might have been consumed
- Attendance at picnics or other outings where food was consumed
- Most recent weight and previous growth pattern
- Medications: Antibiotics, laxatives, antacids, opiates (withdrawal), vitamins (toxicity)
- Pica (metals, plants)
- Chemotherapy
- Recent surgeries (abdominal)

Physical Examination
- Complete a physical examination including vital signs and assessment of behavior/mental status changes
- Assess for dehydration (see Table 32-1)

Diagnostic Studies. Diagnostic studies are ordered if the symptoms (discussed earlier) of more serious infection are present. Some specific diagnostic findings associated with the more common infectious diarrheal illness are found in Table 32-11. Molecular diagnostic tests (e.g., PCR) have greatly improved the ability to diagnose diarrheal illness due to bacteria. The following tests are ordered:
- Stool examination (color, consistency, blood, mucus, pus, odor, volume). In endemic areas, microscopy examination for parasites (e.g., *G. lamblia* and *E. histolytica*).
- Stool: pH (<5.5 suggests carbohydrate intolerance typically seen in viral infections), leukocytes (suggest bacterial invasion), reducing substances (viral infections), and occult blood. Normal stool: pH greater than 5.5, carbohydrate negative.
- Stool cultures should be considered early in the course of illness for bloody or prolonged diarrhea; in the presence of leukocytes; if clinical signs of colitis are present; for suspected food-borne illness outbreaks (especially with *E. coli* O157:H7); in the immunocompromised; or after recent travel abroad.
- Electrolytes, if indicated, to evaluate degree of dehydration and for more serious signs and symptoms of infectious disease
- CBC, as indicated for serious infectious disease

Differential Diagnosis

Gastroenteritis and antibiotic use are the most common causes of diarrhea in all age groups. Systemic infection is a common cause in infants and children, and food poisoning is a common cause in children and adolescents. Overfeeding should also be considered in infants. Rare causes of acute diarrhea in infants include primary disaccharidase deficiency, Hirschsprung toxic colitis, adrenogenital syndrome, and neonate opiate withdrawal; toxic ingestion in children; and hyperthyroidism in adolescents.

Management

The foundation of all treatment of acute diarrhea is fourfold:
- Restore and maintain hydration and correct/maintain electrolyte and acid-base balance (see Table 32-3). Oral rehydration with an oral electrolyte solution should be attempted when dehydration is assessed between 3% and 9% (see p. 746). Administer parenteral hydration if necessary for the following: impaired circulation and possible shock, weight less than 4 to 5 kg or a child younger than 3 months, intractable diarrhea, lethargy, anatomic anomalies, or failure to gain weight or continued weight loss despite oral fluids.
- Maintain nutrition. Resume early refeeding because contents of the bowel stimulate the growth of enterocytes and help facilitate mucosal repair following injury (see Table 32-3).
- Prescribe antibiotics prudently. Antibiotics are recommended for acute diarrhea caused by *G. lamblia*, *V. cholerae*, and *Shigella* species and can be considered for infections caused by enteropathogenic *E. coli* (if infection prolonged), enteroinvasive *E. coli*, *Yersinia* for those with sickle cell disease, and *Salmonella* in young infants with fever or positive blood culture findings (Guandalini et al, 2010) (see Tables 32-11 and 32-12). Children with HIV at risk for acute diarrhea may benefit from cotrimoxazole and vitamin A (Humphreys et al, 2010).
- Treat any related conditions, such as sepsis, and cardiovascular collapse.

Some adjunct medications and treatments have received wider use in countries outside of the U.S. and show efficacy in some studies. Some of these include:
- Antidiarrheals (antimotility agents or adsorbents) are not generally recommended (Bell, 2010). However, a review of literature demonstrated that loperamide in children older than the age of 3 years is safe and decreases the duration and frequency of diarrhea compared with placebo. Children less than age 3 years and those who are malnourished, those with moderate or severe dehydration, those who are systemically ill, or those who have bloody diarrhea should not be treated with this drug (Li et al, 2007; Pulling and Surawicz, 2008). Some over-the-counter products intended for diarrhea contain salicylates (e.g., Pepto-Bismol), and there is concern for Reye syndrome.
- Probiotics: *Lactobacillus casei* strain GG or *S. boulardii* (a yeast) given early in a viral diarrheal illness or antibiotic-associated diarrhea can both treat diarrhea (decrease duration by about 25 hours) (Allen et al, 2010) and ameliorate the risk of antibiotic-associated diarrhea (Johnston et al, 2011; Shane, 2010). Exact doses are undetermined, but Jones cites studies suggesting at least more than 5 billion colony-forming units (CFUs) per day (Jones, 2010).
- Dioctahedral smectite, adsorbent clay, is used in many countries to protect the intestinal mucosa by absorbing viruses, bacteria, and bacterial toxins; there are few reported side effects. Studies have shown that smectite can reduce the duration of diarrhea by 20% to 50% as part of rehydration therapy (Szajewska et al, 2006). Its use is not routinely recommended in the U.S.

TABLE 32-12   Antibiotics More Commonly Used for Diarrheal Infections

Drug	Dosage	Indication
Amoxicillin	25-50 mg divided in 3 doses, PO, for 7-10 days (max daily dose 1.5 g)	*Salmonella, Shigella*
Ampicillin	50-100 mg/kg/day divided into 4 doses for 5-10 days (max daily dose 2 g)	*Salmonella, Shigella*
Azithromycin	10 mg/kg/day first day, then 5 mg/kg/day days 2-5, PO (up to max daily dose of 500 mg on day 1; 250 mg on days 2-5)	*Clostridium jejuni, Escherichia coli* O157:H7
Cefotaxime	IM: 75-100 mg in 3 or 4 doses	*Salmonella*
Ceftriaxone	IM: 50-75 mg in 1 or 2 doses	*Salmonella, Shigella*
Ciprofloxacin	>18 years of age: 20-30 mg/kg/day divided into 4 doses, PO (max daily dose 1 g) for 5-10 days for *E. coli*. Same dosage divided in 2 doses and treated for 7-10 days for *Salmonella* and *Shigella;* for 5-7 days for *Campylobacter*	*E. coli* O157:H7, *Listeria, Shigella, Salmonella, Campylobacter*
Doxycycline	>8 yr: 2-4 mg/kg/day in 1 or 2 doses, PO for 7-10 days (max daily dose 200 mg)	*Yersinia enterocolitis*
Erythromycin	30-50 mg/kg/day in 2 to 4 divided doses, PO, for 5-7 days (max daily dose 2 g)	*C. jejuni*
Metronidazole	15-30 mg/kg/day in 3 divided doses, PO, for 5 days (max daily dose 1.5 g) for *C. difficile*. Refer to pharmacology book for length to treat other pathogens.	*Clostridium difficile* (first-line drug), *Entamoeba histolytica, Giardia lamblia, C. jejuni, E. coli* O157:H7
Tetracycline	>8 yr of age: 25-50 mg/kg/day in 4 divided doses, PO, for 7-10 days (max dose 1-2 g)	*Y. enterocolitis*
TMP-SMX	>2 mo of age: 8 mg/kg/day (TMP component) in 2 divided doses, PO, for 7-10 days (up to 160-320 mg per dose depending on pathogen)	*Y. enterocolitis, Salmonella, Shigella, E. coli* O157:H7, *Cyclospora cayetanensis*
Vancomycin	40 mg/kg/day in 4 divided doses, PO, for 7-10 days (max 500 daily dose)	*C. difficile*

IM, Intramuscular; *PO,* orally; *TMP-SMX,* trimethoprim-sulfamethoxazole.
Data from Bhutta ZA: Acute gastroenteritis in children. In Kliegman RM, Behrman RE, Jenson HB et al: *Nelson textbook of pediatrics,* ed 18, Philadelphia, 2007, Saunders, p 1617; Chen SF: Principles of antiparasitic therapy. In Kliegman RM, Behrman RE, Jenson HB et al: *Nelson textbook of pediatrics,* ed 18, Philadelphia, 2007, Saunders, p 1449; Edmunds MW, Mayhew MS, Bridgers C: *Pharmacology for the primary care provider,* ed 3, St. Louis, 2009, Mosby; Pickering LK, Baker CJ, Kimberlin DW et al: *Red Book: 2009 Report of the Committee on Infectious Diseases,* ed 28, Elk Grove Village, IL, 2009, American Academy of Pediatrics, pp 747-757.

• Oral enteric peppermint oil capsules have been studied for use with diarrhea, cramping, and bloating, especially when related to IBS. It may produce smooth muscle relaxation, slow food transit through the intestines (Goerg and Spilker, 2003), and help with general symptom relief (Pirotta, 2009); its efficacy is still debated (Chang et al, 2006). Essential peppermint oil *(Mentha piperita)* aromatherapy can be used for abdominal pain and relaxation (Loo, 2009). See also Chapter 42 for complementary medicine therapies for diarrhea.

• Zinc is commonly prescribed to shorten the duration of acute diarrhea in children from developing countries. Patel and associates (2010) found that zinc was efficacious for diarrhea caused by *Klebsiella,* not necessarily for *E. coli* or parasitic infections, and was detrimental when used in infections caused by rotavirus. The optimal dose of zinc has not been established and variations may account for varying efficacy. Zinc supplementation might have limited effect if the child is not zinc deficient (Patro et al, 2010). It is added to ORS solutions (along with prebiotics) in many developing countries (Passariello et al, 2011; Mazumder et al, 2010).

Complications
See Table 32-11 for complications associated with some common pathogens.

Prevention
Preventive measures include the following:
• Good handwashing by all individuals (including children and all care providers), especially when handling food. Liquid soap and paper towels are recommended at daycare centers. Use of non-water alcohol hand sanitizers with an ethanol content of at least 60% has also shown efficacy to reduce GI illnesses (Reynolds et al, 2006).
• Good sanitation and appropriate removal of soiled clothing and diapers. The diapering area should be cleaned after changing each child at daycare centers.
• Avoid contaminated sources; meat should be properly cooked.
• Promote exclusive breastfeeding for the first 6 months of life to promote passive immunity and guard against exposure to contaminated food and water.

- Promote appropriate supplemental nutrition starting at 6 months (breastfeeding should continue through the first year or longer in developing countries), food handling, and storage.
- In developing countries, consider addition of vitamin A and zinc in cases of malnutrition.
- With *Shigella,* culture all symptomatic contacts and treat those with positive stool cultures.
- Avoid unnecessary antibiotic usage.
- Promote well-functioning sewage system in developing countries (including latrines, septic tanks, dry-composting toilets), which can cut diarrheal illness by up to 30% (Norman, 2010).
- Promote rotavirus vaccine for all children worldwide (WHO, 2009).

CHRONIC DIARRHEA
Description and Epidemiology

Chronic diarrhea is defined as the passage of three or more watery stools per day for more than 2 weeks (Grishan, 2007). The terms "persistent" or "prolonged" diarrhea have also been used when describing a state of chronic diarrhea; these generally refer to a continuing diarrheal illness that started as acute diarrhea and is affecting growth. Diarrhea that is chronic is the result of intraluminal factors (that influence digestion) or mucosal factors (that influence digestion and transport of nutrients across the mucosa); either factor affects the normal cellular mechanisms of the GI tract. Because "persistent" diarrhea is generally associated with an acute diarrheal onset, it is surmised that there is either persistent infectious colonization with an enteric pathogen or impaired healing and return to the normal intestinal processes/structure (Bhutta et al, 2008). Table 32-13 lists the most common causes of chronic diarrhea by age group. Infants and children have difficulty absorbing volumes of liquid larger than 200 mL/kg/day; an excess can cause diarrhea, a not uncommon finding in toddlers ("toddler's diarrhea").

Clinical Findings
History
- Occurrence of three or more watery stools per day for more than 2 weeks; 10 watery/runny stools per day that often contain undigested food particles is more typical of "toddler's diarrhea"
- Presence of red flags (Keating, 2005)
  - Hematochezia or melena
  - Persistent fever
  - Weight loss or growth arrest
  - Anemia
- Dietary history (including amount of fruit juices or high-carbohydrate fluids ingested per day)
- Stool consistency, blood, mucus, pus, particles of food
- Stool incontinence
- Exposure to illness (including daycare; contact with pets/other animals)
- Teething
- Prior treatments for diarrhea (any dietary manipulation, drug, or home treatments)
- Recent travel

Physical Examination. Look for physical findings associated with the underlying pathologic condition.

TABLE 32-13	Common Causes of Chronic Diarrhea Seen in Children
Age	**Conditions**
0-6 months	• Carbohydrate malabsorption (acquired, congenital) (e.g., cow's-milk protein intolerance) • Protein hypersensitivity • Excessive intake of formula or other fluid (water, juice [especially those containing sorbitol/fructose], high-carbohydrate liquids) • Postenteritis • Infections • Cystic fibrosis or other fat absorption conditions • Neuroblastoma (rare) • Immunodeficiency (e.g., HIV/AIDS and others) • Lymphangiectasia (rare) • Hirschsprung disease • Neonatal or infant enteropathies (rare) • Radiation treatments
7-24 months	First eight bulleted conditions listed above plus: • Chronic nonspecific diarrhea • Small-bowel overgrowth • Celiac disease • Graft-versus-host enteropathy • Autoimmune enteropathy • Radiation treatments
>24 months	• Excessive intake of fruit juice/high-carbohydrate drinks • Infections • Small-bowel bacterial overgrowth • Celiac disease • Munchausen syndrome by proxy • Grant-versus-host enteropathy • Carbohydrate malabsorption • Irritable bowel syndrome • Adult-type hypolactasia • Encopresis • Inflammatory bowel disease (e.g., Crohn disease) • Excessive use of laxatives • Radiation treatments • Acquired lactase deficiency in older children, primarily of African, Asian, or Middle Eastern descent (Keating, 2005) • Perforated appendix

AIDS, Acquired immunodeficiency syndrome; *HIV,* human immunodeficiency virus.
Data from North American Society for Pediatric Gastroenterology, Hepatology and Nutrition (NASPGHAN) book: *Acute and chronic diarrhea,* Chapter 3. Available at www.naspghan.org/wmspage.cfm?parm1=126 (accessed Jan 17, 2011).

- Assessment of hydration status
- Weight and height measurements; any weight loss
- Growth retardation
- Skin and hair condition, color of skin and conjunctivae
- Vital signs (heart rate and blood pressure)
- Palpation of the thyroid for enlargement
- Increased heart rate
- Respiratory symptoms
- Clubbing of fingers

- Abdominal examination
- Rectal examination (skin tags, impaction, tenderness)
  Diagnostic Studies
- Stool: Culture, O&P (best done on three specimens collected on separate days), pH, reducing substances, occult blood, leukocytes, fat. (Normal stool pH greater than 5.5, carbohydrate negative)
- CBC with differential, electrolytes, and albumin
- Urinalysis and culture in young children
  The following are ordered as indicated by the history, physical examination, and consideration of differential diagnoses:
- ESR, CRP
- Hormonal studies to assess for secretory tumors (vasoactive intestinal peptide, gastrin, secretin, urine assay for 5-hydroxytryptamine [5-HT])
- Breath hydrogen test for lactose or sucrose intolerance (difficult to assess in infants)
- Viral serologies, such as HIV or CMV
- Sweat chloride test
- Endoscopy, barium studies

Differential Diagnosis
See Table 32-13.

Management
- Treat the underlying cause.
- Chronic nonspecific diarrhea (toddler's diarrhea) (Grishan, 2007): Normalize the diet; remove offending foods and fluids; eliminate sorbitol and fructose-containing fluids; reduce fluid intake to no greater than 90 mL/kg/24 hours (give half of fluid as milk [whole or 2%]); increase fat to 35% to 40% of the diet; and increase fiber to bulk up stools.
- Treat carbohydrate malabsorption by decreasing lactose or sucrose; add lactase or sacrosidase as indicated by particular carbohydrate intolerance.
- Postgastroenteritis malabsorption syndrome (evidenced in infants with weight loss and fat globules in the stool) can be given a predigested formula (e.g., Pregestimil or Alimentum), if tolerated, for 3 to 4 weeks (elemental formula can be used if those are not tolerated) (Grishan, 2007).
- Refer the following patients to a gastroenterologist: Newborns with diarrhea in first hours of life; patients with growth delay or failure or abnormal physical findings (anorexia, abdominal pain, chronic bloating, vomiting, or weakness); or those with severe illness.

Complications
Malnutrition, growth failure, and cognitive/developmental impairments (found more in developing countries) can occur.

INTESTINAL PARASITES
Description and Epidemiology
Various protozoa and helminths can invade the GI tract and cause disease. In developed countries, such infestations are usually by protozoa. Endemic areas of developing countries are subject to more significant morbidity and mortality from parasitic infestations (Haque, 2007). All can multiply within the human body, are associated with diarrheal symptoms, and are spread by fecal contamination due to poor water and sewage disposal practices. Cysts of these parasites are often resistant to chlorine (Haque, 2007).

Helminths are worms; nematodes (roundworms), cestodes (tapeworms), and trematodes (flatworms) that most commonly reside in the human intestines but do not multiply there. Fecaloral contact with eggs or cysts excreted from the initial vector via ingestion of contaminated food or water is one route of infestation. Some helminths (hookworms and whipworms) release larvae into the soil; humans become infected when they walk barefoot on contaminated soil and the skin is penetrated by the larvae. These larvae then travel to the lungs and intestines. Eggs can also be excreted in the stool; poor sanitary disposal of human waste into soils affords the further potential for ingestion via contamination of food and water. They are found worldwide, principally in tropical and subtropical developing countries. In industrialized countries, infestation is found in those who travel to endemic areas, in the immunocompromised, and immigrants from endemic areas. Their insidious nature causes chronic health and nutritional problems that can impair physical and mental growth of children (Haque, 2007). *Enterobius vermicularis* (pinworm), *Ascaris lumbricoides* (roundworm), and *Taenia* (tapeworm) are some of the more common intestinal parasites that affect the pediatric population.

Clinical Findings, Management, and Differential Diagnosis
See Tables 32-14 and 32-15 for clinical findings and management. The differential diagnosis includes all other causes of infectious and noninfectious diarrhea.

Prevention
Most parasitic infestations can be prevented by good handwashing and good sanitation. The following preventive measures are recommended:
- Travelers to developing countries need to eat only foods that can be peeled or cooked. Ice and "washed" foods and tap water can be contaminated. Bottled or treated water is advised for drinking and brushing teeth. Shoes should be worn when walking on potentially contaminated soil.
- *G. lamblia:* Encourage good hand hygiene. Prevent contamination of water sources. Treat questionable water with iodine, boiling for 20 minutes, or use commercial filters to filter contaminated water. Exclude symptomatic children and staff from school and daycare until asymptomatic.
- *E. vermicularis:* Avoid scratching. Wash sheets and clothing in hot water and detergent.
- *A. lumbricoides:* Appropriate food preparation is necessary to prevent infection. Where human feces is used for fertilizer, thoroughly cook or soak fruit and vegetables in diluted iodine solution before consuming. Periodic, empiric treatment of children may prevent nutritional and cognitive deficits in endemic areas.
- *Taenia:* Avoid raw or undercooked beef or pork.

CONGENITAL GASTROINTESTINAL CONDITIONS
These are discussed in Chapter 38 with other perinatal concerns.

TABLE 32-14 Intestinal Illnesses Due to More Common Parasites (Protozoa and Helminths)

Etiology	Incubation Period	Signs and Symptoms	Duration of Illness	Route of Transmission	Laboratory Testing	Treatment (see Table 32-15 for dosages)
Cryptosporidium parvum	2-10 days	Diarrhea (usually watery), stomach cramps, upset stomach, bloating, slight fever, anorexia, weight loss, flatulence, nausea	May remit and relapse over weeks to months	Fecal-oral route; from uncooked food or food contaminated by an ill food handler after cooking; drinking water (collects on water filters and membranes that cannot be disinfected); reservoirs include cattle, sheep, goats, birds, reptiles, young animals	Request specific testing of the stool for *Cryptosporidium* using antigen-detection tests. May need to examine water or food.	Supportive care, self-limited. If severe, or individual immunocompromised consider paromomycin for 7 days. For children ages 1-11 yr, consider nitazoxanide for 3 days.
Cyclospora cayetanensis	Usually takes about 1 wk, but may be seen as early as 1-4 days after exposure	Diarrhea (usually watery), loss of appetite, substantial loss of weight, stomach cramps, nausea, vomiting, fatigue	May remit and relapse over weeks to months	Fecal-oral from sewage or nontreated water; food (various types of fresh produce [imported berries, lettuce])	Request specific examination of the stool for *Cyclospora*. May need to examine water or food.	TMP-SMX for 7-10 days
Entamoeba histolytica	Commonly 2-4 wk (known to also range from days, months, to years); fecal-oral transmission	Can be asymptomatic with nonspecific complaints of diarrhea, lower abdominal pain. In invasive disease (amebic colitis) symptoms of increasing diarrhea, bloody diarrhea, lower abdominal pain, tenesmus, weight loss progress over a 1-3 wk period; occasional fever. Advanced disease hepatomegaly, liver tenderness.	Weeks to years, depending on response to treatment; no drug is completely effective (Pickering et al, 2009)	Spread by fecal-oral route	Stool exam for trophozoites or cysts; PCR; isoenzyme analysis, monoclonal antibody–based antigen; enzyme immunoassay; ultrasounds and CT scans to identify suspected liver abscess or other extraintestinal infection.	• Asymptomatic cyst excreters: luminal amebicide (iodoquinol, paromomycin, diloxanide). • Mild to moderate or severe involvement/liver abscesses: metronidazole or tinidazole followed by luminal amebicide. • Follow-up stool exam after treatment. Perform stool exams on household members or other suspected contacts. Do not treat with corticosteroids or antimotility drugs. Complications include liver abscess, ameboma.
Giardia lamblia	1-4 wk	Can include bouts of watery diarrhea; abdominal pain, greasy, foul-smelling stools; bloody diarrhea (rare); flatulence; abdominal distention; anorexia; weight loss; failure to thrive; anemia; asymptomatic infection common.	Pending effective treatment	Fecal-oral or contaminated food or water. Water can be contaminated by *Giardia* from dogs, cats, beavers, and other animals.	Stool specimens for trophozoites or cysts using staining methods; antigens using enzyme immunoassay; PCR techniques. Increased sensitivity by obtaining 3 or more specimens every other day and by rapid examination of stool (can be placed in a fixative).	• Correct for any dehydration or electrolyte imbalance. Tinidazole, metronidazole, nitazoxanide drugs of choice. Albendazole, mebendazole effective also in children with fewer side effects. Consult for those immunocompromised. Contact local health departments in cases of outbreaks. Infected individuals should not use recreational water sources for swimming until 2 weeks after symptoms resolve (Pickering et al, 2009). Filtration, boiling, chemical disinfection may be required for drinking water. • Complications: debilitating disease leading to malabsorption; anorexia; weight loss; FTT.

Continued

TABLE 32-14 Intestinal Illnesses Due to More Common Parasites (Protozoa and Helminths)—cont'd

Etiology	Incubation Period	Signs and Symptoms	Duration of Illness	Route of Transmission	Laboratory Testing	Treatment (see Table 32-15 for dosages)
Ancylostoma duodenale (hookworm)	5-8 wk for eggs to appear in feces; 4-12 wk for onset of symptoms	Often asymptomatic or stinging/burning sensation in feet followed by pruritus, papulovesicular rash (lasting up to 2 wk), pharyngeal itching, hoarseness, nausea, vomiting. As migrates through lungs: mild cough, pneumonitis. Chronic infestation: anemia, edema, growth delays, slowed development and cognition in children.	5 yr unless treated	Larvae in feces-contaminated soil penetrate skin (travel to lungs and settle in the intestines) or are directly ingested from contaminated food or water, including human milk (Pickering et al, 2009).	CBC shows hypochronic microcytic anemia, eosinophilia; hypoproteinemia. Stool microscopic exam for ova.	Albendazole, mebendazole, pyrantel pamoate; repeat stool exam in 2 wk recommended. Iron and nutritional supplementation if indicated; severe cases require blood transfusions. Complications: delayed growth, developmental/mental status delays in children
Enterobius vermicularis (pinworm)	1-2 mo from ingestion to migration to perianal area	Perirectal and/or vaginal pruritus; nervous irritability, hyperactivity, insomnia; urethritis, vaginitis, salpingitis, and pelvic peritonitis have been reported	Reinfection common in children	Ingested eggs from soil, water contamination, or direct fecal-oral route from fomites on bedding, clothing, toys, baths; person-to-person. Female lays eggs in perianal area and dies; ingested eggs hatch, become larvae in small intestine and migrate to rectum.	1 cm long white, threadlike worms can be visualized at anus during night after child has been asleep for 2-3 hr. Microscopic exam: use transparent adhesive tape applied to anus to collect any eggs or pinworms present on 3 consecutive nights or mornings before child arises. Direct stool exam usually not productive.	Mebendazole, pyrantel pamoate, albendazole and repeated in 2 wk; also treat family members; vaginitis is self-limiting. Easily spread among family members, in daycare settings, and institutions (up to 50% infestation rates in these populations) (Pickering et al, 2009). Preventive: morning baths, change bedding, hand hygiene, clip fingernails, avoid scratching perianal region, avoid nail biting. Daycare precautions include hand hygiene, proper handling of underwear and diapers.
Ascaris lumbricoides (roundworm)	8 wk from egg ingestion to adult egg-laying capacity	Weight loss, malnutrition; worms can be seen in vomitus and stools; can cause cough, fever, chest discomfort if pass through lungs (not a common occurrence) (Deming, 2009). Children can have large worm burdens. Stressful conditions (fever, illness) and some anthelmintic drugs can cause adults to migrate.	12-18 mo without treatment	Fecal-oral from ingestion of eggs from contaminated food (fruit, vegetables) or soil (where incubation occurs; adult worms live in small intestine and eggs are excreted in feces). Larvae migrate from intestines via portal blood to liver and lungs, ascend through tracheobronchial tree to pharynx, to intestines again to develop into adults. Found in areas where human feces are used for fertilizer.	Stool/vomitus/nares: worms seen via microscopy. CBC: marked eosinophilia. Have laboratory check for all concurrent worm infestations in order to treat all worms appropriately.	Albendazole, mebendazole, ivermectin; surgical intervention if necessary. Complications: impaired nutritional status of children and growth; bowel or biliary obstruction, peritonitis, obstruction of common bile duct (biliary colic, cholangitis, pancreatitis); Löffler syndrome due to allergic response as larvae migrate to the lungs. Reinfection common. Globally, most common human intestinal nematode (Pickering et al, 2009).

Organism	Incubation	Signs and symptoms		Transmission	Diagnosis	Treatment/Complications
Taenia (tapeworm) (*T. saginata* [beef]; *T. solium* [pork])	2-3 mo after larvae ingested to feces excretion	Worm(s) may be seen in perianal region. May be asymptomatic or have abdominal pain, nausea, diarrhea, excessive appetite.	Several years before cysticercosis symptoms evident	Fecal-oral from ingestion of water or food contaminated with eggs or from ingested cysts or larvae in inadequately cooked pork or beef	Stool microscopy: ova seen	Praziquantel, niclosamide, nitazoxanide. Complications: systemic cysticercosis from *T. solium* (viscera, brain, muscle invasion with possible seizures).
Trichuris trichiura (whipworm)	Not fully known; about 90 days after ingestion of eggs prior to passage in feces	Asymptomatic unless infestation is heavy; abdominal pain, tenesmus, bloody diarrhea with mucus; can mimic IBD; growth retardation.		Fecal-oral from contaminated soil (where eggs incubate), water, food (embeds in mucosal lining of large intestines) Not spread person to person	Stool microscopy or concentration techniques	Mebendazole, albendazole, ivermectin for 3 days; can reexamine stools after 2 wk to ensure resolution. Complications: chronic colitis, rectal prolapse, compromised nutritional status, growth retardation

CBC, Complete blood count; *CT,* computed tomography; *FTT,* failure to thrive; *IBD,* inflammatory bowel disease; *PCR,* polymerase chain reaction; *TMP-SMX,* trimethoprim-sulfamethoxazole.

Data from Deming M: Other infectious diseases related to travel: helminths, intestinal. In Centers for Disease Control and Prevention: *Traveler's health—yellow book.* Reviewed 2009, Chapter 5. Available at www.cdc.gov/travel/yellowbook/2010/chapter_5/intestinal-helminths.aspx (accessed Jan 17, 2011); Department of Health and Human Services, Centers for Disease Control and Prevention: Diagnosis and management of food borne illnesses, *MMWR Morb Mortal Wkly Rep* (RR04):1-33, 2004, Table 3; Haque R: Human intestinal parasites, *J Health Popul Nutr* 25(4):387-391, 2007; Pickering LK, Baker CJ, Kimberlin DW et al: *Red Book: 2009 Report of the Committee on Infectious Diseases,* ed 2, Elk Grove Village, IL, 2009, American Academy of Pediatrics.

TABLE 32-15	Medications for Treatment of Parasite Infestations

Drug	Dosage
Albendazole (take with food)	1 yr: 200 mg once >2 yr: 400 mg once *Taenia solium:* 15 mg/kg/day in 2 doses × 8-30 days; can be repeated as necessary (max 400 mg per dose)
Diloxanide furoate*	20 mg/kg/day in 3 doses × 10 days (max 500 mg per dose)
Ivermectin (take on empty stomach)	All ages: 150-200 mcg/kg once
Iodoquinol	30-40 mg/kg/day in 3 doses × 20 days (max 2 g) Adults: 650 mg 3 times daily × 20 days
Mebendazole (take on empty stomach)	All ages: 100 mg twice daily × 3 days or 500 mg once
Metronidazole	35-50 mg/kg/day in 3 doses × 7-10 days (max 500-750 mg per dose) *Giardia lamblia:* 15 mg/kg/day in 3 doses × 5 days (max 250 mg per dose)
Niclosamide (not readily available)	50 mg/kg once (max 2 g)
Nitazoxanide	1-3 yr: 100 mg every 12 hr × 3 days 4-11 yr: 200 mg every 12 hr × 3 days > 11 years to adult: 500 mg twice daily × 3 days
Paromomycin	All ages: 25-35 mg/kg/day in 3 doses × 7 days
Praziquantel	All ages: 5-10 mg/kg once
Pyrantel pamoate (over the counter)	All ages (caution with use in children <2 yr): 11 mg/kg daily (max 1 g) × 3 days
Tinidazole	50 mg/kg once (max 2 g)

*Can be compounded by Panorama Compounding Pharmacy (1-800-247-9767) or Medical Center Pharmacy [New Haven, Conn.] (203-688-6816) and others.
Data from Chen SF: Antiparasitic therapy. In Kliegman RM, Behrman RE, Jenson HB et al: *Nelson textbook of pediatrics,* ed 18, Philadelphia, 2007, Saunders, pp 1448-1458.

Dental and Oral Disorders

PETER M. MILGROM, DONALD L. CHI, OHNMAR K. TUT, MARY ANN DRAYE, AND MICHELE E. ACKER

The mouth serves many functions, including speech, and is richly endowed with special systems that serve complex needs; it is increasingly recognized as a barometer of health and well-being throughout life. For this reason, good oral health is essential for normal growth and development. Saliva is replacing serum and blood as the vehicle for noninvasive diagnostic tests for systemic diseases in some cases. Many of these tests are already on the market.

In children, microbial infections caused by bacteria, viruses, and fungi cause tooth decay (dental caries), periodontal or gum diseases, herpes labialis, and candidiasis. Moreover, inherited and congenital conditions result in impairments and cosmetic defects that have serious effects on children as they grow and develop. Lifestyle choices such as tobacco and drug use, body art, and piercings create challenges for maintaining oral health.

Dental problems, particularly tooth decay, are much more common than asthma and can restrict normal daily activity. Dental caries are the most common infectious disease of children. The unmet dental needs of children 2 to 17 years in the U.S. over the past nine years have been steady at 6% to 7% (Blackwell, 2010; Bloom et al, 2009; U.S. Department of Health and Human Services [USDHHS], 2010). Increased demand for dental services is compounded by an inadequate supply of dentists and a maldistribution of pediatric dentists, especially in underserved areas. In addition, the dentist-to-population ratio continues to decline (Nash, 2009).

Ensuring an adequate workforce to meet the needs of children requires involvement of primary care providers (PCPs). They are in a unique position to play a critical role in preventing oral disease, identifying and minimizing the effects of disease, and providing guidance to parents and children about oral health. And yet, Danielson and colleagues' study (2006) found that although 82% of the physician assistants and nurse practitioners recognized the importance of performing an oral examination, less than half expressed confidence in their ability to do so. These results largely reflect similar findings of a study of physicians that revealed that although 84% knew the importance of oral examinations, only 19% performed the examination routinely; 56% expressed lack of confidence in their skills, and 77% felt their training was insufficient (Morgan et al, 2001).

In response, this chapter offers information and practical answers for providers in everyday practice to ensure they have basic examination competencies; are able to distinguish between normal and abnormal structures, pathology, and common oral diseases; feel competent to educate regarding oral health and prescribe and apply preventive treatment (e.g., fluoride and fluoride varnish); and know when to refer to dentists (Danielson et al, 2006).

◼ Normal Growth and Development

ANATOMY OF THE MOUTH

The structures of the mouth include the mucosa (buccal and gingival), palate, salivary glands, frenula, tongue, and teeth.

The Teeth

Anatomy of a Tooth. Primary and permanent teeth have similar anatomy, differing primarily in the size and external shape of each tooth. Figure 33-1 shows a cross section of the typical tooth including the crown (white part), neck, and root (encased in bone).

Pattern of Tooth Eruption. The first primary tooth (also called baby tooth or deciduous tooth) may be present at birth. Normally the eruption of primary teeth begins with the anterior primary teeth, occurs during the first 6 to 8 months of life, and ends at about 30 to 36 months old with the maxillary second molars. The sequence of eruption and the timing of eruption for each tooth are similar for both sexes. Variability in the age of children at emergence of the individual teeth is small, with a standard deviation of 2 to 3 months. In most children, the 20 primary teeth (10 per arch) erupt in a period spanning about 2 years.

The permanent teeth begin erupting as children reach school age (about 6 years old), and the jaws grow. The eruption of permanent dentition begins with eruption of the mandibular central incisors and ends with the eruption of the maxillary third molars. The primary teeth are shed as the permanent ones erupt. The permanent molars erupt behind the primary molars. The shedding and replacement of the

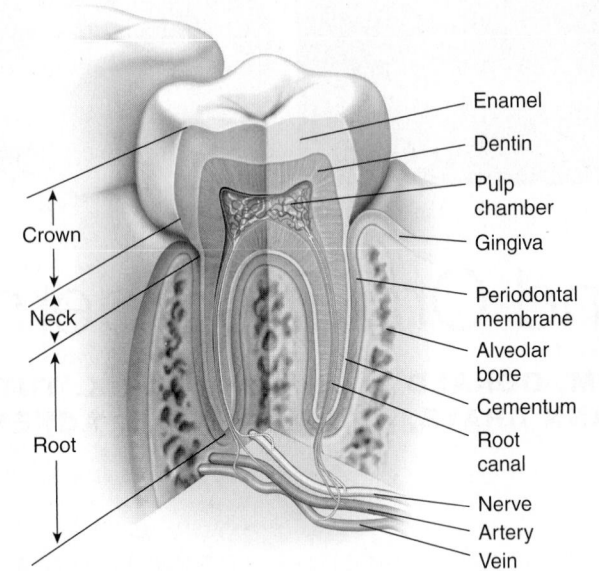

FIGURE 33-1 Anatomy of a tooth. (From Harkreader H, Hogan MA: *Fundamentals of nursing: caring and clinical judgment*, ed 2, 2004, Saunders, p 728.)

TABLE 33-1	Calcification, Crown Completion, and Eruption
Tooth	**Age of Eruption**
Primary Dentition	
Maxillary	
Central incisor	7½ months
Lateral incisor	8 months
Canine	16-20 months
First molar	12-16 months
Second molar	20-30 months
Mandibular	
Central incisor	6½ months
Lateral incisor	7 months
Canine	16-20 months
First molar	12-16 months
Second molar	20-30 months
Permanent Dentition	
Maxillary	
Central incisor	7-8 years
Lateral incisor	8-9 years
Canine	11-12 years
First premolar	10-11 years
Second premolar	10-12 years
First molar	6-7 years
Second molar	12-13 years
Third molar	17-21 years
Mandibular	
Central incisor	6-7 years
Lateral incisor	7-8 years
Canine	9-10 years
First premolar	10-12 years
Second premolar	11-12 years
First molar	6-7 years
Second molar	11-13 years
Third molar	17-21 years

Adapted from Logan WHG, Kronfeld R: Development of the human jaws and surrounding structures from birth to age fifteen years, *J Am Dent Assoc* 20:379, 1993.

primary molars by permanent premolars is usually complete around the fifth grade or by 12 years of age. This period, when both primary and permanent teeth are present, is called transitional dentition. The total period of eruption of permanent teeth (except for the third molars) spans about 6 years in most children.

In general, the variability in eruption times for the permanent dentition is much greater than the variability observed in the primary dentition, with standard deviation of 8 to 18 months (about five times greater than in the primary dentition). The sequence of permanent tooth eruption is almost identical for both sexes. However, all teeth erupt earlier in girls than in boys. The gender difference in eruption times averages approximately 6 months. The tooth eruption pattern for both the primary and permanent dentitions is listed in Table 33-1.

Managing Teeching. Often, teeth pierce the gums without causing any symptoms. However, some children show local symptoms, such as redness and swelling in the oral mucosa overlying the erupting tooth. These symptoms appear a few days before clinical eruption. The child may also show signs of irritation, drooling, and sometimes slight fever.

Recommended treatments for teething discomfort include topical treatments, such as chewing on a cold teething ring, pacifier, or even ice. Massaging the gums with a wet finger or a cold spoon may also be helpful. Topical analgesics containing benzocaine gel are marketed for this purpose and may be recommended. Exercise caution regarding topical benzocaine because of potential sensitivity. Oral acetaminophen is an effective remedy.

A great number of folk remedies are used, especially in communities without good access to medical care (Smitherman et al, 2005). Rubbing whiskey on the gums or tying a penny on a string around the child's neck (creates a potential risk of strangulation) are discouraged, as is using a honey-coated pacifier that might cause tooth decay or introduce

botulism. At least one case of methemoglobinemia has been reported in a 6-year-old after the use of Baby Orajel for a toothache (had symptoms of cyanosis, vomiting, lethargy, and tachycardia) (Chung et al, 2010). Overuse of topical salicylates can cause burns.

The Oral Examination

PERFORMING AN INFANT OR CHILD ORAL EXAM

An infant's teeth and oral tissues are examined most easily by placing the child on his or her back on an examining table with the head toward the end of the table. Have the parent restrain the legs and hands. Stand at the head of the table and use a tongue blade or toothbrush as a mouth prop. Use a penlight and intraoral mirror for optimal visualization. Tip the head back to see the upper teeth. The examination table approach is also useful for looking at the teeth of older children. Trying to examine the mouth and teeth with the child sitting in the parent's lap is not recommended because the provider has to bend over to see the upper teeth, and the crying and movement of the child make visibility very poor.

An alternative for examining a small child is the knee-to-knee approach favored by many dentists. In this approach, the provider and parent sit knee to knee. The parent holds the child facing him or her and then lowers the head into the provider's lap. The child's legs are wrapped around the parent's waist. Again the parent restrains the hands. Small children may cry during the examination, but the crying will stop as soon as the examination is completed.

CLINICAL FINDINGS

An oral and dental examination should be systematic. During the examination, take the opportunity to point out abnormalities (e.g., tooth decay) to the parent.

Oral Mucosa

The soft mucosal tissues are examined before the teeth. This part of the examination should also include an assessment of the tonsils for size and the presence of inflammation or exudate.

Start the examination with the inside of the lips and continue to the mucosa on the inside of the cheeks, including the mucosal surfaces that connect and surround each tooth. Inspect the palate directly by tipping the child's head backward. Use a mirror to help direct light to the soft palate. Examine the dorsal and ventral mucosal surfaces of the tongue and floor of the mouth by retracting the tongue with a tongue blade, a dental mirror, or by holding the tongue with cotton gauze. Ulcerations, changes in color and surface texture, swelling, or fistulae of any of these tissues should be noted.

When examining the gums, give special attention to any swelling or retraction of the gingiva where the gums meet the tooth surface. Such symptoms can be a notable sign of tooth or gingival abnormality typical of periodontal disease in peripubertal children and adolescents. Note the presence and attachment of frenula, with special emphasis on the possible complicating effects of high insertion of such frenula on the periodontal tissues.

Saliva

Salivary flow does not appreciably change over the life span. Note the quantity and quality of the saliva; thick or ropy saliva or a dry mouth may be abnormal. Decreased salivary flow and changes in sensation in the area of the facial nerve can result from infection or tumor in the parotid space or facial musculature, or can be a side effect of dehydration or medications.

Teeth

Examine the teeth systematically by beginning with the upper right buccal or facial surfaces and moving around to the left. Then from left to right, examine the lingual surfaces of the upper teeth. Then examine the biting surfaces in the same systematic manner. After this, move to the lower jaw. The number and types of teeth erupted, color changes, irregularities, and asymmetries should be noted.

Variations in number, morphology, color, and surface structure should be observed under good light after drying the teeth with cotton gauze. Primary teeth may be malformed or have incompletely formed, chalky, or pitted enamel due to other systematic conditions, such as ectodermal dysplasia. In the case of traumatically injured teeth, the color and translucency of the injured tooth or teeth should be evaluated. Slight color changes are often found as one of the first signs of intrapulpal damage after trauma and may lead to an abscessed tooth.

Early tooth decay can be detected most effectively by cleaning the teeth with a toothbrush and then drying them with gauze. Note any surface roughness or loss of surface continuity.

Aberrations in Primary Tooth Eruption

NATAL AND NEONATAL TEETH

The prevalence of natal or neonatal teeth is estimated to be 1:2000 to 3000 births and is equally common in boys and girls. The teeth usually erupt in pairs. Natal and neonatal teeth have been shown to occur in about 50 different syndromes, of which about 10 are associated with chromosomal aberrations. More than 90% of these prematurely erupting teeth are mandibular central incisors belonging to the normal dentition, with normal shape and color. Supernumerary teeth may be abnormal in shape and color and only loosely attached to the gingiva. Natal or neonatal teeth can lead to gingivitis, self-mutilation of the tongue, and trauma to the mother's breast. However, they should be extracted only if they are loose enough to involve risk of aspiration or if feeding is severely disturbed. Most will develop normally with normal root structure (Leung and Robson, 2006).

DELAYED TOOTH ERUPTION

Delayed tooth eruption can result from either systemic or local factors. These include prematurity, low birthweight, genetic syndromes (e.g., Down and Turner syndromes), a diet low in protein, children born to mothers with severe goiter (iodine deficiency), hereditary gingival fibromatosis, and adjacent supernumeraries or dental tissue tumors (odontomes) (Crawford and Aldred, 2005; Hayes and Thornton, 2007). In general, children with chronic diseases who show delay in both physical and dental development experience delayed but otherwise normal tooth eruption. Parents may need reassurance if there is some delay. Once the child is old enough to tolerate dental x-rays, no earlier than 4 years old and often later, diagnostic films can be taken to provide a better assessment of the developing dentition.

OTHER GUM EVENTS

Preeruption Cysts

When a tooth starts erupting through the gingival tissue, a blood-filled cyst may precede it. Alarmed parents may report a purple, reddish, black, or blue bump or bruise in their child's mouth. If the enlargement is on the alveolar ridge, reassurance is all that is required. The symptom will resolve as the tooth erupts (Fig. 33-2).

Congenital Epulis

Congenital epulis is a fibrous, pedunculated, soft-tissue enlargement that occurs on the maxillary alveolar ridge at birth (Fig. 33-3). This condition is more common in female babies. It typically regresses with time, but large lesions should be excised.

Bohn Nodules

Bohn nodules are present at birth and appear as firm nonpainful nodules on the buccal surface of the alveolar ridge (Fig. 33-4). They are remnants of dental lamina connecting the developing tooth bud to the epithelium of the oral cavity. No treatment is required because they will resolve spontaneously. If they appear in the midline of the palate, they are referred to as Epstein pearls.

■ Professional Dental Care

ACCESS TO DENTAL CARE

Numerous studies report considerable disparities in oral health and access to care, with the greatest burden experienced by low-income, ethnic minority children in households with low child or parental education, and in smokers (Beltrán-Aguilar et al, 2005; Edelstein and Chinn, 2009; Klein, 2009; Tinanoff and Reisine, 2009; USDHHS, 2003). Those without insurance are four times as likely to have unmet dental needs as those with some form of public insurance (Bloom et al, 2009).

Although Medicaid-enrolled children have better access to dental care than uninsured children (Bloom et al, 2009), they continue to exhibit low dental utilization rates (less than 60%) (Chi and Milgrom, 2009). This could be due to dentists' unwillingness to accept Medicaid insurance (because of low reimbursements rates) and high no-show rates (Al Agili et al, 2007; Iben et al, 2000). Low preventive care utilization rates can result in a cycle of emergency care with less comprehensive treatment, pain, and then more symptomatic care.

FEAR OF THE DENTIST

Parents' and caregivers' own fear of the dentist can have a negative effect on the oral health of children. As many as one in five adults in North America profess such fear (Smith and Heaton, 2003). Many of the parents of children with whom primary care providers interact may have this fear and consequently avoid dental visits themselves.

Early and consistent primary prevention is the best way to avoid the development of fear and avoidance (Weinstein and Milgrom, 2006). Allowing tooth decay to go untreated until a child is school age results in extensive restorative intervention—a traumatic experience for any child. Dental restorative care is the only area of medicine in which children are expected

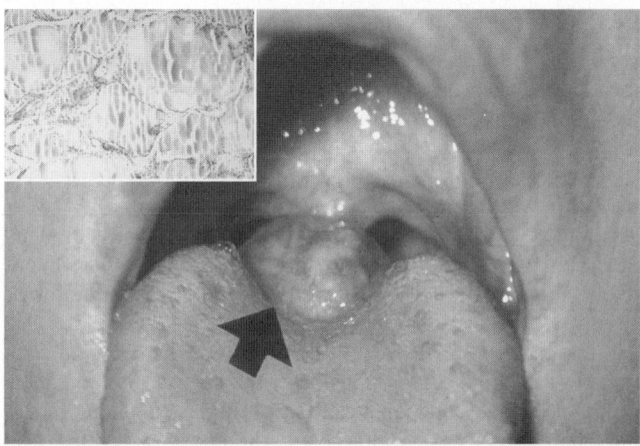

FIGURE 33-3 Congenital epulis. (From Gnepp DR: *Diagnostic surgical pathology of the head and neck,* ed 2, Philadelphia, 2009, Elsevier.)

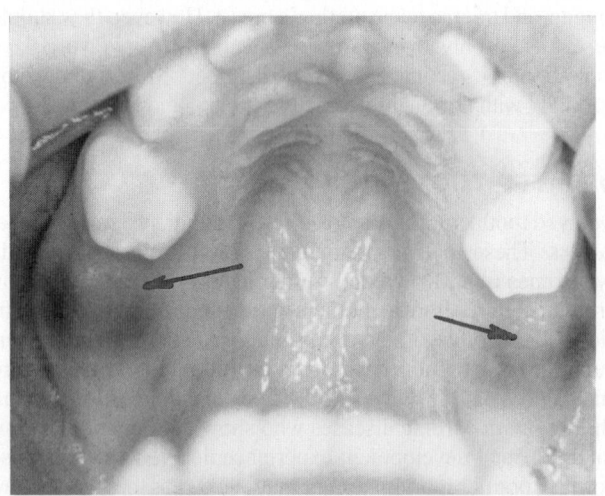

FIGURE 33-2 Preeruption cyst. Eruption hematomas *(arrows)* have developed before the eruption of the second primary molars. (From McDonald RE, Avery DR, Dean JA: *Dentistry for the child and adolescent,* ed 8, 2004, Mosby, p 182.)

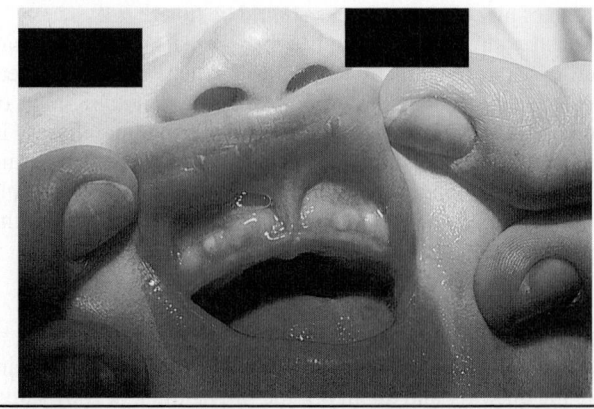

FIGURE 33-4 Bohn's nodule. (From Eichenfield LF, Frieden IJ, Esterly NB: *Neonatal dermatology,* ed 2, Philadelphia, 2008, Mosby.)

to endure extensive surgery while they are awake. Hospitalizing children and performing reparative services under general anesthesia is a scarce, expensive, and risky option. Moreover, the majority of children experience recurrence of disease within 6 months because the surgical treatment does not address the underlying problem.

CHOOSING A DENTIST

The choice of a dentist is critical, especially for children who have had poor previous experiences. Many general dentists are skilled at working with children, so the absence of a pediatric specialist is not a huge barrier. A dentist new to the child should be told about any prior dental experiences. Parents of dentally naive children should be counseled to choose a dentist known to like and work well with children. Parents should be encouraged to ensure that their child has had a good night's sleep and is fed before a visit. The child's teeth should be brushed before any visit to the dentist. A parent or caretaker should accompany the child into the treatment room; avoid dentists who are adverse to such. Counsel parents to avoid dentists who rely only on pharmacology to manage behavior, such as using nitrous oxide, oral antihistamines, or narcotics. The most effective strategies are behavioral. Combinations of behavioral and pharmacologic methods—such as distraction and nitrous oxide—can be effective, whereas the drug alone may not be.

Preparation should focus on helping the child develop coping skills and ways to gain control. Children gain control when the dentist briefly explains procedures and allows them to signal any discomfort. An example of a coping skill is relaxation breathing. Finding a dentist who tells stories and riddles, sings to the children, or otherwise distracts them (e.g., with videos, music, or games) is particularly effective. Directed guidance strategies—specific kinds of direction followed by praise—are also very effective in managing children's behaviors. For fearful children, practitioners can be successful by using structured rehearsals, in which procedures are broken into small steps, and teaching coping strategies. Dentists and parents who rely solely on authoritarian approaches or who are permissive are likely to fail with a fearful child (Weinstein and Milgrom, 2006).

Parents should be cautious about dentists with laser-based diagnostic devices. These devices are often marketed to dentists as being capable of detecting "invisible" cavities. They are being misused to justify unnecessary fillings, often called "preventive resins." The standard method of examination of the teeth is visual, using strong light and transillumination (shining light through the tooth) without using sharp probes, which can damage teeth and transfer potential pathogenic bacteria from one groove or surface to another. Most tooth decay in permanent teeth in children occurs on the biting surface, and x-rays are of limited diagnostic value in such cases. Parents should be urged to seek second opinions whenever eight or more fillings (two for each quadrant of the child's mouth) are recommended.

■ Dental Health Education

Dental health education is a crucial preventive strategy. Tailoring health education messages and instruction to an individual's capacity to "obtain, process, and understand" reflects a health literacy approach to oral health education. Low parental health literacy is most often associated with early childhood caries, low income, and inadequate maternal education. Low reading literacy, combined with low health literacy, is of particular concern given the dual role a parent plays as decisionmaker for self and child. The potential negative consequences for health and safety escalate.

Health information that is accessible to individuals with limited literacy is just beginning to influence dentistry. A review of dental education materials for parents found many required reading skills above the seventh to ninth grades. Additionally, many materials included dental jargon and unnecessarily difficult words (Alexander, 2000). The same study found that more than 80% of secondary school children (spanning a reading level equivalent to that of adults) were unsure of many dental terms, such as "fluoride tablets" and "gum disease." The advice given in published materials often is inconsistent. In addition, there are many oral health myths that should be dispelled by the PCP during conversations on oral health (e.g., caries in baby teeth aren't important since they eventually fall out anyway; it is "impossible" to brush children's teeth; fluoride is unsafe; pregnant women shouldn't see the dentist).

A good source of reference material on the Internet is www.medlineplus.gov, the consumer side of PubMed from the National Library of Medicine. Access is free, and materials are often in multiple languages. The site includes brochures that can be freely downloaded and copied.

REDUCING DISPARITIES THROUGH PREVENTIVE INTERVENTION AND MANAGEMENT

Weinstein and colleagues (2004) have shown that parents of young children are willing and able to change home preventive oral health practices. Using an intervention based on the transtheoretical "stages of change" model of Prochaska and Norcross, individuals overcome self-identified barriers to change, setting goals that are attainable and of personal value (Weinstein and Milgrom, 2006; Weinstein et al, 2004) (see Chapter 9 for discussion of this model).

Parents' toothbrushing skills and oral hygiene education can be improved when staff in the primary care clinic, preschool, Head Start, or Women, Infants, and Children (WIC) program demonstrate proper technique and give parents a chance to practice. Researchers found that oral hygiene and gingivitis scores improved in children when instructions about oral health were reinforced both in the home and at school (Kwan et al, 2005). Davies and colleagues (2005) reported positive benefits of a series of "gifts" by mail to parents of infants 8 through 32 months old. The gifts included written educational pamphlets, a trainer cup, toothpaste, and a toothbrush. Parents who received the repeated mailings versus those who did not were more likely to report favorable feeding behaviors, initiation of toothbrushing before 12 months old, and twice daily toothbrushing.

Beil and Rozier's study (2010) evaluated whether a recommendation by a PCP to see a dentist resulted in more dental checkups in children. They found that children 2 to 5 years who received such a recommendation were more likely to have a dental examination, whereas children from 6 to 11 years of age showed no increase. This supports the efficacy of the recommendation that primary care providers refer children to a "dental home" at an early age.

■ Bacterial Diseases of the Mouth

TOOTH DECAY (CAVITIES, DENTAL CARIES)

Description and Epidemiology

The Centers for Disease Control and Prevention (CDC) notes that of the approximately 50% of children who have had decay, two thirds of these children are in the 12- to 19-year-old range (CDC, 2010a); about one quarter are from 2 to 5 years old. Tooth decay is a bacterial disease that can result in irreversible damage and potential loss of teeth. The decay is caused by lactic acid demineralization of the tooth subsurface enamel. The acid is produced by an alpha hemolytic streptococcus (mutans streptococci), in older literature referred to as *Streptococcus mutans*, after metabolism of carbohydrates in the diet. Unless neutralized and buffered by saliva (remineralized), the demineralization process will lead to cavitation. Active cavities are also frequently infected with lactobacilli. The bacterial species are part of the biofilm adherent to the teeth. The bacteria are usually transmitted when saliva is shared between the child, caregivers, or other children (California Dental Association Foundation, 2010). Infection and colonization peak around the time of the eruption of the primary teeth, but may occur before.

In infants the carbohydrates may be present in the form of prolonged exposure to formula or breast milk, especially if the infant is allowed to sleep with the nipple in his or her mouth (Azevedo et al, 2005; van Palenstein Helderman et al, 2006). Before and after weaning, carbohydrates may also come from milk sweetened with honey or sugar or from juices in baby bottles or training cups, especially when given at bedtime, naptime, or when a child is allowed to take swigs of the fluid throughout the day. In older children, the source of the carbohydrates may be Tang, Kool-Aid, sports drinks, and/or soda. This frequent carbohydrate exposure keeps the pH of mouth fluid near the tooth surface below 5 and results in an environment conducive to demineralization. The neutralization process does not have enough time to increase the mouth pH to a level that would allow remineralization. In patients undergoing chemotherapy or radiation to the head and neck and in patients who are immunocompromised, normal salivary flow and salivary buffering of acids is disrupted. Cavities result. Box 33-1 provides a list of risk factors associated with dental caries in children.

Clinical Findings

Clinical findings can include the following:

- Early caries lesions. These appear as horizontal white or brown lines or spots along the upper central gumline or gingival margin, more commonly in populations using baby bottles because the cavity-causing fluids pool in these areas of the mouth (breastfed babies are not necessarily excluded from such lesions). In cultures where bottle use, especially at night or naptime, is less common the damage may occur in back teeth first as a function of other dietary patterns. When white lesions occur, the dentin is initially damaged. Then, as the lesion progresses, the hard enamel breaks, and a clinical cavity is evident (see Color Plate). Baby teeth are important for chewing food, serve an aesthetic function, and hold space in the mouth so that the permanent teeth can erupt properly. Therefore, it is critical to prevent cavities and intervene early in any decay.

BOX 33-1 Factors That Increase a Child's Risk for Developing Dental Caries

Health and Personal History

- Extra health care need associated with poor motor coordination or cooperation
- Xerostomia
- No dental home
- Previous history of tooth decay
- Braces or orthodontic appliances
- Child's parent or sibling has tooth decay
- Low socioeconomic status
- Frequent exposure to fermentable carbohydrates (e.g., snacking more than three times per day)
- No exposure to topical fluoride

Clinical Evaluation

- Visible plaque on teeth
- Gingivitis (red, swollen gums)
- Demineralized enamel (white spot lesions on teeth)
- Enamel defects (e.g., hypercalcification, deep pits and fissures)

Supplemental Findings

- Radiographic evidence of enamel caries
- High levels of mutans streptococci

Adapted from American Academy of Pediatric Dentistry (AAPD): Reference manual 2009-2010: policy on use of a caries-risk assessment tool (CAT) for infants, children, and adolescents, *Pediatr Dent* 31(special issue):29-33, 2009a.

- Advanced tooth decay. This appears as cavitations in the teeth. Nearly all cavities in permanent teeth in children in the U.S. begin on the biting surface of the molars. The initial lesion appears as a pinhole surrounded by a white, opaque halo. As the lesion enlarges greater damage to the enamel becomes apparent. Lesions typically appear about 1 year after the eruption of the tooth and frequently begin while the tooth is still erupting. A gumboil may form if the tooth becomes abscessed (Fig. 33-5).
- Sensitivity. Cavities can be hot, cold, or sweet sensitive.
- Localized pain. Lesions that progress can begin to hurt all the time, disrupting normal activity, sleeping, and eating.
- Inflammation and abscesses. Bacterial invasion of the pulpal tissue in the tooth causes inflammation and necrosis. In severely decayed primary teeth, a gumboil or draining fistula will form on the gum tissue above the root end of the tooth. This also occurs in permanent teeth, but is a late stage (see Fig. 33-5).
- Facial pain
- Gingival swelling, erythema
- Possible lymphadenopathy
- Possible fever
- Methamphetamine use ("meth mouth") can cause accelerated tooth decay on the facial surfaces of the teeth and between the teeth. In later stages the teeth are blackened, stained, and appear to be crumbling. There may be signs of severe grinding and dry mouth (Klasser and Epstein, 2005). See the discussion on the use of 12% chlorhexidine gluconate oral rinse for this condition.
- Cavities may spontaneously arrest. This is thought to occur, for example, when cavities are exposed to saliva high in fluoride or when the diet changes (such as after

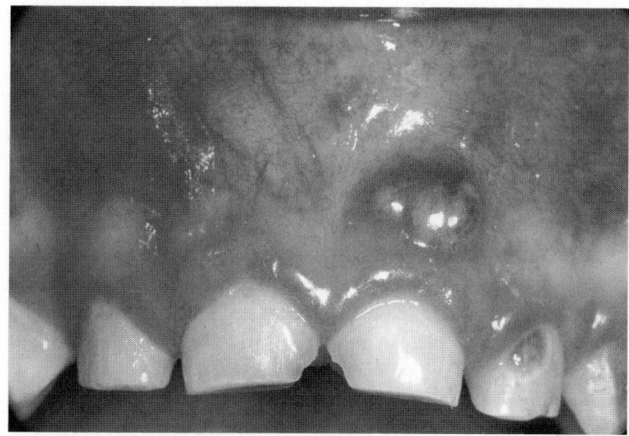

FIGURE 33-5 Advanced tooth decay with gumboil. (Courtesy John Davis, DDS, MSD, Professor Emeritus, University of Washington, Seattle, Department of Pediatric Dentistry.)

weaning). Arrested caries appear as open cavities that are black or dark brown. If the child has such open cavities, is asymptomatic, the teeth are primaries, and access to dental care is problematic, these teeth can be left alone and allowed to shed normally. Ideally, these children should receive dental care. The discoloration also may be the result of previous topical treatment by a dentist with diamine silver fluoride or silver nitrate that was used in an attempt to arrest and prevent carious lesions.

Management and Prevention Strategies in Primary Care

Fluoride Varnish. Early white spot lesions in primary and permanent teeth can be remineralized using topical fluoride varnish. In many states, PCPs and nurses are permitted to apply fluoride. Marketed fluoride varnish preparations contain from 1000 parts per million (ppm) (0.1% silane fluoride) to 22,600 ppm (sodium fluoride, 5%). Typically the 5% varnish preparations are used for children. All of the 5% varnishes for sale in the U.S. are essentially similar, varying in flavor or color. Twice-yearly applications have been shown to reduce tooth decay by about one third. A recent study suggested that four treatments given at the same time as well-child visits before 24 months reduced tooth decay in high risk children (Holve, 2008). Frequent application of fluoridated toothpaste also promotes repair (Do and Spencer, 2007). Plasma fluoride levels following applications of varnish are low and are not associated with toxicity or fluorosis. Fluoride varnish is the agent of choice for young children and has been shown to be more effective than the fluoride gels that are still widely used in the U.S. Fluoride gels are dangerous and difficult to apply in preschool children and are not recommended because of the risk of acute toxicity.

To apply fluoride varnish:

1. Dispense approximately 0.5 mL of varnish into a small well. Prepackaged individual-dose systems come with their own well that is filled with varnish.
2. Lightly dry the teeth with air or gauze to remove moisture.
3. While keeping the teeth isolated from further moisture contamination, paint the varnish onto the teeth with a brush or another type of applicator (Fig. 33-6). The varnish sets on contact with the slightly moist teeth.

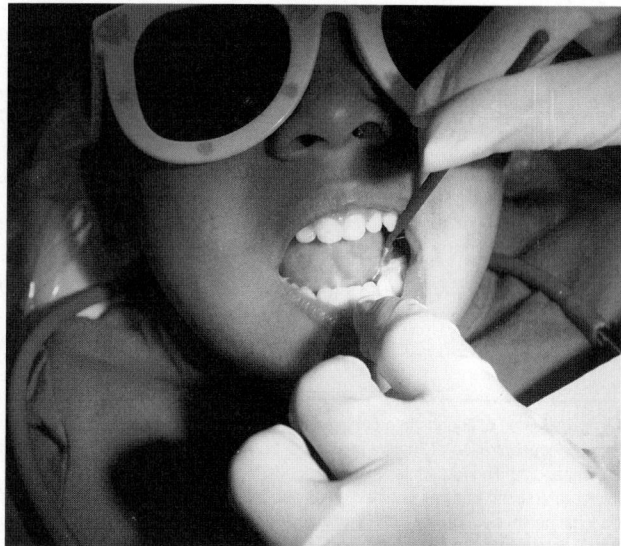

FIGURE 33-6 Applying fluoride varnish. (Courtesy Peter Milgrom, DDS.)

A short training video on the technique for applying varnish is available from the National Maternal and Child Oral Health Resource Center at www.mchoralhealth.org/highlights/flvarnish.html.

Topical Iodine. Polyvinylpyrrolidone iodine (10% PVP-I or povidone-iodine) can be painted on the teeth before the application of fluoride varnish for an additive effect to depress the tooth decay-causing mutans streptococci in children at high risk for dental problems (Milgrom et al, 2011). Application of topical iodine alone at 3-month intervals over 12 months has been shown to cause a significant reduction in the rise of flora from a baseline measurement (Singh et al, 2010).

Fluoride Therapy. The most effective preventive measure against dental caries is optimizing the fluoride content of communal water supplies (a new proposal recommends the optimal level be reset to 0.7 ppm [USDHHS, 2011]). However, only about 50% of children in the U.S. drink fluoridated water. Children who consume fluoride-deficient water supplies and who are at risk for caries will benefit from dietary fluoride supplementation (CDC, 2010b).The fluoride level of public water supplies can usually be ascertained by calling the local health department. If the patient uses a private water supply, the fluoride level should be tested before prescribing fluoride supplements. To prevent potential overdoses, no prescription should be written for more than a total of 120 mg of fluoride. See Table 33-2 for adjusting the dose of fluoride supplements in relation to that found in the community water supply.

Bottled Water. Although some bottled waters marketed in the U.S. contain an optimal concentration of fluoride, most contain less than 0.3 ppm fluoride. Thus, a person who uses bottled water with a low fluoride concentration instead of fluoridated community water may need fluoride supplementation. In the U.S., current U.S. Food and Drug Administration (FDA) regulations require that fluoride be listed on the bottled water label only if fluoride is added during processing, but the concentration does not have to be stated.

Toothbrushing Techniques. Parents should be taught to clean a child's teeth with a brush or washcloth as soon as teeth

TABLE 33-2 Recommended* Fluoride Supplementation Based on Drinking Water Fluoride Concentration

Age	FLUORIDE ION LEVEL IN DRINKING WATER (PPM)[†]			
	None	**<0.3 ppm**	**0.3 to 0.6 ppm**	**>0.6 ppm**
Birth to 6 months	None	None	None	None
6 months to 3 years	0.25[‡] mg/day; drops given directly into mouth or in water *(not in milk)*	0.25 mg/day[‡]	None	None
3 to 6 years	0.50[‡] mg/day; tablet	0.50 mg/day	0.25 mg/day	None
6 to 16 years	1[‡] mg/day; tablet	1 mg/day	0.50 mg/day	None

*Take all sources of fluoride into consideration: from water (including bottled) and amount and frequency of fluoridated toothpaste used in brushing.
†Optimal concentration of fluoride in water supply in mg/L or parts per million (ppm).
‡2.2 mg sodium fluoride contains 1 mg fluoride ion.
Only children living in nonfluoridated areas should receive supplements between 6 months and 16 years old. If the fluoride level is not known, it should be tested first. State and local health departments can provide information on testing drinking water for fluoride levels.
From Centers for Disease Control and Prevention (CDC): *Dietary fluoride supplement schedule*, 2010. Available at www.cdc.gov/fluoridation/other/spplmnt_schdl.htm (accessed Sep 29, 2010).

erupt, using the "lift the lip" method. Simple flip charts are available to teach parents how to do this; a demonstration by the provider during a well-child visit is ideal. The technique involves having a parent lift the child's upper lip and use a wet washcloth, special finger brush, or soft toothbrush to cleanse each tooth surface. As the infant is repeatedly exposed, and if the parent makes it an enjoyable activity, any resistance should decrease. It may be easier to brush a child's teeth if the child lies on the floor, on a couch with the child's head in the parent's lap, or using the knee-to-knee technique. A second adult can help by holding the hands and feet if necessary. Brushing in the bathroom standing up is more difficult. Most children and adults do not brush teeth long enough or miss some teeth surfaces. Toothbrush songs and timers help in teaching children and parents how long to brush. The type of toothbrush, manual or electric, is not clinically relevant. Small soft brushes are widely available for children, and large-handled brushes are available for children with physical disabilities that make holding a regular brush difficult. Child resistance to brushing will disappear with repeated endeavors and perseverance on the part of parents.

Parents should also check monthly to see if dental problems are beginning. Using the "lift the lip" method, they should look closely for the signs of demineralization (see earlier discussion). Early detection allows for more timely intervention.

Toothpaste. Fluoridated toothpaste works by creating a reservoir of fluoride in the fluid layer of the plaque and in the saliva that is available to remineralize or repair teeth that are being damaged by bacterial acids. All fluoridated toothpastes sold in the U.S. are similar. The provider should know the fluoride content level in the community drinking water, other sources of fluoride the child might be consuming (e.g., bottled water), and risk factors for tooth decay prior to recommending the use of fluoride toothpaste (CDC, 2010b). Parents should be encouraged to choose a simple toothpaste with a sweet flavor. Strongly flavored toothpastes and those containing whitening or bleaching agents are contraindicated for children. A small amount of toothpaste (about the size of a pea) should be used. The amount should be controlled by an adult because children can swallow a large amount of what is brushed on; this added systemic intake of fluoride can lead to an increased risk of

enamel fluorosis (a whitish discoloration of the tooth enamel) in children younger than the age of 6 years (CDC, 2010b). In children at very high risk for tooth decay, parents should begin brushing teeth with fluoridated toothpaste with the eruption of the first tooth at 6 to 9 months of age (Altarum Institute, 2009). This is an updated recommendation, and primary care providers may encounter dentists who are unfamiliar with it. Toothpastes and fluoride supplements should be stored out of reach of younger children. If a child ingests a large dose of fluoride, the caregiver should contact 911 immediately.

Diet. Dietary advice is essential to parents. Bottles should only be filled with formula or water, and the child weaned from a bottle at 12 months of age. Nursing mothers should not allow their infants to sleep attached to the nipple. Bottles should never be propped during naps or sleep. Training cups should be started at 4 to 6 months old for water and juices for both breastfed and bottle-fed infants. Some WIC centers in the U.S. distribute training cups to promote appropriate eating behaviors and prevent tooth decay. However, personnel may not be aware of the potential danger of the cups themselves if sugary drinks or juice are available ad lib.

Xylitol Gum and Syrup. Xylitol, a naturally occurring sugar, has been demonstrated to prevent and control tooth decay when used from three to seven times per day with a total dose ranging from 4 to 10 g daily (American Academy of Pediatric Dentistry [AAPD], 2010a). Xylitol is FDA approved and works by reducing the adhesiveness of oral bacteria in the dental plaque and reducing the overall numbers of virulent organisms. The effect is topical, not systemic. Chewing gum and mints are the most frequent sources of xylitol, but it is also available in chewable tablets, lozenges, toothpastes, mouthwashes, cough mixtures, and nutraceutical products. Gum is the recommended delivery vehicle until the other products have been adequately studied for efficacy (AAPD, 2010a), although chewing gum is not appropriate for preschoolers because of the risk of choking. Products should contain at least 50% xylitol, and xylitol should be the first ingredient listed on the label. If using the gum, it should be chewed for about 5 minutes or until the sweetness disappears. In the dosage range used for tooth decay prevention, side effects are rare and usually limited to abdominal cramping (Ly et al, 2006).

More risk of severe abdominal pain and diarrhea can occur in children who use xylitol and who also consume sorbitol in excess from other products. Children whose mothers who used xylitol chewing gum at least three times per day for 2 years after their birth had less tooth decay because of reduced or postponed bacterial colonization (Isokangas et al, 2000).

Xylitol syrups have been shown to reduce cavities in young preschoolers, and a syrup is available by prescription. Children who received at least 8 g per day of xylitol in syrup divided into two or three doses and applied topically to the teeth by a caregiver had 50% to 70% less decay than children who received an ineffective treatment (Milgrom et al, 2009).

Chlorhexidine Oral Rinse. Chlorhexidine gluconate oral rinse, 0.12%, provides antimicrobial activity as long as it is used consistently. After rinsing, 30% of the chlorhexidine gluconate remains in the oral cavity and is released into the oral fluids. It has an important role as part of a professional treatment program for some dental conditions discussed in the rest of this chapter.

Instructions for the chlorhexidine gluconate mouth rinse are as follows: half a capful (0.5 fl oz, undiluted) swished in the mouth for 30 seconds twice daily and then spit out. Individuals should not swallow the rinse, rinse the mouth afterward, or eat for 30 minutes. It is necessary to use it at least 60% of the time to have any clinical effect. Side effects include staining of teeth, restorations, and tongue (can be removed by having the teeth professionally cleaned); calculus formation above the gumline; and an aftertaste that may change taste perception temporarily. Pregnant and nursing mothers should use the product only if clearly needed. The effectiveness and safety of its use have not been established in children younger than 18 years of age.

"Meth Mouth." Methamphetamine users should be encouraged to seek drug treatment. Any dental intervention will fail without control of the underlying condition. Encourage the patient to drink lots of water and switch to artificially sweetened drinks. Over-the-counter fluoride mouth rinse, remineralizing solutions, xylitol chewing gum, and prescription chlorhexidine gluconate mouth rinse 0.12% may be recommended.

Toothache. If tooth decay has resulted in pain and a draining tract, analgesics, warm-water or saline rinses, and a bland diet are recommended. In the presence of cellulitis and fever, antibiotic therapy is appropriate, and follow-up dental treatment is needed. Penicillin is the drug of choice. In the case of penicillin allergy, azithromycin or clindamycin are alternatives. Amoxicillin-clavulanic acid (dose using the amoxicillin component) can also be used in treating dental abscesses, as well as cefoxitin (Gould and Cies, 2010). The child needs an emergency dental visit (not an emergency department visit) after several days if not responding to antibiotic treatment.

Preventing Person-to-Person Spread of Caries-Causing Bacteria

Eating utensils should not be shared between caregivers and their children, especially if the caregiver has untreated cavities in the mouth. Parents should not use their own saliva to clean pacifiers or bottles, and children should be discouraged from sharing beverages using the same cup. Dental visits are especially important for pregnant women because of the association between untreated cavities in the mother and future development of cavities in the child. Pregnant women can safely receive all diagnostic, preventive (including radiograph), and restorative dental treatment (e.g., during second and third trimesters; local anesthesia, fillings, periodontal treatment) during pregnancy.

Management and Prevention Role of the Dentist

The American Academy of Pediatrics (AAP) and the AAPD recommend that children be examined by a dentist by 12 months old or within 6 months of the eruption of the first tooth. Box 33-2 defines some common dentistry terms that are used throughout the rest of this chapter.

The first dental visit commonly involves a cleaning, dental examination, and topical fluoride treatment. For children younger than age 3 years, the caregiver may be asked to help the dentist by securing the child's legs and hands in the knee-to-knee position. Older children frequently use a dental chair that reclines. Sitting next to the child or holding the child's hands during this first visit may help to alleviate the child's stress. Some dentists may not allow parents or caregivers in the treatment area. Encourage parents to inquire about such a policy prior to making the first dental appointment and choose an alternative dentist if such an exclusionary policy is disagreeable to them or the child. Even if the first dental visit is difficult, caregivers should be instructed to praise the child afterward for specific actions (e.g., for opening the mouth or keeping hands on the tummy). This positive reinforcement can help make subsequent dental visits easier.

When tooth decay is present, subsequent dental visits may involve treatment. Larger cavities in primary teeth can be repaired with plastic fillings or with steel or plastic crowns. Deep cavities involving the pulp tissue in primary teeth require a form of therapy called a pulpotomy, removing the inflamed or necrotic pulp tissue, followed by the placement of a stainless steel crown. Teeth with deep cavities and draining gumboils are generally extracted. A decision to repair teeth or remove them depends on the extent of damage and the length of time until the tooth would be normally exfoliated. Retention of primary molars is important because they hold space to allow the normal eruption of permanent successors. Young children may need to be sedated or receive treatment under a general anesthetic to cope with the treatment.

Cavities in permanent teeth are repaired with either silver amalgam or plastic composite resin fillings. About half of a silver amalgam filling is composed of liquid mercury. This binds the other half of the amalgam components (a powdered alloy of silver, tin, and copper) together. Although mercury releases low levels of vapor, the FDA considers silver amalgams safe for adults and children based on scientific evidence. The mercury levels from amalgams (even in those individuals who have 15 or more amalgam surfaces) have been determined by the Environmental Protection Agency and the CDC to be below the lowest levels associated with brain and kidney toxicity. They are also considered safe for use in pregnant and lactating women and children younger than the age of 6 years (FDA, 2009). The longevity of plastic fillings is very much shorter than silver fillings except when small and when not applied to high-stress areas (e.g., chewing surface on a back tooth). Severe cavities resulting in abscess formation in permanent teeth are treated with root canal therapy. Permanent molars either need to be capped (crown) after root canal therapy or treated with large silver fillings.

BOX 33-2 Glossary of Terms Used in Dentistry

Amalgam filling: Metal filling material used to replace tooth structure affected by decay in permanent teeth. Contains silver, mercury, copper, and other metals. Usually referred to generically as amalgam. Not commonly used in primary teeth now.

Composite filling: Tooth-colored acrylic filling material used to replace tooth structure affected by decay. Also used as an aesthetic material for replacing discolored tooth structure. Main filling material used in children's teeth.

Crossbite: Type of malocclusion in which one or more upper teeth are located behind the opposing teeth. Usually caused by premature tooth loss.

Erythroplakia: Matted red plaques located on the soft tissues of the oral cavity in smokers and those using smokeless tobacco; can be a sign of oral cancer.

Extrusion: Condition in which a tooth is loosened from its normal tooth position in the direction of tooth eruption.

Fluoride varnish: An alcohol-based lacquer that is brushed on the teeth to prevent tooth decay; it contains 5% sodium fluoride.

Glass ionomer: Tooth-colored filling material often used in atraumatic restorative procedures in young children.

Gumboil: Fistula associated with an abscessed tooth draining through the gums.

Intrusion: Condition in which a tooth is loosened from its normal position in the opposite direction of tooth eruption.

Leukoplakia: Matted white plaques located on the soft tissues of the oral cavity that can be a sign of oral cancer.

Luxation: Condition in which a tooth is loosened from its normal tooth position.

Malocclusion: A term to describe abnormalities in the way maxillary and mandibular teeth articulate. Includes crossbites, open bites, and abnormal spacing. May or may not have functional significance. Can usually be corrected by a dentist or orthodontist.

Nitrous oxide: Laughing gas. Commonly used as a relaxing agent mixed with oxygen for mildly anxious or nervous patients during conscious sedation. Usually used at less than 50% in an open anesthesia system.

Open bite: Type of malocclusion in which the front teeth do not touch together when the back teeth are biting.

Periapical pathosis: Tooth infection that often presents as a radiolucency on a dental radiograph.

Pericoronitis: Inflammation around the crown of an unerupted tooth.

Pulp: Part of the tooth anatomy containing the nerves and blood vessels. When invaded by bacteria in tooth decay, it swells and necroses, resulting in gumboils and pain and the need for pulpotomy or root canal treatment.

Root canal: Space that houses a tooth's neurovascular bundle. Root canal treatment involves removing the infected neurovascular bundle and replacing it with an inert filling material. Treatment in children is called a pulpotomy.

Sealants: Plastic coatings placed on the chewing surfaces of permanent molars at about 6 to 7 years and again at about 13 to 14 years old, when the tooth is fully erupted. Also called pit and fissure sealants or occlusal sealants.

Xerostomia: Dry mouth that results from reduced salivary flow or production. May be secondary to medications.

Remineralizing creams are used by some dentists to reverse or arrest white or brown tooth decay lesions. These pastes contain casein phosphopeptide-amorphous calcium phosphate and are applied topically multiple times. There are limited data available to assess the effectiveness of this approach, although that which exists is generally positive and encouraging (Bailey et al, 2009).

Pit and fissure (occlusal) sealants are recommended for children at moderate or high risk for tooth decay; sealants are underused in the U.S. Moderate- or high-risk children are those who have experienced a lot of tooth decay in their primary teeth, have poor oral hygiene, or diets with lots of refined carbohydrates and soft drinks. Sealants are polymerizing resin coatings placed on the biting surfaces of permanent molars (Fig. 33-7) at about 6 to 7 years old and 13 to 14 years old, depending on tooth eruption; they are very effective in preventing decay and do not involve drilling.

Complications

Fluorosis. A complication of too much systemic fluoride exposure during the years of tooth development is fluorosis, a defect in tooth enamel. Surveys show that there has been an increase in all levels of fluorosis that range from very mild to moderate-severe. Children 6 to 11 years old have rates of 33%, while those 12 to 15 years old have rates of about 41%. In the 12- to 15-year-olds, the rate represents about an 18% increase since the mid 1980s (Beltrán-Aguilar et al, 2010). Recognizing that children may be overexposed to fluoride, at least occasionally, the USDHHS has recommended adjusting the amount of fluoride being added to community water supplies to achieve an optimal fluoride level of 0.7 milligrams of fluoride per liter of water. This is at the lower limit of the previously recommended range and would apply to community water systems that are currently fluoridating or will initiate fluoridation (USDHHS, 2011) (check the USDHHS website [www.hhs.gov] to determine if these new recommendations were implemented).

In most cases, the fluorosis appears as tiny white specks or streaks that are largely unnoticeable. The advisability of introducing toothpaste for very young children should always depend on the risk of tooth decay. When risk is high (e.g., if the mother and siblings have tooth decay, poor hygiene, and diet), the benefit outweighs the minimal consequences of fluorosis. Nevertheless, toothpaste should always be metered by parents.

Abscesses. Some teeth abscess after fillings are placed in them. Permanent teeth may be sensitive to hot and cold for many weeks after fillings are placed. Untreated abscesses may develop into life-threatening bony facial space infections, requiring surgical drainage and parenteral antibiotic treatment.

AGGRESSIVE PERIODONTITIS
Description and Epidemiology

Periodontitis is an aggressive bacterial infection of the gums and bone with phagocyte abnormalities and hyperresponsive macrophages. It results in loss of periodontal attachment and supporting bone around teeth. The primary infection is by *Actinobacillus* and *Bacteroides* species in younger children and by *Treponema* species and other gram-negative rods in older children. The disease may be localized or generalized, depending on the location of the loss of attachment and which teeth are affected. The incidence is about 0.2% to 0.5% in

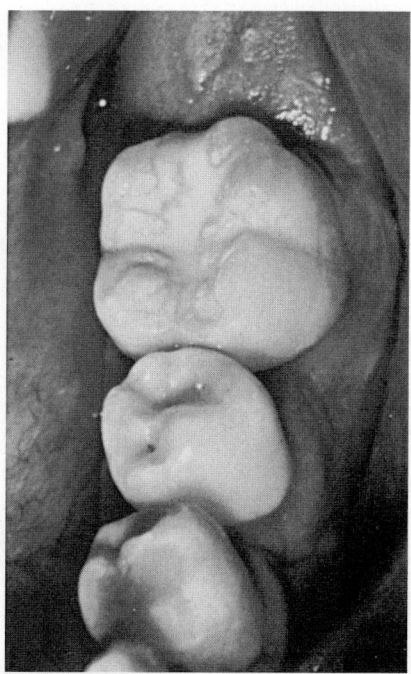

FIGURE 33-7 Sealant. (From Pinkham JR: *Pediatric dentistry: infancy through adolescence,* ed 4, St Louis, 2005, Saunders, p 537.)

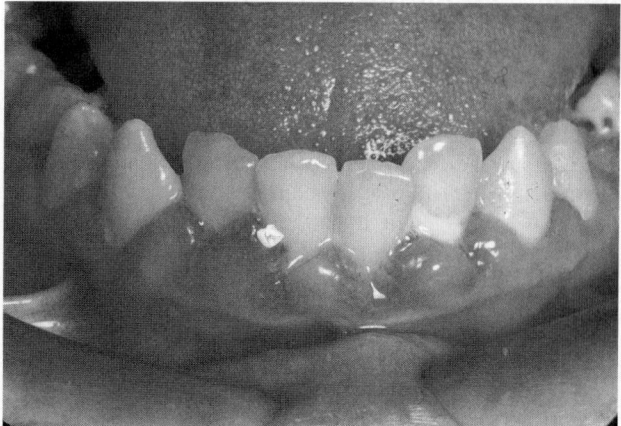

FIGURE 33-8 Periodontitis (gross gingivitis). (From Davis J, Peterson D: *Atlas of pediatric dentistry,* Seattle, 2004, University of Washington.)

children and adolescents, especially those 12 years and older; African-American children are at slightly greater risk. Age of onset is typically circumpubertal, with a familial aggregation of cases (AAPD, 2009b).

Clinical Findings

This condition can be localized (around the primary incisors and molars) or more generalized (all teeth affected). The teeth may become loose, but in the localized form there is generally no inflammatory response, suppuration, or fever. The localized disease is not oral hygiene related, and the damage happens within months.

Individuals with the generalized form of gum disease often have poor oral hygiene. This condition is more common in patients with special health care needs brought about by such systemic diseases as Papillon-Lefevre disease, Down syndrome, and cyclic neutropenia. A history of periodontal disease in parents may be found. Figure 33-8 illustrates this condition.

Management

If gum disease is caught early, local debridement of the teeth and systemic antibiotics are used. Management with tetracyclines or metronidazole in combination with amoxicillin is appropriate. Tetracyclines should not be prescribed while the crowns of the permanent teeth are still developing in the jaws. Individual circumstances may vary, but typically the tetracyclines would be safe for children 8 years and older. For patients with a familial history of gum disease, frequent dental examinations and radiographs during the peripubertal period are essential. Patients should be counseled to avoid tobacco products (they increase the risk of all periodontal diseases); damage to dentition is permanent.

Complications

The major complication of gum disease is loss of bone and tooth attachment, resulting in the loss of teeth. Untreated periodontal diseases may also negatively affect birth outcomes through problems such as preeclampsia or premature labor (Bobetsis et al, 2006; Herrera et al, 2007).

NECROTIZING PERIODONTAL DISEASE

This is an aggressive bacterial disease resulting in damage to the gum tissue between the teeth. The gum tissues harbor high levels of spirochetes, and invasion of the tissues has been demonstrated. Predisposing factors are viral infections (including human immunodeficiency virus [HIV] and other systemic diseases), malnutrition, emotional stress, and lack of sleep. The incidence in North America is less than 1% of children and adolescents; the prevalence is 2% to 5% in those age groups from Africa, Asia, or South America (AAPD, 2009b). Children have severe gingival pain and fever. The triangular area of gums between the teeth is ulcerated and necrotic and covered with a gray film. There may be a fetid mouth odor. If the PCP notes this condition and the patient is febrile, metronidazole and penicillin should be started and a dental referral made. Careful oral hygiene and a bland diet are recommended. Address the predisposing conditions. Loss of teeth is a complication. Early treatment is needed to prevent disfigurement of the gums with chronic infection.

PYOGENIC GRANULOMA

Pyogenic granuloma is an inflammatory hyperplasia that is usually caused by low-grade localized infection, trauma, or hormonal factors. It is usually a small exophytic (outward growing) lesion that is smooth or lobulated and sometimes hemorrhagic. The surface color ranges from pink to red to deep purple, depending on how long the lesion has been present in the oral cavity. A pyogenic granuloma most commonly occurs in pregnant women. Possible treatments include improved oral hygiene, 0.12% chlorhexidine gluconate rinses, surgical excision, cryosurgery, or intralesional injections of corticosteroids. If hygiene or chlorhexidine does not resolve the problem, the patient should be referred.

BRUXISM/GRINDING

Bruxism is a condition of excessive grinding of the teeth. Studies of the prevalence are limited and plagued by poor design and measurement. One well-designed study showed that a group of predominantly Caucasian, well-educated parents estimated the prevalence of bruxism in their 8-year-old children at 38%. Almost all the grinding was at night, and no facial pain or other symptoms were associated with the grinding. Many of the children had a familial history of bruxism or had undefined "psychological disorders" (Cheifetz et al, 2005). Although the conclusions need to be viewed cautiously, this study suggests that underlying stressors may be a cause, and as such, may provide an opportunity for intervention and education.

Primary teeth show marked wear, and parents report that their child grinds his or her teeth during sleep. There may also be an orthodontic problem that needs attention. Some individuals may complain of facial muscle pain and develop temporomandibular joint disorder (discussed later). Clicking of the jaw on opening or closing is not a pathologic condition, and is seen mostly in adults. No treatment is required for most grinding and tooth wear. The use of plastic night guards rarely eliminates grinding. Behavioral methods, such as relaxation training for stress management and other self-management skills including control of gum chewing, have been shown to be effective in helping to manage facial muscle pain and headache.

Children or adolescents who have either limited mouth opening, pain on opening or closing, or deviation of the jaw to one side during opening may have a jaw fracture or another serious problem, such as a tumor or infection. Parents should be told that tooth grinding is not associated with any damage to permanent dentition. Teens may experience headache or facial muscle pain, particularly at stressful times. Parents should be counseled to avoid dentists who routinely prescribe expensive plastic mouth guards or similar appliances for this complaint.

DENTAL EROSION

Description and Epidemiology

Dental erosion is a chemical process that leads to irreversible acid demineralization of tooth structure. Acids that cause dental erosion can be classified as intrinsic or extrinsic. Intrinsic acids include stomach acid introduced into the oral cavity by diagnosed or silent gastroesophageal reflux disorder (GERD), bulimia nervosa, and vomiting. Extrinsic acids include acidic beverages, methamphetamines, citrus fruits (e.g., sucking on lemons), and medications (e.g., chewable vitamin C tablets or hydrochloric acid supplements). Factors that can aggravate dental erosion include xerostomia (dry mouth) secondary to decreased salivary flow; medications that interfere with saliva composition or production (e.g., clonidine); dental attrition; and dental abrasion. Asthmatic children have greater amounts of dental erosion than other children. This may be due to increased gastroesophageal reflux in those with asthma, to acidic long-term medications, or to an increased consumption of erosive beverages taken to counteract the drying effect of inhalers (Hosey and Welbury, 2005). A study in 2000 demonstrated an erosion prevalence rate of 41% to the upper permanent incisors in children 11 to 13 years old in the U.S. (37% in the United Kingdom) (Deery et al, 2000).

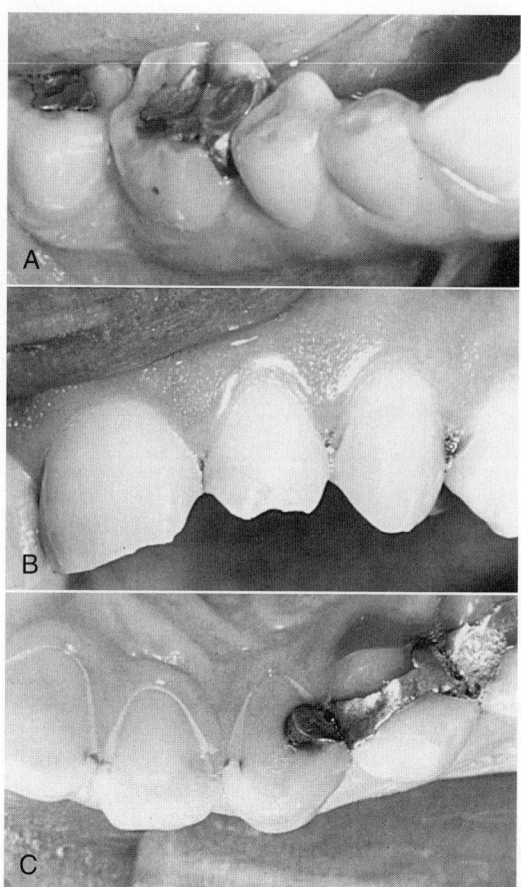

FIGURE 33-9 Dental erosion from bulimia. **A,** Loss of occlusal enamel with exposure of dentin. **B,** Ragged incisal edges. **C,** Lingual exposure of dentin highlighted by outlines of remaining enamel and exposed surfaces of restorations. (From Casamassimo P, Castaldi C: Considerations in the dental management of the adolescent, *Pediatr Clin North Am* 29:648, 1982.)

Clinical Findings

Clinical manifestations of dental erosion include smooth, cupped-out teeth on chewing surfaces; fillings that are raised above the normal level of the tooth; overly shiny silver fillings; enamel cuffing along the gums; and tooth hypersensitivity. Bulimic patients usually have very smooth lingual surfaces of the permanent teeth (Fig. 33-9).

Differential Diagnosis

Consider abrasion caused by gritty substances, such as coarse toothpaste or hard toothbrushes, and attrition caused by mechanical forces, such as tooth grinding (bruxism). Also consider tooth decay.

Management

Early detection, diagnosis, and treatment of dental erosion are critical. Hot and cold sensitivity can be managed by the use of "sensitive teeth" fluoridated toothpastes or topical treatments applied by the dentist. Treatment and/or referral to for suspected GERD or bulimia are warranted in suspected cases of GERD or bulimia. Dietary counseling may be appropriate. Unless the erosion is deep, fillings are not required. Deep grooves in teeth can be repaired by the dentist using atraumatic techniques and materials. Typically the problem can be managed by identifying and eliminating the etiologic agent. Over-the-counter products, such as soft toothbrushes, low-abrasive fluoridated toothpaste, and fluoride rinses, are helpful.

Complications

Patients with mild to moderate dental erosion may report tooth hypersensitivity. Severe dental erosion can lead to dental nerve (pulp) exposures, which can necessitate root canal treatment.

PERICORONITIS ASSOCIATED WITH PARTIALLY ERUPTED WISDOM TEETH

Description

This condition is due to a partially erupted lower wisdom tooth with a tissue flap covering part of the crown. A foreign body, such as a piece of food, is forced under the flap, causing a localized infection. In some cases, upper wisdom teeth will erupt with the crown rubbing against the buccal mucosa and cause pain. The problem is common in college-age students. Partially erupted wisdom teeth can create an environment in which the distal surface of the second molar becomes decayed because it cannot be cleaned.

Clinical Findings

The gum tissue partially covering the tooth is inflamed and painful. The patient may be febrile. The tissue flap may show trauma from biting.

Differential Diagnosis

Aggressive periodontal diseases and severe tooth decay may have similar clinical presentations.

Management

Primary care providers may recommend irrigation of the area with sterile water or saline, prescribe analgesics, and start amoxicillin if the patient is febrile. Not all wisdom teeth need to be removed. Wisdom teeth do not cause other teeth to become crooked. Teeth fully covered in bone do not need to be removed and carry no significant risk. Similarly, if there is space for the erupting teeth, there is no reason to remove them. It is appropriate to wait for the teeth to fully erupt as much as they can. Studies show they may still erupt at 23 or 24 years old. Waiting maximizes the chance they will not need to be removed and minimizes the morbidity associated with the surgery. Impacted teeth and upper teeth that have erupted toward the buccal mucosa should be surgically removed.

Complications

Removal of wisdom teeth always requires a risk-benefit calculation because there is significant morbidity associated with the surgery (Friedman, 2007). Temporary or permanent nerve damage is possible. A common complication of wisdom tooth surgery is alveolar osteitis or dry socket. This painful condition is associated with the loss of the normal clot in the healing socket. The cause of the pain is exposed bone. Smoking and the use of oral contraceptives are risk factors. Pretreatment rinsing with 0.12% chlorhexidine gluconate mouth rinse reduces the risk of complications. Treatment at the time of surgery with a nonsteroidal antiinflammatory may reduce the extent of swelling postoperatively. Pain and foul taste in the mouth are the main symptoms, beginning 4 to 5 days after surgery. The patient should be referred back to his or her dentist. The treatment is symptomatic with analgesics because the problem is self-limiting.

TRAUMATIC INJURIES TO ORAL STRUCTURES

Description

Injuries to the face usually result in trauma to the soft tissues of the mouth, teeth, or jaws. Such trauma is one of the most common presentations of young children to dentists. Dental injuries occur secondary to falls, motor vehicle accidents, violence, abuse, and sporting activities. Fewer traumas are presently seen from supervised, organized sports because most children wear mouth guards; nevertheless, a disproportionate amount of trauma results from leisure activities, such as skateboarding, swimming, and other noncontact sports. Upper incisors are particularly vulnerable to dental injuries. In addition, a child who has received local anesthesia for dental treatment may accidentally injure him- or herself by biting the inside of the cheek, tongue, or lip.

Epidemiology

Age is a significant consideration in trauma to teeth, with most injuries occurring between 7 and 12 years of age. Luxation (loosening) injuries to upper anterior teeth predominate in toddlers because of their frequent falls during attempts at walking. Studies show that males have dental injuries more frequently than females. Other risk factors for trauma-related dental injuries include participation in sports, cerebral palsy, and misaligned bites. Between 25% and 50% of all accidents in children up to 14 years of age involve the head. Children 6 to 15 years old are most likely to go to the emergency department with a sports-related tooth injury (AAPD, 2009c).

It is also important to rule out physical abuse, as the orofacial region is commonly traumatized during such episodes. See Chapter 17 for a discussion of signs of physical abuse in the head area.

Clinical Findings

History. Because a dental injury may become the subject of litigation, a thorough history and examination is mandatory. When possible, an injury should be photographed. The provider should ask the following questions:
- When and how did the trauma occur?
- Were there any other injuries?
- Have there been any injuries in the past?
- Is there any concern for the safety of this child and family?
- Is there any history of abuse, drug or alcohol use in the family?
- Are any problems occurring as a result of the trauma?
- Is tetanus immunization current (within the last 5 years)? This question is especially important with soil-contaminated wounds or with complete displacement of a tooth from its socket. (See Chapter 23 for tetanus prophylaxis treatment.)
- For children presenting with trauma to the inside of the cheek, tongue, or lip, did the child recently receive local anesthetic for dental treatment?

Physical Examination. Blunt trauma tends to cause greater damage to soft tissues and supporting structures, whereas high-velocity or sharp injuries cause luxation and fractures of the teeth. Children with sports-related injuries can have teeth that are avulsed, fractured, luxated, intruded, or extruded. The examination should include:

- Soft tissue. Palpate the jaws and the rest of the facial skeleton to determine if a fracture is possible.
- Skin. Look for extraoral lacerations and facial wounds.
- Intraoral mucosa. Look for wounds, swelling, and bruising of the oral mucosa, gingiva, tongue, cheeks, and/or palate.
- Teeth. Look for:
  - Displacement: A tooth forced from its normal socket position (intrusion, extrusion)
  - Luxation: Loosened, mobile tooth
  - Avulsion: Tooth knocked out
  - Tooth fractures: Classified as complicated (those involving nerve exposure) and uncomplicated (those involving enamel or dentin)
  - Root fracture: Caused by injury to the tooth root
  - Bite problems: Check for abnormalities in occlusion
  - Pulp exposure: Bleeding from the broken stump of the tooth itself
  - Color change: The whole tooth turning dark from internal bleeding when the tooth is intact
  - Jaw movement: Deviation to one side or pain and limitation on opening

Management

Most minor injuries to the oral soft tissues do not require suturing unless bleeding is a problem. Wound care should consist of irrigating the area with sterile saline and prescribing water-based 0.12% chlorhexidine gluconate mouth rinse for 2 to 3 minutes twice daily. Avoid the alcohol-based rinse because its use may be painful. If it is determined that a child self-injured the inside of the cheek, tongue, or lip after receiving dental local anesthesia, the child should be referred to the dentist who provided the dental treatment (Chi et al, 2008).

Children with avulsed and fractured teeth, those unable to bite normally, and those with jaw injuries should be referred promptly. Left untreated, dental injuries secondary to trauma can lead to tooth abscesses, dental pain, and problems with the eruption of permanent teeth.

- Tooth avulsion. Primary teeth cannot be replanted. If permanent teeth are knocked out, timing is important, and the following instructions can be provided over the phone; the child should be referred to a dentist at the same time:
  - Replant an avulsed clean tooth immediately or within 5 minutes. If the tooth is dirty, rinse it gently in cold milk, saline, or room-temperature water, and then replant it. Do not rub the root surface. If the tooth can be replanted, have the child bite gently on a handkerchief or clean cloth to keep the tooth in place; the dentist will be able to ensure that the tooth is in the right position and stabilized. For children age 8 years or older, prescribe tetracycline (doxycycline) 4.4 mg/kg every 12 hours on day 1, then 2.2 to 4.4 mg/kg/day for 7 days. If the child is under age 8, prescribe Pen VK 500 mg four times daily for 7 days (or 25 to 50 mg/kg/day every 6 hours, not to exceed 500 mg per dose).
  - If unable to immediately replant the tooth, it may be kept several hours in cold milk, saline, or room-temperature

tap water while wrapped in plastic wrap to prevent dehydration. The tooth can also be kept in the child's mouth next to the cheek, being careful that the child does not swallow it. If available, the best transport media are Viaspan or Hanks Balanced Salt Solution. The prognosis for successful reimplantation decreases with time. A tooth that is allowed to dehydrate will not be viable after 1 hour. However, it is worth having a dentist evaluate anyway because there are some interventions that can be taken for a tooth that has been out longer than 60 minutes (McIntyre et al, 2009). The dentist should also x-ray to rule out an alveolar fracture and for placement of a flexible plastic splint to maintain proper tooth position. A follow-up dental visit is also indicated within 7 to 10 days of reimplantation.

- Tooth fracture. If possible, have the patient keep the pieces of permanent incisors and place them in saline or water to prevent drying. Sometimes the dentist can temporarily repair the tooth if the fragment is large enough. Tooth fractures with bleeding from the stump are emergencies. Simple fractures not involving the pulp or nerve tissue are not emergencies, but still may be repaired.

The provider should be alert to the possibility of a closed head injury if severe trauma is reported. See Chapter 13 for a discussion of head injuries after sports participation and return-to-play policies. See Chapter 27 for further discussion of head injuries.

Complications

Trauma not only compromises a previously healthy dentition but also may affect self-esteem and quality of life. In some cases, the traumatized tooth may be asymptomatic and appear to be clinically normal. This tooth can subsequently become darker, which is an important indication that the tooth needs assessment by a dental professional. The tooth can also become spontaneously symptomatic, with the patient reporting cold sensitivity, pain on chewing, or unprovoked pain.

Education and Prevention

It is important to identify and educate children who are at high risk for dental trauma–related injuries. Children and teenagers who participate in sports should be encouraged to wear mouth guards and helmets. Parents and coaches should also encourage youths to remove all intraoral piercings (e.g., tongue and lip rings or studs) while engaging in sports.

Parents, coaches, and physical education teachers should be alerted to the importance of making saline part of first-aid kits to treat tooth avulsions. Parents and caregivers with children who are learning to walk should be instructed on how to childproof their homes. To prevent head/dental trauma in motor vehicle accidents, it is important that children be properly placed in car and booster seats. See Chapter 39 regarding child-restraint system recommendations.

TEMPOROMANDIBULAR JOINT DISORDER
Description and Epidemiology

Temporomandibular joint (TMJ) disorder includes chronic facial pain and mandibular dysfunction. In the past, this disorder was evaluated strictly based on the physical state of the jaws or bite. This led to a great many inappropriate, ineffective, and even dangerous treatments. Today the condition is evaluated within the context of a biopsychosocial model. The affected individual adapts behaviorally to the perceived discomfort or pain by being anxious, depressed, avoiding social interaction, developing other physical symptoms, or by seeking treatment or pharmacologic relief (Dworkin and Drangsholt, 2003). Both the pain and other functional and psychological components need to be assessed (LeResche et al, 2007).

An array of studies suggests that onset of most TMJ disorder is in adolescence with prevalence rates higher for females than males (AAPD, 2010b). A well-designed Swedish study of 28,899 youths 12 to 19 years old found a prevalence of 4.2% with a rate of 6% in girls and 2.7% in boys (Nilsson et al, 2005). Similar rates have been found in children in the U.S.

Clinical Findings

Two clinical symptoms are predictive of TMJ disorder: (1) self-reported facial pain once or more per week associated with limitation in normal ability to open the mouth wide, and (2) pain once a week or more in the temples, face, or jaws (Nilsson et al, 2006). Facial muscles are tender to palpation, often unilaterally, but there is usually no swelling or skin bruising. The individual will be afebrile. Tooth pain, if present, is nonspecific. There may be a deviation to the painful side when the mouth is opened.

Differential Diagnosis

Consider infection of the face or teeth, traumatic injury (fracture of the jaw), myositis, dislocation of the jaw, neoplasm, arthritis, collagen diseases (systemic lupus erythematosus [SLE]), congenital and developmental anomalies of the joint (rare), and capsulitis.

Management

Viewed as a biopsychosocial problem, surgical interventions, particularly changes to the teeth, are inappropriate. Treatment recommendations include avoiding extreme jaw movements, soft diet, muscle relaxation and gentle stretching exercises, application of ice packs, analgesics, and antiinflammatory medication (National Institute of Dental and Craniofacial Research [NIDCR], 2010). Evidence does not support the supposition that chewing gum causes TMJ disorder, but it can exacerbate existing jaw pain in sufferers (University of California–Berkeley, 2009). Previously, expensive plastic guards or splints and similar appliances to reposition the bite were used to treat this problem. However, current treatment recommendations are found to be less expensive and as efficient (Truelove et al, 2006). A guide to self-help treatment is available from NIDCR and can be downloaded from the Internet. Patients who do not respond to the basic recommendations need referral to specialized centers where teams of dentists and psychologists work together. Diagnosis involves assessment of physical findings and both Axis I and II dimensions of the mental state.

Complications

Chronic headaches, otalgia, tinnitus, and lost time from work, school, or activities may result.

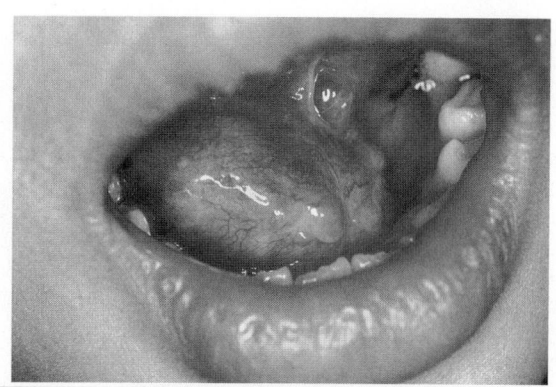

FIGURE 33-10 Ranula of the floor of the mouth. (From Pinkham JR: *Pediatric dentistry: infancy through adolescence,* ed 4, St Louis, 2005, Saunders, p 44.)

GINGIVAL HYPERPLASIA

Gingival hyperplasia is a fibrous enlargement of gingival tissue around the teeth. The enlargement is typically caused by drugs (phenytoin, cyclosporine, nifedipine), hormones, chronic inflammation, leukemia, or heredity. It can be idiopathic. The gingival tissue can be normal, red-blue, or lighter than the surrounding tissue. It may be spongy or firm and dense. The tissue is generally not inflamed, and patients are asymptomatic. Treatment consists of improved oral hygiene and chlorhexidine mouth rinses. In cases in which the overgrowth interferes with chewing, gingivectomy is required.

RANULA

A ranula is a cyst filled with saliva products. It is associated with a major salivary gland in the sublingual area and is caused by lip or cheek biting. A common clinical problem occurring at any age, including infancy, a ranula is evidenced by a large, soft, mucus-containing swelling in the floor of the mouth. The cyst should be excised by an oral surgeon (Fig. 33-10).

MUCOCELE

A mucocele is a salivary gland lesion caused by a blockage of a salivary gland duct. It is most common on the lower lip and has the appearance of a fluid-filled vesicle or a fluctuant nodule with the overlying mucosa normal in color. The patient should be referred to an oral surgeon for surgical excision of the involved tiny accessory salivary gland.

■ Viral Diseases of the Mouth

HERPES STOMATITIS

Herpes gingivostomatitis is a viral disease that results in oral and circumoral ulcers and is caused by herpes simplex virus type 1 (HSV-1) (Fig. 33-11 and Color Plate). It most commonly affects children 6 months to 5 years of age as an initial infection (see also Chapter 36). The classic signs and symptoms of HSV-1 orolabial infection occur in only 10% to 30% of children (Prober, 2008). The clinical findings are described in Chapter 36.

Herpes stomatitis/labialis may be confused with aphthous ulcers (canker sores), ulcerative gingivitis, hand-foot-and

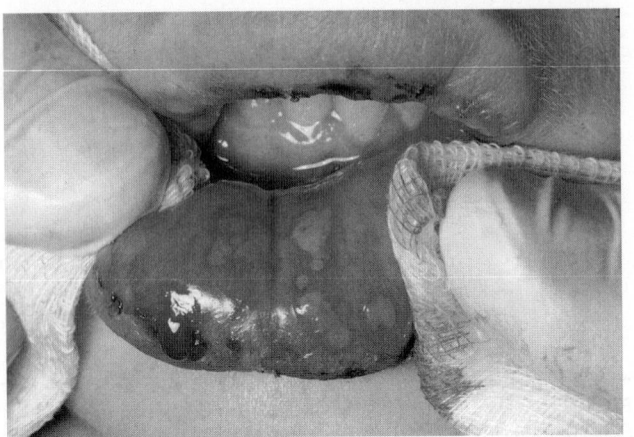

FIGURE 33-11 Herpes stomatitis in an infant. (From Davis J, Peterson D: *Atlas of pediatric dentistry*, Seattle, 2004, University of Washington.)

mouth disease, trauma, herpangina, or chemical burns. Rare conditions that may also cause lesions are neutrophil defects, systemic lupus, Behçet syndrome, and Crohn disease.

Lesions heal without treatment in 7 to 14 days. Supportive therapy is appropriate, such as cold liquids and analgesics. Topical treatment with an equal mixture of diphenhydramine and Maalox may provide symptomatic relief. Antimicrobials are not appropriate. Exclude the child from daycare or school during the drooling phase of the illness. Encourage parents to clean the teeth with a soft toothbrush or cloth. Oral acyclovir is recommended to reduce the degree and length of symptoms if initiated within 72 hours of the onset of the episode (Stanberry, 2007) (see Chapter 36 for dosing information). Topical antiviral agents are not thought to be helpful (Keels and Clements, 2010).

Children are at risk for dehydration. Parents should be instructed to watch for such signs and symptoms and seek medical care in such an event. Careful handwashing should be recommended to the child and the caregivers to prevent autoinoculation or transmission of infection to the eyes.

■ Idiopathic Oral Conditions

APHTHOUS ULCERS

Description and Epidemiology

This is a condition of recurrent, painful oral ulcers (aka canker sores). The etiology is not well understood. Infectious agents, such as *Helicobacter pylori*, HSV-1, or even measles have been implicated in the etiology. Alterations of cell-mediated immunity may be associated with the disease. Emotional and physical stress, local trauma (orthodontic braces, toothbrush abrasion), hormonal factors, and food hypersensitivity have been implicated. Sodium lauryl sulfate in toothpaste has been implicated. Vitamin and mineral deficiencies also can cause recurrent oral aphthae, particularly deficiencies in several B vitamins (1, 2, 6, and 12), iron, folic acid, and zinc. Aphthous ulcers are reported to develop in 20% of the population and are most common in childhood and adolescence (Weiss et al, 2010). There are three forms: minor (the most common), major, and herpetiform.

Clinical Findings

Single or multiple small, shallow mucosal lesions are present on alveolar or buccal mucosa, tongue, soft palate, or the floor of the mouth. The ulcers are surrounded with an erythematous halo and covered by gray, yellow, or white plaques. Minor lesions are less than 10 mm in diameter.

Major lesions (also called Sutton's disease) are generally more than 1 cm in diameter; these may take up to 30 days or more to heal and leave residual scarring. Herpetiform lesions are multiple, clustered, 1 to 2 mm that may coalesce; healing should be complete in about 7 to 10 days. Some individuals may complain of prodromal symptoms, such as tingling or burning (Rizzolo and Sedrak, 2009).

Differential Diagnosis

Consider HSV-1 infection.

Management

The goal of treatment is to decrease the ulcers, relieve pain, and reduce frequency of occurrence. Minor lesions generally resolve spontaneously in 10 to 14 days; they heal without treatment and without scarring. A bland diet and oral analgesics may be appropriate. Vitamin or mineral replacement may prevent recurrence if history suggests a deficiency. Over-the-counter treatments, such as triamcinolone hexacetonide in Orabase paste, fluocinonide gel covered by Orabase paste, or amlexanox 5% oral paste, may be applied four times per day for 3 to 4 days for pain relief and to promote healing. A mild mouthwash, such as sodium bicarbonate dissolved in warm water may provide comfort. Chlorhexidine gluconate mouthwash can reduce the severity of an episode. Thalidomide has been used in severe cases associated with HIV infection (Weiss et al, 2010). Consider additional diagnostic testing should the symptoms and history suggest an infectious agent or gastrointestinal etiology. There are homeopathic and complementary remedies as well (see Chapter 42). Maintaining good oral hygiene is essential.

BENIGN MIGRATORY GLOSSITIS (BMG)

Also known as geographic tongue or erythema migrans, BMG usually presents as asymptomatic, yellowish-white, circular or serpentine-bordered lesions with atrophic red centers varying in intensity. They appear on the anterior two thirds of the dorsum of the tongue (Fig. 33-12). The lesions may heal and reappear on other areas of the tongue. The etiology is unknown, but the result is inflammation affecting the epithelium of the tongue. Approximately 1% to 2.5% of the population is affected, with children and young adults affected more than older individuals (Rozzolo and Sedrak, 2009). Females seem to be affected twice as often as males (Weiss et al, 2010). Occasionally one may experience pain, especially when eating hot or spicy foods. Proposed risk factors for BMG include immunologic factors, hormonal changes, use of oral contraceptives, diabetes mellitus, and stress. Diagnosis is made by appearance; patients can be reassured that the lesions are benign and do not generally require treatment. If treatment is indicated for pain, topical steroids, zinc supplements, and topical anesthetic rinses have been used with varying success (Weiss et al, 2010).

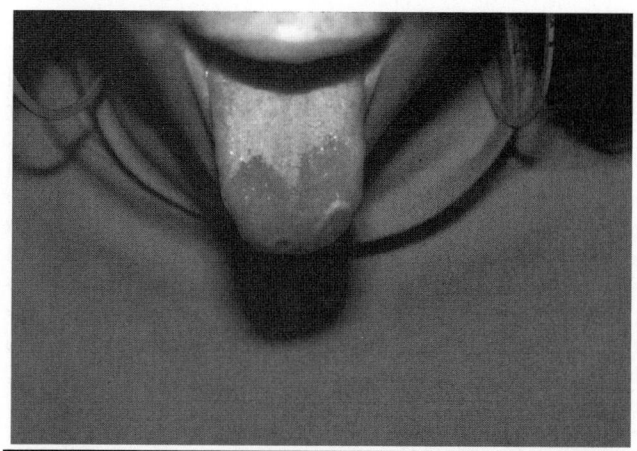

FIGURE 33-12 Benign migratory glossitis/geographic tongue. (From Kliegman RM, Behrman RE, Jenson HB et al: *Nelson textbook of pediatrics*, ed 18, Philadelphia, 2009, Saunders, p 2736.)

HALITOSIS

Halitosis is oral malodor or bad breath. It is primarily associated with poor oral hygiene. It is more common in individuals who are mouth breathers, who suffer from postnasal drip or dry mouth, or who use tobacco products. Encourage proper oral hygiene, including regular brushing, flossing, and dental visits. Provide reassurance and encourage patients to avoid sugar-containing breath mints and other candies that might cause tooth decay or erosion; sugarless gum or mints may be helpful. Patients who have not had their teeth cleaned or an oral examination within the last 6 months should be referred to a dentist. For those with oral dryness, there are bioactive enzyme mouthwashes available over the counter. The patient may also need to be evaluated for systemic disease, sleep apnea, and other airway-related conditions.

MALOCCLUSION

Description and Epidemiology

Dental occlusion is the way the maxillary and the mandibular teeth articulate. From birth to adulthood and beyond, dental occlusion undergoes significant changes. Malocclusions have their basis in hereditary or genetic and/or environmental factors. Prevention of genetic causes for malocclusion is not possible at this time, but the prevention of environmental factors holds much promise. The most current study of malocclusion in the U.S. estimates that 57% to 59% of children younger than 18 years of age need orthodontic treatment for malocclusions; in the U.K. the estimates are 66% of children at 12 years of age. Severe problems related to occlusion and crowding occur in 15% to 20% of children in the U.S. and 33% in the U.K. (Mitchell, 2007; Proffit et al, 1998). Ethnic minorities and the uninsured and underinsured have higher levels of need.

Clinical Findings

The most common malocclusions that may require early diagnosis and interception include an anterior or posterior crossbite or an open bite. Retention of a primary tooth beyond the normal period can deflect the eruption of the permanent successor and lead to a crossbite. Crossbites are classified as follows:

- Anterior crossbite. The most common cause is crowding where one or two teeth are either behind or in front of the teeth in the opposing jaw while the others are in good alignment.
- Posterior crossbite. In the posterior jaw, one or more of the upper teeth is inside the opposing lower tooth. In the upper jaw, the premature loss of a second primary molar in a crowded mouth may result in forward movement of the first permanent molar, forcing the second premolar to erupt palatally.
- Anterior open bite. In the anterior jaw, the front teeth do not touch together when the back teeth are biting. Children with this problem may have a habit of passing their tongues through the space and can have problems speaking or chewing.

In early stages of the mixed dentition period when both primary and permanent teeth are present, a child may have a temporary open bite, usually either a result of the still incomplete eruption of the incisors or a result of mechanical interference from a persistent finger habit (Warren et al, 2005). Sucking habits are normal in infancy, and pacifiers do not normally cause lasting effects. Thumb and finger sucking or long-term use of a pacifier that is not discontinued by the time the permanent teeth erupt may result in an anterior open bite. The upper front teeth will tip and push out. Tongue habits described previously exacerbate the open bite.

Management

Dental health education and improved caries prevention by PCPs and dentists can affect the number of children who develop malocclusion because of the premature loss of primary teeth from necessary extraction of severely decayed teeth. Malocclusion has an important effect on the function and aesthetics of the entire dentition, and can have a lifelong effect on the self-esteem of a child or an adolescent. Most crossbites in the permanent dentition are readily treated by a dentist or orthodontist. A persistent open bite in a school-age or older child is difficult to correct and requires referral to an orthodontic specialist.

DIASTEMA

Spacing issues also affect the dentition. A space between any neighboring two teeth is referred to as a *diastema*. During the mixed dentition stage, when both primary and permanent teeth are present, a midline space between the upper front teeth is normal. If the teeth are not otherwise crowded or malaligned, these spaces usually close by the time the permanent maxillary canines fully erupt, and referral is not needed. Diastemas caused by missing incisors or midline supernumerary tooth or teeth will persist in the permanent dentition stage and require referral.

Another cause of a diastema is a prominent labial frenum, which is the tissue connecting the upper lip to the area of the gums between the front upper teeth. Sometimes the frenum is large and appears to be causing space between the front teeth. Generally the space closes as the jaws grow, and referral is not needed. Unnecessary or premature excision can result in scarring. A prominent labial frenum attachment that persists in the permanent dentition stage may require excision.

ANKYLOGLOSSIA ("TONGUE-TIE")

Ankyloglossia or "tongue-tie" is caused by a short lingual frenum that hinders tongue movement. The frenum may lengthen as the child gets older. Usually no treatment is needed. If the extent of the ankyloglossia is severe, speech may be affected and referral for a surgical correction indicated. In the absence of speech effects, referral can result in unnecessary excision and damage to the gums around the lower teeth.

■ Lifestyle Choices That Affect Dental Health

SMOKELESS TOBACCO: GUM DISEASE AND CANCER

Smokeless tobacco (ST) is a highly addictive substance that is held in the oral cavity, allowing nicotine to enter the bloodstream. Slightly less than 9% of all teenagers nationwide report using this product; its use is more prevalent by rural youth. It is commonly used by individuals who think chewing tobacco is a healthier alternative to smoking cigarettes. Popular cultural events (e.g., baseball) and heroes (e.g., rodeo riders and baseball players) make the habit "look cool." Its popularity has also been attributed to intensive promotion and flavors, being viewed as a way to lose weight, and a way to get nicotine without having to frequent restricted smoking areas (Muscari, 2010). Its use can be detrimental to oral health.

The PCP should examine the posterior buccal vestibule of the lower jaw and the anterior buccal vestibule of the upper jaw. These are the areas where smokeless tobacco is commonly held in the mouth. The intraoral findings of smokeless tobacco include leukoplakia; erythroplakia; gingivitis and gum recession (particularly in the lower jaw); periodontitis; stained teeth; halitosis; and tooth decay, which may be associated with tobacco products that have added sweeteners.

Patients who use tobacco products should be assessed for willingness to undergo tobacco cessation treatments. Results from research studies suggest ways to apply cessation principles in the pediatric patient population (Weinstein and Milgrom, 2006). See Chapter 8 for a discussion of an effective strategy to use with adolescents. Active family involvement in the lives of children can help prevent the start of smokeless tobacco use. If young patients have relatives who use tobacco products, the PCP may need to focus tobacco-cessation efforts on these family members. Complications include lip and oral cancer, gingivitis, gum recession, periodontitis, and stained teeth.

ORAL BODY ART: PIERCING AND INTRAORAL TATTOOS

Studs and other body ornaments pierce the tongue and lower lip. Some patients may also have tattoos on the buccal mucosa of the lips. Tissue around tongue studs may be infected as evidenced by inflammation, swelling, and pain. Some individuals may exhibit inflammation and pain as an allergic response to the metals in the studs or piercings, particularly to nickel. There also may be gum recession or fractures of the lower anterior teeth from metal studs that habitually click against the teeth. Tongues, especially just after stud insertion, are swollen.

The mouth heals quickly, and the inflammatory response should be resolved within 8 to 10 days without treatment.

Swelling beyond this period suggests infection or an allergic response. Infection should be treated with chlorhexidine gluconate mouthwash twice per day for at least 1 week and a broad-spectrum systemic antibiotic, such as penicillin or clindamycin (Jasper et al, 2010). If mouth tissue is infected, the ornament should be removed, at least temporarily. If an allergic reaction to nickel is suspected, have the patient change to gold or silver. Devices that cause chronic allergic reactions should be removed permanently. The patient's immunity to tetanus and hepatitis B should be ensured. Deep neck infection, airway obstruction, bleeding, nerve damage, tooth fracture, and hepatitis have been noted. Systemic infections also have been reported. Adolescents contemplating or who have oral piercings should be counseled about:

- The potential for acquiring an infectious disease
- Using only regulated practitioners
- Ensuring that only sterile equipment and noble metals are used
- Completing a hepatitis B vaccination series before seeking piercing
- The potential damage to the teeth and gums
- Removing studs and piercings during sports

TOOTH WHITENING (BLEACHING)

Description

Patient requests for "whiter and brighter" smiles have resulted in increased demands for tooth whitening. The procedure may be indicated for permanent teeth stained by trauma, fluorosis, tetracycline consumed during tooth development, or colored foods and beverages.

Tooth whitening can involve the use of over-the-counter kits, in-office treatment, or take-home bleaching trays that are customized for each patient. The in-office tooth whitening process involves repeated short-term exposure of teeth to carbamide peroxide (typically in the range of 10% to 38%) until desired results are achieved. Over-the-counter kits include lower concentration carbamide peroxide in trays or hydrogen peroxide in strips. Most are used for 2-week periods. There are also numerous gels, rinses, gums, toothpastes, and paint-on films. Most have been inadequately studied. Higher concentrations of hydrogen peroxide are more effective than lower concentrations.

In all cases, the effect of the treatment is temporary, and the teeth will eventually return to their normal coloring. As far as we know, repeated treatments do not carry great risk for complications, but published aftermarket studies are limited and potentially biased (Hasson et al, 2006). Common side effects associated with tooth whitening include tooth sensitivity and tissue irritation (Donly et al, 2007). The AAPD recommends that tooth bleaching procedures be used judiciously in children and discourages bleaching for children in mixed dentition, when both primary and permanent teeth are present in the mouth (AAPD, 2009d).

Clinical Findings

The most common clinical evidence of tooth bleaching in children and adolescents is a complaint of hypersensitive teeth and gum irritation. In some studies, one third to one half of subjects experienced tooth sensitivity or gingival inflammation or both. There are no studies of these products in children.

Management

Teeth will generally return to their normal sensation, gum status, and color if treatments are not repeated.

Education and Prevention

Health providers can remind parents and caregivers that permanent teeth are naturally darker than primary teeth and in most cases do not need whitening. Unless there are major aesthetic concerns that could affect a child's psychosocial development, tooth whitening should not be undertaken until all permanent teeth have fully erupted. This measure will also prevent shade mismatching that can occur when teeth are whitened during the mixed dentition stage. The potential side effects should be mentioned. The patient or parent should consult with a dental professional.

■ Dental Care of Children With Extra Needs

Children with chronic disease or with congenital or acquired physical and/or mental challenges require extra preventive strategies and individualized dental appointments based upon their particular needs and conditions. Success in treating those children can be enhanced by knowing about particular child's diagnosis and difficulties and about the dental, educational, social, and psychological support systems needed to successfully address the short- and long-term issues.

At-risk children include those with neuropsychological conditions (e.g., mental retardation, autism spectrum); sensory challenges (e.g., blindness, visual impairment, deafness and hearing impairments); musculoskeletal or other structural difficulties (e.g., osteogenesis imperfecta, cerebral palsy, spina bifida, cleft lip/palate, paralysis); and chronic diseases (e.g., asthma, cardiovascular disorders, chronic renal failure, diabetes mellitus, bleeding disorders, malignant disease, and epilepsy). Low birthweight can be associated with structural tooth defects, which can lead to increased risk for tooth decay. Some individuals have a higher incidence of oral disease either because of a systemic problem itself or because of the secondary effects on tooth development, diet, medications, or the inability of caretakers to clean or maintain the teeth. These include the following:

- Diet. A number of conditions, such as congenital heart disease, facial clefts, esophageal defects, generalized hypotonia, muscular dysfunction, or mental retardation involve feeding problems. A child's sucking or chewing problems may lead to meals lasting for an hour or more. Liquid, soft, and high cavity-causing sugary foods are common. Food is often retained in the mouth for a long time before it is swallowed.
- Elimination. Many children with extra needs experience chronic constipation or diarrhea. Sweet remedies, such as dried fruits or sodas and juices, are often used to cure such conditions. Frequent intake of beverages is often recommended for children on medication to prevent kidney failure. To increase hydration, parents often resort to sugar-containing drinks.
- Medications. Long-term use of sweetened medicines or syrups can also present a hazard to dental health. Box 33-3 lists the classes of drugs, such as the antihistamines, that

---

BOX 33-3 Classes and Examples of Drugs Associated with Xerostomia

- Analgesics: NSAIDs, narcotic analgesics
- Antidepressants: fluoxetine, amitriptyline
- Antiemetics: promethazine, metoclopramide
- Antihistamines: diphenhydramine, promethazine
- Antihypertensives: beta-blockers, diuretics, ACE inhibitors
- Antipsychotics: clozapine, chlorpromazine, risperidone

ACE, Angiotensin-converting enzyme; *NSAIDs,* nonsteroidal antiinflammatory drugs.

---

may reduce salivation and thereby increase susceptibility to caries (Lam et al, 2009). Phenytoin commonly causes gingival hyperplasia.
- Cognition. In some children, problems may relate to an inability to understand the meaning behind oral hygiene procedures.
- Muscular function. Hypotonia may influence salivation and cause drooling or chewing problems. Impaired manual dexterity may make it difficult for children to perform preventive oral hygiene routines. Hyperfunction may result in extensive tooth wear as a result of grinding of teeth. This is also seen in some children with mental retardation. Children with feeding tubes face many difficulties.

MANAGEMENT STRATEGIES

The ability of parents to follow recommendations for preventive dental care varies with the difficulties presented by the child's condition. In addition, the ability of parents to take full responsibility over time for the preventive dental care of a child may vary. Therefore, recommendations for professional checkups and preventive services, such as fluoride treatments, should be individualized. If hygiene is poor, preventive treatments need to be provided more often. Counseling parents to maintain good communication involving both medical and dental providers is essential.

The PCP is advised to frequently ask about the status of dental visits and whether routine oral hygiene is both taught to the child and actively supervised in the home and school. In addition, the following topics should be covered:
- Diet. For children with reduced salivary secretion or impaired self-cleaning mechanisms of the oral cavity, parents or caretakers must be especially attentive to the diet. Restrictions in cavity-causing foods are necessary to prevent rampant tooth decay. Chronic use of sweetened medicinal syrups can cause severe decay. If sweetened medicines cannot be replaced by sugar-free alternatives, medicines should be taken at mealtime. Rinsing the mouth and teeth with water after a meal is efficacious if brushing is not feasible. Water or sugar-free beverages should be recommended for drinks between meals.
- Topical fluorides. A child with reduced salivary secretion, impaired muscular function, or with a cavity-causing diet may need an intense fluoride program in addition to careful oral hygiene. PCPs can apply 5% sodium fluoride topical varnish or prescribe a fluoride rinse, gel, or high-fluoride (1.1% sodium fluoride) toothpaste for home use. Carefully monitor the teeth of these patients and make prompt referrals when problems are noted.

- Topical iodine. The teeth and gums can be painted with topical polyvinylpyrrolidone iodine (PVP-iodine) once every 4 to 6 months. There is evidence that topical 10% povidone-iodine suppresses tooth decay–causing flora without major changes in the overall flora (Tut and Milgrom, 2010; Zhan et al, 2006). Children who have had major dental treatment under general anesthesia because of extensive dental caries are obvious candidates for repeated iodine treatments (Berkowitz et al, 2009). Iodine can be painted on the teeth at the same visit in which fluoride varnish is applied with the iodine wiped off with gauze before applying the varnish. The PCP can do this treatment if dental services are lacking.

- Chemical plaque control. When oral hygiene is difficult to perform, chemical plaque control with a 0.12% chlorhexidine gluconate mouth rinse is recommended (Milgrom and Weinstein, 2001). Such rinses can be used daily. They are also recommended for use in children with hemophilia, cardiac disease, or immunodeficiency 7 to 10 days prior to dental procedures in order to minimize bleeding or bacteremia. Gels and toothpastes with chlorhexidine are available outside the U.S.; compounding pharmacists can be asked to create a facsimile within the U.S.

Genitourinary Disorders

NAN M. GAYLORD AND ANN M. PETERSEN-SMITH

The genitourinary system is responsible for maintaining an optimal environment for metabolism, including regulation of water and electrolytes (sodium, potassium, chloride, calcium, phosphate, and magnesium); excretion of waste products (urea, creatinine, poisons, and drugs); acid-base regulation; and hormonal secretion (vitamin D, renin, erythropoietin, and prostaglandins). The male system has both reproductive and excretory functions. Genitourinary problems in children and adolescents range from commonly occurring, easily treated diseases to significant congenital or acquired conditions. Pediatric primary care providers play a significant role in working with children, adolescents, and families to identify problems, manage disorders, maintain optimal function, and provide education and support related to genitourinary function. First-line assessment and management, provision of continuity of care, and referral to and collaboration with pediatric urologists and nephrologists are important components of patient management.

Discussion of related functional health problems—enuresis and dysfunctional voiding—is included in Chapter 12.

■ Standards of Care

The U.S. Preventive Services Task Force (USPSTF) (2009) has concluded that screening for asymptomatic bacteriuria is unnecessary at any age. A urine dipstick is a poor screening test for chronic kidney disease and a cost-ineffective procedure in pediatric primary care (Sekhar et al, 2010). The American Academy of Pediatrics (AAP Committee on Practice and Ambulatory Care, 2007) and the *Bright Futures Practice Guidelines* recommend that a complete urinalysis be done at 5 years of age and once during adolescence (Hagan et al, 2008).

Hypertension is frequently renal in origin in children. Blood pressure (BP) screening is recommended by the AAP Committee on Practice and Ambulatory Care (2007) and *Bright Futures* (Hagan et al, 2008) at every recommended preventive health care visit beginning at 3 years of age. The management and treatment of hypertension is discussed in Chapter 30.

■ Anatomy and Physiology

The renal system is composed of two kidneys, two ureters, a bladder, and a urethra. The kidneys are positioned posteriorly on the abdominal wall. The main features of the kidney are the cortex, the medulla, and the collecting system. The renal medulla and nephrons are present at birth, but the peripheral tubules are small and immature. By adolescence, the kidneys are of adult size and weight. The ureters are muscular tubes that convey urine from the kidneys to the bladder by peristaltic contractions. The bladder is a muscular reservoir to collect the urine. It lies close to the anterior abdominal wall in early childhood. With growth it descends into the pelvis and changes shape from cylindrical to pyramidal. As the bladder nears its capacity, nerve signals are transmitted to the brain to indicate that urination is required. When urination occurs, the sphincter between the bladder and urethra opens and contractions of the bladder create pressure to force urine out the urethral meatus. The male urethra is significantly longer than the female's as it leaves the bladder in the lower pelvis, passes through the prostate with openings for the release of bulbourethral gland fluids and semen with sexual activity, and extends the full length of the penile shaft. The urethral meatus is normally located on the tip of the glans in the male. In the female, the urethra descends from the bladder and exits the body inside the labia minora, midline, just posterior to the clitoris.

Physiologically the kidneys serve to filter, clear, reabsorb, and secrete substances essential to the body's metabolism. The urinary system begins forming and excreting urine at 3 months of gestational age. Glomerular filtration and renal blood flow begin to increase at birth and become stable by 1 to 2 years of age. In infants, total extracellular fluid volume is significantly greater than that of adults, and fluid composition tends to have a lower bicarbonate concentration. Normal urine excretion is 1.5 to 3 mL/kg/hr. The kidneys are still maturing throughout infancy, although all measurable variables of kidney function approach adult values between 6 and 12 months of life.

■ Pathophysiology and Defense Mechanisms

Problems in the urinary system can occur at any point in the system from the kidneys to the urethral meatus. If the kidneys and ureters are involved, the disease is considered to be in the upper tract; if the problem is in the bladder, urethra, or meatus, it is considered a disease of the lower urinary tract. These differentiations can be difficult because frequently disease in one part of the system affects the entire system. Additionally, disease can be relatively silent in clinical presentation or noticeably problematic at any age. The main mechanisms of disorders can be classified as follows: infection, inflammatory response, congenital malformation or condition, and abnormalities acquired from injury, infection, or malfunction within the system.

The urinary tract is normally a sterile system. The mucosal lining of the bladder serves as the first line of defense and inhibits bacterial growth and adherence. The acid pH of the urine also protects the urinary system by inhibiting bacterial growth. Finally, actual flow of urine out of the bladder provides mechanical defense by its flushing action. If these defenses are compromised, the body initiates an inflammatory response within the urinary system.

■ Assessment of the Genitourinary System

HISTORY

- History of the present illness
  - Onset and pattern of symptoms
  - Fever, abdominal pain, or both
  - Preceding injury or illness, especially streptococcal infection
  - Vomiting
  - Voiding pattern: Stream force and direction, any dribbling or discharge
  - Color, odor, frequency, and volume of urine, dysuria, urgency; enuresis, or incontinence
  - Diarrhea or chronic constipation
  - Sexual activity or abuse
- Family history
  - Any familial history of renal disease, deafness, high BP, structural abnormalities, or syndromes involving the genitourinary system
- Past history of urinary tract infection (UTI), hematuria, proteinuria, syndrome associated with genitourinary abnormality, or any other related finding

PHYSICAL EXAMINATION

- Growth parameters—failure to thrive (FTT) can be associated with UTI, renal tubular acidosis (RTA), and chronic renal failure in infants. Unusual weight gain can be associated with nephrotic syndrome or acute renal failure
- BP—often elevated with nephritis and nephrotic syndrome
- Edema, pallor, dehydration
- Ear position and formation—if low-set or abnormal, may have concurrent renal involvement
- Abdominal masses, ascites, flank or suprapubic tenderness
- Costovertebral tenderness
- External genitalia abnormalities
- Other unusual facial features associated with syndrome with related renal disease

DIAGNOSTIC STUDIES

Diagnostic studies are ordered as indicated. The proper collection, transport, and storage of urine are essential to obtain accurate results. Most tests on urine, unless otherwise indicated, are best done on a first morning void. A second morning void, collected before the ingestion of large amounts of fluid, is recommended for microscopic examination. This second void collects fresh urine and increases the likelihood of seeing cellular casts, which can dissolve within 10 to 30 minutes. Urine should be evaluated within 30 minutes and, if stored, kept below 39.2° F (4° C), but not overnight unless in a special preservative (e.g., boric acid).

The following should be noted on urinalysis (UA):

- *Physical characteristics.* Color, clarity, odor, specific gravity, and osmolality are noted.
  - Specific gravity is a measure of hydration and renal concentration ability and varies from 1.003 to 1.030. A random first-voided urine specimen specific gravity of 1.023 or more indicates intact renal concentrating ability. Urine with a specific gravity greater than 1.020 is considered concentrated.
- *Chemical characteristics.* Urine dipsticks are available, are among the waived tests by the Clinical Laboratory Improvement Amendment (CLIA), and are widely used to determine pH, specific gravity, glucose, ketones, protein, bile pigments, hemoglobin, nitrites, and leukocyte esterase. For correct results, strips must remain in their original containers and not be exposed to moisture, light, cold, or heat until used. Urine must be fresh, warmed to room temperature if refrigerated, and read at correct time intervals for each test strip (Table 34-1).
  - Urine pH can vary from 4.6 to 8 and is reflective of the body's ability to maintain acid-base balance.
  - A dipstick positive for blood indicates the presence of hemoglobin. Intact erythrocytes cause spotty changes on the dipstick, whereas free hemoglobin or myoglobin causes uniform changes of color.
  - Leukocyte esterase indicates white blood cells (WBCs) in the urine and, if positive, warrants further investigation.
  - Nitrites: The nitrite test on the dipstick is an indirect measure of bacteria in the urine. Common urinary pathogens contain enzymes that reduce nitrate in urine to nitrite. However, the urine must usually be in the bladder at least 4 hours to show accurate results. Leukocyte esterase and nitrite dipsticks are not reliable in children younger than 3 years of age so a negative dipstick does not rule out a UTI (Hutchings and Jadresic, 2010). A urine culture should be done on any urine sample positive for nitrites or leukocyte esterase, if the child has symptoms of UTI, if the risk criteria as described in section of UTIs is met, or if the child has a high fever without a source. The combination of leukocyte esterase and nitrites is highly predictive of a positive urine culture (Quigley, 2009). Conversely, urine that is negative for leukocyte esterase and nitrites can be used to reasonably rule out a UTI (Cataldi et al, 2010).
- *Microscopic examination of urine.* Urine can be spun by centrifuge and the sediment examined, or it can be examined without being spun. When evaluating results, consideration must be given to which method of collection was used. Urine should be examined under the microscope for red blood cells (RBCs), WBCs, bacteria, casts, and crystals. Microscopic examination of a fresh specimen is essential if blood or protein is found on the dipstick or urinary tract symptoms are present.

TABLE 34-1 Chemical Characteristics of Urine

Constituent	Positives Indicate	False Positives Caused By	False Negatives Caused By
Glucose	Metabolic problem (e.g., diabetes), recent high glucose intake, oral corticosteroids, galactosemia	Antibiotics, delay in reading, myoglobin, oxidizing contaminants	Ascorbic acid intake, ketones, high specific gravity
Ketones	Dehydration, starvation, strenuous exercise, stress, fever, metabolic problems (e.g., diabetes)		If urine left standing, acetone evaporates
Protein	Renal disease, orthostatic proteinuria	Exercise, fever, dehydration, alkaline or concentrated urine (specific gravity >1.02), semi-synthetic penicillin, oxidizing, cleansing agents	Dilute or acidic urine
Blood (hemoglobin)	If concurrent microscopic examination is negative for RBCs: Free hemoglobin secondary to chemicals, illness, or drugs; myoglobin secondary to burns, muscle trauma, physical child abuse, myositis, strenuous exercise If concurrent microscopic examination is positive for RBCs: Renal problems	Menses, oxidizing cleansing agents, dilute urine	Ascorbic acid
Nitrite	Bacteria causing UTI	Rare	Common; urine should be in bladder at least 4 hours
Leukocyte esterase	Pyuria (WBCs in urine); inflammation from irritation or infection of vulva, vagina, or urethra; inflammation of bladder or kidneys with or without infection	Oxidizing agents	Immunocompromised
Urobilinogen	Hemolytic disease; hepatic disease	Rare	Rare
Bilirubin	Hepatic disease; biliary obstruction	Rare	Rare

RBCs, Red blood cells; *UTI,* urinary tract infection; *WBCs,* white blood cells.

○ RBCs. The number of RBCs per high-power field (hpf) that are thought to be abnormal varies; in general more than 2 to 5/hpf (×40) in unspun urine or more than 2 to 10/hpf in spun urine is thought to be abnormal (Elder, 2007d) (Fig. 34-1). If cells are dysmorphic, the origin of the blood is most likely the kidney.

○ WBCs. Fewer than 2 WBCs/hpf should be seen. More than 10 WBCs often indicates an infection (Fig. 34-2).

○ Bacteria. Leukocytes seen in unspun urine are associated with bacterial colony counts of greater than 100,000 (Fig. 34-3).

○ Casts. RBCs, hyaline, waxy, epithelial, leukocyte, or fatty casts are seen in various disease states (Fig. 34-4).

○ Crystals, if amorphous, are not unusual. Calcium oxalate, cystine, tyrosine, leucine, cholesterol, or sulfa crystals are abnormal.

Depending on the results of the UA and/or clinical symptoms, other tests may be indicated, including:

• *Gram stain.* A Gram stain of the urine can be helpful in identifying organisms when examining urine under the microscope. Greater than 10 WBCs/hpf and bacteria on the Gram stain are highly predictive of a UTI, and a urine culture should be performed (Quigley, 2009).

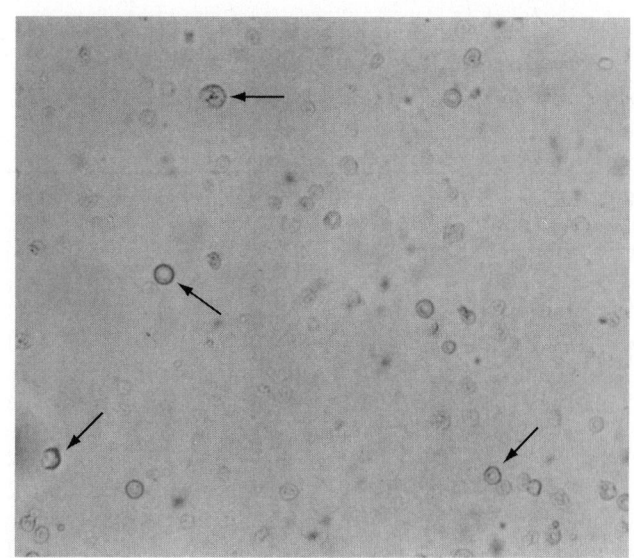

FIGURE 34-1 Red blood cells (RBCs) may originate from any part of the renal system. The presence of large numbers of RBCs suggests a pathologic condition. (From Graff SL: *A handbook of routine urinalysis,* Philadelphia, 1983, Lippincott.)

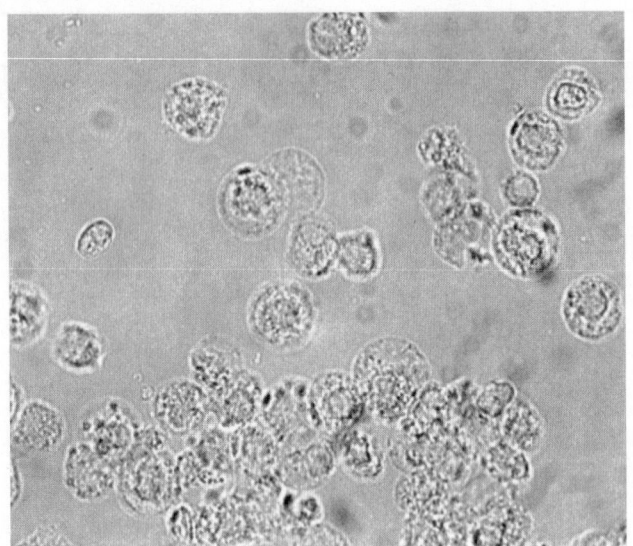

FIGURE 34-2 White blood cells (WBCs) in the urine (pyuria) may originate from any part of the renal system. The presence of more than 5 WBCs per high-power field (hpf) suggests a pathologic condition. (From Graff SL: *A handbook of routine urinalysis*, Philadelphia, 1983, Lippincott.)

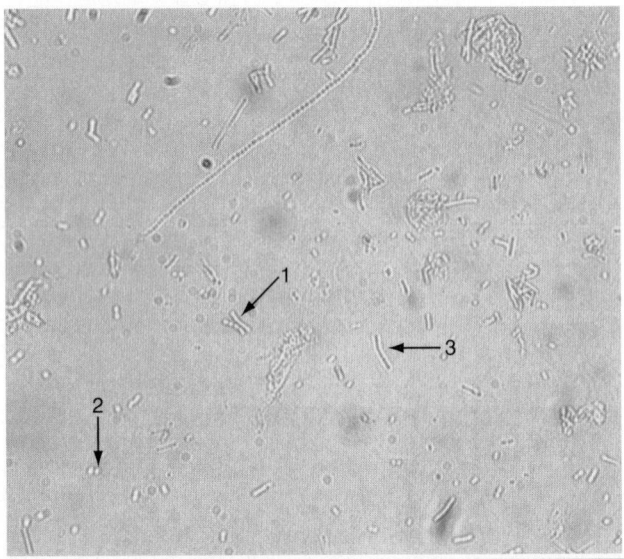

FIGURE 34-3 Bacteria (rods *[1]*, cocci *[2]*, and chains *[3]*) (×500). (From Graff SL: *A handbook of routine urinalysis*, Philadelphia, 1983, Lippincott.)

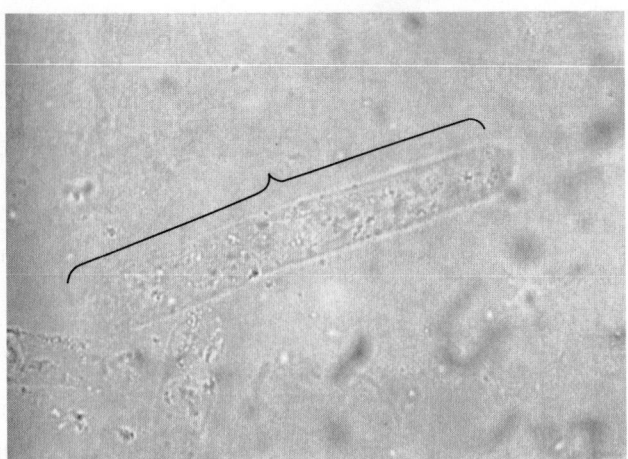

FIGURE 34-4 Hyaline casts. Viewed with an 80A filter (×400). (From Graff SL: *A handbook of routine urinalysis*, Philadelphia, 1983, Lippincott.)

- *Urine culture and sensitivities.* Culture remains the gold standard for diagnosing and treating UTIs. Urine culture can be done by standard culture methods or with a dipslide incubated overnight at room temperature. Urine should be cultured immediately but may be refrigerated for up to 24 hours before plating. Urine specimens unrefrigerated for 2 hours or more are subject to bacterial overgrowth, change in pH, and dissolution of RBC and WBC casts. Bacterial identification and sensitivities need only be performed in complicated or nonresponsive cases.
  - Dipslides with more than 100,000 colony forming units (CFUs) indicate UTI (Quigley, 2009).
  - Urine cultures with any growth of bacteria on a suprapubic aspiration or more than 100,000 CFUs on a voided or catheterized specimen indicate UTI.
- *Urethral swabs.* Either urethral swabs (insertion of the specified sterile swab 1 to 2 cm into the urethral opening with a slow gentle twisting action on removal) or vaginal swabs are accurate methods of culture acquisition for diagnosis of *Neisseria gonorrhoeae* and *Chlamydia trachomatis* and are the only diagnostic methods available in some areas of practice. The culture media are specific for each of those organisms. This method of specimen collection for culture, however, is being replaced with screening tests using a urine nucleic acid amplification test (NAAT) to detect these organisms (AAP, 2009). If the urine test for these organisms is available, the specimen should only be between 10 and 20 mL of the first-catch urine with no cleansing of the perineum or penis. See Chapter 35 for more information.
- *A 24-hour urine collection.* Collecting a 24-hour sample of urine is done to determine calcium excretion, the calcium-creatinine ratio, and quantification of protein.
- *Blood work*
  - Serum or blood urea nitrogen (BUN) estimates the urea concentration in serum or blood and is a measure of toxic metabolites that can cause uremic syndrome.
  - Serum creatinine in combination with creatinine clearance is used to estimate the glomerular filtration rate (GFR) or kidney function.
  - Serum electrolytes and acid-base status can detect renal tubular abnormalities.
  - Serum procalcitonin level of more than 0.5 ng/mL is an accurate and reliable biological marker for renal involvement during a febrile urinary tract infection, pyelonephritis, and renal scarring and may be useful in the clinical diagnosis and treatment of UTIs (Bressan et al, 2009; Cataldi et al, 2010).
- *Ultrasonography* of the renal system provides noninvasive structural information.
- *Voiding urosonography (VUS)* using a second-generation contrast agent is a safe, sensitive, and radiation-free method for detecting and grading vesicoureteral reflux (VUR) and

has been shown to be superior to voiding cystourethrogram (Kis et al, 2010).

- *Dimercaptosuccinic acid (DMSA)* scanning is the most sensitive tool for detecting acute pyelonephritis and renal scarring and should be considered in a young child with febrile UTI (Feld and Mattoo, 2010; Lee et al, 2009). Combined with renal ultrasound scanning, DMSA scanning has high sensitivity for detecting VUR. However, alone the DMSA provides limited information regarding VUR (Fouzas et al, 2010).
- *Voiding cystourethrogram (VCUG).* There is controversy related to the indications for VCUG in children with UTI. According to Lee and colleagues (2009), a VCUG is only indicated if there is an abnormal DMSA scan and voiding urosonography or there is recurrent infection. However, Fouzas and colleagues (2010) suggest that DMSA scanning has limited ability to identify VUR and should not replace VCUG. Feld and Mattoo (2010) suggest that VCUG is the gold standard for diagnosing VUR and should be done as soon as the urine is sterile.

◼ Management Strategies

EDUCATION AND COUNSELING

Education and counseling are essential components in the management of genitourinary tract disorders. Parents and children must be informed about the pathologic condition, etiology, treatment, prevention strategies, and prognosis with and without treatment. A plan of care that the family and care provider are comfortable with must be decided on and initiated. Urinary problems can begin in the neonatal period or occur any time during childhood or adolescence. They vary in severity, chronicity, and disability. The primary care provider must modify appropriate strategies for each individual situation.

MEDICATION, DIET, AND ACTIVITY

Depending on the diagnosis, medications can include antibiotics and steroids. Diet and activity may need to be modified in some chronic renal conditions. These modifications are usually carried out in consultation with appropriate specialists.

REFERRAL

Referral to a pediatric urologist, nephrologist, or surgeon may be required. When a referral is made, the primary care provider retains the essential role of serving as case manager for the child and providing continuity of care over time. The primary care provider is often the one whom the family knows best and is most comfortable with when discussing concerns, potential plans, and long-term management.

◼ Genitourinary Tract Disorders

URINARY TRACT INFECTION AND PYELONEPHRITIS

Description

There are three kinds of UTI in children: asymptomatic bacteriuria, cystitis, and pyelonephritis. Young children may have limited or unusual symptoms; therefore, a high degree of

suspicion must be maintained to diagnose UTI. Inflammation and infection can occur at any point in the urinary tract, so a UTI must be identified according to location. Asymptomatic *bacteriuria* is bacteria in the urine without other symptoms and is benign and does not cause renal injury. *Cystitis* is an infection of the bladder that produces lower tract symptoms but does not cause fever or renal injury (Elder, 2007d). *Pyelonephritis* is the most severe type of UTI involving the renal parenchyma or kidneys and must be readily identified and treated because of the potential irreversible renal damage that can occur. Clinical signs thought to be consistent with pyelonephritis include fever, irritability, and vomiting in an infant and urinary symptoms associated with fever, bacteriuria, vomiting, and renal tenderness. It is the most common cause of serious bacterial infection in infants younger than 24 months of age with fever without a focus (Elder, 2007d). A *complicated UTI* is defined as a UTI with fever, toxicity, and dehydration or a UTI occurring in a child younger than 3 to 6 months of age. The UTI may be classified based on its association with other structural or functional abnormality, such as VUR, obstruction, dysfunctional voiding, or pregnancy. Additionally, a UTI must be identified as a first occurrence, recurrent (within 2 weeks with the same organism or any reinfection with a different organism), or chronic (ongoing, unresolved, often caused by a structural abnormality or resistant organism). Finally, age and gender of the pediatric patient are important factors in determining the method of evaluation and the course of treatment.

Epidemiology

The organism most commonly associated with UTI is *Escherichia coli* (70%), although other organisms, such as *Enterobacter, Klebsiella, Pseudomonas,* and *Proteus* can be found. UTI secondary to group B streptococcus is more common in neonates. Several factors are believed to contribute to the etiology of UTIs. Most UTIs are thought to be ascending (i.e., the infection begins with colonization of the urethral area and ascends the urinary tract). If the infection progresses to the kidney, intrarenal reflux deep into the kidneys can lead to scarring. However, the most important risk factor for the development of pyelonephritis in children is VUR, which can be detected in 10% to 45% of young children who have symptomatic UTIs. Furthermore, reflux of infected urine from the bladder increases the risk of pyelonephritis. This damage to the kidney occurs in the composite papillae, which have wide and gaping openings allowing intrarenal reflux. The composite papillae are located in the upper and lower poles of the kidney, which is the usual site of scarring. Simple papillae have angled, slitlike openings that resist intrarenal reflux (Fig. 34-5).

Host resistance factors and bacterial virulence factors are also important in the etiology of UTIs. Host resistance factors include the presence of a structural abnormality or dysplasia (such as VUR, obstruction, or any other anatomic defect) or the presence of functional abnormalities (such as dysfunctional voiding or constipation). Other factors affecting resistance include female gender (having a short urethra), poor hygiene, irritation, sexual activity or sexual abuse, and pinworms.

Several bacterial factors are known, but the two most important ones are adherence and virulence of the bacteria. Bacteria that have fimbriae or pili are able to anchor or adhere to the surface of the bladder mucosa. This adherence allows the bacteria to resist the bladder's defensive cleansing flow of urine and

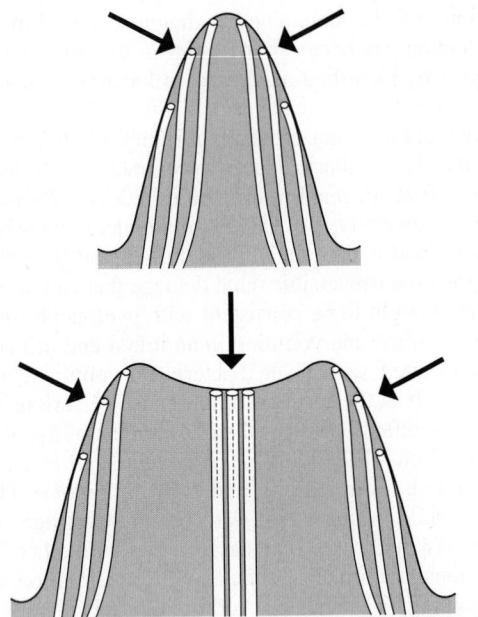

FIGURE 34-5 Most renal papillae are conical, with papillary ducts that open obliquely into the renal pelvis *(top)*. These do not allow intrarenal reflux. But some kidneys have compound papillae, formed by the fusion of conical papillae *(bottom)*. These have papillary ducts with gaping openings at right angles to urine flow and do permit intrarenal reflux. (From Ransley PG: Intrarenal reflux: anatomical, dynamic and radiological studies-part I, *Urol Res* 5:61-69, 1977.)

causes tissue inflammation and cell damage. Adherence may also play a role in bacteria ascending the urinary tract. Virulence refers to the toxicity of substances released by bacteria. The greater the virulence, the greater the damage to the urinary tract. Both of these factors enhance colonization of the urinary tract and aid in the persistence and effect of the bacteria.

The risk of UTI in infants 2-24 months of age is about 5%. The incidence in females is more than twice that of males (2.27%); uncircumsized boys have a rate 4 to 20 times greater than circumsized boys (AAP, 2011). There is a greater frequency in premature and low-birthweight infants. Females older than 12 months of age have 2.1%

prevalence; after the first year of life, it is also more common to find a UTI in females than in males with an overall incidence of 3% to 5% in girls and 1% in boys (Elder, 2007d). Ten percent of girls and 3% of boys will have a UTI by 16 years of age (Hutchings and Jadresic, 2010). The incidence of UTI is often increased in adolescent girls as they become sexually active. Recurrence is common, often within the first year after the initial infection.

Clinical Findings

History. The following information should be obtained:
- Family history of VUR, recurrent UTI, or other kidney problems
- Prenatally diagnosed renal abnormality
- Previous infection: Request records from the evaluation of past infections and diagnostic studies performed
- Circumcision
- Risk factors for infants 2-24 months of age with no other source of infection (AAP, 2011)
  - Female—white race, age <12 months, temperature ≥39°C, fever ≥2 days
  - Male—nonblack race, temperature ≥39°C, fever >24 hours
- Hygiene habits: Wiping front to back
- Voiding patterns: Frequency, abnormal stream, complete emptying, dribbling, and enuresis
- Constipation, perianal itching (pinworms)
- Irritants such as nylon underwear or clothing (spandex, tight pants or shorts that rub); bubble bath
- High blood pressure
- Sexual activity or sexual abuse
- Other infection: Pinworms, diaper rash

Physical Examination. See Table 34-2 for age-related symptoms.
- General appearance (toxic appearing?)
- Vital signs: Temperature, blood pressure
- Growth parameters: Growth may be decreased with chronic UTI or renal insufficiency, especially in infants
- Flank pain or tenderness in the costovertebral angle
- Abdominal examination: Suprapubic tenderness, bladder distention or a flank mass (obstructive signs), mass from fecal impaction

TABLE 34-2	Clinical Findings of Urinary Tract Infection in Children of Various Ages		
Neonates	**Infants**	**Toddlers and Preschoolers**	**School-Age Children and Adolescents**
Jaundice	Malaise, irritability	Altered voiding pattern	"Classic dysuria" with frequency, urgency, and discomfort
Hypothermia	Difficulty feeding	Malodor	
Failure to thrive	Poor weight gain	Abdominal/flank pain*	Malodor
Sepsis	Fever*	Enuresis	Enuresis
Vomiting or diarrhea	Vomiting or diarrhea	Vomiting or diarrhea*	Abdominal/flank pain*
Cyanosis	Malodor	Malaise	Fever/chills*
Abdominal distention	Dribbling	Fever*	Vomiting or diarrhea*
Lethargy	Abdominal pain/colic	Diaper rash	Malaise

*Findings especially likely with pyelonephritis.

- Genitalia: Vaginal erythema, edema, irritation, or discharge; labial adhesions; uncircumcised male, urethral ballooning; weak, dribbling, threadlike stream
- Neurologic examination (if voiding is dysfunctional): Perineal sensation, lower extremity reflexes, sacral dimpling, or cutaneous abnormality

Diagnostic Studies. The method used to collect urine has an effect on the interpretation of results. It is acceptable to collect urine for urinalysis only from a non–toilet-trained child by using a sterile, adhesive bag carefully place over well cleaned genitals. If the bagged urine results in a positive leukocyte esterase or nitrite test, a child younger than 24 months of age has risk factors, or the patient is symptomatic additional urine should be collected by sterile catheterization or suprapubic aspiration. The National Collaborating Center for Women's and Children's Health (2007) recommends that prior to suprapubic tap an ultrasound should be used to confirm urine in the bladder. Older children, who can void on command, should be able to obtain a clean-catch void. Having the female child sit backward on the toilet separates the labia and decreases contamination. See the diagnostic studies section earlier in this chapter for other pertinent information.

- UA should be used only to raise or lower suspicion. Suspicious findings include foul odor, cloudiness, nitrites, leukocytes, alkaline pH, proteinuria, hematuria, pyuria, and bacteriuria.
  - Nitrite chemical tests are reliable on urine specimens when gram-negative bacteria are present and when the urine has been in the bladder for 4 hours or longer. False-positive results are rare, whereas false-negative results are common.
  - Leukocyte esterase chemical tests detect pyuria, but pyuria may arise from causes other than UTI.
- Microscopic evaluation of uncentrifuged urine is helpful if bacteria are seen.
- Urine culture by standard culture methods or by dipslide is essential to confirm the diagnosis. See Table 34-3 for evaluation of culture results.
- Gram stain is helpful if bacteria are identified.
- Bacterial identification and determination of sensitivities are necessary in patients who appear toxic or could have pyelonephritis, have relapses or recurrent UTI, or are nonresponsive to medication.
- Complete blood count (CBC) (elevated WBC count), erythrocyte sedimentation rate (ESR), C-reactive protein (CRP), BUN, and creatinine should be done if the child is less than 1 year of age, appears ill, or if pyelonephritis is suspected.
- Serum procalcitonin level of more than 0.5 ng/mL is an accurate and reliable biologic marker for renal involvement during a febrile urinary tract infection, pyelonephritis, and with renal scarring, so it may be useful in the clinical diagnosis and treatment of UTIs (Bressan et al, 2009; Cataldi et al, 2010).
- Blood culture should be done if sepsis is suspected or if the young child is unimmunized (see Chapter 23).

Differential Diagnosis

The differential diagnosis includes urethritis, vaginitis, viral cystitis, foreign body, sexual abuse, dysfunctional voiding, appendicitis, pelvic abscess, and pelvic inflammatory disease. Any child who has acute fever without a focus, FTT, chronic diarrhea, or recurrent abdominal pain should be evaluated for UTI.

Management

Goals of treatment are to quickly identify the extent and level of infection; to treat appropriately to eradicate infection; to provide symptomatic relief; to find and correct anatomic or functional abnormalities; and to prevent recurrence and new or progressive renal damage (AAP, 2007). When deciding on a treatment plan, the child's age, sex, symptoms, the suspected location of the UTI and antibiotic resistance patterns in the community must be considered. Figure 34-6 outlines treatment of UTI in the child.

Infants 2-24 months of age. To diagnose UTI the child should have both a urinalysis suggesting infection (positive leukocyte and/or nitrite tests) and urine culture from a sterile catheterization or SPA with at least 50,000 cfu/ml. Risk factors have been identified to help steer management. (See AAP, 2011.)

Asymptomatic bacteriuria. If there is an absence of leukocytes on urinalysis, no treatment is indicated.

Uncomplicated cystitis. There is no agreement on the most effective antimicrobial agent or dosage for treating a UTI (Fitzgerald et al, 2010). Some authorities believe that short-term antibiotics can be just as effective in treating bladder infections as standard 7- to 10-day dosing with no increased risk of recurrence (Michael et al, 2003). However, until further studies of efficacy are done in the pediatric population, short-term antibiotics are to be used with caution (Sobel and Kaye, 2009). Children 2-24 months should have

TABLE 34-3	Criteria for Diagnosis of Urinary Tract Infections	
Method of Collection	**Colony Count (Pure Culture)**	**Probability of Infection (%)**
Suprapubic aspiration	Any organism	>99
Catheterization	>10,000	95
	≥10,000 to 100,000	Infection likely, especially if obstruction or if voids frequently
	1000 to <10,000 single organism	Suspicious, repeat
	<1000	Infection unlikely
Clean Voided		
Boy	>10,000 single organism	Infection likely
Girl	Three specimens, >10,000	95
	Two specimens, >100,000	90
	One specimen, >100,000	80
	50,000 to 100,000	Suspicious, infection possible, repeat
	10,000 to 50,000	Suspicious, if symptomatic, repeat
	10,000 to 50,000	Infection unlikely if asymptomatic
	<10,000	Infection unlikely

From Tan JM: Nephrology. In Custer JW, Rau RE: *The Harriet Lane handbook*, ed 18, Philadelphia, 2009, Mosby.

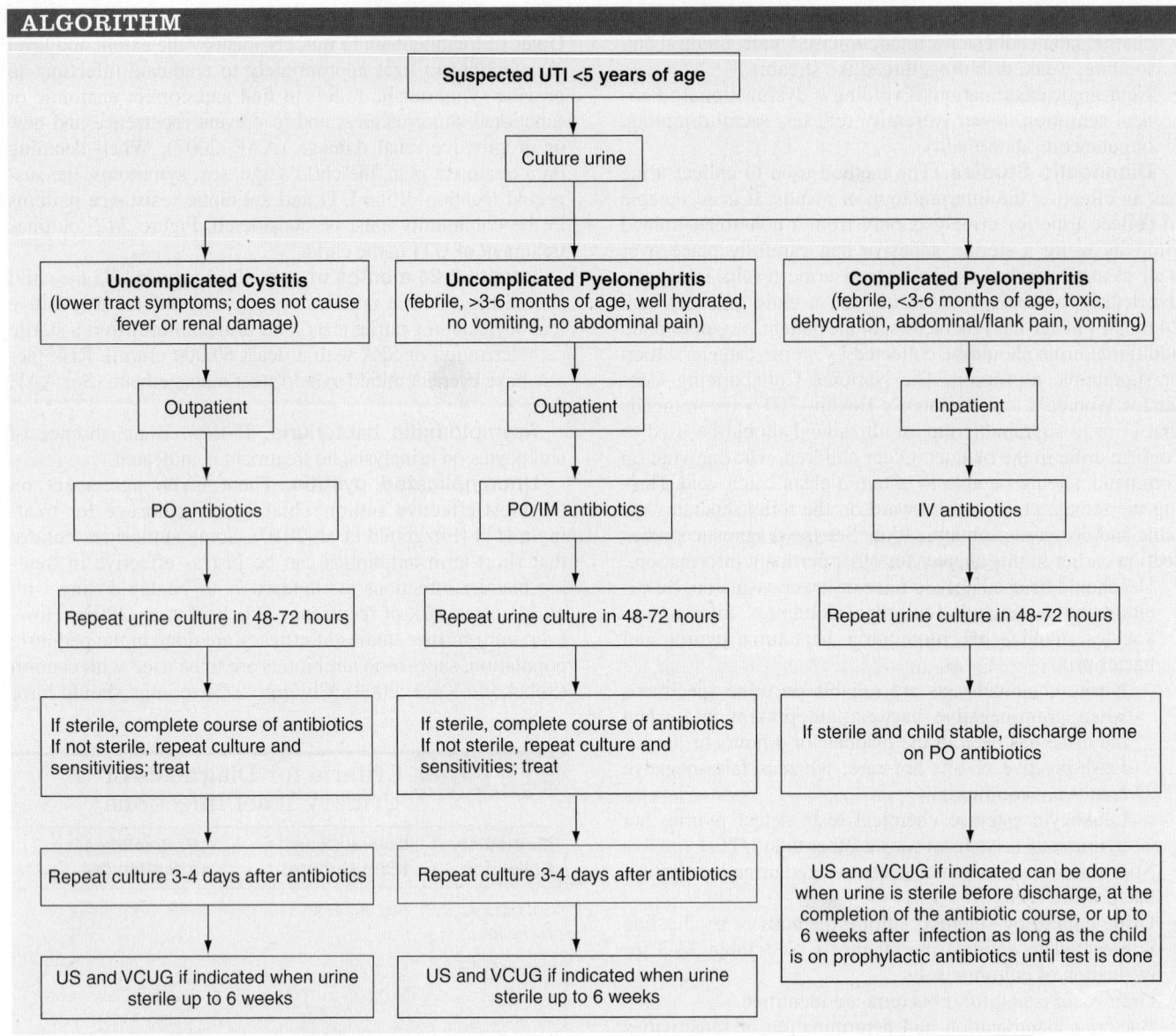

FIGURE 34-6 Suspected urinary tract infection (UTI) less than 5 years of age.

7-14 days of antibiotics. Specific recommendations for the febrile child can be found in the AAP Guideline (AAP, 2011). Choice of antibiotic should be made based on culture and sensitivity results and regional antibiotic resistance patterns. Recommended oral medications include (Custer and Rau, 2009; Edmunds and Mayhew, 2009; Feld and Mattoo, 2010):

○ *Trimethoprim-sulfamethoxazole (TMP-SMX):* More than 2 months old: 6 to 12 mg/kg TMP component in two divided doses; adolescents: 160 mg TMP component every 12 hours. There is increasing resistance to TMP-SMX in the U.S. (20%) (Sobel and Kaye, 2009).

○ *Amoxicillin:* Less than 3 months old: 20 to 30 mg/kg/day in two divided doses every 12 hours; more than 3 months old: 25 to 50 mg/kg/day in two divided doses; adolescents: 250 mg every 8 hours or 500 mg every 12 hours (resistance in U.S. is approaching 35%) (Sobel and Kaye, 2009).

○ *Amoxicillin clavulanate (doses for amoxicillin component):* Less than 3 months old: 30 mg/kg/day in two divided doses; less than 88 pounds (40 kg): 25 to 45 mg/kg/day in two divided doses; adolescents: 875/125 mg every 12 hours.

○ *Cephalexin:* 2-24 months: 50-100 mg/kg divided in four doses; 25 to 50 mg/kg/day divided every 6 hours (maximum dose of 4 g).

○ *Cefixime:* 2-24 months: 8 mg/kg/day in one dose 16 mg/kg/day divided every 12 hours for first day, then 8 mg/kg/day divided every 12 hours to complete treatment; adolescents: 400 mg every 12 to 24 hours.

○ *Cefpodoxime proxetil:* 2 months to 12 years: 10 mg/kg/day divided every 12 hours (maximum dose of 400 mg/day); adolescents: 200 to 800 mg/day divided every 12 hours (maximum dose of 800 mg/day).

- ○ *Ciprofloxacin extended release:* Adolescents older than 18 years: 500 mg once a day for 3 days
- ○ *Nitrofurantoin:* Older than 1 month of age: 5 to 7 mg/kg/day divided every 6 hours (maximum 400 mg/24 hr). Adolescents: 50 to 100 mg/dose every 6 hours (macrocrystals) or 100 mg twice a day (dual release).
- *Recurrent UTI:* Further evaluation required (USN, VCUG if not done). Use of prophylactic antibiotics (Box 34-1) is controversial
- *Acute pyelonephritis:* Oral therapy is equally as effective in treating pyelonephritis and preventing kidney damage as parenteral antimicrobials (Pohl, 2007). Hospitalization (if severity of symptoms warrants): Parenteral regimen for children younger than 12 years is available (Feld and Mattoo, 2010). Outpatient uncomplicated 10-day oral regimen (Feld and Mattoo, 2010):
  - ○ Young children with uncomplicated pyelonephritis (well hydrated, no vomiting, no abdominal pain) can be effectively treated with cefixime, ceftibutin, or amoxicillin clavulanate.
  - ○ Adolescents with uncomplicated pyelonephritis can be treated with either amoxicillin clavulanate (875/125 mg twice a day) or ciprofloxacin (500 mg twice a day or extended release 1000 mg once a day).
  - ○ Amoxicillin and TMP-SMX should not be used due to increasing community resistance (Sobel and Kaye, 2009).
- Follow-up urine culture should be done 48 to 72 hours after initiating treatment, especially if symptoms persist or organism resistance is found in the community. If the culture is sterile, continue antibiotic therapy.
  - ○ If the culture is not sterile or if no clinical improvement is seen, urine should be sent for bacterial identification and sensitivity studies, and an alternative broad-spectrum antibiotic should be used pending those results. Culture should again be repeated after 48 to 72 hours and, if sterile, antibiotic therapy continued.
  - ○ Follow-up cultures should be obtained 3 to 4 days after finishing antibiotic treatment.
  - ○ Repeat urine culture should be done with any fever, illness, dysuria, or frequency.
- Phenazopyridine may be given at 100 mg for 6 to 12 years of age and 200 mg for those older than 12 years three times a day for dysuria.
- Radiologic workup (Table 34-4):
  - ○ Children younger than 5 years of age or any child with a febrile UTI should have a renal and bladder ultrasound as soon as the urine is sterile or when the prescribed antibiotic has been completed (Elder, 2007e; Feld and Mattoo, 2010). Waiting 2 to 6 weeks after infection may be recommended to allow any inflammatory changes to subside. VCUG may be done prior to discharge in a hospitalized child.
  - ○ VCUG does not need to be done routinely with first febrile UTI. However, if US reveals hydronephrosis, scarring or other atypical or concerning findings, VCUG should be completed.
  - ○ DMSA scan may be recommended for children with a febrile UTI or when a diagnosis of pyelonephritis is uncertain; it is ideally done 6 months after the infection (Elder, 2007e; Feld and Mattoo, 2010; Lee et al, 2009).

BOX 34-1 Radiologic Workup and Prophylaxis for Urinary Tract Infections

Why Do a Radiologic Workup?
- To identify any structural or functional abnormality of the urinary tract
- To identify any renal scarring or damage

Who Requires a Workup?
- Recommendations vary among experts. Those who recommend the most aggressive workup do so to identify scarring early and prevent further damage.
- Any child less than 5 years of age with the first infection (Chang and Shortliffe, 2006; Elder, 2007d; Lum, 2009)
- Any child with pyelonephritis as evidenced by fever (Elder, 2007d)
- With no fever, girls with second or third UTI; boys with first UTI (Elder, 2007d)
- Any child with suspicious factors (e.g., HTN, abnormal urine stream, poor growth) or with a positive family history of UTI or abnormal voiding patterns
- Adolescents with pyelonephritis or after a second UTI with documented culture and no history of recent sexual activity

What Test Should Be Done and When?
- Renal and bladder ultrasound and VCUG once urine is sterile
- VCUG if US is positive or concerning clinical picture
- Nuclear imaging scan (DMSA): Done to detect renal scars or parenchymal inflammation and ideally done 6 months after infection when the inflammatory changes in the kidney have resolved (Elder, 2007e; Feld and Mattoo, 2010; Lee et al, 2009)
- IVP: Done if further definition of structure or function of the kidney is needed but is rarely indicated

When Should Prophylaxis Be Used?
- There is controversy about when and whether prophylaxis should be used (AAP, 2011; Feld and Mattoo, 2010).

What Should Be Used for Prophylaxis?
- Depending on the source, between one quarter to one half of the treatment dose of antibiotic may be given at bedtime.
- Nitrofurantoin: >2 months age: 1-2 mg/kg as a single daily dose; expensive; liquid form poorly tolerated; consider sprinkling capsules over applesauce, yogurt, pudding
- TMP-SMX: TMP 2 mg/kg as a single daily dose or 5 mg/kg twice/wk (based on TMP component) if older than 1 month
- Cephalexin 10 mg/kg as a single daily dose
- Amoxicillin 10 mg/kg as a single daily dose; can be used for a newborn or premature infant; not used past the first 2 postnatal months; shelf life for liquid is 14 days

---

DMSA, Dimercaptosuccinic acid; *HTN,* hypertension; *IVP,* intravenous pyelogram; *TMP-SMX,* trimethoprim-sulfamethoxazole; *US,* ultrasound; *UTI,* urinary tract infection; *VCUG,* voiding cystourethrogram; *VUR,* vesicoureteral reflux.

Patient Education, Prevention, and Prognosis

The following should be discussed with parents and/or patients:
- Clear explanation of the cause, potential complications, and overall treatment plan, including both short- and long-term plans.
- Frequent and complete voiding and increased quantities of fluids, especially water. Sometimes scheduled voiding times, voiding with knees spread apart, or double voiding (voiding and then immediately attempting to void again) can be helpful.

TABLE 34-4	Radiologic Studies Done for Evaluation of Urinary Tract Infection			
Study	**Cost**	**Advantages**	**Disadvantages**	**Use**
Ultrasound	Least expensive	Shows structure, shape, and growth Detects structural abnormality, obstruction, pyelonephritis, large scars Painless, low risk, no radiation, noninvasive, available	Does not detect small scars of VUR Poor visualization of ureters Does not measure renal function or transient injury to kidney	Initial evaluation and follow-up
VUS		Uses second-generation contrast agent that is safe, sensitive, and is radiation-free method for detection and grading of VUR Superior to VCUG	None	Initial evaluation and follow-up
VCUG (radiographic)	Least expensive	Detects and grades VUR if high or low pressure, high or low bladder volumes, during voiding, during early or late bladder filling Visualizes bladder and urethra (especially in males) and diverticula	Does not detect obstruction, pyelonephritis, scars Risk of urethral trauma from catheterization Greater radiation than with scan	Initial evaluation in infants and children younger than 5 years of age with abnormal ultrasound or dysfunctional voiding
VCUG (nuclear)	More expensive	Visualizes bladder and reflux Constantly monitors for transient reflux Less radiation	Discomfort of catheterization No urethral visualization Unable to grade reflux	Follow-up of VUR to evaluate siblings of child with VUR Follow-up of surgery
IVP	Less expensive	Detects obstruction, pyelonephritis, large scars, stones, nephrocalcinosis Details pelvicaliceal system, shows ureters Estimates renal function Readily available	Does not detect small scars or VUR Risk of allergic reaction, acute renal failure, pain of injection, radiation Requires good renal function Only identifies structural damage	Better defines level of obstruction Used infrequently
DMSA (nuclear)	Most expensive	Detects acute inflammation, scars, and obstruction Earlier detection of parenchymal damage—large or small scars, permanent or focal—than with IVP (1-3 years of age)	Does not detect VUR or measure renal function Does not evaluate calyces, ureters, bladder, or urethra	Follow-up Fever of unknown origin and negative ultrasound in neonates To diagnose APN To detect renal scars
Tc-DTPA (nuclear)		Good in neonates Shows renal outline, estimates renal and tubular function, measures changes Less radiation		
CT scan (contrast)	Expensive	Detects obstruction, pyelonephritis, large scars	Does not detect small scars or VUR Risk of allergic reaction, acute renal failure	Trauma

APN, Acute pyelonephritis; *CT,* computed tomography; *DMSA,* dimercaptosuccinic acid; *IVP,* intravenous pyelogram; *Tc-DTPA,* technetium-labeled diethylenetriamine-penta-acetic acid; *VCUG,* voiding cystourethrogram; *VUR,* vesicoureteral reflux; *VUS,* voiding urosonography.

- Proper hygiene and avoiding irritants, such as bubble baths and perfumed soaps. Avoid wearing tight pants, especially spandex pants. Wear cotton underwear. Treat perineal inflammation to help prevent UTI.
- Treatment of constipation; pinworms.
- Sexually active females should be encouraged to drink water before intercourse and void immediately afterward.
- Decrease intake of bladder irritants, such as the "four C's" (caffeine, carbonated beverages, chocolate, citrus), aspartame (NutraSweet), alcohol, and spicy foods.

- Importance of prompt medical attention with recurrence of fever and/or duration of fever for more than 48 hours, especially if less than 24 months of age.
- Cranberry juice is considered helpful in preventing the adherence of *Escherichia coli* in the urethra (see Chapter 42).

According to Fitzgerald and colleagues (2009), "The relationship between UTI, renal scarring, and VUR is unclear, as is the progression of uncomplicated UTI to pyelonephritis and subsequent damage to the kidneys." Major risk factors for renal damage include delay in treatment of pyelonephritis,

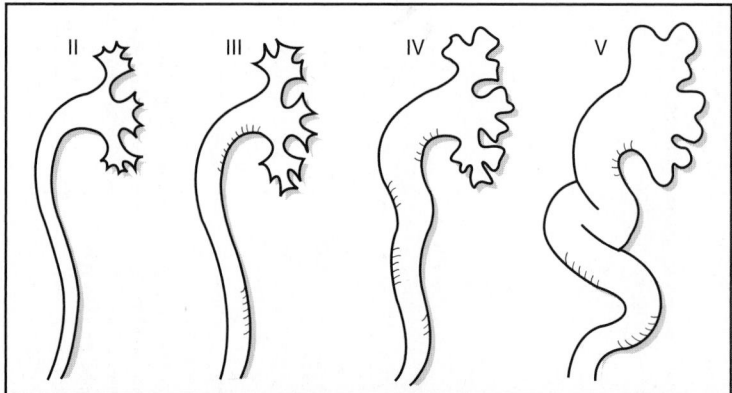

FIGURE 34-7 International reflux grading. *Grade I:* Ureter only. *Grade II:* Ureter, pelvis, and calyces; no dilation, normal calyceal fornices. *Grade III:* Mild or moderate dilation or tortuosity (or both) of ureter, and mild or moderate dilation of renal pelvis but no or slight blunting of the fornices. *Grade IV:* Moderate dilation or tortuosity (or both) of ureter and moderate dilation of renal pelvis and calyces. Complete obliteration of sharp angles of fornices but maintenance of papillary impressions in majority of calyces. *Grade V:* Gross dilation and tortuosity of ureter; gross dilation of renal pelvis and calyces; papillary impressions are no longer visible in majority of calyces. (From Lebowitz RL, Olbing H, Parkkulainen KV et al: International system of radiographic grading of vesicoureteral reflux, International Reflux Study in Children, *Pediatr Radiol* 15[2]:105, 1985.)

younger than 1 year of age, anatomic or neurogenic obstruction, severe reflux, dysplasia, and multiple infections. The same acute inflammatory process responsible for eradication of bacteria is also responsible for damage to renal tissue and subsequent scarring.

VESICOURETERAL REFLUX

Description
VUR is regurgitation of urine from the bladder up the ureter to the kidney. The major concern with VUR is the exposure of the kidney to infected urine (Feld and Mattoo, 2010). Primary VUR is the most common type and is typified by a congenital, abnormally short ureter and ineffective valve. Secondary VUR is due to bladder outlet obstruction and can be functional or structural. It is graded according to an international classification (Fig. 34-7). Grade I does not reach the renal pelvis; grade II extends up to the renal pelvis without dilation; grade III describes reflux to the renal pelvis with mild to moderate dilation of the ureter and the renal pelvis; grades IV and V (high grade) include definite distention of the ureters and renal pelvis and can include hydronephrosis or reflux into the intrarenal collecting system (Elder, 2007e).

Epidemiology
Reflux occurs because of congenital abnormalities and can persist with recurrent infection. Reflux provides a route for bacteria to ascend to the kidney and cause pyelonephritis. VUR is the most common anatomic abnormality found in young infants and children with UTI. Approximately 30% to 40% of siblings of children with reflux also have reflux, and 50% of children whose mothers have reflux also have reflux (Elder, 2007e). A meta-analysis identified that children who have UTIs more often and have associated bladder and bowel dysfunction (BBD) are more at risk for renal scarring (Peters et al, 2010).

Clinical Findings
History. The history may be positive for a previous UTI, abnormal voiding pattern or dysfunction, unexplained febrile illness, chronic constipation, or UTI symptoms.

Diagnostic Studies. The following are ordered, as indicated, to identify obstructive uropathy and dysplasia:
- Ultrasonography (may be normal even in the presence of reflux)
- VCUG establishes the presence of reflux, determines the grade, and gives high detail
- DMSA scan to look for renal scarring

Management
The goal of treatment is the prevention of infection and subsequent scarring. Early identification and appropriate treatment of infection achieve this goal. Table 34-5 presents a summary of the American Urological Association (AUA) guideline on management of primary VUR (Peters et al, 2010). The guideline statements are labeled as standards, recommendations, and options based on the level of evidence and degree of flexibility in application.
- Most children outgrow their reflux, probably secondary to an increase in the intramural length of the ureter. Grades I and II reflux resolve spontaneously in up to 85% of children, grade III in 50%, and grade IV in 30%; however, grade V is unlikely to resolve spontaneously (Greenbaum and Mesrobian, 2006). VUR tends to resolve earlier in African-American children. Older children who present with VUR and those with bilateral VUR tend to have lower rates of spontaneous resolution (Feld and Mattoo, 2010). Very few children with low-grade VUR require surgery.
- Treat underlying comorbidities such as constipation and dysfunctional voiding.
- Prophylactic antibiotics may be used when a child has VUR to prevent UTI, pyelonephritis, renal injury and other

TABLE 34-5 Management of Primary Vesicoureteral Reflux in Children

	Standard (Most Rigid Treatment Policy)	Recommendation (Less Rigid; There Is Sufficient Evidence, Even if Not Highest Quality, to Advocate for a Particular Clinical Approach)	Option (Most Flexible; Evidence of Relatively Equal Strength and Quality Supporting More Than One Approach; With Any Being Acceptable or Justifiable)
Initial Evaluation of a Child With VUR			
General evaluation	• Thorough history and physical examination • Measure weight, height, and blood pressure • Serum creatinine if bilateral renal cortical abnormalities are found	• UA for proteinuria and bacteriuria; if UA indicates infection, obtain urine culture and sensitivities	Baseline serum creatinine may serve as an estimate of GFR
Imaging procedures	None	• Renal US to assess upper urinary tract	DMSA renal imaging to assess the status of the kidneys for scarring and function
Assessment of voiding patterns	Information related to symptoms of bladder and bowel dysfunction (BBD) should be elicited, especially urinary frequency and urgency, prolonged voiding intervals, daytime wetting, perineal/penile pain, holding maneuvers to prevent wetting, and constipation or encopresis		
Family and patient education	Family and patient education should include a discussion of the rationale for treating VUR, the equivalency of certain treatment approaches, assessment of likely adherence to the treatment plan, determination of parental concerns, and accommodation of parental preferences when treatment options offer a similar risk-benefit balance		
Initial Management of the Child With VUR			
Child <1 year of age with VUR		• History of febrile UTI: Low-dose continuous antibiotic prophylaxis (CAP) is recommended because of the increased risk of morbidity from recurrent UTIs in this age group • No history of febrile UTI: CAP is recommended with VUR grades III-V identified through screening	• No history of febrile UTI: CAP may be offered for VUR grades I-II. • Circumcision may be considered. Goal of management of VUR is to prevent febrile UTI and renal injury and circumcised males have a decreased incidence of UTIs • CAP may be considered in the absence of BBD • Observation without CAP with prompt initiation of antibiotic therapy for UTI
Child >1 year of age with UTI and VUR		• If BBD is present, treatment of BBD is indicated before any surgical intervention • Treatment options for BBD include behavioral therapy, biofeedback, anticholinergic medications, alpha-blockers, and treatment of constipation and encopresis. Monitor effectiveness of BBD treatment • CAP is recommended for the child with BBD and VUR due to the increased risk of UTI while BBD is present and being treated	Surgical intervention for VUR (both open and endoscopic methods) may be considered (even as initial therapy)

Follow-up management of the child with VUR	• Ongoing monitoring of weight, height, blood pressure; UA for proteinuria and bacteriuria (including culture and sensitivity if necessary) annually
	• US every 12 months to monitor renal growth and parenchymal scarring.
	• VCUG every 12-24 months with longer intervals in patients with lower rates of spontaneous resolution (grades III-V VUR) in order to limit the overall imaging studies performed
	• DMSA imaging when renal US is abnormal, when there is a greater concern for scarring due to breakthrough UTI or grade III-V VUR, or if serum creatinine is elevated
		• Follow-up cystography may be an option:
		  ○ Grades I-II VUR because of high rate of spontaneous resolution
		  ○ A single normal VCUG can be used to establish resolution
		  ○ DMSA for follow-up of VUR to detect new renal scarring, especially after a febrile UTI

Interventions for the child with breakthrough UTI (BT-UTI)	• Symptomatic BT-UTI (fever, dysuria, frequency, FTT, or poor feeding): A change in therapy is recommended. Treat infection with appropriate antibiotic • Child on CAP with BT-UTI: Consideration should be given for open surgical or endoscopic correction • Child on CAP with a single BT-UTI without evidence of previous or new renal cortical abnormalities: Changing to an alternative antibiotic agent is an option before surgical correction • Child not on CAP with BT-UTI: Initiation of CAP is recommended	• Child not receiving CAP with nonfebrile UTI: Initiation of CAP is an option (not all pyelonephritis presents with fever) • Surgical intervention for VUR may be used. Studies have shown a reduction in the occurrence of febrile UTIs in patients who have had surgical correction compared with those on CAP.
Follow-up management after resolution of VUR	• Following spontaneous or surgical resolution of VUR: General evaluation, including monitoring weight, height, BP, and UA for protein and UTI, is recommended annually through adolescence if either kidney is found to be abnormal by ultrasound or DMSA scanning • With occurrence of febrile UTI following resolution of surgical treatment of VUR: Evaluation for BBD or recurrent VUR is recommended • Long-term concerns of hypertension (especially during pregnancy), renal function loss, recurrent UTI, and familial VUR in the child's siblings and offspring should be discussed with family and child	• Following spontaneous or surgical resolution of VUR, if both kidneys are normal by US or DMSA scanning: General evaluation, including monitoring weight, height, BP, and UA for protein and UTI, annually through adolescence is an option

BBP, Bowel and bladder dysfunction; *BP*, blood pressure; *CAP*, continuous antibody prophylaxis; *DMSA*, dimercaptosuccinic acid; *FTT*, failure to thrive; *GFR*, glomerular filtration rate; *UA*, urinalysis; *US*, ultrasound; *UTI*, urinary tract infection; *VCUG*, voiding cystourethrogram; *VUR*, vesicoureteral reflux.
Data from Peters CA et al: Summary of the American Urological Association guideline on management of primary vesicoureteral reflux in children, *J Urol* 184(3):1134-1144, 2010. The complete guideline is available at www.auanet.org/content/guidelines-and-quality-care/clinical-guidelines.cfm?sub=vur2010.

sequelae. Feld and Mattoo (2010) recommend prophylaxis for any grade of primary VUR although a number of other studies have questioned the efficacy of prophylactic antibiotics for both VUR and recurrent UTI (Dai et al, 2009; Garin et al, 2006; Peters et al, 2010). Recommended medications used for prophylaxis should be given at bedtime and are listed in Box 34-1. The duration of prophylaxis depends on the age of the child, the severity of the VUR, patient compliance, presence of renal scarring, and recurrent infections on prophylaxis.

- Surgery is reserved for failed medical management.
- Interval urine cultures are performed with symptoms of unexplained illness.
- Repeat VCUG once after the diagnosis of reflux at 12 to 18 months to monitor reflux and scarring. Routine follow-up studies are recommended every 1 to 2 years, depending on the reflux grade, sex, and whether both or only one kidney is affected. Blood pressure and growth parameters should be checked at least yearly.
- Nephrology consultation is indicated in the presence of higher-grade reflux, notable scarring, a solitary or atrophic kidney, hypertension, elevated creatinine, or evidence of abnormal kidney function with any grade of reflux.

Patient Education, Prevention, and Prognosis

- VUR does not cause scarring, infection does, but VUR is a risk factor for pyelonephritis and subsequent scarring.
- Screen all siblings younger than 3 years of age for VUR (Menezes and Puri, 2009).
- Management, prevention of UTIs, and compliance must be understood by families. The necessity of urine culture with any suspicious symptoms should also be emphasized. The potential for untreated, chronic UTI leading to chronic renal disease must be explained.
- Other points to emphasize include the following:
  ○ Prompt treatment of UTI should be instituted.
  ○ Prophylactic medicines are best given at night because of urinary stasis while asleep.
  ○ BP and growth should be monitored.
  ○ The guidelines discussed in the Patient Education and Prevention section of UTIs should be reviewed.

Preexisting renal damage may be present, and new renal scarring can occur. Children with grades I and II reflux usually have resolution of the reflux if infections are thwarted or treated early. Ten percent of children with renal scarring develop hypertension. Reflux nephropathy is a complication of VUR. Further complications related to scarring include end-stage renal disease (10%), growth failure, and decreased glomerular filtration rates (90%) (Nguyen, 2009).

HEMATURIA

Description

Hematuria is defined as the presence of five or more RBCs per hpf in three consecutive fresh, centrifuged specimens obtained over several weeks (Massengill, 2008). The number of RBCs per hpf considered to be abnormal varies and ranges from any to more than 5 per hpf in unspun urine to more than 5 to 10 per hpf in spun urine (Davis and Avner, 2007). For management purposes, hematuria in this text is defined as more than 2 RBCs per hpf in unspun or 5 per hpf in spun urine. The term *gross hematuria* is related to the concentration of RBCs rather than to the location or significance of the disorder. Brownish, tea-colored urine with casts or protein is usually glomerular in origin. Clots and red to pink urine with isomorphic RBCs but no protein usually originates from the lower tract. Factors causing hematuria can arise anywhere in the urinary system, from the urinary meatus to the kidneys. Urine can be discolored and urine dipsticks can be positive for RBCs when there is myoglobinuria or hemoglobinuria in which case no RBCs are seen on microscopic examination (Massengill, 2008). It is necessary to confirm the diagnosis of hematuria. Hematuria can be microscopic or macroscopic. Microscopic hematuria may be either persistent or transient.

Epidemiology

The causes of macroscopic hematuria include hypercalciuria (23%), immunoglobulin A (IgA) nephropathy (16%), glomerulonephritis (GN) (9%), and no known cause (38%). UTI, hydronephrosis, tumor, cystitis cystica, polyps, or epididymitis are characterized by macro-hematuria less than 1% of the time (Halverson and Alper, 2006). However, according to Bloom and Kolon (2005), 50% of children with gross hematuria have UTIs. The incidence of hematuria is 0.5% to 2% when confirmed with repeat UA (VanDeVoorde and Bissler, 2006).

Clinical Findings
History
- Previous medical history of cystic kidney disease, sickle cell disease, systemic lupus erythematosus (SLE), malignancy
- Family or previous history of hematuria, nephrolithiasis, cystic kidney, hemoglobinopathy, sickle cell disease or trait, SLE, hypertension, congestive heart disease, malignancy, deafness, renal failure
- Preceding illness: Viral or streptococcal pharyngitis or impetigo
- Onset, duration, pattern, and timing of hematuria; color of urine
- Dysuria, urgency, or frequency
- Presence of pain (back, abdominal, or flank) with voiding
- Straining or squatting with urination (tumor)
- Strenuous exercise or trauma (including bladder catheterization)
- Enuresis
- Trauma, foreign body
- Sexual activity or abuse
- Current menstruation
- Edema, rash, pallor, or arthralgias
- Certain drugs (sulfonamides, nitrofurantoin, salicylates, phenazopyridine, toxins [lead, benzenes]) and foods (food color, beets, blackberries, rhubarb, and paprika) can discolor the urine but test negative for RBCs (Massengill, 2008)
- Symptoms related to chronic renal disease (Box 34-2)
Physical Examination
- Growth parameters: FTT or falling growth curves (chronic renal insufficiency or long-standing acidosis)
- Vital signs, especially BP
- Malformed ears (congenital renal disease)
- Oliguria or anuria

BOX 34-2	Seven "Red Flags" for Chronic Renal Failure

1. Failure to thrive (poor growth, fatigue, anorexia, nausea, gastroesophageal reflux, vomiting)
2. Chronic anemia (normochromic, normocytic, nonresponsive to medication)
3. Complicated enuresis (daytime frequency, urgency, incontinence, chronic constipation, encopresis, infrequent voiding, straining to void, recurrent UTI)
4. Prolonged, unexplained vomiting or nausea (especially in the morning), anorexia, weight loss without diarrhea
5. Hypotension
6. Unusual bone disease (e.g., rickets, valgus deformity, fracture with minor trauma)
7. Poor school performance (e.g., headache, fatigue, inattention, withdrawal from activities)

- Edema, hypertension, and proteinuria, which are suggestive of glomerular disease
- Flank pain, which is suggestive of a lower tract disorder
- Abdominal or flank mass, which suggests an obstruction, such as Wilms tumor, cystic disease, or posterior valves
- External genitalia: Excoriation, bleeding, foreign body, abuse

Diagnostic Studies

- Urine dipstick analysis for pyuria, proteinuria, hematuria, and concentration
  - If greater than 1+ hematuria by dipstick (which equals 3 RBCs/hpf or 0.02 mg/dL hemoglobin), microscopic examination for RBCs is needed to differentiate RBCs from hemoglobinuria or myoglobinuria.
  - If protein is present, refer to the section on proteinuria and nephritis for further workup. NOTE: The most significant differentiating factor is the presence of proteinuria. If present, rapid evaluation and early referral to a nephrologist are essential
- Microscopic examination of the urine includes RBCs, size and shape of the cells, casts, crystals, and WBCs
  - A few RBCs/hpf can be normal in a pediatric patient (see description of hematuria).
  - Distorted, misshapen RBCs of different sizes suggest glomerular disease.
  - Crystalluria is most commonly caused by hypercalciuria.
- Urine culture
- 24-hour urine collection
- First morning UA on first-degree relatives
- Renal US if Wilms tumor or nephrolithiasis are suspected. Spiral helical computed tomography (CT) scan is the most sensitive modality for diagnosing nephrolithiasis but there is a large radiation exposure (Massengill, 2008)
- If there are systemic symptoms (e.g., edema, hypertension, changes in urine output), consider further evaluation as described in the Nephritis and Glomerulonephritis sections (Massengill, 2008; Tan, 2009).
- Renal biopsy is recommended for recurrent gross hematuria and coexisting nephritic syndrome, hypertension, renal insufficiency, systemic illness, and parent anxiety (Massengill, 2008).
- Cystoscopy, which is invasive and costly, is rarely used in children

Differential Diagnosis

There are five categories to be considered in the diagnostic workup for hematuria (Massengill, 2008):

- Gross hematuria
  - Urine color is red or tea-colored; microscopic examination shows RBCs.
  - Common causes are poststreptococcal glomerulonephritis, renal disease, UTI, trauma, coagulopathy, crystalluria, and nephrolithiasis. Recurrent episodes of gross hematuria are rare.
  - Consider Henoch-Schönlein purpura (HSP) when there is gross hematuria in the presence of abdominal pain, with or without bloody stools, arthralgias, and purpuric rash.
  - Consider IgA nephropathy with gross hematuria in the presence of acute illness or strenuous exercise.
  - Sickle cell disease and trait can cause gross hematuria (mostly males, unilateral kidney) and there can be recurrence in up to 40% of cases (Massengill, 2008).
  - Rhabdomyosarcoma causes gross hematuria and voiding dysfunction (Massengill, 2008).
- Symptomatic microscopic hematuria
  - Greatest attention and methodic approach are required (Massengill, 2008). History and physical examination guide the workup.
  - Renal disease is more likely if microscopic hematuria is accompanied by proteinuria on a first morning sample.
  - Other nonspecific symptoms (fever, malaise, weight change), extrarenal symptoms (malar rash, purpura, arthritis, headache, dysuria, abdominal or flank pain, edema, oliguria) may be present.
- Asymptomatic microscopic hematuria
  - Asymptomatic microscopic hematuria rarely indicates significant renal disease.
  - Family history is important to assess for benign familial hematuria.
  - Hypercalciuria is commonly associated with asymptomatic microscopic hematuria which leaves patients prone to symptomatic urolithiasis. The diagnosis is made by laboratory examination of urine. The spot calcium-creatinine ratio done on the first morning specimen is elevated to more than 0.2, or the 24-hour urinary calcium to more than 4 mg/kg/day. Hypercalciuria is also associated with immobilization, diuretics, vitamin D intoxication, hyperparathyroidism, and sarcoidosis (Massengill, 2008).
  - Regularly monitor for hypertension and proteinuria.
- Asymptomatic hematuria with proteinuria
  - Condition is worrisome for renal disease. Finding both abnormalities is not uncommon, and there is usually resolution of one or both features (Massengill, 2008).
  - Consider evaluating for orthostatic proteinuria (see Proteinuria section).
  - Persistent proteinuria is more indicative of a glomerular process.
- Other differential diagnoses to consider include:
  - Pseudohematuria occurs when a false-positive dipstick reading is noted, but no RBCs are found on the microscopic examination. The two most common causes are myoglobinuria and hemoglobinuria (see Table 34-1).
  - Extrarenal hematuria is common with systemic bleeding disorders and is evidenced by macroscopic and microscopic hematuria.

○ Although rare, renal stones (nephrolithiasis) or calcification (nephrocalcinosis) can occur. If suspected, a renal ultrasonogram can be included as part of the workup.

○ Hematuria caused by external irritation of the urinary meatus will resolve with healing and removal of the offending irritant (diaper rash, soaps, bubble bath, lotions) or avoidance of the offending behavior (e.g., scratching, masturbation, sexual activity).

Management

A progressive approach to evaluating hematuria should be undertaken with the goal of not overlooking serious, treatable, progressive conditions while at the same time avoiding unnecessary studies (see Fig. 34-8).

- Gross hematuria: If the cause is unclear, refer to a nephrologist.
- Symptomatic microscopic hematuria: refer to a nephrologist for evaluation and management.
- Asymptomatic hematuria: Periodic evaluation every 1 to 2 years to reevaluate for coexisting conditions or proteinuria and to revisit family history of hematuria or hearing deficits.
- Persistent asymptomatic hematuria and proteinuria: refer to a nephrologist; renal biopsy may be indicated (Massengill, 2008).

Patient Education, Prevention, and Prognosis

Patient education should stress the importance of follow-up for evaluation of the hematuria. Prognosis depends on the cause of the hematuria.

PROTEINURIA

Description

Protein in the urine is commonly detected by dipstick tests. It may be transient, recurrent, or fixed. Proteinuria can be a symptom of disease, or it can reflect a benign, self-limited condition. The quantity of protein and the timing of its presence determine its significance. Qualitative protein in urine, as tested by dipstick, is considered a positive result if it registers 1+ (30 mg/dL) or more in urine with a specific gravity of less than 1.015. Quantitative protein is tested by measuring a volume of urine over a set period. A level of less than 4 mg/m²/hr is considered normal, 4 to 40 mg/m²/hr is abnormal, and greater than 40 mg/m²/hr indicates nephritic disease.

Four groups of proteinuria exist: isolated, transient or functional, glomerular, and tubulointerstitial.

- Isolated proteinuria includes orthostatic proteinuria and persistent asymptomatic proteinuria, which are the most common.
  ○ *Orthostatic proteinuria* accounts for up to 60% (75% in adolescents) of cases of proteinuria (Mahesh and Woroniecki, 2009). In this condition, the child excretes abnormal amounts of protein when upright but normal amounts when lying down. Orthostatic proteinuria is demonstrated by collecting urine as described under diagnostic studies.
  ○ *Persistent asymptomatic proteinuria* is a common, transient phenomenon in which an otherwise healthy child, with normal clinical and laboratory workup, has an abnormally high level of protein in the urine.

- Transient or functional proteinuria is usually caused by some type of stress.
  ○ *Exercised-induced proteinuria* is documented by collecting a urine sample, having the patient exercise vigorously for several minutes, and then collecting another sample. The postexercise sample is usually strongly positive.
  ○ *Fever-induced proteinuria* can accompany any febrile state and usually subsides with resolution of the fever. Other stress-related causes include cold exposure, infection, congestive heart failure, and seizures. This type of proteinuria usually resolves in 1 to 2 weeks, and if resolution has been verified, no further workup is required.
- Glomerular proteinuria and tubulointerstitial proteinuria are the least common types and are characterized by high levels of proteinuria. Some authorities believe that children with persistent proteinuria, even at low levels, should be followed with a high index of suspicion for an underlying, progressive renal disorder.

Epidemiology

Proteinuria originates from problems with glomerular filtration, tubular reabsorption or secretion, or both. The child is often asymptomatic. If proteinuria is significant enough to cause hypoproteinemia, edema is present. The incidence of proteinuria is cited at 30% to 55% in school-age children. It persists, however, in up to 6% of children when four consecutive urine specimens are tested (Mahesh and Woroniecki, 2009).

Clinical Findings
History
- Family history of deafness, visual problems, and renal disease
- Recent strenuous exercise or febrile illness
- Polydipsia or polyuria
- Vague symptoms, such as malaise, fatigue, or pallor
- Symptoms related to chronic renal disease (see Box 34-2)
Physical Examination
- Growth and development parameters (poor weight gain or FTT with chronic disease; weight gain with nephrotic syndrome)
- BP (hypertension), pulse, respiratory rate
- Edema, especially periorbital edema, or symptoms of fluid retention
- Abdominal examination for a mass, enlarged kidney, fluid, tenderness
Diagnostic Studies
- UA (repeated three times over 1 to 2 weeks), preferably done on a first-voided specimen:
  ○ 1+ protein (30 mg/dL) is significant if the specific gravity is less than 1.015; 2+ protein (100 mg/dL) is significant if the specific gravity is greater than 1.015.
  ○ False-positive results occur in highly concentrated or alkaline (pH greater than 5.5) urine. False-negative results occur in dilute or acidic urine.
  ○ At least 75% of asymptomatic patients with proteinuria in a single urine specimen have normal urine on repeated testing.
- A urine sample collected immediately after arising in the morning can be compared with a specimen collected after

several hours of activity to rule out orthostatic etiology. The child must have voided before sleep to obtain accurate results. A typical result yields negative to trace amounts on the first-morning specimen, but 1+ or greater on the second specimen. If the result is equivocal, back-to-back urine samples (from arising to bedtime and bedtime to arising) can be evaluated for quantitative protein.

- Microscopic urine:
  - RBCs or WBCs (or both), casts, bacteria, oval fat bodies, or other abnormalities are present in most pathologic conditions.
- A urine protein-to-creatinine ratio on a first morning voided sample. Normal values are less than 0.5 mg/dL in children younger than 2 years of age and less than 0.2 mg/dL in children older than 2 years; greater than 2 mg/dL is considered nephritic (Lum, 2009). An abnormal urine protein-to-creatinine ratio requires further testing.
- A 12- or 24-hour timed urine collection for creatinine (normal: 14 to 20 mg/kg/24 hr) and protein excretion (normal: less than 4 mg/m^2/hr) is elevated with proteinuria (Lum, 2009). A back-to-back sample collection (see earlier) is done to compare active or upright and resting levels.
- If protein in urine is greater than 4 mg/m^2/hr, check the CBC, electrolytes, BUN, creatinine, albumin/total protein, C3, C4, cholesterol, liver functions, and urine culture. Perform an ultrasonogram, VCUG, and radionuclide scans as indicated. Evaluate for systemic disease as indicated (e.g., ANA, ASO, streptozyme, hepatitis B, HIV, tuberculosis).

Differential Diagnosis

Pseudoproteinuria can be caused by semisynthetic penicillins or benzalkonium chloride.

Management

The persistence, quantity, and presence of other abnormalities (e.g., hematuria) are key in evaluating proteinuria (see Fig. 34-9).
- If protein by dipstick is *trace* or *1+* and specific gravity is greater than 1.015, offer reassurance; do monthly recheck of urine for 4 to 6 months. If protein is persistent, refer the patient to a nephrologist.
- If protein by dipstick is *greater than 1+*, evaluate the child for orthostatic proteinuria (Fig. 34-8).
- If first morning urine protein is *1+ or 2+*, perform either a quantitative 12- to 24-hour urine protein excretion test or a random urine total protein-creatinine ratio and UA with microscope. Proceed as in Figure 34-9.
- If protein by dipstick is *greater than 2+*, evaluate for nephrotic syndrome (see later section).
- If hematuria is present, evaluate for nephritis (see later section).
- Follow-up is important to monitor for any change in status.
- Refer the following to a nephrologist: Persistent unexplained nonorthostatic proteinuria, any hematuria or RBC or WBC casts, polyuria or oliguria, nephrotic levels of protein, elevated BUN or creatinine, elevated BP, systemic complaints (e.g., joint pain, rashes, or arthralgias), or a child with a family history of renal failure, GN, sensorineural hearing loss, or kidney transplantation.

Patient Education, Prevention, and Prognosis

Patient education should stress the importance of follow-up to evaluate the cause of proteinuria. Children with mild asymptomatic proteinuria who have a normal first-morning specimen do not require extensive testing for kidney disease but should be monitored annually.

NEPHROTIC SYNDROME
Description

Nephrotic syndrome is due to excessive excretion of protein in urine as a result of alterations in the integrity of the glomerular filtration barrier. The main mechanism of the massive protein loss is increased glomerular permeability. The loss can be selective (albumin only) or nonselective (including most serum proteins), and such selectivity is an important distinction in diagnosis. The classic definition of nephrotic syndrome is massive proteinuria (greater than 40 mg/m^2/hr and a protein-creatinine ratio on spot urine of greater than 1, hypoalbuminemia (less than 2.5 g/dL), edema, and hyperlipidemia. Edema formation results from a decrease in the plasma oncotic pressure due to a loss of serum albumin, which causes water to extravasate into the interstitial space. This then leads to decreased intravascular volume with decreased renal perfusion and activation of the renin-angiotensin system (Gordillo and Spitzer, 2009). With protein loss, the liver increases its synthesis of protein and thereby causes concurrent hyperlipidemia and lipiduria. Nephrotic syndrome can be congenital, idiopathic, or secondary.
- Congenital (early onset) can be associated with genetic mutation or congenital infection (Lennon et al, 2010). It can be associated with other syndromes and is generally not responsive to corticosteroids.
- Idiopathic nephritic syndrome has three types: minimal change nephrotic syndrome (MCNS), focal segmental glomerulosclerosis (FSGS), and membranous nephropathy. MCNS is the most common (85% in children). FSGS accounts for 10% to 15% of all cases of nephrotic syndrome. Scar tissue develops in the glomeruli, leading to glomerulosclerosis and tubular atrophy. Membranous nephropathy accounts for 4% and is characterized by diffuse thickening of the glomerular walls (Gordillo and Spitzer, 2009).
- Secondary nephrotic syndrome occurs in association with or secondary to systemic disorders (e.g., SLE, HSP), infectious processes (e.g., syphilis, hepatitis B, HIV, or malaria), drug toxicities (e.g., nonsteroidal antiinflammatory drugs [NSAIDs], mephenytoin), allergens, or other renal disorders (e.g., IgA or congenital nephritis). Histopathologic examination shows moderate to severe morphologic abnormality. This type occurs in 10% of cases.

Nephrotic syndrome is a chronic disease characterized by periods of remission (when both the urinary protein excretion and serum albumin normalize) and relapses (recurrence of proteinuria and hypoalbuminemia after complete remission). Most children are "steroid responders," having remission with steroid treatment. Steroid responsiveness is the best prognostic indicator for nephrotic syndrome (Gordillo and Spitzer, 2009). Of the remaining children, most are steroid resistant and show no response to steroid treatment. A small number of cases are either partial responders with minimal response to steroids or are steroid dependent and require high doses of prednisone with frequent relapses.

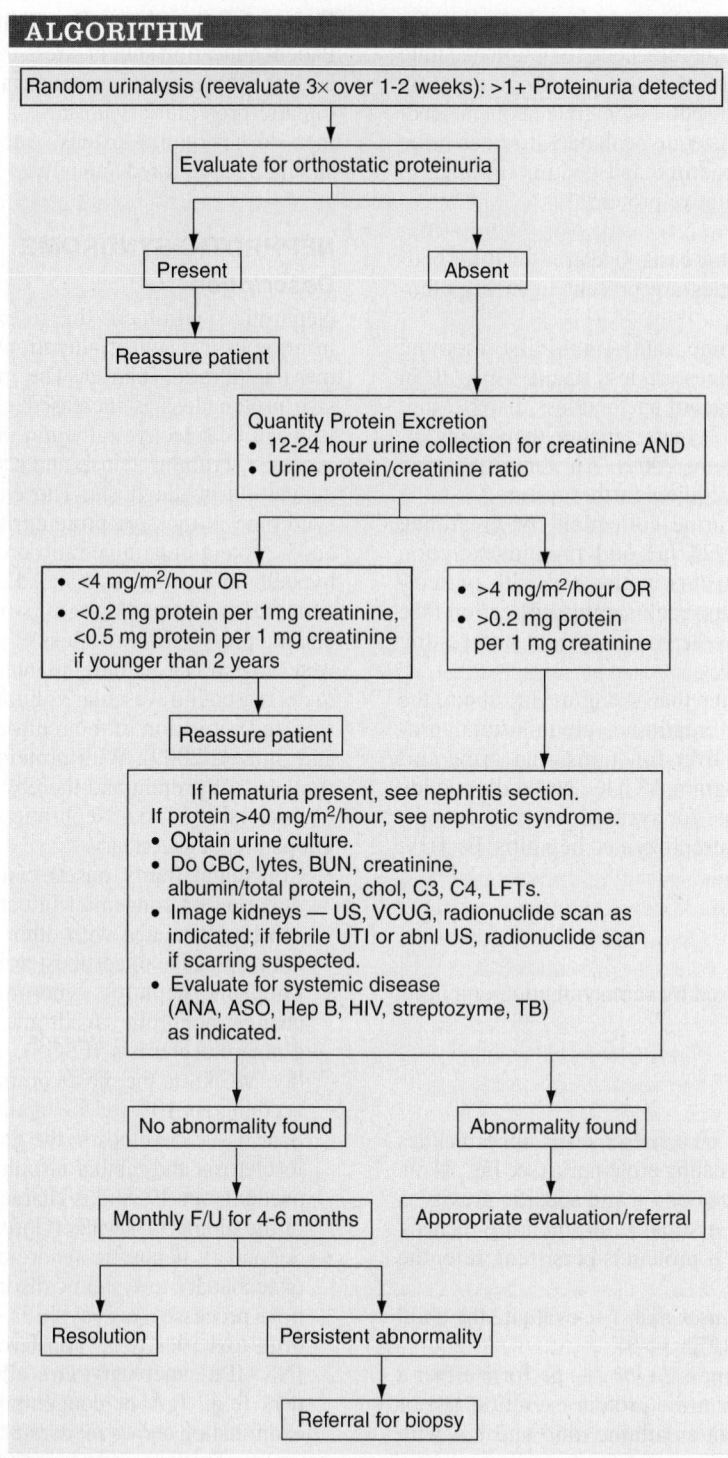

FIGURE 34-8 Evaluation of proteinuria. *abnl,* Abnormal; *ANA,* antinuclear antibody; *ASO,* antistreptolysin O; *BUN,* blood urea nitrogen; *C3,* complement 3; *C4,* complement 4; *CBC,* complete blood count; *chol,* cholesterol; *Cr,* creatinine; *ANA,* antinuclear antibody; *F/U,* follow-up; *Hep B,* hepatitis B; *HIV,* human immunodeficiency virus; *LFTs,* liver function tests; *lytes,* electrolytes; *TB,* tuberculosis; *US,* ultrasound; *UTI,* urinary tract infection; *VCUG,* voiding cystourethrogram. (Adapted from Dershewitz RA, editor: *Ambulatory pediatric care,* ed 3, Philadelphia, 1999, Lippincott-Raven.)

Epidemiology

Nephrotic syndrome occurs as a result of genetic, immune, systemic, nephrotoxic, allergic, infectious, malignant, vascular, or idiopathic processes. Nephrotic syndrome in the neonatal or infancy period is usually caused by genetic

mutations or congenital infection (Lennon et al, 2010). The actual mechanism of nephrotic syndrome has been extensively studied, and the understanding of its histopathology is better than the understanding of its pathogenesis. The primary mechanism is believed to be immunologic rather than

ALGORITHM

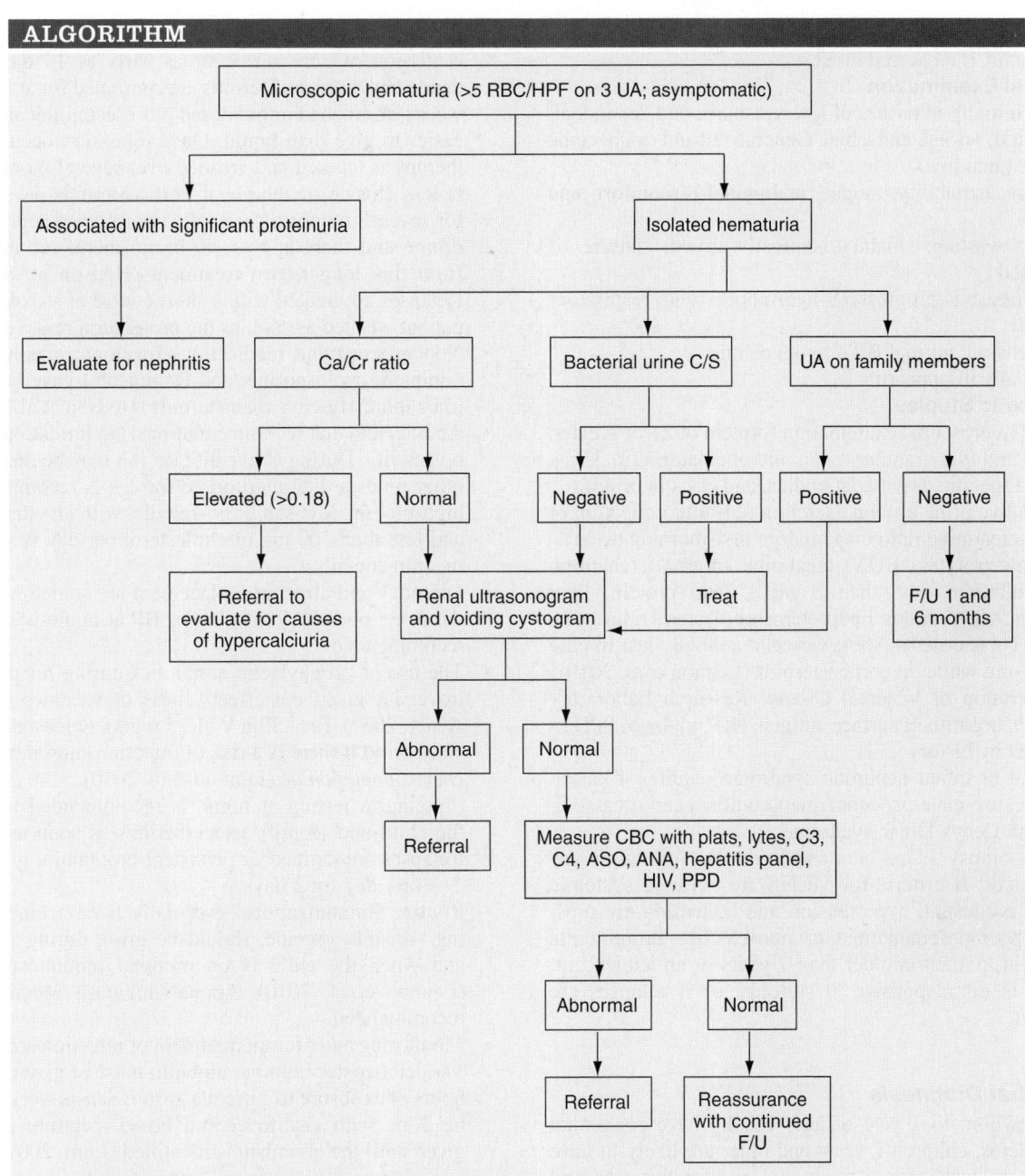

FIGURE 34-9 Management of asymptomatic microscopic hematuria. *ANA,* Antinuclear antibody; *ASO,* antistreptolysin O; *BUN,* blood urea nitrogen; *C3,* complement 3; *C4,* complement 4; *Ca/Cr,* calcium/creatinine ratio; *CBC,* complete blood count; *C/S,* culture/sensitivity; *F/U,* follow-up; *HIV,* human immunodeficiency virus; *lytes,* electrolytes; *plats,* platelets; *PPD,* purified protein derivative; *RBC/HPF,* red blood cells per high-power field; *UA,* urinalysis. (Adapted from Dershewitz RA, editor: *Ambulatory pediatric care,* ed 3, Philadelphia, 1999, Lippincott-Raven.)

renal (Lum, 2009). The most common subtype of nephrotic syndrome is MCNS.

The incidence of idiopathic nephrotic syndrome in the U.S. is 2 to 3 per 100,000 per year, with a 15 times greater incidence in children than in adults. The male-to-female ratio is approximately 2:1 during childhood and equivocal in adolescence, and there is a familial tendency among siblings (Gordillo and Spitzer, 2009). Thirty to 60% of children with nephrotic syndrome have a history of atopic disease and 3% have a family history of a similar nephrotic syndrome (Lennon et al, 2010).

Clinical Findings
History
- History of allergy in up to 50% of children with MCNS
- Edema is the cardinal clinical feature, especially periorbital edema, dependent areas (tight shoes or underwear), and lax tissues (puffy eyes).
- Low urine production
- Gastrointestinal symptoms: Anorexia, paleness, listlessness, diarrhea, vomiting, abdominal pain (right upper quadrant)

- Respiratory difficulties secondary to ascites, effusion, Pneumonia, if advanced disease.
  Physical Examination
- Edema initially in tissues of low resistance and dependent: Periorbital, scrotal, and labial. Generalized and can become massive (anasarca).
- Anorexia, irritability, fatigue, abdominal discomfort, and diarrhea
- Muscle wasting, malnourishment, growth failure if prolonged
- If the disease is progressive, hydrothorax with respiratory difficulty
- Hypertension; normal BP if hypovolemic
- Chronically ill-appearing
  Diagnostic Studies
- UA and microscopic examination (protein of 2+ or greater, hyaline and fine granular casts, microhematuria [in 33%], elevated specific gravity, fat bodies, and casts in urine)
- Quantitative urine protein excretion (24-hour collection or protein-creatinine ratio on a random first-morning urine)
- CBC; electrolytes, BUN, creatinine (normal); calcium; serum albumin (less than 2 g/dL), total protein; liver enzymes; triglycerides, lipoproteins, cholesterol (elevated); C3 and C4 (normal); ANA; varicella antibody test in case of exposure while on corticosteroids (Lennon et al, 2010)
- Consideration of Venereal Disease Research Laboratory (VDRL), hepatitis B surface antigen, HIV, malaria, PPD as indicated by history
- Neonatal or infant nephrotic syndrome requires a karyotype because male pseudohermaphroditism can be associated with Denys-Drash syndrome.
- Kidney biopsy is recommended in the following circumstances: If criteria for MCNS are not met, systemic disease is present, hypertension and hematuria are present, hypocomplementemia or nonselective proteinemia is present, patient is older than 7 years or an adolescent, patient is nonresponsive to steroids, or if relapses are frequent.

Differential Diagnosis

Infants (newborn to 1 year of age) usually have congenital renal problems, children 7 years and older are likely to have focal glomerulosclerosis or mesangial proliferative GN, and teens have membranous nephropathy. The differential diagnosis includes hypoproteinemia from starvation, liver disease, and protein-losing enteropathy; none of these conditions has associated proteinuria. GN should also be considered in the differential diagnosis.

Management

Nephrotic syndrome is a complex, often chronic disorder that responds to careful management with a gratifying long-term positive outcome. The diagnosis is made with 95% certainty on clinical impressions. A major goal is to control edema while awaiting definitive remission.

- Consultation with and/or referral to a nephrologist should occur because of the constantly changing strategies for managing these children.
- Hospitalization may be necessary initially if disease is severe.

- Prednisone (2 mg/kg/day; maximum 60 mg) to induce remission, which can occur as early as 14 days as evidenced by diuresis. Steroids are continued for at least 4 to 6 weeks. A crushed or quartered pill is economical and often easier to give than liquid. Once remission occurs, steroid therapy is tapered and weaned over several months. There is less chance of relapse if corticosteroids are continued for several months after the first episode of nephrotic syndrome and there appears to be no increased side effects from this longer-term treatment (Hodson et al, 2008a). Relapses are treated with a short course of steroids and the patient weaned as soon as the proteinuria resolves.
- Noncorticosteroid medications (cyclophosphamide, chlorambucil, cyclosporine, and levamisole) have been found to be more effective than steroids (Hodson et al, 2008b).
- Activity and diet recommendations: No limitation is placed on activity. During active disease salt may be restricted. At other times a diet appropriate for age is recommended. A high-protein, low-salt or no-salt diet with less than 35% fat and less than 300 mg of cholesterol per day is sometimes recommended.
- Diuretics and albumin replacement are sometimes used in the acute phase. Monitoring of BP at home is sometimes recommended.
- The use of prophylactic antibiotics during relapse is controversial given the effectiveness of vaccines (Vogt and Avner, 2007). Penicillin V (12.5 mg/kg twice a day) can be considered if there is a risk of infection caused by *Streptococcus pneumoniae* (Lennon et al, 2010).
- Proteinuria testing at home is recommended to monitor the child and identify exacerbations as soon as possible. Relapses are defined as persistent proteinuria greater than 2+ every day for 3 days.
- Routine immunizations, especially live vaccines, including varicella vaccine, should be given during remissions and when the child is on minimal immunosuppression (Lennon et al, 2010). Annual influenza vaccine is also recommended.
- Monitoring and prompt treatment of infection are essential. Varicella-zoster immune globulin must be given within 72 hours of exposure to varicella zoster. Sepsis workup should be done with any fever and broad-spectrum antibiotics given until the organism is identified (Lum, 2009).

Complications

Children with nephrotic syndrome are susceptible to pneumococcal, *E. coli, Pseudomonas*, and *Haemophilus influenzae* infection because of stasis of fluid; such infection is seen as peritonitis, pneumonia, cellulitis, or septicemia. Hypertension or hypotension is a possibility. Because the child is in a hypercoagulable state, thromboembolism is possible. Protein losses and compromising edema are also potential complications.

Patient Education, Prevention, and Prognosis

Patient education should stress the importance of continued, regular care to monitor renal function and the early treatment of the disease or concurrent infections. Families must know that relapses are the rule. An understanding of the disease process, side effects of steroids, recognition of infection, and the importance of monitoring proteinuria for relapses is crucial. If chronic steroid treatment is needed, the child and family must understand the side effects of the medication. The prognosis is good in steroid responders, with relapses that decrease in frequency as the child grows older, typically without any residual renal dysfunction.

NEPHRITIS AND GLOMERULONEPHRITIS

Description
Nephritis is a noninfectious, inflammatory response of the kidneys characterized by varied degrees of hypertension, edema, proteinuria, and hematuria that can be either microscopic or macroscopic with dysmorphic RBCs and casts. Nephritis is classified as acute, intermittent, or chronic. Primary GN occurs when the original and predominant structure impaired is the glomerulus. Secondary GN occurs when renal involvement is secondary to systemic disease (e.g., SLE, HSP, primary vasculitis, Goodpasture syndrome, or drug hypersensitivity reactions). Involvement can be in the glomerulus or the interstitium and either localized in one part of the kidney or generalized throughout. GN refers to inflammation primarily in the glomeruli; interstitial nephritis refers to inflammation in the interstitium primarily caused by drug reactions. Poststreptococcal GN (PSGN) is the classic form of GN.

Acute nephritis most commonly occurs as PSGN, which is characterized by a history of streptococcal infection within the prior 2 weeks and an acute onset of edema, oliguria, hypertension, and gross hematuria. Consider an alternative diagnosis if the following findings are present: nephrotic levels of protein, lack of evidence for a postinfection mechanism, rapidly deteriorating renal function, or clinical or laboratory findings suggesting other forms of GN (e.g., rash, positive ANA).

Intermittent gross hematuria and proteinuria syndromes include the following:

- *IgA nephropathy*, or *Berger disease*, is the most common chronic GN in children of European-Asian descent and is uncommon in African Americans; it has a 2:1 male preponderance. It is an immunologic entity causing recurrent gross and microscopic hematuria and often proteinuria. It is present in about one third of persons biopsied for persistent microscopic hematuria. It is often precipitated by viral infections or strenuous exercise, and each episode lasts less than 72 hours. BP is normal, no edema is present, and C3 is normal. Definitive diagnosis is made by biopsy. The prognosis is good in the absence of elevated serum creatinine or nephrotic-range proteinuria, although progression to chronic renal insufficiency can occur.
- Hereditary or familial nephritis involves many disorders, but the best known is *Alport syndrome*. More common and severe in males, with onset before 15 years of age in 75% of children, this condition is inherited as an X-linked dominant trait. The initial manifestation is isolated, persistent, microscopic hematuria with intermittent macrohematuria and variable proteinuria, occurring with an upper respiratory infection or exercise. Laboratory abnormalities are variable; biopsy verifies the diagnosis. Extrarenal abnormalities, including neurogenic deafness, ocular abnormalities, and macrothrombocytopenia, are often found. Vision and hearing screening is essential with referral for any abnormalities. Severe forms of the disease can lead to end-stage renal disease, which is often heralded by hypotension.
- Familial or benign recurrent nephritis, also known as thin-basement-membrane disease, is a disorder inherited as an autosomal dominant trait with unknown etiology. Episodes are characterized by macroscopic and microscopic hematuria and mild proteinuria, often precipitated by upper respiratory tract infection. Laboratory values other than UA are normal. The diagnosis is confirmed by biopsy, which may not be needed if the disease is mild and confirmed in relatives. In the absence of notable proteinuria, deafness, ocular defects, renal failure, and with normal biopsy findings, the prognosis is excellent.

Chronic nephritis is most commonly known as *membranoproliferative GN* (MPGN) and is distinguished by four types based on biopsy. Chronic nephritis can be found after acute nephritis or when investigating nonspecific complaints, such as anorexia, intermittent vomiting, and malaise. It is manifested by diminished renal function that ultimately has detrimental effects on other organ systems. Types I and II may respond to steroids, but the overall prognosis is guarded. Pyelonephritis, discussed earlier in the UTI section, is inflammation of the renal parenchyma, calyces, and pelvis caused by bacteria.

Epidemiology
The inflammatory response of the kidneys results from various causes, such as infection, an immunologic response, a drug or toxin, and vascular or systemic disorders. PSGN is an immune response by the host to a group A beta-hemolytic streptococcal infection, whereas acute postinfectious GN (APGN) can be caused by bacterial, fungal, viral, parasitic, or rickettsial agents.

PSGN is the most common form of nephritis in childhood, occurs most often between 5 and 12 years of age, occurs more often in males (2:1), and is unusual in children younger than 3 years of age. The incidence of APGN is difficult to determine because of the large number of patients with subclinical cases (Varade, 2009).

Clinical Findings
History
- Streptococcal skin (more likely) or pharyngeal infection within the past 2 to 3 weeks (PSGN). Classically a latent period of 7 to 10 days elapses between infection and the onset of symptoms; if fewer than 5 days or more than 14 days, consider other causes.
- Abrupt onset of gross hematuria
- Reduced urine output (with diuresis in 5 to 7 days)
- Lethargy, anorexia, nausea, vomiting, abdominal pain
- Chills, fever, backache (pyelonephritis)
- Medication for any infection taken in the past few weeks

Physical Examination
- Hypertension that is transient and resolves in 1 to 2 weeks
- Edema, especially periorbital edema, or abrupt onset with weight gain
- Circulatory congestion—dyspnea, cough, pallor, pulmonary edema if severe
- Ear malformations
- Flank or abdominal pain or a mass (in polycystic kidney or malignancy [e.g., Wilms tumor])
- Costovertebral angle tenderness (in pyelonephritis)
- Rashes or arthralgias (with SLE, HSP, or impetigo)
- Evidence of trauma or abuse

Diagnostic Studies

- UA with microscopic examination—tea color; elevated specific gravity; macrohematuria and microhematuria; proteinuria not exceeding the amount of hematuria; pyuria in PSGN; granular, hyaline, WBC, or RBC casts, and dysmorphic RBCs
- Serum C3 or C4 (low early in disease, returning to normal in 6 to 8 weeks), total protein and albumin (elevated)
- CBC, ESR, ASO titer (elevated), streptozyme test (positive), anti–deoxyribonucleic acid (DNA) antibody titer
- Electrolytes, BUN, creatinine, and cholesterol
- Fluorescent antinuclear antibody (SLE), hepatitis titers, sickle cell or hemoglobin electrophoresis, tuberculin PPD, and fluorescent treponemal antibody absorption (syphilis)

Differential Diagnosis

Acute nephritis also occurs as part of systemic illnesses, such as SLE, HSP, hemolytic-uremic syndrome, vasculitis, or as a reaction to drugs or irradiation.

Management

See Figure 34-10. Consultation with a nephrologist is recommended in all cases.

PSGN treatment is supportive because resolution occurs spontaneously 90% of the time within 6 to 24 months. The course does not seem to be affected by corticosteroids, immunosuppression, or other treatment modalities. During the peak of oliguria and hypertension in the first few days of illness, hospitalization may be required with fluid and sodium limitation and diuretic, antihypertensive, and antibiotic treatment if cultures are positive. Resolution occurs once diuresis begins. Gross hematuria persists for 1 to 2 weeks, urine can be abnormal for 6 to 12 weeks, and microscopic hematuria can persist for up to 2 years. Complement levels return to normal in 3 to 6 weeks.

- Acute nephritis—possible hospitalization with treatment, as described previously.
- IgA nephropathy—annual follow-up with BP, UA, and determination of renal function.
- Benign familial or hereditary nephritis—perform audiometry and review family medical history. Hereditary markers are being developed for this disease.
- Benign recurrent nephritis—monitor UA and renal function every 1 to 2 years.
- Chronic nephritis—a team approach is required to adequately provide care.

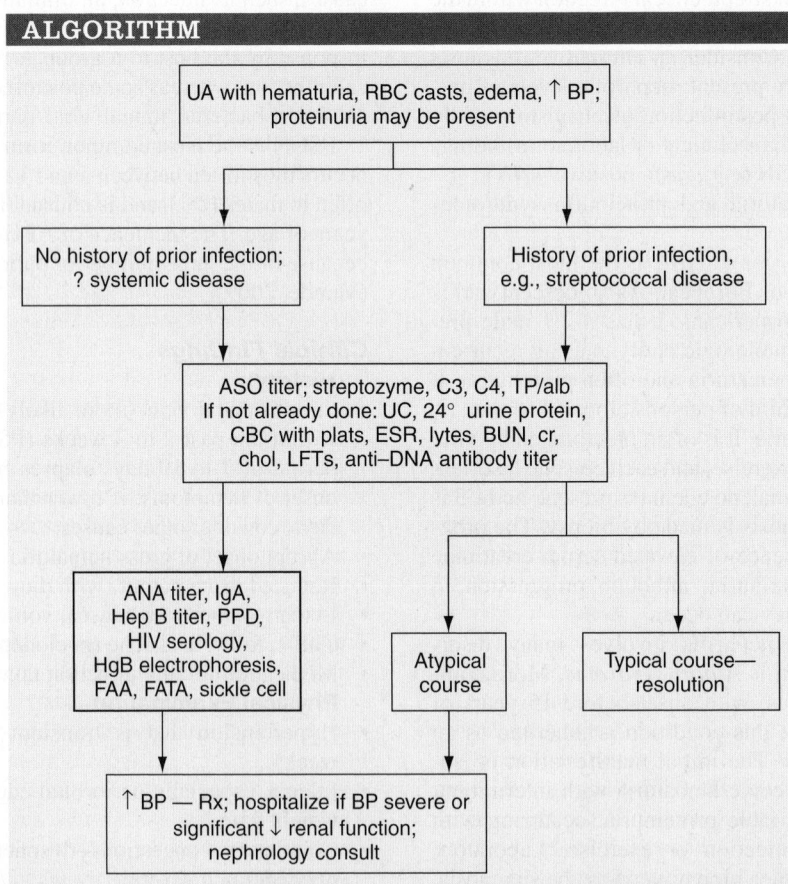

ALGORITHM

UA with hematuria, RBC casts, edema, ↑ BP; proteinuria may be present

No history of prior infection; ? systemic disease

History of prior infection, e.g., streptococcal disease

ASO titer; streptozyme, C3, C4, TP/alb
If not already done: UC, 24° urine protein,
CBC with plats, ESR, lytes, BUN, cr,
chol, LFTs, anti–DNA antibody titer

ANA titer, IgA,
Hep B titer, PPD,
HIV serology,
HgB electrophoresis,
FAA, FATA, sickle cell

Atypical course

Typical course— resolution

↑ BP — Rx; hospitalize if BP severe or significant ↓ renal function; nephrology consult

FIGURE 34-10 Evaluation of nephritis. *alb*, Albumin; *ANA*, antinuclear antibody; *ASO*, antistreptolysin O; *BP*, blood pressure; *BUN*, blood urea nitrogen; *C3*, complement 3; *C4*, complement 4; *CBC*, complete blood count; *chol*, cholesterol; *cr*, creatinine; *DNA*, deoxyribonucleic acid; *ESR*, erythrocyte sedimentation rate; *FAA*, fluorescent antinuclear antibody; *FATA*, fluorescent treponemal antibody absorption; *Hep B*, hepatitis B; *HgB*, hemoglobin; *HIV*, human immunodeficiency virus; *IgA*, immunoglobulin A; *LFT*, liver function test; *plats*, platelets; *PPD*, purified protein derivative; *RBC*, red blood cell; *Rx*, prescribe; *TP*, total protein; *UA*, urinalysis.

Complications

Prolonged oliguria and renal failure can occur if acute nephritis progresses. Hypertensive encephalopathy or congestive heart failure can occur secondary to PSGN. Irreversible parenchymal damage causes hypertension and renal insufficiency.

Patient Education, Prevention, and Prognosis

Patients with PSGN may have macrohematuria or microhematuria for up to 6 to 12 months, but the long-range outcome is excellent. Thin-basement-membrane disease has a good outcome. IgA nephropathy with severe histologic findings has a poor outcome, especially if the child is African-American. Patient education should stress the importance of continued, regular care to monitor renal function.

RENAL TUBULAR ACIDOSIS
Description

Dysfunction of renal tubule transport capability results in a condition known as renal tubular acidosis (RTA). Several distinct types of RTA have been identified. Type I, classic or distal RTA (dRTA), occurs when the defect is in the distal tubule. When the defect occurs in the proximal tubules, it is known as proximal RTA (pRTA), type II, or bicarbonate-wasting RTA. Type III has been reclassified as a subtype of type I that occurs primarily in preterm infants. Type IV, also known as hyperkalemic RTA, occurs with problems in the functioning of aldosterone most commonly following relief of obstructive uropathy (Dell and Avner, 2007).

The diagnosis depends on a combination of clinical features, laboratory values, and response to treatment.
- RTA is suggested by a serum carbon dioxide level less than 20, especially if the anion gap is normal (12 ± 4 mEq/L). Anion gap = $Na^+ - (Cl^- + HCO_3^-)$.
- dRTA (type I) is suggested by hypokalemia, hyperchloremia with a serum CO_2 less than 16, and urine pH greater than 5.5.
- pRTA (type II) is suggested by hypokalemia, hyperchloremia with a serum CO_2 less than 16, and urine pH less than 5.5.
- Type IV is suggested by hyperkalemia.

Fanconi syndrome is an uncommon and more complex form of pRTA (type II) with associated glycosuria, phosphaturia, aminoaciduria, and a defect in vitamin D metabolism manifested as nausea, anorexia, intermittent vomiting, and possibly rickets.

Epidemiology

RTA is often an isolated and primary problem with unknown cause. It can also be associated with systemic disease or intoxication. It is seen most typically in children evaluated for growth failure and is often revealed when illness, dehydration, or starvation stresses a child. RTA is more common in males than females, with pRTA being the most common form seen in children.

Dysfunction in the transport capability of the renal tubules affects either the reabsorption of filtered bicarbonate, excretion of hydrogen ion, or both and results in a metabolic acidosis. The proximal tubule, which normally absorbs 85% of bicarbonate, is able to reabsorb only 60% of bicarbonate from filtered urine in patients with pRTA. The distal tubule continues to function and reabsorbs approximately 15% of the bicarbonate, and the urine is acidified (pH less than 5.5). However, a large amount of bicarbonate is wasted. As the body adapts, a new threshold for serum bicarbonate is set, usually around 14 to 16 mEq/L (Dell and Avner, 2007).

A defect in the ability of the distal renal tubule to excrete hydrogen is the cause of dRTA. This defect causes complete loss of reabsorption of the final 15% of bicarbonate and an inability to acidify urine (pH greater than 5.5). Type IV RTA is characterized by a deficiency in the production or responsiveness of aldosterone and impaired ammonia production. Type IV RTA is often associated with an obstructive uropathy or other transient phenomenon in infancy (Dell and Avner, 2007).

Clinical Findings
History
- Failure to gain weight (especially) and height—the most common symptoms
- Polyuria and polydipsia
- Muscle weakness (caused by hypokalemia)
- Irritability before eating, satiation after eating, vomiting, diarrhea, or constipation in dRTA
- Preference for liquids over solid foods, poor appetite, or anorexia, especially with type IV

Physical Examination
- Arrested growth curve toward the end of the first year with prior consistent growth
- Normal physical examination and development

Diagnostic Studies
- Serum electrolytes, including CO_2 (hypokalemia, hyperchloremic metabolic acidosis), renal function tests (BUN, creatinine), calcium, phosphorus, alkaline phosphatase, and UA (first-morning void) to test for glucose and pH

If any of the laboratory findings are abnormal, consider the following:
- A 24-hour creatinine clearance to establish the normal GFR, calcium (normal less than 4 mg/kg/24 hr), and calcium-creatinine ratio
- Renal ultrasonography to determine the anatomy and rule out nephrocalcinosis, nephrolithiasis, hydronephrosis, obstructive uropathy, and parenchymal damage

Differential Diagnosis

Primary RTA must be differentiated from secondary RTA, which can be due to many disease states or conditions, such as other causes of growth failure (e.g., FTT), hypothyroidism, and systemic acidosis.

Management

Goals of management include correcting the acidosis and maintaining normal bicarbonate (greater than 20 mEq/L), thereby restoring growth and minimizing complications.
- Oral alkalizing medications are given to achieve these goals. Dosing is determined by the type of RTA. dRTA requires low doses, often between 2 and 5 mEq/kg/day. pRTA requires high doses, often between 5 and 15 mEq/kg/day and sometimes as high as 20 mEq/kg/day. The dose

must be titrated to the child's response as determined by weight and laboratory results (CO_2 and electrolytes). Initiate medication at 3 mEq/kg/day and check laboratory results in a few days. Titrate the dose until a serum bicarbonate level of 20 to 22 mEq/L is achieved (Dell and Avner, 2007). To maintain as normal a bicarbonate level as possible, doses should be given frequently throughout the day (with meals) and as late as possible at night (at bedtime). A larger dose at bedtime has been advocated to coincide with growth hormone secretion at night to maximize growth (Kallen, 2009).

○ Bicitra (sodium citrate and citric acid or Shohl solution), which equals 1 mEq bicarbonate/mL and is relatively pleasant tasting

○ Polycitra (sodium and potassium citrate and citric acid), which equals 2 mEq bicarbonate/mL and is less palatable. Giving it in juice, water, or formula may ease its administration. Polycitra is especially useful if the child is hypokalemic or requires an excess quantity or if compliance is an issue.

○ $NaHCO_3$ tablets, available in 325-mg strength (4 mEq bicarbonate) and 650-mg strength (8 mEq bicarbonate)

○ 8 oz baking soda mixed with 2.65 L of distilled water; equals 1 mEq/mL of bicarbonate

- The response to medication helps confirm the diagnosis and type of RTA. dRTA has a rapid response to treatment, and normal bicarbonate levels are maintained with little difficulty. pRTA requires higher doses to normalize bicarbonate and is less easily maintained. Type IV RTA requires mineralocorticoid treatment if aldosterone is deficient.
- Maximizing caloric intake to enhance growth can be accomplished by emphasizing solid foods for all meals and snacks, and avoiding water and noncaloric foods. Providing nutritional supplements is also ideal.
- Meticulous follow-up is imperative. Weight and laboratory results should be monitored biweekly to monthly until weight gain is established and CO_2 is stabilized. Weighing on the same scale and by the same person is essential.
- Pseudoephedrine should be avoided because it is minimally excreted in alkalinized urine and associated with a risk of intoxication.
- Referral to a pediatric nephrologist is necessary for any child who is not growing well despite treatment, or whose laboratory values are not normalizing with treatment, has unusual laboratory results, has type IV RTA, or has any complication of RTA.

Complications

It is rare to have complications with pRTA. Hypercalciuria can occur with dRTA, leading to nephrocalcinosis, nephrolithiasis, renal parenchymal destruction, and occasionally renal failure. Rickets are sometimes found in type IV RTA.

Patient Education, Prevention, and Prognosis

Patient education should stress the importance of continued, regular care to monitor renal function and growth. Isolated pRTA responds quickly to treatment, with children showing catch-up growth and obtaining normal maximum height. pRTA resolves spontaneously without recurrence of

symptoms, often within 1 to 2 years but at worst over the first decade of life (Dell and Avner, 2007). dRTA usually lasts a lifetime; type IV resolves with correction of the underlying problem.

NEPHROLITHIASIS AND UROLITHIASIS
Description

Urinary stones can be found anywhere in the urinary tract. In North America most children with stones have stones that are found in the kidneys; bladder stones occur in less than 10% of the pediatric cases and are most often related to urologic abnormalities. Bladder stones are endemic to other parts of the world and are likely related to diet.

Epidemiology

The prevalence of urinary stones varies by region, with a higher incidence in the Southeast U.S. and in Caucasians, with a slightly higher incidence in males than in females. Seventy-five percent of children who have nephrolithiasis have an identifiable predisposition to stone formation. Metabolic risk factors account for more than 50% of cases, structural abnormalities account for 32%, and infections account for 4%. Hypercalciuria is the most common metabolic cause (accounts for 30% to 60%) of urinary calculi and is a condition with many causes including renal tubular dysfunction, endocrine disturbances, bone metabolic disorders, UTI, familial idiopathic hypercalcemia, and medications (Elder, 2007c). Hyperoxaluria is found in up to 20% of children with nephrolithiasis. Hyperuricosuria has been documented in 2% to 10% of children with stone formation. Cystine stones account for less than 1% of urinary stones.

Clinical Findings
History
- Family history of nephrolithiasis, arthritis, gout, or renal disease
- Stones or fragments passed in urine
- Dietary history high in protein, sodium, calcium, and oxalate intake
- Colic in an infant
- History or symptoms suggestive of a UTI in a preschooler

Physical Examination
- Abdominal, flank, or pelvic pain (occurs at all ages, but present in 94% of adolescents)

Diagnostic Studies
- UA and culture shows gross or microscopic hematuria in 33% to 90% of children and stone or stone fragments with chemical analysis.
- Abdominal radiography, abdominal ultrasound, and/or CT

Differential Diagnosis

Other diagnoses causing flank pain should be considered (e.g., UTI or pyelonephritis and trauma). Just slightly more than half of preschool children with nephrolithiasis have flank pain, so other afebrile illnesses including gastrointestinal viral syndromes and early appendicitis, chronic recurrent abdominal pain of no known cause, and emotional stress should be considered in the preschool child.

Management

Increased fluid intake is the first line of therapy for all stone types regardless of the cause. In adolescents, a goal of 2 L of urine output per day is helpful. Stone removal may be required if the stone is not passed and severe symptoms continue for a significant amount of time. Extracorporeal shockwave lithotripsy (ESWL) is safe in children; long-term kidney damage has not been validated in follow-up studies. Skin bruising and hematuria are almost universal side effects of ESWL. Stones may also be removed by using rigid or flexible endoscopes passed through the urethra into the bladder or ureter. Renal calculi may also be removed percutaneously, and open surgical lithotomy is still an option if other techniques fail.

Refer to a dietary expert for nutritional advice. Dietary restrictions control stone formation and renal injury in most metabolic disorders contributing to stone formation. Refer to urologist for a complete metabolic evaluation if stone or fragments are passed or seen in the urinary system on imaging studies.

Patient Education, Prevention, and Prognosis

Recurrence rates are high if left untreated, and patients with hyperuricosuria may continue to have symptomatic or asymptomatic calculi. Despite an excellent response to therapy, children with nephrolithiasis require long-term follow-up with a nephrologist because of the potential for renal insufficiency and end-stage renal disease.

WILMS TUMOR

Description

Wilms tumor, the most common malignancy of the genitourinary tract, is typically recognized as a firm, smooth mass in the abdomen or flank. It is staged according to the National Wilms Tumor Study as follows:

- Stage I: The tumor is limited to the kidney and can be completely excised with the capsular surface intact.
- Stage II: The tumor extends beyond the kidney but can still be completely excised.
- Stage III: There is postsurgical residual nonhematogenous extension confined to the abdomen.
- Stage IV: There is hematogenous metastasis, most frequently to the lung.
- Stage V: There is bilateral kidney involvement.

Epidemiology

This malignancy manifests as a solitary growth in any part of either or both kidneys. There are approximately eight cases of Wilms tumor per million children less than 15 years of age (Jaffe and Huff, 2007). Most Wilms tumors occur in children between 2 and 5 years of age. The peak incidence and median age at diagnosis is 3 years of age. About 1% to 2% of children with Wilms tumor have a family history, and the tumor is inherited in an autosomal dominant manner (Jaffe and Huff, 2007). An important feature of Wilms tumor is the occurrence of associated congenital anomalies including renal abnormalities, such as cryptorchidism, hypospadias, duplication of the collecting system, ambiguous genitalia, hemihypertrophy, aniridia, cardiac abnormalities, and Beckwith-Wiedemann, Denys-Drash, and Perlman syndromes. Wilms tumor develops in 15% to

20% of children with neurofibromatosis. It occurs with equal frequency in both sexes and has a 3:1 African-American–to–Caucasian incidence; 55% of tumors occur on the left side.

Clinical Findings

History

- The most frequent finding is increasing abdominal size or an actual palpable mass.
- Pain is reported if the mass has undergone rapid growth or hemorrhage.
- Fever, dyspnea, diarrhea, vomiting, weight loss, or malaise may be reported.

Physical Examination

- A firm, smooth abdominal or flank mass that does not cross the midline may be noted.
- BP is elevated if renal ischemia is present (rare).
- A left varicocele is found in males if the spermatic vein is obstructed.
- A careful examination is needed to rule out congenital anomalies.

Diagnostic Studies

- Chest and abdominal radiography is performed to differentiate neuroblastoma, which is usually calcified.
- Abdominal ultrasonography is used to differentiate a solid from a cystic mass or hydronephrosis and multicystic kidney.
- UA demonstrates hematuria in 25% to 33% of children.
- A CBC, reticulocyte count, and liver and renal chemistry studies are performed.
- A CT scan of the chest, abdomen, and pelvis to stage the disease and bone marrow is done by the oncology team.

Differential Diagnosis

Neuroblastoma is the main differential diagnosis (the mass often crosses the midline). Multicystic kidney, hydronephrosis, renal cyst, or other renal malignancies are additional conditions to consider.

Management

Diagnostic workup is the initial urgent priority, with concurrent referral to a pediatric cancer center for treatment. Surgery is scheduled to remove the affected kidney and possibly the ureter and adrenal gland; combined chemotherapy and radiotherapy are instituted if the disease is advanced or histologic findings are unfavorable. Close follow-up after the initial treatment should be coordinated with the cancer team.

Complications

The lungs and liver are the most common sites of metastasis. High BP is possible because of renal ischemia and occasionally leads to cardiac failure. Scoliosis resulting from radiation therapy is uncommon because radiation exposure is carefully controlled.

Patient Education, Prevention, and Prognosis

The prognosis is determined by the histology of the neoplasm, by the patient's age (the younger the better), the size of the tumor, positive nodes, and, most significantly, the extent or stage of the disease. A pediatric urologist should determine if a child should be allowed to participate in sports on an individual basis (American Association of Family Physicians [AAFP] et al, 2010). Use of kidney protectors is highly recommended during sports. New information on the long-term sequelae for the treatment of Wilms tumors and the present trials and treatment recommendations can be accessed at the National Wilms Tumor Study.

■ Common Genitourinary Conditions in Males

HYPOSPADIAS

Description

Hypospadias is a common congenital abnormality in which the urethral meatus is located anywhere from the proximal glans to the perineum on the ventral surface (underside) of the penis. Chordee, a ventral bowing of the penis, occurs when a tight band of fibrous tissue pulls on the penis. Torsion refers to rotation of the penis to the right or left.

Epidemiology

The etiology of hypospadias is unknown. It is believed that the endocrine system probably has an important role, but what that role is remains unclear. The primitive gonad in the eighth week of embryonic development differentiates into male or female. As the genital tubercle enlarges, developmental arrest occurs along the line of urethral fusion and causes hypospadias.

Hypospadias occurs in 1 in 250 male infants (Elder, 2007a). There was a major increase in incidence in the 1990s, especially in low-birthweight babies and babies whose mothers had taken fertility drugs or undergone in vitro fertilization. The cause of this may be due to genetic factors (e.g., endocrine abnormalities) or environmental factors (e.g., androgen blockers and estrogen or endocrine disruptors), and it probably occurs early in gestation. Risk is increased if family members have hypospadias: 8% if the father, 14% if a sibling, and 21% if two family members. Hypospadias occurs more commonly in Caucasians, in Italians and Jews, and in winter conceptions. Ten percent of boys with hypospadias also have undescended testicles, inguinal hernia, or hydrocele (Elder, 2007a).

Clinical Findings

History

- A family history of a male relative with genitourinary problems may be reported.
- The child sits to void or urinates on the floor in front of the toilet unless he holds his penis to direct the stream.

Physical Examination. In a newborn the classic finding is a dorsally hooded foreskin. It is essential to visualize the urethral meatus. Pulling the ventral shaft skin in a downward and outward direction facilitates visualization. Anatomic classification is made by location:

- Anterior (70%), glanular, coronal, or anterior penile
- Middle (10%)
- Posterior (20%), scrotal, penoscrotal, or posterior penile
  Other findings include:
- Urinary stream that aims downward rather than straight
- Inguinal hernia or undescended testicles (9%)
- Chordee

Differential Diagnosis

The differential diagnosis includes intersex abnormalities.

Management

The goal of surgical repair is to have a functional penis that appears normal. Circumcision must not be done because the foreskin may be used in the surgical repair. Referral should be made to a pediatric urologist at birth for evaluation. Surgery to correct hypospadias is best done at around 6 to 18 months of age. Considerations in scheduling surgery at this age include the following: it is psychologically less damaging; a caudal block is easily performed; the wound heals more rapidly; and there is more time to repair complications before toilet training begins. Surgery scheduled after 18 months of age minimizes anesthesia risk, the larger anatomy makes surgery easier, and the patient can participate in the decision-making process. Repair is usually accomplished in a one-stage outpatient procedure unless it is a complex defect.

Complications

With unrepaired hypospadias, peer taunting of boys and problems with erections are possible complications. Intersex abnormalities are possible if associated with cryptorchidism.

Patient Education, Prevention, and Prognosis

Education and reassurance regarding etiology, repair, and outcome should be provided. Careful assessment of the newborn should be done when hypospadias is reported in a family member. Hypospadias is usually an isolated anomaly, but it does require further workup to assess the anatomy of the urinary system for other anomalies.

CRYPTORCHIDISM (UNDESCENDED TESTES)

Description

Cryptorchidism describes a testis that does not reside in and cannot be manipulated into the scrotum. A retractile testis is out of the scrotum, but can be brought into the scrotum and remains there. A gliding testis can be brought into the scrotum, but returns to a high position in the scrotum once released. An ectopic testis lies outside the normal path of descent. An ascended testis is one that has fully descended, but has spontaneously re-ascended and lies outside the scrotum. A trapped testis is one dislocated after herniorrhaphy. Any testis that is not in the scrotum is subject to progressive deterioration. Undescended testes are a common disorder that often causes great anxiety for parents.

Epidemiology

Testes develop in the abdomen and descend in the seventh fetal month to the upper part of the groin, subsequently progressing through the inguinal canal into the scrotum. Failure of the testes to descend can be caused by mechanical lesions or can be secondary to hormonal, chromosomal, enzymatic, or anatomic disorders.

Undescended testis is the most common genitourinary disorder in boys, occurring in 3 per 1000 newborns (Mahesh and Woroniecki, 2009). It is more common in preterm, low-birthweight, and twin infants. The incidence of cryptorchidism is 0.2% to 1.8% in young adults, 0.5% to 0.8% in children 0 to 1 year of age, 2.5% to 4% in term infants, and 20% to 30% in premature infants. More than 60% of infants with a birthweight less than 1500 g and nearly 100% of 900-g neonates have undescended testes (Elder, 2007b). A great majority of undescended testes descend spontaneously by 6 months of age. After 6 months of age, it is rare for them to descend. The frequency of bilateral occurrence is 10% to 25%; unilateral involvement (55% to 66%) is more likely to be right sided. Retractile testes are bilateral and most common in boys 5 to 6 years of age.

Clinical Findings
History
- Family history of undescended testes or testicular malignancy
- Testes not consistently descended during the infant's bath
- Associated urinary problems
- Risk factors include prematurity, being first born, cesarean section, toxemia, hypospadias, congenital subluxation of the hip, low birthweight, winter conception, Down syndrome, maternal age less than 20 and more than 35 years of age
- Other congenital, endocrine, chromosomal, or intersex disorders

Physical Examination. Having the child sit cross-legged or frog-legged, squat, or stand can facilitate testicle descent and palpation.
- Scrotal rugae less fully developed
- Bilateral or unilateral absence of a testicle
- Retractile testes, which move between the scrotum and external ring, but can be manipulated to the lower part of the scrotum and remain there; in children 3 months to 7 years old, retraction is especially common with tactile stimulation of the area or cold
- Gliding testes that lie between the scrotum and external ring and can be manipulated to the lower part of the scrotum, but return to the high position
- Location:
  ○ Prescrotal (at the external inguinal ring)
  ○ Canalicular, high or low (between the external and internal rings), the most common type
  ○ Ectopic (superficial inguinal, femoral, or perineal)
  ○ Intraabdominal (above the internal inguinal ring), not palpable, occurring in less than 15% of males with undescended testes
  ○ Indirect inguinal hernia

Diagnostic Studies. None are indicated except in newborns with potential sex abnormalities, hypopituitarism, Down syndrome, or congenital adrenal hyperplasia. The risk of intersex abnormality is 27% if hypospadias and unilateral or bilateral cryptorchidism are present.

Differential Diagnosis
Anorchism and chromosomal abnormalities are the differential diagnoses.

Management
The goals of treating undescended testes are to improve fertility outcome, decrease malignancy potential, and minimize the psychological stress associated with an empty scrotum.

Management has come full circle from an initial recommendation for surgery, to treatment with hormonal therapy, and back to early surgical intervention. Both forms of treatment are still options. The best time for surgical repair remains a controversy. One belief is that the optimal timing for repair is 6 months of age because the critical time for maturation and transformation of gonocytes to adult dark spermatogonia is before 6 months of age. However, others believe that surgical management within the first 2 years of life improves future fertility.
- If the testes are undescended by 6 months of age with the peak of postnatal testosterone, they are unlikely to descend spontaneously. If the testes have not descended by 1 year of age, an orchiopexy should be performed by a skilled pediatric urologist or surgeon with an attendant, skilled pediatric anesthesiologist. A laparoscopic orchiopexy is the surgical procedure of choice, although repair can be done by inguinal incision or the intraabdominal route, depending on placement of the testes.
- Hormonal therapy can be used to differentiate a retractile testis from a true cryptorchid testis. Human chorionic gonadotropin (hCG) by the intramuscular route is the only approved method in the U.S., although intranasal gonadotropin-releasing hormone (GnRH) is used in other countries.
- In a child younger than 1 year of age, regular examination to assess the position of the testes should be performed at every well-child care visit. If the testes remain undescended, referral to a pediatric urologist or surgeon should occur by 1 year of age. Referral should also occur if a retractile testis does not retain scrotal residence.
- If undescended testes are found after 1 year of age, the child should be immediately referred to a pediatric urologist or surgeon for treatment.

Complications
Poor testicular development, infertility, malignancy, vulnerability to trauma, testicular torsion, and inguinal hernia are possible complications of undescended testicles.

Patient Education, Prevention, and Prognosis
Histologic changes have been shown in an undescended testis as early as 6 months of age, with irreversible changes shown by 2 years of age that contribute to infertility and are associated with malignancy (Elder, 2007b). Infertility as a complication of cryptorchidism has been reported in as many as 15% of men with unilateral undescended testes and 35% to 50% if bilateral (Elder, 2007b). Testicular malignancy in males with cryptorchidism is reported to have an incidence 4 to 10 times higher than the general population. Correction of undescended testes does not diminish the incidence of testicular cancer (North and Gearhart, 2009), although an increased incidence in testicular tumors has been observed if orchiopexy is done at later ages. Malignancy is more common with an intraabdominal testis. A testicular neoplasm in one child mandates examination of his male siblings.

Testicular self-examination should be taught to all adolescents but especially to these young men (Fig. 34-11). The website for the Testicular Cancer Awareness Week has a patient handout sheet on testicular self-examination and provides the opportunity to sign up to receive monthly reminders to perform testicular self-examination.

In the realm of "if it ain't broke, don't fix it," there has been a substantial increase in information about prostate cancer. However, testicular cancer is the most common cancer in men 15 to 35 yr old, an age when we do not want to admit the possibility of illness. If detected early, it is among the easiest to cure. For men in this age group, a once-a-month simple self-examination is suggested. This can help catch this cancer at an early stage.

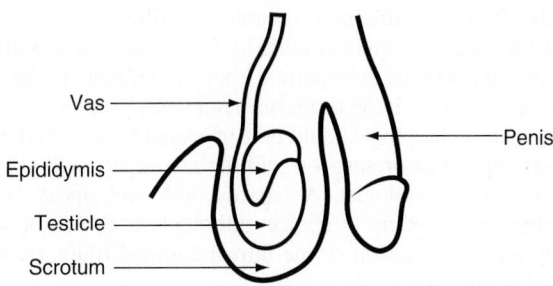

The most convenient time to examine yourself is while taking a shower or bath. The warm water causes the skin to relax, making the examination of the underlying tissues easier.

First:

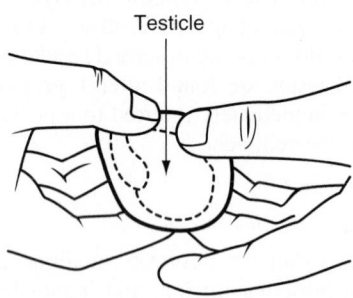

Examine your testicles. Slowly roll each testicle between thumb and forefingers. Try to find any hard, nonsensitive bumps.

Second:

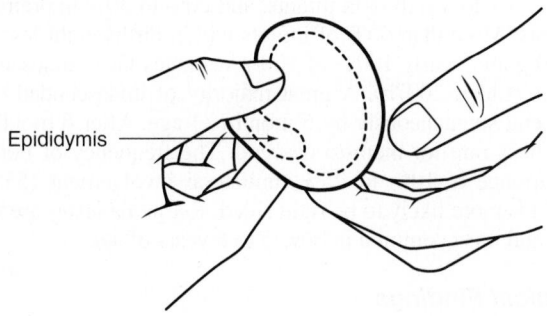

Examine the epididymis for lumps. This crescent-shaped cord is behind each testicle. This area is tender so do not be alarmed.

Third:

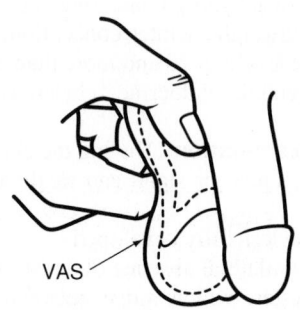

Examine the vas deferens, the sperm carrying tube that extends from the epididymis of each testicle.

Symptoms:
In early stages, testicular cancer may be symptomless. When symptoms do occur, they include:
* Lump on testicle, epididymis, or vas deferens
* Enlargement of a testicle
* Heavy sensation in groin area or testicles
* Dull ache in groin or abdomen area
If you find a lump or have any of the above symtoms, see your physician or NP immediately for an accurate diagnosis.

FIGURE 34-11 Self-examination for testicular cancer. (From National Men's Resource Center: *Self exam for testicular cancer: "in the shower" guide,* San Anselmo, CA, 1994, The Center.)

No evidence has indicated that undescended testes resolve with puberty; retractile testes generally settle into the scrotum by puberty. Open discussion of the problem, management, and potential complications is essential, initially as well as over time. Participation in contact sports is discouraged because of the risk of losing the one viable testicle to trauma.

HYDROCELE

Description

A common cause of painless scrotal swelling is a hydrocele, a collection of serous fluid in the scrotal sac. A noncommunicating hydrocele has a collection of fluid only in the scrotum. If the processus vaginalis remains patent so that fluid moves from the abdomen to the scrotum, it is called a communicating hydrocele and is more likely to be associated with a hernia (Fig. 34-12).

Epidemiology

Incomplete closure of the processus vaginalis through which the testes descend into the scrotum allows a hydrocele to develop. Incidence is 0.5% to 2% of males, appearing primarily in those younger than 1 year of age (Schnitzer, 2006).

Clinical Findings

Hydroceles that persist beyond 1 year of age are assumed to be in conjunction with a hernia. In older children, hydroceles appear after trauma, with an inflammatory illness or neoplasm.

History

* Intermittent or constant bulge or lump in the scrotum, often more distally placed. Scrotal size increases with activity and decreases with rest.
* Overlying skin may be tense.
* No distress or vomiting

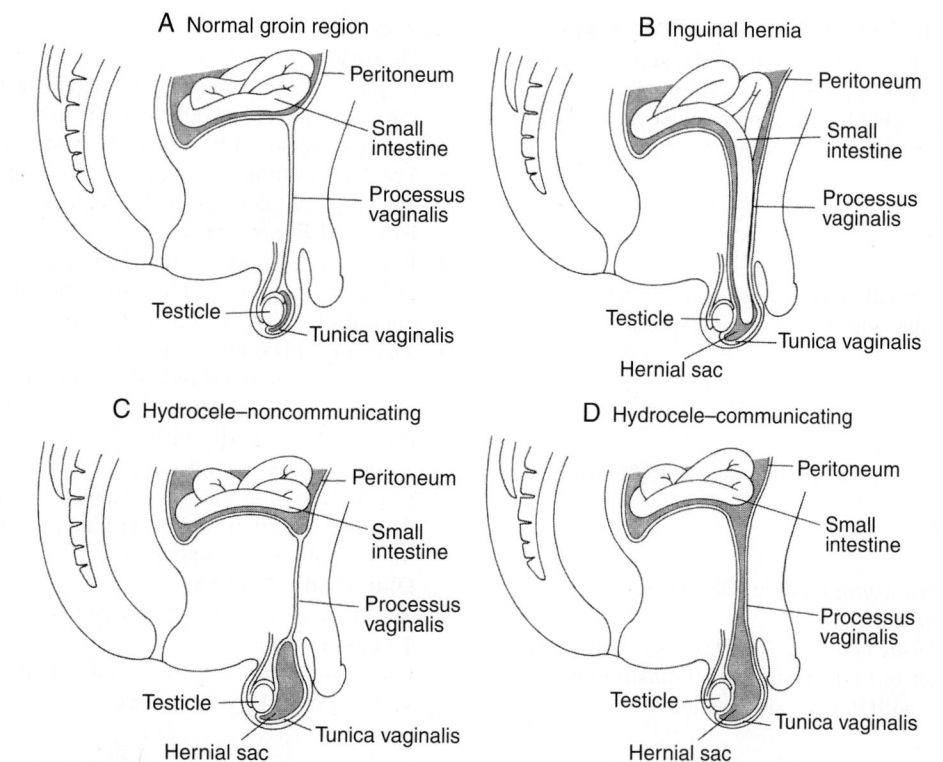

FIGURE 34-12 Hydroceles and hernias. **A,** Groin region of the normal male infant. **B,** An inguinal hernia is the protrusion of bowel into the groin region. **C,** A hydrocele is a collection of fluid within the processus vaginalis. In a noncommunicating hydrocele, the scrotal swelling does not change in size or shape because there is no connection with the abdominal cavity. **D,** In a communicating hydrocele, the processus vaginalis remains open from the scrotum to the abdominal cavity, and scrotal swelling may vary in size during the course of an infant's day. (From Betz CL, Hunsberger M, Wright S: *Family-centered nursing care of infants*, ed 2, Philadelphia, 1994, Saunders.)

Physical Examination

- Asymmetry or a scrotal mass present; if swelling is present in the inguinal area, a hernia is probable; swelling is usually unilateral (Table 34-6)
- Testes descended
- Translucent on transillumination (pink or red glow)
- Noncommunicating hydrocele—scrotal sac tense, slightly blue tinged, fluctuant, and does not reduce; no swelling in the inguinal region
- Communicating hydrocele—fluid in the scrotal sac comes and goes (probably flat in the morning, swollen later in the day)

Differential Diagnosis

Hernia, undescended testicle, retractile testicle, and inguinal lymphadenopathy are the differential diagnoses.

Management

- Noncommunicating hydrocele—fluid is generally absorbed spontaneously; no treatment is indicated unless the hydrocele is so large that it is uncomfortable or persists longer than 1 year.
- Communicating hydrocele—Many communicating hydroceles will resolve without surgery and deserve observation (Koski et al, 2010). If the hernia persists for more than 1 year, surgical intervention is generally recommended.
- Surgery is usually done on an outpatient basis.

TABLE 34-6 Physical Findings in Scrotal Swellings

Condition	Tender	Red	Blue	Cremasteric Reflex	Transillumination
Chronic					
Hydrocele	−	−	+	+	+
Tumor	−	−	−	+	−
Varicocele	−	−	−	+	−
Acute					
Torsion of newborn	−	−	+	−	−
Torsion of older child	+	+	−	−	−
Torsion of appendage	+	+	−	+	−
Epididymitis	+	+	−	+	−
Trauma	+	−	+	±	−

From Kaplan GN: Scrotal swelling in children, *Pediatr Rev* 21(9):312, 2000.

Patient Education, Prevention, and Prognosis

Reassure parent that the increased size of the scrotal sac will resolve, usually by 1 year of age and involves no danger. Signs of hernia must be explained, and parents must be alerted to observe and report any abnormal findings.

SPERMATOCELE

Description

A benign, painless scrotal mass or cyst on the head of the epididymis or testicular adnexa containing sperm is called a *spermatocele*.

Epidemiology

A spermatocele is an uncommon, generally benign finding.

Clinical Findings

History
- Scrotal swelling but asymptomatic otherwise

Physical Examination
- Painless, mobile cystic nodule usually less than 1 cm in size, superior and posterior to the testicle that transilluminates
- No change in size with the Valsalva maneuver

Differential Diagnosis

A varicocele and an epididymal cyst (identical in appearance, but not containing sperm) are the differential diagnoses.

Management

No treatment is required unless the cyst is large and bothersome or painful. Refer the patient for an ultrasound or to a urologist.

Patient Education, Prevention, and Prognosis

Any pain or discomfort should be reported. Testicular self-examination assists in early detection of this disorder in later adolescence.

VARICOCELE

Description

A varicocele is a benign enlargement or dilation of testicular veins causing a painless scrotal mass of varying size that may feel like a "bag of worms." It is usually found on the left side.

Epidemiology

The etiology of varicoceles is probably multifactorial, with the physiologic changes associated with puberty playing some role. A varicocele is caused by valvular incompetence of the spermatic vein resulting in dilated or varicose veins. Varicoceles are rare before 10 years of age and may be indicative of malignancy. They occur in 5% of adolescent males and 15% of adult males (Elder, 2007b, Palmer, 2009). Up to 85% to 95% arise on the left side because the left spermatic vein drains into the left renal vein and arterial compression of the renal vein obstructs blood flow from the vein. In contrast, the right spermatic vein drains into the vena cava. However, 22% of varicoceles occur bilaterally.

Clinical Findings

History
- Usually a painless swelling is noted in the left side of the scrotum, occasionally a "dull ache" or "heavy" feeling if large.
- Pain can occur with strenuous physical activity.
- Scrotal swelling with prolonged standing causes pain; swelling and pain resolve on reclining.

Physical Examination
- In the standing position, a "bag of worms" can be felt posterior and superior to the testis that collapses on lying and enlarges with the Valsalva maneuver.
- Measure and compare the size of both testes (length, width, and depth) using a standard orchidometer.
- Grade 3 varicocele, the classic "bag of worms," is larger than 2 cm and easily visualized; grade 2 varicocele is 1 to 2 cm in diameter and is easily palpable when the adolescent is standing, but not visualized; grade 1 varicocele is the most common, very small, and difficult to palpate (the Valsalva maneuver may help).

Diagnostic Studies
- Serial ultrasonography to measure testicular size every 6 to 12 months of age
- Ultrasonography to rule out malignancy in children younger than 10 years of age

Differential Diagnosis

Varicoceles must be differentiated from other testicular masses, such as lipoma, hernia, hydrocele, spermatocele, and tumors.

Management

Asymptomatic grade 1 varicocele with normal testicular volumes usually does not require intervention in adolescence. Ultrasonographic monitoring of testicular size can be done every 6 months. Any change in comfort level should be reported. Referral to a surgeon or urologist should be made if the varicocele is grade 2 or 3, if the varicocele is painful, if the difference in testicular volume is marked (greater than 2 mm by ultrasound), if the varicocele is right sided or bilateral, or if testicular growth becomes retarded over a 6- to 12-month period (Elder, 2007b). Treatment by spermatic vein embolization or ligation may be attempted in adolescents. Ligation is the usual procedure, completed on an outpatient basis with few complications.

Complications

Atrophy or testicular growth arrest, as noted by a discrepancy in testicular size, can occur. Lower fertility rates with decreased sperm concentration and motility have been noted and are factors in an aggressive surgical approach for the adolescent male with grade 2 or 3 varicocele. Hydrocele may be an insignificant, self-limiting complication following surgery.

Patient Education, Prevention, and Prognosis

A varicocele is the most common cause of infertility. Because of this, early identification is essential. All patients should be counseled about the long-term risks to fertility. Correction of testicular atrophy and an improved sperm count and fertility have been noted in 80% to 90% of those undergoing surgery early in adolescence. Testicular self-examination assists in early detection of this disorder.

INGUINAL HERNIA

Description

A scrotal or inguinal swelling (or both) that includes abdominal contents is an inguinal hernia (see Fig. 34-12). In females, inguinal hernias cause swelling in the inguinal area and labia majora.

Epidemiology

Incomplete closure of the processus vaginalis through which the testes descend into the scrotum allows the presence of abdominal contents in the inguinal canal or scrotum (labia majora in females) and thus the development of a hernia. Males who are obese or weight lifters or have a family history of undescended testes are at high risk for hernias.

Inguinal hernias are much more common in males than in females (8 to 10:1), occurring in 1% to 5% of boys. Premature infants are at increased risk (7% to 30% of males, 2% of females). More than 50% of hernias are diagnosed during the first year of life, with the peak incidence in the first 3 months of life. Bilateral hernias are common (10% to 20%). Unilateral hernias are more likely to occur on the right side (50% to 60%) than the left (30%) (Aiken and Oldham, 2007). Indirect hernias are a congenital condition and are the most common type in children younger than 3 years of age. Direct hernias increase in incidence after 3 years of age and are usually acquired. Incarceration is more likely to occur within 2 weeks of initial diagnosis of the hernia. There does not seem to be any increased risk of incarceration based on age (Gholoum et al, 2010).

Clinical Findings
History
- Family history of undescended testes
- Swelling in the inguinal area, scrotum, or both that comes and goes and increases with crying or straining
- Weight lifting or obesity
- Prematurity
Physical Examination
- Swelling is found in the inguinal area, scrotal area (labia majora in females), or both.
- The hernia is reducible with pressure on the distal end.
- Transillumination does not occur unless the bowel is filled with fluid.
- Direct hernias push outward through the weakest point in the abdominal wall.
- Indirect hernias push downward at an angle into the inguinal canal.
- The child is fussy and has a distended abdomen if the hernia is incarcerated.
- Silk glove sign—a sensation of two surfaces rubbing against each other while one palpates the spermatic cord as it crosses the pubic tubercle.

Diagnostic Studies. An abdominal radiograph can be helpful if air is present below the inguinal ligament. Ultrasonography can differentiate a hernia from a hydrocele and is especially helpful if an incarcerated hernia is suspected.

Differential Diagnosis

Hydrocele, undescended testes, and inguinal lymphadenopathy are included in the differential diagnosis.

Management

If a child is seen with a hernia, an attempt should be made to reduce it, and the child should be referred to a surgeon or urologist for repair within 1 to 2 weeks. Even if no swelling is seen at the visit but is elicited by the history, the child should be referred to a surgeon or urologist. Inguinal hernias do not resolve spontaneously. Premature infants should have the hernia repaired prior to discharge. If the hernia is not easily reduced, if it is painful, or if a hard, tender, or red mass is present, refer immediately. If reduction has been difficult and ischemia is ongoing, hospitalization and surgical repair within 24 to 48 hours are indicated.

Complications

Incarceration and strangulation of a hernia cause pain, irritability, erythema, vomiting, and abdominal distention. The overall incidence of incarceration is 12% to 17%, and two thirds of incarcerated hernias occur during the first year of life (Aiken and Oldham, 2007). Either of these conditions should be treated as a surgical emergency. Bowel ischemia is of immediate concern, and testicular injury can occur from torsion as a result of the direct pressure of the incarcerated hernia or as a result of ischemia from cord compression. Because of the 40% to 60% contralateral occurrence of hernias in children, bilateral exploration is usually done at the time of surgery in infants younger than 1 year of age.

Patient Education, Prevention, and Prognosis

If surgery is deferred, parents must be aware of the signs and symptoms of incarceration (tenderness, redness, crying, nausea, vomiting, abdominal distention) and be cautioned to seek immediate evaluation by a medical provider should they occur.

TESTICULAR MASSES

Description

A mass located on the testicle is most often a malignancy.

Epidemiology

Testicular tumors can occur at any age; 35% of prepubertal testicular tumors are malignant. Most of the tumors are yolk sac tumors; however, rhabdomyosarcoma and leukemia can appear in this age group; 98% of painless testicular tumors in adolescents are malignant (Elder, 2007b).

Clinical Findings
History
- Family history of testicular cancer
- Sensation of fullness or heaviness
- Possibly no complaints because testicular masses cause little or no pain and are often small
- Cryptorchidism, trauma, and atrophy
Physical Examination
- A hard, painless testicular mass that does not transilluminate

- There may be an associated hydrocele
- The abdomen and supraclavicular areas should be assessed for any palpable nodes.
Diagnostic Studies
- If a tumor is suspected, levels of alpha-fetoprotein, β-hCG, and lactate dehydrogenase are indicated.
- Scrotal sonography to establish the exact location of the mass and differentiate a cystic from a solid mass
- CT scan to evaluate for metastasis

Differential Diagnosis

Intratesticular masses, which are almost always malignant, must be differentiated from extratesticular masses, such as hernia, varicocele, hydrocele, or spermatocele.

Management

Any child or adolescent with a testicular mass must be referred immediately for further evaluation. Treatment is dependent on the stage and type of tumor and can include orchiectomy, irradiation, and chemotherapy.

Patient Education, Prevention, and Prognosis

Metastasis may have occurred before the initial tumor is noticed. Pay attention to complaints about back or abdominal pain, unexplained weight loss, dyspnea (pulmonary metastases), gynecomastia, supraclavicular adenopathy, urinary obstruction, or a "heavy" or "dragging" sensation. Early detection and therapeutic intervention can lead to a 90% survival rate; 90% of relapses occur in the first 12 months after treatment. Testicular examination must be routinely done during physical examinations and must also be taught to adolescent males (see Fig. 34-11).

PHIMOSIS AND PARAPHIMOSIS
Description

Phimosis refers to a foreskin that is too tight to be retracted over the glans penis. Physiologic or primary phimosis occurs over the first 6 years of life when the glans has not completely separated from the epithelium. Pathologic or secondary phimosis occurs when the foreskin cannot be retracted after previously being retracted or after puberty. Paraphimosis is the opposite—a retracted foreskin that cannot be reduced to the normal position.

Epidemiology

Phimosis can be congenital or acquired from infection and inflammation under the foreskin. Paraphimosis causes constriction of the penis and results in pain, edema of the glans, and possible necrosis. Paraphimosis is most common in adolescents and can follow masturbation, sexual abuse, or forceful retraction.

Clinical Findings
History
- May be a history of infection or inflammation of the penis
- Retraction of the foreskin with an inability to reduce it (paraphimosis)
- Pain and dysuria

- Signs of urinary obstruction
  - Ballooning of the foreskin with urination
  - Abnormal intermittent urinary stream
Physical Examination
- Phimosis—a tight, pinpoint opening of the foreskin with minimal ability to retract the foreskin; foreskin flat and effaced
- Pathologic phimosis—thickened rolled foreskin
- Paraphimosis—edema and bluish discoloration of the glans and foreskin

Management
- Phimosis
  - Normal cleansing with gentle stretching of the foreskin until resistance is felt. Most foreskins are retractable by 5 or 6 years of age. Never forcefully retract the foreskin.
  - Circumcision is indicated if urinary obstruction or infection is present.
  - Persistent phimosis can be treated with a 0.1% mometasone furoate cream for 2 to 6 weeks (Pileggi and Vincente, 2007). This frequently allows successful retraction of the foreskin and promotes awareness of improved hygiene.
- Paraphimosis
  - A trial of ice may be done to reduce the swelling and allow reduction of the foreskin. Reduction may be accomplished by using the index and third fingers to hold the penis with gauze proximal to the foreskin and by pushing the glans penis back with the thumbs. If this technique is not successful, surgical release of the constricting band must be done to prevent necrosis of the glans.
  - Severe paraphimosis is a surgical emergency.
  - Investigation of events leading to the paraphimosis is needed to rule out sexual abuse.

Patient Education, Prevention, and Prognosis

Infection, urinary obstruction, and reflux can occur with phimosis; however, a tight foreskin in uncircumcised males is normal and usually resolves by 6 years of age. It is not an indication for circumcision. Necrosis of the penis is possible with paraphimosis. The foreskin of infants and children should never be forced back.

BALANITIS AND BALANOPOSTHITIS
Description

Balanitis is an inflammation of the glans; balanoposthitis is an inflammation of the foreskin and glans penis occurring in males with phimosis or in uncircumcised males.

Epidemiology

Accumulation of debris under the foreskin, probably resulting from poor hygiene, irritates the foreskin and glans and leads to infection. If purulent discharge with fiery-red erythema and moist translucent exudates is present, streptococcal etiology should be considered. Normal skin flora are the usual causes of infection, but gram-negative bacteria can be involved. If a urethral discharge is present, an STI must be considered. Occasionally trauma or allergy can be the cause.

Clinical Findings
History
- A fussy infant
- Pain and dysuria in an older child
Physical Examination
- Edema and inflammation are noted on the foreskin and glans.
Diagnostic Studies
- Cultures

Management
Antibiotics, both topically and orally, as directed by the cultures, along with warm soaks in the bathtub are prescribed. Depending on the swelling, topical steroids might also be prescribed.

Patient Education, Prevention, and Prognosis
Paraphimosis can occur with severe infections; however, forcible retraction of the foreskin is to be avoided. A review of proper hygiene and the removal of irritants are needed. Occurrence is not an indication for circumcision.

SCROTAL TRAUMA
Description
Trauma to the scrotum most often occurs as a result of sports participation or play.

Epidemiology
Direct blows to the scrotum and straddle injuries are the most common causes of trauma. In a prepubertal child the testicle is often spared damage because of the small size and mobility of the testes. Damage can occur when the testicle is forcibly compressed against the pubic bones. Significant symptoms (swelling, discoloration, and tenderness) from minor trauma suggest an underlying tumor.

Clinical Findings
History
- Pain after some type of injury; older children and adolescents usually report a specific mechanism of injury, time, and place.
Physical Examination
- Swelling, discoloration, ecchymosis, and tenderness of the scrotum
- Clear transillumination is compromised if a hematoma is present.
Diagnostic Studies.
Ultrasound is useful to differentiate the degree and type of injury and assess for testicular rupture.

Differential Diagnosis
Urethritis, epididymitis, orchitis, and prostatitis should all be included in the differential diagnosis. Degrees of injury include the following:
- Traumatic epididymitis—inflammation, but no infection. Pain and tenderness with scrotal erythema and edema and a tender indurated epididymis develop within a few days after injury. UA and Doppler ultrasonographic findings are normal. The course is usually acute, but short-lived.

- Intratesticular hematoma
- Hematocele with contusion and ecchymosis of the scrotal wall with severe scrotal injury
- Testicular torsion

Management
NSAIDs, cool compresses, scrotal support or elevation, and bed rest are modalities used to help relieve pain. An enlarging scrotum merits immediate surgical exploration, as does hematocele.

Complications and Patient Education
On rare occasion, testicular rupture can occur and be manifested by massive swelling and ecchymosis. An athletic cup should be worn when participating in any sport in which injury could occur. A testicular mass should be considered cancer until proved otherwise.

TESTICULAR TORSION
Description
Testicular torsion is the result of twisting of the spermatic cord, which subsequently compromises the blood supply to the testicle. Generally, there is a 4- to 8-hour window following a testicular torsion before significant ischemic damage and alteration in spermatic morphology and formation occurs (Gatti and Murphy, 2008).

Epidemiology
Normal fixation of the testis is absent, so the testis can rotate and block lymphatic and then blood flow. Torsion can occur after physical exertion, trauma, or on arising. Torsion can occur at any age but is most common in adolescence. The left side is twice as likely to be involved because of the longer spermatic cord.

Clinical Findings
History
- Sudden onset of unilateral scrotal pain, often associated with nausea and vomiting. The pain is unrelenting (Gatti and Murphy, 2008).
- History of bouts of intermittent testicular pain. Prior episodes of transient pain are reported in about half of patients.
- Minor trauma, physical exertion, or onset of acute pain on arising is possible.
- May be described as abdominal or inguinal pain by the embarrassed child
- Fever is minimal or absent.
Physical Examination
- Ill-appearing and anxious male, resisting movement
- Gradual, progressive swelling of involved scrotum with redness, warmth, and tenderness
- The ipsilateral scrotum can be edematous, erythematous, and warm.
- Testis swollen larger than opposite side, elevated, lying transversely, exquisitely painful
- Spermatic cord thickened, twisted, and tender
- Slight elevation of the testis increases pain (in epididymitis it relieves pain).

- Transillumination can reveal a solid mass.
- The cremasteric reflex is absent on the side with torsion.
- Neonate—hard, painless, nontransilluminating mass with edema or discolored scrotal skin

Diagnostic Studies
- Doppler ultrasound
- CBC (possible elevated WBC count); probably not useful
- UA is usually normal and pyuria and bacteriuria indicate UTI, epididymitis, or orchitis.
- Radiographic imaging (Doppler ultrasonography or nuclear scintigraphy) to measure intratesticular blood flow if the diagnosis is in question (Palmer, 2009)

Differential Diagnosis

Torsion of the testicular or epididymal appendage, acute epididymitis (mild to moderate pain of gradual onset), orchitis, trauma (pain is better within an hour), hernia, hydrocele, and varicocele are included in the differential diagnosis.

Management

Testicular torsion is a surgical emergency, and identification with prompt surgical referral must occur immediately. Occasionally manual reduction can be performed, but surgery should follow within 6 to 12 hours to prevent retorsion, preserve fertility, and prevent abscess and atrophy. Contralateral orchiopexy may be done because of a 50% occurrence of torsion in nonfixed testes. Rest and scrotal support do not provide relief.

Complications

Testicular atrophy, abscess, or decreased fertility and loss of the testis as a result of necrosis can occur if the torsion persists more than 24 hours.

TORSION OF THE APPENDIX TESTIS

Description

Torsion of the appendix testis (appendix epididymis) is a common cause of acute scrotal pain and is often misdiagnosed (Gatti and Murphy, 2008). It most commonly occurs in the prepubertal age group and may be a response to hormonal stimulation. Recurrence is not uncommon because there are a number of appendages.

Epidemiology

This condition is the most common cause of testicular pain in boys 2 to 10 years of age (Elder, 2007b).

Clinical Findings
  History
- Gradual onset of scrotal pain
  Physical Examination
- "Blue dot" sign, which is a subtle blue mass visible through the scrotal skin (Gatti and Murphy, 2008)
- Early in process there may be a 3- to 5-mm tender indurated mass on the upper pole (Elder, 2007b).
  Diagnostic Tests
- Doppler ultrasonography
- Testicular flow scan

Differential Diagnosis

Testicular torsion, acute epididymitis, orchitis, trauma, hernia, hydrocele, and varicocele are included in the differential diagnosis.

Management

Testicular torsion is a self-limited condition; inflammation resolves in 3 to 5 days. Management includes NSAIDs, limited activities until pain is gone, and warm compresses to the scrotum. Surgery is rarely indicated but might be necessary if testicular torsion cannot be ruled out or if symptoms do not resolve spontaneously in a few days.

EPIDIDYMITIS
Description

Epididymitis is an inflammation of the epididymis that is painful and acute.

Epidemiology

Epididymitis is commonly caused by *N. gonorrhoeae* or *C. trachomatis* in the sexually active adolescent, with infection initially present in the urethra or bladder. However, it can also be caused by a viral, coliform bacterial, or tubercular infection; by chemical irritation; by anomalies of the genitourinary tract; or by dysfunctional voiding. It is rare before puberty, but does occur in children younger than 2 years of age with genitourinary tract abnormalities (Elder, 2007b).

Clinical Findings
  History
- Sexual encounters within past 45 days
- Painful scrotal swelling, usually gradual but can be acute in onset
- Dysuria and frequency or obstructive voiding
- Trauma
- Fever, nausea, vomiting
  Physical Examination
- Scrotal edema and erythema are noted.
- The epididymis is hard, indurated, enlarged, and tender; the spermatic cord is tender.
- The testis has normal position and consistency.
- The cremasteric reflex is normal (not present in older adolescents).
- Prehn sign can be elicited—elevation of testis relieves pain (in torsion it increases pain).
- Hydrocele may be present as a reaction to inflammation.
- Urethral discharge may be present, purulent in gonorrhea, and scant and watery in chlamydial infection.
- Rectal examination reveals prostate tenderness and can produce a urethral discharge.
  Diagnostic Studies
- UA (pyuria and occasional bacteria may be present)
- CBC (elevated WBC count)
- Urethral culture and Gram stain (urine nucleic acid amplification tests may be done for gonococci and chlamydia)
- Testing for other STIs and HIV if there is a history of sexual activity
- Doppler ultrasonography or radionuclide imaging to differentiate torsion of the testis

- Follow-up VCUG, ultrasonography, or both in prepubertal children and in those who deny sexual activity, to identify urogenital problems

Differential Diagnosis

The differential diagnosis includes testicular torsion of the spermatic cord or appendix testis, hernia, hydrocele, varicocele, spermatocele, trauma, tumor, or concomitant urethritis. Testicular cancer has been confused with epididymitis.

Management

Management is directed toward symptom relief and treatment of a causative organism if found. Bed rest, scrotal support, and elevation is indicated; apply ice packs as tolerated. Sitz baths and analgesics or NSAIDs are administered to relieve pain. Antibiotic treatment includes (APA, 2009):

- *First line:* Ceftriaxone (250 mg intramuscularly one time) plus doxycycline (100 mg twice a day for 10 days)

- *Alternative treatments:* Ofloxacin (300 mg twice a day for 10 days) or levofloxacin (500 mg once a day for 10 days)
- Referral to a urologist is indicated if a solitary testicle is involved, if a prompt response to treatment does not occur, or if a question about the diagnosis remains. Treatment of sexual partner(s) from the last 60 days is indicated if caused by an STI. Intercourse should be avoided until cured. Follow-up is needed within 3 days if no improvement is seen or if symptoms recur after treatment. Follow-up after antibiotics is recommended to ensure that no palpable mass remains.

Complications and Patient Education

Infertility, abscess formation, testicular infarction, and late atrophy are possible but rare complications of epididymitis. Because epididymitis is usually caused by an STI, partners must be evaluated and treated. Patients must understand the sexually transmitted etiology of this disease. Pain and edema usually resolve within 1 week.

Gynecologic Disorders

TERAL GERLT AND NANCY BARBER STARR

Pediatric gynecology can provide the health care provider with varied and interesting challenges. Knowledge, sensitivity, and comfort with gynecology aid the pediatric provider in working with the child or adolescent and the parent. Educating children and adolescents about their bodies as they mature is essential. Approaching issues that may be considered personal or embarrassing openly and directly allows more comprehensive care and an opportunity for anticipatory guidance. Establishing and maintaining a good relationship with parents and adolescents helps ease the transition during which adolescents take an increasingly larger role in determining their own care.

Gynecologic issues range from normal transitions that may be perceived as abnormal to serious systemic diseases or abnormalities. The provider should have an elevated index of suspicion in all cases so as to not overlook significant signs and symptoms. At the same time, most conditions are normal and can be easily addressed, reassuring the child, adolescent, and/or parent that all is well and that her body is developing normally.

Standards of Care

Healthy People 2020 (U.S. Department of Health and Human Services [USDHHS], 2009) has multiple objectives that are applicable to children and adolescents. Those that fall into pediatric gynecology are to promote responsible sexual behaviors, and reduce teen pregnancies, sexually transmitted infections (STIs), and human immunodeficiency virus (HIV) infections in adolescents. These objectives remain mostly unchanged from the *Healthy People 2010* (USDHHS, 2000).

Bright Futures (Hagan et al, 2008) recommends as a routine part of annual health supervision asking all adolescents about sexual health behaviors that place them at risk for pregnancy, STIs, and HIV. Further, they should receive counseling about responsible sexual behavior, including abstinence and the use of contraception and condoms to prevent pregnancy and infection with STIs and HIV. All sexually active adolescents should be screened for STIs (gonorrhea [GC], chlamydia, and syphilis if living in an endemic area) and HIV infection. The *Guide to Clinical Preventive Services* (U.S.

Preventive Services Task Force [USPSTF], 2009) also recommends screening all sexually active women 24 years old and younger for chlamydia.

Anatomy and Physiology

For the first 6 to 7 weeks of gestation, male and female fetuses are sexually undifferentiated, both having two bipotential gonads and bilateral paramesonephric (müllerian) and mesonephric (wolffian) ducts. At this point testicular differentiation begins at the direction of the testes-determining factor on the Y chromosome. In the male gonad, the Sertoli cells produce antimüllerian hormone (AMH) that inhibits müllerian duct development, and the Leydig cells produce testosterone, which maintains wolffian duct development and causes them to differentiate into the epididymis, vas deferens, and the seminal vesicles.

Without the influence of the Y chromosome, the female gonads develop into ovaries by about 8 weeks' gestation, and by 20 weeks the fetal ovary reaches mature compartmentalization. The müllerian ducts become the uterus and fallopian tubes, and the wolffian ducts regress. By week 22 of gestation, canalization to create the uterine cavity, cervical canal, and the vagina is complete.

The external genitalia are neutral primordial and able to develop into either male or female structures. The presence of testosterone from the testes masculinizes the external genitalia, whereas the lack of androgens allows female genitalia to form.

In utero, maternal estrogen thickens and enlarges the female genital structures. After birth, maternal hormones are withdrawn resulting in the desquamation of the hypertrophic walls of the uterus. The mucus from the cervix results in the physiologic leukorrhea of the newborn period. As the hormonal influences continue to decrease, the endometrial shedding may be accompanied by bleeding.

Between 8 weeks and 7 years of age, without maternal or endogenous estrogens, the labia majora are flat, the labia minora are thin, and neither offers protection to the genitalia. The absence of fat pads results in an open labia whenever the child is in the squatting position. In addition, this thin atrophic genital epithelium is readily traumatized.

The function of the reproductive system is controlled by the hypothalamic-pituitary-ovarian (HPO) axis. This complex process begins in the neurologic system (the hypothalamus), involves the endocrine system (the anterior pituitary), and completes its cycle with the gonads (ovaries). Initially this cycle causes sexual maturation, and once that is completed the ongoing release of hormones controls the menstrual cycle, pregnancy, and lactation.

PUBERTY

Puberty is the "coming together of multiple systems and influences, including genetic, metabolic, and hormonal factors" (Speroff and Fritz, 2005, p 178). It is a process usually starting with early breast development (thelarche), then growth of pubic and axillary hair (pubarche), and finally the first menses (menarche).

What sets this all in play is the reactivation of the HPO axis that has been suppressed since shortly after birth. The catalyst for this is unknown; however, there is a reduction of gonadotropin-releasing hormone (GnRH) suppression and decreased sensitivity of the negative feedback to estrogen, which leads to increasing GnRH pulsations to the anterior pituitary. This stimulates the anterior pituitary to release the gonadotropins, follicle-stimulating hormone (FSH) and luteinizing hormone (LH). These in turn stimulate the ovaries to synthesize estrogen (gonadarche). Increasing estrogen stimulates breast development, vaginal and uterine growth, skeletal growth, and female fat distribution. Independent of the HPO axis, increasing levels of adrenal androgens (adrenarche) lead to the growth of pubic and axillary hair. Finally, by midpuberty there is enough estrogen to cause endometrial proliferation, and the first menses occurs (menarche). Because early cycles are anovulatory 50% to 80% of the time in the first 2 to 3 years after menarche, menstrual irregularities and 21- to 45-day cycle lengths are common. Anovulatory cycles may continue 10% to 20% of the time up to 5 years after menarche (Harel, 2005).

On average it takes approximately 4.5 years to traverse all the pubertal stages. The mean age of menarche in Caucasian American girls is between 12 and 13 years and slightly earlier for African-American girls. This age has remained unchanged for more than 50 years. If a girl has not started breast development by 13 years of age or had menarche by 16 years of age, she is experiencing delayed puberty and should be evaluated for medical or genetic conditions. Likewise, precocious puberty, the early development of secondary sex characteristics, needs further evaluation. However, the age at which a further workup is recommended varies by source. Traditionally the definition of precocious puberty is breast or pubic hair development in girls younger than 8 years old. In 1999 the Lawson Wilkins Pediatric Endocrine Society developed revised guidelines in response to research findings. Their recommendation, which remains unchanged since 1999, is to evaluate only if secondary sexual characteristics develop before 7 years old in Caucasian American girls and before 6 years old in African-American girls (Kaplowitz and Oberfield, 1999). Others argue that lowering the age of workup will miss girls with significant pathology. Mansfield and Neinstein (2008) recommend that girls with both breast development and pubic hair at age 7 to 8 should have a review of history and growth and bone age testing for height prediction.

MENSTRUAL CYCLE

The menstrual cycle is controlled by the HPO axis. It is essential that pediatric providers have an understanding of this complicated feedback system for the evaluation of menstrual disorders.

The average adult menstrual cycle is 28 days with a range of 21 to 34 days. Figure 35-1 illustrates the female reproductive cycle. The four phases of the cycle are:

- Menses—4 days plus or minus 2 days
- Follicular—10 to 14 days
- Ovulation—10 to 12 hours after LH surge
- Luteal—consistently close to 14 days plus or minus 3 days

The Follicular Phase

Initial follicular development occurs without hormonal influence. However, it is the stimulation by FSH that moves the follicles to the preantral stage.

Antral Follicle. The dominant follicle is established during cycle days 5 to 7, leading to increased levels of estradiol by day 7 (Figs. 35-1 and 35-2). The increasing estradiol suppresses FSH and leads to LH secretion. Estrogen also modifies the gonadotropin molecule, increasing the quality and the quantity of FSH and LH midcycle. LH levels rise steadily during the late follicular phase, stimulating the theca in the production of androgen. The action of FSH in the granulosa permits the dominant follicle to use androgen to make estrogen, further increasing estrogen production. FSH also stimulates LH receptors to form on the granulosa cells.

It is not the gonadotropins alone acting on the follicle; growth factors and autocrine and paracrine peptides also influence the feedback loop. Inhibin B, which is secreted by the granulosa cells in response to FSH, suppresses pituitary FSH. Activin, from the pituitary and the granulosa, augments FSH secretion and action, and insulin-like growth factor (IGF) acts to enhance all actions of FSH and LH (Speroff and Fritz, 2005).

Preovulatory Follicle. When the estrogen levels are sufficient to induce the LH surge, the increasing LH initiates luteinization and progesterone production in the granulosa. This rise in progesterone assists the positive feedback action of estrogen and may be needed to stimulate the FSH peak midcycle. An increase in local and peripheral androgens also occurs midcycle from the thecal tissue of lesser follicles (Fig. 35-3).

Ovulation

The LH surge stimulates continuation of miosis in the oocyte, luteinization of the granulosa, and production of progesterone and prostaglandins within the follicle. Progesterone augments the activity of the proteolytic enzymes that, together with prostaglandins, are responsible for the digestion and rupture of the follicular wall. The progesterone-influenced midcycle rise in FSH assists to free the oocyte from follicular attachments, to convert plasminogen to the proteolytic enzyme, plasmin, and to guarantee that adequate LH receptors are present to allow a normal luteal phase.

The Luteal Phase

A normal luteal phase requires both consummate preovulatory follicular development and the continued support of LH. Centrally, progesterone, estrogen, and inhibin A suppress new

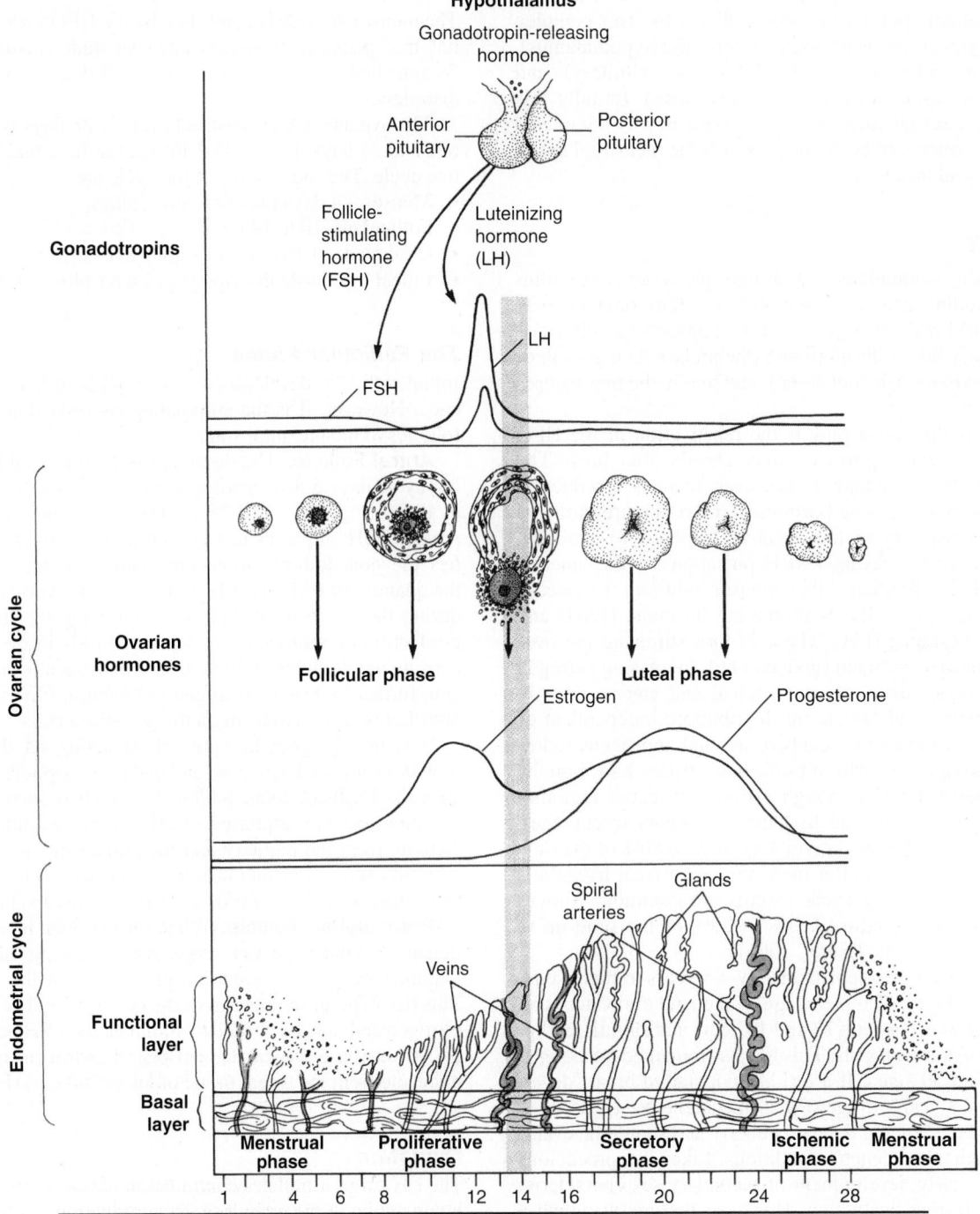

FIGURE 35-1 Female reproductive cycle showing changes in hormone secretion and in the ovary and the uterine endometrium. (From Gorrie T, McKinney E, Murray S: *Foundations of maternal newborn nursing,* ed 2, Philadelphia, 1998, Saunders.)

follicular growth. The regression of the corpus luteum may involve the luteolytic action of estrogen produced by the corpus luteum itself and is interceded by a modification in local prostaglandin and endothelin-1 concentrations (Fig. 35-4).

Luteal-Follicular Transition. The loss of the corpus luteum causes a fall in circulating levels of estradiol, progesterone, and inhibin A. The decreasing inhibin A eliminates the suppression of FSH secretion in the pituitary. The decrease in estradiol and progesterone permits a rapid increase in the

frequency of GnRH pulsatile secretion and the elimination of negative feedback on the pituitary. The loss of inhibin-A and estradiol and the increasing GnRH pulsations join to permit greater secretion of FSH as compared with LH, which in turn increases in the frequency of episodic secretion of FSH. This increase in FSH is influential in rescuing an approximately 70-day-old group of follicles from atresia. This allows a dominant follicle to begin its emergence, and the cycle begins again (Fig. 35-5).

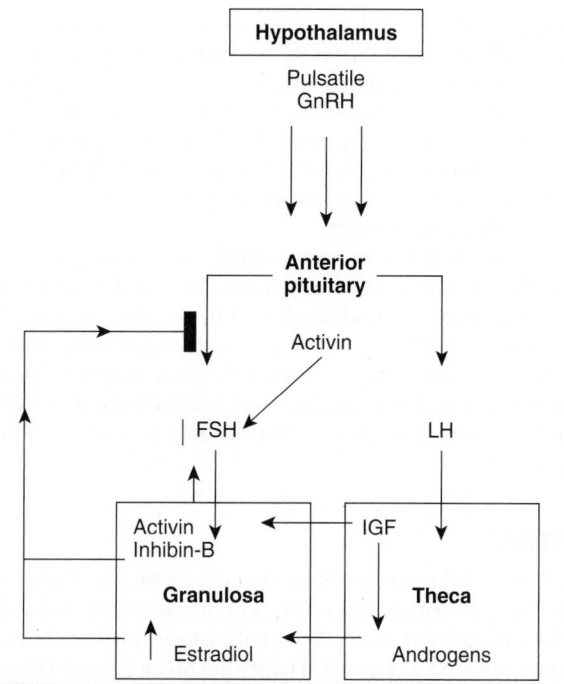

FIGURE 35-2 Early follicular to midfollicular phase. *FSH,* Follicle-stimulating hormone; *GnRH,* gonadotropin-releasing hormone; *LH,* luteinizing hormone; *IGF,* insulin-like growth factor; dark box represents negative feedback. (Data from Speroff L, Fritz MA: *Clinical gynecologic endocrinology and infertility,* ed 7, Philadelphia, 2005, Lippincott Williams & Wilkins.)

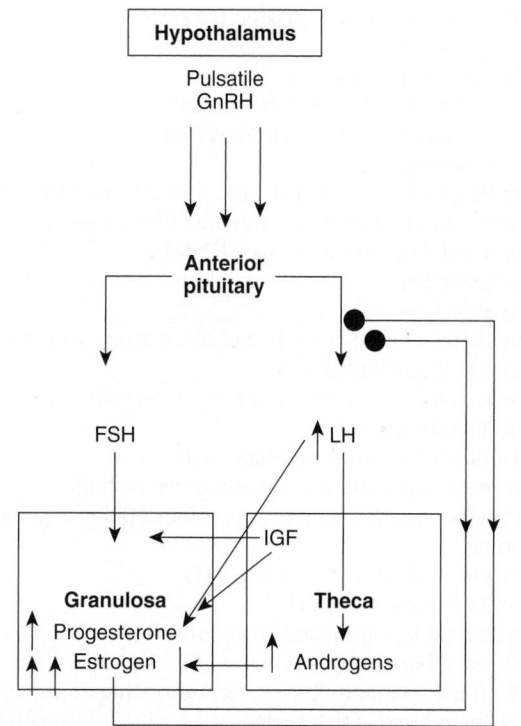

FIGURE 35-3 Late follicular phase to ovulation. *FSH,* Follicle-stimulating hormone; *GnRH,* gonadotropin-releasing hormone; *LH,* luteinizing hormone; *IGF,* insulin-like growth factor; dark circle represents positive feedback. (Data from Speroff L, Fritz MA: *Clinical gynecologic endocrinology and infertility,* ed 7, Philadelphia, 2005, Lippincott Williams & Wilkins.)

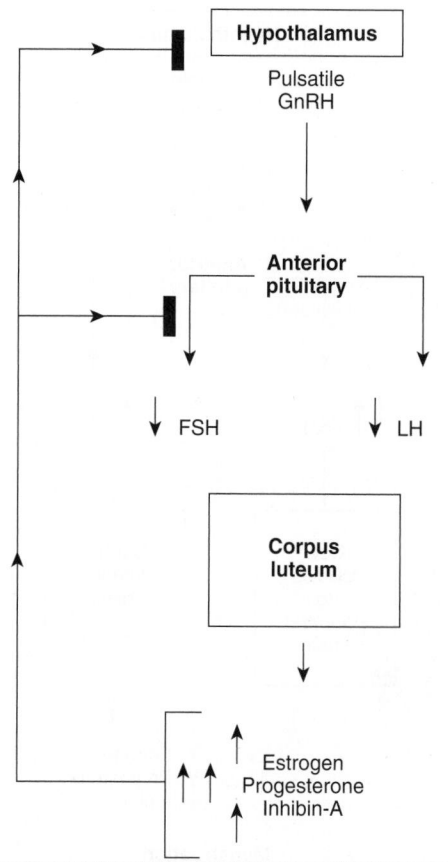

FIGURE 35-4 Early luteal to midluteal phase. *FSH,* Follicle-stimulating hormone; *GnRH,* gonadotropin-releasing hormone; *LH,* luteinizing hormone; dark boxes represent negative feedback. (Data from Speroff L, Fritz MA: *Clinical gynecologic endocrinology and infertility,* ed 7, Philadelphia, 2005, Lippincott Williams & Wilkins.)

■ Pathophysiology and Defense Mechanisms of the Gynecologic System

The primary disorders of the gynecologic system can be classified as menstrual cycle disorders, inflammatory reactions, infection, and reproductive problems. Pubertal development is a complex but normal process. Adolescents may be seen with common menstrual problems, such as mittelschmerz or dysmenorrhea. Abnormal uterine bleeding, endometriosis, and amenorrhea are three less common menstrual cycle disorders that require the provider to differentiate normal growth and developmental variations from systemic disorders or disease (especially neurologic, endocrine, and reproductive problems). The female athlete is especially prone to exercise-related menstrual problems.

An inflammatory response can occur in either the external or internal genitalia. Local reactions involve the external genitalia and can be caused by dermatologic disorders or skin irritation from such factors as normal leukorrhea, chemical or allergic reactions, or nonspecific causes. Internal inflammation caused by infection is not always as obvious.

The warm, moist environment of the reproductive tract provides an ideal place for infection. Viral pathogens, such as herpes simplex virus (HSV) and human papillomavirus (HPV), or fungal infection can manifest as vulvitis or a vaginal infection. Trichomonas, a protozoal infection, colonizes the

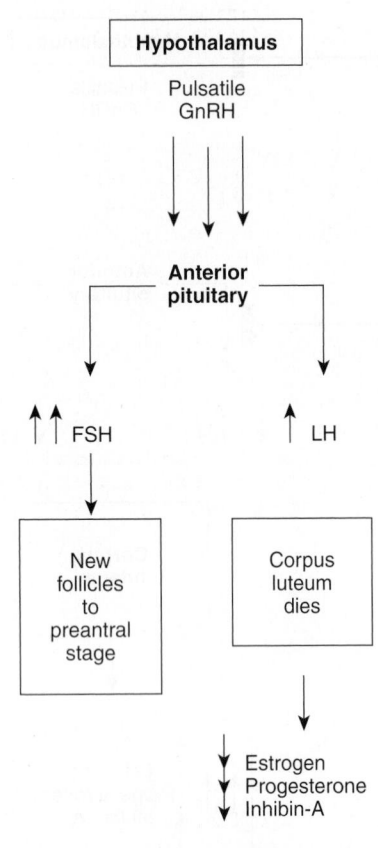

FIGURE 35-5 Luteal-follicular transition. *FSH,* Follicle-stimulating hormone; *GnRH,* gonadotropin-releasing hormone; *LH,* luteinizing hormone. (Data from Speroff L, Fritz MA: *Clinical gynecologic endocrinology and infertility,* ed 7, Philadelphia, 2005, Lippincott Williams & Wilkins.)

vaginal vault. By contrast, bacterial infections caused by chlamydia and GC can ascend into the upper genital tract where pelvic inflammatory disease (PID) can cause tubal damage.

Reproductive problems occur as a result of structural, hormonal, or endocrine disorders or as sequelae of infection. Refer to a gynecologic or endocrine text for further information.

The gynecologic system has both anatomic and physiologic defense mechanisms. The labia majora and the pubic hair provide a barrier that serves as the first line of defense. The vagina, serving as an exit for mucosal secretion, menstrual fluids, and products of conception, also provides a means of defense with its natural downward and outward flow of secretions. Additionally, with increasing estrogen exposure, the vaginal epithelial tissue thickens and an acid pH develops, discouraging infection. The small external cervical os, a thick mucous plug, and the downward flow of cervical secretions provide barriers to entry to the uterus. A chemical barrier is also established by the cervical enzymes and antibodies.

■ Assessment of the Gynecologic System: Health Supervision Visits for Female Adolescents

The American Congress of Obstetricians and Gynecologists (ACOG) recommends that young female adolescents have an initial reproductive health visit between 13 and 15 years old to provide preventive care, anticipatory guidance, and screening (ACOG, 2010b). This visit includes discussions of sexual development and reproductive issues rather than problem-focused care (Holland-Hall et al, 2005). Counseling and education about normal menses and patterns, pregnancy prevention, STIs, and HIV are essential; a pelvic examination is performed only if concerning (discussed later).

This visit is the perfect opportunity to discuss confidentiality with the patient and her parents. All need to understand the importance of confidentiality in the health care provider–patient relationship and the limits to confidentiality imposed by state and local statutes and/or medical necessity. A relationship of trust and mutual respect is extremely important to establish so that the adolescent is willing to discuss intimate matters.

HISTORY

The history taken depends on the age of the child and chief complaint. Histories for specific conditions are included later in this chapter. An in-depth sexual history for the adolescent can be found in Chapter 18. The sexual history should be completed with the parent out of the room.

- Family history
- Maternal age at menarche and any problems encountered
- Dysmenorrhea, dysfunctional uterine bleeding (DUB), or endometriosis
- Diabetes mellitus
- Thyroid disease
- Bleeding or clotting disorders
- Cancer of the female reproductive system
- Genetic disorders
- Pubertal development
- Knowledge of pubertal development
- Age at breast and pubic hair development
- Age at menarche
- Length of cycles, longest and shortest interval between menses, duration of flow, estimated blood loss
- Last normal menstrual period (LNMP)
- Dysmenorrhea
- Sexual history
- Knowledge about sexuality and discussions with parent or guardian (see Chapter 18)
- Age at first intercourse (voluntary or forced)
- Current sexual activity
- Type of activity (oral, vaginal, anal)
- Partners of opposite sex, the same sex, or both
- Number of sexual partners in previous 60 days, 12 months, lifetime
- Previous vaginal infections or STIs
- Current exposures to STIs
- Papanicolaou (Pap) test date and results
- Contraceptive history
  - Current method—type, duration, frequency of use, problems and satisfaction
  - Past methods—type, duration, frequency of use, problems and satisfaction
- Obstetric history, as appropriate
- Review of systems: Urinary, gastrointestinal, endocrine, dermatologic, general health, growth, stressors, medications, allergies, and substance use

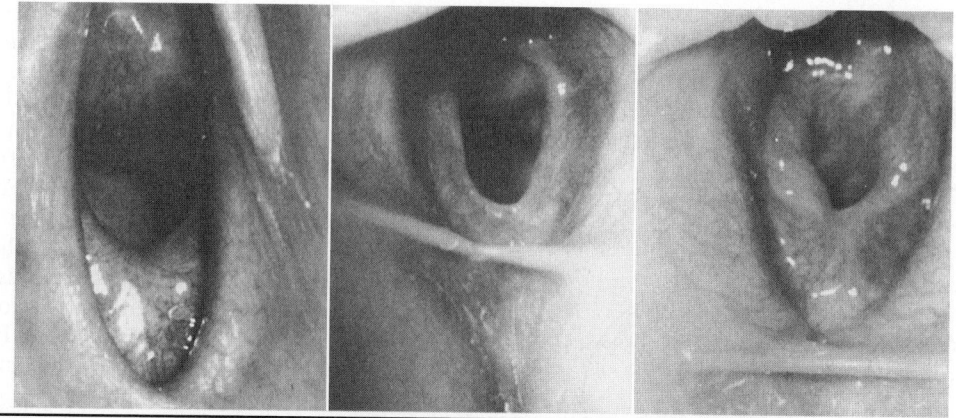

FIGURE 35-6 Types of hymens, photographed through a colposcope. **A,** Crescentic hymen. **B,** Annular hymen. **C,** Redundant hymen with crescent appearance after retraction. (From Emans SJ: Vulvovaginal problems in the prepubertal child. In Emans SJ, Laufer MR, Goldstein DP, editors: *Pediatric and adolescent gynecology,* ed 5, Philadelphia, 2005, Lippincott Williams & Wilkins.)

PHYSICAL EXAMINATION

A girl's first gynecologic examination can influence her attitude toward future gynecologic care. When a gynecologic examination is performed, the child or adolescent should maintain a feeling of being in control. It is important that the provider take the time to establish rapport, preserve modesty, give choices, and obtain consent to examine. It is also important that the parent understands what the examination entails and why it is necessary.

The adolescent should be given as many choices as possible; if she would like someone else in the room with her; the position of the table; use of a hand mirror to observe; and when possible, the timing of the examination. This requires flexibility and time from the care provider, but demonstrates respect for the adolescent.

Prepubertal Child

There are a variety of positions in which to examine the vulva, vestibule, and lower vagina of a prepubescent girl. Lying on a table, supine, with feet together and knees out ("frog legged") is generally the most comfortable for patients and provides ease of examination and obtaining of cultures if necessary. Another alternative is sitting up in the parent's lap with feet and knees frog legged. Putting the parent on the examination table with feet in the stirrups and the child on his or her lap with feet to the outside of the parent's legs is another alternative. If examination of the entire vagina is necessary, putting the child in knee-chest position on the examination table is the best position for noninvasive, internal examination of the vulva and vagina.

Examine or note the following:

- Breasts, abdomen, and inguinal area
- Presence and distribution of pubic hair
- Presence and distribution of body hair: Face, chest, back, abdomen, legs, arms
- Skin lesions
- State of hygiene
- Anus for cleanliness, excoriation, or erythema
- Sexual maturity rating (SMR) or Tanner staging (see Chapter 8 and Fig. 8-3)
- Genital examination with gentle traction on the labia majora
- Size of clitoris (approximately 3 × 3 mm prepubertal)

- Signs of estrogenization (prepubertal vaginal mucosa—moist, thin, and red; postpubertal vaginal mucosa—moist and dull pink)
- The hymen is normally smooth and continuous.
  - Described as crescent shaped, annular, or redundant (Fig. 35-6)
  - Presence of notches or tags—normal variation (Sugar and Graham, 2006)
  - Presence of hymenal ridge—usually without sequela (Sugar and Graham, 2006)
  - Imperforate hymen
  - Periurethral bands

The significance of the diameter of the hymenal opening as a diagnostic finding is debated. Both transverse and anteroposterior diameters are dependent on age, relaxation, method of examination, and type of hymen. In general, the older and more relaxed the child, the larger the opening. It is also larger with retraction and in the knee-chest position. In the 3- to 6-year-old, a range of normal findings for the transverse diameter is 1 to 6 mm and for the anteroposterior diameter, 1 to 7 mm. Obesity in young children is associated with hymenal openings larger than average for age (e.g., a 2-year-old with a 4-mm opening when average is 2 mm).

Adolescent

- Inspect the skin for acne.
- Examine the breasts; note Tanner stage.
- Palpate the thyroid.
- Inspect hair distribution on face, chest, back, arms, legs, and abdomen.
- Inspect the external genitalia and determine the Tanner stage.
- Vaginal examination alone may be adequate to assess for irregular bleeding, severe dysmenorrhea, vaginal discharge, and amenorrhea. However, a speculum and a bimanual examination may be necessary based on symptoms and history.

DIAGNOSTIC STUDIES

The routine care of the child and adolescent without gynecologic complaints does not require diagnostic studies.

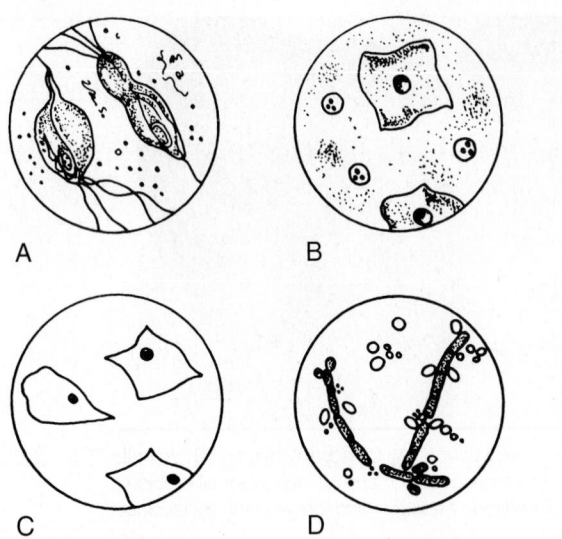

FIGURE 35-7 Drawings of vaginal smears showing **A,** *Trichomonas*; **B,** clue cells of bacterial vaginosis; **C,** leukorrhea; **D,** *Candida*. **A, B,** and **C** are saline preparations; **D** is a potassium hydroxide (KOH) preparation. (From Emans SJ: Vulvovaginal problems in the prepubertal child. In Emans SJ, Laufer MR, Goldstein DP, editors: *Pediatric and adolescent gynecology,* ed 5, Philadelphia, 2005, Lippincott Williams & Wilkins.)

The following studies can be helpful as diagnostic tools. Specific studies and techniques are discussed with each diagnosis. Collection of specimens must be done with care. Techniques that are helpful include using a small amount of saline as a vaginal wash, using a soft plastic eyedropper or feeding tube, or using a moistened cotton swab.

- Wet mounts of vaginal secretions
- Saline for microscopic examination to look for white blood cells (WBCs), clue cells, trichomonads, and bacteria
- 10% potassium hydroxide (KOH) for whiff test and microscopic examination to look for yeast (branching hyphae and spores) (Fig. 35-7)
- pH of vaginal mucus (neutral in prepubescent; less than 4.5 once pubertal)
- Urine-based nucleic acid amplification test (NAAT), cultures, and/or serologic blood tests for STIs
- Other tests as indicated including pregnancy test by urine or serum, BiGGY agar culture (suspected yeast infection), or ultrasound

Cervical Cancer Screening

The American Cancer Society recommends that cervical cancer screening with Pap testing should begin approximately 3 years after a young woman has initiated vaginal intercourse and no later than 21 years old. After the initiation of cervical screening, the young woman should have annual Pap testing with conventional cytology or every 2 years with liquid-based cytology. However, the ACOG (2010a) released its latest committee opinion on screening, evaluation, and management of cervical cancer in adolescents in August 2010. The college recommends not starting Pap testing until 21 years of age unless the adolescent is sexually active and immunocompromised. As part of this publication, ACOG gives guidelines on how to follow up with young women who have had abnormal

cervical cytology prior to this latest practice change (see ACOG, 2010a, for complete recommendations).

The rationale for this recommendation is the increasing understanding of the natural history of HPV infections, the causative agent of most cervical cancer. The Centers for Disease Control and Prevention (CDC) (2009) reports the overall prevalence of high-risk HPV at 23%. For adolescents the rate is 29%, whereas, for women in their twenties the rate has decreased to 13%. There is evidence that the majority of low-grade HPV lesions regress spontaneously and the risk of a young woman having a high-grade lesion leading to cervical cancer is extremely rare. Therefore, Pap annual testing led to overdiagnosis of cervical pathologic conditions and unnecessary interventions.

■ Management Strategies

ANTICIPATORY GUIDANCE, COUNSELING, AND EDUCATION

Anticipatory guidance related to gynecologic issues is important to both the child or adolescent and parents. Attention to appropriate genital hygiene can help prevent some potential childhood problems. The transition to puberty and establishment of menses is eased with appropriate education and counseling beforehand. With the advent of puberty and the increasing interest in sexuality, a great deal of guidance is needed to help the adolescent and her parents through these transitions. See Chapters 8 and 18 for further discussion of these topics.

Counseling and education related to normal gynecologic conditions and disorders of the gynecologic system need to be tailored to the child or adolescent and the parents. See Chapter 18 for more information on sexuality counseling. Confidentiality is a matter to be established with both the parents and the adolescent. Some states have specific laws that allow providers to treat adolescents for obstetric and family planning conditions without parental knowledge or consent.

ADOLESCENT PREGNANCY PREVENTION

There are several common goals in adolescent pregnancy prevention. These goals can be achieved by supporting a positive or protective environment, connecting the adolescent to an intervention program, and providing appropriate health care services. Prevention goals include the following:

- Maintain sexual health and promote sexual responsibility.
- Assist adolescents to make informed choices, recognizing educational, social, and economic effect of choices.
- Encourage abstinence and delay onset of intercourse.
- Provide contraceptive counseling and selection of a contraceptive device for any adolescent who has recently experienced a spontaneous abortion, as part of third-trimester health teaching before delivery, or at the time of an elective termination of pregnancy.

Appropriate health care services are important in preventing adolescent pregnancy. This care should include confidentiality with minimal or no financial barriers; easy availability (e.g., timed for easy access, on site at school, or easy transportation to site); and a full range of contraceptive services for male and female adolescents (see section on contraception for specific methods).

BOX 35-1 Common Components of Successful Adolescent Pregnancy Intervention Programs

- Intensive individualized attention
- Early identification of at-risk children
- Early intervention to prevent high-risk behavior
- Youth empowerment
- Social skills training
- Parental involvement and training in parenting
- Community-wide multiagency collaborative approaches

BOX 35-2 What Parents Can Do to Protect Against Pregnancy

- Be clear about your sexual values and attitudes.
- Talk with your children early and often about sex, and be specific.
- Supervise and monitor your children and adolescents.
- Know their friends and families.
- Discourage early, frequent, and steady dating.
- Discourage dating of older persons.
- Encourage education and future goals.
- Know what your kids are watching, reading, and listening to.
- Build a strong, close relationship from an early age.

BOX 35-3 Factors Predicting Success or Failure With Contraception

- Age. Adolescents 15 years old and younger are at highest risk for pregnancy because 35% report using no method of contraception at their first episode of intercourse. In comparison, only 17% of females 19 years or older report using no method (Abma et al, 2004).
- Noncompliance with the first method chosen (previous method failure).
- Not acquiring a method of contraception at the first reproductive health visit.
- Frequency of family planning visits in the preceding 12 months. Increased compliance with clinic attendance appears to correlate with effective contraceptive use by client.
- Coital frequency. Adolescent females who have sexual intercourse more than six times per month are at greater risk of becoming pregnant.
- Length of time between first coitus and initiation of birth control use. The longer adolescents delay seeking services for contraception, the less likely they are to use a highly reliable method consistently and correctly.

BOX 35-4 Risk Factors for Unintentional Pregnancy

- Early onset of sexual activity, especially before 15 years old
- Early onset of substance use, including cigarettes, alcohol, and illicit drugs
- Lesbian or bisexual; these females are as likely to have sex with males as heterosexuals, but their pregnancy rate is more than doubled (Meininger and Remafedi, 2008)
- Low educational expectation
- Low perception of life options
- Poor grades and academic achievement
- Behavior problems, including truancy and delinquency
- Negative peer influence
- Poor contraceptive compliance or failure with a contraceptive device
- Nonintact families (those without both biologic mother and father present)
- Depression
- Cultural values that favor adolescent pregnancy
- Prior history of sexual or physical abuse or violence at home (Cox, 2008)

Common components of successful intervention programs identified by Dryfoos (1998) are listed in Box 35-1. The National Campaign to Prevent Teen Pregnancy (2008) has also outlined actions that parents can take to help protect against pregnancy (Box 35-2).

CONTRACEPTION

Contraceptive Counseling and Education

Significant and specific knowledge is required for pediatric providers to offer reproductive health and contraceptive services to adolescents. An in-depth discussion is beyond the scope of this text; however, excellent management references are available. The authors recommend *Contraceptive Technology* by Hatcher and colleagues (2007), *A Clinical Guide for Contraception* by Speroff and Darney (2010), and Gupta and associates (2008).

Contraceptive counseling needs to be individualized and at the adolescent's developmental level. It is also important not to overwhelm the patient with too much information at one time. Ascertain what methods she knows about or is thinking about using. Frequently the provider needs to dispel misconceptions about risks related to various methods and educate on the menstrual and health benefits. It may take more than one visit to find a compatible contraceptive method. However, the adolescent should not leave the office without understanding the risk of pregnancy and STIs and HIV with unprotected sex. She should have education about and a prescription for emergency contraception (EC) and know that condoms are a must for safer sex.

Factors identified as predictive of failure or success with contraception are listed in Box 35-3. Antecedent risk factors to unintentional pregnancy are listed in Box 35-4.

Initial Screening to Assess for Appropriate Contraception

History. For the most part adolescent women are healthy with no contraindications for hormonal contraceptive methods. However, it is important to get a personal history related to cardiovascular and peripheral vascular disease, diabetes, headaches, liver and gallbladder disease, and current medications (including prescription, over-the-counter [OTC], herbal, and dietary supplements). The World Health Organization (WHO), using evidence-based methodology, has developed medical eligibility criteria for starting contraceptive methods (2009). The authors recommend using the WHO website to access the most recent updates.

Physical Examination

- Height and weight; body mass index (BMI)
- Blood pressure
- Thyroid examination
- Breast examination, including Tanner staging
- Auscultation of heart and lungs
- Abdominal examination
- Pelvic examination (not a requirement to start oral contraceptive pills [OCPs])

Diagnostic Studies

- Pap smear if indicated by current guidelines
- NAAT on urine or cultures for GC and chlamydia
- Wet mounts when indicated by presence of abnormal vaginal discharge
- Complete blood count (CBC) or hemoglobin or hematocrit and rubella titer as indicated
- Syphilis serology with known STI, particularly condylomas or genital ulcers and if residing in endemic areas
- HIV

Hormonal Methods of Contraception (Coitus-Independent Methods)

Oral Contraceptive Pills

Types of Preparations. Two basic preparations are available: a combination formulation (COC) that contains estrogen (less than 50 mcg) and progestin in a low dose, and a progestin-only minipill. Most women in the U.S. use the combination formulation, in either monophasic or triphasic formats. Progestin-only pills (POPs) are prescribed for women in whom estrogens are contraindicated (e.g., lactating women or women with medical contraindications to estrogen). Generally they are not the first choice for nonlactating adolescents because of irregular bleeding and higher failure rates. Mechanism of action, theoretic and use effectiveness, benefits, disadvantages, and side effects are listed in Table 35-1. The initial use of an OCP requires special attention to dosing, preparation, timing, patient education, and follow-up.

Dosing. Initial dosing for a combination OCP should be at 30 to 35 mcg estrogen, with low progestin potency per tablet. Most providers have one or two OCPs that are favorites for first-time use in women without special conditions. There are 20-mcg combination OCPs available, should an ultra-low dose estrogen formulation be desired. The selection of an OCP can also be individualized based on menstrual characteristics or patient sensitivity. For example, a client with a history of cystic acne can be tried on an OCP in which the progestins are desogestrel or norgestrel, or on Ortho Tri-Cyclen or Estrostep, the only OCPs with U.S. Food and Drug Administration (FDA) approval for use in acne. For clients with hirsutism or polycystic ovary syndrome (PCOS), a low androgenic potency pill is used, such as Ortho-Cyclen, Desogen, or Ovcon-35. For clients who miss pills, using a monophasic 30- to 35-mcg pill provides more protection against escape ovulation than a 20-mcg estrogen, progestin only, or triphasic pill. Adolescents who demonstrate estrogen sensitivity can be tried on a more androgenic pill, such as Lo/Ovral, Nordette, or Loestrin or a 20-mcg preparation, such as Alesse.

Preparation. Given the vast selection of products available to the health care provider, Hatcher and colleagues (2007) developed a four-step flow chart to assist clinicians in choosing a combined OCP with low-dosage estrogen (Box 35-5).

BOX 35-5 Steps in Choosing a Combined Oral Contraceptive With Low-Dose Estrogen

1. Does the adolescent have a contraindication to estrogen use?
2. If yes, consider the use of a progestin-only formulation.
3. If the client can use estrogen, the provider can select from among numerous products, considering the following:
   - The number of micrograms of estrogen in the preparation
   - Availability of the pill on formulary
   - Ease of understanding the packaging of the pill
   - Price of the pill to the adolescent and possibly the clinic
   - Previous adverse event or experience the adolescent may have had with a specific preparation
4. Consider other clinical factors, such as acne, nausea or vomiting, spotting or breakthrough bleeding, and absence of withdrawal bleeding.

Timing. Ideally, OCPs should not be started until the adolescent has had three to six regular periods after menarche, but sexually active or other high-risk teens can be put on OCPs even before menarche. OCPs can be started 3 to 4 weeks postpartum (if breastfeeding, POPs) or after a first-trimester therapeutic abortion (Hatcher et al, 2007; Nelson and Neinstein, 2008).

There are several ways in which OCPs can be initiated:

- Quick start—same day start in certain circumstances
  - If within 72 hours of unprotected sex, use EC now and start OCPs the next day.
  - If pregnancy can be ruled out or there was no unprotected sex since the last menses, may start same day and use backup (condoms) for 7 days or until menses starts. This is a preferable method for adolescents because it is less complicated and has a higher rate of continuation.
- Start first day of menses
- Start within 5 days after menses and use backup (condoms) for 7 days
- First Sunday after menses started and use backup (condoms) for 7 days

Another timing issue is the pattern of COC use. The majority of pill packs come with 28-day cycling: 21 days of active tablets and 7 days of placebo tablets, with the woman having a monthly withdrawal bleed during the placebo week. For years, providers have recommended various patterns of monophasic COC use to prevent withdrawal bleeds. Women can skip the placebo week of their pill packs for one, two, or three cycles to decrease the number of withdrawal bleeds per year. This is particularly helpful in women with endometriosis, menorrhagia, severe dysmenorrhea, and menstrual migraines. In 2003 extended-cycle COCs came on the market, packaged with 84 active pills and 7 inactive pills, giving women only four withdrawal bleeds per year.

Patient Education

- Provide clear instructions on how to start OCPs.
- Emphasize correct and consistent use of the OCP.
- Take the pill every day in the order presented in the pill pack—no matter what your body is doing or what your friends say.
- How to make up missed or forgotten pills and the use of a backup method
  - One missed pill—take as soon as possible (ASAP) and take next pill as usual.

| BOX 35-6 | The Mnemonic ACHES Used to Teach and Assess for Risks of Oral Contraceptive Pills |

- **A**bdominal pain. Have you experienced abdominal pain (severe)?
- **C**hest pain. Have you noticed chest pain (severe), cough, or shortness of breath?
- **H**eadaches. Do you have headaches (severe), dizziness, weakness, or numbness?
- **E**ye problems. Have you had a change in vision (loss or blurring) or other eye problems or speech problems?
- **S**evere leg pain. Have you had any severe leg pain, especially in the calf or thigh?

○ Two missed pills—take one pill ASAP and one pill in 12 hours. Then continue with the remainder of the pack and use backup for 7 days. Additionally, offer emergency contraception (EC) if pills missed in first week of pack.
○ If more than two pills are missed—take EC and restart OCPs the next day and use backup for the next 7 days. If declines EC, skip missed pills and continue the rest of the pack and use backup until next menses (Hatcher et al, 2007.)
- Explain common side effects and the need to call if questions or concerns arise.
- Stress the importance of dual methods for protection from STIs and HIV.
- All adolescents should use condoms along with any other method used for contraception.
- All adolescents should have a prescription for EC and understand how to use them.

Follow-up Management. Provide an emergency follow-up number and instruct the client on indications for calling. Schedule a return appointment. The return visit gives the health care provider an opportunity to assess the physiologic effects of the OCP and the adolescent's acceptance and use of this particular contraceptive method.

Adolescents tend to be acutely aware of and sensitive to body changes and processes. As a result they may incorrectly interpret physical signs, exaggerate the effects of OCPs on their bodies, and discontinue the OCP use without consulting their health care provider. At the follow-up visit, the provider should reemphasize the noncontraceptive benefits of the OCP, have the client discuss concerns about the OCPs, discuss the lower risks of OCPs compared with those of pregnancy, and review and reclarify directions and side effects.

Interview the client for STI exposure, compliance, satisfaction with medication, and perceived side effects. The use of the mnemonic ACHES (Box 35-6) can help guide assessment questions, and can be used carefully to help the teenager understand more clearly the risks of OCPs without unduly concerning her.

Physical examination parameters during the return visit include weight and blood pressure measurements and any laboratory follow-up.

Other Methods of Hormonal Contraception. Hormonal contraception can also be delivered in other preparations. Three of these methods are listed in Box 35-7.

| BOX 35-7 | Other Methods of Hormonal Contraception |

Contraceptive Patch
The contraceptive patch (Ortho Evra) is a 20-cm^2 transdermal adhesive patch consisting of progestin (17-deacetylnorgestimate) and ethinyl estradiol placed on the trunk, buttock, or arm once a week for 3 weeks and removed for 1 week to allow for a withdrawal bleed. The advantage of the patch is that it does not require the user to remember a daily oral contraceptive pill (OCP). Disadvantages include the visibility of the patch, which precludes privacy of method, and the need to remember to replace the patch when indicated. The patch also has decreased efficacy in women who weigh more than 198 pounds (90 kg). It costs about the same as OCPs (except for generic forms) and has the same precautions and side effects as OCPs. There is some evidence that the patch may have an increased risk of nonfatal venous thromboembolism (VTE) over OCPs in some women. Careful screening of VTE risk is recommended.

Vaginal Ring
The vaginal contraceptive ring (NuvaRing) is a self-administered contraceptive, consisting of a soft, flexible, 2-inch transparent plastic ring with a hole in the middle. It is 0.125 inch thick and is impregnated with estrogen and progestin. It is inserted vaginally once a month on or before the fifth day of menses, left in place for 3 weeks, removed for 1 week to allow for a withdrawal bleed, and then a new ring inserted. Placement over the cervix is not necessary. As long as it is in contact with the vagina, it is working. The failure rate is the same as OCPs: typical use 8%, and perfect use 0.3%. Advantages include that it is coitus independent, does not involve the use of messy creams or gels, and is only dealt with once a month. It does not provide protection against sexually transmitted infections (STIs); there is some initial breakthrough bleeding, and the user must be comfortable inserting and removing the device and be able to adhere to the usage schedule.

Subdermal Implant Contraception
Implanon is currently the only implanted form of progestin-only contraception on the market in the U.S. Implanon is a one-rod, 3-year subdermal implant that has a newer form of progestin (etonogestrel). The method of action is the same as other progestin-only methods. The advantage of an implant is that it provides long-acting contraception. Disadvantages include surgical insertion and removal procedures and side effects, such as irregular bleeding, weight gain, and acne. It is a more successful method for mature adolescents committed to long-term contraception.

Injectable Contraception: Medroxyprogesterone Acetate (Depo-Provera)

Protocol for Initial Use. Always evaluate for pregnancy before giving the initial dose. A single 150-mg injection inhibits ovulation for 13 weeks. Dosage adjustment for body weight is not necessary. It is preferable to deliver the initial injection before day 5 of the menstrual cycle to minimize pregnancy potential. Injections are usually given at 12-week intervals. If more than 13 weeks have transpired between injections, evaluate for pregnancy before giving the injection. Mechanism of action, theoretic and use effectiveness, benefits, and disadvantages are listed in Table 35-1.

Patients Appropriate for Medroxyprogesterone Acetate. Medroxyprogesterone acetate is a contraceptive method of choice for patients with the following characteristics:
- Seeking a long-term, reversible, highly reliable, private method of contraception

TABLE 35-1   Hormonal Methods of Contraception: Mechanism of Action, Theoretic and Use Effectiveness, Benefits, Disadvantages, Side Effects, Failure and Efficacy

Method	Mechanism of Action	Theoretic and Use Effectiveness	Benefits	Disadvantages	Side Effects, Failure and Efficacy
Oral contraceptive pills	• Suppression of ovulation (90% to 95% with COC and 50% with POP) • Thickening of cervical mucus, blocking penetration of sperm • Alteration of endometrial lining • Alteration of tubal motility	• Perfect use failure rate is 0.3% • Typical first-year failure rate in all women is 8%	• High rate of effectiveness • Simple method to use • Ease of discontinuing use • Rapid reversal of effects after discontinuing medication • Beneficial effects on the menstrual cycle • Reduction of premenstrual symptoms • Decreased dysmenorrhea • Decreased flow Medical benefits: • For women younger than 20 years old, the estimated death rate while on an OCP is 0.3 per 100,000 nonsmoking users (2.2 per 100,000 smoking users), as compared with that of childbirth, for which the estimated maternal death rate is 7 per 100,000 live births (Emans, 2005b). Other health benefits: • Reduction of anemia risks • Decreased incidence of gonorrheal PID, resulting in less morbidity (chronic pelvic pain, decreased incidence of ectopic pregnancies, and less infertility) • Protection against formation of ovarian cysts (COCs) • Reduction of ovarian and endometrial cancer (COCs) • Ortho Tri-Cyclen and Estrostep are approved by FDA for treatment of acne	• No protection from STIs—need to use condoms • Daily use difficult for some women Triphasic OCPs: • Confusion about color of package • Less flexibility of use by the prescriber (e.g., difficult to use for periods greater than 21 days or for management of ovarian cysts, endometrial bleeding, or DUB) • Some adolescents find triphasic preparation confusing, especially if they forget to take a pill Progestin-only OCPs: • Irregular bleeding • Effectiveness decreases dramatically if even one pill is missed; manufacturer recommends that POPs be taken at the same time every day and that a backup method of birth control be used if even one pill is missed or taken more than 3 hours late (Hatcher et al, 2007). • May increase acne • No protection from STIs—need to use condoms	• Nausea and vomiting • Breakthrough bleeding (spotting) • Breast tenderness • Headaches • Mood changes OCP failure: • Method failure or method ineffectiveness • Patient failure/user effectiveness—68% still use OCPs 1 year after initiation; most discontinuance is for nonmedical reasons • Concurrent drug interaction, such as with anticonvulsants, tetracycline, St. John's wort and possibly oral antifungals • OCPs can increase the action of diazepam, tricyclics, chlordiazepoxide, and theophylline

| Injectable contraception | • Inhibits ovulation by inhibiting LH surge (normal ovulation occurs within 6 months after the last injection in approximately 50% of women; however, 25% will take up to 1 year to return to a normal menstrual pattern) (Speroff and Darney, 2010)
• Creates shallow, atrophic endometrium, unsuitable for implantation
• Increases thickening of cervical mucus, decreasing sperm penetration | • The lowest expected pregnancy rate is 0.3 per 100 women-years with the typical failure rate of 3%. | • One-time dosing every 3 months
• Good method for adolescents who want to keep contraception private from family and friends
• Gynecologic benefits (e.g., decreases in PID, ectopic pregnancy, and endometriosis) | • Menstrual irregularities (including amenorrhea or decreased menstrual flow)
• Weight gain
• Headache
• Breast tenderness
• Acne
• Hirsutism
• Psychological effects, such as moodiness, depression, change in libido
• Evidence of bone density loss in adolescents; osteopenia
• Intramuscular injection
• Need to use condoms to prevent STIs
• Increased risk for low birth-weight in infants exposed in utero |
| Postcoital hormonal contraception OR emergency contraception (EC) | • Inhibits ovulation
• May affect tubal transport | | | • Nausea, vomiting, breast tenderness, headache, and dizziness
• The progestin-only methods have fewer side effects (Speroff and Darney, 2010)
• Plan B has a 1% failure rate
• Yuzpe method has a 2% to 3% failure rate |

COC, Combination oral contraceptive; *DUB*, dysfunctional uterine bleeding; *FDA*, Food and Drug Administration; *LH*, luteinizing hormone; *OCP*, oral contraceptive pill; *POP*, progestin-only pill.

- Those for whom use of estrogen is contraindicated (e.g., patients with a previous thromboembolic episode, lupus, sickle cell anemia)
- Those with seizure disorders—improves control (Speroff and Darney, 2005)
- Those with poor compliance using other contraceptive methods
- Those with menstrual hygiene issues, such as individuals who are mentally retarded, because medroxyprogesterone acetate often causes amenorrhea after two injections

Postcoital Hormonal Contraception or Emergency Contraception

Preparation. EC is designed to be used after unprotected intercourse to prevent an unwanted pregnancy. Plan B was the only FDA-approved oral emergency contraceptive marketed in the U.S. and is approved for purchase without a prescription for women older than 18 years. Plan B is a two-tablet progestin-only method that should be taken within 72 hours of unprotected intercourse for the highest efficacy. The dosage is either one tablet taken immediately with the second tablet taken in 12 hours or both tablets taken at one time. The FDA has approved a second emergency contraceptive (Ella) that can be taken up to 5 days after unprotected intercourse. Ella requires a prescription in all cases. Regular OCPs (combination) may also be used at recommended dosages; this regimen is referred to as the Yuzpe method. POPs are another alternative (see Hatcher et al, 2007, for specifics). There are no contraindications to EC for progestin-only formulations.

Clinical Management. All adolescents should have a prescription, in advance, for self-administration as needed. The prescription is intended for such times as when a condom breaks or there has been a lapse in birth control method. An emergency contraceptive is more effective the earlier it is taken after unprotected intercourse. Studies have shown that when readily available, the use of EC does not increase unprotected sex (Speroff and Darney, 2010).

If a client has a need for EC:

- Assess for pregnancy using a rapid high-sensitivity urine pregnancy test. If LNMP has been within 1 month, a pregnancy test is not necessary.
- Instruct patient to return for a pregnancy test if no menses occurs within 3 weeks.
- Instruct patient to abstain from intercourse until the start of her next cycle or use condoms 100% of the time.
- Discuss a long-term birth control method; review current method and effectiveness for client.
- Schedule return visit in 3 to 4 weeks.

Barrier Methods of Contraception (Coitus-Dependent Methods)

Mechanism of action, theoretic and use effectiveness, and benefits and disadvantages of barrier methods of contraception are listed in Table 35-2.

Condoms. Condoms are the most common barrier method of contraception. Used effectively they can prevent pregnancy and decrease STI transmission. In the CDC's 2009 Youth Risk Behavior Surveillance System data, 61% of high school students stated they used condoms for their last act of sexual intercourse (CDC, 2010b).

More than 100 brands of condoms are available in an array of sizes (most are 170 × 50 mm), textures, lubricants, colors, and scents. Ninety-nine percent use latex condoms, and less than 1% use either natural skin or the newer polyurethane condoms. The polyurethane condoms are not subject to breakdown by petroleum-based lubricants, are latex-free, and have an improved taste over latex. However, they are less elastic, which increases slippage and breakage. They should be reserved for those with latex allergies. *Protocol for use includes:*

- Use every time!
- Apply correctly, allowing for 0.5-inch tip at end and removing any trapped air.
- Remove correctly after intercourse. Hold on to the condom while withdrawing the penis from the vagina to prevent the condom from coming off in the vagina. Replace if used for oral or anal sex before intravaginal intercourse.
- Avoid use of petroleum-based lubricants, such as petroleum jelly, shortening, and oil-based vaginal therapeutics, such as Monistat or Femstat.
- Check expiration date on the package and make sure package is intact.
- Use only once and discard.
- Keep a prescription for an emergency contraceptive handy.

Diaphragm. Available for more than 100 years, there are three types of diaphragms in sizes from 50 to 95 mm, available by prescription only. For most adolescents, the 65- to 75-mm sizes are commonly prescribed. These are:

- Arching spring (Koroflex, Allflex, Ramses Bendex)
- Coil-spring rim (Koromex, Ortho, Ramses)
- Wide-seal rim (Milex) available only from the manufacturer

Protocol for use includes placing the diaphragm in the vagina over the cervix up to 1 hour before intercourse. It can be left in place for 24 hours, but it must be left a minimum of 6 to 8 hours. Reapplication of spermicide is required with subsequent intercourse.

Cervical Cap. The cervical cap, like the diaphragm, is available by prescription only. It may be left in place for 48 hours; however, subsequent intercourse within 6 hours or more requires additional intravaginal spermicide. The cervical cap should probably be reserved for those adolescents who are older, more motivated to comply with contraception, and able to place and remove the device (Speroff and Darney, 2010). Protocol for use: use every time!

Female Condom. The female condom is a device with an inner ring or dome that fits next to the cervix. An outer ring fits around the external opening to the vagina. The single-use condom acts as a barrier to prevent sperm from entering the vagina and may reduce the risk of STIs. *Protocol for use: use every time!*

Contraceptive Sponge. The sponge is made of soft, disposable polyurethane foam and contains the spermicide nonoxynol-9. After it is moistened with water and inserted into the vagina, it becomes effective immediately and protects against pregnancy for the next 24 hours without the need to add spermicidal cream or jelly—even with repeated acts of intercourse. *Protocol for use: use every time!*

Spermicides. Spermicides are marketed in various formats:

- Foams, creams, or jellies that can be used alone or in combination with a condom or diaphragm
- Spermicidal suppositories that are intended for use alone or with a condom; require a 10- to 15-minute wait before intercourse to allow the product to effervesce

TABLE 35-2 Barrier Methods of Contraception: Mechanism of Action, Theoretic and Use Effectiveness, Benefits, and Disadvantages

Method	Mechanism of Action	Theoretic and Use Effectiveness	Benefits	Disadvantages
Condoms	• Prevent sperm from entering vagina	• First-year failure rate among typical users is 15% • First-year failure rate among perfect users is 2% • Concomitant, perfect use of condoms with a spermicide has an estimated probability of contraceptive failure of 0.3%. This is equivalent to perfect-use failure rate with an OCP.	• Encourages male participation • Appeals to those who have episodic intercourse and for sexual debuts (Lohr, 2008) • Is inexpensive and accessible • Use of lubricated condoms reduces mechanical friction and vaginal or penile irritation • Decreases the risk of transmitting STIs • Eliminates postcoital vaginal discharge • Helps maintain erection for some men • Has few contraindications	• Condom breakage or slippage; approximately 2% to 6% of condoms fail as a result of breakage or slippage. • Natural-skin condoms are contraindicated if there is a risk of infection by sexually transmitted viruses (e.g., hepatitis B virus, HPV, HSV, and HIV). • Either partner may be allergic to latex. • Male partner may fail to accept responsibility for use. • Some men cannot maintain an erection when a condom is used.
Other barrier methods (diaphragm, cervical cap, female condom, contraceptive sponge)		• Effectiveness of any of these methods is influenced by the patient's ability to use the method consistently and correctly, along with her own personal fertility characteristics • Patients who are younger than 30 years and have intercourse four or more times a week experience higher failure rates • Diaphragm failure rate is 16% in typical users • Cervical cap failure rate averages 16% to 32% • Female condom pregnancy rates are reported to be 21% • Sponge failure rate with typical use is 14% to18%	• Diaphragms and female condoms help prevent transmission of STIs and decrease risk of PID, bacterial and viral infection, and cervical neoplasia • Female condoms and the sponge are accessible over the counter	• Barrier methods are contraindicated if there is a history of toxic shock syndrome. • Female condoms cost $3 versus $1 for male condoms and have a visible outer ring. • Sponges cost about $3 per sponge. • Cervical caps are contraindicated if there has been a full-term delivery within the last 6 weeks, if there has been a recent spontaneous or induced abortion, or if there is vaginal bleeding from any cause, including menstrual flow. • Allergic reaction may occur in those sensitive to rubber, latex, or polyurethane. • Abnormalities in vaginal anatomy can interfere with satisfactory fit or placement of any of the devices. • Diaphragm can cause recurrent urinary tract infections. • For diaphragms and caps, trained personnel may not be available to fit device or lack the time to instruct patient adequately on use of method. • Patient must be able to learn correct insertion and extraction techniques. • Patient may not feel comfortable touching self or may find procedure messy and unpleasant.

Continued

TABLE 35-2			Barrier Methods of Contraception: Mechanism of Action, Theoretic and Use Effectiveness, Benefits, and Disadvantages—cont'd	

Method	Mechanism of Action	Theoretic and Use Effectiveness	Benefits	Disadvantages
Spermicides	A combination of an inert base or carrier (foam, cream, jelly, suppository, or tablet) with active spermicidal agent nonoxynol-9 or octoxynol, which kills sperm by permeating the cell membrane	• Estimated 15% failure rate among perfect first-year users • Among typical users, failure rate is about 29%	• Medically safe, with same efficacy as barrier methods or condoms • Available over the counter without a prescription; no need to access medical system • No need for partner involvement with decision-making or implementation • Used as backup option while waiting to start OCPs, for missed OCPs, or between relationships	• Can cause allergic reaction in those sensitive to spermicidal agent or base • Can be difficult for some people to learn correct insertion technique • Abnormalities in vaginal anatomy can prevent correct placement or product retention (e.g., septum, prolapse, double cervix)

HIV, Human immunodeficiency virus; *HPV,* human papillomavirus; *HSV,* herpes simplex virus; *OCP,* oral contraceptive pill; *PID,* pelvic inflammatory disease; *POP,* progestin-only pill; *STI,* sexually transmitted infection.

• Vaginal contraceptive film that can be used alone or with a condom or diaphragm; film contains 72 mg of nonoxynol-9 in a thin sheet that is placed next to the cervix 15 minutes before intercourse

Protocol for use: Use every time, keep adequate supply and store properly, be alert to timing of product placement before intercourse, place in vagina at appropriate time, and insert new application of product before every episode of repeated intercourse.

Less Useful Contraceptive Methods for Adolescents

Most methods may be considered for use in the mature and motivated adolescent. However, the following methods are usually not recommended for use with sexually active adolescents because of higher failure rates, the need for more maturity, and proven and committed use of contraceptives:

• Periodic abstinence
• Fertility awareness or rhythm method because of the more irregular cycles of adolescents
• Implanted contraception, as a result of intolerance of side effects and costs associated with early removal
• Progestin only pills unless indicated
• Intrauterine devices, as a result of increased risk of STIs and irregular bleeding

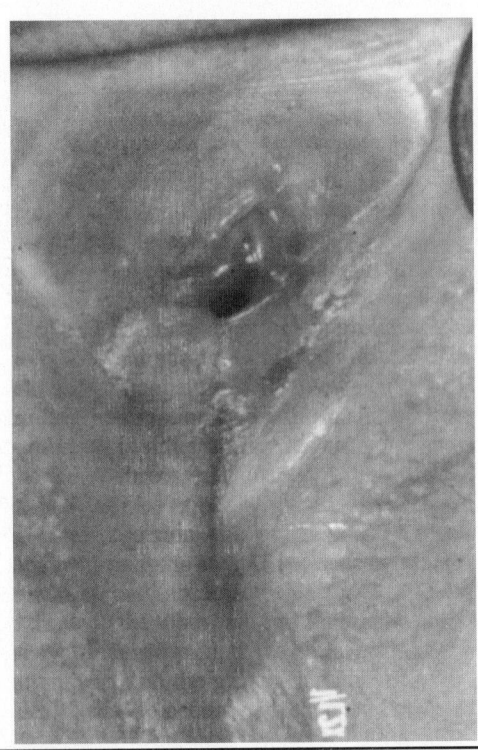

FIGURE 35-8 Labial adhesions that are thinned and almost translucent inferiorly following topical estrogen therapy. (From Craighill MC: Pediatric and adolescent gynecology for primary care pediatricians, *Pediatr Clin North Am* 45:1668, 1998.)

■ Specific Gynecologic Conditions of Children

LABIAL ADHESIONS

Description

The fusion of tissue between the labia minora that appears to cover the vaginal opening is a common, benign condition in infants and prepubertal girls. It is also called agglutination, synechia vulvae, or vulvar adhesion if only the lower half of the labia minora is involved (Fig. 35-8).

Epidemiology

Before puberty the vaginal tissues are in a hypoestrogenized state and are prone to inflammation and denudation. As the tissues heal, adhesion of the labia can occur. Mechanisms for the initial insult are irritation, infection, and trauma. The most common precipitant is an asymptomatic, nonspecific vulvovaginitis caused by poor hygiene. There is debate about whether lack of hygiene, masturbation, fondling, and

TABLE 35-3	Treatment of Labial Adhesions		
Degree of Involvement	**Treatment**	**Prognosis**
No urinary tract infection, no obstruction, no parental concern	No treatment. Reassure and observe.	Resolution with puberty and estrogenization of tissue.
Opening ensures urinary and vaginal drainage, but treatment desired	Apply ointment (e.g., A&D or petroleum jelly) nightly with cotton-tipped swab with gentle pressure. Following separation, maintain good hygiene and mild ointment (e.g., Vaseline) nightly for 6-12 mo.	Separation within 8 wk. If not, double-check technique to ensure gentle pressure is being applied. If persists, see use of estrogen cream below.
Urinary and vaginal drainage impaired	Apply estrogen-containing 1% cream (e.g., Premarin) bid for 3 wk with cotton-tipped swab then at bedtime for another 2-3 wk. Use gentle pressure until separation occurs. Following separation, use petroleum jelly nightly as outlined above.	Separation occurs 50% of the time within 2-3 wk. If not, check technique to ensure pressure is being applied and continue for another 3 wk. If unresponsive, may anesthetize with 5% lidocaine ointment or EMLA cream, then gently tease the adhesions with a Calgiswab (Emans, 2005d). Always avoid forceful separation.

subsequent irritation from sexual abuse are potential causes in older females. Labial adhesions occur primarily in girls 3 months to 6 years old, but can persist until puberty (Emans, 2005d). They typically resolve spontaneously—50% within 6 months, 90% within 12 months, and 100% within 18 months (Nield, 2009).

Clinical Findings
History
- Concern about rash in genital area
- Parental concern about vaginal opening
- Dysuria, difficulty voiding, or local discomfort

Physical Examination. Physical examination reveals a thin, flat membrane of varying length from the posterior fourchette to the clitoris. The degree of opening near the clitoris varies. The vulva appears flat with a central line of fusion. The urethra may or may not be visualized, and there may be urinary dribbling.

Differential Diagnosis

Scarring, imperforate hymen, clitoral hypertrophy, and intersex problems are the differential diagnoses.

Management

The treatment of labial adhesions is somewhat controversial. Table 35-3 outlines steps that are generally accepted. In asymptomatic labial adhesions, observation is often the best treatment. If treatment is desired, applying A&D ointment or petroleum jelly at bedtime may be helpful. The presence of symptoms of urinary tract infection, pain with activity, and change in behavior dictates treatment. Forceful separation is always contraindicated because it may result in trauma to the child and recurrence of adhesions.

Complications

Urinary tract infections and readhesion following mechanical lysis can occur.

Patient Education

Premarin cream can cause breast tenderness, transient breast enlargement, and vulvar pigmentation or erythema, which resolves after discontinuing the cream. The incidence of recurrence can be decreased with careful attention to perineal hygiene and the daily application of A&D ointment until puberty.

VULVOVAGINITIS

Description

Vulvovaginitis refers to inflammation, often with discharge, from infection or irritation. Vulvitis refers to inflammation of the vulva alone, whereas vaginitis refers to vaginal discharge, often with pruritus and irritation that may be secondary to the vulvitis (Hamel-Teillac, 2004).

Epidemiology

Age is important in differentiating the etiology of vulvovaginitis. In prepubescent children several factors make vulvovaginitis a common problem. The lack of estrogen stimulation leaves the vulvar skin thin and the vaginal mucosa atrophic and contributes to minimal vaginal secretions with neutral pH. The lack of pubic hair and labial fat pads diminishes barrier protection, and the proximity of the vaginal opening to the anus predisposes prepubertal females to irritation and infection of the vulva and vagina. Poor hygiene, including wiping technique and lack of handwashing, and irritants such as bubble bath, harsh soaps, sand from playtime, or tight-fitting clothing provide additional insults. Being overweight is also a risk factor.

Prepubescent vulvovaginitis most commonly is nonspecific (up to 80%). Other causes include foreign bodies (most often toilet paper), bacterial infection (often group A betahemolytic streptococci), or pinworms (Emans, 2005d).

Clinical Findings

The clinical findings pertaining to vulvovaginitis are found in Table 35-4.

TABLE 35-4	Evaluation and Treatment of Vulvovaginitis				
	Signs and Symptoms	**Vaginal Discharge**	**Etiology**	**Laboratory Data**	**Treatment**
Nonspecific vaginitis	Itching, burning; dysuria; varied vulvitis	Scant to copious; brown to green; mucoid; foul smelling, poor hygiene	Irritation from contact with various substances; normal UA	pH variable; no odor on whiff test; micro: leukocytes, bacteria, debris	Refractory cases may need topical estrogen or antibiotics
Physiologic leukorrhea	None or minimal itch or burn; minimal vulvitis; 6-12 mo before menarche; possible mild erythema	Scant to moderate; clear to white; odorless; nonirritating	Endogenous hormones 6-12 mo before menarche	pH <4.5; no odor on whiff test; micro: epithelial cells, lactobacilli; normal UA	No treatment needed; explain and reassure
Chemical or mechanical	Itch, erythema, vulvar inflammation, dysuria	Scant amount; yellow to white	Bubble bath, perfumed soap, lotion; tight-fitting clothes, sand or dirt from playground, overweight	pH <4.5; no odor on whiff test; micro: leukocytes, epithelial cells	Remove irritant; topical steroids
Foreign body	Dysuria, discomfort, bleeding, minimal vulvar excoriation; history of foreign body in other orifices	Purulent, persistent, dark brown, foul smelling (18%), bloody (82%)	Toilet paper (prepubescent); tampons (adolescent); condoms or object used for masturbation	pH >4.5; odd odor on whiff test; micro: WBCs, epithelial cells with bacteria and debris; UA normal	Remove foreign body with forceps or by irrigating with saline and small feeding tube; knee-chest position may work best
Bacterial	Acute respiratory, enteric, or skin infection	Green color, foul, copious with possible bleeding	*Streptococcus* (most common), *Escherichia coli, Enterococcus, Shigella, Staphylococcus,* or other bacteria	Strep test positive; culture positive	Penicillin, erythromycin, amoxicillin, broad-spectrum cephalosporin or other antibiotic as indicated
Candidiasis	Itching, burning, vulvar inflammation, external dysuria, dyspareunia	Thick, white, curdy cottage cheese–like, adherent, odorless; vulva red, edematous with satellite lesions	*Candida albicans;* recent antibiotic or steroid use; diabetes or immunodeficiency; pregnancy	pH <4.5; no odor on whiff test; micro: fungal hyphae and buds or spores; culture positive for *Candida* (see Fig. 35-2)	Azole cream topically or intravaginally; or fluconazole 150-mg oral tab—single dose
Pinworms	Recent exposure to pinworms; perineal itching, especially at night; anal excoriation, erythema, and lesions from scratching	No discharge	*Enterobius vermicularis* spread from anus	Normal UA; tape test reveals eggs	Mebendazole 100 mg once; repeated in 2 wk; treat family members
Bacterial vaginosis	Foul odor, especially after menses or intercourse; often asymptomatic; no inflammation; abdominal pain or irregular prolonged bleeding	Homogeneous, thin milky white discharge adherent* to vaginal walls and pools in posterior fornix; increased amount	*Gardnerella vaginalis,* mycoplasmas, and anaerobic bacteria; caused by replacement of normal vaginal flora; may or may not be sexually transmitted	pH >4.5*; fishy odor on whiff test*; micro: clue cells,* few lactobacilli, gram-negative rods, no WBCs	Treat if symptomatic with metronidazole 500 mg orally twice a day for 7 days or metronidazole gel 0.75% 5 g intravaginally at bedtime for 5 days or clindamycin cream 2% 5 g intravaginally at bedtime for 7 days

*Three of these findings needed to diagnose bacterial vaginosis.
Micro, Microscopic examination; *UA,* urinalysis; *WBC,* white blood cell.

History. The history for the prepubertal child includes the following:

- Onset—less than 1 month usually associated with specific diagnosis, whereas a longer period of time more likely nonspecific (Emans, 2005d)
- Characteristics:
  - Genital irritation, itching, pain, inflammation
  - Vaginal discharge—note onset, quantity, color, type (bloody, mucoid), odor, consistency, and duration
  - Nighttime perianal itching
  - Urinary complaints, including dysuria and enuresis
- Recent medications, especially antibiotics
- Possible trauma, foreign body, pinworm infestation, or sexual abuse
- Previous occurrences and treatment used
- Underlying illnesses (e.g., streptococcus infection, dermatosis, diabetes, immunosuppression)
- Perineal hygiene
- Use of harsh soaps and bubble bath
- Tight-fitting or nylon underwear or clothing
- Superabsorbent diapers

Physical Examination. A good light and magnifying glass may aid in the physical examination. Prepubertal examination includes inspection, possible vaginal otoscopy in frog-leg or knee-chest position, and rectal examination.

Diagnostic Studies

- pH of vaginal secretions
- Wet mounts of vaginal secretions
- Saline for microscopic examination to look for WBCs, clue cells, trichomonads, and bacteria
- 10% KOH for whiff test and microscopic examination to look for yeast (branching hyphae and spores) (see Fig. 35-7)
- Bacterial culture of vaginal secretions
- Slide with 20% KOH of skin scraping for yeast
- Pinworm eggs visualized on tape slide under microscope
- Cultures for GC and chlamydia if suspected sexual abuse

Differential Diagnosis

Atopic dermatitis, psoriasis, seborrhea, lichen sclerosus, or other dermatosis; labial adhesions; polyps or tumors; systemic diseases, such as Kawasaki or Crohn; STIs; and sexual abuse are included in the differential diagnosis.

Management

General treatment measures for any type of vulvovaginitis are listed in Box 35-8. Specific recommendations include the following (see also Table 35-4):

Prepubertal Nonspecific Etiology

- If persistent, prescribe antibacterial cream at night (e.g., Bactroban, Sultrin, or clindamycin) for 2 weeks.
- If persistent after 3 weeks, prescribe a trial of amoxicillin, amoxicillin and clavulanate, or one of the cephalosporins.
- If symptoms still persist, use estrogen cream at bedtime for 2 to 3 weeks, then every other night at bedtime for 2 weeks to thicken vulvar epithelium.
- If recurrent vulvovaginitis, a 1- to 2-month course of low-dose cephalexin or trimethoprim-sulfamethoxazole (TMP-SMX) at bedtime should be tried.

BOX 35-8 General Treatment Measures for Vulvovaginitis

1. Hygiene
   - Wash hands frequently
   - Wipe front to back
   - Change underwear every day
   - Blow-dry perineal area with cool to warm air (especially if overweight)
2. Clothing
   - Wear absorbent white underwear, changing once or twice daily; do not wear underwear at night
   - Wear loose clothing—no pantyhose or tight clothes
   - Avoid spandex and sleeper pajamas
   - Change out of swimsuit after swimming
3. Comfort and healing measures
   - Take sitz bath with thorough drying
   - Blow-dry for 10 to 15 minutes once or twice daily with cool to warm air or pat dry with towel
   - Apply hydrocortisone cream 1% once or twice daily for itching
   - Use oral diphenhydramine or hydroxyzine if itching is severe
4. Protective measures
   - Avoid bubble baths and perfumed lotions or powder
   - Use mild soap (e.g., Dove, Basis, Neutrogena)
   - Avoid shampoo in bath water
   - Use protective ointment twice a day (e.g., petroleum jelly, A&D, Aquaphor)
   - Avoid bleach or fabric softener in wash, double rinse
   - Urinate with knees spread apart to minimize urinary reflux

---

- If a specific infection is found, treat as outlined here or refer to appropriate section.
- If therapy fails, refer to a pediatric gynecologist.
- If an STI is found in a child, a complete workup for sexual abuse is indicated.

Contact Dermatitis

- Steroids and hormonal cream can be used to thicken vaginal skin and minimize irritation.

Foreign Body

- Prepubertal: Irrigate with warm normal saline with a small feeding tube at the hymenal opening with the child in the frog-leg position. If foreign body remains after irrigation, refer to a pediatric gynecologist.
- A broad-spectrum antibiotic, such as amoxicillin or a cephalosporin, may be indicated if infection is apparent.

Bacterial Infection

- Obtain cultures and prescribe appropriate treatment; penicillin or erythromycin is usually used.

Candida Infection

- Topical antifungal creams are usually successful.
- Treatment failure or recurrence may indicate a resistant organism.
- If appropriate, evaluate for STIs.
- Complicated candidal infections (severe local, recurrent in an immunocompromised host) require documentation by culture, workup for predisposing conditions, longer duration of treatment.

Pinworms

- Mebendazole (one chewable 100-mg tablet, repeated in 2 weeks)
- Handwashing is important to minimize the spread of infection.

- See Chapter 32 for further discussion.
- GC, chlamydia, or trichomoniasis in prepubescent children needs to be treated and evaluated as suspected child abuse. See the section on STIs in this chapter and 2010 CDC guidelines for treatment of STIs (CDC, 2010a) for more specifies.

Complications

Labial adhesions can occur.

Patient Education, Prognosis, and Prevention

- Follow up in 5 days if there is no improvement.
- Recurrence is common, especially with poor hygiene, in overweight girls, and during upper respiratory infection.

■ Normal Gynecologic Variations

MITTELSCHMERZ

Description

Pelvic pain that occurs at the time of ovulation, midway between menstrual periods, is referred to as mittelschmerz (middle pain).

Epidemiology

The etiology is unclear, but pain is probably caused by follicular rupture and the irritation of the peritoneum from the follicular fluid. The incidence is unknown, although some ultrasonographic studies have detected follicular fluid midcycle in 40% of women with normal cycles (Laufer and Goldstein, 2005).

Clinical Findings

History

- Pain occurs midway between cycles, although not with irregular cycles.
- Dull, achy pain in lower abdomen lasting a few minutes to several hours
- Recurrent discomfort at same time in each cycle
- Pain occasionally severe and crampy, persisting up to 3 days

Physical Examination. Pain with palpation on either or both sides of lower abdomen overlying the ovaries may be present.

Differential Diagnosis

Included in the differential diagnosis is appendicitis, torsion or rupture of an ovarian cyst, and ectopic pregnancy.

Management

- The etiology and benign nature of the pain should be explained to the adolescent and parent.
- A heating pad may provide some relief, and analgesics, especially prostaglandin inhibitors (ibuprofen, naproxen), may be used. Box 35-9 lists the dosages.
- Rarely oral contraceptives (OCs) may be prescribed to suppress ovulation.

> **BOX 35-9** Common Prostaglandin Inhibitors Used to Treat Adolescent Menstrual Disorders
>
> 1. Ibuprofen: 400-800 mg three times a day with a loading dose of 800 mg; maximum dose of 2400 mg/24 hr
> 2. Naproxen: 500 mg at onset followed by 250-500 mg every 6-12 hr; maximum dose of 1250 mg/24 hr
> 3. Naproxen sodium: 550 mg at onset followed by 275 mg every 6-12 hours; maximum dose of 1375 mg/24 hr
> 4. Mefenamic acid: 500 mg at onset followed by 250 mg every 6 hr
> 5. Meclofenamate: 100 mg initially; 50-100 mg every 6 hr

Patient Education

Provide reassurance and comfort measures as outlined in the management section. The adolescent should be encouraged to return if the pain worsens or changes or if she is concerned.

DYSMENORRHEA

Description

Painful menstruation with cramping in the lower abdomen or pelvis is the most common gynecologic problem seen in adolescence. Primary dysmenorrhea has no pelvic pathologic condition identified, whereas secondary dysmenorrhea is due to a pelvic pathologic condition.

Epidemiology

Primary dysmenorrhea is painful menses caused by an exaggerated production of prostaglandins, primarily prostaglandin $F_2\alpha$, in the secretory endometrium. This causes uterine contractions and vasoconstriction leading to ischemia and pain. The elevation of prostaglandins is brought about by falling progesterone levels during the luteal phase of ovulatory cycles.

Secondary dysmenorrhea may be prompted by endometriosis; complications of pregnancy; outflow obstruction; ovarian cysts, fibroids, or other uterine abnormalities; or infection. Dysmenorrhea is present in more than 50% of adolescents and has been reported in up to 93%. It is the leading cause (greater than 10%) of absenteeism from school or work, with increasing incidence in those who describe the pain as severe (Braverman, 2008; Laufer and Goldstein, 2005).

Clinical Findings

History

- Primary dysmenorrhea
- Menstrual history
- Attitudes and beliefs about menstruation
- Onset—usually 6 to 24 months after menarche
- Location—lower midabdominal area radiating to back, thighs
- Duration and timing of pain—usually begins with menses and lasts less than 2 days
- Character—mild to severe cramping
- Associated symptoms—nausea, vomiting, diarrhea, headache, fatigue, nervousness, dizziness, urinary frequency, lower back or thigh pain
- Ameliorating or aggravating factors

- Treatments or medications tried, including complementary and alternative medicine (CAM)
- Sexual activity
- Number of days of school or activities missed
- Cigarette smoking
- Family history of dysmenorrhea
- Secondary dysmenorrhea (add the following history)
- Onset (with menarche or 2 to 3 years postmenarche)
- Pelvic pain at times other than menstruation (worsens over time)
- Character of pelvic pain (dull and constant rather than crampy)
- History of infection, menorrhagia, intermenstrual bleeding, or abnormal vaginal discharge
- Dyspareunia
- History of sexual abuse
- Family history of endometriosis

Physical Examination. A complete physical examination is recommended and required for secondary dysmenorrhea. A speculum and bimanual examination may be deferred if the adolescent is not sexually active, if the dysmenorrhea is mild, if it does not interfere with daily activities, or if the dysmenorrhea is responding to treatment and without suspicion of pathologic condition (Braverman, 2008; Durain, 2004). However, the external genitalia should be examined and a cotton swab inserted into the vagina to rule out hymenal abnormalities and/or a vaginal septum. A rectoabdominal examination also helps rule out adnexal tenderness and masses (Laufer and Goldstein, 2005).

Diagnostic Studies. The following are ordered only if indicated:

- NAATs or cervical cultures for GC and chlamydia
- CBC with sedimentation rate if PID is suspected
- Pregnancy test
- Pelvic ultrasound if abnormalities are suspected

Differential Diagnosis

Endometriosis, PID, chronic pelvic pain, obstructive malformations and/or other pathologic conditions of the reproductive tract are included in the differential diagnosis. Nongynecologic causes of pelvic pain, such as constipation, Crohn disease and irritable bowel syndrome should be considered.

Management

Primary Dysmenorrhea

- Prostaglandin synthetase inhibitors provide relief in 70% to 80% of patients (Laufer and Goldstein, 2005; Mama, 2010; Speroff and Fritz, 2005). They should be administered at onset of menses or, if cramping precedes menses, at onset of symptoms. Treat the patient for the duration of the pain, usually 1 to 2 days. The trial period should extend for three cycles; if no relief is experienced, an alternative prostaglandin inhibitor should be tried. See Box 35-9 for specific prostaglandin inhibitors. Nonsteroidal antiinflammatory drugs (NSAIDs) are advantageous as first-line therapy because they need to be taken for only 2 to 3 days. Ibuprofen and naproxen are widely used in clinical practice, are available OTC, and are relatively inexpensive. If ineffective, move on to one of the fenamates. Taking NSAIDs with food helps prevent abdominal complaints.

- OCs are widely used for dysmenorrhea. Because they suppress ovulation, total progesterone-induced prostaglandin production is decreased in the endometrium. A 30- to 35-mcg estrogen-progestin combination pill may be used for a 3- to 6-month trial if prostaglandin inhibitors are not successful. The Cochrane Review Group (Wong et al, 2009) found OCs may be more effective for dysmenorrhea than placebo; however, interpretation was limited due to the variable quality of the randomized controlled trials (RCTs) reviewed. OCs have the additional advantages of contraception, cycle regulation, protection from endometrial and ovarian cancer, decreased iron deficiency anemia, and slowing the progression of endometriosis.
- CAM is likely to be beneficial per Cochrane Review Group (Proctor and Farquhar, 2004) (see Chapter 42 for further CAM therapies).
  - Application of topical heat
  - Thiamine 100 mg/day
  - Toki-shakuyaku-san (herbal remedy) 2.5 g three times daily
  - High-frequency transcutaneous electrical nerve stimulation (TENS)
  - Vitamin E, 500 units/day
  - Magnesium
- Follow up by telephone or visit to adjust dose or change medication as needed; the adolescent should be seen again in 3 to 4 months. If failure to respond after 6 months of treatment or if pain worsens over time, a further workup is warranted.

Secondary Dysmenorrhea

Secondary dysmenorrhea requires a full diagnostic workup and often referral for gynecologic care.

Patient Education and Prevention

- Encourage exercise and stress reduction, which may help decrease pain.
- A well-balanced diet with ample amounts of fiber and water, in addition to decreasing caffeine, chocolate, and salt intake, may be useful to control dysmenorrhea (Durain, 2004).
- Smoking cessation may help decrease dysmenorrhea. A longitudinal study of women found that 41% of smokers compared with 26% of nonsmokers experienced moderate or severe dysmenorrhea (Chen et al, 2000).

ADOLESCENT PREGNANCY

Description

Adolescent pregnancy occurs in girls or young women between 13 and 19 years old, although pregnancy is possible for any girl who has ovulatory cycles. Pregnancy has been seen in girls before their first menstrual cycle and in those as young as 10 or 11 years old.

Epidemiology

Except for a slight increase in 2006 and 2007, the rate of teen pregnancy has been declining or remained steady, with the highest rate of pregnancy occurring in Hispanics, followed by African-American adolescents (CDC, 2011). The decline has been regarded as evidence of more effective contraceptive practices, delayed sexual debuts, and a decrease in sexual activity.

Social factors that correlate with adolescent pregnancy are poverty (83% of adolescents giving birth and 61% of those having abortions are from low-income households); being the product of an adolescent pregnancy themselves (one third of cases); history of childhood physical or sexual abuse (as many as 50% to 60% of early adolescent or midadolescent girls who become pregnant); and having a child already (25% of teen births are to adolescents who have had another child) (Klein, 2005). Having a sibling who is a teen parent, decreased parental monitoring of the adolescent, academic underachievement, poor sense of personal efficacy, depression, and substance abuse have been associated with teen pregnancy (Nicoletti, 2005).

Assessment

History

- Menstrual history
- Menarche
- Cycle regularity—normally how many days apart, how many days of flow
- LNMP and/or last bleed
- Contraceptive use—method, consistency of use. If on a hormonal method—any missed pills, late patch or ring replacement, late medroxyprogesterone acetate injection, etc.
- Sexual history (see Chapter 18)
- Associated symptoms: Breast sensitivity, nipple tenderness (1 to 2 weeks after conception), fatigue, nausea, urinary frequency (2 weeks after conception)
- Patients often have vague complaints (e.g., headache, abdominal discomfort, dizziness, and vaginal and urinary symptoms).

Physical Examination. There are three classic signs of pregnancy, each of which may be observed during the pelvic examination:

1. Hegar sign—softening of the isthmus of the uterus (the area between the cervix and the uterine body). This may be observed before there is uterine enlargement.
2. Chadwick sign—dark bluish or purplish discoloration of the vaginal and cervical epithelium, the result of increased blood supply to the pelvis. This is usually observed before uterine growth.
3. Uterine enlargement—occurs at 5 to 6 weeks and initially is a result of changes in the uterine muscle rather than growing gestation. Uterine sizing is traditionally done by bimanual examination and recorded in weeks of estimated gestation.

Fetal heart tones may be auscultated by Doppler at 10 to 12 weeks' gestation.

Diagnostic Studies. Pregnancy testing is done in cases of suspected pregnancy. Urine testing is the chosen test for the ambulatory setting because results can be obtained rapidly, and the test is accurate and inexpensive. Current urine tests can detect human chorionic gonadotropin (hCG) in the urine down to 25 international units/L. Normal serum levels at the time of the first missed menses are between 50 and 100 international units/L.

Serum testing is of two types; a qualitative test can detect hCG down to 5 international units/L, but will not measure the exact amount. A quantitative ß-hCG can measure the exact amount of ß-hCG in the serum and is indicated for serial measurements to evaluate for ectopic pregnancy, molar pregnancy, or to rule out gestational trophoblastic neoplasia (GTN) following a molar pregnancy.

If the pregnancy test result is positive, routine laboratory diagnostics include the following:

- Cervical cultures for GC and chlamydia
- Cervical cytology
- Vaginal pH with saline and KOH wet mounts
- Urinalysis and culture
- Routine prenatal blood work includes blood type and Rh, syphilis serology, rubella titer, CBC with differential, and screening for hepatitis B and HIV. Another test to consider is an abnormal hemoglobin screen in women of African-American, Asian, and Mediterranean descent for sickle cell trait and thalassemias. Women of Ashkenazi Jewish and French-Canadian descent should be referred for testing for Tay-Sachs.
- Possibly vaginal and/or pelvic ultrasonography to determine gestation accurately

Differential Diagnosis

The differential diagnoses for pregnancy are amenorrhea from another etiology, nonviable intrauterine pregnancy, ectopic pregnancy, and molar pregnancy.

Management and Education

Prompt diagnosis assists with pregnancy planning, early onset of prenatal precautions (e.g., avoidance of OTC medications and herbal preparations without provider approval; the dangers of alcohol, smoking, and illicit drug use), and prenatal care. Early care also allows women considering an abortion ample time for counseling, decision-making, and obtaining an abortion in the first trimester, when the procedure is safest. The health visit should include a pregnancy test, physical examination, and health counseling.

If the pregnancy test result is negative, the provider should talk with the adolescent about her situation. Is she in a steady relationship, was this date rape, were drugs and alcohol involved, was this forced or consensual sex, how old is the partner, etc? The counseling should be tailored to her individual needs, in addition to general education regarding the risk of unprotected intercourse, the potential for pregnancy and STIs and HIV, and reliable methods to protect her in the future.

If the pregnancy test result is positive, the visit should include the following:

- Dating parameters and pelvic examination to determine gestational age
- Counseling for pregnancy options, including continuing pregnancy and retaining custody of child, continuing pregnancy and placing child for adoption, or termination
- Assessment of the involvement of her social support system including family, partner, and any significant others. The provider should encourage parental involvement in the decision-making and may need to role-play and/ or serve as mediator for the teenager in informing others. Some states have parental notification laws in place around the issue of abortion, and in most, health care providers are mandatory reporters of statutory rape. Providers must be aware of laws of the state in which they practice.

Initiation of referrals as appropriate for the decision made:

- If the choice is continuing the pregnancy and prenatal care is not part of the provider's practice, the adolescent should be referred to another provider or, if available in the community, a comprehensive adolescent pregnancy program to initiate medical, nutritional, psychosocial, and educational services
- If adoption is the option of choice, refer to the appropriate legal or social service agency, or both. Look for agencies in the community that offer comprehensive preadoption and postadoption counseling
- If the choice is terminating pregnancy, refer to an appropriate resource for abortion counseling and the procedure
- Make additional referrals as indicated for Women, Infants, and Children (WIC) program, Medicaid coverage, and community health nurse. Public health–based research indicates that there is a significant positive effect on pregnancy, parenting, and childrearing outcomes if home visits are made by public health nurses.

Complications

Young age in a pregnant woman is an inherent risk factor, even with good prenatal care. Adverse outcomes are common in pregnant teenagers and include the following:

- Maternal anemia, preeclampsia, excessive weight gain or poor weight gain, puerperal complications, and potential social consequences (e.g., educational, economic, and occupational delay)
- Fetal and neonatal low birthweight, intrauterine growth retardation, prematurity, and minor acute infections

■ Specific Gynecologic Problems of Adolescents

AMENORRHEA

Description

Amenorrhea is lack of menstruation and is described as either primary or secondary. *Primary amenorrhea* is defined as either absence of menarche by 16 years old with normal pubertal growth and development or absence of menarche by 14 years old in the absence of secondary sexual characteristics. *Secondary amenorrhea* is defined as the absence of menstruation for at least three cycles or more than 6 months in females who have an established menstrual pattern.

Epidemiology

There are multiple etiologies for primary and secondary amenorrhea. When evaluating a young woman for amenorrhea, pregnancy should be ruled out first, regardless of sexual history given. Amenorrhea is usually categorized by clinical findings and laboratory results into broad areas of causation. Speroff and colleagues (1973) devised a compartmental system to categorize amenorrhea that is still in use today (Speroff and Fritz, 2005). They distinguish between compartment 1, disorders of the outflow tract or uterine target organ; compartment 2, disorders of the ovary; compartment 3, disorders of the anterior pituitary; and compartment 4, disorders of the CNS (hypothalamic). Emans (2005a) uses the organs in

the HPO axis to categorize etiology. Others (Wilson et al, 2005), using the lab results of the gonadotropins and prolactin, categorize etiology into hypogonadotropic, hypergonadotropic, normogonadotropic, hyperprolactinemic, and anatomic. Grouping in some manner assists the provider to delineate the origin of an individual adolescent's amenorrhea (Table 35-5).

Clinical Findings

History

- Maternal and sibling age of menarche
- Family history of menstrual irregularities, eating disorders, diabetes, thyroid disease, or genetic disorders
- Any prenatal exposure to hormones
- Detailed history of growth and pubertal development (sequence and tempo)
- Menstrual calendar (last menses, number and pattern of cycles, age at menarche)
- Chronic systemic disease or illness or previous surgery, radiation, or chemotherapy

TABLE 35-5 Differential Diagnosis of Amenorrhea

	Primary	Secondary
Hypogonadotropic		
Compartment IV	Delayed puberty	Psychological disorder
Hypothalamic	Chronic illness	Depression
	Eating disorders	Eating disorders
	Excessive exercise	Excessive exercise
	Kallmann syndrome	
Compartment III Pituitary	Pituitary disease	Pituitary disease
	Hyperprolactinemia	Hyperprolactinemia
		Sheehan syndrome
Thyroid		Hypothyroid
Hypergonadotropic		
Compartment II	Premature ovarian failure	Premature ovarian failure
Ovaries	Gonadal dysgenesis	PCOS
	PCOS	
Adrenals	Adrenal hyperplasia	Adrenal hyperplasia
Anatomic	Müllerian agenesis	Asherman syndrome
Compartment I Outflow	Androgen insensitivity	
	Imperforate hymen	
	Vaginal septum	
Hyperprolactinemia		
Compartment III Pituitary	Medication/drugs	Medication/drugs
	Macroadenoma	Macroadenoma
	Tumor	Tumor
		Lactation

PCOS, Polycystic ovary syndrome.
Data from Emans SJ: Amenorrhea in the adolescent. In Emans SJ, Laufer MR, Goldstein DP, editors: *Pediatric and adolescent gynecology,* ed 5, Philadelphia, 2005a, Lippincott Williams & Wilkins; Speroff L, Fritz MA: *Clinical gynecologic endocrinology and infertility,* ed 7, Philadelphia, 2005, Lippincott Williams & Wilkins; Wilson GR, Haddad JE, Haddad CJ: Amenorrhea: common causes and evaluation, *Compr Ther* 31:270-278, 2005.

- Nutrition, including eating habits, dieting, weight fluctuations
- Exercise patterns, including amount and intensity, level of participation, weigh-ins, or standards for weight that must be kept
- History of stress fractures
- Bowel patterns or abdominal pain
- Headache or visual change
- Galactorrhea, hirsutism, acne
- Medication use (contraceptives, phenothiazines, antihypertensives)
- Sexual activity, contraceptive use
- Stress, recent change in environment, or depression
- Substance use

Physical Examination
- Height, weight, BMI, nutritional status, blood pressure, pulse
- Sexual maturation rating
- Complete neurologic examination, including cranial nerves, funduscopic examination, and visual fields
- Midline facial defects or other congenital anomalies or stigmata of Turner syndrome

- Palpation of thyroid
- Breast examination with gentle compression to identify galactorrhea
- Palpation of abdomen and groin for masses, tenderness
- Examination of skin, hair distribution, and genitalia for signs of virilization
- External genital examination for estrogenization of vaginal mucosa (indicates ovarian function), vaginal and hymenal patency, and clitoromegaly (androgen excess)
- Digital vaginal examination and speculum examination if any abnormality is suspected
- Bimanual examination

Diagnostic Studies
Initial laboratory studies include pregnancy test regardless of sexual history, thyroid-stimulating hormone (TSH), FSH, and prolactin. Follow the algorithm (Fig. 35-9) for complete evaluation.

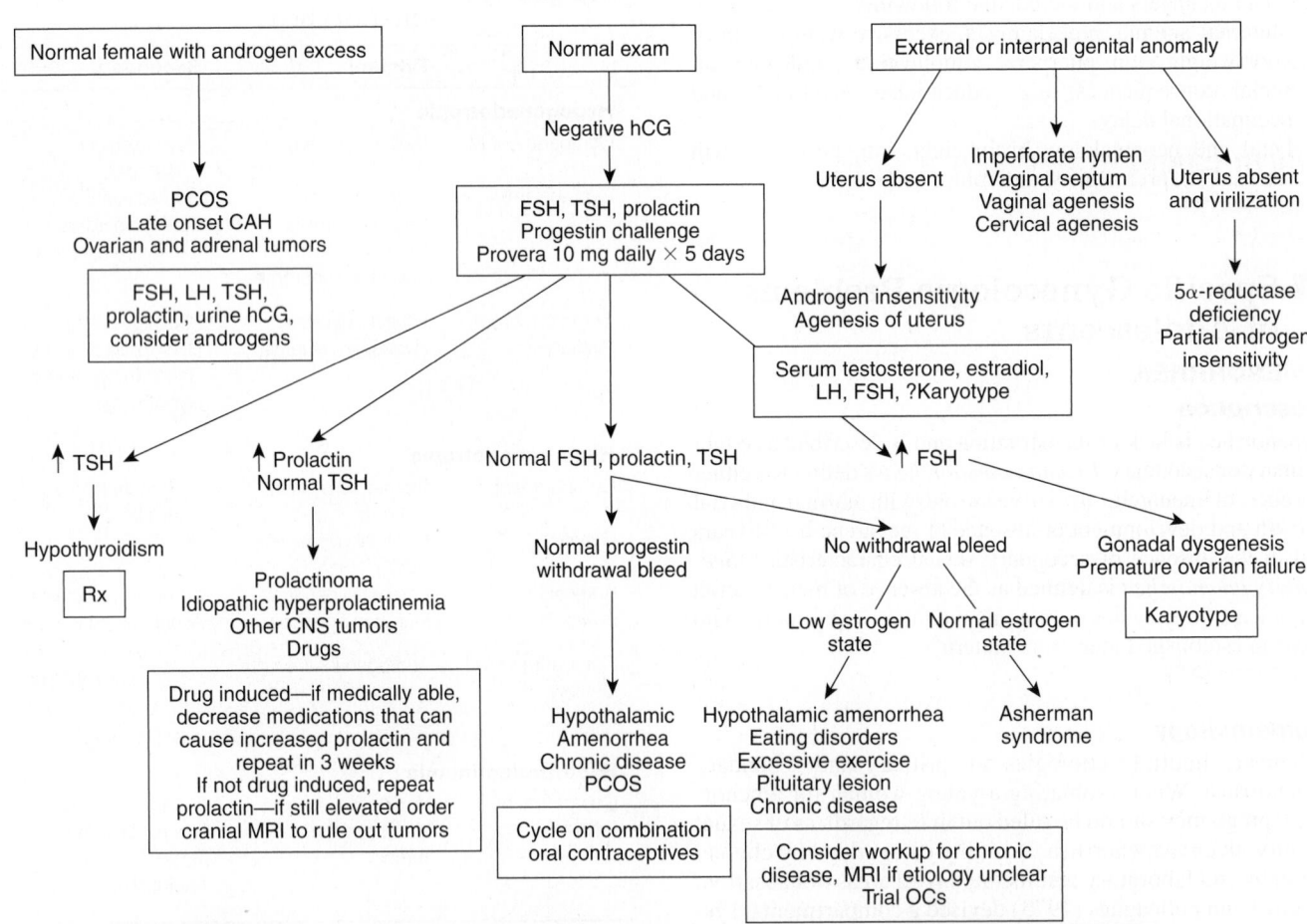

FIGURE 35-9 Evaluation and management of amenorrhea. *CAH,* Congenital adrenal hyperplasia; *CNS,* central nervous system; *FSH,* follicle-stimulating hormone; *hCG,* human chorionic gonadotropin; *LH,* luteinizing hormone; *MRI,* magnetic resonance imaging; *OC,* oral contraceptive; *PCOS,* polycystic ovary syndrome; *Rx,* medication; *TSH,* thyroid-stimulating hormone. (Adapted from Emans SJ: Amenorrhea in the adolescent. In Emans SJ, Laufer MR, Goldstein DP, editors: *Pediatric and adolescent gynecology,* ed 5, Philadelphia, 2005, Lippincott Williams & Wilkins.)

Differential Diagnosis

The differential diagnoses for primary amenorrhea and secondary amenorrhea have considerable overlap (see Table 35-5). The exceptions are a few genetic conditions that cause primary amenorrhea (e.g., Turner syndrome). The most common causation of amenorrhea in the adolescent falls within the hypogonadotropic-hypothalamic category. An important marker of hypogonadotropic hypogonadism is the female athlete triad of amenorrhea, eating disorder, and osteoporosis (Emans, 2005a), especially common in gymnasts, figure skaters, ballet dancers, and long-distance runners at elite or highly competitive levels. The pressure for the ideal body for the sport and the intense exercise required may lead to this triad (also see Chapter 13 for a discussion of this triad).

Management

The treatment of amenorrhea obviously depends on its cause. Restoration of ovulatory cycles leads to the best long-term prognosis, and this is often accomplished through estrogen-progestin therapy. The primary care pediatric provider may need to consult and/or refer to a pediatric gynecologist or endocrinologist depending on the etiology. Anxiety about amenorrhea is common, and frequent reassurance is necessary. Young women should be made aware of the long-term skeletal effects of amenorrhea and instructed on adequate diet, reasonable exercise, and calcium supplementation to prevent osteoporosis.

DYSFUNCTIONAL UTERINE BLEEDING

Description

DUB refers to abnormal uterine bleeding that is excessive, prolonged, or unpatterned. It can be described as follows:

- *Polymenorrhea:* Fewer than 21 days between menses
- *Menorrhagia:* Normal intervals with excessive flow or duration of menses
- *Metrorrhagia:* Irregular frequency of cycles with bleeding between cycles
- *Menometrorrhagia:* Excessive amount of bleeding with irregular frequency of cycles

DUB is a diagnosis of exclusion, so any other causes of pathologic conditions must first be ruled out. DUB can be classified as mild, moderate, or severe based on hemoglobin level, duration of cycle, and quantity of bleeding.

Epidemiology

The mechanism of DUB appears to be a delay in the maturation of the negative feedback cycle and is not related to structural pathologic conditions or medical illness (Emans, 2005c). Estrogen production continues without the balancing decrease in FSH, which would suppress estrogen. This results in abnormal endometrial thickening. The abnormal endometrium then sheds in a disorderly manner manifested by heavy, irregular, or prolonged bleeding. There is great variation in what is considered to be a normal menstrual cycle, especially in adolescents. Normal can range from 21 to 45 days between periods, with duration of flow from 3 to 7 days and 30 to 40 mL of blood loss (10 to 15 soaked tampons or pads) per cycle. Periods that last longer than 8 to 10 days with blood loss in excess of 80 mL are considered excessive (Emans, 2005c).

Abnormal uterine bleeding is frequently seen in adolescents (Emans, 2005c; Harel, 2005; Matytsina, 2006). Anovulation is the most common cause of DUB in the adolescent; however, not all anovulatory cycles result in DUB. Adolescents with sustained anovulation (e.g., as a result of eating disorders, weight fluctuations, competitive athletics, chronic illness, or endocrine disease) have an increased incidence of DUB. Anovulation can also be due to stress or illness, thus appearing in adolescents after several years of regular cycles (Emans, 2005c).

Clinical Findings

History

- Family history of bleeding disorders or dyscrasias, thyroid dysfunction, diabetes mellitus, or diethylstilbestrol (DES) exposure
- Menstrual history: Onset, pattern, duration, quantity, and color; last menstrual period; breakthrough bleeding; dysmenorrhea; passing of clots, number of tampons or pads used; longest and shortest intervals between cycles
- Associated menstrual symptoms (e.g., premenstrual syndrome [PMS])
- Sexual activity and contraception used
- Postcoital bleeding
- Previous infection or STIs
- Vaginal discharge, pelvic pain
- Galactorrhea, hirsutism (endocrine disease), or other chronic disease
- Bleeding gums, nosebleeds, bruises, hemorrhage (bleeding disorders)
- Hair loss, sleep disorders, cold intolerance, constipation (thyroid symptoms)
- Recent stressors, medications, or substance use
- Exercise and eating patterns, weight, weight fluctuations, laxative use, body image
- Genital trauma, sexual abuse
- Effect of bleeding on lifestyle

Physical Examination

- Height, weight, BMI, body type, and fat distribution
- Vital signs (temperature, pulse, respiratory rate), orthostatic blood pressures
- Observation for acne, hirsutism, clitoromegaly (evidence of androgen excess)
- Breast examination for galactorrhea
- Thyroid palpation
- Observation for petechiae, bruising, pale color
- Abdominal examination for mass or tenderness
- Pelvic examination, including digital and speculum examination for foreign bodies, cervical lesions. In young, nonsexually active girls, the speculum examination may not be necessary per provider discretion.
- Tanner staging
- Bimanual and rectoabdominal examination

Diagnostic Studies. The following are ordered as indicated:

- Pregnancy test regardless of sexual history
- CBC with differential, platelet count, reticulocyte count
- Sedimentation rate or C-reactive protein (CRP) (if infection or inflammation is suspected)
- Coagulation studies: Prothrombin time, partial thromboplastin time, bleeding time (if bleeding disorder is suspected or there has been a significant drop in hemoglobin)

- Thyroid function test, blood sugar, prolactin level (if systemic disease is suspected), markers for PCOS (free and total testosterone, sex hormone-binding globulin and androstenedione)
- Wet preparations and cultures for GC, chlamydia, if patient is sexually active
- Ultrasound of pelvis if mass is palpated, anomaly is suspected, bimanual examination cannot be completed, or condition is unresponsive to treatment

Differential Diagnosis

The differential diagnoses include pregnancy or pregnancy-related complications (postabortion, ectopic pregnancy); stress; excessive participation in athletics; eating disorders, including overweight; drug use; systemic diseases, such as blood dyscrasias (20% of patients with coagulation defects have excessive menstrual bleeding especially with first menses); infection (e.g., STIs); trauma, including forceful intercourse or rape; foreign bodies, including intrauterine device; tumors; anomalies; endometriosis; endocrine disorders (e.g., thyroid disorder, diabetes mellitus, prolactinoma); debilitating or chronic diseases (especially lupus, hepatic or renal diseases); reproductive tract disorders, including malignancy; and medications, including OCs, progesterone implants, and injectables (Emans, 2005c; Harel, 2005; Mama, 2010; Mitan and Slap, 2008).

Management

The goals in managing DUB include controlling bleeding, preventing endometrial hyperplasia, preventing and treating anemia, restoring quality of life, and preventing recurrence. The following will enable the provider to manage DUB (Emans, 2005b; Levine, 2006; Mitan and Slap, 2008):

Mild DUB: A shortened cycle or menses longer than normal with flow slightly to moderately increased or unpredictable; hemoglobin greater than 12 g/dL:
- Observe and reassure.
- Have patient start and maintain a menstrual calendar.
- Prescribe iron supplementation and dietary interventions to prevent anemia.
- Use prostaglandin inhibitors to reduce heavy bleeding (see Box 35-9).
- Consider OCs for 3 to 4 months to decrease menorrhagia and stabilize menses.
- Reevaluate in 3 months.

Moderate DUB: Shortened (1 to 3 weeks), irregular cycle with moderate to heavy bleeding, hemoglobin between 10 and 12 g/dL:
- Prescribe 35 mcg monophasic combination OCs.
  - If not currently bleeding, use same day start (see contraception section).
  - If currently bleeding, start with one OC bid for 3 to 4 days until bleeding stops. Then continue with one daily until finished with that pack, skip the placebo week, and start another pack without a withdrawal bleed. If bleeding resumes when OCs are decreased to one per day, again take one bid until first pack is completed and start a second pack, taking one OC daily without a withdrawal bleed. Occasionally the bid dose will not stop the bleeding. Add one OC every 3 to 4 days up to

four OCs per day. After the bleeding stops, decrease the dose by one pill every 3 to 4 days until down to one per day. Continue OCs without a withdrawal bleed until the patient is completing a regular pill pack at one pill per day. If unable to control bleeding with four OCs per day, consult and/or referral is necessary.
- Add antiemetic to control the nausea of higher doses of estrogen.
- Usual length of treatment with OCs is 6 months.
- Alternatively, prescribe a progestin, such as medroxyprogesterone acetate (5 to 10 mg every day for 10 to 14 days started on the fourteenth day of cycle for 1 to 2 months). OCs are more effective at stopping active bleeding.
- Have patient start and maintain a menstrual calendar.
- Prescribe iron supplementation plus 1 mg folic acid per day.
- Reevaluate at least monthly until condition is stable.
- Reassess after 6 months.

Severe DUB: Irregular, prolonged, heavy bleeding; hemoglobin less than 10 g/dL:
- Refer to gynecologist and hospitalize if active bleeding is heavy and adolescent is hemodynamically symptomatic; treatment may include transfusion, intravenous hormonal therapy, and dilation and curettage (D&C).
- Manage as moderate DUB if not actively bleeding.

Complications

Anemia, profuse bleeding, shock, and side effects of OCs can occur. A long history of anovulation and DUB increases the risk of infertility and endometrial carcinoma.

Patient Education and Prognosis

Encourage individual to keep a calendar of bleeding days and amounts. This includes keeping track of the number of pads or tampons used to increase accuracy. Educate the patient and her parents about the use of OCs as a medication in the treatment of DUB. It is important that it be taken as directed. Suddenly stopping it midcycle will result in resumed bleeding. Prognosis is excellent if DUB is due to anovulation and immaturity of the HPO axis; these adolescents respond well to treatment, and most will develop regular menstrual patterns within 4 years of menarche (Matytsina, 2006).

ENDOMETRIOSIS
Description

Endometriosis is the proliferation of ectopic endometrial tissue outside the pelvic cavity. It is primarily manifested by dysmenorrhea that progressively worsens. Other symptoms include acyclic pelvic pain, gastrointestinal complaints, and dyspareunia. Adolescents usually experience pain, and as many as 62% of adolescents with endometriosis have both cyclic and acyclic pain.

Epidemiology

The cause of endometriosis is unknown. A risk factor is early menarche. Several theories have been developed to explain the possible cause of endometriosis, including retrograde menstruation; embryonic müllerian remnants, coelomic metaplasia; lymphatic, vascular, and iatrogenic dissemination; genetic factors; and immunologic or hormonal problems or defects.

The incidence rate in adolescents is difficult to obtain because endometriosis is rarely studied in this age group. Estimates of 7% in the population with a first-degree relative with endometriosis, and 1% otherwise, are reported. Between 50% and 70% of adolescents with untreatable dysmenorrhea or pelvic pain are found to have a diagnosis of endometriosis on laparoscopy. This incidence of endometriosis on laparoscopy in adolescents increases with age, from 12% among 11- to 13-year-olds to 54% among 20- to 21-year-olds (Laufer and Goldstein, 2005).

Clinical Findings
History
- First-degree relative with endometriosis
- Deep unilateral or bilateral pain described as sharp or dull
- Chronic pelvic pain that is cyclic and/or acyclic and mildly to severely disabling, disrupting routine and causing missed school days or emergency department visits without definitive diagnosis
- Bladder and bowel dysfunction; rectal pain
- Dyspareunia
- Cyclic leg pain
Physical Examination
- Tender, enlarged, or fixed ovaries
- Adnexal masses, thickening, or tenderness
- The pelvic examination is most often unremarkable, with mild to moderate pelvic tenderness on palpation
Diagnostic Studies.
The following are ordered as indicated:
- CBC, urine testing, or cervical cultures for GC and chlamydia to rule out infectious cause
- Ultrasound (helpful to evaluate anatomic structures; however, nonspecific for diagnosing endometriosis)

Differential Diagnosis
Primary dysmenorrhea, PID, appendicitis, ovarian cysts, müllerian anomalies, eating disorders, lactose intolerance, irritable bowel syndrome, chronic constipation, and depression are included in the differential diagnosis.

Management
- Have adolescent keep pain diary.
- Proceed with trial of cyclic OCs and NSAIDs.
- If unresponsive and the patient is younger than 18 years, refer for a laparoscopic evaluation. If older than 18 years, may try empiric trial of GnRH agonist. If pain improves, a diagnosis of endometriosis can be made (ACOG, 2005).
- Supportive phone follow-up for side effects of medications and painful flare-ups is essential.
- See at 1- to 3-month intervals to provide support and reevaluate.
- Diet and exercise are important aspects in coping with chronic pain.
- Stress reduction techniques and support groups may also be helpful.

Complications
Miscarriage and infertility can occur. Endometriomas are rare in the adolescent age group. Gastritis, which may be treated with histamine-2 blockers, is seen frequently.

Prognosis and Prevention
Endometriosis is a chronic disease, and remission and exacerbation are to be expected. Stressful events often cause exacerbation. The goals of treatment are to control pain and prevent infertility.

VAGINITIS AND VAGINAL DISCHARGE
Description
Vaginitis refers to an inflammation or infection of the vulva and vaginal wall with or without discharge from the vagina.

Epidemiology
At puberty, the pH changes from 7 to 4.5, vaginal mucosa thickens, acidogenic bacteria predominate, and lactobacillus stabilizes the environment, all offering protection from infection. Adolescent vaginitis is most often due to a specific cause, often secondary to sexual contact. Normal physiologic leukorrhea occurs 6 to 12 months before puberty. Yeast, group A beta-hemolytic streptococci or other infections, foreign bodies (toilet paper fragments, tampon), and pinworms are possible causes. Bacterial vaginosis (BV), trichomoniasis, or other STIs (discussed later in this chapter) must also be considered. Up to one half of female gynecologic complaints are related to vaginitis. *Candida vaginitis,* BV, and *Trichomonas* are the most common infecting agents (Syed and Braverman, 2004).

Clinical Findings
The clinical findings pertaining to vaginitis are found in Table 35-4.
History
- Onset—How long have the symptoms been present?
- Location—vulva, vagina, perineum, and/or anus
- Characteristics:
  - Genital irritation, itching, pain, and inflammation
  - Vaginal discharge—note onset, quantity, color, type (bloody, mucoid), odor, consistency, and duration
  - Urinary complaints, including dysuria
  - Pelvic pain and/or dyspareunia
  - Ameliorating or aggravating factors
- Treatments or medications tried including CAM
- Previous occurrences and treatment used
- Recent medications, especially antibiotics
- Use of contraception
- Possible trauma, foreign body, or sexual abuse
- History of sexual activity or menstrual irregularities
- History of or recent exposures to STIs
- Perineal hygiene
- Use of harsh or perfumed soaps and bubble bath
- Use of tampons or pads, with deodorant
- Douching, personal sprays, or any other hygiene measures
- Underlying illnesses (e.g., streptococcus infection, dermatosis, diabetes, immunosuppression)

Physical Examination. The examination of the adolescent should include the careful inspection of the perianal area and a speculum examination to visualize the cervix and vaginal walls. If the adolescent has not initiated vaginal intercourse, vaginal secretions can be collected with a saline-moistened cotton swab. See Table 35-4 for physical examination findings.

Diagnostic Studies. The following should be considered:
- pH of vaginal secretions
- Wet mounts of vaginal secretions
- Saline for microscopic examination to look for WBCs, clue cells, trichomonads, and bacteria
- 10% KOH for whiff test and microscopic examination to look for yeast (branching hyphae and spores) (see Fig. 35-7)
- NAATs on urine or cultures for GC and chlamydia if indicated
- Urinalysis and culture if UTI suspected

Differential Diagnosis

The differential includes normal physiologic discharge, yeast vaginitis, BV, trichomoniasis and other STIs, foreign body, and contact or allergic dermatitis.

Management

See Table 35-4 for treatment.
CAM recommendations:
- For yeast: Decrease foods high in simple carbohydrates; avoid foods with yeast or mold; increase fiber, garlic, ginger, cinnamon; live lactobacillus (1 to 2 billion live organisms per day) and acidophilus in diet
- For BV: Lactobacillus in the diet, and vaginal boric acid capsules

Complications

BV can contribute to PID, endometritis, postsurgical infection (abortion), and adverse pregnancy outcomes, such as preterm labor and birth, premature rupture of the membranes, and chorioamnionitis. Trichomoniasis has been linked with premature rupture of membranes and preterm delivery.

Patient Education, Prognosis, and Prevention
- Follow up in 5 days if there is no improvement.
- For the sexually active adolescent, recommend not using diaphragm or condom until 3 days after treatment with topical vaginal cream or tablet.
- Recommend frequent changes of tampons and use of a pad, especially at night, or ceasing the use of tampons.

SEXUALLY TRANSMITTED INFECTIONS
Description

Multiple organisms are responsible for STIs in adolescents and children. GC, chlamydia, syphilis, HSV, and HPV are the most common STIs affecting the lower female reproductive tract.

Trichomonas (discussed in previous section), hepatitis B, and HIV also are recognized as STIs. See Chapter 23 for discussion of hepatitis B and HIV (systemic STIs). The term *sexually transmitted infection* is often used instead of sexually transmitted diseases (STDs). Diagnosis can also be made in terms of the location of the infection (e.g., vaginitis, cervicitis, or urethritis) if causal organism is unknown.

STIs are a significant public health problem, placing a heavy financial health burden on society, having a tremendous effect on individuals' lives, and playing an important role in the transmission of HIV. Much progress has been made in treating STIs, with historic low incidence rates for GC and syphilis. However, the highest STI rates in the industrial world still occur in the U.S.

Epidemiology

Considered an epidemic, STIs have the highest rates in adolescents. The CDC reports that of the 19 million new STIs per year almost half occur in adolescents and young adults 15 to 24 years of age. Furthermore, young women between 15 and 19 years old have the highest rates of *Neisseria gonorrhoeae* and *Chlamydia trachomatis* (CDC, 2010b). Adolescents at highest risk for acquiring STIs include youth in detention facilities, male homosexuals, and injection drug users. Minorities, especially African-Americans, are disproportionally affected.

Factors contributing to this epidemic are the increasingly early age and frequency of sexual activity, inconsistent use of contraceptive and protective devices, physiologic characteristics that predispose adolescents to infection, adolescents' lack of access to and use of health care, and societal influences (Box 35-10). Another factor that may contribute to higher reported numbers of STIs is the increased use and availability of accurate screening tests for diseases, especially chlamydia.

BOX 35-10 Risk Factors for Sexually Transmitted Infections

1. Adolescent younger than 15 years
2. Sexually active adolescent, especially with two or more partners in 6 months, high frequency of intercourse, or high rate of new partners
3. Use of drugs or alcohol or other high-risk behaviors
4. Pregnancy or abortion
5. Homosexuality
6. Victim of abuse, rape, or incest
7. Incarcerated, runaway, homeless, in group shelter or detention home
8. Clients in sexually transmitted infection (STI) clinics or with any other STI or previous history of STI
9. Lack of family availability; low level of parental support and monitoring
10. Beliefs about normative behaviors among peers
11. Inappropriate health care behaviors (e.g., not seeking medical care, not adhering to treatment regimen, failure to recognize symptoms, delay in notifying partners, nonuse of barrier contraceptive)

Data from Fortenberry JD, Neinstein LS: Overview of sexually transmitted diseases. In Neinstein L, editor: *Adolescent health care: a practical guide*, ed 5, Philadelphia, 2008, Lippincott Williams & Wilkins; Shrier LA: Bacterial sexually transmitted infections: gonorrhea, chlamydia, pelvic inflammatory disease, and syphilis. In Emans SJ, Laufer MR, Goldstein DP, editors: *Pediatric and adolescent gynecology*, ed 5, Philadelphia, 2005, Lippincott Williams & Wilkins.

Most STIs must be reported, and the provider must be aware of each state's specific rules. All 50 states allow adolescents to be evaluated and to receive treatment for STIs confidentially. Management of children younger than 13 years old with STIs requires a coordinated effort between the pediatric provider and child protective authorities.

GC, caused by *N. gonorrhoeae*, a nonmotile, gram-negative diplococcus, is often found in carriage with chlamydia or other STIs. The GC rate is steadily declining and for 2009 was 99.1 cases per 100,000, which is the lowest it has been since data collection was started in 1941. However, this still far exceeds the 19 cases per 100,000 *Healthy People 2010* objective (CDC, 2009, 2011). However, the rate for adolescent females in the 15- to 19-year-old group was 405.4 per 100,000 population. There are more reported cases of GC in African-Americans than Caucasians (20.5:1). The infection is often asymptomatic, with an estimated 25% to 90% of young women infected with GC reporting no symptoms (Blythe, 2008). Untreated GC can progress to PID.

C. trachomatis infection is the most frequently reported bacterial STI, with a rate of 409.2 cases per 100,000 reported in 2009 (CDC, 2011). This rate is increasing, but the increase is thought to reflect more effective screening. Adolescent females have the highest percentage of these cases, with a reported rate of 876.5 per 100,000 in 15- to 19-year-olds and 1094.2 per 100,000 in 20- to 24-year-olds. All sexually active young women in this age group should be screened at least annually because chlamydia is frequently asymptomatic. Untreated chlamydia can progress to PID; as many as 20% to 40% of the women with untreated infections develop PID, and 20% of those may loose their fertility (CDC, 2009).

Syphilis, caused by *Treponema pallidum*, is a motile spirochete with a rate of 4.6 cases per 100,000 in 2009. Though the rate continues to increase, the good news is that there has been no increase among women. The rate for 15- to 19-year-olds is 405.4 per 100,000, and for 20- to 24-year-olds the rate is 479.1 per 100,000. The stabilization in women has also kept the rate of congenital syphilis stable (CDC, 2011).

There are two identified serotypes of HSV: HSV-1 and HSV-2. Although either type may infect any part of the body, most recurrent genital herpes is a result of HSV-2. Asymptomatic HSV infections are responsible for the transmission of most cases of genital herpes. Type 2 in prepubescent children is reportable in some states.

HPV is a small deoxyribonucleic acid (DNA) virus. More than 30 types of HPV can infect the genital tract. Visible warts are usually caused by HPV types 6 or 11. A person may be infected with multiple types of HPV. Types 16, 18, 31, 33, and 35 have been strongly associated with cervical cancer and vulvar, penile, and anal squamous intraepithelial neoplasia (CDC, 2006). Kahn and associates (2007) found that 20% of 14- to 17-year-olds and 38% of 18- to 21-year-olds were HPV positive.

Clinical Findings

History. Many patients are asymptomatic. The history should assess the following:

- Type of sexual activity (including oral, vaginal, anal sex/intercourse) and contraceptive use
- Number of sexual partners over 60 days, 12 months, and lifetime; heterosexual or homosexual (or both) activity
- Known exposure or previous STIs
- Use of drugs or alcohol

- Vaginal discharge (amount, color, odor), pruritus, irregular or painful bleeding, dysmenorrhea, dyspareunia
- Dysuria, urinary urgency or frequency
- Abdominal or pelvic pain
- Skin rashes or lesions, ulcers, warts
- Systemic symptoms, such as fever, malaise, headache

See Box 35-10 for risk factors for STIs; Box 35-11 for CDC's five P's (*P*artners, *P*revention of pregnancy, *P*rotection from STIs, *P*ractices, *P*ast history of STIs), and Table 35-6 for history specific to each STI. See Chapter 18 for further details on obtaining history.

Physical Examination

- General examination—skin rashes and lesions, lymphadenopathy
- Abdominal examination—hepatic or splenic enlargement or tenderness in right upper quadrant
- Pelvic examination—inspection of external genitalia and vaginal mucosa, vaginal pH and discharge, cervical erythema, friability and mucopus, bimanual examination for cervical motion tenderness, uterine size, adnexal tenderness
- Rectal examination
- See Table 35-6 for physical findings specific to each STI.

BOX 35-11 CDC's the Five P's: Partners, Prevention of Pregnancy, Protection from STIs, Practices, Past History of STIs

1. Partners
   - "Do you have sex with men, women, or both?"
   - "In the past 2 months how many partners have you had sex with?"
   - "In the past 12 months how many partners have you had sex with?"
2. Prevention of pregnancy
   - "Are you or your partner trying to get pregnant?" If no, "What are you doing to prevent pregnancy?"
3. Protection from STIs
   - "What do you do to protect yourself from STIs and HIV?"
4. Practices
   - "To understand your risks for STIs, I need to understand the kind of sex you have had recently."
   - "Have you had vaginal sex, meaning 'penis in vagina sex'"? If yes, "Do you use condoms: never, sometimes, or always?"
   - "Have you had anal sex, meaning 'penis in rectum/anus sex'?" If yes, "Do you use condoms: never, sometimes, or always?"
   - "Have you had oral sex, meaning 'mouth on penis/vagina'?"
   For condom answers:
   - If "never": "Why don't you use condoms?"
   - If "sometimes": "In what situations or with whom, do you not use condoms?"
5. Past history of STIs
   - "Have you ever had an STI?"
   - "Have any of your partners had an STI?"
6. Additional questions to identify HIV and hepatitis risk:
   - "Have you or any of your partners ever injected drugs?"
   - "Have any of your partners exchanged money or drugs for sex?"
   - "Is there anything else about your sexual practices that I need to know about?"

CDC, Centers for Disease Control and Prevention; *HIV,* human immunodeficiency virus; *STI,* sexually transmitted infection.

(From Centers for Disease Control and Grevention: *Sexually transmitted diseases treatment guidelines 2010,* 2011. Available at www.cdc.gov/std/treatment/2010/clinical.htm. Accessed Jan 3, 2012)

TABLE 35-6 Sexually Transmitted Disease: History, Physical Examination, and Initial Treatment

	History	Physical Examination	Treatment
Gonorrhea (GC) *Neisseria gonorrhoeae*	Often asymptomatic (33%); dysuria; vaginal discharge or bleeding; dyspareunia	Profuse, thick, green discharge, urethritis, cervicitis; Skene or Bartholin gland abscess; exudative pharyngitis	Ceftriaxone 250 mg IM one time *or* Cefixime 400 mg PO one time *or* Cephalosporin injectable single-dose regimens *plus* Azithromycin 1 g PO in a single dose *or* Doxycycline 100 mg PO bid for 7 days* Report to state health department Follow up cultures not needed if ceftriaxone used
Chlamydia *Chlamydia trachomatis*	Often asymptomatic (30%-70%); spotting, vaginal discharge; dysuria, pyuria; mild abdominal pain or foreign body sensation in eyes possible	Clear to white or yellow discharge, mucopurulent cervicitis with edema, erythema, hypertrophy; Fitz-Hugh–Curtis syndrome (right upper quadrant pain); conjunctivitis	Azithromycin 1 g PO in a single dose *or* Doxycycline 100 mg PO bid for 7 days* Alternative medications: Erythromycin base 500 mg PO qid for 7 days *or* Erythromycin ethylsuccinate 800 mg PO qid for 7 days *or* Ofloxacin 300 mg PO bid for 7 days *or* Levofloxacin 500 mg PO for 7 days Report to state health department Test of cure not recommended unless pregnant
Syphilis *Treponema pallidum*	Primary: vaginal, anal, or oral chancre Secondary: copper-penny rash especially on palms and soles, lymphadenopathy, mucocutaneous lesions	Single painless papule with serous discharge, smooth base, raised edges; painless regional lymphadenopathy	Benzathine penicillin G 2.4 million units IM in a single dose *or* If penicillin allergy and not pregnant: Doxycycline 100 mg PO bid for 14 days* *or* Tetracycline 500 mg PO qid for 14 days* Test for GC, chlamydia, and HIV at time of infection and in 3 mo Follow with RPR or VDRL titers at 6, 12, and 24 mo; should have fourfold decline by 6 mo Report to state health department
Herpes simplex virus (HSV)	Painful rash, blisters and ulcers; burning and irritation 24 hr before outbreak; dysuria; other systemic complaints	Clear to white to yellow discharge; vesicles on erythematous base that become ulcers in 1-3 days; extragenital lesions; lymphadenopathy	*Primary*—Acyclovir 400 mg tid for 7-10 days (*or* 200 mg 5 times a day for 7-10 days) *or* Famciclovir 250 mg tid for 7-10 days *or* Valacyclovir 1 g bid for 7-10 days *Recurrent*—Acyclovir 400 mg tid for 5 days *or* Acyclovir 800 mg bid for 5 days *or* Acyclovir 800 mg tid for 2 days *or* Famciclovir 125 mg bid for 5 days *or* Famciclovir 1 g bid for 1 day *or* Famciclovir 500 mg once followed by 250 mg bid for 2 days *or* Valacyclovir 500 mg bid for 3 days or 1 g once a day for 5 days *Comfort measures*—sitz bath, dry heat, lidocaine jelly 2%
Human papillomavirus (HPV)	Asymptomatic or subclinical unrecognized; can be painful	Warts, friable or pruritic (or both); moist, cauliflower-like anogenital and inguinal 4-6 wk after exposure	*Patient-applied treatment* (see text): Podofilox or imiquimod 5% cream *Provider-applied treatment* (see text): Cryotherapy, podophyllin resin, trichloroacetic acid or bichloroacetic acid, or surgical removal

†Contraindicated if younger than 8 years of age.
HIV, Human immunodeficiency virus; *IM,* intramuscular; *RPR,* rapid plasma reagin; daily; *VDRL,* Venereal Disease Research Laboratory.
Data from Centers for Disease Control and Prevention (CDC): Sexually transmitted diseases: treatment guidelines, *MMWR Morb Mortal Wkly Rep* 55(RR-11):1-100, 2006; Centers for Disease Control and Prevention (CDC): Update to CDC's sexually transmitted diseases treatment guidelines, 2006, fluoroquinolones no longer recommended for treatment of gonococcal infections, *MMWR Morb Mortal Wkly Rep* 56(14):332-336, 2007.

Diagnostic Studies. In deciding which studies to order, the provider needs to know the difference in and accuracy of tests. Methods that are sufficiently accurate for adolescents (presumptive tests) are not adequate for children who are being evaluated for possible abuse.
- *GC.* Culture on selective media with determination of penicillin resistance is the definitive test for GC in women. Nucleic acid hybridization tests (DNA probes) and NAATs are also available for GC testing. NAATs are more reliable when done by cervical swab testing than with urine testing for GC (Shrier, 2005). Gram stains of vaginal discharge or cervical secretions are not recommended (CDC, 2010a).
- *Chlamydia.* Culture is the only acceptable method to diagnose possible sexual abuse cases; many family planning clinics use direct immunofluorescent smears; however, DNA probes and NAATs are acceptable in adolescents, especially in high-prevalence populations. Only NAATs

can be done on either a cervical swab or urine and are therefore preferable for adolescents.

- *Syphilis.* Direct visualization with darkfield microscopy or direct immunofluorescent antibody (DFA) test is definitive. Serologic nontreponemal tests (Venereal Disease Research Laboratory [VDRL], rapid plasma reagin [RPR], or automated reagin test) correlate with disease activity, decline after treatment, and are used to monitor disease progress. Treponemal tests (fluorescent treponemal antibody absorption [FTA-ABS] and microhemagglutination test for *T. pallidum* [MHA-TP]) are confirmatory, but once positive they usually remain so for years.
- *Herpes.* Culture of scraped vesicle or ulcer is the preferred method. Type specific serologic testing is available; however, not recommended for the general population
- *HPV.* Testing is not recommended in the adolescent.

Differential Diagnosis

Chancroid, lymphogranuloma venereum, cytomegalovirus, hepatitis, granuloma inguinale, and molluscum are included in the differential diagnosis.

Management

The guidelines identified in this section are those recommended by the CDC (2010) for uncomplicated, initial treatment of STIs. Other recommendations and options for children weighing less than 45 kg and for recurrent and complex cases are found in that CDC resource and in adolescent gynecology or child abuse literature. The goals of treatment include making a prompt diagnosis, determining the mode of acquisition, instituting appropriate treatment, preventing complications, contacting appropriate authorities, ensuring appropriate follow-up, and educating the adolescent and partner about risk reduction. All adolescents in the U.S. can consent to confidential diagnosis and treatment of STIs.

Several options for treatment are given for each disease (see Table 35-6). When determining appropriate treatment, consideration should be given to the site of infection, the resistance patterns in the community, concurrent infections, side effects of the medication, and cost. See Box 35-12 for general treatment measures for STIs.

1. *GC* (uncomplicated, patient weighing more than 99 pounds [45 kg]) (see Table 35-6):
   - Cefixime 400 mg orally in a single dose is recommended as the single-dose treatment.
   - Fluoroquinolones should not be used for treatment of GC if the infection was acquired in Asia, the Pacific Islands (including Hawaii), or California because the prevalence of fluoroquinolone-resistant *N. gonorrhoeae* is high in these areas.
   - Evaluate and treat all partners exposed in the previous 30 to 60 days and treat last sexual partner if more than 60 days since last intercourse.
2. *Chlamydia* (uncomplicated genital infection) (see Table 35-6):
   - Treat last partner and any partner exposed within the 60 days before the onset of symptoms.
   - Rescreen 3 to 4 months after positive test result because a high prevalence of *C. trachomatis* infection is found in women who had a chlamydial infection in the preceding

several months. Reinfection is usually the cause of infection and elevates the risk for PID.

3. *Syphilis* (primary or secondary) (see Table 35-6):
   - The same laboratory tests (RPR or VDRL) should be used for follow-up and should decrease fourfold by 6 months and become nonreactive 1 year after treatment in primary cases. If still reactive after 12 months, retreat and reevaluate for HIV.
   - Treat all partners exposed during symptomatic period and for the 3 months before onset of infection.
   - An acute febrile reaction (Jarisch-Herxheimer reaction) with myalgia, headache, and other symptoms can occur within 24 hours after treatment.
   - Refer if symptoms of secondary or tertiary syphilis is present.
4. *Genital herpes.* No treatment will eradicate the disease. Treatment or prevention of acute outbreaks is the goal of therapy (see Table 35-6):
   - Use daily suppressive treatment if episodes occur six times or more in a year. This reduces the frequency of episodes by more than 70% to 80%.
   - Test for other STIs as indicated.
   - Counsel to abstain from sexual activity when active lesions are present and inform sexual partners.
   - Inform that transmission of HSV can occur during asymptomatic periods.
   - Stress the risk of perinatal infection and follow pregnancies closely.
   - Educate regarding course of disease, self-inoculation, transmission, and asymptomatic viral shedding.
   - Suggest dietary modifications including increased intake of vitamin C, B-complex and B_6 vitamins, zinc, and calcium to boost the immune system. A diet high in lysine and low in arginine (e.g., eating fish, chicken, cheese, and most fruits and vegetables and avoiding chocolate, peanuts, and white and wheat flour) may be helpful.

BOX 35-12 General Treatment Measures for Sexually Transmitted Infections

1. Have patient abstain from sexual intercourse until patient and partner are cured (treatment complete and symptoms resolved). Consequences of untreated STIs should be explained.
2. Test for other STIs, including hepatitis B, HIV, BV, and *Trichomonas.*
3. Notify, examine, and treat all partners of patient for any STI identified or suspected.
4. Report STIs to state health department. Reporting to appropriate authorities is important to identify those at risk, recognize new strains, and assess extent of infection in community and the effect of prevention efforts.
5. Provide regular sex health assessment including vaginal examination and testing for STIs.
6. Give hepatitis B, HPV vaccines if not done already.
7. Discuss safer sex practices, including abstinence and use of condoms.
8. Educate and counsel about complications and transmission of STIs and perinatal consequences.

BV, Bacterial vaginosis; *HIV,* human immunodeficiency virus; *HPV,* human papillomavirus; *STI,* sexually transmitted infection.

5. **HPV.** No treatment will eradicate this disease. The goal should be to remove visible warts and reduce symptoms. The benefit of identification and treatment of subclinical infections has not been established. Patient preference and treatment availability should guide treatment course; spontaneous resolution occurs in most cases. Warts on moist surfaces respond better to topical treatment than do warts on drier surfaces.

   • Patient-applied treatment: Treat with (1) podofilox 0.5% solution or gel twice a day for 3 days, no treatment for 4 days, for a total of four cycles (safety in pregnancy has not been established) or (2) imiquimod 5% cream applied with finger at bedtime three times a week for up to 16 weeks. Wash treated area with mild soap and water 6 to 10 hours after application. Warts should clear after 8 to 10 weeks. Safety in pregnancy is not determined

   • Provider-applied treatment: Treat external visible warts with (1) cryotherapy with liquid nitrogen or cryoprobe every 1 to 2 weeks or (2) 10% to 25% podophyllin resin in benzoin washed off in 1 to 4 hours to decrease local irritation, repeated weekly (safety in pregnancy not established), or (3) trichloroacetic acid (TCA) or bichloroacetic acid (BCA) applied in small amounts, dried to frosting consistency, followed by baking powder or baking soda to remove unreacted acid, repeated weekly, or (4) surgical removal with scissors, shave, curette, or electrosurgery.

   • Change treatment if there is no response after three patient-applied treatments or six provider-applied treatments.

   • Use only one treatment modality at a time to prevent increased complications.

   • Advise patient that an inflammatory reaction is common before resolution.

   • After cryotherapy, pain, necrosis, and blistering are common.

   • Refer patients with cervical warts, suspected abuse, or extensive lesions in difficult areas for gynecologic treatment. Intralesional interferon or laser surgery may be necessary in severe cases.

   • No change in the schedule for Pap testing is necessary with clinical warts.

   • Advise patient that recurrence is common, most often in the first 3 months following treatment.

Complications

In general, perinatal transmission, disseminated infection, and increased risk for chronic hepatitis are possible. PID, ectopic pregnancy, and infertility are possible sequelae to GC and chlamydia. Tertiary disease is a risk with syphilis. An increased risk of HIV transmission has been found with other STIs. HPV infection is linked with cervical dysplasia and cancer.

Patient Education and Prevention

Prevention occurs at a variety of levels and in a variety of ways. The following approaches are recommended:

   • Primary prevention seeks to reduce the number of new cases of STIs. This best occurs before sexual debut by delaying initiation of sexual intercourse. If the adolescent currently is, or plans to become sexually active, promoting the use of condoms and partner communication skills to avoid exposure to STIs is imperative. Addressing these topics specifically, using knowledge, attitudes, and behaviors to guide education as well as considering developmental needs, cultural values, misperceptions, and social skills. Peer facilitators are useful. Hepatitis B, HPV, and possibly hepatitis A immunizations are recommended.

   • Secondary prevention seeks to reduce the numbers of existing cases by early detection and treatment through well-woman care and STI screening (recommended every 6 months for those at risk). Access to health care for treatment and follow-up, monitoring for sequelae, partner notification, and evaluating risk behaviors are important aspects to successful secondary prevention.

   • Tertiary prevention seeks to minimize the psychological and biologic sequelae of STIs including minimizing perinatal complications, infant morbidity and mortality rates and reducing the frequency of PID and its complications. Identifying coping strategies and means of increasing self-esteem are also important aspects.

   Treatment of any STI in a child should be coordinated with the laboratory, child protective services, and the state authorities. Important family factors that reduce risk behaviors include perceived parental support, degree of family closeness, communication among family members, parenting style, and parental supervision and monitoring.

PELVIC INFLAMMATORY DISEASE

Description

Considered an ascending infection, PID refers to infection and inflammation involving the upper genital tract (uterus, fallopian tubes, ovaries, or peritoneal tissue). PID is either acute (less than 3 weeks' duration) or chronic. The classic picture is acute salpingitis that causes lower abdominal pain, vaginal discharge, and fever with an onset after menses. However, PID is difficult to diagnose because symptoms are widely varied.

Epidemiology

PID is often a polymicrobial infection, with GC and chlamydia being the two most common STIs causing PID. Vaginal flora, other aerobic and anaerobic organisms, group B streptococcus, genital mycoplasma, and gram-negative bacteria also are implicated. Approximately 33% of cases of PID are in adolescents. The two risk factors considered to be most significant among teenagers are multiple sexual partners and the high prevalence of STIs in this age group. Other risk factors include increased susceptibility of adolescents to infection, cervical ectopy and thinner cervical mucus, recent instrumentation or intrauterine device use, previous PID, history of lower genital tract infection (including GC, chlamydia, trichomoniasis, and BV), and nonuse of contraceptives of any type.

Clinical Findings

PID in adolescents is often subtle and can go undiagnosed, contributing to the inflammatory sequelae. Criteria for diagnosis of PID have been identified, including a set of minimal,

BOX 35-13 Criteria for Diagnosing Pelvic Inflammatory Disease

Minimum criteria for treating pelvic inflammatory disease (PID) in sexually active adolescents with pelvic or lower abdominal pain and no other cause for illness identified include one or more of the following pelvic examination findings:
- Cervical motion tenderness
- Uterine tenderness
- Adnexal tenderness

Additional lower-genital-tract inflammatory findings that support the diagnosis:
- Cervical friability
- Cervical exudates
- Predominance of leukocytes in the vaginal secretions

Additional criteria that support a diagnosis of PID:
- Oral temperature >101° F (>38.3° C)
- Abnormal mucopurulent cervical or vaginal discharge
- Presence of abundant WBCs in saline microscopy of vaginal secretions
- Elevated erythrocyte sedimentation rate
- Elevated C-reactive protein
- Laboratory documentation of cervical infection with GC or chlamydia

Most specific criteria for diagnosing PID, warranted in selected cases:
- Endometrial biopsy with histopathologic evidence of endometritis
- Transvaginal sonography or magnetic resonance imaging showing thickened fluid-filled tubes with or without free pelvic fluid or tubo-ovarian complex
- Laparoscopic abnormalities consistent with PID

GC, Gonorrhea; *WBC,* white blood cell.
Data from Centers for Disease Control and Prevention (CDC): Sexually transmitted diseases: treatment guidelines, *MMWR Morb Mortal Wkly Rep* 59(RR-12):63-64, 2010.

low-threshold criteria prompting early intervention (Box 35-13).

History
- Sexual history, including number of partners and type of activity
- Last menstrual period, contraceptive use, and previous STI or PID
- Lower abdominal pain or tenderness (acute onset with GC, subtle with chlamydia)
- Intermenstrual bleeding
- Malaise, dysuria, nausea, vomiting, chills, dyspareunia

Physical Examination
- Abdominal examination—bilateral lower quadrant tenderness (most common initial symptom) and possibly right upper quadrant pain (Fitz-Hugh–Curtis syndrome: inflammation of liver capsule); occasional peritoneal signs
- Speculum examination—cervical or vaginal mucopurulent discharge
- Bimanual examination—cervical motion tenderness, uterine or adnexal tenderness (may be unilateral)

Diagnostic Studies
- CBC (WBCs greater than 10,000), erythrocyte sedimentation rate (greater than 15 mm/hr), CRP (elevated)
- Microscopic examination of cervical discharge

- NAATs or culture for GC and chlamydia
- Serologic test (syphilis)
- Pregnancy test (ectopic)
- Urinalysis and culture if symptoms of pyelonephritis or cystitis
- Pelvic ultrasound (if adnexal enlargement or tubo-ovarian abscess suspected)

Differential Diagnosis
Acute appendicitis, ectopic pregnancy, torsion of an ovarian cyst, ruptured corpus luteal cyst, salpingitis, tubo-ovarian abscess, endometritis, acute pyelonephritis, gastroenteritis, vaginitis, and functional pain are included in the differential diagnosis.

Management
Outpatient treatment regimens are delineated in Table 35-7a.

Goals of treatment include the relief of acute discomfort and prevention of infertility and other sequelae. More than one diagnosis is possible. Empiric treatment should be initiated in sexually active young women if the minimal criteria are met. Treatment should be initiated as soon as possible with broad-spectrum coverage to minimize long-term sequelae. Follow-up should occur within 72 hours. Patients should demonstrate clinical improvement as evidenced by defervescence, decreased abdominal tenderness, and decreased uterine, adnexal, and cervical motion tenderness. If no clinical improvement, the patient will need hospitalization.

Hospitalization is also recommended in the following situations: surgical emergency cannot be excluded; pregnancy; lack of response to oral antibiotics; inability to tolerate oral antibiotics; severe illness with nausea, vomiting, or high temperature; or tubo-ovarian abscess (CDC, 2010a).

Other recommendations include:
- Treatment of any sexual partners exposed within 60 days of onset of symptoms. Abstinence from intercourse until partners have been treated.
- Follow up 7 to 10 days after treatment.
- Rescreen for chlamydia and GC 3 to 6 months after treatment. HIV screening should be offered.
- PID is a reportable STI in some states.

Complications
Infertility (13% to 50% attributable to PID, a higher percentage with subsequent episodes); tubo-ovarian abscess; ectopic pregnancy (6-fold to 10-fold increased risk); perihepatitis (Fitz-Hugh–Curtis syndrome); chronic pelvic pain; dyspareunia; and repeated PID (Shrier, 2008) can occur.

Prevention
Decrease prevalence and transmission of STIs by promoting abstinence and barrier methods (condoms, diaphragms, cervical caps, and spermicidal foams). Screen sexually active adolescents for GC and chlamydia every 6 months.

TABLE 35-7	Outpatient Treatment Regimens for Pelvic Inflammatory Disease	
Regimen A	**Regimen B**	**Regimen C**
Ceftriaxone 250 mg IM in a single dose	Cefoxitin 2 g IM in a single dose **And** Probenecid 1 g orally administered concurrently in a single dose	Other parenteral third-generation cephalosporin (e.g., ceftizoxime or cefotaxime)
Plus	**Plus**	**Plus**
Doxycycline 100 mg orally bid for 14 days	Doxycycline 100 mg orally bid for 14 days	Doxycycline 100 mg orally bid for 14 days
With or Without	**With or Without**	**With or Without**
Metronidazole 500 mg twice daily for 14 days	Metronidazole 500 mg twice daily for 14 days	Metronidazole 500 mg twice daily for 14 days

IM, Intramuscular.

Data from Centers for Disease Control and Prevention (CDC): Sexually transmitted diseases: treatment guidelines, *MMWR Morb Mortal Wkly Rep* 59(RR-12):66, 2010.

Dermatologic Disorders

PEGGY VERNON, MARGARET A. BRADY, NANCY BARBER STARR, AND ANN M. PETERSEN-SMITH

The skin is the body's largest organ and one of its most important. The condition of the skin reflects physical and emotional health, plays a major role in defining identity and supporting survival, and often gives clues to underlying conditions. Skin functions are multiple. Beauty is often defined by the appearance of the skin. Emotions are expressed by blushing and sweating. Skin conveys many impressions through its sensory functions, including reaction to touch, heat, cold, pressure, and pain. Additionally, the skin provides a protective physiologic covering, the first line of defense against injury from chemical, physical, and microorganic invaders. Homeostasis is maintained through fluid regulation and thermoregulation.

Disruptions in the skin account for a significant percentage of all pediatric office visits. The primary care provider plays an essential role in maintaining skin integrity, identifying and minimizing skin disruptions, maximizing healing, and educating parents and children about skin care.

Skin development is constant from embryogenesis throughout life. During the embryonic period (the first 2 months of gestation), the skin differentiates into several layers. The skin changes and develops throughout childhood and adolescence, achieving adult skin thickness and characteristics in the late teenage years. Melanin in the skin reaches adult levels by 1 year of age. Vascularization is well developed by the end of the second year of life. Cutaneous nerves develop until puberty and beyond. Sebaceous glands cease production between 6 and 12 months of age, but become active again at around 7 years old. Eccrine sweat function begins between 2 and 18 days of age, although full function is not in place until 2 or 3 years old. The apocrine glands become active at puberty. Hair grows approximately 1 cm per month. Nails are spoon shaped and thin from infancy until 2 to 3 years old.

■ Anatomy and Physiology

The skin is composed of three layers: the epidermis, the dermis, and the subcutaneous layer (Fig. 36-1). Skin, including its epidermis and dermis, varies from 1.5 to 4 mm in thickness (Weston et al, 2007).

The epidermis, the thinner outer layer, functions as a protective barrier between the body and the environment and is comprised of five layers of stratified squamous epithelium. Most epidermal cells are keratinocytes, and the replication and maturation of the keratinocytes is called keratinization. New keratinocytes of the basal layer mature and shed approximately every 28 days. The outer horny layer, the stratum corneum, is responsible for much of the barrier protection against microorganisms and irritating chemicals. It impedes the exchange of fluids and electrolytes with the environment and provides strength for the skin. Melanin protects deoxyribonucleic acid (DNA) from damage by ultraviolet (UV) light irradiation. It is produced in the basal layer of the epidermis and contributes to the color of the skin, eyes, and hair. The water content of the environment influences the epidermal barrier, with either excess or inadequate amounts contributing to microscopic and macroscopic breaks.

The thicker middle layer, the dermis, contributes strength, support, and elasticity to the skin. It is a tough, leathery mechanical barrier that also regulates heat loss, provides host defenses of the skin, and aids in nutrition and other regulatory functions. The dermis is primarily composed of fibrous connective tissue (made up of fibroblasts and collagen), with some elastic fibers and a mucopolysaccharide gel. It includes mast cells, inflammatory cells, blood and lymph vessels, and cutaneous nerves that elicit sensations (touch, pain, pressure, itch, warmth, and cold). These specialized receptors are a defense mechanism to protect the skin surface from environmental trauma.

Underlying the dermis is subcutaneous tissue primarily composed of adipose tissue. It contains arteries and arterioles that assist in skin thermoregulation. The subcutaneous tissue insulates, cushions against trauma, provides energy, and metabolizes hormones.

Skin appendages include the hair, nails, sweat glands, and sebaceous glands. Hair follicles are found over the entire body except for the palms, soles, knuckles, distal and interdigital spaces, lips, glans and prepuce of the penis, and areolae and nipples. Two types of hair can be found on the body. Terminal hair is thick and visible and found on the scalp, axillae, and pubis. Very fine vellus hair is found over the remainder of the body. The visible portion of the hair is the shaft. The hair root is embedded in the dermis as a pilosebaceous unit, consisting of a hair follicle and a sebaceous gland. The hair shaft may be straight, wavy, helical, or spiral. Following an acute febrile illness or stress, there may be hair thinning for several months.

Nails are epidermal cells converted to keratin that grow continually. The nailbed, underneath the nail plate, is composed

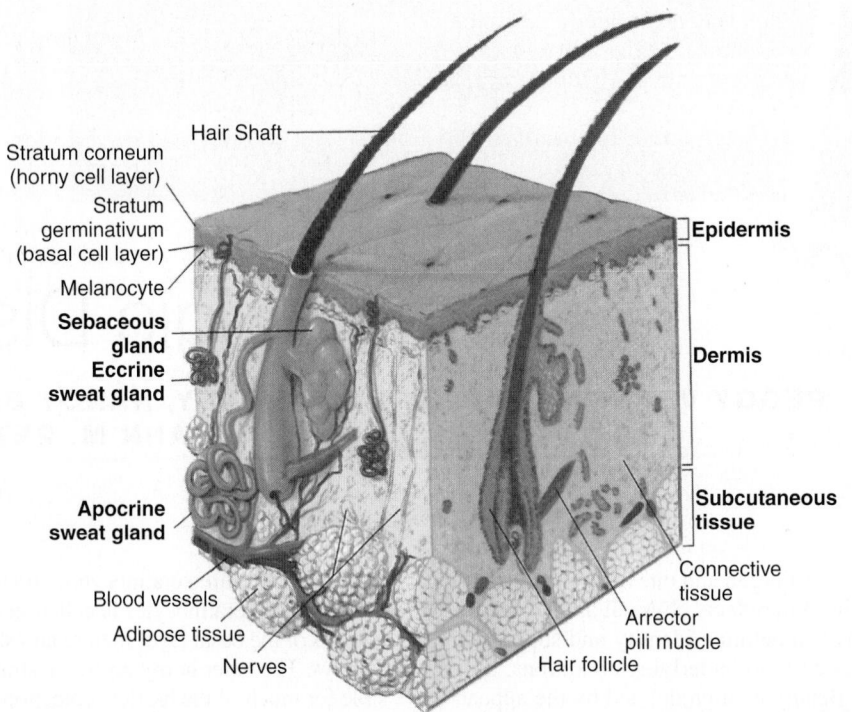

Stratum corneum
(horny cell layer)

Stratum
germinativum
(basal cell layer)

Melanocyte

**Sebaceous
gland**

**Eccrine
sweat gland**

**Apocrine
sweat gland**

Blood vessels

Adipose tissue

Nerves

Hair Shaft

Epidermis

Dermis

**Subcutaneous
tissue**

Connective
tissue

Arrector
pili muscle

Hair follicle

FIGURE 36-1 Structure of the skin. (From Jarvis C: *Physical examination and assessment,* ed 2, Philadelphia, 1996, Saunders.)

of layers of epidermis and dermis, which serve as structural support. The nail root lies just under the epidermis.

There are three types of sweat glands. Eccrine glands are distributed over the entire body. They help maintain fluid and electrolyte balance and body temperature, and provide some excretory function. Ceruminous glands are located in the external ear canal and secrete a waxy pigmented substance, cerumen. Apocrine glands are located primarily in the axillary, genital, and periumbilical areas. They open into hair follicles, require androgens to stimulate their secretions, and are thought to be responsible for body odor.

Sebaceous glands, found in conjunction with hair follicles, are distributed over the entire body except the soles, palms, and dorsa of the feet and contribute to the epidermis protection. These glands secrete sebum (oil) when stimulated by androgen and function to prevent excessive water evaporation, minimize heat loss, and lubricate the skin and hair.

Pathophysiology and Defense Mechanisms

Disruption of the skin and subcutaneous tissue occurs through a variety of assaults. These include:

- Bacterial, fungal, and viral infections
- Allergic and inflammatory reactions
- Infestations
- Vascular reactions
- Papulosquamous and bullous eruptions
- Congenital lesions
- Hair and nail disorders

The skin's outer layers provide the body's first line of defense from chemical, physical, and microorganic injury. The epidermis provides a functional barrier, the dermis provides

strength and protection through the cutaneous nerves, and the subcutaneous tissue ensures insulation, is a cushion to prevent injury, is an energy source, and functions in hormonal metabolism. These layers, in turn, protect the other body systems. The water content of the skin enhances the protective barrier of the skin. If the skin becomes too dry or too wet, breaks in the barrier elicit an inflammatory response. As a continuously growing system, the skin not only heals itself but controls growth or colonization of microorganisms by continual shedding.

There are three identified cutaneous reactions to trauma, infection, or inflammation: pigment lability, follicular response, and mesenchymal response. Pigment lability occurs as postinflammatory hypopigmentation or hyperpigmentation. If superficial, with changes in the epidermis only, normal pigmentation returns in about 6 months (e.g., in diaper rash, seborrhea, tinea, pityriasis alba). If dermal changes happen, dermal tattooing may occur, causing long-term or permanent changes (e.g., excoriated acne, impetigo, varicella, contact dermatitis). The exaggerated follicular response results in prominent papule and follicle formation, especially with atopic dermatitis, pityriasis rosea (PR), syphilis, or tinea versicolor. The mesenchymal response causes scars and keloids (that extend beyond the edge of the scar), often following varicella, ear piercing, burns, or any surgical procedure.

Special Dermatologic Considerations in Children With Dark Skin or from Diverse Cultural or Ethnic Groups

Knowledge of the normal variations in children both with different levels of pigmentation of the skin and from diverse ethnic or cultural groups is important for assessing and treating dermatologic conditions. Skin reactions to injury, inflammation, common skin conditions, and cultural practices are varied. A wise pediatric health care provider listens to parents because they are often the first to detect subtle changes in color or texture of the skin. This section discusses some of the dermatologic differences of children with dark skin.

Preventive care for patients with dark skin should be implemented in routine well-child care. The following are initial areas to include:

- Prevent acne or contact dermatitis.
- Avoid pomades.
- Prevent traction alopecia.
- Immunize against varicella to prevent scarring.
- Use insect repellents to minimize insect bite reactions.
- Treat early signs and symptoms of pruritic or inflammatory conditions (acne, eczema) and infections.
- Use moisturizing agents and eliminate soaps for dry, itchy skin.
- Use oral antipruritics for dry, itchy skin.
- Caution about the use of topical medications, especially high-potency steroids, benzoyl peroxide, and isotretinoin.
- Avoid trauma and any procedures that can induce keloids.

CUTANEOUS REACTION PATTERNS

Pigment lability is common and tends to be more obvious in dark-skinned individuals regardless of race. People of color are especially prone to the development of keloids and hypertrophic scars, sometimes from relatively minor skin trauma. Other exaggerated responses common in darker-skinned individuals include lichenification and vesicular or bullous reaction to bites or staphylococcal infection. African-American children may have an exaggerated cutaneous response to common disorders of the skin. Of note, erythema of inflamed black skin may be difficult to detect and may appear as a purplish tinge (Paller and Mancini, 2011).

NORMAL VARIATIONS AND COMMON PROBLEMS

The following are normal variations or common problems in children with dark skin:

- Variation in color and texture of skin from one part of the body to another
- Pigmentation of gingiva, mucous membrane, sclerae, and nails correlates with degree of cutaneous pigmentation.
- Increased areas of melanin in thicker-skinned areas (elbow, knee)
- The term, *Futcher's* or *Ito line,* describe the vertical line that separates the hyperpigmented dorsal and extensor surfaces from less-pigmented ventral surfaces. This line of differentiation follows Voigt lines and is most noticeable on the extremities.
- Mongolian spots and increased numbers of café au lait spots (see later discussion)
- Normal exfoliation produces a fine layer of gray scales.
- Color alterations (jaundice, anemia, cyanosis) are difficult to assess.
- Kinky, wooly, tightly curled hair with closely knit growth that tangles when dry and mats when wet
- Atopic dermatitis (see Chapter 24) with prominent follicular pattern with pityriasis alba and postinflammatory hypopigmentation

CULTURAL OR ETHNIC PRACTICES WITH SKIN SEQUELAE

Grooming, cosmetic, or healing practices of cultural or ethnic groups contribute to various conditions that may be seen. These include the following:

- Hair pomade—acne
- Bleaching creams—discoloration and erythematous nodules
- Chemical or thermal hair straighteners—alopecia, fragile hair shaft, scalp contact dermatitis
- Tightly braided, twisted, locked hair (dreadlocks), and tight ponytails—traction folliculitis followed by traction alopecia that can be permanent and cause scarring (Putgen, 2008)
- Henna for superficial tattooing—orange discoloration of skin, increased bilirubin levels in infants
- Decorative practices—scars or tattoos
- Healing practices used during significant illness that produce burns—circular 1- to 2-cm scars on chest, periumbilicus, wrists, ankles, or back
- Coining—petechiae and ecchymoses, especially on chest and back
- Cupping—circular ecchymoses on neck, chest, back, and arms

◼ Assessment of the Skin and Subcutaneous Tissue

HISTORY

The history should assess the following:
- History of present illness
  ○ Onset and duration of present or recent illness (e.g., respiratory or gastrointestinal [GI])
  ○ Most common concerns: Pruritus, scaling, and alterations in cosmetic appearance
  ○ Symptom analysis—questions to ask about an eruption or lesions include:
    - What did the rash or lesion(s) originally look like?
    - How has it changed in appearance?
    - Where did the eruption first begin, and has it spread to other locations (pattern of spread)?
    - How long has the rash or lesion been present?
    - Is the way it looks today typical of its appearance?
    - Does the rash come and go?
    - Has the lesion blistered, bled, or had discharge?
    - Does it itch?
    - What have you used to treat it and what was the effect?
  ○ What parts of the body are not affected by the rash or lesions (e.g., face, soles, or palms)?
  ○ Associated systemic symptoms: Fever, malaise, pain associated with lesion or eruption
  ○ Factors that alleviate or worsen skin symptoms or seem to trigger them
  ○ Exposures or allergies: Medication, foods, animals, plants? Known allergens? New substances? Persons with similar symptoms or illness? What soaps, hair products (shampoos, gels, pomade, etc.), lotions, and detergents are used?
  ○ All medication (prescription and over-the-counter) taken over the last few days, including creams, ointments, powders, or lotions (it is often helpful to have patients bring medications they have used to the appointment)

- ○ Prior incidents of similar rash
- ○ Recent travel
- Family review of systems
  - ○ Similar symptoms
  - ○ Skin disorders or history of atopy disorders (asthma, seasonal or drug allergies or atopic dermatitis)
  - ○ Chronic illnesses with related dermatologic findings
- Client review of systems and past medical history
  - ○ Usual state of health and recent illnesses
  - ○ Skin, hair, and nails: Skin type (dry or oily), recent and long-term changes, previous incidence of skin disease
  - ○ Eyes, ears, nose, and throat: Swelling, itching, crusting, discharge or circles around eyes, nasal mucus discharge, patency or irritation, dry mouth, lesions, or pain
  - ○ Chest: Wheezing, coughing, or respiratory difficulty
  - ○ Chronic illnesses with related dermatologic findings

PHYSICAL EXAMINATION

When seeing a child with a dermatologic condition, it is essential to assess whether the child is ill. This clinical impression helps the provider differentiate serious illnesses from the majority of dermatologic conditions. The entire body, not just exposed skin, needs to be examined. Attention should be given to the eyes, nose, mouth (mucous membranes, teeth), lymph nodes, and lungs because a skin disorder may be a cutaneous manifestation of other disease. The dermatologic examination includes a thorough look at the skin, scalp, hair, palms and soles, nails, and anogenital region.

Special techniques for examination of the skin may be required. Good light (daylight is best) is essential to a good examination. A source of direct light, such as a gooseneck lamp, is the best alternative. Other helpful tools include a magnifying glass, a ruler, a glass slide, and a Wood's lamp (UV light). A glass slide gently pressed on the skin (diascopy) allows viewing of the skin with and without capillary filling. A Wood's lamp is used to examine fluorescent-positive fungal infections and depigmenting skin disorders, such as vitiligo.

Identification of the type of lesion and correct use of terminology are essential to good dermatologic care. Essential documentation includes the following:

- Location and type of lesion
- Color, color changes, size, and shape
- Arrangement (e.g., isolated, grouped, linear, annular, zosteriform)
- Pattern (e.g., sun-exposed area, symmetry)
- Distribution of lesion (e.g., regional, generalized, crops)
- Border (e.g., indistinct, well circumscribed)
- Consistency (e.g., firm, soft, mobile)

Primary skin lesions (Box 36-1) include changes that arise from previously normal skin. These descriptions should be memorized and used. *Secondary* skin lesions (Box 36-2) result from changes in primary lesions. *Vascular* skin lesions (Box 36-3) involve the blood supply. Other useful descriptive terms are listed in Box 36-4. Vesicles, pustules, scaling, and color changes should be noted when considering differential diagnoses.

DIAGNOSTIC STUDIES

A few simple laboratory tests are helpful in identifying or excluding dermatologic disorders. Proper procurement of the sample is important. Lesions can be scraped with a no. 15

BOX 36-1 Primary Skin Changes to Lesions

Bulla—vesicle larger than 1 cm
Comedo—plugged, dilated pore; open (blackhead), closed (whitehead)
Cyst—palpable lesion with definite borders filled with liquid or semi-solid material
Macule—flat, nonpalpable, discolored lesion, 1 cm or smaller
Nodule—raised, firm, movable lesion with indistinct borders and deep palpable portion, 2 cm or smaller
Papule—solid, raised lesion of varied color with distinct borders, 1 cm or smaller
Patch—macule, larger than 1 cm
Plaque—solid, raised, flat-topped lesion with distinct borders, larger than 1 cm
Pustule—raised lesion filled with pus, often in hair follicle or sweat pore
Tumor—large nodule, may be firm or soft
Vesicle—blister filled with clear fluid
Wheal—fleeting, irregularly shaped, elevated, itchy lesion of varied size, pale at center, slightly red at borders

---

BOX 36-2 Secondary Skin Changes to Lesions

Atrophy—thinning skin, may appear translucent
Crusts—dried exudate or scab of varied color
Desquamation—peeling sheets of scale
Erosion—oozing or moist, depressed area with loss of superficial epidermis
Excoriation—abrasion or removal of epidermis; scratch
Fissure—linear, wedge-shaped cracks extending into dermis
Keloid—healed lesion of hypertrophied connective tissue
Lichenification—thickening of skin with deep visible furrows
Scales—thin, flaking layers of epidermis
Scar—healed lesion of connective tissue
Striae—fine pink or silver lines in areas where skin has been stretched
Ulcer—deeper than erosion; open lesion extending into dermis

BOX 36-3 Vascular Skin Lesions

Angioma or hemangioma—papule made of blood vessels
Ecchymosis—bruise, purple to brown, macular or papular, varied in size
Hematoma—collection of blood from ruptured blood vessel, larger than 1 cm
Petechiae—pinpoint, pink to purple macular lesions that do not blanch, 1 to 3 mm
Purpura—purple macular lesion, larger than 1 cm
Telangiectasia—collection of macular or raised, dilated capillaries

---

blade or a toothbrush and scales or debris placed on a glass microscope slide or in culture material. The No. 15 blade is also useful for exfoliating a blister. It is important to scrape under any scabs to get a sample of the organisms. Moistening the lesion may facilitate this. Scrapings can be obtained from the edges of skin lesions, from plucked hair (getting the root is essential), from the nail plate, or from

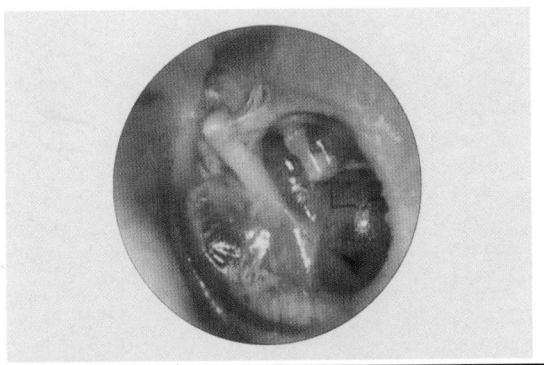

Left ear with posterior retraction. (Photograph courtesy Sylvan Stool, MD, The Children's Hospital, Denver, CO.)

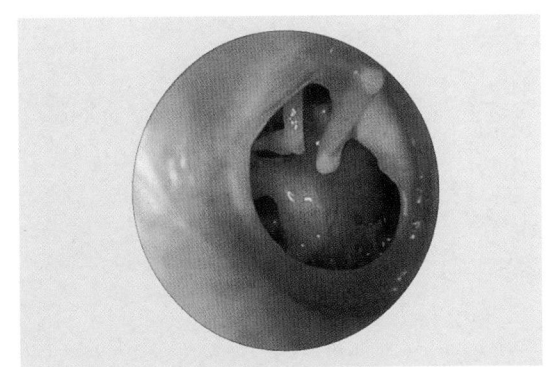

Near total perforation of the right ear. (Photograph courtesy Sylvan Stool, MD, The Children's Hospital, Denver, CO.)

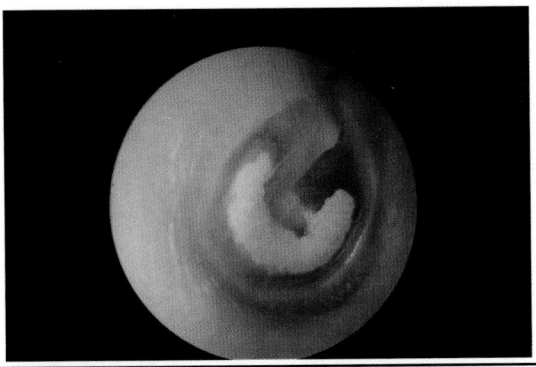

Tympanosclerosis of the right ear. (Photograph courtesy Sylvan Stool, MD, The Children's Hospital, Denver, CO.)

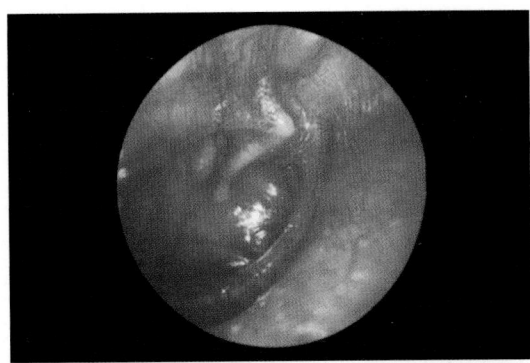

Severely retracted, opaque right tympanic membrane in otitis media with effusion. (From Bluestone CD, Klein JO: *Otitis media in infants and children*, ed 2, Philadelphia, 1995, Saunders.)

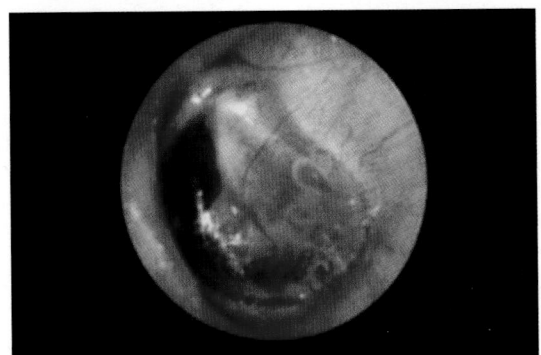

Serous effusion. (From the American Academy of Pediatrics Online Learning in Otitis Media: www.aap.org/otitismedia. Developed by the University of Colorado Health Sciences Center, Department of Pediatrics.)

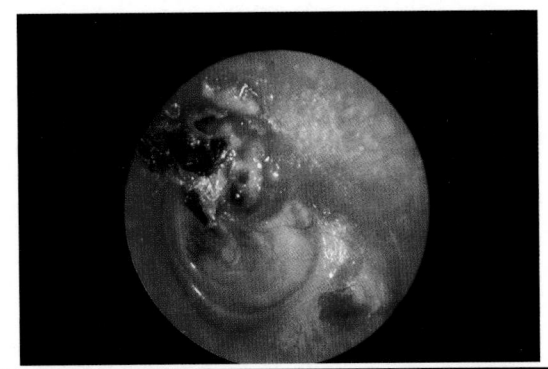

Cholesteatoma of the left ear. (Photograph courtesy Sylvan Stool, MD, The Children's Hospital, Denver, CO.)

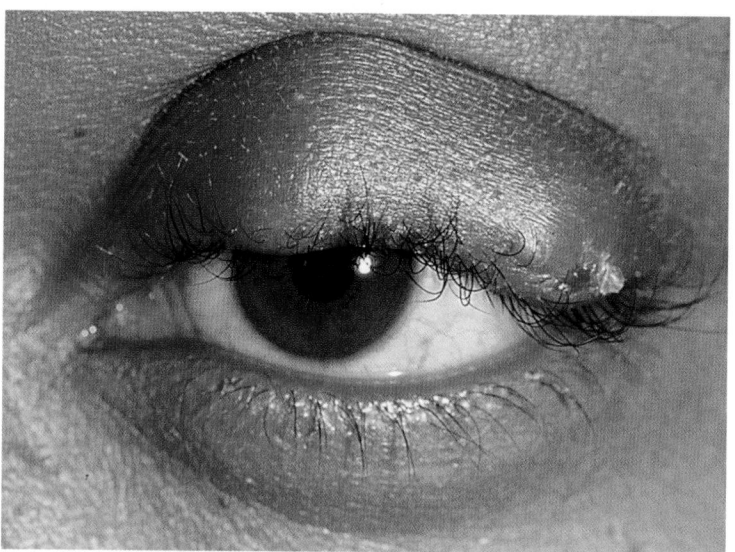

Chalazion and external hordeolum. The medial lesion of the upper eyelid appeared as a firm, painless nodule, consistent with a chalazion. The lateral lesion caused pain and eyelid erythema, subsequently becoming more localized, with drainage of purulent material through the skin surface. (From Yanoff M, Duker JS: *Ophthalmology*, ed 3, Philadelphia, 2009, Mosby.)

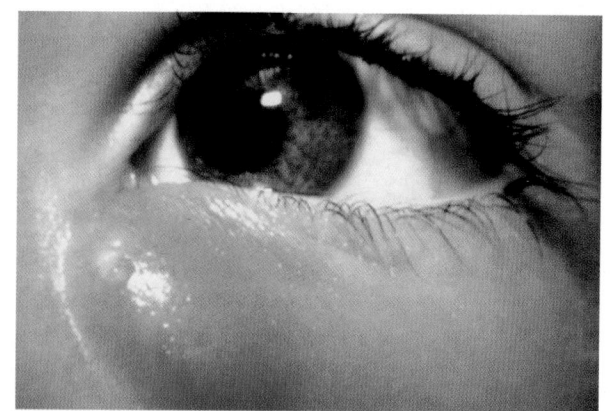

Dacryocystitis. (From Marx JA, Hockberger RS, Walls RM, et al, editors: *Rosen's emergency medicine*, ed 7, Philadelphia, 2010, Mosby.)

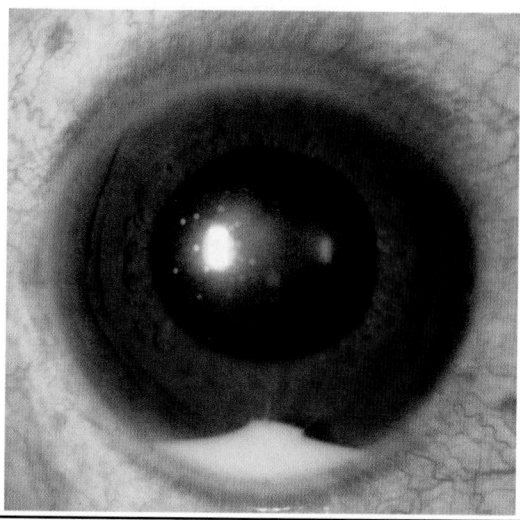

Uveitis. Accumulation of inflammatory cells forming a hypopyon in the anterior chamber. (From Palay DA, Krachmer JH: *Primary care ophthalmology*, ed 2, Philadelphia, 2005, Mosby.)

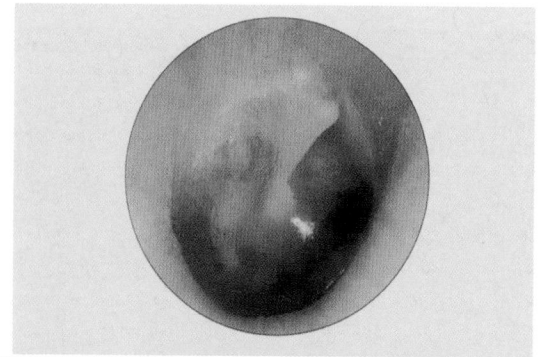

Normal right tympanic membrane. (Photograph courtesy Sylvan Stool, MD, The Children's Hospital, Denver, CO.)

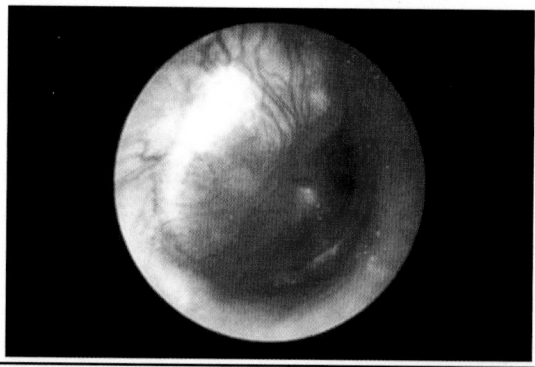

Acute otitis media of the right ear. (From the American Academy of Pediatrics Online Learning in Otitis Media: www.aap.org/otitismedia. Developed by the University of Colorado Health Sciences Center, Department of Pediatrics.)

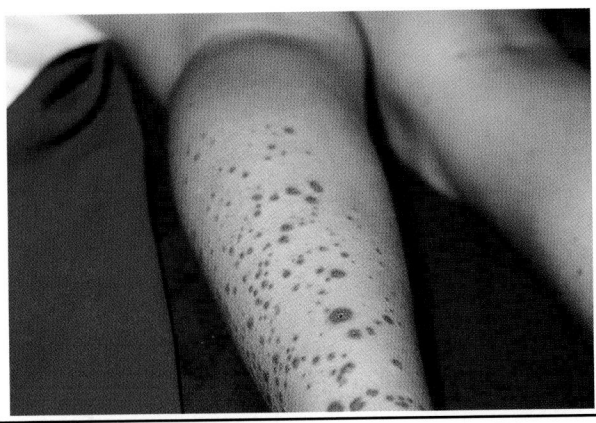

Henoch-Schönlein purpura. (From Paller AS, Mancini AJ: *Hurwitz clinical pediatric dermatology: a textbook of skin disorders of childhood and adolescence,* ed 3, Philadelphia, 2006, Saunders, p 558.)

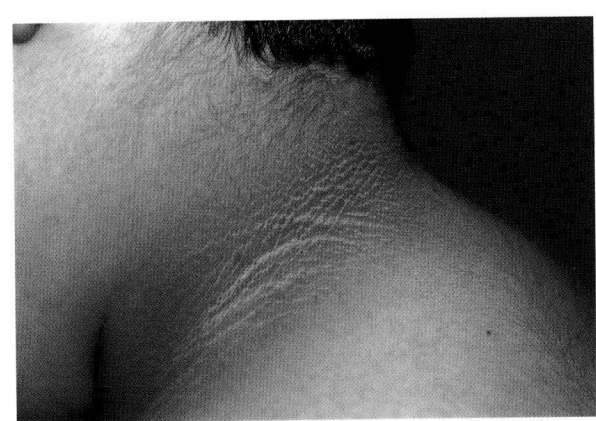

Acanthosis nigricans of a child's neck. (From Weston WL, Lane AT, Morelli JG: *Color textbook of pediatric dermatology*, ed 4, St Louis, 2007, Mosby, p 331.)

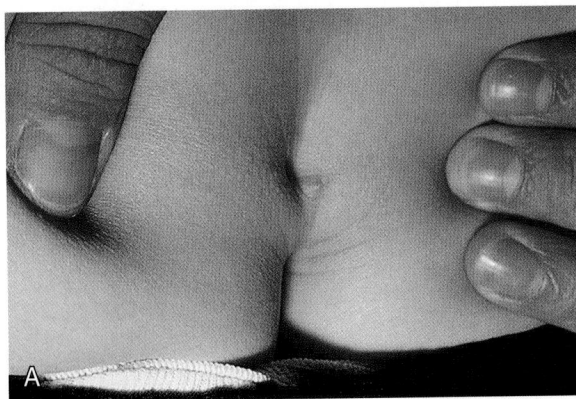

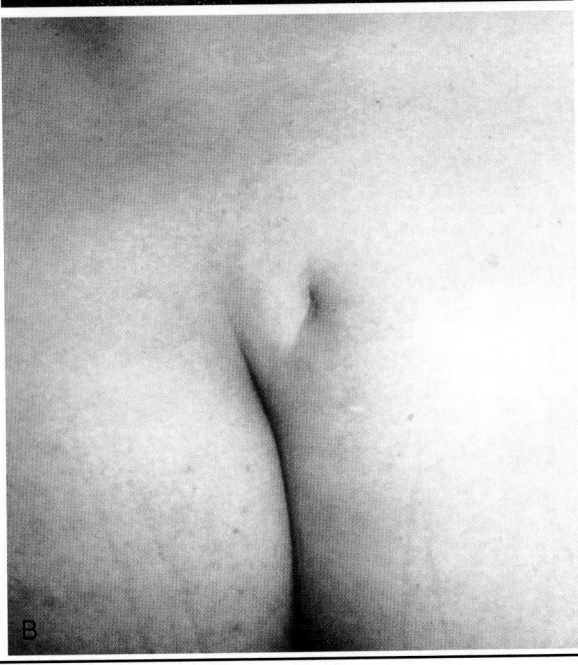

A, Deep sacral dimple above the gluteal crease. Most sacral dimples that fall within the gluteal crease are normal. Dimples that are deep, large (>0.5 cm), located in the superior portion or above the gluteal crease (>2.5 cm from the anal verge), or that are associated with a deviated gluteal crease or other cutaneous markers should be radiologically imaged. **B,** Buttocks of teenage boy with tethered cord secondary to lipomeningocele. Note sacral dimple and deviation of gluteal fold to the left. (**A,** From Eichenfield LF, Frieden IJ, Esterly NB: *Neonatal dermatology*, ed 2, Philadelphia, 2008, Saunders. **B,** From Kliegman RM, Stanton BF, St. Geme III JW, et al, editors: *Nelson textbook of pediatrics*, ed 19, Philadelphia, 2011, Saunders.)

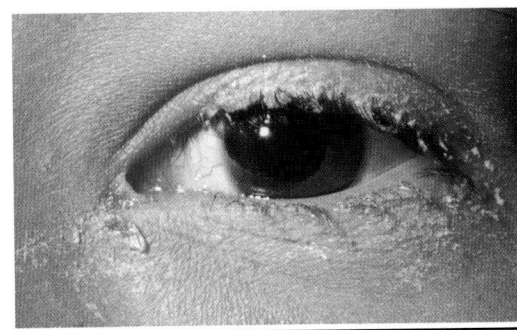

Bacterial conjunctivitis. In this case, the purulent material has dried, creating a thick crust of material on the lid and lid margin. (From Palay DA, Krachmer JH: *Primary care ophthalmology*, ed 2, Philadelphia, 2005, Mosby.)

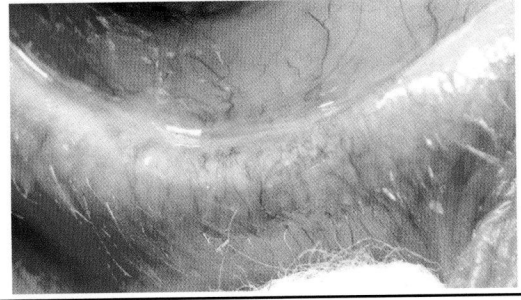

Allergic conjunctivitis. (From Palay DA, Krachmer JH: *Primary care ophthalmology*, ed 2, Philadelphia, 2005, Mosby.)

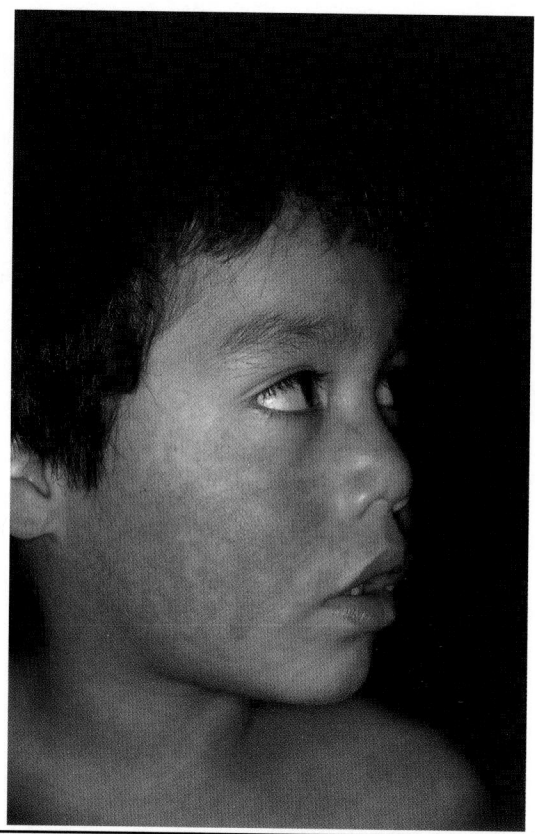

Slapped-cheek appearance of a child with parvovirus B19 infection (erythema infectiosum). (From Weston WL, Lane AT, Morelli JG: *Color textbook of pediatric dermatology*, ed 4, St Louis, 2007, Mosby, p 119.)

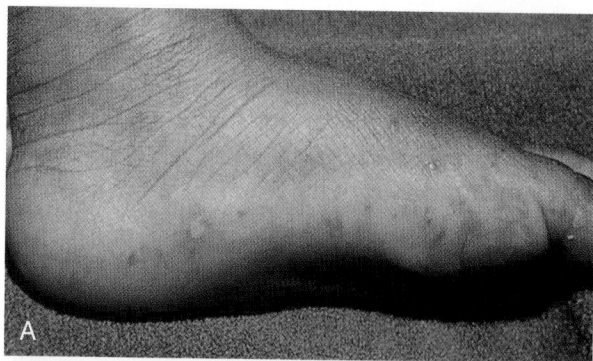

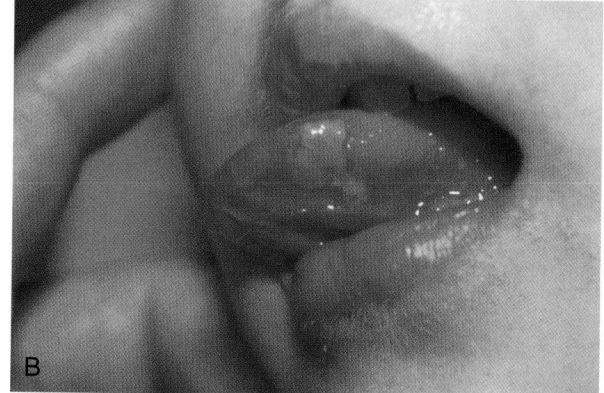

A, Oval blisters on the feet of a child with hand-foot-and-mouth syndrome. **B**, Erosion of the tongue in a child with hand-foot-and-mouth syndrome. (**A** and **B** from Weston WL, Lane AT, Morelli JG: *Color textbook of pediatric dermatology*, ed 4, St Louis, 2007, Mosby, pp 109, 201.)

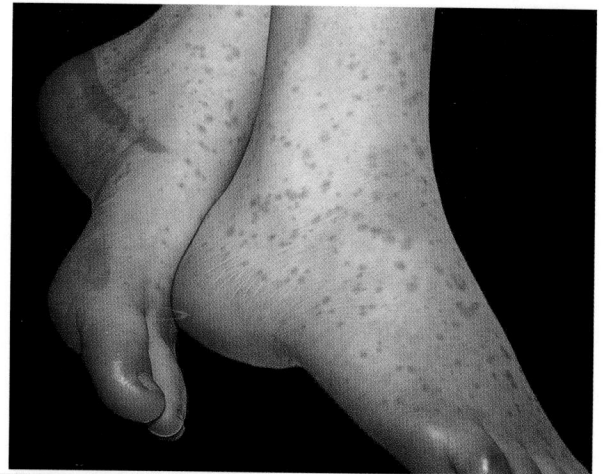

Meningococcemia. Petechiae may be located in the center of lighter-colored macules. Confluence of lesions may then result in hemorrhagic patches, often with central necrosis. (From Habif TP: *Clinical dermatology*, ed 5, Philadelphia, 2010, Mosby.)

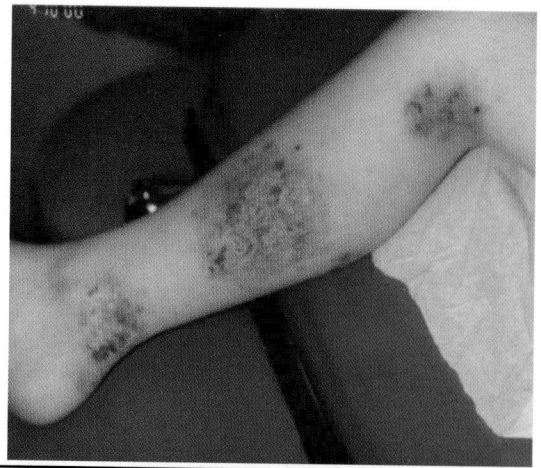

Acute atopic dermatitis. (Photograph courtesy of Peggy Vernon, RN, MA, CPNP, Aurora/Parker Skin Care Center, CO.)

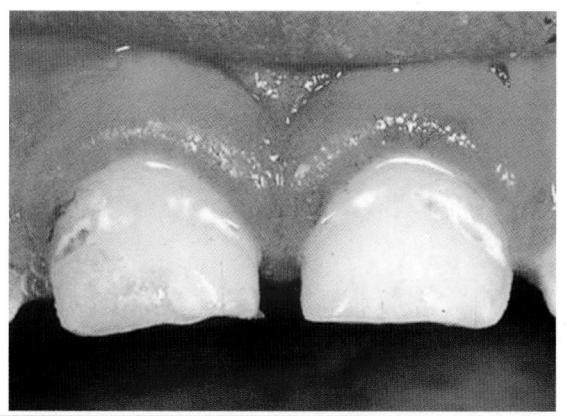

Early childhood caries. Upper incisor white spots. (Courtesy John Davis, DDS, MSD, Professor Emeritus, University of Washington, Seattle, Department of Pediatric Dentistry.)

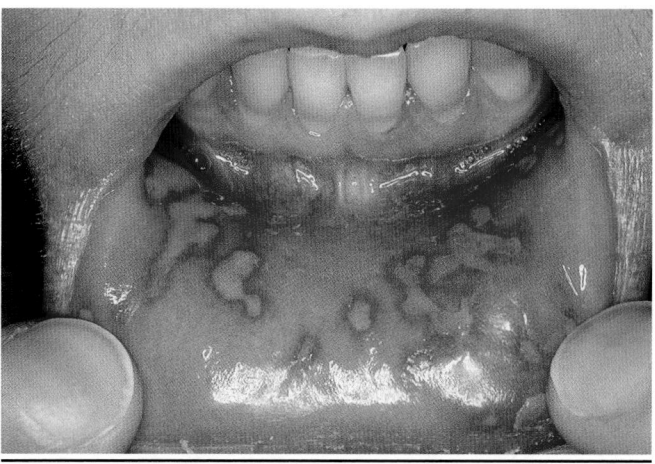

Herpetic gingivostomatitis, extensive erosions of the oral mucosa. (From James WD, Berger TG, Elston DM: *Andrews' diseases of the skin: clinical dermatology*, ed 11, Philadelphia, 2011, Saunders.)

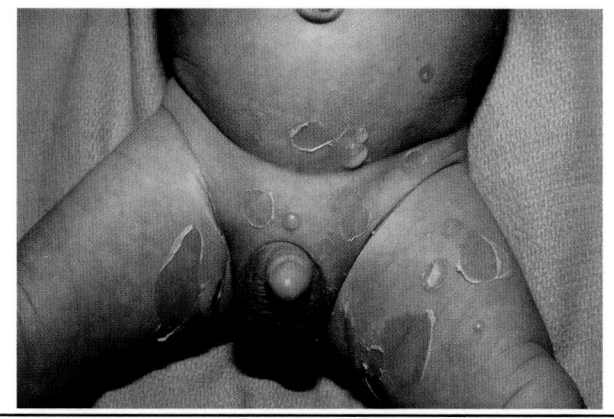

Bullous impetigo in a newborn. Multiple areas of flaccid blisters and shallow erosions on a red base. (From Weston WL, Lane AT, Morelli JG: *Color textbook of pediatric dermatology*, ed 4, St Louis, 2007, Mosby, p 62.)

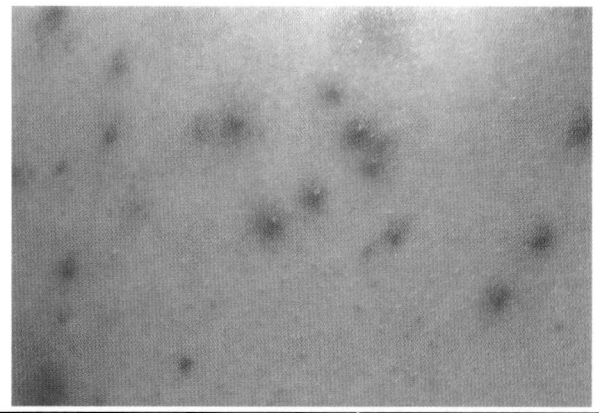

Staphylococcal superficial folliculitis. Multiple pustules on a red base. (From Weston WL, Lane AT, Morelli JG: *Color textbook of pediatric dermatology*, ed 4, St Louis, 2007, Mosby, p 69.)

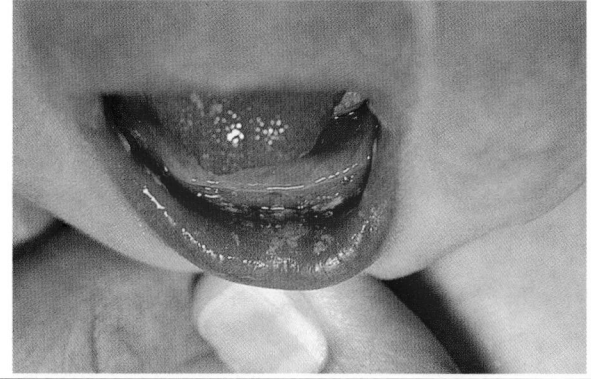

White plaques of oral thrush. (From Eichenfield LF, Frieden IJ, Esterly NB: *Neonatal dermatology*, ed 2, Philadelphia, 2008, Saunders.)

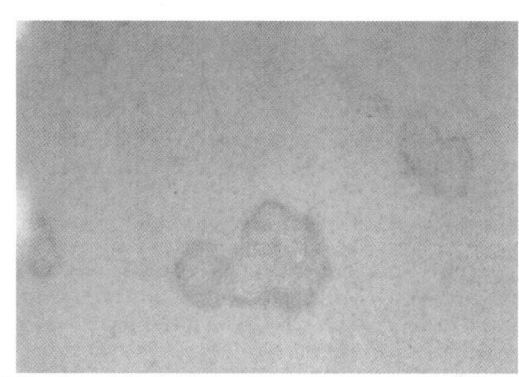

Tinea corporis. Lesions are annular with a raised inflammatory edge and central clearing. (From Aly R, Maibach H: *Atlas of infections of the skin*, Philadelphia, 1999, Saunders, p 23.)

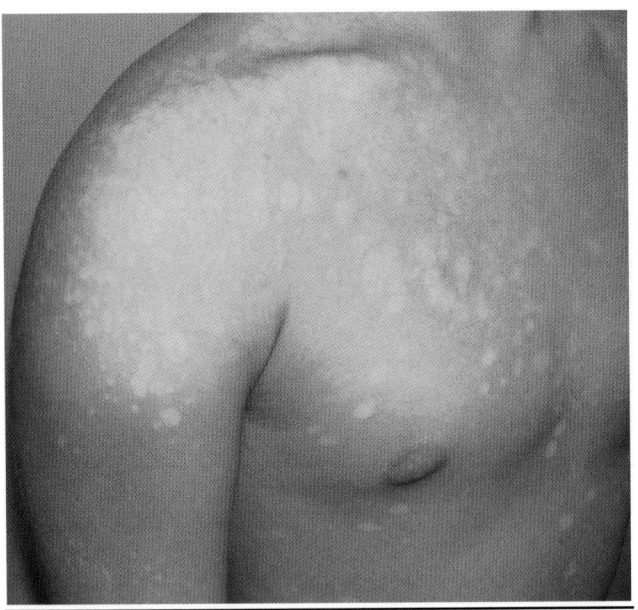

Tinea versicolor—hypopigmented patches. (From Marks JG, Miller JJ: *Lookingbill and Marks' principles of dermatology*, ed 4, Philadelphia, 2006, Saunders.)

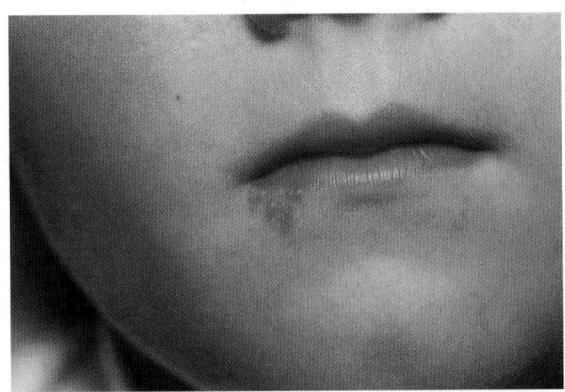

Recurrent herpes labialis of the lower lip and adjacent skin in a child. (From Weston WL, Lane AT, Morelli JG: *Color textbook of pediatric dermatology*, ed 4, St Louis, 2007, Mosby, p 128.)

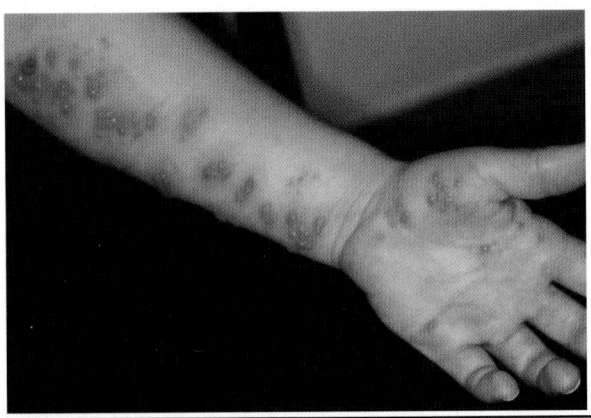

Many groups of blisters occurring over the arm of a child with herpes zoster. (From Weston WL, Lane AT, Morelli JG: *Color textbook of pediatric dermatology*, ed 4, St Louis, 2007, Mosby, p 134.)

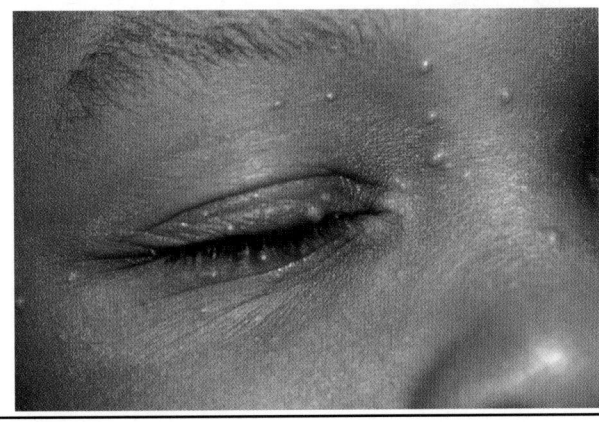

Multiple molluscum papules on an infant's face. (From Weston WL, Lane AT, Morelli JG: *Color textbook of pediatric dermatology*, ed 4, St Louis, 2007, Mosby, p 144.)

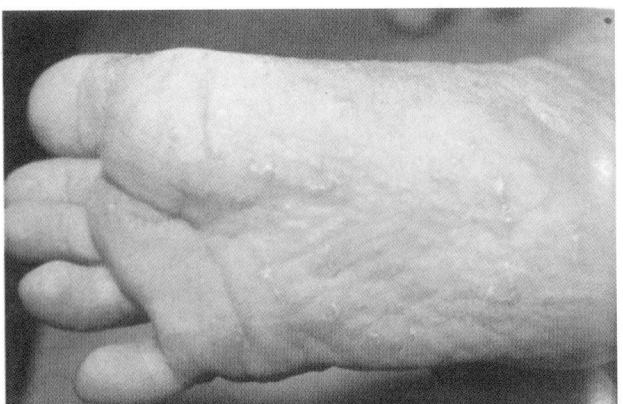

Scabies in an infant with multiple burrows and pustules on soles. (From Aly R, Maibach H: *Atlas of infections of the skin*, Philadelphia, 1999, Saunders, p 176.)

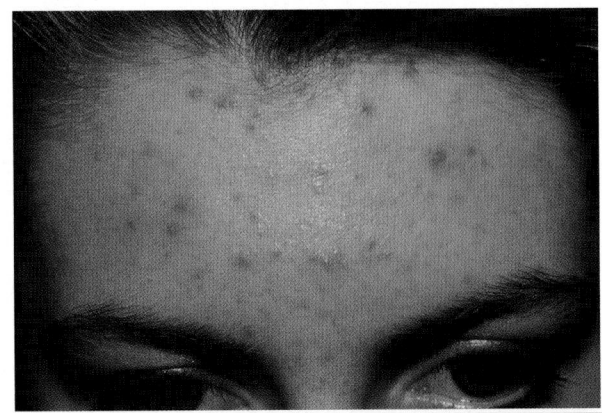

Mild inflammatory acne. Several inflammatory papules. (From Weston WL, Lane AT, Morelli JG: *Color textbook of pediatric dermatology*, ed 4, St Louis, 2007, Mosby, p 27.)

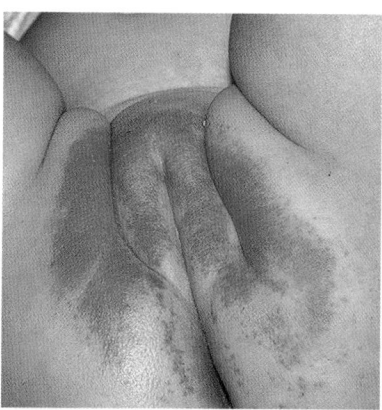

Irritant diaper dermatitis. (Adapted from White G, Cox N: *Diseases of the skin*, ed 2, St Louis, Mosby, 2006.)

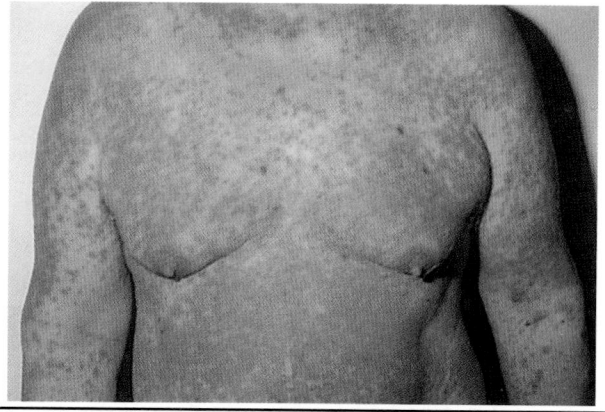

Allergic drug eruption in an erythematous and symmetric rash, usually generalized. (From Lookingbill DP, Marks JG: *Principles of dermatology*, ed 2, Philadelphia, 1993, Saunders, p 218.)

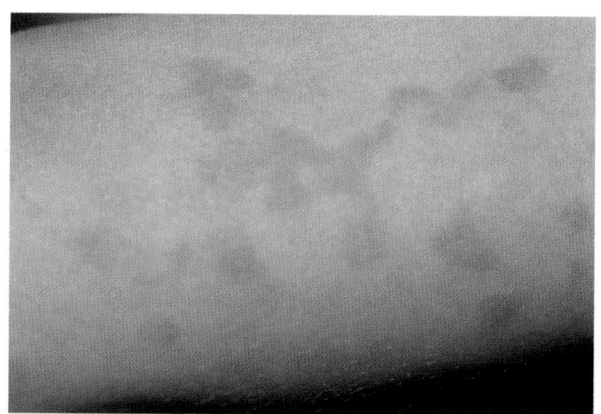

Urticaria. (From Weston WL, Lane AT, Morelli JG: *Color textbook of pediatric dermatology*, ed 4, St Louis, 2007, Mosby, p 259.)

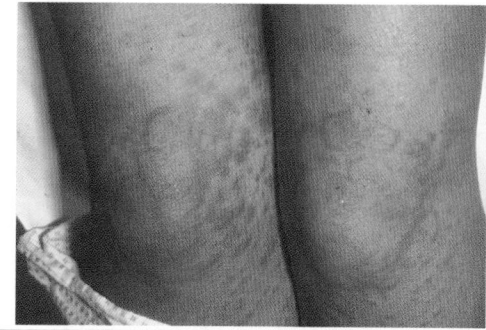

Erythema multiforme secondary to herpes simplex. (From Arndt KA, Wintroub BU, Robinson JK, et al: *Primary care dermatology*, Philadelphia, 1997, Saunders.)

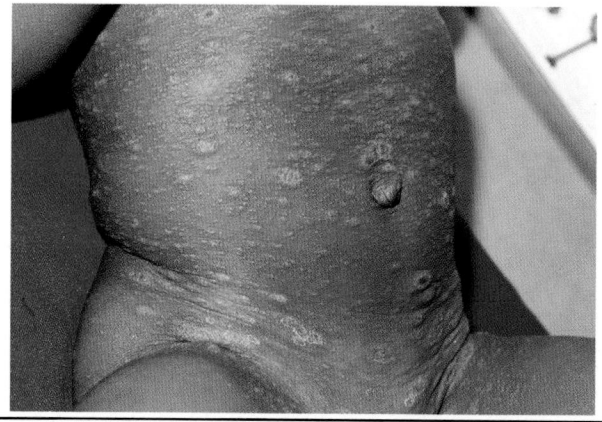

Pityriasis rosea. Truncal involvement with larger plaques and predominantly round papular lesions, most commonly seen in young children and African-Americans. Note the peripheral scale and distribution along skin lines. (From Paller AS, Mancini AJ: *Hurwitz clinical pediatric dermatology: a textbook of skin disorders of childhood and adolescence,* ed 3, Philadelphia, 2006, Saunders, p 101.)

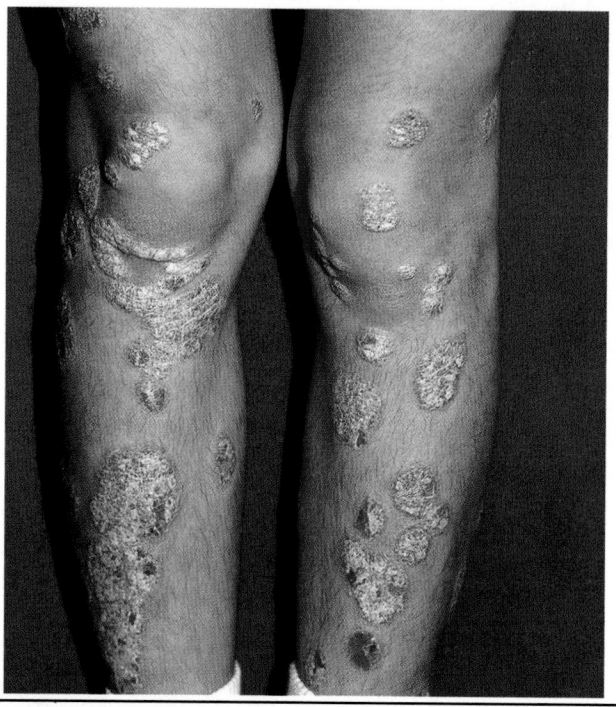

Psoriasis. Typical plaques of psoriasis with thick, micaceous scale overlying erythema. (From Paller AS, Mancini AJ: *Hurwitz clinical pediatric dermatology: a textbook of skin disorders of childhood and adolescence,* ed 3, Philadelphia, 2006, Saunders, p 86.)

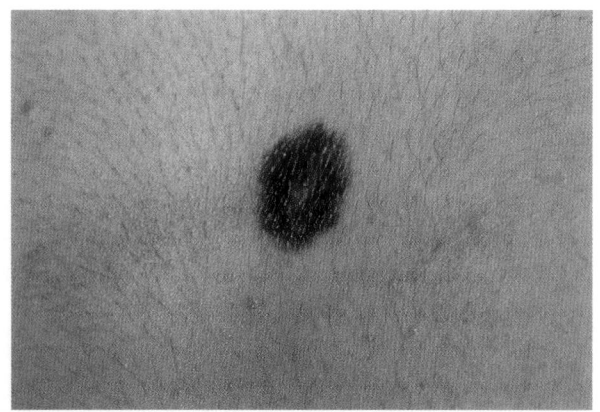

Halo nevus. Loss of pigment around regressing central intradermal nevus. (From Weston WL, Lane AT, Morelli JG: *Color textbook of pediatric dermatology*, ed 4, St Louis, 2007, Mosby, p 329.)

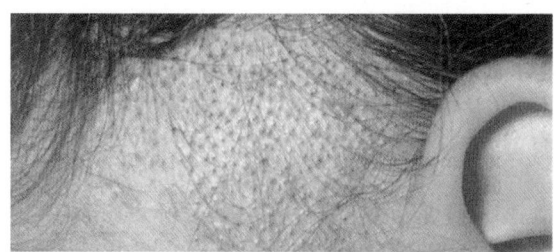

Tinea capitis showing a black dot variety with minimal inflammation. (From Aly R, Maibach H: *Atlas of infections of the skin*, Philadelphia, 1999, Saunders, p 20.)

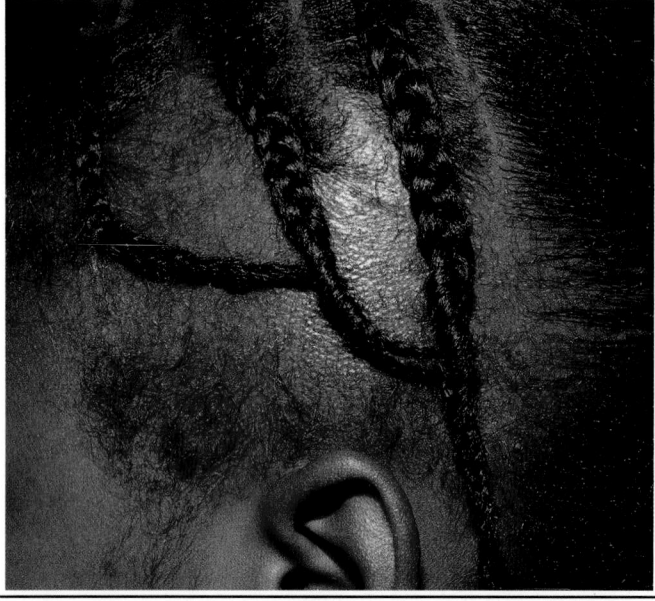

Traction alopecia. (From James WD, Berger TG, Elston DM: *Andrews' diseases of the skin: clinical dermatology*, ed 11, Philadelphia, 2011, Saunders.)

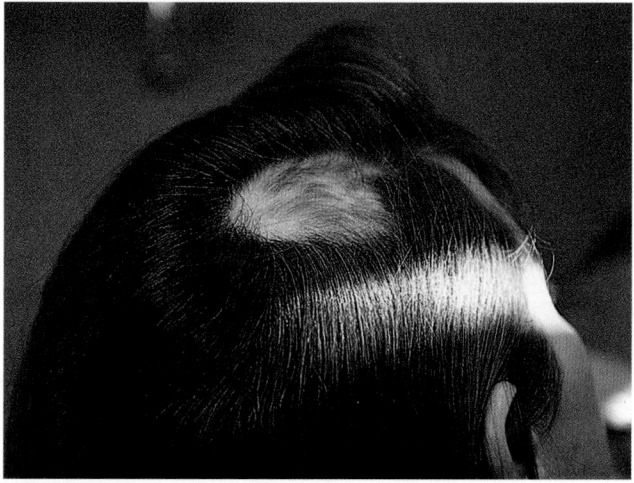

Alopecia areata. (From Thibodeau GA, Patton KT: *The human body in health & disease*, ed 5, St Louis, 2010, Mosby.)

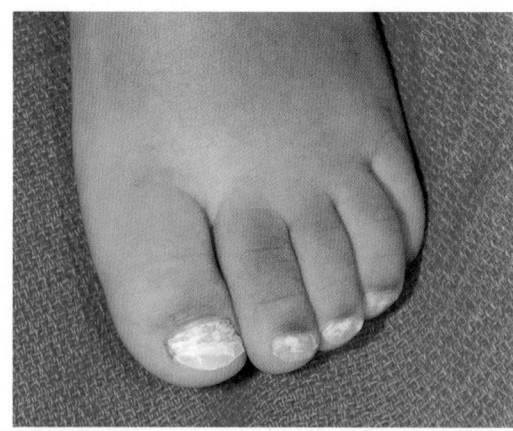

Onychomycosis, proximal subungal type. White discoloration of the nail plate, with the process originating in the proximal nail fold regions. (From Paller AS, Mancini AJ: *Hurwitz clinical pediatric dermatology: a textbook of skin disorders of childhood and adolescence,* ed 3, Philadelphia, 2006, Saunders, p 461.)

BOX 36-4	Descriptive Terms for Dermatologic Lesions

Acral—involving extremities (hands, feet, ears, etc.)
Annular—ring-shaped
Arcuate—arc-shaped
Circinate—circular
Confluent—running together
Contiguous—touching or adjacent
Diffuse or generalized—scattered, widely distributed
Discrete—distinct and separate
Eczematous—referring to vesicles with oozing crust
Grouped—arranged in sets
Guttate—small, droplike
Herpetiform—referring to grouped vesicles resembling those of herpes
Iris—arranged in concentric circles, one inside the other
Linear—arranged in a line
Localized—in a limited area
Nummular—coin-shaped
Pedunculated—having a stalk
Polycyclic—oval with more than 1 ring
Reticular—netlike
Serpiginous—snakelike, creeping
Symmetric—balanced on both sides
Target lesion—(iris or targetoid) erythematous papule or plaque characterized by a red to violet dusky center surrounded by a raised, edematous pale ring and red periphery
Telangiectatic—referring to dilated terminal vessels
Umbilicated—depressed or shaped like a navel
Verrucous—wartlike
Zosteriform—resembling shingles, following a nerve root or dermatome

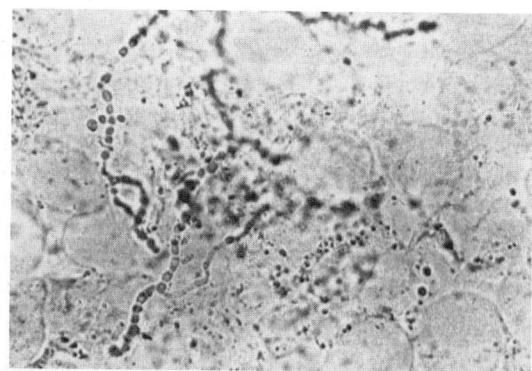

FIGURE 36-2 Fungal elements (hyphae) as seen on microscopic examination of a potassium hydroxide preparation. (From Hurwitz S: *Clinical pediatric dermatology*, ed 2, Philadelphia, 1993, Saunders, p 374.)

subungual debris. Laboratory tests that can be used include the following:

- Microscopic examination of skin scrapings:
  - Potassium hydroxide (KOH) can be used to examine for fungal disorders (hyphae or spores; Fig. 36-2). Scrape fine scales from the edge of the lesion onto a glass slide. Add a drop of KOH 20% to dissolve debris, and cover with a coverslip. Let sit for 20 to 30 minutes or heat gently (do not boil). Use × 10 magnification to examine.
  - Wright, Giemsa, or Gram stains are used to examine for bacteria or herpes simplex or herpes zoster (HZ) giant cells. Allow scrapings to air-dry, then stain with Wright or Giemsa stain. Use × 40 magnification to examine for bacteria.
- Tzanck smear for herpes, varicella, or zoster
- Microbial culture of lesions for bacteria, viruses, or fungi. Simple, inexpensive culture methods for fungal organisms include the dermatophyte test medium [DTM] and InTray CCD [includes *Candida*]. Skin or nail scrapings or hairs, including the root, are applied so that they break the agar surface. A color change is noted in 1 to 5 days.
- Patch or skin testing for allergic or contact reactions is usually done by dermatologists or allergists.
- Skin biopsy following local anesthesia may be by punch or shave method for any tumor, palpable purpura, persistent dermatitis, or blister that is not otherwise definitively diagnosed. Such procedures often require referral to a dermatologist.
- Complete blood count (CBC) and erythrocyte sedimentation rate (ESR) may evaluate infection or inflammation.

■ Management Strategies

HYDRATION AND LUBRICATION

Adequate skin hydration is essential to prevent and treat skin conditions. If the skin is overhydrated, the bonds between cells at the stratum corneum loosen and the barrier is broken. If the skin is too dry, it cracks, again breaking the barrier.

Bathing

Bathing is an efficient means of hydrating and lubricating the skin, especially with dry skin or in dry climates. Luke-warm, not hot, water should be used. The bath should last long enough for skin to become moisturized without becoming supersaturated or "pruned." Bubble-bath solutions are especially irritating and should be avoided. Soaping and shampooing should be done at the end of the bath followed by thorough rinsing. The skin should be gently dried and a lubricating agent applied immediately. See Chapter 24 for further information on lubricating baths. Baths containing baking soda or colloidal oatmeal may help relieve pruritus. Bathing and other heat exposures can make a rash seem worse temporarily.

Environmental Considerations

Because water is essential to skin integrity, environmental humidity also plays a role. Excessive humidity (greater than 90%) or deficient humidity (less than 10%) can cause disruption of the skin. Macerated skin, for example, benefits from less humidity. Itching from excessively dry skin is often relieved by increased humidity provided by using a vaporizer or humidifier. In hot temperatures, itching can be alleviated by air conditioning. Water consumption also plays a role in maintaining proper skin hydration, and children should be encouraged to drink plenty of water.

Skin Care Agents

Soaps, Oils, and Colloids. Mild soaps are best and include Dove, Aveeno, Neutrogena, Basis, Alpha Keri, and Lubriderm. Cetaphil cleanser and Purpose Gentle Cleansing Wash are soap substitutes. Bath oils include Alpha Keri and Domol. Colloids include Aveeno.

Moisturizers and Lubricants. Moisturizers and lubricants treat chronic dryness and inflammation of the skin by retaining water in the skin. Composed of petrolatum or a mixture of petrolatum and lanolin, moisturizers and lubricants are most effective when applied to damp skin. Petrolatum-based lubricants include Moisturel, Purpose, Dermasil cream, Vaseline pure petroleum jelly, and Vaseline Dermatology Formula Lotion. Petrolatum and lanolin combinations include Aquaphor ointment, Eucerin cream and lotion, Lubriderm lotion, and Keri Creme. Glycerin preparations without lanolin or petrolatum include Corn Huskers Lotion, Cetaphil, Keri Light, and Neutrogena.

Sunscreens and Sunblocks. Sunscreens and sunblocks protect the skin from UV light and are graded by their ability to provide sun protection. Daily application of a fragrance-free sunscreen with a minimum sun protection factor (SPF) greater than 30 is recommended (American Academy of Dermatology, 2010). Children who are extremely photosensitive should use sunscreen with levels of SPF 30 or higher. Sunscreens that act by absorbing UV light in the B range include para-aminobenzoic acid (PABA) or PABA esters, cinnamates, salicylates, benzophenones, and anthranilates. Only benzophenones protect from UV rays in the longer UVA range. Sunblocks, including titanium dioxide, zinc oxide, and talc, scatter light and act as protective barriers. They are especially useful on the nose, ears, and lips (see Box 36-10).

Chemical-containing sunscreens should be applied 30 minutes before exposure to the sun to allow binding of the agents to the stratum corneum. Sunblocks can be applied immediately before sun exposure. Reapply sunscreens after swimming, excessive periods of perspiration, or after washing or showering. Sunscreen is never a substitute for sensible sun protection, which includes limiting exposure to intense sun rays. Other protective strategies include wearing protective clothing, hats with visors, and sunglasses with UV protection.

Wet Dressings

For acute oozing, crusting, or itching skin, wet dressings are useful to help dry the skin, decrease itching, and remove crusts. Thin cloths, such as diapers, handkerchiefs, or strips of sheets, make the best wet dressings. Dressings should be moderately wet but not dripping, with lukewarm water and applied for 10 to 20 minutes two to four times daily over a period of 48 to 72 hours. During the treatment dressings must be kept wet either by removing and rewetting or by applying water directly to the dressing. Alternative solutions include saline (1 teaspoon salt with 1 pint of water) or Burow solution (one Domeboro tablet [aluminum acetate; calcium acetate] with one pint of cool or tepid water). The medication in creams or ointments applied following wet dressings is absorbed more effectively. A slightly more intense technique involves applying a steroid ointment or cream to the skin, then covering the skin with a wet dressing and then a dry dressing (e.g., a sleeper, pajamas, or long johns are wetted, put on, and covered with a dry sleeper or long johns) (Weston et al, 2007). The dressing is changed every 6 hours for 24 to 72 hours or is used overnight for 5 to 10 nights. When using this technique, care must be taken to prevent excessive steroidal absorption by applying steroid only to areas needing it, especially in infants and young children.

BOX 36-5 Preparations of Topical Medications

Creams—contain more water than oil and therefore are less occlusive; better used with less dry skin, in high-humidity areas, in summertime, and on parts of body that naturally cause occlusion (body folds); often accepted better by patient, but must be applied every 2 to 3 hours

Gels—alcohol based, provide good penetration of skin, but can burn on application; primarily used for acne and in hairy areas

Lotions—mixtures of powder and water, useful for drying, cooling, and soothing actions; *emulsion lotions* contain some oil, so are not as drying as lotions; lotions come in suspension or solution

Oils—fluid fats that hold medication to the skin as barriers or occlusive agents

Ointments—best used with dry skin; composed primarily of oil with little or no water; provide most potent concentration of medication because of their occlusive action on skin; generally need to be used only every 12 hours; tend to leave a greasy feeling and can cause heat retention from decreased evaporation

Pastes—made of a combination of powder and oil, which makes them somewhat difficult to apply and remove, but effective in providing dryness and protection for skin

Powders—absorb moisture and reduce friction, provide cooling, decrease itching, increase evaporation

Shampoos—liquid soaps or detergents for cleaning the hair and skin (e.g., tar for psoriasis or seborrhea, antifungal shampoos for tinea versicolor or tinea corporis)

Occlusive Dressings

Occlusive dressings decrease water evaporation from the skin and enhance hydration and absorption of topical medications. Plastic wrap is placed over the affected area after hydrating the skin and applying cream or ointment; these dressings should not be left on longer than 8 hours. Ointments, oils, urea compounds, and propylene glycol used alone are occlusive. Skinfolds serve as naturally occurring occlusive areas. Lichen simplex chronicus, dyshidrotic eczema, and psoriasis are skin conditions that benefit from occlusion.

Other Considerations

- Irritants and sensitizing agents, such as wool, sweat, and saliva, should be avoided.
- Allergens and foods that most commonly cause skin reactions include milk, eggs, wheat, tomatoes, citrus, chocolate, fish, and nuts.

MEDICATIONS

Topical treatments are most commonly used for dermatologic conditions. Topical therapy restores hydration, alleviates symptoms, reduces inflammation, protects the skin, reduces scale and debris, cleanses, and eradicates causative organisms.

Thought must be given not only to the medication used in treating skin conditions but also its preparation (Box 36-5) and vehicle (Fig. 36-3), including stabilizers, preservatives, and perfumes. Occasionally an individual is sensitive to a medication vehicle or preparation, and symptoms are aggravated rather than relieved. Common agents that cause sensitization include ethylenediamine, lanolin, parabens, thimerosal, diphenhydramine, propylene glycol, "caines," and neomycin.

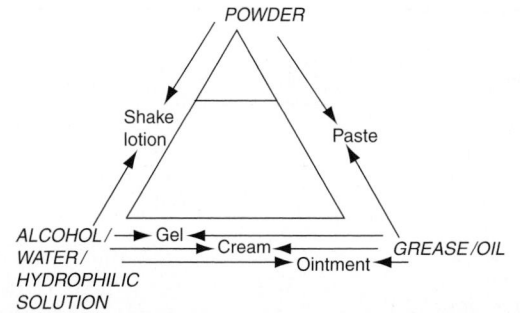

FIGURE 36-3 Vehicles for dermatologic therapy. See Box 36-5 for description.

The following guidelines for use of preparations may be helpful:

- Acute inflammation—wet dressings, powders, suspension lotions, alcohol- or water-based lotions, or aerosols
- Chronic inflammation—creams, oil-based lotions or gels, ointments
- Patient's tolerance for and willingness to use certain vehicles
- Patient's environment (dry or humid)

All topical medications except powders have enhanced absorption if applied to skin immediately after it has been saturated with water. Occlusion enhances absorption (skinfolds or plastic wraps; see previous discussion). Application of the topical medication is best done in one direction, preferably along the hair follicles, without rubbing, applied with a single motion. Use an adequate but not excessive amount.

Antibacterial Agents

Topical antiseptics, soap, and antibacterial soap reduce the number of bacteria on the skin and provide thorough cleansing. Examples of antiseptics include povidone-iodine, chlorhexidine gluconate, and pHisoderm. Topical antibiotics, such as bacitracin, polymyxin B, mupirocin, or retapamulin applied directly to the skin, are used to treat minor skin infections. Products containing neomycin should be avoided because of the high incidence of contact sensitization. Oral antibiotics used to treat more significant bacterial infections include penicillins, erythromycin, cephalosporins, and tetracycline. If methicillin-resistant *Staphylococcus aureus* (MRSA) is suspected, obtain a culture and sensitivity of the drainage (see Chapter 23).

Antifungal Agents

Many topical antifungals are over-the-counter medications. Oral antifungals are used for hair and nail infections or refractory skin infections. Because of concerning side effects and minimal clinical experience in children, oral antifungals should be used with caution in children; many of these drugs are not U.S. Food and Drug Administration (FDA) approved for pediatric use (antifungal agents are listed in Table 36-4).

Antiviral Agents

Topical antivirals are used to control cutaneous herpes infections. Oral antivirals, such as acyclovir, can shorten the course of the infection and should be used in children with acute or recurrent herpetic skin infections.

Wart therapy agents destroy keratinocytes. These include salicylic acid and lactic acid collodion, salicylic plaster, salicylic solution, liquid nitrogen, cantharidin, podophyllum, and trichloroacetic acid.

Antiacne Agents

Topical keratolytics are used in acne to relieve follicular obstruction by inhibiting bacteria and promoting peeling of the skin. The two most common keratolytics are benzoyl peroxide and retinoic acid. They are the first line of treatment for mild acne and are used in combination with other agents for moderate or severe acne. Topical antibiotics have few side effects and are most effective in maintaining control of acne. Clindamycin, erythromycin, and sulfacetamide are the most commonly used topical antibiotics. Systemic antibiotics such as tetracycline, doxycycline, minocycline, and erythromycin, are effective in treating inflammatory acne. Antibiotics work by decreasing the population of *Propionibacterium acnes*. The oral retinoid, isotretinoin, is effective in nodulocystic acne that is not responsive to other combination treatments. Patients taking isotretinoin should be monitored by a dermatologist, with tightly controlled follow-up and prescriptions. The use of isotretinoin is contraindicated in pregnancy because of teratogenic effects. Some estrogen containing oral contraceptives are being combined with antiandrogen for treating acne. Studies have shown ethinyl estradiol-drospirenone and ethinyl estradiol-cyproterone to be most effective (Thielitz and Gollnick, 2009). Photodynamic therapy is also an option.

Antiinflammatory Agents

Topical glucocorticoids are frequently used to reduce inflammation, decrease itching, and promote vasoconstriction without causing the widespread systemic effects of oral steroids. They are subdivided into three categories: high potency, moderate potency, and low potency (Table 36-1). It is important to note that steroids are classified as fluorinated or nonfluorinated. Nonfluorinated steroids are less potent and have fewer side effects.

Primary care providers should rarely use high-potency topical steroid preparations. Only low-potency steroids should be used on the face, buttocks, groin, and axillae. Always use the lowest potency available, use them sparingly, and for the shortest length of time. The key to using topical steroids is to be familiar with a few low-, medium-, and high-potency steroids and use them consistently. Brand-name preparations often have a more consistent base and potency. Ointments are more potent than creams, creams are more potent than lotions, and foams are better in hairy areas. Absorption is enhanced in areas that are traumatized or denuded. Potential side effects of prolonged topical steroid use include skin atrophy, striae, increased fragility of the skin, hypopigmentation, secondary infection, acneiform eruption, folliculitis, miliaria, hypertrichosis, telangiectasia, and purpura.

Oral glucocorticoids (prednisone) are used only in acute situations and are limited to short courses. Intralesional steroid injections may be used by a dermatologist to control localized eczema, lichen planus, or psoriasis.

TABLE 36-1	Topical Corticosteroids		
Class	**Generic Name**	**Trade Name**	**Potency**
1	Betamethasone dipropionate, augmented 0.05% Clobetasol propionate 0.05%	Diprolene 0.05% Diproline AF 0.05% Temovate 0.05% Dermovate 0.05%	High potency
	Diflorasone diacetate 0.05% Halobetasol propionate	Psorcon 0.05% Ultravate 0.05%	↑↑↑↑
2	Amcinonide Betamethasone dipropionate Diflorasone diacetate	Cyclocort ointment 0.1% Diprosone ointment 0.05% Florone ointment 0.05% Maxiflor ointment 0.05%	
	Halcinonide Fluocinonide	Halog cream 0.1% Halciderm 0.1% Lidex cream 0.05% Metosyn 0.05%	
	Desoximetasone Mometasone furoate	Lidex ointment 0.05% Topicort cream 0.25% Elocon ointment 0.1%	↑↑↑
3	Betamethasone dipropionate Betamethasone benzoate Betamethasone valerate	Diprosone cream 0.05% Benisone gel 0.025% Valisone ointment 0.1% Betacap 0.1%	
	Fluticasone propionate	Cutivate ointment 0.05%	↑↑
4	Triamcinolone acetonide	Aristocort ointment 0.1% Kenalog ointment 0.1% Adocortyl 0.1%	
	Flurandrenolide Fluocinolone acetonide	Cordran ointment 0.05% Synalar cream 0.025%	↑
5	Desonide Flurandrenolide Fluocinolone acetonide	Tridesilon ointment 0.05% Cordran SP cream 0.05% Fluonid cream 0.01% Synalar 0.025% Synalar cream 0.01%	Medium potency ↓ ↑
	Clocortolone pivalate Betamethasone valerate Hydrocortisone valerate Hydrocortisone butyrate Prednicarbate 0.1%	Cloderm cream 0.1% Valisone cream 0.1% Westcort cream 0.2% Locoid cream 0.1% Dermatop cream/ointment	
6	Hydrocortisone 1%, urea 10% Flumetasone pivalate Desonide 0.05%	Alphaderm cream 1% Locorten cream 0.03% Tridesilon cream 0.05% DesOwen cream Aclovate cream 0.05%	↓↓
	Alclometasone dipropionate	Modrasone 0.05% Desonide 0.05%	
7	Hydrocortisone 1%	Hytone cream 1%; Cobadex 1%; Dioderm 0.1%; Mildison 1%; Hydrocortisyl 1%; Hytone ointment 1%	↓↓↓
	Dexamethasone Methylprednisolone acetate Prednisolone	Hexadrol cream 0.04% Medrol ointment 0.25% Meti-Derm cream 0.5%	
8	Hydrocortisone 0.5%	Cortaid cream	Low potency

From Cohen BA: *Pediatric dermatology*, ed 3, Philadelphia, 2005, Mosby, p 11; Taketomo CK, Hodding JH, Kraus DM: *Pediatric dosage handbook*, ed 17, Hudson, OH, 2011, Lexi-Comp; Weston WL, Lane AT, Morelli JG: *Color textbook of pediatric dermatology*, ed 4, St Louis, 2007, Mosby.

TABLE 36-2	Diagnosis and Treatment of Common Bacterial Infections

	Causative Organism	Presentation	Area of Involvement	Treatment	Prevention
Impetigo	*Staphylococcus aureus* or *Streptococcus pyogenes*	Honey-colored crust on erythematous base, or blisters that rupture, leaving varnish-like coat	Superficial layers of skin (epidermis)	Topical antibiotic if minor, oral antibiotics (amoxicillin clavulanate or cephalexin) if more significant infection	Moisturize skin; thoroughly cleanse any break in skin
Cellulitis	Most commonly group A streptococcus (GAS) or *S. aureus*	Erythema, swelling, tenderness; irregular borders with significant induration resembling an orange peel is associated with GAS	Dermis and subcutaneous tissue	Oral antibiotic depending on likely organism; amoxicillin clavulanate (first-line) or cephalexin or dicloxacillin	Same as above
Folliculitis	*S. aureus*	Pruritus, erythematous papule or pustule at hair follicle	Hair follicle	Warm compresses, topical keratolytics, topical antibiotics, or antistaphylococcal antibiotic if severe	Same as above; good hygiene and antibacterial soap

Antipruritic Agents

Antihistamines are used both for sedation and to relieve itching. The most commonly used antihistamines are hydroxyzine, cetirizine, fexofenadine, and diphenhydramine. Topical antihistamines, especially diphenhydramine HCl and "caine" medications, should be avoided because of the possibility of contact sensitization. Menthol and pramoxine are topical anesthetics that do not cause sensitization (Patel et al, 2007).

Topical Calcineurin Inhibitors

This class of immunosuppressive, nonsteroidal antiinflammatory topical medication is used for short-term or intermittent long-term treatment of atopic dermatitis when conventional therapy is inadvisable, ineffective, or not tolerated. Immunomodulators are expensive and cannot be used in children younger than 2 years of age (see Chapter 24).

Scabicides and Pediculicides

These agents are toxic to mites and lice. Crotamiton (Eurax), permethrin (Elimite, Nix), and pyrethrin plus piperonyl butoxide are used in children but should be used sparingly. Lindane (Kwell) is no longer recommended for use in children.

Hair and Scalp Preparations

Antimicrobial, tar, keratolytic, and detergent shampoos are used on the hair and scalp.

COUNSELING AND ANTICIPATORY GUIDANCE

It is essential to spend adequate time with the patient and parents to discuss the child's skin condition and the family's concerns and needs. Education regarding the disease, plan of treatment, and potential risks and benefits should be provided. Because disorders of the skin are so visible, time must be spent discussing the short- and long-term prognoses and potential plans to prevent complications, recurrence, and spread.

■ Bacterial Infections of the Skin and Subcutaneous Tissue

Diagnosis and treatment of common bacterial infections are listed in Table 36-2.

IMPETIGO

Description

Impetigo is a common contagious bacterial infection of the superficial layers of the skin. It has two forms: nonbullous, with honey-colored crusts on the lesions, and bullous (see Color Plate).

Epidemiology

Impetigo is usually caused by group A streptococcus, *Staphylococcus aureus,* or MRSA. Often streptococcus and staphyloccus can be cultured from an impetigo lesion. Nonbullous impetigo accounts for more than 70% of cases, with *S. aureus* as the most common pathogen rather than group A streptococcus as had occurred in the past, and usually follows some type of skin trauma (e.g., bites, abrasions, varicella) or another skin disease such as atopic dermatitis. Bullous impetigo occurs sporadically, develops on intact skin, and is more common in infants and young children. Certain epidermal types of *S. aureus* produce a toxin that causes bullous skin lesions.

Bacterial colonization of the skin occurs several days to months before lesions appear; the organism usually spreads from autoinoculation via hands, towels, clothing, nasal discharge, or droplets. Impetigo occurs more frequently with poor hygiene; during the summer months; in warm, humid climates; and in lower socioeconomic groups. Streptococci that cause pharyngitis rarely cause impetigo and vice versa.

Secondary bacterial infections of underlying skin problems (dermatitis, varicella, psoriasis) are most commonly caused by staphylococci (Weston et al, 2007).

Clinical Findings

History

- Pruritus, spread of the lesion to surrounding skin, and earlier skin disruption at the site
- Weakness, fever, diarrhea may accompany bullous impetigo

Physical Examination. The following can be found:

- Nonbullous, classic, or common impetigo—begins as 1- to 2-mm erythematous papules or pustules that progress to vesicles or bullae, which rupture, leaving moist, honey-colored, crusty lesions on mildly erythematous, eroded skin; less than 2 cm in size; little pain but rapid spread
- Bullous impetigo—large, flaccid, thin-wall, superficial, annular, or oval pustular blisters or bullae that rupture, leaving thin varnish-like coating or scale
- Lesions are most common on face, hands, neck, extremities, or perineum; satellite lesions near the primary site, although they can be found anywhere on the body
- Regional lymphadenopathy

Diagnostic Studies. Gram stain and culture are ordered if identification of the organism is needed in recalcitrant or severe cases.

Differential Diagnosis

Herpes simplex, varicella, nummular eczema, contact dermatitis, tinea, kerion, and scabies are included in the differential diagnosis.

Management

Management involves the following:

- Topical antibiotics may be used if the impetigo is superficial, nonbullous, or localized to a limited area. Topical treatment alone provides clinical improvement, but may prolong the carrier state (Weston et al, 2007). Mupirocin and retapamulin are the best choices for topical treatment (Koning et al, 2008; Weinberg and Tyring, 2010; Weston et al, 2007; Yang and Kearn, 2008). Polymyxin B, gentamicin, and bacitracin are less effective (Parish and Parish, 2008).
- Oral antibiotics are recommended for multiple lesions or nonbullous impetigo with infection in multiple family members, childcare groups, or athletes. Treat for *S. aureus* and *Streptococcus pyogenes* because coexistence is common (Cole and Gazewood, 2007; Weston et al, 2007).
  - Amoxicillin/clavulanate: 90 mg/kg/day for 10 days
  - Cephalexin: 40 mg/kg/day for 10 days
  - Dicloxacillin: 15 to 50 mg/kg/day for 10 days
  - Cloxacillin: 50 to 100 mg/kg/day for 10 days
  - Clindamycin: 10 to 25 mg/kg/day for 10 days
- For widespread infection with constitutional symptoms and deeper skin involvement, use an oral antibiotic active against beta-lactamase–producing strains of *S. aureus,* such as amoxicillin/clavulanate, dicloxacillin, cloxacillin, or cephalexin.
- If an infant has bullous impetigo, use parenteral beta-lactamase–resistant antistaphylococcal penicillin, such as methicillin, oxacillin, or nafcillin.

- If there is no response in 7 days, swab beneath the crust and do Gram stain, culture, and sensitivities. Community-acquired MRSA should be considered. This organism is more susceptible to clindamycin and trimethoprim-sulfamethoxazole (TMP-SMX) (see Chapter 23 for treatment of MRSA).
- Educate regarding cleanliness, handwashing, and spread of disease.
- Exclude from daycare or school until treated for 24 hours.
- Schedule a follow-up appointment in 48 to 72 hours if not improved.

Complications

- Cellulitis may occur with nonbullous impetigo and present in the form of ecthyma (infection involving entire epidermis) or erysipelas (spreading cellulitis with induration).
- Lymphangitis, suppurative lymphadenitis, guttate psoriasis, erythema multiforme (EM), scarlet fever, or glomerulonephritis may occur following infection with some strains of *Streptococcus*. Acute rheumatic fever is a rare complication of streptococcal skin infections.
- Staphylococcal scalded skin syndrome (SSSS) is a blistering disease that results from circulating epidermolytic toxin–producing *S. aureus*. SSSS is most common in neonates (Ritter disease), infants, and young children less than 5 years of age. It manifests abruptly with fever, malaise, and tender erythroderma, especially in the neck folds and axillae, rapidly becoming crusty around the eyes, nose, and mouth. Nikolsky sign (peeling of skin with a light rub to reveal a moist red surface) is a key finding. Treatment may include hospitalization and parenteral antibiotics, especially for young children (Berk and Bayliss, 2010). Antibiotics of choice are intravenous (IV) or oral dicloxacillin, a penicillinase-resistant penicillin, first- or second-generation cephalosporins, or clindamycin. Quicker healing without scarring results if steroids are avoided, there is minimal handling of the skin, and ointments and topical mupirocin are used at the infection site (Aronson and Florin, 2009; Berk and Bayliss, 2010). Severe cases may need treatment similar to extensive burn care.

Patient Education and Prevention

- Thorough cleansing of any breaks in the skin helps prevent impetigo.
- Postinflammatory pigment changes can last weeks to months.
- The patient should not return to school or day care until 24 hours of antibiotic treatment is completed.

CELLULITIS

Description

Cellulitis is a localized bacterial infection often involving the dermis and subcutaneous layers of the skin. It is commonly seen following a disruption of the skin surface from an insect or animal bite, trauma, or a penetrating wound. Cellulitis is more common in children with diabetes and immunosuppression. Periorbital cellulitis is discussed in Chapter 28.

Epidemiology

In children cellulitis is often periorbital, perivaginal, perianal, or buccal, or it involves a joint or an extremity. *Streptococcus pneumoniae* and *S. aureus* are the most common causes (Fisher et al, 2009; Morelli, 2007). Buccal cellulitis and infections over joints are most commonly caused by *Haemophilus influenzae* and occur in 3-month-olds to 3-year-olds (Weston et al, 2007). Periorbital and orbital cellulitis are most commonly caused by streptococcal species (*S. pneumoniae* and group A beta-hemolytic streptococcus [GABHS]). Most cases of cellulitis of the extremities and perianal area are caused by streptococci or *S. aureus* (Fisher et al, 2009). MRSA can also cause cellulitis with pus accumulation. Rarely, other aerobic, anaerobic, and fungal organisms can cause cellulitis in immunocompromised individuals.

Clinical Findings
History
- A previous skin disruption at the site or recent upper respiratory infection *(H. influenzae)*. Note that edema that occurs within 24 hours of an insect bite is most likely to be inflammatory, whereas edema that occurs between 48 to 72 hours is more likely to be infectious.
- Fever, pain, malaise, irritability, anorexia, vomiting, and chills can be reported.
- Recent sore throat or upper respiratory infection
- Anal pruritus, stool retention, constipation, and blood-streaked stools

Physical Examination
- Erythematous, indurated, tender, swollen, warm areas of skin with poorly demarcated borders
- Blue to purple tinge to the cellulitis is often associated with *H. influenzae* (Weston et al, 2007)
- Regional lymphadenopathy
- Well-demarcated perianal erythema up to 2 cm around the anus. The erythema may extend to the vulva and vagina (Gerber, 2007).
- Erysipelas—a superficial variant of cellulitis—presents with rapidly advancing lesions that are tender, bright red, have sharp margins and an "orange peel" look and feel.

Diagnostic Studies.
CBC and blood culture are done if the child is febrile, appears ill or toxic, or is less than 1 year of age. Leukocytosis is common. Blood cultures are positive in less than 5% of cases (Fisher et al, 2009). Perform gram stain and culture of the erythematous area if unusual organisms are suspected, pus is present (which is more typical of MRSA), or the child looks toxic. An aspirate at the point of maximum inflammation is more likely to yield a causative organism than one taken from the leading edge, though the bacterial counts tend to be low with either method (Morelli, 2007; Weston et al, 2007). Gram stains and cultures lead to identification of the causative organism in less than 25% of cases (Fisher et al, 2009).

Differential Diagnosis

Pressure erythema, giant urticaria, contact dermatitis, Popsicle panniculitis, early erythema nodosum, subcutaneous fat necrosis, herpetic whitlow, and diaper dermatitis are included in the differential diagnosis.

Management

Immediate antibiotic therapy is needed.
- Hospitalization is recommended if the child is a febrile neonate or infant, is acutely ill or toxic, or has periorbital cellulitis.
- Neonates with cellulitis require a full septic workup and initiation of empiric therapy with methicillin or vancomycin and gentamicin or cefotaxime (Morelli, 2007).
- Antibiotic therapy
  ○ Prompt administration of antibiotics is essential.
  ○ If a streptococcal infection is suspected, penicillin is the drug of choice.
    - A hospitalized febrile acutely ill infant or child should have penicillin up to 2 million units per day.
    - Benzathine penicillin: 600,000 to 1,200,000 units IM for one dose
    - Penicillin V: 30 to 60 mg/kg/day orally for 10 days
    - If allergic or concern for multiple organisms a third-generation cephalosporin, such as 50 to 75 mg/kg ceftriaxone intramuscularly (IM) once a day
  ○ If suspected organism is staphylococcus:
    - An initial IM dose of ceftriaxone 50 to 75 mg/kg/dose, then dicloxacillin 50 to 75 mg/kg/day orally, divided four times a day for 10 days or cephalexin 50 to 100 mg/kg/day orally, divided three times a day for 10 days
    - If MRSA suspected, clindamycin 10 to 30 mg/kg/day orally divided three times a day for 10 days
  ○ If suspected organism is *H. influenzae*:
    - Amoxicillin clavulanate 50 to 80 mg/kg/day orally for 10 days
    - Methicillin or a third-generation cephalosporin is also an option.
- Follow up in 24 hours to assess response and observe toxicity. Continue daily visits until child is recovering. Counsel parents to call the provider immediately or return for an urgent visit if the infection is not improving or getting worse.

Complications

Recurrent perianal streptococcal infection, septicemia, necrotizing fasciitis (NF), and toxic shock syndrome (TSS) are possible complications.
- NF is a rare infection in children and has two subtypes. Type I is generally a polymicrobial infection that usually affects children who have an underlying disease. Type II, commonly referred to as flesh-eating strep, is an acute, rapidly progressing necrotic invasion of GABHS through the skin and subcutaneous tissue to the fascial compartments. It is more common in otherwise healthy children or children with varicella. NF is more common in boys less than 5 years of age and children with diabetes, skin injury, surgery, immunodeficiency, IV drug use, malnutrition, and obesity (Leung et al, 2008; Weston et al, 2007). NF begins as cellulitis (usually on the leg or abdomen in infants) with severe pain, edema, fever, and bullae on an erythematous surface. It quickly progresses to ulcer, eschar, and gangrene within 2 days. Prompt treatment (hospitalization, surgical debridement, and fluid management), prolonged antibiotic treatment (penicillin), and IV immunoglobulin (IVIG) may be lifesaving because the overall mortality rate is high.

• TSS is an acute febrile illness with rapid onset that causes significant fever, vomiting and diarrhea, engorged mucous membranes, hypotension, a diffuse macular or sunburn-like rash, conjunctival injection, and multiple organ system involvement. *S. aureus* or *S. pyogenes* (group A streptococci) are the causative agents associated with TSS, and incubation can be as little as 14 hours. Both organisms can be associated with invasive infection (e.g., pneumonia, osteomyelitis, bacteremia, or endocarditis) or focal tissue invasion that is rapidly progressive (American Academy of Pediatrics [AAP], 2009). Initially recognized in menstruating adolescents, TSS is also found in males and younger children. *S. aureus* is usually the causative agent in menstruating females. Nasal packing, surgical procedures, and postpartum condition are some factors linked to nonmenstrual TSS. Treatment is intensive, requires hospitalization, and consists of fluid management, antibiotics, and other supportive measures. Staphylococcal TSS has a mortality rate of 3%, whereas streptococcal TSS has a mortality rate of 30% to 60% (Berk and Bayliss, 2010). It is a reportable disease in most states.

Prevention

• Thorough cleansing of any break in the skin helps prevent cellulitis.
• Keep bites, scrapes, and rashes clean and bandaged until healed to prevent them from being infected by staphylococcal bacteria.
• Frequent handwashing is essential; immunize against *H. influenzae*.
• Perianal spread can occur through shared bath water.
• See Chapter 23 regarding treatment of children and families with MRSA infection.

FOLLICULITIS AND FURUNCLE

Description

A superficial bacterial inflammation of the hair follicle is called *folliculitis*; a deeper infection with involvement of the base of the follicle and deep dermis is called a *furuncle* (boil) (see Color Plate that illustrates staphylococcal superficial folliculitis).

Epidemiology

Obstruction of the follicular orifice is the most important factor contributing to the development of folliculitis, but a moist environment, maceration, poor hygiene, occlusive emollients, and prolonged submersion in contaminated water are also factors. *S. aureus* is a common causative organism as is *Pseudomonas aeruginosa*, which causes hot-tub folliculitis. *Escherichia coli* is also implicated. These infections are more common in males than in females.

Clinical Findings
History
• Pruritus with folliculitis; tenderness with furuncle
• Hot-tub exposure
• Irritating surface agent
• Occasional fever, malaise, or lymphadenopathy

Physical Examination. The child often is asymptomatic, but the following can be seen:
• Discrete, erythematous 1- to 2-mm papules or pustules on an inflamed base centered around a hair follicle
• Involvement of face, scalp, extremities (typically thighs and upper arms), buttocks, and back
• Nodules with larger areas of erythema and tenderness (furuncle)
• Pruritic papules, pustules, or deep red to purple nodules, most dense in areas covered by swimsuit 8 to 48 hours after exposure (hot-tub folliculitis)

Diagnostic Studies. Gram stain and culture are occasionally ordered (e.g., in the case of persistent or difficult-to-treat folliculitis, consider the possibility of MRSA).

Differential Diagnosis

Cellulitis, *Candida* infection, tinea, acne pustules, and chemical folliculitis constitute the differential diagnosis.

Management

The following steps are taken:
• Warm compresses after washing with soap and water several times a day
• Topical keratolytics, such as benzoyl peroxide 5% to 10% twice a day for 5 days, especially if chronic or recurrent
• Topical antibiotic, such as erythromycin or clindamycin, in cream, gel, solution, or ointment twice a day for 10 to 14 days for superficial folliculitis
• Antistaphylococcal beta-lactamase–resistant antibiotics, such as dicloxacillin 15 to 50 mg/kg/day divided four times a day for 7 to 10 days or cephalexin 40 to 50 mg/kg/day divided three times a day for 7 to 10 days in severe or widespread cases
• Review of good personal hygiene habits. Avoid shaving until resolved.
• Follow-up treatment in 1 week for folliculitis, in 1 day for furuncle or abscess, which may need incision and drainage
• Identify and eliminate predisposing factors.
• If recurrent, look for nasal or skin carrier state.

Complications

Deep abscess formation or carbuncles can occur. Sycosis barbae occurs on the chin, upper lip, and jaw, especially in adolescent African-American males.

Patient Education and Prevention

Good personal hygiene and an antibacterial soap minimize spread to other household members. Hot-tub folliculitis resolves in 5 to 14 days but can recur up to 3 months after exposure.

■ Fungal Infections of the Skin

Diagnosis and treatment of common fungal infections are listed in Table 36-3.

TABLE 36-3	Diagnosis and Treatment of Common Fungal Infections			
Infection	**Causative Organism**	**Clinical Findings**	**Management**	**Complications**
Candidiasis	*Candida albicans*	Moist, bright-red diaper rash with sharp borders, satellite lesions; may have associated white spots in mouth, mucous membranes, or corner of mouth	Topical or oral antifungal, generally nystatin; diaper area hygiene	Paronychia or onychomycosis
Tinea corporis	*Trichophyton tonsurans, T. rubrum, Microsporum canis*	Pruritic, slightly erythematous circular lesion with a slightly raised border and central clearing; well demarcated	Topical antifungals; identify and treat source; exclude from daycare until treated; use oral medications for resistant cases	Tinea incognita from steroid treatment
Tinea cruris	*Epidermophyton floccosum, T. rubrum, T. mentagrophytes*	Raised-border, scaly lesion on upper thighs and groin; penis and scrotum spared; symmetric	Same as for tinea corporis; loose clothes, absorbent medicated powder	Possible secondary infection
Tinea pedis	*T. rubrum, T. mentagrophytes*	Vesicles and erosions on instep; fissure between toes with scaling and erythema; diffuse scaling on weight-bearing surfaces with exaggerated scaling in creases; pruritus	Same as for tinea corporis; absorbent medicated powder; cotton socks; open-toed shoes; moisturize	Reinfection common
Tinea versicolor	*Malassezia furfur (Pityrosporum orbiculare, P. ovale)*	Multiple scaly, discrete oval macules on neck, shoulders, upper back, and chest; hypopigmented to hyperpigmented areas; fail to tan in summer	Selenium shampoo; ketoconazole shampoo; topical imidazoles	50% recurrence rate

CANDIDIASIS (MONILIASIS)

Description

Candidiasis is a fungal infection of the skin or mucous membranes commonly called a *yeast infection* or *thrush*. See Chapter 35 for discussion of vaginal candidiasis.

Epidemiology

Candida albicans, a yeastlike fungus, is commonly found on skin and oral, vaginal, and intestinal mucosal tissue. Although *Candida* is part of the normal flora, overgrowth, and penetration of inflamed skin or mucous membranes can occur when there is a localized or systemic alteration in host defenses. Candidiasis is more common in infants, obese children, adolescents, and chronically ill or immunocompromised children. It also is often seen as a secondary infection in persistent diaper rashes or with antibiotic, oral steroid, or oral contraceptive use. Systemic infection with candidiasis is not discussed in this text.

Clinical Findings

History. The history often includes antibiotic or steroid use over the previous weeks and occurrence of a rash in a moist, warm area.

Physical Examination
- Mouth—friable, adherent white plaques on an erythematous base on the mucous membranes (thrush); cracked lips (cheilitis); fissured and inflamed corners of the mouth (angular cheilitis)
- Intertriginous areas (neck, axillae, or groin)—bright erythema in flexural folds
- Diaper area—moist, beefy-red macules and papules with sharply marked borders and satellite lesions; erosions may also be present

- Vulvovaginal area—thick, cheesy, yellow discharge; erythema; edema; and itching
- Nail plates—transverse ridging of the nail plate, loss of cuticle, and mild proximal lateral periungual erythema (chronic paronychia)

Diagnostic Studies. If treatment failure or questionable diagnosis occurs, KOH-treated scrapings of satellite lesions or mucosa reveal yeast cells and pseudohyphae (see Fig. 36-2).

Differential Diagnosis

The differential diagnoses include erythema toxicum, miliaria, staphylococcal pustulosis, transient neonatal pustulosis, neonatal herpes simplex, and congenital syphilis.

Management

The following steps are taken:
- Thrush: Oral nystatin suspension four times a day or gentian violet 1% to 2% aqueous solution applied twice a day until 1 to 2 days after white adherent patches are gone. If breastfeeding, the mother should put the solution on her nipples to eliminate reinfection. A second course is sometimes needed to clear the infection.
- If resistant to treatment, oral fluconazole 6 mg/kg the first day in a single dose; then 3 mg/kg/dose daily for 14 days (Taketomo et al, 2011)
- Thrush (in older children), cheilitis and angular cheilitis: clotrimazole troche 10 mg dissolved slowly five times a day for 14 days (Taketomo et al, 2011)
- Skin infection: Topical antifungals (Table 36-4), such as nystatin, miconazole, clotrimazole, ketoconazole, ciclopirox, or econazole applied to skin every diaper change until the rash is gone plus an additional 1 to 2 days

TABLE 36-4	Antifungal Medications		

Drug (Trade Name)	Strength and Formulation	Application	Mode of Action, Indications, Side Effects, and Comments
Topical Medications Imidazoles			
Clotrimazole	1% C, L, S, P	Twice daily	Fungistatic; erythema, stinging, blistering, peeling, edema, pruritus, hives, burning
Econazole nitrate	1% C	Daily/twice daily	Fungistatic; burning, pruritus, stinging, erythema; may have antibacterial effects
Ketoconazole	2% C, Sh	Daily/twice daily	Fungistatic; irritation, dry skin, pruritus, stinging
Miconazole nitrate	2% C, P, L	Daily/twice daily	Fungistatic; irritation, maceration, urticaria, allergic contact dermatitis, pruritus; economical
Oxiconazole nitrate	1% C, L	Daily/twice daily	Fungistatic; pruritus, burning, irritation, erythema, folliculitis
Sulconazole nitrate	1% C, S	Daily/twice daily	Fungistatic; pruritus, burning, stinging
Allylamines			
Butenafine HCl	C	Daily	Fungicidal; irritation, burning
Naftifine HCl	1% C, G	Daily/twice daily	Fungicidal; burning, stinging, erythema, pruritus, irritation
Terbinafine HCl	1% C, S	Daily/twice daily	Fungicidal; pruritus, irritation, burning
Ethanolamine			
Ciclopirox olamine	1% C, L, G (Penlac Nail Lacquer 8% solution)	Twice daily Penlac applied daily preferably at bedtime	Fungicidal; irritation, erythema, burning
Others			
Gentian violet	1%-2% S	Twice daily	Topical antiseptic/germicide; staining, burning, vesicle formation
Nystatin (Mycolog-II,* Mycostatin, Nilstat, Mytrex*)	100,000 units/g C, P, O, Su	Twice or four times a day	Fungistatic; rare adverse reactions; effective against yeast only
Selenium sulfide (Excel; Head & Shoulders Intensive Treatment Dandruff Shampoo; Selsun Blue)	1% and 2.25% Sh, 2.5% L	Daily for lotion Twice weekly for shampoo for 2 weeks then once every 1 to 4 weeks as needed	Thought to block the enzymes involved in growth of epithelial tissues; discoloration of hair, alopecia; used for tinea capitis (reduces transmission), tinea versicolor, and seborrheic dermatitis (shampoo may be used as lotion)
Tolnaftate	1% C, P, S, G	Two to three times daily	Fungistatic; rare adverse reactions; pruritus, stinging
Oral Medications			
Clotrimazole	10 mg troche	1 troche five times a day dissolved slowly in mouth	Treatment of oral candidiasis; gastrointestinal symptoms; hepatotoxicity
Fluconazole	10 to 40 mg/mL; 50-, 100-, 150-, 200 mg tablets	3 to 6 mg/kg/day in single dose for 2 wk for oropharyngeal candidiasis; day one dosage is 6 mg/kg (children) and 200 mg/dose (adults) followed by daily therapy of 3 mg/kg/dose (pediatric) and 100 mg/dose (adults)	Approved for pediatric use for oropharyngeal, esophageal, or disseminated candidiasis; possible drug interactions; elevated AST, ALT, or alkaline phosphatase; hepatitis

TABLE 36-4	Antifungal Medications—cont'd		
Drug (Trade Name)	**Strength and Formulation**	**Application**	**Mode of Action, Indications, Side Effects, and Comments**
Griseofulvin	Ultramicrosized Microsized	>2 yr: 5 to 15 mg/kg in single or in two divided doses; max dose 750 mg/day 10 to 20 mg/kg/day given daily or two divided doses	Fungistatic; mainstay of therapy; excellent safety profile and extensive use; monitor CBC LFTs, renal function at 8 wk and every 8 wk while on treatment; possible drug interactions Duration of treatment: tinea corporis: 2 to 4 wk; tinea capitis: 4 to 6 wk or longer; tinea pedis: 4 to 8 wk; tinea unguium: 4 to 6 mo or longer
Itraconazole		Consult pediatric dermatologist	Not approved for pediatric use; used in treatment failures or for onychomycosis by some; monitor CBC, LFTs; pulse doses often used
Ketoconazole	100 mg/tab Su; Su 200 mg tablets	3.3 to 6.6 mg/kg/day in single dose	Less effective than griseofulvin and higher risk of hepatotoxicity
Nystatin	100,000 units/mL	Infants: 2 mL four times a day after meals Children/adolescents: 400,000 to 600,000 units four times a day—swished about mouth	Treatment of oral candidiasis

Terbinafine	125 mg/packet of granules
	
	250 mg tablets
		Granules: tinea capitis in children >4 yr:
		  <25 kg, 125 mg once daily for 6 weeks;
		  25-35 kg, 187.5 mg once daily for 6 weeks;
		  >35 kg, 250 mg once daily for 6 weeks
		Onychomycosis dosage once daily for 6 wk (fingernails) or 12 wk (toenails) as follows:
		  10-20 kg, 62.5 mg; 20-40 kg, 125 mg;
		  >40 kg, 250 mg
			Treatment of tinea capitis in children >4 yr; costly; possible drug interactions

*Nystatin; triamcinolone acetonide.

ALT, alanine aminotransferase*; AST,* aspartate aminotransferase*; C,* cream*; CBC,* complete blood count*; G,* gel*; L,* lotion*; LFTs,* liver function tests*; max,* maximum*; O,* ointment*; P,* powder*; S,* solution*; Sh,* shampoo*; Su,* suspension*; tab,* tablet.

Data from Paller AS, Mancini AJ: *Hurwitz clinical dermatology: a textbook of skin disorders of childhood and adolescence,* ed 4, Philadelphia, 2011, Saunders; Taketomo DK, Hodding JH, Kraus DM: *Pediatric dosage handbook,* ed 17, Hudson, OH, 2011, Lexi-Comp; Weston WL, Lane AT, Morelli JG: *Color textbook of pediatric dermatology,* ed 4, St Louis, 2007, Mosby.

(Weston et al, 2007). Avoid antifungal/corticosteroid combination medications.

- If inflammation is severe, 1% hydrocortisone can be applied simultaneously to the diaper area for 1 or 2 days (Liptack, 2009). Topical mupirocin applied four or five times a day may be effective (Weston et al, 2007).
- Keep area dry and cool. Minimize skin irritation:
  ○ Frequent diaper changes.
  ○ Leave diaper area open to air.
  ○ Blow-dry with warm air (low setting) for 3 to 5 minutes at diaper change (especially helpful in intertriginous areas in infants and obese children).
  ○ Avoid rubber pants.
  ○ Use mild soap and water; rinse well; avoid diaper wipes.
  ○ Avoid powders and other medications not prescribed.
  ○ Discontinue oral antibiotics and steroids when possible.
  ○ Discard or sterilize pacifiers.
  ○ Educate about avoiding underlying predisposing factors (e.g., lip licking).
  ○ Add topical or oral antibiotic if secondary infection is suspected.

- Nail involvement (chronic paronychia) can be treated with topical application of antifungal cream twice daily, but it will take several months for the nail plate to grow out normally; oral fluconazole may be needed for severe or resistant involvement.

Complications

Chronic mucocutaneous candidiasis resulting from immunologic deficit can occur and is heralded by widespread involvement (oral, skin, nails). Paronychia may occur with thumb sucking.

Patient Education

Emphasize good handwashing. Treatment failure is usually due to lack of compliance.

TINEA CAPITIS

See later section on alopecia.

TINEA CORPORIS

Description

Tinea corporis, commonly called *ringworm*, is a superficial fungal skin infection found on the non-hairy skin of the body. It is also identified by the part of the body affected (e.g., tinea manuum [hand], tinea barbae [beard], tinea faciei [face]) (see Color Plate).

Epidemiology

Tinea corporis is most commonly caused by the dermatophytes *Microsporum canis*, *Trichophyton rubrum*, and *Trichophyton tonsurans* (Theos, 2007). Transmission comes as the stratum corneum is invaded following direct contact with infected humans, animals, or fomites. The exact mechanism is unknown but is probably due to a toxin causing an inflammatory response. Infection is common in children. Contact sports (especially wrestling), hot and humid climates, crowded living conditions, and immunosuppression increase the incidence of tinea corporis. Auto-inoculation accounts for spreading lesions (Weston et al, 2007).

Clinical Findings

History. Contact with a person or animal with ringworm is sometimes reported.

Physical Examination
- Classical appearance of lesions: Annular, oval, or circinate with one or more flat, scaling, mildly erythematous circular patches or plaques with red, scaly borders
- Lesions spread peripherally and clear centrally or may be inflammatory throughout with superficial pustules.
- Often prominent over hair follicles
- Multiple secondary lesions may merge into a large area several centimeters in diameter.

Diagnostic Studies. If treatment failure or questionable diagnosis occurs:
- KOH-treated scrapings of border of lesion reveal hyphae and spores (see Fig. 36-2).
- Fungal culture
- Wood's lamp does not fluoroesce most tinea infections (*T tonsurans*).
- Fungal culture of the lesion

Differential Diagnosis

PR herald patch, nummular eczema, psoriasis, seborrhea, contact dermatitis, tinea versicolor, granuloma annulare, and Lyme disease are in the differential diagnosis.

Management

Management involves the following:
- For superficial or localized tinea corporis, topical antifungals (see Table 36-4) such as miconazole or clotrimazole are generally effective. Antifungal and steroid combinations should be avoided. Apply cream to the lesion, including a zone of normal skin, twice a day until clinical resolution, which can take 1 to 4 weeks (Theos, 2007). Prescription antifungals (e.g., econazole, ciclopirox) penetrate the skin more effectively but are more expensive.

- Tinea faciei (face), extensive infection, immunosuppression, coexisting tinea infections on scalp or nails, or infection that is unresponsive to topical treatment may require systemic treatment. Griseofulvin (see Table 36-4) is the systemic drug of choice for children older than age 2. Treatment typically lasts for 2 to 4 weeks and the medications should be taken with fatty foods for better absorption. Because of the risk of hepatotoxicity, nephrotoxicity, and neutropenia, patients requiring extended therapy should have a CBC, liver and renal function 8 weeks after initiating therapy and every 8 weeks until treatment is stopped. Tinea corporis gladiatorum may require systemic therapy because it is endemic among wrestling team members.
- Identify and treat contacts.
- Educate about communicability of lesions and length of treatment.
- Exclude from daycare or school until 24 hours after treatment has begun.
- Follow up in 2 weeks or sooner if lesions are not responding. If unresponsive, diagnosis is incorrect or resistance is possible. Culture to confirm diagnosis and change class of antifungal used.

Complications

Tinea incognito is a dermatophyte infection that has been altered by the use of topical calcineurin inhibitors (tacrolimus and pimecrolimus) or steroid creams, either alone or in combination with a topical antifungal. The lesions improve but there is a rapid relapse when the creams are stopped and chronic infection persists (Theos, 2007). Occasionally a pruritic papulovesicular rash on the trunk, hands, or face that is caused by a hypersensitivity response to the fungus may occur and is known as an *id response* or *dermatophytic reaction* (AAP, 2009).

Patient Education

Find the source of infection and treat or eliminate it to prevent recurrence. Keep skin dry following application of antifungal.

TINEA CRURIS

Description

Tinea cruris, commonly called *jock itch*, is a superficial fungal skin infection found on the groin, upper thighs, and intertriginous folds.

Epidemiology

Caused by the dermatophyte *Epidermophyton floccosum*, *Trichophyton rubrum* or *Trichophyton mentagrophytes*, tinea cruris rarely occurs before adolescence and is more common in males, obese individuals, or those with hyperhidrosis or experiencing chafing from tight clothes or moisture. It is extremely common.

Clinical Findings

History
- Hot, humid weather, tight clothing, vigorous physical activity and chafing, or contact sport, such as wrestling
- Often associated with tinea pedis

Physical Examination

- Erythematous to slightly brown, sharply marginated plaques with a raised border of scaling, pustules or vesicles; central clearing may be present
- Usually bilateral and symmetric, but not always
- Occurs on inner thighs and inguinal creases; penis, scrotum, and labia majora generally spared
- Occasionally occurs in perianal region or on the buttocks and/or abdomen

Diagnostic Studies. If treatment failure or questionable diagnosis occurs:

- KOH-treated scraping reveals hyphae and spores.
- Fungal culture

Differential Diagnosis

Psoriasis, candidiasis, contact dermatitis, seborrhea, intertrigo, and erythrasma are in the differential diagnosis.

Management

Management is the same as for tinea corporis. Duration of topical treatment is usually 4 to 6 weeks. Antifungal and steroid combinations are to be avoided. Advise the patient to wear cotton underwear and loose clothing and to use absorbent antifungal powder. If tinea pedis is suspected, advise the patient to put socks on before underwear to prevent the spread of the infection.

- Maintain good hygiene following a wrestling event (e.g., bathing as soon as possible, sole use of towel; dry thoroughly).
- Do not use steroids because of risk of atrophy and striae.

TINEA PEDIS

Description

Tinea pedis is a superficial fungal skin infection found on the feet, commonly called *athlete's foot*. There are three clinical forms: (1) vesicles and erosions on the instep of one or both feet; (2) an occasional fissure between the toes with surrounding scale and erythema; and (3) rare diffuse scaling on the weight-bearing surface of the foot with exaggerated scaling in creases (moccasin foot) often extending to lateral foot margins.

Epidemiology

Caused by the dermatophytes *T. rubrum* or *T. mentagrophytes*, tinea pedis is uncommon in preadolescent children and is more common in males (Theos, 2007; Weston et al, 2007). It is acquired through direct contact with contaminated surfaces (e.g., warm moist environment of showers and locker room floors) and often occurs with tinea cruris.

Clinical Findings

History

- Sweaty feet
- Use of nylon socks or nonbreathable shoes
- Exposure in family or at school
- Itching, intense burning, stinging, foul odor
- Microtrauma to feet—cracks, abrasions, nicks, cuts
- Contact with damp areas (e.g., swimming pools, locker room, showers)

Physical Examination

- Red, scaly, cracked rash on soles or interdigital spaces and instep, especially between the third, fourth, and fifth toes
- Infection initially presents as white peeling lesions becoming erythematous, vesicular, macerated, or fissured, and scaly
- Dorsum of foot remains clear
- Chronic infection manifested by a moccasin pattern with diffuse scaling (plantar hyperkeratosis) and mild erythema

Diagnostic Studies. Laboratory studies are the same as those for tinea corporis.

Differential Diagnosis

Contact dermatitis, atopic dermatitis, dyshidrotic eczema, psoriasis, pitted keratolysis and juvenile plantar dermatosis (red, dry fissures of weight-bearing surface) are in the differential diagnosis.

Management

Management is the same as that for tinea corporis. Antifungal medication should be applied 1 cm beyond the borders of the rash twice daily until 7 days after clearing. Usual treatment is 3 to 6 weeks. In rare cases, griseofulvin may be required, and treatment for 6 to 8 weeks is usually recommended. Additionally:

- Advise patient to keep feet dry, use absorbent antifungal powder or sprays, wear cotton socks, avoid scratching, and wear shoes that allow the feet to breathe or go barefoot when home. Thoroughly dry feet and between toes after using a commercial showering facility.
- Rinse feet with plain water or water and vinegar; dry carefully, especially between the toes. Moisturize and protect feet to prevent splitting and cracking.
- Aluminum chloride (Drysol, CertainDri, Xerac AC, Arrid Extra Dry antiperspirant spray) may be used for hyperhidrosis.
- Acute vesicular lesions may need to be treated with wet compresses two to four times daily for 10 to 15 minutes in addition to application of topical antifungals.
- Moccasin-type tinea pedis may need the addition of a keratolytic agent (lactic acid or urea) with the application of antifungals.
- Tennis shoes may be washed in the machine with soap and bleach.
- Physical education or sports may be continued.
- Follow up in 2 to 3 weeks or sooner if lesions are not responding.

Complications

A secondary bacterial infection, indicated by foul odor, can occur. An allergic reaction to fungus, called an *id response*, is manifested by a vesicular eruption on the palms and sides of fingers and occasionally on the trunk and extremities.

TINEA VERSICOLOR

Description

Tinea versicolor is a superficial fungal infection, also called *pityriasis versicolor*, that tends to be persistent and occurs predominantly on the trunk. The lesions do not tan in the summer and become relatively darker in winter months. (See Color Plate.)

Epidemiology

This infection is caused by a yeastlike organism, *Malassezia furfur* (referred to as *Pityrosporum orbiculare* and *P. ovale*) and occurs more commonly in adolescents than in younger children, in chronically ill and immunocompromised children, and in warmer seasons and humid climates. Breastfeeding infants can acquire the organism from their mother and exhibit facial lesions.

Clinical Findings

History. The infection is associated with warm, humid weather. Occasional mild itching may occur.

Physical Examination. Multiple, annular, scaling, discrete macules or patches, ranging from hypopigmented in dark-skinned individuals to hyperpigmented (salmon-colored to brown) in light-skinned individuals, are seen on the neck, shoulders, upper back and arms, chest midline, and face (especially in children). They tend to have a guttate or raindrop pattern.

Diagnostic Studies. KOH scrapings, though not necessary, reveal short curved hyphae and circular spores ("spaghetti and meatballs"). Scrapings fluoresce yellow-orange under Wood's lamp if not cleansed recently.

Differential Diagnosis

Pityriasis alba, PR, vitiligo, postinflammatory hypopigmentation or hyperpigmentation, seborrhea, and secondary syphilis are included in the differential diagnosis.

Management

The following steps are taken:
- Selenium sulfide 2.5% lotion or 1% shampoo applied in a thin layer from face to knees for 30 minutes daily for a week followed by monthly applications for 3 months to help prevent recurrences (AAP, 2009).
- Older adolescents and adults can use ketoconazole 2% shampoo as a daily application for 5 days.
- Hyposulfite or thiosulfate 15% to 25% concentrations applied twice a day for 2 to 4 weeks.
- For small areas of infection, topical imidazoles (clotrimazole, miconazole, ciclopirox, or terbinafine solution) or topical azoles (ketoconazole or oxiconazole) applied twice daily for 2 to 4 weeks can be used.
- Resistant or severe cases in older adolescents sometimes require oral antifungal treatment, such as ketoconazole, fluconazole, or itraconazole. Dosing recommendations include multiple administrations as continuous, intermittent, and single-dose approaches. A single dose of ketoconazole (400 mg) or itraconazole 200 mg daily for 5 days can be used as an alternative. Follow up in 1 month.

Patient Education

- Sun exposure makes lesions appear hypopigmented as the surrounding skin tans.
- Repigmentation takes several months.
- If the patient is taking oral antifungal medication, encourage exercise to induce sweating because this may enhance concentration of medication in the skin.
- Skin irritation occurs with overnight application.
- Absence of flaking when skin is scraped is a sign of effective treatment.

■ Viral Infections of the Skin

HERPES SIMPLEX

Description

In the active state, herpes simplex virus (HSV) causes contagious infections of the skin and mucous membranes ranging from mild to life threatening. HSV infection can be either primary or recurrent. Primary infection occurs in individuals without circulating antibodies after direct contact with secretions or mucocutaneous lesions of an infected individual. Incubation takes days to weeks and then manifests itself anywhere from subclinical to severe infection. The virus then becomes dormant in certain nerve cells until reactivated by triggering factors, such as stress, menses, illness, sunburn, windburn, and fatigue. Recurrent infection occurs in individuals previously infected who had either clinical or subclinical manifestations of infection.

HSV type 1 (HSV-1) usually affects the oral mucosa, pharynx, lips, and occasionally the eyes, causing a herpes labialis infection, commonly called *cold sores* or *fever blisters* (see Color Plate). HSV-2 infection commonly occurs as a neonatal infection (see Chapter 38) or herpetic vulvovaginitis (see Chapter 35) or progenitalis. Type 1 can also be found in the genital area, and type 2 can be found on the lips and mouth. Herpetic keratoconjunctivitis is discussed in Chapter 28; other information may be found in Chapter 23.

Epidemiology

HSV is transmitted by close contact with skin, mucous membranes, and body fluids, often through a break in the skin or by autoinoculation. Lesions occur in children of all ages, are contagious as long as they are present, and have an incubation period of 2 to 12 days. Primary lesions usually occur before 5 years old, are more painful and extensive, and last longer.

Clinical Findings

History. In primary herpes, fever, malaise, sore throat, and decreased fluid intake can occur. Primary genital HSV presents with painful vesicles in genital areas. In recurrent HSV infection there is often a painful prodrome of burning, tingling, paresthesia, and itching at the involved site. Recent acute febrile illness or sun exposure may also be reported.

Physical Examination. The following are seen on physical examination:
- HSV-1
  ○ Gingivostomatitis—pharyngitis with grouped vesicles on an erythematous base that ulcerate and form white plaques on mucosa, gingiva, tongue, palate, lips, chin, and nasolabial folds; lymphadenopathy and halitosis are present
  ○ Herpes labialis—cluster of small, clear, tense vesicles with an erythematous base that become weepy and ulcerated, progressing to crustiness, usually only on one side of the mouth and on the vermillion border—classic cold sore
  ○ Hand or fingers—deep-appearing vesicles

TABLE 36-5	Diagnosis and Treatment of Herpes Simplex and Herpes Zoster			
Presentation		**Clinical Findings**	**Treatment**	**Education**
Herpes simplex	Gingivostomatitis as primary infection; herpes labialis or herpes facialis as recurrent infection	Pharyngitis with erythematous vesicles, near, on, and/or in mouth; small, clear vesicles on erythematous base progressing to crusting	Burow solution; acyclovir in primary case or underlying disorder; antibiotics if secondary infection; oral anesthetics; supportive care	Degree and duration of contagion; triggers to infection
Herpes zoster	Reactivation of latent varicella virus, especially after mild cases or in infants <1 year old or immunocompromised host	Two or three clustered groups of vesicles on erythematous base, especially over thoracic or lumbosacral dermatomes; pain (can be severe), itch, tingle is minimal in children	Burow solution; antihistamine; drying lotions; possible acyclovir; silver sulfadiazine; antibiotics if secondary infection	New vesicles occur for up to 1 week; takes 2 to 3 weeks to resolve; contagious until lesions stop erupting and are crusted over; varicella vaccine to prevent

- Common sites of involvement: Lips, hand, fingers, nose, cheek, forehead, and eyes; can also occur in the genital area
- HSV-2
  - Grouped vesicopustules and ulceration with edema
  - Primary lesions on vaginal mucosa, labia, or perineum in females and on the penile shaft or perineum in males; females may have cervical involvement; oral lesions are possible
  - Recurrent lesions on labia, vulva, clitoris, or cervix in females and on the prepuce, glans, or sulcus in males; generally less severe cutaneous lesions
  - Regional lymphadenopathy

Diagnostic Studies. A Tzanck smear can be done on fluid from the lesions to identify epidermal giant cells; however, it does not distinguish HSV-1 from HSV-2. Viral cultures are the gold standard for definitive diagnosis. Direct fluorescent antibody (DFA) tests, enzyme-linked immunosorbent assay (ELISA) serology, and polymerase chain reaction (PCR) tests are usually only used with severe forms of HSV infection.

Differential Diagnosis

The differential diagnosis includes aphthous stomatitis, hand-foot-and-mouth disease, varicella, impetigo, folliculitis, and EM.

Management

Management can be guided by considering the host (e.g., age, area and extent of involvement, and immune status), the organism (is it definitely HSV?), and the drug needed (Table 36-5).
1. Burow solution compresses three times a day to alleviate discomfort
2. Acyclovir 20 to 40 mg/kg/day orally five times a day for 5 days or 200 mg every 4 hours five times a day for 7 to 10 days may be indicated to help shorten the course and alleviate symptoms for children older than 2 years with the following conditions:
   - Any underlying skin disorder (e.g., eczema)
   - A severe case
   - An immunocompromised disease
   - Systemic symptoms with primary genital infection
   - Occasionally for initial severe gingivostomatitis
   Acyclovir is most effective if started within 3 days of disease onset. Famciclovir or valacyclovir are additional antiviral agents approved for use in adults.
3. Topical acyclovir ointment may help for initial genital herpes infections, but is often not beneficial for recurrent infections.
4. Antibiotics for secondary bacterial (usually staphylococcal) infection:
   - Mupirocin: Topically three times a day for 5 days
   - Erythromycin: 40 mg/kg/day for 10 days
   - Dicloxacillin: 12.5 to 50 mg/kg/day for 10 days
5. Oral anesthetics for comfort; use with caution in children (need to be able to rinse and spit).
   - Viscous lidocaine 2% topical
   - Liquid diphenhydramine alone or combined with aluminum hydroxide or magnesium hydroxide as a 1:1 rinse (maximum of 5 mg/kg/day diphenhydramine in case it is swallowed); it can also be applied with cotton-tipped swabs to the lesions
6. Newborn infant, immunosuppressed child, child with infected atopic dermatitis, or child with a lesion in the eye or on the eyelid margin: Consult with or refer to an appropriate provider.
7. Offer supportive care, such as antipyretics, analgesics, hydration, and good oral hygiene.
8. Exclude from daycare only during the initial course (gingivostomatitis) and if the child cannot control secretions.
9. Recurrent, frequent, and severe HSV infection may be treated with acyclovir prophylaxis for 6 months.

Complications

Herpetic whitlow, occurring on a finger or thumb, is a swollen, painful lesion with an erythematous base and ulceration resembling a paronychia. It occurs on fingers of thumb-sucking children with gingivostomatitis or adolescents with genital HSV infection. Therapy with oral acyclovir 200 mg five times a day for 5 to 10 days may speed healing. *Eczema herpeticum* or *Kaposi varicelliform eruption* is discussed in Chapter 23. HSV has also been implicated as a possible cause of EM and Stevens-Johnson syndrome (SJS).

Patient Education, Prognosis, and Prevention

Recurrence of infection, possible triggering factors, and avoidance measures should be discussed. Triggers can include physical and psychological stress, trauma, fever, exposure to UV light, illness, menses, and extreme weather. Contagiousness of lesions and oral secretions must be understood. Explanation of the course of primary disease, with fever lasting up to 4 days and lesions taking at least 2 weeks to heal, is important.

HERPES ZOSTER

Description

HZ is a recurrent varicella infection commonly called *shingles* (see Color Plate).

Epidemiology

Caused by reactivation of the latent varicella zoster infection from the sensory root ganglia, HZ occurs in 10% to 20% of all individuals, is rare in childhood, and occurs more frequently with increasing age (three times more common in adolescents than preschoolers). HZ is more common following mild cases of varicella infections before 1 year old (3-fold to 20-fold increased risk), after varicella vaccination, and in immunocompromised children.

Clinical Findings

History. Burning, stinging pain, tenderness to light touch, hyperesthesia, or tingling precedes eruption by about 1 week, though this is less common in children. The lesions can be extremely itchy and painful.

Physical Examination

- Two or three clustered groups of macules and papules progress to vesicles on an erythematous base. These vesicles become pustular, rupture, ulcerate, and crust.
- Lesions develop over 3 to 5 days and last 7 to 10 days. Lesions may develop for up to 1 week followed by crusting and healing during the next 2 weeks. In children delayed chronic pain, known as postherpetic neuralgia, is rare.
- Lesions commonly follow the dermatomes of the second cervical to lumbar nerves and the fifth to seventh cranial nerves with scattered lesions outside these areas.
- Lesions do not cross midline (key to diagnosis); sharp demarcation at the midline with occasional contralateral involvement.
- Lymphadenopathy may occur.

Diagnostic Studies. The diagnosis is clinical. If needed, Tzanck smear or viral culture can distinguish from HSV infection. Bacterial culture or Gram stain can be used to distinguish from impetigo. A DFA stain of vesicle base scrapings is beneficial in the difficult to diagnosis case and results are timely.

Differential Diagnosis

Local cutaneous HSV infection and impetigo are differential diagnoses.

Management

Management steps include the following:
1. Apply Burow solution compresses three times a day to alleviate discomfort.

2. Warm, soothing baths
3. Antihistamines for itching
4. Analgesics for discomfort. Do not use salicylates.
5. Ointment such as Aquaphor or Vaseline moisturizes the lesions and decreases itching.
6. Antiviral medications are not recommended for use in all children with HZ.
   - Acyclovir 30 mg/kg/day divided four times a day for 5 days may be useful for children who are immunosuppressed, have ocular herpes, or have Ramsay-Hunt syndrome (Weston et al, 2007).
7. Antibiotics for secondary bacterial (usually staphylococcal) infection
   - Mupirocin topically twice daily
   - Dicloxacillin 12.5 to 25 mg/kg/day for 7 to 10 days
8. Refer for immediate ophthalmologic examination if eyes, forehead, or nose is involved.

Complications

Complications are rare except in immunocompromised children. Occasionally HZ is the initial finding in acquired immunodeficiency syndrome (AIDS), especially if more than one dermatome is involved. Eczema herpeticum may occur.

Patient Education, Prevention, and Prognosis

- New vesicles appear for up to 1 week and take 2 to 3 weeks to resolve. Illness is usually mild.
- The child is contagious for varicella until lesions are crusted. If the lesions can be covered, the child does not need to be excluded from school or childcare. If the lesions cannot be covered, the child should avoid contact with others until the lesions are crusted (AAP, 2009).

MOLLUSCUM CONTAGIOSUM

Description

A benign common childhood viral skin infection with little health risk, molluscum contagiosum often disappears on its own in a few weeks to months and is not easily treated (see Color Plate).

Epidemiology

This poxvirus replicates in host epithelial cells. It attacks skin and mucous membranes and is spread by direct contact, by fomites, or by autoinoculation (typically scratching). It is commonly found in children and adolescents. The incubation period is about 2 to 7 weeks but may be as long as 6 months (AAP, 2009). Infectivity is low but the child is contagious as long as lesions are present.

Clinical Findings

History

- Itching at the site
- Possible exposure to molluscum contagiosum

Physical Examination

- Very small, firm, pink to flesh-colored discrete papules 1 to 6 mm in size (occasionally up to 15 mm)
- Papules progressing to become umbilicated (may not be evident) with a cheesy core; keratinous contents may extrude from the umbilication

- Surrounding dermatitis is common.
- Face, axillae, antecubital area, trunk, popliteal fossae, crural area, and extremities are the most commonly involved areas; palms, soles, and scalp are spared.
- Single papule to numerous papules; most often numerous clustered papules and linear configurations
- Sexually active or abused children can have genitally grouped lesions.
- Children with eczema or immunosuppression can have severe cases; those with human immunodeficiency virus (HIV) infection or AIDS can have hundreds of lesions.

Differential Diagnosis

Warts, closed comedones, small epidermal cysts, blisters, folliculitis, and condyloma acuminatum are included in the differential diagnosis.

Management

- Untreated lesions usually disappear in a year but may take up to 4 years to completely go away (AAP, 2009).
- There is no consensus on the management of molluscum. Genital lesions should be treated to prevent spread to sexual partners. Nongenital lesions resolve spontaneously. Therapy may be necessary to alleviate discomfort, reduce itching, minimize autoinoculation, limit transmission, and for cosmetic reasons (AAP, 2009).
- Mechanical removal of the central core is to prevent spread and autoinoculation. Using eutectic mixture of local anesthetics (EMLA) cream (lidocaine; prilocaine) 30 to 45 minutes before the procedure reduces discomfort. Curettage is done with a sharp blade to remove the papule. Piercing the papule and expressing the plug is an option, but is painful.
- There are reports that irritants like surgical tape, adhesive tape, or duct tape applied each night and can result in lesion resolution.
- Topical medications may prove beneficial. Recheck the patient in 1 to 2 weeks to determine need for retreatment.
  - Liquid nitrogen may be applied for 2 to 3 seconds (easiest but also painful).
  - Trichloroacetic acid 25% to 50% applied by dropper to the center of the lesion, followed by alcohol (use with caution). Surround the lesion first with petroleum jelly.
  - Cantharidin 0.7% in collodion applied by dropper to the center of the lesion, followed by alcohol. Salicylic or lactic acid or potassium hydroxide or podophyllin can also be used.
  - Podofilox 0.5% topical solution or gel, or imiquimod 5% applied daily with a toothpick or cotton-tipped swab
  - Tretinoin or tazarotene cream or gel applied to lesion each night
  - Silver nitrate, iodine 7% to 9%, or phenol 1% applied for 2 to 3 seconds
- Cimetidine 30 to 40 mg/kg/day in two divided doses orally if topical treatment fails
- Sexual abuse of children with genitally grouped lesions should be suspected and evaluated.
- Evaluate for HIV infection if hundreds of lesions are found.
- Wait and see approach—spontaneous clearing occurs over years

Complications

Molluscum dermatitis, a scaly, erythematous, hypersensitive reaction, can occur and will respond to moisturizer; avoid hydrocortisone because it causes molluscum to flare. Impetiginized lesions, inflammation of the eyes or conjunctiva, and scarring can occur.

Patient Education and Prevention

Patients are contagious, but there is no need to exclude them from daycare or school. Children with impaired immunity, atopic dermatitis, or traumatized skin are at greater risk for broader spread. Severe inflammation is possible several hours after application of cantharidin. Scarring is unusual.

WARTS

Description

Warts are a common childhood skin infection characterized by a proliferation of the epidermis; they can also cause mucosal infection. There are four basic types of warts: verruca vulgaris, verruca plana, verruca plantaris, and condyloma acuminatum. Trauma to cutaneous warts promotes inoculation of the human papillomavirus (HPV) (Koebner phenomenon); therefore, most warts are on the hands, fingers, elbows, and plantar surfaces of the feet. With koebnerization, a line of warts develops in a linear constellation of lesions where the skin was excoriated. Cutaneous warts are rarely a serious health concern but present cosmetic problems for children and their families.

Epidemiology

Warts are viral-induced epithelial tumors caused by DNA-containing HPV. There are basically two groups of HPV genotypes: cutaneous and mucosal. Certain types of HPV are associated with cutaneous and genital oncogenesis. Warts are among the most common skin disorders in children. The transmission of warts from person to person depends on viral and host factors, such as quantity of virus, location of warts, preexisting skin injury, and cell-mediated immunity. Transmission is from fomites or skin-to-skin contact, and autoinoculation is frequent. Incubation is from 1 to 6 months.

Although a large percentage of all warts resolve spontaneously within 2 years, there is a high recurrence rate.

Clinical Findings

History. The history can include exposure to someone with warts. Though most common on the extremities, warts can occur anywhere on the body, including the face, scalp, and genitalia.

Physical Examination

- Common warts (verruca vulgaris) are usually elevated flesh-colored single papules with scaly, irregular surfaces and occasionally black pinpoints, which are thrombosed blood vessels. They are usually asymptomatic and multiple and are found anywhere on the body, although most commonly on the hands, nails, and feet. They may be dome shaped, filiform, or exophytic (Fig. 36-4). Filiform warts project from the skin on a narrow stalk and are usually seen on the face, lips, nose, eyelids, or neck. Periungual warts are common, occurring around the cuticles of the fingers or toes.

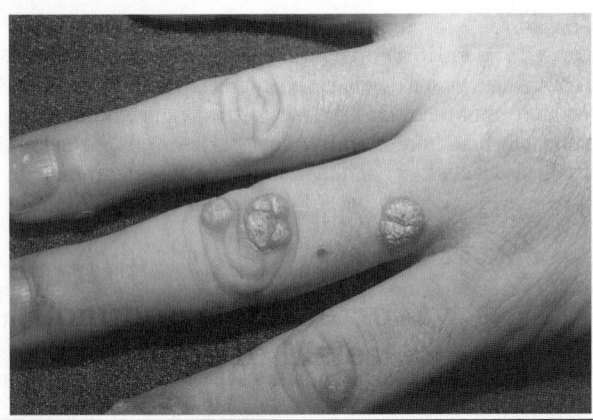

FIGURE 36-4 Multiple common warts (verruca vulgaris). (From Weston WL, Lane AT, Morelli JG: *Color textbook of pediatric dermatology*, ed 4, St Louis, 2007, Mosby, p 139.)

- Plantar warts (verrucae plantaris or mosaic) are commonly found on weight-bearing surfaces of the feet. They grow inward and disrupt skin markings.
- Flat warts (verruca plana or juvenile warts) are seen commonly on the face, neck, and extremities. They are small, slightly elevated papules and number from few to several hundred.
- Condylomata acuminata on genital mucosa and adjacent skin are multiple, confluent warts with irregular surfaces, light color, and cauliflower-like in appearance.

Differential Diagnosis

The differential diagnosis includes calluses, corns, foreign bodies, moles, comedones, and squamous cell carcinoma.

Management

There is no single effective treatment for warts; watchful waiting is an option. The recurrence rate is high; they typically do not resolve with just a single treatment. No treatment is necessary if the warts are asymptomatic. The decision to treat should be based on location, number and size of lesions, discomfort, and whether they are cosmetically objectionable. Treatment should not be harmful, and scarring should be avoided. Genital warts found in young children or in adolescents who are not sexually active should create suspicion of sexual abuse. Specific treatment options are outlined in Box 36-6. Follow up in 2 to 3 weeks to evaluate response.

Complications

Scarring from removal can occur. A ring of satellite warts may develop at the edge of the blister following treatment with cantharidin. Immunocompromised hosts can have extensive involvement.

Patient Education

A blister, sometimes hemorrhagic, may form 1 to 2 days after liquid nitrogen treatment. Redness and itching may herald regression of a wart. Parents and patients must be warned that multiple or prolonged treatment is often necessary.

■ Infestations of the Skin

PEDICULOSIS

Description

Pediculosis (lice infestation) can affect the scalp, body, or pubic area. Pediculosis capitis (head) is most common, pediculosis corporis (body) is uncommon, and pediculosis pubis (pubic area) is considered a sexually transmitted disease. Infestation is defined by some as presence of either nits (eggs) or lice and by others as presence of lice alone.

Epidemiology

Lice infestation is caused by three subspecies, *Pediculus humanus corporis* and *capitis* (head and body) or by *Phthirus pubis* (pubic). The adult female louse, which survives by sucking human blood, deposits 6 to 10 eggs per day on a glue-like substance about 4 mm from the scalp on the hair shaft within a waterproof shell. Nits incubate for about 1 week, hatch and grow into adult lice over another 1 to 2 weeks, then begin laying eggs. Head lice live approximately 30 days on a host and lay up to 100 nits. Transmission is by direct or indirect contact, often by sharing hairbrushes, caps, clothing, or linen or through close living quarters, poor hygiene, or sexual activity (pubic lice).

Pediculosis capitis is common in children. Head lice are not considered a health hazard because they do not spread disease. All socioeconomic groups are affected, but lice are most common in school-age Caucasian females, with the peak season occurring from August to November. Lice are uncommon in African-Americans (AAP, 2009).

Pediculosis corporis is uncommon in childhood. The louse is rarely seen on the body; rather it attaches to clothing and intermittently pierces the skin. It is the only louse that can carry human disease (e.g., epidemic typhus and trench fever). If pediculosis pubis is found in a child, sexual abuse must be considered.

Pubic lice may involve the scalp, eyebrows, or eyelashes, but primarily are found in the pubic area. Clothing and bed linens are a source of residence.

Lice are growing resistant to available pharmacologic treatment options mainly in children who have been treated multiple times. This has led to the trial of many alternative treatments.

Clinical Findings
History
- A history of infestation in a family, friend, or daycare contact
- Dandruff-like substance in the hair
- Itching of the scalp, scratching, and irritability if infestation has been present for a few weeks
- Reports of a crawling sensation in the scalp

Physical Examination
- Head lice
  - Lice can be visualized; nits can be seen as small white oval cases attached tightly to a hair shaft. Nits are usually laid within 4 mm of the scalp; as the hair grows, the nits and empty shells are found farther from the scalp, indicating more long-term infestation.
  - Care must be taken to differentiate hair casts, epithelial cells, and other debris from nits.

BOX 36-6 | Treatment Options for Warts

- Keratolytics eliminate the wart by causing an inflammatory response and topical peeling. They are often available over the counter, cause little pain, and are low in cost and risk, but are slow to work.
  - Salicylic acid paints with a concentration of greater than 20% are applied with a toothpick once or twice a day for 4 to 6 weeks. On thick skin, a combination of 16.7% salicylic acid and 16.7% collodion is more effective. This method is useful for common or periungual warts, but it is not effective with warts larger than 5 mm in diameter.
  - Salicylic acid plasters with 40% concentration are cut to size and taped in place for 3 to 5 days. After the plaster is taken off, the area should be soaked for 45 minutes and the dead epidermis removed. A new plaster is then applied. Treatment can last 3 to 6 weeks. This method is useful for plantar warts.
  - Retinoic acid gel 0.025% to 0.05% applied once or twice daily brings resolution in 4 to 6 weeks. This method is useful for flat warts, but it does not work for common, plantar, or periungual warts.
  - Occlusion with duct tape. Place on for 12 hours a day for 6 days in a row, followed by soaking and scraping of epidermis; is easy, painless, and inexpensive.
- Destructive agents eliminate the wart by causing necrosis and blister formation. Most techniques are painful and require patient cooperation.
  - Cryotherapy. Liquid nitrogen is applied for 2 to 10 seconds until an area 1 to 3 mm beyond the wart turns white or patient complains of pain; goal is to induce blister formation above the dermal-epidermal junction. Take care not to freeze the wart too vigorously. Caution should be used when freezing warts over joints and the lateral aspects of digits. This method is uncomfortable and often not tolerated by children.
  - Retreatment is often necessary.
  - Cantharidin 0.7% is applied directly to the wart with a toothpick and covered with tape for 24 hours. This is a potent blistering agent that creates a blister in 2 to 3 days that is sloughed after 7 to 14 days. This method is useful for periungual and some plantar warts. Do not use on other body surfaces.
  - Podophyllum 25% solution in compound benzoin tincture is applied to the wart with a toothpick; it should be washed off in 4 hours; may be repeated in 1 week. Podofilox, available over the counter for home use, is applied twice a day for 3 days. After a 4-day rest period, the 3-day cycle may be repeated as necessary. This technique is useful for common or genital warts.
  - Surgical excision of warts can lead to scarring that can be more painful than the wart itself, but can be highly effective for large individual warts. Surgery by snipping with scissors, not scalpel, is useful for filiform warts.
  - Laser treatments are often as effective as cryosurgery, but can be painful and require several treatments for complete resolution.
- Immunotherapy modalities stimulate an immune response to HPV. These newer treatment modalities do not have controlled studies evaluating their effectiveness.
  - Oral cimetidine, a histamine 2–receptor-blocking agent, may improve immunity to HPV. It is used in conjunction with other modalities at a dose of 20 to 30 mg/kg divided twice a day for 3 to 4 months.
  - Imiquimod cream creates cell-mediated immunity in surrounding areas and is often effective as a home treatment. It is applied daily for 1 to 2 months.
  - Contact sensitization and interferon injection are methods used by dermatologists, usually in adult patients.

HPV, Human papillomavirus.

- Common sites are the back of the head, nape of the neck, and behind the ears; eyelashes can be involved. Scalp excoriations and occipital or cervical adenopathy can be present.
- Body lice
  - Excoriated macules or papules may be present (secondary bacterial infection of the skin may develop).
  - Belt line, collar, and underwear areas are common sites.
  - A hemorrhagic pinpoint macule is seen where the louse extracted blood.
  - Axillary, inguinal, or regional lymphadenopathy can be present.
- Pubic lice
  - Excoriation and small bluish macules and papules may be present.
  - Eyelashes can be involved; spread to other short-haired areas (thighs, trunk, axillae, beard) may occur.

Diagnostic Studies

- Microscopic examination of a hair shaft can more clearly identify nits.
- Test for other sexually transmitted diseases if pubic lice found; specifically gonorrhea and syphilis.

Differential Diagnosis

Scabies (Table 36-6), dermatitis herpetiformis, and necrotic excoriations are in the differential diagnosis. Rule out sexual abuse if pubic lice are found.

Management

Treatment options are varied and controversial. Standard over-the-counter medications, prescription medications, and dangerous substitutes are often used by parents. Correct diagnosis is imperative to accurate management. Nonviable nits can persist on the hair shaft for several months, so treatment is recommended when live lice and viable nits are observed. Table 36-6 outlines recommended treatment. The AAP discourages "no-nit" policies in schools because such policies have been ineffective in controlling head lice transmission and result in excessive lost school and workdays (Frankowski et al, 2010).

Pediculicides are toxic substances and should be used only as directed and with care. Pregnant women and nursing mothers should not be exposed to pediculicides; they should not be used to treat lice in babies (National Pediculosis Association [NPA], 2009). The NPA also advises caution in children

TABLE 36-6 Diagnosis and Treatment of Pediculosis and Scabies

	Clinical Findings	Treatment
Pediculosis (head lice)	History of infestation; itchy scalp, scratches; postoccipital nodes; occasional visualization of lice or nits (small white oval cases), commonly on back of head, nape of neck, behind ears, possibly eyelashes	Key to treatment is proper technique! *First step:* Apply pediculicide: permethrin *or* pyrethrin plus piperonyl butoxide *Second step:* Remove nits: comb hair with fine-toothed comb in 1-inch sections with special attention to nape of neck and behind ears *Third step:* Cleanse the environment: check family, friends, day-care/school contacts; clean sheets, towels, clothing, headgear; store other items in plastic for 2 weeks; vacuum; soak brushes and combs; follow up in 2 weeks with daily recheck at home by parent. May return to school after pediculicide treatment; "no nit" policies are not recommended
Scabies	Key finding: itching, worse at night, and complaints are more significant than physical findings; fitful sleep, crankiness; curving burrows, especially in webs of fingers, sides of hands, folds of wrist, armpits, forearms, elbows, belt line, buttocks, proximal half of foot and heel; secondary excoriation; infants may have lesions on palms, soles, scalp, face, posterior auricle and axilla, folds, red-brown; may be <10 lesions total or may be dozens (typical of infants); lesions may occur in the form of firm nodules in infants	Treat with permethrin 5%, repeated in 1 week; use antihistamine, hydrocortisone, or nonsteroidal antiinflammatory drugs for itching; simultaneously treat family members (even if asymptomatic), friends, school/daycare contacts Cleanse environment: linens and clothing, vacuum, store anything else in plastic bags for 1 week; rash and itch persist for up to 3 weeks after treatment; return to school 24 hours after treatment

with allergies, asthma, epilepsy, other chronic illness, or open wounds; and those undergoing chemotherapy, using other medications, or already overexposed to pediculicides (NPA, 2009). Treatment failure is common, whether as a result of poor technique or actual medication resistance (AAP, 2009). Recommendations are to follow local resistance patterns when determining treatment.

1. Proper pediculocide application is key to success. Prior to use do not use a shampoo that contains conditioner or cream rinse, or petrolatum products on the hair or scalp. Keep the pediculicide out of the eyes. If applying solution to damp hair, make sure the hair is damp, not wet (dilutes the pediculicide). Do not rewash the hair for 1 to 2 days following treatment. Retreatment is recommended in 7 to 10 days.
   - Permethrin 1% cream rinse, also called pyrethrum, is the treatment of choice for head lice because of its safety, efficacy, and 10-day residual. Hair should be shampooed and towel dried, permethrin applied, left on for 10 minutes, and then rinsed. Hair should not be rewashed for at least 24 to 48 hours. Many advise retreatment in 7 to 10 days.
   - Benzyl alcohol, a prescription medication that is not ovicidal, is applied to the dry hair and left on for 10 minutes before rinsing. Repeat application 7 days later is recommended in order to kill newly hatched lice. It is contraindicated in children less than 6 months of age.
   - Pyrethrin, a natural extract from the chrysanthemum plant, is effective as a pediculicide but not as an ovicide. It is usually a 10-minute shampoo applied to dry hair, with repeat application in 7 to 10 days. It is contraindicated in children with allergy to ragweed. Because pyrethrin does not kill both lice and eggs, treatment failures are more common than with permethrin.

- Lindane is a prescription organochloride that effectively kills lice and nits. It is a neurotoxin and there are safety concerns because of potential central nervous system effects on the child and long-term environmental contamination. Many countries have banned the use of lindane because of these safety concerns. The AAP (2009) recommends that it be used only in patients who have failed to respond to adequate doses of other approved agents. For head lice, a 1% lindane shampoo is used, left on the hair for 4 minutes, then rinsed; for body lice, cream or lotion may be applied for 8 to 12 hours (overnight) and then rinsed off; for pubic lice, a 1% shampoo is applied for 10 minutes, then rinsed off. Retreatment is not recommended (AAP, 2009; Diamantis et al, 2009).
- Malathion lotion 0.5% is an organophosphate with a pine-needle-oil base that is available only by prescription. The AAP does not recommend its use in children younger than the age of 2 years (AAP, 2009). It is a potent lice killer that binds to the hair shaft for 4 weeks and it is considered the most effective therapy for killing lice and nits (Diamantis et al, 2009). The drug is flammable, and if ingested causes severe respiratory distress. Malathion 0.5% lotion should be applied to dry hair, be allowed to dry, and then carefully rinsed off 8 to 12 hours later. The treatment should be repeated in 7 to 10 days if live lice are still seen.

2. The second step is removal of nits, although this is not an absolutely necessary step. Proper technique is the key to success. A good light, a magnifying glass, and tweezers are useful. A wide-toothed comb may be used initially to straighten the hair.
   - Some products claim to dissolve the substance (cement) that attaches the nit to the hair to facilitate removal. A 1:1 vinegar-to-water solution applied to the scalp,

then covered with a warm, moist towel for 30 minutes before beginning to comb, may also help.

- Use a proper nit-removal comb with fine teeth (included in most pediculicide kits).
- Comb damp hair for a minimum of 20 to 30 minutes, working from the top of the scalp down in 1-inch sections. Pay special attention to the nape of the neck and behind the ears.
- If eyelashes are involved, coat with petroleum jelly two or three times a day for 8 to 14 days and manually remove nits.
- Comb-outs and inspection should be repeated every night for 2 to 3 weeks to ensure cure.

3. The third step is thorough cleansing of the environment.
- Examine family members, friends, school, and daycare contacts. Do not treat family members if nothing is found because of the emergence of treatment-resistant lice and pediculicide toxicity.
- Launder sheets, towels, clothing, and headgear in hot water and machine dry on hot cycle for 20 minutes, iron, or dry clean.
- Any item that cannot be washed or dry-cleaned should be stored in a plastic bag for 2 weeks.
- Hot iron or vacuum play areas, floors, rugs, and furniture.
- Soak brushes, combs, and hair accessories in pediculicide, alcohol, or Lysol for 1 hour, followed by hot-water rinse.
- Spraying or fumigating the house is not recommended.

4. Alternative treatments include herbal or essential oils, such as olive oil, pine oil, tea-tree oil, margarine, mayonnaise, dog shampoo, styling gels, and petroleum jelly, all of which suffocate and kill the lice. Further studies are needed regarding these practices. Definitely avoid wrapping the hair in plastic and putting the child under a hair dryer or washing the hair with gasoline or kerosene. The LouseBuster is a nonchemical treatment for head lice that has demonstrated effectiveness in initial studies (Goates et al, 2006). Because it is expensive, cost is an issue for individual use. Topical application of Cetaphil cleanser also works.

5. Treatment failure is not unusual. However, with proper use of a pediculicide, reinfection from contact with an untreated individual is more common (AAP, 2009). Common mistakes include misdiagnosis; improper use of pediculicide; dilution of pediculicide by applying to wet hair, not damp hair; use of a shampoo with conditioner or cream rinse; inadequate combing techniques; not cleansing personal care items; and not screening and treating family members and close contacts.

6. There are neither formal recommendations nor FDA approval for dealing with resistance. Some methods for treating resistant lice include the following:
- Use Nix creme rinse for 4 to 8 hours instead of 10 minutes.
- Use Nix creme rinse under a shower cap overnight.
- Use Elimite cream (five times stronger than Nix) overnight.
- Use TMP-SMX to kill symbiotic bacteria on which lice survive (studies inconclusive to date) (Diamantis et al, 2009).
- Use oral ivermectin 200 mcg/kg as a single dose, repeated in 10 days if the child weighs more than 15 kg. This is an off-label use and its effectiveness is unclear (Diamantis et al, 2009).

7. Body lice are treated by improving hygiene and cleaning clothes. Wash infested clothing and dry at hot temperatures on a weekly basis for several weeks. Pediculicides are not necessary (AAP, 2009).
8. Pubic lice are treated as pediculosis capitis.

Complications
Secondary bacterial infection can occur.

Patient Education and Prevention
Items for discussion include the following:
- Daily to weekly checks or combing for lice or nits should be carried out at home.
- Educate family members about the expected course, that lice infestation is not a social disease, and about the need to avoid excessive or unnecessary retreatment. Do not use extra amounts; do not treat more than three times with the same medication without being seen by a care provider; do not mix pediculicides.
- Children should not be excluded or sent home from school because of lice. Parents should be notified and informed that the child should be treated. No-nit policies are ineffective in controlling head lice transmission and are not recommended.

SCABIES
Description
Scabies is caused by the mite, *Sarcoptes scabiei*, which is an obligate human parasite that burrows into the epidermis and causes intense itching (see Color Plate).

Epidemiology
Scabies is a highly contagious infestation spread through close contact and shared clothing or linen. The female mite burrows into the skin, laying up to three eggs a day as she travels. The eggs hatch in about 3 to 4 days and mature into adult mites in 10 to 14 days. The female mite has a life span of 15 to 30 days. Sensitization, which causes intense itching, occurs approximately 3 weeks after infestation. Scabies occurs in all socioeconomic groups and in all age groups. However, infestation of African-Americans is rare.

Clinical Findings
History
- Key finding: Itching, worse at night, initially mild but progressively more intense
- Fitful sleep, crankiness, or rubbing of hands and feet (infants)

Physical Examination
- Complaints are significantly greater than examination findings.
- Characteristic lesions include curving S-shaped burrows, especially on webs of fingers and sides of hands, folds of wrists and armpits, forearms, elbows, belt line, buttocks, genitalia, or proximal half of foot and heel.
- Vesiculopustular lesions tend to be found in infants and young children. They classically have vesicular lesions on palms, soles, scalp, face, posterior auriculae, and axillae,

concentrated in the folds; head and neck lesions typically are red-brown vesiculopustules or nodules. However, any child younger than 2 years can have an unusual manifestation.
- Secondary lesions include itchy papules, red-brown nodules from inflammatory response, crusting, excoriation, and other signs of secondary infection.
- Infants classically have dozens of lesions; older children may have fewer than 10.

Diagnostic Studies
- Microscopic examination of scrapings from an unscratched burrow in saline or mineral oil can reveal an eight-legged mite, eggs, or feces. Do not use KOH because it dissolves the mites, eggs, and feces. Burrows and fresh papules are best for specimen collection.
- Burrow ink test: Apply a drop of ink or rub a washable felt-tipped pen across suspected burrow. Wipe off excess ink and examine with magnifying glass for an ink-stained burrow.

Differential Diagnosis
Papular urticaria; atopic, seborrheic or contact dermatitis; insect bites; folliculitis; lichen planus; and dermatitis herpetiformis are included in the differential diagnosis.

Management
Management involves the following:
1. Pharmacologic treatment begins with applying a thin layer of scabicide to the entire body, excluding the eyes. Areas of special importance are under the fingernails, the scalp, behind the ears, all folds and creases, and the feet and hands. In general, the scabicide should be reapplied in 7 days on all symptomatic patients.
   - Permethrin 5% cream is the drug of choice for treating scabies because of its safety and efficacy. It can be used on infants as young as 2 months old. Apply as a thin, even coat and rub in well from the neck down. Leave on for 8 to 14 hours, then thoroughly rinse off. Retreat in 1 week. In infants special application is needed to head, postauricular area, and hands and feet; be sure to avoid the areas around the eyes and mouth. This medication is safe for use in infants, young children, pregnant women, and nursing mothers (AAP, 2009).
   - Ivermectin 200 mcg/kg/dose orally for two doses is effective for crusted (Norwegian) scabies or severe infection. Ivermectin is not FDA approved for this, nor is it recommended for use in children less than 5 years old or those who weigh less than 15 kg (AAP, 2009).
2. Antihistamines (hydroxyzine or diphenhydramine) or topical 1% hydrocortisone can be helpful for itching, which can last for several weeks after successful treatment.
3. Simultaneous treatment of family members, friends, and school and daycare contacts, even if asymptomatic, is essential.
4. At time of treatment, linens and any clothing worn during the past 48 hours should be washed with hot water, put into a hot dryer for 20 minutes, or dry-cleaned. The house should be vacuumed.
5. Store nonwashable items in sealed plastic bags for 1 week.
6. Reasons for treatment failure include an incorrect diagnosis, not applying medication to the whole body, or not treating all members of the household.
7. The child may develop postscabetic eczema that can be misdiagnosed as treatment failure. Evaluate and treat with topical corticosteroids.
8. Resistance to medication is not common and continued infestation is usually due to treatment failure rather than resistance.

Complications
A secondary bacterial infection is possible and should be treated. Postscabetic syndrome is common, with visible lesions and pruritus persisting for days to weeks following treatment; nodular lesions can persist for weeks to months. Norwegian scabies is a nonpruritic, crusted, scaling infestation with thousands to millions of mites occurring in immunosuppressed or institutionalized patients.

Patient Education, Prognosis, and Prevention
- Educate the family about the course of disease. Rash and itching persist for up to 3 weeks following treatment. Avoid overbathing and further irritation of the skin.
- The child should not be infectious 24 hours after treatment and may return to school or daycare.

■ Allergic and Inflammatory Reactions of the Skin

ACNE VULGARIS
Description
Acne is an inflammatory disorder of the pilosebaceous unit in which excess sebum, keratinous debris, and bacteria accumulate, producing microcomedones. The microcomedones may be noninflamed or inflamed lesions. Although rarely a serious disorder, acne may cause permanent scarring and decreased self-esteem, and occasionally heralds underlying disease. It is often of significant concern to the adolescent, having a serious effect on social development (see Color Plate).

Epidemiology
Acne is the most common skin disorder and affects approximately 80% to 85% of individuals between 11 and 30 years old in the U.S. (Paller and Mancini, 2011). Four mechanisms contribute to this sebaceous follicle disorder:
- Sebaceous follicules become plugged with keratinous material.
- Colonies of anaerobic bacteria grow deep in the follicle, primarily *P. acnes,* but coagulase-negative staphylococci, and *M. furfur* can be involved.
- Sebum is overproduced and androgen production increases, resulting in expansion of the follicle.
- Inflammation occurs and pustules form secondary to trapped *P. acnes* and sebum. The bacteria release chemotactic factors that attract neutrophils to ingest the bacteria and release hydrolytic enzymes.

Acne usually begins at the onset of puberty, occurring earlier in girls (12 to 13 years old) than boys (14 to 15 years old). It tends to improve in the summer and worsens with menses and stress. The pathogenesis of acne is multifactorial; gender, age, genetic factors, and environment are significant factors. Although not a serious physical disorder, acne has been associated with psychosocial morbidity and decreased emotional well-being. "Patients with even mild to moderate acne have demonstrated high scores on the Carrol Rating Scale for Depression and an increased prevalence of suicidal ideation" (Paller and Mancini, 2011, p 167).

Neonatal acne occurs in about 20% of normal newborns; infants are occasionally affected by acne. Neonatal acne is thought to be related to either stimulation of sebaceous glands by maternal androgens or transient adrenal and gonadal androgen production. Infantile acne may occasionally be associated with hyperandrogenism.

Clinical Findings

History
- Family history of acne
- Stage of pubertal development and menstrual history
- Facial products used, especially occlusive products or pomades
- Oral and topical prescription medication, especially oral contraceptives, antibiotics, or steroids
- Current or previous acne treatment and results
- Sports participation, especially if wearing football pads, helmets, headbands, or other protective devices
- Jobs, such as cooking at a fast-food grill or working at a gas station
- Other medical conditions

Physical Examination. Lesions most commonly are found on the face, back, and chest.
- Noninflammatory lesions:
  - Microcomedone—a follicular plug as a result of obstruction of the pilosebaceous unit (hair follicle and sebaceous gland) typically localized on the face and trunk.
  - Open comedone (blackhead)—a noninflammatory lesion or papule, firm in consistency, caused by blockage at the mouth of the follicle and occurring on the face, upper back, shoulders, and chest. The black color is thought to come from oxidized keratinous material at the follicular opening. This is the main lesion in early adolescence.
  - Closed comedone (whitehead)—a noninflammatory lesion, semisoft in consistency, caused by blockage at the neck of the follicle. This is a precursor to inflammatory acne.
- Inflammatory lesions occur secondary to rupture of noninflamed lesions into the dermis and can include papules, pustules, excoriation, lesion crusting, nodules, cysts, scars, and sinus tracts (confluent nodules likely to scar).

The severity of acne is determined by the quantity, type, and spread of lesions (Table 36-7). It is helpful to use a diagram of the face or a grading graph to identify the number and type of lesions to allow more precise patient follow-up. If only open and closed comedones are found, the disorder is called *comedonal acne*. Most adolescents have a combination of comedones, red papules, and pustules called *papulopustular acne*, which can be mild or severe. *Nodulocystic acne* is the most severe form and requires more intensive intervention. Specific types of acne include *frictional*, occurring from rubbing of bras, tight clothes, or headbands; *pomadal*, along the temple and forehead, as a result of pomades or oil-based

TABLE 36-7	Grading Scale for Acne Severity
Scale	**Definition**
0	None: skin is clear
1	Few comedones
2	Mild comedones, few papules, minimal erythema
3	Comedones, papules, pustules, erythema
4	Moderate comedones, greater number of papules, pustules extending over wider area of face, chest, shoulders, back, increasing erythema
5	Comedones, increasing number of papules, pustules, nodules with erythema
6	Comedones, papules, pustules, nodules, cysts; scarring may or may not be present with hyperpigmentation

cosmetics; *athletic*, on forehead, chin, or shoulders, caused by helmets and pads; and *hormonal*, with a beard distribution.

Differential Diagnosis
Cosmetic, mechanical, environmental, or drug-induced acne; rosacea; flat wart; milia; perioral dermatitis; and folliculitis are included in the differential diagnosis.

Management
The goals of acne management are to (1) reduce the excess production of sebum, (2) counteract the abnormal desquamation of epithelial cells, (3) decrease the proliferation of *P. acnes*, and (4) prevent or decrease scarring. Choice of treatment depends on the extent, severity, and duration of disease; type of lesions; and psychological effects the adolescent is experiencing (Table 36-8 and Box 36-7).
1. *Education* is the first priority. The adolescent must have realistic expectations and understand the pathophysiology and the process of treatment, including the fact that the acne often worsens before improving. Reading materials about acne and its treatment may support them in their self-management efforts.
   - Wash face twice a day with a mild soap, such as Dove, Neutrogena, or Aveeno Cleansing bar. Avoid scrubbing, rubbing, picking, and squeezing. Medication should be applied lightly.
   - Use of a comedone extractor can cause scarring and should be discouraged. Hot soaks applied to pustules may help their resolution.
   - All products used on the face should be labeled as *noncomedogenic*.
   - Identify aggravating substances, such as oil-based cosmetics, pomades, hair spray, mousse, and face creams.
   - Identify possible aggravating factors, such as stress; hot, humid weather; and jobs involving frying oil or grease.
   - Reassure that no scientific evidence indicates that any particular foods adversely affect acne; however, a well-balanced diet is important to maintaining healthy skin.
   - Discuss psychosocial concerns and provide support.

TABLE 36-8 Treatment of Acne

Type of Acne	Lesions	Initial Treatment	If Not Improving
Comedonal	Open or closed comedones	Choose one: • Benzoyl peroxide: 5% gel daily (if mild) • Tretinoin: 0.025% cream daily (if moderate) • Adapalene: 0.1% gel	Combine benzoyl peroxide with tretinoin or increase strength of tretinoin to 0.05%
Mild papulopustular	Red papules, few pustules	Option 1. Choose one: • Benzoyl peroxide: 5% to 10% daily • Adapalene: 0.1% gel • Azelaic acid: twice a day (if mild) *Plus* topical antibiotic twice a day Option 2. Choose one: • Erythromycin: 3% with 5% benzoyl peroxide daily to twice a day (if moderate) • Clindamycin: 1% with 5% benzoyl peroxide daily to twice a day	Increase benzoyl peroxide to twice a day *or* Combine benzoyl peroxide with tretinoin (for comedones) Substitute topical antibiotic twice a day (for inflammatory acne)
Moderate to severe papulopustular	Red papules, many pustules	Choose one: • Benzoyl peroxide: 5% and tretinoin 0.025% • Adapalene: 0.1% gel • Azelaic acid (if comedonal) • Topical antibiotic twice a day (if no comedones) *Plus* oral antibiotic twice a day	Increase strength of treatment *or* Refer to dermatologist
Nodulocystic, scarring, or unresponsive	Red papules, pustules, cysts, and nodules	Choose one: • Oral antibiotics twice a day and tretinoin 0.05% daily • Adapalene: 0.1% gel and benzoyl peroxide: 10% gel twice a day (if comedonal) • Adapalene: 0.1% gel and topical antibiotic	Refer to dermatologist for oral isotretinoin

BOX 36-7 Medications Commonly Used in Treating Acne

Topical Keratolytic or Comedolytic Agents
Retinoids
  Tretinoin: 0.01% to 0.025% gel; 0.025% to 0.1% cream; 0.1% microgel
  Tretinoin/clindamycin (combination topical)
  Tazarotene: 0.05% to 0.1% cream; 0.05% to 0.1% gel
  Adapalene: 0.1% gel or cream; 0.3% gel
Benzoyl peroxide: 2.5% to 20% gel; 5% and 10% cream; 5% to 20% lotion or wash
Azelaic acid: 20% cream; 15% gel

Topical Antibiotics
Clindamycin: 1% solution, lotion, gel, pledget, foam
Erythromycin: 1% to 2% solution, 3% gel or swabs
Erythromycin: 3% with benzoyl peroxide 5% gel
Clindamycin: 1% with 5% benzoyl peroxide

Oral Antibiotics (Paller and Mancini, 2011)
Tetracycline: 250 to 500 mg per dose twice a day
Erythromycin: 250 to 500 mg per dose twice a day
Minocycline: 50 to 100 mg per dose twice a day (associated with more side effects)
Doxycycline: 50 to 100 mg per dose twice a day

• Remind the patient that results take months and that adherence to treatment is essential to improvement.
• Sun exposure helps clear acne for some adolescents, but may worsen it for others. Sunscreen use is recommended, and caution about sun exposure should be given if using medication that increases photosensitivity.

2. *Medications* used in treatment of acne vary by action, route of administration, and strength. They include topical and systemic preparations; keratolytic or comedolytic agents; those with antibacterial or antibiotic effects; hormonal agents; and preparations that have a combination of actions.

3. *Topical keratolytic* or *comedolytic agents*, used to minimize follicular obstruction and break up microcomedones, are the first line of acne treatment. They may be dispensed in a combination form with a topical antibacterial agent. Many strengths and forms are available, the strongest being the gels, if tolerated; creams are the least drying. A general rule is to start low (in strength) and slowly (in frequency) and advance as tolerated or needed. A useful technique to decrease the incidence of irritation is to start therapy only for three nights weekly and slowly increase to a nightly application over a few weeks. A minimum of 4 to 6 weeks of treatment is required before improvement is seen.

There are three topical retinoids (tretinoin, adapalene, and tazarotene) and two agents that possess both antibacterial and keratolytic properties (benzoyl peroxide [BPO] and azelaic acid). Each works by a different mechanism. They can be used together and interchangeably. Dryness, erythema, irritation, and scaling can occur with these products, and the strength and frequency of use must be adjusted for this.

- Tretinoin is a keratolytic that causes sun sensitivity. A pea-sized application should be made 20 minutes after washing the face. Initially it is used every other night, advancing to every night. Sensitivity to tretinoin is worst in the first 2 weeks of use and decreases thereafter.
- Adapalene seems to cause less irritation and less photosensitivity, and has better efficacy.
- Tazarotene is a keratolytic to be used once daily.
- Azelaic acid is antibacterial and keratolytic. It is useful in individuals with sensitive or dark skin and is also effective in treating acne rosacea.
- BPO, the most frequently used topical preparation for acne, is used once or twice a day, depending on the severity of acne and dryness of skin. It is a powerful antimicrobial with comedolytic and antiinflammatory effects. Use in combination with topical antibiotics causes less antibiotic resistance.

4. *Topical antibiotics* are used to control the inflammatory process, usually most helpful in moderate inflammatory acne. They are used to maintain control after treatment with oral antibiotics, and are applied to the entire skin surface, not just to problem areas. They should not be applied within 30 minutes of shaving. Erythromycin can have up to a 51% resistance rate (Paller and Mancini, 2011).

- Topical clindamycin, erythromycin, or sulfacetamide is used once or twice a day, either alone or in combination with other topical medications.
- Topical erythromycin with BPO and clindamycin with BPO are combination products that are more effective than either drug alone and have less resistance from *P. acnes*. This combination is especially effective in mild to moderate inflammatory acne or as an adjunct to oral therapy (Paller and Mancini, 2011).

5. *Oral antibiotics* are used in addition to topical agents to decrease the concentration of *P. acnes* and to decrease the degree of inflammation if there is no response to topical agents. Systemic antibiotics should be used for the shortest time possible, rarely longer than 6 months and often require 3 to 4 weeks to see improvement. Once improvement is noted, the dose should be tapered to a daily dose, then discontinued.

- Tetracycline should be taken with 8 ounces of water 1 hour before or 2 hours after eating. Tetracycline should not be used by pregnant or breastfeeding females or in children less than 9 years old. Photosensitivity reactions can occur. Usual dose: 250 to 500 mg twice daily.
- Erythromycin can be taken with food, but GI upset is common, and vulvovaginal candidiasis can be problematic. Usual dose: 250 to 500 mg twice daily.
- Minocycline can be taken with food although dairy products decrease absorption. Side effects include blue-black discoloration in scars, photosensitivity, and hypersensitivity reactions. Usual dose: 50 to 100 mg twice daily.
- Doxycycline can be taken with food (dairy products decrease absorption), but has the highest rate of photosensitivity reactions. Usual dose: 50 to 100 mg twice daily.
- *Oral retinoids* are used for severe, recalcitrant nodulocystic acne. Isotretinoin is contraindicated in pregnancy (pregnancy Category X drug known for its teratogenic effect) and requires evaluation by a dermatologist before use. Its association with depression and suicide is controversial. The usual course is 20 weeks; there are many side effects, and CBC, liver function tests (LFTs), human chorionic gonadotropin (hCG), and urinalysis for pregnancy must be monitored every month while the patient is taking the medication. The *iPledge* program creates a registry for all patients being treated with isotretinoin. The FDA requires health care providers, female patients, and pharmacists to access the *iPledge* website monthly after office visits and before filling their prescription for documentation regarding pregnancy, blood donation, and contraceptive counseling.

- *Hormonal and other therapies.* Hormonal therapies can be used in females to oppose effects of androgen on sebaceous glands, such as antiandrogens (e.g., spironolactone, flutamide) and androgen receptor blockers; OCPs provide estrogen and a progestin with some FDA-approved to treat acne vulgaris. Intralesional steroid therapy for large cysts or nodules is sometimes used; resurfacing lasers and dermabrasion are used for acne scarring.
- *Noncomedogenic moisturizers* can be used for dryness, which is common with treatment. Noncomedogenic makeup is also available and helpful in treating these patients.

6. Follow-up visits should occur at least every 4 to 6 weeks until control is established, defined as when lesions clear or only a few new lesions appear every 2 weeks. Refer to a dermatologist for nonresponsive or severe cases.

Mild cases of neonatal or infantile acne are best treated with a plan of watchful waiting and gentle daily cleansing with soap and water. In mild comedonal acne, sparing use of topical tretinoin is recommended. Use 2.5% BPO or topical antibiotics for mild inflammatory acne. Have the parents apply these agents every other night. Severe acne may need an oral antibiotic.

Complications

Failure can be due to lack of patient motivation, lack of education, inappropriate treatments, initial treatment that was too strong, or expectations of a quick fix. Psychological effects include decreased self-esteem and poor body image, problems with interpersonal relationships, self-consciousness, embarrassment, depression, and decreased athletic participation, especially in gymnastics, swimming, and wrestling. Resistance of *P. acnes* to tetracycline, erythromycin, and minocycline is increasing.

ATOPIC DERMATITIS

See Chapter 24. (See Color Plate.)

CONTACT DERMATITIS
Description

Contact dermatitis is an acute or chronic inflammation resulting from a hypersensitive reaction to a substance (either irritants or allergens). Common types of contact dermatitis include the following:

- *Dry skin dermatitis* caused by extremely low humidity (less than 30%), excess soap or cleansing cream use, or inadequate rinsing of soap products

- *Nickel* dermatitis from contact with jewelry, belts, snaps, or eyeglasses
- *Lip-licker dermatitis* caused by frequent lip licking, most often in dry, cold weather
- *Phytophotodermatitis* occurs with sun exposure following contact with plants or juices, such as limes, lemons, carrots, celery, figs, parsnips, or dill; manifests as a blistered lesion on an erythematous base and may be confused with a burn
- *Plant oleoresins*, such as poison ivy, oak, or sumac; contact can be direct or indirect (exposure to burning plant material); oils may be inhaled, causing damage to lung tissue
- *Juvenile plantar dermatosis*, manifested as dryness, cracking, and erythema of weight-bearing surfaces of the feet, initially the big toes. It mimics tinea pedis, often found in children with atopic dermatitis
- *Latex dermatitis*, associated with the use of products containing latex, such as protective gloves

Epidemiology

The most common form of contact dermatitis is caused by an irritant, a chemical or substance with a toxic effect on the skin. The severity of the rash depends on the length of exposure and the concentration of the irritant. Substances such as saliva, urine, and feces; baby wipes; bubble bath; agents that dry the skin; and adhesives often cause irritation. Diaper dermatitis is the most common form (see following section). Contact dermatitis can also be caused by allergens. Allergic reactions occur as an immunologic response to an antigen penetrating the skin. There are two phases: sensitization and elicitation. Allergic dermatitis is seen only after sensitization to an allergen has occurred and a subsequent type IV delayed hypersensitivity response has activated an immune cascade. Common causes are contact with shoes (components, such as rubber and potassium dichromate), nickel, clothes with woolen or rough textures, topical medications (e.g., neomycin and lanolin), perfumed soaps or cosmetics (including lanolin), preservatives, or poison ivy, oak, or sumac. Sometimes the cause is obvious; often no specific cause can be identified. Although it occurs at any age, contact dermatitis is extremely common in children.

Clinical Findings

History
- Contact with any new or unusual substances
- Repeated exposure to any substance or item
- Diarrhea or infrequently changed diapers
- Rash localized to specific area(s)

Physical Examination. The area of involvement offers clues to the causative agent. Often the rash is localized to one area and has sharp borders. Common examples include a linear-type rash secondary to wearing a necklace or bracelet, circular areas from snaps on clothing, or inflammation of the earlobes from jewelry or a reaction pattern on the toes and dorsum of the foot from shoes. The duration and concentration of exposure also affect the intensity of the rash. Minimal contact may produce only mild erythema, whereas prolonged or concentrated contact may produce significant erythema, edema, and blistering with possible crusting and secondary infection. Irritant reactions tend to be immediate, whereas allergic ones are delayed.
- A chafed appearance with shiny, mild to severely erythematous, peeling, or dry, fissured skin or red patches and plaques with secondary scales may be seen if the reaction is due to an irritant. For example, the dorsum of the hand may exhibit the above characteristic appearance with frequent handwashing with irritating soaps.
- Erythema, vesicles, and weeping may be present in the acute stage of allergic contact dermatitis. The lesions are pruritic.
- Hyperpigmentation and lichenification are seen in chronic conditions.

Differential Diagnosis

The differential diagnosis includes atopic dermatitis, impetigo, herpes simplex, psoriasis, and seborrhea.

Management

Appropriate skin care, recognizing and eliminating offending agents, and treating inflammation are key to managing contact dermatitis successfully.
- Identify and avoid the substance (irritant or allergen) causing the dermatitis.
  - Urushiol, the allergen in poison ivy, oak, and sumac, can remain on contaminated items, such as clothing, animal hair, toys, and sports equipment resulting in sequential outbreaks due to reexposures.
  - A generalized id (idiosyncratic) reaction can develop to an allergen. An id reaction occurs as a secondary or "sympathy" rash distant from the primary site of exposure.
- Burow solution soaks or oatmeal baths and cool compresses (1 teaspoon salt/pint water) applied for 20 minutes every 4 to 6 hours soothe vesicular rashes.
- Apply water and either petrolatum-based or lanolin-and-petrolatum-based emollients to the skin to restore moisture to areas of dryness and chafing.
  - Petrolatum-based emollients include dimethicone, white petrolatum, and Vaseline Dermatology Formula.
  - Lanolin-and-petrolatum-based emollients should not be used if there is inflammation.
- Topical corticosteroids used two or three times daily give relief in 2 or 3 days, although it may take 2 or 3 weeks for complete healing. Occasionally oral corticosteroids are used for short periods if the area of allergic involvement exceeds 10% of the skin surface (10 to 14 days, tapered the last 7 days).
- Do not use flavored lip creams in cases of lip-licker dermatitis. Emollient lotions and petroleum-based emollients can moisturize the skin and discourage lip licking because of their bad taste.
- Oral antihistamines are helpful if itching and scratching are problems.
- Resolution may take 2 to 3 weeks. Refer to a dermatologist or an allergist for patch testing if the dermatitis worsens, fails to respond, or recurs.
- Chronic allergic contact dermatitis should be treated with medium potency topical corticosteroids twice daily until resolved (Ghali, 2006).

DIAPER DERMATITIS

Description

Diaper dermatitis is the most frequent contact dermatitis seen in children. It is a skin inflammation caused by an irritant that breaks down the skin's natural defense barrier (Table 36-9;

TABLE 36-9 Diagnosis and Treatment of Diaper Dermatitis

Type	Cause	Presentation and Location	Other Characteristics	Treatment
Irritant contact dermatitis	Related to wearing diapers; contact with urine and feces	Chapped, shiny, erythematous, parchment-like skin with possible erosions on convex surfaces; creases spared	Peaks at 9-12 months old; may progress to involve creases; skin may be dry	Frequent diaper changes, gentle cleansing; greasy lubricant; sitz bath, air-dry; 0.5%-1% hydrocortisone for inflammation
Candidiasis	Related to wearing diapers; a superinfection with *Candida*	Shallow pustules, fiery-red scaly plaques on convex surfaces, inguinal folds, labia, and scrotum	Satellite lesions, oral thrush; recent antibiotic or diarrhea; occurs at any age	Antifungal cream plus same measures as for contact dermatitis
Miliaria or intertrigo	Related to wearing diapers; a result of heat and occlusion	Discrete vesicles or papules (miliaria); erythematous, scaly, maceration in skinfolds	Sweat retention or friction associated	Self-limited (miliaria); avoid precipitating factors; care as for contact dermatitis
Seborrhea	Exaggerated by wearing diapers; overgrowth of *Malassezia* yeast in areas of sebaceous gland activity	Greasy, erythematous scales, well circumscribed in creases of skin, groin; spared convex surfaces	Onset at 3 to 4 weeks old; also occurs on face or body; often superinfected with *Candida*	Ketoconazole and/or hydrocortisone is treatment of choice
Atopic dermatitis (AD)	Exaggerated by wearing diapers; exact cause unknown	Increased number of lines in skin; areas of excoriation in folds and convex surfaces and buttocks; less widespread	AD in other areas; usually begins in first year of life; scratches skin with diaper change; hyperlinear skinfolds with diffuse borders	Skin care as for contact dermatitis and as indicated for AD (see Chapter 24); antibiotics for bacterial infection
Psoriasis	Exaggerated by wearing diapers; psoriasis evolves in response to chronic trauma	Erythematous, well-defined sharp, scaly plaques on convex surfaces and inguinal folds; less widespread	Psoriasis affects other places; rare occurrence if found, usually at 6 to 18 months old	Treatment often required for weeks or until toilet trained; steroids; ketoconazole if *Candida* present
Bacterial dermatitis	Usually caused by staphylococcal or streptococcal infection	Red, denuded areas or fragile blisters; crusting and pustules in suprapubic area and periumbilicus	Usually in newborn, can occur anywhere	Nystatin if yeast is present as well; mupirocin if minimal; amoxicillin clavulanate or cephalexin

see Color Plate). The initial rash is termed *irritant contact diaper dermatitis*. A variation of this is called *tidewater* or *tidemark dermatitis* and is found at the diaper edges. *Jacquet dermatitis*, a severe form manifested by punched-out lesions or erosions primarily on the labia and buttocks, is especially prone to secondary infection.

Epidemiology

Diaper dermatitis is one of the most common skin disorders of infancy. Factors contributing to diaper dermatitis include the following:

- Improper hygiene and cleansing methods
- Chemical irritation caused by prolonged contact with skin products, urine, feces, or breakdown products. Feces and its breakdown products are the major factors
- Mechanical irritation from diapers or skinfolds
- Occlusion of skin with use of diapers and plastic or rubber pants
- Other skin dermatoses aggravated by wearing diapers (e.g., seborrhea, atopic dermatitis, or psoriasis)
- In the diaper area around the anus, the rash is often due to diarrhea; if the skin is affected but the folds are spared, urine is often responsible

Clinical Findings

History

- Type of diapers and diaper covering used; recent change in brand or laundering products
- Frequency of diaper changes and methods of cleansing used
- Any new baby care products used
- Frequency of wet diapers and stools
- Medication taken (particularly antibiotics) or used on rash
- Present or recent use of antibiotics

Physical Examination. Erythema, edema, and vesiculation are typically the first characteristic changes observed. Chronic changes include scale, lichenification, and increased or decreased pigmentation. Other findings associated with specific causative factors can include the following:

- Chemical causes
  - Shiny, peeling, erythematous macular or papular rash confluent in the diaper area, sparing folds
  - Head of penis erythematous and dry
  - Erythema primarily on buttocks and around anus (fecal irritation)
- Mechanical causes
  - Erythematous, macerated (acute) or dry (chronic), hyperpigmented area prominent along edges of diaper or plastic or rubber pants

○ Erythematous, macerated folds caused by overlapping skin
- Hygiene problems
  ○ Any finding listed previously
  ○ Poor hygiene in general

Differential Diagnosis

Differential diagnosis includes contact dermatitis; bacterial, viral, or monilial infection; atopic dermatitis; psoriasis; seborrhea; scabies; and congenital syphilis.

Management

The best treatment is prevention!
1. Keep diaper area dry, clean, and aerated.
   - Frequent diaper changes are essential; every 1 to 2 hours is recommended with one change at night and a minimum of eight changes in a 24-hour period for infants. Cleanse the area well with water at every diaper change and use mild soap, rinsing well following a stool. Avoid vigorous cleansing because this can worsen matters. Avoid using wipes.
   - Use a greasy lubricant if skin is dry.
   - Use a protective barrier ointment or cream, such as Desitin (cod liver oil with zinc oxide), A&D ointment, Aquaphor, petrolatum, or zinc oxide at the first sign of irritation.
2. Proper use of diapers
   - Frequent changes are essential, and use thick or absorbent diapers.
   - Avoid use of rubber or plastic pants.
   - Cloth diapers should be soaked, prerinsed, washed in a mild soap, double rinsed with ¼ cup of vinegar, and dried in the sun if possible.
   - Disposable diapers must be large enough not to bind and should never be worn with rubber pants.
3. Treatment of diaper rash
   - Sitz baths in warm water for 10 to 15 minutes four times a day
   - Expose diaper area to air by leaving diaper off or by blow-drying with low heat three or four times a day.
   - Burow solution soaks or compresses four times a day if skin is weepy
   - Undecylenic acid or zinc oxide containing diaper cream to decrease the friction and moisture
   - Hydrocortisone 0.5% or 1% applied as a thin layer three times a day for no more than 5 days, especially if skin is dry, for moderate to severe diaper dermatitis. Do not use fluorinated steroids.
   - Increase intake of fluids to dilute urine. In older infants, 2 to 3 ounces of cranberry juice acidifies the urine.
   - If the rash has been present for more than 3 days or if there is no response to the aforementioned measures, add a topical antifungal cream, such as clotrimazole or miconazole. If there is still no response, a trial of oral antifungal is indicated (see section on monilial dermatitis).
   - Any recalcitrant rash should be referred to a dermatologist.
   - Follow up by phone in 1 to 2 days. If not improved, reassess within 1 week.

Complications

Secondary infection with bacteria, viruses, or fungi can occur (see previous sections). Red flags that could indicate systemic disease or require consultation with a dermatologist include severe erosions or ulcers; bullae or pustules; large papules or nodules, purpura, or petechiae; and redness or scaliness over entire body.

SEBORRHEIC DERMATITIS

Description

Seborrhea is a chronic inflammatory dermatitis commonly called *cradle cap* in infants or *dandruff* in adolescents.

Epidemiology

The condition is thought to be related to overproduction of sebum because it commonly occurs in areas with large numbers of sebaceous glands. It may be an overgrowth of *M. ovalis* (formerly *P. ovale*), a saprophytic yeast, which is universally present on the human body. Seborrhea occurs most often in early infancy and adolescence, is associated with blepharitis, and is more common in spring and summer.

Clinical Findings

History. Note age of onset (infancy or adolescence).

Physical Examination. In infants, erythematous, flaky to thick crusts of yellow, greasy (waxy appearance) scales occur predominantly on the scalp, but also on the face, behind the ears, on the neck and trunk, and in the diaper area. In adolescents there are mild flakes with some erythema and yellow, greasy scales on the scalp, forehead, nasal bridge, and eyebrows; behind the ears; on the face and flexural surfaces; and in intertriginous areas. The dermatitis is not pruritic and has no pustules.

Differential Diagnosis

Atopic dermatitis, psoriasis, *Candida* infection, contact dermatitis, tinea, scabies, and PR are included in the differential diagnosis.

Management

Seborrhea in infants may be self-limited, typically resolving in the first year of life. However, in adolescents, it is usually chronic and recurring.
- Four main categories of treatment may be helpful in either age group (Poindexter et al, 2009)
  ○ Antifungal: Azoles, selenium sulfide
  ○ Antiinflammatory: Topical steroids, topical calcineurin inhibitors
  ○ Keratolytic (remove excess scale): Topical salicylic acid, urea
  ○ Alternative: Tar-based topical preparations, tea-tree oil
- Treatment of infantile seborrheic dermatitis (Poindexter et al, 2009)
  ○ Emphasize that the dermatitis will resolve spontaneously
  ○ Remove thick scale with emollients or nonprescription shampoos. Note that there are no FDA-approved treatments for seborrheic dermatitis in children younger than 2 years old (Poindexter et al, 2009).
    - Mineral oil, P&S liquid are commonly used in infants, baby oil, or petroleum jelly can be placed on

thick crusts 10 to 15 minutes before washing to soften them. Follow by gentle brushing during shampooing to remove crusts.
- ○ Off label treatments for severe cases include ketoconazole 2% shampoo selenium sulfide shampoos, low-potency topical steroids, and topical antifungal agents.
- Treatment for adolescents with seborrheic dermatitis (Poindexter et al, 2009)
  - ○ Facial dermatitis
    - Daily ketoconazole 2% topical preparations (cream, shampoo, gel, or foam)
    - Intermittent use of low-potency topical corticosteroids (0.05% desonide cream or lotion)
    - Calcineurin inhibitors are good for face and ears.
  - ○ Scalp dermatitis
    - Medicated shampoos (tar, salicylic acid, ketoconazole, or selenium sulfide) two or three times a week (one to four times per month for African-Americans) alternated with prescription-strength shampoos (ketoconazole 2.5%, selenium sulfide 2.5%) (Connelly and Schachter, 2009). Shampoo should be left on the scalp for 5 to 10 minutes before scrubbing crusts and then rinsing.
    - Topical corticosteroids added weekly for recalcitrant dermatitis (leave-in foams or solutions work best)
    - Body and *skinfold seborrheic dermatitis: The same regimens mentioned previously can be used on the body.*

Educate parents about the etiology, control measures, and the need to continue treatment for a few days after resolution, and arrange for follow-up in 1 to 2 weeks.

Complications

Secondary infection with bacteria or *Candida* can occur. Severe, generalized seborrhea is commonly found in persons infected with HIV.

SUNBURN

Description

Sunburn is an injury to the skin occurring from overexposure of the skin to the UV rays of the sun. The incidence of skin cancer is increasing as a result of overexposure to the sun and the use of tanning beds.

Epidemiology

Excessive sun exposure causes a change in the skin's blood flow, cell kinetics, and pigment products. Damage to the skin by sun (primarily ultraviolet B [UVB]) includes erythema, pigmentary or texture changes, and potential carcinogenesis. Injury to the skin begins as quickly as 30 minutes after exposure, peaks at 24 hours, and may last for 72 hours. Other factors that contribute to sun sensitivity are medications (especially griseofulvin, NSAIDs, oral contraceptives, tetracycline, topical diphenhydramine, and tretinoin and other keratolytics) and some illnesses.

Children are at increased risk for sunburn because of the greater amount of time they spend outdoors. They are also particularly susceptible to UV radiation during their first two decades of life because of age-related structural and immunologic skin differences. Blistering sunburns before 20 years old more than double the chance of skin cancer. Factors contributing to the degree of burn include the coloring of skin and hair

BOX 36-8	Skin Types (I-VI) and Photosensitivity

Type I: Very sensitive—always burns easily and severely, never tans; has fair skin, blond hair, blue or brown eyes, and freckles

Type II: Very sensitive—usually burns easily, minimally tans; has fair skin; red, blond, or brown hair; and blue, hazel, or brown eyes

Type III: Moderately sensitive—sometimes burns, gradually and uniformly tans; average Caucasian individual

Type IV: Moderately sensitive—minimally burns, always tans easily; has dark brown hair, dark eyes, and white or light brown skin

Type V: Minimally sensitive—rarely burns, profusely tans; brown-skinned (middle Eastern and Hispanic)

Type VI: Heavily pigmented—rarely burns, tans deeply; African-Americans and other heavily pigmented individuals

Adapted from Paller AS, Mancini AJ: *Hurwitz clinical pediatric dermatology: a textbook of skin disorders of children and adolescence,* ed 4, Philadelphia, 2011, Elsevier, p 437.

(Box 36-8) and amount of previous sun exposure. Burns are less common in children with darker hair and skin because of their increased amount of melanin. Timing of sun exposure, latitude, and altitude affect skin sensitivity because UV rays are strongest between 10 AM and 2 PM, at higher altitudes, and nearer the equator. Sunburn can occur on cloudy days, and reflection from sand, water, snow, and concrete increases the risk.

Clinical Findings
History
- Length and time of sun exposure and tanning bed use
- Previous sunburns, especially blistering ones
- Any medications currently taken
- Chills, headache, and fatigue with moderate to severe burn
- Family history of melanoma or other skin cancer
Physical Examination
- Mild or first-degree burns are evidenced by erythema, tenderness, and mild pain.
- Moderate or second-degree burns involve a greater degree of erythema, increased pain, edema, and blisters.
- Severe or third-degree burns involve greater areas of skin and include systemic symptoms of headache, fever, and fatigue.
- Erythema and tenderness are evident from 30 minutes to 4 hours after exposure; 2 to 7 days later, affected layers of the epidermis are shed.

Differential Diagnosis

The differential diagnosis includes photosensitization from medication, xeroderma pigmentosum, lupus erythematosus, viral exanthem, dermatomyositis, and porphyrias.

Management

Prevention is the best intervention. The degree of burn helps determine which of the following strategies is most appropriate.
- Use cool water, saline compresses, or ice packs at least four times a day to ease pain and reduce swelling: Baking soda or cornstarch baths help cool skin. White vinegar or milk compresses help initiate healing.

- Administer ibuprofen 5 to 10 mg/kg/dose or acetaminophen 10 to 15 mg/kg dose as soon as possible and every 6 to 8 hours for the next 2 to 3 days for fever and pain relief.
- Low-dose cortisone creams 0.5% or 1% two or three times a day, used with caution because of the increased absorption through damaged skin, help reduce inflammation and pain.
- Local anesthetic sprays or first-aid creams with benzocaine are contraindicated because of the risk of sensitization.
- Skin emollients, such as aloe vera gel or moisturizer, are helpful if skin is dry. Jojoba oil and vitamin E creams are sometimes helpful. Avoid petrolatum, butter, or any occlusive ointment because their occlusive properties intensify the burn.
- Extra fluid intake prevents dehydration and restores natural moisture balance.
- If blisters break, dead skin needs to be trimmed and an antibiotic ointment, such as polymyxin B sulfate and bacitracin zinc, applied.

Complications

In addition to skin cancer, photoaging, including telangiectasia and actinic keratosis, cataracts, retinal damage, heat stroke, and a triggering or aggravation of disorders, such as acne rosacea, EM, and herpes labialis, to name a few, are possible complications of sunburn.

The incidence of skin cancer (basal cell carcinoma, squamous cell carcinoma, and malignant melanoma) is increasing rapidly, with 1% to 3% of malignant melanomas occurring in those younger than 20 years of age (Paller and Mancini, 2011). Risk factors for skin cancer include fair skin, history of multiple blistering sunburns, presence of multiple atypical moles, development of new nevi, and family history of melanoma. Basal and squamous cell carcinomas are slow-spreading cancers, directly linked with chronic exposure to UV light. Basal cell carcinomas occur in varied forms, as nodular, pearly, pigmented lesions often on the hand, neck, or head. Squamous cell carcinomas are quickly growing, firm, indurated nodules with or without ulceration on sun-exposed areas, especially the rim of the ear, face, lips, and mouth.

Malignant melanoma has become the most rapidly increasing type of cancer with an alarming increase in the incidence of this deadly skin cancer seen in adolescence. Melanomas manifest as new, pigmented lesions or as changes in existing moles. In preadolescents, melanoma often is nodular, grows rapidly, and itches or bleeds. Typically, melanomas in adolescents are enlarging or changing lesions with irregular color or borders (Weston et al, 2007). There is a link to multiple severe, blistering sunburns, but family history is a more important factor. Any change in a mole, especially with rapid asymmetric growth, crusting, ulceration, or color variation, needs immediate evaluation. All school-age children and adolescents should be taught to do a monthly skin examination (Box 36-9).

Patient Education and Prevention

- Suntanned skin is not a sign of good health, but of skin injury. There is no such thing as a healthy tan. Never seek a tan; seek the shade. Avoid tanning devices or parlors.
- Know your skin type and protection needs (see Boxes 36-8 and 36-10).

BOX 36-9 | Monthly Skin Examination

The **ABCDE**s of skin examination:
  Asymmetry
  Border irregularity or notching
  Color variation, especially if multicolored
  Diameter greater than 6 mm
  Elevation, especially if asymmetric (also **E**volution)
Note any new growths, itchy patches, nonhealing sores, changes in size of old nevus, irritability, or different sensation in any moles.

Process of Skin Examination

Use a full-length mirror, a hand mirror, and a brightly lit room.
Examine the following areas:
  Front and back, right and left sides with arms raised
  With elbows bent, forearms, back of arms and palms
  Back of legs and feet, toes and soles
  Back of neck and scalp
  Back and buttocks

From Starr NB: Skin smarts: the essentials of skin protection, *J Pediatr Health Care* 13(3):136-138, 1998.

- Avoid the sun between 10 AM and 2 PM. Learn the "shadow rule"—seek shade if your shadow is shorter than you are tall. Most newspapers print in the weather section the predicted index of UV exposure (1 to 10) as prepared by the National Weather Service.
- Cover up with hats, sunglasses, and clothing.
  ○ Hats with a wide (3-inch) brim are recommended.
  ○ Sunglasses should be worn beginning in infancy. Large-framed, wraparound lenses provide the best protection. UV protection is provided by a chemical added to the lenses and is indicated by one of the following labels: UV absorption to 400 nm, special purpose, meets American National Standards Institute (ANSI) UV requirements.
  ○ Tight-weave, long-sleeved, long-pants clothing with sunscreen applied to the skin underneath provides maximal protection. Color, weight, stretch, wetness, and quality of material all affect the amount of protection offered. Solumbra and SunSkins offer clothes that provide an SPF of 30 and block 97% of UV rays. Shades offer clothes that provide 81% UV protection. Stingray offers swimwear that blocks 99% of the sun's rays.
- Use a sunscreen that is broad spectrum and provides protection from both UVB and UVA light (see Box 36-10).
- Teach sun protection early on by example and words. "Play Smart When It Comes to the Sun" is an educational program sponsored by the American Academy of Dermatology (AAD) and the Major League Baseball Players Association. The program's goal is to educate the public to reduce sun exposure and increase protective behaviors.
- "Choose Your Cover" is a Centers for Disease Control and Prevention (CDC) program to increase awareness and change social norms related to skin protection and tanned skin.
- Do monthly skin checks (see Box 36-9).

BOX 36-10 Sunscreen, Clothing, Sunglasses, and Outdoor Activity Time Recommendations

Sunscreens block the rays of the sun. Sun protection factor (SPF) is the length of time an individual can be exposed to sun without burning if sunscreen is used appropriately. The substantivity of a sunscreen describes its adherence. Sweat resistant (effective for up to 30 minutes of heavy, continuous perspiration), water resistant (effective for up to 40 minutes of swimming), and waterproof (effective for up to 80 minutes of immersion) are different types of substantivity. Specific recommendations include the following:

- Use SPF 30 or greater, nonalcohol base, without lanolin, paraben, or fragrance. Use a waterproof product when in water, but reapply every 80 minutes with continuous water exposure.
- Apply at least 30 minutes before exposure to sun; reapply at least every 2 hours while in the sun, and after swimming, toweling, or heavy perspiration.
- Apply liberally (1 oz for an adult) and use cream instead of lotion for better coverage.
- Pay special attention to eyelids, nose, cheeks, ears, neck, scalp, shoulders, hands, and feet. Use a lip balm with SPF 30 or greater.
- Do not use sunscreen on infants younger than 6 months old, but keep baby out of the sun completely, using shade, brimmed hat, and protective clothing.
- Use sunscreen daily in summer or in warm climates. Use even on overcast or cloudy days.
- Extra protection is needed with increasing altitude, closer location to the equator, and sand, snow, concrete, or water reflection.
- Set an example for children by using sunscreen.

Sunscreens are available in various chemical combinations (e.g., para-aminobenzoic acid [PABA], PABA esters, cinnamates, benzophenes, salicylates, octocrylene, dibenzoylmethane) and vehicles (e.g., emollient for dry skin, gel or lotion for oily skin, noncomedogenic for acne-prone skin). If a child is sensitive to one, try a sunscreen with different ingredients. A PABA-free sunscreen is recommended for children. Dibenzoylmethane provides the most protection from ultraviolet A.

Sunblocks scatter and reflect light. Zinc oxide, titanium oxide, or a combination product, such as Sportz Bloc, is useful for especially sensitive areas, such as the nose or previously burned areas.

Clothing can help increase protection against the sun's rays. Caps and hats with visors or wide brims help protect the face. Wear clothing made of cotton rather than synthetic fibers—long-sleeved shirts and pants. Children at particular risk for skin cancer may benefit from clothing treated with protection (Solumbra). Cotton T-shirts can be laundered with Rit Sunguard, which provides additional protection from the sun's rays.

Children should wear well-fitted UV protective *sunglasses* when outdoors.

Avoid lengthy *outdoor activities* during peak sun times from 10:00 AM to 3:00 PM on sunny days; beware that reflective surfaces (water, sand, snow, cement) can reflect up to 85% of sunlight.

Data from Baumann LS, Schucluter LA: Sun protection in the pediatric patient. In Burg FD, Polin RA, Gershon AA et al, editors: *Current pediatric therapy*, ed 18, Philadelphia, 2006, Saunders, pp 1091-1093; Starr NB: Skin smarts: the essentials of skin protection, *J Pediatr Health Care* 13(3):136-138, 1998.

DRUG ERUPTIONS

Description

Drugs taken systemically can result in a variety of skin reactions or rashes. The two most common types of drug-related eruptions found in children are morbilliform (measles-like) rash (also called an exanthematous reaction manifested by erythematous macules and/or papules) and urticaria typified by erythematous wheals (Table 36-10). Morbilliform rash is discussed first and urticaria is discussed later in the section on vascular reactions. Although not described in this chapter, other drug-related reactions manifested by significant dermatologic eruptions include acute generalized exanthematous pustulosis, drug hypersensitivity syndrome, serum sickness-like reaction, vasculitis, fixed drug eruption, acneiform eruptions, and SJS.

Epidemiology

The morbilliform rash, also called an exanthematous rash, is the most common allergic skin reaction to a drug. The rash may be an immunologic or nonimmunologic reaction to the drug. The most common drugs causing reactions are the penicillins; sulfonamides; cephalosporins, especially cefaclor; erythromycin; NSAIDs; anticonvulsants, barbiturates; isoniazid; carbamazepine; phenytoin; and fluconazole, ketoconazole, and itraconazole (Weston et al, 2007). The risk of this type of eruption is increased if the patient also has a viral infection (e.g., the rash that appears after giving penicillin to a patient with Epstein-Barr virus). Exanthematous rashes typically have their onset within 1 to 2 weeks of starting a new medication and can occur after the medication has been

stopped. If there is a rechallenge of that medication, the reaction can occur within a few days (Paller and Mancini, 2011). Repeated exposure can progress to anaphylaxis.

Clinical Findings
History
- Medication taken within the past 3 weeks
- Varying degrees of itching—can be intense
- Rash worsens even after medicine is discontinued for up to 5 days
- Possible systemic symptoms—low-grade fever, arthralgia, arthritis, lymphadenopathy, edema

Physical Examination. Findings include the following (see Color Plate):
- Condition often begins as a fairly symmetric, macular erythematous rash that becomes papular and confluent.
- Patches of normal skin are scattered throughout areas of involvement.
- Rash begins on the trunk, where it is a brighter red, more confluent, and extends distally to the extremities, including the palms and soles.
- Rash may turn brownish red and desquamate in 7 to 14 days.
- The face often has confluent areas of erythema.
- Mucous membranes are typically spared.

Diagnostic Studies. The following are ordered if necessary for differential diagnosis:
- CBC, monospot test, C reactive protein (CRP), antinuclear antibodies, antistreptolysin-O (ASO), cold agglutinins
- Chest radiograph

TABLE 36-10	Differentiating Drug Eruptions, Urticaria, and Erythema Multiforme		
	Etiology	**Clinical Findings**	**Treatment**
Drug eruption	Reaction to medication, especially penicillin, cephalexin, erythromycin, sulfa drugs, NSAIDs, barbiturates, isoniazid, carbamazepine, phenytoin	Symmetric, macular, erythematous to papular, confluent morbilliform rash; intense itching; patches of normal skin throughout; begins on trunk, extends distally, including palms and soles; face with confluent erythema	Stop drug and label as allergen to the child; give antihistamine, antipruritic, prednisone if severe; lubricate skin; rash can last 7 to 14 days; use medical alert bracelet
Urticaria	Hypersensitive reaction; immunologic antigen-antibody response to release of histamines; often unknown cause; possible reaction to food, drug, insect bite or sting, pollen; possible reaction to infection, especially streptococcal, sinus, mononucleosis, hepatitis	Key finding: appears suddenly, fades from 20 minutes to 24 hours. Family history of hives; possible atopy; intense itching; mild erythema, annular, raised wheals with pale centers; lesions scattered or coalesced; blanch with pressure; associated edema of eyelids, lips, tongue, hands, feet	Quick resolution; identify and remove offending agent if possible and treat; stop antibiotic; give oral antihistamines; topical antipruritics; epinephrine or prednisone if anaphylactic, angioedema, or refractory; refer if >6 weeks' duration
Erythema multiforme	Immune-mediated hypersensitivity reaction often to infection, especially HSV; also to many other agents	Key finding: target or iris lesions: lesions fixed, symmetric, typical distribution on hands, feet, elbows, knees, also face, neck, trunk. History of infection, especially herpes labialis; variety of lesions on skin and mucous membranes—macules, papules, vesicles, early lesions, such as urticaria; possible oral mucous membrane involvement	Identify, treat, discontinue trigger if possible; treat infection; supportive measures for hydration, prevention of secondary infection, relief of pain; oral antihistamines, cool compresses; oral lesions—mouthwash, topical anesthetics; lesions last 5 to 7 days, recur in batches over 2 to 4 weeks, resolve without scarring or sequelae

HSV, Herpes simplex virus; *NSAIDs,* nonsteroidal antiinflammatory drugs.

Differential Diagnosis

Viral exanthem; measles; toxic erythema, such as in scarlet fever, staphylococcal scarlatina, or Kawasaki disease; morbilliform rash (if the patient has mononucleosis and is taking amoxicillin); TSS; roseola; and erythema infectiosum are included in the differential diagnosis.

Management

Decisions about whether a drug is to be implicated depend on the patient's previous history of taking the drug, the experience of the general population with the drug, the morphology and timing of the rash, and other possible explanations for the rash (e.g., viral illness). The following steps are taken:

1. Discontinue the suspected drug.
2. Label the patient's medical record with the potential allergen.
3. Prescribe antihistamines if itching is present; recommend a lubricant and antipruritics as adjuncts.
4. Systemic steroids not usually indicated in a morbilliform drug eruption (Newell and Horii, 2010). If severe reaction, prednisone 1 to 2 mg/kg/day for 5 to 7 days.
5. Schedule follow-up visit as determined by severity of reaction and other illness.
6. Refer to allergist for skin testing to confirm allergy if there are limited or no alternative medications, for desensitization, to clarify drug allergy, for severe parental anxiety, or if symptoms are severe and life threatening.

Complications

Body heat and water loss can occur if the rash is severe. Progression of the rash if medicine is continued can lead to toxic epidermal necrolysis or SJS (see section on EM) or allergic interstitial nephritis.

Patient Education and Prevention

- The rash can last 7 to 14 days with itching, and worsening before getting better.
- There is potential risk from further exposure to that drug or related ones; alternative therapies should be explained.
- Identification and communication of the child's allergy are imperative. In life-threatening allergies, wearing a medical alert bracelet or necklace is essential.

■ Vascular Reactions of the Skin

URTICARIA AND ANGIOEDEMA

Description

Urticaria and angioedema are hypersensitivity reactions (usually a type I reaction—IgE mediated) commonly called *hives* (see Color Plate). Transient or acute urticaria lasts less than 6 weeks; chronic, recurrent, or persistent urticaria lasts more than 6 weeks. Angioedema involves the deeper dermis and subcutaneous tissue; in contrast, urticaria involves the superficial dermis. Patients who get both angioedema and urticaria tend to have more severe reactions.

Epidemiology

Urticaria and angioedema are the result of a complex interplay of immunologically mediated antigen-antibody responses to the release of histamine from mast cells and other vasoactive mediators, such as leukotrienes and prostaglandins. Vasodilation and increased vascular permeability cause erythema and the characteristic wheal of urticaria. Onset is usually rapid, and resolution occurs within a few days of onset. The cause often remains a mystery (idiopathic). Possible causative factors include the following:

- Reactions to foods (e.g., nuts, eggs, shellfish, strawberries, tomatoes), drugs (salicylates and penicillins are the two most common), stings (e.g., bees, wasps, scorpions, spiders, jellyfish), bites (e.g., mosquitoes, fleas, mites), or pollen
- Reaction to skin contact with antigens such as chemicals, latex, fish, or caterpillars
- Response to bacterial, viral, or fungal infections, especially streptococcal or sinus infection, mononucleosis, hepatitis, adenoviruses and enteroviruses, or parasites
- Cholinergic response to physical stimuli (e.g., heat or cold, sun or water [aquagenic urticaria], tight clothing, vibrations) or stress
- Genetic origin
- Concurrent with inflammatory systemic diseases (e.g., collagen-vascular or inflammatory bowel disease)

Urticaria occurs sometime in the lives of about 15% of the population. Portals of entry include infection (most common), ingestion, injection, inhalation, immunologic (rare), and idiopathic. Drugs are responsible for about 10% of the episodes of urticaria, which are generally acute in nature (Paller and Mancini, 2011).

Urticaria and angioedema are more common in children, and about 50% of patients with urticaria also have angioedema. Angioedema is an extension of the reaction into the subcutaneous tissue and tends to involve the face (especially the eyes), hands, and feet (Weston et al, 2007). It is gradual in onset and often involves reactions to medication. Hereditary angioedema is a rare autosomal dominant disorder that results from either a deficiency or dysfunction of the first component of complement (C-esterase inhibitor). It is life threatening and usually manifests before 10 years old, typically with exacerbations in adolescence, often following trauma (e.g., dental work, surgery, accident). It is manifested by repeated episodes of swelling of the extremities, face, and throat, accompanied by abdominal pain that becomes progressively more severe (Paller and Manicini, 2011). Severe airway edema, if untreated, is often the cause of death.

Clinical Findings
History

- Family or previous history of hives, angioedema, connective tissue disease, juvenile arthritis
- Possibility of atopy
- Intense itching and scratching
- Ingestion (within 4 hours) of nuts, shellfish, chocolate, berries, spices, egg white, milk, fish, sesame
- Ingestion or injection of medicines (penicillin, sulfa drugs, sedatives, diuretics, analgesics, acetylsalicylic acid), additives, or preservatives
- Injection of diagnostic agents, vaccine, insect venom, blood, medicine

- Infection with upper respiratory infectious agent, virus, streptococcus, mononucleosis; hepatitis; parasites
- Inhalation of animal dander, pollen, dust, smoke, or aerosols
- Flea or mite bites
- Cold, heat, exercise, sun, water, pressure, or vibration

Physical Examination. Location of lesions may help determine the cause (e.g., a lesion around the mouth or tongue is likely due to an ingested agent). Findings can include the following:

- Urticaria is seen as mildly erythematous, annular, raised wheals or welts with pale centers from 2 mm to several centimeters in diameter; however, they can be of various shapes. Such lesions typically:
  - Are scattered or coalesced but generalized
  - Appear suddenly as individual lesions and fade in anywhere from 20 minutes to less than 24 hours, reappearing in other areas later; if fixed more than 48 hours, it is not urticaria
  - Blanch with pressure
  - Seem to be intensified with heat
  - Appear as wheals after rubbing or stroking the skin (dermatographism)
  - Occur most commonly as papulovesicular lesions with central punctate lesion and wheals in toddlers (papular urticaria)
  - Can appear as large, blotchy, erythematous lesions with 1- to 3-mm central wheals (cholinergic urticaria)
- Angioedema is seen as asymmetric, localized, nondependent and transient edema.
- Typically less pruritic than urticaria
- May involve the upper airway and progress to life-threatening obstruction
- Can cause associated edema of eyelids, lips, tongue, hands, feet, and genitalia

Diagnostic Studies. If urticaria with possible anaphylaxis from an insect bite is suspected, refer to an allergist for testing and hyposensitization. If fever is present, evaluate for underlying disease.

Differential Diagnosis

Contact dermatitis, atopic dermatitis, scabies, EM (lesions are fixed with dusky centers and appear within 72 hours—see Color Plate), mastocytosis, reactive erythemas, vasculitis, psoriasis, and juvenile arthritis are also included in the differential diagnosis (see Table 36-10).

Management

The following steps are taken:

1. Identify and remove the offending substance if possible. Stop all antibiotics. Avoid any possible food or environmental trigger.
2. Test for dermatographism by stroking the skin, for cholinergic urticaria by applying heat or observing immediately after exercising, for cold urticaria by applying cold packs, for pressure urticaria by applying weighted bands for several minutes, and for water urticaria by applying wet compresses.
3. Administer medications as indicated.
   - Oral antihistamines, such as diphenhydramine 0.5 to 1 mg/kg/dose every 4 to 6 hours as needed (maximum 50

mg/dose and 300 mg/day) or hydroxyzine 0.6 mg/kg/dose every 6 hours as needed (400 mg/day maximum) until itching and urticaria are resolved. Nonsedating antihistamines are less effective, but if needed, astemizole, cetirizine, or loratadine are best. Urticaria is less likely to recur if the antihistamine is continued for 1 to 2 weeks after resolution.
- Topical antipruritics may be helpful.
- Aqueous epinephrine 1:1000 (subcutaneously 0.01 mL/kg up to 0.3 mL) may be needed if anaphylaxis or significant angioedema with swelling of the face, mucous membranes, and airway is present.
- Prednisone 1 to 2 mg/kg/day for 1 week with rapid taper only if refractory to other measures or if angioedema is present with swelling of lips and face.
4. Follow-up visit if not improved within 48 hours
5. Chronic urticaria persisting longer than 6 weeks needs evaluation for infection or systemic causes or referral for further evaluation.
6. An emergency epinephrine kit (EpiPen Jr, 0.15 mg or adult, 0.3 mg) should be prescribed for children after the first episode or with recurrent episodes of life-threatening urticaria or angioedema.

Complications

Angioedema or anaphylaxis occurs by the same mechanism as urticaria.
- Anaphylactic symptoms require emergency intervention.
- Serum sickness begins with hives, but has other systemic symptoms (e.g., fever, arthralgias, malaise, lymphadenopathy, proteinuria).
- If urticaria is from a drug reaction, rechallenge with the drug is more likely to cause anaphylaxis.

Patient Education and Prevention

The following are needed:
- Explanation of causes (often unknown), course, and treatment. Control of symptoms is the main goal of treatment. The entire episode usually resolves in 24 to 48 hours, rarely extending beyond 3 to 4 weeks. Further evaluation is needed only if urticaria lasts longer than 8 weeks.
- Papular urticaria hypersensitivity often declines within 6 to 12 months.
- Physical urticarias last 2 to 4 years in most cases, but occasionally persist into adulthood.
- Occasionally macular blue-brown lesions are found on resolution of urticaria.
- Avoid allergen if known; wear a medical alert bracelet in case severe reaction occurs; refer for hyposensitization if life-threatening symptoms occur.
- Carry an epinephrine kit if indicated.

ERYTHEMA MULTIFORME, STEVENS-JOHNSON SYNDROME, TOXIC EPIDERMAL NECROLYSIS

Description

EM minor is an acute, usually benign, self-limiting eruption of targetoid papules with varying bullae formation. In the past, EM, SJS (also know as erythema multiforme major), and toxic epidermal necrolysis (TEN) were thought to be related disorders. EM minor is a distinct disorder that does not progress to TEN or SJS. EM is rarely associated with complications and has a benign course characterized by the development of target lesions and minor mucosal involvement. SJS and TEN are considered to represent a distinct syndrome that occurs with variable expression along a continuum. SJS and TEN are associated with significant risk of morbidity and mortality.

Epidemiology

EM usually follows an infection with approximately 80% of cases of classic EM attributed to HSV. Herpes labialis or progenitalis lesion(s) are commonly associated with the onset of EM. The herpetic lesion may have healed or had a subclinical presentation. EM tends to be recurrent as do herpes lesions. The herpes infection is believed to be caused by a precipitating mechanism and results in an immune response. EM may also be associated with other viruses such as EBV, cytomegalovirus (CMV), and other herpesviruses (Weston et al, 2007).

Clinical Findings
History
- With EM
  - Recent or current infection with herpes virus (herpes labialis or progenitalis)
  - Exposure to UV light or trauma to area
  - Low-grade fever, malaise, and myalgia
- With SJS or TEN
  - SJS usually caused by medication or viral illness; TEN nearly exclusively caused by medication (Treat, 2010)
  - TEN begins with a fever, sore throat, malaise, and generalized sunburn-like erythema.
  - SJS can have a prodrome of high fever, cough, sore throat, vomiting, diarrhea, chest pain, and arthralgia that usually lasts 1 to 3 days (but can last from 1 to 14 days) followed by the onset of lesions.

Physical Examination. It is important to differentiate the clinical findings of EM from SJS and TEN.
- In EM
  - Lesions vary from patient to patient, within a single episode, and with recurrence.
  - Lesions initially appear dusky, as red macules or edematous papules that evolve into target lesions with multiple, concentric rings of color change.
  - Lesions are fixed (another diagnostic clue), tend to be symmetric, and have a typical distribution predominantly on the face, extensor surface of the arms and legs, dorsum of the hands and feet, and the palms and soles.
  - Mucous membranes may be involved with erythema and erosions noted (Weston et al, 2007).
- In SJS or TEN
  - SJS skin lesions typically are erythematous macules on the head and neck and can spread to the trunk and extremities with blister formation (within hours) that is often hemorrhagic, extensive, and confluent; mucosal involvement of eyes, nose, and mouth is widespread.
  - The TEN rash has rapidly coalescing target lesions and widespread bullae that become full-thickness epidermal peeling or sloughing within 24 hours; Nikolsky sign (peeling of skin with a light rub that reveals a moist red surface) is present.

○ Conjunctivae, urethra, rectum, oral and nasal mucosa, larynx, and tracheobronchial mucosa may or may not be involved with TEN.

Diagnostic Studies. Studies are ordered as indicated by the clinical condition of the child.

Differential Diagnosis

Urticaria can be differentiated by lack of itching, lability of lesions, and shorter-lasting hives that are pale centrally, not target or iris lesions (see Table 36-10). Viral exanthems are more centrally located, confluent, and less erythematous. Purpura is present in vasculitis. In SSSS, the skin peels superficially (not full thickness) and is significantly red. Also included in the differential diagnosis are Kawasaki disease and lupus erythematosus.

Management

Care for EM is generally supportive because the condition is self-limited.

- Symptomatic and supportive care: maintain hydration, prevent secondary infection, and relieve pain.
  - ○ Mild analgesics, cool compresses, and oral antihistamines, such as diphenhydramine
  - ○ Soothing mouthwashes or topical anesthetics, such as Kaopectate or Maalox, mixed in equal parts with diphenhydramine
  - ○ Topical intraoral anesthetics, such as dyclonine liquid or viscous lidocaine, are sometimes used with caution in older children and adolescents.
  - ○ Debridement of oral lesions with half-strength hydrogen peroxide
  - ○ Wound care
  - ○ IV fluids if oral hydration is not adequate
  - ○ Systemic antihistamines, analgesics, and antimicrobials as needed
- Prevention of herpes simplex: Avoid sun exposure and use sunscreen and protective clothing.
- Prophylaxis for recurrent EM treatment:
  - ○ Oral acyclovir, for child weighing less than 40 kg, 20 mg/kg/day divided twice daily, or weighing greater than 40 kg, 400 mg/day divided twice daily, for a 6- to 12-month trial with periodic stopping to reassess
  - ○ Acyclovir during an acute episode of EM does not alter its course.

SJS and TEN are potentially life-threatening diseases. Children are typically admitted to the pediatric intensive care unit (PICU) or burn unit for wound care, management of hydration and electrolyte issues, nutritional support, and pain control. IVIG should be started as quickly as possible in order to reverse the blistering and sloughing. The use of systemic corticosteroids is contraindicated in the treatment of SJS and TEN because of the increased risk of sepsis (Treat, 2010).

Complications

EM is typically a self-limiting condition. SJS and TEN are associated with significant morbidity including pneumonitis, sepsis, GI bleeding, renal disease, keratitis, and other ophthalmologic disorders.

Patient Education and Prevention

EM lesions can erupt in crops that last 1 to 3 weeks, but resolve without scarring or sequelae, except for transient desquamation, scaling, or hyperpigmentation. Recurrence of EM is common.

■ Papulosquamous Eruptions of the Skin

PITYRIASIS ROSEA

Description

PR, meaning rose-colored flaking, is a common, mild, self-limited papulosquamous disease (see Color Plate).

Epidemiology

The etiology of PR has not been established. There is debate as to whether PR is caused by human herpesvirus 6 or 7 (HHV-6 or HHV-7). It is minimally contagious and occurs most commonly in the fall, early winter, and spring in temperate climates. Fifty percent of all cases occur before 20 years old, most commonly in adolescence, with males and females equally affected. Approximately 98% of cases result in life-long immunity (Paller and Mancini, 2011).

Clinical Findings

History. Although most are otherwise well, a small percentage (5%) of patients experience a prodrome of mild symptoms including malaise, pharyngitis, lymphadenopathy, and headache before onset of rash. Those that have prodromal symptoms tend to have a more florid rash.

Physical Examination

- Herald spot or patch (70% of presentations)—a 2- to 5-cm solitary, ovoid, slightly erythematous lesion with a finely scaled slightly elevated border that enlarges quickly with central clearing); typical locations for the herald patch include the trunk, upper arm, neck, or thigh
- Secondary generalized lesions appear that are symmetric, small macular to papular, thin and round to oval. The lesions have thin scales centrally with thicker scales peripherally ("collarette" scales surround the lesions). They are also pale pink; more common on trunk and proximal extremities from neck to knees; typically spare the face, scalp, and distal extremities; and usually occur 2 to 21 days after the appearance of the herald patch (key finding).
- Christmas tree pattern—rash, especially on back, follows dermatome skin lines with oval lesions running parallel and wraps around the trunk horizontally.
- Itching occurs in about 25% of cases particularly with secondary lesions.
- Oral lesions have punctate hemorrhages, erosions or ulcerations, erythematous macules, or annular plaques; such lesions occur in about 16% of patients.
- The face and neck are frequent areas of involvement in young children especially if African-American.
- Atypical disease occurs in an inverse distribution to PR lesions with involvement of usually spared areas (lesions on the face, axilla, groin), most occurring in young children, typically African-American children (Paller and Mancini, 2011).

Diagnostic Studies. If needed, a KOH preparation of a skin scraping is done to rule out tinea.

Differential Diagnosis

Include psoriasis, guttate psoriasis, nummular eczema, scabies, tinea (especially the herald patch), secondary syphilis, drug eruptions, or viral exanthems in the differential diagnosis.

Management

The following steps are taken:
- Application of calamine lotion (or other lotions containing menthol and/or camphor or pramoxine), tepid baths with Aveeno, antihistamines, and emollients as needed for itching
- Topical steroids do not change the lesions or hasten recovery.
- Minimal sun exposure can help lesions resolve more quickly. Prevent sunburn.
- Early administration of oral erythromycin has been demonstrated as beneficial in shortening the course of PR (Dyer, 2007; Weston et al, 2007).

Patient Education and Prevention

PR is a benign, self-limited, and noncontagious disease that has three cycles (emerging, persisting, and fading) with spontaneous resolution in 6 to 12 weeks. Transient pigmentary changes can occur, especially in African-Americans. Recurrence is common.

PSORIASIS

Description

Psoriasis, a chronic papulosquamous skin disorder with spontaneous remissions and exacerbations, is characterized by thick silvery scales, varied distribution patterns, and an isomorphic (Koebner phenomenon) response (see Color Plate). Types of psoriasis include guttate psoriasis (following a streptococcal infection), psoriasis vulgaris, napkin psoriasis (occurring in the diaper area), inverse psoriasis (limited to areas that are normally spared), localized pustular psoriasis, generalized pustular or psoriatic erythroderma, and psoriatic arthritis.

Epidemiology

Psoriasis is an immune-mediated disorder associated with genetic predisposition and environmental risk factors. Though the exact cause is unknown, chromosome 6p21.3 is linked to the development of psoriasis, and the contributing gene is termed PSORSI. The disease results from keratinocyte proliferation and dermal vascular abnormalities. Trigger factors include infection, local trauma, stress (physical and psychological), and certain drugs (corticosteroids, lithium, beta-blockers, NSAIDs).

Psoriasis occurs at all ages; 30% of cases have onset in childhood (Lyon, 2011). Guttate psoriasis is often the first sign of psoriasis in children.

Clinical Findings
History
- There is often a family history of psoriasis. Genetic factors are involved in the development of psoriasis (Weston et al, 2007).

- Streptococcal infection of the oropharynx or perianal area before onset (guttate)
- Trauma before onset
- Itching (variable)

Physical Examination
- The scalp (encircling the hairline and external ears), elbows, knees, and buttocks (especially the diaper area in infants) are the most common sites of involvement. In children the face may also be involved. Lesions are often found around areas of trauma (e.g., genitalia, palms, soles).
  - *Plaque psoriasis.* Discrete, initially erythematous, symmetric, well-marginated rash becoming papular with silver scales that may be trivial to widespread
  - *Guttate (teardrop) psoriasis.* Widespread, symmetric, round, or oval 0.5- to 2-cm lesions occurring primarily on the trunk and proximal extremities, occasionally on the face, scalp and ears and rarely on the palms or soles. There is less scaling than in psoriasis vulgaris.
  - *Psoriasis vulgaris.* Well-circumscribed, erythematous plaques with thick, silvery white scales concentrated on elbows, knees, scalp, and hairline, but also seen on eyebrows, around ears, and in intergluteal fold and genital area.
  - *Koebner phenomenon (isomorphic response).* The occurrence of psoriasis lesions several days after trauma (e.g., bites, scratch, abrasion, sunburn, pressure) is characteristic (Weston et al, 2007).
  - *Auspitz sign.* Bleeding occurs when a scale is removed.
  - *Nail signs.* Nails have "ice pick" pits and ridges, are thick and discolored (yellowing), and can have splinter hemorrhages or subungual hyperkeratosis, and be separated from the nailbed (Lyon, 2011).
  - *Napkin or diaper area psoriasis.* Appears eczematous with sharply defined plaques, bright red coloration, shiny with large drier scales, affecting inguinal and gluteal folds.

Diagnostic Studies
- ASO if guttate pattern
- KOH-treated scrapings and culture to rule out fungal infection
- VDRL to rule out secondary syphilis

Differential Diagnosis

PR, seborrhea, *Candida* infection, contact or irritant dermatitis, atopic dermatitis, tinea, dyshidrosis, secondary syphilis, and other nail-pitting conditions are included in the differential diagnosis.

Management

In children, treatment should be as conservative as possible. Medications and treatments should be rotated for best effectiveness. The following are options for management:
- Sun exposure in moderate amounts alleviates lesions. Prevent sunburn.
- Emollient creams, such as petrolatum, Eucerin, Aquaphor, or Cetaphil for dry skin can minimize trauma and subsequent psoriasis and may improve psoriasis.
- Apply topical steroids two or three times a day for 2 to 3 weeks. They should be used intermittently, but not discontinued spontaneously because worsening can occur. Monitoring of the patient during use is important. Small

localized lesions can be treated with topical fluorinated steroids. A moderate-potency steroid can be used on thick plaques and larger areas. Severe plaques on the elbows and knees may need a higher-potency steroid (see Table 36-1). Systemic steroids are not indicated and may worsen the condition, causing pustular flare. Consultation with a dermatologist is often indicated.

- Tar or keratolytic shampoos (ketoconazole, anthralin, salicylic acid) can be used on the scalp.
- Mineral or olive oil and warm towels to soak and remove thick plaques
- Keratolytic agents, such as sulfur 3% or salicylic acid 3% to 6%, to reduce thick, unresponsive plaques. Salicylic acid blocks UVB and should not be used in combination with phototherapy.
- Anthralin ointment for plaques that are resistant to steroids and tar. In high strengths (1% and higher), apply ointment for 10 to 30 minutes once a day, then wash off. In lower strengths, leave on for 8 hours. Strength used is determined by tolerance. Anthralin stains skin and clothing and can irritate skin.
- Calcipotriol, a vitamin D analogue, is effective for mild to moderate plaque psoriasis in adults and children. Available in cream, ointment, and lotion, it is safe, effective, and well-tolerated for short- and long-term treatment. Hypercalcemia is reported with application of excessive quantities over large areas.
- Tazarotene is a retinoid that may be effective in management of plaque psoriasis, but is often too irritating for use in childhood psoriasis (Paller and Mancini, 2011).
- Tacrolimus ointment, a calcineurin inhibitor, has demonstrated benefit when used for facial and intertriginous psoriasis in children (Paller and Mancini, 2011).
- Balneo-phototherapy combines magnesium-rich Dead Sea salt baths with UV light treatments for 4 to 6 weeks or 15 to 25 treatments. This natural treatment may bring 80% to 85% clearance of skin lesions or remission (Mikula, 2003).
- Cyclosporine and methotrexate are systemic therapies used for recalcitrant and severe disease.
- Follow up every 2 weeks until psoriasis is controlled and during exacerbations and then as needed.
- Refer to a dermatologist if psoriasis is not responsive. Other treatment options include UV light treatment, psoralens, intralesional steroids, retinoids, cyclosporine, biologic therapy, and immunotherapy.

Complications

The following complications are possible and require referral to a dermatologist:
- *Candida* infection. As a secondary infection in the diaper area.
- Erythrodermic and pustular psoriasis. Unusual in childhood; characterized by generalized or local multiple 1- to 2-mm pustules with erythema and scaling also involving palms and soles; accompanied by malaise, fever, electrolyte and fluid imbalances, temperature instability, and leukocytosis; can be fatal.
- Exfoliative erythroderma. Rare manifestation, including desquamation and loss of hair and nails with previous history of psoriasis.

- Psoriatic arthritis. An inflammatory arthritis that is rare but increasing in frequency, most common in females 9 to 12 years old. Prognosis is good but should be referred to a rheumatologist.

Patient Education and Prevention

Emotional support and education are the most important aspects in dealing with psoriasis. Areas for discussion include the following:
- Psoriasis is chronic and involves spontaneous remissions and exacerbations. Control and relief are sought, but cure is not available. Treatment may require up to 1 month to determine effectiveness.
- Guttate psoriasis often resolves with antibiotic treatment for streptococcal infection. Psoriasis vulgaris may persist for months to years.
- Lifestyle changes help prevent recurrence. These include avoiding cutaneous injury, streptococcal infection, sunburn, stress, itching, bites, tight clothes and shoes, some medications (e.g., oral steroids, NSAIDs), and occlusive dressings. Good skin care, including regular use of emollients and avoiding irritating underarm deodorants and harsh soaps, may improve psoriasis and minimize recurrences. With nail involvement, avoid long fingernails or toenails and use of nail polish. Do not vigorously brush or comb hair if scalp area affected.
- Psoriasis tends to improve during summer and with pregnancy.
- Psoriasis is considered stable if there are either no new plaques or if existing plaques are not enlarging.
- Refer patients to the National Psoriasis Foundation (www. psoriasis.org).

LICHEN STRIATUS
Description

Lichen striatus (LS) is peculiar to childhood, characterized by unilateral shiny papules along embryonic lines, or lines of Blaschko.

Epidemiology

Although the etiology is unknown, it is thought to be related to a cutaneous defect from an embryologic mutation of somatic cells. It is most common in school-age children and affects girls more than boys. LS is typically located on the extremities, upper back, or neck, but can be found on the palms, soles, nails, genitals or face. Lesions spontaneously disappear after 3 to 12 months, but may last up to 3 years. Short relapses occur on occasion.

Clinical Findings
History. Lesions appear spontaneously without prodrome.
Physical Examination
- Linear, shiny hypopigmented or flesh-colored, flat-topped papules with adherent scale
- Limited to one extremity, initially lesions coalesce in a linear distribution down an extremity
- Lesions involving a nailbed result in nail deformity.
- Rarely are lesions noted on the face.
- May be asymptomatic or may be intensely pruritic
- May resolve with hypopigmentation that lasts several months

Diagnostic Studies. A skin biopsy is diagnostic when in doubt.

Differential Diagnosis

The unilateral linear lesions are characteristic. However, differential diagnosis includes lichen planus, lichen nitidus, psoriasis, epidermal birthmarks, and linear Darier disease.

Management

Lesions are resistant to treatment, and treatment is unnecessary for asymptomatic cases. However, pruritus may be relieved with the use of group I or group II topical steroids or topical tacrolimus ointment (Morelli, 2007; Weston et al, 2007).

Patient Education and Prevention

LS is a benign, self-limited, noncontagious disorder that results in complete resolution.

KERATOSIS PILARIS

Description

Keratosis pilaris is a common finding on the extensor aspects of the extremities, buttocks, and occasionally the cheeks. The skin has a typical appearance of "chicken skin" with small bumps at the hair follicle.

Epidemiology

The etiology is unknown. It is not present at birth but is common in early childhood onward. Some believe it to be a disorder of abnormal keratinization; others believe it to be a response to drying of the skin surface. Keratosis pilaris is more common in children with atopic disorders; in those living in cold, dry climates; and in winter months.

Clinical Findings

History. Keratosis pilaris appears spontaneously, without prodrome. It is usually asymptomatic, although most patients are bothered by the appearance and seek treatment.

Physical Examination
- Rough dry skin on the posterior upper arms, anterior thighs, buttocks, and cheeks
- Small papules with follicular plugs of stratum corneum
- Occasional diffuse eruption with small sterile pustules

Diagnostic Studies. Skin biopsy reveals inflammation outside the hair follicle; however, this is typically not needed because the diagnosis is easy to determine.

Differential Diagnosis

Microcomedones of acne, molluscum contagiosum, warts, milia, and folliculitis are often confused with keratosis pilaris.

Management

It is important to recognize keratosis pilaris as a benign disorder to avoid detrimental treatment. Management includes the following:
- In mild cases lubricants and emollients to moisturize skin are sufficient for improvement.

- Topical keratolytics combined with lactic acid 12%, salicylic acid, urea creams, retinoids, and lubricants are applied several times daily.
- Antibiotics active against *S. aureus* are useful for folliculitis.

Patient Education and Prevention

The chronic but benign nature of keratosis pilaris should be stressed. Treatment takes weeks to months, and recurrence is common.

◼ Congenital Lesions of the Skin

VASCULAR AND PIGMENTED NEVI

Description

Nevi are a common finding in children. The two most common types are vascular nevi (vascular malformations and hemangiomas) and pigmented nevi (mongolian spots, café au lait spots, acquired melanocytic nevi, AN, and lentigines).

Epidemiology

Vascular nevi are caused by a structural abnormality (malformations) or by an overgrowth of blood vessels (hemangiomas) and are flat, raised, or cavernous. Flat lesions or vascular malformations include salmon patches (also called macular stains), an innocent malformation that is a light red macule appearing on the nape of the neck, upper eyelids, and glabella. Approximately 40% of newborns have a salmon patch on the back of the neck. Port-wine stains occur in 3 per 1000 newborns (Weston et al, 2007). At 1 year old, 10% to 12% of Caucasian infants have a hemangioma—females three times more likely than males. There is also an increased incidence of hemangioma in premature neonates. Vascular lesions are always present at birth and do not resolve spontaneously. Precursor lesions of hemangiomas are present at birth 50% of the time. They undergo rapid growth (proliferative stage), stability (plateau phase), and regression (involution phase); 90% are completely resolved by 9 to 10 years old (Paller and Mancini, 2011).

Pigmented nevi are caused by an overgrowth of pigment cells. Pigmented nevi most commonly seen are mongolian spots (up to 90% in African-Americans, 62% to 86% in Asians, 70% in Hispanics, and less than 10% in Caucasians), café au lait spots (found in up to 33% of normal children and in 50% of patients with McCune-Albright syndrome), and acquired melanocytic nevi, the most common tumor of childhood. Atypical nevi, also called dysplastic nevi, are potential precursors for malignant melanoma. Dysplastic nevi are uncommon under 18 years of age but have a higher incidence in melanoma-prone families (Paller and Mancini, 2011).

Clinical Findings

History
- Presence from birth, or age first noted
- Progression of lesion
- Familial tendencies for similar nevi, especially for history of melanoma

Physical Examination. Findings include the following (Box 36-11):
- Vascular malformations or flat vascular nevi are present at birth and grow commensurate with the child's growth.

| **BOX 36-11** | Common Vascular and Pigmented Lesions |

I. Vascular malformations or flat vascular nevi
  A. Salmon patch or nevus flammeus
    1. Light pink macule of varying size and configuration
    2. Commonly seen on the glabella, back of neck, forehead, or upper eyelids
  B. Port-wine stain or nevus flammeus
    1. Purple-red macules that occur unilaterally, tend to be large
    2. Usually occur on face, occiput, or neck, although they may be on extremities
II. Hemangiomas
  A. Superficial (strawberry) hemangiomas are found in the upper dermis of the skin and account for the majority of hemangiomas.
  B. Deep cavernous hemangiomas are found in the subcutaneous and hypodermal layers of the skin; although similar to superficial hemangiomas, there is a blue tinge to their appearance.
    1. With pressure, there is blanching and a feeling of a soft, compressible tumor.
    2. Variable in size, they can occur in places other than skin.
  C. Mixed hemangiomas have attributes of both superficial and deep hemangiomas.
III. Pigmented nevi
  A. Mongolian spots
    1. Blue or slate-gray, irregular, variably sized macules
    2. Common in the presacral or lumbosacral area of dark-skinned infants; also on the upper back, shoulders, and extremities
    3. The majority of the pigment fades as the child gets older and the skin darkens.
    4. Solitary or multiple, often covering a large area
  B. Café au lait spots
    1. Tan to light brown macules found anywhere on the skin; oval or irregular shape; increase in number with age
  C. *Acquired melanocytic nevi* are benign, light brown to dark brown to black, flat, or slightly raised, occurring anywhere on the body, especially on sun-exposed areas, above the waist
    1. *Junctional nevi* represent the initial stage, with tiny, hairless, light brown to black macules.
    2. *Compound nevi*—a few junctional nevi progress to more elevated, warty, or smooth lesions with hair.
    3. *Dermal nevi* are the adult form, dome shaped with coarse hair.
    4. *Atypical nevi* usually appear at puberty, have irregular borders, variegated pigmentation, are larger than normal nevi (6 to 15 mm); usually found on trunk, feet, scalp, and buttocks.
    5. *Halo nevi* appear in late childhood with an area of depigmentation around a pigmented nevus, usually on trunk (see Color Plate).
  D. *Acanthosis nigricans* is velvety brown rows of hyperpigmentation in irregular folds of skin, usually the neck and axilla; tags may also be present.
  E. *Lentigines* are small brown to black macules 1 to 2 mm in size appearing anywhere on the body in school-age children.
  F. *Freckles:* 1 to 5 mm light brown pigmented macules in sun-exposed areas

---

- Hemangiomas are classified as superficial, deep (cavernous), or mixed. They may or may not be present at birth, but usually emerge by 2 to 3 weeks of life. They may manifest as a pale macule, a telangiectatic lesion, or a bright red nodular papule. Involution occurs slowly (10% per year) but spontaneously (30% by 3 years old, 50% by 5 years old, 70% by 7 years old, and 90% by 9 to 10 years old). Average involution is between 12 and 24 months old, heralded by gray areas in the lesion followed by flattening from the center outward. Most hemangiomas appear as normal skin after involution, but others may have residual changes, such as telangiectasias, atrophy, fibrofatty residue, and scarring (Paller and Mancini, 2011). During the proliferative phase, hemangiomas grow rapidly and form nodular compressible masses, ranging in size from a few millimeters to several centimeters. Occasionally they may cover an entire limb, resulting in asymmetric limb growth. Rapidly growing lesions may ulcerate.
- Pigmented nevi may be present at birth or acquired during childhood.
- Atypical nevi are larger than acquired nevi; have irregular, poorly defined borders; and have variable pigmentation.

Differential Diagnosis

Hematomas or ecchymoses of child abuse are occasionally confused with some nevi. Non–insulin-dependent diabetes mellitus (NIDDM) often causes AN.

Management

1. Flat vascular nevi
   - Salmon patches: Fade with time, usually by 5 or 6 years old
   - Port-wine stains: A permanent defect that grows with the child, so cosmetic covering is often used. If forehead and eyelids are involved, there is potential for multiple syndromes, including Sturge-Weber, Klippel-Trenaunay-Weber, and Parkes Weber. Neurodevelopmental and ophthalmologic follow-up is needed. Requires referral to a dermatologist for possible laser treatment or corrective cosmesis.
2. Hemangiomas
   - Reassure and educate the family about the nature and course of these nevi and that they are not related to anything the mother did during pregnancy.
   - Frequent follow-up, especially during the growing phase. Sequential photographs are helpful.
   - If the lesions are strategically placed (eye, lip, oral cavity, ear, airway, diaper area), ulcerating, multiple, very large, or grow very quickly, prompt referral to a dermatologist is indicated because early treatment is most effective. Steroids (intralesional and oral) are prescribed during the proliferative stage until growth is stabilized, then gradually tapered. Indications for steroid treatment are interference with physiologic functions (e.g., breathing, hearing, eating, vision), recurrent bleeding or ulceration, high-output congestive heart failure,

Kasabach-Merritt syndrome, rapid growth that distorts facial features, or presence in the diaper area. Interferon-alpha may also be used. Treatment by surgery, cryotherapy, radiation, or injecting sclerosing agents often leads to scarring. Large, deep lesions can cause cardiovascular complications, disseminated intravascular coagulation, or compression of internal organs.

- Regression (without treatment) occurs at a rate of 10% per year. Scarring may be present if ulceration occurs; fibrofatty masses, atrophy, and telangiectasis can occur following involution. Laser therapy is effective management for residual telangiectasias (Paller and Mancini, 2011).

3. Pigmented nevi. Educate family about the nature of these lesions.
   - *Mongolian spots:* Document to distinguish from bruise; fade with time, usually no traces by adulthood
   - *Blue nevus:* Heavily pigmented melanocytes in papule or nodule that can develop melanoma
   - *Café au lait spots:* If six or more lesions larger than 0.5 cm in diameter are present in children younger than 15 years old and more than 1.5 cm in diameter for older individuals or if axillary freckling or tumors are also present, refer child to rule out neurofibromatosis, McCune-Albright syndrome, or other genetic disorder (Weston et al, 2007).

4. Other disorders of hyperpigmentation that can appear in early childhood
   - *Acquired melanocytic nevi*: Giant nevi (e.g., bathing trunk nevus) are at increased risk of developing melanoma and need referral to a dermatologist.
   - *Atypical nevi* appear most commonly in adolescents and require regular follow-up because of increased risk for melanoma. However, melanoma often manifests with new lesions rather than from transformation of current ones (see section on sunburn complications).
   - *Halo nevus*: A depigmented ring around a pigmented nevus
   - *Spitz nevus*: A smooth, pink to brown, dome-shaped papule often occurring on head and neck
   - *Nevus spilus* is a light-brown speckled lentiginous nevus with darker papules within it; it can be congential or acquired and has potential to develop melanoma.

5. Guidelines for when a child with a nevus should be referred to a dermatalogist are listed in Box 36-12.

Complications

Ulceration, infection, platelet trapping, airway or visual obstruction, or cardiac decompensation can occur with large vascular nevi. Kasabach-Merritt syndrome occurs when thrombocytopenic hemorrhage occurs in a large, deep hemangioma. Melanoma in congenital nevi (see discussion in complications of sunburn) is possible, and monitoring these lesions is important. Changes of particular concern are development of an off-center nodule or papule, color change, bleeding, persistent irritation, erosion, ulceration, and rapid growth.

An autosomal dominant, familial, atypical mole and melanoma syndrome has been identified genetically. Children with multiple atypical nevi and family members with melanoma are at risk for childhood melanoma.

BOX 36-12   When to Refer Nevi to a Dermatologist

- Suspicious appearing nevus (as identified by ABCDE signs [see Box 36-9])
- Rapidly growing or changing nevus
- More than 50 nevi
- One or more atypical nevi
- History of one or more first-degree relatives with melanoma
- Presence of a giant or large congenital nevus
- Signs of excessive sun exposure (increased nevi and freckles in exposed areas)
- History of immunosuppression and multiple nevi on examination

---

Patient Education and Prevention

Monitoring nevi that are at risk for developing melanoma is important as is teaching the family to watch nevi for any changes. See sunburn complications section for more information.

■ Cutaneous Manifestations of Underlying Disease

ACANTHOSIS NIGRICANS
Description and Epidemiology

AN is not a skin disease per se; rather it is typically a sign of an underlying problem. It may be related to factors of heredity; endocrine disorders (e.g., insulin resistance, hypothyroidism, hyperandrogenic states, Cushing syndrome; obesity [more commonly seen in darker-pigmented individuals]); drug administration (e.g., oral contraceptives, stilbestrol use in young males, high levels of nicotinic acid); and malignancy (e.g., adenocarcinoma, Wilms tumor, and less commonly lymphoma). All but the malignant form of AN result in papillary hypertrophy, hyperkeratosis, and an increase in the number of melanocytes from keratocyte and dermal fibroblast changes. Insulin resistance and obesity are most commonly associated with the benign form of AN. When it occurs in the hereditary form (autosomal dominant trait with no associated obesity), it may appear at birth or during childhood with proliferation during adolescence. There is no sex predominance. It occurs in Native Americans (40%), African-Americans (13%), Hispanics (6%), and Caucasians (less than 1%) (Baron and Levine, 2006).

Clinical Findings

AN is characterized by symmetric, brown thickening of the skin; as time progresses the skin develops a velvety, leathery, warty, or papillomatous surface. The axillary areas (most commonly), neck, groin, belt line, dorsal surfaces of the fingers, in the mouth, around the areola of the breast, and umbilicus can be affected. In areas of maceration, odor or discomfort may be reported. (See Color Plate.)

Differential Diagnosis

Terra firma-forme dermatosis, a condition with lamellar hyperkeratosis, resembles AN but can occur anywhere on the body. Although it can look like dirt, terra firma-forme dermatosis is not related to hygiene, and cannot be washed off with soap and water. Unlike AN, however, the darkened skin of terra firma-forme dermatosis can be removed with vigorous rubbing with isopropyl alcohol. It is important to diagnose terra firma-forme dermatosis in order to avoid an extensive and expensive workup for an endocrine or metabolic disorder.

Management

Treatment consists of addressing the underlying causes of AN. This most commonly includes management of overweight (diet changes and weight loss) and correction of metabolic abnormality (hyperinsulinemia). In nonoverweight individuals, an underlying malignancy must be considered. The skin lesions themselves are benign, usually asymptomatic, and do not require intervention. Thicker lesions may cause discomfort and respond to topical retinoic acid cream or gel once daily. Dermabrasion and long-pulsed alexandrite laser therapy have also been used. Lac-Hydrin (12% lactic acid cream) can help soften lesions.

Patient Education

It is important for patients to understand that AN may be a cutaneous marker for an underlying disorder (e.g., for hyperinsulinemia in overweight individuals or for a malignancy [AN can precede clinical symptoms of some cancers]) (Morelli, 2007). AN may completely resolve with adequate treatment of the underlying disorder.

LENTIGINES

Lentigines are small, tan, dark brown or black, flat, oval or circular, sharply circumscribed lesions that appear in childhood and may increase in number until adulthood. They may also be seen on mucous membranes and may fade or disappear with time. Lentigines can be associated with various syndromes, such as Peutz-Jeghers, which is related to an increased risk of GI and genitourinary carcinomas (Weston et al, 2007).

■ Other Common Dermatologic Issues in Pediatrics

VITILIGO AND HYPOPIGMENTATION DISORDERS

Description

Lack of skin pigment, leaving white or light-colored areas, can be either hypopigmentation or vitiligo. It is congenital or acquired and appears in a diffuse or localized pattern. Vitiligo is a patterned pigmentation loss with great variation in location, size, and shape of individual lesions. Hypopigmentation following inflammation of the skin is common. Other less common disorders are incontinentia pigmenti achromians and piebaldism. Albinism and progressive vitiligo are examples of generalized pigmentary disturbances.

Epidemiology

Vitiligo is presumed to be an immune disorder that has a genetic component. It occurs in about 1% of the U.S. population, with 50% of cases appearing before 20 years old. It is more common

in children with systemic or immune disorders (Paller and Mancini, 2011; Weston et al, 2007). Hypopigmentation follows inflammation or injury to the melanocytes in the skin resulting from diseases such as atopic dermatitis, psoriasis, or PR, or from abrasions, burns, injury from liquid nitrogen, or severe sunburn.

Clinical Findings
History
- Family history of vitiligo, halo nevi, traumatic depigmentation of skin, or markedly premature graying of the hair (Paller and Mancini, 2011)
- Onset of depigmentation (birth or more recent)
- Presence of any systemic or skin diseases
- Any recent trauma to the skin; Koebner phenomenon is noted in about 15% of children with vitiligo

Physical Examination
- Vitiligo
  - Flat milk-white macules or papules with scalloped, distinct borders of varied size
  - Symmetric or asymmetric, possibly following a nerve segment
  - Few to multiple, seen most commonly on face and trunk
- Hypopigmentation
  - Macules and patches with irregular mottling and borders
  - Linear or patterned
  - Possibly associated hyperpigmented areas

Diagnostic Studies. For vitiligo, a skin biopsy and CBC, fasting glucose, thyroid function and antithyroid antibodies, early-morning serum cortisol, and VDRL are sometimes indicated. A Wood's light may be helpful in fair-skinned individuals to delineate a contrast between the normal and depigmented skin of vitiligo.

Differential Diagnosis

PR, pityriasis alba, tinea versicolor, and albinism (which is seen at birth and affects eye color) are included in the differential diagnosis.

Management
The following steps are taken:
- Vitiligo
  - Broad-spectrum sunscreens are used to decrease the tanning of normal skin.
  - Cover-up agents, such as skin dyes and walnut oil, may be used.
  - Mild to moderate steroids may show success in some patients. Topical calcineurin inhibitors (tacrolimus ointment, pimecrolimus cream) eliminate atrophy, with 40% to 90% of pediatric patients showing a response to these treatments (Paller and Mancini, 2011).
  - Refer for treatment with psoralens. May be used in combination with UVA radiation (best used in children less than 9 years old). UVB may also be used.
  - Support groups help families because this is a highly disfiguring condition, especially for those with dark complexion.
- Hypopigmentation
  - Reassure family that repigmentation will occur. Postinflammatory hypopigmentation is self-limited and lasts only a few months.

Complications

Vitiligo may be associated with other immune disorders or their symptoms, such as thyroid disease, diabetes mellitus, pernicious anemia, Addison disease, uveitis, and alopecia areata. Patients are at risk for severe sunburn.

■ Hair and Nail Disorders

Alopecia, hair loss from areas of skin normally producing hair, can be limited to one area or scattered over the scalp, and can be complete or leave residual hairs of differing lengths. The three main causes of hair loss are tinea capitis, traumatic alopecia, and alopecia areata (Table 36-11).

TINEA CAPITIS

Description

Ringworm of the scalp and hair may be seen in four different manifestations: (1) diffuse fine scaling without obvious hair breaks and with subtle to significant hair loss; (2) discrete areas of hair loss with stubs of broken hairs (black-dot ringworm) (see Color Plate); (3) "classic" patchy hair loss and scaly lesions with raised borders; and (4) scaly, pustular lesions, or kerions. Tinea capitis occurs in a noninflammatory stage for 2 to 8 weeks, then becomes inflammatory.

Epidemiology

The fungus invades the scalp and hair shaft, causing an inflammatory response and fragile hair shaft. *T. tonsurans* and *M. canis* are the most common causes in the U.S. (Weston et al, 2007). Tinea capitis is transmitted by fomites when humans share hats, combs, and brushes, or by cats, dogs, or rodents. Tinea capitis is the most common dermatophyte infection of childhood, typically found in 3- to 7-year-old children (Connelly and Friedlander, 2006; Paller and Mancini, 2011). It is more common in boys and in African-American children.

Clinical Findings

History. Hair loss, itching, and contact with another person or pet with ringworm are sometimes reported.

Physical Examination
- Scaling, erythema, or crusting usually occurs.
- Bald patches or areas of broken hairs are noted.
- *T. tonsurans* manifests as black-dot tinea, with tiny black dots that are the remainder of hair that has broken off at the shaft; no scalp scale is present (most common).
- *M. canis* leaves the hair broken and lusterless with a fine gray scale on the scalp.
- Occipital or posterior cervical adenopathy may be significant.
- A kerion is a boggy, inflamed mass filled with pustules. It results from a delayed inflammatory reaction. There may be regional lymphadenopathy, fever, and leukocytosis. The contents of the kerion are sterile.

Diagnostic Studies. Examine hair scrapings as follows:
- Wood's light fluoresces yellow-green (positive with *M. canis,* negative with *T. tonsurans*).
- KOH examination of scraped hair: Wait 20 to 40 minutes after application of KOH to examine. If Wood's light was positive, under microscopy the KOH-prepared outer surface of hair is coated with tiny mats of spores; if Wood's light was negative, hyphae and spores are present in hair shaft.
- Fungal culture of a completely plucked hair with its root (use a Kelly clamp) is most reliable.

TABLE 36-11	Diagnosis and Treatment of Alopecia		
	Etiology	**Clinical Findings**	**Treatment**
Tinea capitis	*Trichophyton tonsurans* 90%-95%; *Microsporum canis;* others	Fine diffuse scaling without obvious hair breaks and subtle to significant hair loss; hair loss discrete with stubs of broken hair; patchy hair loss with scaling and raised borders to lesions; scaly, pustular lesions or kerions	Griseofulvin taken with fatty food until 2 weeks after negative culture; monitor CBC, LFTs, renal function at 8 weeks and every 8 weeks; prednisone if kerion present; culture family members; sporicidal shampoo; follow up in 2 weeks; launder sheets, clothes, vacuum house
Traumatic alopecia	Chemical, thermal, traction (hairstyling), friction (trichotillomania)	Traumatic: incomplete hair loss with varying lengths Traction: erythema and pustules, hair thins and breaks in certain areas, especially linear Trichotillomania: circumscribed hair loss with irregular borders and broken hair of varied lengths, no erythema or scarring, especially frontal, parietal, or temporal	Traction: avoid hairstyles that precipitate; use mild shampoo, gentle brushing; short course of antibiotics if pustules are present Trichotillomania: discussion with parents, oil at night, counseling, behavioral modifications
Alopecia areata	Autoimmune mechanism	Family history; single or multiple round or oval patches of complete or near-complete hair loss; no erythema or scaling, scalp smooth with fine new hair growth, usually frontal or parietal; "exclamation hairs" present; nail ridging or pitting; occasional loss of body or pubic hair	Discussion and support; often self-limited course; if extensive, refer to dermatologist for alternative treatments; supportive care; prescription for wig; refer to National Alopecia Foundation

CBC, Complete blood count; *LFTs,* liver function tests.

Differential Diagnosis

Traumatic alopecia, alopecia areata, hypothyroid and hyperthyroid hair loss, seborrhea, atopic dermatitis, psoriasis, impetigo, and folliculitis are included in the differential diagnosis.

Management

Topical antifungals are ineffective. Antibiotic treatment is not indicated. The following steps are taken:

- Griseofulvin ultramicrosize at 5 to 15 mg/kg/day once daily or in two divided doses or griseofulvin microsize at 20 to 25 mg/kg/day once daily or 2 divided doses for 6 to 8 weeks; taken with fatty food, such as ice cream, to enhance absorption. Treatment should be continued until clinical and mycologic cure (Taketomo et al, 2011).
- In addition to griseofulvin therapy, shampoo with selenium sulfide 2.5% or econazole or ketoconazole 2% (two or three times per week for 4 weeks) to decrease spore viability and keep other household members from being infected.
- If a long-standing kerion with severe inflammation is present, give prednisone 1 to 2 mg/kg/day for 5 to 14 days.
- Family members and pets should be checked for infection by fungal culture and treated if positive. Do not rely on lack of symptoms as asymptomatic carriers are common.
- A follow-up visit should be scheduled after 2 weeks to evaluate response to treatment. Medication should be continued until 2 weeks after culture is negative. Follow-up should be continued every 2 to 4 weeks until new hair growth is evident.
- Monitoring of CBC, LFTs, and possibly renal function tests is recommended at 8 weeks and every 8 weeks thereafter if griseofulvin is continued (Weston et al, 2007).
- If resistance to griseofulvin is encountered, oral itraconazole, terbinafine, fluconazole, and ketoconazole have been used, but are not all approved for use in children less than 18 years old. Terbinafine is not FDA approved for this indication. However, some studies in children show it to be effective for resistant cases (see Table 36-4 for dosing).

Complications

An id reaction to the fungus, not to the medication, can occur. It manifests either as a red, superficial edema or as scaly, red plaques and papules on the scalp and is treated with 1 to 2 weeks of topical or systemic steroids. Permanent hair loss and scarring can occur with an untreated kerion.

Patient Education and Prevention

- Sites and modes of transmission are identified (*M. canis,* animal source; *T. tonsurans,* human source) and treated.
- Side effects of medication should be explained and monitored; griseofulvin typically may result in GI disturbances, photosensitivity, skin eruptions, and headache.
- Hair regrowth is slow (3 to 12 months), and, if a kerion was present, hair loss can be permanent.
- Laundering sheets and clothes in a hot water wash and hot dryer cycle and vacuuming may decrease spread in the family.
- Grooming practices (e.g., hair traction, greasy pomades, infrequent shampooing) may be predisposing factors.
- There is a high rate of asymptomatic carriers; culture is the only definitive means of identification.

TRAUMATIC ALOPECIA

Description

Traumatic hair loss, characterized by incomplete hair loss with hair of varying lengths, can be due to chemical or thermal traction or friction. The most common forms are traction alopecia and trichotillomania. Trichotillomania is considered a behavior disorder. (See Color Plate.)

Epidemiology

Traction alopecia, commonly seen in African-American females, is due to hair styling. Common causes are cornrows, ponytails, or braids; tight curlers; or excessive brushing.

Trichotillomania (TTM) is a common disorder seen in children of all ages after infancy. Hair loss is varied and is caused by repeated pulling and/or excessive twisting of hair with fracturing of the longer hair shafts. Research indicates etiology is multifactorial, including genetic predisposition and environmental and behavioral variables. In preschoolers it is associated with habitual behaviors and situational stress. It is often seen in children with other obsessive-compulsive habits, such as thumb sucking or nail biting (Bloch, 2009). TTM after the preschool years is classified as an impulse control disorder.

Clinical Findings

History

- Various methods of hair styling with tight pull on hair
- Habits, such as nail biting, finger sucking, or hair twirling
- Any recent life changes or stressors
- Medications (anticonvulsants, antithyroids, beta-blockers, isotretinoin, lithium, oral contraceptives, vitamin A supplements, warfarin)
- Excess time spent lying supine

Physical Examination. The following findings are present due to different causes:

- Traction alopecia
- Possible erythema and pustules
- Thinning and breaking in certain areas, tending to occur in a linear pattern related to hairstyle
- TTM
- Circumscribed hair loss with irregular borders and broken hairs of varied length
- No erythema or scaling of the scalp
- Commonly found on frontal eyelashes, parietal, and temporal areas with peripheral sparing, but also eyebrows

Differential Diagnosis

The differential diagnosis includes tinea capitis, alopecia areata, neonatal occipital alopecia, and child abuse (make sure no one but the child is pulling out the hair).

Management

The following steps are taken:

1. Traction alopecia
   - Avoid any hairstyle or device that causes traction on the hair, including cornrows, ponytails, braids, and curlers.
   - Use only mild shampoo, shampoo infrequently, use wide-toothed combs with rounded ends, and brush gently.
   - A short course of antibiotics is prescribed if pustules are present.

2. TTM

- A straightforward discussion and ongoing support of the child and parents are essential. In very young children TTM is usually benign and resolves spontaneously. Older children and adolescents may require individual and family therapy. Attempt to relieve stress and cope with any traumatic events.
- Applying oil to the hair at night makes it slippery and harder to pull.
- Medication, behavior therapy, habit reversal, relaxation, and hypnosis are often used in combination (Bloch, 2009).

Complications

Trichobezoars (hairballs) in the child with TTM can cause GI symptoms. Some children with TTM have extensive psychopathologic conditions.

Patient Education and Prevention

The cause of the hair loss must be discussed and support offered to resolve issues. New hair growth can take 3 to 6 months.

ALOPECIA AREATA

Description

Alopecia areata is an asymptomatic, complete hair loss occurring primarily in frontal or parietal areas (see Color Plate).

Epidemiology

The cause of alopecia areata is unknown, but is thought to be an autoimmune mechanism. It is unusual in children younger than 2 years of age, but can be seen anytime throughout childhood, with 24% to 65% experiencing their first episode before 16 years old. There is an 8% to 52% familial occurrence (Paller and Mancini, 2011; Weston et al, 2007).

Clinical Findings

History. The history can include other family members with alopecia areata.

Physical Examination

- Single or multiple (up to three) round or oval patches of complete or nearly complete hair loss without erythema or scaling. Scalp is smooth with fine new hair growth.
- The frontal and parietal areas are involved 90% of the time.
- "Exclamation hairs" are narrower at the base, short, and broken off.
- Nail ridging or pitting (a helpful distinguishing factor)
- Occasional loss of body or pubic hair, or eyelashes or eyebrows
- Possible atopic dermatitis or vitiligo

Diagnostic Studies. The following are sometimes performed:

- KOH examination or fungal culture to rule out tinea
- Skin biopsy
- Thyroid screening because it can be associated with autoimmune thyroiditis

Differential Diagnosis

Tinea capitis versus traumatic alopecia is the differential diagnosis.

Management

The following steps should be taken:

1. Open discussion and support of the child and parents. If only one or two patches are present, reassure that regrowth will occur.
2. If extensive involvement, refer to a dermatologist for treatment options. These include potent topical steroids, intralesional steroids, minoxidil, anthralin, or Excimer laser therapy (Paller and Mancini, 2011; Weston et al, 2007).
3. Recommend wearing a wig, depending on the severity of involvement; prescribing the wig as a medical treatment helps defray the cost. Locks of Love is an organization that provides hairpieces to financially disadvantaged children less than 21 years old, and the National Alopecia Areata Foundation (www.naaf.org) is a national support group for affected children and families.

Complications

Self-esteem issues are common. *Ophiasis* is a form of alopecia areata that begins in the frontal or occipital hairline and spreads along the hair margins. *Alopecia totalis* is a loss of all the hair on the scalp. *Alopecia universalis* is a loss of all the hair on the body.

Patient Education, Prognosis, and Prevention

All families should be put in touch with the National Alopecia Areata Foundation. The condition is self-limited in most school-age children and adolescents. Full recovery, often within 1 year, is more likely if three or fewer areas are involved and if onset is in late childhood. However, the greater the hair loss, the longer it takes for regrowth. Prognosis is guarded in infants and toddlers. Approximately one third of patients have a recurrence within months to years, with a worsening prognosis with each episode.

ONYCHOMYCOSIS

Description

Onychomycosis is a fungal infection of the nail(s) typically with *T. rubrum* or *Candida* (see Color Plate). When the nail infection is due to a dermatophyte, it is often called tinea unguium. One or two nails are often involved. The infection may be superficial, hypertrophic (onychauxic), or cause separation of the nail plate from the tissue (onycholytic).

Epidemiology

The infecting organism invades the nail, proliferates, and destroys the nail integrity, causing separation of the nail plate from the nailbed. The infection originates at the distal edge of the nail. It is uncommon during the first two decades of life, limited most commonly to adolescents and adults. When it occurs in children, there is often a concurrent tinea pedis or tinea manuum. There may be a relationship to the use of occlusive shoes. The causative organisms include *T. rubrum*, *T. mentagrophytes*, *E. floccosum*, and *C. albicans*. However, 50% of the time another condition is responsible for dystrophic nail.

Clinical Findings

History. The patient may report a thickened, discolored nail.

Physical Examination

- Opaque white or silvery nail that becomes thick, yellow, with subungual debris
- Toenails are involved more often than fingernails with tinea.
- Fingernails are involved more often than toenails with *Candida.*
- Seldom symmetric; it may be one to three nails on one extremity

Diagnostic Studies. KOH preparations and fungal cultures of the material under the nail are helpful in confirming the diagnosis.

Differential Diagnosis

Psoriasis (involves all nails and includes pitting), hereditary nail defects, dystrophy secondary to eczema or chronic paronychia, lichen planus, and trauma are the differential diagnoses.

Management

1. Successful treatment is difficult and requires oral medication. Griseofulvin can be used, but side effects, length of treatment, low cure rates, and high recurrence rates following treatment make successful management uncommon (Paller and Mancini, 2011).
2. Oral terbinafine, fluconazole, and itraconazole have a better short-term success rate than griseofulvin and a lower relapse rate. Treatment recommendations for onychomycosis are based on the site of infection (Connelly and Friedlander, 2006; Taketomo, 2011):
   - Toenails
     - Itraconazole: 5 mg/kg/day for 12 weeks; or as pulse therapy, 5 mg/kg/day for one week each month for three months (Connelly and Friedlander, 2006)
     - Terbinafine: >40 kg, 250 mg tab once daily for 12 weeks
     - Griseofulvin: 15 to 20 mg/kg/day (decrease dose if using ultramicronized form) for 6 to 18 months
     - Fluconazole: 6 mg/kg/wk for 8 months
   - Fingernails
     - Itraconazole: 5 mg/kg/day for 6 weeks or one week each month for two months (Connelly and Friedlander, 2006)
     - Terbinafine: 4 to 6 mg/kg/day for 6 weeks
     - Fluconazole: 6 mg/kg/wk for 4 months
3. Ciclopirox in nail lacquer used daily has high cure rates in adults, but has not been studied in children. It has been used as monotherapy and adjunctive therapy (Paller and Mancini, 2011).
4. If triazoles are used, a careful history of current medications must be taken because there are many interactions. Monitoring of CBC and hepatic function is recommended at onset of therapy and every 4 to 6 weeks.
5. *Candida* infection is treated with topical application of ketoconazole under occlusion (plastic glove covered by a cotton sock at bedtime) for 3 to 4 weeks.
6. Follow-up visits at 1-month intervals to monitor laboratory values are recommended; long-term follow-up every 6 months is suggested.

Patient Education, Prognosis, and Prevention

The unfortunate truth to communicate is that cure is difficult to obtain, and relapse is common.

PARONYCHIA
Description

Chronic or acute inflammation and infection around a fingernail or toenail is called *paronychia.*

Epidemiology

Paronychia is a common disorder seen in childhood and adolescence caused by a bacterial infection of a nail with bacteria (often *S. aureus,* occasionally *Streptococcus* or *Pseudomonas*), *Candida* (in infants with thrush or thumb sucking or when hands are frequently immersed in water), or herpes. It is more common with tight shoes or when nails are malaligned, cut with rounded edges, or too short.

Clinical Findings

History. Tenderness and drainage are reported and discomfort, especially with walking.

Physical Examination

- Proximal nailfold erythematous, swollen, and tender; if chronic, may not be tender
- Purulent exudate expressed
- Cuticle broken or absent
- Nontender erythema and edema with thickened, disrupted nail (*Candida* infection, often with secondary bacterial infection)

Diagnostic Studies. A culture of the exudate is occasionally done.

Differential Diagnosis

Herpetic whitlow (grouped vesicles on an erythematous base) and eczematous inflammation should be ruled out.

Management

Management includes the following:

- Systemic oral antibiotic if acute infection; coverage for staphylococcal infection may be required
- If *Candida* is suspected, nystatin cream under occlusion (a plastic glove covered by a cotton stocking) every night for 3 to 4 weeks
- If purulent area is full, loosen cuticle from nail with a no. 11 blade to allow exudate to escape.
- Frequent warm soaks, after which cotton pledgets are inserted beneath the nail to lift it.
- Instruction on proper trimming of nails and care of toenails:
  - Wear wide-toed shoes.
  - Trim nails straight across and not too short.
  - If condition is recurrent, refer for surgical removal of lateral portion of nail. Do a follow-up visit in 1 month.

Complications

Recurrent infection is possible.

■ Body Art

TATTOOS AND BODY PIERCING

Description

A tattoo is an indelible mark fixed on the body by insertion of pigment under the skin. Body piercing is the creation of a hole anywhere in the body (typically the ear, eyebrow, lip, naris, tongue, navel, nipple, or genitalia) to insert jewelry. Both are considered forms of *body art*, or embellishment of one's appearance, that have been practiced throughout the ages in many cultures as rites of passage, as means of showing status or membership in a particular group, or as proof of virility.

Epidemiology

Most tattoos or piercings are done in unregulated, unlicensed tattoo parlors, although some adolescents may tattoo or pierce themselves or their peers. Some states have legislation preventing tattooing of minors in tattoo parlors or requiring parental consent.

Adolescents obtain tattoos for any number of reasons including making a personal statement, seeing it as a form of art or a fashion statement, or wishing to be daring. Piercing is considered less permanent than a tattoo. Adults and parents may see piercing or tattooing as a deviant behavior, a strange new trend, a fetish, a fad, or a fashion.

Tattooing and piercing have an increased incidence, especially in the adolescent population. Approximately 22% of undergraduate college students have tattoos, and 51% have piercings (Mayers and Chiffriller, 2008). Teens who participate in piercing, tattooing, and branding were also more likely to engage in other risk-taking behaviors, such as eating disorders, drug use, increased sexual activity, and suicide.

Clinical Findings

History. Questions to discuss include the following:
- When and where was the body art obtained?
- Where is it located, and what care is being given?
- Were there any complications?

Physical Examination. Any symptoms of infection—erythema, crusting, or scabs?

Differential Diagnosis

Branding, the burning of the skin to create a permanent scar in a desired design via blowtorch or wire coat hanger in hot oil, is one differential diagnosis. *Self-mutilation*, a self-directed violence that ranges from altering physical appearance (e.g., ear piercing) to extreme forms (e.g., amputation), is another. Some forms are considered normal, but deviant forms are physically damaging, done in response to crisis, and demonstrate disconnectedness and alienation from others.

Management

1. Aftercare for tattoos:
   - Perform basic wound care, including not touching for 24 hours.
   - A moderate amount of oozing and local swelling is normal for 48 hours.
   - Scab should be left alone except for the application of ointment.
   - Protect from rough surfaces that can traumatize; protect from sunburn.
   - Review signs and symptoms of infection.
2. Aftercare for body piercings
   - Wash hands before touching; wash area with soap twice daily.
   - A moderate amount of oozing and swelling is normal; if crusts appear, remove with wet swab.
   - Tongue
     - Use ice to minimize swelling.
     - Rinse mouth 10 to 12 times a day with half-strength Listerine, twice a day with carbamide peroxide.
     - No deep kissing for 48 hours; once healed, use dental dams for dental work and avoid smoking.
   - Navel
     - Slowest to heal, most likely area to reject jewelry
     - Cleanse twice a day with antibacterial soap.
     - Avoid handling; avoid clothing that rubs for up to 1 year.
   - Nipples and genitalia
     - Cleanse twice a day with antibacterial soap.
     - Avoid manipulation and tight garments; cotton clothes are ideal.
     - Latex barriers must be used with sexual activity.
3. Healing times are variable and should be considered. A tattoo may take 2 to 3 weeks to heal. Body piercing, depending on the site, can take from 4 to 8 weeks for ears to 6 to 12 months for navel and genital piercings (Table 36-12).

TABLE 36-12	Healing Time for Body Piercings
Type of Piercing	**Time to Heal**
Cheek	2 to 4 months
Clitoris	4 to 10 weeks
Ear cartilage	2 months to 1 year
Earlobe	6 to 8 weeks
Eyebrow	6 to 8 weeks
Frenum (underneath tongue)	2 to 6 months
Inner labia	4 to 8 weeks
Lip	2 to 3 months
Male genitalia	4 weeks to 6 months
Nasal septum	6 to 8 months
Nasal bridge	8 to 10 weeks
Navel	2 months to 1 year
Nipple	2 to 6 months
Nostril	2 months to 1 year
Outer labia	2 to 4 months
Tongue	4 to 6 weeks

Data from Martel S, Anderson JE: Decorating the "human canvas": body art and your patient, *Contemp Pediatr* 19(8):86-102, 2002; Schnare SM: Tattooing, branding, and body piercing, *Womens Health Care* 1(4):21-28, 2002.

4. Infection can be treated with dicloxacillin 500 mg four times a day for 10 days. The decision to remove jewelry during an infection should be based on whether leaving it in place will provide a route for drainage, become an obstacle to healing, or be an ongoing source of infection.
5. Screen for high-risk behaviors.
6. Discuss the need to remove dangling ornaments during contact sports.

Complications

Common complications of tattooing or body piercing include infections, allergic reactions to the dyes or jewelry, and the transmission of blood-borne diseases, primarily hepatitis B and C, and, potentially HIV. Other reported complications of tattoos include skin neoplasms, syphilis, leprosy, cutaneous tuberculosis, tetanus, hyperplasia, and granuloma annulare. Complications of piercings also include excessive bleeding, nerve damage, keloids, dental fracture, soft-tissue damage, and speech impediments.

Patient Education, Prognosis, and Prevention

Provide information and encouraging teenagers to thoroughly research and consider the idea of getting a tattoo or body piercing. Removing tattoos is expensive, not necessarily completely successful, and fraught with complication (scarring, rashes) (Box 36-13). Maintaining an open, nonjudgmental attitude in discussing the options and in caring for adolescents who have body art is essential. Alternatives to discuss include temporary stick-on tattoos and use of henna or other body paints.

BOX 36-13 So You're Thinking About Getting a Tattoo or Body Piercing

Know the Facts: Make an Informed Decision

- Unsterile tattooing and piercing equipment and needles can spread serious infections, hepatitis, or possibly even HIV.
- The law in many states prohibits the tattooing of minors.
- Asking a friend to apply a tattoo may ruin a friendship if the tattoo does not look like you thought it would.
- Tattoos and permanent makeup are not easily removed and in some cases may cause permanent discoloration. Think carefully before getting a tattoo.
- Tattoo removal is very expensive. A tattoo that costs $50 to apply may cost more than $1000 to remove.
- Blood donations cannot be made for 1 year after getting a tattoo, body piercing, or permanent makeup.

Before You Get a Tattoo or Body Piercing:

First: Talk to your friends or others who have been tattooed or pierced. Ask them about their experience, the cost, pain, healing time, and so on. Ask them what they would do if they had a chance to do it over again.
Second: Understand that you do not have to tattoo or pierce your body to belong. Remember that you are directly involved in decisions that affect your health and body. You can always change your mind or wait if you are not sure.
Third: Because of potential complications, if you decide to get a tattoo or body piercing, never tattoo or pierce your own body or let a friend do it.

Health Risks to Consider Before You Act

- Both tattooing and piercing involve puncturing the skin to introduce a foreign material, jewelry, or ink, and the procedures carry similar risks. The primary health concern is introducing blood-borne germs or viruses into your body.
- Blood-borne illnesses, such as hepatitis B and C, tetanus, tuberculosis, and HIV infection, can lead to serious health problems or death.
- Make sure you have had the three series hepatitis B vaccination and a tetanus booster within 10 years.
- Localized infections, such as *Staphylococcus* or *Pseudomonas*, can lead to illness, deformity, and scarring.
Tattoo troubles: Tattoos are open wounds that may become infected. Keep the new tattoo clean and moist with an ointment to prevent a scab from forming. If you are allergic to the inks in the tattoo, the site will not heal properly and scarring may occur.
Piercing problems: Complications depend on the location of the piercing. Navel infections are the most common; it takes approximately 1 year for navel piercings to heal. Ear cartilage heals slowly. Tongue piercings may lead to tooth and enamel damage from biting on the jewelry and jewelry knocking against a tooth, partial paralysis if the jewelry pierces a nerve, and extreme inflammation during the first few days.

Selecting a Tattoo Artist or Piercer

- Visit several piercers or tattooists. The work area should be kept clean and have good lighting. If they refuse to discuss cleanliness and infection control with you, go somewhere else.
- Consent forms (which the customer must fill out) should be handled before tattooing. Reputable piercing and tattoo studios will not serve a minor without signed consent from parents. Check the laws in your state about tattooing of minors if you are less than 18 years old.
- The tattooist or piercer should have an *autoclave*—a heat sterilization machine used to sterilize equipment between customers.
- Packaged, sterilized needles should be used only once and then disposed of in a biohazard container.
- Immediately before tattooing or piercing, the tattooist or piercer should wash and dry his or her hands and wear latex gloves. These gloves should be worn at all times while the tattoo or piercing is being done. If the tattoo artist or piercer leaves or touches other objects, such as the telephone, new gloves should be put on before the procedure continues.
- Only jewelry made of a noncorrosive metal, such as surgical stainless steel, niobium, or solid 14-karat gold, is safe for a new piercing.
- Leftover tattoo ink should be disposed of after each procedure. Ink should never be poured back into the bottle and reused.

HIV, Human immunodeficiency virus.
Information adapted from Akron Children's Hospital: *Tattoos and body piercings.* Available at www.akronchildrens.org/cms/tips/59f2a3e4b43f4752/index.html (accessed Jan 13, 2011).

Musculoskeletal Disorders

JAN BAZNER-CHANDLER AND MARGARET A. BRADY

Musculoskeletal complaints are reported in 4% to 30% of young people. In most cases the causes of pediatric musculoskeletal symptoms are benign and self-limiting (Jandial et al, 2009). Sports-related injuries are found to be the highest causative factor of musculoskeletal complaints in 5- to 24-year-olds (Benjamin and Hang, 2007). Common musculoskeletal disorders include athletic injuries, back pain, foot injuries, knee disorders, shin splints, and stress factors. Inborn problems include spinal deformities, hip and foot anomalies, growth disorders and developmental delay, metabolic disorders, and neuromuscular disorders ranging from cerebral palsy to muscular dystrophy. A variety of other conditions can cause musculoskeletal findings, including child abuse, trauma, cancer, and juvenile idiopathic arthritis. Iatrogenic deformities that result from cultural practices, such as using a cradleboard, or from in utero packing problems can also cause deformities. Disorders of the musculoskeletal system present unique problems because growth and development of this system contribute to the evolution of pathologic conditions over time. Limited mobility, pain, and deformity can interfere with the lifestyle of the child. Children with functional disabilities may not be able to fully participate in all activities with peers and family or have access to various occupations. They may also face challenges related to self-esteem. Primary care providers must be vigilant and seek to help children and their families prevent these problems.

Primary care providers play a significant role in the early identification and management of children with orthopedic problems. Primary care providers assess development of the musculoskeletal system, identifies problems for early intervention, focus on lifestyle and injury prevention, and monitor the long-term outcomes of orthopedic care. They are often the first to refer to specialists as needed for early diagnosis and treatment. When necessary, primary care providers help families integrate orthopedic care within the daily living activities at home and school and assist families to cope with the issues of disability, deformity, and long-term care.

■ Anatomy and Physiology

Limb formation occurs early in embryogenesis (4 to 8 weeks of gestation); primary ossification centers are present in all the long bones of the limbs by the twelfth week of gestation.

Limb abnormalities occur in approximately 6 in 10,000 live births (Koifman et al, 2008). Development of the skeletal system begins around the fourth week of gestation, with ossification of the fetal skeleton beginning during the fifth month of gestation. The clavicles and skull bones are the first to ossify, followed by the long bones and spine. The epiphyses of the newborn's long bones are composed of hyaline cartilage. Soon after birth the cartilage along the epiphyseal plate begins secondary ossification. The shape of the spine also changes from a C shape at birth to a double S curve by late adolescence. As the child starts to walk, the lumbar curve develops. The sacrum starts out as five separate bones at birth only to become fused as one large bone by 18 to 20 years old (Duderstadt and Schapiro, 2006).

Bone age, measured by radiographs of the left hand and wrist, can be used to quantitatively determine somatic maturation and serves as a mirror that reflects the tempo of growth. In adolescents, the skeletal growth spurt begins at about Tanner stage 2 in girls and Tanner stage 3 in boys. Growth peaks around stage 4 and then ends with stage 5. The growth spurt lasts longer in boys than in girls. The pelvis widens early in pubescent girls. In both sexes the legs usually lengthen before the thighs broaden. Next the shoulders widen, and the trunk completes its linear growth. Bone growth ends when the epiphyses close.

Long bones have a growth plate, or physis, at each end that separates the epiphysis from the diaphysis or shaft. Openings through this plate allow blood vessels to penetrate from the epiphysis. In the growth plate, chondrocytes produce cartilage cells, dead cells are absorbed, and the calcified cartilage matrix is converted into bone. The entire growth plate area is weaker than the remaining bone because it is less calcified. Because the blood supply to the growth plate comes primarily through the epiphysis, damage to epiphyseal circulation can jeopardize the survival of the chondrocytes. If chondrocytes stop producing, growth of the bone in that area stops (Fig. 37-1).

There are two ways that children's bones grow. Longitudinal growth occurs in the ossification centers; changes in bone width and strength take place via intramembranous ossification. The length of long bones comes from growth at the epiphyseal plates while their diameter increases as a result of deposition of new bone on the periosteal surface and resorption on the surface of the medullary cavity. Growth of the

928

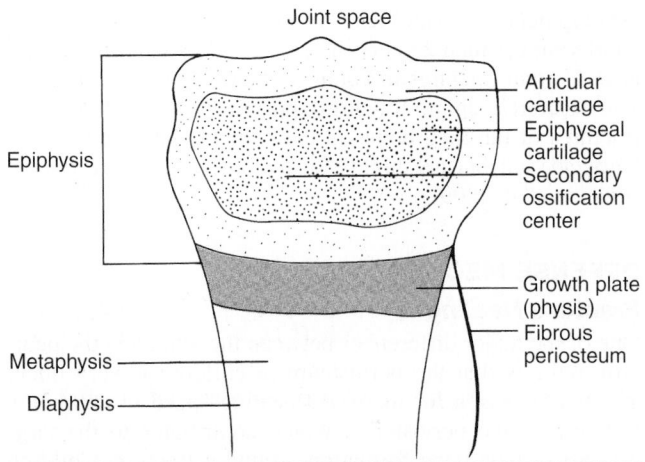

FIGURE 37-1 Anatomy of long bones. (Modified from Shapiro F: Epiphyseal disorders, *N Engl J Med* 317:1702-1710, 1987.)

small bones, hip, and spine comes from one or more primary ossification centers in each bone. Apophyses are the sites for connection of tendons to bone. In children these sites, similar to epiphyses, allow for growth and are weaker than bone. These sites can become inflamed with stress.

The development of bones and muscles is influenced by use. Thus in infants and toddlers, the legs straighten and lengthen with the stimulus of weight bearing and independent walking. The infant is born with the full complement of muscle fibers. Growth in muscle length results from lengthening of the fibers, and growth in bulk comes from hypertrophy. Length of muscles is related to growth in length of the underlying bone. If a limb is not used, it grows minimally. Furthermore, if muscles and bones are not used in their intended normal manner, such as occurs with spastic diplegia, the forces for development tend to stimulate growth in abnormal patterns. Thus scoliosis can develop or bowlegs may increase in severity. Muscle contractures occur if muscles are not used regularly and put through their full range of motion. The growth of fibrous tissue, tendons, and ligaments is also dependent on mechanical demands.

Nutritional, mechanical, and hormonal factors during the growth process influence the thickness of bones and the health of the marrow. Adequate protein, calcium, and vitamin D in the diet are key nutritional elements that affect the growth and development of a child's musculoskeletal system.

The muscle structures originate from the embryonic mesoderm and include tendons, ligaments, cartilage, and joints. Muscle fibers are developed by the fourth or fifth month of gestation and grow in tangent with their respective bones. The rate of muscle growth (muscle mass and cell sizes) speeds up dramatically around 2 years old, with girls exhibiting a greater rate of growth than boys until this gender trend is reversed at puberty (Duderstadt and Schapiro, 2006).

Pathophysiology and Defense Mechanisms

PATHOPHYSIOLOGY
Muscles and bones can be affected by localized or systemic problems. Thus the initial orthopedic problem can be symptomatic of a larger problem.

Systemic Problems
Musculoskeletal presentation in children and adolescents can be a feature of potentially life-threatening conditions such as sepsis, malignancy or nonaccidental injury, and chronic pediatric conditions such as inflammatory bowel disease, cystic fibrosis, and juvenile idiopathic arthritis.

Systemic problems can include chronic conditions such as hemophilia, sickle cell disease, and arthritic diseases; neurologic problems such as cerebral palsy; and various cancers, including osteosarcomas and leukemias. Children with metabolic problems, such as vitamin D–resistant rickets, have bony deformities. Acute systemic problems can also affect the musculoskeletal system. For example, viruses and bacteria can infect joints and bones. In developing countries, tubercular infections of bones are common and devastating. Thus the pediatric provider must assess patients from a broad perspective, asking questions about other body systems and ordering appropriate laboratory studies that might identify systemic problems.

Genetic Problems
Many genetic problems have an orthopedic component. Osteogenesis imperfecta (OI) is a genetic disorder characterized by decreased levels of collagen, the major protein of the body's connective tissue. Children with OI have bones that break easily, even from minor trauma. Down syndrome is a consequence of a genetic anomaly of chromosome 21. The main orthopedic pathology is hypotonia and the possibility of loose capsule and ligaments. Children with Down syndrome have a higher incidence of scoliosis, dislocation of the hip, Legg-Calvé-Perthes disease (LCPD), instability of the patella, and pes planus (flat feet). Children with Marfan syndrome may have long spider-like fingers, low muscle tone, and lax joints that are prone to dislocate. Severe scoliosis may develop in children with neurofibromatosis, Turner syndrome, and Noonan syndrome. Girls with Turner syndrome may present with webbed neck, short stature, valgus deformity of the elbow, and short fourth metacarpal deformity. Children with Noonan syndrome can present with webbed neck, clumsiness, poor coordination, and motor delay.

Many orthopedic problems have a multifactorial inheritance pattern. Thus if one child in a family has a dislocated hip or scoliosis, the risks increase for other children. The pediatric provider needs to understand the genetic disorder to monitor related orthopedic problems, consider the genetic implications, and provide families with appropriate genetic information or refer them for genetic counseling (see Chapter 40).

Uterine Packing Deformations
The developing fetus moves its body parts frequently, and this movement influences musculoskeletal development. When the baby fills the uterine space, movements are restricted and body parts begin to assume a shape in which they are fixed. With in utero positioning, joints and muscle contractions can develop and are considered generally physiologic in nature. Orthopedic deformities of uterine compression include clubfoot, torticollis, hip dislocation, metatarsus adductus, equinovarus foot, calcaneovalgus foot, tibial bowing, hyperflexed hips, hyperextended knees, contractures, and internal tibial torsion (Wynshaw-Boris and Biesecker 2007). Fetal movement is required for proper development of

the musculoskeletal system, and anything that restricts fetal movement can cause deformation from intrauterine molding. Two major intrinsic causes for deformations are neuromuscular disorders and oligohydramnios. Extrinsic causes are related to fetal crowding that restricts fetal movement. For a fetus in the breech position the incidence of deformations is increased 10-fold (Wynshaw-Boris and Biesecker, 2007). Infants with deformations caused by extrinsic causes have an excellent prognosis with corrections occurring spontaneously. Torsional and angular alignment issues can affect the long bones, most commonly those of the lower extremities. Because much of the bony structure is cartilaginous, molding occurs with relative ease. Thus in normal newborns, the tibias are normally bowed, and the hips have a 20- to 30-degree flexion (Hosalkar and Wells, 2007). Occasionally, a foot may be turned awkwardly, the legs might be fixed straight up with the feet near the ears, or the neck may be tipped to one side. Such positioning issues are outside the range of normal. The outcomes are deformities in various degrees. The longer the position is maintained, the more severe the problems are. In general, there is a tendency for bowing and late deformations to straighten; however, the effects related to in utero positioning may not fully abate until the child is 3 to 4 years old. More severe deformities (i.e., those significantly outside the range of normal) need to be referred to orthopedists for treatment as soon as they are found because a softer skeleton is easier to realign in a positive direction.

Injuries

There are approximately 2.6 million emergency department visits annually in the U.S. for sports-related injuries in children ages 5 to 24 years, with the highest percentage occurring in the 5- to 14-year-old male. This does not account for the children who present to their primary care physician for evaluation and treatment (Soprano and Fuchs, 2007). The unique differences in the pediatric skeletal system predispose children to injuries unlike those seen in adults. The important differences are the presence of periosseous cartilage, physes, and a thicker, stronger, more osteogenic periosteum that produces new bone called callus more rapidly and in great amounts. Joint injuries, dislocations, and ligament disruptions are infrequent in children (Gholve et al, 2007). Physeal fractures in preadolescent children are the most common musculoskeletal injuries seen. Clavicular fractures are seen at all ages ranging from a newborn birth injury to trauma in adolescence. They can occur as a result of direct or indirect injury and are most commonly associated with a fall (Benjamin and Hang, 2007). Tendinoses are seen infrequently in children but may occur in the young athlete in the rotator cuff from throwing motions and swimming, in the iliopsoas in dancers, and in the ankle of dancers, gymnasts, and figure skaters. Shoulder injuries can be acute or result from chronic overuse. Overuse injuries are common chronic injuries in children that are related to repetitive stress on the musculoskeletal system without sufficient time to recover. The repetitive use overwhelms normal reparative processes (Soprano and Fuchs, 2007). Management of traumatic injuries is discussed in Chapter 39.

The possibility of child abuse should always be considered when orthopedic injuries, especially fractures, are present. The rule of thumb is that the injury history should match the appearance of the problem and be consistent with the child's developmental capabilities. An unexplained fracture in a child younger than 2 years of age should be carefully evaluated. Certain fractures in younger children such as metaphyseal fractures, spiral fractures, posterior rib fractures, and fractures of the long bones in the nonambulatory child may be accidental but are highly suspicious for abusive trauma (Legano et al, 2009).

DEFENSE MECHANISMS
Fracture Healing

One of the major differences between the adult and the pediatric bone is that the periosteum in children is very thick. The major reason for increased healing speed of children's fractures is the periosteum, which contributes to the largest part of new bone formation around a fracture. Children have significantly greater osteoblastic activity in this area because bone is already being formed beneath the periosteum as part of normal growth. This already active process is readily accelerated after a fracture. Periosteal callus bridges a fracture in children long before the underlying hematoma forms a cartilage anlagen that goes on to ossify. Once cellular organization from the hematoma has passed through the inflammatory process, repair of the bone begins in the area of the fracture. In most children, by 10 days to 2 weeks after fracture, a rubber-like bone forms around the fracture and makes it difficult to manipulate. As part of the reparative phase, cartilage formed as the hematoma organizes is eventually replaced by bone through the process of endochondral bone formation. The remodeling phase of fracture healing may continue for some time and is accelerated by motion of the adjacent joints and use of the extremity (Green and Swiontkowski, 2008).

Growth Plate Fractures. Fractures of the long bones can produce permanent deformities in children if the fracture occurs through the growth plate. The outcomes depend on the fracture location and type, the age of the child, the status of the blood supply to the physis, and the treatment. The Salter-Harris classification is based on the mechanism of injury, the relationship of the fracture line to the layers of physis, and the prognosis with respect to subsequent growth disturbance. There are five classifications (Fig. 37-2). Type I is the most frequent type of fracture that involves a fracture through the zone of hypertrophic cells of the physis with no fracture of the surrounding bone. Type II fractures are similar to type I except that a metaphyseal fragment is present on the compression side of the fracture. Growth disturbance in types I and II is rare.

Type III fracture involves physeal separation with fracture through the epiphysis into the joint. The fracture requires anatomic reduction, occasionally through an open approach. Type IV fracture involves the metaphysis, physis, and epiphysis. Type V fracture involves a compression or crushing injury to the physis. Type V fractures are rare and are difficult to diagnose initially due to the lack of radiologic signs. Types IV and V require anatomic reduction to prevent articular incongruity and osseous bridging across the physis. There are additional rare types of Salter-Harris fractures, types VI through IX. Type VI is an injury to the perichondral ring of LaCroix, a fibrous band that is continuous with the periosteum and a potential reservoir for growth-plate germ cells. Type VI fracture is seen in injuries about the medial malleolus

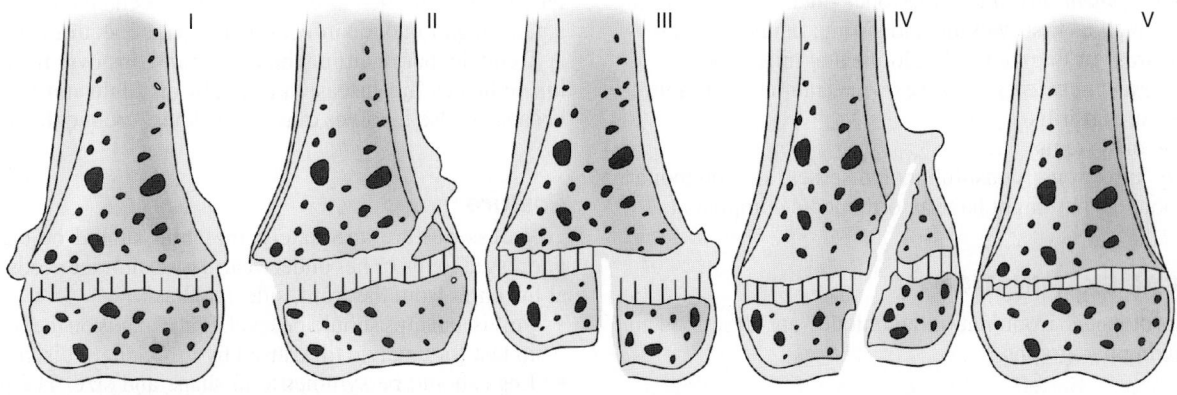

FIGURE 37-2 The types of growth plate injury as classified by Salter and Harris. (From Salter RB, Harris WR: Injuries involving the epiphyseal plate, *J Bone Joint Surg Am* 45:587, 1963.)

and often requires later reconstructive surgery (Green and Swiontkowski, 2008).

Although 30% of Salter-Harris fractures result in growth disturbances, only 2% result in significant functional disturbance (Moore and Smith, 2009).

Shaft Fractures. The mechanism of injury is an important part of the history in evaluating a child for a traumatic injury. Closed pediatric fractures are largely caused by low-energy activities and play; open fractures are generally caused by more violent accidents. Open fractures in children younger than school age are rare because of their small body mass, large amount of protective subcutaneous fat, and their limited exposure to high-risk activities (Sabharwal and Bhrens, 2008).

There are a variety of shaft fractures. In children between 9 months and 6 years of age, torsion of the foot may produce an oblique fracture of the distal aspect of the tibial shaft without a fibula fracture. These fractures are usually the result of tripping while walking or running, stepping on a ball or toy, or falling from a modest height. The child is typically seen due to failure to bear weight, a limp, or pain when asked to stand on the involved extremity. Physical findings may be minimal and radiographs may show the characteristic faint oblique fracture line crossing the distal tibial diaphysis and terminating medially. Treatment is immobilization. Fractures of the forearm represent 40% of all fractures in children (Dolan and Waters, 2008). Fractures of the forearm in children most often result from a fall on an outstretched hand. This results in forceful axial loading with resultant bony failure in compression and bending. These forces generally cause a plastic deformity or partial fracture (greenstick fracture). The rotational malalignment may not be identified and may be undertreated. During physical examination the provider should observe for subtle rotational deformities and compare with the contralateral limb. Plain radiograph remains the gold standard for musculoskeletal evaluation and should be performed on all patients with a physical examination suggestive of fracture or dislocation (Dolan and Walters, 2008). Malrotation is indicated on x-ray by malalignment of the elbow in relation to the wrist. Failure to diagnose and treat rotational malalignment is the most common cause of loss of forearm rotation in children.

■ Assessment of the Orthopedic System

HISTORY

- History of present illness
  - *Onset:* Appearance of first symptoms; insidious or sudden; association with injury or strain; accompanied by any constitutional symptoms or signs (e.g., fever, malaise, swelling, ecchymosis)
  - *Pain:* Location and character, course of radiation, severity, extent of disability produced, effect of various activities including weight bearing, relief measures, changes from day to night or from day to day, child's refusing to move the painful part or assuming a pain-relieving position, effects of previous treatment, presence of pain or discomfort in other parts of the body
  - *Deformity:* Character (swelling, inflammation, contracture, joint stiffness, unusual positioning, appearance); first appearance and who noted it; association with injury or disease; rate of change; extent of disability; a cosmetic problem or a cause of embarrassment
  - *Injury:* How, when (time and date), why, and where; mechanism or manner in which injury was produced; involvement in organized or competitive sports
  - *Altered function:* Weakness, limp, decreased range of motion
  - *Altered gait patterns:* Toe walking, in-toeing or out-toeing
  - *Other factors or constraints:* Type of shoe worn (e.g., platform shoes); use of backpack and amount of weight in backpack, amount of time spent at repetitive tasks or at computer station; sitting in TV squat or "W" position
  - *Medication use:* Steroids, antiinflammatories
- Family history
  - Any family members with musculoskeletal problems; many orthopedic problems have a genetic component
- Medical history
  - *Pregnancy history and birth history:* Breech delivery, shoulder presentation, multiple births, oligohydramnios, asphyxia at birth; maternal alcohol or substance abuse

○ *Development history:* Milestones met at appropriate age, such as first walking and sitting; delays in achieving gross or fine motor developmental milestones
○ *Illnesses, accidents, or surgeries:* Trauma, meningitis, juvenile arthritis
• Review of systems
○ Any infections, constitutional diseases, or congenital problems that might have an orthopedic component

PHYSICAL EXAMINATION

Special orthopedic examination techniques are described in the following paragraphs.

Range-of-Motion Examination

Range of motion is the normal range, flexion, extension, and rotation of a joint. Joint hypermobility is the ability of the joint to move beyond its normal range. Hypermobility of joints generally does not cause problems, although there is a slight increase in dislocation and sprain of the involved joint. The normal values of joint motion are age related, which must be kept in mind (e.g., external hip rotation is greatest in early infancy). Passive range of motion, in which the examiner moves the joint, provides information about joint mobility and stability. It can also provide information about the limits of tendons and muscles that are contracted. Active range of motion, in which the child moves the joint, provides information about both muscle and bony structures working together for functional movement.

Limited range of motion can be the result of mechanical problems, swelling, muscle spasticity, pain, infection, injury or arthritis. Note pain, stiffness, limitations or deviations, and rigidity.

Gait Examination

A normal gait cycle consists of the stance phase, during which the foot is in contact with the ground, and the swing phase, during which the foot is in the air. The stance phase is further divided into three major periods: the initial double-limb support, followed by the single-limb stance, then another period of double-limb support. The gait undergoes developmental changes. Walking velocity, step length, and duration of the single-limb stance increase with age, whereas the number of steps taken per minute decreases. A mature gait pattern is well established by 3 years of age. By 7 years of age the gait is that of an adult (Sawyer and Kapoor, 2009).

Observe the child walking without shoes and minimal covering. The stance and swing phases should be compared in both legs, and the range of motion of each joint should be evaluated. Inspect from the front, side, and back as the child walks normally, on his or her toes, and then on the heels. The gait should be smooth, rhythmic, and efficient. Ankle, knee, and hip movements should be symmetric and full with little side-to-side movement of the trunk.

Limping is a disturbance in gait. Abnormal gait can be antalgic or non-antalgic. An antalgic gait is characterized by a shortening of the stance phase to prevent pain in the affected leg. Painful or antalgic gaits serve to reduce stress or pain at the affected area. The trunk shifts to the opposite side to keep balance and reduce stress; the stance phase and stride

length are shortened as compensatory mechanisms. Causes of a painful gait include infection, trauma, or acquired disorders. A Trendelenburg gait in which the trunk tips over the affected hip indicates hip disease and might or might not be painful because it also involves muscle weakness around the hip joint.

Posture

To assess posture adequately, the child should be examined undressed to his or her underwear. The examiner needs to look at the child from the front, side, and back.
• Pelvis and hips should be level. Place hands on the iliac crest to test for a pelvic tilt caused by limb length discrepancy.
• Legs should be symmetric in shape and size. The patellae should be straight ahead.
• The feet should point straight ahead, with an imaginary line from the center of the heel through the second toe. There should be an arch (except in babies, in whom a fat pad obscures the arch) and straight heel cords.
• The spine should be straight, and the back should look symmetric, with shoulder and scapula heights and waist angles equal. There should be slight lordotic curves at the cervical and lumbar areas.

■ Special Examinations

HIP EXAMINATIONS
Galeazzi Maneuver

The Galeazzi sign can signal conditions that cause leg length discrepancies. The Galeazzi maneuver includes flexing the hips and knees while the infant or child lies supine, placing the soles of the feet on the table near the buttocks, and then looking at the knee heights for equality (Fig. 37-3, *A*). The Galeazzi sign is positive if the knee heights are unequal. However, it is not reliable in children with dislocatable but not dislocated hips or in children with bilateral dislocation.

Barlow Maneuver

The Barlow maneuver dislocates an unstable or dislocatable hip posteriorly (Fig. 37-4, *A*). The infant is placed in the supine position with knees flexed. The hip is flexed, and the thigh is brought into an adducted position applying downward pressure. With hip instability the femoral head slips/drops out of the acetabulum or can be gently pushed out of the socket; this is termed a positive Barlow. The dislocation should be palpable as this maneuver is performed. The maneuver needs to be done gently in a noncrying neonate to keep from damaging the femoral head. The hips should be examined one at a time. The hip generally spontaneously relocates after release of the posterior force.

Ortolani Maneuver

The Ortolani maneuver can be done after the Barlow maneuver or separately (see Fig. 37-4, *B*). The Ortolani maneuver reduces a posteriorly dislocated hip. It is done to reduce a recently dislocated hip and is not done forcefully. The infant is in the supine position with both knees flexed and supported by the thumb and forefinger of the examiner. The thumb is placed near the lesser trochanter, and the pad of the second finger is positioned on the bony prominence of the greater

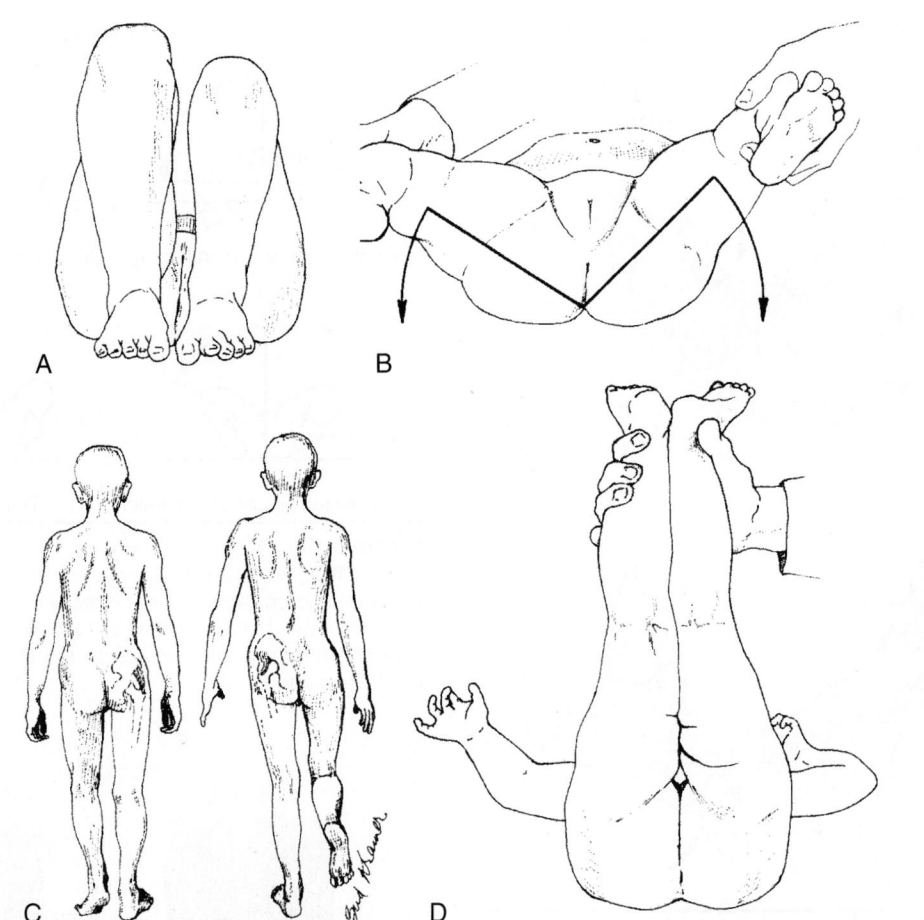

FIGURE 37-3 Physical findings in congenital hip dislocation. **A,** Leg length inequality is a sign of unilateral hip dislocation (Galeazzi sign). **B,** Limitation of hip abduction is often present in older infants with hip dislocation. Abduction of greater than 60 degrees is usually possible in infants. Restriction or asymmetry indicates the need for careful radiologic examination. **C,** Trendelenburg sign. In single-leg stance the abductor muscles of the normal hip support the pelvis. Dislocation of the hip functionally shortens and weakens these muscles. When the child attempts to stand on the dislocated hip, the opposite side of the pelvis drops. **D,** Thigh-fold asymmetry is often present in infants with unilateral hip dislocation. An extra fold can be seen on the abnormal side. The finding is not diagnostic, however. It may be found in normal infants and may be absent in children with hip dislocation or dislocatability. (From Scoles P: *Pediatric orthopedics in clinical practice*, ed 2, St Louis, 1988, Mosby.)

trochanter. The leg is flexed at the hip and then abducted while pushing up with the fingers located over the trochanter posteriorly. The femoral head is lifted anteriorly into the acetabulum. A clunk and a palpable jerk are obtained as the femoral head is relocated. A mild clicking sound is not a positive Ortolani sign. These are common and normal sounds radiating from the knee or ankle that are fine, of short duration, and high pitched (Duderstadt and Schapiro, 2006). Of note, the hip may be dislocated easily only during the first month or two of life. The Ortolani maneuver is most likely to be positive in infants 1 to 2 months old. The examiner should not still be charting "no hip click" on examinations at 6 months old. Dislocation can occur late in infancy. However, if this occurs, the provider will note limited abduction on the side of the dislocation (Fig. 37-5).

Klisic Test

The Klisic test provides an observational sign of hip placement. The examiner places the tip of the third finger of one hand over the greater trochanter and the index finger of the

same hand on the anterior superior iliac spine. An imaginary line is then drawn between the index and third fingers. Normally, the imaginary line points to the umbilicus. If the hip is dislocated, the imaginary line points halfway between the umbilicus and the pubis (i.e., the line points below the umbilicus). The Klisic sign is another physical assessment marker of dislocation (Hosalkar et al, 2007b) (Fig. 37-6).

Trendelenburg Sign

The Trendelenburg test can be used to identify conditions that cause weakness in the hip abductors. The Trendelenburg sign is elicited by having the child stand and then raise one leg off the ground. If the pelvis (iliac crest) drops on the raised leg side, the sign is positive and indicates weak hip abductor muscles on the side that is bearing the weight. Normally the muscles around a stable hip are strong enough to maintain a level pelvis if one leg is raised (see Fig. 37-3, *C*). With bilaterally dislocated hips, a wide-based Trendelenburg limp is noted.

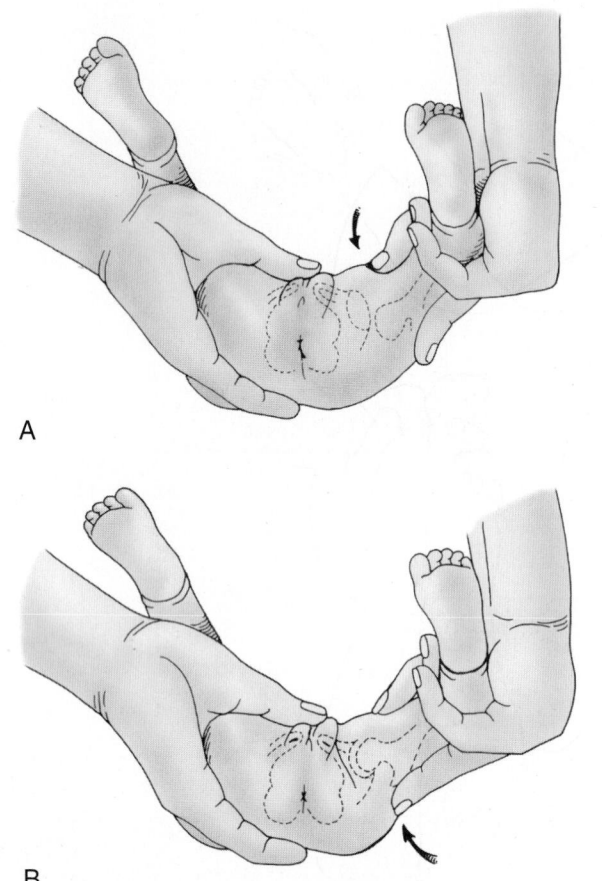

A

B

FIGURE 37-4 **A,** Barlow (dislocation) test. The "stabilizing hand" is positioned with the thumb on the symphysis and the fingers on the sacrum. The thumb of the abducting hand is placed on the inner aspect of the thigh and gives lateral pressure to the adductor region while the hand (wrapped around the knee with the index finger on the lateral side of the thigh) provides gentle downward pressure. If there is hip instability, dislocation is palpable as the femoral head slips out of the acetabulum. Diagnosis is confirmed with the Ortolani test. **B,** Ortolani (reduction) test. With the infant relaxed on a firm surface, the hips and knees are flexed to 90 degrees. The hips are examined one at a time. Grasp the infant's thigh with the middle finger over the greater trochanter and lift the thigh to bring the femoral head from its dislocated posterior position to opposite the acetabulum. Simultaneously the thigh is gently abducted, reducing the femoral head in the acetabulum. In a positive finding, the examiner senses reduction by a palpable, nearly audible "clunk." Test one hip at a time for both of these tests. (From Marcdante KJ, Kliegman RM, Jenson HB et al, editors: *Nelson essentials of pediatrics*, ed 6, Philadelphia, 2011, Saunders.)

Medial (Internal) and Lateral (External) Rotations

The child is placed prone, and the knees are flexed 90 degrees. Medial rotation is measured as the legs are allowed to fall apart as far as possible, using gravity alone or with light pressure. The angle between vertical (0 degree) and the leg position is the medial rotation. It is measured for each leg (Fig. 37-7, *A*). Asymmetric hip rotation is abnormal. Lateral rotation is measured by allowing the legs to cross while the child is still prone. The angle between vertical and the leg position is measured for each leg (see Fig. 37-7, *B*). Again, asymmetric hip rotation is abnormal. By 1 year old, a normal child has approximately 45 degrees of internal and external hip rotation.

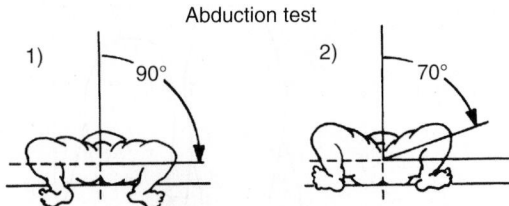

Abduction test

1) 90° 2) 70°

Normal at birth to 1 month of age Often normal, 1 to 9 months of age

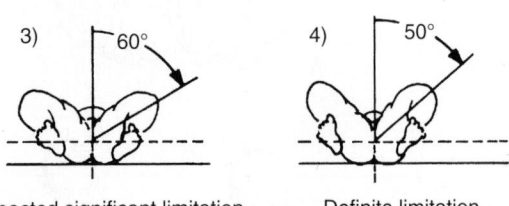

3) 60° 4) 50°

Suspected significant limitation Definite limitation

FIGURE 37-5 Hip abduction test. The child is placed supine, and the hips are flexed 90 degrees and fully abducted. Although the normal abduction range is quite broad, one can suspect hip disease in any patient who lacks more than 35 to 45 degrees of abduction. (From Chung SMK: *Hip disorders in infants and children*, Philadelphia, 1981, Lea & Febiger.)

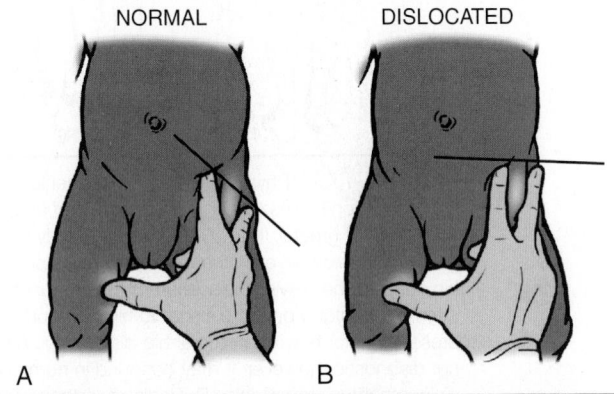

NORMAL DISLOCATED

A B

FIGURE 37-6 Klisic test. (From Kliegman RM, Stanton BF, St. Geme JW et al, editors: *Nelson textbook of pediatrics*, ed 19, Philadelphia, 2011, Saunders.)

BACK EXAMINATION

Adams Test or the Adams Forward Bend Position

The Adams forward bend test (Adams test) looks for asymmetry of the posterior chest wall on forward bending. This position allows for evaluation of structural scoliosis. The child bends at the waist to a position of 90 degrees back flexion with straight legs, ankles together, and arms hanging freely or with palms together (in a diving position) but not touching the toes or floor (Fig. 37-8). The back is inspected for asymmetry of the height of the curves on the two sides or rib hump; the provider inspects the child's back by looking at it from the rear and side positions. The examiner should be seated in front of the child to best visually scan each level of the spine. If a rib hump is present, a scoliometer, if available, can be used to measure the angular tilt of the trunk. A spinal rotation

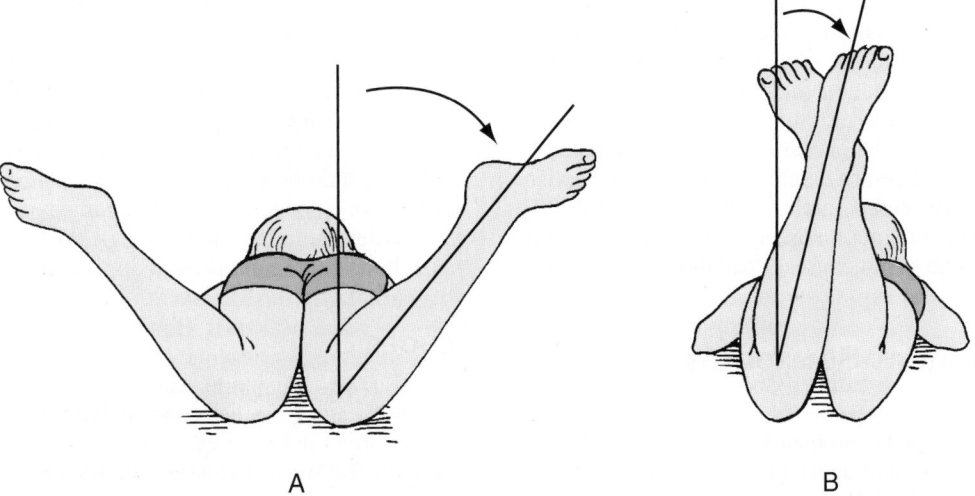

A   B

FIGURE 37-7 Hip rotation in extension. This is measured with the child in prone position and the knee flexed 90 degrees. The lower leg is vertically oriented. This is considered the neutral position. On outward rotation **(A),** the leg produces internal hip rotation, and on inward rotation **(B),** the leg produces external hip rotation. (From Thompson GH: Gait disturbances. In Kliegman RM, editor: *Practical strategies in pediatric diagnosis and therapy*, Philadelphia, 1996, Saunders.)

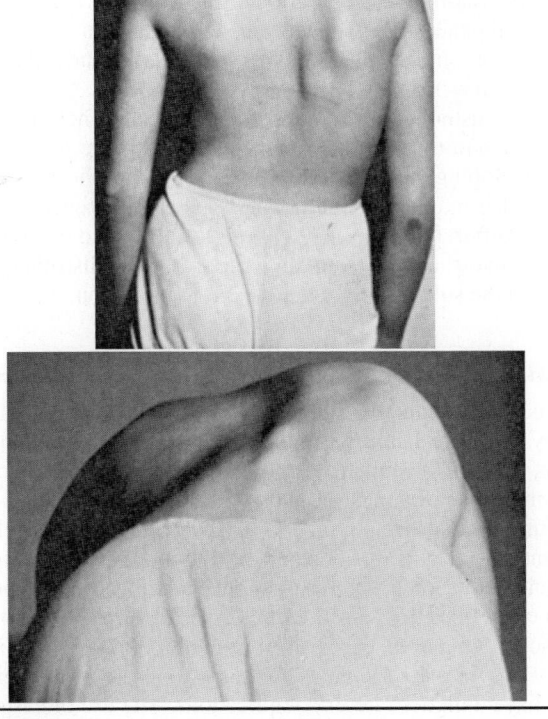

FIGURE 37-8 Adams position with rib hump of structural scoliosis. Lateral curvature of thoracic and lumbar segments of the spine, usually with some rotation of involved vertebral bodies. Functional scoliosis is flexible; it is apparent with standing and disappears with forward bending. It may be compensatory for other abnormalities, such as leg length discrepancy. Structural scoliosis is fixed; the curvature is visible both on standing and on bending forward. *Note rib hump with forward flexions*. At greatest risk are females 10 years old through adolescence. (From Delp MH, Manning RT: *Major's physical diagnosis: an introduction to the clinical process*, ed 9, Philadelphia, 1981, Saunders.)

greater than 5 degrees measured by placing the scoliometer at the peak of the curvature indicates the need for further evaluation (Duderstadt and Schapiro, 2006). Other characteristics of scoliosis to look for include unequal scapula heights, unequal waist angles, unequal iliac crests or shoulders, asymmetry of the elbow to flank distance, and some deviation of the spine from a straight head-to-toe line. Looking primarily at the straightness of the spine, however, can be misleading because scoliosis involves both rotation and misalignment of the vertebrae. The Adams forward bending position accentuates the rotational deformity of scoliosis.

■ Diagnostic Studies

Radiographs are an important diagnostic tool for the musculoskeletal system. Imaging should begin with standard radiographs of the area of concern. Anteroposterior and lateral views of the affected area, bone, or joint are typically ordered to analyze the anatomic structures. Views of both extremities may be ordered so that comparisons can be made. Computed tomography (CT) scans augment radiographs to detail specific areas of the body, especially in identification of soft-tissue lesions. CT is useful in detailing the relationship of bones to their contiguous structures. Magnetic resonance imaging (MRI) gives excellent visualization of joints, soft tissues, cartilage, and medullary bone. It can distinguish among various physiologic changes that occur in bone marrow related to age and disease process. Ultrasonography can provide information about cartilaginous areas or tissues not visible on radiograph. The test is highly sensitive for detecting effusion of the hip joint. Bone scans (scintigraphy) are more sensitive than radiographs, demonstrate abnormal uptake earlier than conventional radiographs, and are useful in detecting causes of obscure skeletal pain.

Laboratory studies can help to identify systemic disease, infection, or inflammation. Erythrocyte sedimentation rate (ESR), C-reactive protein (CRP), complete blood count (CBC), blood cultures, rheumatoid factor, and antinuclear antibodies are hematologic tests that can assist in the diagnosis and management of bone disorders. Other laboratory tests also can provide an understanding of muscle metabolism (e.g., lactic acid, pyruvates, carnitine). Some bony lesions may need to be biopsied, and muscle tissue frequently needs to be sampled to determine specific disease pathologic conditions.

■ Management Strategies

COUNSELING

Counseling for orthopedic problems involves several components. The family should understand and have time to ask questions about all of the following issues:
- The pathologic condition, including possible etiologies
- The treatment plan
- The prognosis with and without treatment
- Any genetic implications of the diagnosis
- Long-term care issues

Counseling helps families cope with a poor or challenging diagnosis and its short-term and long-term implications. Congenital problems are often identified prenatally, at birth, or shortly thereafter. Families need to be given the diagnosis truthfully, humanely, and as soon as possible. Issues of etiology need to be discussed to address parents' feelings of guilt for causing the problem and to discuss genetic implications, if any. A plan of care that is mutually agreed on by the family and the health care provider must be developed before the infant is discharged from the hospital or clinic.

EXERCISE

With childhood obesity on the rise, there is a push to improve fitness and activity levels in children and adolescents. Physical activity needs to be promoted at home, in the community, and at school. Toddler and preschool-age children should participate in unorganized, supervised play including running, swimming, tumbling, throwing, and catching. School-age children can be encouraged to increase activity by unorganized outdoor free play, personal fitness (dance, yoga, running), recreational activities, and organized sports. During late childhood and adolescence, strength training may be added. Even children with disabling conditions can exercise in some way. (Refer to Chapter 13 for more in-depth discussion about activities and sports. Tables 13-2 and 13-5 provide some guidance regarding some specific medical conditions and sports participation.) Exercise for children should be fun and perceived as play, not work. Often physical therapists or the child's orthopedist can provide ideas for safe, therapeutic play or sports activities. At school, children with orthopedic problems should engage in physical activities that are as much a part of the regular physical education class as possible.

ANTICIPATORY GUIDANCE: MUSCULOSKELETAL DEVELOPMENT

Families are sometimes concerned about problems that providers believe are within normal limits and do not require an orthopedic referral. The provider should provide the child's family with a description of the child's predicted musculoskeletal development. Timelines and markers that parents can use to monitor their child's development are particularly helpful in allowing families to understand their child's pattern of growth. Misperceptions about the implications of minor variations need to be clarified, and the family should always be given the opportunity to return for further assessment or discussion if concerns remain. Examples of common concerns are flat feet in infants and toddlers, "bowed" legs in toddlers, and "knock-knees" in preschool children.

SHOES

The use of therapeutic shoes to correct orthopedic problems is controversial. Studies confirm that therapeutic shoes do little to correct deformities. Shoes for the average child should keep the feet warm and protected from injury. Shoes should be selected to fit properly and comfortably with room for growth. High-top shoes for toddlers may have the advantage of staying on pudgy little feet better, but they do not provide additional support. Toddler feet do not need extra support. Features of a good shoe are as follows:
- Flexible sole—to allow as much free motion as possible; for young children, test to see if the shoe can be flexed in the parent's hand
- Flat—do not allow high heels
- Foot shaped—avoid pointed toes or other shapes that are not the normal configuration of the foot
- Fitted generously—better to be too large than too small
- Friction similar to skin—the soles should have the same friction as skin so that they are not slippery

Well cushioned, shock-absorbing shoes are helpful in the child or adolescent athlete in order to decrease the chances of developing overuse syndrome. Shoe modifications may be needed in certain conditions. Shoe lifts are needed if limb length differences exceed 2.5 cm. Orthotics also can be used in certain orthopedic situations to more evenly distribute pressure on the sole of the foot and facilitate function.

CARE OF CHILDREN IN CASTS AND SPLINTS

Casts and splints serve to immobilize orthopedic injuries. They promote healing, maintain bone alignment, diminish pain, protect the injury, and help compensate for surrounding muscular weakness (Boyd et al, 2009a). Splints are noncircumferential immobilizers that accommodate swelling. Splints are used in orthopedic conditions where swelling is anticipated: acute fractures or sprains and for initial stabilization of reduced, displaced, or unstable fractures before orthopedic intervention. Casts are circumferential immobilizers. They provide superior immobilization but are less forgiving and have a higher rate of complications. The use of casts and splints is generally limited to a short period of time. Excessive immobilization can lead to chronic pain, joint stiffness, and muscle atrophy (Boyd et al, 2009b).

The child's cast should be kept cool, clean, and dry. Cover the cast with plastic wrap or a plastic bag when the child bathes or is in a situation in which the cast may get wet. The only cast that can go in water is a Gore-Tex cast. If the cast becomes wet, a hair dryer set on cool setting can be used for drying small areas. If the cast becomes soiled it can be cleaned with a slightly damp washcloth and cleanser.

The family should be taught how to do a circulatory inspection to check the function of nerves and blood vessels. The child's toes or fingers below the cast should be pink and warm to touch. The child should be able to feel all sides or his or her fingers or toes when touched and should be able to wiggle the fingers or toes.

The family needs to know when to call the provider: if the toes or fingers are cold to touch and appear pale or blue, complaints of tingling or numbness, inability to move fingers or toes, and excessive swelling. Additional problems with casts, such as foul smell, breakage, or loosening, should be reported.

PHYSICAL THERAPY

Children with developmental delays, cerebral palsy, spine disorders, and torticollis may benefit from physical therapy. Treatments focus on improving gross and fine motor skills, balance and coordination, strength and endurance, as well as cognitive and sensory processing. Structured physical therapy postorthopedic injury can be helpful.

■ Orthopedic Problems Specific to Children

ARM PROBLEMS

BRACHIAL PLEXUS INJURIES

Description

Brachial plexus injuries are typically classified using Narakas criteria types I through IV (Table 37-1). Brachial plexus injuries can also be classified as type I (Erb-Duchenne paralysis) with C5 through C6 involvement that includes the shoulder and upper arm; type II (Erb-Duchenne-Klumpke paralysis) involves the entire brachial plexus (i.e., C5 through T1 involvement) affecting the shoulder, arm, and hand; or type III (Klumpke paralysis) caused by injury to C8 through T1 with involvement of the lower arm and hand (Zafeirious and Psychogious, 2008).

Epidemiology

Obstetric brachial plexus palsy results from injury to the cervical roots C5-C8 and thoracic root T1. Most injuries are transient, with full return of function occurring in 70% to 92% of cases and prolonged and permanent disability in a small percentage (Zafeirious and Psychogious, 2008). Risk factors for brachial plexus palsies may be divided into three categories: neonatal, maternal, and labor-related factors. Maternal characteristics include diabetes, obesity, maternal age (more than 35 years), and maternal pelvic anatomy. Vacuum extraction or direct compression of the fetal neck during delivery by forceps can cause stretching of the cervical nerve roots and eventually brachial plexus injury. Other causes may include induction of labor, epidural anesthesia, and postdate gestation (Zafeirious and Psychogious, 2008).

Clinical Findings

History. History should include obstetric history, mode of delivery, and postnatal health of the infant.

Physical Examination. All limbs should be examined for fractures and postnatal neurologic deficit and comprehensive

TABLE 37-1	Brachial Plexus Injury Using Narakas Classification	
Name	**Nerve and Muscle Involved**	**Prognosis**
Narakas type I	C5 and C6; shoulder and biceps	Recovery usually complete
Narakas type II	C5-C7; shoulder, biceps, and forearm extensors	Recovery usually complete
Narakas type III	C5-T1	Variable with complete paralysis of limb; shoulder and biceps recovery is fair to poor with hand recovery variable
Narakas type IV	C5-T1	Complete paralysis of the limb and Horner syndrome; shoulder and biceps recovery is fair to poor with hand recovery variable

examination of the entire body to identify any other injures that may have occurred during delivery (Zafeirious and Psychogious, 2008). Passive range of motion of involved arm, forearm, hand, and shoulder is assessed. Findings may include:
- Erb palsy, presenting with an adducted arm, which is internally rotated at the shoulder. The wrist is flexed, and the fingers extended, resulting in a characteristic "waiter's tip" posture.
- Absent bicep reflex with absent Moro reflex on the affected side
- Limp wrist and hand with absent grasp reflex (lower plexus involvement)
- Horner syndrome (ipsilateral ptosis, miosis, enophthalmos, anhidrosis) if the sympathetic fibers of the T1 nerve root are involved
- Occasionally hand paralysis with normal shoulder movement, which is a rare occurrence of an isolated C8 through T1 injury
- Ruptured intraabdominal structures, especially the liver and spleen, which require careful abdominal examination
- Limited neck movement due to damage to the sternocleidomastoid muscle; skull fracture
- Impaired respiratory effort as a result of diaphragmatic paralysis and flaccidity

Diagnostic Studies. Radiologic examination, electrophysiologic studies, and MRI are useful to confirm clinical diagnosis and the extent of the injury. X-rays of the chest and upper limbs are important because they reveal associated injuries such as rib, transverse process, clavicle, or humeral fractures. Chest x-ray is necessary to rule out phrenic nerve injury. Electrodiagnostic studies with electromyography and nerve conduction velocities are used to determine severity of the neural lesion.

Differential Diagnosis

The differential diagnosis of upper extremity paralysis in a newborn includes epiphyseal separation of the humeral head, fracture of the clavicle or humerus, septic arthritis of the upper extremity, spinal cord injury, cervical cord lesions, and congenital varicella of the upper limb (Zafeirious and Psychogious, 2008).

Management

A multidisciplinary team approach is ideal with referral to health professionals who specialize in treating brachial plexus injuries. Referral should be made in the first week of life. Therapy is initially conservative; 95% of infants born with obstetric brachial plexus palsy recover complete function with physical therapy only (Zafeirious and Psychogious, 2008). The initial goal of therapy is to maintain passive range of motion, supple joints, and muscle strength. Radiographs should be taken twice yearly for persistent upper plexus palsy. Indications for surgical exploration and reconstruction of the brachial plexus include failure of recovery of elbow flexion and shoulder abduction from the third to the sixth month of life. The spectrum of nerve surgery includes neurolysis neuroma resection, nerve grafting, and nerve transfers.

Complications

Late sequelae include internal rotation contractures, hypoplasia of the arm, altered sensibility, flexion contractures of the elbow, dislocations of the radial head, and psychological and social consequences.

Prognosis

Complete recovery may take up to 2 years. Infants should be examined regularly until either total recovery or an absence of improvement for 2 to 3 years is documented (Zafeirious and Psychogious, 2008).

SHOULDER PROBLEMS

CLAVICLE FRACTURE

Epidemiology

Clavicle fractures are seen in newborns, as a result of birth trauma and in very young children as a result of child abuse. They can occur as a result of a direct hit or indirect trauma and are most commonly associated with a fall. Approximately 80% to 85% of these fractures occur in the middle third of the clavicle and 12% to 15% in the distal third. Although the clavicle is the first bone to ossify, the physis does not close until 23 to 25 years of age (Benjamin and Hang, 2007).

Clinical Findings

History. In the neonate:
- Difficult delivery, birthweight, midforceps delivery, and shoulder dystocia
- Irritability when infant is moved or lifted
  In the older child:
- History of fall or trauma with focus on mechanism of injury
  Physical Examination. In all children, look for the following:
- Pain with shoulder movement
- Decreased arm movement on affected side (asymmetric spontaneous arm movements) or absent Moro reflex

- Swelling, bony abnormality, discoloration and/or crepitus elicited over fracture site
- Callus felt over fracture site within a few days
- Spasm of sternocleidomastoid muscle on affected side
- An associated Erb palsy
  Diagnostic Studies. Imaging studies are recommended. Radiography with routine clavicle views is sufficient.

Differential Diagnosis

Brachial palsy, shoulder dislocation, or other bony problem should be considered.

Management

Management involves the following:
- Neonate
  - Incomplete fractures that do not cause pain need no treatment.
  - Immobilization of the shoulder is an option when movement results in a painful arm (usually with a complete fracture). Pin the sleeve of the infant's arm to the front of the shirt for 1 to 2 weeks.
- Older child
  - Sling immobilization for comfort to support the affected extremity is often sufficient. Generally sling immobilization can be discontinued at 3 to 4 weeks.
  - A figure-eight clavicle brace can be used if displacement results in a decreased shaft length. However, it is uncomfortable to wear, and its effectiveness is questionable.
  - Protection for 4 to 5 weeks is generally sufficient because union requires about 4 weeks of healing.
  - An older child may need analgesics or a nonsteroidal antiinflammatory drug (NSAID) for pain.
  - The need for surgical intervention is uncommon with clavicle fractures. Surgery may be needed in open fractures, neurovascular compromise, multiple trauma, rib cage fractures, and those with greater than 100% displacement with severe skin tenting.

Prognosis

The prognosis is excellent. Often the injury in neonates is identified only at later primary care visits, when the callus lump is palpated, though the child may be irritable until the fracture is stable. The infant is usually asymptomatic within 7 to 10 days. Parents need information and emotional support. In older children general healing time is 6 to 8 weeks with average return to noncontact sports in 4 to 6 weeks. Bony callus appears approximately 10 days postinjury as a painless, firm "lump." Follow-up radiographs are not necessary to monitor healing (Benjamin and Hang, 2007).

RIB PROBLEMS

COSTOCHONDRITIS AND STERNOCHONDRITIS
Description

Costochondritis is a common cause of chest pain in children and adolescents. The condition is characterized as an inflammatory process of one or more of the costochondral cartilages that causes localized tenderness and pain of the anterior chest wall. Most are idiopathic (Garry and Myones, 2010).

Epidemiology

Trauma to the area and unaccustomed physical effort (lifting heavy objects or coughing) are factors known to cause costochondritis. Inflammation is the underlying problem.

Clinical Findings

History. Pain localized to the costosternal or costochondral junction is the major symptom. It often presents with tenderness over more than one rib as a result of referred pain. The primary rib that is inflamed and usually responsible for the symptoms is most often the one that exhibits the greatest sensitivity to palpation. Characteristics of the pain include the following:

- Acute or gradual onset; typically insidious occurring over several days or weeks
- Sharp, darting, or dull quality
- Radiation from chest to upper abdomen or back
- Occasional complaints of a feeling of tightness caused by muscle spasm
- Exacerbating factors may include coughing, sneezing, deep inspiration, movement of the upper torso and upper extremities

Physical Examination. Palpation reveals tenderness over the costochondral junction. The tenderness should be localized and is most common at the sternocostal cartilage of the second through the seventh ribs. The presence of pain, swelling (a unique bulbous enlargement of the joint) with or without redness, and tenderness at the costal cartilage is referred to as Tietze syndrome. Ecchymosis may be seen in cases of trauma. Respiratory effort is normal. Auscultation of the lungs, heart, and abdomen is normal (Garry and Myones, 2010).

Diagnostic Studies. No diagnostic studies are needed because history and physical findings are the key to the diagnosis. Chest radiography may exclude other possible causes but offers no diagnostic value. A CT scan can demonstrate swelling of the costal cartilage.

Differential Diagnosis

Rib fractures are the key differential diagnosis if pain is associated with an injury. Childhood rheumatic diseases also can have complaints similar to costochondritis but generally have other characteristic physical findings. Costochondritis is one of the differential diagnoses of pediatric chest pain (see Chapter 30).

Management

Treatment consists of using mild analgesia and NSAIDs to relieve discomfort and avoiding strenuous activity. Cough suppressants may be beneficial if cough is an aggravating factor. Stretching exercises and use of ice to the area can be useful. Parents and children need to be reassured that this is a benign self-limited condition and is not related to cardiac disease.

BACK PROBLEMS

BACK PAIN
Description

Children do not commonly complain of severe back pain. Most episodes of back pain in pediatric patients are brief with nonspecific findings and history. Back pain that warrants immediate attention includes children younger than 4 years, persistent symptoms, self-imposed activity limitations, systemic symptoms, increasing discomfort, persistent nighttime pain, and neurologic symptoms (Bernstein and Cozen, 2007). The older the child, the more likely the etiology of back pain is musculoskeletal in origin. Younger children who have such complaints should be carefully evaluated for occult pathologic conditions, and the provider's index of suspicion about underlying pathologic conditions should be raised. The young athlete is especially susceptible to back injury. Intense training can cause repetitive microtrauma. Back pain can result from sprains of the ligaments or muscles (or both) of the back caused by injury.

Clinical Findings

History. Onset, duration, location, frequency, and intensity of the pain are key questions to ask to form an initial impression.

The following findings should alert the pediatric provider to possible pathologic conditions:
- Night pain
- Pain that prohibits play or activities
- Pain that persists or worsens
- History of trauma (vertebral fracture)
- Positive neurologic or musculoskeletal signs on examination
- System signs such as fever, chills, weight loss, and malaise
- Presence of any radicular symptoms, gait disturbances, muscle weakness, altered sensation, and changes in bowel and/or bladder function.

In school-age children and adolescents, back pain can be associated with a history of the following:
- Muscle strain as a result of "overuse syndrome" from excessive muscular exertion, usually related to sports, commonly in sedentary children who recently increased their activity level
- Wearing high heels or platform shoes (females)
- Neck/shoulder, low back, and arm pain in relation to computer or video game use; excessive TV watching

Physical Examination. The examination should include a complete musculoskeletal and neurologic assessment with the child adequately exposed for the clinical examination. Inspect for any changes in alignment in the frontal or sagittal plane, and range of motion should be assessed in flexion, extension, and lateral bending. Younger children may be asked to pick up an object off the floor to assess spinal flexion. Palpation will reveal any areas of tenderness and/or muscle spasm. Palpate the top of the iliac wings while the child is standing to assess leg lengths. A careful neurologic examination should be performed.

Diagnostic Studies. A CBC with differential, ESR, and CRP are useful screening tests, particularly in young children with constitutional symptoms or those complaining of night pain (Spiegel et al, 2007). Initially anteroposterior and lateral radiographs of the involved region of the spine are recommended. With lumbar back pain, right and left oblique views are recommended. MRI is most helpful when neurologic symptoms or findings are present. CT is the study of choice for defining lesions (Bernstein and Cozen, 2007).

Differential Diagnosis

Occult pathologic conditions should be ruled out. Diskitis, vertebral osteomyelitis, vertebral fracture, or tumor can cause significant back pain in toddlers. Older children can experience these same problems in addition to intervertebral disk herniation, vertebral endplate fractures, low back stress fracture, and spondylosis. Back pain is a commonly reported symptom in somatizing children. Athletes with a history of low back pain lasting more than 1 month deserve careful evaluation. A low-back stress fracture or spondylosis needs to be included in the differential diagnoses.

Management

Treatment is determined by the findings on history and physical examination and can include referral for radiographs (anteroposterior and lateral views) and imaging studies or referral to a subspecialist physician or pediatrician. If the back pain is due to injury, pain management and physical therapy may be part of the treatment plan.

SCOLIOSIS

Description

Scoliosis is a three-dimensional deformity most commonly described as a lateral curvature of the spine in the frontal plane (Spiegel et al, 2007). There are seven principal classifications for scoliosis:

- *Idiopathic*: Etiology is unknown and is likely multifactorial. A positive family history does not help predict the behavior of the individual curve. Abnormalities identified in connective tissue, muscle, and bone appear to be secondary. There are three types divided by age at manifestation:
  - Infantile (0 to 3 years old)
  - Juvenile (3 to 10 years old)
  - Adolescent (puberty to maturity)

Idiopathic scoliosis is the most common of all forms of lateral deviation of the spine and is a lateral curvature of the spine. It is defined as a curvature greater than 10 degrees according to the Cobb method in which the angle between the superior and inferior end vertebrae (tilted into the curve) is measured by a radiologist (see diagnostic studies in the following text).

- *Paralytic*: Secondary to muscle imbalance in the growing spine caused by primary neuromuscular problems (e.g., cerebral palsy or muscular dystrophy); can worsen rapidly
- *Congenital*: A structural anomaly present at birth (e.g., hemivertebrae), often associated with other congenital abnormalities, such as renal and cardiac anomalies; can worsen slowly, rapidly, or stay the same
- *Mesenchymal*: Associated with connective tissue problems (e.g., Marfan syndrome or diastrophic dwarfism)
- *Posttraumatic*: Following injury, thoracoplasty, or irradiation
- *Tumors*: Secondary to bone tumors or other lesions constricting the spine

- *Functional*: There is the appearance of a lateral curvature but no structural change in the vertebral column.
- *Other causes, miscellaneous*: Examples include metabolic disturbances or dystrophies.

Epidemiology

Secondary or functional scoliosis (i.e., the appearance of a lateral curvature but no structural change in the vertebral column) is a result of such problems as leg length inequality, poor posture, or muscle spasm. Congenital scoliosis is due to bony deformities caused by failure in formation or segmentation of vertebrae during fetal development (e.g., neural tube disorders). Paralytic or neuromuscular scoliosis is caused by myopathies and upper or lower neuron diseases (e.g., muscular dystrophy, cerebral palsy, and polio). Mesenchymal or constitutional scoliosis is associated with genetic syndromes (e.g., Marfan syndrome or diastrophic dwarfism). Miscellaneous scoliosis has numerous etiologies that do not fit one of the other classifications.

Idiopathic is the most common type of scoliosis. Its etiology is unknown, but often has a familial or genetic pattern. The overall incidence of idiopathic scoliosis is approximately 2% to 3% with between 0.3% and 0.5% having curves greater than 20 degrees on radiography and less than 0.1% demonstrating curves greater than 40 degrees Cobb's angle.

Hormonal changes play a role in the disease process, and a rapid growth period is believed to be a significant factor in the progression of curvature associated with idiopathic scoliosis. Females with this type of scoliosis are more likely than males to have lateral curvatures that progress (Spiegel et al, 2007). The most common type of idiopathic scoliosis is found in adolescents and is the major focus of the remaining discussion.

Small to moderate scoliotic curves do not increase significantly after skeletal growth is complete. Double S curves and more severe curves are more likely to progress during the growth years. For a given child, however, the ability to predict progression is difficult because even small curves can progress to severe deformity. Thus regular monitoring of the curve is important (Table 37-2).

The female-to-male ratio increases with increasing curve magnitude. For curves less than 20 degrees, the risk for progression of the curve is low; these curves generally just need to be observed. However, for curves between 20 and 45 degrees, the risk for progression is high during growth, and early intervention is of paramount importance. Young premenarchal females with large curves are a vulnerable group because their spines are skeletally immature with growth remaining. The majority of adolescents with idiopathic scoliosis have a right thoracic curve. Juvenile manifestation is uncommon, and infantile scoliosis is rare in the U.S.

Clinical Findings

History. Scoliosis is generally painless, and insidious onset is typical. Generally there is no significant history. The provider should assess the following:

- Family history of scoliosis
- Age of menarche
- Etiologic factors related to the various causes of structural scoliosis

The presence of pain with a lateral curvature of the spine suggests an inflammatory or neoplastic lesion as the cause of

TABLE 37-2 Scoliosis, Kyphosis, and Lordosis

	Curve	Etiology	Clinical Findings	Radiographs	Management	Prognosis
Scoliosis	Lateral	Classifications: idiopathic (most common); neuromuscular; constitutional; secondary; congenital; miscellaneous; functional (leg length discrepancy—not scoliosis)	Hx: positive family Hx; related to etiologies (classifications); painless curvature; typically have right thoracic curve	AP and lateral standing views to identify degree of curve; >10 degrees abnormal; may have 1 curve (C) or 2 curves (S); vertebrae show lateral deviation and rotation	Referral to orthopedic surgeon; brace or surgery; need to monitor progression of curve	Most curves do not increase after growth complete; females with idiopathic scoliosis more likely to have curve progression
Kyphosis	AP curve of thoracic spine	Familial (Scheuermann disease); secondary to tumor, trauma, etc.; congenital; postural, not true kyphosis	Postural roundback	Narrow disk space and loss of normal anterior height of vertebrae	Postural: PT, dancing, and swimming can be helpful; if structural: refer to an orthopedic surgeon for observation, bracing, or surgery	
Lordosis	AP curve of lumbar spine	As a result of hip contractures; physiologic; family and racial groups; before puberty	Abdomen and buttock protuberant; if result of hip contractures, lordosis disappears when sitting	Standing lateral views	If lumbar spine flattens and lordosis disappears when child bends forward, it is physiologic and no treatment; if fixed, refer to an orthopedist	

AP, Anteroposterior; *Hx*, history; *PT*, physical therapy.

the scoliosis. Some children with idiopathic scoliosis complain of mild pain that is activity related. Severe, constant, or night pain and point tenderness indicate some other pathologic condition (Bernstein and Cozen, 2007).

Physical Examination. The child is evaluated in the standing position, from both the front and the side, to identify any asymmetry in the chest wall, trunk, and shoulders. Adams test looks for asymmetry of the posterior chest wall on forward bending, the earliest abnormality seen. Rotation of the vertebral bodies toward the convexity results in outward rotation and prominence of the attached ribs posteriorly. The anterior chest wall may be flattened on the concavity due to inward rotation of the chest wall and ribs. Associated findings may include elevation of the shoulder, lateral shift of the trunk, and an apparent leg-length discrepancy. Additional physical findings include:
- Unequal shoulder height
- Unequal scapula prominences and heights. Note that the muscle masses may be somewhat unequal, especially if the child uses one shoulder more than the other as in carrying books. Look for bony, not muscular, prominence.
- Unequal waist angles—the hip touches one arm, and the contralateral arm hangs free.
- Unequal rib prominences and chest asymmetry.
- Unequal rib heights when the child stands in the Adams forward bend position (see Fig. 37-8)

Congenital scoliosis may be visible in the infant lying prone; it is sometimes more prominent if the infant is suspended prone. Inspect for skin abnormalities, sacral dimple, and hairy patches.

The physical examination should also include the following:
- Observation for equal leg lengths
- Examination of the skin for hairy patches, nevi, café au lait spots, lipomas, dimples
- Neurologic examination checking for weakness or sensory disturbance
- Cardiac examination for Marfan syndrome

Diagnostic Studies. Standing anteroposterior (AP) and lateral radiographs of the entire spine are recommended at the initial evaluation for patients with clinical findings suggestive of a spinal deformity. On the PA radiographs, the degree of curvature is determined by the Cobb method. An MRI is helpful when an underlying cause for the scoliosis is suspected based on age (infantile, juvenile curves), abnormal findings in the history and on physical examination, and atypical radiographic features. Atypical radiographic findings include uncommon curve patterns, such as the left thoracic curve, double thoracic curves, high thoracic curves, widening of the spinal canal, and erosive or dysplastic changes in the vertebral body or ribs. On the lateral radiograph, an increase in thoracic kyphosis or an absence of segmental lordosis may be suggestive of an underlying neurologic abnormality (Spiegel et al, 2007).

Differential Diagnosis

Structural scoliosis must be differentiated from functional scoliosis. The latter disappears when the child is placed in the Adams forward bending position, whereas the former is enhanced in this position. Persistent functional scoliosis to one side in a child with a neuromotor problem can eventually become structural and must be managed with physical therapy or other means to prevent progression. Consider systemic problems, such as neurofibromatosis, cerebral palsy, multiple sclerosis, Rett syndrome, rickets, tuberculosis, and tumor.

Management

The primary aim of scoliosis management is to stop curvature progression and improve pulmonary function. Guidelines for conservative treatment are based on the progression of the curvature. The three modalities of treatment for scoliosis include physical therapy by a therapist certified in scoliosis-specific interventions, bracing, and surgical intervention. Brace treatment has been found to be effective in preventing curvature progression. Brace treatment may reduce the need for surgery, restore the sagittal profile, and change vertebral rotation. Surgery is indicated for children who have progressive spinal deformity that cannot be controlled by nonoperative means, such as bracing, and where there is significant spinal growth remaining (Smith, 2009).

Idiopathic Scoliosis

- Treatment varies depending on age at manifestation. Infantile scoliosis often involves a left thoracic curvature in males and resolves spontaneously in 90% of children. Nonresolving and progressive infantile curves are treated with bracing. Juvenile scoliosis occurs more often in females, is generally progressive, and commonly is a right thoracic curvature.
- Adolescent scoliosis has a 3:2 female-to-male ratio and can resolve, remain static, or increase.
- Key considerations for the management of scoliosis are:
  - *For Cobb angle less than 15 degrees:* Observation at 6- to 12-month intervals
  - *For Cobb angle 15 to 20 degrees:* Outpatient therapy with a combination of therapist guided sessions and home exercise program
  - *For Cobb angle 21 to 25 degrees:* Outpatient physiotherapy, scoliosis intensive rehabilitation (SIR) program where available. A brace may be indicated.
  - *For Cobb angle greater than 25 degrees:* Outpatient physical therapy, SIR program, and brace wear. Rationale for surgical intervention is discussed below.

Referral to an orthopedist or a center that specializes in working with infants and children with scoliosis is essential. Support must be given to the child and family through the diagnostic and treatment phases, considering school and peer factors. The primary care provider will need to assist the child with psychological adjustment issues that arise if casting, bracing, or surgery is recommended and instituted. Some specific concerns of the child can include self-esteem problems, managing hostility and anger, learning about the disease and its care, wondering about the long-term prognosis, and concerns about clothing and participation in sports and other activities.

Other Classifications of Scoliosis.
For congenital, constitutional, paralytic, tumor, mesenchymal, posttraumatic, or miscellaneous causes of scoliosis, treatment depends on the etiology and severity of the curve and the rate of its progression. Bracing may be tried, is controversial, and is generally not effective. Bracing may help reduce compensatory curves

in congenital scoliosis. Rapidly increasing curves need early operative treatment (e.g., spinal fusion and instrumentation). Supervision needs to be maintained until growth is complete. Exercises are not helpful. Paralytic scoliosis with neuromuscular-related curves greater than 20 degrees is treated with surgery.

Complications

Progressive scoliosis can result in a severe deformity of the spinal column. Severe deformities can result in impairment of respiratory and cardiovascular function and limitation of physical activities and decreased comfort. The psychological consequences of an untreated scoliosis deformity can be severe.

Prevention

Prevention is not possible; however, early identification of children with scoliosis can help them avoid more expensive, invasive care and prevent the long-term consequences of the disorder. School screening clinics are recommended by the American Academy of Orthopaedic Surgeons and the Scoliosis Research Society. Screening is effective, however, only if identified children are referred for care. Their parents must be notified, a referral arranged, and follow-up ensured.

KYPHOSIS

Description

The thoracic spine normally has between 20 and 45 degrees of posterior curvature, which is considered physiologic. Kyphosis is the term used to describe the condition when the normal posterior curvature of the thoracic spine becomes excessive or exaggerated and is outside the physiologic range of normal. With kyphosis there is an anteroposterior (AP) forward curve of the thoracic spine with the apex posterior (i.e., the back is prominent). The most common clinical type of kyphosis is postural (postural roundback). The curvature of the spinal column points backward, and when viewed from the side, gives the appearance of being humpbacked. In postural kyphosis the Adams forward bending test demonstrates normalization of the lateral spine profile when viewed from the side (see Table 37-2), and the child can reverse the roundback appearance with active extension. Postural kyphosis is the most common type and is more common in girls than boys. It rarely causes pain, and the curvature is flexible.

Scheuermann kyphosis is an osteochondrosis that presents as an abnormality of the vertebral epiphyseal growth plates. Onset generally occurs in adolescence. The kyphosis is rigid and the pain is located over the deformity and is worse at the end of the day. In Scheuermann kyphosis, radiograph findings may include vertebral wedging of 5 degrees or more on three adjacent vertebral bodies, endplate changes, or disk-space narrowing (Bernstein and Hang, 2007).

Management

Depending on cause and severity of the kyphosis, there are different treatment options. Postural kyphosis may be improved with an exercise and physical therapy program that strengthens the supporting muscles. Activities, such as dancing or swimming, that require a full range of motion of the shoulders, back, and arms, can be helpful. Adolescent kyphosis may be treated with a combination of a back brace, exercise, and physical therapy. Surgery may be required in children with structural problems that cause kyphosis and in adolescents with curvature of the back that exceeds 50 to 60 degrees. Kyphosis caused by infections or tumors may also require surgery.

LUMBAR LORDOSIS

Description

Lumbar lordosis, or hyperlordosis, is an AP curve of the lumbar area of the spine (i.e., the child stands with the abdomen and buttocks protuberant). It is the least common of the congenital spinal deformities and is often associated with kyphosis or scoliosis. Congenital lordosis deformity is usually progressive. Lordosis can be a secondary result of a hip problem in which full extension is limited by hip flexion contractures or from lumbosacral deformities.

Management

If the pediatric provider suspects lumbar lordosis, have the child bend forward. If the lumbar spine flattens and the lordosis disappears in the forward bending position, it indicates that the spine is flexible and the lordosis is only physiologic. This child should be seen for follow-up in 6 to 12 months, and the examination repeated to ensure continued physiologic findings. If the lordosis persists in the forward bending position, this indicates a fixed structural deformity and needs referral to an orthopedist. Lordosis resulting from hip flexion contractures is absent while sitting; it is commonly seen in children with cerebral palsy, spina bifida, and developmental dysplasia of the hip (see Table 37-2).

HIP PROBLEMS

DEVELOPMENTAL DYSPLASIA OF THE HIP

Description

Developmental dysplasia of the hip (DDH) represents a spectrum of anatomic abnormalities in which the femoral head and the acetabulum are in improper alignment and/or grow abnormally. This includes dysplastic, subluxated, dislocatable, and dislocated hips. Dysplasia is characterized by a shallow more vertical acetabular socket with an immature hip/acetabulum. In subluxation, the hip is unstable, and the head of the femur can slide in and out of the acetabulum. DDH occurs congenitally or develops in infancy or childhood. Dysplasia may be diagnosed many years after the newborn period.

Epidemiology

Physiologic, mechanical, and genetic factors are implicated in DDH. Physiologic factors include the hormonal effect of maternal estrogen and relaxin that are released near delivery and produce a temporary laxity of the hip joint. Mechanical factors include constant compression in utero with restriction of movement late in gestation if the fetal pelvis becomes locked in the maternal pelvis. This is seen with first pregnancy,

oligohydramnios, and breech presentation. In cultures that swaddle infants in an extended position or place them on cradleboards, the incidence of DDH is greater than normal because of such neonatal positioning.

In the unstable hip, the femoral head and the acetabulum may not have a normal tight, concentric anatomic relationship, which can lead to abnormal growth of the hip joint and result in permanent disability. In the newborn the left hip is most often involved because this hip typically is the one in a forced adduction position against the mother's sacrum.

The hip can dislocate noncongenitally or in utero in children with certain muscular or neurologic disorders that affect the use of the lower extremities, such as cerebral palsy, arthrogryposis, or myelomeningocele. Dislocation results from the abnormal use of the extremity over time.

The incidence of DDH is estimated to range from 1.5 to 20 per 1000 live births in the U.S. The reported incidence has increased significantly since the advent of clinical and sonographic screening, which suggests possible overdiagnosis (Shipman et al, 2006). It is found more commonly with breech births and is four times more common in girls than boys. A positive family history (genetic risk factors) increases the risk for having a child with this problem. Other risk factors seen in infants that are associated with DDH include oligohydramnios, torticollis, and lower limb deformities, such as clubfoot, metatarsus adductus (MA), and dislocated knee.

Clinical Findings

History. Risk factors for DDH include female gender, family history, high birthweight, breech positioning, and utero postural deformities (Shipman et al, 2006).

Physical Examination. A hip examination should be performed on children as part of their well-child supervision until they are 2 years old. Findings of DDH include the following:

- Screening tests are serial physical examinations of the hip and lower extremities using the Barlow, Ortolani, and Klisic procedures and ultrasonography.
- Sixty to 80% of abnormal hips of newborns identified by physical examination resolve by 2 to 8 weeks. Around 2 months old, soft-tissue contractures develop, which prevents manual reduction of the dislocated hip.
- In the older infant, 6 to 18 months:
  - Limited abduction of the affected hip and shortening of the thigh is a reliable sign (see Fig. 37-3, *B* and Fig. 37-5).
  - Normal abduction with comfort is 70 to 80 degrees bilaterally. Limited abduction includes those cases with less than 60 degrees of abduction or unequal abduction from one side to the other (see Fig. 37-5).
  - Positive Galeazzi sign (see Fig. 37-3, *A*)
- Other findings include asymmetry of inguinal or gluteal folds (thigh-fold asymmetry is not related to the disorder [see Fig. 37-3, *D*]) and unequal leg lengths, shorter on the affected side.

In the ambulatory child who was not diagnosed earlier or was not corrected, the following might also be noted:

- Short leg with toe walking on the affected side
- Positive Trendelenburg sign (see Fig. 37-3, *C*)
- Marked lordosis or toe walking
- Painless limping or waddling gait with child leaning to the affected side

If the hips are dislocated bilaterally, asymmetries are not observed. Limited abduction is the primary indicator in this situation (see Fig. 37-5). Also in the subluxed hip (not frankly dislocated), limited abduction again is the primary indicator. A waddling gait may also be noted.

Diagnostic Studies. Radiologic evaluation of the newborn to detect DDH is unreliable because so much of the hip joint is cartilaginous in the young infant. Ultrasound is widely used to assess the infant hip. Ultrasound evaluation of the cartilaginous and osseous components of the infant hip at rest and during dynamic maneuvers provides information about morphology, position, and stability (Torres and DiPietro, 2009). By around 3 months old, radiography is reliable. AP and Lauenstein (frog-leg) position lateral radiographs of the pelvis are adequate.

Differential Diagnosis

The condition is relatively unique.

Management

The goal of management is to restore the articulation of the femur within the acetabulum.

- Refer to an orthopedist promptly while the infant is still in the newborn nursery, if possible. Infants ages 7 weeks and younger have a higher rate of success than those ages 8 weeks and older (Atalar et al, 2007). The treatment of choice for subluxation and reducible dislocations identified in the early phase is a Pavlik harness. The harness is applied with hips having greater than 90 degrees of flexion, and with adduction of the hip limited to a neutral position. The line of pull of the flexion straps must be lateral enough to affect flexion in a relatively abducted rather than an adducted position (Atalar et al, 2007).The success rate of Pavlik harness treatment is reported to be between 80% and 97%. Radiographic or ultrasound documentation can be used during treatment to verify the position of the hip. If the infant does not respond to treatment with the harness, surgical treatment may be needed. The 6- to 18-month-old infant with a dislocated hip is likely to require either closed manipulation or open reduction. Preoperative traction, adductor tenotomy, and gentle reduction are especially helpful in preventing osteonecrosis of the femoral head. After the closed or open reduction, a hip spica cast is applied with the hip joint in 95 degrees of flexion and 40 to 45 degrees of abduction (Beaty, 2007).
- Triple diapering is not helpful because the musculoskeletal forces far outweigh the force that can be exerted by the diaper material.
- The majority of neonatal hip instability cases resolve spontaneously by 6 to 8 weeks of age. Close observation of these children is recommended.
- The child with a Pavlik harness should be seen weekly to ensure that it fits properly and the femur is properly seated in the socket. It is worn 24 hours a day except for bathing. Ultrasonography can be performed while the Pavlik harness is worn to assess hip position. Radiographs have been suggested at 8 to 18 months after completion of therapy to determine whether there is any evidence of residual dysplasia or avascular necrosis (Atalar et al, 2007).
- The earlier treatment is started with the Pavlik harness, the better the prognosis for a successful outcome. Generally the harness is worn full time for 2 months and then worn during waking hours for decreasing periods of time.

- Support the child and family through the treatment phases. Explain management goals clearly. For a child in a Pavlik harness or spica cast, cast care, skin care, and car safety when the child cannot easily be placed in a car seat are issues to be addressed (see Chapter 39). Furthermore, the child needs special attention to maintain developmental stimulation while immobilized.
- An orthopedist should be immediately consulted for any infant seen in a primary care setting who is in a Pavlik harness and exhibits excessive hip flexion (beyond 100 degrees) or abduction (beyond 60 degrees). These degrees of flexion or abduction can be harmful (Atalar et al, 2007).

Complications

The Pavlik harness and other positional devices may cause skin irritation, and a difference in leg length may remain. There may be delay in walking if the child is put in a body cast. The long-term outcomes depend on the age at diagnosis, the severity of the joint deformity, and the effectiveness of therapy. Untreated cases may result in a permanent dislocation of the femoral head so that it lies just under the iliac crest posteriorly. Clinically the child has limited mobility of this pseudo joint and related short leg. Forceful reduction can result in avascular necrosis of the femoral head with permanent hip deformity. Redislocation or persistent dysplasia can occur. Adult degenerative arthritis is associated with acetabular dysplasia.

Prevention

The condition cannot be prevented, but early identification resulting in early treatment significantly reduces the long-term consequences of the problem. Screening of all neonates and infants should include full hip abduction, examination for unequal inguinal and gluteal folds and unequal leg lengths, and Barlow, Ortolani, and Galeazzi maneuvers at every examination. The hip can dislocate at any point in early development, even up to the point of first ambulation. In older children, limited abduction, gait, and standing position, including the Trendelenburg position, add important information. Charting should always include notation about hip findings because these can change at subsequent visits.

LEGG-CALVÉ-PERTHES DISEASE
Description

Legg-Calvé-Perthes (LCPD) disease is a childhood hip disorder that results in infarction of the bony epiphysis of the femoral head. It presents as avascular necrosis of the femoral head. The basic underlying cause of LCPD is insufficient blood supply to the femoral head.

Epidemiology

There is an initial ischemic episode of unknown etiology that interrupts vascular circulation to the capital femoral epiphysis. The articular cartilage hypertrophies, and the epiphyseal marrow becomes necrotic. The area revascularizes, and the necrotic bone is replaced by new bone. This process can take 18 to 24 months. There is a critical point in these dual processes when the subchondral area becomes weak enough that fracture of the epiphysis occurs. At this time the child becomes symptomatic. With fracturing, further reabsorption and replacement by fibrous bone occurs, and the shape of the femoral head is altered. Articulation of the head in the hip joint is interrupted. The bone reossifies with or without treatment, but without treatment the femoral head flattens and enlarges, causing joint deformity. Lateral subluxation of the femoral head is associated with poor outcomes.

Etiology is unclear, but certain risk factors have been identified in children. These include gender, socioeconomic group, and the presence of an inguinal hernia and genitourinary tract anomalies. Boys are affected three to five times more often than girls; incidence increases in lower socioeconomic groups and in children with low birthweights. The disease is bilateral in 10% to 20% of children. It affects children ages 4 to 8 years. There is a familial history in 6% of children (Khan et al, 2008).

Clinical Findings

History. There can be an acute or chronic onset with or without a history of trauma to the hip, such as jumping from a high place.

- The earliest sign is an intermittent limp (abductor lurch) especially after exertion, with mild or intermittent pain in the anterior part of the thigh.
- Some children may present with limited range of motion of the affected extremity.
- The most common symptom is persistent pain.
- Pain may be referred to the medial aspect of the ipsilateral knee or to the lateral thigh.

Physical Examination. Findings may include the following:

- Antalgic gait with limited hip movement
- Trendelenburg gait resulting from pain in the gluteus medius muscle
- Muscle spasm
- Atrophy of quadriceps and thigh muscle
- Decreased abduction, internal rotation, and extension of the hip
- Adduction flexion contracture
- Pain on rolling the leg internally

Diagnostic Studies. Routine AP pelvis and frog-leg lateral views are used to confirm the diagnosis, stage the disease, and follow disease progression and response to treatment. Radiographic alterations can include smaller epiphysis, increased epiphyseal density, subchondral fracture line, lateralization of the femoral head, and other features. Changes in the epiphysis margin are discerned by the orthopedist and radiologist (Fig. 37-9). However, there may be no radiographic findings early in LCPD. Ultrasonography is useful in the preliminary diagnosis; capsular distention can be seen on sonographic images. Bone scans and MRI allow for precise localization of the bone involvement, but changes seen as bone marrow edema and joint effusions are nonspecific. CT scans allow early diagnosis of bone collapse and curvilinear zones of sclerosis early in the disease process, but the use is limited due to high radiation dosing (Khan et al, 2008).

Differential Diagnosis

Acute and chronic infections, sickle cell disease, toxic synovitis, Gaucher disease, slipped capital femoral epiphysis (SCFE), osteomyelitis, juvenile rheumatoid arthritis, hemophilia, and neoplasm are included in the differential diagnosis.

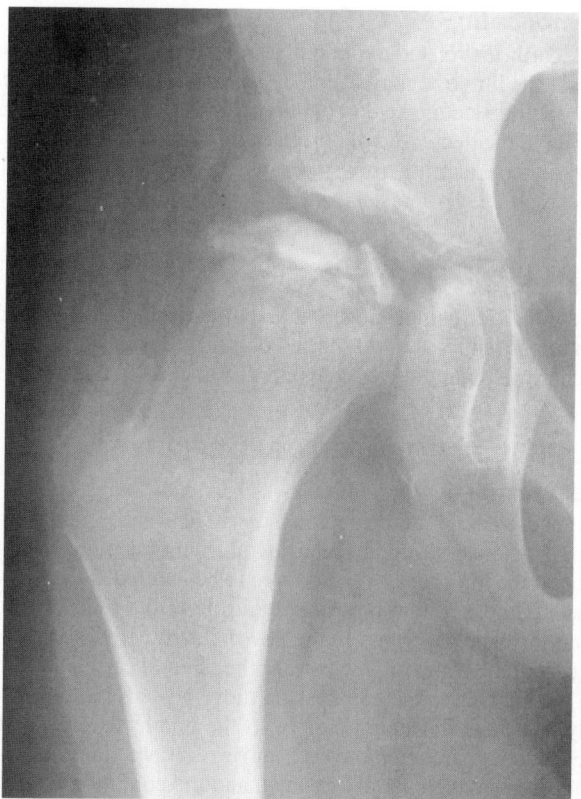

FIGURE 37-9 Anteroposterior (AP) radiograph of the right hip of an 8-year-old boy with Legg-Calvé-Perthes disease (LCPD). There is a collapsed yet dense capital femoral epiphysis with early fragmentation. The small medial triangle of the capital femoral epiphysis is uninvolved in the disease process. (From Behrman RE, Kliegman RM, Jenson HB editors: *Nelson textbook of pediatrics*, ed 17, Philadelphia, 2004, Saunders.)

Management

The following steps are taken (Harris, 2009):

- Consult with an orthopedist. The goals of treatment include eliminating hip irritability, restoring and maintaining good range of motion, preventing femoral epiphyseal collapse, and attaining a spherical femoral head when the hip heals (Harris, 2009). Initial bed rest and possibly femoral abduction traction (to relieve muscle spasms) may be used to eliminate or reduce hip irritability (1 to 2 weeks). Physical therapy may then be needed to reduce residual stiffness. For moderate to severe cases, bracing and surgical intervention are the treatment options. With both, the goal is abduction and rotation of the femur. Bracing is continued 24 hours a day for 6 to 18 months. Surgical treatment includes either femoral osteotomy to redirect the involved portion within the acetabulum or innominate osteotomy. Both procedures produce equal results, but femoral osteotomy may cause shortening of the limb, leading to a chronic limp (Harris, 2009). Surgery does not speed healing of the femoral head, but it does cause the head to reossify in a more spherical fashion.
- Support and monitor the child throughout treatment and recovery, including during interruption of school or other activities. Treatment and monitoring of LCPD can last from 12 to 40 months.

Complications

Osteoarthritis related to femoral head deformity and decreased use of the hip joint may occur, depending on the femoral head remodeling status. Older children have a poorer prognosis owing to the decreased opportunity for femoral head remodeling in the remaining growth period. Females with LCPD also have a poorer prognosis.

Prevention

The condition is not preventable, but early identification and treatment reduce the long-term complications of the disorder, such as premature degenerative arthritis in early adult life.

SLIPPED CAPITAL FEMORAL EPIPHYSIS

Description

Slipped capital femoral epiphysis (SCFE) is a Salter-Harris type I fracture through the proximal femoral physis. Stress around the hip causes a shear force to be applied at the growth plate. Although trauma may play a role in the fracture, there is an intrinsic weakness in the physeal cartilage. The fracture occurs at the hypertrophic zone of the physeal cartilage. Stress on the hip causes the epiphysis to move posteriorly and medially. Because the blood supply to the epiphysis crosses the weakened area, the epiphysis is at risk for avascular necrosis. The slippage is generally gradual, and the condition is classified as stable or unstable based on the continuity of the capital femoral epiphysis and the femoral neck (Adler, 2008).

Epidemiology

SCFE typically occurs just after the onset of puberty, often in overweight and slightly skeletally immature boys. It is seen in children in whom puberty is delayed. African-American children are affected slightly more than others. The incidence is slightly greater in boys than girls. Additional underlying risks include malnutrition, endocrine abnormalities, and prior developmental dysplasia of the hip (Adler, 2008). It can also be seen following chemotherapy, irradiation, and renal failure. Slippage is bilateral in 20% to 37% and synchronous in 9% to 18% (Adler, 2008). The most exclusive incidence of SCFE during the adolescent growth spurt indicates a hormonal role. Obesity is the other key predisposing factor.

Clinical Findings

Clinical presentation is often misleading and can result in delay of diagnosis and treatment.

History
- A vague history of antecedent trauma
- Pain in affected hip, groin, thigh, or knee
- Some have complaints of limping or gait abnormalities.

Physical Examination
- Obesity
- Delayed puberty
- Pain in the groin or diffusely over the knee or anterior thigh
- Pain and decreased internal rotation
- Antalgic limp with short leg component (50% are up to 1 inch shorter on affected side)
- As the epiphysis continues to slip there may be a more pronounced limping and external rotation of the toes when walking.

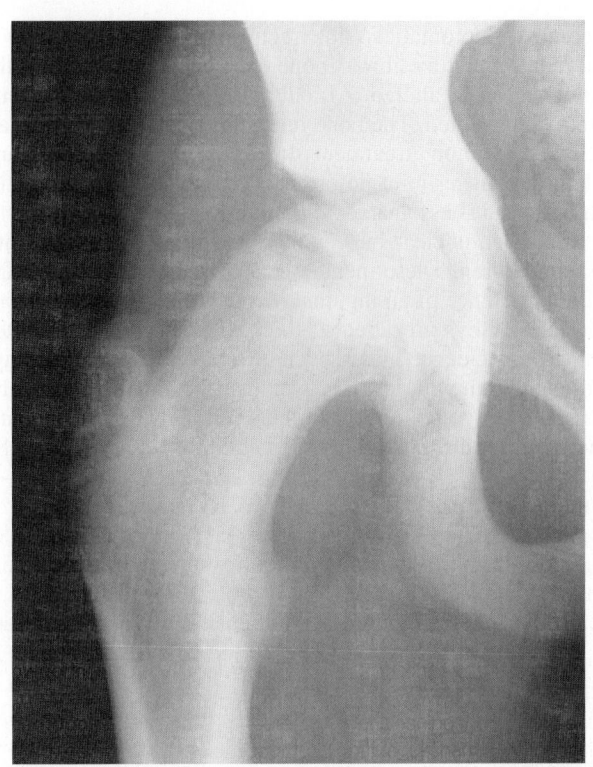

FIGURE 37-10 Anteroposterior (AP) radiograph of the right hip of a 13-year-old boy with a moderately severe chronic slipped femoral epiphysis. Notice the physeal widening and the distorted relationship between the capital femoral epiphysis and femoral neck. (From Behrman RE, Kliegman RM, Jenson HB et al, editors: *Nelson textbook of pediatrics*, ed 17, Philadelphia, 2004, Saunders.)

- External rotation of the thigh when the hip is flexed; lack of internal rotation of the hip with range of motion
- Mild atrophy of the thigh and gluteal muscles
- Limited abduction and extension
- With unstable SCFE the child is unable to bear weight.

Diagnostic Studies. AP pelvis, frog-leg lateral, and true lateral views of the pelvis are obtained. Radiographic findings include flattening of the epiphyseal prominence, widening or irregularity of the growth plate, and narrowing of the area if the epiphysis has slipped posteriorly. The varus angle between the femoral head and the shaft is also assessed (Fig. 37-10). Radiographically the slippage can be classified as mild (less than 33% slippage of the epiphysis or less than a 30-degree slip angle), moderate (33% to 50% slippage of the epiphysis or 30- to 60-degree slip angle), or severe (greater than 50% slippage of the epiphysis or greater than 60 degree slip angle) (Hart et al, 2007).

Differential Diagnosis

LCPD, sepsis of the hip joint, and osteoarthritis should be considered.

Management

The goal of treatment is to prevent further slippage and to stabilize the epiphysis (Hart et al, 2007):
- Refer immediately to an orthopedic surgeon or to the emergency department for definitive treatment.
- Place child on crutches or a wheelchair. Non–weight bearing needs to be emphasized to prevent further slippage.

- Standard treatment for a stable SCFE involves percutaneous pinning and placement of a single cannulated screw through the femoral neck into the central aspect of the proximal femoral epiphysis.
- If the slippage is more severe or unstable, a more involved procedure or corrective osteotomy may be necessary.
- There is a high incidence of contralateral SCFE within 6 to 12 months. The hip(s) need to be monitored until skeletal maturity is achieved.
- Support and monitor the child throughout the treatment phase, which includes interruption of school and activities during the recovery period. Contact sports are usually restricted by the orthopedist until growth is complete.

Complications

The two most severe complications of SCFE are avascular necrosis (AVN) and chondrolysis. AVN is loss of blood supply to the proximal femoral physis resulting in death of a portion of the bone. It is the most serious complication and has a higher incidence of occurring if the slip is severe or unstable. Chondrolysis is acute cartilage necrosis and represents a loss of articular cartilage.

Prevention

SCFE is not a preventable condition. However, identification of the condition during the preslip period, when complaints of hip or referred knee pain, loss of motion, or weakness in the hip are present, allows early intervention. This can prevent deformity and long-term sequelae, such as premature degenerative arthritis in early adult life. If the child is overweight, advise about the need for weight reduction.

FEMORAL ANTEVERSION

Description

Everyone has some degree of femoral anteversion. By 10 to 12 years old, the normal angle of anteversion is 10 to 15 degrees. Younger children have a somewhat wider angle. Increased femoral anteversion (more than 2 standard deviations [SD] from the mean) is called femoral torsion and can be either medial or lateral. Medial femoral torsion or medial antetorsion generally occurs around 2 to 3 years old and lasts until about 5 years old. It is a condition in which the head and neck of the femur are rotated at an increased angle anteriorly in relation to the femoral shaft. Femoral anteversion is also called *internal femoral torsion* (Gholve et al, 2007).

Epidemiology

A family history is often identified, and it occurs more commonly in girls. "W" sitting (TV squat) can increase the deformity. Physiologically the condition produces an in-toeing gait because the anteriorly directed femoral neck internally rotates to a more neutral position and the head of the femur fits neatly into the acetabulum. This results in internal rotation of the lower femur and leg with the feet in-toeing. Increased femoral anteversion generally is more severe between 4 and 6 years old, but resolves as the child grows, and the tibia rotates laterally.

Clinical Findings
History
- In-toeing gait, perhaps more severe with fatigue
- Runs awkwardly (looks like an "eggbeater"); may actually trip as a result of crossing the feet while walking or running.
- Possible family history
- Usually a history of "W" sitting
Physical Examination
- In-toeing gait with patellae medial
- Internal (medial) rotation normally less than 70 degrees (mild deformity—70 to 80 degrees; moderate—between 80 and 90 degrees; severe—greater than 90 degrees [see Fig. 37-7])
- External (lateral) rotation decreased (limited to 0 to 10 degrees)
- Knees medially rotated ("kissing patella") when standing

Diagnostic Studies. Radiographs are not merited unless surgery is contemplated.

Differential Diagnosis

Consider other rotational deformities, such as internal tibial torsion or MA. Cerebral palsy with a "scissoring gait" might be mistaken for severe femoral anteversion.

Management

Management includes observation of the child and referral to an orthopedist if medial rotations are significant (no external rotation of the hip in extension) or the child or family has significant concerns. Nonoperative management strategies, such as shoe modifications, twister cables, and night splints, are ineffective. Operative correction is successful, but carries the risk of complications. Osteotomy is rarely performed and is done only in the child older than 8 years with significant cosmetic and functional deformity. The natural history of the condition is for the medial, or internal, rotation to decrease, providing some improvement.

Complications

Studies have shown that the condition does not cause flatfoot, bunions, knee problems, back difficulties, difficulties in running, or degenerative arthritis of the hip in adults. It is primarily a cosmetic problem unless severe enough to interfere with activities. Self-esteem can be affected.

Prevention

The condition cannot be prevented, but its aggravation can be minimized by discouraging "W" sitting, which places the weight of the upper body directly on the femoral neck, thus increasing the molding in the abnormal direction. Ballet lessons or activities such as skating, bicycle riding, or skiing can help mildly affected children learn to point their feet straight ahead, but such activities do not modify the bony structures (Sawyer and Drendel, 2006).

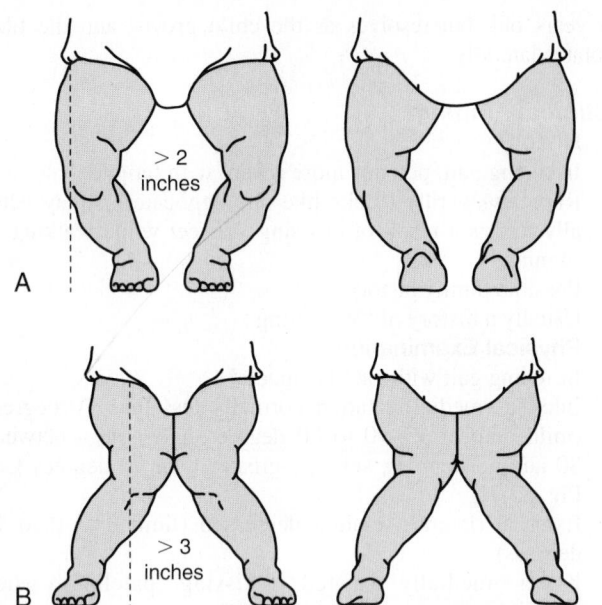

FIGURE 37-11 Genu varum and genu valgum. In genu varum **(A)** the knees are titled away from the midline; measure the intercondylar (knee) distance with the ankles together. In genu valgum **(B)** the knees are tilted toward the midline; measure the intermalleolar distance with knees approximated.

KNEE PROBLEMS

GENU VARUM

Description

Genu varum, or bowing of the legs, can be a physiologic or developmental variation of normal or a pathologic condition that involves a rotational deformity (Fig. 37-11). The term *bowlegs* is used to describe physiologic variations of the normal knee angle resulting in bowing of the legs that is typically seen in children up to 2 years old, but can be considered normal until 3 years old. The typical pattern of normal bowing seen in children is a symmetric lateral bowing of both tibias in the first year followed by bowlegs in the second year. Most bowing resolves spontaneously but can progress to persistent or pathologic varus. The angle between the tibia and femur is in pronounced varus (up to 15 degrees) in normal children before 1 year old. This is considered a uterine packing effect. The angle approaches neutral by 18 months old and then proceeds to a valgus angle, with an average angle of 12 degrees from 2 to 3 years old. The angle then gradually decreases to 8 degrees in females and 7 degrees in males by adulthood. If the varus angle is greater than 15 degrees in infants, does not begin to decrease in the second year, is asymmetric, is associated with short stature, or is rapidly progressing, the condition is considered pathologic. Knee angle variations that fall 2 SD beyond the mean are outside the normal range of varus and are considered pathologic.

If the varus persists after 30 months of age or increases, it may represent Blount disease, rickets, tumor, neurologic problems, infection, or other conditions. A Salter fracture through the tibial growth plate can result in later genu varum as growth across the plate progresses unevenly.

With Blount disease (idiopathic tibia vara that affects the proximal tibia), there is an abnormal growth of the medial aspect of the proximal tibial epiphysis that results in progressive varus angulation of the tibia. Blount disease is rare, but can occur in infancy (18 months to 3 years old), school years (4 to 10 years old), and during adolescence (11 years and older). It is seen more frequently in African-American, Hispanic, and Scandinavian populations, is associated with obesity and early walkers, and commonly has a positive family history. Onset in infancy presents the highest risk for greatest deformity (Stevens, 2010).

Clinical Findings

History. Family history is important because certain heritable conditions—Marfan syndrome, osteogenesis imperfecta, or vitamin D–resistant rickets—may predispose a child to this condition. Additional history may include progression since birth; increasing deformation is problematic.

Physical Examination
- Tibial-femoral angle greater than 15 degrees
- Associated internal tibial torsion
- Lower extremity length discrepancy
- Intercondylar (knees) distance with the ankles together—measurement greater than 4 to 5 inches suggests the need for additional evaluation
- Joint laxity of the lateral collateral ligaments in older children

Diagnostic Studies. The standard radiograph for the older child is an AP of the lower extremities with the patellae facing forward and a lateral radiograph of the involved extremity. The length of each femur and tibia is measured and any diaphyseal deformities are noted. The mechanical axis is a line drawn from the center of the head of the femur to the center of the ankle; this line should bisect the knee (Stevens, 2010). In physiologic bowing the deformity is gentle and symmetric, with a metaphyseal-diaphyseal angle less than 11 degrees, and normal appearance of the proximal tibial growth plate. In Blount disease the bowing is asymmetric, abrupt and with sharp angulation, metaphyseal-diaphyseal angle greater than 11 degrees; there is medial sloping of the epiphysis and widening of the physis (Hosalkar et al, 2007a).

Differential Diagnosis

Physiologic, persistent, and pathologic genu varum must be differentiated. Metabolic (rickets) or neurologic problems, Blount disease, infections, tumor, osteochondrodysplasias, and internal tibial torsion should be ruled out.

Management

- In physiologic genu varum (no increasing deformity):
  - No active treatment and resolves spontaneously. Corrective shoes and splinting are unnecessary.
  - Reassure parents; provide information about the natural progression of the problem.
  - Observe the child's condition over time (in 3 to 6 months) to be sure the problem is resolving, especially during the second year of life. Photographs of the legs for the chart can be helpful.
- In pathologic genu varum (increasing deformity):
  - Refer to an orthopedist. Blount disease may be treated with bracing in children younger than 3 years. Bracing

is effective and can prevent progression in 50% of these children. In children older than 4 years of age, a proximal tibial valgus osteotomy and associated fibular diaphyseal osteotomy are the procedures of choice.

○ Monitor to be sure braces are used consistently with good fit.

○ Observe to be sure the problem is not worsening.

Complications

Knee degeneration and deformity result if pathologic genu varum is not treated.

Prevention

Early identification and referral reduce the complexity and expense of treatment and the residual deformities.

GENU VALGUM
Description

Genu valgum is commonly referred to as *knock-knees* (see Fig. 37-11). Females tend to have a somewhat higher degree of valgus knee posture than males, leveling off by 7 years old at 5 to 9 degrees compared with 4 to 7 degrees for boys. Physiologic genu valgum tends to peak at around 24 to 36 months old and lasts until about 7 to 8 years old.

Epidemiology

Normal valgus is achieved by 4 years of age. Variation up to 15 degrees is possible until 6 years of age. The condition can be considered developmental or physiologic. Pathologic conditions leading to valgus are metabolic bone disease (rickets, renal osteodystrophy), skeletal dysplasia, posttraumatic physeal arrest, tumors, and infection (Hosalkar et al, 2007a).

Clinical Findings
History
- Progression of the deformity
- Risk factors as listed under epidemiology
- Joint pains or stiff gait
- Older child may report knee pain due to the stretching of the medial aspect of the knee.

Physical Examination
- Bilateral tibial-femoral angle less than 15 degrees of valgus in the child up to 7 years old is considered normal; a valgus angle greater than 15 degrees is outside the range of normal.
- Unilateral deformity
- Awkwardness of gait
- Subluxing patella
- Intermalleolar (ankles) distance with the knees together—measurement greater than 4 to 5 inches suggests the need for additional evaluation (Hosalkar et al, 2007a).
- Short stature (genu valgum associated with short stature should be referred)

Diagnostic Studies. No radiographic studies are needed unless a pathologic condition is suspected. Long length anteroposterior radiographs of the leg in a weight-bearing stance are used for preoperative planning.

Differential Diagnosis

Rule out pathologic conditions of genu valgum.

Management

Deformities greater than 15 degrees and occurring after 6 years of age are unlikely to correct with growth and require surgical management. In the skeletally immature, medial tibial epiphyseal hemiepiphysiodesis is the surgical procedure. In the skeletally mature, osteotomy is necessary at the center of rotation of angulation.

Prevention

Preventive measures are the same as those for genu varum.

OSGOOD-SCHLATTER DISEASE
Description

Osgood-Schlatter disease (OSD) is caused by microtrauma in the deep fibers of the patellar tendon at its insertion on the tibial tuberosity. The diagnosis is usually based on history and physical examination.

Epidemiology

The quadriceps femoris muscle inserts on a relatively small area of the tibial tuberosity. Naturally high tension exists at the insertion site. In children, additional stress is placed on the cartilaginous site as a result of vigorous physical activity, leading to traumatic changes at insertion.

OSD is often seen in the adolescent years after undergoing a rapid growth spurt the previous year. It occurs more frequently in boys than girls, with a male-to-female ratio as high as 7:1. This difference is probably related to a greater participation in specific risk activities by boys than by girls (Joshi, 2010).

Clinical Findings
History
- Recent physical activity, such as playing track, soccer, or football or surfboarding commonly produces the condition.
- Pain increases during and immediately after the activity and decreases when the activity is stopped for a while.
- Running, jumping, kneeling, squatting, and ascending/descending stairs exacerbate the pain.
- The pain is bilateral in 25% of cases.
- Approximately 25% of patients give a history of precipitating trauma.

Physical Examination. Characteristic findings include the following (Chang, 2010):
- Pain may be reproduced by extending the knee against resistance, stressing the quadriceps, or squatting with the knee in full flexion.
- Focal swelling, heat, and point tenderness at the tibial tuberosity
- Possibly reduced knee range of motion

Diagnostic Studies. The diagnosis is based on history and physical examination. Radiographs are not needed unless another pathologic condition is suspected.

Differential Diagnosis

Other knee derangements, tumors (osteosarcoma), and hip problems with referred pain should be considered. The referred pain of hip problems is diffuse across the distal femur without point tenderness at the tibial tubercle.

Management

OSD is a self-limiting condition, with symptom management the key consideration. The following steps are taken:

• Avoid or modify activities that cause pain until the inflammation subsides.
• Ice or cold therapy to reduce pain and inflammation.
• Once the acute symptoms have subsided, quadriceps-stretching exercises, including hip extension for complete stretch of the extensor mechanism may be performed to reduce tension on the tibial tubercle. Stretching of the hamstrings may also be useful.
• Use of NSAIDs is recommended by some, but thought ineffective by others. Because this condition may last up to 2 years, their chronic use may be problematic.
• A neoprene sleeve over the knee may help stabilize the patella.
• A patella tendon strap that wraps around the joint just below the knee reduces the strain on the tibial tuberosity.
• Cylinder casting for 2 to 3 weeks may be used in severe cases.

Complications

In the postpubertal child a residual ossicle in the tendon next to the bone may cause persistent pain. Surgical removal is indicated and will relieve the pain.

Prevention

The condition cannot be prevented, but earlier management may decrease the length of disability and the discomfort associated with it. Avoid overuse and encourage balanced training and adequate warm-up before exercise or sports participation. The use of kneepads may help protect the tibial tuberosity from direct injury for those who engage in sports that result in knee contact.

TIBIAL TORSION

Description

Tibial torsion is a common problem in children that involves the twisting of the long bone along its long axis. *Tibial version* is the term used to describe the normal variation in tibial rotation. At birth the tibias have a mean lateral rotation of 2.2 degrees and rotate laterally over time, with an adult mean lateral tibial rotation of about 23 degrees. Tibial torsion describes those rotations that are outside the range of normal. Medial tibial torsion (MTT), also known as internal tibial torsion, consists of abnormal medial rotation or twisting, resulting in in-toeing of the feet; lateral tibial torsion (LTT) consists of abnormal lateral rotation resulting in out-toeing (Hosalkar et al, 2007a).

Epidemiology

Tibial torsion may be congenital, developmental, or acquired. MTT is the most common cause of in-toeing during the second year of life and is often noted around

6 to 12 months of life. In most cases it is a physiologic condition that is the result of in utero positioning. In 90% of cases internal tibial torsion gradually resolves on its own by the time the child reaches 8 years old. LTT is a cause of out-toeing in late childhood and is usually an acquired deformity. Contracture of the iliotibial band is the underlying problem.

Clinical Findings

Physical Examination. Observe the child's gait for in-toeing. The thigh-foot angle (TFA) is used to assess tibial rotation. With the child prone and the knees flexed 90 degrees, the foot and thigh are viewed from directly above (looking downward at the angle of the thigh and foot). The foot should be relaxed. MTT exists if the TFA is negative by more than 10 to 20 degrees (−10 to −20 degrees), bearing in mind the child's age. In-toeing is expressed in negative values (Fig. 37-12). The normal range at 13 years old is −5 to +30 degrees. Abnormal lateral torsion is associated with forward-pointing patellae and outward-pointing feet. A TFA measurement of greater than +30 degrees indicates abnormal LTT (Hosalkar et al, 2007a).

Diagnostic Studies. Radiographs are usually not necessary.

Differential Diagnosis

Genu varum in which the problem originates at the knee with a tibial-femoral angle, femoral torsion (femoral anteversion), adducted great toe, and MA also produce in-toeing gaits. Adducted great toe (the searching toe) is a benign condition that resolves spontaneously. Lateral femoral torsion also causes an out-toeing gait. Screen for associated hip dysplasia and neuromuscular problems (cerebral palsy).

Management

• Treatment of tibial version (the normal variation in tibial rotation) is observation and monitoring.
• MTT should be referred to an orthopedist if the problem is significant (TFA greater than −20 by 3 years old). Stretching exercises or external rotational splints may be recommended. Surgical intervention may be needed for severe cases that persist into late childhood and cause significant functional problems.
• Shoes are ineffective for the treatment of MTT. The avoidance of certain postures that are thought to exacerbate MTT is controversial (e.g., sleeping in the knee-chest position and sitting with the feet tucked under the buttocks).
• LTT with TFA greater than +30 degrees should be referred to an orthopedist because it usually worsens with growth and does not correct spontaneously. Medial femoral torsion with pain also should be referred.

Complications

There are no complications with normal tibial version and no interference with activities. Tibial torsion (the TFA is outside the acceptable range of normal) can lead to significant functional problems in severe cases.

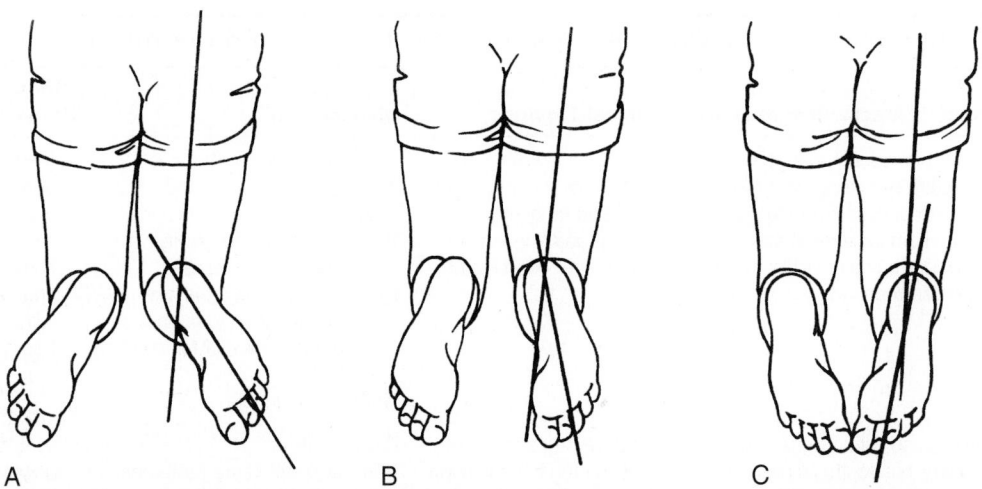

FIGURE 37-12 Thigh-foot angle. With the child in the prone position and the knees flexed and approximated, the long axis of the foot can be compared with the long axis of the thigh. The long axis of the foot bisects the heel and the second toe or lies between the second and third toes. External tibial torsion **(A)** produces excessive outward rotation. Normal alignment **(B)** is characterized by slight external rotation. Internal tibial torsion produces inward rotation of the foot and is a negative angle **(C)**. (From Thompson GH: Gait disturbances. In Kliegman RM, Nieder ML, Super DM, editors: *Practical strategies in pediatric diagnosis and therapy*, Philadelphia, 1996, Saunders.)

POPLITEAL CYSTS

Description

Popliteal cysts, or Baker cysts, result from egress of fluid through a normal communication of a bursa or may be caused by herniation of the synovial membrane through the joint capsule. Baker cysts appear much less frequently in children than adults.

Clinical Findings

The major findings are swelling behind the knee with or without discomfort. Cysts are generally located at or below the joint line.

Diagnostic Studies. Ultrasonography can distinguish between a fluid-filled cyst and solid tumor. Radiographs will show if there is soft calcification in the mass.

Differential Diagnosis

Rule out lipomas, xanthomas, vascular tumors, and fibrosarcomas.

Management

Observation is the treatment of choice. The cyst usually resolves in 10 to 20 months. Ice, NSAIDs, and assisted weight bearing if the child is experiencing discomfort are helpful (Bui-Mansfield and Youngberg, 2009).

■ Knee Injuries and Foot Problems

KNEE INJURIES

Chapters 13 and 39 discuss issues related to the musculoskeletal examination and common sports injuries. Table 37-3 outlines the etiology, assessment, management, and differential diagnosis of common knee injuries that are seen in children and young adults.

FOOT PROBLEMS

PES PLANUS

Description

Physiologic or flexible pes planus (flatfoot) is commonly seen in neonates and toddlers and is due to a fat pad in the arch that makes the appearance of the arch seem flat. This generally resolves by 2 to 3 years old, but in a small percentage of cases, can persist into adulthood. Flexible flatfoot is often familial, common, and benign. The arch is seen when the foot is suspended, but flattens with weight bearing. Rigid flatfoot is pathologic.

Epidemiology

There are three types of flatfeet: a flexible flatfoot, a flexible flatfoot with a tendo-Achilles contracture, and a rigid flatfoot. Flatfeet in neonates and toddlers are associated with physiologic ligamentous laxity. Flexible flatfeet persisting into adolescence are usually associated with familial ligamentous laxity because there is often a familial tendency toward the problem. Flatfoot also is associated with certain syndromes (Marfan and Down syndromes), myelodysplasia, cerebral palsy, and obesity. Flatfeet may be secondary to muscle imbalance or weakness, a bony abnormality, or shortened heel cords (Hosalkar et al, 2007c).

History. Onset is noticed with weight bearing. The flexible flatfoot is painless and asymptomatic. Examine the shoes to see if there is abnormal wear on the inner side.

Physical Examination. Clinical manifestations include (Hosalkar et al, 2007c):
- There is a normal longitudinal arch when examined in a non–weight-bearing position, but the arch disappears when standing.

TABLE 37-3	Characteristics of Various Types of Knee Injuries and Conditions			
Condition	**History, Mechanism of Injury**	**Clinical Findings**	**Management**	**Differential Diagnosis, Prognosis, Comments**
Quadriceps contusion	Typically a sports injury that results in bruising/contusion of the quadriceps muscle. Injury can sometime result from minor trauma or indirectly from tensile overload.	Acute pain, swelling, and restriction of active and passive range of motion of hip and knee; tenderness over quadriceps	Rest not to exceed 48 hr, ice, compression wrap, and elevation (RICE) Progressive leg and gravity-assisted ROM after rest Flexion of the knee is the last function to return to normal, so it is a good indicator for return to sport NSAID for pain relief	In teens, rule out rhabdomyosarcoma of the quadriceps, Ewing sarcoma, and osteosarcoma if there is swelling and pain in thigh without clear history of trauma
Meniscal tear (torn cartilage)	Associated with a significant injury in a youth; results from axial loading with rotation Tear of a normal meniscus is rarely seen in children <12 yr Congenital abnormal cartilage (diskoid) can tear at any age	Pain, swelling and limping Joint line tenderness and positive McMurray sign May report a sensation of a clicking or catching in the knee or a locking of the knee Can be isolated or occur in combination with ACL or MCL injuries	RICE initially MRI if suspected tear; arthrography with MRI to rule out nerve injury with a prior tear Pain management Surgical intervention: meniscectomy generally relieves symptoms	75% of patients develop degenerative articular changes on x-ray by 30 yr A small percentage of youths develop degenerative changes 3 to 5 yr after injury Chondral fractures or injuries to articular cartilage have similar history and physical findings
Sprain of the anterior cruciate ligament (ACL)	Acute injury; typically there is a twisting or hyperextension while the foot is planted and knee extended Report of a "popping" feeling and knee shifting or pulling apart	Swelling/effusion and pain Instability with lateral movement Positive Lachman test	Following the injury, a knee brace or immobilizer is used until swelling and pain subside ACL reconstruction Pain management Neuromuscular training to prevent injury	Associated with MCL and meniscal tears
Sprains of the medial collateral ligament (MCL)	Most commonly injured ligament of the knee Valgus stress to an extended knee Reports tearing sensation with medial pain, swelling, stiffness	Instability with lateral movement and medial knee pain Tenderness over the MCL If tenderness extends along the distal femoral physis, suspect physeal fracture	Ice, elevation, compression, splint or hinged knee brace to protect against valgus stress Pain management Plain radiographs to look for physeal and epiphyseal fractures in skeletally immature children Surgical repair on an isolated collateral ligament is not beneficial; nonoperative treatment is the standard of care	Combined ACL and MCL injuries are common Physeal fractures are more common than MCL sprains in youths
Osteochondritis dissecans	Juvenile and adolescent types Common 10-15 yr; boys more common than girls Isolation and sometimes sequestration of an osteochondral fragment without significant trauma May be caused by microtrauma, trauma, or may involve metabolic or genetic factors Pain increased with activity and diminished with rest plus intermittent effusions Locking and catching are unusual findings but may be present if bone fragments are detached	Activity-related pain and swelling Tenderness of the femoral condyle	Plain radiographs or MRI; 4-6 wk on immobilization and non–weight bearing if <12 yr Youths >12 yr: arthroscopic surgery Eliminate high-impact activities—non–weight bearing for several wk until symptoms abate About 50% heal spontaneously with rest and protected weight bearing Surgical intervention if still symptomatic despite 6-12 mo of conservative treatment, symptomatic loose body, or nonunion	Mimics symptoms of a torn meniscus Articular cartilage transplantation for selected patients

TABLE 37-3	Characteristics of Various Types of Knee Injuries and Conditions—cont'd			
Condition	**History, Mechanism of Injury**	**Clinical Findings**	**Management**	**Differential Diagnosis, Prognosis, Comments**
Dislocation of the patella	Associated with patellar malalignment Most cases involve lateral dislocation Pain and swelling Most occur in youths <20 yr Family history in 20%-30% More frequently in girls than boys	Massive and tense effusion Tenderness at the medial border of the patella and medial retinaculum Guarding with gentle pressure on the medial patella with lateral displacement	Nonoperative management: 2-3 wk of joint rest with splint or knee immobilizer (patella-stabilizing sleeve), then intensive rehabilitation Isometric exercises, especially of quadriceps 80%-85% of cases are successfully managed with nonoperative treatment Surgical correction for recurrent dislocations or chronic instability	Outcomes with nonoperative therapy vs. acute surgery are similar Patellar dislocation tends to recur (recurrence is more frequent in younger child) but decreases over time Degenerative arthritis is common with or without surgery with recurrent dislocations

MRI, Magnetic resonance imaging; *NSAID,* nonsteroidal antiinflammatory drug; *ROM,* range of motion.

Data from Anderson SJ: Lower extremity injuries in youth sports, *Pediatr Clin North Am* 49:627-641, 2002; Hosalkar HS, Wells L: The knee. In Kliegman RM, Behrman RE, Jenson HB et al, editors: *Nelson textbook of pediatrics,* ed 18, Philadelphia, 2007, Saunders; Landry GL: Management of musculoskeletal injury. In Kliegman RM, Behrman RE, Jenson HB et al, editors: *Nelson textbook of pediatrics,* ed 18, Philadelphia, 2007, Saunders; McMahon P, editor: *Current diagnosis and treatment: sports medicine,* New York, 2007, Lange Medical Books/McGraw-Hill; Staheli LT, editor: *Pediatric orthopaedic secrets,* ed 2, Philadelphia, 2003, Hanley & Belfus.

- On standing the hindfoot collapses into valgus, and the midfoot sag becomes evident.
- Generalized ligamentous laxity is commonly observed.
- Range of motion should be normal in flexible flatfoot.

Differential Diagnosis

Congenital vertical talus should be considered if the foot is rigid and no arch can be molded or if the foot has a rocker-bottom appearance. Calcaneovalgus foot might be considered also.

Management

Management involves the following:
- Only symptomatic feet and rigid flatfoot should be treated; refer to an orthopedist.
- For painful, flexible flatfoot, a removable, longitudinal arch support may be recommended by the orthopedist.
- If the Achilles tendon is tight, passive stretching may be helpful.
- Routine radiographs are not indicated unless pathologic flatfoot is suspected.

Complications

Flatfoot should be considered a variation of normal unless there is pain or rigidity. Congenital vertical talus is difficult to treat and should not be missed. Some cases of flatfeet are symptomatic in adulthood, and in severe cases the bones of the feet adapt to abnormal position with pronation and possible development of bunions.

Patient Education

Parents need to understand that special shoes do not cure the problem, and arch supports do not help the foot to "grow" an arch.

METATARSUS ADDUCTUS
Description

Metatarsus adductus (MA) involves adduction of the forefoot relative to the hindfoot. When the forefoot is supinated and adducted, the deformity is termed metatarsus *varus.*

Epidemiology

The most common cause is intrauterine molding; the deformity is bilateral in 50% of cases (Hosalkar et al, 2007c). A nonflexible foot, especially with heel valgus, or persistence may indicate a more serious problem.

Clinical Findings
History. There can be a family history.
Physical Examination
- The forefoot is adducted, whereas the midfoot and hindfoot are normal.
- The lateral border of the foot has a convex shape with the base of the fifth metatarsal appearing prominent. Normally this border should look straight. Sometimes spreading of the toes is noted with a wider space between the first and second toes.
- The foot should normally be straight. If one draws a line from the middle of the heel, it should pass through the second toe or between the second and third toes. In MA, the forefoot has an increased angle (greater than 15 degrees) or resists stretching (Fig. 37-13).
- To determine whether the foot is flexible or rigid, the heel is grasped with one hand while the forefoot is abducted with the other hand. In flexible MA the forefoot can be abducted past midline.

Diagnostic Studies. Radiographs are not performed routinely. AP and lateral weight bearing are indicated in toddlers or older children with residual deformities. The AP radiographs demonstrate adduction of the metatarsals at the tarsometatarsal articulation and an increased intermetatarsal angle between the first and second metatarsals.

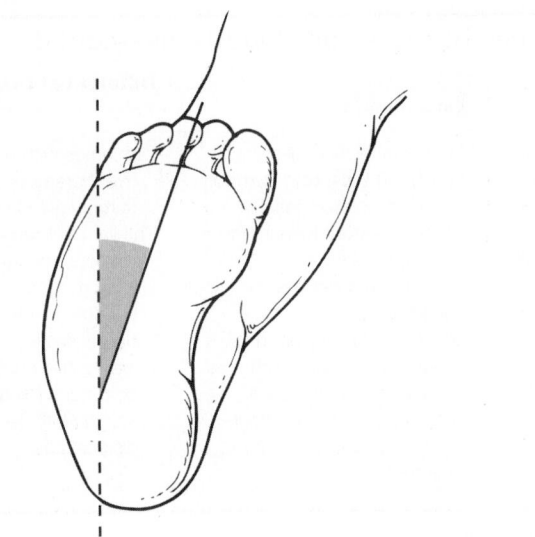

FIGURE 37-13 Metatarsus adductus (MA) angle. An angle (created by the intersecting lines) that is greater than 15 degrees indicates MA.

Differential Diagnosis

Consider congenital vertical talus, which will be rigid, or clubfoot, in which the foot is inverted and in the pointed-toe position. A careful hip examination should be performed to rule out DDH.

Management

Management is based on the rigidity of the deformity; most children respond to nonoperative treatment:

- For the flexible foot that can be brought past midline, the soft tissues can be stretched by the parents with each diaper change. Stretching is done as described under physical examination when the examiner determines whether the foot is flexible. Instruct the parents to hold the hindfoot in one hand and stretch the midfoot to overcorrect the deformity to the count of five and repeat five times. The soft tissues should blanch with each stretch. Be sure that the parent is not just pushing on the great toe. Feet that correct just to the neutral position may benefit from stretching exercises and retention in a slightly overcorrected position by a splint or reverse shoe. If there is no improvement in 4 to 6 weeks, serial plaster casts should be considered. Once flexibility and alignment are restored, orthoses or corrective shoes are generally recommended. Surgical treatment may be considered in the small subset of children with symptomatic residual deformities. Surgery is generally delayed until 4 to 6 years of age (Hosalkar et al, 2007c).
- For the nonflexible foot:
  - Refer to an orthopedist.
  - Educate the family that the treatment for infants may include serial short-leg casts or braces to stretch the foot (two or three casts for 2 weeks per cast) or other management if the bones of the foot are more severely affected. If the child is more than 2 to 3 years old, surgery may be needed to correct the problem.
  - Surgical treatment may be considered in patients with symptomatic residual deformities that have not responded to conservative treatment. Surgery is generally delayed until the child is 4 to 6 years of age.

Complications

Early intervention can prevent more intensive therapeutic measures to correct the deformity.

TALIPES EQUINOVARUS
Description

Talipes equinovarus (clubfoot) has three elements: the ankle is in equinus (the foot is in a pointed-toe position), the sole of the foot is inverted as a result of hindfoot varus or inversion deformity of the heel, and the forefoot has the convex shape of MA (forefoot adduction). The foot cannot be manually corrected to a neutral position with the heel down.

Epidemiology

The etiology of clubfoot may be idiopathic (which tends to be hereditary), neurogenic (as seen with myelomeningocele), or associated with certain syndromes, such as arthrogryposis and Larsen syndrome. It varies in severity, with uterine positioning a factor in mild clubfoot. The incidence is 1:1000 live births, with approximately 50% of cases being bilateral. The etiology is thought to be multifactorial and likely involves the effects of environmental factors in a genetically susceptible host (Hosalkar et al, 2007c). The problem is congenital and can be identified in neonates. It is more common in boys.

Clinical Findings

History. Clubfoot is present at birth.

Physical Examination. The foot appears as described previously. A complete physical examination should be performed to rule out coexisting musculoskeletal and neuromuscular problems.

Diagnostic Studies. AP and lateral radiographs are recommended, often with the foot held in a maximally corrected position. Radiographic measurements can be made to describe malalignment between the tarsal bones. A common radiographic finding is "parallelism" between lines drawn through the axis of the talus and the calcaneus on the lateral radiograph, indicating hindfoot varus. Radiographs are not required as an infant to diagnosis the anomaly.

Management

The following steps are taken:

- Refer to an orthopedist as early as possible, ideally in the newborn nursery, because the joints are most flexible in the first hours and days of life. Nonoperative treatment should be initiated as soon as possible after birth. The treatments include taping and strapping, manipulation and serial casting. The Ponseti method of clubfoot treatment involves a specific technique for manipulation and serial casting. Weekly cast changes are performed; 5 to 10 casts are usually required. Up to 90% of children will need a percutaneous tenotomy of the heel cord as an outpatient followed by a long leg cast with the foot in maximal abduction and dorsiflexion. This is followed by a full-time bracing program for 3 months and then nightly bracing for 3 to 5 years. For older children with untreated clubfeet or for those who have residual deformity, osteotomies may be required in addition to the soft-tissue surgery (Hosalkar et al, 2007c).

- Stiffness remains a concern at long-term follow-up. Although pain is uncommon in childhood and adolescence, symptoms may appear during adulthood.

Complications

With growth, the abnormality can become increasingly distorted, making correction more difficult. Calf hypoplasia and a shorter than normal foot can occur even with correction.

OVERRIDING TOES

Overriding toes are generally identified at birth. Efforts to tape them into a correct position or otherwise modify their position are usually futile. Overriding of the second, third, and fourth toes generally resolves with time. Occasionally, if severe, they can be surgically improved. Shoe fit can be a problem.

IN-TOEING AND OUT-TOEING ROTATIONAL PROBLEMS

When a child has an in-toeing or out-toeing gait, the degree of rotation and source of the rotational deformity must be assessed (Fig. 37-14). These include internal femoral torsion (femoral anteversion), internal tibial torsion, and MA. The causes of in-toeing usually are physiologic, are related to age, and resolve as the child grows (Table 37-4). In addition, in-toeing in children can vary with activities and from step to step.

Clinical Findings
History
- Onset, progression, functional limitations, previous treatment, evidence of neuromuscular disorder, and significant family history
Physical Examination
- Observe the gait. Note that the slightly older child may consciously or unconsciously improve or worsen the gait for the examiner. Asking the child to run may also be helpful.
- Lay the child prone on the examining table.
- Examine for femoral anteversion (medial and lateral rotations).
- Examine for internal or external tibial torsion (TFA).
- Examine for MA or other deformity.

The child may have a combination of any or all of the aforementioned problems.

Management
See the individual diagnoses for management strategies.

■ Other Common Musculoskeletal System Findings Needing Attention

TOE WALKING
Description
Most young children walk on their toes until they establish the heel-toe pattern, usually within the first 6 months of walking. Consistent toe walking is frequently associated with neurologic problems, such as cerebral palsy. Autistic children or those with early muscular dystrophy may toe walk. Children with tight heel cords may toe walk. Unilateral toe walking can be associated with a short leg, as found with a dislocated hip. Toe walking

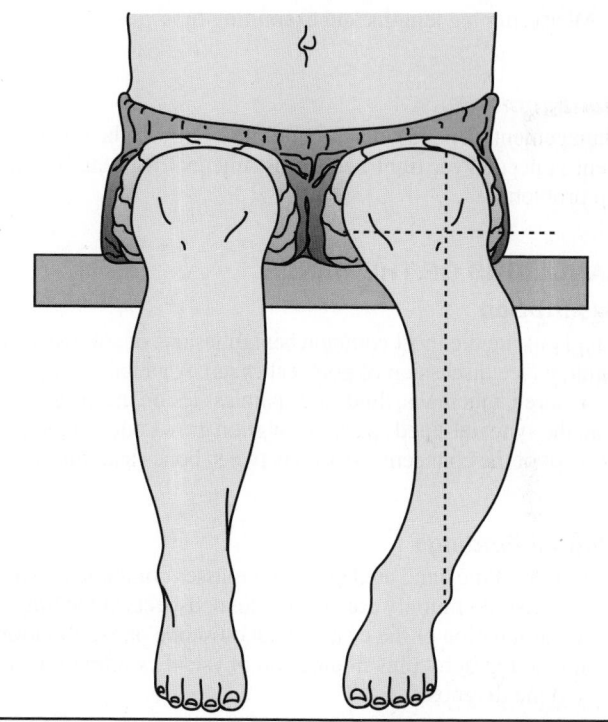

FIGURE 37-14 In-toeing from internal (medial) tibial torsion.

TABLE 37-4	Typical Cause of In-Toeing and Out-Toeing Rotational Problem		
Cause	**Possible Diagnoses**	**Typical Finding**	**Age at Manifestation**
In-toeing	Equinovarus	Plantar foot flexion, forefoot adduction, and hindfoot varus	At birth
	Metatarsal adductus	Curved foot—refer if not flexible	Birth-6 months
	Abducted great toe	Searching toe—resolves spontaneously	Toddler period
	Medial tibial torsion	Refer if thigh-foot angle (TFA) more than −10 to −20 degrees	12-18 months
	Internal femoral torsion	Refer if >70 degrees medial and <10 degrees lateral hip rotation	2-5 years
Out-toeing	Physiologic infantile out-toeing	Feet may turn out when infant is positioned upright— resolves spontaneously	Early infancy
	Lateral tibial torsion	Refer if TFA >+30 degrees	Late childhood
	Lateral femoral torsion	Refer if >2 SD of the mean	Late childhood

SD, Standard deviation.

also can be a habit, especially in children who used walkers. In these children, toe walking generally resolves before 3 years old and is not associated with any musculoskeletal deformity. It is important to differentiate between the idiopathic toe walker and the child who toe walks because of a neuromusculoskeletal condition associated with tight heel cords and contractures.

Clinical Findings

History. The provider should assess:
- Onset
- Severity
- Neurologic history
- Use of a walker

Physical Examination. The examination should include:
- Looking at shoe wear to assess extent of toe walking. For example, is the heel worn?
- Assessing for tight heel cords. The foot should be brought beyond a 90-degree angle.
- Conducting a neurologic assessment
- Measuring leg lengths and examining hips

Management

Management depends on the etiology. Orthopedic management is needed for tight heel cords, unequal leg lengths, and hip problems.

GANGLIONS OF THE HANDS

Description

Ganglions are the most common benign lesions of soft tissue in children (see discussion of popliteal cysts). A ganglionic cyst is an acquired, mucinous, fluid-filled painless lesion that originates from the synovial-lined space. A ganglion grows out of a joint. It rises out of the connective tissues between bones and muscles.

Clinical Findings

Ganglions of the hand are hard, fixed masses commonly found on the wrist (commonly dorsal) and flexor aspects of the finger. Transillumination of the cyst with an otoscope or examination by ultrasonography plus findings on physical examination are keys to the diagnosis.

Management

Ganglionic cysts in children are rarely symptomatic and usually regress spontaneously. The likelihood of recurrence with any form of treatment is higher in children than the recurrence rate in adults with such lesions. Conservative care with rest and splinting can be tried. If conservative care fails to result in partial or complete resolution, refer for needle aspiration or surgical excision (the most reliable method to eliminate a ganglion because the tract that extends into the joint is removed). Steroid injections are not advised.

LEG ACHES OF CHILDHOOD

Description

Extremity pain, often referred to as "growing pains" by the layperson, is a frequent clinical presentation. The pain is usually nonarticular; in two thirds of children it is described as

being located in the shins, calves, thighs, or popliteal fossa. It is almost always bilateral. The pain appears late in the day or is nocturnal, often awaking the child. The pain can last from minutes to hours. By morning the child is almost always pain-free. Because it occurs late in the day and is often reported on days of increased activity, it may represent a local overuse syndrome, and may be associated with decreased bone strength. Leg aches of childhood are generally not associated with serious organic disease, and usually resolve by late childhood; 15% of school-age children have occasional limb pain (Uziel and Hashkes, 2007). However, it is important to differentiate these pains from more serious pathologic conditions.

Clinical Findings

History. Pain or leg aches are typically described as:
- Occurring characteristically in the evening or late in the day; may wake child up from sleep
- Pain gone in the morning with no limitation of activity
- Poorly localized and bilateral
- Occurring commonly in the front of the thighs, in the calves, and behind the knees
- Transient and occurring over a period of time as long as several years
- Not associated with a limp or disability (Uziel and Hashkes, 2007)
- No reported fevers or swelling

Physical Examination
- Have the child stand on tiptoes and heels.
- Measure leg lengths.
- Evaluate range of motion.
- Assess for swelling, erythema and tenderness.
- Observe for limping.

Findings include normal physical examination with no tenderness, guarding, or reduced range of joint motion.

Diagnostic Studies. There is no single diagnostic test. It is a diagnosis of exclusion.

Differential Diagnosis

Neoplastic lesions, leukemia, sickle cell anemia, juvenile arthritis, and subacute osteomyelitis must be ruled out (Owens, 2007).

Management

Reassure the parents that these are common complaints that are benign and generally resolve spontaneously. Symptomatic treatment with heat and analgesic may be of benefit. Stress the need for parents to bring the child in for reevaluation if there is a change in symptoms or other signs emerge. Refer a child if the pain is localized to one region, is associated with swelling or other constitutional symptoms, is increasing in severity, or alters gait.

LIMPS

Description

Deviations from normal age-appropriate gait pattern can be caused by a wide variety of conditions. A limp is usually mild and self-limited and caused by contusion, strain, or sprain. In some cases the cause can be a sign of a serious inflammatory or infectious process. The incidence is unknown (Sawyer and Kapoor, 2009). Age is an important factor in diagnosing the many causes of limping. Table 37-5 describes the various types of limps commonly seen in children.

Clinical Findings

History. A careful history is needed, including:
- Presence of pain
- History of trauma, past medical history
- Presence of fever, night sweats
- Weight loss or anorexia
- Type of limp
- Interference with activities
- Review of systems

Physical Examination
- Child should be unclothed during examination.
- Observe for areas of erythema, swelling, and deformity.
- Identify limp type: Have the child walk and run while distracted.
- Observe each limb segment.
- Stance and swing phase should be compared in both legs.
- Range of motion of each joint should be evaluated, especially the hip.
- Complete a neurologic examination, including strength, reflexes, balance, and coordination.
- Assess Trendelenburg sign for hip stability.

Diagnostic Studies. A CBC with differential and measurement of ESR and CRP levels should be obtained to rule out infection, inflammatory arthritis, or malignancy. Imaging should include radiographs of the area of concern. When imaging the hip, frog-leg lateral views should be obtained. Ultrasound may be used to detect effusion of the hip joint. If radiographs and ultrasound are positive a CT may be indicated.

Differential Diagnosis

Fracture, DDH, LCPD, SCFE, tumor, infection, juvenile arthritis, and others should be considered (Table 37-6).

Management

Refer the patient to an orthopedist immediately unless the etiology is a mild strain or a local lesion that can be managed conservatively by the primary care provider.

OVERUSE SYNDROMES OF CHILDHOOD AND ADOLESCENCE

Description

Overuse injuries, overtraining, and burnout among child and adolescent athletes are a growing problem. It is estimated that 30 to 45 million children and youth, ages 6 to 18 years of age, participate is some form of athletic activity (Brenner and Council of Sports Medicine and Fitness, 2007). An overuse injury is microtraumatic damage to a bone, muscle, or tendon that has been subjected to repetitive stress without sufficient time to heal or undergo the natural reparative process. The risk of overuse injuries is more serious in the pediatric population because the growing bones cannot handle as much stress as the mature adult bone. Typical overuse injuries of childhood are varus overload of the elbow ("Little League elbow"), OSD, proximal humeral epiphysiolysis ("Little League shoulder"), patellofemoral pain syndrome, shin splints, and stress fractures (Table 37-7).

Clinical Findings

History. In-depth history about the sport played and hours played per week, including games and practice, needs to be determined. What makes the pain better or worse?

Overuse injuries can be classified into four stages (Brenner and Council of Sports Medicine and Fitness, 2007):
- Pain in the affected area after physical activity
- Pain during the activity, without restricting performance
- Pain during the activity that restricts activity
- Chronic, unremitting pain even at rest

Physical Examination. The examination is dependent on the joint or limb involved. Check for deformity, warmth, swelling, range of motion, and ecchymosis. Observe for guarding of an extremity or limping.

TABLE 37-5	Types of Limp			
Type of Limp	**Cause**	**Characteristics**	**Examples**	
Antalgic	Pain: typically due to infection, fracture, or trauma	Walking on a painful extremity results in an attempt to get weight quickly off affected side; gait has shortened stance phase*	Sore knee: walks with fixed knee. Sore toe: tries not to roll off toe at toe-off phase of the stride. Appendicitis causes slight slumping posture and shortened stride on the right side due to psoas muscle irritation.	
Trendelenburg gait/ abductor lurch	Hip problems: typically developmental, congenital, or muscular disorders	Tilts over affected hip to decrease mechanical stresses; unaffected leg is off the ground during swing-through phase of gait	Hip dysplasia	
Equinus/toe-to-heel gait	Neurologic incoordination	Unsteady, wide-based gait	Cerebral palsy: toe-to-heel sequence to gait during stance phase due to heel-cord contractures	
Circumduction	Functionally longer leg; knee or ankle stiffness	Longer leg progresses forward in swing motion	Leg length inequality/knee injury with hyperextension/ankle problems	

*Stance phase: represents 60% of the gait cycle; swing about 40%.

TABLE 37-6 Differential Diagnosis of Limping

Condition	Age	Pain ±	Historical Findings	Clinical Findings	Causative Factors	Management
Developmental dysplasia of the hip	I, T, C, A	−	Breech delivery; metatarsus adductus; torticollis; poor treatment outcomes if not diagnosed at birth or shortly thereafter	Limited abduction; Trendelenburg; radiography at 2-3 mo; shortening of leg; acetabular dysplasia	Familial; joint laxity, positioning, maternal hormones	Newborn: no triple diapers; Pavlik harness to hold hips in flexion—see weekly; after 6 mo, traction or open reduction; after 18 mo old, osteotomy
Leg length inequality	T, C, A	−	None	Circumduction gait; joint contracture; >1 cm discrepancy in leg lengths	Congenital; neurogenic; vascular; tumor; trauma; infection	Shoe lifts; epiphysiodesis (fusion of growth plate to arrest growth of the opposite side), if discrepancy 2-6 cm
Neuromuscular (NM) disease	T, C, A	−	Depends on cause	Depends on cause; equinus or abductor gait	Cerebral palsy, muscular dystrophy, and other NM diseases	Referral to appropriate specialists
Diskitis	T, C, A	+	Varied: fever, malaise, unwilling to walk, backache	Stiff back, ↑ ESR; positive x-ray 2-3 wk—narrow disk space, irregular vertebral body endplate; bone scan, CT, MRI show early findings early bone scan has typical findings	Bacterial infection in disk space (*Staphylococcus aureus*) or inflammatory response	Immobilization and antistaphylococcal antibiotic therapy
Septic arthritis	T, C, A	++	Moderate to high fever, malaise, arthralgias; irritability; progressive course	Redness, warmth and swelling of joint—knee or hip; limited hip motion; ESR >25 mm/hr	*S. aureus* likely organism	Appropriate antibiotic coverage (7 days, IV; 3-4 wk total)
Acute hematogenous osteomyelitis	T, C, A	+	Varied: malaise, low-grade to high fever; may have severe constitutional symptoms; toxicity	Refusal to walk or move limb; point tenderness; limp; 7-10 days to see radiographic bony changes; 25% ↑WBCs; ↑CRP	*S. aureus* likely organism	Appropriate antibiotic coverage (generally 7 days, IV; 4-6 wk total or until ESR normal)
Neoplasm	T, C, A	+	Depends on type of neoplasm	Varied	Neoplasm—benign or malignant	Referral to oncologist
Trauma	T, C, A	+	Depends on type (fractures, strains, sprains)	Varied	Varied	Rule out physical abuse if discrepancy related to developmental capabilities, injury history, and type of injury
Occult trauma: toddler fracture	T	+	Well child	Commonly radiograph shows spiral fracture of tibia; refusal to walk, mild soft tissue swelling	Trauma	See trauma above
Transient synovitis	3-8 yr	+	Mild to moderate fever, mild irritability; resolves within 1 wk	Limited hip motion; ESR <25 mm/hr	Inflammatory reaction; unknown etiology; often URI (50%) prior	Rest
Juvenile arthritis (JA)	Childhood until 16 yr	+	Fever, rashes, ↑ WBCs; some iritis; joint stiffness and swelling; S&S >3 mo	Mono-/polyarticular arthropathy; + ANA (25%- 88%); ↑ ESR in moderate/severe JA	Unknown; genetic (HLA) or environmental	Treat with NSAIDs initially; may need sulfasalazine, methotrexate; corticosteroids; joint replacements when older

TABLE 37-6 Differential Diagnosis of Limping—cont'd

Condition	Age	Pain ±	Historical Findings	Clinical Findings	Causative Factors	Management
Slipped capital femoral epiphysis	9-15 yr	+	>90th percentile weight; African-American; male	Limited abduction and extension; external rotation of thigh if hip flexed	Multifactorial: mechanical; endocrine; trauma; familial	Needs immediate surgery; non–weight-bearing crutches until admitted; bilateral involvement does occur
Legg-Calvé-Perthes disease	4-8 yr	+	Acute or chronic onset; pain in hip, groin, knee; stiffness; male	+ Trendelenburg, shortening; ↓ abduction, internal rotation, hip extension; + radiographs but not early	Familial; breech birth; prior trauma (17%)	In female tends to be more serious problem; bed rest, traction, then PT; bracing and surgery may be needed; bilateral involvement does occur

A, Adolescent (≥11 yr); *ANA,* antinuclear antibody; *C,* child (4-10 yr); *CRP,* C-reactive protein; *CT,* computed tomography; *ESR,* erythrocyte sedimentation rate; *HLA,* human leukocyte antigen; *I,* infant (newborn to 12 mo); *IV,* intravenous; *JA,* juvenile arthritis; *MRI,* magnetic resonance imaging; *NSAIDs,* nonsteroidal antiinflammatory drugs; *PT,* physical therapy; *S&S,* signs and symptoms; *T,* toddler (1-3 yr); *URI,* upper respiratory infection; *WBC,* white blood cell.

TABLE 37-7 Overuse Injuries of Childhood: Characteristic Features and Their Treatment

Condition	Clinical Findings	Treatment	Comments
Osgood-Schlatter disease	Swelling and tenderness/pain over tibial tubercle	NSAIDs, kneepad, knee immobilizer if severe pain for 1-2 weeks	Most resolve with time (12-18 months); x-ray only if pain persists (shows soft tissue swelling and possible residual ossicle); if pain persists, consider surgical incision of ossicle
Patellofemoral pain syndrome	Anterior knee pain	Rest, NSAIDs, retraining, and strengthening of quadriceps muscles	Arthroscopic surgery only if recurring problems
Proximal humeral epiphysiolysis ("Little League shoulder")	Shoulder pain—gradual onset; pain ↑ with throwing, especially curve ball	Modify activity; gradual restart, but limit intensity and frequency of throwing with retraining and muscle strengthening	Seen in skeletally immature children; radiographs show widening proximal humeral physis
Shin splints	Pain along medial border of tibia; child has a history of prolonged running	NSAIDs; ice after running; retraining and muscle strengthening after inflammation ↓; gradual return to running	Associated with poor running technique, hard running surface, muscle weakness; inadequate running shoes; sudden increase in running; is an inflammatory response; may need to consider exertional compartment syndrome (see Chapter 39)
Stress fractures	Tenderness and swelling at site	Reduce or eliminate activity that caused injury for 10-14 days; may need to cast	Caused by microtrauma; most commonly seen in active teens, but can occur during childhood; proximal tibia most common site
Varus overload of the elbow ("Little League elbow")	Elbow pain with activity; locking and ↓ extension of elbow; medial humeral epicondyle tenderness	Rest; NSAIDs; ice; when pain-free, gradual return to activity with retraining; surgery if elbow instability	Leads to osteochondral lesions and stress fractures if severe; radiographs reveal widening proximal physis; also seen in gymnasts

NSAIDs, Nonsteroidal antiinflammatory drugs.

Differential Diagnosis

Depending on the presenting symptoms, a plain film, CT, MRI, or bone scan may be indicated.

Management

Most of the injuries can be managed conservatively with proper and timely diagnosis. Treatment often involves resting and icing the extremity or joint, doing retraining and strengthening exercises, gradually reintroducing activities, and using analgesics. NSAIDs help reduce the inflammatory component of the trauma. Patient and parent education is important to prevent further injury and disability and to allow the child to return to safe sport participation. If not managed properly and effectively, overuse injuries can affect normal physical growth and maturation (Brenner and Council of Sports Medicine and Fitness, 2007).

MUSCLE DISEASES

Description

The muscular dystrophies are a group of hereditary disorders of skeletal muscle that produces progressive degeneration of skeletal muscle leading to weakness. The muscular dystrophies are autosomal dominant, sex-linked, and can appear in several children in a family. The X-linked dystrophies are the most common with the most common dystrophy being Duchenne. The incidence of Duchenne is 1 in 3500 births with 70% having a family history of the disease (Canale and Beaty, 2007).

Clinical Findings

History.

- Disease becomes evident between 3 and 6 years of age.
- Family history of muscle disease
- Failure to achieve motor milestones, especially independent ambulation
- Toe walking
- Loss of motor skills, such as the ability to climb stairs easily
- Easy fatigue with physical activity
- A history of good days and bad days in relation to ability to accomplish physical activities
- Increasing difficulties with motor activities

Physical Examination

- Toe walking
- Large firm calf muscles
- Fibrotic or "doughy" feel to the muscles
- Widely based lordotic stance
- Waddling Trendelenburg gait
- Lower extremities show early weakness of gluteal muscle strength.
- Positive Gowers sign. Gowers sign is obtained by asking the child to get up off the floor without help. The sign is positive if the child uses his or her arms to push off from the legs, gradually standing in a segmented fashion.

Management

Referral is necessary. These conditions may need to be handled by an interdisciplinary team with orthopedic, metabolic, and physical therapy, social service, and nursing care. Genetics counseling may be necessary, depending on the diagnosis.

The use of prednisone and deflazacort has been shown to preserve or improve strength, but each has significant side effects, including weight gain, osteopenia, and myopathy. Between ages 8 and 14 years, children with Duchenne muscular dystrophy typically develop contractures of the lower extremity and may require early orthopedic treatment to prolong the child's ability to ambulate (Canale and Beaty, 2007).

Patient and family support is needed. Muscle diseases are chronic, debilitating, and sometimes fatal conditions. Helping the child to lead as normal a life as possible, while coping with his or her condition, is a major task.

Perinatal Disorders

NAN M. GAYLORD AND ROBERT J. YETMAN

The neonatal period is remarkable for the vast array of physiologic changes that occur as the infant transitions from the intrauterine to extrauterine life. This period is a highly vulnerable time for the infant. In the U.S., about two thirds of all deaths in the first year of life occur among infants less than 28 days old with the highest risk being in the first 24 hours of life (Stoll, 2007a). Because serious health problems can arise for the infant in the hours after the initial transition to extrauterine life, the primary care provider must be prepared to manage these problems while providing psychosocial support and education for the families. An understanding of the physiology of fetal development, risk factors for potential problems, and pertinent physical findings is necessary to effectively assist the newborn's transition to extrauterine life.

■ Standards of Care

The *Healthy People 2020* objectives (U.S. Department of Health and Human Services [USDHHS], 2010) related to maternal, infant, and child care are available online. The overall goal of these objectives is to improve maternal health and pregnancy outcomes and reduce rates of disability in infants, thereby improving the health and well-being of women, infants, children, and families in the U.S. Since its inception in 1979, the *Healthy People* program suggests that the health of a population is reflected in the health of its most vulnerable members. A major focus of many public health efforts, therefore, is improving the health of pregnant women and their infants, including reductions in the rate of birth defects, risk factors for infant death, and death of infants and their mothers. Included among these goals are improvements in the rates of breastfeeding, ensuring that all newborns are screened for state-mandated diseases, reducing the proportion of children with a metabolic disorder who experience developmental delay requiring special education services, and increasing the percentage of healthy full-term infants who are put down to sleep on their backs.

The *Guide to Clinical Preventive Services* (U.S. Preventive Services Task Force [USPSTF], 2009) recommends the following preventive services for neonates:

- Prenatal screening for Rh(D) incompatibility; human immunodeficiency virus (HIV); hepatitis B; syphilis; chlamydia and gonorrhea
- Promotion of breastfeeding

- Neonatal screening for sickle hemoglobinopathies to identify infants who may benefit from antibiotic prophylaxis to prevent sepsis
- Screening for congenital hypothyroidism for all newborns during the first 4 days of life
- Screening for phenylketonuria (PKU) for all newborns before discharge from the nursery. Infants who are tested before 24 hours old should receive a repeat screening test by 2 weeks old.
- Ocular antibiotic prophylaxis of all newborn infants to prevent gonococcal ophthalmia neonatorum
- Routine newborn hearing screening for all infants in the first month of life and an audiologic evaluation for hearing loss in the first 3 months of life

Bright Futures: Guidelines for Health Supervision of Infants, Children, and Adolescents (Hagan et al, 2008) and the American Academy of Pediatrics (AAP) Committee on Practice and Ambulatory Medicine (AAP, 2007) have detailed anticipatory guidelines for the newborn, first-week, and 1-month health supervision visits. *Guidelines for Perinatal Care* from the AAP and the American College of Obstetricians and Gynecologists (Lemnos and Lockwood, 2008) is another thorough compendium of standards of caring for the newborn.

■ Anatomy and Physiology

INTRAUTERINE-TO-EXTRAUTERINE TRANSITION

The infant's intrauterine-to-extrauterine transition requires an extraordinary number of biochemical and physiologic changes. In utero, the placenta provides metabolic functions for the fetus. Oxygenated blood from the placenta arrives to the fetus through the umbilical vein. Because of high pulmonary vascular pressure, this blood is shunted from the right to the left side of the fetus's heart through the foramen ovale or to the systemic circulation through the ductus arteriosus. At birth the umbilical cord is severed. Simultaneously, the infant begins to breathe and the high pulmonary vascular pressure drops, allowing blood flow to the lungs for oxygenation. The foramen ovale and ductus arteriosus are no longer necessary and close after birth. The newborn becomes dependent on gastrointestinal tract function to absorb nutrients, renal function to excrete wastes and maintain chemical balance, liver function to metabolize and excrete toxins, and the functions of the immunologic system to protect against infection. Many newborn problems are related to poor transition to extrauterine life as a result of asphyxia, premature birth, congenital anomalies, or adverse effects of delivery.

A predictable series of changes or reactivities in vital signs and clinical appearance take place after the delivery of most normal infants (Fig. 38-1). The first period of reactivity includes sympathetic system changes, such as tachycardia, rapid respirations, transient rales, grunting, flaring and retractions, a falling body temperature, hypertonus, and alerting exploratory behavior. Parasympathetic system changes during the first period of reactivity include the initiation of bowel sounds and the production of oral mucus. After an interval of sleep, the infant enters the second period of reactivity. During this time the oral mucus production again becomes evident, the heart rate becomes labile, the infant becomes more responsive to endogenous and exogenous stimuli, and meconium is often passed.

■ Pathophysiology

HIGH-RISK PREGNANCY

High-risk pregnancies are defined as those in which factors exist that increase the chances of abortion, fetal death, premature delivery, intrauterine growth retardation, fetal or neonatal disease, congenital malformations, mental retardation, and other handicaps. Identification of a high-risk pregnancy is the first step toward prevention of neonatal problems (Box 38-1). Comprehensive and frequent prenatal visits for women with high-risk pregnancies are aimed at preventing complications in the newborn.

ACQUIRED HEALTH PROBLEMS

In utero exposure to poor nutrition, alcohol, drugs, viruses or bacteria, and maternal conditions, such as hypertension and diabetes, can result in prematurity and abnormalities at birth. The risk of neonatal problems increases with maternal age younger than 20 years and older than 35 years (see Box 38-1).

GENETIC PROBLEMS

The presence of chromosomal abnormalities, congenital anomalies, inborn errors of metabolism, mental retardation, and familial diseases increases the risk of the same condition in the infant. Because many conditions are not easily identifiable on physical examination, exploring family histories to identify newborns at risk for any inheritable diseases is important. Anticipation of various inherited conditions leads to their early identification and management of potential problems.

PERINATAL COMPLICATIONS AND INJURIES

Perinatal complications occur immediately before or during birth. Prolonged or dysfunctional labor increases the risk of fetal distress. Prolonged rupture of the membranes and chorioamnionitis increase the risk of infant infection, and ruptured placenta previa increases the risk of infant blood loss. Cesarean deliveries, the use of forceps or vacuum extraction, and the type of maternal anesthesia used also pose risks. The term *birth injury* includes mechanical and anoxic trauma incurred by an infant during labor and delivery. Predisposing

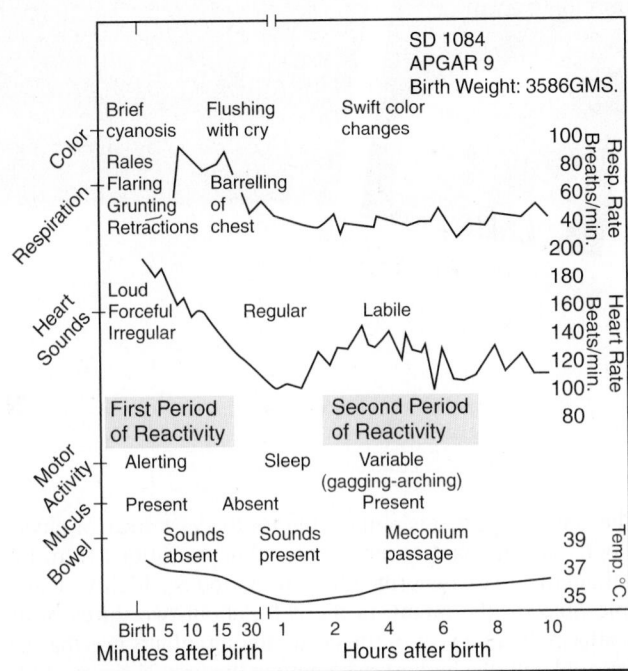

FIGURE 38-1 Summary of normal transition. (From Desmond MM, Rudolph AJ, Phitaksphraiwan P: The transitional care nursery, *Pediatr Clin North Am* 13:651-668, 1966.)

risk factors for birth injury include macrosomia, prematurity, cephalopelvic disproportion, dystocia, prolonged labor, and breech presentation. Birth injuries include caput succedaneum, cephalhematoma, subcutaneous fat necrosis of the face or scalp, fractures of the skull, subconjunctival and retinal hemorrhages, intracranial hemorrhage, peripheral nerve palsies (brachial, phrenic, facial), fractured clavicle or humerus, ruptured liver or spleen, and hypoxic-ischemic insults. Proper steps to monitor and treat an infant with perinatal complications and injuries must be undertaken immediately after birth. The provider must be familiar with perinatal conditions that subject the newborn to a higher risk and be prepared to intervene quickly based on the available perinatal information.

■ Assessment of the Neonate

HISTORY

- Past maternal health history
- Past obstetric history
  - Number of previous pregnancies; number of infants born alive or stillborn
  - Number of elective or spontaneous abortions; number of preterm and term deliveries
  - Cesarean deliveries and indications for them
  - Health status of living children; if deceased, age and cause of death
- Family history
  - Genetically acquired conditions, birth defects, mental retardation, or other diseases
  - Hypertension, hyperlipidemias, heart disease, or familial cancers
  - Age and health status of living relatives
  - Causes of death of family members

BOX 38-1 Factors Associated With High-Risk Pregnancies

Demographic Social Factors
Maternal age less than 20 years or greater than 35 years
African-American race
Developmentally delayed mother or low educational status
Illicit drug, alcohol, cigarette use
Poverty, unemployed, homelessness
Unmarried or lack of support
Emotional or physical stress including depression and other mental health problems
Poor access to or use of prenatal care, underinsured or uninsured

Medical History
Diabetes mellitus
Hypertension, maternal hypercoagulable state, sickle cell disease, congenital heart disease
Asymptomatic bacteriuria
Autoimmune disease including rheumatologic illness (SLE)
Chronic medication
Sexually transmitted infections (colonization: herpes simplex, GBS, syphilis, HIV)

Prior Pregnancy
Intrauterine fetal demise or neonatal death
Previous infertility
Prematurity or low-birthweight infant
Intrauterine growth retardation
Congenital malformation
Incompetent cervix
Blood group sensitization, neonatal jaundice
Neonatal thrombocytopenia
Hydrops
Inborn errors of metabolism

Present Pregnancy
Uterine bleeding (abruptio placentae, placenta previa)
Inception by reproductive technology
Poor weight gain or abnormal fetal growth
Multiple gestation, parity more than 5
Preeclampsia or eclampsia
Premature rupture of membranes
Short interpregnancy time
Polyhydramnios or oligohydramnios
High or low maternal serum alpha-fetoprotein

Labor and Delivery
Premature labor (<37 weeks) or prolonged labor
Postdates (>42 weeks) or prolonged gestation
Fetal distress
Immature L/S ratio: absent phosphatidylglycerol
Breech presentation
Meconium-stained fluid
Nuchal cord
Forceps or Cesarean delivery
Apgar score less than 4 at 1 minute

Neonate
Birthweight less than 2500 g or greater than 4000 g
Birth before 37 or after 42 weeks of gestation
Small or large for gestational age
Hypoglycemia
Tachypnea, cyanosis
Congenital malformation
Pallor, plethora, petechiae

GBS, Group B streptococcus; *HIV*, human immunodeficiency virus; *L/S*, lecithin-sphingomyelin ratio; *SLE*, systemic lupus erythematosus.
Adapted from Stoll BJ: High-risk pregnancies. In Kliegman RM, Behrman RE, Jenson HB et al, editors: *Nelson textbook of pediatrics*, ed 18, Philadelphia, 2007, Saunders, p 684.

- Current obstetric history
  - Present health and medical history including depression or other mental health conditions
  - Age of mother
  - Prenatal care—duration of
  - Medications used during pregnancy including prescription, over-the-counter, and natural health products
  - Use of pregnancy-enhancing drugs or technology
  - Infections (including group B streptococcus [GBS] status and results of other screening tests) and illnesses during pregnancy
  - Alcohol, cigarettes, or other drugs used during pregnancy
  - Hypertension or glucose intolerance
  - Duration of labor, duration of ruptured membranes, analgesia, anesthesia, presentation and route of delivery, use of forceps
  - Polyhydramnios (excessive fluid) or oligohydramnios (little to no fluid)
  - Infant meconium stained or amniotic fluid foul smelling
  - Fever
- Social history
  - Emotional stressors during pregnancy including homelessness
  - Unplanned or unwanted pregnancy
  - Financial and emotional support
  - Dietary considerations (e.g., strict vegan diet)
  - Educational background of parents
  - Father's anticipated involvement in raising infant
  - Age of other children in the home

PHYSICAL EXAMINATION
Immediately After Birth
Apgar Score. Immediate evaluation of the newborn infant at 1 and 5 minutes old can be a valuable routine procedure. An Apgar score is assigned to the baby based on the criteria in Table 38-1.
- Apgar score 8 to 10
  - Vigorous, pink, and crying
  - Requires only warming, drying, gentle stimulation
  - Occasionally requires oxygen for a short period
- Apgar score 5 to 7
  - Cyanotic
  - Slow, irregular respirations
  - Good muscle tone and reflexes
  - Responds to bag-and-mask ventilation
- Apgar score 4 or less
  - Limp, pale, or blue
  - Apneic, slow heart rate
  - Maximal resuscitative efforts with bag and mask, chest compressions, intravenous (IV) volume expansion, and drug therapy

TABLE 38-1	Apgar Scores		
	SCORE		
Sign	**0**	**1**	**2**
Heart rate (beats per minute)	Absent	Slow (<100)	>100
Respiratory effort	Absent	Weak cry; hypoventilation	Good; strong cry
Muscle tone	Limp	Some flexion of extremities	Well flexed
Reflex irritability (response of skin stimulation to feet)	No response	Some motion	Cry
Color	Blue; pale	Body pink; extremities blue	Completely pink

The 5-minute Apgar score is an indication of how well the resuscitation efforts have succeeded. Caution must be exercised when using the Apgar score to predict long-term outcomes of mortality and developmental delay. Only when combined with other factors, such as fetal status, umbilical cord or scalp blood pH, evidence of organ injury, or seizures, can the Apgar score be useful in determining long-term outcome (AAP, 2006). In actual practice, the decision to resuscitate an infant typically is based on a quick assessment of the heart rate, color, and respiratory rate rather than the full 1-minute Apgar score (Fig. 38-2).

Gestational Age. Maturational assessment of an infant's gestational age is based on the physical examination (Fig. 38-3). The assessment is done promptly after birth to confirm maternal estimated dates, and interpreted with information on the mother's menstrual history, obstetric milestones achieved during pregnancy, and prenatal ultrasonograms. An infant's length, weight, and fronto-occipital head circumference are measured and plotted on growth curves based on gestational age (Fig. 38-4). Infants whose weights fall above the 90th percentile for age are classified as large for gestational

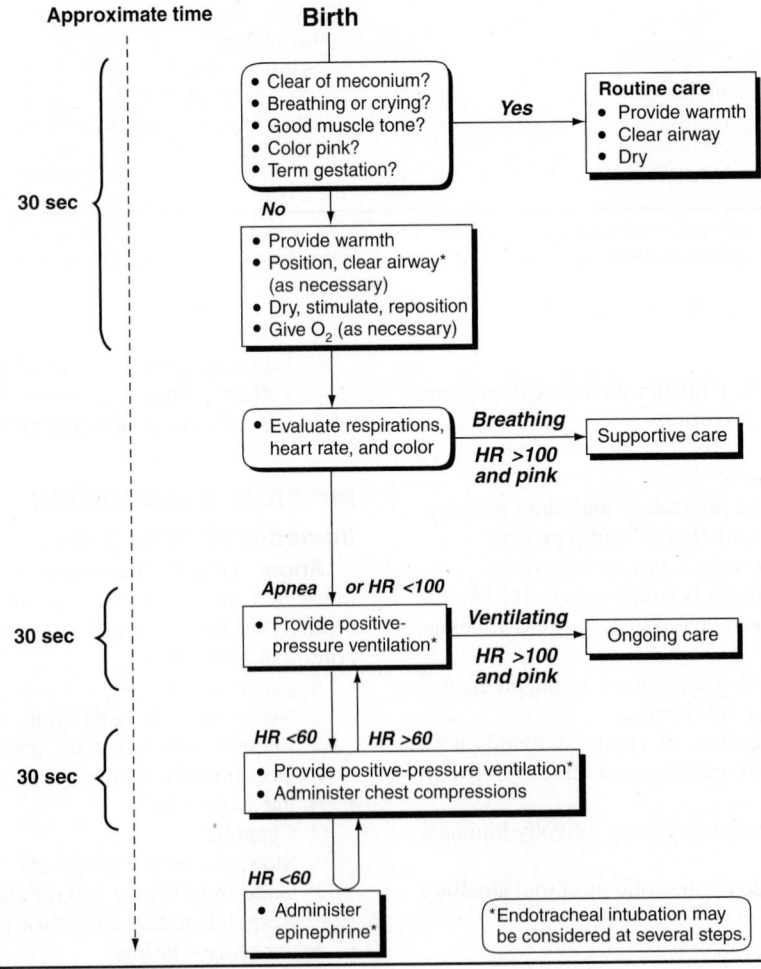

FIGURE 38-2 Resuscitation in the delivery room. (From Niermeyer S, Kattwinkel J, Van Reempts P: International guidelines for neonatal resuscitation: an excerpt from the Guidelines 2000 for Cardiopulmonary Resuscitation and Emergency Cardiovascular Care: International Consensus on Science, *Pediatrics* 106[3]:29, 2000.)

age (LGA); those whose measurements fall below the 10th percentile for age are classified as small for gestational age (SGA). Those whose measurements fall between the 10th and 90th percentiles are classified as appropriate for gestational age (AGA).

Temperature. Body surface area of the newborn infant relative to its weight is approximately three times that of the adult. Estimated rate of heat loss in the newborn is four times that of an adult (Stoll, 2007a). Body temperature falls precipitously in a cool environment unless adequate precautions are taken. Towel

MATURATIONAL ASSESSMENT OF GESTATIONAL AGE (New Ballard Score)

NAME _____ SEX _____

HOSPITAL NO. _____ BIRTH WEIGHT _____

RACE _____ LENGTH _____

DATE/TIME OF BIRTH _____ HEAD CIRC. _____

DATE/TIME OF EXAM _____ EXAMINER _____

AGE WHEN EXAMINED _____

APGAR SCORE: 1 MINUTE _____ 5 MINUTES _____ 10 MINUTES _____

NEUROMUSCULAR MATURITY

NEUROMUSCULAR MATURITY SIGN	SCORE -1	0	1	2	3	4	5	RECORD SCORE HERE
POSTURE								
SQUARE WINDOW (Wrist)	>90°	90°	60°	45°	30°	0°		
ARM RECOIL		180°	140°-180°	110°-140°	90°-110°	<90°		
POPLITEAL ANGLE	180°	160°	140°	120°	100°	90°	<90°	
SCARF SIGN								
HEEL TO EAR								

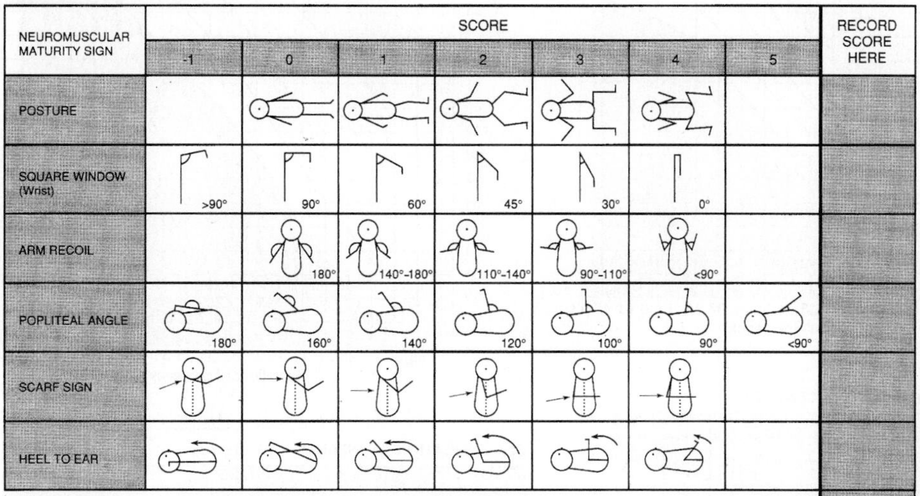

TOTAL NEUROMUSCULAR MATURITY SCORE

PHYSICAL MATURITY

PHYSICAL MATURITY SIGN	SCORE -1	0	1	2	3	4	5	RECORD SCORE HERE
SKIN	sticky friable transparent	gelatinous red translucent	smooth pink visible veins	superficial peeling &/or rash, few veins	cracking pale areas rare veins	parchment deep cracking no vessels	leathery cracked wrinkled	
LANUGO	none	sparse	abundant	thinning	bald areas	mostly bald		
PLANTAR SURFACE	heel-toe 40-50 mm:-1 <40 mm:-2	>50 mm no crease	faint red marks	anterior transverse crease only	creases ant. 2/3	creases over entire sole		
BREAST	imperceptible	barely perceptible	flat areola no bud	stippled areola 1-2 mm bud	raised areola 3-4 mm bud	full areola 5-10 mm bud		
EYE/EAR	lids fused loosely: -1 tightly: -2	lids open pinna flat stays folded	sl. curved pinna; soft; slow recoil	well-curved pinna; soft but ready recoil	formed & firm instant recoil	thick cartilage ear stiff		
GENITALS (Male)	scrotum flat, smooth	scrotum empty faint rugae	testes in upper canal rare rugae	testes descending few rugae	testes down good rugae	testes pendulous deep rugae		
GENITALS (Female)	clitoris prominent & labia flat	prominent clitoris & small labia minora	prominent clitoris & enlarging minora	majora & minora equally prominent	majora large minora small	majora cover clitoris & minora		

TOTAL PHYSICAL MATURITY SCORE

SCORE

Neuromuscular _____

Physical _____

Total _____

MATURITY RATING

score	weeks
-10	20
-5	22
0	24
5	26
10	28
15	30
20	32
25	34
30	36
35	38
40	40
45	42
50	44

GESTATIONAL AGE (weeks)

By dates _____

By ultrasound _____

By exam _____

Reference
Ballard JL, Khoury JC, Wedig K, et al: New Ballard Score, expanded to include extremely premature infants. *J Pediatr* 1991; 119:417-423. Reprinted by permission of Dr Ballard and Mosby-Year Book, Inc.

FIGURE 38-3 Classification of newborns by intrauterine growth and gestational age. (From Ballard JL, Khoury JC, Wedig K et al: New Ballard score, expanded to include extremely premature infants, *J Pediatr* 119: 417-423, 1991.)

CLASSIFICATION OF NEWBORNS (BOTH SEXES)
BY INTRAUTERINE GROWTH AND GESTATIONAL AGE [1,2]

NAME_____ DATE OF EXAM_____ LENGTH_____

HOSPITAL NO._____ SEX_____ HEAD CIRC._____

RACE_____ BIRTH WEIGHT_____ GESTATIONAL AGE_____

DATE OF BIRTH_____

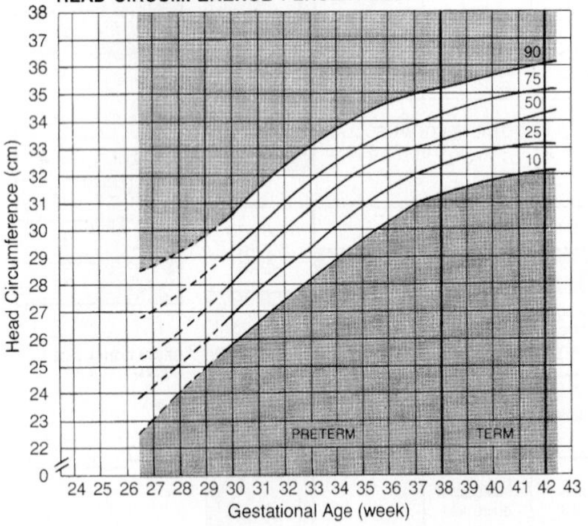

CLASSIFICATION OF INFANT*	Weight	Length	Head Circ.
Large for Gestational Age (LGA) (>90th percentile)			
Appropriate for Gestational Age (AGA) (10th to 90th percentile)			
Small for Gestational Age (SGA) (<10th percentile)			

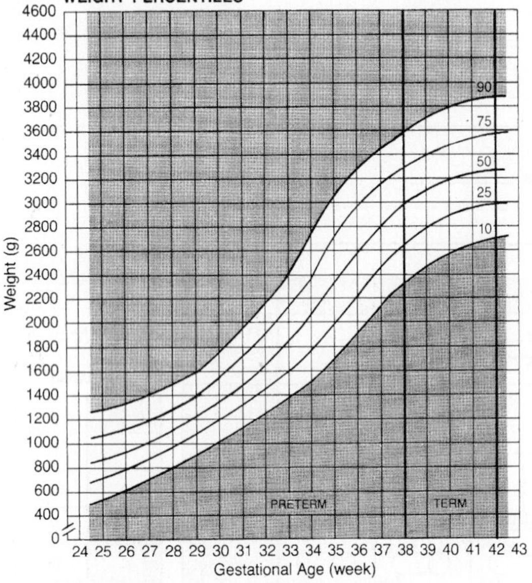

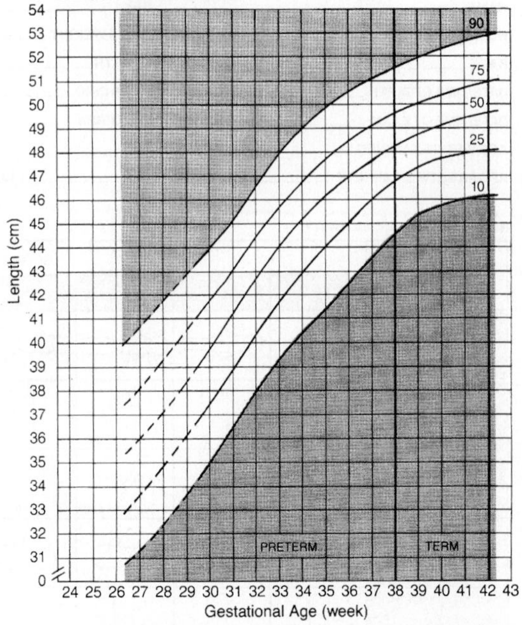

*Place an "X" in the appropriate box (LGA, AGA or SGA) for weight, for length and for head circumference.

References
1. Battaglia FC, Lubchenco LO: A practical classification of newborn infants by weight and gestational age. J Pediatr 1967; 71:159-163.
2. Lubchenco LO, Hansman C, Boyd E: Intrauterine growth in length and head circumference as estimated from live births at gestational ages from 26 to 42 weeks. Pediatrics 1966; 37:403-408.

Reprinted by permission from Dr Battaglia, Dr Lubchenco, Journal of Pediatrics and Pediatrics.

A service of **SIMILAC® WITH IRON** Infant Formula

The Ross Hospital Formula System

A5860(0.05)/JULY 1993

ROSS ROSS PRODUCTS DIVISION ABBOTT LABORATORIES COLUMBUS, OHIO 43215-1724

LITHO IN USA

FIGURE 38-4 Newborn maturity rating and classification. (From Ross Hospital Formula System, Ross Products Division, Abbott Laboratories, Columbus, OH; adapted from Battaglia FC, Lubchenco LO: A practical classification of newborn infants by weight and gestational age, J Pediatr 71:159-163, 1967; Lubchenco LO, Hansman C, Boyd E: Intrauterine growth in length and head circumference as estimated from live births at gestational ages from 26 to 42 weeks, Pediatrics 37:403-408, 1966.)

dry the infant after birth to prevent evaporative heat loss, use radiant warmer, and wrap infant in warm blankets and cover the head to reduce heat loss when the baby will be held by parents.

Lungs. During a vaginal delivery the squeezing action on an infant's chest as it passes through the pelvis and vagina assists in expulsion of amniotic fluid from the lungs. Further expulsion of amniotic fluid from the lungs and reversal of high pulmonary vascular resistance ensue with an infant's first large breaths. Careful bulb suctioning assists in clearing the amniotic fluid from the oropharynx. An infant born by cesarean delivery does not experience the squeezing action of a vaginal birth and is dependent on respiratory efforts and appropriate bulb suctioning to adequately clear the amniotic fluid. Auscultation of the newborn's lungs reveals bronchovesicular or bronchial breath sounds. Fine crackles can be present during the first few hours of life and is a variant of normal.

Umbilical Cord. The normal umbilical cord contains two thick-walled arteries and a single thin-walled vein. Vessel numbers other than this are abnormal and can be associated with congenital anomalies. The umbilical cord is clamped using sterile technique to prevent infection and bleeding.

After Stabilization

After a quick initial assessment in the delivery room to evaluate for obvious problems, a more complete physical examination is done (Table 38-2). When performing the physical examination, the infant's gestational age, age in hours, and stage of transition must be considered.

DIAGNOSTIC STUDIES

All states in the U.S. require screening of infants for a variety of congenital abnormalities, although the screening tests performed vary from state to state (see Chapter 40). Infants should be screened before they are discharged and before the seventh day of life; if initial screen was before 24 hours of life, rescreening should be done by 14 days old. Although most infants require no special screening tests, some are at risk for predictable complications in the newborn period. Infants born to mothers with poorly controlled diabetes and LGA or SGA infants are at higher risk for hypoglycemia and usually require serum glucose level screening. Similarly, infants demonstrating Coombs test positivity because of maternal-child blood incompatibility are screened for evidence of hemolysis. Some nurseries screen both mothers and infants for syphilis; mothers should be screened for HIV and hepatitis B unless done prenatally. Universal hearing screening is recommended by 1 month of age (see Chapter 29), and special attention is paid to any newborn at higher risk for hearing loss as a result of low birthweight, rubella or other infection, malformation, trauma, asphyxia, prematurity, intensive care unit stay, or antibiotic use.

◼ Management Strategies

INITIAL CARE

Following birth, newborns require special care and observation as they master the transition to the extrauterine environment. Additional components of care at this period include prophylaxis for eye infection with antibiotic ointment and vitamin K injection for hemorrhagic disease.

ESTABLISHING FEEDING

Regardless of the route of feeding the family has chosen, the provider must ensure that the infant and parents have well-established feeding patterns before discharge. Follow-up care is scheduled in 2 or 3 days to ensure adequate ongoing nutrition. See Chapters 10 and 11 for more detailed information on breastfeeding and formulas.

ANTICIPATORY GUIDANCE BEFORE DISCHARGE
Physical Care

Umbilical Cord. Applying alcohol to the base of the cord traditionally has been recommended to aid in cord separation, although the utility of this practice has been questioned, especially in industrialized areas; air-drying by tucking the diaper below the cord may be preferable (Lin et al, 2005; Zupan et al, 2004). After cord separation, which usually occurs at 10 to 14 days of life, a slight bloody discharge can be seen for 1 to 2 days. Bellybands or coins to cover the navel are avoided because these increase the chance of infection. If a foul-smelling discharge or erythema appears around the umbilicus, the infant should be evaluated immediately for sepsis. If a granuloma appears after the cord falls off, an application of silver nitrate helps to heal it.

Circumcision. Circumcision, the removal of the foreskin that normally covers the glans penis, is a controversial surgical procedure. The decision to circumcise is the parents' responsibility, although the provider can supply factual information on the risks and potential benefits of the procedure.

Proponents of circumcision claim that it keeps the glans cleaner; the chance for developing urinary tract infections is reduced (although the chance of urinary tract infections in uncircumcised males is only 1%); it reduces the incidence of penile cancer, phimosis, balanitis, adhesions, and occlusion of the urethral meatus; and the boy may look more like his peers. The opponents of circumcision claim that it does not prevent sexually transmitted infection; that good hygiene prevents penile cancer; that circumcision leaves the glans open to the chance of cautery burns and meatal stenosis; and that because fewer boys are being circumcised, these boys will not be different from many of their peers. In 2012 the American Academy of Pediatrics (American Academy of Pediatrics: Circumcision policy statement, *Pediatrics* 130(3):585-586, 2012.) issued a policy statement on circumcision stating that there is no evidence for routine circumcision, but that the benefits of the procedure are greater than its risks. Additionally, this statement advocates for circumcision access for all families desiring the procedure.

Contraindications to circumcision include epispadias or hypospadias, ambiguous genitalia, exstrophy of the bladder, familial bleeding disorders, and illness. Complications of circumcisions include infections, bleeding, gangrene, scarring, meatal stenosis, cautery burns, urethral fistula, amputation or trauma to the glans, and pain. For infants who undergo circumcision, procedural anesthesia is recommended. A variety of anesthesia techniques are available, including application of topical anesthetics (eutectic mixture of local anesthetics [EMLA] cream), dorsal penile nerve block, and subcutaneous ring block. Postoperative pain relief measures in the form of sucrose on a pacifier, acetaminophen, soft music, and physiologic positioning of the infant in a padded environment are helpful (Brady-Fryer et al, 2004).

Care of the uncircumcised baby includes gentle cleaning around the genital area. The skin normally adheres to the penis

TABLE 38-2	Physical Examination Findings

System	Findings
Vital signs and measurement	Check vital signs frequently in the first hours after birth, then every 6-8 hr when stable. Evaluate ability to maintain temperature (97.7° to 99.3 ° F [36.5° to 37.4° C]) in open crib after transition to extrauterine environment. *Failure to maintain temperature* requires evaluation for other problems, particularly sepsis. Respirations should remain between 30 and 60 breaths/min. Heart rate should remain between 100 and 160 bpm. Significant molding of the head requires repeated measurements to verify size. Daily weight losses of up to 10% in the first 2-3 days of life are not abnormal because normal infants excrete a large amount of water in the first days of life. *Weight loss of greater than 10%* is unexpected and is often due to poor intake or excessive losses.
Skin	*Lanugo and vernix.* Lanugo is fine dark hair, prominent over the trunk and shoulders. It is seen in infants born prematurely, becoming less prominent as the gestation approaches term. Thick, greasy, white vernix is more common on prematurely born infants' skin. *Dry and cracked skin.* This is normal over the first several days of life. If associated with thin subcutaneous fat (parchment-like), it is suggestive of a postmature infant, fetal growth retardation, or both. *Cyanosis.* Acrocyanosis, bluish changes in the color of the hands and feet, and generalized mottling of the skin are frequently noted in the first several days of life when an infant loses body heat. Central cyanosis beyond the first few moments of life is abnormal and can represent a significant problem with oxygenation. *Pallor.* Many perinatal events can result in pallor, indicating a significant disruption of the infant's circulatory system. Specific causes include anemia, sepsis, cold stress, hypoglycemia, and seizures. *Plethora.* An excessively reddish discoloration to the skin can be caused by polycythemia or hyperthermia. Infants born to diabetic mothers can be plethoric. *Meconium staining.* Antenatal stress can cause the first stool to pass in utero. If this greenish black meconium remains in the amniotic fluid for a prolonged period, staining of the infant's skin and fingernails results. *Jaundice.* See the discussion of jaundice in the text under Hematologic Conditions.
Head	*Sutures and molding.* Vaginally delivered infants demonstrate some degree of molding, usually elongation of the anteroposterior diameter of the skull; if delivered by cesarean method, there are minimal alterations to the shape of the head. *Fontanelles.* The anterior fontanelle is usually about 2-3 cm in diameter; the posterior fontanelle is about 1 cm in diameter. Both are usually slightly depressed (see Fig. 38-5).
Face	Symmetric structures of the face should be apparent, although unilateral facial edema as a result of delivery conditions can occur normally. Overall view of the face may reveal maxillary or mandibular hypoplasia, distortion, or hemifacial hypoplasia.
Eyes	Too small or large, too widely spaced, or abnormal upward or downward slanting of palpebral fissures should alert the practitioner to potential congenital problems. *Uncoordinated eye movements.* Intermittent uncoordinated eye movements (disconjugate gaze) during the first weeks after birth are common, improving by 2-4 months old and resolving by 6 months old. *Fixed disconjugate gaze* is abnormal, even in the neonate. *Conjunctivae.* Reddening in the first 24-48 hours of life caused by chemical irritation of the eyes from silver nitrate drops or erythromycin ointment is normal. *Purulent discharge* in the first days or weeks of life can be associated with gonococcus, chlamydia, or herpes. Conjunctival hemorrhages secondary to delivery resolve spontaneously over the first weeks of life. *Sclerae.* Yellowing is associated with hyperbilirubinemia. Small hemorrhages secondary to delivery resolve spontaneously over the first weeks of life. Thinning of the sclera, common in African-Americans, is manifested by dark blue or black patches. Blue sclerae are associated with osteogenesis imperfecta. *Red reflex.* Shining an ophthalmoscope's white light through the pupil reveals the "red reflex," a disk ranging from pearly gray to orange. *Absence of a red reflex* may indicate the presence of lens opacities secondary to cataracts, congenital infection (rubella), or calcium metabolism abnormality. A *white reflex* can indicate retinoblastoma. Absence of the expected red reflex indicates the need for an immediate ophthalmologic evaluation.
Ears	Identify normalcy in the size, rotation, shape, position, and patency of the external auditory canal. Presence of low-set ears should prompt careful examination for other dysmorphic features. Abnormalities in shape require thorough physical examination, especially of the genitourinary system. Assessment of hearing is done by noting a startle response to a loud noise, avoiding any tactile sensations, such as a wind current on the face as a result of clapping near the ear. Auditory brain response testing should be ordered for any infant in whom a question of hearing exists. Screening for universal detection of infants with hearing loss is recommended and is especially important for high-risk infants (e.g., family history, in utero infection, craniofacial anomalies, syndromes associated with hearing loss). Preauricular skin tags or significant pits should be noted (can be a genetic red flag). See text section on skin dimpling.
Nose	Patency of the nasal passages can be tested by closing the mouth and one nostril at a time or by passing a small catheter into the nasopharynx to see if the passage is clear. Nasal flaring is a sign of respiratory distress that can be caused by any number of abnormalities, including mechanical obstruction, parenchymal lung disease, or acidosis.

TABLE 38-2	Physical Examination Findings—cont'd
System	**Findings**
Mouth	*Size and symmetry of the lips* • Thin lips with a smooth philtrum (the area between lips and nose) are associated with fetal alcohol syndrome. • Asymmetric movements while crying can be due to nerve palsies or absence of perioral muscles. Cleft lip and palate can be associated with midline CNS abnormalities. Incomplete cleft palates are recognized by digital examination of the mouth for bony defects of the hard palate in the presence of normal palatal mucosa. Excessive salivation can be related to reflux of gastric contents or esophageal atresia. Epstein pearls are small white epithelial inclusion cysts on the palate and gums. An excessively large tongue can be associated with genetic or metabolic abnormalities, such as hypothyroidism or Down syndrome. Natal teeth are sometimes seen at birth (approximately 1 in 3000 live births). If they are extremely loose, aspiration is a concern. Consultation with a pediatric dentist is indicated.
Neck	Short neck indicates the possibility of Klippel-Feil syndrome or other vertebral problems. *Webbing.* Redundant skin is seen in trisomy 21, Turner syndrome, and Noonan syndrome. *Masses* • Thyroglossal duct cysts (midline) or branchial cleft cyst (along the edge of the sternocleidomastoid muscles) can be found. • Other masses that can be seen include a hematoma in the sternocleidomastoid muscle, cystic hygromas, and, rarely, goiters. *Torticollis.* Asymmetric shortening of the sternocleidomastoid muscle results in preferential turning of the head to one side, not to be confused with irritability of neck movement associated with meningitis or subarachnoid hemorrhage. Hematoma of the sternocleidomastoid muscle can result in the development of torticollis and requires early management.
Thorax	*Shape, symmetry.* Rounded appearance measuring about 2 cm less than the fronto-occipital head circumference (approximately 33 cm): • *Minimization of rounding* occurs with RDS, atelectasis, and other diseases of decreased expansion of the chest. • Accentuation is seen in meconium aspiration. Wide-spaced nipples and a shieldlike appearance are characteristic of Turner syndrome. Chest movement on inspiration should be symmetric and unlabored. Movement of the abdomen with respirations is normal. *Asymmetric movement* occurs with unilateral pneumothorax. *Intercostal, subcostal, or supracostal retractions* indicate respiratory distress. *Clavicles.* Vaginally delivered LGA babies are especially prone to fractures of the clavicle (see perinatal injury section in text). *Breast bones.* Pectus excavatum (concave chest) and pectus carinatum (pigeon chest) are occasionally seen. If severe both can lead to restrictive lung disease later in life. *Nipples* • Fullness and sometimes secretion of a white milky substance are normal and are secondary to maternal hormonal stimulation. • Supernumerary and inverted nipples are not uncommon. • Redness surrounding the nipple, especially with purulent drainage, occurs in neonatal mastitis.
Lung	*General.* Coughing, retractions, and an intermittently increased respiratory rate occur immediately after birth, resolving by about 12 hours of life to smooth and unlabored respirations at a rate of 30 to 60 breaths/min. *Respiratory distress.* Tachypnea, apnea (pauses in respiration >15 seconds), *grunting* (an infant's attempt to increase functional residual capacity, thereby improving gas exchange), *interclavicular, subclavicular, or supraclavicular retractions, nasal flaring,* and *central cyanosis* all indicate distress. *Auscultation* • Rales or crackles are commonly heard immediately after birth as lung fluid is resorbed. Beyond the immediate postpartum period, rales can indicate pneumonia, delayed resorption of lung fluid, meconium aspiration, or pulmonary edema. • *Unilateral absence of breath sounds* occurs in pneumothorax, atelectasis, and pleural effusion. • *Bowel sounds over the chest,* especially with a scaphoid abdomen and significant respiratory distress, indicate a diaphragmatic hernia with displacement of abdominal contents into the chest.
Heart	*Inspection.* Observe neonate for adequacy of perfusion. Respiratory distress is common with cardiac abnormalities. Edema as a result of cardiac failure is rarely seen in the newborn. *Palpation* • *Point of maximal impulse is displaced* from the fourth left intercostal space with pneumothorax, situs inversus, or dextrocardia. • *Thrills or heaves* are associated with murmurs and cardiac abnormalities. *Auscultation.* Heart rate is normally 100 to 160 bpm. Detection of skipped beats warrants electrocardiogram. *Heart sounds may be muffled or displaced* in the infant with a pneumothorax. *Murmurs.* Common in the newborn period, many murmurs disappear after a few hours or a few days. Significant murmurs should be investigated. *Pulses.* Brachial or radial pulses are compared with femoral or dorsalis pedis pulses for symmetry of impulse and strength in pulse. Delay or relative weakness of lower extremity pulses occurs in coarctation of the aorta. *Blood pressure.* By Doppler device using a 2.5-4 cm wide and 5-9 cm long cuff, compare with normals for age and gestation. Systolic blood pressures greater than 96 mm Hg are considered significant hypertension in the newborn, and systolic blood pressures exceeding 106 mm Hg are considered severe hypertension.

Continued

TABLE 38-2	Physical Examination Findings—cont'd
System	**Findings**
Abdomen	*General* • Normal abdomen is slightly protuberant, is soft, moves smoothly with respirations, and has fine bowel sounds scattered throughout. *Absent bowel sounds* can indicate ileus. • The liver is usually palpated 1-2 cm below the right costal margin; the spleen tip is sometimes felt at the left costal margin; kidneys, deep within lateral aspects of the abdomen measuring 3-4 cm in size, may be palpated. • Pain is indicated by crying, grimacing, or forceful resistance with palpation. *Umbilical hernias.* Midline outpouching from the sternum to the umbilicus is seen with weak abdominal musculature (diastasis recti); a large and protuberant umbilicus occurs with an umbilical hernia. *Umbilical vessels.* The normal cord contains two arteries and a single vein. Absence of the second artery can be associated with congenital abnormalities. *Vomiting and abdominal distention.* Regurgitation of large volumes of feeding is not expected. • *Bilious vomiting* is always abnormal and usually a sign of obstruction. • *Abdominal distention* with enlargement of any of the organs of the abdomen or failure to pass stool is abnormal. • Meconium ileus with failure to pass stool in the first 24-48 hours of life is associated with cystic fibrosis.
Genitalia	*Male* • The penis should have the urethral opening at the tip of the phallus with completely developed foreskin. Chordee means that the distal end of the penis is bent. • Testes not located in the scrotal sac or inguinal canal but retrievable to the scrotum are normal. Testes not located in or relocated in the scrotal sac from the canal are considered to be undescended. • Hydrocele is identified by transilluminating fluid collection around the testis and is regarded as normal unless it is associated with inguinal hernia or it lasts more than 12 months. • Inguinal hernia with displacement of intestines into the scrotal sac is frequently nontransilluminating and is associated with bowel sounds. Inguinal hernias are sometimes apparent and reduced at other times. A surgical consultation is indicated. *Female* • Labia majora are large and completely surround the labia minora. • Labia and vagina should be open, often with a white discharge. • Blood-tinged fluid in small amounts by day 2-3 is normal. *Ambiguous genitalia* are genitalia that do not appear to be completely masculinized or feminized. An endocrine referral is essential. *Anus and rectum.* Patency of the rectum and placement of the anus should be noted. A small amount of blood streaking in the diaper, especially with a small anal fissure, is common.
Extremities, back, hip	*Molding.* Intrauterine constraint and resultant molding cause mild curvatures of the forefeet (metatarsus adductus vs. varus [in-toeing or out-toeing]) or the tibia (genu varum [bowleg], genu valgum [knock-knee]), or both. See Chapter 37 for more information. *Contractures of the joints and molding of the bones* occur if amniotic fluid was decreased and is abnormal. *Fractures* • Skull fractures can occur as a result of extensive molding of a large head. • *Clavicle.* Femora and humeri can fracture with difficult deliveries and use of instrumentation. • *Multiple fractures* can indicate osteogenesis imperfecta. *Spine.* Dimples, hemangiomas, tufts of hair, or other lesions along the spine may be associated with spinal abnormalities, such as spina bifida occulta. *Hips.* See Chapter 37 for information about eliciting Ortolani and Barlow signs. Both are indicators of dislocated or dislocatable hips.
Neurologic examination	*Muscle tone.* Observe tone, movement, and symmetry of the extremities while the infant is awake. *Reflexes.* Elicit the following: • Rooting • Sucking • Palmar grasp • Moro reflex • Ankle clonus (3 or 4 beats of clonus at ankle is normal) • Stepping and placing response • Galant reflex • Asymmetric tonic neck reflex *Cranial nerves.* Cranial nerve (CN) I (olfactory) is rarely tested. Vision (CN II) is tested by an infant's response to a bright light. CNs III, IV, and VI are tested by noting an infant's ability to gaze in all directions, although intermittent disconjugate gaze is normal through 6 months old. Adequate sucking and swallowing confirm presence of CNs V, IX, X, and XII. Symmetric movement of the face with crying confirms presence of CN VII. Hearing (CN VIII) is assessed by startle to loud noise.

bpm, Beats per minute; *CNS,* central nervous system; *LGA,* large for gestational age; *RDS,* respiratory distress syndrome.

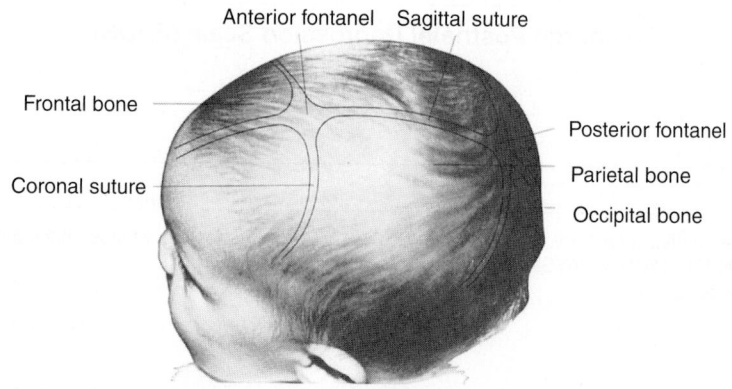

Anterior fontanel   Sagittal suture

Frontal bone

Coronal suture

Posterior fontanel

Parietal bone

Occipital bone

FIGURE 38-5 Fontanelles and sutures. (From Betz CL, Hunsberger M, Wright S: *Family-centered nursing care of children*, ed 2, Philadelphia, 1994, Saunders, p 124.)

and is not retractable at birth, but loosens as the baby grows. The parents are counseled not to force the foreskin back. If the baby is circumcised, the penis should be cleansed daily with cotton balls dipped in tap water followed by the application of a small amount of petroleum jelly to the tip of the penis with each diaper change to prevent discharge from the penis sticking to the diaper. The petroleum jelly is needed only for the first 2 to 3 days after the circumcision.

Bathing, Oils, and Powders. Tradition favors that the infant not be immersed in a tub of water, but rather should be sponge bathed until the umbilical cord separates and the navel appears healed. Mild cleansing agents, such as Dove, Caress, Neutrogena, and Basis, are gentle enough for infants' skin—oils and powders are not recommended. Oils and greasy substances tend to clog the skin's pores and can cause acne or rashes. Powders should be avoided because inhaling the talc could lead to respiratory problems. For dry skin, a lotion such as Keri, Eucerin, Aveeno, or Cetaphil is recommended.

Diapers. There is much controversy about whether disposable or cloth diapers are the better choice for infants. The need for frequent changing and proper cleansing is the important message to deliver.

Sleep Position

By 1992 the preponderance of available evidence suggested that the prone sleeping position was associated with an increased incidence of sudden infant death syndrome (SIDS). Recommendations for healthy infants include (AAP, 2005, 2009a):

- Placing infant in a supine position (side-lying is not recommended)
- Avoiding soft surfaces and gas-trapping objects in an infant's sleeping environment
- Advising that co-sleeping can be hazardous, but sleeping in the same room as the caregiver for the first 6 months of life may be beneficial
- Avoiding overheating
- Offering pacifiers
- "Tummy time" during the awake period—recommended for developmental reasons and to help prevent flat spots on the occiput

Encourage parents to ensure that their childcare center and other caregivers (e.g., grandparents) are following these guidelines. SIDS is discussed later in this chapter.

Injury Prevention

The appropriate use and installation of a crash-tested safety seat are essential. The best child safety seat is the one that fits the child properly, is easy to use, and fits in the parent's vehicle correctly. The National Highway Traffic Safety Administration rated scores of infant child restraint systems for ease of parental use. Correct installation of the infant safety seat can be checked at a child safety seat inspection station (often located in fire stations) or by a certified child passenger safety technician. Most hospitals have a certified person on-site who can assist parents when the infant leaves the hospital, or one can be located by searching the Internet. At the first visit it is ideal to have a trained staff member check for appropriate positioning and belt use. It is disconcerting that 80% of car seats are used inappropriately (AAP, 2002) (see Chapter 39).

The house should be childproofed before the infant is taken home. Falls and burns are the most common injuries to neonates. Parents should be counseled to avoid shaking their baby for any reason (refer to Chapters 9 and 39 for more information).

Parenting

The parenting role is stressful, even if all goes well. Fatigue and maternal depression resulting from hormonal shifts are common. Encourage parents to identify and make use of supportive people, arrange time for rest and time alone, and keep their expectations reasonable. When a mother seems to be having significant difficulty in adjusting to her new infant, it is imperative that the provider also keep in mind the possibility of severe postpartum depression and be ready to intervene on the behalf of the infant, the mother, and the family. The 10-question Edinburgh Postnatal Depression Scale (EPDS) is an easy-to-administer tool that is a valuable and efficient way of identifying mothers at risk for perinatal depression (Fig. 38-6). Women with postpartum depression need not feel alone; intervention, with possible referral for mothers whose score indicates a depressive illness, should be individualized.

EARLY DISCHARGE AND FOLLOW-UP

Newborns are often discharged after a relatively short period of hospital observation. Although "early discharge" is a common

Edinburgh Postnatal Depression Scale (EPDS)

Name: _____ Address: _____

Your date of birth: _____

Baby's date of birth: _____ Phone: _____

As you are pregnant or have recently had a baby, we would like to know how you are feeling. Please check the answer that comes closest to how you have felt IN THE PAST 7 DAYS, not just how you feel today.

Here is an example, already completed.

I have felt happy:
- ○ Yes, all the time
- X Yes, most of the time
- ○ No, not very often
- ○ No, not at all

This would mean: "I have felt happy most of the time" during the past week.

Please complete the other questions in the same way.

In the past 7 days:

1. I have been able to laugh and see the funny side of things
   - ○ As much as I always could
   - ○ Not quite so much now
   - ○ Definitely not so much now
   - ○ Not at all

2. I have looked forward with enjoyment to things
   - ○ As much as I ever did
   - ○ Rather less than I used to
   - ○ Definitely less than I used to
   - ○ Hardly at all

*3. I have blamed myself unnecessarily when things went wrong
   - ○ Yes, most of the time
   - ○ Yes, some of the time
   - ○ Not very often
   - ○ No, never

4. I have been anxious or worried for no good reason
   - ○ No, not at all
   - ○ Hardly ever
   - ○ Yes, sometimes
   - ○ Yes, very often

*5. I have felt scared or panicky for no very good reason
   - ○ Yes, quite a lot
   - ○ Yes, sometimes
   - ○ No, not much
   - ○ No, not at all

*6. Things have been getting on top of me
   - ○ Yes, most of the time I haven't been able to cope at all
   - ○ Yes, sometimes I haven't been coping as well as usual
   - ○ No, most of the time I have coped quite well
   - ○ No, I have been coping as well as ever

*7. I have been so unhappy that I have had difficulty sleeping
   - ○ Yes, most of the time
   - ○ Yes, sometimes
   - ○ Not very often
   - ○ No, not at all

*8. I have felt sad or miserable
   - ○ Yes, most of the time
   - ○ Yes, quite often
   - ○ Only occasionally
   - ○ No, never

*9. I have been so unhappy that I have been crying
   - ○ Yes, most of the time
   - ○ Yes, quite often
   - ○ Only occasionally
   - ○ No, never

*10. The thought of harming myself has occurred to me
   - ○ Yes, quite often
   - ○ Sometimes
   - ○ Hardly ever
   - ○ Never

Administered/reviewed by _____ Date _____

SCORING

QUESTIONS 1, 2, and 4 (without an *) are scored 0, 1, 2 or 3 with top box scored as 0
QUESTIONS 3, 5, 6, 7, 8, 9, and 10 (marked with an *) are reverse scored, with the top box scored as a 3
   Maximum score: 30
   Possible depression: 10 or greater
   Always look at item 10 (suicidal thoughts)

Instructions for using the Edinburgh Postnatal Depression Scale:
1. The mother is asked to check the response that comes closest to how she has been feeling in the previous 7 days.
2. All the items must be completed.
3. Care should be taken to avoid the possibility of the mother discussing her answers with others. (Answers come from the mother or pregnant woman.)
4. The mother should complete the scale herself, unless she has limited English or has difficulty with reading.

Users may reproduce the scale without further permission providing they respect copyright by quoting the names of the authors, the title and the source of the paper in all reproduced copies.

FIGURE 38-6 Edinburgh Postnatal Depression Scale (EPDS). (From Cox JL, Holden JM, Sagovsky R: Detection of postnatal depression: development of the 10-item Edinburgh Postnatal Depression Scale, *Br J Psychiatry* 150:782-786, 1987; Wisner KL, Parry BL, Piontek CM: Postpartum depression, *N Engl J Med* 347[3]:194-199, 2002.)

- No ongoing medical issues that require continued hospitalization
- Term (37 to 41 completed weeks) baby
- Stable vital signs for at least 12 hours before discharge:
  ○ Axillary temperature of 97.7° to 99.3° F (36.5° to 37.4° C) in open crib
  ○ Heart rate 100 to 160 beats per minute
  ○ Respiratory rate less than 60 breaths/minute
- Regular passage of urine and at least one stool
- Two successful feedings have been accomplished
- Normal physical examination
- No excessive bleeding at circumcision site
- The clinical significance of jaundice has been determined and appropriate follow-up plans made
- Evaluation and monitoring for sepsis based on maternal risk factors have been accomplished
- Infant laboratory data, including maternal syphilis, hepatitis B, and human immunodeficiency virus (HIV), and infant blood type and Coombs testing (as indicated) completed
- Appropriately timed neonatal metabolic and hearing screenings completed
- Initial hepatitis B administered
- Social support and continuing health care identified
- Social situation adequate: screen for drug abuse, previous child abuse, mental illness, lack of social support, lack of permanent home, history of domestic violence, communicable diseases in the household, teenage mother, inadequate transportation or communication abilities
- Appropriate medical home identified with early follow-up care achievable preferably within 48 hours of discharge but no later than 72 hours in most cases
- Mother knowledgeable in the care of the infant, including the following:
  ○ Feeding, with breastfeeding encouraged
  ○ Normal stool and urine frequency
  ○ Skin, genital, and cord care
  ○ Ability to identify illness (especially jaundice)
  ○ Proper safety (car seat, sleeping position, smoke-free environment, room sharing)
  ○ Smoke alarms in the home

Data from American Academy of Pediatrics (AAP): Policy statement-hospital stay for healthy term newborns, *Pediatrics* 125:405-409, 2010.

BOX 38-3 Guidelines for 48- to 72-Hour Follow-up Visit of the Normal, Healthy Newborn

- Review delivery and discharge summary for any identified follow-up needs (e.g., hearing screening, specialty referrals)
- Assess the infant's general health, weight, hydration, and jaundice; identify any new problems; review feeding, stooling, and urination
- Assess quality of bonding
- Reinforce maternal and family education
- Review outstanding laboratory data
- Perform neonatal screen or other tests (such as bilirubin), if indicated
- Develop plan for health care maintenance, including emergency care, preventive care, immunizations, and periodic screenings
- Evaluate mother for post-partum depression
- Refer to Women, Infants, and Children (WIC) program eligibility screening as appropriate.

practice, infants can experience difficulty with breastfeeding, poor weight gain, jaundice, and dehydration (Madden et al, 2004). Guidelines for early discharge of normal, healthy newborns are listed in Box 38-2. Plans for follow-up care within 48 to 72 hours and plans for ongoing health maintenance should be confirmed before discharge (Box 38-3). Even newborns who are hospitalized longer may need follow-up care within the first few days of life. All parents leaving the hospital with a newborn should have a confirmed time and place for follow-up, in addition to contacts in case of an emergency or questions.

PREMATURE INFANTS AND NEWBORNS WITH SPECIAL NEEDS

Premature infants have special needs that must be addressed before discharge (Box 38-4). Newborns with special needs (e.g., anomalies, disease states, social situations) require early assessment, intervention, and referral before discharge to ensure that support, education, and follow-up are in place.

◼ Common Neonatal Conditions
SKIN CONDITIONS

MILIA
Description and Epidemiology
Milia are multiple, firm, pearly, opalescent white papules scattered over the forehead, nose, and cheeks. Their intraoral counterparts are called Epstein pearls. Histologically, milia represent superficial epidermal inclusion cysts filled with keratinous material associated with the developing pilosebaceous follicle.

Management
No treatment is necessary because milia exfoliate spontaneously in most infants over the first few weeks of life.

SEBACEOUS HYPERPLASIA
Description and Epidemiology
Sebaceous hyperplasia is characterized by prominent yellow-white papules at the opening of each pilosebaceous follicle, predominantly over the nose, forehead, upper lip, and cheeks. The overgrowth of sebaceous glands in response to the same androgenic stimulation that occurs in adolescence causes sebaceous hyperplasia.

Management
No treatment is required. These tiny papules diminish in size and disappear entirely within the first few weeks of life.

ERYTHEMA TOXICUM
Description and Epidemiology
Firm, yellow-white 1- to 2-mm papules or pustules with a surrounding erythematous flare characterize erythema toxicum. Lesions are clustered in several sites. These lesions usually develop at 24 to 48 hours old. The cause is unknown, although

---

BOX 38-4 Guidelines for Discharge and Follow-up of the High-Risk Neonate

Discharge Planning

- Demonstrate adequate weight gain, temperature control in open crib, adequate feeding without cardiorespiratory compromise, and mature and stable cardiorespiratory function.
- Ensure adequacy of immunizations based on infant's chronologic age and appropriate metabolic screenings.
- Screen for anemia and nutritional risks; begin therapy, if indicated.
- Conduct funduscopic evaluation if necessary.
- Ensure appropriate hearing screen has been completed.
- Identify all active medical or social problems through a review of the medical record and physical examination of infant; ensure home readiness has been evaluated, especially for the technologically dependent child.
- Complete car seat evaluation.
- Review with family member medications, feeding schedules, well-child care, signs of illness, safety instruction, and appropriate response and follow-up for infants with active medical conditions.
- Identify family and community resources if infant is to be discharged on home oxygen therapy.
- Ensure adequate training of appropriate family members in cardiopulmonary resuscitation (CPR) and, if applicable, home apnea monitor or other equipment use.
- Consider need for visiting nurse, social service, respite care, support groups, early intervention services, or referral to the Women, Infants, and Children (WIC) program.
- Ensure that follow-up care is arranged to include a primary care provider and surgical or other subspecialty providers, if indicated.

Follow-up Planning

- Schedule follow-up hearing screen (if necessary) for infants with:
  - Craniofacial abnormalities
  - In utero infections
  - Birthweight less than 1500 g
  - Meningitis
  - Exchange transfusion for hyperbilirubinemia
  - Use of ototoxic medications
  - Apgar score of 0 to 4 at 1 minute or 0 to 6 at 5 minutes
  - Mechanical ventilation for 5 days or longer
  - Stigmata of syndrome associated with hearing loss
  - Failed initial screening
  - Family history of deafness
- Ensure that by about 4 to 6 weeks of chronologic age a dilated binocular indirect ophthalmoscopic examination has occurred for neonates with:
  - A birthweight of 1500 g or less or with a gestational age of <32 weeks
  - A birthweight between 1500 and 2000 g or gestational age of more than 32 weeks with an unstable clinical course including cardiorespiratory support, especially if infant is thought to be at high risk for retinopathy of prematurity (see Chapter 28)
- Additional examinations may be recommended based on the results of this first evaluation.
- Follow-up visits every 1 to 2 weeks, especially if infant is on oxygen therapy
- Growth and development should be of prime interest at each routine outpatient visit with referral for formal developmental assessment if any concerns are identified.

Data from American Academy of Pediatrics (AAP): Hospital discharge of the high-risk neonate, *Pediatrics* 122:1119-1126, 2008; Section on Ophthalmology American Academy of Pediatrics; American Academy of Ophthalmology, American Association for Pediatric Ophthalmology and Strabismus: Screening examination of premature infants for retinopathy of prematurity, *Pediatrics* 117:572-576, 2006.

---

examination of a Wright-stained smear of the lesion reveals numerous eosinophils. Up to 50% of infants develop erythema toxicum, with a higher incidence in term than in premature infants.

Differential Diagnosis

Pyoderma, candidiasis, herpes simplex, transient neonatal pustular melanosis, and miliaria should be considered (Table 38-3).

Management

No treatment is required because the course is brief and transient.

TRANSIENT NEONATAL PUSTULAR MELANOSIS

Description and Epidemiology

Transient neonatal pustular melanosis is characterized by superficial vesiculopustules that rupture easily and leave a halo of white scales around a central pinhead-sized macule of hyperpigmentation. Pustular melanosis is caused by increased melanization of the epidermal cells, with sites of predilection being the trunk, limbs, palms, and soles. It is more common in African-American than in Caucasian infants.

Differential Diagnosis

Pyoderma and erythema toxicum are the differential diagnoses.

Management

No treatment is required. The pustular phase rarely lasts more than 2 to 3 days; hyperpigmented macules can persist for as long as 3 months.

SUCKING BLISTERS

Description and Epidemiology

Sucking blisters are solitary or scattered superficial bullae on the upper limbs and lips of infants at birth, commonly found on the radial aspect of the forearm, the thumb, and the index finger. These blisters result from vigorous sucking on the affected part in utero.

Management

No treatment is required. These bullae resolve rapidly without sequelae.

CUTIS MARMORATA

Description and Epidemiology

Cutis marmorata is a lacy, reticulated, red or blue cutaneous vascular pattern appearing over most of the body surface. The vascular change is a response to exposure to low environmental temperatures. It represents an accentuated physiologic vasomotor response that disappears with increasing age. Persistent and pronounced cutis marmorata occurs in Down and trisomy 18 syndromes.

TABLE 38-3 Comparison of Erythema Toxicum and Herpes Simplex Virus

Erythema Toxicum	Herpes Simplex Virus
Benign, self-limited	Pathologic, progressive
No specific maternal history	Frequently a history of maternal disease
Usually seen only in term infant	Can occur in infants of any gestational age
Begins on the second or third day of life, lasting as long as 1 week	Often begins late in the first week of life or early in the second week of life
Rash is evanescent, often involving the face, trunk, and extremities	Can be superficial and localized only to the presenting part (vertex or buttocks) or widespread and disseminated with or without cutaneous involvement
1- to 2-mm white papules or pustules on an erythematous base that occasionally may become somewhat vesicular	May manifest similar to sepsis without cutaneous findings or as grouped vesicles on an erythematous base on the presenting part about days 9-11 of life
Wright or Giemsa stain of lesion scraping demonstrates large numbers of eosinophils and no organisms; cultures are sterile	DFA staining or ELISA detection of HSV antigens of vesicle scrapings or growth of the organism from vesicle fluid is diagnostic
No specific therapy necessary	Acyclovir and other antiviral agents

DFA, Direct fluorescent antibody; *ELISA*, enzyme-linked immunosorbent assay; *HSV*, herpes simplex virus.

Management

Cutis marmorata usually resolves with warming of the infant.

HARLEQUIN COLOR CHANGE
Description and Epidemiology

Harlequin color change is a division of the body skin coloring from forehead to pubis into red and pale halves. The cause is unknown.

Management

No treatment is indicated with this transient and benign condition.

MONGOLIAN SPOTS, CAFÉ AU LAIT SPOTS, SALMON PATCH (NEVUS SIMPLEX), AND PORT-WINE STAIN (NEVUS FLAMMEUS, PORT-WINE NEVUS)

See Chapter 36 for a discussion of these skin conditions.

NEVUS SEBACEOUS
Description and Epidemiology

Nevus sebaceous is a yellowish, hairless, sharply demarcated smooth plaque usually on the head and neck. Histologically these nevi contain an abundance of sebaceous glands. With maturity, usually during adolescence, the lesions become verrucous with large rubbery nodules. During adulthood the lesions are complicated by secondary malignancies, most commonly basal cell carcinoma.

Management

Total excision before the onset of adolescence is recommended. Referral to a pediatric dermatologist is warranted.

SKIN DIMPLING
Description and Epidemiology

Deep skin dimples, in addition to pits and creases, can occur over bony prominences and in the sacral area. They occur in normal infants and in those with dysmorphologic syndromes, such as congenital rubella, deletion of the long arm of chromosome 18, and cerebrohepatorenal syndromes.

Management

No treatment is indicated if isolated and not associated with other findings.

PREAURICULAR SINUS TRACTS AND PITS
Description and Epidemiology

Sinus tracts and pits occur anterior to the pinna and can be unilateral or bilateral. They result from imperfect fusion of the tubercles of the first and second branchial arches during gestational development, are familial, are more common in females and African-Americans, and occasionally are associated with other anomalies of the ears and face.

Management

Excision rarely is required and only if tracts and pits are chronically infected and draining.

AMNIOTIC CONSTRICTION BANDS
Description and Epidemiology

In utero fibrous strands that encircle fetal parts can cause permanent depression of the underlying tissue, producing defects in the extremities and digits. Found in otherwise normal infants, these bands are thought to result from intrauterine rupture of the amnion with formation of fibrous strands. Sometimes there are associated abnormalities, including craniofacial anomalies and thoracic or abdominal wall defects.

Management

Treatment depends on the severity of deformities produced. Constriction bands on the limbs are often managed in consultation with plastic surgery.

SUPERNUMERARY NIPPLES
Description and Epidemiology

Solitary or multiple accessory nipples and sometimes areolae occur in unilateral or bilateral distribution along a line from the midaxilla to the inguinal area. The cause is unknown. Urinary tract anomalies do occur, but are very rare.

Management

Usually no treatment is necessary.

BRANCHIAL CLEFT AND THYROGLOSSAL CYSTS AND SINUSES

Description and Epidemiology

Cysts and sinuses in the neck can be unilateral or bilateral and can open onto the cutaneous surface or drain into the pharynx. Thyroglossal cysts and fistulas are similar defects located in or near the midline of the neck, extending to the base of the tongue. Thyroglossal cysts occasionally contain aberrant thyroid tissue and mucinous material. Cysts and sinuses in the neck can be formed along the course of the first and second branchial clefts as a result of improper closure during embryonic life. These anomalies can be inherited as autosomal dominant traits.

Management

Antibiotic therapy is indicated for infections of the cysts or sinuses, which are rare in the neonatal period. Surgical excision is recommended for thyroglossal cysts.

HEAD, FACE, AND EYE CONDITIONS

CAPUT SUCCEDANEUM

Description and Epidemiology

Caput succedaneum is a diffuse swelling of the soft tissue of the scalp with possible underlying bruising; the swelling usually crosses the suture lines (Fig. 38-7). Caput succedaneum originates from trauma as the baby descends through the birth canal.

Clinical Findings
History and Physical Examination
- Primigravida and traumatic delivery
- Obvious swelling and bruising in the parietal regions of the scalp
- Swelling that crosses suture lines
- Frequently associated with molding

Differential Diagnosis

Cephalhematoma is the differential diagnosis.

Management

No treatment is necessary because swelling resolves spontaneously over a few days. If the lesion is large, observe the baby for the development of jaundice as the blood from bruising is reabsorbed.

CEPHALHEMATOMA

Description and Epidemiology

Cephalhematoma is a collection of blood in the subperiosteal area of the scalp that does not cross the suture lines. Frequently no noticeable bruising of the area is seen (Fig. 38-8). Cephalhematoma results from trauma occurring during a difficult delivery. The swelling appears hours to days after delivery.

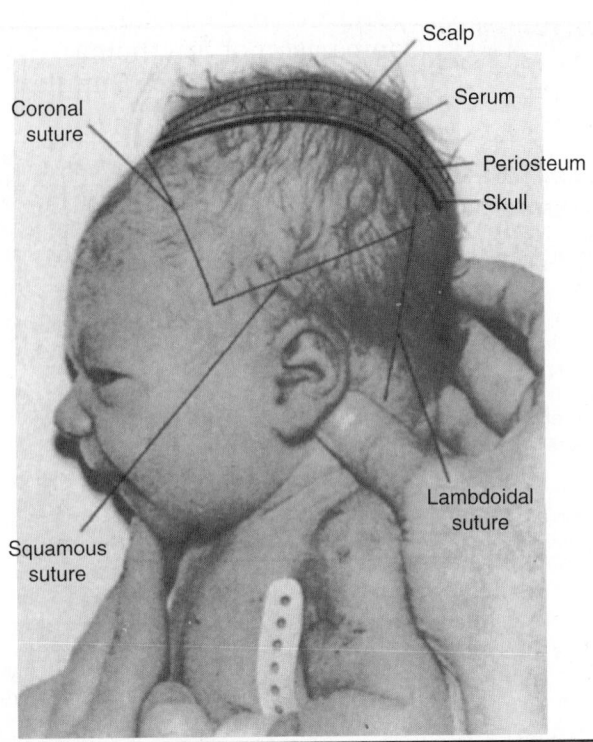

FIGURE 38-7 Caput succedaneum. (From Betz CL, Hunsberger M, Wright S: *Family-centered nursing care of children*, ed 2, Philadelphia, 1994, Saunders, p 124.)

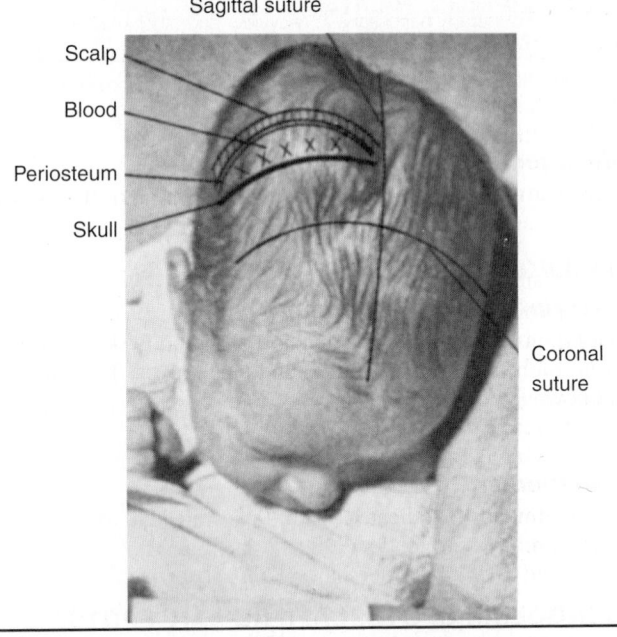

FIGURE 38-8 Cephalhematoma. (From Betz CL, Hunsberger M, Wright S: *Family-centered nursing care of children*, ed 2, Philadelphia, 1994, Saunders, p 124.)

Clinical Findings
History and Physical Examination
- Primigravida and traumatic delivery may be part of the history
- Swelling in the parietal area that does not cross suture lines
- Rarely associated with a skull fracture, coagulopathy, or intracranial hemorrhage

Differential Diagnosis

Caput succedaneum and cranial meningocele should be considered.

Management

No treatment is indicated because the condition resolves in a few weeks to months. Calcification of the hematoma can occur, which will be felt as bony prominences on the cranium. Observe for hyperbilirubinemia.

CRANIOTABES

Description and Epidemiology

Craniotabes is thinning of the bone of the scalp. This is a normal variation of the parietal bone, usually near the sagittal suture line.

Clinical Findings
History and Physical Examination
- Prematurity
- A "ping-pong ball" effect when pressing on the parietal bone

Management

No treatment is necessary because craniotabes resolves spontaneously. If persistent, pathologic causes, such as rickets, should be investigated.

CLEFT LIP AND PALATE

Description and Epidemiology

Cleft lip results from failure of embryonic structures surrounding the oral cavity to join. Cleft palate appears when the palatal shelves fail to fuse. There are various degrees of clefts. Genetic factors influence the development of cleft lip more than cleft palate; however, both occur sporadically. A combination of cleft lip and cleft palate is more common than one without the other. Cleft lip with or without cleft palate occurs in about 1 in 750 Caucasian births. Cleft palate alone occurs in 1 in 2500 Caucasian births (Tinanoff, 2007). Clefts are more common in males. In most cases, a genetics consultation is warranted.

Clinical Findings
Physical Examination
- A varying degree of cleft, from a small notch to a complete separation
- Unilateral or bilateral cleft
- Involvement of the soft palate, hard palate, or both
- A bifid uvula, which may indicate a submucosal cleft palate

Management and Complications

Surgical repair is indicated, and the timing is individualized. Special nipples and feeding techniques are used until surgery can be performed. Breastfeeding and bottle feeding may be successful depending on the severity of the cleft. Speech evaluation and perhaps therapy are necessary in later years. Dental restoration is often needed. Team management is beneficial. Middle ear, nasopharyngeal, and sinus infections, as well as associated hearing loss can occur.

TABLE 38-4 Clinical Comparison of Transient Tachypnea of the Newborn and Respiratory Distress Syndrome

Transient Tachypnea of the Newborn	Respiratory Distress Syndrome (RDS)
Seen only in infants delivered at or near term; often in infants born by cesarean section	Found almost always in premature infants, with the greatest incidence in infants weighing <1500 g
Increased respiratory rate is invariably present; grunting and intercostal retractions are not always present	Usually, respiratory rate is increased, infants grunt at expiration, nasal flaring is noted, and sternal and intercostal retractions are commonly seen
Cyanosis is not a prominent feature	Cyanosis in room air is a prominent feature
Air exchange is good; rales and rhonchi are usually absent	Auscultation reveals diminished air entry
Begins at birth, usually resolving in the first 24 to 48 hours of life	Progressive respiratory distress in the first hours of life
Chest radiograph shows central perihilar streaking with slightly enlarged heart with fluid in the fissure	Chest radiograph demonstrates reticulogranular, ground-glass appearance and air bronchograms
Typical course involves gradual decrease in respiratory rate with resolution in about 72 hours	Course variable depending on infant's gestational weight and age; usually, RDS begins to improve after about 5 days of life
No specific therapy other than maintaining oxygenation is usually necessary	Artificial surfactant and antenatal administration of steroids to the mother can reduce the severity of this disease; mechanical ventilation is commonly needed

CONGENITAL CATARACTS, GLAUCOMA, AND RETINOPATHY OF PREMATURITY

See Chapter 28.

CARDIAC CONDITIONS

See Chapter 30.

RESPIRATORY CONDITIONS

RESPIRATORY DISTRESS SYNDROME

Description and Epidemiology

Respiratory distress syndrome (RDS), formerly called hyaline membrane disease, occurs secondary to atelectasis of the lungs. This is the most common pulmonary disease in the newborn (Table 38-4). Surfactant deficiency is the underlying cause of the disease, resulting in alveolar atelectasis and decreased lung compliance. The incidence is 1% of all live births, but only 0.5% of term births. The incidence rises rapidly at less than 33 to 34 weeks of gestational age. An estimated 50% of all neonatal deaths result from RDS or its complications (Dudell and Stoll, 2007). The incidence increases with decreasing gestational age and/or weight.

Clinical Findings
History
- Diabetic mother (incidence increased at older gestational ages in infants of diabetic mothers)
- Preterm delivery
- Multiple births
- Cesarean delivery
- Precipitous delivery
- Asphyxia
- Cold stress
- Previously affected siblings
Physical Examination
- Tachypnea
- Grunting
- Intercostal retractions
- Nasal flaring
- Duskiness, cyanosis
- Breath sounds may be normal but often are diminished with harsh tubular quality
- Fine rales on deep inspiration

Diagnostic Studies. A radiograph of the chest shows a fine reticular granularity of the parenchyma and air bronchograms. Blood gas results indicate hypoxemia, hypercarbia, and mixed metabolic/respiratory acidosis.

Management, Prognosis, and Prevention
Supportive care and mechanical ventilation are used as indicated. The immediate use of exogenous surfactant has been found to reduce mortality rates and improve short-term respiratory status in preterm infants. The prognosis depends on the severity of the disease and the birthweight of the infant. The only fully effective preventive measure is elimination of prematurity. Administration of synthetic corticosteroids to women expected to deliver prematurely is also used to reduce the severity of the problem (Roberts and Dalziel, 2006).

TRANSIENT TACHYPNEA OF THE NEWBORN
Description and Epidemiology
Transient tachypnea of the newborn (TTN) is a respiratory condition that results from incomplete evacuation of fetal lung fluid in full-term infants. TTN results from decreased pulmonary compliance and tidal volume and increased dead space secondary to slow absorption of fetal lung fluid. It is more common in cesarean deliveries.

Clinical Findings
History and Physical Examination
- Usually disappears within 24 to 48 hours
- Tachypnea
- Expiratory grunting
- Auscultation without findings
- Intercostal retractions
- Occasionally responding to minimal oxygen

Diagnostic Studies. A chest radiograph shows prominent pulmonary vascular markings, fluid lines along fissures, overaeration, flat diaphragms, and occasionally pleural fluid.

Differential Diagnosis
The differential diagnosis is RDS (see Table 38-4).

Management and Prognosis
If the infant is not in significant respiratory distress, close observation and transcutaneous oxygen saturation monitoring can be sufficient until the tachypnea resolves. The need for supplemental oxygen therapy provided in a hood should be based on close oxygen monitoring. The use of mechanical ventilation in TTN is rare. Infants usually recover rapidly within 24 to 48 hours with no intervention.

MECONIUM ASPIRATION SYNDROME
Description and Epidemiology
Meconium aspiration syndrome occurs in term or postterm infants. This syndrome is a serious pulmonary disorder characterized by small airway obstruction, chemical pneumonitis, and secondary respiratory distress. In utero fetal distress and anoxia increase intestinal peristalsis and relax the anal sphincter resulting in release of meconium into the amniotic fluid. Thick meconium is aspirated either in utero or with the first breath. Approximately 10% to 15% of all newborns are meconium stained, but only 5% of these infants develop respiratory problems (Dudell and Stoll, 2007).

Clinical Findings
History and Physical Examination
- Meconium in the amniotic fluid and below the vocal cords on resuscitation
- Tachypnea
- Intercostal retractions
- Grunting
- Cyanosis within hours of delivery

Diagnostic Studies. A chest radiograph shows patchy infiltrates, coarse streaking of both lung fields, and flattening of the diaphragm.

Management, Prognosis, and Prevention
An infant born with meconium in the amniotic fluid but who is vigorous (strong respiratory effort, good muscle tone, and a heart rate of higher than 100 beats per minute [bpm]) does not need intubation and suctioning. Meconium-stained depressed infants do benefit from intubation and suctioning before the initiation of positive pressure ventilation (Vain et al, 2004). Ongoing treatment includes supportive care and standard management of respiratory distress. Severe meconium aspiration cases are managed by extracorporeal membrane oxygenation (ECMO). The mortality rate of meconium-stained infants is higher than that of nonstained infants. Meconium aspiration accounts for a significant proportion of neonatal deaths. Residual lung problems are possible. Ultimate prognosis depends on the extent of central nervous system (CNS) injury from asphyxia. DeLee suctioning after the infant's head is delivered was previously felt by some to reduce the risk

of meconium aspiration, especially if the baby had not yet breathed deeply. However, it is no longer recommended.

GASTROINTESTINAL AND ABDOMINAL CONDITIONS

ESOPHAGEAL ATRESIA AND TRACHEOESOPHAGEAL FISTULA

Description and Epidemiology
In esophageal atresia, a blind pouch occurs in the esophagus with or without an associated fistula. Most infants (90%) have a proximal pouch, with the associated fistula connecting the distal esophagus and the trachea (Fig. 38-9). This defect occurs in 1 in 3500 births. Approximately one third of affected infants are born prematurely (Orenstein et al, 2007).

Clinical Findings
History. The history includes maternal polyhydramnios and inability to pass a nasogastric tube into the stomach during resuscitation at birth or afterward in the nursery, especially in a child with vomiting.

Physical Examination
- Excessive oral secretions that require frequent suctioning
- Choking, coughing, and cyanosis, particularly during feedings
- Spitting or vomiting

Diagnostic Studies. Chest and abdominal radiographs show the nasogastric tube coiled in the thoracic region. Carefully performed water-soluble x-ray evaluation of the upper esophagus demonstrates the exact location of the atresia and rules out tracheoesophageal fistula.

Differential Diagnosis
RDS, meconium aspiration, and congenital heart disease should be considered.

Management, Complications, and Prognosis
This is a surgical emergency requiring immediate intervention. A nasogastric tube can be inserted into the blind pouch to prevent aspiration until surgical repair can be accomplished. Preoperatively the infant should be placed in a prone position and suctioned frequently. Pneumonia, atelectasis, aspiration, postoperative strictures, and repeated surgery are possible complications. The survival rate postoperatively is almost 100% unless other congenital anomalies are present. Approximately 50% to 70% of affected infants have other congenital anomalies (Orenstein et al, 2007; Ulshen, 2006).

DUODENAL ATRESIA

Description and Epidemiology
Duodenal atresia is a complete obstruction of the duodenum, ending blindly just distal to the ampulla of Vater. Duodenal atresia occurs in 1 in 10,000 to 30,000 births. It is associated with prematurity in 50% of cases, Down syndrome in 40% of cases, and other anomalies in up to 20% of cases (Ulshen, 2006; Wyllie, 2007).

Clinical Findings
History
- Maternal polyhydramnios
- Down syndrome
- Premature birth

Physical Examination
- Bilious vomitus
- Abdominal distention
- Jaundice

Diagnostic Studies. Abdominal radiographs show a "double-bubble" pattern in the upright position secondary to air in the stomach and a distended duodenum.

Differential Diagnosis
Malrotation, duodenal obstruction, and annular pancreas should be considered.

Management, Complications, and Prognosis
Surgical intervention is indicated. Feedings should be discontinued and gastric suctioning applied. The prognosis depends on early identification and treatment and other associated anomalies. Aspiration of gastric contents can occur as a complication of this condition.

VOLVULUS

Description
Volvulus is the twisting of a loop of bowel, causing intermittent or acute pain and obstruction, occurring in 1 in 6000 live births (Ulshen, 2006).

Clinical Findings
Physical Examination. Findings include abdominal distention and bilious vomiting.

Diagnostic Studies. Intestinal obstruction is demonstrated on abdominal radiograph.

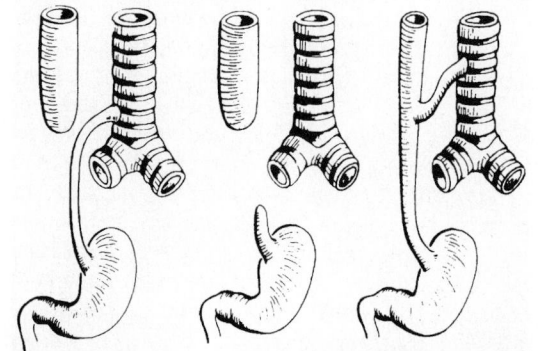

FIGURE 38-9 The three most common types of esophageal atresia and tracheoesophageal fistula (TEF). (From Ein SH: Congenital malformations of the esophagus. In Wyllie R, Hyams JS, editors: *Pediatric gastrointestinal disease,* Philadelphia, 2006, Saunders.)

Differential Diagnosis
Duodenal obstruction or atresia and annular pancreas are in the differential diagnosis.

Management, Complications, and Prognosis

Surgical repair and fluid replacement are indicated. The prognosis depends on identification of the volvulus and the urgency of surgery. Perforation, necrosis of the bowel, sepsis, and peritonitis are possible complications.

PYLORIC STENOSIS

Description and Epidemiology

Pyloric stenosis is characterized by hypertrophied pyloric muscle, causing a narrowing of the pyloric sphincter. Pyloric stenosis occurs in 3 per 1000 live births, with a fourfold increase in males compared with females (Wyllie, 2007). It tends to be familial and is seen more commonly in Caucasian first-born males.

Clinical Findings

History

- Regurgitation and nonprojectile vomiting during the first few weeks of life
- Projectile vomiting beginning at 2 to 3 weeks old
- Insatiable appetite with weight loss, dehydration, and constipation
- An association of pyloric stenosis with the early administration of erythromycin has been demonstrated (Mahon et al, 2001).

Physical Examination

- Weight loss
- Vomitus that is nonbilious and can contain blood
- A distinct "olive" mass that is often palpated in the epigastrium to the right of midline
- Reverse peristalsis visualized across the abdomen

Diagnostic Studies. An upper gastrointestinal series demonstrates a "string sign," indicating a fine, elongated pyloric canal. Ultrasound, with measurement of the pyloric muscle thickness, is used in most centers.

Management and Prognosis

Surgical intervention (pyloromyotomy) is indicated after correction of fluid and electrolyte imbalance. Vomiting can continue for a few days after surgery, although it is not as significant as it was preoperatively; feedings should be introduced gradually. The prognosis is excellent.

HIRSCHSPRUNG DISEASE (CONGENITAL AGANGLIONIC MEGACOLON)

Description and Epidemiology

Hirschsprung disease is an absence of ganglion cells in the bowel wall, most often in the rectosigmoid region, resulting in a portion of the colon having no motility. This disorder occurs in 1 in 5000 births. It is the most common cause of neonatal obstruction of the colon and accounts for approximately 33% of all neonatal obstructions. The disease is familial, affects males four times more commonly than females, and is common in children with trisomy 21. Additional anomalies are sometimes present (Middlesworth and Kadenhe-Chiweshe, 2006; Wyllie, 2007).

Clinical Findings

History

- Failure to pass meconium within the first 48 hours of life
- Failure to thrive
- Poor feeding
- Chronic constipation
- Down syndrome

Physical Examination

- Vomiting
- Abdominal obstruction
- Failure to pass stools
- Diarrhea, explosive bowel movements, or flatus

Diagnostic Studies. Radiographs indicate dilated loops of bowel (Fig. 38-10). A biopsy determines the absence of ganglion cells.

Differential Diagnosis

The differential diagnosis includes acquired functional megacolon, colonic inertia, chronic idiopathic constipation, obstipation, small left colon syndrome, meconium plug syndrome, and ileal atresia with microcolon.

Management

Surgical resection of the affected bowel is indicated, with or without a colostomy.

IMPERFORATE ANUS

Description and Epidemiology

Imperforate anus is the lack of a rectal opening. This condition occurs in about 1 in 4000 births, about half associated with another anomaly (often the VACTERL syndrome consisting of *v*ertebral dysgenesis, *a*nal atresia [imperforate anus], *c*ardiac anomalies, *t*racheo*e*sophageal fistula, *r*enal anomalies, and *l*imb anomalies (Klein and Thomas, 2007).

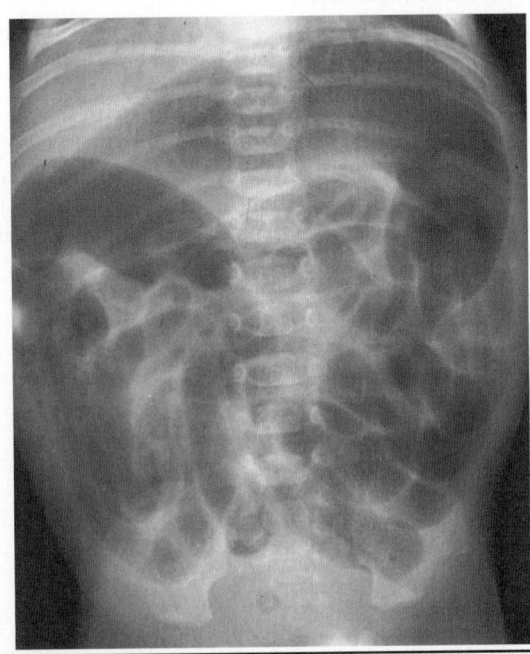

FIGURE 38-10 Dramatic dilation of bowel consistent with Hirschsprung disease. (Photo courtesy Lawrence H. Robinson, professor of Radiology and Pediatrics, University of Texas Medical School, Houston.)

Clinical Findings

History and Physical Examination. The history includes lack of passage of meconium. Findings include no obvious opening in the rectal area.

Diagnostic Studies. Endoscopic examination and ultrasound indicate the degree of malformation.

Associated Conditions

Congenital heart disease, esophageal atresia, intestinal atresia, annular pancreas, intestinal malrotation or duplication, bilateral absence of the musculus rectus abdominis, trisomy 21, finger and hand anomalies, omphalocele, bladder exstrophy, and exstrophy of the ileocecal area are associated conditions (Klein and Thomas, 2007).

Management

Immediate surgical repair with or without performing a colostomy is indicated. Long-term management related to bowel functioning may be needed because some children will have trouble with bowel emptying or incontinence.

OMPHALOCELE AND GASTROSCHISIS

Description and Epidemiology

An omphalocele is a protrusion of the sac of intestines into the base of the umbilical cord. The intestines are covered by the peritoneum without overlying skin. Occurrence is 1 in 5000 to 10,000 births (Stoll, 2007b). Gastroschisis is similar in appearance with intestinal contents protruding through the abdomen with no protective peritoneal covering. Gastroschisis occurs in about 1 in 10,000 to 20,000 live births when there is failure to close the lateral ventral folds of the developing abdominal wall.

Clinical Findings

Physical Examination. Examination reveals a saclike protrusion covered by the peritoneum without overlying skin at the midabdomen.

Associated Conditions

With omphalocele, serious associated conditions occur in 50% of newborns including chromosomal abnormalities (trisomy 13 and 18), congenital diaphragmatic hernia, and a variety of cardiac problems. Concomitant hypoglycemia and macroglossia suggest Beckwith syndrome (Stoll, 2007b). Associated congenital anomalies are rare with gastroschisis.

Management and Complications

Maintain body temperature. Apply protective gauze and wrap abdomen with cellophane to prevent heat and fluid loss. When the infant is stable, surgical repair is indicated. Ileus is a common complication.

NECROTIZING ENTEROCOLITIS

Description and Epidemiology

Necrotizing enterocolitis (NEC) is characterized by varying degrees of mucosal or transmural necrosis of the intestine. The usual onset is in the first 2 weeks of life, but can be later in very-low-birthweight infants. The cause is unknown, but it is much less common in infants who are breastfed and have minimal feeds before bolus feeds. High-risk infants are found to have immature colons that become necrosed from trauma or injury. NEC occurs in 3% to 5% of neonates in the NICU, with the vast majority (90% to 93%) of these cases occurring in premature infants, especially those between 500 and 750 g (Brown and Neu, 2006; Piazza and Stoll, 2007).

Clinical Findings

History
- Prematurity, SGA
- Maternal hemorrhage, preeclampsia
- Cocaine exposure in utero
- Exchange transfusions, umbilical catheters
- Asphyxia
- Polycythemia

Physical Examination
- Abdominal distention
- Vomiting
- Bloody stools (25%)
- Lethargy
- Apnea
- Disseminated intravascular coagulation
- Rapid progression of shock

Diagnostic Studies
- Sepsis workup should be done.
- An abdominal radiograph shows pneumatosis intestinalis, a specific air pattern.

Differential Diagnosis

The differential diagnosis includes sepsis, intestinal obstruction, volvulus, Hirschsprung disease, anal fissures, and neonatal appendicitis.

Management, Complications, and Prognosis

- Prescribe systemic antibiotics following sepsis workup.
- Stop feedings, initiate gastric suctioning, maintain electrolyte balance, give oxygen as needed, and initiate surgical consultation.
- Obtain serial abdominal radiographs to follow course of disease.
- Delay oral feedings in very-low-birthweight infants for at least 1 week after definitive diagnosis; when feedings are begun, they should be continuous slow drip before advancing to bolus.

The mortality rate is 10% to 50%, causing 1000 deaths per year. Ileus and perforation are early complications. Sequelae to NEC include feeding intolerance, stricture formation, and short-bowel syndrome, especially after intestinal resection (Brown and Neu, 2006; Piazza and Stoll, 2007).

MECONIUM ILEUS

Description and Epidemiology

Meconium ileus is an impaction of the bowel with meconium, causing intestinal obstruction. Meconium ileus is associated with cystic fibrosis and maternal polyhydramnios. About 80% to 90% of patients with meconium ileus have cystic fibrosis; about 10% to 20% of patients with cystic fibrosis have meconium ileus (Piazza and Stoll, 2007).

Clinical Findings

History and Physical Examination

- There is a failure to pass meconium within 48 hours of life.
- Findings include abdominal distention and persistent vomiting.

Diagnostic Studies. A radiograph shows bowel loops of varying width. There is a grainy appearance at points of heaviest meconium concentration.

Associated Conditions

Infants with complicated meconium ileus may have associated intestinal disorders, including atresia, stenosis, volvulus, or perforations, and symptoms suggestive of cystic fibrosis (Wyllie, 2007).

Management and Prognosis

Treatment is individualized; high enemas (with water-soluble contrast material) or laparotomy can be used. The survival rate is good. Identification of any underlying disorders should be undertaken, and referral to a gastrointestinal specialist may be necessary.

DIAPHRAGMATIC HERNIA

Description and Epidemiology

In diaphragmatic hernia, abdominal contents herniate into the thoracic cavity. A diaphragmatic hernia is caused by failure of the pleuroperitoneal canal to close completely during embryologic development. It occurs on the left side 80% to 90% of the time with a frequency of about 1 in 2000 to 5000 live births and is more common in females (Ehrlich and Coran, 2007).

Clinical Findings

History. After birth, immediate respiratory failure occurs secondary to pulmonary hypertension or pulmonary hypoplasia. The amount of respiratory distress depends on the amount of functional lung capacity. Any newborn with respiratory distress should be evaluated for diaphragmatic hernia.

Physical Examination

- Respiratory distress with tachypnea
- Cyanosis
- Scaphoid abdomen
- Rarely, bowel sounds heard in the chest
- Absence of breath sounds
- Heart tones best heard in the contralateral chest

Diagnostic Studies. A chest radiograph shows fluid and air-filled loops of intestine in the chest. The mediastinum is displaced toward the unaffected side, usually to the right.

Management

- As soon as the diagnosis is suspected, the infant should be positioned with the head and chest higher than the abdomen.
- Intensive respiratory support, which often includes ECMO
- Surgery, with intensive respiratory and metabolic support

Prognosis

The mortality rate is about 30%, depending on the degree of hypoplastic lung (Ehrlich and Coran, 2007).

HYDROCELE AND INGUINAL HERNIA

See Chapter 34.

UMBILICAL HERNIA

Definition

Umbilical hernia is a weakness or imperfect closure of the umbilical ring.

Clinical Findings

Physical Examination. Findings include a soft swelling in the umbilical area that can be reduced, often associated with diastasis recti.

Management, Prognosis, and Education

Surgery is not required unless the hernia persists beyond 5 years old, strangulates, is nonreducible, or dramatically enlarges. Most umbilical hernias resolve spontaneously by 1 year old, but can take up to 4 to 5 years; those with fascial defects greater than 1.5 cm in diameter have a lower rate of spontaneous closure. Incarceration is extremely rare. Counsel parents to avoid taping coins or placing bellybands over the umbilicus because these efforts do not help and can contribute to infection.

RENAL CONDITIONS

ACUTE RENAL FAILURE

Description and Epidemiology

The newborn normally produces 1 to 3 mL/kg/hr of urine and urinates within the first 48 hours of life, most within the first 24 hours of life. A stressed neonate may develop decreased renal function. Urine output less than 0.5 mL/kg/hr can indicate acute renal failure and puts the infant at risk for disrupted body fluid homeostasis. Multiple causes of renal failure can be identified, including stress during the prenatal period, dehydration, sepsis, anoxia, shock, administration of nephrotoxic drugs, renal dysgenesis, obstructive uropathy, congenital heart disease, hemorrhage, and renal vein thrombosis.

Clinical Findings

History and Physical Examination

- Neonatal history of decreased or no urinary output; maternal oligohydramnios
- Abdominal mass
- Pallor, edema, lethargy, vomiting, seizures, coma
- High blood pressure
- Pulmonary edema, congestive heart failure, or arrhythmias
- Myelomeningocele
- Prune-belly syndrome

Diagnostic Studies. Order the following, as indicated:

- Bladder tap or catheterization to confirm inadequate urinary output
- Urinalysis to identify hematuria or pyuria
- Urine osmolarity, sodium, and potassium values to indicate kidney filtration ability
- Serum blood urea nitrogen, creatinine, sodium, and potassium values to indicate poor filtration (although in the first days of life these values may be reflective of maternal renal function)
- Complete blood count (CBC) including differential and platelets for evidence of thrombocytopenia, sepsis, or renal vein thrombosis

Management and Prognosis

- Replace fluid loss (approximately 30 mL/kg/24 hr), then restrict fluid and diet.
- Maintain strict intake, output, and fluid and electrolyte balance.
- Monitor blood pressure.
- Peritoneal dialysis is sometimes indicated.
- The prognosis depends on the cause and the degree of renal failure.

HYDRONEPHROSIS
Description and Epidemiology
Hydronephrosis is a dilation of one or both kidneys frequently caused by an obstruction of the ureteropelvic junction, posterior urethral valves, ectopic ureterocele, prune-belly syndrome, or ureteral or ureterovesical obstructions. Obstructive uropathy is slightly more common in males.

Clinical Findings
History and Physical Examination
- Decreased urinary output
- Findings on prenatal ultrasonogram
- Asymptomatic in early stages
- Findings include an abdominal mass.

Management and Prognosis
Surgical repair may be necessary depending on the cause of the hydronephrosis and if spontaneous resolution does not occur by 6 to 12 months old. The longer the obstruction lasts, the less likely renal function will return to normal.

CYSTIC KIDNEY DISEASE
Description and Epidemiology
The presence of multiple cysts of various sizes and shapes in the kidney can be either an autosomal dominant or autosomal recessive disease. The autosomal dominant form usually appears in the fourth or fifth decade of life and can be associated with hepatic cysts or cerebral aneurysms. In the autosomal recessive form, which also usually has hepatic cysts, the infant has abdominal masses at birth. The adult form (autosomal dominant) occurs in 1 per 500 to 1000 individuals; the juvenile form (autosomal recessive) occurs in 1 per 10,000 to 40,000 live births (Davis and Avner, 2007; Suchy, 2007).

Clinical Findings
History and Physical Examination
- Maternal oligohydramnios in the juvenile form
- Abdominal lobular mass
- Hematuria
- Hypertension
  Diagnostic Studies. A renal ultrasonogram is done to document the disorder.

Differential Diagnosis
Multicystic dysplastic kidney, hydronephrosis, von Hippel-Lindau disease, tuberous sclerosis, Wilms tumor, and renal vein thrombosis are included in the differential diagnosis.

Management and Prognosis

Monitor kidney function and check for enlargement of cysts (with a renal ultrasound) or infection. Nephrectomy may be necessary if no regression is seen or a complication occurs. Dialysis or transplantation is sometimes considered. With severe involvement, the neonate dies from pulmonary or renal insufficiency. Hypertension may be difficult to control.

RENAL ARTERY OR VEIN THROMBOSIS
Description
There is decreased blood flow to the kidney because of thrombus formation.

Clinical Findings
History and Physical Examination. In the newborn this condition is often associated with asphyxia, dehydration, shock, and sepsis. Maternal diabetes is a rare cause. Sudden onset of gross hematuria may be noted. Findings include a firm flank mass.

Diagnostic Studies. Ultrasonography shows marked enlargement of the kidney. The hematocrit is low. The urine contains protein and often blood.

Differential Diagnosis
Other causes of hematuria, such as hydronephrosis, cystic disease, Wilms tumor, hemolytic-uremic syndrome, and renal abscess, are included in the differential diagnosis.

Management
- Maintain fluid and electrolyte balance.
- Monitor blood pressure.
- Prophylactic anticoagulation therapy is occasionally given to prevent thrombosis in the other kidney.
- Nephrectomy is not necessary unless chronic infection or uncontrollable hypertension occurs.

NEUROBLASTOMA
Description and Epidemiology
A neuroblastoma is a solid tumor that originates from neural crest tissue along the craniospinal axis. The majority of neuroblastomas develop in the abdomen, usually in the adrenal gland. The cause is unknown. About 500 new cases of neuroblastoma are diagnosed each year; it is the most commonly diagnosed neoplasm in neonates (Ater, 2007).

Clinical Findings
History and Physical Examination
- An unexplained fever, mass, and symptoms related to the site of the tumor
- Firm, irregular, nontender mass in abdomen
- Pallor
- Hypotension
- Ascites
- Irritability
- Possible external tumors in newborn
  Diagnostic Studies. The following help assess and stage the disease:
- CBC, basic chemistry panel
- Renal radiographs to detect calcifications

- Ultrasound, computed tomography (CT) or magnetic resonance imaging (MRI) of abdomen
- Radiograph or CT scan of chest
- Skeletal survey or bone scan
- Urine catecholamines, homovanillic acid (HVA) and vanillylmandelic acid (VMA)
- Bone marrow aspirate and biopsy

Differential Diagnosis

Wilms tumor, hydronephrosis, renal vein thrombosis, and lymphoma are included in the differential diagnosis.

Management and Prognosis

Although some neuroblastomas regress without therapy, usually only those in children younger than 1 year old, treatment generally involves surgical removal followed by radiation therapy or chemotherapy. The prognosis depends on the age of the patient and the stage of the tumor.

RENAL AGENESIS

Description and Epidemiology

Renal agenesis is failure of the kidney to form normally. Bilateral agenesis is incompatible with life, and occurs in 1 in 3000 births (Elder, 2007).

Clinical Findings

History. Maternal oligohydramnios is noted in bilateral agenesis. Unilateral renal agenesis usually is detected on prenatal ultrasound or when the child is evaluated for other congenital anomalies or for urinary tract infection.

Physical Examination

- Single umbilical artery associated with unilateral agenesis
- Associated anomalies involving the gastrointestinal or urinary tract and skeleton, especially with Potter syndrome (bilateral agenesis)
- Low-set ears, senile appearance, broad nose, and receding chin consistent with Potter syndrome

Management and Prognosis

Monitor for proteinuria and hypertension. Patients with bilateral disease die within a few months of life.

ENDOCRINE CONDITIONS

CONGENITAL HYPOTHYROIDISM AND CONGENITAL ADRENAL HYPERPLASIA

See Chapter 25.

METABOLIC CONDITIONS

HYPOGLYCEMIA

Description and Epidemiology

In the term infant serum glucose levels rarely fall below 35 mg/dL in the first 3 hours of life, below 40 mg/dL between 3 and 24 hours of life, or below 45 mg/dL thereafter. Infants at higher risk of developing hypoglycemia include SGA infants and those with diabetic mothers, asphyxia at birth, sepsis,

erythroblastosis fetalis, glycogen storage disease, or galactosemia (Table 38-5).

Clinical Findings
History
- Risk factors for sepsis or asphyxia
- Infant of a diabetic mother
- SGA

Physical Examination
- Lethargy
- Poor feeding and regurgitation
- Apnea
- Jitteriness
- Pallor, sweating, cool extremities
- Seizures

Management and Prognosis

See Management in Table 38-5. Infants with symptomatic hypoglycemia, particularly low-birthweight infants and infants of diabetic mothers, are less likely to have normal intellectual development than are asymptomatic infants. Prognosis for normal intellectual function is guarded in infants with prolonged and severe hypoglycemia.

INFANT OF A DIABETIC MOTHER

Description and Epidemiology

An infant born to a mother whose pregnancy is complicated by poorly controlled gestational or insulin-dependent diabetes mellitus is referred to as an infant of a diabetic mother (IDM). Maternal hyperglycemia causes fetal hyperglycemia and hyperinsulinemia, leading to increased hepatic glucose uptake and glycogen synthesis, accelerated lipogenesis, and augmented protein synthesis (Hendricks-Munoz, 2006) (see Table 38-5).

Clinical Findings
History and Physical Examination
- History of a mother with diabetes, especially those who are poorly controlled
- Large and plump neonate with large viscera
- Puffy facies
- Plethora
- Hyperexcitability during the first 3 days of life, although hypotonia, lethargy, and poor sucking also occur

Management, Complications, and Prevention

See Table 38-5. Cardiomegaly is common (30%), and heart failure occurs in 5% to 10% of infants. Congenital anomalies are increased threefold; cardiac malformations (15 times greater) and lumbosacral agenesis are most common (Hendricks-Munoz, 2006). There is a predisposition to obesity in childhood that can extend into adult life. Symptomatic hypoglycemia increases the risk of impaired intellectual development. Strict management of blood glucose levels in mothers with diabetes decreases the risk of severe problems in the infant.

ORTHOPEDIC CONDITIONS

FRACTURED CLAVICLE AND BRACHIAL PALSY

See Chapter 37.

TABLE 38-5	Identification and Management of Hypoglycemia, Infant of Diabetic Mother, and Polycythemia in the Newborn		
Condition	**Clinical Finding**	**Workup**	**Management**
Hypoglycemia	Blood glucose <30 mg/dL Infant with history of SGA; poorly controlled diabetic mother (IDDM); at risk for sepsis; asphyxia; erythroblastosis fetalis Lethargy Poor feeding and regurgitation Apnea Jitteriness Pallor, sweating, cool extremities Seizures	Serum glucose—measure within 1 hr of birth, every 2 hr until 6-8 hr of life, then every 4-6 hr until 24 hr of life	Give normoglycemic high-risk infants oral or gavage feedings with breast milk or formula at 1-3 hr of life and continue every 2-3 hr for 24-48 hr; IV glucose at 8 mg/kg/min if serum glucose less than 30-35 mg/dL and oral feedings poorly tolerated (Custer and Rau, 2009).
Infant of diabetic mother (IDM)	IDDM: large, plump infant with large viscera; puffy facies; plethora; hyperactivity first 3 days; ± hypotonicity, lethargy, poor suck; ± cardiomegaly and murmur	Intensive observation and care Serum glucose—measure within 1 hr of birth, then frequently for the next 6-8 hr, especially for macrosomia or growth restriction	If clinically well and normoglycemic, initially give oral or gavage feedings with infant formula or breast milk started within 2-3 hr old and continued at 3-hr intervals. If infant is unable to tolerate oral feeding, discontinue feeding and give 10% glucose by peripheral IV infusion at a rate of 4-8 mg/kg/hr (Custer and Rau, 2009). Treat hypoglycemia, even in asymptomatic infants, with IV infusions of glucose.
Polycythemia	Cyanosis, tachypnea, respiratory distress; hyperbilirubinemia; infant with history of diabetic mother; IUGR, postmaturity, SGA exposed to chronic hypoxia; recipient of twin-twin transfusion; delayed clamping of umbilical cord Plethora Feeding disturbance	Hematocrit ≥65%	Phlebotomy and replacement with saline or albumin or partial exchange transfusion to reduce hematocrit to 50% (Custer and Rau, 2009)

IDDM, Insulin-dependent diabetes mellitus; *IUGR*, intrauterine growth retardation; *IV*, intravenous; *SGA*, small for gestational age.

POLYDACTYLY AND SYNDACTYLY

Description and Epidemiology
Polydactyly is a condition that varies from a skin tag to a formed finger or toe with a nail that extends most commonly from the postaxial side. Polydactyly occurs in 2 per 1000 births, more commonly in the African-American population (Cornwall, 2007; Hosalkar et al, 2007). In contrast, syndactyly can be identified by finding fingers or toes fused by skin and sometimes bone. Syndactyly can be seen as part of a variety of syndromes.

Clinical Findings
History and Physical Examination. There is a positive family history in 30% (Cornwall, 2007; Hosalkar et al, 2007). In polydactyly, a floppy digit is seen on the foot or hand. It varies in degree of formation. Syndactyly is webbing of two digits, partially or to the tip of the digit.

Management
For polydactyly, surgical removal of the floppy extra digit is indicated. If the digit is stabilized by bone, surgical removal is deferred until the patient is older, when function can be assessed. For patients with syndactyly, treatment is not indicated in the neonate. Surgical separation is recommended at 2 to 3 years old.

CENTRAL NERVOUS SYSTEM CONDITIONS

CONGENITAL HYDROCEPHALUS

Description and Epidemiology
Congenital hydrocephalus is an accumulation of cerebrospinal fluid (CSF) in the brain's ventricles at birth, occurring in 1 of 1000 live births (Feldstein and Anderson, 2006). Malformations, infections, intraventricular hemorrhage, and disorders in brain development can lead to congenital hydrocephalus. The incidence varies depending on which of these conditions is causative.

Clinical Findings
History and Physical Examination
- Head circumference enlarging or rapidly increasing in size
- Cranial sutures separated by large, tense fontanelles

Diagnostic Studies. Cranial ultrasonography shows dilated ventricles. Often an MRI is obtained to further define anatomy.

Management
Medications that decrease CSF production (e.g., acetazolamide), a ventriculoperitoneal shunt, or both are used. Referral should be prompt.

INTRAVENTRICULAR HEMORRHAGE

Description and Epidemiology

Intraventricular hemorrhage (IVH) occurs within the ventricles of the brain, usually within the first 72 hours of life. Risk factors include prematurity, RDS, hypoxic-ischemic or hypotensive injury, increased or decreased cerebral blood flow, hypertension, hypervolemia, and reduced vascular integrity. The incidence of IVH decreases with increasing gestational age. Infants weighing less than 1000 g are especially prone to severe IVH (Adams-Chapman and Stoll, 2007).

Clinical Findings

History and Physical Examination

- Risk factors include SGA, prematurity, and others mentioned above.
- Diminished or absent Moro reflex
- Poor muscle tone, lethargy, somnolence
- Apnea
- Periods of pallor or cyanosis
- Failure to suck well
- High-pitched, shrill cry; seizures

Diagnostic Studies. Ultrasonography is used to classify IVH into grades I to IV based on the presence and quantity of blood in the ventricles or brain tissue. Screening cranial ultrasounds are routinely performed on all small premature infants. Recommendations include screening infants between 1250 and 1500 g at 3 to 5 days and before discharge; on infants weighing between 1000 and 1250 g at 3 to 5 days, at 28 days, and before discharge; and on infants less than 1000 g at 3 to 5 days, at 10 to 14 days, at 28 days, and before discharge (Perlman, 2006).

Management and Prognosis

Treatment may include the following:
- Glucocorticoid given antenatally to reduce severe IVH
- Supportive management and minimal stimulation
- Indomethacin to reduce the severity of IVH
- Acetazolamide to decrease CSF production
- Repeated lumbar punctures
- Ventriculoperitoneal shunt or external ventriculostomy

Outcome is related to white matter involvement, with grade IV being associated with the most adverse outcome (Perlman, 2006).

HYPOXIC-ISCHEMIC INSULTS

Description and Epidemiology

Hypoxic-ischemic insult in the newborn is divided into three stages of injury (stages I, II, and III, or mild, moderate, and severe) (Table 38-6). Brain damage results from fetal hypoxia or ischemia over an extended period. The initial hypoxic or ischemic insult is followed by metabolic and respiratory acidosis. Compensatory mechanisms, such as shunting blood through the ductus to maintain perfusion of the brain, heart, adrenals, kidneys, liver, and intestines, ultimately fail if the insult is severe enough. Depending on the organ most damaged, a variety of signs and symptoms can be seen; 15% to 20% of infants with hypoxic-ischemic encephalopathy die in the neonatal period, and up to 30% develop permanent neurodevelopmental disabilities. Causes of the initial hypoxic or ischemic insult include abruptio placentae, hemorrhage, cord compression, mechanical injury, severe maternal hypertension or diabetes, and inadequate resuscitation of the infant (Adams-Chapman and Stoll, 2007).

Clinical Findings

Physical Examination

- Seizure activity
- Pallor
- Cyanosis, apnea
- Bradycardia and unresponsiveness to stimulation

Management and Prognosis

The prognosis depends on the effectiveness of managing the underlying symptoms. Severe complications (hypoxia, hypoglycemia, shock) and encephalopathy characterized by flaccid coma, apnea, and seizures are associated with a poor prognosis (Adams-Chapman and Stoll, 2007). An infant who remains neurologically abnormal after the initial recovery phase (2 weeks) likely has suffered permanent neurologic impairment. A low Apgar score at 20 minutes, absence of spontaneous respirations, and persistence of abnormal neurologic signs at 2 weeks old predict death or severe cognitive and motor

TABLE 38-6	Hypoxic-Ischemic Encephalopathy in Term Infants		
Signs	**Stage 1**	**Stage 2**	**Stage 3**
Level of consciousness	Hyperalert	Lethargic	Stuporous, coma
Muscle tone	Normal	Hypotonic	Flaccid
Posture	Normal	Flexion	Decerebrate
Tendon reflexes/clonus	Hyperactive	Hyperactive	Absent
Myoclonus	Present	Present	Absent
Moro reflex	Strong	Weak	Absent
Pupils	Mydriasis	Miosis	Unequal, poor light reflex
Seizures	None	Common	Decerebration
Electroencephalograph	Normal	Low-voltage changing to seizure activity	Burst suppression to isoelectric
Duration	<24 hours if progresses, otherwise may remain normal	24 hours to 24 days	Days to weeks
Outcome	Good	Variable	Death, severe deficits

Adapted from Sarnat H, Sarnat M: Neonatal encephalopathy following fetal distress: a clinical and electroencephalopathic study, *Arch Neurol* 33:696, 1976; cited in Kliegman R, Behrman RE, Jenson HB et al, editors: *Nelson textbook of pediatrics*, ed 18, Philadelphia, 2007, Saunders.

deficits; Apgar scores done at 1 and 5 minutes are far less predictive of outcome (AAP, 2006).

MYELOMENINGOCELE

Description and Epidemiology

A myelomeningocele is the result of failure to close the posterior neural tube and the vertebral column. This is the most severe form of neural tube defect occurring in 1 per 4000 live births (Kinsman and Johnston, 2007). Genetic and environmental factors are believed to play a causative role (see Chapter 27 for more information).

Clinical Findings

History and Physical Examination

- Poor intake of folic acid and exposure to hyperthermia or valproic acid
- Saclike cyst containing meninges and spinal fluid covered by thin layer of partially epithelialized skin; 75% found in the lumbosacral area
- Flaccid paralysis of lower extremities
- Absence of deep tendon reflexes
- Lack of response to touch and pain
- Constant urinary dribbling

Management, Prognosis, and Prevention

Surgical repair and multidisciplinary supportive management are indicated. The mortality rate is 10% to 15% in aggressively treated children with most deaths occurring before 4 years old. At least 70% have normal intelligence, but seizure disorders, hydrocephalus, learning disabilities, and neurogenic bowel and bladder are more common than in the general population (Kinsman and Johnston, 2007). Folic acid supplementation (400 mcg/day) with a daily multivitamin is helpful in preventing neural tube defects and should be taken by all females of childbearing age. Prenatal vitamins have at least 400 mcg/vitamin; however, additional folic acid supplementation (4000 mcg) is recommended for those women who have had a child with a neural tube defect (AAP, 2010; Centers for Disease Control and Prevention [CDC], 1991, 2010a).

HEMATOLOGIC CONDITIONS

POLYCYTHEMIA

Description and Epidemiology

Polycythemia is characterized by a central hematocrit of 65% or higher. Polycythemia can occur in a variety of conditions, including IDM, cyanotic congenital heart disease, and infants with growth retardation who were exposed to chronic fetal hypoxia that stimulated erythropoietin production and increased red blood cell production. Polycythemia occurs in 1% to 2% of term AGA births, depending on the etiology (see Table 38-5).

Clinical Findings

History

- Diabetic mother
- Recipient of a twin-twin transfusion
- Delayed clamping of umbilical cord
- Postmature infant
- SGA

Physical Examination

- Infants with polycythemia may be asymptomatic
- Feeding disturbances
- Hypoglycemia
- Cyanosis (persistent fetal circulation), tachypnea, respiratory distress
- Hyperbilirubinemia

Management and Prognosis

See Table 38-5. Long-term problems may include speech deficits, abnormal fine motor control, reduced IQ, and other neurologic abnormalities as a result of the decreased brain tissue perfusion both with and without intervention.

HEMORRHAGIC DISEASE IN THE NEWBORN

Description and Epidemiology

Severe transient deficiencies of vitamin K–dependent clotting factors lead to bleeding. Hemorrhagic disease is caused by a lack of free vitamin K in the mother and absence of bacterial intestinal flora normally responsible for synthesis of vitamin K in the infant. Vitamin K–dependent clotting factors (factors II, VII, IX, X) are normal at birth, but decrease within 2 to 3 days. Breast milk is a poor source of vitamin K; late-onset bleeding (occurring 1 to 3 months after birth) is rare, but may be seen in exclusively breastfed infants. A particularly severe form of deficiency of vitamin K–dependent coagulation factors occurring in the first day of life has been reported in women receiving the anticonvulsants phenytoin and/or phenobarbital.

Clinical Findings

History and Physical Examination

- Anticonvulsant (phenytoin or phenobarbital) use by the mother
- Prematurity
- Exclusive breastfeeding without vitamin K supplementation
- Failure to administer parenteral vitamin K at birth
- Neonatal hepatitis or biliary atresia
- Gastrointestinal, nasal, subgaleal, or intracranial bleeding or bleeding at the site of an injection or circumcision

  Diagnostic Studies. Prothrombin time, blood coagulation time, and partial thromboplastin time are prolonged.

Differential Diagnosis

This disorder may be the result of disseminated intravascular coagulation or congenital bleeding disorders unrelated to vitamin K.

Management, Prevention, and Prognosis

- IV infusion of 1 to 5 mg of vitamin K is needed. Improvement of coagulation defects and cessation of bleeding should occur within a few hours.
- If a newborn is delivered at home, confirm vitamin K was given.
- Prevention of early- and late-onset bleeding is achieved by routinely giving 1 mg of natural oil-soluble vitamin K intramuscularly within 1 hour of birth. Prognosis depends on the site and extent of bleeding.

ANEMIA

Description and Epidemiology

Anemia is characterized by less than the normal range of hemoglobin for birthweight and postnatal age. Anemia occurs secondary to acute blood loss before or during delivery. Acute blood loss after delivery can be external (gastrointestinal, circumcision site, umbilical stump), internal (fracture site, cephalhematoma, pulmonary hemorrhage, injured internal organ), or secondary to hemolysis or congenital aplastic or hypoplastic anemia.

Clinical Findings
History and Physical Examination
- Twin-twin transfusion
- Unexpected tearing or delayed clamping of umbilical cord resulting in neonatal blood loss
- Internal hemorrhage (caused by fracture, cephalhematoma, or internal organ trauma)
- Umbilical stump or circumcision bleeding
- Pallor, congestive heart failure, and shock possible

Management and Prognosis

Treatment depends on the cause. An asymptomatic full-term infant with a hemoglobin level of 10 g/dL can be observed, whereas a symptomatic neonate born after abruptio placentae or with severe hemolytic disease of the newborn warrants transfusion. Treatment with blood should be balanced by concern about transfusion-acquired infection with cytomegalovirus (CMV), HIV, and hepatitis B and C viruses. Prognosis depends on the cause and severity of the anemia.

BLOOD IN VOMITUS OR STOOL

Description and Epidemiology

Bright red or dark red blood in the vomitus or stool can be seen without clinical evidence of blood loss. This problem often is caused by ingestion of maternal blood during delivery.

Clinical Findings
Physical Examination. Bright red or dark red blood is seen in vomitus or stool.

Diagnostic Studies. Blood of maternal origin can be differentiated from infant blood by testing for fetal hemoglobin using the Apt test.

Differential Diagnosis

The differential diagnosis includes infant gastrointestinal bleeding caused by trauma, duplication of bowel, intussusception, volvulus, hemangioma or telangiectasia of bowel, rectal prolapse, vitamin K deficiency, or anal fissure.

Management

No treatment is necessary if blood is of maternal origin, although breakdown of maternal blood may exaggerate neonatal jaundice.

JAUNDICE

Description and Epidemiology

Jaundice, a clinically apparent accumulation of bilirubin in the skin, causes a yellowish orange or sometimes green hue to the skin. Jaundice becomes apparent when serum bilirubin levels exceed 5 to 7 mg/dL and usually advances in a pattern from the infant's head to the toes (Table 38-7). Physiologic jaundice is the most common type of jaundice in the newborn period with the infant showing no signs of illness. Classic physiologic jaundice is characterized by a rise in bilirubin from 1.5 mg/dL in cord blood to 5 to 6 mg/dL on the third day of life, declining to a normal adult level (less than 1.3 to 1.5 mg/dL) by 10 to 12 days in Caucasian and African-American infants. Asian infants reach 8 to 12 mg/dL on day 4 to 5 and decline more slowly; 2% of Asian newborns and 1% of Caucasians and African-Americans have serum bilirubin higher than 20 mg/dL in the first week of life. Breast milk jaundice can be divided into early-onset and late-onset types. Early-onset breast milk jaundice develops within 2 to 4 days of birth and is believed to occur as a result of infrequent breastfeeding and insufficient intake leading to decreased intestinal motility. Late-onset breast milk jaundice develops 4 to 7 days after birth, peaks at 10 to 15 days of life, and frequently persists. See Chapter 11 on breastfeeding for more information.

Nonphysiologic (pathologic) jaundice appears at less than 24 hours old and may last longer than 8 days. The rate of increase in total bilirubin is rapid at greater than 0.5 mg/dL/hr. Total bilirubin levels are frequently greater than 12.5 mg/dL before 48 hours old, or the direct bilirubin exceeds 1.5 to 2 mg/dL. Kernicterus or bilirubin encephalopathy involves toxicity of the nervous system resulting from very high levels of bilirubin. The estimated minimal level of risk for kernicterus and thus considering exchange transfusion is probably at 25 to 30 mg/dL in healthy term infants (AAP, 2004).

Jaundice is observed during the first week of life in approximately 60% of term infants (Piazza and Stoll, 2007). Causes include:
- Increased rate of hemolysis: ABO incompatibility, Rh incompatibility, abnormal red blood cell shapes (spherocytosis, elliptocytosis, pyknocytosis, and stomatocytosis), red blood cell enzyme abnormalities (glucose-6-phosphate dehydrogenase deficiency, pyruvate kinase deficiency)
- Decreased rate of conjugation: Immaturity of bilirubin conjugation (physiologic jaundice), congenital familial nonhemolytic jaundice (inborn errors of metabolism affecting glucuronyl transferase system and bilirubin transport), breast milk jaundice
- Abnormalities of excretion or absorption: Sepsis, hepatitis (viral, parasitic, bacterial, toxic), metabolic abnormalities (galactosemia, glycogen storage disease, IDM, cystic fibrosis), biliary atresia, choledochal cyst, obstruction of ampulla of Vater (annular pancreas), drugs

Clinical Findings
Family History. The following are risk factors for the development of hyperbilirubinemia:
- Significant hemolytic disease, anemia
- Inborn errors of metabolism
- Early or severe jaundice
- Ethnic or geographic origin associated with hemolytic anemia
- Hepatobiliary disease
- Previous sibling received phototherapy
History
- ABO or Rh incompatibilities in previous pregnancies
- Sepsis risk for the infant, such as prolonged rupture of maternal membranes
- Macrosomic infant of a diabetic mother

TABLE 38-7 Diagnostic Features of the Various Types of Neonatal Jaundice

Diagnosis	Nature of Van Den Bergh Reaction	JAUNDICE		PEAK BILIRUBIN CONCENTRATION		Bilirubin Rate of Accumulation (mg/dL/day)	Remarks
		Appears	Disappears	mg/dL	Age (days)		
Physiologic jaundice							Usually relates to degree of maturity; infant shows no signs of illness
Full-term	Indirect	2-3 days	4-5 days	10-12	2-3	<5	
Premature	Indirect	3-4 days	7-9 days	15	6-8	<5	
Hyper-bilirubinemia caused by metabolic factors							Metabolic factors: hypoxia, respiratory distress, lack of carbohydrate
Full-term	Indirect	2-3 days	Variable	>12	First week	<5	Hormonal influences: cretinism
Premature	Indirect	3-4 days	Variable	>15	First week	<5	Genetic factors: Crigler-Najjar syndrome, transient familial hyperbilirubinemia Drugs: vitamin K, novobiocin
Hemolytic states and hematoma	Indirect	May appear in first 24 hours	Variable	Unlimited	Variable	Usually >5	Erythroblastosis: Rh, ABO Congenital hemolytic states: spherocytic, nonspherocytic Infantile pyknocytosis Drugs: vitamin K; enclosed hemorrhage—hematoma
Mixed hemolytic and hepatotoxic factors	Indirect and direct	May appear in first 24 hours	Variable	Unlimited	Variable	Usually >5	Infection: bacterial sepsis, pyelonephritis, hepatitis, toxoplasmosis, cytomegalic inclusion disease, rubella Drugs: vitamin K
Hepatocellular damage	Indirect and direct	Usually 2-3 days	Variable	Unlimited	Variable	Variable; can be >5	Biliary atresia; galactosemia; hepatitis, infection

From Brown AK: Diagnostic features of the various types of neonatal jaundice, *Pediatr Clin North Am* 9:589, 1962; cited in Kliegman R, Behrman RE, Jenson HB et al, editors: *Nelson textbook of pediatrics*, ed 18, Philadelphia, 2007, Saunders.

Physical Examination

- Jaundice at birth or at any time during the neonatal period, depending on the underlying condition, with face affected first, followed by the shoulders, chest, and abdomen. Jaundice from deposition of indirect bilirubin in the skin tends to appear bright yellow or orange; jaundice of the obstructive type (direct bilirubin) appears greenish or muddy yellow, with the difference apparent only in severe jaundice. There is no dependable relationship between the intensity of jaundice and the degree of hyperbilirubinemia.
- A crude estimate of the level of jaundice can be based on the dermal zone in which the jaundice is noticed. This estimate should not be used to determine bilirubin levels or management, but it can help determine whether acquiring a total serum bilirubin (TSB) or a transcutaneous bilirubin (TcB) is warranted.
  - Head and neck—a mean bilirubin of 6 mg/dL
  - Trunk and umbilicus—a mean bilirubin of 9 mg/dL
  - Groin including the upper thighs—a mean bilirubin of 12 mg/dL
  - Knees and elbows (including the ankles and wrists) or to the feet and hands (including the palms and soles)—a mean bilirubin of 15 mg/dL
- Petechiae, bruising, hepatosplenomegaly, or signs of infection
- Lethargy, hypotonia, poor feeding, and loss of the Moro reflex are common initial signs of bilirubin toxicity to the brain (kernicterus). These symptoms are subtle and indistinguishable from those of sepsis, asphyxia, hypoglycemia, intracranial hemorrhage, and other acute illnesses in the neonate.
- Diminished tendon reflexes, respiratory distress, failure to suck, opisthotonos, bulging fontanelle, twitching of face or limbs, seizures, and a shrill, high-pitched cry are later signs of kernicterus.

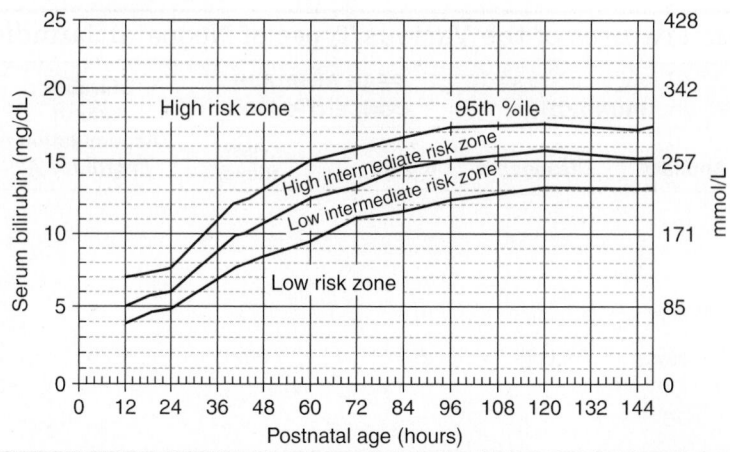

FIGURE 38-11 Nomogram for designation of risk in 2840 well newborns at 36 or more weeks' gestational age with birthweight of 2000 g or more or 35 or more weeks' gestational age and birthweight of 2500 g or more based on the hour-specific serum bilirubin values. (From the Academy of Pediatrics Subcommittee on Hyperbilirubinemia: Clinical practice guideline: management of hyperbilirubinemia in the newborn infant 35 or more weeks of gestation, *Pediatrics* 114:297-316, 2004.)

Diagnostic Studies

- TcB
- TSB level (indirect and direct) for infants who have a TcB more than 15, for darker skinned infants, or for infants under phototherapy
- If the provider suspects that the total bilirubin is significantly elevated for the age of the infant, extra blood can be drawn and held for further testing, eliminating a return visit, stick, and/or unnecessary expense if all of the tests are not later indicated. Tests that may be indicated include:
  - ABO, Rh, blood type, isoimmune antibodies of mother (should be available at prenatal and delivering hospital), Coombs test on infant (many times this is done at delivery and held in the hospital's laboratory)
  - Hemoglobin, hematocrit, reticulocyte count

Elevated indirect (unconjugated) serum bilirubin with a normal reticulocyte count and negative Coombs test indicates conditions such as physiologic jaundice, breast milk jaundice, or congenital familial nonhemolytic jaundice. Elevated indirect serum bilirubin with an increased reticulocyte count indicates increased hemolysis secondary to conditions such as isoimmunization (positive Coombs test, such as caused by ABO or Rh incompatibility), abnormal red blood cell shape, or red blood cell enzyme abnormalities. Elevated indirect and direct serum bilirubin with a negative Coombs test and a normal reticulocyte count indicates hepatitis, metabolic abnormalities, biliary atresia, choledochal cyst (in the bile duct), gastrointestinal or pancreatic obstruction, sepsis, or drugs.

Pathologic jaundice requires a more in-depth workup for the cause. Risk factors include:

- Appearance of jaundice in first 24 hours of life
- Rise of bilirubin greater than 0.5 mg/dL/hr
- Conjugated bilirubin greater than 2 mg/dL

Management and Prevention

Prevention of severe hyperbilirubinemia and bilirubin encephalopathy in infants requires the promotion and support of successful breastfeeding, systematic assessment of the newborn for the risk of hyperbilirubinemia, early and focused follow-up based on the risk assessment, and treatment when indicated.

- Promote breastfeeding by advising mothers to put the baby to the breast 8 to 12 times per day for the first several days and discourage the use of routine supplementation of water or dextrose water.
- In the healthy full-term (greater than 35 weeks) infant, physical findings, bilirubin level according to age and designation of risk are helpful in determining the course of treatment (Figs. 38-11, 38-12, and 38-13).
- Phototherapy is used to treat elevated indirect hyperbilirubinemia. Home phototherapy can be used for those infants without risk factors and with TSB levels 2 to 3 mg/dL less than those shown in Figure 38-12. Phototherapy is contraindicated with elevated direct bilirubin. The infant should be dressed only in a diaper and should be wearing eye shields. Three types of phototherapy are used:
  - Banks of overhead lights placed close to the infant requires eyepatch removal at regular intervals, taking care to prevent corneal abrasions; monitoring of temperature; increased fluid intake in response to evaporative water losses; and avoidance of oral drugs because of decreased absorption
  - Biliblanket (fiberoptic pad) allows ongoing interaction between mother and infant
  - Bilibed
- If the breastfeeding infant requires phototherapy, breastfeeding should be continued. It is also an option to temporarily interrupt breastfeeding (have the mother pump to maintain her supply) and substitute formula for 24 hours. In breastfed infants receiving phototherapy, supplementation with expressed breast milk or milk-based formula is appropriate if the infant's intake is inadequate, weight loss is excessive (greater than 10% of birthweight), or the infant seems dehydrated (AAP, 2004).
- Rebound bilirubin testing (measurement of bilirubin after phototherapy is discontinued) is not required in full-term newborns with physiologic jaundice (AAP, 2004).

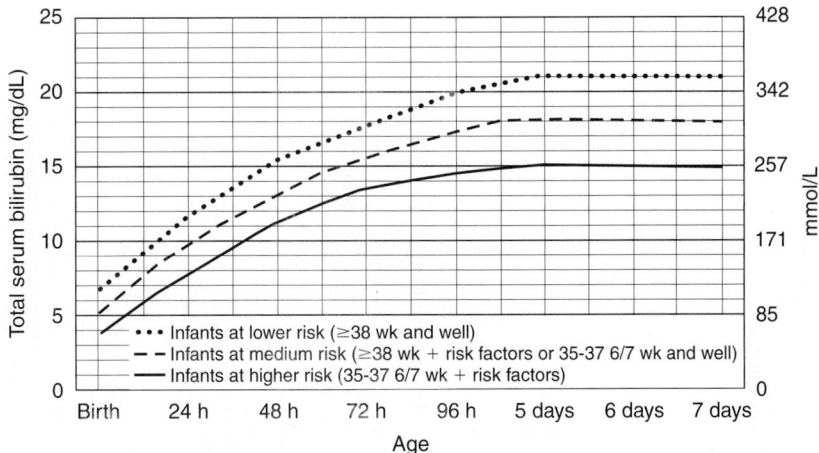

- Use total bilirubin. Do not subtract direct-reacting or conjugated bilirubin.
- Risk factors = isoimmune hemolytic disease, G6PD deficiency, asphyxia, significant lethargy, temperature instability, sepsis, acidosis, or albumin <3 g/dL (if measured)
- For well infants 35-37 6/7 weeks can adjust TSB levels for intervention around the medium risk line. It is an option to intervene at lower TSB levels for infants closer to 35 wks and at higher TSB levels for those closer to 37 6/7 weeks.
- It is an option to provide conventional phototherapy in hospital or at home at TSB levels 2-3 mg/dL (35-50 mmol/L) below those shown but home phototherapy should not be used in any infant with risk factors.

FIGURE 38-12 Guidelines for phototherapy in hospitalized infants of 35 or more weeks of gestation. (From the Academy of Pediatrics Subcommittee on Hyperbilirubinemia: Clinical practice guideline: management of hyperbilirubinemia in the newborn infant 35 or more weeks of gestation, *Pediatrics* 114:297-316, 2004.)

- Guidelines for exchange transfusion levels are available in the AAP practice parameter on the management of hyperbilirubinemia.

INFECTIONS OF THE NEWBORN

Three mechanisms for acquiring neonatal infections exist:
- Transplacental, when the mother acquires an organism that invades her bloodstream and passes through the placenta
- Vertical, when organisms in the vagina invade the amniotic fluid within the uterus
- Horizontal, when the newborn is exposed to environmental agents after birth

Syphilis is transplacentally acquired; herpes, gonorrhea, GBS, *Listeria, Escherichia coli,* and *Chlamydia trachomatis* are typically vertically acquired (Fanaroff and Martin, 2006; Remington and Klein, 2005). Staphylococcal infection is the most common horizontal infection. The most common means for horizontal transmission are the unwashed hands of health care providers.

Risk factors for sepsis (systemic infection) in the newborn include early rupture of amniotic membranes followed by preterm labor, prolonged rupture of membranes, maternal fever, maternal diagnosis of chorioamnionitis, maternal tachycardia, fetal tachycardia, and malodorous amniotic fluid. The neonate with sepsis can be asymptomatic or have nonspecific symptoms (Fanaroff and Martin, 2006; Remington and Klein, 2005). This is in part caused by a delayed immune response to local infection, allowing the neonate to bypass the typical signs and symptoms of infection (e.g., fever). Organisms quickly invade the systemic circulation,

and significant deterioration occurs before it can be clinically recognized. Because of the serious nature of neonatal sepsis, significant risk factors or a clinically unstable neonate without perinatal risk factors warrants investigation and initiation of appropriate antibiotics (Box 38-5 lists an overview of neonatal sepsis).

TOXOPLASMOSIS
Description and Epidemiology
Toxoplasmosis is an infection caused by *Toxoplasma gondii,* an obligate intracellular protozoan. *T. gondii* infects most species of warm-blooded animals, particularly cats. Cats excrete oocysts in their stools; intermediate hosts include cattle, pigs, and sheep. Humans become infected by consumption of poorly cooked meat or by accidental ingestion of oocysts from soil or in contaminated food. Depending on the timing of the infection, 17% to 65% of untreated women who acquire toxoplasmosis during gestation transmit the parasite to their fetuses (McLeod and Remington, 2007).

Clinical Findings
History and Physical Examination
- Prematurity and low Apgar scores
- Infants with congenital infection are asymptomatic at birth in 70% to 90% of cases (AAP, 2009b).
- Jaundice
- Anemia
- Hepatosplenomegaly
- Chorioretinitis
- Microcephaly

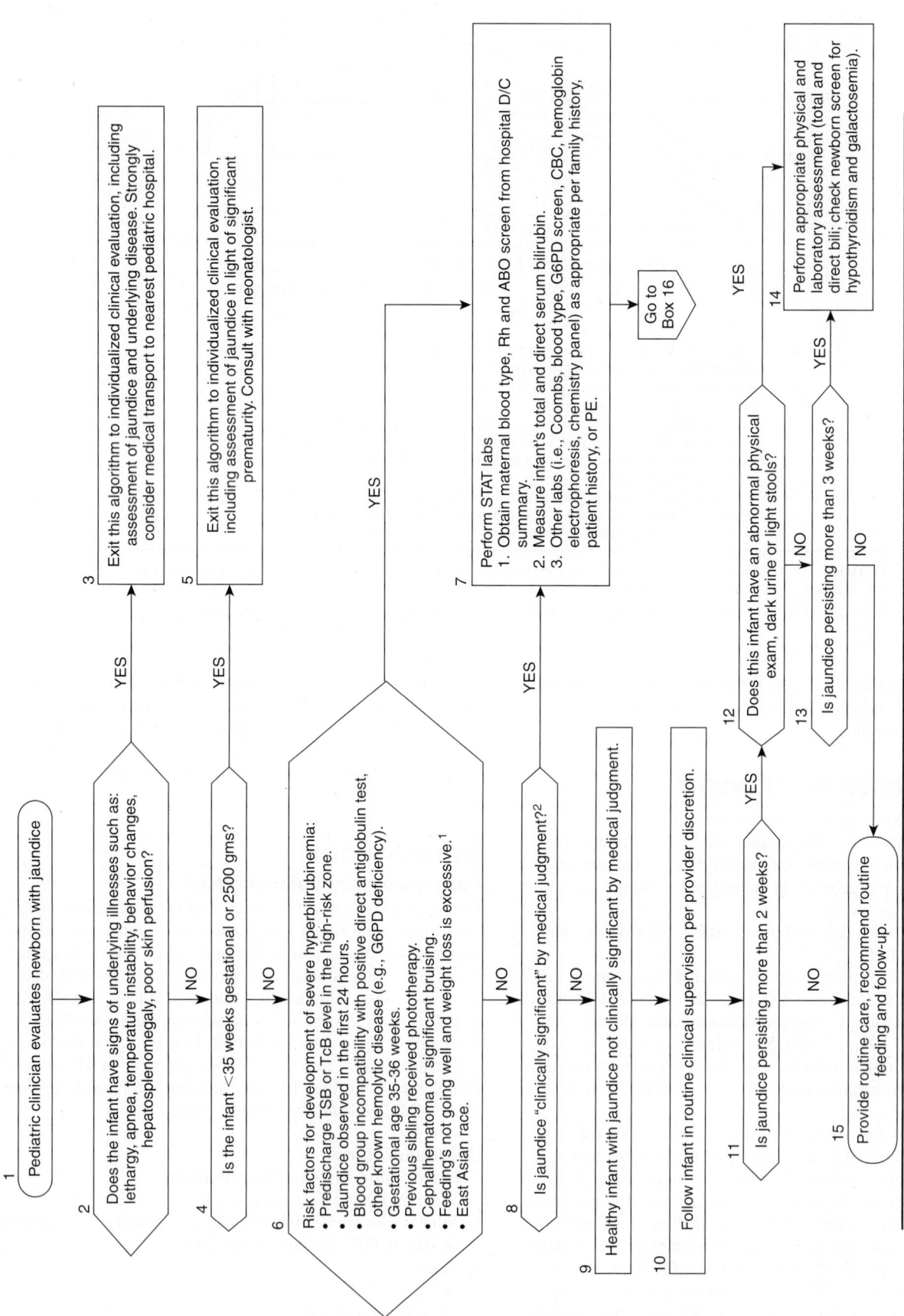

FIGURE 38-13 Algorithm for the management of neonatal hyperbilirubinemia in the outpatient setting. (Modified and used with permission of the Multnomah County Health Department, Primary Care Division, Portland, OR.)

1 Pediatric clinician evaluates newborn with jaundice

2 Does the infant have signs of underlying illnesses such as: lethargy, apnea, temperature instability, behavior changes, hepatosplenomegaly, poor skin perfusion?

YES → 3 Exit this algorithm to individualized clinical evaluation, including assessment of jaundice and underlying disease. Strongly consider medical transport to nearest pediatric hospital.

NO

4 Is the infant <35 weeks gestational or 2500 gms?

YES → 5 Exit this algorithm to individualized clinical evaluation, including assessment of jaundice in light of significant prematurity. Consult with neonatologist.

NO

6 Risk factors for development of severe hyperbilirubinemia:
- Predischarge TSB or TcB level in the high-risk zone.
- Jaundice observed in the first 24 hours.
- Blood group incompatibility with positive direct antiglobulin test, other known hemolytic disease (e.g., G6PD deficiency).
- Gestational age 35-36 weeks.
- Previous sibling received phototherapy.
- Cephalhematoma or significant bruising.
- Feeding's not going well and weight loss is excessive.[1]
- East Asian race.

YES → 7 Perform STAT labs
1. Obtain maternal blood type, Rh and ABO screen from hospital D/C summary.
2. Measure infant's total and direct serum bilirubin.
3. Other labs (i.e., Coombs, blood type, G6PD screen, CBC, hemoglobin electrophoresis, chemistry panel) as appropriate per family history, patient history, or PE.

→ Go to Box 16

NO

8 Is jaundice "clinically significant" by medical judgment?[2]

YES → (to Box 7)

NO

9 Healthy infant with jaundice not clinically significant by medical judgment.

10 Follow infant in routine clinical supervision per provider discretion.

11 Is jaundice persisting more than 2 weeks?

YES → 12 Does this infant have an abnormal physical exam, dark urine or light stools?

YES → 14 Perform appropriate physical and laboratory assessment (total and direct bili; check newborn screen for hypothyroidism and galactosemia).

NO → 13 Is jaundice persisting more than 3 weeks?

YES → (to Box 14)

NO

NO → 15 Provide routine care, recommend routine feeding and follow-up.

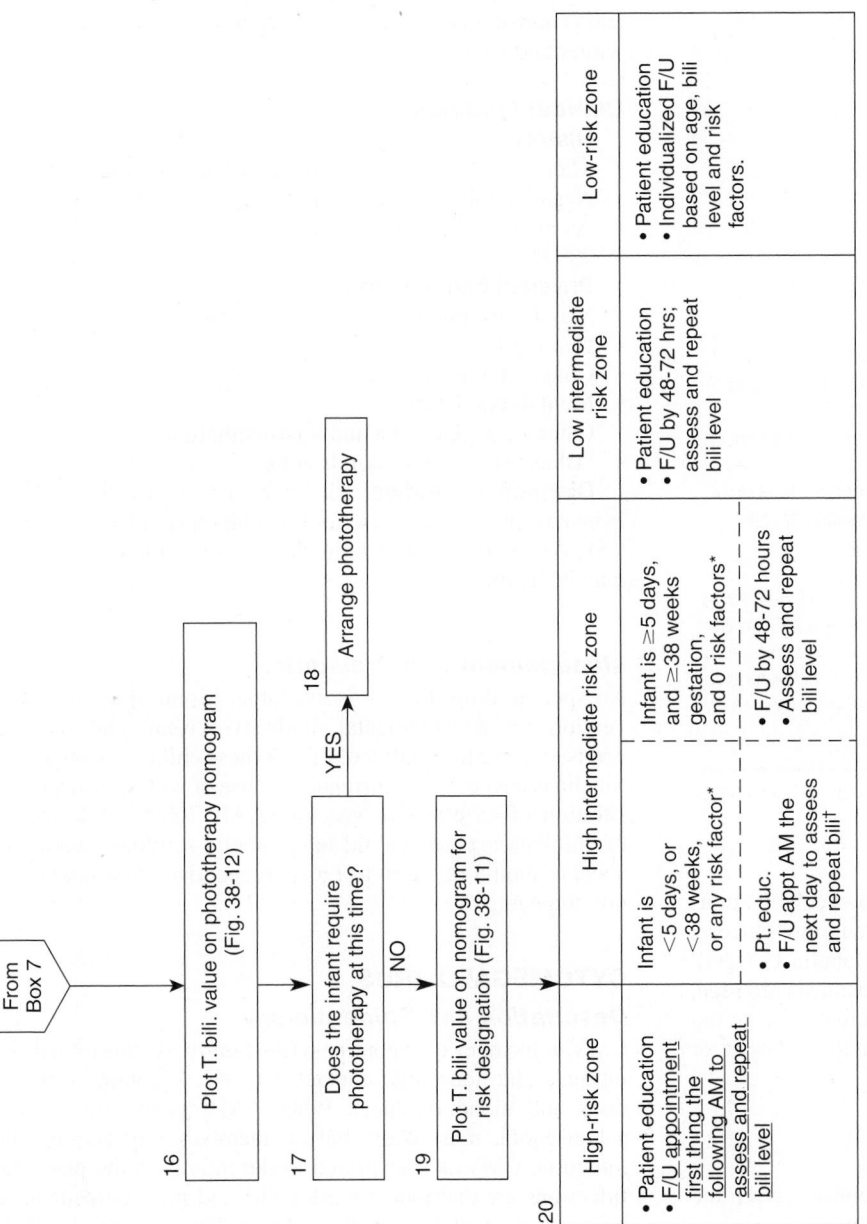

From Box 7

16 Plot T. bili. value on phototherapy nomogram (Fig. 38-12)

17 Does the infant require phototherapy at this time?

YES → 18 Arrange phototherapy

NO

19 Plot T. bili value on nomogram for risk designation (Fig. 38-11)

20

High-risk zone	High intermediate risk zone	Low intermediate risk zone	Low-risk zone
• Patient education • F/U appointment first thing the following AM to assess and repeat bili level	Infant is (<5 days, or <38 weeks, or any risk factor* • Pt. educ. • F/U appt AM the next day to assess and repeat bili†	Infant is ≥5 days, and ≥38 weeks gestation, and 0 risk factors* • F/U by 48-72 hours • Assess and repeat bili level	• Patient education • F/U by 48-72 hrs; assess and repeat bili level	• Patient education • Individualized F/U based on age, bili level and risk factors.

* Risk factors as defined in Box #6

† If infant's bilirubin levels have stabilized at the high intermediate risk zone or below, follow up can be slightly later than the above recommendations

¹ Weight loss of >10% of birth weight is excessive at 72-96 hrs, or >12% after 96 hrs. Breastfed babies usually reach their maximum weight loss on day three. To additionally assess adequacy of intake in breastfed infants consider normal 4-6 wet diapers/24 hours; 3-4 stools/day by day four. Change from meconium to yellow soft breast stool by day four.

² Severely jaundiced infants should be referred immediately to the ED for assessment in order to expedite medical intervention.

ABO, Blood types; *AM*, morning; *bili*, bilirubin; *CBC*, complete blood count; *D/C*, discharge; *ED*, emergency department; *F/U*, follow-up; *G6PD* glucose-6-phosphate dehydrogenase; *hr*, hour; *PE*, physical exam; *Rh*, rhesus; *T.bili*, total bilirubin; *TcB*, transcutaneus bilirubin; *TSB*, total serum bilirubin; *wk*, week.

FIGURE 38-13—cont'd

BOX 38-5 Neonatal Sepsis

History
"Not doing well"
Temperature instability (often hypothermia)
Jitteriness
Poor feeding, vomiting
Irritability or lethargy
Apnea or respiratory distress
Seizures

Physical Examination
Jaundice
Pallor
Petechiae or purpura
Rash
Hepatosplenomegaly
Poor tone and perfusion
Tachycardia or bradycardia
Tachypnea
Cyanosis, grunting, flaring, retractions

Laboratory Evaluation
Blood for CBC with differential, platelet count, and culture—looking for anemia; increase or decrease in WBC count with left shift; thrombocytopenia; serum ammonia for urea cycle defects
  Urine—culture usually not done in the first 72 hours of life because of low yield
  CSF often obtained for protein, glucose, cell count, and culture—looking for elevated protein and WBC count; depressed glucose

Management
Combination broad-spectrum antibiotic coverage for gram-positive cocci, gram-negative bacilli, and *Listeria* is recommended. Consider adding coverage for herpes infection when suspected. *Listeria* is treated with ampicillin; *GBS* can be treated with the penicillins and the cephalosporins; gram-negative organisms are well covered by aminoglycosides and some cephalosporins.

CBC, Complete blood count; *CSF,* cerebrospinal fluid; *GBS,* group B streptococcus; *WBC,* white blood cell.

Diagnostic Studies. CT of the brain shows calcifications or hydrocephalus. The CSF shows high protein, low glucose, and evidence of *T. gondii.* Serum immunoglobulin G (IgG), IgM, IgA, and IgE antibodies against toxoplasmosis are seen. The organism can be isolated by inoculation into mice or tissue culture of blood from the placenta, the umbilical cord, or the infant.

Differential Diagnosis

Sepsis, syphilis, and hemolytic disease are considered in the differential diagnosis.

Management, Prognosis, and Prevention

Pyrimethamine plus sulfadiazine (with folic acid supplementation) for up to 1 year is often recommended. Treatment usually eliminates the manifestations of toxoplasmosis, such as active chorioretinitis, meningitis, encephalitis, hepatitis, splenomegaly, and thrombocytopenia. However, infants with extensive involvement at birth have mild to severe impairment of vision, hearing, cognitive function, and other neurologic

functions. No protective vaccine is available. Pregnant women should be informed not to handle raw meat or contaminated cat litter, to wash fruits and vegetables before consumption, to cook meat and eggs well, and to drink pasteurized milk.

CONGENITAL RUBELLA
Description and Epidemiology

Rubella is a ribonucleic acid (RNA) virus. Rubella is transmitted by person-to-person contact; the virus infects the placenta and is transmitted to the fetus. It occurs more frequently in the winter and spring.

Clinical Findings
History
- Maternal infection before 16 weeks of gestation
- Negative rubella titers in mother
- As many as 50% of infected women asymptomatic (AAP, 2009b)

Physical Examination
- May be asymptomatic in the newborn period
- Hearing loss
- Congenital heart disease
- Mental retardation
- Cataract or glaucoma and microphthalmia
- "Blueberry muffin" skin lesions

Diagnostic Studies. The rubella virus can be isolated from nasopharyngeal secretions, conjunctiva, urine, stool, and CSF. Alternatively, measurement of serum immunoglobulins may be helpful.

Management and Prevention

No specific drug therapy is available. Monitoring and intervention for developmental, auditory, visual, and medical needs improve the quality of life for these children. Congenital rubella is now a rare occurrence because of widespread administration of an effective vaccine (AAP, 2009b). All women of childbearing age should have rubella serology titers, and vaccine should be given to IgG-seronegative women who are not pregnant.

CYTOMEGALOVIRUS
Description and Epidemiology

CMV, a member of the herpesvirus family, is transmitted via intimate and household contact with virus-containing secretions and blood products. When CMV is introduced into a household, it is likely that all members will acquire the infection. CMV is transmitted to the infant via the placenta. Infections are distributed worldwide, and most humans have become infected by the time they reach adulthood. CMV causes congenital infection in 1% to 2% of all live births in the U.S. When pregnant women acquire the virus, there is a 30% to 40% transmission rate to the fetus (AAP, 2009b; Fanaroff and Martin, 2006; Remington and Klein, 2005).

Clinical Findings
History and Physical Examination
- Maternal infection (though many women are asymptomatic)
- As many as 90% of infected newborns asymptomatic
- SGA and/or intrauterine growth retardation

- Hepatosplenomegaly
- Jaundice
- Petechial rash
- Chorioretinitis
- Cerebral calcifications
- Microcephaly

Diagnostic Studies. CMV is isolated in cell cultures from urine, saliva, or other body fluids. Techniques for detection of viral deoxyribonucleic acid (DNA) by polymerase chain reaction (PCR) are available from selected reference laboratories. Proof of congenital infection requires obtaining specimens within 3 weeks of birth. Viral isolation or a strongly positive test for serum IgM anti-CMV antibody is considered diagnostic.

Management, Prognosis, and Prevention

Limited data in infants suggest that ganciclovir may be helpful in decreasing progression of hearing impairment; consultation with an expert is recommended (AAP, 2009b). Monitor urine for CMV for 18 to 24 months. The outcome of symptomatic congenital CMV infection is poor; there is a 20% to 30% mortality rate and a 90% to 95% morbidity rate, characterized by psychomotor retardation, microcephaly, hearing loss, seizures, chorioretinitis, optic atrophy, mental retardation, and learning disabilities. At greatest risk are susceptible pregnant women exposed to the urine and saliva of CMV-infected children who attend daycare centers (AAP, 2009b). Handwashing and simple hygienic measures should be reinforced in this population.

GROUP B STREPTOCOCCUS

Description and Epidemiology

GBS, a gram-positive diplococcus, is the leading cause of sepsis in infants from birth to 3 months old resulting in significant perinatal morbidity and mortality rates. Early-onset disease usually occurs at birth or within the first 24 hours of life; late-onset disease occurs during the second week of life.

The organism forms colonies in the maternal genitourinary and gastrointestinal tracts. Pregnant women are usually asymptomatic, but can manifest chorioamnionitis, endometritis, or urinary tract infection. Infants born of women who are highly colonized are more likely to become colonized. GBS is acquired by newborns following vertical transmission (e.g., ascending infection through ruptured amniotic membranes or contamination following passage through the colonized birth canal). As many as 50% of infants with early-onset disease are symptomatic at birth, indicating an intrauterine infection. The highest attack rate of early-onset GBS is in high-risk deliveries, premature SGA infants, very-low-birthweight infants, or those with prolonged ruptured membranes; full-term infants account for 50% of cases. Colonization of pregnant women and newborns ranges from 15% to 40%. Incidence of early-onset GBS disease has been reduced from about 1 to 4 cases per 1000 live births to about 0.3 cases per 1000 live births owing to widespread chemoprophylaxis (AAP, 2009b).

Clinical Findings
History
- Infants who are less than 37 weeks of gestation
- Rupture of membranes (ROM) of 18 hours or greater

TABLE 38-8 Gentamicin Doses

Gestational Age (weeks)	Age (days)	Dose
≤29 or asphyxia, decreased renal function	0-7	5 mg/kg every 48 hours
	8-28	4 mg/kg every 36 hours
	>28	4 mg/kg every 24 hours
30-33	0-7	4.5 mg/kg every 36 hours
	>7	4 mg/kg every 24 hours
≥34	0-7	4 mg/kg every 24 hours
	>7	4 mg/kg every 12-18 hours

- Maternal fever during labor of greater than 100.4° F (40° C) oral
- Previous delivery of a sibling with invasive GBS disease
- Maternal chorioamnionitis to include ROM and maternal fever with at least two of the following:
  - Maternal tachycardia (heart rate greater than 90 bpm)
  - Fetal tachycardia (heart rate greater than 170 bpm)
  - Maternal leukocytosis (white blood cell count greater than 15,000)
  - Uterine tenderness
  - Foul-smelling amniotic fluid

Physical Examination
- Poor feeding
- Temperature instability
- Cyanosis, apnea, tachypnea, grunting, flaring, and retracting
- Seizures, lethargy, bulging fontanelle
- Rapid onset and deterioration

Diagnostic Studies. Cultures of blood, CSF, or both are definitive; antigen identification tests are available, but have poor specificity.

Differential Diagnosis

RDS, amniotic fluid aspiration syndrome, persistent fetal circulation, meningitis, osteomyelitis, septic arthritis, sepsis from other infections, and metabolic problems are included in the differential diagnosis.

Management, Prognosis, and Prevention

Initiate antibiotic therapy with a penicillin (usually ampicillin) and an aminoglycoside, often gentamicin, until GBS has been differentiated from *E. coli* or *Listeria* sepsis or meningitis (AAP, 2009b).
- Ampicillin IV:
  - Infant less than 7 days old: Give 200 to 300 mg/kg/day in three divided doses
  - Infant older than 7 days: Give 300 mg/kg/day in four divided doses
- Gentamicin doses are found in Table 38-8.
- IV penicillin G is the treatment of choice for documented GBS infection.
  - Infant less than 7 days old: Give 250,000 to 400,000 units/kg/day in three divided doses

○ Infant older than 7 days: Give 450,000 to 500,000 units/kg/day in four divided doses
○ Duration of therapy is 10 (bacteremia without focus) to 14 days (uncomplicated meningitis)
- Consultation with pediatric infectious disease specialists is recommended.

Screening of all pregnant women for GBS at 35 to 37 weeks of gestation is recommended. Antepartum treatment of asymptomatic mothers carrying GBS is not recommended. The mortality rate of early-onset disease ranges from 10% to 40%; mortality rate is highest in very-low-birthweight infants and in those with low neutrophil count (less than 1500), low Apgar scores, hypotension, apnea, and a delay in starting antimicrobial therapy. Chemoprophylaxis of high-risk, colonized, pregnant women is an effective method of preventing early-onset GBS infection. Consensus guidelines developed by the CDC are under review. The guidelines outline steps for a screening-based and risk-factor strategy to prevent GBS (AAP, 2009b; CDC, 2002). Treatment consists of IV penicillin or ampicillin given to high-risk women at the onset of labor, repeated every 4 hours until the infant is born.

LISTERIOSIS

Description and Epidemiology

Listeria monocytogenes is a small gram-positive rod isolated from soil, streams, sewage, certain foods, silage, dust, and slaughterhouses. The food-borne transmission of disease is related to Mexican (soft ripened) cheese, whole and 2% milk, uncooked hot dogs, undercooked chicken, raw vegetables, and shellfish. The newborn infant acquires the organism transplacentally or by aspiration or ingestion at the time of delivery.

Clinical Findings
History and Physical Examination
- Brown-stained amniotic fluid
- Generalized symptoms of sepsis
- Whitish posterior pharyngeal and cutaneous granulomas
- Disseminated erythematous papules on skin

Diagnostic Studies. Blood, CSF, meconium, and urine are cultured. The CSF shows elevated protein, depressed glucose, and a high leukocyte count. Cultures of the placenta and amniotic fluid also may be helpful.

Management and Prognosis
- Administer IV ampicillin and an aminoglycoside (gentamicin) as initial therapy for severe infections.
- After clinical response occurs or for less severe infections in normal hosts, administer ampicillin alone.
- The duration of therapy is 10 to 14 days for infections without meningitis and 14 to 21 days for infections with meningitis (AAP, 2009b).

Transplacentally acquired listeriosis often results in spontaneous abortion. The death rate of premature infants with *Listeria* pneumonia noted within 12 hours of birth approaches 100%. Mortality rate varies from 20% to 50% if disease develops between 5 and 30 days of birth, and is especially high in premature infants. Mental retardation, paralysis, and hydrocephalus have been noted in survivors of *Listeria* meningitis (Fanaroff and Martin, 2006; Remington and Klein, 2005).

CONGENITAL VARICELLA

Description and Epidemiology

Varicella-zoster virus (VZV) is a herpesvirus. Humans are the only source of infection for this highly contagious virus. The infectivity rate for congenital varicella syndrome in infants born to mothers with chickenpox during the first trimester is 2% when infection occurs between 12 and 20 weeks of gestation (Myers, et al, 2007).

Clinical Findings
History and Physical Examination
- History of maternal chickenpox infection
- Limb atrophy
- Scarring of the skin
- Eye manifestations

Diagnostic Studies. Diagnosis of VZV is made by immunofluorescent staining of vesicular scrapings.

Management, Prognosis, and Prevention

Some experts recommend acyclovir for pregnant women with varicella, especially in the second or third trimester (AAP, 2009b). Varicella-zoster immune globulin (VZIG) is recommended for the term newborn infant whose mother had an onset of chickenpox within 5 days before delivery or within 48 hours after delivery. All exposed premature infants less than 28 weeks of gestation or less than 1000 g birthweight should receive VZIG; exposed premature infants more than 28 weeks of gestation whose mothers lack serologic evidence of disease or a reliable history of disease also require VZIG (AAP, 2009b). VZIG is not indicated if the mother has varicella-zoster (shingles) only. Airborne and contact precautions are recommended for neonates born to mothers with varicella. If still hospitalized, such precautions are continued until 21 days old or 28 days if they received VZIG.

Prevention efforts are targeted to potential mothers. Varicella vaccination is recommended for nonpregnant women of childbearing age who have no history of varicella infection (AAP, 2009b; CDC, 2010b).

SEXUALLY TRANSMITTED INFECTIONS

GONORRHEA

Description and Epidemiology

Neisseria gonorrhoeae is a gram-negative diplococcus that occurs only in humans. The organism lives in exudate and secretions of infected mucous membranes. The organism is transmitted primarily through sexual contact and parturition. Gonococcal infections in the newborn are acquired primarily during delivery.

Clinical Findings

History and Physical Examination. There is a history of maternal gonococcal infection. Findings include conjunctivitis.

Diagnostic Studies. Culture of eye exudate is positive for *N. gonorrhoeae*.

Management and Prevention

Administer a single dose of intramuscular ceftriaxone 25 to 50 mg/kg (not to exceed 125 mg) for prophylaxis of infants born to mothers with active gonorrhea. Because gonorrheal conjunctivitis can rapidly lead to blindness, all infants are given eye prophylaxis at birth with either 1% silver nitrate, 1% tetracycline ophthalmic ointment, or erythromycin 0.5% ophthalmic ointment (AAP, 2009b; CDC, 2006).

CHLAMYDIA

Description and Epidemiology

Chlamydial infection is caused by an obligate intracellular parasite, *Chlamydia trachomatis,* and is the most common sexually transmitted infection in the U.S. Acquisition occurs in approximately 50% of infants born vaginally to infected mothers and in some infants delivered by cesarean section with intact membranes. Of infants acquiring *C. trachomatis* infection, the risk of developing conjunctivitis is 25% to 50% and pneumonia is 5% to 20% (AAP, 2009b).

Clinical Findings

History and Physical Examination

- History of maternal chlamydial infection
- Conjunctivitis a few days to several weeks after birth
- Infant commonly afebrile with normal activity level
- Pneumonia 2 to 19 weeks after birth

Diagnostic Studies

- Tests for detection of *C. trachomatis* without cell culture include DNA probe, direct fluorescent antibody (DFA) staining, enzyme immunoassay (EIA), and nucleic acid amplification (PCR, ligase chain reaction [LCR]).
- Routine bacterial cultures are not helpful.
- Gram stain and culture of discharge from the eye (must include epithelial cells from the palpebral conjunctival sac because chlamydia is an obligate parasite) are necessary for diagnosis.

Management and Prevention

Oral erythromycin suspension (50 mg/kg/day in four divided doses for 10 to 14 days) is given for both conjunctivitis and pneumonia (AAP, 2009b; CDC, 2006). Appropriate treatment of the pregnant woman before delivery prevents disease in the newborn. Prophylaxis with oral erythromycin of the asymptomatic infant born to an untreated but *Chlamydia*-positive woman generally is contraindicated because of the increased risk of developing hypertrophic pyloric stenosis in the infant exposed to erythromycin.

SYPHILIS

Description and Epidemiology

Syphilis is caused by the spirochete *Treponema pallidum,* which crosses the placenta in an infected mother. Routine maternal serologic testing is legally required during prenatal care in all states.

Clinical Findings

History and Physical Examination

- Maternal infection and positive serologic testing
- The majority of neonates are asymptomatic at birth.
- Hepatosplenomegaly
- Persistent rhinorrhea
- Maculopapular or bullous dermal lesions
- Failure to thrive, restlessness, fever

Diagnostic Studies. Evaluation needs to be individualized depending on the adequacy of maternal treatment and

follow-up for syphilis. Consultation with infectious disease may be indicated. CSF evaluation shows high protein, low glucose, high white blood cell count, and positivity on Venereal Disease Research Laboratory (VDRL) test; serum liver enzymes are elevated with liver involvement, and serum rapid plasma reagin (RPR) test is positive.

Management and Prognosis

For proven or highly probable congenital syphilis, the CDC (2010) recommends 10 consecutive days of crystalline penicillin G 100,000 to 150,000 units/kg/day, given as 50,000 units/kg/dose IV every 12 hours during the first 7 days of life and every 8 hours thereafter. Procaine penicillin G 50,000 units/kg IM/dose daily in a single dose for 10 days is the only acceptable treatment regimen for congenital syphilis and for all infants born to seropositive mothers without a documented history of adequate treatment. If more than 1 day is missed, the entire course must be restarted. For infants with less certain evidence of syphilis, alternative regimens are available; referral to the latest CDC guidelines is recommended (CDC, 2006). Untreated congenital syphilis can lead to severe multiorgan involvement. Infants who are appropriately treated have a good prognosis.

HERPES SIMPLEX VIRUS

Description and Epidemiology

Three clinically distinguishable categories of herpes simplex virus (HSV) infection exist: (1) disseminated disease, (2) CNS disease, and (3) disease restricted to the skin, eyes, and mouth (AAP, 2009b) (see Table 38-3). HSV is transmitted by direct contact with infected maternal genitalia during the birth process. Transplacental transmission occurs, but has been reported in only a few cases. The risk of neonatal infection is highest with primary genital infection (see Chapter 23 for further discussion).

Clinical Findings

History and Physical Examination. The mother may have active lesions and deliver vaginally. Vesicles in the skin, eye, and mouth are found. Signs or symptoms of encephalitis, pneumonia, or sepsis can also be present.

Diagnostic Studies. The virus is isolated in tissue cultures obtained from vesicles, nasopharyngeal or conjunctival swabs, urine, stool, and tracheal secretions; alternatively, vesicle scrapings can be evaluated for antigens with rapid diagnostic tests.

Management, Prognosis, and Prevention

Acyclovir 60 mg/kg/day IV given every 8 hours for 14 days (skin, eyes, and mouth infection) or 21 days (disseminated or involving the CNS) (AAP, 2009b; CDC, 2010). Additionally, treatment with ophthalmic drugs (1% trifluridine, 0.1% iododeoxyuridine, or 3% vidarabine) is used for infants with ocular involvement (AAP, 2009b). Despite effective antiviral therapy, disseminated neonatal HSV infections and localized encephalitis are associated with considerable morbidity and mortality. Some obstetricians provide antiviral therapy in the final weeks of life for women with a history of HSV. The risk of acquiring this serious infection is lowered by performing cesarean delivery before rupture of membranes in any pregnancy in which signs or symptoms of HSV infection occur.

HUMAN IMMUNODEFICIENCY VIRUS

HIV, a retrovirus, is transmitted to the newborn via the placenta or at birth secondary to exposure to maternal blood (see Chapter 23 for further discussion).

DRUG-EXPOSED INFANTS

COCAINE (CRACK) EXPOSURE

Description

Cocaine is a local anesthetic and CNS stimulant that is believed to be a teratogen that crosses the placenta.

Clinical Findings

History and Physical Examination. Maternal exposure to cocaine or crack and positive maternal and/or infant urine drug screen for cocaine are found. Premature labor, abruptio placentae, and fetal asphyxia are possible. Many infants will show no adverse affects from maternal use of cocaine. Findings may include the following:

- Low birthweight, intrauterine growth retardation (IUGR) or prematurity
- Fetal distress and meconium staining
- Microcephaly
- Anomalies of the urinary or gastrointestinal tract
- Rarely, feeding difficulties, including voracious appetite, poorly coordinated sucking and swallowing, and vomiting
- CNS symptoms of transient irritability, abnormal sleeping patterns, tremors, hypertonia, and lability of mood

There is no clinically documented neonatal withdrawal syndrome for cocaine (Stoll, 2007c).

Management, Complications, and Prevention

Take the following steps:

- Offer quiet and pacification techniques, such as swaddling and decreased environmental stimuli.
- If symptoms suggest that further treatment is indicated, see the section on Heroin and Methadone Exposure.
- Because cocaine is detectable in breast milk, mothers who use cocaine should not breastfeed.
- Involvement of the department of child and family services is essential.

In one study, authors found that mothers who stated they had used cocaine or had a positive drug screen had a significantly higher risk of infections, including syphilis, gonorrhea, hepatitis, and HIV; psychiatric, nervous, and emotional disorders; and abruptio placentae. The prevalence of serious and life-threatening medical outcomes is low in drug-abusing pregnant women; however, the disadvantaged social and environmental conditions that are often characteristic of the lifestyle of these women may compound the risk for infection and poor neurodevelopmental outcome (Bauer et al, 2002). Prenatal cocaine exposure has been associated in some studies with long-term changes in IQ or behavior, including neurobehavioral dysfunction, hyperactivity, aggression, and short attention span, but the data are inconsistent (Frank et al, 2001; Singer et al, 2004); further research is underway. Elimination of in utero exposure to cocaine can occur only if there is identification of a potential problem in a high-risk mother and referral to a substance abuse prevention program.

HEROIN AND METHADONE EXPOSURE

Description

Heroin and methadone are narcotics that cross the placenta.

Clinical Findings

History

- Maternal exposure to heroin or methadone
- Urine drug screen positive for opiates in mother and/or infant
- Increased incidence of stillbirths and SGA infants, but probably not congenital anomalies

Physical Examination

- Tremors and hyperirritability often more coarse than those with hypoglycemia
- Limbs rigid and hyperreflexic
- Skin abrasions secondary to hyperactivity
- Tachypnea
- Poor feeding
- Diarrhea
- Vomiting
- High-pitched cry
- Fist sucking
- Low birthweight or SGA in 50% (Stoll, 2007c)

Symptoms of heroin withdrawal occur in up to 75% of infants, usually beginning in the first 48 hours of life, depending on the daily maternal dose, duration of addiction, and time of last maternal dose. Symptoms of methadone withdrawal occur in up to 90% of infants. A higher incidence of symptomatology is seen if the last dose was taken within 24 hours of birth. Overall the withdrawal syndrome is more severe and more prolonged with methadone than with heroin (Stoll, 2007c).

Differential Diagnosis

The differential diagnosis includes hypoglycemia and hypocalcemia.

Management and Prevention

Supportive management, such as swaddling, frequent feedings, and protection from external stimuli, is needed. Education regarding SIDS is imperative because these infants are at increased risk. The department of child and family services must be involved before discharge. Medications such as phenobarbital, tincture of opium and methadone can be used if symptoms such as severe irritability, vomiting and diarrhea, seizures, temperature instability, or severe tachypnea are noted. Pregnant women who are addicted to heroin should be encouraged to enter a treatment program.

FETAL ALCOHOL SYNDROME

See Chapter 40.

■ Sudden Infant Death Syndrome and Apparent Life-Threatening Events

Description and Epidemiology

The accepted definition of SIDS is the sudden death of an infant less than 1 year old that remains unexplained after a complete case investigation, including performance of a complete autopsy, examination of the death scene, and review of the clinical history (Hunt and Hauck, 2007). SIDS rarely occurs in the first month of life, with 90% of deaths occurring between 1 and 6 months old, peaking at 12 weeks old (85% occur between 2 and 4 months old). SIDS is the most common cause of death in infants between 1 and 6 months old, accounting for 5000 deaths per year. African-American infants are at twice the risk, and there is a higher frequency of SIDS in male infants and in the winter months, although the seasonal difference in rates is decreasing (AAP, 2005; Hunt and Hauck, 2007). An apparent life-threatening event (ALTE) is defined as an episode that is frightening to the observer and that is characterized by some combination of apnea (central or occasionally obstructive), color change, marked change in muscle tone, choking, or gagging. In some cases the observer fears that the infant has died.

The diagnosis is one of exclusion because the specific cause of SIDS remains unknown. It cannot be predicted or prevented, although placing the infant in a supine position has been shown to decrease the incidence of SIDS and is the recommended sleep position for infants. The National Institutes of Health has monitored sleep position since 1992, and prone sleeping has decreased from 70% to less than 15%. At the same time, the SIDS death rate has fallen by about 53% in the U.S. (AAP, 2010).

Three main pathophysiologic mechanisms are considered to contribute to SIDS: decreased arousal, asphyxia and rebreathing, and thermal stress. Experts have considered as possible causes respiratory obstruction, restrictive clothing, and hyperthermia. Factors associated with SIDS include ALTE, poverty, lack of prenatal care, low birthweight, SGA, preterm birth, young maternal age, high parity, maternal smoking and drug use, and co-sleeping.

Clinical Findings

History

- Maternal: Cigarette smoking, drug or alcohol use; no or poor prenatal care; bottle feeding; poor education; unmarried; multiparity; maternal age less than 20 years; short intervals between pregnancies; anemia
- Infant: Prematurity (less than 37 weeks); low birthweight (less than 2500 g) or SGA; twins or other multiple births; Apgar score less than 6 at 5 minutes; apnea; poor weight gain; anemia; intensive care unit stay; neonatal respiratory abnormality, bronchopulmonary dysplasia, previous ALTE; previously healthy infant with or without recent upper respiratory infection (URI) symptoms
- Socioeconomic, other: Low-income family; crowded living conditions; poor housing conditions; prior SIDS in family; prone sleeping position, soft bedding, overheating; co-sleeping, especially with smoke, alcohol, or mind-altering drug use; race, ethnicity, culture (higher rates in African-American and American Indian and Alaska Native children).

Physical Examination

- No sign of injury (nonaccidental trauma must be ruled out)
- Frothy blood-tinged secretions in mouth and nares
- Intrathoracic petechiae on autopsy
- Retention of periadrenal brown fat on autopsy

Diagnostic Studies. Autopsy and death scene evaluation must be done. A skeletal bone survey may be done if there is concern about abuse.

Differential Diagnosis

Aspiration; suffocation; infant botulism or poisoning; cardiac or respiratory disease; hypoxemia; infection; metabolic disorders; child abuse, Munchausen syndrome, or shaken baby syndrome; and CNS abnormalities should be ruled out. Bed sharing,

especially if the parent is large, appears to be associated with an increased likelihood of some SIDS-like deaths (AAP, 2005).

Management and Prevention

Management is aimed at assisting the family to cope with the loss of the child. The first response of the family is disbelief and shock.

- Obtain a thorough history from the caretaker within a short period of time after the death. Do not accuse the family of any wrongdoing. Focus the questioning on the cause of death to better understand the circumstances.
- Reassure caretaker and family that it was not their fault and the death could not have been prevented.
- Offer support and counsel to families as soon as possible after death.
- Supply names of different support groups to help the family overcome grief.
- Provide follow-up for 1 year.
- Assist surviving siblings. Observe their reaction to the death and refer for counseling if necessary. Help them understand that it was not their fault and alleviate their feelings of guilt. Allow children to verbalize their feelings. Assist parents to deal with their other children; suggest that parents give extra love, attention, and reassurance to their other children.
- Evaluate need for home monitoring. Because the rate of SIDS in succeeding children is low (less than 2%) and because monitoring a child cannot prevent a SIDS episode from occurring, controversy remains about whether to monitor succeeding children (AAP, 2005). Monitors are recommended by some in the following instances: when more than one child in a family has died from SIDS; in infants with ALTEs; in infants with tracheostomy or other airway problems; in infants with neurologic problems affecting respiratory control; and in infants with chronic lung disease. Box 38-6 lists measures that aid in the prevention of SIDS.

BOX 38-6	**Measures That Aid in Preventing Sudden Infant Death Syndrome**

- Breastfeeding is recommended.
- Infants should be immunized (reduces risk by 50%).
- Place infants on their backs to sleep until at least 6 months old. The National Institutes of Health has a "Back to Sleep" program with parent information, stickers, and video.
- Use a firm mattress. Do not use bumper pads or soft bedding or have stuffed animals in bed. Infants should not sleep on a sofa or chair, or on a waterbed or in bed with an adult.
- Avoid overheating and overbundling; room temperature should be 68° to 72° F (20° to 22.2° C).
- Avoid alcohol and drugs (including smoking) while pregnant and breastfeeding, and while in bed.
- Do not allow cigarette smoking within the house or car.
- Avoid bed sharing and co-sleeping.
- Separate but proximate caregiver sleeping environments are recommended.
- Consider pacifier use at naptime and bedtime (but not in breastfed infants until after the first month of life when feedings are established).
- A variety of products to maintain an infant's sleep position are commercially available; their efficacy and safety have not been thoroughly investigated and cannot be recommended.
- For at-risk infants, educate parents and caregivers regarding pros and cons of apnea monitor use. Cardiopulmonary resuscitation instruction is recommended.

Common Injuries

DAWN LEE GARZON, SARA D. DeGOLIER, AND CONSTANCE B. BREHM

Injuries are major pediatric health problems that are best managed with treatment as well as prevention strategies. A child with an injury might respond best to (1) a simple home treatment by the parent, caregiver, or supervising adult; (2) intervention by the provider in the primary care setting; (3) referral to a medical specialist or inpatient facility; or (4) a combination of these. Addressing the potential for injury before it has occurred is a key factor of injury management. Health care professionals have a responsibility to educate families to prevent injuries from occurring.

Due to the importance of injury prevention, the term "accident" has been replaced by the term "unintentional injury." "Unintentional injury" implies that the resulting injury was predictable and preventable, whereas "accident" does not (Hagan et al, 2008). For children older than 1 year of age, injuries (defined as unintentional injury, violence, and suicide) cause more deaths than the next five causes combined (National Center for Health Statistics, 2010). Unintentional injury is also the leading cause of pediatric hospitalization and disability, resulting in more than 9 million emergency department visits each year and more than $17 billion in health care expenditures (Borse et al, 2008).

Prevention of unintentional injuries involves anticipatory guidance to help parents provide a safe environment and necessary supervision. Strategies to prevent injuries in children and adolescents focus on understanding and modifying risk factors, developing community-wide program approaches, and promoting health policy legislative agendas that focus on injury prevention. When implementing prevention strategies, it is important to consider that injury occurrence and severity vary depending on several factors including age, race, gender, and socioeconomic status.

■ Principles of Injury Control

In the past, there was an underlying assumption that children were simply "accident prone" because of their highly active and impulsive nature. Earlier prevention efforts often focused on these childhood characteristics. Emphasizing accident proneness is now considered a counterproductive strategy. Injury control and prevention guidance strategies focus on "the development and age of the child, the environment in which the safety concern or injury takes place, and

the circumstances surrounding the event" (Hagan et al, 2008, p 178). This new approach evaluates injury and safety more closely, focusing not just on the injury itself, but all associated factors including, but not limited to, culture and economics. Information gathered from these three domains helps to customize education for families and communities and create safe environments for children.

The most effective injury prevention education focuses on specific, usable information to decrease injury risk rather than broad, nonspecific recommendations. For example, teaching children and parents how to purchase and size a bicycle helmet is more effective than telling children, "always use a bike helmet." Anticipatory guidance provided by health providers at well-child visits should be geared to the developmental stage of the child. Written materials, audiovisual presentations, peer counseling, and one-to-one interaction with a health professional are all effective teaching and learning strategies. However, safety information should be provided in moderate doses, with reinforcement or repetition at subsequent visits. This strategy helps ensure that the prevention education points are well received and used by caregivers, patients, and their families.

For infants, preschoolers, and school-age children, active adult supervision is key because young children are not able to identify risk, are developmentally impulsive, and cannot consistently remember safety rules. Active supervision involves proximity (close enough to intervene should risk occur), consistency (adult does not stop supervising to engage in other activities like cooking or cleaning), and freedom from distraction or impairment (the adult is not distracted by a book or phone call, for example, and is not under the influence of alcohol or prescription or recreational drugs that cause impairment).

Passive injury prevention is the implementation of safety measures that do not require caregivers to constantly change their behavior to make the environment safer for their children. This prevention strategy is the most effective intervention and includes modification of everyday items in the child's environment. Examples include the use of child-resistant caps on medicines and cleaning products, and safety designs in toys. Other safety implementations include environmental modification such as the use of smoke and carbon monoxide detectors, safe roadway design to reduce traffic volume and speed in residential neighborhoods, window locks, and firearm safety locks. Providers can advocate for local and national prevention strategies and support such programs as the Safe Kids USA campaign. They can also play a key role by supporting injury prevention legislation or initiatives. Public and consumer awareness is crucial for successful prevention programs.

Although most children with serious injuries are seen first in emergency departments (ED), primary care providers have a professional obligation to remain current in basic life support techniques. Competence in performing emergency cardiopulmonary resuscitation and emergency intervention for choking (whether it be for infants, children, or adults) should be a requirement of all licensed health professionals employed in clinical practice settings. Likewise, all parents and caregivers should be encouraged to enroll in a basic pediatric life support program, especially parents and caregivers of infants and children at risk for cardiopulmonary arrest.

APPROACH TO TRAUMA

Three main components essential in the management of an injured child include history, mechanism of the injury, and a thorough physical examination. If the injury is life-threatening, or there has been any deterioration in the child's condition, a trauma severity assessment must immediately be performed. Primary assessment of the injured child should occur within the first 5 minutes of initial contact and includes the assessment of the airway, breathing, circulation, evaluation of vital signs, obtaining a brief history (allergies, medications, past medical history, and events surrounding the injury), and rapid assessment of essential organ status. Cardiopulmonary resuscitation must be initiated if indicated. Once the patient is stabilized, a secondary assessment should include complete physical examination and laboratory and radiographic studies as indicated. Assessment of the patient's vital signs, physical exam, and laboratory tests should be repeated as indicated based on the injury and initial study results. The definitive care phase includes stabilization of local injuries and preparation of the patient and family for transport to the ED if necessary (Table 39-1).

The practitioner should always consider non-accidental trauma (child abuse) when a child presents with an injury, especially when the history of the injury given by the caregiver fails to adequately explain the child's injury (Hisea and Sirotnak, 2009).

■ Common Pediatric Injuries

TRAUMA TO THE SKIN AND SOFT TISSUE

ABRASIONS

Description

Abrasions are superficial skin injuries that involve epidermal trauma. The depth of skin tissue involvement varies depending on the amount of force and friction the skin encounters at the time of injury. The most serious form of abrasion is an avulsion, a trauma that results in loss of the epidermal, dermal, and subcutaneous layers.

Epidemiology

Abrasions often result from falls or friction accidents.

Clinical Findings

History. Seek information about the cause and type of injury and the presence of a foreign object or dirt at the accident scene.

Physical Examination. Determine the extent of the abrasion and the presence of dirt, grime, or other foreign body (e.g., tar). Findings include an area of skin that appears scraped off and may include oozing of serous fluid and blood. Increasing pain, swelling, warmth, redness, and red streaking of the injured area might indicate secondary infection. Assess the surrounding tissue and extremity (if the injury is located on an extremity) for circulation, sensation, motion, and function.

Differential Diagnosis

The injury history and physical findings are the keys to diagnosis. Any other skin condition that can cause loss of epidermis, such as a burn, is included in the differential diagnosis.

Management

Appropriate first-aid care is important to prevent infection. Most abrasions of the skin can be managed at home unless the abrasion is deep, involves a large area, is associated with severe pain, or has a significant amount of dirt, grime, tar, or

TABLE 39-1	Classification and Disposition of Trauma by Severity				
				PHYSICAL EXAMINATION	
Category	**History**	**Vital Signs**	**Local Findings**	**Laboratory/Radiologic Studies**	**Probable Disposition**
Mild	Minimal force	Normal	Superficial only	Few	Discharge
Moderate	Significant force	Normal	Suspicious for internal injury	Intermediate	Evaluate
Severe	Critical force	Abnormal	Indicative of internal injury	Many	Immediate therapy; admit

From Ruddy RM, Fleischer GR: An approach to the injured child. In Fleischer GR, Ludwig S, Henretig FM, editors: *Textbook of pediatric emergency medicine*, ed 5, Philadelphia, 2006, Lippincott Williams & Wilkins, p 1340.

a foreign body in the wound. A child who is immunocompromised may need to be seen due to increased risk of infection.

Management of an abrasion includes the following:

- Thoroughly cleanse the wound. The area can be scrubbed with soap or an antibacterial cleanser using a wet gauze or soft surgical nail brush. Gentle irrigation with copious amounts of water or normal saline (300 to 1000 mL) is the preferred method to thoroughly cleanse a wound and prevent infection. Povidone-iodine, alcohol, and peroxide should not be used on open wounds. If dirt or dark-colored matter is not adequately removed, new skin may grow over the particles, resulting in a permanent tattoo. A secondary infection may occur as well if all debris is not removed from the wound. Remove pieces of loose skin with a sterile scissors and remove foreign particles with tweezers. If tar particles are present, rub the wound area with petrolatum, and then repeat normal saline or water irrigation.
- Small abrasions can be left open to the air or may require a small bandage.
- Cover larger abrasions with a sterile nonadherent dressing. Double antibiotic ointment such as bacitracin/polymyxin B may be applied, especially to abrasions of the elbows or knees to prevent cracking or reopening of the wound because of constant movement and stretching of the joints.
- Protect abrasions of the hands, feet, or areas overlying joints from friction and dirt until a protective dry scab is formed.
- Instruct the caregiver to wash the abrasion at least every 24 hours and reapply the dressing and antibiotic ointments until a protective dry scab is formed. Instructions regarding the signs and symptoms of infection should also be provided.
- Tetanus prophylaxis should be administered if the wound is significant. The use of Tdap is the preferred vaccination for children 10 to 11 years of age and older (see Chapter 23).

PUNCTURE WOUNDS

Description

Puncture wounds result from varying levels of the skin and underlying tissue penetration. These wounds are typically classified as superficial or deep. Because of the potential for serious infection, puncture wounds must be carefully evaluated and treated if indicated. The location and depth of the wound and the presence of a foreign object are key risk factors for the subsequent development of infection. For example, deep penetrating injuries to the forefoot with a dirty object, especially if they involve the plantar fascia, have a higher risk of infection than wounds to the arch or heel area. The forefoot has less overlying soft tissue than other plantar surfaces and is the major weight-bearing area of the foot; therefore, cartilage and bone can be involved. The metatarsophalangeal joint region is also at high risk for infection due to the same principles. Puncture wounds through the soles of tennis shoes can transfer bacteria into the tissue, where minimal drainage is possible, placing the child at higher risk for a secondary infection.

Epidemiology

Puncture wounds are common pediatric injuries and may occur at any age. Glass, wood splinters, toothpicks, needles, nails, metal, staples, and thumbtacks are common sources of injury. Bites also produce puncture wounds and are especially infection-prone.

Although the majority of puncture wounds heal without problems, a sizable minority of these injuries are complicated by infections that may lead to cellulitis, fasciitis, septic arthritis, or soft-tissue abscesses. *Staphylococcus aureus* and beta-hemolytic streptococci are normal flora of the skin and are common causative agents in secondary infections from puncture wounds. *Pseudomonas aeruginosa* colonizes on the rubber soles of tennis shoes and is a common pathogen for plantar puncture wounds when the puncture occurs through the sole of a tennis shoe and into the foot. Osteomyelitis can occur if the puncture wound penetrates a bone or joint. The most common pathogens that cause osteomyelitis secondary to a puncture wound are *P. aeruginosa* in nondiabetic patients, and *S. aureus* in diabetic patients (Baddour, 2009). Cat and dog bites can cause wound infection from *Pasteurella multocida*.

Clinical Findings

The assessment of a child with a minor wound includes first excluding more serious and sometimes occult injuries.

History. Important information to elicit after a report or suspicion of a puncture wound includes the following:

- Date and time of injury and history of wound care provided at time of injury and thereafter
- Identification of and the type and estimated depth of object penetration. If it is not known what object penetrated the skin, the likelihood of an imbedded foreign body is high.
- Location and condition of the penetrating object. Was the object clean or rusty, jagged or smooth?
- Whether all or part of the foreign object was removed
- Type and condition of footwear that was being worn (pertinent to injuries to the foot) or if the child was barefoot
- Immunization status for tetanus coverage (see Chapter 23)
- Presence of any medical condition that increases the risk for infectious complications

Physical Examination. To ensure a thorough examination, a good light source is necessary when assessing and treating a puncture wound. Note circulation, movement, and sensation of the area next to the injury. Determine the amount of involvement of underlying tissue or bone structures. For plantar puncture wounds, have the child lie prone with the feet positioned at the head of the examining table and the knees slightly flexed to assist in proper examination positioning (Buttaravoli, 2007). Assess the wound for length and depth, presence of debris or penetrating object, and signs of infection.

Examination findings consistent with *cellulitis* include:

- Localized pain or tenderness, swelling, and erythema at the puncture site (may be more obvious at dorsum of the foot for plantar puncture wounds)
- Possible fever
- Pain with flexion or extension of the extremity involved
- Decreased ability to bear weight
- For plantar puncture wounds, pain along the plantar aspect of the foot during extension or flexion of the toes may indicate deep tissue injury.

Examination findings consistent with *osteomyelitis-osteochondritis* include:

- Extension of pain and swelling around the puncture wound and to the adjacent bony structures
- Exquisite point tenderness over the bone
- Fever

- Increasing erythema
- Decreased use of the affected extremity

Examination findings consistent with *pyarthrosis* (septic arthritis) include:

- Pain, swelling, warmth, and erythema over the affected joint
- Decreased range of motion and weight bearing of the affected joint

Diagnostic Studies

- Plain film radiograph should be ordered if any of the following are true:
  - A retained foreign object is suspected.
  - There is tremendous amount of pain at the puncture site with localized tenderness or questionable mass underneath the skin surface (Baddour, 2009).
  - There was penetration of a joint space, bone or growth cartilage, or the plantar fascia of the foot.
  - The puncture site has signs of infection and is from a nail injury.
- Most metal and glass foreign bodies can be seen on a plain radiograph. However, if the foreign object is not radiopaque or if the x-ray is negative despite suspicion of foreign object in the wound, computed tomography (CT), ultrasound, and magnetic resonance imaging (MRI) are useful diagnostic tools (Buttaravoli, 2007).
- Bone scans are sensitive, but not specific for osteomyelitis. Radiographs are specific, but findings for osteomyelitis are noted late. Clinical examination and laboratory studies and imaging should be considered early in the diagnosis of osteomyelitis (Polousky and Eilert, 2009).
- A complete blood count (CBC) and blood culture may be needed. An elevation in the white blood cell count might indicate infection.
- An erythrocyte sedimentation rate (ESR) and C-reactive protein (CRP) are nonspecific inflammatory markers and are helpful in the diagnosis and management of bony inflammation and infection.
- A wound culture is indicated prior to starting antibiotics if the wound appears infected.

Differential Diagnosis

The circumstance surrounding the penetrating injury and the presenting symptoms are the best indicators of whether the injury represents a superficial wound that will heal uneventfully or develop infectious complications.

Management

Buttaravoli (2007) suggests the following practical and straightforward approach to the management of puncture wounds:

- Irrigate with copious amounts of normal saline for puncture wounds caused by small, clean, slender nonrusty objects (e.g., thumbtack or needle) after confirmation of complete removal of the intact object, and when signs of infection are absent.
- Larger puncture wounds require profuse irrigation. Wound debridement may also be necessary. A No. 10 scalpel may be used to gently shave off the cornified epithelium surrounding the puncture wound to aid in the removal of debris that collected around the point of entry of the puncture wound. If debris is found in the wound, gently slide the plastic sheath

of an over-the-needle catheter down the wound track and move the catheter sheath in and out while irrigating with copious amounts of normal saline until debris no longer flows from the wound. A local anesthetic agent may be necessary for debridement and irrigation procedures.

- Obtain imaging studies as indicated for proper management of the puncture wound. If imaging studies demonstrate that the foreign object has invaded bone, growth cartilage, or a joint space, refer the child immediately to an orthopedic surgeon. Always suspect a retained foreign object if the puncture wound is infected, the infection is not responding to antibiotic therapy, or if pain or aching of the injured site is still present weeks after the injury. In order to prevent a catastrophic outcome, wounds that are deep or highly contaminated should be referred to an orthopedic surgeon so that debridement can take place in an operating room (Buttaravoli, 2007).
- Following careful wound cleansing, the wound can be covered with a simple bandage. Deeper wounds that require more extensive exploration should have a small sterile wick of iodoform gauze placed in the wound tract in order to keep the edges open, thus aiding in granulation tissue growth and wound healing. Remove the gauze 2 to 3 days after placement (Selbst and Attia, 2010).
- Children with simple, uncomplicated puncture wounds do not need antibiotics; however, if there are signs of infection, the puncture is the result of a cat bite, or if the wound is deep or contained debris, antibiotics should be part of the treatment plan. Appropriate antibiotics for puncture wounds include amoxicillin clavulanate or cephalexin. Clindamycin should be used when children are allergic to penicillins. Plantar puncture wounds require ciprofloxacin. If methicillin-resistant *Staphylococcus aureus* (MRSA) is cultured from the wound or pus is present at the puncture site, then trimethoprim-sulfamethoxazole (TMP-SMX) or clindamycin is recommended until sensitivities are known. All antibiotics should be prescribed for 7 to 14 days depending on severity of infection (Baddour, 2009).
- Schedule a recheck appointment within 48 hours. If pain, erythema, and swelling have not improved or symptoms have worsened within the first 48 hours of outpatient treatment, hospitalization and intravenous antibiotics are indicated (Baddour, 2009).
- Treatment for severe infections secondary to puncture wounds such as septic arthritis and osteomyelitis includes surgical debridement and parenteral antibiotics (Hosalkar et al, 2007).
- Tetanus prophylaxis is indicated if it has been more than 5 years since the last tetanus vaccine or if the date of the last tetanus vaccine is unknown. Consider passive immunization with tetanus immune globulin (TIG) or initiation/continuation of a primary tetanus series (DTaP, Tdap, or Td as appropriate) for children who may have never been immunized or are behind in their vaccinations (see Chapter 23).

Patient and Parent Education

Home care management for a puncture wound includes:

- No weight bearing for 3 or 4 days if the injury was a puncture to the foot
- Warm compresses to the affected area three or four times daily

- Wound elevation
- Close observation for signs and symptoms of infection and if infection is suspected, rapid re-evaluation is necessary. Further evaluation is required if a puncture wound continues to cause localized or spreading pain or discomfort.

INGROWN TOENAILS AND NAIL HEMATOMA

Description

Onychocryptosis (ingrown toenail) and nail hematomas are common occurrences in pediatrics. Ingrown toenails are caused by several factors including abnormal position of the toenail on the nailbed, tight and improperly fitting shoes, trauma to the nail, and improper toenail trimming. The lateral nail edges of the toenail impinge on the adjacent skin tissue causing erythema and edema. This constant impingement causes granulation tissue to build up at the site of the impingement and presses the toenail into the nail base and corner edge of the adjacent skin structure, which causes pain and potentially infection (Jacome et al, 2008).

Subungual hematomas are blood accumulations under the intact nail. Nail injuries that involve lacerations or a fracture of the distal phalanx should be referred to an orthopedist. Uncomplicated nail hematomas can be drained (nail trephination) by primary care providers. Tuft fractures (distal phalanx) are commonly associated with fingertip crush injuries and are often able to be managed in the primary care setting with orthopedic consult if needed.

Management

- Ingrown toenail
  - Pack cotton under the nail edge to elevate the nail, and educate the patient to repack the cotton daily to prevent infection.
  - Epsom salt mixed with warm-water foot soaks for 20 minutes, three times a day. Keep the foot or affected toenail clean and dry. Encourage frequent elevation of the affected toe as well as minimal activity to aid in healing.
  - Educate about the importance of clipping nails straight across with extension of toenail just over the edge of the nailbed. Properly fitting shoes are also important.
  - Systemic antibiotics are rarely needed and should be reserved for severe cases.
  - For persistent ingrown toenails with or without infection, consider a referral to a podiatrist for partial or complete toenail removal.
- Subungual hematoma
  - Determine whether a digital or regional nerve block is needed (proper training is required).
  - Attempt to lift the nail to examine for the presence of significant nailbed injuries.
  - Irrigate nail surface with saline solution, then clean with chlorhexidine or isopropyl alcohol.
  - Make one or more holes in the area of the nail hematoma with either a portable heat cautery device or the end of an untwisted heated-to-red paperclip (heated to melt the nail). Ensure the holes are large enough to drain the hematoma. Remove the cautery device immediately after creating a hole to ensure that the underlying tissue is not cauterized subsequently blocking the drainage of fluid.

  - Antibiotics generally are not needed.
  - Home care includes educating patient and parent to monitor for signs of infection (increased redness, swelling, pain, or purulent drainage) and to return for further care if infection is suspected. Instruct soaking of affected nailbed three times per day with antibacterial soap until the drainage has stopped and the underlying skin has healed.
  - An aluminum splint can be used to immobilize a Tuft fracture for 2 to 3 weeks.

LACERATIONS

Description

Lacerations are second only to contusions as the most common soft-tissue injury managed in the ED, resulting in approximately 112 million visits annually (Garcia-Gubern et al, 2010). Lacerations are deep cuts to the skin caused by a wide variety of mechanisms and are most common on the face, scalp, and hands. Lacerations often require more complicated treatment than other minor wounds because they can be associated with occult injuries to the deeper tissues and require careful exploration.

Shear, tension, and compression injuries are the three most common types of lacerations (Sullivan, 2009). Shear injuries are caused by sharp objects that tend to cause minimal, if any, damage to the tissues surrounding the injury. The biggest danger of shear injuries is the potential for damage to nerve, tendon, and vascular structures that may require more complicated repair that should only be attempted in the ED or operating room by a skilled surgeon. Shear injuries heal quickly and have the lowest potential for wound infection.

Tension lacerations are caused from stresses on the skin, usually secondary to the force of a blunt object at less than a 90-degree angle. The skin tears due to the stress and causes an irregularly shaped edge to the injury. These types of lacerations are accompanied by damage to surrounding tissues. A classic example is when a child falls and bumps his or her head on the dull edge of a piece of furniture, causing the skin to break open in the appearance of a laceration.

Compression lacerations are caused by a crush injury, usually involving blunt force of an object at a 90-degree angle. This type of laceration usually has irregular, often stellate wound edges. Compression injuries can cause significant injury to adjacent tissues and have the highest incidence of wound infections.

Epidemiology

Lacerations are caused by various forms of trauma and are a very common reason for pediatric health care visits.

Clinical Findings

History. Key questions when assessing a laceration include:
- How did the injury happen? Determining the mechanism of injury is essential in identifying the potential extent of tissue damage, the presence of contaminants, and the possible presence of a foreign body, such as dirt, debris, glass, and splinters.
- How long ago (number of hours) did the injury occur? Length of time since injury is a critical factor to consider and can influence the treatment plan for the patient.

- Does the child have allergies to antibiotics or anesthetics?
- What is the child's tetanus immunization status? Is there a need for further immunization?

Physical Examination. Key points in the examination of a laceration include:

- Perform a neurovascular examination, including evaluation of pulses, motor function, and sensation distal to the laceration.
- Evaluate the range of motion, especially with wounds involving the distal forearm, wrist, and hand due to the high potential for tendon injury.
- Determine whether the wound edges approximate and note the degree of tension at the wound site.

Differential Diagnosis

The history and physical examination provide the diagnosis.

Management

Providers may repair the wound using sutures, staples, glue, or tape, as indicated. Minor lacerations to the scalp, arms, and legs are commonly managed by primary care providers. Significant wounds to the face, hands, or genital areas should be referred to a specialist, such as an orthopedic surgeon that specializes in hand repair, or a plastic surgeon for plastic and reconstructive surgery (particularly for the face).

The steps in wound management are summarized as follows (Selbst and Attia, 2010):

1. *Decision to close the wound.* Compared with adults, children are less likely to get wound infections. In fact, the infection rate from sutured lacerations in children is 2%. Most wounds may be closed using a primary wound closure (i.e., bringing the edges of the skin together, known as "approximation") as soon after the injury as possible to speed healing, prevent infection, and improve the cosmetic result. Delayed closure increases the risk of infection. Some researchers suggest a "golden period" for wound closure of 6 hours. However, wounds considered low risk for infection, such as a clean knife wound to an extremity, can be closed even 12 to 24 hours after the injury. Other guidelines to consider in wound closure include the following:
   - Most facial wounds may be closed up to 24 hours after initial injury in order to provide the child with the most optimal cosmetic outcomes. Depending on the severity of the laceration or potential for infection (such as a dog bite), repair and management may be best performed in the operating room.
   - Risk of infection is inversely related to the blood flow to the body part where the laceration is present. The lower the blood flow, the higher the infection risk. For example, a hand or foot laceration is far more likely to become infected than a scalp laceration because the extremities of the body have lower blood perfusion than the head and scalp.
   - Contaminated wounds, crush wounds, and lacerations in children who are immunocompromised are at high risk for infection and should be closed within 6 hours of injury.
   - Animal, human, or barnyard animal bites should be left open for healing by secondary intention, which is a process of healing by granulation and reepithelialization.

The potential of scar formation increases with this method, but the benefits of improved healing and decreased infection outweigh the cosmetic negative.

   - Delayed primary closure consists of closing of a wound 3 to 5 days after initial injury when the risk of infection has decreased. This type of closure is recommended for selected heavily contaminated wounds and those associated with extensive damage, such as high-velocity missile injuries, crush injuries, and explosion injuries. Initial management of such an injury should include wound cleansing, debridement, and a sterile dressing. Close follow-up is recommended in order to check for infection and for wound closure (Selbst and Attia, 2010).

2. *Anesthesia.* Appropriate use of local anesthetic and conscious sedation is essential for successful repair of lacerations in children. Proper wound care includes wound exploration and careful cleansing, both painful procedures made worse by fear and anxiety. Infiltration of the wound with local anesthetic, such as 1% lidocaine with or without epinephrine (depending on location of laceration) can also help control bleeding. LET (lidocaine, epinephrine, tetracaine), LAT (lidocaine, adrenaline, tetracaine), and TAC (tetracaine, adrenaline, cocaine) are topical solutions placed on minor wounds 20 to 30 minutes prior to cleansing or repair procedures to help with pain management and to control bleeding. Topical solutions such as these cannot be used on eyes, ears, nose, fingers, genitals, or toes. Texts are available that address procedures in primary care that include excellent information on local anesthetic and wound closure. Attendance at workshops that focus on wound management is also helpful.

3. *Hair.* Hair near the wound usually creates minimal difficulty during repair and generally does not need to be removed. In any case, hair should not be shaved because to do so can damage hair follicles and increase the risk of infection. Instead, the hair should be clipped with scissors when necessary. Alternatively, petroleum jelly can be used to keep unwanted scalp hair away from the wound while suturing. Eyebrow hair should not be removed because this may lead to abnormal or slow regrowth.

4. *Wound cleansing.* Chlorhexidine or povidone-iodine surgical scrub preparations may be used to clean the skin surrounding the wound but are not recommended for use in the wound itself. Other agents not recommended for wound cleansing include hydrogen peroxide and alcohol. These agents may be irritating to tissues, causing slow healing times, and may increase infection by damaging white blood cells. The preferred method of wound cleansing is *irrigation* to reduce bacterial contamination and prevent subsequent infection. Normal saline or tap water is a safe and cost-effective choice for irrigation (Garcia-Gubern et al, 2010). A good rule of thumb for volume needed for saline irrigation is to use 50 to 100 mL of normal saline per centimeter of the wound or laceration. More solution may be needed if the wound is unusually large or contaminated. A large irrigating syringe (20 to 50 mL) is needed to provide enough force to cleanse the wound. A splash guard attached to the syringe is recommended to reduce splatter during irrigation. *Scrubbing* the wound should be reserved only for particularly "dirty" wounds when irrigation does not remove contaminants completely. Forceps may also be required to remove foreign

debris from the wound when saline irrigation is unsuccessful. It is important to remove all foreign debris to decrease infection risk and prevent tattooing of the skin.

5. *Exploration of the wound.* The wound must be explored for presence of foreign bodies, deep tissue layer damage, injury to nerve or blood vessel, or joint involvement. It is imperative that the depth of the wound be determined. Wound probing is done with a cotton-tipped swab, a hemostat, or a needle holder. Deep lacerations should be referred to an ED for layered closure. If tendon injury is suspected or if bone is exposed, referral to an orthopedist is the standard of care.

6. *Wound debridement.* Gentle removal of unattached loose tissues may be done with sterile instruments. Debridement is advantageous because it helps to remove contaminant from the wound and creates more approximated wound edges. The approximation of wound edges allows for easier wound repair and cosmetic acceptability after the wound is healed for the patient. Although it is helpful to excise necrotic skin, excessive trimming of irregular lacerations should not be attempted. Excessive removal of tissue can create a defect that is difficult to close or that may increase tension at the wound margin, making scarring more likely.

7. *Wound closure.* Several methods are available for wound closure.
   - *Traditional stitches* (or sutures) are often used to close lacerations. This involves "sewing" the skin together with a needle and surgical thread. This procedure usually requires an injection of anesthetic and a bandage applied to the wound afterward. Simple, uncomplicated lacerations to the scalp, trunk, arms, or legs may be closed with sutures (called *primary closure*). Choice of suture material and type of stitch used is dependent on the wound itself. In general, an absorbable suture material is used for closure of structures deeper than the epidermis and nonabsorbable sutures are used to close the outermost layer of a laceration. Deep sutures promote more efficient healing of the wound by relieving skin tension and decreasing dead space.
   - *Staples* can be used for the scalp, trunk, and extremities (not including the hands and feet) and provide a more rapid closure time than with sutures. Laceration repair with staples is associated with a lower infection rate but can be more painful to remove and also not as cosmetically appealing after the wound has healed. Staples should not be used if MRI or CT is going to be necessary.
   - *Surgical tape* such as Steri-Strips is used for small superficial wounds. Surgical tape cannot be used on wounds in moist areas or in areas of tension such as flexor or extensor surfaces. Surgical tape should also be avoided in wounds on small children, who will most likely remove the tape prematurely.
   - *Topical skin adhesive*, also known as skin glue, is used for simple lacerations. The adhesive is applied on top of the skin while the edges of the wound are held together. Usually two or three applications of the adhesive are applied to ensure adequate closure. Adhesive in the wound or between wound margins should be avoided. Skin glue takes less time to apply than stitches and forms a strong, flexible bond over the top of the wound. A bandage is not required for cover after tissue repair with skin glue. The topical skin adhesive sloughs off the wound as it heals, usually in 5 to 10 days and does not

TABLE 39-2	Advantages and Disadvantages of Common Wound Closure Techniques	
Technique	**Advantages**	**Disadvantages**
Suture	Time honored Meticulous closure Greatest tensile strength Lowest dehiscence rate	Requires removal Requires anesthesia Greatest tissue reactivity Highest cost Slowest application Highest risk of needlestick
Staples	Rapid application Low tissue reactivity Low cost Low risk of needlestick	Less meticulous closure May interfere with imaging techniques
Tissue adhesive	Rapid application Patient comfort Resistant to bacterial growth No need for removal Low cost Low or no risk of needlestick	Lower tensile strength than sutures Dehiscence over high-tension areas Not useful on hands
Surgical tape	Least reactive Lowest infection rate Rapid application Patient comfort Low cost No risk of needlestick	Frequently falls off Lower tensile strength than sutures Highest rate of dehiscence Requires use of toxic adjuncts to adhere to skin Cannot be used in areas with hair Cannot get wet

From Sullivan DM: Soft tissue injury and wound repair. In Strange GR, Ahrens W, Schafermeyer R, et al, editors: *Pediatric emergency medicine,* ed 3, New York, 2009, McGraw-Hill, p 335.

require a return visit to the physician for suture removal. Infection risk is minimal due to antimicrobial properties of the adhesive. Minimal scarring is associated with this method of laceration repair. Table 39-2 compares wound closure techniques.

8. *Dressing.* A simple repaired laceration may be covered with an adhesive bandage. For more complex repaired injuries, dress the wound with nonadherent gauze for the first layer followed by a second layer of plain gauze if needed and secured in place with adhesive tape or elasticized gauze (tubular net bandage).

9. *Immunization.* Give tetanus booster or tetanus immunoglobulin as indicated.

10. *Antibiotic controversy.* Antibiotic prophylaxis of clean wounds is not indicated. Its use in contaminated wounds may be helpful, but careful wound cleaning with extensive irrigation followed by prompt wound closure (when indicated) are the most effective safeguards in preventing infection.

11. *Suture and staple removal.* Remove sutures or staples depending on their location (a useful guide can be found in Table 39-3).

TABLE 39-3 Suture and Staple Removal Guide

Location of Sutures	Length of Time Before Removal
Facial	3-5 days
Scalp	7-10 days
Upper extremity	7-10 days
Trunk	10 days
Lower extremity	8-10 days
Over a joint	10-14 days

Patient and Parent Education

Instructions for wound care at home are best given in writing and should include the following information:

- Patient can briefly shower 48 hours after sutures are in place without worrying about the risk of possible infection. However, dry the area well and keep it dry at all times.
- Note signs and symptoms of infection that warrant an early recheck (redness, swelling, discharge, increasing pain).
- Give instructions about cleansing and bandaging the wound; instructions vary based on severity of the wound. For surgical tape and topical skin adhesive, do not use topical antibiotic ointment because it will remove the adhesive.
- List any restrictions on activities.
- Identify a date for a return appointment.

BURNS

Description

A burn injury to one or more layers of the skin and underlying tissues causes varying degrees of damage. Burns are classified by depth of injury, percent of body surface area involved, location of the burn, and association with other injuries. Although traditional classification of the depth of burns as first, second, third, or fourth degree are still in use, the designations of superficial, partial thickness (superficial or deep partial thickness), and full thickness are more commonly used based on recommendations from many experts (Tsarouhas and Agosto, 2008).

- Superficial, or first-degree, burns involve only the epidermis. The skin is erythematous, inflamed, and painful, but there are no blisters. Superficial burns typically heal in 3 to 7 days, have little risk of scarring, and require only symptomatic treatment. A common example of a superficial burn is a sunburn.
- Partial-thickness, or second-degree, burns involve the epidermis and the dermis to a variable degree. Superficial partial-thickness burns involve less than 50% of the dermis, and deep partial thickness burns involve more than 50% of the dermis (Tsarouhas and Agosto, 2008). The dermal appendages are always preserved and provide a source for regeneration.
  - Superficial partial-thickness burns are red, very painful, mottled, moist, and blistered. These burns usually heal in 7 to 14 days, and scarring may occur.
  - Deep partial-thickness burns appear pale and yellow. These burns are less painful and weepy than superficial partial thickness burns. Deep partial-thickness burns take longer to heal (3 weeks) and scarring is more likely to occur.
- Full-thickness or third-degree burns are major thermal injuries in which the epidermis and dermis are completely destroyed. The skin appears whitish (a waxy white appearance) or leathery. The surface is dry and nontender to palpation. Fluid losses can be profound with this degree of burn. Full-thickness burns usually require skin grafting, are associated with permanent scarring, and take several weeks to heal.
- Full-thickness burns with extension into deep tissues, also known as fourth-degree burns, involve destruction and/or extensive injury of muscle, fascia, nerves, tendons, vessels, and bone. They typically require surgical intervention and skin grafting.

Burns involving large surfaces of the body generally vary as to their degree of depth. Burn wounds are dynamic, and the effect of dermal ischemia (affected by infection, exposure, and dehydration) may not be readily apparent at first. Their depth can also change from day to day. The percentage of body surface area (BSA) and the part(s) of the body affected are also key factors to determine treatment, disposition, and prognosis (Table 39-4). Multiple methods have been devised to estimate the BSA affected. For example, the area covered by a child's palm (from wrist crease to finger crease), also called the "rule of the palm," is considered to represent 1% of total BSA and may be used for estimating the extent of small burns covering less than 10% of BSA (Antoon and Donovan, 2007). Free software to calculate BSA in pediatric burn victims is available at http://www.sagediagram.com/.

Determining the need for admission to a hospital or burn center involves many factors including burn depth, percentage of body surface area injured, and mechanism of the burn injury. Other factors that influence hospital or burn center admission include risk of infection, pain control, functional and cosmetic outcomes, and social considerations. Children with burn injuries who meet the following criteria should be admitted to a children's hospital or a burn center (Reddy and Parke Maier, 2009; Tsarouhas and Agosto, 2008):

- Partial-thickness burns involving 10% to 25% of BSA
- Partial-thickness burns, or superficial burns of concern involving the hands and feet, genitalia, perineum; circumferential burns and burns overlying joints
- Full-thickness burns involving 2% to 15% of BSA
- Chemical burns, electrical burns (including lightning injury), inhalation injury
- Burns associated with another injury (e.g., motor vehicle accident) or in a child with a preexisting medical disorder
- Very young child
- Inability of caregiver to care for a child with a burn at home or suspicion of child abuse or neglect

Children with any sign of airway compromise should immediately be placed on 100% oxygen and sent to the hospital for further care and management. Airway complications and inhalation injuries should be suspected if there is loss of consciousness, presence of facial burns, burns over nasal passages or oral cavity, hoarseness, change in voice, or presence of cough or wheezing (Antoon and Donovan, 2007).

TABLE 39-4 Estimation of Surface Area Burned Based on Age*

Area	AGE (YEARS)					
	Birth to 1	1-4	5-9	10-14	15	Adult
Head	19	17	13	11	9	7
Neck	2	2	2	2	2	2
Anterior trunk	13	13	13	13	13	13
Posterior trunk	13	13	13	13	13	13
Right buttock	2.5	2.5	2.5	2.5	2.5	2.5
Left buttock	2.5	2.5	2.5	2.5	2.5	2.5
Genitalia	1	1	1	1	1	1
Right upper arm	4	4	4	4	4	4
Left upper arm	4	4	4	4	4	4
Right lower arm	3	3	3	3	3	3
Left lower arm	3	3	3	3	3	3
Right hand	2.5	2.5	2.5	2.5	2.5	2.5
Left hand	2.5	2.5	2.5	2.5	2.5	2.5
Right thigh	5.5	6.5	8	8.5	9	9.5
Left thigh	5.5	6.5	8	8.5	9	9.5
Right leg	5	5	5.5	6	6.5	7
Left leg	5	5	5.5	6	6.5	7
Right foot	3.5	3.5	3.5	3.5	3.5	3.5
Left foot	3.5	3.5	3.5	3.5	3.5	3.5

*This modification by O'Neill of the Brooke Army Burn Center Diagram shows the change in surface area of the head from 19% in an infant to 7% in an adult. Proper use of this chart provides an accurate basis for subsequent management of the burned child.

From Joffe MD: Burns. In Fleisher GR, Ludwig S, Henretig FM, editors: *Textbook of pediatric emergency medicine*, ed 6, Philadelphia, 2010, Lippincott Williams & Wilkins, p 1285.

Epidemiology

Although the incidence of pediatric burn injuries has declined with the help of legislative action and public education, burn injuries continue to be a major source of morbidity and mortality for children (Tsarouhas and Agosto, 2008). Nearly 34% of all fatal injuries in children younger than 16 years are due to burns (Antoon and Donovan, 2007). In 2006, 553 children younger than age 20 died from burns, and 133,000 children were treated in EDs for nonfatal burns in 2007 (Quinlan et al, 2010). Modern technology such as the use of microwaves has increased the exposure of children to potentially injurious thermal energy in their environment. Common modes of injury include scalding, flash injuries from ignition of volatile substances, and electrical and flame injuries. The house fire is by far the most lethal cause of burns in children and typically results in thermal and concomitant inhalation injury.

Overall, scald-related burns account for 85% of total injuries and occur most commonly in children younger than 5 years of age, with a peak between 9 and 33 months of age (Antoon and Donovan, 2007; Quinlan et al, 2010). Scald injuries are usually caused from accidental tipping of a container holding hot liquid that spills on a child. Burn injuries sustained from hot liquid can be deeper and more severe with less contact time in children than in adults (Reddy and Parke Maier, 2009).

The intentional inflicting of burns to a child is unfortunately a common form of abuse. Every burn injury in a child should be evaluated for a potential etiology of abuse or neglect. Intentionally inflicted burn injuries often leave a characteristic pattern.

Clinical Findings

History. The following information should be obtained:
- Description of how the burn occurred, including agent of injury and length of time agent was in contact with the skin, circumstances surrounding the injury, when it occurred, and likelihood of other injuries, such as trauma or smoke inhalation
- Initial and subsequent treatment of the burn
- Previous history of burn injuries
- Other current medical problems, medications, allergies, and tetanus status
- Suspicion of child abuse if the injury does not match the history and mechanism described (see Chapter 17).

Physical Examination. The physical examination should begin by conducting a primary assessment of the airways.

The most common cause of death during the first hour after a burn injury is respiratory impairment. Inhalation injury produces upper airway edema that can proceed with alarming speed to complete airway obstruction. Inhalation injury should be suspected if there is hoarseness, wheezing, cough, rales, singed nasal hairs, carbonized sputum, cyanosis, or altered mental status. Inhalation injury may also be associated with facial or neck burns. In such cases immediate emergency intervention (paramedics and immediate transport to the ED) is warranted. Once the patient is stable, a thorough physical examination requires the following determinations:

- Percentage of BSA affected (see Table 39-4)
- Type of burn and associated injuries
- Distribution and pattern of the burn with particular concern for circumferential burns to the thorax that may cause poor chest expansion and declining oxygen saturation
- Burn depth—classified as superficial, partial thickness, or full thickness
- Assessment of the vascular status of extremities
- Presence of any complicating medical condition

Diagnostic Studies
- A CBC is indicated to establish baseline levels. The hematocrit is often elevated secondary to fluid loss. Initial elevation of the white blood cell count is most always secondary to an acute phase reaction, but later may be an indicator of infection.
- A basic metabolic panel may reveal elevated potassium due to cell breakdown. Blood urea nitrogen (BUN) and creatinine are used to assess renal function and tissue perfusion.
- A urinalysis, particularly the specific gravity, helps determine hydration status, and presence of myoglobin may suggest acute tubular necrosis secondary to muscle tissue destruction and breakdown.
- Baseline clotting studies and typing and crossmatching may be indicated if there is associated trauma or if surgical intervention, such as grafting, is considered.
- Pulse oximetry, arterial blood gases, carboxyhemoglobin (for inhalation or suspected inhalation injury), and chest radiographs are indicated if there is airway involvement or vascular instability.
- Cardiac monitoring may be needed for electrical burn injury and as indicated.
- Culturing of critical burn wounds may need to be done weekly or more frequently if infection develops.

Differential Diagnosis

Chapter 17 discusses intentional burn injuries resulting from child abuse. Scalded skin syndrome caused by staphylococcal infection can cause skin exfoliation, but the clinical presentation clearly differentiates it from an accidental burn injury. Management is similar to that used for burn management.

Management

Most children with major burns require treatment in the hospital setting and management by a burn specialist team. Electric and chemical burns also require hospitalization for observation and management. Children with a burn injury associated with inhalation injury, fractures, suspicion of abuse, uncertainty of follow-up by the parent, or severe pain should also be admitted. The outpatient treatment of minor burns is an option only for superficial burns (first degree) and partial-thickness burns (second degree) to less than 10% of BSA. Referral and consultation with a burn specialist should be made depending on severity and location of the burn. Box 39-1 outlines the primary care management of superficial and partial-thickness burns. Partial-thickness burns covering greater than 10% of BSA, full-thickness burns covering more than 2% of BSA, and any partial- or full-thickness burns of the face, hands, feet, perineum, or genitalia should be referred for hospital management by burn specialists (Reddy and Parke Maier, 2009; Tsarouhas and Agosto, 2008).

Patient and Parent Education

The following points are important components of patient and parent education:

- Emphasize use of sunscreen protection to prevent sunburn. This is also very important for skin that is recovering from a burn because the skin is prone to hyperpigmentation from sunlight for up to a year following the burn injury. All skin that has been burned should be protected from sun for at least 12 months. Encourage parents to avoid sun exposure as much as possible and to use a sunscreen with a sun protection factor (SPF) of 30 (or higher) if sun exposure is unavoidable.
- Discuss home and environmental safety issues related to burn prevention at health maintenance visits. Effective strategies include the use of anti-scald temperature devices for the tub and shower, turning pot handles, making the area around the stove a "kid-free zone," avoiding carrying children with lit cigarettes or hot liquids in hand, keeping appliance cords away from counter edges, installing working smoke detectors, changing the batteries at the start and end of daylight saving time, and keeping fire extinguishers in homes and cars (Quinlan et al, 2010).
- Reinforce safety issues after a burn injury has occurred (e.g., scald prevention, use of smoke detectors, safekeeping of matches and cigarette lighters, safe use of electric cords and outlets).
- Teach first-aid measures for burns (e.g., submerge minor burned area in tepid water; do not use butter, margarine, and oil-based creams and lotions; rinse chemical burns in cold water, and flush skin thoroughly for at least 20 minutes).
- Inform parents of serious or long-term consequences of burns: frequent and significant sunburns during early childhood can predispose to skin cancers in later life; electric burns cause thermal injury to skin [contact burn]; if an arc is created and there is passage of electrical current through the body, there is a potential for cardiac dysrhythmias and neurologic impairment following the burn.
- Inform parents that the extent of scarring is difficult to predict with certainty; that scarring depends on depth of the burn, length of time needed for healing, whether grafting was done, and the child's age and skin color; and that scars remain immature for the first 12 to 18 months and go through color and texture changes as the child grows. Most minor scald injuries from hot liquids heal quickly with little or no scarring.

BOX 39-1 Management of Superficial and Partial-Thickness Burns in the Primary Care Setting

1. Maintain proper nutrition and hydration to enhance healing.
2. Management of superficial burns (Sheridan, 2008):
   - Cleanse the burn and surrounding skin with lukewarm water and soap once a day. Then apply a topical antibiotic such as bacitracin.
   - A nonadherent dressing followed by a gauze dressing may be applied for larger more severe superficial burns and changed once per day or when soiled.
   - Administer analgesics, such as acetaminophen or ibuprofen as directed for pain relief.
3. Management of superficial partial-thickness burns (Antoon and Donovan, 2007):
   - Administer adequate analgesic medication. Acetaminophen with codeine may be needed before wound care is performed and during the day. Switch to over-the-counter acetaminophen or ibuprofen as the pain subsides.
   - Cleanse the wound by generous irrigation with normal saline solution.
   - Monitor the burn daily for the first few days to ensure proper healing, and assess for infection. Dressing changes and wound cleansing with debridement should be performed twice a day until the burn has healed.
   - Treat very small areas, especially facial wounds with bacitracin ointment and leave area open to air.
   - If bullae or blisters are present and intact, leave them intact. They act as a natural bandage to keep bacteria out. Most bullae or blisters open eventually on their own, but while left intact they protect the underlying skin from infection and allow time for internal healing.

- Gently debride open blisters to remove devitalized tissue and residue from prior dressing changes.
- Apply bacitracin or 1% silver sulfadiazine cream to the clean debrided area followed by the application of sterile petrolatum gauze. Next apply a dry gauze outer dressing. Do not apply a circumferential gauze wrap because of the risk of impaired circulation if swelling occurs. Instead, a tubular stretch gauze netting may be used to hold the dressing in place.
- Do not use 1% silver sulfadiazine if the patient has a sulfa allergy or if the burn is on the face. This product is an antimicrobial and soothing agent, but has the potential to stain skin, which is why its use should be avoided on facial burns.
- Use mittens for young children to prevent scratching if itching occurs as the burn heals. If needed, administer an antihistamine such as diphenhydramine.
- If a partial-thickness burn involves an extremity, keep it elevated to reduce edema and compromise of blood flow to the burned area. Individuals with circumferential burns of an extremity may need to be admitted to the hospital for observation so that compartment syndrome does not develop.
- Another option for partial thickness burn management is the use of Aquacel Ag dressing (ConvaTec). Aquacel Ag is a dressing that is impregnated with silver ion, which helps prevent infection. Apply the Aquacel Ag after cleansing and debridement of the burn is complete. Cover the burned area with sterile gauze and leave in place for 10 days, checking the wound twice a week.
- For deep partial-thickness burns, Papain/urea ointment (Accuzyme) ointment is a debridement agent that can be used once daily.

CONTUSIONS AND HEMATOMAS

Description

A contusion, or bruise, is an injury in which the skin is not broken but trauma has caused effusion into muscle and subcutaneous tissue with injury to the vessels and possibly the nerves. In children, contusions can occur anywhere on the body, but are most often seen on the extremities.

Epidemiology

Contusions are common in children and are caused by blunt trauma, most often as a result of falling or bumping into objects during play. Participation in contact sports puts children at increased risk for contusions. Bruises to the trunk, face, or head should raise a red flag for possible child abuse. A careful history must be taken to determine whether the explanation of the injury is consistent with the child's condition and his or her independent report of what happened.

Hematomas are localized collections of extravasated blood that are relatively or completely confined within a space or potential space. In essence, a hematoma is a raised, palpable ecchymosis or bruise. Hematomas can be associated with most types of minor and major wounds; they must be observed closely for signs of infection and, in some instances, drained.

Clinical Findings

History. The following should be assessed:
- Cause of bruise
- Treatment given
- History of easy bleeding or bruising, or slow healing

Physical Examination. The following should be determined:
- Circulatory status and discoloration
- Motor and sensory function: Reduced mobility or range of motion
- Involvement of underlying structures
- Presence of swelling
- Pain or point tenderness
- Limited mobility

If there is any evidence of circulatory compromise, such as lack of pulse, it is important to seek care in the ED immediately.

Differential Diagnosis

Hemophilia, von Willebrand disease, and purpura should be considered. Myositis ossificans, a complication of contusions rarely seen in children, can be confused with osteogenic sarcoma.

Management

With contusions involving extremities:
1. Acute phase, first 24 hours (Toy, 2009):
   - Prescribe rest, ice, compression, and elevation (RICE):
     o Rest and immobilize the affected part (this is best achieved with a splint in extremity injuries).
     o Ice (or cold compress with an ice bag wrapped in a towel) applied to the injury for 10 to 20 minutes per hour for the first 24 hours

○ Compression: Application of a pressure bandage to help prevent swelling

○ Elevation of the affected part (ideally, above the level of the heart) to prevent swelling

• Provide appropriate analgesia. A nonsteroidal antiinflammatory drug (NSAID), such as ibuprofen, is a good choice.

2. From *24* to *48* hours after the acute phase of tenderness and swelling:
   • Apply warm compresses or soaks.
   • Stretch.
   • Do range-of-motion and strengthening exercises.

3. For *5* to *7* days, avoid exercise that involves the contused area.

4. Key management points to remember:
   • Reserve radiographs for suspected foreign bodies or bone fracture.
   • Refer severe injuries for orthopedic management.

Complications

Most contusions heal quickly without sequelae, but severe trauma to the quadriceps muscle can lead to myositis ossificans if not treated properly or, with large hemorrhage, to compartment syndrome.

Patient and Parent Education

Explain to parents the expected color changes of ecchymosis from the purple discoloration to greenish and that the ecchymosis may also migrate to other surrounding tissues. Arrange for follow-up if discomfort continues or increases. Encourage parents to provide their children with a physical environment that minimizes risk of injury. Return to activities is determined by the degree of injury and resolution of subjective symptoms. A program of rehabilitation may be needed (Toy, 2009).

SPRAINS AND STRAINS

Description

Ligaments act to help stabilize a joint. A sprain is a tear of a ligament joining bone to bone around the joint and is caused most commonly by outside forces, especially contact sports. Strains are tears of the muscle or of fascia joining muscle to bone, often resulting from a dynamic injury and usually not a contact sport.

Sprains and strains may occur concurrently, and both can be graded by severity as a first-degree, second-degree, or third-degree injury. A grade I sprain involves minimal stretching of a ligament with no major change in the affected joint. However, small hemorrhagic areas are noted on histologic examination. A grade II sprain results in more tearing and hemorrhaging of the ligament than seen with a grade I sprain. There is mild to moderate functional loss and bleeding but the ligament is still holding. A grade III sprain is a complete disruption of the ligament with ligamentous instability and often requires casting (Toy, 2009).

Ankle injuries are the most common acute sports-related injury. Ankle sprains account for 85% of ankle injuries and are the result of an inversion injury, eversion injury, or a combination of the two (Landry, 2007). Eighty-five percent of ankle sprains are caused from inversion injuries alone (Anderson, 2010; Landry, 2007).

Epidemiology

Sprains are a common athletic injury in children. They most commonly affect the ankle, knee, shoulder, elbow, or wrist and are caused by falls or contact in which the extremity is immobile or moving on one plane and a countervailing force is applied to the joint. In general the degree of disability immediately after the injury correlates with the severity. For example, if an athlete is injured during a game and cannot walk off the playing field, he or she is more likely to have a serious injury than one who is able to continue playing. The incidence of ankle sprains increases as children age (Staheli, 2008). Ankle sprains are less common than fractures in children and preadolescents because ligaments are stronger compared with growth plates and growing bones in this age group. Associated avulsion fractures are commonly seen in children with an open growth plate who have sustained a ligamentous injury.

Muscle strain is a common injury and may occur with delayed muscle soreness (muscle pain 24 to 72 hours after intense physical activity) and partial or complete muscle tears. This injury is commonly seen in fatigued muscles that are not able to lengthen in a controlled fashion (Toy, 2009).

Clinical Findings

History. The following are assessed (McMahon, 2007):

• Detailed history of the mechanism of injury (e.g., fall, collision, twisting of joint)

• Description of symptoms (e.g., onset, location, duration, characteristics, aggravating and relieving factors)

• Type of first-aid treatment given

• Sprain complaints depend on the site of ligamentous injury:
   ○ Calf—some children may describe an immediate sharp pain, hear or feel a "pop" or "snap," and are unable to raise their lower leg, or complain of calf pain when raising their leg.
   ○ Knee—for the anterior cruciate ligament sprain (becoming more common in older children and adolescents due to increase in sports participation), a "pop" or "snap" heard or felt at time of injury (Shea et al, 2008).
   ○ Ankle—inversion injury. In younger children, tears of the lateral ankle ligament often disrupt the open growth plate of the distal fibula. In contrast, with skeletal maturity, classic lateral ankle sprain is more common in an adolescent than a Salter-Harris I fracture of the distal fibula
   ○ Wrist—swelling and pain along the dorsum of the wrist; positive Watson sign (pain and an audible click heard when dorsal pressure is placed over the distal scaphoid while performing ulnar and radial deviation)
   ○ Lumbar—midline tenderness because these sprains are often due to injury to the interspinous process ligament; low back pain and paraspinal muscle spasm are common; neurologic symptoms are absent

• Strain complaints depend on the site of muscular injury (McMahon, 2007):
   ○ Calf—may describe an immediate sharp pain, hear or feel a "pop" or "snap," and are unable to raise the lower leg or complain of pain when raising the lower leg
   ○ Cervical—limited range of motion and tenderness over the involved neck muscles
   ○ Lumbar—either acute or chronic back pain; pain is limited to the back or paraspinal muscles and there is no radiating pain to the lower extremities; may have a painful trigger point with palpation

An orthopedic injury should be suspected if there is a history of significant trauma (fall from height, motor vehicle accident, etc.) or if the patient complains of immediate pain after an injury. However, the cause may have been unwitnessed or not noticed so that an injury is not suspected until significant swelling becomes apparent. Toddlers and young children may present with crying after an unwitnessed fall. Younger children may self-splint an extremity for many reasons, including infection, tumor, inflammation, or neurologic etiology, but trauma is the most common cause of decreased arm movement.

Physical Examination. The approach to the physical examination depends on the joint involved, the severity of the injury, and the child's ability to cooperate. If the injury is acute, it can be difficult to distinguish the extent of damage. The child may require additional visits for a more careful examination as the swelling and pain subside. Always examine the joints and structures located above and below the injury for possible involvement, check function of the injured part, and check circulation and sensation. Any circulatory compromise or notable reduction in sensation (numbness or paralysis) suggests a more serious injury and should be referred to the ED or an orthopedist. Use the corresponding joint and muscle mass in the other extremity as a control for comparison. Inspect for degree of swelling and ecchymosis over the affected side of the injured extremity, especially in ankle injuries. Physical examination findings can be helpful to differentiate ankle sprain from ankle fracture. Ankle sprains are marked by tenderness over the anterior talofibular, posterior talofibular, or calcaneofibular ligament; tenderness over the distal fibula or tibia physis is associated with a fracture (Anderson, 2010).

Diagnostic Studies. Radiographs are indicated if there is gross deformity, serious impairment in mobility, point tenderness on examination, or moderate to severe swelling. Simple radiographs of extremities or other major joint systems are relatively inexpensive and can be useful in distinguishing a sprain or strain from a fracture. Table 39-5 identifies the grading system for sprains and strains. With ankle injuries, if there is significant tenderness over the lateral malleolus, x-rays should be performed to rule out a physeal fracture (Staheli, 2008) (for evaluation of knee injuries, refer to Chapter 37). To rule out fractures and dislocations of the cervical spine, two orthogonal radiographic views from the occiput to the T1 junction are needed. MRI is necessary if there is cervical instability or neurologic compromise.

Stiell and colleagues (1995) developed the Ottawa Ankle Rules (OAR) to guide clinical decision-making regarding when radiographs are indicated for certain foot and ankle injuries. Figure 39-1 depicts the OAR. These rules have been applied successfully in adult populations and are shown to save time and money in the health care system without compromising quality of care.

Dowling and colleagues (2009) published a systematic review of the accuracy of using the OAR in children (18 years and younger) with blunt foot and/or ankle injury. They found that the use of the OAR in children 5 years of age and older with acute blunt ankle and/or midfoot injury had a 98.5% pooled sensitivity in identification of fractures. The researchers concluded from their findings that the OAR is a reliable ankle fracture exclusion tool used in children 5 years of age and older with ankle and midfoot injuries. A limitation of the study was that the types of clinically significant fractures included in the sensitivity and specificity calculations varied among

TABLE 39-5	Grading of Sprains and Strains	
Severity	**Sprain**	**Strain**
Grade I	Injury involves ligament stretching, and very mild if any tearing of ligament fibers; mild swelling and pain with evaluation of stress testing, no laxity in joint noted	Muscle or tendon stretched with mild tearing; strength of muscle intact, mild pain on evaluation
Grade II	Partial tearing of ligament; moderate swelling and pain and some laxity of joint on evaluation	Partial tearing of muscle or tendon; moderate pain and weakness on evaluation
Grade III	Complete tear of ligament fibers; severe swelling and pain with significant laxity of joint on evaluation	Complete tear of muscle and or tendon; severe pain and weakness on evaluation

the 12 studies included in the meta-analysis. Some studies included all fractures in their statistical analysis, whereas others excluded all Salter-Harris 1 fractures. This variation in the inclusion criteria could have altered the meta-analysis sensitivity and specificity results, thus influencing the reliability and applicability of the OAR use within the pediatric population. In light of current research, the OAR should be used with caution and only in children older than the age of 5 years who are verbal and without neurologic impairment or multiple trauma.

The Ottawa Knee Rules (OKR) can also be used as guides for when to order radiographs in cases of acute knee injury in patients more than 5 years old. The OKR criteria, which are used as indicators for the presence of a fracture, tenderness at the head of the fibula (it must be the only area of bone tenderness), isolated tenderness of the patella, inability to flex 90 degrees, and inability to bear weight (take four steps) immediately and in the ED. For the pediatric population, the rule of age greater than 5 years is not used for radiograph criteria. Vijayasankar and associates (2009) conducted a systematic review and meta-analysis of observational studies regarding the use of the OKR in children with knee injuries to identify fractures. They reported 99% sensitivity and 46% specificity, concluding that the OKR is a great diagnostic tool to use in children older than age 5 years. Their systemic review and meta-analysis included studies using the OKR in children and found limited evidence to support use of the OKR in children younger than 5 years, attributing verbal skills and challenges of assessing the younger child as barriers for use of the rules. Although the evidence to support use of the OKR in children older than 5 years was noted, a limited number of studies were included in the meta-analysis. Therefore, until greater certainty is established about the use of OKR in children, liberal referral for radiograph in cases of knee injury in children is still recommended.

Differential Diagnosis

If there is excessive swelling or discoloration around the joint, suspect a fracture, especially of the epiphysis, or dislocation. The degree of pain or pain behavior (e.g., dramatic) does not

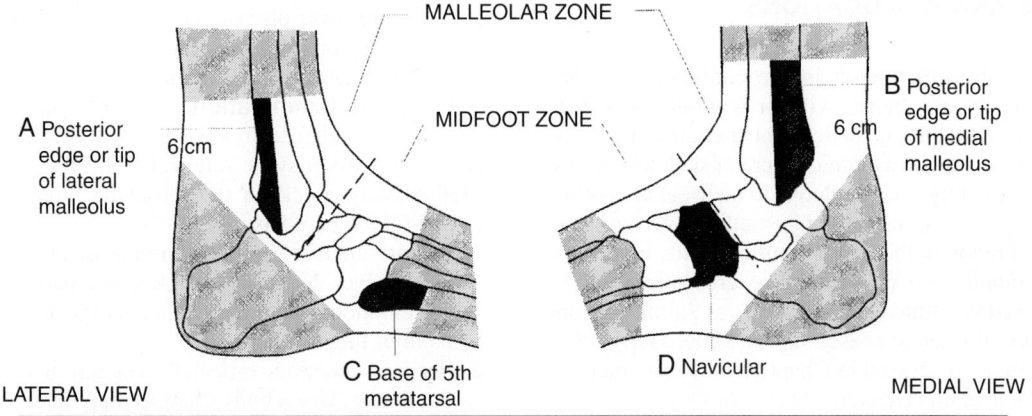

MALLEOLAR ZONE

MIDFOOT ZONE

A Posterior edge or tip of lateral malleolus

6 cm

B Posterior edge or tip of medial malleolus

6 cm

C Base of 5th metatarsal

D Navicular

LATERAL VIEW

MEDIAL VIEW

FIGURE 39-1 The use of radiography in acute ankle injuries: Ottawa Ankle Rules.
An ankle x-ray series is required only if there is any pain in the malleolar zone and any of these findings:
- Bone tenderness at A
- Bone tenderness at B
- Inability to bear weight both immediately and in emergency department

A foot x-ray series is required only if there is any foot pain in midfoot zone and any of these findings:
- Bone tenderness at C
- Bone tenderness at D
- Inability to bear weight both immediately and in emergency department

(From Stiell IG, Greenberg GH, McKnight RD et al: A study to develop clinical decision rules for the use of radiography in acute ankle injuries, *Ann Emerg Med* 21:384-390, 1992, with permission from the American Academy of Emergency Physicians.)

distinguish a sprain or strain from a fracture. Preverbal children, in particular, may have difficulty localizing pain, may complain of generalized pain, or may experience referred pain in one area caused by injury in an adjacent area. Although trauma is the most common cause of joint pain in children, infectious, rheumatologic, inflammatory, neoplastic, and hematologic abnormalities also should be considered, especially with fever, joint effusion, swelling, or erythema.

Management

Care of sprains and strains differs depending on the grade of injury. Children with grade III sprains or strains should always be referred to an orthopedist. Management for lesser injuries is as follows:
1. Acute management for grade I or II sprains and strains
   - RICE for the injured part. Apply ice immediately for 15 to 20 minutes, and then, depending on the severity of the injury, every 2 to 6 hours for the first 24 to 48 hours. Ice may be applied using massage (a paper cup filled with water and frozen is ideal), ice packs, or immersion of the injured part in an ice-water bath. A pressure bandage, preferably an adhesive tape athletic wrapping, may then be applied with gentle, steady pressure. An Ace wrap is less effective. Take care not to allow impairment of circulation. Elevate the limb. No weight-bearing activity on the injured limb should occur until pain diminishes.
   - Give NSAID with food. Initially, NSAIDs can be used for 7 to 10 days without affecting muscle healing, but longer use may interfere with muscle healing at a later stage.
   - Heat may be used after 48 hours for mild sprains to facilitate healing.

2. Nonacute or chronic management
   - May bear weight as tolerated
   - Apply stabilizer or brace for unstable joint; may be needed for 3 to 6 weeks.
   - Recommend rehabilitation exercises, including range of motion, stretching, and strengthening. Rehabilitation should be gradual, beginning with isometric exercises of muscles and progressing to fuller range of motion and strengthening exercises. There should be no pain or swelling as exercise progresses. A general rule of thumb for return to sport activities for ankle sprains is 1 month for grade I, 2 months for grade II, and up to 3 months for grade III sprains. Ultrasound therapy may be beneficial.
   - Apply ice after exercise.
   - Athletes should not return to competition after a sprain until they are pain-free and can perform all sports-specific activities.
3. For grade II and III sprains, consultation with an orthopedist is needed. Severe sprains may need casting or surgery (Latterman et al, 2007).

Patient and Parent Education

Prevention of injury is key. Teach children and parents the importance of using protective gear (e.g., wrist guards for skaters). Children should also be encouraged to maintain a continuous level of physical activity to maximize muscle strength.

Prevention of strains can be achieved with consistent stretching, warm-up exercises, and maintenance of muscle strength through regular activity. Strength training may reduce the incidence and severity of overuse injuries. For children who wish to participate in sports activities, advise them to structure a period of conditioning into their schedules.

FRACTURES AND DISLOCATIONS

Description

A fracture involves a disruption in the continuity of bone tissue, with bowing or a break, with or without separation. Pediatric patients have unique patterns of fractures due to the immaturity of bone and the dynamic nature of skeletal growth. Due to the strength of ligaments relative to the weakness of the physis, fractures are common among youth sports activities (Canty, 2009). Fractures that occur in the physis, epiphysis, metaphysis, or diaphysis may be complete, greenstick, buckle, comminuted, avulsed, transverse, oblique, or spiral. Various types of epiphyseal fractures based on the Salter-Harris classification system are discussed in Chapter 37. Stress fractures are discussed later in this chapter.

Dislocations are characterized by displacement of bone ends from their normal position in a joint. There can be wide variation in degree of displacement.

Epidemiology

Fractures are relatively common in children, accounting for 15% of all childhood injuries (Staheli, 2008). The frequency and severity of sports injuries increase with age, with boys more likely to be injured than girls; 20% of all pediatric ED visits secondary to sports injuries are caused from fractures (Landry, 2007). Clavicular fractures may be due to birth trauma (see Chapter 37). Accidents in which the child tries to break a fall using outstretched arms can result in fractures of the wrist, ulna, radius, or humerus. Direct trauma to bones or joints (e.g., resulting from contact sports, auto accidents, falls) can cause fractures or dislocations.

Clinical Findings

History. A description of the acute trauma, and the signs and symptoms occurring at the time of trauma, provides useful data. An accurate history of the time of the event, mechanism of injury, and direction of forces is important and helps define the type of injury. Often such orthopedic injuries are not witnessed. A child may be too frightened, in too much pain, or too immature to articulate what happened to give a reliable history. However, children rarely complain about persistent pain unless there is an abnormality. Be sure to ask about any history of previous injury and aggravating disease processes, such as preexisting bleeding abnormality, rickets,

renal failure, liver disease, or malignancy. A delay in seeking medical care or a history that is vague or inconsistent with injuries is suggestive of child abuse.

Physical Examination. Carefully inspect the injured part and the adjacent body parts, keeping in mind that pain and tenderness may be referred from injury in another area. Meticulously check for the following three functions, which can be remembered as MSV:

1. **M**otor function, including range of motion, both passive and active. Note any limitations, particularly problems with tendon functioning. This is especially important with hand or finger injuries.
2. **S**ensory function, especially for any loss of sensation or numbness. Use a body chart to map the location. The existence of point tenderness, produced by palpating over a particular area, is suggestive of possible fracture.
3. **V**ascular function, especially for evidence of any vascular compromise.

Carefully document findings before and after any manipulation that is done. Significant findings include the following:
- Deformity
- Swelling
- Ecchymosis
- Bone or joint misalignment
- Loss of function or mobility (especially with dislocation); limping or inability to bear weight
- Muscle spasm
- Discoloration (pallor or cyanosis)
- Decrease in vascular function, such as capillary refill, diminished or absent pulses

Lacerations with open fractures must be treated promptly in the ED. Dislocations are rare, but when they do occur, they most commonly involve the radial head or patella. Fractures often accompany dislocations because ligamentous structures are more resistant to trauma (Table 39-6).

Diagnostic Studies. Because of pain, anxiety, and the possibility of an unreliable or incomplete history, the health care provider must maintain a high index of suspicion for possible fracture. Radiography must be considered for findings of deformity, marked swelling, persistent pain of the injured site at rest or during motion, ecchymosis, point tenderness, numbness, and loss of function. Figure 39-1 shows the use of radiography in acute ankle injuries using the OAR for children ages 5 years and older.

TABLE 39-6	Assessment and Management of Fractures		
Injury	**Clinical Findings**	**Diagnostic Studies**	**Management**
Fracture/ dislocation	Point tenderness over site, generalized pain, deformity, misalignment of bone or joint, loss of function or mobility (especially in dislocation), muscle spasm, discoloration, swelling, lacerations (if open fracture) *Clinical pearl:* tenderness below the lateral malleolus is typically ankle sprain, not fracture; if excessive swelling or discoloration along the joint, suspect fracture or dislocation, especially of epiphysis	Lateral and anteroposterior radiographs (for ankle radiographs, also obtain a mortise view); may need to repeat in 10-14 days because early and Salter I fractures may not appear on first films	Referral for casting or other orthopedic interventions
Stress fracture (repeated microtrauma)	Gradual onset of pain with activity that decreases with rest, point tenderness; distal atrophy and local swelling may be noted	Radiograph; if normal, do a bone scan/ ultrasonography	Rest and eliminate activity that caused microtrauma for 10-14 days; casting if complete fracture; retraining

Lateral and anteroposterior radiographic views should be obtained along with radiographs of the joint above and below an injury. If a fracture of the ankle is suspected, obtain a mortise view as well. Because of the growth plates, comparison views may be obtained on a selective basis. Contralateral radiographs, though not routinely recommended, can be helpful for diagnosing suspected fracture sites where bone ossification is not complete and radiograph interpretation is challenging (Staheli, 2009). This is especially helpful for elbow fractures in children. Early fractures and Salter I fractures do not always appear on radiographs at the time of injury. However, follow-up radiographic studies 7 to 10 days after the trauma may reveal a fracture line. Guidelines for ordering radiography after ankle injuries are discussed earlier in this chapter.

A CT scan may be necessary to delineate articular fractures or for complex physeal fractures (e.g., in the area of the distal tibia). Toddler's fracture (an oblique fracture of the distal one third of the tibia without a fibula fracture) may not be seen radiographically. An oblique view may help to visualize the fracture.

Differential Diagnosis

The cause of a fracture should be determined because fractures can also be a result of pathologic conditions such as genetic or metabolic bone disease (osteogenesis imperfecta, osteoporosis), benign bone tumors (bone cysts, cartilage or fibrous tumor), skeletal sarcoma or skeletal metastases, nutritional deficit, or environmental causes (rickets) (Schwartz and Holt, 2008). Conditions such as hyperparathyroidism and copper deficiency have also been linked to causing pathologic fractures. Careful review of the child's medications should be performed because some medications can cause pathologic fractures as well. Children who are physically abused may have multiple fractures at different stages of healing or have a history of repeated fractures. The fractures typically seen in cases of child abuse involve the skull, ribs, or vertebrae, or spiral, oblique, or transverse fractures in the long bones (especially in children before the age of walking) (see Chapter 17).

Management

All suspected fractures should be splinted promptly. This stabilizes the fracture, prevents damage to the surrounding soft tissues, and reduces pain by reducing movement. If the injury is to an extremity, immediate intervention includes application of ice and elevation of the body part to prevent swelling. Uncontrolled swelling can cause neurovascular compromise if confined to a compartment.

Simple fractures can usually be easily reduced and immobilized. They typically heal quickly with no disruption in the child's growth. The potential for impairment to growth plates, joints, tendons, or neurovascular structures following trauma is of serious concern. All children with fractures, other than simple fractures or dislocations, need immediate referral to an orthopedic specialist for management. Open reduction is often necessary with severe fractures. Pediatric elbow fractures are often difficult to diagnose and are prone to complications. Referral of these fractures to a pediatric orthopedist is usually needed. Children with fractures involving the growth plate (Salter-Harris) or those that are pathologic in etiology should also be referred to an orthopedist.

Because dislocations often involve fractures in addition to the stretching and deforming of the ligaments, it is best to have an orthopedist involved for the dislocation reduction procedure. Analgesia is usually required before the reduction, and radiographic studies should be obtained before and after the reduction. Open dislocations or those associated with neurovascular compromise are true emergencies and must be referred immediately for emergency care. Patients recovering from fractures and dislocations should be provided with appropriate and adequate analgesia because fractures and dislocations are painful.

General indications for emergency referral and immediate orthopedic consultation include (Landry, 2007):
- Open fracture
- Displaced, severely angulated fractures (depending on severity and location of fracture)
- Vascular or nerve compromise surrounding the injured site
- Deep laceration over a joint
- Unreducible dislocation
- Grade III muscle-tendon tear

Specific indications requiring emergency referral and immediate orthopedic consultation include:
- Upper extremity (Harley, 2009)
  - Carpometacarpal joint or shoulder dislocation
  - Supracondylar fracture
- Lower extremity (Canty, 2009)
  - Pelvis or femur fracture
  - Hip or knee dislocation

Patient and Parent Education

Provide information concerning cast care or application of compression bandages, use of ice to minimize swelling, and keeping the injured part immobilized and elevated as much as possible. Parents should also be cautioned to carefully observe the injury for signs of worsening pain, circulatory compromise, or delayed healing and should promptly notify their health care provider if any such signs occur. As with strains and sprains, injury prevention through use of protective devices, proper conditioning, and attention to the child's physical environment is essential.

STRESS FRACTURES
Description

Stress fractures are classified as overuse injuries and are becoming more common in children and adolescents. They are caused by repeated muscular action on a bony insertion site or repetitive direct trauma. Bone remodeling cannot keep up with the repeated microtrauma, which leads to bone resorption and fracture. Stress fractures in athletes are typically associated with too much training and minimal recovery time. Amenorrheic athletes are at higher risk for stress fractures (see information on the female athlete triad in Chapter 13).

Epidemiology

Stress fractures occur in typical locations and are associated with activities and sports. Common sites and causes include the following:
- Metatarsal shaft—running, marching, and ballet
- Tarsal navicular—running, high-impact aerobics

- Distal fibula and proximal tibia—running
- Ribs—coughing and golf
- Neck and shaft of the femur—running, ballet, and gymnastics

Clinical Findings

Characteristic history includes:
- Gradual onset of pain (insidious) with activity that decreases with rest
- Point tenderness over the fracture site, and occasionally local swelling
- Distal atrophy may be noted

The typical history is that of excessive exercising or beginning an aggressive exercise program without preconditioning (see Table 39-6).

Diagnostic Studies. Most stress fractures typically show normal radiographic findings or a zone of radiolucency. Only 10% of stress fractures are initially positive on radiograph. A bone scan or MRI may be needed to identify the fracture if radiographs are normal. With bone scans, a "hot spot" is noted at the fracture site and helps identify other bones at risk (Latterman et al, 2007).

Management

Management includes rest and eliminating the repetitive activity that is the source of the microtrauma for 3 to 16 weeks, depending on the severity of the stress fracture (Toy, 2009). Noncompliant patients may need to be casted for immobilization, usually for 6 to 8 weeks. For fractures of the forefoot (metatarsal fracture), a hard-soled shoe (e.g., cast shoe) or removable boot with a rocking sole can be used. A tarsal fracture can be treated by being protected or with non–weight bearing for 6 to 8 weeks. Complete fractures need to be referred to an orthopedic surgeon and most likely will be casted or may require surgical intervention. Retraining is necessary to eliminate the source of the problem, with a gradual return to activity. For amenorrheic patients, review dietary and exercise regimens with modification as needed. Also consider lab testing and referral to a gynecologist if amenorrhea persists (see Chapter 35). Consultation with an orthopedist may be needed if symptoms persist or reappear.

SUBLUXATION OF THE RADIAL HEAD

Description

Subluxation of the radial head, also known as "nursemaid's elbow" or "pulled elbow," occurs frequently in infants and children from 1 to 5 years old. There is a 30% recurrence rate of nursemaid's elbow in younger children (Harley, 2009). After 5 years of age, radial head subluxation is rare (Cornwall, 2007). The injury occurs when abrupt longitudinal (axial) traction is applied to the wrist or hand of the extended, pronated forearm of the young child. This action causes the annular ligament to slide off the head of the radius, landing in between the radius and capetellum where it becomes entrapped (Harley, 2009).

Epidemiology

Often subluxation results from an unintentional injury when a child's arm is suddenly tugged when stepping off a curb, when roughhousing with older siblings, if a child falls from playground equipment and reaches out to break the fall, or when the child is swung by the forearm. It can be a recurrent problem (not related to child maltreatment). It can also occur if the arm of an infant is trapped beneath the child's trunk as the child is rolled over. The injury is occasionally reported as the result of a fall. However, pulling of the child's arm, especially if this is a recurrent problem, may be the result of inappropriate disciplining, ignorance, or child maltreatment.

Clinical Findings

History. Often the history is nonspecific as to a report of an injury, and the parent may not have been aware of when the injury occurred. Commonly a caregiver will report the child cried, complaining of arm pain after being pulled up by his or her arm, or swung by the arms. The caregiver will also report that since the incident the child has refused to bend or use the affected arm, crying out in pain if the arm is moved, particularly the elbow. The toddler with nursemaid's elbow may be comfortable, but refuses to actively flex the elbow.

Physical Examination. Common findings in children include the following:
- The child uniformly holds the arm in pronation with the elbow slightly flexed. The degree of distress may appear minimal, but range of motion of the elbow elicits pain.
- Mild tenderness may be noted with palpation of the radial head, and pain is localized to the lateral aspect of the elbow.
- Swelling of the injured elbow is usually absent (Cornwall, 2007).

Diagnostic Studies. Radiographs are not routinely recommended when the history and clinical presentation are classic. However, if obtained, radiography of the elbow is normal.

Differential Diagnosis

Subluxation has a classic history and presentation. If the child does not improve after the reduction procedure (see next section), a fracture of the elbow or clavicle should be considered. The clinical presentation of a fracture may be similar to that of a subluxation injury. Consider maltreatment if recurrent dislocations or other symptoms or signs are present.

Management

Two techniques can be used to reduce the radial head: supination and flexion or pronation and flexion. The steps to correct the subluxation involve the following:
- Approach the child in a slow, nonthreatening way and distract the child by talking or other diversionary tactics.
- Use either the supination and flexion technique as illustrated in Figure 39-2 or the pronation and flexion technique. With the pronation and flexion technique, the provider hyperpronates the child's forearm and then flexes the elbow (Burge and ten Napel, 2008). Do not attempt this procedure if epitrochlear tenderness is present.
- A palpable or audible "pop" or "click" usually signals successful reduction. Typically the patient will begin reaching for objects again with the affected arm within 15 minutes of reduction. If reduction is successful, no further treatment is necessary.

Several attempts (up to three at reduction) may be necessary before the patient resumes normal use of the arm. If normal use does not follow reduction attempts, alternative

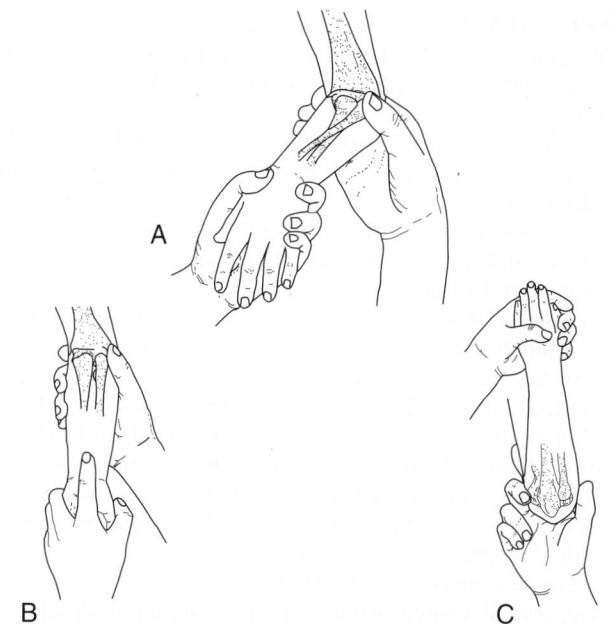

FIGURE 39-2 Reduction of radial head subluxation by supination and flexion technique. **A,** Grasp the palm of the child's hand as if to shake it. Axial traction is applied to the forearm with the wrist adducted to the ulnar side. Pressure is also applied directly over the radial head at the elbow. **B,** The forearm is supinated while axial traction and pressure are maintained over the forearm and radial head; flex the elbow to the shoulder while supination and pressure are maintained over the radial head **(C).** (From Shah B: Reduction of radial head subluxation. In Finberg L, Kleinman RE, editors: *Saunders manual of pediatric practice,* ed 2, Philadelphia, 2002, Saunders, p 1162.)

diagnoses should be considered. In these cases, immobilization with prompt orthopedic follow-up is indicated.

Patient and Parent Education

Key points to cover include the following:

- Instruct parents not to lift or pull the child by the hand or elbow.
- Parents should be taught to reduce the subluxation if it happens again.
- Subluxation of the radial head can recur in children, but is usually not seen after 5 years of age.

COMPARTMENT SYNDROME

Description

Compartment syndrome is a complication of increased pressure in an enclosed tissue space. Compartment syndrome can occur secondary to soft-tissue injuries, such as those associated with fractures, crush injuries, burns, and strenuous running. It has also been known to occur secondary to a circumferential cast.

Compartment syndrome generally affects the leg and forearm; however, it can develop in any muscle that is contained by fascia. This complication tends to occur after supracondylar fractures at the distal humerus and tibial shaft fractures. Compartment syndrome develops when there is bleeding or soft-tissue swelling within a closed fascial space (compartment), producing progressive swelling and an increase in

intracompartmental pressure. As the pressure increases venous blood flow is impaired and followed by ischemia, which if prolonged results in cellular death of the surrounding muscle and nerves. In the case of a circumferential cast, the injured soft tissue is unable to expand due to the artificially created compartment space by the cast, thus causing ischemia and tissue necrosis if the cast is not removed promptly.

Clinical Findings

Using the traditional "six P's" (pain, pallor, paresthesia, pulselessness, poikilothermia, and paralysis) in clinical identification of compartment syndrome (with the exception of pain and paresthesia) is unreliable (Jarjosa, 2009). The strongest clinical indicators of the presence of compartment syndrome are increasing pain and need for analgesia, pain on passive stretching of the involved muscle, and numbness or tingling of the muscle or extremity (Jarjosa, 2009; Vaillancourt and Shrier, 2008).

Chronic exertional compartment syndrome can be seen in athletes who participate in running, jumping, and skating sports. It is associated with a history of a local dull ache or pain confined to the muscle (not the bone) with exercise and relief of pain noted with rest. The affected compartment may be tender and feel significantly swollen. The pain can be reproduced after a period of time following onset of the activity or intensity of the exercise. Children will complain of pain with passive stretch and numbness or weakness of the site of chronic exertional compartment syndrome, and the area may feel significantly swollen. Medial tibial stress syndrome presents similar to chronic exertional compartment syndrome with the exception of no swelling at the site of pain, and pain after exercise is described as a "dull ache" (Landry, 2007; Toy, 2009).

Management

Prompt recognition of acute compartment syndrome and referral are important. The diagnosis is made by direct measurement of compartment pressures. If the syndrome is confirmed, it is treated by immediate fasciotomy. Without treatment, irreversible damage to the compartment structures occurs within 6 to 8 hours after onset of symptoms and leads to muscle necrosis, fibrosis, and ischemic contracture. With chronic exertional compartment syndrome caused by running, pain usually prevents resumption of exercise and limits the risk of muscle and nerve damage. Resting of the involved muscle until pain resolves should be stressed to the patient and parent. Physical therapy should also be considered as a treatment option for chronic exertional compartment syndrome.

BITES

ANIMAL AND CHILD BITES

Description

Children can be bitten by pets, stray animals, or humans, especially other children. Most bites are to the hand, although pet ferrets may attack a child's face. Human bites (10% to 15%), cat bites (50%), dog bites (10% to 15%), and bites to the hand carry the greatest risk of infection (American Academy of Pediatrics [AAP], 2009).

Epidemiology

An estimated 1% of ED visits annually in the U.S. are due to mammalian bites (AAP, 2009; Brook, 2009). About 80% of bites are dog bites (both provoked and unprovoked). Boys are attacked more often than girls. Dog bites are often caused by animals known to the child; in contrast, cat bites are more commonly caused by strays. The risk of infection from a dog bite is between 10% and 15%. By contrast, the risk of infection from a cat bite (despite early medical attention) is at least 50%. Cat bites cause puncture wounds and tend to be deeper than dog bites. Dog bites can cause abrasions, puncture wounds, and lacerations, with or without an associated avulsion of tissue. Limited data define the incidence of human bite injuries, but it is suspected that human bites are the leading cause of injury in child care centers. All human bite wounds, regardless of mechanism of injury, should be considered at high risk for infection. Other animal bites, such as rat bites, are not reportable, so there is a paucity of information about their epidemiology (Ginsburg, 2007). Clenched-fist bites are the most serious of human bites and typically are the result of fighting. In this type of injury, the closed fist hits the teeth of another with laceration(s) of the skin typically over the third and fourth metacarpals. These human bite injuries are high risk for infection and joint compromise.

Clinical Findings

History. Ask about the circumstances surrounding the bite, including the type of animal, domestic or sylvatic (forest-dwelling) animal, provoked or unprovoked attack, and location of the attack. History of drug allergies and immunization status of the child also should be ascertained.

Physical Examination. The wound should be assessed for the type, size, and depth of injury. Explore for the presence of foreign material and the status of underlying structures. If the bite is on an extremity, assess its range of motion and sensory intactness. Likewise, assess functioning of the facial nerve with deep facial bite injuries. A diagram of the injury should be recorded in the child's chart (Ginsburg, 2007). The provider may be wise to consider photographing the injury for documentation.

Secondary infection is the most common complication of mammalian bites and can lead to cellulitis and lymphangitis, requiring hospitalization. *Streptococcus* and *Staphylococcus* are common organisms associated with infected animal and human bites; anaerobic infection is also possible. Species of gram-negative bacteria, such as *Pasteurella*, *Moraxella*, and *Enterococcus* from dog and cat bites, and *Eikenella corrodens* and *Corynebacterium* from human bites can also cause infections (Brook, 2009). The potential for rabies exposure must also be considered.

Diagnostic Studies. Obtain wound cultures if indicated to look for aerobic and anaerobic microorganisms. A roentgenogram of the affected part should be obtained if it is likely that a bone or joint could have been penetrated or fractured or if retained foreign material is present.

Differential Diagnosis

The differential diagnosis includes lacerations or puncture wounds from other causes.

Management

Management involves both physical and psychological care of the child and includes the following (AAP, 2009; Brook, 2009):

- Administer tetanus booster and rabies prophylaxis if indicated (consult with local animal control or public health department).
- Swab the wound with moistened gauze to remove gross debris and culture the wound if indicated.
- Superficial wounds not extending farther than the epidermis need cleansing with normal saline or standard agents.
- Anesthetize, clean, and vigorously irrigate the wound that extends through the epidermis with copious amounts of normal saline under pressure. Puncture wounds should be thoroughly cleaned and gently irrigated using at least 150 mL of normal saline or lactated Ringer's solution via a 19-gauge angiocatheter (Brook, 2009).
- If rabies is a possibility, cleansing with soap and water after initial irrigation is recommended.
- Debride avulsed or devitalized tissue.
- Superficial wounds that do not involve high-risk structures, such as the fingers, cartilaginous tissue, tendons, bones, and joints generally do not need to be treated with prophylactic antibiotics.
- Culture the wounds of clearly infected bites and those that involve deep tissues, the hands, or are at high risk for infection.
- Prescribe prophylactic antibiotics for all human and cat bites, and for the following types of bite or wound characteristics: hand, puncture, overlying bone fracture, substantial crushing tissue injuries or if requiring debridement, or those involving tendons, muscles, or joint spaces. In addition, antibiotic coverage is needed for wounds in children who are immunosuppressed. For outpatients, prescribe a broad-spectrum antibiotic such as amoxicillin clavulanate (first choice). Penicillin-allergic individuals should be treated with an extended spectrum cephalosporin or trimethoprim-sulfamethoxazole plus clindamycin (Hodge, 2010). Prescribe a 3- to 5-day course of prophylactic antibiotics. Clindamycin needs to be added to the regimen if symptoms of infection, particularly methicillin-resistant *Staphylococcus aureus* (MRSA), are present (Brook, 2009). Some sources recommend prophylactic antibiotics for facial wounds only because of the potential for scarring from infection.
- Rabies exposure prophylaxis should also be considered if there is any question about possible exposure. Refer to *Human Rabies Prevention—U.S. Recommendations of the Immunization Practices Advisory Committee (ACIP)* available though the Centers for Disease Control and Prevention (CDC) at www.cdc.gov/vaccines/vpd-vac/rabies.
- Some controversy exists over whether bite wounds should be closed primarily with delayed closure (3 to 5 days after injury) or allowed to heal by secondary intention (leaving the wound open). Factors to consider are the type, size, and depth of the wound; the anatomic location; presence of infection; the time interval since the injury; and the potential for cosmetic disfigurement. Surgical consultation should be obtained for all deep or extensive wounds and those involving the bones, joints, or hands. Because of the excellent blood supply to the face, facial lacerations are at

less risk for infection. Many plastic surgeons advocate primary closure of facial bite wounds that have been brought to medical attention within 5 to 6 hours and have been thoroughly irrigated and debrided. Because of concern about scarring, the provider may refer facial wounds for plastic surgery repair.

- There is consensus that bites involving the hand or foot should not be sutured but allowed to drain. Hand and foot bites less than 1.5 cm are best left to heal by secondary intention; bites greater than 1.5 cm should have delayed primary closure.
- Bite wounds more than 8 to 12 hours old should not be sutured except for facial wounds that can be sutured up to 24 hours, maximum.
- A single layer of nonabsorbable sutures is best (avoid multiple closure layers).
- Refer children with severe bites. Obtain a surgical consult if evidence of or concern about nerve, tendon, and/or ligament injury or if a joint space was involved. Hospitalization, reconstructive surgery, and long-term follow-up can also be indicated.
- Discuss the child's fears and management of any behavioral problems that may result.
- Report dog and wild animal bites to animal control.

Patient and Parent Education

Preventive education and actions should include the following:
- Teach children to avoid stray animals, be cautious around domesticated animals, and not tease or provoke any animal.
- Emphasize the importance of parental supervision of children as they play with pets.
- Do not keep typically wild animals as pets in families with very young children.
- Do not allow pets to roam freely.
- Never leave infants or young children alone with dogs or cats; animals with histories of aggression are inappropriate in households with children.
- Report stray animals promptly to animal control officials.

HYMENOPTERA

Description

Bees, hornets, yellow jackets, fire and harvester ants, and wasps belong to the Hymenoptera order of insects and have common antigens in their venom. Bees and wasps ordinarily do not sting unless frightened, bothered, or hurt. Yellow jackets are aggressive. Fire ants may cause multiple, painful stings. Reactions to stings by these insects are caused by the Hymenoptera venom and can vary from mild, local responses to life-threatening anaphylaxis with wheezing and urticaria. Most children experience only a local reaction, but some children suffer severe systemic reactions, which can progress to medical emergencies unless prompt intervention is initiated.

Epidemiology

Immunoglobulin E–dependent hypersensitivity is the underlying cause of reactions. Histamines, leukotrienes, prostaglandins, and other inflammatory factors are released, causing local or systemic symptoms. The venom of bees, wasps, and yellow jackets is different and can cause cross-reactivity (Diaz, 2009).

Clinical Findings

History. The child usually reports being bitten or stung. There may be a past history of a local or systemic reaction following an insect bite.

Physical Examination. Findings include the following:
- Mild reaction consists of local redness, pruritus, pain, edema, and possibly generalized urticaria.
- Severe reactions, including anaphylaxis, are characterized by local signs plus any of the following:
  - Watery eyes
  - Hives
  - Difficulty in breathing, wheezing
  - Difficulty swallowing
  - Hoarseness, thickened speech
  - Gastrointestinal disturbances, abdominal pain
  - Dizziness, weakness, confusion
  - Collapse, unconsciousness, even death
  - Fire ant bites are characterized by vesicles that develop into sterile pustules.

Diagnostic Studies. Skin testing is not necessary and can be dangerous if there is a history of an allergic response to a Hymenoptera sting.

Differential Diagnosis

Other insect bites or dermatologic eruptions that produce similar symptoms are included in the differential diagnosis.

Management

The following steps are taken:
- For *mild local* reactions:
  - If the stinger is visible, flick it off with the edge of a sharp object (e.g., knife blade or credit card), taking care to not squeeze the attached venom sac.
  - Apply cool compresses locally or cool baths.
  - Administer an antihistamine such as diphenhydramine at 5 mg/kg per day, in divided doses every 6 to 8 hours (300 mg/day maximum), or hydroxyzine 2 mg/kg/day, in divided doses every 6 to 8 hours daily (50 mg/day maximum under 6 years; 50-100 mg/day maximum over 6 years), for treatment of pruritus.
  - Complementary treatments like vinegar and salt poultices and meat tenderizers have no supporting scientific evidence but may help relieve discomfort (Diaz, 2009).
- For *moderate* to *severe* allergic reactions:
  - Moderate reactions may need to be treated with oral antihistamines, corticosteroids, and inhaled bronchodilators (if wheezing).
  - Institute emergency measures for treatment of anaphylactic reactions and transport to the ED as quickly as possible.
    - Epinephrine: 0.01 mg/kg (0.01 mL/kg/dose of 1:1000 aqueous epinephrine per dose intramuscularly, repeated at 5- to 15-minute intervals up to three times, not to exceed 0.5 mg every 20 minutes) (Taketomo et al, 2011). Intramuscular administration of epinephrine into the lateral aspect of the thigh results in

more rapid absorption and higher peak plasma levels than does administration in the arm and is now recommended over subcutaneous administration (Diaz, 2009; Linzer, 2011).

- Antihistamines should be given immediately following epinephrine, but not as a substitute for epinephrine; give both histamine type 1 (H_1) and H_2 blockers parenterally every 6 hours. The H_2 class of antihistamines may be helpful in reducing histamine-induced cardiac arrhythmias in selected cases. Give intravenous (IV) famotidine 1 to 2 mg/kg (50 mg maximum) slowly (Russell et al, 2010).
- Glucocorticoids are not helpful in treating acute reactions, but may help in the late-phase inflammatory response and in preventing serum sickness. Give IV hydrocortisone (5 mg/kg every 6 hours) or methylprednisolone (1 to 2 mg/kg every 6 hours to a maximum of 60 mg), or for less severe reactions oral prednisolone (1 mg/kg; 50 mg maximum) (Covar et al, 2011).
- Nebulized albuterol (2.5 to 5 mg/dose) may be used for bronchospasm not responding to epinephrine (Linzer, 2011).
- Persistent hypotension is treated with vasopressors (e.g., dopamine); glucagon is preferred in the treatment of persistent hypotension in individuals taking beta-blocking agents.
- IV fluids should be administered if the child is hypotensive as a result of anaphylactic shock.
- Administer high-flow oxygen (warm humidified) by nonbreather mask.
- Tracheostomy should be performed if laryngeal edema is life threatening.
- Hospitalize for anaphylactic shock.

Referral to an allergist is indicated for any child who has life-threatening respiratory symptoms (e.g., stridor or wheezing) or hypotension. Venom immunotherapy desensitization is highly effective (98% protective) in preventing further systemic reactions. Children less than 16 years old who have only urticaria or angioedema do not require venom immunotherapy because only 10% of these children will have systemic reactions with subsequent stings.

Patient and Parent Education

Key issues to discuss with moderate to severe reactions include the following:

- Importance of wearing a medical alert tag or bracelet
- Proper use of an insect sting kit that includes a self-injectable epinephrine pen and need to have a kit always readily available for emergency use
- Prevention of stings by avoiding areas likely to be infested with these insects, not wearing bright-colored clothing, and not using perfumed products

MOSQUITOES, FLEAS, AND CHIGGERS (RED BUG MITES)

Description

Mosquitoes are the vectors of many important diseases in humans (see Chapter 23) and cause irritating local skin reactions when they bite. Similarly, flea and chigger bites produce local skin eruptions. The chigger is also known as a red bug mite or harvest mite.

Epidemiology

Mosquito bites are the most common insect bites of infants and children. Fleas that commonly attack humans in the U.S. include the human flea, cat flea, and dog flea. The six-legged larvae of harvest mites are responsible for the skin eruption characteristic of chigger bites. Harvest mites live on grain stems, shrubs, grass, and vines. As humans or animals pass by, the larvae attach themselves to the skin and inject an irritating secretion. The harvest mites then drop to the ground or are scratched off within 1 to 2 days. There is a seasonal pattern to mosquito, flea, and chigger bites.

Clinical Findings

History. The following may be reported:

- Mosquito or flea bites
  - Known mosquito or flea bite or seasonal time
  - Presence of cat or dog in child's environment
  - Complaints of a brief stinging sensation followed by itching after mosquito bite
- Chigger bites
  - Complaints of itching followed by dermatitis after chigger bite
  - History of playing or walking in grassy areas, parks, or other harvest mite habitat near woods and water

Physical Examination. Mosquito bites are characterized by the following:

- Local irritation in unsensitized children
- Urticarial wheals that itch and last several hours to days in sensitized children or firm papules or nodules that last a long time
- Central punctum (sometimes noted)
- Secondary impetigo from scratching of skin lesions

Flea bites are characterized by the following:

- Urticarial wheal or papule surrounded by redness in a sensitized person
- Often, central hemorrhagic punctum
- Progression of wheals into bullae in highly sensitized individuals, especially young children
- Grouping of multiple lesions, commonly found on arms, ankles, legs, feet, thighs, waist, buttocks, and lower abdomen
- Bites are commonly in a classic linear configuration, which is referred to as the "breakfast, lunch, and dinner" sign

Chigger bites are characterized by the following:

- Discrete, bright-red papules 1 to 2 mm in diameter that often have hemorrhagic puncta
- Lesions mainly seen on legs (sock area) and belt line but can be widespread
- Wheals, papules, or papulovesicles in sensitized individuals
- Blisters if a secondary hypersensitivity reaction; purpuric lesions or bullae
- Intense pruritus reaching a peak on the second day and decreasing over the next 5 to 6 days, but can persist for months
- Possible secondary impetigo from scratching lesions
- May see the embedded chiggers

Diagnostic Studies. The presence of fleas or harvest mites is diagnostic; otherwise, no studies are done.

Differential Diagnosis

The diagnosis is often obvious, but the differential diagnosis can include insect bites that produce similar papular, vesicular lesions, or other skin conditions.

Management

Management consists of controlling pruritus and can include such measures as the following:

- Cool compresses
- Topical corticosteroids (e.g., 1% hydrocortisone cream)
- Topical antipruritic agents such as calamine lotion; avoiding topical diphenhydramine
- Oral antihistamines (e.g., diphenhydramine) if topical corticosteroids do not provide relief
- Removal of embedded chiggers (can be withdrawn by covering the insect with alcohol, mineral oil, nail polish, or ointment)
- Colloidal oatmeal baths (clean tub thoroughly after to avoid fall risk from oil residue left behind)
- Treatment of secondary skin lesions as indicated
- Elimination of fleas by treating animals and cleaning carpets, bedding, upholstered furniture; avoid areas that are potentially infested with mosquitoes, fleas, or chiggers
- Insecticides should be used with caution.

Patient and Parent Education

Prevention of insect bites is a key component in education. Bites can be prevented by eliminating mosquitoes, fleas, and chiggers from the environment or by preventing their contact with the skin.

- Use insect repellents (generally effective against mosquitoes and harvest mites).
- Wear protective clothing to cover the body and tuck pants into shoes or socks.
- Wear neutral-colored clothes (white, green, tan, and khaki do not attract mosquitoes).
- Avoid scented hair sprays, powders, soaps, lotions, creams, and perfumes because they can attract all forms of stinging insects.
- Mosquitoes are attracted to bright clothing and sweaty skin and are drawn to humans by scent.
- Treat suspected animal carrier for fleas, and spray carpets and other infested areas; spray yards and grassy places for fleas in those environments that the child frequents.
- Vacuum carpets daily if fleas are seen on household pets.
- Avoid playing in areas of harvest mite habitat.

TICKS

Description

Ticks are blood-sucking arachnids and are classified into three families: Ixodidae (hard ticks), Argasidae (soft ticks), and Nuttalliellidae (soft ticks). They are vectors of significant diseases such as rickettsial infection (e.g., Rocky Mountain spotted fever and Q fever), Colorado tick fever, erlichiosis, tularemia, and Lyme disease (see discussion of Lyme disease in Chapter 23).

Epidemiology

Ticks are found in grass, shrubs, vines, and brush and attach themselves to various animals and humans. The female tick sucks blood from the skin and can inject a toxin while sucking blood. Lyme disease transmission in the U.S. is primarily by the *Ixodes scapularis* (deer) tick. However, *I. ricinus* is the vector of Lyme disease in northern California and Oregon.

Transmission of Lyme disease requires at least a 24-hour tick attachment. Tick bites are most common from early spring to early fall and are associated with both acute and chronic dermatoses. Rocky Mountain spotted fever occurs throughout the United States but is most common in the southeastern and central regions. Erlichiosis, caused by *Erlichia chaffeensis,* is endemic to the southern U.S. and common in the Midwest and northeast coast of the U.S. (Zivna and Ellison, 2009).

Clinical Findings

History. Assess for a report of known tick bite and exposure to a tick habitat. However, many individuals may have no recall of tick bites. Research indicates that as many as half of patients with confirmed Rocky Mountain spotted fever have no recollection of being bitten by a tick (Elston, 2010).

Physical Examination. Findings include the following:

- The initial bite is painless and innocuous; thus the tick is frequently undetected or detected only after several days of attachment.
- Hypersensitivity reactions are common and can include papules, nodules, bullae, ulceration, and necrosis.
- In Lyme disease an infiltrated lesion with a distinct surrounding erythematous halo develops and can last for 1 to 2 weeks.
- Rickettsial infections most often present with fever and headache (Elston, 2010).
- A small pruritic nodule, lasting for months or years, can result if the tick's mouthparts are left in the skin.
- Tick bite pyrexia or tick paralysis, occurring about 6 days after attachment, can result. Tick paralysis results in symptoms approximately 4 to 7 days after the initial bite and is characterized by restlessness, irritability, and ascending paralysis. Both disorders are reversible, and symptoms quickly resolve if the tick is removed (Hodge, 2010).
- Other signs depend on the tick-related illness that can develop; erythema chronicum migrans can develop around the bite in 2 to 3 weeks and progress to a disseminated rash and Lyme disease.

Diagnostic Studies. Identification of the tick is diagnostic. Diagnostic studies are ordered depending on the disease for which the tick is the vector.

Differential Diagnosis

The differential diagnosis of local reactions to simple tick bites includes other insect bites. Many different diseases result from tick bites and their sequelae. The presentation of tick-related diseases is variable and depends on the illness for which the tick is the vector.

Management

The most effective means of managing tick-borne infection is through prevention. This is best accomplished through avoiding tick-infested areas (especially brush and grassy areas), using DEET-containing insect repellents, and prompt tick removal (Elston, 2010). Although intervention varies with the specific disease, illnesses resulting from tick bites are best managed with prompt introduction of antibiotics, such as amoxicillin or doxycycline. Antibiotic prophylaxis for asymptomatic tick bites is generally not recommended especially if the tick has been attached for less than 24 hours.

Complete removal of the tick is essential. If fragments of mouthparts or the proboscis are left in the skin, local symptoms can continue. To remove ticks, wear gloves and firmly grasp the tick with forceps, tweezers, or gloved fingers as close to the skin as possible (try to grasp its head and not crush the tick). Avoid placing pressure on the tick's abdomen. Gently pull straight upward with steady, even pressure. Wash the area with soap and water and save the tick for identification. If any part remains, a skin punch biopsy will remove the rest. Symptoms of tick bite paralysis can resolve within 24 hours after the tick is removed.

Patient and Parent Education

The following key points should be made:

- Avoid areas known to be infested with ticks.
- Wear protective clothing—preferably light colored to see ticks better (e.g., long-sleeved shirts tucked into pants and pants tucked into socks).
- Use of insect repellents sprayed onto clothes and hats or directly on the skin can help prevent tick bites, but should not be applied to the face or nonintact skin. Also inform parents that repellents occasionally cause allergic or toxic effects. Skedaddle 7.25% and OFF 10% are effective agents and have a good safety profile. Use a higher sun protection factor (SPF) of sunscreen if applying insect repellents because the SPF may be decreased.
- Inspect for ticks after exposure or walking in areas likely to be infested; check for ticks every 2 to 3 hours during a hike; carefully check the scalp, hairline, neck, behind the ears, armpits, legs, back of knees, and groin because these areas are favorite hiding places of ticks.
- Take a brisk shower after a hike to help remove ticks that are not firmly attached. Wash off tick repellents with soap.

SPIDERS AND SCORPIONS

Description

Most spider bites are innocuous and do not cause reactions. If reactions occur, they are generally a minor, localized response that can be mistaken for a flea, bedbug, or some other insect bite. Most spiders cannot bite humans because of their short and fragile fangs, and almost all avoid humans unless provoked. There are two main spiders common in the North American continent that can cause serious complications: the black widow (*Latrodectus mactans*) and the brown recluse (*Loxosceles reclusa*). The black widow spider has a globular body about 1 cm across that is shiny black with a red or orange hourglass marking on its underside. It is found throughout the U.S. The black widow has a neurotoxic venom. The brown recluse, one of the most dangerous spiders in the U.S., has an oval light fawn to dark chocolate-brown body; it is approximately 1 cm long (adults range from 1 to 5 cm in total length), with a dark brown violin-shaped band extending from its eyes partially down its back. It bites humans only in self-defense. The brown recluse is found in southern and midwestern states but can be found anywhere in the U.S.

There are multiple species of scorpions, but only a few are dangerous to humans (Hodge, 2010). Scorpions have a stinging apparatus in their tail. They are nocturnal and found in the southwestern and southern U.S. Scorpions commonly live in cool, dark places during the day and are known to crawl into sleeping bags, shoes, and discarded clothing.

Epidemiology

The black widow spider prefers to live in cool, dark, dry places in buildings and little-used structures, such as woodpiles, garages, basements, and tool sheds (less frequented outbuildings). It often spins its web on outdoor furniture, which explains why many black widow spider bites are received around the genital and buttock areas. The brown recluse spider typically lives in dark, dry places (attics, basements, boxes) and storage closets among clothes; when living outdoors it resides in grasses, rocky bluffs, and barns. The brown recluse prefers dark recesses and bites only in self-defense. The venom of the brown recluse can be hemolytic and necrotizing with extension caused by a spreading factor. Scorpions come out at night and hide by day; they are nonaggressive unless disturbed (Hodge, 2010).

Clinical Findings

History. Assess the known history of a spider bite or activities in, or travel to, an environment that is frequented by these spiders. The characteristic appearance of the spider helps in its identification. Children are more vulnerable to spider and scorpion bites.

Physical Examination. The characteristic features are identified for each type of spider bite (Hodge, 2010):

- Black widow spider bites
  - Bites generally do not cause local symptoms.
  - Severe, muscle-cramping pain starts from 10 minutes to 1 hour after the bite and increases to maximum intensity within 3 hours. Cramping is typically felt in the abdomen, flank, thighs, and chest.
  - Sweating, irritability, agitation, nausea, and vomiting occur in children.
  - Central nervous system symptoms include headache, anxiety, salivation, lacrimation, sweating, hypertension, and tachycardia.
  - Chills, priapism, and urinary retention can occur.
  - Most children recover in 2 to 3 days. The mortality rate in young children is as high as 50%.
- Brown recluse spider bites
  - Localized reaction is characterized by mild itching or stinging at the time of bite; however, the bite is usually painless. Mild to severe pain typically follows the bite by 2 to 8 hours and is accompanied by redness around the puncture with a central pustule or blister (Hodge, 2010). This is followed by swelling, itching, tenderness, a hemorrhagic vesicle (a red ring followed by blue-purple discoloration) 12 to 24 hours later, and finally a gangrenous eschar. Lymphangitis is common if a bite is on an extremity. The lesion frequently takes weeks to months to resolve.
  - Systemic reactions, when present, occur 24 to 48 hours after the bite and may include nausea, vomiting, chills, fever, malaise, muscle aches and pains, weakness, a petechial morbilliform rash, thrombocytopenia, hematuria, renal failure, and hemolysis (Hodge, 2010).
- Scorpion bites (Hodge, 2010)
  - Severe, local, and painful burning sensation with redness, discoloration, edema, and severe necrosis.

○ Systemic reactions include restlessness, hyperactivity, abnormal eye movements, uncontrolled jerking, muscle fasciculation, facial twitching, hypersalivation, diaphoresis, and respiratory paralysis.
○ Death is usually caused by respiratory failure, pulmonary edema, or shock.

Differential Diagnosis

Other spider bites and conditions that result in similar cutaneous manifestations or systemic findings, or both, are included in the differential diagnosis.

Management

In cases in which venomous spider bites are suspected or confirmed, refer to the appropriate medical specialist. Treatment for black widow spider bites for children less than 88 pounds (40 kg), younger than age 16 years, who have respiratory symptoms, or who have significant hypertension includes administration of specific antivenin (usually 2.5 mL), muscle relaxants, pain medications, tetanus prophylaxis, and antibiotics if secondary infection develops (Hodge, 2010). Most brown recluse bites tend to heal without incident. Bites with necrotic centers generally require tetanus prophylaxis, pain medication, application of ice or cold compresses, and elevation of the extremity. Surgical excision and skin grafts may be needed if extensive necrosis occurs. Children are at greatest risk of developing severe scorpion envenomation. Scorpion stings may be managed immediately with application of a restrictive bandage above the sting area and application of ice or cold water. Intensive care is needed in severe cases for sedation and management of cardiorespiratory and neurologic complications.

Patient and Parent Education

The focus of patient and parent education is prevention. Careful monitoring of environments in which these spiders tend to live and prompt treatment, if bitten, are important. Use caution when near woodpiles and attics, and always shake out shoes and sleeping bags before using them.

SNAKEBITES

Description

Only about 15% of snakes in the U.S. are venomous (Hodge, 2010). However, approximately 2500 children per year receive poisonous snakebites causing approximately 5 to 15 deaths. Poisonous snakes include indigenous pit vipers (Crotalinae), such as rattlesnakes, cottonmouths, water moccasins, and copperheads, and the Elapidae (coral snake). The Crotalinae cause 99% of venomous snakebites occurring in the wild and Elapidae and exotic pet snakes are responsible for the other 1% (Hodge, 2010).

Epidemiology

The highest incidence of snake bites occurs in the southeastern and southwestern regions of the U.S., and males between 5 and 15 years old have the highest snakebite rates (Hodge,

2010). The snake injects venom that contains a variety of toxins into the soft tissue; the venom can be carried throughout the body via the blood and lymph systems. Snake venom reactions can be divided into three types: cytotoxic, hemotoxic, and neurotoxic. Cytotoxic envenomation presents with localized pain, swelling, and ecchymoses; compartment syndrome may develop in severe cases. Hematologic effects include hemolysis, fibrinogen activation, and thrombocytopenia. Neurologic toxicity can include taste abnormalities, local paresthesias, and in severe cases, bulbar and respiratory muscle weakness. Respiratory failure can result from pulmonary edema or as a complication from shock (Hodge, 2010).

Clinical Findings

History. Assess for report of a snakebite. It is helpful to determine the type of snake. Pit vipers have a large triangular head and vertically oriented elliptical pupils, unlike the round pupils of nonvenomous snakes. Copperheads and rattlesnakes have diamond-shaped patterns of varying colors. Coral snakes have black heads, followed by yellow and red bands that are followed by black bands.

Physical Examination. Characteristic features indicating the presence of venom include the following:

- Severe local reaction soon after the bite, with intense pain, burning, discoloration, edema, and hemorrhagic effects
- Proximal extension of ecchymosis and swelling during the first few hours after the bite with later fluid-filled or hemorrhagic bullae and necrosis
- Peripheral and central neurologic symptoms including worsening weakness, numbness or tingling of the face and/ or extremities, diplopia, and lethargy
- Increased salivation, metallic taste in the mouth, sweating, nausea, and vomiting
- Evidence of hematologic coagulopathy, such as hematemesis, melena, and hemoptysis
- Respiratory distress and shock that can lead to death

Diagnostic Studies

Coagulation studies and other laboratory tests are ordered as indicated by the child's condition.

Management

For nonvenomous bites, simply clean the wound, give tetanus prophylaxis if necessary, and administer appropriate pain medication. Give oral antibiotic therapy for 5 days with amoxicillin/clavulanic acid. If there is any uncertainty about the identity of the snake, contact poison control, and observe for venomous symptoms for at least 3 to 4 hours.

If a venomous snakebite is suspected, the effects (including possible death) will depend on the size of the child, site of the bite, type of snake, and degree of envenomation, plus the effectiveness of treatment. Up to 20% of venomous snake bites are "dry" bites and are therefore asymptomatic. In the case of a rattlesnake bite there is a period of 6 to 8 hours between the bite and death in which effective treatment can be instituted to reverse the effects of the venom. Treatment of all snakebites includes rapid transportation to a medical center, referral to appropriate medical specialists, antivenin therapy, and treatment for shock and respiratory difficulties.

Patient and Parent Education

Prevention of snakebite is important. Parents and patients who live or vacation in areas where pit vipers are found should be familiar with emergency first-aid treatment of snakebites. First-aid measures include the following (Hodge, 2010):

- Splint the affected extremity and minimize the patient's movements.
- Remove any jewelry that could cause a tourniquet effect.
- Do not elevate the affected extremity; lay or sit the person down with the bite below the level of the heart.

- Do not give the person alcohol as a pain killer or a caffeinated beverage to drink.
- Cover the bite with a clean, dry dressing.
- Do not use a tourniquet or ice packs.
- Do not cut the bite area and attempt to suction out the venom.
- Transport immediately to a medical facility.

HEAD INJURIES

Description

An evolving body of research indicates that young children are particularly vulnerable to mild traumatic brain injury (TBI), also known as concussion. Most TBIs occur secondary to acceleration-deceleration or rotational forces, and long-term sequelae are much more likely in children with developing brains (Halstead et al, 2010). The CDC defines mild traumatic brain injury (MTBI) as a complex pathologic brain process that results from primary or secondary forces on the head that disrupt brain processes and functioning (CDC, 2010). MTBI results in physical, cognitive, emotional and sleep symptoms (CDC, 2010; Halstead et al, 2010) (Table 39-7).

See Chapter 27 for an in-depth discussion of the brain and its functions and Chapter 13 for a discussion on the evaluation, management, and return-to-play policies for athletes.

The discussion of head injury in this chapter is limited to minor traumatic brain injuries and is based on a joint American Academy of Pediatrics and American Academy of Family Physicians practice parameter titled "The Management of Minor Closed Head Injury in Children," and other current documents. In addition, indications of impending central nervous system compromise are presented. Head injuries can also be classified as mild, moderate, and severe. Table 39-8 identifies key characteristics that are used in this classification system.

Epidemiology

TBI is a common cause of trauma in pediatrics, resulting in almost 2200 deaths, 35,000 hospitalizations, and 474,000 ED visits annually in the U.S. for children 0 to 14 years old (Faul et al, 2010). Approximately 2 to 5 million children sustain head traumas of varying intensities each year in the U.S. when all ages during childhood and adolescence are considered. Common causes of ED-treated TBI include falls, sports-related injuries, motor vehicle accidents, violence and assaults, and being struck by or against objects (Faul et al,

---

TABLE 39-7 Mild Traumatic Brain Injury (Concussion) Symptoms

Physical	Cognitive	Emotional	Sleep
Headache	Confusion	Abnormal irritability	Drowsiness
Nausea/vomiting	Altered concentration	Feelings of sadness or being "emotional"	Insomnia or hypersomnia
Difficulty with balance	Mental torpor	Abnormal feelings of being nervous	Difficulty falling asleep
Changes in vision	Altered memory		
Dizziness	Forgetfulness (especially conversations or recent events)		
Light or sound sensitivity	Needs to repeat or slowly answer questions		
Paresthesias			
Feelings of being dazed or stunned			

Adapted from Centers for Disease Control and Prevention: *Heads Up: facts for physicians about mild traumatic brain injury.* Available at www.cdc.gov/concussion/headsup/pdf/Facts_for_Physicians_booklet-a.pdf (accessed Nov 29, 2010); Halstead ME, Walter KD, the Council on Sports Medicine and Fitness: Clinical report—sport-related concussion in children and adolescents, *Pediatrics* 126: 597-615, 2010.

TABLE 39-8 Classification of Head Injuries Based on Key Characteristics

Classification	Glasgow Coma Scale*	Neurologic Focal Deficit†	Loss of Consciousness	Other Neurologic Findings
Mild	13-15	No	No or brief loss (<30 minutes)	May have linear skull fractures
Moderate	9-12	Focal signs	Variable loss	May have depressed skull fracture or intracranial hematoma
Severe	≤8	Focal signs	Prolonged loss	Often have depressed skull fractures and intracranial hematoma

*Either initial or subsequent scores.
†Neurologic focal deficit (e.g., hemiparesis, reflex asymmetry, Babinski sign, abnormal cranial nerve findings).

2010). Boys experience head injury twice as frequently as girls. Many children die each year from head trauma, and children who survive their injuries can have significant long-term disability. Children can also experience subtle symptoms of TBI that may not appear until days or weeks after the injury. Various types of head injuries can result in pathologic conditions: skull fracture, concussion, posttraumatic seizure, cerebral contusion, epidural hematoma, subdural hematoma, cerebral edema, and penetrating injury.

Clinical Findings

History. Symptoms of TBI can mimic those of other medical conditions, thus making the diagnosis challenging. It is recommended that providers use an evidence-based assessment tool like the CDC's Acute Concussion Evaluation (ACE) tool (available at www.cdc.gov/concussion/headsup/pdf/ACE_care_plan_school_version_a.pdf) (CDC, 2010).

The following information should be obtained:

- History of how injury occurred; if injury involved a fall, the height from which the child fell needs to be determined. Specifically, providers should ascertain injury cause, body part affected, forces, and circumstances.
- Loss of or alteration in consciousness or memory, confusion, irritability, inappropriate behavior, repetitive questioning
- Presence of vomiting and frequency
- Presence of headache, description of the headache pain
- Presence of blurred vision, diplopia, or other vision problem
- Numbness or loss of sensation, loss of balance, or difficulty walking
- Specify symptoms occurring at the time of injury and interval changes

Child abuse should be strongly suspected when a head injury is present in a child without a history of a fall or with a history of a fall from a relatively low height of less than 4 feet. It is also recommended that a skeletal survey be obtained in children younger than 3 years when inflicted head injuries are suspected because younger children are at higher risk for skeletal trauma as well (Christian and Blum, 2011).

Physical Examination. Check vital signs (temperature, blood pressure, pulse, and respiration) and compare findings with normal parameters expected for children of varying ages. Changes in vital signs can indicate shock or intracranial hypertension. Perform a thorough physical examination (including a careful oral examination) and a careful neurologic examination including level of consciousness, mental status, motor function (both gross and fine motor), sensory function, cranial nerve functioning, and reflexes. Be alert to any signs of central nervous system involvement. Evaluation of mental status can be based on the Glasgow Coma Scale (GCS) (Table 39-9). Always remember to examine the entire child for other signs of trauma such as neck injury, internal abdominal injuries, or bone fractures. Periorbital hemorrhage ("raccoon-eyes"), ecchymosis behind the ear (Battle sign), blood behind the eardrum, and bleeding from the ears or nose indicate a basilar skull fracture.

Diagnostic Studies. The severity of the head trauma dictates the need for investigative studies. All children with moderate (GCS 9 to 12) and severe (GCS 3 to 8) acute trauma should have a cranial CT scan. In addition, the need for skull radiographs and other views is determined by the severity of the head trauma. Schutzman (2010) recommends including plain radiographs (cervical spine and a series of skull views) with significant head injury, loss of consciousness, focal neurologic signs (GCS 3 to 8), and further neurologic study. Indications for obtaining a CT scan include any of the following:

- Penetrating trauma
- Altered level of consciousness (excessive irritability or lethargy)
- History of loss of consciousness (exceeding 1 minute)
- Amnesia about the injury
- Focal neurologic signs or deficit
- Depressed skull fracture or signs of basilar injury
- Seizures
- Persistent vomiting
- History of coagulopathy

CT is the preferred imaging technique because it can be obtained rapidly, and the child can be monitored easily during the study. Skull fractures are better visualized on skull radiographs. Acute hemorrhage is detected more easily by CT (order without contrast) than by MRI. If CT is ordered after several days (3 or more days past injury), it should be done both with contrast (to pick up extravasated blood) and without. CT can demonstrate brain edema, midline displacements, hydrocephalus, loss of brain tissue, and most skull fractures. Although CT itself is a safe procedure, some healthy children require sedation or anesthesia (with some risk), so the benefits gained from CT should be carefully weighed against the possible harm of sedating or anesthetizing a child. In addition, CT scans obtained for asymptomatic children may show incidental findings that lead to subsequent unnecessary medical or surgical interventions.

CT scans, MRI, or skull radiographs are generally not indicated for mild or minor closed head trauma without focal neurologic signs or loss of consciousness (CDC, 2010; Schutzman, 2010).

TABLE 39-9	Glasgow Coma Scale	
Category	**Best Response**	**Score***
Eye opening (E)	Spontaneous	4
	To speech (command)	3
	To pain	2
	None	1
Motor (M)	Obeys (command)	6
	Localizes	5
	Withdraws	4
	Abnormal flexion	3
	Extensor response	2
	None	1
Verbal (V)	Oriented	5
	Confused conversation	4
	Inappropriate words	3
	Incomprehensible sounds	2
	None	1

*Total score (E + M + V): maximum 15; minimum 3.
From Coulter DL: Head trauma. In Finberg LL, editor: *Saunders manual of pediatric practice*, Philadelphia, 1998, Saunders, pp 883-885.

Differential Diagnosis

History of a head injury is the key to diagnosis. Differentiating minor head trauma that will resolve on its own from more extensive brain injury is problematic at times. Head trauma may cause injuries of the scalp, skull, dentition, and intracranial contents. Remember that these injuries may occur alone or in combination (Schutzman, 2010). Children with intracranial lesions after minor closed head injury are not easily distinguishable clinically from the large majority with no intracranial injury. Children with mild nonspecific signs such as headache, vomiting, or lethargy after minor closed head injury may be more likely to have intracranial lesions than children without such signs. However, these clinical signs are of limited predictive value, and most children with headache, lethargy, or vomiting after minor closed head injury do not have demonstrable intracranial injury. In addition, some children with intracranial injury do not have any such signs or symptoms, showing a normal neurologic assessment. Because of these findings, some experts recommend a liberal policy on the ordering of cranial CT scans following any head trauma; however, there are drawbacks to routine CT scanning (see discussion in prior section).

Management

Management issues related to only mild and moderate head injuries are discussed in this chapter. The level of consciousness is a key determinant of the child's prognosis. Prompt identification of a deteriorating level of consciousness and quick medical and/or surgical intervention are essential components of the management plan.

Management of the Child With Minor Closed Head Injury and No Loss of Consciousness. Observation in the clinic, office, ED, or home, under the care of a competent caregiver, who understands what signs and symptoms to watch for, is able to closely and reliably monitor, and can quickly bring the child back for treatment or access emergency medical services if necessary, is recommended for children with minor closed head injury and no loss of consciousness. Observation implies regular monitoring by a competent adult who would be able to recognize abnormalities and seek appropriate assistance.

Management of the Child With Minor Closed Head Injury and Brief Loss of Consciousness. For children with minor closed head injury and brief loss of consciousness (several minutes) and no other neurologic or physical deficits reported or detected on examination, observation in the office, clinic, ED, hospital, or home, when under the care of a competent caregiver (see definition in preceding paragraph), may be used to evaluate such a child. The use of CT scan, skull radiographs, or MRI in the initial management of children with minor closed head injury and loss of consciousness is not routinely recommended. However, CT scanning along with observation is also accepted. If the provider is not assured that the child will be closely and reliably monitored at home, hospitalization is indicated.

Management of the Child With Moderate Head Injury or Worrisome Symptoms. Children with moderate head injuries (GCS 9 to 12) may require admission or prolonged observation in the ED until their mental status stabilizes; children with severe head injuries (GCS less than 8 or coma and physical findings) need immediate hospital admission and consultation with a neurologist. Children with any of the following should be hospitalized (CDC, 2010):

- Changing vital signs
- Seizures
- Altered mental status
- Slurred speech
- Prolonged unconsciousness (greater than 30 seconds)
- Persisting memory deficit or focal neurologic signs
- Depressed or basilar skull fractures
- Persistent headache (particularly with stiff neck)
- Recurrent vomiting or unexplained fever
- Unexplained injury (suspected child abuse)
- CT scan or MRI findings that are worrisome

A child with a skull fracture or transient neurologic findings whose level of consciousness is normal may be admitted for overnight observation.

Complications

Complications of head injury can include concussion, posttraumatic seizures, cerebral contusion, epidural hematoma, subdural hematoma, intracerebral hematoma, subarachnoid hemorrhage, acute brain swelling, and penetrating injuries. Second impact syndrome is described in Chapter 27. Intracranial lesions, particularly epidural hematomas, are life-threatening and have significant complications. Features indicative of serious injury include loss of consciousness (longer than 1 minute), persistent vomiting, depressed level of consciousness, seizures, unequal pupil size, severe headache, and GCS less than 15.

Patient and Parent Education

Give caregivers a "head injury sheet," and make every effort to ensure that they understand the instructions and will comply with them. Salient points to cover in a pediatric head injury information sheet include instructions about when to contact the health care provider or take the child to an ED. Indications for such actions are the following:

- Increased drowsiness, sleepiness, inability to wake up, unconsciousness
- Vomiting more than twice
- Neck pain
- Watery or bloody drainage from ear or nose
- Seizures, "fit," or fainting
- Unusual irritability, personality change, confusion, or any unusual behavior
- Headache that gets worse or lasts more than a day
- Unequal pupils
- Trouble with vision (blurred), hearing, or speech
- Trouble with walking (e.g., clumsiness or stumbling) or weakness of any muscle of arms, legs, or face

In addition, parents or caregivers should be given the following specific instructions:

- Wake child every 2 to 4 hours for the first 24 hours after injury; child should wake easily and be able to stay awake for a few minutes.
- Make sure child is moving his or her arms and legs normally.
- Give only acetaminophen, if needed for headache or relief of soft tissue pain.

Parents should also be informed that sometimes symptoms from head trauma occur days, weeks, or months after the initial trauma.

Neurologic sequelae following mild head injury in children often improve or resolve within 9 to 12 months. These sequelae include the following:
- Headache
- Vertigo or dizziness
- Difficulty concentrating or loss of memory
- Depression, fatigue
- Poor school performance and neurobehavioral problems

Postconcussive Syndrome and Return to Contact Sports

Typical postconcussive syndrome in adolescents is manifested by headache, dizziness, irritability, and impaired ability to concentrate. In younger children it is manifested as aggression, disobedience, behavioral regression, inattention, and anxiety. See Chapter 13 for a discussion of return to play guidelines.

HEAT AND COLD INJURIES

FROSTBITE

Description

Frostbite occurs when ice crystals form within the soft tissues as a consequence of exposure to cold. The freezing of tissue impairs circulation to the affected area and results in constriction and vaso-occlusion. This causes microvascular changes leading to cellular destruction and the release of inflammatory mediators that also cause damage. Frostbite most commonly involves distal, relatively poorly perfused regions of the body, such as fingertips, toes, earlobes, and the nose. In children, areas that have poor heat-generating ability and insulation, including the cheeks and chin, are also at high risk for frostbite. However, any area of skin that is exposed to prolonged cold can be affected.

Epidemiology

Exposure to temperatures ranging from 28.4° to 14° F (−2° to −10° C) can cause frostbite. Factors such as duration of exposure, increased wind velocity, dependency of the extremity (limb in a dependent, not elevated position), application of emollients, fatigue, injury, high altitude, immobility, and general health can potentiate the effects of cold. Exposure to very cold chemicals (e.g., liquid nitrogen or oxygen) also produces instant frostbite.

Clinical Findings

History. The provider should assess the following:
- Exposure to cold temperatures
- Sensory changes (initially painful, then numbness if deeply frostbitten)
- Complaints of throbbing pain after thawing

Physical Examination. Typical initial findings include the following:
- Frozen area is cold.
- Skin is red at first, then appears pale or waxy white or slightly yellow or may have a bluish tint if deeply frostbitten.

- In early stages, tissue blanches; in later stages, it feels doughy or rock hard.

On rewarming, the extent of tissue damage becomes apparent. Deep frostbite occurs when tissues are icy hard and without deep tissue resilience. With deep frostbite the following signs and symptoms appear with rewarming:
- Cyanosis or mottling
- Erythema and swelling
- Numbness that evolves into complaints of burning pain
- Vesicles and bullae that appear within 24 to 48 hours
- Gangrene in severe frostbite

Table 39-10 describes the four levels of frostbite.

Differential Diagnosis

The differential diagnosis includes other conditions that produce similar cutaneous manifestations and injury; a history of exposure to extreme temperatures is the key to the diagnosis.

Management

Severe frostbite should be managed by medical specialists. Treatment includes rapid rewarming procedures, pain management, medical and surgical management of tissue necrosis, prevention of infection, and amputation if needed. Damaged skin should never be massaged or rubbed with snow or ice. Early treatment of mild frostbite includes the following:
- Cover affected area with other body surfaces and warm clothing.
- Avoid pressure or any rubbing of the affected area.
- Control pain initially with opioids and then with ibuprofen to decrease prostaglandins and discourage platelet aggregation and vasoconstriction (Singer and Dagum, 2008).
- *Do not use local dry heat*; this practice is dangerous and can cause tissue damage.

TABLE 39-10	The Four Categories of Frostbite	
Category by Degree	**Description**	**Complication**
First (frostnip)	Redness, edema, transient discomfort; reversible within a few hours	Normal skin appearance within a few hours; may have mild desquamation
Second	Notable redness and swelling; numbness becomes burning pain in 12-24 hours; bullae and vesicles form	Sensory neuropathy and cold sensitivity are residuals after healing
Third	Hemorrhagic bullae or waxy, mummified skin	Extensive tissue loss
Fourth	Involvement of full-thickness skin, muscle, tendon, bone	Amputation is likely

Patient and Parent Education

Education of children and parents about the prevention and initial management of frostbite is important. Essential points include the following:

- Use of appropriate clothing when exposed to extreme cold temperatures
- Survival skills for travelers, hikers, or winter sports participants who are exposed to cold temperatures or who could become lost
- Immediate rewarming of skin that is white by covering with warm clothing or another body surface
- Danger of rubbing affected area with snow or ice or massaging; these practices are contraindicated because they lead to mechanical trauma

HYPOTHERMIA

Description

Hypothermia is the condition in which body core temperature falls below 95° F (35° C). At less than 95° F (35° C), the human body loses its ability to generate sufficient heat to maintain bodily functions. Predisposing factors include malnutrition, physical disability, hypoglycemia, major trauma, hypothyroidism, Addison disease, and drug use or abuse (Ewald and Baum, 2010). Although most cases of accidental exposure are seen in winter, hypothermia can occur in other seasons during wet, windy weather. It can also come on quickly in the case of cold-water emersion.

Epidemiology

Hypothermia can be the result of environmental exposure. Body heat is lost by radiation of heat to nearby objects, evaporation of moisture from the skin and respiratory system, convection of heat from the skin's surface into cooler air, or conduction of heat to objects in direct contact with the body. The effect of cool ambient temperatures is exacerbated by wind, moisture, and lack of appropriate clothing or shelter.

Children are at increased risk of hypothermia because of their relatively larger body surface area, proportionately larger head, smaller body fluid volume, less developed temperature-regulating mechanisms, and decreased amount of protective body fat. Children are also less able to escape on their own from a cold environment and are more likely to wander off from adult supervision. Newborns, particularly low-birthweight or premature infants, very young children, and children who are ill, fatigued, poorly nourished, or have experienced trauma are at high risk.

Hypothermia results in cutaneous vasoconstriction and increased heat production by shivering and thyroxine releases. Hypothermia, not associated with environmental exposure, may be a sign of other life-threatening illnesses or injuries (e.g., near-drowning in cold water). This secondary hypothermia is not discussed here.

Clinical Findings

History. The following are assessed:
- Exposure to low ambient temperatures
- Risk factors (e.g., age, physical condition)

Physical Examination. Signs of hypothermia progress from early to late stages and include the following:
- Decreasing body temperature
- Shivering that disappears in late hypothermia

- Pallor or blue lips and skin
- Disorientation, listlessness, sleepiness
- Decreased pulse and respiration
- Decreasing neurologic status and eventually coma and death

Diagnostic Studies. No studies are done if hypothermia is mild and responds to basic treatment measures.

Differential Diagnosis

Shock is the differential diagnosis.

Management

For mild hypothermia (greater than 89.6° F [32° C] body temperature), in early stages of cooling, remove the child from the cold environment, replace wet clothing, and provide warm liquids. Placing the child in a warm water bath can be effective. As the body cools further, it can no longer generate adequate heat itself, so external sources of heat must be provided. Remove the child from the cold environment, replace wet clothing, and provide heat with warm blankets, heat lamps, hot-water bottles, or, if none of these is available, use the classic technique of placing the child skin-to-skin with a warm person of normal temperature in a sleeping bag or blanket.

Active rewarming by external or core-rewarming techniques (e.g., warmed, humidified oxygen and warmed IV fluids) is necessary for children with severe hypothermia (less than 89.6° F [32° C] body temperature) who are in danger of cardiovascular instability (Ewald and Baum, 2010). Children who require external or core rewarming should be transferred to an ED because of the risk of cardiovascular instability and death.

Patient and Parent Education

Instruct parents on the risks of hypothermia in young children. Emphasize the need to monitor children's activities in cold weather and to provide adequate supervision and protection from exposure. The higher metabolic rate of normal, healthy children keeps them warm, and they may not feel the effects of short-term exposure to the cold. Thus they may not want a jacket, sweater, hat, or mittens when their parents believe they need them. Having a survival kit along with families or teens on camping trips or traveling in uninhabited areas may save a life.

HYPERTHERMIA: COMMON HEAT-RELATED ILLNESS

Description

Hyperthermia is a life-threatening increase in body core temperature. Heat cramps, heat exhaustion, and heat stroke are types of hyperthermia. Heat cramps are painful muscle cramps that are probably caused by electrolyte depletion associated with insufficient blood supply to an exercising muscle. Heat exhaustion is caused by excessive sweating associated with inadequate intake of water and salt in a hot environment. Heat stroke is associated with core temperatures of more than 105.8° F (41° C) (Ewald and Baum, 2010). Heat cramps and heat exhaustion often occur during sports activities (see

Chapter 13). They are reversible changes; in contrast, heat stroke is a life-threatening condition. This section more specifically discusses heat stroke.

Etiology

Heat-related illness results from an ineffective response of the body's thermoregulatory mechanisms to environmental conditions. Hyperthermia causes cutaneous vasodilation, sweating, and decreased heat production by inhibiting shivering. Children with some genetic myopathies have malignant hyperthermia, a pathologic reaction to anesthetic. All children are at risk for hyperthermia or heat stroke when exposed to high air temperature, especially if the heat is combined with high humidity and if steps are not taken to keep the child cool. Evaporation through sweating is the body's primary cooling mechanism with activity. If air temperature is higher than body temperature, if humidity is high, or if the body is dehydrated, the body's cooling mechanisms and the process of evaporation are compromised. Internal body temperature then increases. Age, exertion, illness, obesity, and poor nutrition also exacerbate the risk of hyperthermia. Compared with adults, children sweat less, begin to sweat at a higher internal temperature (or set-point), have a higher metabolic rate thus producing more body heat and lower cardiac output, and are more susceptible to dehydration because of proportionately larger body surface area.

Clinical Findings

History. Assess the following:

- Exposure
- Excessive exercise
- Wearing inappropriate clothing
- Inadequate fluid intake or the use of water or other low-sodium fluids during prolonged and strenuous exercise
- Previous episode of heat stroke
- Heat cramps: Complaints of intermittent muscle cramping (no rigidity)
- Heat exhaustion: Complaints of thirst, weakness, headache, fatigue, dizziness, malaise, myalgias and muscle cramps, nausea, and vomiting; core temperature is normal or slightly elevated and the patient still sweats
- Heat stroke: Delirium, stupor, or coma—central nervous system dysfunction

Physical Examination. Signs of heat exhaustion include the following:

- Appears anxious and diaphoretic
- Tachycardia
- Temperature less than 105.8° F (41° C)
- Orthostatic hypotension

Signs of heat stroke, include all the symptoms of heat exhaustion listed above, are progressive, and also include the following:

- Body temperature greater than 105.8° F (41° C)
- Hot, dry, red skin
- May or may not sweat
- Initially a rapid, strong pulse that becomes progressively weaker
- Initially constricted pupils, progressively dilated
- Initially a deep, rapid "snorelike" breathing that becomes progressively weaker
- Tremors, increasing dizziness, and weakness

- Confusion, irritability, anxiety (central nervous system dysfunction)
- Headache
- Loss of appetite, nausea, vomiting
- Decreasing blood pressure, tachyarrhythmia
- Seizures, collapse
- Renal insufficiency, coma, and death

Diagnostic Studies. CBC and urinalysis, along with electrolyte monitoring may be necessary for significant heat cramps and heat exhaustion. Heat stroke requires extensive laboratory studies and monitoring of physiologic parameters.

Differential Diagnosis

Fever differs from hyperthermia in that it is an alteration of the body's hypothalamic set-point in response to a pathologic illness or condition.

Management

The management of heat-related illness includes the following:

- Heat cramps—usually mild
  - Cooling measures
  - Rest
  - Oral sodium replacement with electrolyte fluids or liberally salted foods
- Heat exhaustion
  - Rest in a cool or well-ventilated environment
  - Oral sodium replacement with electrolyte fluids or liberally salted foods
  - If weak or impaired level of consciousness, administer IV replacement of electrolytes (initial bolus of 10 to 20 mL/kg normal saline)
- Heat stroke—focuses on cardiovascular support and normalizing body temperatures
  - All individuals with heat stroke die without treatment and require intensive or emergency care. Heat stroke patients should be transported to a medical facility as quickly as possible. The goal of treatment is to reduce the temperature to 101.3° F (38.5° C) or by about 5.4° F (3° C).
  - First-aid management includes the following steps:
    - Remove the child from the source of heat.
    - Apply cold packs, wet sheets, or towels, or spray the body with lukewarm water. The body responds quickly to cooling of the neck, head, abdomen, and inner thighs.
    - Use a fan to cool and circulate air over the child and to facilitate evaporation.
    - Be alert for vomiting; prevent aspiration.
    - Administer IV lorazepam to prevent shivering, which generates heat.
    - When the body temperature is lowered to the desired level, stop cold packs, monitor, and be prepared to reapply cold packs if temperature increases.
    - Alcohol baths are contraindicated due to the potential for alcohol poisoning.
    - Acetaminophen and ibuprofen have no role in the treatment of heat stroke.
    - Other therapies are instituted based on the child's condition—IV hydration and therapy for myoglobinuria (Ewald and Baum, 2010).

Patient and Parent Education

Instruct parents on the risks of hyperthermia (e.g., never leave an infant or a child in a closed car or continuously exposed to direct sunlight) and that children who suffer heat stroke are at a higher risk for subsequent heat-related illnesses. Teach ways to prevent hyperthermia:

- Keep children well hydrated. Offer water often during active play and athletic events or practices. Water is the primary replacement fluid, although children can also use some electrolyte-based sports drinks.
- Make sure children are well rested and have good nutritional intake.
- Provide appropriate clothing (e.g., sunshades, hats, and light-reflective shirts that allow ventilation).
- Regulate children's activity levels to the conditions (e.g., limit active play if it is very hot or humid).
- Acclimatize child gradually to changes in environment.

MOTOR VEHICLE TRAUMA

Motor vehicle trauma continues to be the leading cause of death among children in the U.S., with significant mortality and morbidity rates in all age groups. In 2009, 1314 children birth to 14 years old died in motor vehicle crashes, and approximately 179,000 were injured. Fortunately, these data represent a 7% decrease in motor vehicle accident (MVA) injuries in children of similar age from 2008 statistics. Alcohol impairment was a factor in 181 (14%) of these pediatric fatalities, with 92 of the deaths occurring in a car with a driver whose blood alcohol concentration was .08 or higher (National Highway Traffic Safety Administration [NHTSA], 2009a).

Positioning young children in rear seats and correctly using child restraint systems (CRSs) can prevent fatalities from motor vehicle trauma and can reduce the number and severity of injuries to children. The NHTSA noted that child safety seats used correctly reduced the risk of fatal pediatric injuries in passenger vehicles by 71% in infants younger than 12 months and by 54% in the 1- to 4-year-old group (NHTSA, 2009b). Nonetheless, many children ride unrestrained or incorrectly restrained with 40% of the children who died in motor vehicle accidents in 2009 unrestrained (NHTSA, 2009b). Serious injury or death caused by airbags is also more likely if a child is not properly restrained or if a child in a rear-facing child safety seat is incorrectly placed in the front seat (NHTSA, 2009b). In states with primary seat belt enforcement laws (i.e., drivers can be stopped and cited by law enforcement officials for failure to wear a seat belt) versus those with secondary enforcement laws (i.e., drivers can be cited if they are stopped for another traffic violation and are not wearing a seat belt), seat belt usage is significantly higher.

In addition to not using restraints, a number of common errors have been found in the way CRSs are used (Box 39-2). The most common errors are loose vehicle safety straps attached to the CRS and loose harness straps securing the child to the CRS. Providers should assess the parents' use of CRSs and correct errors. This may mean accompanying parents to the parking lot to observe how children are placed in the restraint. Use of CRSs should be reviewed at each well-child visit, and children should be involved in the discussion from a very early age. Both parents and children should receive positive reinforcement for proper use of CRSs. Information from

---

BOX 39-2 Common Errors in the Use of Child Restraint Systems

- Seat belt is not tight enough.
- Rear-facing seat is not positioned at a 45-degree angle.
- Harness straps are not snug (infant may be wrapped in a "cocoon" of blankets).
- Harness straps in infant, rear-facing seat are not at or below shoulders of infant.
- Harness straps in child, forward-facing seat are not at or above shoulders of child.
- Retainer clip in child, forward-facing seat is not at armpit level.
- Seat belt is not in locked mode.
- Infants and toddlers less than 2 years old are placed in forward-facing position.

---

the NHTSA on which restraint system is appropriate for the size, age, and condition of the child should be shared with parents (Fig. 39-3).

The 2011 NHTSA guidelines are based on emerging evidence and research related to child restraint technologies and now include recommendations that take both the child's age and size into consideration (NHTSA, 2011). Parents should be advised to register their child's car seat online with the manufacturer to receive notification in the event of a safety recall. There are child car seat inspection stations where a certified technician can inspect the safety seat and demonstrate how it should be correctly installed and used. NHTSA's website provides an inspection station locator for parents seeking information about the closest station to their home.

Pedestrian injuries or injuries involving bicycles, skateboards, and automobiles are common among children. Providers should discuss this issue with parents at each well-child visit, ask children about their pedestrian safety habits during the well-child visit, and support educational efforts to instruct children on pedestrian safety and age-appropriate safe use of cycles or boards. Children of all ages need adult supervision related to motor vehicles. Adult supervision is especially important for younger children who are unaware of the dangers.

Adolescents, especially new drivers, are often involved in MVAs because of their inexperience, immature judgment, or tendency to take risks. Legislation has been passed in all but one state to restrict adolescent driving. Enactment of "graduated driver" licensing (learner, intermediate, and fully licensed stages) laws began in the 1990s. From 1998 to 2007 fatalities involving young drivers decreased by 13% (NHTSA, 2009c). Successful implementation of the law depends on parents acting as advocates for safety and supporting their adolescents' compliance with the regulations. Providers also can reinforce the message to teenagers that driving is a privilege that requires skill and maturity.

Graduated driver licensing legislation may require some or all of the following:

- Teens must complete driver education classes.
- Teens with learner permits may drive only with a fully-licensed adult.
- Driving is restricted to certain times of day and/or without other teenagers in the car.

As adolescents gain experience with age, restrictions on driving decline (NHTSA, 2009c).

Car Seat Recommendations for Children

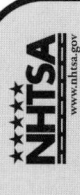

- Select a car seat based on your child's age and size, and choose a seat that fits in your vehicle and use it every time.
- Always refer to your specific car seat manufacturer's instructions; read the vehicle owner's manual on how to install the car seat using the seat belt or LATCH system; and check height and weight limits.
- To maximize safety, keep your child in the car seat for as long as possible, as long as the child fits within the manufacturer's height and weight requirements.
- Keep your child in the back seat at least through age 12.

AGE

 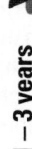

Birth – 12 months

Your child under age 1 should always ride in a rear-facing car seat. There are different types of rear-facing car seats: Infant-only seats can only be used rear-facing. Convertible and 3-in-1 car seats typically have higher height and weight limits for the rear-facing position, allowing you to keep your child rear-facing for a longer period of time.

1 – 3 years

Keep your child rear-facing as long as possible. It's the best way to keep him or her safe. Your child should remain in a rear-facing car seat until he or she reaches the top height or weight limit allowed by your car seat's manufacturer. Once your child outgrows the rear-facing car seat, your child is ready to travel in a forward-facing car seat with a harness.

 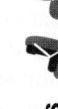

4 – 7 years

Keep your child in a forward-facing car seat with a harness until he or she reaches the top height or weight limit allowed by your car seat's manufacturer. Once your child outgrows the forward-facing car seat with a harness, it's time to travel in a booster seat, but still in the back seat.

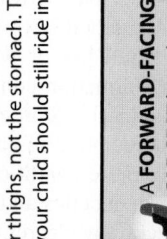

8 – 12 years

Keep your child in a booster seat until he or she is big enough to fit in a seat belt properly. For a seat belt to fit properly the lap belt must lie snugly across the upper thighs, not the stomach. The shoulder belt should lie snug across the shoulder and chest and not cross the neck or face. Remember: your child should still ride in the back seat because it's safer there.

DESCRIPTION (RESTRAINT TYPE)

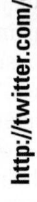 A **REAR-FACING CAR SEAT** is the best seat for your young child to use. It has a harness and in a crash, cradles and moves with your child to reduce the stress to the child's fragile neck and spinal cord.

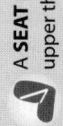 A **FORWARD-FACING CAR SEAT** has a harness and tether that limits your child's forward movement during a crash.

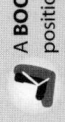 A **BOOSTER SEAT** positions the seat belt so that it fits properly over the stronger parts of your child's body.

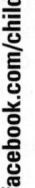 A **SEAT BELT** should lie across the upper thighs and be snug across the shoulder and chest to restrain the child safely in a crash. It should not rest on the stomach area or across the neck.

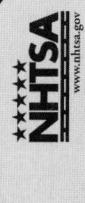
www.nhtsa.gov

www.facebook.com/childpassengersafety

http://twitter.com/childseatsafety

March 21, 2011

FIGURE 39-3 Car seat recommendations for children. (From National Highway Traffic Safety Administration: *Child safety: which car seat is the right one for your child?*, 2011. Available at http://www.nhtsa.gov/DOT/NHTSA/Traffic%20Injury%20Control/Articles/Associated%20Files/4StepsFlyer.pdf. Accessed October 27, 2011.)

Genetic Disorders

CATHERINE E. BURNS

The science of the human genome is transforming the field of genetics as we understood it from a mendelian inheritance perspective into a new genomics paradigm. In the new paradigm the focus is no longer on single genes and chromosomes, but on the influence of individual genes, the effects of many genes working in concert with one another, and with environmental exposures via epigenetics pathways to influence health outcomes. The issues involve identification of genome sequences of interest, interpretation of how those genes affect health, and use of that information to improve the health of children and their families (McBride and Guttmacher, 2009).

Genetic factors are linked to many disorders found in children. Some of these disorders are considered to be classic genetic diseases. Examples include cystic fibrosis, Down syndrome, and Duchenne muscular dystrophy. However, many of the most prevalent disorders of childhood have some genetic components. The chance that a child has or will develop a single-gene, chromosomal, or malformation condition during his or her life is between 3.2% and 7.3% (Jorde et al, 2006). The Human Genome Project is helping researchers identify the genetic markers for many more conditions. With this knowledge the intersection between genetics and environment (i.e., the field of epigenetics) is becoming clearer, and newborn screening has expanded, allowing for earlier identification of genetic conditions, and new therapies are being developed.

The manifestations of genetic diseases can appear immediately after birth or after many years, such as in patients with Huntington chorea; and can present in biochemical, reproductive, growth, developmental, or behavioral ways. Therefore, the primary health care provider must be constantly vigilant for the possibility of genetic disease. Furthermore, once a genetic condition is suspected, referral to a medical geneticist is not always required or possible. Primary care providers need to be knowledgeable, yet know their own limitations and set personal criteria for referral to specialists.

Caring for children with significant long-term problems confers enormous responsibilities on the provider, family, community, and society. Primary care providers assume a variety of roles related to the care of children with genetic disorders. These roles include promoting health of individuals with genetic conditions, assisting children and families to reduce risk for medical problems by helping families make decisions about childbearing, screening for early detection to prevent disability, assisting parents to use specialized services, teaching health principles, monitoring and evaluating clients with genetic diseases, and working with families under the stress of caregiving. Ethical decision-making has a particularly important role in the area of genetics and genetic counseling.

Cellular and Molecular Genetics

Humans have 46 chromosomes arranged in 23 pairs. Twenty-two pairs are autosomes (the same in males and females) and are homologous because their deoxyribonucleic acid (DNA) is very similar. The remaining pair is the sex chromosomes, with two X chromosomes for females and one X and one Y chromosome for males. They are not homologous. Each chromosome has a long arm (q) and a short arm (p) and is numbered according to its distinct appearance from the largest to the smallest. The gametes (egg and sperm) have half the chromosome complement from the parents (23). During meiosis (formation of the haploid with 23 chromosomes from the egg or sperm), the original paired chromosomes from paternal and maternal sides cross over and exchange genetic material, resulting in genetic diversity. Fusion at fertilization restores the 46-chromosome (23-pair) complement, with one of each chromosome pair from each gamete. As a result of genetic variation, a gene may differ from one individual to another in its DNA sequence. These differences in sequencing are called *alleles*. If the two alleles at any given location of a pair of homologous chromosomes are identical, the locus is *homozygous*. If the two alleles are different, the locus is *heterozygous*.

Genes, which carry the information about inherited characteristics from parent to child, are arranged linearly on the chromosomes, each with a specific locus. Thousands of genes are located on each chromosome. Not all genes are active at once; certain mechanisms activate them at various developmental points. In homozygous loci, the genes from a pair of chromosomes carry similar instructions regarding the trait of interest; in heterozygous loci, the instructions are different for

Thanks to Robyn Robinson, PNP, for her help with the Klinefelter discussion.

each gene. In the latter case, one gene may be dominant, with its instructions manifested in the phenotype, as in Huntington disease, or the genes can be co-dominant, as in the case of individuals with blood type AB.

The human genome contains approximately 25,000 to 30,000 genes. Genes are composed of DNA. Each DNA molecule includes pairs of nitrogenous bases—adenine, cytosine, guanine, and thymine (labeled A, C, G, T)—wound around a histone protein core in a double helix. There are more than 3 billion base pairs in the human genome for an individual. From the four nitrogenous bases, 64 triple-base combination sequences (codons) of A, C, G, and U (uracil is substituted for thymine in the messenger ribonucleic acid [mRNA] at this point) such as GUA, UUG, and CGG are possible (Jorde et al, 2006). Three codons signal the end of a gene (stop codons) and 61 define the 20 amino acids. Thus each amino acid may be specified by more than one codon. The sequence of the amino acids directs the synthesis of proteins in the cell cytoplasm (Fig. 40-1). Telomeres at the tips of each chromosome protect the chromosome from breaking down. These deteriorate with age.

Now that the genome has been defined, geneticists are working to understand the functions of individual genes. In the case of conditions such as Down syndrome, which has been identified as a chromosomal disorder, understanding of the functions of the many genes on chromosome 21 may help clarify how some of the various phenotypes of the condition are controlled and, ultimately, might be able to provide therapies for some of the problems such as leukemia or cataracts, which emerge later in life (Patterson, 2009). Similar progress may offer new perspectives and options for other genetic conditions.

Epigenetics

Epigenetics is defined as the study of heritable changes in genome function that occur without a change in DNA sequence. This includes the study of how patterns of gene expression are passed from one cell to its descendants, how gene expression changes during the differentiation of one cell type into another, and how environmental factors can change the way genes are expressed (Bagot and Meaney, 2010; Epigenome Network of Excellence, 2009).

In the nucleus of nondividing cells, genomic DNA is highly folded and compacted with histone and nonhistone proteins into a polymer called chromatin (DNA does not normally look like the nice double helix strands seen in many diagrams). The *epigenome* is the group of proteins around the genome that tells genes when to turn on and off. An analogy could be made to computers: the genome is the computer's hardware; the epigenome is the software that tells it what to do.

There are several recognized mechanisms for epigenetic inheritance, not all of which are discussed here. DNA methylation is the most studied. When DNA material is methylated, the gene is turned off. Methylation is involved with cellular differentiation in utero but the same process occurs throughout life. A second mechanism for epigenetic modifications to DNA functioning involves the way DNA attaches to histones. It is called chromatin modification. DNA is wrapped around a series of proteins called histones. If these proteins are tightly joined to the DNA, the DNA is hidden from exposure and cannot express itself. If the histone wrap is loosened, often through acetylation, enzymes, or certain forms of RNA, then the gene may be expressed

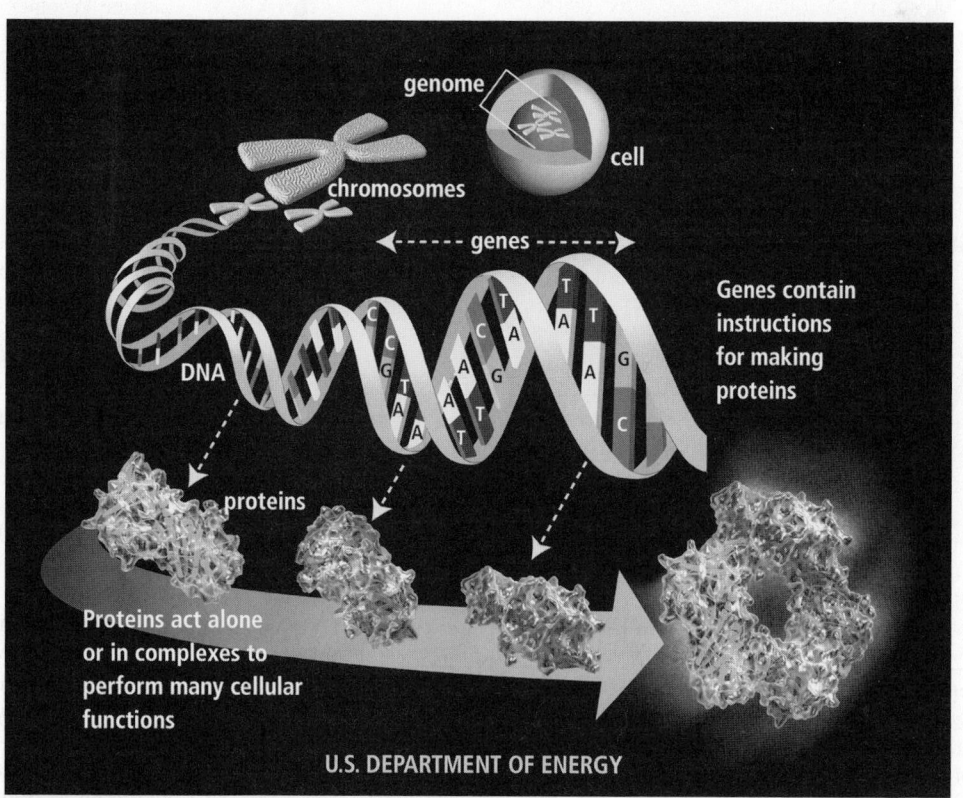

FIGURE 40-1 Genetic diagram. (From the U.S. Department of Energy, Washington, DC.)

(Fig. 40-2). In general, when chromatin is tightly folded, gene expression is restricted while more open chromatin allows gene expression. In other words, gene regulation varies depending on the type of histone linkage. Certain RNA proteins are also transmitted with reproduction and are involved with epigenetic inheritance (Jablonka and Raz, 2009).

Genes are regulated when the histone allows signals to reach the gene. These signals may come from one cell touching another as in neurologic growth, when a cell releases factors that are picked up by neighboring cells as happens at cell synapses, through hormones that are broadcast to the whole body (cells that are tuned in will respond), or by signals coming from environmental factors. Some of these environmental factors reach cells directly and others indirectly (mediated, for example, by stress), and cause responses that are transmitted across body systems. Signals are passed to a gene regulatory protein that attaches to a specific sequence of DNA molecules. Once the protein is attached to the DNA molecule, the gene turns off. The epigenetic tags allow the cell to "remember" what to do over time and over many replications. Some tags are passed on to later generations. Certain enzymes can be recruited to remove epigenetic tags, the histones, or both, and cells are stripped of many of their tags with reproduction of sperm and egg. The tags that remain to be passed along to the next generation are referred to as *imprinted*. More than 80 genes can be imprinted (Weinhold, 2006). Chemical

exposures can cause methylation of DNA and transmission to future generations—altering the function of cells but not the DNA itself (Jablonka and Raz, 2009).

An individual normally has one copy of an imprinted gene (it came along on the sperm or egg chromosome). Improper imprinting can cause an individual to have two copies of active, imprinted genes, or two inactive copies. Prader-Willi and Angelman syndromes come from the same imprinting area on chromosome 15. If the individual is missing gene activity that normally comes from the father or there are two active copies from the mother, Prader-Willi will result; if the imprinting defect results in failed gene activity that normally comes from the mother, Angelman will result.

The study of epigenetics is revolutionizing our understanding of many conditions (e.g., autism spectrum disorders, which are known to have both genetic and environmental etiologic factors; epigenetics may explain how the various factors interrelate to cause these disorders). Rett, fragile X, Prader-Willi, Angelman, and all demonstrate dysregulation of normal epigenetic mechanisms (Grafodatskaya et al, 2010). It is thought that many cancers may result from epigenetic control of gene expression rather than defective genes themselves, or may be caused by a mixture of the two factors. Cancer epigenetics may involve disruption of the stem cells, sometimes when they have replicated many times over years and no longer seem to be able to function properly (Feinberg, 2007; NOVA, 2007). Some of the endocrine disruptor toxins

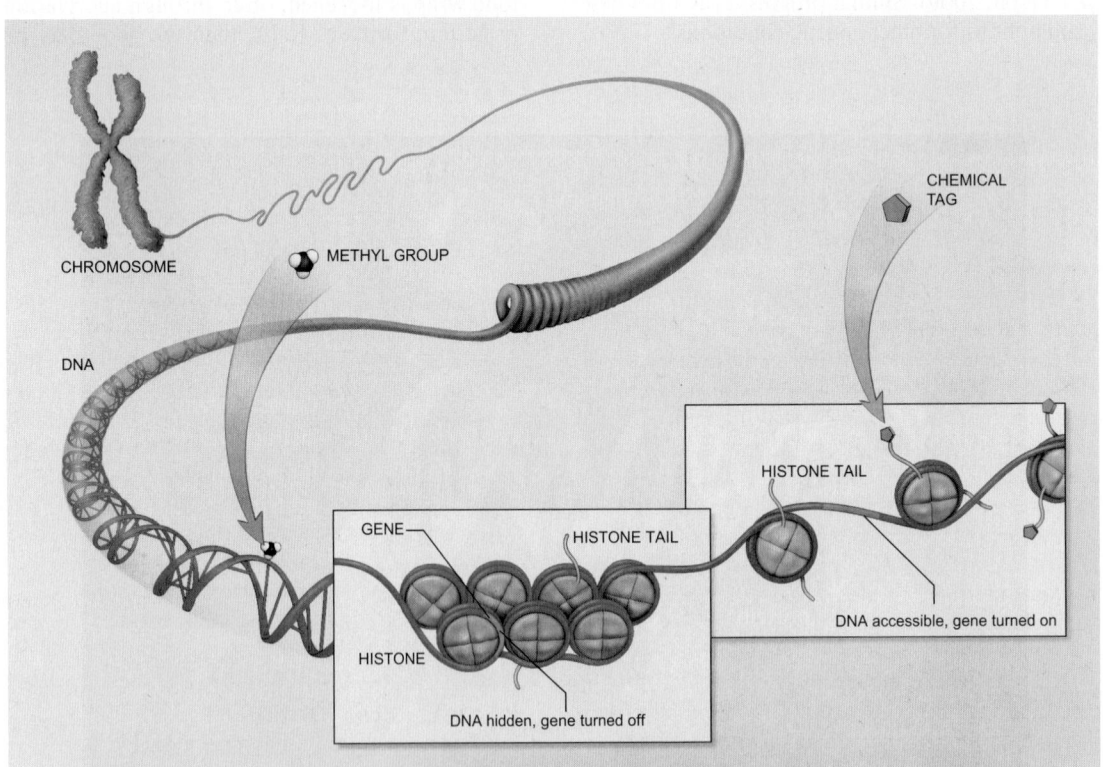

FIGURE 40-2 Epigenetic diagram. Chromatin modification: deoxyribonucleic acid (DNA) is wrapped around a series of proteins called histones. If these proteins are tightly joined to the DNA, the DNA is hidden from exposure and cannot express itself. If the histone wrap is loosened, often through acetylation, enzymes, or certain forms of ribonucleic acid (RNA), then the gene may be expressed. Methyl groups attached to the DNA also affect gene expression. (From The National Institutes of Health Common Fund, Division of Program Coordination, Planning, and Strategic Initiatives, National Institutes of Health.)

in the environment cause epigenetic trangenerational effects, meaning that the germline is affected and this change is transmitted to future generations (Guerrero-Bosagna and Skinner, 2009).

Epigenetic research has contributed to the development of new epigenetic therapy in which instructions to cells are changed, allowing them to reactivate in a normal way after having been silenced by cancer cells (Issa, 2010).

■ Ethical Issues

Since 1990, largely due to the work of the Human Genome Project (HGP), the technical capability to diagnose a hereditary condition for those who are presymptomatic or currently symptomatic, to identify those who are carriers of a genetic condition, and to determine susceptibility to a genetic condition has increased dramatically. However, the availability of this technology raises significant ethical issues. The HGP was concerned about these issues from the beginning and has a branch specifically devoted to oversight of these concerns (the Ethical, Legal, and Social Initiative [ELSI]). Issues involve the rights to privacy and confidentiality, rights to know and right not to know, and whether there is a duty to warn third parties (Ross, 2008).

Maintenance of confidentiality is a challenge. The presence of genetic information in the medical record, health insurance diagnostic database, or in DNA databases such as newborn screening specimens mandates policies to maintain the confidentiality and integrity of these records. The Health Insurance Portability and Accountability Act (HIPAA) of 1996 specifies the duty for clinicians not to disclose medical information without the signed consent of the patient or the child's parents (U.S. Department of Health and Human Services [USDHHS], 2010).

As genetics tests are conducted, it is also possible to discover unanticipated information, for instance, data regarding the parentage of the child being tested. Situations such as misattribution of paternity and children being raised by nonbiologic parents may be discovered. There is disagreement about whether these findings should be routinely disclosed. Prior agreement in the consent process can assist in the decision about whether to disclose this information.

The ability to screen for a large number of genetic disorders via the tandem mass spectrometry newborn screening process has increased the number and types of conditions that can be included. Because these programs are organized by and paid for through state governments, there is some variability in required tests between states. Congenital hypothyroidism, sickle cell disease, sickle-C, sickle-beta thalassemia, classical galactosemia, and phenylketonuria are mandated in newborn screening programs in all U.S. states. An additional sixty-one conditions are included in individual state newborn screening programs (National Newborn Screening & Genetics Resource Center, 2006). Three principals have been suggested by the Institute of Medicine (IOM) to be used in making decisions about the introduction or continuation of tests:

- Identification of the genetic condition must provide a clear benefit to the child.
- A system must be in place to confirm the diagnosis.
- Treatment and follow-up must be available for affected infants.

Predictive genetic testing is another area for ethical consideration. The availability of presymptomatic testing for conditions that may not become apparent until adulthood, such as Huntington disease and breast cancer, has raised another set of questions. Should children and adolescents be tested for such conditions? Arguments related to the issue of predictive genetic testing generally fall into four categories: potential provision of good news (i.e., the child is found not to have the genetic markers); unbearability of knowing (if the child has the markers); identity and adjustment (if the child has the markers); and parental anxiety and uncertainty (Borry et al, 2008). Generally it is recommended that genetic testing for late-onset conditions be deferred until adulthood when individuals, rather than their parents, can make the decision, unless there is evidence that early diagnosis can result in treatment strategies that will alter the progression of the disease (American Academy of Pediatrics [AAP] Committee on Bioethics, 2001). If predictive testing is considered, parents should have the right to decide whether to have their child tested and to receive counseling regarding the disease including diagnostic workup, ongoing research, associations, resources available, and clinical trials in progress or registering for trials in the future (Trott and Matalon, 2009).

Biobanks including many thousands of genetic samples from children are being collected to study genetic-environmental influences on disease. Should participants have access to the data? To what extent do those children have a right to privacy?

Families also face issues of disclosure of genetic information within their own families. What information should be disclosed? When? To whom? Disclosure is influenced by the perceived risks and benefits of doing so, the sense of closeness among the family members, concerns about reactions from those receiving the information, their sense of personal risk, and readiness to disclose information (Gallo et al, 2009). Disclosure to children is also an issue many families face. Families worry about psychological harm, the child's lack of autonomy in deciding whether to be tested, and concerns that the child won't understand the information given. The child's developmental age is a key factor. For preschoolers there may only be a dawning awareness of symptoms, treatments, or physical differences. Parents will want to choose whether they disclose information, choose to wait, or want a health care professional to begin the dialogue with the child about the genetic condition of interest. School-age children may question parents about the implications of a particular diagnosis or become aware of reproductive risks. Adolescents are aware of conditions and want information in more depth. They may have very specific questions about reproductive risks. Health care professionals need to assist patients and families to disclose information as is appropriate, Questions such as, "Have you ever talked with your child about his condition?" may start a helpful discussion.

These are only a few of the ethical issues under discussion. Primary care providers must be part of the ongoing debate and be aware of the issues, policies, and laws as they work with families who are trying to make decisions.

■ Genetics Testing in the Future

Genetics testing will become more complex in the future and primary care providers will need to be knowledgeable in all these areas. First, universal screening can be expected to expand as therapies evolve, making it possible to prevent or modify significant pathology in affected individuals. Second, screening will be expanded for diagnosis of common conditions. For example, more than 50% of sensorineural hearing loss is due to genetic conditions. When infants are identified through newborn hearing screening, they will then undergo genetic testing to ascertain possible causes. Some autism and obesity cases are now connected to certain genetic profiles in children. Hypertension, diabetes, heart disease, and cancer are adult conditions in which greater genetic information will affect identification of and management of those at risk (Lose, 2008). Third, additional screening will be done to identify those at risk for future problems, such as the breast cancer and Parkinson disease tests that are already available. Finally, pharmacogenetics will involve genetic testing to ascertain drug responses in individuals with different genetic profiles (Cheng et al, 2008). Primary care providers will serve as translators for patients needing and receiving genetic information over their lifetime (Lose, 2008).

Causes of Genetic Variation and Genetic Disorders

Mutations occur when genetic material is permanently changed through alteration, deletion, duplication, or misplacement. Sometimes mutations arise spontaneously, but once the change occurs in the germ cells, it is transmitted to future generations. Mutations are defined as characteristics being present in less than 1% of the population. A change in greater than 1% is called a *polymorphism*. Mutations and polymorphisms may be benign, beneficial, or detrimental.

Genetic disorders are classified as chromosomal disorders, in which the entire chromosome or large segments of it are duplicated or missing; single-gene disorders, in which single genes are altered; and multifactorial problems, in which multiple genetic and environmental factors interact. Although the majority of genetic conditions fit in these categories, other patterns of inheritance, such as mitochondrial inheritance may lead to genetic disorders. Conditions that result from mutation in mitochondrial DNA are inherited through the maternal line. Some epigenetic changes can also be inherited, at least to the next generation and perhaps more. This is an emerging area of research.

▪ Chromosomal Disorders

Chromosomal disorders are present in 0.6% to 0.9% of the general population (Jorde et al, 2006). There is also a high frequency of chromosomal disorders in spontaneous abortions and stillbirths. Such disorders are commonly linked to alterations in cognitive development; linear growth, usually short stature; and congenital anomalies. The chromosomal disorders include problems of chromosome number (increase or decrease in the number of chromosomes), structure, or both.

The prevalence of chromosomal disorders due to nondisjunction (failure of homologous pairs to separate properly

during meiosis) increases with advancing maternal age. Testing to diagnose a chromosome disorder is done through cell culture and chromosome analysis. In addition to the more traditional method of karyotype analysis, in which the total number of each chromosome is identified, staining techniques to identify chromosomal banding assist in the identification of deletions and duplications of chromosomal material. Techniques such as fluorescence in situ hybridization (FISH) provide the ability to identify missing, additional, or rearranged chromosomal material for some of the more common abnormalities but must be ordered for the specific location of interest.

▪ Single-Gene Disorders

Mendelian theory describes four patterns of inheritance: autosomal dominant, autosomal recessive, X-linked dominant, and X-linked recessive. Dominant inheritance disorders occur in heterozygotes, where one gene dominates its counterpart from the other parent. Recessive inheritance disorders occur only when a person is homozygous, when the gene with a disease-causing mutation appears on both of the chromosomes of the pair. However, genetic mutations for some conditions have reduced *penetrance*, in which a person may have the affected gene (genotype) without expressing the observable characteristics (phenotype), and variable *expressivity*, in which the severity of the disease condition varies greatly. The result is that some children have clinically severe disease, whereas others, with mutations in the same gene, are more mildly affected.

▪ Multifactorial or Multiple-Gene Disorders

Multifactorial problems result from the complex interaction of multiple genes in various sites and/or interaction of genes with the environment. Several terms are used for this group of conditions (e.g., *multifactorial, multiple gene,* and *polygenic*). Cleft lip and palate, spina bifida, hypertension, schizophrenia, pyloric stenosis, diabetes, hypercholesterolemia, Hirschsprung disease, and asthma fall into this category.

Multifactorial problems are more likely to cluster in families. The exact recurrence risk is more difficult to predict because the precise genetic and environmental risks are usually not known. However, in general, the risk for the condition increases if more family members are affected, and if the disease has a more severe expression. It is likely that epigenetics will provide explanations for many of the multifactorial disorders, identifying those combinations of genes, gene mutations, or expression or silencing of genes that result in disease.

▪ Nontraditional Inheritance

Three additional patterns of transmission of genetic material from generation to generation have been identified—germline mosaicism, uniparental disomy, and mitochondrial inheritance.

GERMLINE MOSAICISM

In this pattern a mutation occurs in a cell of the developing organism sometime after fertilization. As cells multiply, some begin to reproduce with the mutation, whereas others do not. The outcome is a person with "mosaicism"—some normal and some abnormal cells. Whether the gametes are affected will dictate inheritance to the next generation, and the cells involved determine whether the condition is clinically relevant. Thus the term *germline mosaicism* is used to indicate inheritability of the trait. With germline mosaicism, parents appear normal but have some gametes with the gene mutation. The challenge, clinically, is to identify the condition as inheritable. If normal-appearing parents have a first child with a condition such as achondroplasia, which is normally autosomal dominant, the clinician would deduce that the achondroplasia was not inherited in an autosomal dominant manner (in which case one parent would have had the disorder), so a new mutation, and the possibility of germline mosaicism, must be considered. If germline mutation is present, the risk of recurrence in a second offspring is increased. It is because of such situations that genetic counseling for parents is important to help determine the risk to subsequent children.

UNIPARENTAL DISOMY

Generally, children receive one chromosome from each parental pair at the time of fertilization. If, by some chance, the child receives two copies of one chromosome of a pair from one parent and none from the other parent, uniparental disomy has occurred. The result is that the child will be homozygous for every gene located on that chromosome, which increases the possibilities of an autosomal recessive disorder in the child. The process has been described in some patients with cystic fibrosis. The same process also may result in either Prader-Willi or Angelman syndrome, diseases that involve the same gene loci but differ depending on whether the copies are from the mother or the father. Beckwith-Wiedemann and Russell-Silver syndromes are also examples of uniparental disomy.

MITOCHONDRIAL DNA INHERITANCE

Mitochondria in cells also have DNA (mtDNA). Unlike chromosomal DNA, mtDNA is circular. All inherited mtDNA comes from the ovum—thus it has a maternal transmission pattern. Because each cell has more than one mitochondrion, there are more opportunities for mutations and also for variable expressivity; if many normal mitochondria are present, the effects from the aberrant mtDNA may be minimal. Several biopsies of different tissues will be subjected to both enzymatic and DNA analyses for diagnosis of mtDNA-related diseases. Although rare, mitochondrial diseases do play a role in some more common conditions such as deafness and non–insulin-dependent diabetes (Jorde et al, 2006).

■ Teratogens

Although not strictly genetic in origin, teratogens are often discussed with genetic disorders because the differential diagnosis includes factors that affect the embryo after fertilization and those that affect the DNA of the germ cells or their joining with fertilization. Fetal alcohol syndrome is an example of a condition in this category. Viral diseases, such as rubella, certain drugs, and environmental toxins—such as mercury—are also considered teratogens. The Pregnancy Exposure InfoLine (www.thepeil.org) contains current information on potential teratogenic effects of specific environmental substances.

Assessment

Primary care providers identify possible genetic disorders by using the same skills as those for other pediatric health problems: knowledge of risk factors, collection of a good history, and a complete physical examination augmented with appropriate laboratory or other studies. After the assessment, providers determine the operative genetic mechanism and develop and implement a plan of care for the patient and family with consideration of individual, family, and cultural factors. Box 40-1 identifies some common features of children or family members with genetic disorders that should lead providers to explore issues of possible genetic problems.

■ Risk Factors

Risk factors that may be identified in the child or family members include the following:

- Family history of known genetic disorder or recurrent pathologic condition
- Malformations
- Mental retardation
- Metabolic disorders
- Delayed development of secondary sex characteristics
- Sensory deficits
- Progressive disorders
- Neuromuscular disorders
- Affective disorders (e.g., schizophrenia)
- Presence of birth defects
- Developmental delays or learning problems
- Repeated spontaneous abortions or stillbirths

BOX 40-1 Features Suggesting a Genetic Disorder

Mental retardation/developmental delays
Seizures with mental retardation
Severe hypotonia in infancy
Loss of developmental milestones
Short stature
Failure to thrive/growth retardation
Microcephaly
Dysmorphic features
Two or more physical malformations
Ambiguous genitalia
Pigmentary skin lesions
Ocular findings such as colobomas or blindness
Deafness

TABLE 40-1	Genetic Risks Associated With Ethnic Background

Ethnic Background	Genetic Disorder at Higher Risk
Northern European	Cystic fibrosis, phenylketonuria
Jewish (Ashkenazi descent)	Tay-Sachs, Canavan, Gaucher
West African	Sickle cell, sickle cell–hemoglobin C
Mediterranean	Beta-thalassemia, sickle cell
French-Canadian	Tay-Sachs, branched-chain ketoaciduria

- Maternal factors, including alcohol or drug exposure, medication exposure, age older than 35 years, environmental or occupational toxin exposure
- Family ethnic background (Table 40-1)

History

The history of genetic diseases usually includes the following main areas (Dolan and Moore, 2007):
- Family history of the disease using a pedigree format. A family history is needed to identify family members with conditions that may be genetically transmitted. The pedigree provides a visual map of the occurrence of specific traits and identifies other family members who might be at risk. Providers can see the potential pattern of inheritance and the relationships among affected family members. Past and current health of each person in the pedigree, birth histories of other family members, and mental retardation or learning problems of family members are all important areas to explore. Consanguinity should be noted; persons who have a common ancestor may each be carriers of a gene mutation present in that family.
- Environmental and occupational history. The environmental and occupational history may provide information about specific teratogenic factors that might be involved.
- Reproductive history. The mother's reproductive history may give information about malformations, genetic conditions, or infectious diseases transmitted to other offspring. Her pregnancy and delivery of the child in question may give other information to determine whether the condition was the result of genetic factors or whether the condition was a result of trauma, infection, or some other factor occurring during the pregnancy or delivery.
- Dietary history
- Medical history of the child
- Developmental data

Figures 40-3 and 40-4 illustrate the pedigree notation format. Screening questions for genetic disorders that should be asked of all patients are included in Table 40-2. Families can be encouraged to record their own family history information by using programs such as the U.S. Surgeon General's Family History Initiative (USDHHS, 2005). Parents and children should be encouraged to learn about the health of members of their family, which may, in turn, provide clues as to specific health

TABLE 40-2	General Screening for Genetic Conditions: The History

Question	Rationale/Comments
Has anyone in the family had a birth defect?	To identify conditions that affect others in the family. If answer is yes, try to get more information about the nature of the defect.
Is there anyone in the family with a stillborn baby or baby who died early in life?	To identify unrecognized genetic disorders. Babies who died very early may have inheritable metabolic disorders. Distinguish from sudden infant death syndrome.
Is there any chance that you and your partner are blood-related? Is this pregnancy a product of incest?	Consanguinity of partners closer than first cousins is a risk factor for autosomal recessive disorders. If yes, recommend genetics consultation.
Are there any diseases or traits that run in your family?	Significant if early onset, two or more close relatives affected. Genetic heart disease and genetic cancer risks are important. If yes, recommend genetic consultation and monitoring.
Have you or any of your parents or siblings had three or more miscarriages?	May indicate a chromosome translocation. If yes, order a karyotype of the mother or father (or both).
Does anyone in the family have mental retardation?	Look for multiple members affected and associated with dysmorphic features. If yes, recommend genetic consultation.
What is your ethnic background? Your partner's?	Consider ethnic risk factors and screen if at risk.

risks for themselves. When a genetic disorder is suspected, the history must become more specific, as outlined in Table 40-3.

Physical Examination

When a genetic disease is being considered, the physical examination focuses on growth, major and minor anomalies, and comparisons with family members. Any major anomaly can have a genetic cause. A known genetic cause is identified in approximately 30% of newborn infants with a congenital malformation (Nelson and Holmes, 1989). Three minor anomalies or more should raise the suspicion of a major anomaly and a genetic disorder.

First, general appearance and familial similarities are assessed. Note if a parent with similar physical features has specific health problems. Body size and proportions, measurements and percentiles, and a careful assessment of all systems constitute the remainder of the examination.

Common minor anomalies are identified in Box 40-2. For major anomalies, Smith's Recognizable Patterns of Human Malformations includes tables on the size, length, and shape of various body parts that can be used to validate observations presumed to represent pathology (Jones, 2006). About 3% of

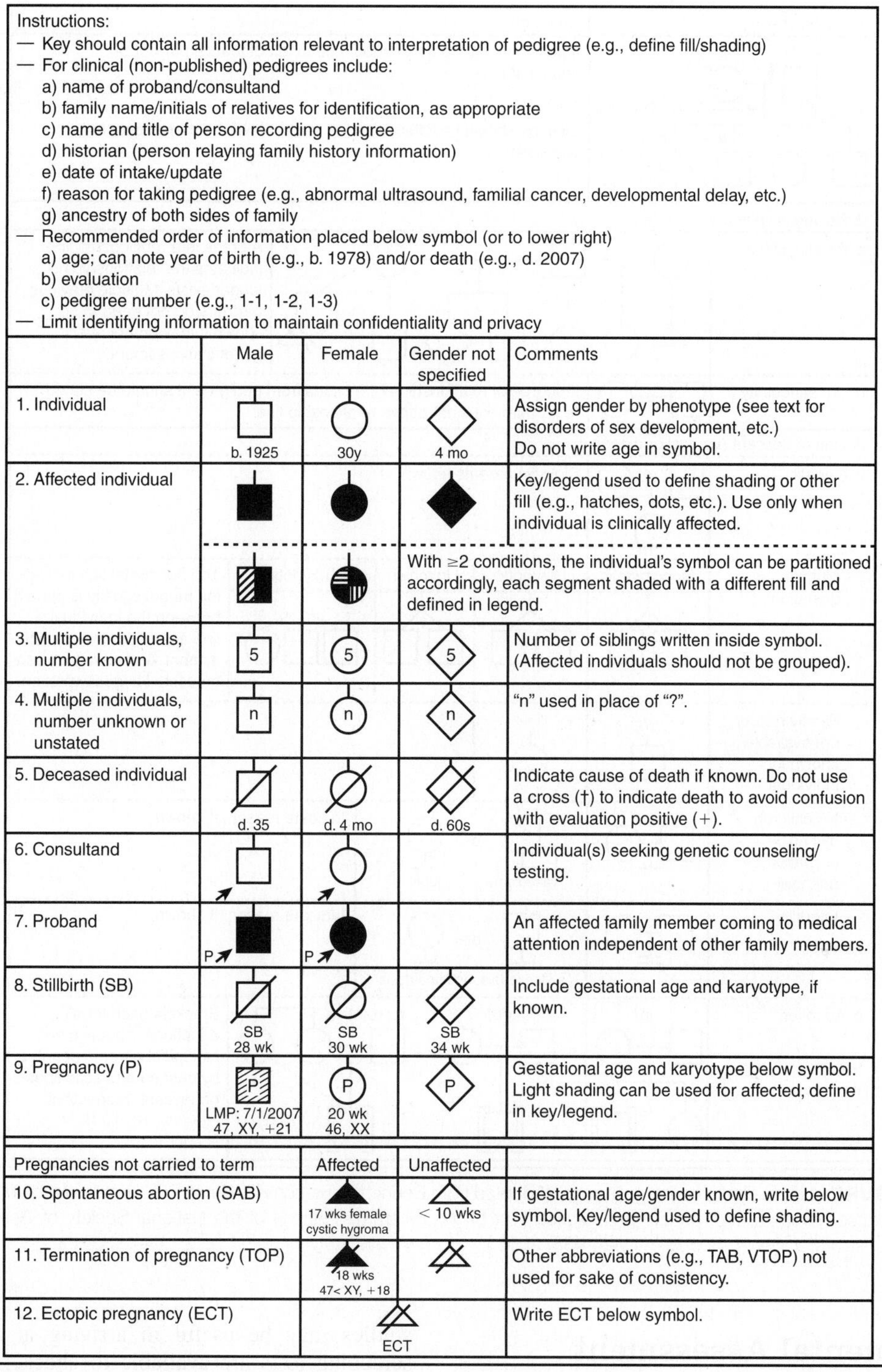

Instructions:
— Key should contain all information relevant to interpretation of pedigree (e.g., define fill/shading)
— For clinical (non-published) pedigrees include:
  a) name of proband/consultand
  b) family name/initials of relatives for identification, as appropriate
  c) name and title of person recording pedigree
  d) historian (person relaying family history information)
  e) date of intake/update
  f) reason for taking pedigree (e.g., abnormal ultrasound, familial cancer, developmental delay, etc.)
  g) ancestry of both sides of family
— Recommended order of information placed below symbol (or to lower right)
  a) age; can note year of birth (e.g., b. 1978) and/or death (e.g., d. 2007)
  b) evaluation
  c) pedigree number (e.g., 1-1, 1-2, 1-3)
— Limit identifying information to maintain confidentiality and privacy

	Male	Female	Gender not specified	Comments
1. Individual	□ b. 1925	○ 30y	◇ 4 mo	Assign gender by phenotype (see text for disorders of sex development, etc.) Do not write age in symbol.
2. Affected individual	■	●	◆	Key/legend used to define shading or other fill (e.g., hatches, dots, etc.). Use only when individual is clinically affected.
	(partitioned square)	(partitioned circle)		With ≥2 conditions, the individual's symbol can be partitioned accordingly, each segment shaded with a different fill and defined in legend.
3. Multiple individuals, number known	□ 5	○ 5	◇ 5	Number of siblings written inside symbol. (Affected individuals should not be grouped).
4. Multiple individuals, number unknown or unstated	□ n	○ n	◇ n	"n" used in place of "?".
5. Deceased individual	⊘ d. 35	⊘ d. 4 mo	⊘ d. 60s	Indicate cause of death if known. Do not use a cross (†) to indicate death to avoid confusion with evaluation positive (+).
6. Consultand	□↗	○↗		Individual(s) seeking genetic counseling/testing.
7. Proband	P↗ ■	P↗ ●		An affected family member coming to medical attention independent of other family members.
8. Stillbirth (SB)	⊘ SB 28 wk	⊘ SB 30 wk	⊘ SB 34 wk	Include gestational age and karyotype, if known.
9. Pregnancy (P)	P LMP: 7/1/2007 47, XY, +21	P 20 wk 46, XX	P	Gestational age and karyotype below symbol. Light shading can be used for affected; define in key/legend.

Pregnancies not carried to term	Affected	Unaffected	
10. Spontaneous abortion (SAB)	▲ 17 wks female cystic hygroma	△ < 10 wks	If gestational age/gender known, write below symbol. Key/legend used to define shading.
11. Termination of pregnancy (TOP)	▲ 18 wks 47< XY, +18	△ (slashed)	Other abbreviations (e.g., TAB, VTOP) not used for sake of consistency.
12. Ectopic pregnancy (ECT)	△ (slashed) ECT		Write ECT below symbol.

FIGURE 40-3 Pedigree model. Common pedigree symbols, definitions, and abbreviations. (Adapted from Bennett R, French KS, Resta RG: Standardized human pedigree nomenclature: update and assessment of the recommendations of the National Society of Genetic Counselors, *J Genet Counsel* 17:424-433, 2008.)

infants are born with any one of 45 birth defects (Centers for Disease Control and Prevention [CDC], 2006).

Dysmorphic features may be recognized and can result from the following:
• *Deformation:* Abnormal shape or position of body part caused by external mechanical forces (e.g., clubfoot)
• *Disruption:* Defect of organ or large body part caused by external disruption of originally normal process (e.g., amniotic bands)
• *Dysplasia:* Abnormal organization of cells into tissues (e.g., polycystic kidneys)
• *Malformation:* Abnormal development of an organ or large body part from an intrinsically abnormal process (e.g., cleft palate)

Visual recognition, combined with family history evaluation, is a major skill in diagnosing genetic diseases. Providers can hone their abilities by reviewing pictures of patients with various disorders and consulting with experts.

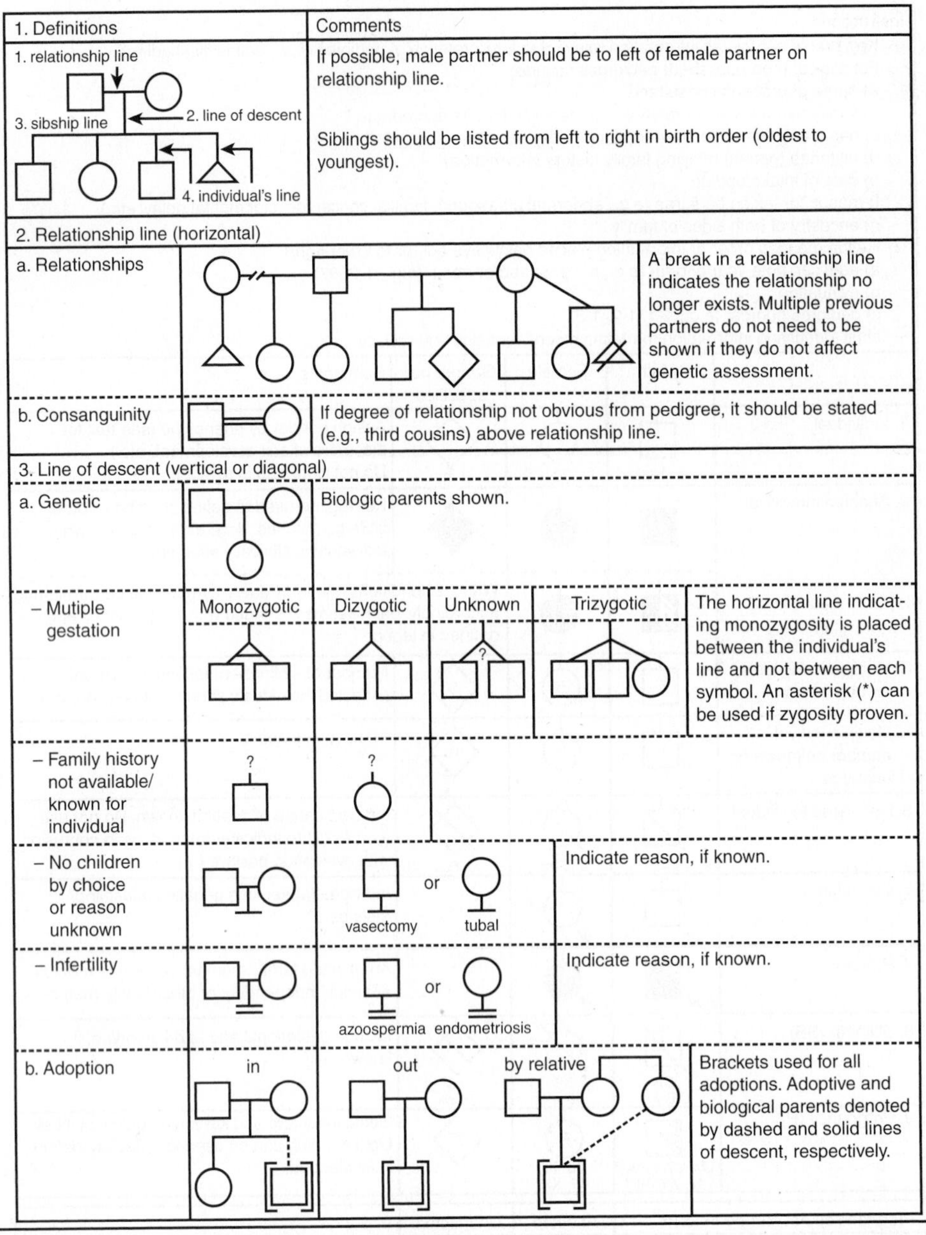

FIGURE 40-4 Pedigree line definitions. (Adapted from Bennett R, French KS, Resta RG: Standardized human pedigree nomenclature: update and assessment of the recommendations of the National Society of Genetic Counselors, *J Genet Counsel* 17:424-433, 2008.)

■ Developmental Assessment

Many genetic disorders have central nervous system (CNS) effects and cause some degree of mental retardation. Other affected tissues are associated with neuromotor delays. Developmental assessment is a key component in the evaluation of a child with a possible genetic disorder. The genetic evaluation of a child with mental retardation is diagrammed in Figure 40-5.

■ Diagnostic Studies

BIOCHEMICAL STUDIES

Based on findings from the family history, physical examination, and developmental assessment, specific laboratory studies may be useful in arriving at a diagnosis. Many screening tests are available to check for inborn errors of metabolism. Such tests include those for phenylketonuria (PKU), galactosemia, and others. See Chapter 38 for further discussion.

CYTOGENETICS AND CHROMOSOME STUDIES

Blood tests are commonly used to screen for sickle cell disease, thalassemias, and Tay-Sachs disease. Molecular genetics methods are increasingly being used for many disorders, such as cystic fibrosis. Generally the tests must be ordered with some specificity. Linkage analysis, direct mutation analysis, and molecular cytogenetic analyses are types of DNA studies. Each has its own advantages and disadvantages.

TABLE 40-3 Specific Genetic History Questions

Topic	Specific Items of History
Family history: helps identify family with conditions that may be genetically transmitted	• The pedigree should focus on at least three generations and look for individuals with similar characteristics. • Consanguinity of partners (closer than first cousins) is very important. • Note the past and current health of each person listed on the pedigree. • Note the age of onset for family members' illnesses. • Note multiple miscarriages, stillbirths, and anomalies within family. • Family members with learning disabilities or mental retardation are important to document.
Environmental and occupational history	Exposure to environmental toxins, alcohol, cigarette smoke, drugs, or radiation that might affect offspring
Reproductive history: helps identify malformations, genetic conditions, or infectious diseases transmitted from mother to child	Maternal medical history • Uterine anomalies • Maternal illnesses and diseases (e.g., phenylketonuria, diabetes) • Immunization status Prenatal history: The reproductive history should list every pregnancy, stillbirth, and abortion. Fetuses with significant chromosomal disorders are often aborted, and 5% to 7% of stillbirths and perinatal deaths are related to genetic problems. Pregnancy and delivery history • Parity • Advanced maternal or paternal age • Complications of pregnancy • Polyhydramnios or oligohydramnios • Fetal movements • Fetal growth assessments • Prenatal screening results • Breech position • Birth measurements • Gestational age • Results of newborn screening tests • Presence of three or more minor anomalies in neonate • Failure of neonate to adapt to extrauterine life • Complications of delivery
Dietary history: helps identify infants with single-gene–related metabolic disorders	• Infant feeding behavior • Formula or food intolerance • Temporal relation of symptoms to meals • Relation of signs and symptoms to types of food
Medical history of affected child	Use routine past medical history questions—history and current status of illnesses, hospitalizations, surgeries, allergies, injuries, immunizations. List all health care providers involved with the child's care.
Developmental history	• Achievements of milestones • Speech and language development • School performance • Developmental evaluations • Growth

BOX 40-2 Minor Malformations and Variations of Normal

Large fontanelle
Epicanthal folds
Hair whorls
Widow's peak
Low posterior hairline
Preauricular tags or pits
Minor ear anomalies
Protruding ears
Rotated ears
Low-set ears
Darwinian tubercle (blunt point protruding from upper edge of helix)
Digital anomalies
Clinodactyly (curved finger)
Camptodactyly (bent finger)
Syndactyly (webbed finger)
Transverse palmar crease
Shawl scrotum
Redundant umbilicus
Widespread nipples
Supernumerary nipples

Chromosome tests may be needed to identify specific genetic diseases. FISH combines elements of standard cytogenetic technique with molecular technology; probes for specific, extremely small chromosome abnormalities are used. For instance, FISH analysis might identify the deletion of chromosome site 15q11-q13 associated with Prader-Willi. Comparative genomic hybridization (CGH) microarray chip methods are used to look at changes in chromosomal and subchromosomal levels but need to be interpreted with care because polymorphisms not previously identified may be picked up (Tsai et al, 2009).

IMAGING STUDIES

Radiographs and other imaging studies are used to identify skeletal, CNS, cardiac, and other anomalies.

PHOTOGRAPHY

Photographs provide a visual record of facial and other anatomic variations. They may also be useful in identifying other family members with similar characteristics.

Management Strategies

Primary care management of children with genetic disorders includes a variety of strategies, depending on what diagnosis has been made.

■ Prenatal Screening and Diagnosis

Prenatal evaluations can be done for many diseases if the family history indicates the possibility of a specific disease appearing in offspring. Prenatal carrier tests of parents can be conducted if these parents are at risk to be carriers of gene

ALGORITHM

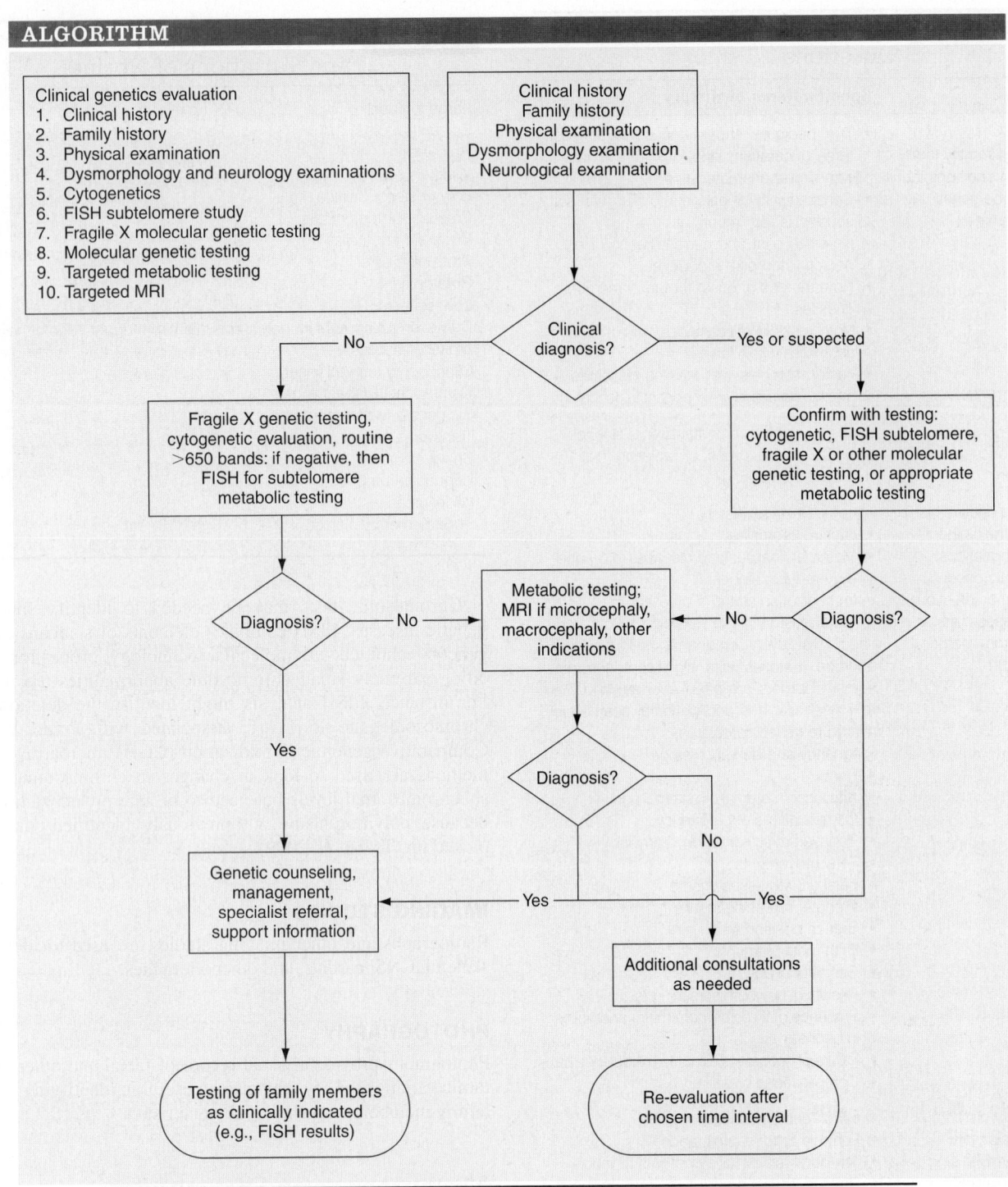

Clinical genetics evaluation
1. Clinical history
2. Family history
3. Physical examination
4. Dysmorphology and neurology examinations
5. Cytogenetics
6. FISH subtelomere study
7. Fragile X molecular genetic testing
8. Molecular genetic testing
9. Targeted metabolic testing
10. Targeted MRI

Clinical history
Family history
Physical examination
Dysmorphology examination
Neurological examination

Clinical diagnosis?

No → Fragile X genetic testing, cytogenetic evaluation, routine >650 bands: if negative, then FISH for subtelomere metabolic testing

Yes or suspected → Confirm with testing: cytogenetic, FISH subtelomere, fragile X or other molecular genetic testing, or appropriate metabolic testing

Diagnosis? → No → Metabolic testing; MRI if microcephaly, macrocephaly, other indications ← No ← Diagnosis?

Yes

Diagnosis?

Genetic counseling, management, specialist referral, support information ← Yes ← Yes

No

Additional consultations as needed

Testing of family members as clinically indicated (e.g., FISH results)

Re-evaluation after chosen time interval

FIGURE 40-5 Clinical genetic evaluation of the child with mental retardation or developmental delays. (From Moeschler JB, Shevell M, AAP Committee on Genetics: Clinical genetic evaluation of the child with mental retardation or developmental delays, *Pediatrics* 117:2304-2316, 2006.)

BOX 40-3 Indications for Karyotype Analysis

Suspected chromosomal problem
Two major malformations
One major and two minor malformations
Ambiguous genitalia
Congenital heart disease
Hypotonia

Malformed stillborns and normal stillborns when demise is of undetermined etiology
Mental retardation or developmental delay
Growth retardation or short stature
Couple with two or more miscarriages or infertility

mutations for sickle cell disease, Tay-Sachs disease, the thalassemias, cystic fibrosis, or other conditions based on the couple's family history. Childbearing women who screen positive for a genetic problem should be referred to obstetric or genetic clinics for prenatal genetic counseling, testing, and diagnosis. For diagnosis of some conditions, chorionic villus biopsy sampling may be performed at 8 to 12 weeks of gestation and amniocentesis in the second trimester. By the fourteenth to sixteenth week of gestation, many imaging studies can also be done to look for structural anomalies. A combination of tests including maternal serum alpha-fetoprotein, ultrasound, and maternal serum markers may be offered during the end of the first trimester and early weeks of the second trimester. Efficacy of prenatal testing options continues to be evaluated, and prenatal diagnostic centers may vary regarding screening procedures. These tests can identify fetuses likely to have chromosome abnormalities, neural tube defects and other prenatally identifiable disorders. Prenatal diagnosis gives the family information to make decisions regarding reproductive alternatives, such as possible termination of pregnancies with affected fetuses, artificial insemination, egg donor, deferral of childbearing, or special preparations at childbirth.

Newborn Genetic Screening

Newborn genetic screening for a variety of metabolic diseases is done routinely. As mentioned, different states include different groups of diseases in their panels. The provider should be sure that the routine newborn statewide screening panel blood test is completed correctly, and that infants who have a presumptive positive result on their screening test are promptly referred for further evaluation. The provider can help parents understand that a positive result from a screening test indicates that further testing is needed to determine if their child has the condition in question. Providers need to be aware of resources for appropriate care because infants affected by disorders detected by newborn screening usually require lifelong management.

Benefits of screening include detection of serious, treatable disease before symptoms are present, treatment to prevent serious problems including mental retardation and death, and detection of carriers of some genetic disorders. Risks include failure to identify children who have the condition, parental anxiety caused by false-positive tests, identification of misattributed paternity, or detection of conditions for which treatment is not effective (Kaye and Committee on Genetics, 2006).

Newborn Screening Fact Sheets are available from the American Academy of Pediatrics.

Genetic Disorder Diagnosis

Careful history taking and physical examinations of children help providers identify children with genetic diseases. Newborn infants with malformations or dysmorphic features should be evaluated. Children with two major, one major and two minor, or three minor anomalies with other indicators as noted in Box 40-3 should be referred for further genetic evaluation.

In the case of a stillbirth or neonatal death, the infant's features should be documented—preferably photographed. A karyotype on blood and establishment of a fibroblast culture are also important. Head and renal ultrasound should be done if no autopsy is performed.

Children and their families should be referred for diagnosis if a genetic disease is suspected. Establishing the correct diagnosis is important for the family and the provider. The recurrence risk, prognosis given the natural history of the condition, guide to appropriate laboratory testing, plan of treatment and management, and facilitation of family coping require knowledge of the nature of the disorder.

Telling new parents that their child may have a genetic disorder needs to happen as soon as possible—even if a diagnosis cannot be confirmed. It should be done in a quiet, comfortable place when both parents are present, by someone with credibility. When the diagnosis is made in a newborn, the infant should be present and referred to by name if possible. The discussion should include some positive points and the problems to be faced. Accurate, up-to-date information and sources of information, support organizations, clinical resources, and/or opportunities to contact other parents need to be given to the parents. The parents should have some uninterrupted time with their baby. A follow-up phone call should be planned to review the findings and information provided, answer questions, and assess the family's responses and needs after the information about their baby has settled in for them (Skotko et al, 2009). Genetic counseling is essential.

Genetic Counseling

Genetic counseling involves open communication with families who are at risk for, or who have a genetic disease. A nondirective approach is used to allow families to determine what decisions, especially regarding reproductive plans, are best for them. However, when management or ongoing surveillance is discussed for some conditions, (e.g., for familial cancers), the family may expect health care providers to be more directive regarding recommended screening or treatment options. Genetic counseling goals include helping the family to do the following:

- Understand the diagnosis, its course, and its management
- Appreciate the way heredity influences the disorder and the risks of recurrence and carrier status to specific family members
- Understand the alternatives available to reduce the risk of recurrence
- Choose the course of action that is appropriate in view of the risks, family ethics and values, and family goals
- Adjust as well as possible to the disorder, its prognosis, and the risks of recurrence

The process takes time and may require many visits. Generally genetic counseling is provided by specialists. Ethical genetic counseling takes into consideration the principles of beneficence (helping the patient and family) and nonmaleficence (do no harm).

The primary care provider's role in genetic counseling is to perform the following:

- Identify individuals at risk for genetic disorders
- Teach children and families about the genetic counseling process
- Initiate referrals with screening pedigrees, medical records, and appropriate histories and physical examinations
- Evaluate the family's understanding of genetic counseling and provide support as the family makes decisions based on genetic testing information
- Provide health care as indicated

All families with genetic diseases should receive genetic counseling. The extent of counseling needed, and the ongoing needs of the child and family determine when the primary care provider can manage the child and family and when referral to a genetic or specialty clinic is necessary.

Primary Health Care of Children With Genetic Disorders

Primary care and chronic disease management of children with genetic disorders need to be integrated. Health supervision, screening for complications, and management of the health of the child with the genetic condition are essential. The AAP has developed health supervision guidelines for children with Down syndrome that incorporate developmental, psychological, educational, and medical components (AAP Committee on Genetics, 2001a). Monitoring for high-risk conditions, including congenital heart disease, thyroid disorders, hearing loss, atlantoaxial subluxation, ophthalmic abnormalities, and growth and development, needs to be integrated into the plan for primary health care. There are similar guidelines for the care of children with neurofibromatosis type 1 (Hersh and AAP Committee on Genetics, 2008), Turner syndrome (Frias et al, 2003), achondroplasia (Trotter et al, 2005), sickle cell disease (AAP Committee on Genetics, 2002), Marfan syndrome (AAP, 1996b), Williams syndrome (AAP, 2001b), and fragile X syndrome (AAP Committee on Genetics, 1996a). (Key features for several genetic disorders are listed later in Table 40-5.) These guidelines illustrate the integration of monitoring for the physiologic, developmental, and psychological consequences that may occur (see Box 40-4).

Families with a child with a genetic condition or chronic disease face many challenges and stresses. Stresses can be emotional, social, and financial, and demand that families deal with bureaucracies in the health care delivery, education, and health insurance systems. The family's adjustment is a long-term process that requires monitoring and support with new information and resources as the child grows and changes. Some areas to include in planning care are as follows:

- Health education
  - Educate the family about the condition and its management, including family responsibilities.
  - Answer questions about health care services, and respect the confidentiality of the patient and parents so that information is not shared with insurance companies, employers, or other family members without the client's consent.
  - Assist the child and family to evaluate information they obtain from Internet, print, and other sources.
  - Provide children who have genetic conditions, within developmental limits, with health education and support to understand and manage their own care.
- Health care services
  - Provide primary care for health promotion and disease prevention services.
  - Monitor the child for growth, development, emergence of new disease manifestations, and complications.
  - Assess the child's developmental age, and recommend appropriate interventions.
  - Work with the family regarding long-term planning for the child's care, including attention to psychologic, developmental, social, and sexual factors.

- For conditions unresponsive to known medical therapies, help families with support for ongoing management, decision-making related to experimental treatments that may be offered, and assistance in deciding when residential care or withdrawal of supportive care might be considered.
  - Be an advocate for the family with schools, insurance companies, and others.
  - Support and monitor the care of children with inborn errors of metabolism who need treatment to decrease the offending substrate, increase a deficient substance, provide an enzymatic cofactor, or a combination of these.
- Resources
  - Know community resources for specific problems that the family may face.
  - Direct the family to financial resources or social services to be sure that necessary care is provided.
  - Direct the family to support groups and local resources.
  - Provide the family with written materials from disease-related organizations.
  - Refer to early intervention and other special educational programs as needed.
  - Direct the family to respite care services as needed.
- Family coping
  - Evaluate all family members, including siblings and grandparents, for their responses to the child with the diagnosed condition.
  - Support the family through the grief process.
  - Evaluate the parents' coping skills, family dynamics, and psychosocial responses.
  - Assess the adjustment of siblings.

Care needs to be especially vigilant during times of transition. Parents need a support person who will listen to their concerns, joys, and sorrows over time. The primary care provider can be that person.

Genetic Disorders

Various genetic disorders are described in this section. Information is summarized in Tables 40-4 and 40-5.

Chromosomal Disorders

As described earlier, chromosomal disorders are problems of chromosome number or structure. Thus with thousands of genes involved for a given chromosome, chromosomal disorders usually result in major, multisystem problems. Only the most common of the many chromosomal disorders are described here. Chorionic villus sampling or amniocytes is used for prenatal diagnosis of chromosomal disorders. FISH techniques are used for postnatal diagnosis.

CHANGES IN CHROMOSOME NUMBER

The trisomies are the most common chromosomal disorders involving a change in chromosome number; three copies of a chromosome are present instead of two. Trisomies usually result from a nondisjunction that occurs during meiosis or mitosis.

TABLE 40-4 Inheritance Patterns With Examples

Inheritance Pattern	Characteristics	Examples
Chromosomal Abnormalities		
Changes in number of chromosomes	Generally major anomalies and multisystem problems with the trisomies. Sex chromosome disorders cause sterility and changes in growth patterns. Other changes may be more subtle.	Trisomies 21, 18, 13 XXY (Klinefelter) XO (Turner)
Changes in structure of chromosomes	Changes may include deletions, duplications.	Cri du chat (46, XY, deletion [5p]), Cornelia de Lange (duplicated 3q segment), fragile X
Single-Gene Defects		
Autosomal dominant	Person with condition has parent with condition. Sexes equally affected. Normal offspring will have normal children.	Neurofibromatosis, osteogenesis imperfecta, achondroplasia, Huntington chorea, familial hypercholesterolemia
Autosomal recessive	Both parents heterozygous for trait. Sexes equally affected. Newborn screening may pick up these disorders. Family history usually negative except that siblings may be affected.	Cystic fibrosis, sickle cell, Tay-Sachs, phenylketonuria
X-linked recessive	Males have condition. Female carriers usually do not have condition unless they are homozygous for the abnormal gene.	Hemophilia, Duchenne muscular dystrophy, glucose-6-phosphate dehydrogenase deficiency
Multifactorial	Familial clustering. Sex difference in frequency. No clear biochemical or molecular defect Considerable variation in expression. Both genetic and environmental components are important.	Cardiac defects, cleft lip/palate, clubfoot, scoliosis, dislocated hip
Germline Mosaicism	Two or more cell lines with differing genotypes in an individual. Consider if parents seem normal but offspring has an autosomal dominant condition.	Achondroplastic siblings from normal-appearing parents
Uniparental Disomy	Proband has two copies of a chromosome from one parent and none from the other.	Prader-Willi, Angelman
Mitochondrial	Circular, double-stranded mitochondrial DNA defect, not in nuclear DNA.	Leber hereditary optic neuropathy, myoclonic epilepsy
DNA Disorder	Variable expression depends on how many mitochondria carry defect.	Kearns-Sayre syndrome

TRISOMY 21

Trisomy 21 (also called Down syndrome [DS]) occurs in 1.10 per 1000 live births (Morris and Alberman, 2009). There is a third chromosome 21 in most cases, although the syndrome can occur through a translocation of extra chromosome material attached to another chromosome, usually 14 or 21 (4% of cases) or through a mosaic pattern in which some cells have the extra chromosome but not all (2% of cases) (Cohen, 2009).

Clinical Findings

A person with trisomy 21 may not have all of the features that are found in this condition. Common characteristics include brachycephaly; hypotonia; hyperlaxity; oblique palpebral fissures; protruding tongue; flat nasal bridge; small ears; Brushfield spots on the iris; short, wide hands with palmar simian creases; epicanthal folds; wide gap between the first and second toes; growth retardation; and mental retardation. Complications may include cardiac anomalies (40% to 50%), ocular abnormalities (20%), myopia (70%), serous otitis media (60% to 80%), hearing loss (66% to 75%), thyroid disease including hypothyroidism (15%), gastrointestinal tract anomalies including duodenal stenosis and Hirschsprung disease (12%),

psychiatric disorders, delayed sexual development, and leukemia (close to 1%), among others (Korenberg, 2009). Renal and urinary tract anomalies occur commonly (Kupferman et al, 2009). Refractive errors, strabismus, nystagmus, and blepharitis are common but cataract and glaucoma are less common (Creavin and Brown, 2009). The likelihood that a person with DS will develop leukemia is 10- to 20-fold higher than in a non-DS child (Xavier et al, 2009). Musculoskeletal abnormalities, including reduced muscle strength, low bone density, and atlantoaxial instability, are also more common with DS (Hawli et al, 2009). Approximately 5% to 10% of children with DS develop autistic disorders (Cohen, 2009).

Screening

Ultrasonography and maternal serum screening are done to determine the likelihood that a fetus has DS. All pregnant women should be screened via first-trimester beta-human chorionic gonadotropin and an ultrasound examination for nuchal translucency. Those not screened in the first trimester should be screened with an alpha-fetoprotein, estriol, human chorionic gonadotropin, and inhibin-alpha determinations (American College of Obstetricians and Gynecologists

TABLE 40-5	Characteristics of Common Chromosomal Disorders
Chromosomal Disorder	**Principal Clinical Findings of the Diagnosis***
Down syndrome (trisomy 21)	Short stature, brachycephaly, small midface with upturned nose, hypoplastic frontal sinuses, speckled iris, epicanthal folds with palpebral fissures that slant down to midline, small mandible with resulting appearance of large tongue, myopia, small ears, lax joints (including atlantoaxial articulation), short broad hands and feet and digits, single palmar crease, clinodactyly, exaggerated space between great and second toes, developmental delays, hypotonia as infant, congenital heart disease At risk for leukemia, Alzheimer disease, hypothyroidism
Turner syndrome (XO)	Fetal edema—neonatal carpal or pedal edema (or both), short stature, sexual infantilism, low hairline, webbed neck, increased carrying angle of arms (cubitus valgus), wide-spaced nipples, horseshoe kidney At risk for bicuspid aortic valve, coarctation of aorta, problems with spatial relationships and visual problem-solving, hypertension Difficulties with arithmetic Social development often impaired secondary to not understanding nonverbal communications
Klinefelter syndrome (XXY)	Mean IQ in the normal range but may have ADHD or language-processing problems. Physical findings include decreased testicle size, long limbs, decreased muscle tone, fifth finger clinodactyly, tremor, gynecomastia. Postpubertal males will become infertile and exhibit hypogonadism.
Neurofibromatosis	At risk for pheochromocytoma, skeletal dysplasia, renovascular hypertension, mental retardation, scoliosis, compromised organs and neurologic system from neurofibroma invasion More than five café au lait spots greater than 5 mm, axillary freckles, Lisch nodules, neurofibromas, optic glioma, megalencephaly
Fragile X syndrome	Large ears, macro-orchidism, long narrow face, mental retardation, autistic behavior
Fetal alcohol syndrome	Growth deficiencies, decreased adipose tissue, mental retardation, infant irritability/child hyperactivity, poor coordination/hypotonia, microcephaly, short palpebral fissures, ptosis, retrognathia in infancy, maxillary hypoplasia, hypoplastic long or smooth philtrum, thin vermilion border of upper lip, short upturned nose, micrognathia in adolescence At risk for heart defects, myopia, small teeth with poor enamel, hypospadias, hydronephrosis, hernias

*Not all children will exhibit all findings.
ADHD, Attention-deficit/hyperactivity disorder.

[ACOG], 2007). Although prenatal screening has identified more children with DS and more pregnancies have been terminated, there are also more women having babies at later ages, so the prevalence of infants born with DS has changed by only 1% in the past 20 years (Morris and Alberman, 2009).

Management

Health care guidelines developed and revised by the AAP are summarized in Box 40-4. Early intervention begins in infancy and continues throughout childhood. Education in integrated classrooms in a neighborhood school has been shown to be successful (McKusick-Nathans Institute of Genetic Medicine, Johns Hopkins University and National Center for Biotechnology Information, National Library of Medicine, 2010). Many people with DS enter the workforce after high school and may live in group homes as adults. Immunizations are important because these children are more susceptible to infections. Cardiac care, hearing screening, growth monitoring, and prevention of overweight are important roles for providers. Thyroid screening; gastrointestinal care for disorders such as pyloric stenosis, duodenal atresia, Hirschsprung disease, or imperforate anus; atlantoaxial instability screening for those involved in sports; and awareness that leukemia may emerge as a problem are further issues that the provider should monitor (AAP Committee on Genetics, 2001a). Thyroid screening from 1 to 18 years has led to increased rates of thyroid disease management in these children (Carroll et al, 2008), but in some regions of the U.S.

only 14% of children are being screened (Ferguson et al, 2009) despite the fact that thyroid screening is part of the guidelines for care of children with DS (AAP, 2001a).

Long-Term Follow-Up

As teens enter early adulthood, their care needs to continue and transition to adult providers needs to occur. Atlantoaxial subluxation; hypothyroidism; cardiac findings such as mitral valve prolapse and aortic regurgitation; early dementia; adult-onset epilepsy; spinal stenosis; mental health problems such as depression, obsessive-compulsive disorder (OCD), abuse, and conduct disorder; cataracts; hearing loss; osteoporosis; and sleep apnea are more common in adults with DS and must be considered in assessing and planning for these patients (Wilson, 2010). Social-sexual education is also needed.

TRISOMY 18

Trisomy 18, or a third chromosome 18, occurs in 1 in 3500 live births (Tsai et al, 2009). It is the second most common autosomal chromosomal disorder. Features of trisomy 18 include mental and growth retardation, failure to thrive, rocker-bottom feet, prominent occiput, small features, short sternum, low-set malformed ears, hypoplasia of the nails, horseshoe kidneys, hernias, flexed and overlapping fingers, micrognathia, and other deformities. More than 50% of individuals with trisomy 18 have cardiac defects, and only about 5% survive the first

BOX 40-4 Primary Care Monitoring of Children With Common Genetic Disorders

This box highlights some of the specific monitoring that can be done by primary care providers. It does not serve as a comprehensive guide and assumes the following:

- General health supervision guidelines for all children will be followed as much as possible.
- Genetic counseling will be provided to all families.
- Family support and counseling services will be provided.
- Support groups that might be helpful will be identified for the family.
- Long-term planning will occur.
- Sexual and reproductive issues will be addressed when the child approaches adolescence, including information/referrals for both the child directly and the parents.
- School placement and ongoing educational evaluations will occur.
- Care will be coordinated with a clinic specializing in services for children with the specific condition.
- Developmental and behavioral issues will be addressed, with referrals as needed.
- Intrafamily relationships will be assessed.

Down Syndrome

- Cardiac echocardiography: At diagnosis and follow-up as needed if defects identified*
- Screen for mitral valve prolapse at adolescence.[†]
- Hearing: At 9 months (or sooner if concerns) and follow-up as needed* (50% to 70% have hearing loss). Review risks of serous otitis media (50% to 70%)
- Ophthalmologic: At 4 months (sooner if concerns), 12 months, 24 months, then every 2 years and follow-up as needed.* Check for strabismus, cataracts, nystagmus by 6 months
- Thyroid: Screen as newborn, 6 months, 12 months, then annually.
- Cervical spine for atlantoaxial instability at 3 to 5 years; Down clinic assessment at 4 months, 12 months, then annually to 6 years, then biannually[‡]
- Early intervention services for developmental delays and ongoing assistance with development of age-appropriate self-help skills, sense of responsibility socialization, speech, Supplemental Security Income referral[†‡]
- Use Down syndrome growth charts to evaluate shorter stature and increased weight[†] and manage obesity.
- Screen for hip dislocation through 10 years old.[†]
- Administer pneumococcal vaccine as well as all other vaccines recommended for children unless there are specific contraindications.
- Discuss symptoms related to obstructive sleep apnea.
- Encourage families to establish optimal dietary and physical activity routines to prevent obesity.
- Discuss skin problems because very dry skin and other skin problems are very common.

Neurofibromatosis[‡]

To be done at initial evaluation with follow-up as indicated:
- DNA analysis, phenotype review
- Growth, blood pressure, skin examination, bone/scoliosis, neurologic examination
- Hearing, vision, sexual maturation
- Psychosocial evaluation, development and behavioral, preschool and school placement

Turner Syndrome[§]

Cardiac evaluation at diagnosis:
- Evaluation by cardiologist with expertise in congenital heart disease
- Blood pressure in all four extremities, clear imaging of heart, aortic valve, aortic arch, pulmonary veins (echocardiography in infants and young girls or MRI and echo in older girls and adults), ECG

- Imaging every 10 years and before attempting pregnancy
- Treatment for girls with cardiac pathology

Screening at diagnosis:
- Renal ultrasound, hearing evaluation, kyphosis screening
- Evaluation for growth and pubertal development
  - Ages 0 to 4 years: Evaluate for hip dislocation, eye examination
  - Ages 4 to 10 years: Thyroid function tests, celiac screen, educational and psychosocial evaluations
  - Age older than 10 years: Thyroid function tests (T_4, TSH) and celiac screen (TTG Ab), educational and psychosocial evaluations, orthodontic evaluation, ovarian function/estrogen replacement, LFTs, FBG, lipids, CBC, Cr, BUN, BMD

Ongoing monitoring:
- Cardiac evaluations as indicated
- Blood pressure annually
- ENT and audiology every 1 to 5 years
- Less than 5 years: Social skills assessment at 4 to 5 years
- School age: Liver and thyroid screens annually, celiac screen every 2 to 5 years, educational and social progress annually, dental and orthodontics as needed
- Older girls and adults: Fasting lipids, blood sugar, liver and thyroid screens annually; celiac screen as indicated, age-appropriate evaluation for pubertal and psychosexual development

Klinefelter Syndrome[∫]

- Testosterone replacement around 12 years to maintain age-appropriate serum concentrations of testosterone, estradiol, FSH, LH
- Speech and behavioral evaluation and therapy to improve speech impairments, academic difficulties, and other psychosocial and behavioral problems
- Physical and occupational therapy for boys with hypotonia or delayed gross motor skills—occupational therapy is helpful for boys with motor dyspraxia.
- Treatment for infertility
- Genetic and reproductive counseling

Achondroplasia[¶]

- MRI of foramen magnum at diagnosis; if small, repeat at 3 to 6 months and similarly thereafter; if normal, repeat at 1 year
- Ultrasonography/CT or MRI of brain at diagnosis; repeat if head growth exceeds achondroplasia growth curves or if symptoms of increased intracranial pressure are present
- Physical therapy to focus on development of gross and fine motor skills
- Monitoring of upper airway restriction, obstructive sleep apnea, and potential for cor pulmonale
- Orthopedic evaluation if bowing of lower extremities progresses because of fibular overgrowth

Hemophilia and von Willebrand Disease[**]

- Developmental screen and neuro examination as follow-up to head trauma
- Adequate protein and calcium intake for bone formation
- Safety: Protective helmets and knee pads as needed
- ID bracelet with diagnosis, treatment product, blood type; remember to update annually
- Noncontact sports participation
- Regular dental hygiene care; may need clotting replacement products for dental extractions
- Annual screening for hematocrit and microscopic hematuria
- Hemophilia management through a regional hemophilia treatment center with copy of active bleed plan shared with primary care provider and family

Continued

BOX 40-4 Primary Care Monitoring of Children With Common Genetic Disorders—cont'd

Sickle Cell Disease[††]
- Penicillin prophylaxis and immunizations including pneumococcal
- Urgent evaluation and parenteral antibiotics for febrile illness >38.5 C
- Risks for bacterial infections, pain, acute chest syndrome, splenic sequestration, aplastic crisis, stroke, priapism
- Coordinate care with comprehensive sickle cell program and acute care facility access

- Baseline CBC and retic counts, blood typing
- Screen for proliferative retinopathy beginning at 10 years
- Follow specific health management guidelines per published recommendations with visits q 2-4 months in first year and then every 6 months to 1 year.

Ab, antibody; *BMD,* bone mineral density; *BUN,* blood urea nitrogen; *CBC,* complete blood count; *Cr,* creatinine; *CT,* computed tomography; *ECG,* electrocardiogram; *ENT,* ear, nose, throat; *FBG,* fasting blood glucose; *FSH,* follicle-stimulating hormone; *LFTs,* liver function tests; *LH,* luteinizing hormone; *MRI,* magnetic resonance imaging; *TSH,* thyroid-stimulating hormone; *TTG,* tissue transglutaminase

*American Academy of Pediatrics (AAP), Committee on Genetics: Health supervision for children with Down syndrome, *Pediatrics* 107:442-449, 2001. Reaffirmed 9/1/2007.
†Jackson Allen P, Vessey J, Shapiro N: *Primary care of the child with a chronic condition,* ed 5, St Louis, 2010, Mosby
‡§Hersh J, AAP Committee on Genetics: Health supervision guidelines for children with neurofibromatosis, *Pediatrics* 121(3):633-642, 2008.
§Bondy C: Care of girls and women with Turner syndrome: a guideline of the Turner Syndrome Study Group, *J Clin Endocrin Metab* 92(1):10-25, 2007.
∫Chen H: *Klinefelter syndrome: treatment and medication.* Available at emedicine.medscape.com/article/945649-treatment (accessed Dec 29, 2010).
¶Trotter TL, Hall JG, AAP Committee on Genetics: Health supervision for children with achondroplasia, *Pediatrics* 116:771, 2005.
**World Federation of Hemophilia, *Guidelines for Management of Hemophilia* (2005). Available at wfh.org/2/docs/Publications/Diagnosis_and_Treatment/Guidelines_Mng_Hemophilia.pdf. (accessed Nov 26, 2011).
††American Academy of Pediatrics, Section on Hematology/Oncology and Committee on Genetics: Health supervision for children with sickle cell disease. Reaffirmed on May 1, 2006. *Pediatrics* 109(3):526-535, 2002.

---

year of life. The potential for scoliosis, deafness, and central apnea needs to be monitored.

TRISOMY 13

Children with *trisomy 13* have problems so severe that 50% die in the first month of life and 95% die by 1 year old, usually from fatal heart anomalies. Characteristics include mental retardation, growth retardation, capillary hemangiomas, persistent fetal hemoglobin, microcephaly and brain malformations, cleft lip or cleft palate (or both), microophthalmia, colobomas, apparent deafness, cardiac septal defects, polycystic kidneys, polydactyly, omphalocele, and other features. The incidence is about 1 in 5000 live births (Tsai et al, 2009).

OTHER TRISOMIES

Generally, other trisomies are not compatible with life.

■ Sex Chromosome Disorders

Sex chromosome disorders involve changes in the number or structure of X or Y chromosomes. Turner syndrome and Klinefelter syndrome are examples of changes in number, and fragile X syndrome (discussed later in greater detail) involves change in a gene on the X chromosome leading to an apparent fragility of a portion of the chromosome.

TURNER SYNDROME

Turner syndrome (45, XO) is a disorder of girls in which one X chromosome is present instead of two.[2] The diagnosis is also used for girls who have the phenotypic features of the syndrome but have other structural abnormalities of the X

chromosome such as deletions of part of the long or short arm, a ring X chromosome, or isochromosomes. Five percent to 10% of women with Turner syndrome have some Y genetic material and are at increased risk for gonadoblastomas (Tsai et al, 2009). There can also be mosaicism with a 46,XY line and a 45,XO line (Loscalzo, 2008).

The incidence is 1 in 2500 girls. However, about 25% of chromosomally abnormal spontaneous abortions are XO.

Clinical Features

Girls with Turner syndrome have short stature and absence of ovarian function. Other features that may be present include a broad chest, webbed neck, cubitus valgus, congenital heart disease (30%), urinary tract anomalies (greater than 60%), and a low hairline. Some newborns do not exhibit any signs of the condition or they may have neck webbing from the cystic hygroma, shield chest, coarctation of the aorta, and edema of hands and feet. Many come to attention through the characteristic heart anomaly. Anomalies of the left outflow system of the heart are most common and need to be addressed throughout life. Girls may develop aortic dissection, abnormalities of the aortic valve, systemic hypertension, and coarctation of the aorta. This occurs in 75% of those with cardiac malformations (Morgan, 2007). Hyperopia and strabismus occur in 25% to 35% of patients (Loscalzo, 2008). Girls with Turner syndrome are at higher risk for learning disabilities but generally have normal intelligence.

Screening

Turner syndrome is increasingly being identified prenatally, via chorionic villus sampling or amniocentesis. Karyotyping takes 1 week; X-specific FISH screening can be done more quickly.

Management

Growth hormone, estrogen, and androgen therapies are important to help with both growth and development of female characteristics and normal height (Bondy, 2009; Denson, 2008). Cardiac care is essential (Loscalzo, 2008). Audiometry at diagnosis,

---

[2]46 XX and 46, XY are normal chromosome configurations. A notation of 45 XO means that there are 45 chromosomes, including one X chromosome but no second sex chromosome.

ultrasound to identify renal abnormalities, periodic testing for celiac disease, and scoliosis screening all need to be done. Type 2 diabetes, obesity, hypothyroidism, hypertension, scoliosis, and hearing and vision impairments occur with relative frequency in adulthood. Orthodontia may be needed. Girls with Turner syndrome will be infertile, but some may be able to successfully complete a pregnancy through assisted reproductive technology using a donor egg, although with considerable risk.

47,XXX can also occur. It is estimated that only 10% of these girls are identified during their lifetimes. They may have some difficulties with language-based learning, attention-deficit/hyperactivity disorder (ADHD), and behavioral difficulties (Tsai et al, 2009). Turner syndrome may cause psychological problems due to infertility, short stature, lack of development of sexual characteristics, and lack of libido (Morgan, 2007).

KLINEFELTER SYNDROME

Klinefelter syndrome (47,XXY) is the most common sex chromosome abnormality, occurring in 1 in 660 boys. Variations, including 48,XXXY and 49,XXXXY are more affected than those with 47,XXY. Less than 10% of affected males are diagnosed before adolescence when testes fail to enlarge (Bojesen and Gravholt, 2007) and up to 70% are never diagnosed throughout their life span (Tsai et al, 2009).

Clinical Features

Physical presentation includes decreased testicular size, long limbs, decreased muscle tone, fifth finger clinodactyly, tremor, gynecomastia, and decreased body hair. In postpubertal males, infertility and hypogonadism become more important features of the condition. Boys with Klinefelter syndrome are not feminine in behavior or sexual orientation and usually have normal sexual function. Although puberty begins normally, testicular failure progresses during adolescence, as evidenced by increased follicle-stimulating hormone (FSH) and luteinizing hormone (LH) and decreased testosterone levels. After early spermatogenesis, boys with Klinefelter syndrome always become sterile, although viable sperm can be found in 50% of males and successfully used with in vitro fertilization (Paduch et al, 2009; Wikstrom et al, 2006). Boys with Klinefelter syndrome may have language processing and learning disabilities associated with enlarged ventricle volumes and reduced cerebellar hemispheres (Itti et al, 2006).

Management

Early diagnosis and intervention can address the wide variability in potential physical, psychosocial, psychoeducational, and endocrine problems associated with Klinefelter syndrome (Bojesen et al, 2006a; Ishikawa et al, 2008; Simm and Zacharin, 2006). The longer the delay in diagnosis, the greater effect on long-term health and disability. Treatment with testosterone beginning in early to mid-adolescence normalizes mood, focus, confidence, and psychosexual development (Morris et al, 2009). In adulthood, boys with Klinefelter syndrome are at increased risk for autoimmune diseases, diabetes, leg ulcers, osteopenia, osteoporosis, and tumors of the breast and germ cells. Metabolic syndrome is more frequent, so obesity, hypertension, and hypercholesterolemia need to be addressed (Bojesen et al, 2006b). Cryopreservation can be used to preserve viable sperm in postpubescent boys who have not yet undergone apoptosis of the sperm and resulting sterility.

Depression and anxiety may be improved by mood stabilizers and testosterone supplementation (Patwardhan et al, 2000). The mean IQ is within the normal range (Boada et al, 2009) with magnetic resonance imaging (MRI) findings supporting ADHD and language processing problems (Giedd et al, 2007).

Other changes in the number of sex chromosomes such as 47,XYY may or may not have clinical implications. The most common feature of 47,XYY is tall stature which has an incidence of 1:1000 male births. There is an increased rate of developmental delays, ADHD, and autism spectrum disorders (10%) (Tsai et al, 2009).

CHANGES IN CHROMOSOME STRUCTURE

Structural chromosome defects are rearrangements of genetic material within and between chromosomes; they can be of several types (Tsai et al, 2009). First, *deletions* can occur in which a part of a chromosome is lost. Cri du chat syndrome involves loss of the 5p segment. Some deletions are called *microdeletions* because they can only be identified with high-quality studies. Prader-Willi syndrome is a condition in which a small segment of chromosome 15q11.2-q13 inherited from the father is missing. Children with Prader-Willi syndrome have mental retardation and obesity, with small hands and feet, among other characteristics. If the problem stems from the chromosome 15 inherited from the mother, Angelman syndrome occurs. Characteristics of this disorder include mental retardation, progressive hypotonia, microcephaly, seizures, ataxia, excessive laughter, and others that are very different from those of Prader-Willi syndrome (Proud and Elias, 2009). Prader-Willi and Angelman syndromes may also be caused by uniparental disomy as described previously. Prader-Willi children treated with growth hormone achieve greater height and improved body composition, motor function, and lipid profiles (Carrel et al, 2010).

Duchenne muscular dystrophy, Williams syndrome, and DiGeorge syndrome have been found to include some microdeletions.

Duplications of sections of chromosomes can occur, such as a duplication of the 3q segment resulting in a Cornelia de Lange–like syndrome. Unbalanced inversions, or the wrong order of genes, are not usually compatible with life. However, children with *translocations* in which genetic material is exchanged between nonhomologous pairs may survive. Some children with DS (3.3%) have a translocation rather than a duplication of chromosome 21.

Inversions, rings, insertions, and *isochromosomes* can also occur. Chromosomes can also have breakage and fragile sites such as in fragile X syndrome.

FRAGILE X SYNDROME

Fragile X syndrome is an X-linked disorder as a result of an *expansion repeat*. It is the most common inherited cause of mental retardation and is responsible for about 40% of cases of X-linked mental retardation (Fig. 40-6). It is also the most common single-gene disorder associated with autism. Fragile X occurs in both boys (1 in 4000) and girls (1 in 8000), but is more common in males. It is named for the fragile site on the long arm at Xq27.3. The specific site is identified

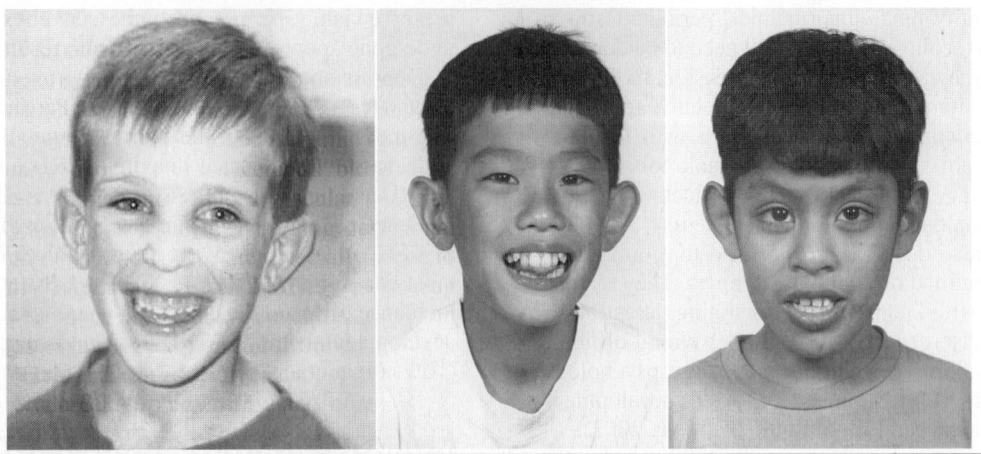

FIGURE 40-6 Children with fragile X syndrome. (From Jorde L, Carey J, Bamshad M: *Medical genetics*, ed 4, St Louis, 2010, Mosby.)

as *FMR-1*. The DNA of a normal person contains 10 to 60 copies of the CGG trinucleotide repeat in the region of the *FMR-1* gene. A small increase in the number of repeats to between 61 and 200 increases the instability of the area and is called a *premutation*. A man who carries the premutation is a phenotypically normal male and has normal intelligence, but passes the premutation to all of his daughters. If these daughters have sons, there is a likelihood of further increases in the number of repeats of the CGG/CGG sequence. When the number of repeats exceeds 200, a full mutation (called *symptomatic*) causes moderate to severe mental retardation. The increase in number of CGG repeats is called *repeat expansion* and may be associated with *anticipation,* a progressively earlier and more severe expression of a disease in more recent generations. It may take several generations of expansion in females to finally reach the symptomatic point.

Clinical Features

Males with the syndrome are likely to have a long face, large ears, prominent forehead and jaw, high-arched palate, macrocephaly, and single palmar crease. Macro-orchidism is significant in postpubescent males. Thirty percent have no dysmorphic physical features, so DNA testing should not be dependent on observed features of the disorder (Tsai et al, 2009). Mental retardation with an IQ in the range of 30 to 60 is common with the full mutation, although the problem may be milder in females (IQ of 70 or higher). About 15% of men exhibit ADHD and learning disability characteristics. Thirty percent of fragile X boys have autism (Tsai et al, 2009). Many boys with the premutation also have ADHD. Behavioral features are important and include hyperactivity, short attention span, perseveration of speech, hand flapping, hand biting, poor eye contact, excessive chewing on clothes, tactile defensiveness, mood instability, shyness, and social anxiety. Seizures occur in approximately 20% of individuals. Females with the syndrome show varying degrees of mental retardation.

Management

Children with fragile X syndrome and their families need follow-up for connective tissue dysplasias including pectus excavatum, scoliosis, flatfoot, and cardiac valve dysplasia;

multidisciplinary team assessment of developmental issues; treatment of behavioral problems such as autistic symptoms and ADHD; hearing and vision deficits; and genetic counseling (long-term depression and seizures can be controlled and decrease cognitive deficits). Some of the adults with premutation develop tremor and ataxia and women may experience premature ovarian failure or early menopause (Tsai et al, 2009).

■ Single-Gene Disorders

Single-gene disorders follow mendelian rules of inheritance. The online catalog, *Online Mendelian Inheritance in Man (OMIM)*, describes more than 17,000 entries (McKusick-Nathans Institute of Genetic Medicine, Johns Hopkins University and National Center for Biotechnology Information, National Library of Medicine, 2010). Inherited biochemical (metabolic) disorders are generally single-gene defects. The reported incidence of inborn errors of metabolism is thought to be 1% to 2% of live births, but this may be underreported because not all are apparent at birth.

AUTOSOMAL DOMINANT DISORDERS

Chromosome pairs 1 to 22 are the autosomes, and pair 23 consists of the sex chromosomes. In autosomal dominant disorders, a mutation in only one gene of a pair is needed for the problem to appear. The risk for recurrence is 50% if one parent has the gene mutation. Offspring who inherit the normal gene from the parent who has the gene mutation will not have the condition, nor would they be able to pass the mutated gene on to their children; males and females are equally likely to inherit the gene mutation. A Punnett square is used to diagram the inheritance risk for the genotype for each pregnancy and is shown in Figure 40-7, *A*. Often vertical transmission of the disease phenotype through several generations is identified by a family history, although wide variability in expression can occur. It is also possible that nonpenetrance can be observed in a family where there are several people with an autosomal dominant condition. This is illustrated when a grandparent and a grandchild have the same autosomal dominant disorder, yet the condition is not apparent in the parent who has inherited the gene mutation

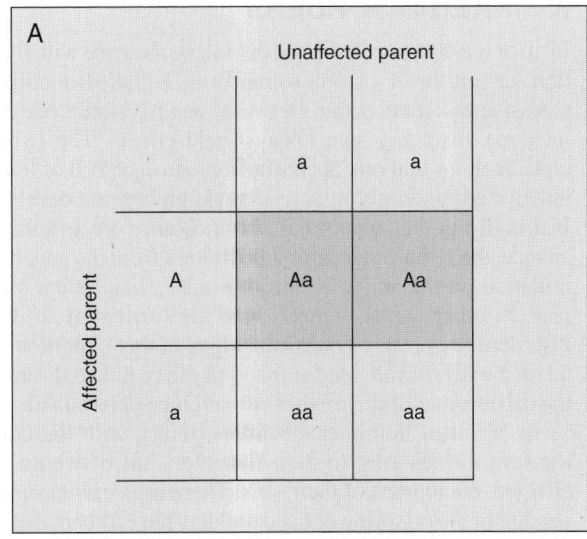

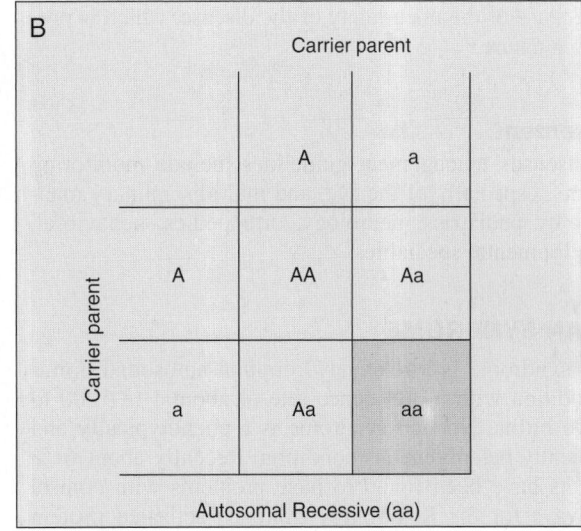

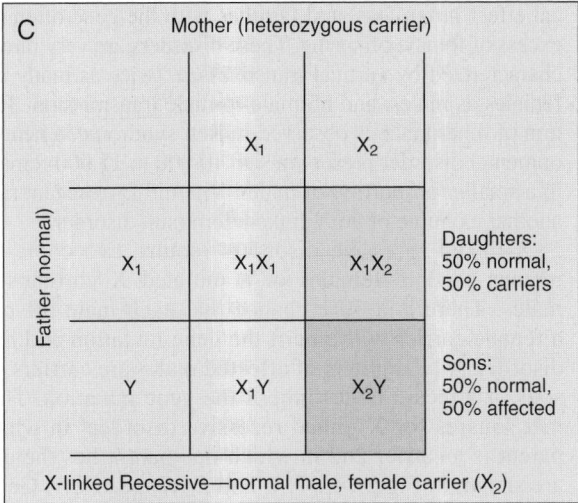

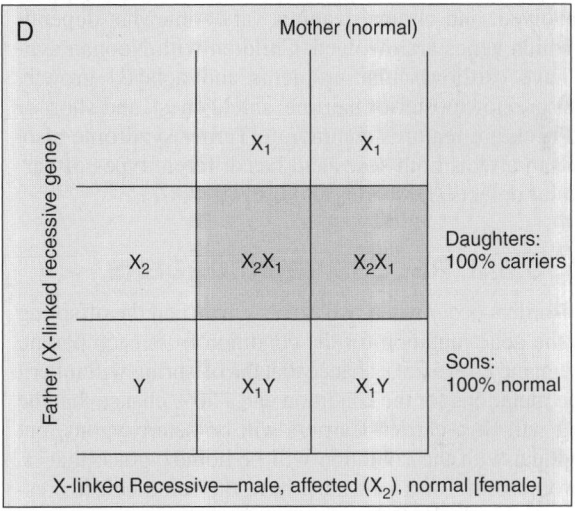

FIGURE 40-7 Punnett squares. (Adapted from Jorde L, Carey J, Bamshad M: *Medical genetics*, ed 4, St Louis, 2010, Mosby.)

and has passed it on to his or her child. Although it can appear that the gene mutation has "skipped a generation," this can be explained by the principle of nonpenetrance. If DNA testing is available for the condition, a DNA test would confirm that the parent has the gene mutation, even though there are no signs of the disease. This parent could pass the gene mutation on to other offspring. When there is no evidence of an autosomal dominant condition in either parent, the cause may be a new mutation in the child. Increased paternal age can be associated with the likelihood of a new mutation (Jorde et al, 2006). Neurofibromatosis, tuberous sclerosis (1 in 10,000 live births), achondroplasia (1 in 6000), Huntington chorea (1 in 20,000), osteogenesis imperfecta (1 in 10,000), and familial hypercholesterolemia (1 in 500) are examples of autosomal dominant disorders.

NEUROFIBROMATOSIS

Neurofibromatosis is one of the most common genetic disorders seen in children (1 in 3500 live births). About two thirds of affected individuals have only mild disease manifestations (café au lait spots and cutaneous neurofibromas).

Clinical Findings

Neurofibromatosis I is diagnosed if an individual has at least two of the following symptoms from National Institutes of Health (NIH) clinical guidelines (Hersh and AAP Committee on Genetics, 2008):

- Six or more café au lait spots greater than 5 mm in diameter
- Axillary or inguinal freckling (20% to 50% of cases)
- Lisch nodules on the iris in individuals more than 10 years of age
- Skin neurofibromas or a plexiform neurofibroma of the subcutaneous tissues
- A distinctive osseous lesion, such as sphenoid dysplasia or scoliosis
- Optic gliomas (15% of cases)
- Bony pseudarthrosis, especially of the tibia
- A first-degree relative diagnosed with neurofibromatosis or who meets the previously listed characteristics for diagnosis.

Children may have learning disabilities (50% of cases) or ADHD. Speech abnormalities may occur and need to be screened for periodically. Malignancies occur in less than 10% of cases (see Table 40-5). Psychological problems can occur because of the uncertainty of the disease, which is progressive in nature.

Management

NIH consensus management guidelines include monitoring for tumors, especially of the eye, and multidisciplinary management by pediatrics, neurology, orthopedics, behavioral, and developmental specialties.

NOONAN SYNDROME

Noonan syndrome is a relatively common autosomal dominant condition with a prevalence rate of about 1 in 1000 to 2000 live births. Noonan syndrome is a phenotypically and genotypically heterogeneous condition. Recently about 61% of patients have been found to have problems with control of pathways for the Ras/MAPK (mitogen-activated protein kinase) signal transduction pathway. Six main genes appear to be involved, and clinical features vary somewhat depending on which genes are involved. Children with Noonan syndrome have cardiovascular problems and delayed growth. Short stature, low posterior hairline, shield chest, and short or webbed neck are features common to Turner syndrome also, but Noonan affects both sexes and has different types of cardiovascular defects (Descartes and Carroll, 2007).

AUTOSOMAL RECESSIVE DISORDERS

These disorders occur when two carriers mate and the offspring inherits the gene mutation for the condition from each parent. Each pregnancy has a 25% chance that the offspring will inherit two gene mutations for the condition and a 50% chance that the offspring will be a carrier. Carriers will be heterozygous, but an individual with the condition will be homozygous; that is, both chromosomes of a pair must have the same defect present for expression. The Punnett square for autosomal recessive disorders is shown in Figure 40-7, *B*. Males and females are affected in equal numbers. The family history is usually negative, although siblings from the same parents may have the condition. Consanguinity increases the risk for autosomal recessive disorders, and fresh gene mutations are rare. The disease usually presents in infancy and often involves an enzyme deficiency or defect; these diseases may be severe. Prenatal diagnosis and carrier detection are often available. Ethnicity risk factors are most significant for autosomal recessive disorders (see Table 40-1). Uniparental disomy may also result in an autosomal recessive condition (see discussion earlier in this chapter).

Examples of these disorders include cystic fibrosis (1 in 2000 U.S. Caucasians), Tay-Sachs disease (1 in 3900 Ashkenazi Jews), Fanconi anemia (1 in 100,000 ethnic group), and sickle cell disease (1 in 400 African-Americans). Congenital adrenal hyperplasia, which may produce ambiguous genitalia in females and adrenal crises in males and females, is also autosomal recessive (Robin, 2007).

Newborn blood screening tests are used to identify children with some of these disorders. A metabolic disorder may need to be included in the differential diagnosis in any child with developmental delay or regression, seizures or other neurologic abnormalities, psychosis, failure to thrive, hypoglycemia, unusual odor, abnormal eating patterns, liver disease, or metabolic acidosis (see Chapter 25).

X-LINKED DISORDERS

In all of the 400-plus X-linked disorders, the gene with the mutation lies on the X chromosome. Both X-linked dominant and recessive disorders occur. Because men have only one X chromosome, disorders here always yield effects. The Lyon principle explains that one X chromosome in each cell of females is inactivated randomly in early female embryonic development. If a high number of normal chromosomes are inactivated by chance, the female can exhibit pathology from the gene with the mutation on the active X chromosomes, which then predominate. In other words, females who are carriers of an X-linked disorder may or may not exhibit signs of that condition. Prenatal diagnosis is available for many of the X-linked diseases, and the carrier state of the mother can often be determined.

In X-linked dominant disorders, males with the condition transmit the disorder to their daughters, all of whom will be affected, but to none of their sons. There is no carrier state. Fifty percent of the offspring of the daughters have a chance of receiving the gene with the mutation. X inactivation lessens the clinical effect in females, and families with the gene often have an excess of female offspring. These disorders are very rare but are characterized by vertical transmission, twice as many affected females as males, and no male-to-male transmission. This pattern of inheritance is observed in Rett syndrome, a neurodevelopmental disorder present in 1 in 10,000 to 15,000 females and in a smaller proportion of males. Vitamin D–resistant rickets is another example of an X-linked dominant disorder.

X-linked recessive disorders require two copies of the mutant gene in females or a mutated X chromosome in males. There is a 50% chance that each male offspring of a female carrier will inherit the gene mutation and have the disorder. All daughters of affected males are carriers, and no sons of affected males inherit the gene mutation. The Punnett squares for X-linked recessive disorders in which one parent is a carrier and in which one parent has the disorder are shown in Figure 40-7, *C* and *D*, respectively. Generally, females who are homozygous for the gene mutation will have the disorder; those in whom the majority of X chromosomes with the normal gene are inactivated may have milder signs of the condition. X-linked recessive disorders are characterized by much greater prevalence in males, lack of male-to-male transmission, and transmission through carrier females. Some of the X-linked recessive disorders include hemophilia A (1 in 5000 to 10,000 males), Duchenne muscular dystrophy (1 in 3500 males), and glucose-6-phosphate dehydrogenase deficiency (1 in 10 African-American males).

■ Multifactorial Conditions

Cleft lip and palate, congenital heart disease, and CHARGE syndrome are considered multifactorial genetic conditions. CHARGE syndrome is an acronym for *c*oloboma, *h*eart anomaly, choanal *a*tresia, *r*etardation, and *g*enital and *e*ar anomalies.

■ Other Conditions with Repeat Expansion

Expansions can occur at other sites on autosomes as well, causing problems such as myotonic dystrophy and Huntington disease.

■ Teratogens

A variety of drugs and diseases, as well as irradiation, can have significant effects on the developing fetus. Congenital infections include syphilis, rubella, and many others. Maternal PKU and diabetes can also affect fetuses. Fetal alcohol, fetal hydantoin, and fetal warfarin effects are described. Alcohol is the most common human teratogen. Some environmental toxins such as lead and mercury discussed in Chapter 41 can also be teratogenic.

FETAL ALCOHOL SPECTRUM DISORDER

Fetal alcohol spectrum disorder (FASD) is severe and occurs in approximately 0.3 to 1.5 per 1000 children or 40,000 children per year. Fetal alcohol syndrome (FAS) is the most severe. Other conditions that fall within the spectrum include partial fetal alcohol syndrome, alcohol-related neurodevelopmental disorder, and alcohol-related birth defects (Defendi, 2010). Alcohol-related neurodevelopmental disorder occurs at a higher rate, estimated to be at 1% of live births.

Etiology

There is no clear dose-related response relationship between the amount of alcohol consumed and the clinical features. Rather, certain maternal and fetal characteristics are key variables. Risks are greater for older mothers, those with high parity, those with compromised nutritional status, and of African-American or Native American descent. Binge drinking seems to be more harmful than consuming one drink per day.

Clinical Findings

Characteristics of FAS include intrauterine and postnatal growth retardation; CNS abnormalities including microcephaly, structural brain abnormalities, and other neurologic signs such as developmental delays, retardation, poor motor control, attention deficits, hyperactivity, and muscle weakness; and a specific facial dysmorphology with an underdeveloped philtrum, thin upper lip, flat midface, short or upturned nose, low nasal bridge, ear anomalies, short palpebral fissures, ptosis, micrognathia, and epicanthal folds (Fig. 40-8). The average IQ is 65 with a range from 20 to 120 (Jones, 2006). Many other anomalies have also been described, including scoliosis, clubfoot, renal and hepatic defects, cardiac defects, cleft lip and palate, ophthalmic abnormalities, hearing loss, and limb reduction.

Differential Diagnosis

Differential diagnoses include Williams syndrome, Noonan syndrome, Dubowitz syndrome, Bloom syndrome, Russell-Silver syndrome, fetal hydantoin syndrome, and maternal PKU fetal effects. Fragile X syndrome, Turner syndrome, and other syndromes may also have some similar physical, CNS, or behavioral features.

Management

Management includes evaluation of growth and nutrition, management of medical problems related to the birth defects, and identification of other medical issues. Educational evaluation

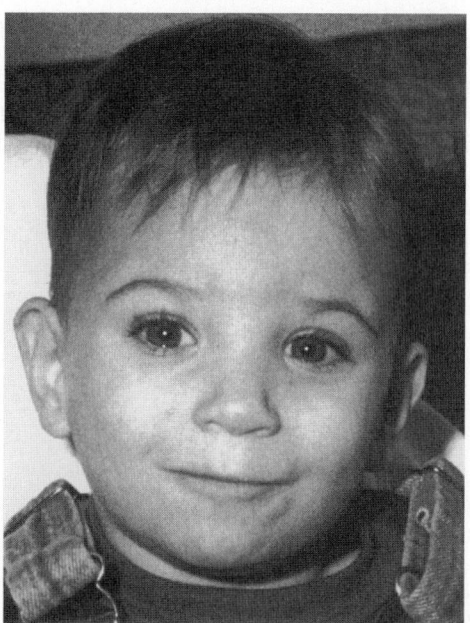

FIGURE 40-8 Child with fetal alcohol syndrome. (From Jorde L, Carey J, Bamshad M et al: *Medical genetics*, ed 3, St Louis, 2006, Mosby, p 321.)

and support with community resources can help the child reach his or her potential. Maternal and family help may be useful when children live in homes with continued alcohol use. Other siblings may also be diagnosed with one of the alcohol-related conditions. Abstinence from alcohol during pregnancy is the best prevention for the problem (Defendi, 2010).

Genetics and Cancer

Most cancers are a mixture of genetic and epigenetic changes, though some probably occur from genetic changes and some from epigenetic ones. Cells have the ability to recognize alterations in DNA and, in most instances, cells correct the change before it is passed on to subsequent cells through cell division. Cells' capacities to repair damage from gene mutations may diminish over time, leading to an accumulation of genetic changes, some of which can lead to disease (ACOG Committee on Genetics, 2007). Cancer is a genetic disease because alterations in the genetic material of somatic and/or germ cells can result in aberrant cellular growth.

Cancer genes are classified into three categories: (1) tumor suppressors, which inhibit cellular proliferation; (2) oncogenes, which activate cellular proliferation; and (3) defects in DNA repair, which lead to an increase in the number of somatic mutations. Errors in any of these areas result in abnormal cell growth. Epigenetic mechanisms can alter how cells grow and repair. Myelodysplastic syndrome is probably an epigenetic cancer. Studies are underway to see if the instructions to the genes can be reset to restore normal function (Issa, 2010). Genetic changes such as chromosomal instability associated with specific conditions also put the child at risk for certain cancers; for example, Down syndrome is associated with a risk of acute leukemia. Rhabdomyosarcoma, Ewing sarcoma, lymphoma, neuroblastoma, and other cancers are under study. In some cases the risk for cancer can be associated with cancer susceptibility mutations, which are passed from parent to child. Conducting a thorough family history can help providers identify which children may be at risk for a familial form of cancer (i.e., children from families in which several members have the same cancer diagnosis). For example, familial adenomatous polyposis is an example of an autosomal dominant subtype of colon cancer, and it is recommended that adolescents with this gene mutation have colonoscopies to detect the presence of polyps.

Environmental Health Issues

CATHERINE E. BURNS AND ARDYS M. DUNN

"All things are connected. Whatever befalls the earth befalls the children of the earth."

Chief Seattle, *The Soul of an Indian*

The environment is a basic determinant of human health and illness. It is estimated that 13% to 37% of the global burden of disease can be attributed to three major categories of environmental risk factors: water, sanitation, and hygiene; indoor air quality; and outdoor air quality (Prüss-Üstün et al, 2008). Children between birth and 14 years old bear nearly half the burden of disease in low- and middle-income countries (World Health Organization [WHO], 2008). Environmental factors are estimated to contribute to 100% of lead poisoning, 30% of asthma, 5% of cancers, and about 10% of neurobehavioral disorders. In a classic study based on these estimates, the *annual* cost of environment-related illness in children in the U.S. in 2002 was calculated to be $54.9 billion (Landrigan et al, 2002). Since then, individual states have estimated costs that are at least as high or higher.

Chemicals, natural as well as synthetic, constitute a large part of the environmental risk to health, contaminating water, soil, and air. Naturally-occurring elements like radon cause lung cancer. There is sufficient scientific evidence of a causal link between prenatal or childhood exposure to methyl mercury, polychlorinated biphenyls, polychlorinated dibenzofurans, active maternal smoking (during pregnancy), environmental tobacco smoke (ETS) (during childhood), and 2,3,7,8-tetrachlorodibenzo-p-dioxin and adverse health outcomes in children and adults (Wigle et al, 2008). Research indicates that chemical exposure of the father or mother prior to conception, at the time of conception, and (for the mother and fetus) during pregnancy results in a gene-environment interaction that accounts for most adverse developmental outcomes of pregnancy (Mattison, 2010). Concern has been raised that human exposure to genetically modified organisms (GMOs) and to hormones fed to animals may contribute to cancers, hepatorenal toxicity, and long-term reproductive problems (de Vendômois et al, 2009). In 2009 the U.S. Department of Health and Human Services (USDHHS) and the Centers for Disease Control and Prevention (CDC) released the Fourth National Report on Human Exposures to Environmental Chemicals, showing that almost all subjects studied had measurable levels of many industrial toxins in their blood and urine (USDHHS and CDC, 2009). Yet despite the known effects of many environmental agents and despite the presence of toxins in almost all humans, a great deal of uncertainty about the relationship between the environment and disease and illness remains. Many providers are at a loss when confronted with questions about environmental health, do not know how to best approach it, or feel overwhelmed by the volume and complexity of environmental health information. The challenge lies in several areas:

- Some providers may believe the effect of environmental agents is negligible, that lifestyle choices, genetic conditions, and/or infectious agents are responsible for most disease.
- There is not always definitive evidence that exposure to an environmental agent causes a particular disease. Is the condition being seen clinically caused by environmental exposure or something else?
- Exposure to some environmental agents may cause disease if there are preexisting or genetic conditions, or agents working together may cause problems (e.g., tobacco smoke and radon combined). It is often difficult for the provider to sort out the many variables.
- Research findings vary as to the type of problem caused by an environmental agent. What effect does an environmental agent have on the human body? Using the Multiple Exposure-Multiple Effects model (Briggs, 2003), some agents can cause several problems, and many different agents may cause the same problem (e.g., cancer). Sometimes the effect may be so subtle as to be missed: a decline in IQ scores after exposure to lead may still leave the child within the range of "normal" IQ.
- To what environmental agents has this individual been exposed? When? The health effect of an agent may be delayed for years and the exposure forgotten or unnoticed at the time it occurred (e.g., asbestosis, melanoma).
- Some providers may believe that correcting environmental health problems is beyond their purview. Exposure to disease-causing agents, they think, is a systemic not an individual issue, so beyond treating the illness, they may feel they can do nothing to help their patients or change the system.

Our sincere thanks to Marilee Dea, CPNP, Portland, OR, for her help with the reference search for this chapter.

- Providers feel inadequate to the task; they are not prepared well to manage environmental health concerns. Many providers state they lack knowledge and confidence in managing children's environmental health issues, failing, for example, to know about and use available resources (e.g., the Pediatric Environmental Health Specialty Unit [PEHSU] in their region) (Trasande et al, 2010). Nursing and medical schools do not devote sufficient time to teaching about environmental health, and continuing education may be limited.

To complicate matters, this uncertainty on the part of providers and in the field of pediatric environmental health is taking place in a social and economic context where profit, not concern for health, drives corporate development. Companies that produce chemicals or GMOs often conduct their own safety testing, and the results may not need to be made public. Approximately 83,000 chemicals are registered for use in the U.S.; however, less than half of these have any laboratory testing at all. Almost 3000 of these chemicals are produced in quantities of 120 tons or more annually and 80% of these have no information available about developmental or pediatric toxicity. Further, the information available almost never considers interactions among chemicals or genetic susceptibility (Grandjean and Landrigan, 2006). Though corporations state they do not intend to cause health problems with their products, examples of environmental contamination, advertising to vulnerable groups (e.g., cigarettes to adolescents), cover-ups of harmful findings (e.g., tobacco company assertion that nicotine is not a health risk), and regulatory violations occur frequently (Shrader-Frechette, 2007).

Regulation of chemical toxins is difficult. The Toxic Substances Control Act (TSCA) of 1976 authorizes the U.S. Environmental Protection Agency (EPA) to require testing and reporting of some chemicals and to restrict mixing of some toxic substances. However, the requirements of regulation are high: the EPA must demonstrate that the chemical in question represents an "unreasonable risk" to human health in order to ban its use. Also, many chemicals used in cosmetics, foods, drugs, and pesticides are exempt from the law (Duderstadt, 2009).

Because it is difficult to establish direct cause and effect in the area of environmental health, it would be prudent to adopt a precautionary approach to environmental toxins. Many European nations operate using the precautionary principle, which stipulates that chemicals should not be introduced into the environment until they have been proven to be safe. In the U.S., unfortunately, a "cost-benefit" approach is used, in which the burden of proof falls on regulatory agencies (e.g., the EPA) to show that the chemical represents an "unreasonable risk" to health. The cost of testing and regulating chemicals to ensure they are safe is balanced against the health problems those chemicals might cause, and, to date, U.S. industry has successfully been able to argue that it can be "too costly" to control pollution and restrict exposure for many chemicals (Schapiro, 2007). As a result, many people are unnecessarily exposed. Health care providers across the U.S. must advocate for use of the precautionary principle to control exposure to environmental toxins nationally and internationally.

The current situation is grim, but it is important to note that health care providers are increasingly aware of the problem, and many efforts are being made to address environmental health in pediatric practices. A network of regional PEHSUs has been created to provide information, clinical consultation, and support for pediatric providers (see www.aoec.org/PEHSU.htm). In 1999, the American Academy of Pediatrics (AAP) published a pediatric environmental health manual for providers (Etzel and Balk, 2003). Educators are developing curricula and preparing materials for students in health disciplines (Beitz and de Castro, 2010; Jamil et al, 2010); some are suggesting a medical specialty in environmental medicine (le Moal and Reis, 2011), and tools for assessment and management of environmental variables continue to be written (Cohen Hubal et al, 2010; Judson et al, 2008; Kavlock and Dix, 2010). New technology allows for more sophisticated assessment of how chemicals affect the human body, and intricacies of the environment-health relationship are better understood. Lack of strong evidence for a cause-effect relationship is not due to absence of an effect; rather, more research is needed to clearly establish the connections (Wigle et al, 2008). In 2000, the U.S. Congress authorized the National Children's Study to investigate the root causes of many childhood and adult diseases. It is proposed that 100,000 children be followed from before conception until 21 years old, examining environmental influences on health, including diet, ambient air, and home and school environments as well as interactions with various genetic traits. As of 2010, 37 regional participation sites had been identified; the challenge is to develop a recruitment plan, assessment tools, and protocols to coordinate, administer, and conduct the research (Savitz and Ness, 2010).

Health care providers need to be able to give their clients the most accurate information available about environmental health issues. Parents may suspect that an illness is associated with environmental conditions, or express concern about the risk of exposure to untested substances. The provider who is knowledgeable about the potential hazards of environmental exposure will be able to explain the possible connections, collect clear assessment data, and work closely with families to make appropriate treatment choices, including referral and consultation with public health authorities. If not personally knowledgeable, the provider should know where to get information. A core competency for all nurse practitioners (NPs) states that the NP "recognizes environmental health problems affecting patients and provides health protection interventions that promote healthy environments for individuals, families, and communities" (USDHHS, 2002). This chapter is designed to help prepare providers to meet this competency. In addition to direct patient care and education, primary health care providers can collaborate with other health care providers, conduct research to identify environmental problems, and advocate in the public arena (e.g., industry, policy, funding, and regulation) for more responsible management of environmental agents that affect health.

■ Principles for Understanding Children's Environmental Health

CHILDREN'S INCREASED RISK FOR ENVIRONMENT-RELATED ILLNESS

Children, because of their developmental immaturity, rapid growth, size, and behavior, are particularly susceptible to environmental threats (Table 41-1). Exposure to toxins or other harmful substances affects growth and damages organs

TABLE 41-1	Environmental Risk Factors for Children at Different Stages of Development			
Developmental Stage	**Developmental Characteristics**	**Exposure Pathways (Physical Environment)**	**Biologic Vulnerabilities**	**Appropriate Responses in the Social Environment**
Preconception	Maternal and paternal health status	Maternal/paternal reproductive organs may be compromised. Maternal stores of toxicants in bones and fatty tissue can be mobilized during pregnancy.	Problems with fertilization, implantation of ovum Damage to ovum or sperm	Research and education regarding long-term effects of environmental contaminants on reproductive system and subsequent offspring
Prenatal	Fetal development dependent on maternal health status and environmental exposure	Maternal blood supply via placenta Radiation Noise Heat	Tissue differentiation Rapid cell division and growth Organ development Metabolic pathways incomplete	Prenatal education, programs, and regulations regarding: • Alcohol • Cigarettes • Drugs • Metals
Newborn (0-2 months)	Nonambulatory Restricted environment High calorie, water intake High air intake Highly permeable skin Alkaline gastric secretions (low gastric acidity)	Food: breast milk, infant formula Dyes in clothing Soaps and shampoos Indoor air Tap/well water in home	Brain: cell migration, neuron myelination, creation of neural synapses Lungs: developing alveoli, rapid air exchange, narrow airways Bones: rapid growth and hardening Other organs: rapid growth Poor enzyme detoxification	Newborn-sensitive programs and regulations regarding: • Polychlorinated biphenyls (PCBs) • Lead in drinking water and dust particles • Environmental tobacco smoke Educate parents and policy makers concerning environmental hazards
Infant/toddler (2 months-2 years)	Beginning to walk Oral exploration (mouthing) Restricted environment and near floors Increased time away from parents Minimal variation in diet: high intake of fruits, vegetables, and milk products per body weight	Food: baby food, food additives, milk and milk products Air indoor layer effects: air near floor contains more toxicants Tap/well water in home and daycare Surfaces: rugs, floors, lawns, playgrounds	Brain: creation of synapses Lungs: developing alveoli, rapid air exchange, narrow airways	Child-sensitive programs and regulations regarding: • Radon in the home • Residential pesticide use • Lead abatement • Environmental tobacco smoke Educate parents and policy makers concerning environmental hazards
School-age child (6-12 years)	Beginning school Playground activities Increased involvement in group activities	Food at home and school Air: school, outdoor Water: school water fountains, tap/well water, swimming areas Playgrounds: wood preservatives, pesticides, and fertilizers Other: arts and crafts supplies, personal electronic equipment	Brain: specific synapse formation, dendritic trimming Lung: volume expansion Metabolic enzymes more active than in younger child	Child-sensitive programs and regulations regarding: • Asbestos abatement • Lead in school drinking water • Hazards in arts and crafts materials • Environmental tobacco smoke Educate parents and policymakers concerning environmental hazards
Adolescent (12-18 years)	Development of abstract thinking Puberty Growth spurt Increased adherence to peer norms	Food Air Water Personal electronic equipment Other occupation Self-determination: smoking, inhalations	Brain: continued synapse formation Lung: volume expansion Gonad maturation: ova and sperm maturation Breast development Bone growth and calcification Muscle growth	Adolescent-sensitive programs and regulations regarding child labor and other issues, especially environmental tobacco smoke Educate parents and policymakers concerning environmental hazards

Adapted from Gitterman BA, Bearer CF: A developmental approach to pediatric environmental health, *Pediatr Clin North Am* 48(5):1071-1083, 2001.

or body systems during critical developmental periods or *windows of vulnerability,* prenatally and during childhood. It is known, for instance, that a 50-mg dose of thalidomide, administered during the 26th day of gestation will likely result in major malformations to an embryo but that same dose taken at the 10th week of gestation will have no effects (Brent, 2004). Toxicants that cross the placenta (e.g., drugs, carbon monoxide [CO], mercury, lead, and cotinine [from environmental tobacco smoke]) can contribute to low birth-weight, spontaneous abortion, intrauterine growth retardation, increased risk of cancer, poor cognitive and behavioral development, and birth defects. Approximately 3% of all babies born in the U.S. have a serious birth defect. The rate of some birth defects is increasing (Brent, 2004), and about 10% appear to be related to environmental exposure (Chervenak et al, 2010).

Children's rapidly growing tissues more readily absorb environmental toxins; the lungs, skin, and gastrointestinal (GI) tract of newborns are highly permeable and gastric pH is high, facilitating absorption. At the same time, newborns' immature organ systems more slowly metabolize drugs, making it more difficult for infants to detoxify and excrete harmful substances. Children consume more fresh fruit, water, milk, and juice per pound of body weight than adults; many of these products are treated with pesticides or other chemicals. Children engage in more outdoor activities than adults, breathe more pollutants per pound of body weight, and are physically closer to many potentially harmful substances. Crawling on floors, chewing on objects, and running and rolling in grass are behaviors that expose children to environmental toxins and can result in lead poisoning, pesticide poisoning, and respiratory problems, including asthma. Adolescents are particularly susceptible to environmental tobacco smoke and occupational hazards. Children living in poorer communities are at higher risk than others. Poor housing and nutrition, high levels of lead, toxic waste deposits, and limited access to health screening and treatment contribute to increased risk.

In addition to the immediate risk during childhood, children have a longer time span for exposure to environmental toxins, and with some conditions children are more likely to suffer health problems than adults exposed to the same substance.

UNDERSTANDING ENVIRONMENTAL HEALTH HAZARDS

As noted, a direct cause-effect relationship between health and the environment may be impossible to determine because (1) the extent of exposure may be unclear; (2) there can be a long latency period between exposure and appearance of illness; (3) an individual may have exposure to multiple confounding agents; (4) exposure may need to occur during a "window of vulnerability" (e.g., during the period when a particular body system is forming prenatally) for the agent to have an effect; (5) some individuals may have a genetic susceptibility to an exposure, whereas others do not; and (6) much research in environmental health has been short term, or conducted on animals, so results may not translate to human development. Using principles of epidemiologic relationships and toxicology, however, providers can better understand and explain to their patients the relationship between environment and health.

EPIDEMIOLOGIC MODEL: RISK ASSESSMENT APPROACH

A first step in an epidemiologic approach (Fig. 41-1) identifies the interactive factors in the environment, including *receptors* (i.e., hosts or living things that are susceptible or exposed to environmental agents); *toxins,* or harmful substances that might cause damage (i.e., the agent); and the environmental *medium,* or route by which exposure could occur (e.g., air, water, or food).

A second step of risk assessment using an epidemiologic model is to determine the possibility that harm could occur. A number of questions are asked when making this determination:

- How *susceptible* is the receptor to the agent (e.g., age, sex, genetics, diet, and general health)?
- At what quantity (i.e., dose) will the agent present a problem or cause a response in this receptor? This amount is called the *applied action* or dose-response level. For some agents, *any* exposure represents a risk.
- What is the concentration of the toxic agent? How much is there? How strong is it? How long will it stay around? What is the extent of contact of the toxic agent with the receptor?

A final step in this process compares the actual environmental condition with the applied action level, asking the following question: With the amount of exposure present, is the individual at risk for health problems?

TOXICOLOGIC PRINCIPLES

Toxicologic principles are those the primary care provider has learned related to pharmacologic therapy: exposure, absorption, distribution, metabolism, tissue sensitivity, and effects—therapeutic or toxic. In fact, Paracelsus (1493-1541), considered the "father of toxicology," is reputed to have said, "All substances are poisons; there is none that is not a poison. The right dose differentiates a poison from a remedy."

Exposure

Contact of a biologic, chemical, or physical agent with the outer boundary of an organism (e.g., skin, lungs, GI tract) constitutes exposure. The extent to which exposure creates a problem is an epidemiologic issue and depends on factors such as frequency and duration of exposure, concentration of the agent at the point of contact, and the susceptibility of the organism (e.g., an infant's skin burns much more easily than an adult's).

Absorption

Absorption is the process by which an agent is taken into the organism. It occurs in the skin, mucous membranes, lungs, or GI tract. Absorption involves active or passive transport (e.g., lipid-soluble chemicals such as polychlorinated biphenyls [PCBs] are passively absorbed through the gut and stored in fat; lead is taken up through active transport in the GI tract and stored in bone or other tissues).

Distribution

Toxic agents are distributed throughout the organism via the blood or lymph systems. The ability of an agent to cross the blood-brain barrier, the amount of blood flow to an organ, and

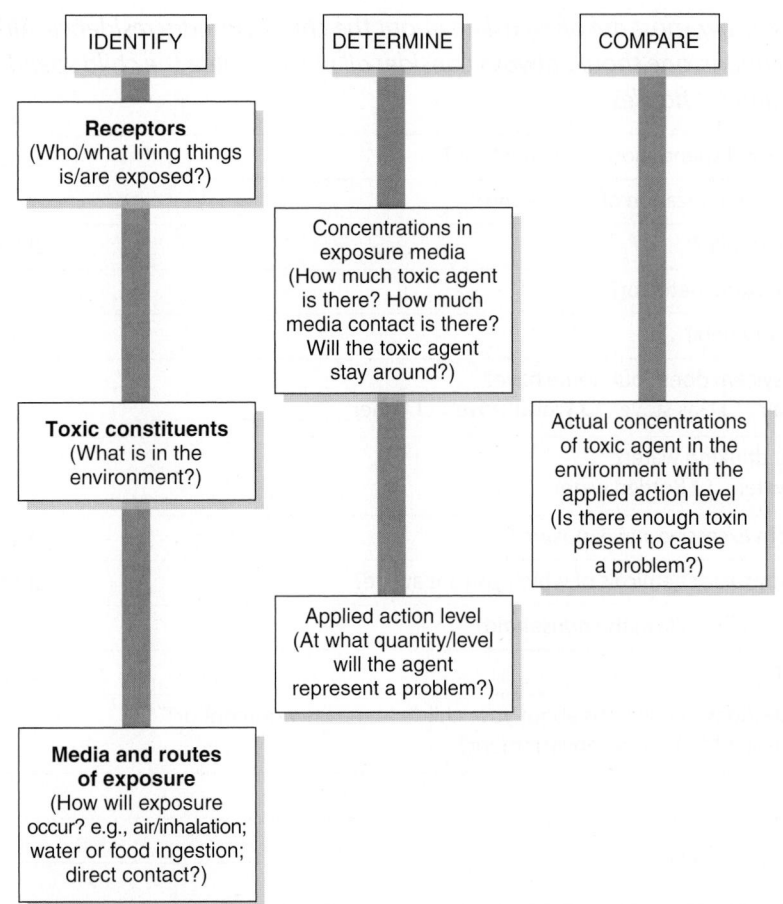

FIGURE 41-1 Risk assessment of environmental hazards. (Adapted from Oregon Poison Center and Health Division, Oregon Department of Human Resources: *Environmental hazards in perspective: seminar syllabus and environmental health resource notebook,* Portland, 1994, Oregon Department of Human Resources.)

the affinity of tissues to take up a particular agent (e.g., lipid-soluble chemicals are found in fatty tissues) all influence the degree to which a toxicant will be distributed throughout the body.

Metabolism

Metabolic enzymes in the body interact with toxic agents in several ways: (1) oxidation, reduction, and hydrolysis of the agent—the agent can be detoxified, but chemicals can also be activated and made more toxic; and (2) conjugation and breakdown to promote elimination, usually through the kidney. Metabolism is influenced by the individual's age, sex, nutritional status, genetic makeup, presence of other drugs, and disease or illness.

Tissue Sensitivity

Susceptibility and reaction of tissue to a particular agent can vary. The thalidomide example illustrates increased tissue susceptibility during a critical point of gestation.

Toxic Effects

Toxic effects vary by agent, dose, and organ or system affected. They include a wide range of pathologic conditions. Prenatal exposures can result in sterility, infertility, miscarriage, stillbirth, congenital malformations, fetal growth retardation, prematurity, and chronic illnesses. Paradoxically, for some environmental toxins, such as endocrine disruptors, small doses may have deleterious effects, whereas large doses do not; the larger doses simply kill the exposed cells rather than being used by the cells in an abnormal fashion.

■ Primary Care Approach to Children's Environmental Health

ASSESSMENT

Assessment of environmental health hazards should be integrated into regular health appraisals, as well as examinations of ill children. Figures 41-2, 41-3, and 41-4 list essential questions to ask for an environmental history, including questions related to asthma.

Physical Examination

The physical examination should cover all body systems thoroughly. Evaluate agent-specific findings (e.g., burns caused by chemicals and neurotoxicity caused by mercury), but also look for subtle, nonspecific signs and symptoms (e.g., skin rashes and headaches). The effects of toxicants on the body can be subclinical in many cases, and effects can occur long after exposure.

For all of the questions below, most are often asked about the child's primary residence. Although some questions may specify certain locations, one should always consider all places where the child spends time, such as daycare centers, schools, and relative's houses.

Where does your child live and spend most of his/her time?	_____
What are the age, condition, and location of your home?	_____
Does anyone in the family smoke?	❏ Yes ❏ No ❏ Not sure
Do you have a carbon monoxide detector?	❏ Yes ❏ No ❏ Not sure
Do you have any indoor furry pets?	❏ Yes ❏ No ❏ Not sure
What type of heating/air system does your home have? ❏ Radiator ❏ Forced air ❏ Gas stove ❏ Wood stove ❏ Other_____	
What is the source of your drinking water? ❏ Well water ❏ City water ❏ Bottled water	
Is your child protected from excessive sun exposure?	❏ Yes ❏ No ❏ Not sure
Is your child exposed to any toxic chemicals of which you are aware?	❏ Yes ❏ No ❏ Not sure
What are the occupations of all adults in the household?	_____
Have you tested your home for radon?	❏ Yes ❏ No ❏ Not sure
Do you have any other questions or concerns about your child's home environment or symptoms that may be a result of his or her environment?	_____

Follow up/ Notes

_____

_____

_____

This screening environmental history is designed to capture most of the common environmental exposures to children. The screening history can be administered regularly during well-child exams as well as to assess whether an environmental exposure plays a role in a child's symptoms. If a positive response is given to one or more of the screening questions, the primary care provider can consider asking further questions on the topic provided in the Additional Categories and Questions to Supplement the Screening Environmental History.

The Screening Environmental History is taken in part from the following sources:

■ Etzel RA, Balk SJ, ed: *Pediatric Environmental Health*, 2nd ed: How to take an environmental history, Elk Grove Village, IL, 2003, American Academy of Pediatrics.

■ Balk SJ: The environmental history: asking the right questions. *Contemp Pediatr* 13:19-36, 1996.

■ Frank A, Balk S, Carter W et al: Case studies in environmental medicine: Taking an exposure history, Atlanta, GA, 2000, Agency for Toxic Substances and Disease Registry.

FIGURE 41-2 Pediatric environmental history (0 to 18 years of age): The screening environmental history. Used with permission of the National Environmental Education Foundation, Washington, DC. Available at www.neefusa.org/pdf/PedEnvHistoryScreening/pdf (accessed Apr 4, 2011).

Diagnostic Studies

Laboratory studies can be performed on patients as indicated, based on signs and symptoms. Agent-specific laboratory studies, if available and reliable, can be helpful in determining treatment plans. However, few tests are appropriate for use in primary care settings because of the following limitations:

• For most toxins, valid and reliable tests have not been developed.

• For those toxins that do have tests, not all laboratories are capable of performing them. The provider should consult with individual laboratories regarding their capabilities.

• Many tests show a wide range of reference levels at which "toxicity" appears.

• There may be little correlation between exposure and levels present in the body at the time the test is done. Levels may have returned to normal, despite damage done to the body; or a one-time sample can reflect recent active exposure, but not measure the total body burden of the contaminant.

Some available tests include the following:

• Plasma lead levels

• Gas-liquid chromatography (for PCBs)

• Atomic absorption spectrometry (for mercury)

• Carboxyhemoglobin (for CO poisoning)

For all of the questions below, most are often asked about the child's primary residence. Although some questions may specify certain locations, one should always consider all places where the child spends time, such as daycare centers, schools, and relative's houses.

General Housing Characteristics (For lead poisoning, see Fig. 41-2, Management recommendations for lead poisoning)

Do you own or rent your home?	_____
What year was your home built? (Or: Was your home built before 1978? 1950?)	_____
Has your child been tested for lead?	❏ Yes ❏ No ❏ Not sure
Is there a family member or playmate with an elevated blood lead level?	❏ Yes ❏ No ❏ Not sure
Does your child spend significant time at another location? (e.g., baby sitters, school, daycare?)	_____

Indoor home environment (For asthma, refer to *Environmental History Form for Pediatric Asthma Patient*)

If a family member smokes, does this person want to quit smoking?	❏ Yes ❏ No ❏ Not sure
Is your child exposed to smoke at the baby sitters, school, or daycare center?	❏ Yes ❏ No ❏ Not sure
Do regular visitors to your home smoke?	❏ Yes ❏ No ❏ Not sure
Have there been renovations or new carpet or furniture in the home during the past year?	❏ Yes ❏ No ❏ Not sure
Does your home have carpet?	❏ Yes ❏ No ❏ Not sure
Is the room where your child sleeps carpeted?	❏ Yes ❏ No ❏ Not sure
Do you use a wood stove or fire place?	❏ Yes ❏ No ❏ Not sure
Have you had water damage, leaks, or a flood in your home?	❏ Yes ❏ No ❏ Not sure
Do you see cockroaches in your home daily or weekly?	❏ Yes ❏ No ❏ Not sure
Do you see rats and/or mice in your home weekly?	❏ Yes ❏ No ❏ Not sure
Do you have smoke detectors in your home?	❏ Yes ❏ No ❏ Not sure

Air Pollution/Outdoor Environment (For asthma, refer to *Environmental History Form for Pediatric Asthma Patient*)

Is your home near an industrial site, hazardous waste site, or landfill?	❏ Yes ❏ No ❏ Not sure
Is your home near major highways or other high traffic roads?	❏ Yes ❏ No ❏ Not sure
Are you aware of Air Quality Alerts in your community?	❏ Yes ❏ No ❏ Not sure
Do you change your child's activity when an Air Quality Alert is issued?	❏ Yes ❏ No ❏ Not sure
Do you live on or near a farm where pesticides are used frequently?	❏ Yes ❏ No ❏ Not sure

Food and Water Contamination

If you use well water for drinking, when was the last time the water was tested?
Coliform bacteria_____ Other microbials_____ Nitrites/nitrates_____ Arsenic_____ Pesticides_____

For all types of water sources:

Have you tested your water for lead?	❏ Yes ❏ No ❏ Not sure
Do you mix infant formula with tap water?	❏ Yes ❏ No ❏ Not sure

Which types of seafood do you normally eat?	_____
How many times per month do you eat that particular fish or shellfish?	_____

How many times a week do you eat any of the following types of fish?
Shark_____ Swordfish_____ Tile fish_____ King mackerel_____ Albacore tuna_____ Other_____

How often do you wash fruits and vegetables before giving them to your child? _____

What type of produce do you buy? ❏ Organic ❏ Local ❏ Grocery store ❏ Other

FIGURE 41-3 Pediatric environmental history (0 to 18 years of age): additional categories and questions to supplement the screening environment history. (Used with permission of the National Environmental Education Foundation, Washington, DC. Available at www.neefusa.org/pdf/PEHIhistory.pdf. Accessed April 4, 2011.)

Continued

Toxic Chemical Exposures			
Consider this set of questions for patients with seizures, frequent headaches, or other unusual or chronic symptoms			
How often are pesticides applied inside your home?			_____
How often are pesticides applied outside your home?			_____
Where do you store chemicals/pesticides?			_____
Do you often use solvents or other cleaning or disinfectant chemicals?			_____
Do you have a deck or play structure made from pressure treated wood?	❏ Yes	❏ No	❏ Not sure
Have you applied a sealant to the wood in the past year?	❏ Yes	❏ No	❏ Not sure
What do you use to prevent mosquito bites to your children?			_____
How often do you apply that product?			_____

Occupations and Hobbies			
What type of work does your child/teenager do?			_____
Do any adults work around toxic chemicals?	❏ Yes	❏ No	❏ Not sure
If so, do they shower and change clothes before returning home from work?	❏ Yes	❏ No	❏ Not sure
Does the child or any family member have arts, crafts, ceramics, stained glass work or similar hobbies?	❏ Yes	❏ No	❏ Not sure

Health Related Questions			
Have you ever relocated due to concerns about an environmental exposure?	❏ Yes	❏ No	❏ Not sure
Do symptoms seem to occur at the same time of day?	❏ Yes	❏ No	❏ Not sure
Do symptoms seem to occur after being at the same place every day?	❏ Yes	❏ No	❏ Not sure
Do symptoms seem to occur during a certain season?	❏ Yes	❏ No	❏ Not sure
Are family members/neighbors/co-workers experiencing similar symptoms?	❏ Yes	❏ No	❏ Not sure
Are there environmental concerns in your neighborhood, child's school, or day care?	❏ Yes	❏ No	❏ Not sure

Has any family member had a diagnosis of any of the following?
❏ Asthma ❏ Autism ❏ Cancer ❏ Learning disability

Does your child suffer from any of the following recurrent symptoms?
❏ Cough ❏ Headaches ❏ Fatigue ❏ Unexplained pain_____

FIGURE 41-3, cont'd Pediatric environmental history.

- Twenty-four-hour urine (for heavy metals)
- Urinary cotinine assays (for tobacco metabolites)
- Plasma cholinesterase (ChE) levels (for pesticide metabolites, organophosphates)

MANAGEMENT OF ENVIRONMENTAL CONDITIONS

Management of illness related to environmental factors uses a public health model of primary, secondary, and tertiary prevention. A multidisciplinary approach that includes epidemiology, pediatrics, toxicology, public health, and health economics is necessary to treat specific conditions, as well as to prevent exposure to toxins. In addition to caring for acute exposures, providers should inform patients and families about health risks and the nature of environmental contaminants, advocate for healthy environments in the creation of public policy, and work with other professionals to report, monitor, and control exposures. The regional PEHSUs and many online sources provide information and support for clinical, toxicologic, educational, and policy work.

Primary Prevention

The goal of primary prevention is to keep a problem from occurring and to maintain a level of wellness. Education of individuals and the public to help them identify health hazards and prevent exposure is a form of primary prevention. Providers can find a wealth of information about specific toxins, patient support groups, advocate activities, and safety practices and regulations on the Internet. Primary prevention also includes assessment of communities and populations. Safety inspections in industry and public areas (e.g., school playgrounds); monitoring of lead or radon in homes, schools, and workplaces; and scientific research to determine connections between environmental agents and disease are examples of early assessment. It is important to conduct research on children, adapt research methodologies to the unique characteristics of children, and develop biologic markers to better assess the effect of environmental hazards on children as the National Children's Study proposes to do.

Primary prevention also takes place at the public policy level. Regulations or legal restrictions can prevent health problems (e.g., through implementation of air and water

Specify that questions related to the child's home also apply to other indoor environments where the child spends time, including school, daycare, car, school bus, work, and recreational facilities.

				Follow up/ Notes
Is your child's asthma worse at night?	❏ Yes	❏ No	❏ Not sure	
Is your child's asthma worse at specific locations? If so, where? _____	❏ Yes	❏ No	❏ Not sure	
Is your child's asthma worse during a particular season? If so, which one? _____	❏ Yes	❏ No	❏ Not sure	
Is your child's asthma worse with a particular change in climate? If so, which?_____	❏ Yes	❏ No	❏ Not sure	
Can you identify any specific trigger(s) that makes your child's asthma worse? If so, what? _____	❏ Yes	❏ No	❏ Not sure	
Have you noticed whether dust exposure makes your child's asthma worse?	❏ Yes	❏ No	❏ Not sure	
Does your child sleep with stuffed animals?	❏ Yes	❏ No	❏ Not sure	
Is there wall-to-wall carpet in your child's bedroom?	❏ Yes	❏ No	❏ Not sure	
Have you used any means for dust mite control? If so, which ones? _____	❏ Yes	❏ No	❏ Not sure	
Do you have any furry pets?	❏ Yes	❏ No	❏ Not sure	
Do you see evidence of rats or mice in your home weekly?	❏ Yes	❏ No	❏ Not sure	
Do you see cockroaches in your home daily?	❏ Yes	❏ No	❏ Not sure	
Do any family members, caregivers or friends smoke?	❏ Yes	❏ No	❏ Not sure	
Does this person(s) have an interest or desire to quit?	❏ Yes	❏ No	❏ Not sure	
Does your child/teenager smoke?	❏ Yes	❏ No	❏ Not sure	
Do you see or smell mold/mildew in your home?	❏ Yes	❏ No	❏ Not sure	
Is there evidence of water damage in your home?	❏ Yes	❏ No	❏ Not sure	
Do you use a humidifier or swamp cooler?	❏ Yes	❏ No	❏ Not sure	
Have you had new carpets, paint, floor refinishing, or other changes at your house in the past year?	❏ Yes	❏ No	❏ Not sure	
Does your child or another family member have a hobby that uses materials that are toxic or give off fumes?	❏ Yes	❏ No	❏ Not sure	
Has outdoor air pollution ever made your child's asthma worse?	❏ Yes	❏ No	❏ Not sure	
Does your child limit outdoor activities during a Code Orange or Code Red air quality alert for ozone or particle pollution?	❏ Yes	❏ No	❏ Not sure	
Do you use a wood burning fireplace or stove?	❏ Yes	❏ No	❏ Not sure	
Do you use unvented appliances such as a gas stove for heating your home?	❏ Yes	❏ No	❏ Not sure	
Does your child have contact with other irritants (e.g., perfumes, cleaning agents, or sprays)?	❏ Yes	❏ No	❏ Not sure	

What other concerns do you have regarding your child's asthma that have not yet been discussed?

FIGURE 41-4 Environmental history form for pediatric asthma patient. (Used with permission of the National Environmental Education Foundation, Washington, DC. Available at www. neefusa.org/health/asthma/historyform/htm. Accessed December 1, 2011.)

quality standards, restaurant and food handling regulations, or bans on the use of hydrofluorocarbons). Various U.S. federal agencies function to regulate development and use of hazardous materials (e.g., the EPA, the U.S. Consumer Product Safety Commission, and the Occupational Safety and Health Administration [OSHA]). In 1997, the U.S. joined seven other countries (the G-8) in creating the 1997 Declaration of the Environment Leaders of the Eight on Children's Environmental Health, raising the issue of protection of children from environmental threats to an international level (EPA, 1997).

Secondary Prevention

Secondary prevention involves early detection, treatment, and referral for identified diseases. Testing for serum lead levels is one form of early detection. Reporting exposures to county and state public health officials helps prevent further contact by removing the child from the contaminant and implementing abatement procedures. Poisoning due to environmental contaminants is reportable in most states.

Tertiary Prevention

Tertiary prevention seeks to rehabilitate and restore the environment to a healthful state (e.g., asbestos and lead abatement, Superfund and "brownfields" cleanup, restoration of wetlands). Individually, patients can take steps to end exposure to a contaminant (e.g., stop using pesticides in the home and follow directions on pesticide usage exactly) or change other behaviors that exacerbate adverse effects (e.g., radon in combination with tobacco smoke is more harmful). Clinical treatment of the individual exposed and follow-up is essential because effects of environmental agents can be severe and may not appear for months or years.

PREVENTION AND PATIENT EDUCATION

The "unknowns" of the relationship between health and environment can be frustrating for both providers and parents. Even though providers may not know of a connection, it is important to listen to and validate patient concerns; this gives the message that the provider is also concerned and will work with patients to best manage the situation. Blanket reassurances are inappropriate, but clinicians can provide perspective to patients by explaining the process of environmental effects on health and encouraging patients to actively control their environment. Providers should also serve as liaisons and advocates between the family and environmental, community, and specialty health care resources.

■ Common Environmental Agents and Adverse Effects

This section presents a brief discussion of general pediatric poisoning and some common environmental agents that are particularly hazardous to children.

GENERAL PEDIATRIC POISONING

Description

Poisoning is the process in which a substance that interferes with the body's normal function is taken in by ingestion,

inhalation, absorption, or injection. Medications, plants, and chemicals are common causes of poisoning in children.

Epidemiology

Poisoning is a major cause of pediatric injury. The mouthing behavior of infants and normal curiosity of toddlers and preschoolers put infants and young children at high risk for accidental ingestion of toxic materials. Cultural factors and beliefs about medications and vitamins may influence storage practices. More than 2.4 million poisonings occurred in 2008 in the U.S. and more than 50% are among children 6 years old or less (Bronstein et al, 2009). Almost 60% involved prescription or nonprescription drugs or supplements and 13% were related to cleaning products (Franklin and Rodgers, 2008).

Assessment (Rodgers et al, 2007)

History. The following are assessed:
- Type of substance taken in. Name of product and ingredients from label
- Amount of intake
- Exact time of intake or exposure
- Route or method of intake
- Reaction or signs and symptoms and their progression over time
- Emergency care given
- Child's health status before poisoning (e.g., any significant chronic illness? Is child taking prescription medication?)
- Contact information including phone and address if the assessment is via phone

Physical Examination. Findings vary greatly depending on the type and amount of poisonous substance, time since exposure, and susceptibility of the child. Consulting with a poison control center can provide the provider with the information needed to proceed with the physical examination. Reactions can be local or systemic. Questions to consider while conducting the physical examination include the following:
- When did exposure occur?
- Which body system or systems does the poison affect?
- What are specific signs of the poison's effect?
- How quickly does the poison have an effect?
- How susceptible is the child?
- What is the child's age and weight?

Diagnostic Studies. Analysis of specimens (e.g., emesis) can be helpful in determining the type of poison, if unknown. Serum levels of the poison can be assessed for some toxins to determine appropriate treatment of the hospitalized child. In general, however, toxicology screens are not necessary, and diagnosis is made on the basis of history and in consultation with a poison control or pediatric environmental health center.

Differential Diagnosis

A history of exposure distinguishes poisoning or potential poisoning from acute-onset illness. Because there is not always an obvious episode of exposure, the provider should be suspicious of poisoning in otherwise well children who experience sudden seizures, GI distress, or cardiorespiratory collapse.

Basic Decontamination Protocol

- Determine the need for decontamination by calling the poison control center in your area.
- If clothing has been contaminated, strip the patient and double-bag clothing, then flush the entire body with plain water for 2 to 5 minutes. If contaminated with dust, keep clothing dry; remove carefully to minimize dust becoming airborne; if possible, apply dust mask or respirator to patient before removing clothing (brush dust from face first).
- Chemical contamination
  - Scrub or irrigate open wounds for 5 to 10 minutes or longer using lukewarm water.
  - Irrigate eyes with sterile saline, balanced salt solution, or Ringer's lactate for at least 15 to 30 minutes.
  - Irrigate face, nose, and ear canals with normal saline using frequent suction.
  - Wash appendages (if that is only body part contaminated) without wetting the whole body, if possible.
  - Clean under nails with scrub brush and nail cleaner.
- Oily or greasy contamination
  - Cleanse with soap or shampoo, followed by water flushing.

Management

Management approaches for ingested poisons vary with the type of poison, amount of exposure, time lapse since exposure, and susceptibility of the child. Initial management focuses on airway, breathing, and circulation (the ABCs). No matter what poison was taken in, vital body functions must be maintained. Consultation with a poison control center is recommended.

If the patient is to be treated at home initially, the provider needs to talk with the parent or caregiver approximately ½, 1, and 3 hours after the ingestion. Changes in the child's condition will dictate changes in the plan of care. If the child requires hospital care, an ambulance may be necessary and the emergency department personnel informed so that they can be prepared appropriately (Rodgers et al, 2007).

Subsequent management involves counteracting or neutralizing the effects of the poison (administration of antidotes), decreasing the amount of poison in the system (gastric decontamination), and providing life-support measures while the body detoxifies itself. For some poisons (e.g., warfarin), observation alone may be sufficient.

Basic decontamination guidelines for contact contaminants are listed in Box 41-1. Prompt action to remove the toxin from the skin (e.g. insecticide exposure) or from the eye may prevent major absorption. With ingested toxins, most liquid products are absorbed completely within 30 minutes and solids within 1 to 2 hours. Thus timing is critical, and because decontamination procedures also contain risks, one must consider whether the technique chosen is likely to be of sufficient value to merit its use. Activated charcoal, an adsorbent agent, has been demonstrated to have good efficacy for many, but not all, toxins. The toxins adhere to its surface, rather than being absorbed from the GI mucosa. The use of gastric lavage is coming into question more and more because it only removes a small portion of gastric contents. Syrup of ipecac is not recommended for use in poisoning (American Academy of Pediatrics [AAP], 2003; Rodgers et al, 2007). Cathartics are often used with activated charcoal but without good evidence to

support use. Whole-bowel irrigation with a polyethylene glycol electrolyte into the stomach to cleanse the entire GI tract has been shown to be somewhat successful for substances that are absorbed slowly, such as iron or sustained-release medications (Rodgers et al, 2007).

Other strategies that can be used in the hospital setting include diuresis, dialysis, and hemoperfusion.

Prevention and Patient Education

Prevention is the best management for poisonings. Teach parents how to "poison-proof" their home, pointing out connections between the developmental stages of children and sources of poisoning. If a child is exposed to a toxic or potentially toxic substance, instruct parents to call the poison control center *before* instituting treatment.

HEAVY METALS

Several heavy metals, including lead, mercury, and arsenic, can cause severe toxic effects in children. Intoxications affect multiple organs in a variety of ways through widespread disruption of cellular functioning. Lead and mercury are particularly well known for their neurodevelopmental effects.

LEAD
Description

Lead poisoning is the presence of blood lead levels (BLLs) that cause toxic effects on multiple organ systems. The major pathway of exposure is via ingestion although lead dust is absorbed through the lungs. Absorption depends on the route of exposure and the age and nutritional status of the individual (Agency for Toxic Substances and Disease Registry, 2010). One hundred percent of lead inhaled into the lower lungs is absorbed; in children, up to 70% of lead in the GI tract can be absorbed, in contrast to about 20% in adults. Once ingested, lead circulates through the body attached to erythrocytes. It affects heme production, competes with calcium for calcium-binding sites on proteins, and may affect any calcium-mediated process. It affects certain enzyme functions (e.g., ferrochelatase in bone marrow) and damages the nervous system, both through direct nerve cell damage and interference with nerve conduction. It also affects brain development as it inhibits the normal pruning process that eliminates multiple intercellular connections (Markowitz, 2007). Exposure to lead is linked with many conditions and diseases, including ADHD, reading problems, school failure, delinquent and criminal behavior, tooth decay, renal disease, and cardiovascular disease (Froehlich et al, 2009; Lanphear et al, 2005; Wright et al, 2008). Prenatal lead exposure has been associated with schizophrenia (Opler et al, 2008).

Children and adults differ in lead exposure sources, absorption, metabolism, and specific ways in which toxicities are expressed. Children are more likely to be exposed via hand-to-mouth behaviors; the fraction of lead absorbed from the gut is higher in infants and children, and the amount absorbed increases in children when nutritional deficiencies, such as iron and calcium, are present. Temporary peripheral neuropathies from lead toxicities predominate in adults, whereas permanent central nervous system effects predominate in children. If children have higher BLLs at age 6 years than they did at age 2 years, they are more likely to have IQ deficits and behavior problems than children who have a higher BLL at age 2 than at age 6 (Hornung et al, 2009).

Over the past 30 years, the definition of the BLL considered to be toxic has been revised downward. The toxic level for clinical assessment in the U.S. is 10 mcg/dL or more, but even at lower levels, impairment of cognitive function occurs. Studies show clear, persistent intellectual impairments at levels of less than 7.5 mcg/dL (Lanphear et al, 2005). Some experts are calling for a toxic level of 2 mcg/dL, recognizing that no level is totally safe (Gilbert and Weiss, 2006; Wigle et al, 2008).

Epidemiology

Although environmental lead sources have decreased in the U.S., lead poisoning continues to be a serious environmental health problem for young children. Approximately 1% of children tested in 2007 had elevated BLLs, and it is estimated that more than 310,000 children 1 to 5 years old in the U.S. have lead levels above 10 mcg/dL (Warniment et al, 2010). A recent study of more than 200,000 children found a positive association between poverty and pre-1950s housing and lead toxicity, with 17.3% of the children having BLLs greater than 10 mcg/dL (Vivier et al, 2010). Boys may be more susceptible than girls to the effects of prenatal exposure to low levels of lead (Jedrychowski et al, 2009).

The major source of lead poisoning in children is dust and chips from deteriorating paint on interior surfaces. Before 1950, much white house paint was 50% lead and 50% linseed oil. Limits on the lead content of paint began in 1955 and were augmented in 1971 and 1977. The prevalence of lead hazards in homes built before 1960 is five to eight times greater than in homes built between 1960 and 1977, and 14 to 23 times greater than in homes built between 1978 and 1998 (Jacobs et al, 2002). Children are at greatest risk in houses where paint is peeling or those where renovation with paint removal is occurring. Lead dust is more readily absorbed than chips. Soil near deteriorating homes, mines, lead-using industries, and smelters can have high lead levels. Acidic water with low mineral content can leach lead from lead pipes or solder. Hot water leaches more lead than cold. Brass fixtures also contain lead. Food can be a source of lead. For example, lead from soil can contaminate root vegetables. Some other sources of lead are listed in Table 41-2. Lead crosses the placenta so that the fetal and newborn blood level is close to that of the mother's, but little lead is transferred in breast milk.

Clinical Findings

Screening. Providers should use state and local recommendations or policies, based on CDC guidelines, to guide their practice (CDC, 1997). Children who have any sign of lead toxicity or are at risk should be screened. Although routine screening of all children for lead is not recommended, the AAP (2005) notes that most children are at sufficient risk to have their BLL measured at least once. All Medicaid-eligible children should be screened. All children who have recently emigrated from other countries should be screened on arrival to the U.S. Screening for lead poisoning involves two processes: (1) assessing the risk of high-dose exposure through history-taking, and (2) testing BLLs.

In addition to questions found in the environmental assessment screening tools (see Figs. 41-2 and 41-3), assessment for lead risk should include questions such as:
- How does the family control dust or dirt particles that might be contaminated with lead?
- Does the child live near a lead smelter, battery recycling plant, or other industry likely to release lead?
- Does the parent or guardian have a job or hobby that uses lead?
- Does the family use ceramic pottery for cooking or storing food?
- Does the family use traditional or folk healing remedies?
- Does the child demonstrate pica behavior?
- Does the child have a retained lead bullet?

In 2006, the U.S. Food and Drug Administration (FDA) approved a rapid screening test that gives results in as little as 3 minutes. If this preliminary screening test is positive, a follow-up test is required, but the second sample can be drawn immediately rather than having the patient return (FDA, 2009a). If the screening BLL is 10 mcg/dL or greater, additional assessment and management are required (Fig. 41-5).

Physical Examination. Most lead retained by the body is stored in the bones and is not measured by BLLs. Although lead affects almost all organ systems, the nervous system, kidneys, and blood are particularly susceptible. Toxicity is a function of both dose and duration of exposure, but clinical signs of toxicity may not accurately reflect the amount of lead in the body. A child can have high BLLs (e.g., 45 mcg/dL) with no obvious clinical signs. Another child may complain of severe GI problems with a lower lead level (e.g., 15 to 20 mcg/dL). Low-level chronic exposure is very difficult to identify.

Subclinical Effects. In most cases, changes caused by lead toxicity are subtle enough not to be identified as a clinical problem (see Table 41-2). Studies indicate that IQ is affected significantly by lifetime BLLs less than 10 mcg/dL. In one study, children with lifetime BLLs as low as 2.1 mcg/dL demonstrated an inverse relationship between BLL and IQ (Jusko et al, 2008). In another study, the IQ deficit was steeper in children with lifetime BLLs less than 10 mcg/dL than it was for all children; IQ decreased by 7.4 points as BLLs increased from 1 to 10 mcg/dL (Canfield et al, 2003).

Clinical Effects. Many children do not demonstrate signs of acute toxicity until late in the disease. At higher levels, lead affects vitamin D metabolism, nerve conduction velocities, and hemoglobin synthesis. See Table 41-2 for clinical signs and symptoms.

Diagnostic Studies. Blood lead level is the measure used to diagnose lead toxicity. A capillary sample can be used, but venous blood should be drawn to confirm the diagnosis. Assessment of free erythrocyte protoporphyrin (FEP) and zinc protoporphyrin (ZPP) can be helpful because these are elevated in the presence of lead. Evaluate iron deficiency, including serum ferritin or low ratio of serum iron to iron-binding capacity. Screening for BLL should be done by a laboratory that has a low range of error (±2 mcg/dL).

Differential Diagnosis

GI infections, other causes of anemia, growth retardation, behavior disorders, attention-deficit/hyperactivity disorder (ADHD), and central nervous system (CNS) infections are included in the differential diagnosis.

Text continued on p. 1071

TABLE 41-2 Common Pediatric Toxicants and Relationship to Disease

Substance	Source	HEALTH EFFECTS Systems Affected	Signs and Symptoms	Prevention Strategies
Lead	Lead-based paint, caulk Dust, soil, water (lead pipes) Cosmetics Solder, ammunition Bearings, fishing weights Folk medicine remedies (e.g., greta, azarcon, pay-loo-ah) Pottery, lead crystal Some dyes used in paper, magazines, plastic wrappers Lead-based insecticides Industries that use/process lead (e.g., smelters, battery manufacturers) Hobbies, stained glass, jewelry Some imported toys, candies Some dietary supplements Some vinyl lunchboxes Polyvinyl chloride (PVC) and artificial turf	Central nervous system (CNS) Cardiac Gastrointestinal (GI) Renal Some enzymes Thyroid	Anemia Constipation Abdominal pain Anorexia, vomiting Learning disabilities; lower IQ scores Impaired hearing Delayed growth and development Hyperactivity or other behavior problems Agitation or clumsiness Myocardial excitability (with high levels) Headache, increased intracranial pressure Seizures, coma (usually above 70-100 mcg/dL), and death	Test blood for lead levels Test soil, water, dust for lead Begin lead abatement as required, using professional experts Repair/replace deteriorating paint Keep children away from remodeling or demolition projects where lead dust could be released Clean surfaces with cleaning solution; do not dry dust Teach handwashing Keep children from chewing on painted surfaces, eating dirt Use fresh, cold water from taps; when faucet has not been used for 2 hours or more, flush 30-60 seconds until water is noticeably colder Make sure diet has adequate iron, calcium, zinc, and ascorbate because deficiencies in these enhance lead absorption, retention, and toxicity Use lead-free paints, gasoline, materials for hobbies Do not store or cook food in lead crystal, old or imported pottery Be sure folk remedies are lead-free Change work clothes before returning home if job is lead-related Avoid use of products that contain lead
Mercury	Food chain; accumulated and concentrated in animals (especially fish), grains, and flour Fungicides Antiseptics Medications Latex paints (added to paints until 1991; older paints still contain Hg) Thermometers and thermostats Fluorescent lights Button/disk batteries Folk medicine remedies or religious practices (e.g., azogue) Burning fossil fuels Mining Smelting Incineration (especially of medical wastes) Industrial discharge Natural seepage from rocks	CNS; GI, respiratory, renal	Five manifestations (see text): *Acrodynia* 　Erythema of palms and soles 　Pruritus *Chronic inorganic mercury intoxication* 　Tremors 　Irritability 　Memory loss 　Metallic taste in the mouth 　Gingivostomatitis 　Renal dysfunction *Methyl mercury intoxication* 　Impaired vision or hearing 　Numbness or pain in extremities 　Birth defects 　Hypotonia 　Ataxia *Acute inhalation of elemental mercury* 　Necrotizing bronchitis 　Pneumonia 　Fever *Acute ingestion of inorganic mercury salts* 　Nausea and vomiting 　Intestinal pain 　Bloody diarrhea 　Renal necrosis and failure 　Seizures, coma, and death	Do not eat fish or other food sources suspected of being contaminated with mercury; limit intake of freshwater fish caught by family or friends: 6 oz cooked fish per week for pregnant women, women of childbearing years, and nursing mothers; 2 oz for young children (EPA, 2004) Pregnant women should avoid eating swordfish, shark, king mackerel, and tile fish; can eat up to 12 oz of other fish per week; should not eat >6 oz albacore tuna per week (EPA, 2004) Do not allow children to play with glass thermometers, electrical wires, paints, or other materials with mercury Replace mercury thermometers and thermostats *Never* vacuum up mercury spills (this vaporizes and spreads the mercury) Call hazardous materials officials for advice on mercury spills Safely store and dispose of products containing mercury Be sure folk remedies are mercury free. Advise families from cultures that use elemental mercury in religious ceremonies of the danger, especially to children

Continued

TABLE 41-2 Common Pediatric Toxicants and Relationship to Disease—cont'd

Substance	Source	HEALTH EFFECTS		Prevention Strategies
		Systems Affected	Signs and Symptoms	
Environmental tobacco smoke (ETS)	Side stream smoke from tobacco products being used by others (child is inhaling unfiltered smoke)	Respiratory Cardiac Growth Neurologic	Bronchitis Pneumonia Asthma Otitis media Middle ear effusion Premature coronary artery disease Low birthweight Sudden infant death syndrome Cognitive delays	Adults and siblings in child's environment stop smoking Enroll child in daycare that is smoke free Prevent child from starting smoking Recommend smoking cessation programs Health care provider recommendation of and support for decision to stop smoking
Radon	Air Water Is concentrated in basements and low areas	Respiratory	Lung cancer May be some other health effects	Test air in basements and first floor of home for radon levels (see text) Avoid having children play in basements of homes with radon Reduce amount of radon in basements: Seal cracks in foundation of house Cover dirt crawl spaces with impermeable plastic Seal drains Pour concrete floors Provide good ventilation Stop smoking (tobacco smoke acts as a vehicle for radon to enter the body)
Particulate matter	Outdoor: Industrial pollution Gasoline and diesel exhaust Pollens Natural phenomena Forest fires Volcanic activity Indoor: Wood-burning stoves Dust mites Animal dander Cockroach particles Molds Tobacco smoke	Respiratory Cardiovascular	Bronchitis Pneumonia Wheezing Chronic cough Decreased lung function Asthma Cardiovascular conditions Lung cancer	When outdoor air pollution is high, keep children indoors, decrease outdoor playtime Air-condition the home (HEPA systems are most effective) Check heating system to ensure it is clean Cover mattresses, wash bedding frequently Launder or discard stuffed animals
Molds	Damp areas in the home or school (leaking roofs or plumbing, flooding in basements, backed-up sewers) Humidifiers Steam from shower, bath, or cooking Wet clothes House plants Dry leaves	Respiratory Skin CNS	Allergic reactions: Cough Wheezing or shortness of breath Sinus congestion Watery, itchy, light-sensitive eyes Sore throat Skin rash Headaches, memory loss, mood changes Aches and pains Fever	Maintain dry, clean environment: Clean with hot water and detergent Clean surfaces where mold grows with solution 1 part bleach: 4 parts water If unable to thoroughly clean, discard moldy materials to prevent spores from being released when materials dry
Asbestos	Construction materials: Insulation Ceiling and floor tiles Shingles	Respiratory	Lung irritation Lung disease later in life with repeated exposure	Prevent exposure to asbestos products: If buildings that contain asbestos are in good repair, it may be best to leave asbestos in place; if there is a question, contact a certified asbestos professional to check it Use asbestos abatement measures as appropriate when renovating If parents' workplace is a source of asbestos exposure, remove clothing and bathe before coming in contact with children

Substance	Source	HEALTH EFFECTS		Prevention Strategies
		Systems Affected	Signs and Symptoms	

Pesticides	Food
	Water
	Direct contact with plants, grass, and other areas treated with pesticides, insecticides, herbicides, or fungicides
	Direct contact with pesticide through dust, mists, sprays
		CNS
		Immune
		Endocrine
		Skin
		GI
			Skin rash
			Increased risk of cancer
			Developmental delay
			Neurotoxicity: Impaired sensation
			  Dizziness
			  Restlessness, confusion, irritability
			  Impaired coordination
			May disrupt endocrine function
			May contribute to immune dysfunction
			Nausea/vomiting
			Seizures
			Death by poisoning
				Use few or no pesticides in the home; use nonchemical treatments
				Use only amount recommended for purpose stated
				Protect skin from exposure when using; wash thoroughly after use
				Do not inhale or use on windy day
				Keep children and pets from treated areas
				Clean up any spills
				Keep pesticides from food/dishes
				Store pesticides safely out of children's reach, in original container
				Do not mix pesticides
				Dispose of pesticides at a registered disposal site
				Keep a copy of the label handy
				Decrease exposure in foods: Vary kinds of fruits and vegetables children eat. Grow your own.
				Buy organically grown foods; check USDA labels: "100% organic," "organic" (at least 95% organic content), "made with organic" (70% organic content for up to 3 ingredients), and "organic components" (products with less than 70% organic content)
				Wash and peel fruits and vegetables (many pesticides are in the product itself; washing and peeling will not remove them)
				Try to use in-season fruits and vegetables to avoid those sprayed for transport and preservation

Polychlorinated biphenyls (PCBs)	Foods and cooking oil
	Fish; concentrated in fatty tissues of animals
	Prenatal exposure via maternal ingestion of contaminated food
	Breastfeeding
	Older and deteriorating electrical equipment or wiring; transformers
	Hydraulic fluids, plasticizers, caulking compounds, paints, adhesives, and flame retardants
	Pesticides
	Inks and carbonless paper
		CNS
		Respiratory
		Hepatic
		Skin
			Low birthweight
			Growth delay
			Developmental delay
			Decreased IQ scores
			Neurologic and intellectual impairment
			Increased respiratory infections
			Increased behavior problems
			Smaller male genitalia
			Chloracne, including cysts (1-10 mm diameter), comedones, papules, hyperpigmentation, conjunctiva, gingiva, and nail changes
			Childhood exposure leads to:
			  Developmental delays
			  Premature pubertal changes in both boys and girls
			  Acute dermatologic and neurologic problems
			  Chronic liver disease
			  Tooth enamel defects (Jan et al, 2007)
				Avoid PCB-contaminated foods, especially prenatally
				Avoid environmental exposure from electrical leakage
				Use professional abatement procedures to dispose of or clean up contaminated materials

HEPA, High-efficiency particulate air; *USDA,* U.S. Department of Agriculture.

Data from American Academy of Pediatrics, Committee on Environmental Health: *Handbook of pediatric environmental health,* ed 2, Elk Grove Village, IL, 2003, American Academy of Pediatrics; Landrigan PJ: Pesticides and PCBs: does the evidence show that they threaten children's health? *Contemp Pediatr* 18:110-126, 2001; Reigert JR, Roberts JR: Pesticides in children, *Pediatr Clin North Am* 48:1185-1198, 2001; Reigert JR, Roberts JR: *Recognition and management of pesticide poisonings,* ed 5, Washington, DC, 1999, U.S. Environmental Protection Agency.

Child has risk factor from screening criteria		
Yes: Draw venous blood sample and complete laboratory assessment		**No:** Routine screening not recommended; provide caregiver dietary and environmental education

Screening sample: blood lead levels (BLLs)	Actions to be taken*	Follow-up BLL monitoring
<10 mcg/dL	Not considered lead poisoning: • Provide caregiver dietary and environmental education • Refer to social services if necessary	If high risk, retest in 6 months If low risk, no further testing needed
10-14 mcg/dL	Borderline: Confirmatory venous blood testing within 3 months	Early follow-up within 3 months If follow-up level is 15-19 mcg/dL or higher in two tests taken 3 months apart, retest every 1-2 months until results <15 mcg/dL for at least 6 months, then retest every 6-9 months
15-19 mcg/dL	Confirmatory venous blood testing within 3 months Proceed according to actions for 20-44 mcg/dL if: • A follow-up BLL is in this range at least 3 months after initial venous testing or • BLLs increase	Early follow-up within 2 months If levels continue >15 mcg/dL, retest every 1-2 months until results <15 mcg/dL for at least 6 months, then retest every 3 months until child is 36 months old
20-44 mcg/dL	Confirmatory venous blood testing shortly (within 1 week to 1 month; the higher levels in the shorter time) Complete history and physical exam Neurodevelopmental monitoring Lab work: Hgb or Hct and iron status (FEP or ZPP) Abdominal x-ray (if particulate lead ingestion is suspected) with bowel decontamination if indicated	Early follow-up in 1-3 months for BLLs 20-24 mcg/dL; in 2 weeks to 1 month for BLLs 24-44 mcg/dL Retest every 1-2 months until results <15 mcg/dL for at least 6 months, then retest every 3 months until child is 36 months old
45-69 mcg/dL	Diagnostic venous blood testing within 24-48 hours Complete history and physical examination Complete neurologic exam Lab work: Hgb or Hct and iron status (FEP or ZPP) Abdominal x-ray with bowel decontamination if indicated Chelation therapy	Early follow-up as soon as possible Retest every month until results <15 mcg/dL for at least 6 months, then retest every 3 months until child is 36 months old
>70 mcg/dL	Medical emergency: Retest immediately as an emergency lab test with venous blood sample Hospitalize for intravenous chelation Proceed according to action for 45-69 mcg/dL	Early follow-up as soon as possible Retest every month until results <15 mcg/dL for at least 6 months, then retest every 3 months until child is 36 months old

*In all cases of lead toxicity:
• Provide caregiver dietary and environmental education
• Remove child from source of lead if known
• Report to Public Health Department
• Initiate environmental investigation
• Initiate lead hazard control/abatement
• Refer to social services
Hgb, Hemoglobin; *Hct,* hematocrit; *FEP,* free erythrocytes protoporphyrin, *ZPP,* zinc protoporphyrin.

FIGURE 41-5 Management recommendations for lead poisoning. (Adapted from Centers for Disease Control and Prevention [CDC]: *Screening young children for lead poisoning: guidance for state and local public health officials,* Atlanta, 1997, CDC; CDC: *Managing elevated blood lead levels among young children: recommendations from the Advisory Committee on Childhood Lead Poisoning prevention,* Atlanta, 2002, CDC.)

Management

Management involves preventing the child's exposure to lead in the environment, treating the child for toxicity, monitoring lead levels, correcting dietary deficiencies (if any), and removing lead from the environment (see Table 41-2 and Fig. 41-5). Other children in the same household or environment where exposure could have occurred should be tested and treated as appropriate. Chelation is indicated to treat acute, severe, and life-threatening poisoning, but there is controversy about its use for long-term exposure or chronic intoxication because the therapy itself may be deleterious and may outweigh the benefits of clearing the metal (Kosnett, 2010). There is no evidence that chelation reverses cognitive impairments, so prevention is critical (AAP, 2005). It is also critical that providers do follow-up testing for children with positive lead screens. Lack of follow-up testing is a common error of omission that can lead to permanent damage in the child (Kemper et al, 2005).

Prevention and Patient Education

Table 41-2 outlines prevention strategies. Parents need to know that lead abatement is absolutely essential; treatments such as chelation therapy and dietary changes are ineffective unless the child is returned to a clean house. Until lead abatement can be implemented, however, parents can work to control lead dust and paint chips in older homes. Conventional vacuums can be used to help control lead dust and high-efficiency particulate air (HEPA) filtering vacuum cleaners can temporarily reduce lead loads, but levels soon rise if the source of lead remains (Yiin et al, 2002). Other strategies parents can use include the following:

- Block access to areas of the room where large peeling paint areas are found.
- Cover smaller peeling areas with sticky-backed paper.
- Damp-mop and damp-dust with household cleaners or lead-specific cleaning products (e.g., Ledizolv) twice weekly to decrease lead dust in the air; do not dry mop or sweep.
- Pick up and dispose of paint chips with a disposable rag or paper towel soaked in phosphate cleaner.

Inform parents that chelation therapy leads to a rapid fall in BLL, but that most children have a rebound increase within days or weeks of treatment, and repeated treatment may be necessary.

MERCURY

Description

Mercury, like lead, is a heavy metal, and is the second most common cause of heavy metal poisoning. Mercury exists in elemental forms (liquid or vapor), inorganic mercury salts, and organic forms. Organic mercury compounds, such as methyl mercury, are the most toxic and are found in the food chain. CNS tissue is the main target organ for mercury in humans. Once absorbed into the brain, mercury metabolizes to its inorganic form and cannot cross the blood-brain barrier to exit the brain; significant neurologic symptoms can result. The fetus and child are more susceptible to mercury toxicity than are others. Permanent damage to the developing fetal brain can occur. Reductions in IQ due to methyl mercury exposure have been estimated to affect between 300,000 and 600,000

U.S. children each year with economic costs due to loss of productivity amounting to an estimated $8.7 billion annually (Trasande et al, 2005). Offspring of pregnant women who ingested methyl mercury have been affected by a severe, irreversible central and peripheral neurologic condition known as Minamata disease. The kidney is another major target organ, especially for inorganic mercury poisoning; and mercury can be corrosive to the GI system.

Epidemiology

Each year 7.8% to 15% of the annual birth cohort is born with cord blood methyl mercury levels greater than 5.8 mcg/L (Trasande et al, 2005). Blood levels are higher in women from Asian, Pacific Islander, Native American, and multiracial populations—groups that include more fish in their diets. Approximately 16.6% of women in these ethnic groups who were sampled through the National Health and Nutrition Examination Survey (NHANES) study for 1999-2002 had levels greater than 5.8 mcg/L. This is of concern because cord blood levels of fetuses are 70% higher than maternal concentrations (Hightower et al, 2006). Follow-up of the NHANES population found that mercury accumulated in the body over time: 2% of the subjects had detectable inorganic mercury in 1999-2000, compared with 30% of the same subjects in 2005-2006 (Laks, 2009).

Mercury is pervasive in the environment. Common sources are listed in Table 41-2; exposure and contamination varies for each type of mercury. Coal-fired electric utilities are a major source of mercury pollution in the U.S.

Children can be exposed to *elemental mercury* through accidents, magico-religious rituals, and vapors from industrial activity. Elemental mercury is found in thermometers and used in dental amalgams; it can be absorbed (although poorly) through skin and in the GI tract. Elemental mercury can vaporize or be atomized (e.g., heating during industrial processing releases vapors; vacuuming up spills can spread the mercury through airborne particles), be inhaled, and is readily absorbed through the lungs. In the body it is oxidized to the inorganic form that is toxic to the kidneys and nervous system. *Inorganic mercury,* found in some fungicides, antiseptics, and medications, is poorly absorbed by the gut or through the skin, and does not readily cross the blood-brain barrier. It can be absorbed through inhalation and will cross the placenta. It is excreted in breast milk and urine and affects the kidneys.

Organic mercury (e.g., methyl mercury, ethyl mercury) accumulates in the biologic organism, is concentrated in food products (especially fish), and is readily absorbed from the GI tract (90%) and through the skin. Methyl mercury easily enters the brain, crosses the placenta, and has been found in breast milk. It bioaccumulates up the food chain, is a neurotoxin and teratogen, and is the most widespread source of mercury toxicity. Ethyl mercury (EtHg) is less toxic. It is not thought to be actively transported across the blood-brain barrier or to bioaccumulate, has a larger molecular size, and decomposes at a faster rate than methyl mercury. It is a metabolite of thimerosal, a vaccine preservative, now out of use in the U.S. except in influenza vaccine. Multiple international studies have shown that there is "no substantial evidence that EtHg in the amounts contained in vaccines is associated with neurodevelopmental disorders, including autism spectrum disorder" (Counter and Buchanan, 2004, p 219). There are no reliable data of an association between thimerosal and autism and thimerosal is not used in most vaccines; however, a gene-environment (i.e., epigenetic) interaction that could make some individuals susceptible remains a theoretical possibility (Aschner and Ceccatelli, 2010).

Clinical Findings

History. A thorough history is essential to identify the source of exposure because signs and symptoms can be very confusing. Questions should focus on potential exposure, workplace environment, diet, and whether others in the family are experiencing similar symptoms.

Physical Examination. Five syndromes of mercury poisoning are found clinically (Mahajan, 2007):
1. Acrodynia ("pink disease"), rare, most often seen in children
   - Hypersensitivity reaction with generalized pain, paresthesias
   - Pink, papular, pruritic rash that may involve face, hands, and feet
   - May have morbilliform, vesicular, or hemorrhagic rash
   - Anorexia
   - Weakness, hypotonia, especially of pelvic area
   - Good prognosis when mercury source is removed
2. Chronic inorganic mercury intoxication (signs and symptoms may also be seen with chronic exposure to elemental and organic mercury)
   - Classic triad: Tremor, neuropsychiatric disturbance, gingivostomatitis
   - May have sensorimotor neuropathy and visual disturbances
   - Renal dysfunction, nephrotic syndrome
3. Methyl mercury intoxication (Minamata disease)
   - Delayed neurotoxicity, ataxia, paresthesias, tremors, sensory impairment, dementia, death
   - Fetal involvement most severe: Low birthweight, profound developmental delays, cerebral palsy, deafness, blindness, seizures
4. Acute inhalation of elemental mercury vapor
   - Cough, dyspnea, chest pain, fever, headache, GI disturbance (metallic taste)
   - Younger children more susceptible to pulmonary toxic effects
   - Can be self-limited
   - Can progress to necrotizing bronchiolitis; may be fatal
5. Acute ingestion of inorganic mercury salts
   - Corrosive gastroenteritis within hours, severe GI pain, hematemesis, cardiovascular collapse, renal failure
   - Often from ingestion of button battery
   - Can be fatal

Diagnostic Studies. Blood mercury levels can be used to determine acute mercury exposure, but the blood half-life is short, and levels may not reflect toxicity. A blood level of less than 2 mcg/L is considered normal. A 24-hour urine sample in an acid-washed container gives the optimal sample of mercury contamination (less than 10 mcg/L is the reference range of "normal"), but a first-morning void may give good information. Hair or nail analysis provides a measure of long-term exposure but is not adequate for diagnosing individual patients (Ng et al, 2007).

Differential Diagnosis

The differential diagnosis includes other poisonings, infections of the CNS, and CNS conditions.

Management

Patients should be referred to a center for clinical management of acute poisoning. Chelation is the treatment of choice and needs to be conducted at a center where supportive therapy can stabilize the patient during the procedure. Decontamination through gastric lavage may be appropriate to remove ingested inorganic mercury, depending on how recently exposure occurred. Because of the corrosive effects of inorganic mercury salts, treatment to induce emesis is not recommended.

Prevention and Patient Education

For all forms of mercury, stopping exposure is essential.

Methyl Mercury. Women of childbearing age, pregnant women, nursing mothers, infants, and young children should not eat shark, swordfish, king mackerel, or tilefish. They should limit their intake of albacore tuna to no more than 4 to 6 oz per week, and other fish to no more than 12 oz per week (EPA, 2004). A list of fish and seafood with levels of mercury is found in Table 41-3.

Elemental Mercury. Children have been known to innocently play with mercury (e.g., from a broken thermometer). If exposure is short-term and cleanup is thorough, there may be no demonstrable harm (Lee et al, 2009). But parents need to be reminded of the deadly effect of mercury and encouraged to keep all materials that contain mercury out of children's reach. Mercury spills should be handled by a professional abatement team or cleaned with wet, occlusive materials. Porous materials that are contaminated by spills (e.g., clothing) should be discarded at a toxic waste facility. Any mercury switches, mercury thermometers, sphygmomanometers, switches containing mercury, or fluorescent light bulbs should be recycled at appropriate recycling centers. Elemental mercury is being removed from the manufacturing of instruments and switches so that it does not enter the environmental waste stream. In 2009 the FDA issued final rules recognizing the potential health effects of elemental mercury from dental amalgams and regulating those dental products (FDA, 2009b). Parents should discuss alternatives to amalgams if their children need dental fillings.

ARSENIC

Description

Arsenic is a highly poisonous chemical element, a heavy metal that occurs naturally in the environment in organic and inorganic forms. Arsenic is found in many different compound forms and salts, such as arsenic acid, arsenic trioxide, and arsenate; some compounds (e.g., arsine) are gaseous, colorless, nonirritating substances with an odor of garlic. Arsenic acts as an enzyme poison in the body and can affect all systems. Long-term, low-level exposure can lead to chronic poisoning and cancer. Acute poisoning is usually paralytic or gastrointestinal in nature. Infant mortality is higher in mothers exposed to arsenic (Rahman et al, 2010).

TABLE 41-3	Levels of Mercury in Fish and Shellfish	
Fish and Shellfish Source	**Average Hg Concentration (mcg/4 oz*)†**
Shark‡	151
Swordfish‡	147
Tilefish (Gulf of Mexico)‡	219
Tilefish (Atlantic)	22
Mackerel, king‡	110
Mackerel: Atlantic and Pacific, not King	8-13
Pollock: Atlantic and walleye	6
Haddock and hake	2-5
Lobster: Northern, American	47
Tuna: bluefin and albacore‡	54-58
Tuna: yellowfin and skipjack	31-49
Tuna: light, canned	13
Tuna: albacore, canned	40
Catfish, channel and flathead	7
Trout: Freshwater	11
Cod: Atlantic and Pacific	14
Crab: blue, king, snow, queen, and dungeness	9
Tilapia	2
Sardines: Atlantic and Pacific	2
Shrimp	0
Scallops: bay and sea	8
Squid	11
Salmon: Pink, sockeye, Atlantic, chinook, coho	2
Clams	0
Oysters: Pacific	2
Anchovies, herring, and shad	5-10

*Mercury values taken from 4 oz cooked fish, assuming 25% moisture loss in cooking; except for tuna, canned fish varieties not included.
†A total of 39 mcg of mercury per week would reach the EPA reference dose limit (0.1 mcg/kg/d) for a woman who is pregnant or breastfeeding and who weighs 124 pounds (56 kg).
‡These varieties should not be eaten by pregnant or breastfeeding women; pregnant or breastfeeding women should also limit white albacore tuna to 6 oz per week.
Adapted from U.S. Department of Agriculture (USDA) and U.S. Department of Health and Human Services (HHS): *Dietary Guidelines for Americans, 2010,* ed 7, Washington, DC, 2010, U.S. Government Printing Office. Available at www.cnpp.usda.gov/DGAs2010-PolicyDocument.htm. Accessed February 10, 2011.

Epidemiology

In addition to its natural occurrence, arsenic is used commercially in pesticides, herbicides, rodenticides, and wood preservatives. Arsenic trioxide is also used in glassmaking and some pigments. Exposure to arsenic occurs primarily through drinking water and contaminated foods. Children can also be exposed through contact with wood used to construct playgrounds that has been treated with chromated copper arsenate (CCA) to prevent decay. Leaching of arsenate into soil and sand of playground areas from treated wood presents a further danger to children. Burning treated wood releases arsenic into the air, where it can be inhaled.

Clinical Findings

History and Physical Examination. An exposure history is essential in determining whether arsenic poisoning has occurred. Physical signs and symptoms depend on the type of exposure and include the following:

- Acute exposure to high levels of arsine gas results in massive hemolysis after a latent period of 2 to 24 hours. Malaise, headache, weakness, abdominal pain, nausea, vomiting, diarrhea, hepatomegaly, pallor, jaundice, hemoglobinuria, and renal failure occur. Ingestion leads to GI symptoms of pain, nausea, vomiting, and diarrhea, either in minutes or hours. Cardiovascular and neurologic toxicity may include cardiogenic shock, arrhythmias, delirium, and coma (Mahajan, 2007).
- Chronic exposure to low levels results in some of the effects listed: cancer, often in the skin; other dermatologic lesions; encephalopathy; peripheral neuropathy; hepatomegaly; splenomegaly; noncirrhotic portal fibrosis; and portal hypertension (Mahajan, 2007).

Diagnostic Studies. A 24-hour urine sample is the preferred specimen, but serum levels can also be measured. Concentrations greater than 50 mcg/L indicate arsenic intoxication.

Management

Prevent exposure by keeping children away from products that contain arsenic. Parents and providers can work with schools and communities to assess for and clean up arsenic contamination of playground areas. If there is a possibility of arsenic in the water supply, testing is recommended. Bottled water, distilled water, or home treatment units that remove arsenic should be used if drinking water is contaminated. Providers should also support standards for use and production of arsenic products, such as a 2001 EPA action that lowers the allowable arsenic in drinking water from 50 to 10 parts per billion, and the voluntary agreement by the pressure-treated wood industry to phase out use of CCA in wood produced for residential use as of 2003. Chelation may help with acute toxicity.

■ Ambient Air Pollution: Indoor and Outdoor

Air quality is an important environmental factor in childhood illness, especially respiratory conditions. Since the 1970s, outdoor air quality has improved in many areas as a result of local, state, and federal regulations, but outdoor, or ambient, air pollution continues to contribute significantly to adverse health effects. Both children and adults are affected by CO, sulfur oxides, hydrocarbons, ozone, nitrogen oxides, and particulate matter, including ultrafine particles that are especially toxic because they penetrate cells. Diesel engines are potent polluters of the environment. The exhaust contains ultrafine, fine, and coarse particles plus a mixture of toxic chemicals and respiratory irritants that chemically promote expression of the T-helper cell type 2 associated with developing asthma (Gilmour et al, 2006).

The effects of ambient air pollution are sometimes studied by individual components and sometimes as a mixture of CO, nitrogen dioxide, particulate matter, sulfur dioxide, polycyclic aromatic hydrocarbons, ozone, and others. Ambient air pollution increases episodes of asthma, sometimes with a lag of 2 days (Akinbami et al, 2010; Mar and Koenig, 2009; Schildcrout et al, 2006). Other studies looking at CO and particulates are mentioned in those sections of this chapter.

Indoor air quality has declined in the same time period, largely due to an increase in the use of carpets, wood stove heating, and synthetic and chemically formulated building materials (e.g., pressed wood made with formaldehyde) coupled with more "energy-conserving" construction that makes new homes more "airtight" and reduces ventilation. Because up to 90% of an individual's time is spent indoors, exposure to airborne toxicants has increased markedly.

As discussed earlier, children are especially susceptible to air quality problems because of their rapid lung development, smaller, narrower airways, more rapid respiration rate, high level of physical activity, and more time spent on the floor. Very young children spend notably more time indoors. This section discusses several of the more common indoor and outdoor airborne toxicants that influence children's health status: environmental tobacco smoke, CO, radon, particulate matter, asbestos, and molds.

ENVIRONMENTAL TOBACCO SMOKE

Description

Environmental tobacco smoke (ETS), the presence of tobacco smoke in the air that smokers and nonsmokers breathe, has been associated with a wide range of health problems during pregnancy and among infants and children. A major Surgeon General's report highlights these problems (USDHHS, 2006). Effects can be grouped into several categories (Samet and Sockrider, 2010):

- Quality of life and costs
- Prematurity and prenatal mortality—spontaneous abortion is higher among women who smoke
- Fetal growth and development—neonates born to smoking mothers are more likely to have low birthweight and cleft lip and palate. The respiratory and growth outcomes are related to smoking in the second and third trimesters (Prabhu et al, 2010).
- Childhood growth and development—ETS affects physical growth and is associated with cognitive and behavioral problems in children. Effects include hypertonicity and irritability in newborns and behavioral problems in older children including oppositional defiant disorder, conduct disorder, delinquency, and ADHD. Maternal prenatal smoking of 10 or more cigarettes per day has been associated with a 4.35 decrease in IQ of offspring (Herrmann et al, 2008).
- Sudden infant death syndrome

- Respiratory symptoms and illness, especially lower respiratory illness including bronchitis and pneumonia, chronic respiratory symptoms, asthma, reduced lung function—prenatal ETS exposure affects the respiratory health of children after birth. Increased asthma rates are still seen in 17-year-olds after prenatal smoke exposure (Goksor et al, 2007).
- Atherosclerosis—pubertal children with a history of long-term exposure to passive cigarette smoke, especially Caucasian males, are at increased risk of premature coronary artery disease.
- Middle ear disease—children who live with ETS have more recurrent otitis media, and middle ear effusions (Bhattacharyya and Shapiro, 2010).
- Childhood cancer
- Infant gastroenteritis

Epidemiology

ETS is perhaps the most hazardous of children's environmental exposures, causing an estimated 6000 excess deaths among American children less than 5 years old annually, and there are no levels at which exposure to ETS can be considered safe. ETS contains more than 4000 chemicals that cause a variety of illnesses. Nicotine, CO, formaldehyde, hydrogen cyanide, sulfur dioxide, nitrogen dioxide, ammonia, polycyclic aromatic hydrocarbons, and nitrosamines are the most common (Kum-Nji et al, 2006). Nicotine, CO, oxidant gases, and polycyclic aromatic hydrocarbons of ETS contribute to cardiovascular disease. Combined, they accelerate atherogenesis and are implicated in sudden cardiac death. Thrombosis, endothelial dysfunction, inflammation, lipid abnormalities, and platelet activation are all involved (Benuck, 2006).

At least four different reasons for increased respiratory infections among children exposed to ETS have been proposed:

- Nicotine suppresses or inhibits phagocytic activity of neutrophils or macrocytes in alveolar pulmonary cells and the oral mucosa.
- Nicotine suppresses Th1 cells responsible for Ig production and stimulates Th2 cell function to produce cytokines and interleukins responsible for clinical symptoms of atopic diseases, including asthma, eczema, allergic rhinitis, and others.
- Nicotine allows pathogenic bacteria to adhere more easily to mucociliary epithelial tissue.
- ETS exposure causes prolonged inflammation and congestion of airways and decreased ciliary action (Kum-Nji et al, 2006).

In addition, ETS may have an epigenetic effect on the fetus, causing adverse changes in the developing organism. More than 241 genes (p <0.05) tested from the placentas of smoking and nonsmoking mothers showed a change in genetic expression in those mothers who smoked (Bruchova et al, 2010). In some conditions tobacco may be a complicating rather than causal factor and other variables such as socioeconomic status and diet must also be considered.

Children, especially very young children, are exposed to tobacco smoke primarily through cigarettes, cigars, or pipes used by parents, other family members, or visitors in the home. Daycare providers or teachers also may smoke. Although smoking has decreased in the U.S., in 2007, 7.6% of U.S. children lived in households where someone smoked in the home

(Singh et al, 2010). About 12% of all pregnant women smoke and 20% of teen mothers smoke (Kum-Nji et al, 2006). ETS is also absorbed into clothing, so even if smokers abstain in the house or around children, their clothes may present a hazard (Sleiman et al, 2010).

Ninety percent of adult smokers tried their first cigarette before the age of 21 years. Every day about 4000 children and adolescents younger than age 18 smoke their first cigarette and an estimated 1200 children and adolescents become daily cigarette smokers (Fiore et al, 2008). More than 2.6 million youth ages 12 to 17 years are estimated to be cigarette smokers. The Youth Risk Behavior Survey (2009 data) revealed that 19.5% of high school students across the U.S. smoked at least once in the past 30 days and 7.3% smoked on more than 20 of the past 30 days (Eaton et al, 2010). Older, Caucasian students tend to smoke more than younger students and those from other ethnic groups. Boys tend to be heavier smokers, with 28% of twelfth-grade males smoking currently. About 9% of students reported using smokeless tobacco at least once in the 30 days before the survey and 14% reported smoking cigars. In total, 26% of students reported current cigarette, smokeless tobacco, or cigar use. Data from these studies indicate that it is easy for children to purchase cigarettes. About 15% of students who currently smoke purchased cigarettes as underage consumers from stores or gas stations (Eaton et al, 2010).

Assessment

Assessment of the extent to which ETS affects a child's health requires a thorough and accurate history. The physical problems for which children are treated vary, and the pediatric health care provider should suspect tobacco smoke as a factor in children who have recurrent respiratory and ear infections.

History. Collect data about the following:

- The amount of smoke in the child's environment. Three screening questions have proven effective for identifying risks of ETS for children:
  - ○ "Does the mother smoke now or did she smoke while pregnant?"
  - ○ "Do others smoke?"
  - ○ "Do others smoke inside?" (Groner et al, 2005)
- The amount of time the child spends in ETS environments: How long is the child exposed to ETS? Is the child ever in a car with a smoker?
- Any symptoms related to ETS: Has the child experienced health problems that may be associated with ETS (cough, colds, ear infections, etc.)?

Physical Examination and Diagnostic Studies. These will be specific to the physical signs and symptoms of the child (see Table 41-2).

Management

The best treatment for adverse affects of ETS is prevention; every effort should be made to ensure that the child's environment begins and stays smoke-free (see Table 41-2). Pregnant women should be strongly advised not to smoke at any time during their pregnancy. Children should be discouraged from starting to smoke, and those who do smoke should be helped to quit. All children should be informed about the dangers associated with smoking, and nonsmoking

---

BOX 41-2	Tobacco Use Prevention: Clinical Practice Guidelines for Children and Adolescents

Clinical Practice Recommendations

Recommendation 1	Clinicians should ask pediatric and adolescent patients about tobacco use and provide a strong message regarding the importance of totally abstaining from tobacco use. (Strength of evidence = C)
Recommendation 2	Counseling has been shown to be effective in treatment of adolescent smokers. Therefore, adolescent smokers should be provided with counseling interventions to aid them in quitting smoking. (Strength of evidence = B)
Recommendation 3	Secondhand smoke is harmful to children. Cessation counseling delivered in pediatric settings has been shown to be effective in increasing abstinence among parents who smoke. Therefore, to protect children from secondhand smoke, clinicians should ask parents about tobacco use and offer them cessation advice and assistance. (Strength of evidence = B)

From Fiore et al: *Treating tobacco use and dependence: 2008 update, clinical practice guideline.* Rockville, MD, 2008, USDHHS, Public Health Service, p 157. Available at www.ahrq.gov/path/tobacco.htm#Clinicians. Accessed April 3, 2011.

---

youth should be praised for their decision to not smoke. Young people vastly underestimate the addictive qualities of tobacco. About half of the students questioned in the Youth Risk Behavior Survey had tried to quit in the year before the study (Eaton et al, 2010). Smoking cessation is a difficult process for youth, just as it is for adults, and depends on a number of biologic, behavioral, and psychosocial factors. A complicating factor is the developmental level of most adolescents—they do not have the cognitive, emotional, and social skills of adults who themselves struggle with tobacco cessation issues.

Health care workers need to help youth and their families with decision-making regarding tobacco use and cessation. Family-based smoking prevention can be effective—parents need to be nonsmoking role models, for instance. Parental monitoring is useful. School-based smoking prevention programs could be more successful than they are, especially when managed by school nurses (Tercyak et al, 2008). In the general population, many providers ask their patients about smoking and urge them to stop, but do not provide support and follow-up intervention. Key recommendations related to children and adolescents from the Agency for Healthcare Research and Quality (AHRQ) guidelines, *Treating tobacco use and dependence: 2008 update,* are found in Box 41-2. Pediatric providers can use AHRQ guidelines to structure their smoking cessation counseling (Fiore et al, 2008). These include the "five *A*'s":

- *Ask about us:* Systematically identify tobacco users and document their status.
- *Advise to quit:* Strongly urge all smokers to quit.
- *Assess willingness to quit:* Identify smokers willing to make an attempt to quit.

- *Assist in quit attempt:* Aid the patient in quitting by offering a plan, providing education and support with nicotine replacement therapy as needed, or referring to a smoking cessation program in the community.
- *Arrange follow-up:* Schedule follow-up contact.

Because it is difficult to stop smoking, the environment in which there is a smoker must be altered to protect the child. If parents continue to smoke, smoking outside the home, not smoking in cars, and using adequate ventilation are essential. Alternative daycare arrangements should be explored if there is smoking at the child's care center.

CARBON MONOXIDE
Description
CO is a colorless, odorless, tasteless, nonirritating poisonous gas. It is formed by incomplete combustion of any fossil fuel. Improperly vented natural gas water heaters, kerosene space heaters, charcoal grills, hibachis, and Sterno stoves emit CO, as do wood stoves, gas stoves, pool heaters, and gas-powered engines (e.g., car exhaust fumes). Methylene chloride, a paint-stripping agent, is metabolized in the liver to CO. Cigarette smokers also have measurable CO blood levels of 3% to 10%.

Epidemiology
Because of its characteristics, CO is not easily detected. In the body it binds to hemoglobin 200 to 250 times more easily than oxygen does, thus diminishing oxygen-carrying capacity. It crosses the placenta and has a particular affinity for fetal hemoglobin so that the fetus of a pregnant woman exposed to CO is affected more than is the mother. In all cases the net result is tissue hypoxia. CO exposure is responsible for up to 40,000 emergency department visits and 5000 to 6000 deaths per year (Clardy et al, 2009).

Assessment
CO may affect the body in other complex ways, and children often have nonspecific neurologic and GI symptoms, including headache, drowsiness, loss of consciousness, seizure, confusion, nausea, vomiting, blurred or double vision, shortness of breath, chest pain, and palpitations. Infants and toddlers may be fussy or have feeding difficulties. Because of their higher oxygen use and higher minute ventilation, children may experience symptoms sooner than do adults around them. Because the symptoms are vague, a key indicator is similar symptoms in more than one person in a specific setting. Long-term, low-level exposure symptoms that have been reported include chronic headaches, learning difficulties, and behavioral problems. A syndrome of delayed neurologic sequelae can occur 3 to 240 days after apparent recovery from exposure (Clardy et al, 2009). Autism, blindness, seizures, urinary and fecal incontinence, psychosis, and paralysis have been reported. Cardiac symptoms may appear as the cardiovascular system tries to supply adequate oxygen to the body. Multiorgan failure can occur with acute, severe poisoning (Clardy et al, 2009). Women exposed to increased CO in their last 6 weeks of pregnancy have been found to experience more preterm births; in this study, CO was due to air pollution from automobile traffic (Ritz et al, 2007).

Management
Acute CO poisoning is treated with 100% oxygen, which shortens the half-life of carboxyhemoglobin of 5 to 6 hours to 40 to 60 minutes. Hyperbaric oxygen therapy is also used.

Prevention and Patient Education
CO detectors are available for installation in homes and are the best assurance against CO exposure. Some states require CO detectors for all new homes. Family and community education should include warnings against using space heaters, barbeques, or gas stoves in unventilated areas. Determination of the source should be paramount for all exposures to prevent risk to others.

RADON
Description
Radon is a colorless, odorless, radioactive gas that enters homes through soil or water (e.g., basement floors, cracks in concrete foundations, sumps, or drains) (see Table 41-2). As radon decays, some of its products change to an isotope of polonium, which when inhaled can cause lung damage leading to cancer. In the atmosphere, radon is diluted and has no health effect. When concentrated in an enclosed area, it represents a risk. Tobacco smoke provides a vehicle for radon to enter the lungs, adding to the risk of radon-induced cancer for smokers and individuals exposed to ETS. Water that has been filtered through the soil can contain radon (e.g., well water), and about 2% to 5% of radon in homes is found in the water supply.

Epidemiology
Radon is the second leading cause of lung cancer in Americans. Radon in water has been associated with a slightly increased incidence of gastric cancer and leukemia, and occupational exposure leads to changes in chromosomal structure. Radon is more prevalent in certain geographic areas. Local health departments can be consulted to determine if radon is a local health risk.

Assessment
In 1988, the Surgeon General recommended that all homes, except residences above the second floor in multilevel buildings, be tested for radon. Radon detector kits can be purchased in hardware, home improvement, or department stores and are available from the National Safety Council. Short-term (2 to 7 days) or long-term (3 to 12 months) testing can be done. The long-term testing gives a more accurate measure of the average radon exposure, because levels fluctuate over time and with changes in seasons; however, the EPA recommends using the short-term test.

Management
Radon mitigation involves decreasing the amount of radon entering the home and removing radon that is present (see Table 41-2). Although the EPA does not yet have standards for safe radon levels in water, it recommends that homes with a radon level of 4 picocuries per liter (pCi/L) or higher in indoor air be repaired immediately. Mitigation companies

may be certified by the National Environmental Health Association (NEHA) or the National Radon Safety Board (NRSB). Children and families should not spend significant amounts of time in high-risk areas of the home (e.g., basements). Parents need education to understand the risks because radon is not a widely known contaminant. In one study, only 21% of parents correctly understood their family's risk status from radon exposure, despite the fact that 32% of the homes in the area studied had radon levels greater than 4 pCi/L (Hill et al, 2006).

PARTICULATE MATTER

Description

Particulate matter (PM) is one of a cluster of indoor and outdoor air pollutants that have an adverse effect on respiratory and cardiovascular function. Other outdoor air pollutants include ozone, sulfur dioxide (SO_2), nitrogen oxides (NO and NO_2), and CO. The diameter of PM is measured in micrometers, and standards have been set for concentrations of PM_{10} and $PM_{2.5}$. Coarse PM (2.5 to 10 micrometers in diameter) can be filtered by the nasal mucosa or trachea and removed by coughing or sneezing. Fine PM (2.5 micrometers in diameter or smaller) is of concern because it can be inhaled and carried deep into lung tissue. Ultrafine particles also represent a serious health problem. These particles are so small (less than 100 nanometers) that they can penetrate cells, carrying toxic compounds into the individual's DNA and other critical areas. To date, they are not regulated. They cause allergic inflammation of the lung (Alessandrini et al, 2006; Grigg, 2009) and are prevalent near major roadways, exacerbating asthma in children (McConnell et al, 2010).

Epidemiology

Eighty percent of alveoli are developed after birth, so the infant and young child's developing lungs are highly susceptible to environmental toxins with demonstrated effects on both lung function and lung growth. Exposure to PM creates an inflammatory response in the body and, in combination with other pollutants, is associated with increased hospitalization rates for respiratory or cardiovascular problems. The anatomic structure of the lung may contribute to differential distribution of PM in the pulmonary tree, with subsequent cancer in particular sites. Studies have shown relationships between ambient air pollution and/or CO and infant mortality, low birthweight, and preterm birth (AAP, 2004). A 2009 study also found a relationship between $PM_{2.5}$ and onset of juvenile idiopathic arthritis (Zeft et al, 2009).

PM is a pervasive by-product of industrial production, gasoline and diesel engines, wood-burning stoves, and natural phenomena (e.g., volcanic activity, grass and forest fires, and blowing dust). Residents of urban and industrial areas are exposed to high levels of PM, and concentrations increase in summer months and when there is more combustion present (e.g., rush-hour traffic). The amount of indoor PM, including dust, mites, cockroach particles, and animal dander, varies among households, but many low-income urban residences have high levels of dust, mouse, and cockroach residue.

Assessment

Parents can keep a record of their child's illness episodes to determine if increased air pollution, dust, insects, or pets in the home are associated with illness.

Management

The goal of management is to decrease the amount of PM in the environment and limit the child's contact with PM (see Table 41-2). Minimizing exposure to diesel exhaust is one measure that families and schools can take; limiting outdoor activities in late afternoon or on hot days when pollution is highest is one strategy.

AIRBORNE POLYCYCLIC AROMATIC HYDROCARBONS

Polycyclic aromatic hydrocarbons (PAHs) are common air pollutants released from combustion of coal, diesel, and gasoline-powered engines. They are found in home heating sources, stoves, and tobacco smoke, and are listed by the EPA as probable human carcinogens. PAHs cross the placenta. The fetus and infants are more susceptible to PAH exposure with the CNS particularly affected during prenatal development (Wang et al, 2010). Studies show an average decrease of 3.8 IQ points at age 5 years for children whose mothers had higher than average exposures while pregnant (Edwards et al, 2010; Perera et al, 2009). Prenatal ambient air exposure to PAHs is positively related to increased respiratory symptoms (cough, wheezing, sore throat, ear infection) in infants. This is thought to result from impaired immune functioning (Jedrychowski et al, 2005). A newly identified source of PAH contamination is coal-tar–based pavement sealants, of which more than 59 million gallons were used in Texas in 1 year (Van Metre et al, 2009). Sealant-related dusts have also been found in apartments located near sealed pavements (Mahler et al, 2010).

MOLDS

Description

Molds are microscopic organisms in the class of bioaerosols, living organisms that can affect health through immune or nonimmune mechanisms. The cell walls of mold and the enzymes and metabolites produced during fungal growth cause allergic reactions (immune mechanism) and elicit irritant and toxic responses (Mazur and Kim, 2006). Molds thrive in damp spaces, but spores can be found in dust, dry leaves, and storage areas. *Aspergillus* (black mold), *Alternaria, Penicillium, Streptomyces, Epicoccum,* and *Cladosporium* are the most common household molds.

Epidemiology

Children have an increased risk of cough and wheezing when exposed to damp and mold. Allergic rhinitis, conjunctivitis, and asthma are common responses to mold. Pneumonitis, sinusitis, and bronchopulmonary aspergillosis are also seen with mold exposure (Mazur and Kim, 2006). Mycotoxins produced by mold spores can also cause GI, skin, neurologic, or renal problems. Infants are especially susceptible to the effects of mycotoxins and children exposed to visible mold in infancy are seven times more likely to develop asthma at age 3 years (Iossifova et al, 2009; Karvonen et al, 2009). Water damage is related to year-round asthma, and visible mold is more strongly related to winter and spring asthma (Han et al, 2009). Common sources of mold exposure for children are listed in Table 41-2.

Assessment

Assessment questions clarify the nature of symptoms, usually a spectrum of allergic reactions (see Table 41-2), and identify the cause of the symptoms:

- Is there a pattern to the symptoms?
- Are they aggravated by any particular environment?
- Are they relieved when the child changes environments?
- What has the family done to remediate the environment?

Laboratory tests to measure antigens and antibodies or to conduct immunoassays do not reliably indicate exposure or establish causal relationships between mold and illness.

Differential Diagnosis

The differential diagnosis includes other causes of allergic reactions and upper respiratory infections. Reaction to molds can be confused with pesticide poisoning.

Management

Treatment involves control of allergic symptoms (e.g., antihistamines to control itching or sneezing) (see Chapters 24 and 36 for discussion of allergies and their management) and removal of mold. The source of moisture must be eliminated because maintaining a dry (<50% humidity), clean environment minimizes the growth of molds (see Table 41-2). Ozone air cleaners are not effective against molds and may cause respiratory problems by creating ozone. Removing contaminated carpets and wiping down showers and garbage pails with a detergent and 5% bleach solution will reduce molds. Dehumidifiers can help reduce humidity in damp rooms and basements (Atkins and Leung, 2007). Children's sleeping areas should be as dry and clean of mold as possible. Provide information regarding the connection between exposure to molds, allergic reactions, and respiratory and other health problems. Parents may need support during cleanup because it may be difficult or nearly impossible to do a thorough job.

ASBESTOS

Description

Asbestos is the name given to a group of incombustible fibrous magnesium silicate minerals used most often in construction materials. Chrysolite is the only asbestos product still on the market; other forms are found in older buildings. Contamination by asbestos is measured in fibers per cubic centimeter of air. The OSHA workplace standard is 0.1 fibers per cubic centimeter averaged over an 8-hour shift or 1.0 fibers over a 30-minute period (OSHA, 2008). Levels in schools may range from 0.05 to 0.2 fibers per cubic centimeter, placing schoolchildren at relatively low risk.

Epidemiology

Asbestosis is considered an occupational problem of adults, and smokers are at higher risk of asbestos-induced lung disease than nonsmokers. Any exposure to asbestos fibers is a risk, but repeated inhalation of the fibers is associated with significant lung disease later in life. There may be a latency period of 10 to 40 years or more before conditions

such as pleural effusion, lung fibrosis, lung cancer, and mesothelioma in the pleura or peritoneum appear. Childhood exposure to asbestos may contribute to serious illness as an adult. Children can be exposed through direct contact with air in a contaminated building or with material or clothing parents bring home from their worksite. Although asbestos is found in many buildings (e.g., tiles, pipes, and insulation), it is considered a hazard only if the material is disrupted through deterioration or renovation and fibers become airborne.

Assessment

Assessment of disease is based on a history of exposure and signs and symptoms of respiratory distress. Exposure to asbestos does not typically produce acute symptoms, although high concentrations of asbestos dust can cause lung irritation, including cough, dyspnea, fatigue, and chest pain in both children and adults. The earliest symptom is usually breathlessness with exertion.

Management

There is no treatment for asbestosis. Preventing unnecessary exposure to asbestos fibers reduces the risk of inhalation and subsequent disease (see Table 41-2). If asbestos is present in the workplace, OSHA standards (not always enforced) require employers to provide workers with full-body suits and shoe covers that are left at the worksite; parents should be encouraged to work with their employers to minimize the possibility of bringing fibers into the home. Parents who work with asbestos should shower and change clothes before returning to the home. Parents should be informed of the adverse effects of asbestos exposure and reassured that their children are at low risk unless they spend significant amounts of time in older buildings that are in poor repair or undergoing renovation.

PESTICIDES

Description

Pesticides are chemicals used to kill or control unwanted pests, including plants; among these products are herbicides, fungicides, and insecticides. Pesticides are classified as "general-use" or "restricted-use" depending on their toxicity to humans or the environment. Restricted-use pesticides require special handling by certified applicators. Labeling of pesticides varies by toxicity, with a skull and crossbones and the statement "DANGER-POISON" on the most toxic; "WARNING" on less toxic; and "CAUTION" on the labels of the least toxic pesticides. All pesticides are hazardous and, although they have improved lives, they also carry significant health risks. The EPA is responsible for regulating pesticides.

Epidemiology

Approximately 5 billion pounds of pesticides are used in the U.S. annually; chlorine and hypochlorites are the major category in use (52% of all pesticides) (EPA, 2006). About 600 pesticide products are registered with the EPA (Landrigan and Forman, 2007). They are used in agriculture; in forests to control insects; on boat hulls to control fungi and growth; in and around houses, schools, and commercial and office buildings to control insects and rodents; in landscaping and recreational areas to control weeds and insects; and in aquatic areas to control mosquitoes. Wood products may be impregnated with chemicals to retard decay and insect damage. Humans and animals may be treated with insecticides.

Herbicides are the most widely used pesticide, and contaminated food products are a major source of exposure. Because of children's small size and large fruit and vegetable intake per unit of body weight, they ingest pesticides in foods at a disproportionately higher rate than adults. Farm workers and children who live on or near farms are exposed to agricultural pesticides. Garden and lawn use increases risks to children playing outdoors in treated areas. Pesticide routes of exposure are oral, inhalation, and dermal. Incidental exposure via residues is most common among children.

Pesticides are increasingly implicated in fetal development and childhood illness (Landrigan and Forman, 2007). Polyneuropathy, CNS dysfunction, hormonal disruption, cancer and pulmonary fibrosis have been linked to various pesticides. Childhood leukemia has also been linked to prenatal maternal occupational exposure to pesticides (Wigle et al, 2008). Bouchard and associates (2010) report increased ADHD among children with increased organophosphate pesticide residues in their urine, especially malathion. Although they are being phased out, chlorpyrifos and diazinon, which are organophosphate insecticides, have been heavily used in inner cities. They are transferred to the fetus if the mother is exposed, and both have been linked to decreased birth weight and birth length. If both pesticides are present, a synergistic effect has been found (Perera et al, 2005). A study of clinical exposures to agricultural pesticides and birth defects in South Africa found that babies born to women exposed to chemicals used in gardens and fields were seven times more likely to have birth defects than babies of women who reported no exposures. A study of children's developmental capacity has demonstrated significant developmental differences in native Yaqui children from Mexico exposed to pesticides versus a cohort not exposed (Guillette, 2000). Chemicals labeled as "inert" are also raising concerns in the U.S. One might interpret "inert" to mean "harmless," but many hazardous inert ingredients have been shown to present risks of injury to humans. These include coal tar, dibutyl phthalate, hydrochloric acid, kerosene, naphthalene, nitric acid, and others. The EPA is considering changes to require industry to disclose more of the ingredients in products, but industry officials worry that having their secret formulations disclosed will affect their market share (Weinhold, 2010).

Assessment

Adverse effects of pesticide exposure can be acute or chronic, and all body systems can be affected, depending on the nature of the toxin and the extent of exposure. Assessment must be comprehensive (see Table 41-2). In acute exposure, assessment is the same as with general poisoning. Acute poisoning with organophosphates or carbamates results in clinical signs of cholinergic excess (i.e., bradycardia, tearing, salivation, bronchospasm, urination, emesis, diarrhea, diaphoresis).

Neurologic disorders may occur 24 to 96 hours after exposure and delayed neurotoxicity may occur 1 to 3 weeks after exposure (Bird, 2009).

Much data about pesticide poisoning are based on studies in adults, so chronic exposure in children presents a more complicated picture. There is concern that the effect of pesticides on children differs, and the risk children face for long-term health problems is seriously underestimated.

Management

Specifics of management depend on the type and amount of pesticide taken in and the route of absorption. Information on treatment is available on product labels. When treating an individual who may have been exposed to pesticides, health care providers, by law, are entitled to access information about the implicated pesticides. The EPA's Worker Protection Standard (WPS) also ensures that providers will be able to access information on general- and restricted-use pesticides. Under the WPS this information can be obtained from employers or manufacturers. Patients may be able to provide the clinician with the pesticide label. Treatment focuses on supporting life functions:

- ABCs (airway, breathing, circulation)
  - Maintain gas exchange; may need to intubate.
  - Prevent aspiration of vomitus.
- Consult with a poison control center for direction in management (refer to a center or provider with expertise in this area as soon as possible; see previous discussion for management of general poisonings).
- Control seizures.
- Report pesticide exposure to the state health department.
- Work with parents, schools, and community agencies to prevent pesticide exposure.

Prevention and Patient Education

The risks pesticides present to children are immense. Pesticide exposure occurs in a number of ways and is additive. Regulating the amount of pesticide children take in from any one source is good, but the pattern of multiple contaminations must be recognized and a plan to regulate overall exposure developed. Education of parents is key in preventing pesticide poisoning in children (Table 41-4). Steps can be taken to reduce pesticide use, which in turn reduces exposure. Integrated pest management combines physical, cultural, biologic, and other means of pest control with minimal use of pesticides. For example, farms might encourage cats to catch mice rather than using rodenticides, or school cafeterias might use bait traps for cockroaches rather than chemical spray. Herbicides on athletic fields could be applied as spot treatments rather than broadcast widely. Pregnant women need to avoid occupational levels of pesticides if at all possible. To reduce pesticide ingestion by children, fruits and vegetables should be washed with water to remove surface residues. But pesticides used in growing the products may be incorporated throughout the plant, so families should choose foods that are local, in season, and organically grown as much as possible. A list of hazardous and safer fruits and vegetables is found in Table 41-4. Organic diets significantly lower children's dietary exposure to organophosphorus pesticides (Lu et al, 2006).

TABLE 41-4	Pesticide Content of Common Fruits and Vegetables
"Dirty Dozen" **(Buy These Organic)**	**"Clean 15"** **(Lowest in Pesticides)**
Celery (Worst)	Onions (Best)
Peaches	Avocados
Strawberries	Sweet corn
Apples	Pineapple
Blueberries	Mangos
Nectarines	Sweet peas
Bell peppers	Asparagus
Spinach	Kiwi
Cherries	Cabbage
Kale/collard greens	Eggplant
Potatoes	Cantaloupe
Grapes (imported)	Watermelon
	Grapefruit
	Sweet potato
	Honeydew melon

Adapted from *FoodNews* Environmental Working Group. Available at www.foodnews.org/executive.php (accessed Oct 26, 2010).

ENDOCRINE DISRUPTORS

Description

Endocrine disruptors are chemicals that may have the most serious effects on living organisms on our planet. The book, *Our Stolen Future,* by Colborn and colleagues (1996), brought their existence to public awareness. Endocrine disruptors are found extensively in the environment including in food, water, soil, air, plastics, cosmetics, and drugs. They alter the function of endocrine hormones through a variety of mechanisms, including binding to hormone receptors to mimic natural hormones, blocking hormone receptors, or altering the production or metabolism of endogenous hormones. It is hypothesized that a "U"-shape effect occurs: extremely low doses and extremely high doses have significant effects, thus traditional toxicologic concepts such as "dose-response" may not apply. Concentrations as low as one tenth of a trillion of a gram can alter the womb environment. Endocrine disruptors can interfere with gene expression, changing developing tissues in permanent ways. Polychlorinated biphenyls, bisphenol A, and phthalates are only three of the many endocrine disruptors present in the environment.

Epidemiology

Many conditions and illnesses that are affected by endocrine function have increased in the past few decades. Abnormal gonadal development, infertility, ADHD, autism, intellectual

BOX 41-3	Hormonal Determinants of Behavior in Humans

- Sexual differentiation of the brain
- Sexual behavior
- Courtship, mating, motivation
- Maternal behavior
- Aggressive and attack behaviors
- Sensory-motor function
- Stress responses
- Cognitive function
- Learning and performance
- Play behavior

impairment, diabetes, thyroid disorders, and some child and adult cancers have been linked to fetal exposures (TEDX, 2010). Between 1973 and 1999, rates of prostate cancer rose about 80% in Americans. The rate of hypospadias and related disorders, such as cryptorchidism and testicular cancer, collectively referred to as testicular dysgenesis syndrome, has also risen significantly. Male fertility has declined over the past 50 years with sperm counts 50% less than they were 50 years ago in some agricultural states. Female reproductive disorders of the ovaries, uterus, breast, and pubertal timing are negatively affected by endocrine disruptors (Crain et al, 2008).

Cancer caused by diethylstilbestrol is a classic example of disease following prenatal exposure to an endocrine disruptor. Phthalates have been linked to asthma symptoms in children. Reduced anogenital distance in male infants (Marsee et al, 2006) and altered semen quality in subfertile men (Hauser et al, 2006) are also associated with exposure. A list of cognitive and behavioral characteristics of humans that are affected by endocrine hormones is found in Box 41-3. Some common endocrine disruptors, their sources, effects, and alternatives for use are found in Table 41-5.

POLYCHLORINATED BIPHENYLS

Description

Polychlorinated biphenyls (PCBs), a family of up to 209 chemicals, are one type of extremely stable organochlorines. Many organochlorines are endocrine disruptors. PCBs used commercially are always mixtures of the various types and are frequently contaminated with furans and dioxins. PCBs are structurally similar to thyroid hormones. They probably work through changes in hormonal function, altering concentrations of hormones or affecting receptor numbers or affinity. PCBs have been shown to affect levels of circulating thyroid hormones, especially T4. Effects have also been found on the human immune system.

Epidemiology

Although banned from production since 1977, PCBs are so stable that they are still commonly found in the environment, even in Arctic mammals (Colborn et al, 1996). Low levels are found throughout the world, evaporating and returning

TABLE 41-5	Endocrine Disruptors			
Type Agent	**Chemical Group**	**Products Containing the Chemical**	**Known Toxic Effects**	**Alternatives**
Industrial chemicals	Bisphenol A (BPA)	Plastics: polycarbonates and polystyrene used in flame retardants and plastic food containers, bottles, dental sealants, linings for metal cans; most baby bottles may leach BPA	Rodent studies: mammary tissue, reduced sperm production, increased prostate weight, accelerated growth, early puberty in females	High density polyethylene (HDPE) (opaque or translucent plastics such as milk bottles) Avoid use of products with BPA or wash with mild detergent, rinse well. Use glass or ceramic containers for storage and reheating of food.
	Polychlorinated biphenyls (PCBs), dioxins, furans	Electrical capacitors, transformers, carbonless copy paper, produced with some manufacturing of paper and plastic, chemicals Recently found in caulking for old windows	*PCBs:* decreased birth weight, increases weight in adolescent females. No effect on pubertal development. Changes thyroid utilization; neurodevelopmental delays and learning problems; increased breast cancer risk. *Dioxins:* cancer, birth defects, learning disabilities, infertility, endometriosis, immune suppression	No longer manufactured in U.S. but may be found in fish that lived in contaminated waters Limit fish consumption of fish at risk. Bioaccumulates
	Phthalates	Plastics: polyvinyl chloride and other plastic products, nail polish, hair spray, inks, adhesives	Premature thelarche, endometriosis, shorter gestation; lower serum testosterone levels in infants exposed to high phthalates from breast milk. Animal studies: testicular dysgenesis in males, suppression of endogenous testosterone, suspected carcinogen	Do not use polyethylene terephthalate (PETE or PET) found in clear containers such as soda bottles, bottled water; do not use PVC cling wraps. Do not reheat foods in Styrofoam. Low density polyethylene (LDPE) used in many food storage bags is okay. Polypropylene (PP) found in storage containers such as Rubbermaid, Ziploc, Gladware, Tupperware is considered safe.
	Polybrominated phenyls (PBB, PBDEs)	Fire retardants	Early onset of menstruation following in utero exposure	Avoid using these materials
	Persistent aromatic hydrocarbons (PAHs)	Industrial pollution, tobacco tar, charred foods	Carcinogen	
Pesticides	DDT/DDE, dieldrin, alachlor, atrazine, malathion, pentachlorophenol, benomyl, aldrin	Insecticides, fungicides, herbicides, wood preservatives	DDT/DDE: possible links to breast cancer; alachlor: probable carcinogen; alachlor and atrazine: antiestrogenic activity with decreased semen quality	Vary food intake of produce to limit exposure; wash produce before eating; choose organic and local, in-season produce if possible. Use traps for insects rather than spraying. Avoid pesticide-sprayed areas for a few days. For pest prevention indoors, clean up food and spills, don't leave pet food out overnight, keep lids on trash, clean dirty dishes right away, eat at the table only, get rid of stacks of paper.

Adapted from DiDiego ML et al: Unmasking the truth behind endocrine disruptors, *Nurse Pract* 30:54-59, 2005.

to earth by rainfall and settling in dust particles. PCBs are not very water soluble, and as a result are not found in high concentrations in drinking water. They dissolve readily in oils, accumulating in the fatty tissues of fish, birds, and mammals. Human exposure comes primarily through ingestion of contaminated foods. Channel catfish, large lake trout, and carp may have high levels. Yellow perch, lake whitefish, smelt, sunfish, and wild ocean salmon have low levels. For children, fetal and neonatal exposures are common, usually via maternal ingestion of contaminated food. Schoolchildren can be exposed through deteriorating building materials since PCBs are found in fluorescent light fixtures and caulking material for windows in older buildings (Herrick et al, 2004). In the U.S., the workplace is a major source of exposure to PCBs.

Assessment
History
- History of maternal ingestion of contaminated food
- Skin disorders, including hyperpigmentation, nail changes, and chloracne
- Hepatic dysfunction
- Low birthweight and developmental delays
- Behavioral symptoms
- Frequent respiratory infections

Physical Examination. Clinical effects are listed in Table 41-2.

Diagnostic Studies. Increased liver enzymes with severe exposure, although these findings are nonspecific.

Differential Diagnosis
The differential diagnosis includes acne vulgaris, other causes of developmental delay, lead poisoning, and hypothyroidism.

Management
Avoid contact with PCB-contaminated food and environmental sources, especially prenatally. Do not stop breastfeeding.

PHTHALATES
Phthalates are industrial compounds used in the production of soft plastics; they subsequently leach from the plastic into the environment. Di(2-ethylhexyl)phthalate (DEHP) is the most commonly used compound. Phthalates are found in cosmetics and fragrances of personal care products (Engle et al, 2010). They are also found in polyvinyl chloride (PVC) toys, vinyl shower curtains, car seats, wallpaper, floor coverings, and many other products (Hall, 2006). In utero phthalate exposure has been associated with preterm birth. It is believed that phthalates interfere with the way the mother uses essential fatty acids that are critical to fetal development (Latini et al, 2006; Whyatt et al, 2009). They also interfere with thyroid homeostasis. Phthalates are associated with testicular dysgenesis (decreased sperm counts, testicular cancer, cryptorchidism, and hypospadias) in male offspring (Goldman, 2010; Hauser et al, 2006), and have been linked to decreased semen quality and endometriosis.

Humans are exposed through dermal, ingestion, and inhalation routes. Many hospitals are removing all DEHP-containing products from patient care, especially from neonatal units. This includes intravenous (IV) tubing, IV bags, umbilical catheters, and other soft plastic materials.

BISPHENOL A
Description
Bisphenol A (BPA) is a chemical that mimics estrogen. It is used in production of polycarbonate plastics and epoxy resins. Polycarbonates are the rigid plastics used in kitchen appliances, reusable water bottles, baby bottles, compact disks, and water coolers. Epoxy resins are strong adhesives and are used as coatings (e.g., liners for food and beverage cans), paints, dental sealants, and water main filters.

Epidemiology
Many studies have linked low-dose BPA exposure to developmental, reproductive, behavioral, and neurologic sequelae (Vogel, 2008). In adults, BPA exposure is linked to cardiovascular disease and diabetes (Lang et al, 2008). The U.S. produced more than 2 billion pounds of BPA in 2004. In response to public concerns, some companies are eliminating BPA from their products. Baby bottle manufacturers use BPA-free products. Infant formula makers and some canned food producers are also eliminating BPA from their products.

Management
The USDHHS has recommended the following actions to decrease exposure of children to BPA:
- Breastfeed.
- Use BPA-free bottles.
- Discard scratched infant feeding cups.
- Do not use boiling water in plastic dishes or bottles, or heat formula or water in plastics.
- Make sure to use "dishwasher safe" and "microwave safe" containers.
- Avoid use of plastic food storage containers with #7 stamped on the bottom (USDHHS, 2010).

NOISE
Description
Noise is defined as any sound, but is usually considered loud, harsh, unpleasant, or unwanted. Noise pollution is the presence of irritating, distracting, or physically dangerous noise. Sound has qualities of frequency or pitch (measured in cycles per minute and stated in hertz [Hz]), intensity or loudness (measured in decibels [dB]), periodicity, and duration (either continuous, short-term, or episodic). The human voice is approximately 50 dB sound pressure levels (Etzel and Balk, 2003). The National Institute for Occupational Safety and Health (NIOSH) defines hazardous noise as 85 decibels for an average of 8 hours of sound exposure (Chepesiuk, 2005), and the WHO sets 55 dB as a safe noise level guideline (Berglund, 1999). "White noise" or very low-level background noise may also be unwanted, though it does not necessarily cause

TABLE 41-6	Noise in the Environment
Noise Source	**Decibels**
Quiet room	28-33
Computer	37-45
Refrigerator	40-43
Normal conversation	40
Forced-air heating system	42-52
Dishwasher	54-85
Microwave oven	55-59
Alarm clock	60-80
Vacuum cleaner	62-85
Telephone	66-75
Inside car, windows closed, 30 mph	68-73
Electric shaver	75
Gas-powered lawn mower	87-92
Average motorcycle	90
Leaf blower	95-105
Maximum output of stereo	100-120
Average snowmobile	120
Average rock concert	140

Data from Chepesiuk R: Decibel hell: the effects of living in a noisy world, *Environ Health Perspect* 113(1):A34-A47, 2005.

hearing loss; in fact, it appears to have a positive effect on some children with attention disorders, improving their cognitive performance (Söderlund et al, 2010). (See Chapter 15, Cognitive-Perceptual Disorders for further discussion of children with hearing loss. Chapter 29 also discusses ear disorders and Table 41-6 lists decibels for common sounds.)

Epidemiology

The effect of noise on human health is varied. Noise-induced hearing loss (NIHL) and tinnitus are the most obvious effects. Hearing loss is a growing problem in the pediatric population, especially among adolescents. NHANES data from 2005 to 2006 indicate that 19.5% of children 12 to 19 years old have demonstrable hearing loss, mostly at higher frequencies, and often unilateral. This is a significant increase from the 1988-1994 NHANES finding that 14.9% of the same age cohort had hearing loss. Children from families below the federal poverty level are more likely to suffer hearing loss (Shargorodsky et al, 2010).

Humans are subject to NIHL from exposure to continuous noise or to sudden acoustic trauma that causes damage to the hair cells of the cochlea due to excessive vibration; extreme noise can rupture the tympanic membrane. Noise of more than 85 dB but less than 140 dB leads to temporary hearing loss, most often in the 4000 Hz range. Permanent hearing loss can result from one exposure to a sudden, extreme noise (greater than 120 dB in children) of short duration, or from ongoing lower levels of noise. Permanent loss is often in the 3000 to 6000 Hz range. Music listened to on headphones, earbuds, and at concerts; firecrackers; electrical tools; and airport noise can cause hearing loss. Chronic, everyday noise causes sleep disturbance, distraction, decreased concentration, and an increased stress response (e.g., increased heart rate, blood pressure, adrenaline, and cortisol production); these in turn result in personality changes, irritability, poor coping, and lower achievement in children. Studies show, for example, that highway and aircraft noise are directly associated with impaired cognition on reading comprehension and cognitive tasks (Clark et al, 2006; van Kempen et al, 2010). The AAP Committee on Environmental Health Policy notes that excessive noise exposure results in high-frequency hearing loss in newborns and that excessive noise in intensive care units may disrupt the natural growth and development of premature infants (Etzel et al, 1997). Though language acquisition is a complex process, young children who are exposed to chronic or excessive noise may have difficulty perceiving clearly the language sounds necessary to master speech well.

Noise and hearing loss are often associated with tinnitus (Mazurek et al, 2010). Tinnitus in adolescents contributes to mental health stress, increased alcohol and illicit drug consumption, and school problems (Brunnberg et al, 2008).

Assessment

History. A careful history looks at the following:
- Type of noise in child's environment
- Exposure to chronic noise
- Episodic acoustic trauma
- History of ear disease
- History of prematurity or exposure to ototoxic drugs

Physical Examination. The CDC recommends universal screening of all newborns for congenital or birth-related hearing loss. Automated auditory brainstem response (AABR) or otoacoustic emissions (OAE) testing are commonly used. This testing establishes a baseline; newborns with hearing loss should be seen by a specialist no later than 3 months of age. Thereafter all children should be assessed for hearing using a pure-tone audiometer at the 4-, 5-, 10-, 12-, and 18-year-old well-child examinations. Visual examination of the tympanic membrane with insufflation should be done at every well-child visit. Tympanography can help rule out otitis media and middle ear effusion.

Management

Noise-induced hearing loss is virtually 100% preventable. The goals of management are to:
- Increase awareness of the health hazard noise represents. Parents and children need to understand the relationship between noise and the auditory system. Every well-child visit should include questions related to the child's noise environment, and both children and parents should be given information on the dangers of excessive noise and how to avoid them. Primary care providers can work with parents and schools to offer a hearing loss management curriculum.

- Decrease noise in the environment. Parents and children should be encouraged to minimize noise in their environment, including efforts to:
  ○ Reduce volume on television and radios; turn off "background" TVs and radios.
  ○ Use headphones cautiously, keeping the volume low enough to hear normal conversation.
  ○ Avoid loud music, firecrackers and other sources of episodic, extreme noise.
  ○ Avoid loud noises; for example, do not vacuum or use appliances (e.g., blender) with infants nearby.
  ○ Create a "quiet" place in the home.
- Mitigate exposure to noise. Wear earplugs and earmuffs to protect against "unavoidable" noise. Commercial-quality ear protectors are available for use in the home (e.g., when electrical saws or other loud tools are used). Earplugs can be purchased at any pharmacy.

- Implement standards to regulate noise. The Federal Noise Control Act of 1972 provides the mechanism to set standards, rules, and regulations for occupational, industrial, and residential noise (e.g., automobiles and construction). States and municipalities have also established standards for noise control. Pediatric providers can be a resource to policymakers by providing information about the health effects of excessive and chronic noise.

Complementary Medicine

CATHERINE G. BLOSSER

National dialogue and legislative action occurred in 2010 that addressed health care reform. This reform focused largely on who would pay for health care, how much it would cost, services covered, who would have health care, and the role of insurance companies as a vehicle for accessing much of it. Less visible was the conversation taking place in health care clinics among providers and their patients, and among academicians, researchers, and economists. This dialogue is not new; it is gaining momentum and causing a paradigm shift. It is about the underlying clinical, academic, and philosophical foundations that drive conventional Western medicine, and it is causing the institutionalization of what was once regarded to be unconventional therapy into the mainstream education and practices of nursing and medicine.

The realization that change was needed is eloquently described by many conventional practitioners: "What we have now is a 'sick care' system that is reactive to problems. The integrative approach flips the system on its head and puts the patient at the center, addressing not just symptoms, but the real causes of illness. It is care that is preventive, predictive, and personalized" (Snyderman, 2010). For example, the health care system must "take account of the insufficiency of science and technology alone to shape the ideal practice of medicine" (Snyderman and Weil, 2002, p 5). "If clinicians understand this concept, they will recognize that they must start their relationship with their patient from an entirely new place" (Gaudet, 2010, p 29).

What follows will bring the reader to a better understanding of how the health care system model may be changing as a "gathering" of human wisdom endeavors to join rather than continue to divide a patient into small pieces.

◼ Use of Complementary Therapies

It is estimated that in some Asian and African countries, 80% of the population rely on non-Western or indigenous traditional medicine for primary health care. In many developed countries, 70% to 80% of individuals have used some form of alternative or complementary treatment (World Health Organization [WHO], 2008). According to an analysis of the 2007 U.S. National Health Interview Survey (NHIS) (Barnes et al, 2008), 38% of adults and 12% of children younger than the age of 18 years (with or without congruent conventional medicine) reported using some form of complementary or alternative medicine (CAM) within the prior 6 months. Vitamins and minerals were not included in these statistics. It is surmised that the reported rates in children may be higher in immigrant communities, where cultures using nontraditional medicine regard such practices as mainstream rather than "alternative" (Lazar, 2008). Birdee and colleagues (2010) found that nearly five times as many children used CAM if a parent also reported using CAM.

COMPLEMENTARY MEDICINE USE IN CHILDREN

For the first time, the 2007 NHIS elicited information regarding CAM use by specific age groups younger than the age of 18 years. Results revealed use rates at 7.6% in those birth to 4 years old; 10.7% for 5- to 11-year-olds; and 16.4% of those 12 to 17 years. For those between 18 and 29 years, CAM use was 36%. In those less than 18 years the most commonly used therapies were *natural products* (most commonly echinacea, fish oil/omega 3, combination herb pills, and flaxseed oil/pills), chiropractics, deep breathing, yoga, homeopathic treatment, traditional healers, massage, meditation, diet-based therapies, and progressive relaxation. CAM therapies were used predominantly for back and neck pain; head or chest colds; anxiety and stress; other musculoskeletal conditions; attention-deficit/hyperactivity disorder (ADHD); and insomnia. *Mind-body therapies* were most commonly used for anxiety and stress, insomnia, and nausea and vomiting; *biologically based therapies* were used for symptoms of fever, insomnia, reflex, and sinusitis; and *manipulation/body-work* was used for abdominal pain, musculoskeletal conditions, and nausea and vomiting. Additional common medical conditions or symptoms for which CAM was used included allergies, asthma, dermatological conditions, developmental disorders, gastrointestinal (GI) conditions, headaches, insomnia, learning disabilities, overweight, and psychological conditions. These treatment modalities were not broken down by age group.

Further analysis of the 2007 NHIS led to a more complete description of the child population using CAM. Use was higher among adolescents, non-Hispanic Caucasians, and those living in households earning more than $65,000, who had a college-educated parent, and who lived in states other than the South. Use was higher in those with private medical insurance and in those who also took prescription medicines in the last 3 months. The chosen therapies were used not only to treat illness but also to prevent it. CAM use in children was often predicated on difficulties accessing medical care; also they experienced higher school absenteeism because of illness. The higher the number of health conditions and clinic visits in the past year, the more likely the child was to seek CAM treatment. There was little difference between CAM use and gender or race except when biologically based and manipulation/bodywork therapies were chosen (Birdee et al, 2010).

A literature review by Kemper and colleagues found that approximately 20% to 40% of general pediatric patients had used CAM therapies. The number increased to 50% for children with chronic, recurrent, and incurable conditions (Kemper et al, 2008a); to 64% for children with special needs, as defined by the Maternal and Child Health Bureau of the U.S. Department of Health and Human Services (Sanders et al, 2003); up to 79% for adolescents (Wilson et al, 2006); and up to 70% for homeless adolescents (Kemper et al, 2008a). The use of dietary supplements (multivitamins, minerals, iron, ergogenic agents) by young children was greater than 50% and from 27% to 30% by adolescents (Gardiner et al, 2004; 2008).

Little has been known about the use of *homeopathic* products (HP) remedies in children. Notable is a study that was administered to the same cohort of children at seven different times from their birth to 8.5 years of age. Slightly less than 12% used HP, with the most common time for administration around 7 years of age. Parents were self-treating children with HP 46% of the time versus having the remedy prescribed by a general practitioner (10%). Ten percent of the parents voiced uncertainty in the definition of HP. Chamomilla for teething and colic and arnica for soft-tissue bruising or cuts were the most commonly used products (Thompson et al, 2010).

Adolescents and their CAM use patterns have received some focus. Reznik and coworkers (2002) revealed that 80% of adolescents reported using CAM therapies for asthma. Wilson and colleagues (2006) showed a correlation between being female, having a positive attitude about CAM use, and being 16 to 17 years of age. Ginseng, zinc, echinacea, ginkgo, weight loss supplements, and creatine were commonly cited supplements in use, with 9% being taken at the same time as prescription medicines in the previous month. A desire to alter body shape was linked with the use of weight loss products and creatine. Those who suffered from chronic headaches reported increased use rates; those reporting fair or poor health status were less likely to use supplements (Gardiner et al, 2008).

Reasons cited by parents for choosing an array of CAM therapies for their children include the following (Barnes et al, 2008; Gardiner et al, 2004):

- Cost
- Maintenance of health and prevention of diseases
- Limited access to or dissatisfaction with traditional care; ready access to CAM practitioners
- Failure of traditional medicine to have an effect on chronic conditions (six or more concurrent health conditions are associated with higher CAM use) (Barnes et al, 2008)

- Awareness of complications and side effects produced by pharmaceuticals
- Discomfort associated with invasive procedures or diagnostics
- Ethnic and cultural beliefs
- Belief that alternative practices are more natural, less harmful, and more effective
- Parents are CAM users
- Belief that by combining conventional and nonconventional treatment a more effective approach to health care is achieved than either practice alone affords
- Awareness of the mind-body connection to affect the immune system response
- Desire for more parental, active participation in their child's treatment

■ History of Complementary Medical Practices in The United States

Before 1910, many different medical and apprenticeship schools allowed graduates to be licensed and referred to as "doctors." With acceptance of the 1910 Flexner report, all medical training, licensure, and regulation in the U.S. became standardized with "approved" medical education based on science and research. Only medical training schools that could meet the rigorous Flexner standards were accredited; graduates were recognized as legitimate medical doctors. Although these standards effectively put many charlatans and snake oil medical practitioners out of work, many other nonconventional medical practitioners were also disqualified or their practices severely limited. The philosophies and practices of chiropractic, naturopathy, osteopathy, homeopathy, herbal treatments, and others fell into the unaccredited category. By excluding these disciplines, the medical community failed to consider the efficacy, benefits, and applications of the healing and treatment theories that these other practices had to offer. Rapid advances in immunology, pathology, and the seduction of technology solidly secured the dominance of the rational-empirical approach, which became known as Western, allopathic, conventional, biomedical, scientific, rational, regular, orthodox, or mainstream medicine. All ailments were expected to fit within a scientific conceptual framework (Janiger and Goldberg, 1993).

In the 1960s a number of doctors and patients began to express disillusionment with the strict limitations of accepted medical practices. The "holistic" health care movement of the 1970s evolved as patients and disaffected medical providers began to refocus health care toward healing, prevention, and the spiritual and environmental factors that affect health. From these contexts, the current trend toward combining the best of Western and nontraditional medicine grew.

Certain basic principles are common to all nonconventional treatment modalities (Micozzi, 1997). These principles include the following:

- A focus on wellness, that, in turn, prevents illness
- Self-healing—focusing external manipulations that stimulate the body's internal healing processes
- Bioenergy—ensuring that the body's energy forces are balanced

- Nutrition, plants, and other natural products—obtaining nutrients from natural food sources to maintain or return to health
- Individuality—recognition and use of the individual's unique constitution, inner resources, and so forth to achieve health

Moving Towards an Integrated Health Care Model

Various phrases have been used to describe health practices that are not fully embraced by conventional Western medicine practices. These terms include *alternative, complementary, contemporary, holistic, integrative, folk, irregular, mind-body medicine, natural, New Age, new medicine, nonconventional, nontraditional, quackery,* and *vernacular medicine.* Representatives of both the dominant and nondominant medical practices more routinely use the terms *complementary* and *integrative* instead of *alternative.* Dr. Wayne Jonas, the first Director of the Office of Alternative Medicine at the National Institutes of Health (NIH), observed that these terms represented "practices that aren't part of the politically dominant medical system of a country" (Wysocki, 1997, p 4). To be acknowledged as a component of the dominant medical system, a particular medical practice must be taught in medical schools, be available in hospitals or conventional health clinics, and be reimbursable by third-party payers (Wysocki, 1997). A Bravewell Collaborative report summarizes the position of integrative medicine practitioners and educators: "Integrative health care is derived from lessons integrated across scientific disciplines and it requires scientific processes that cross domains. The most important influences on health, for individuals and society, are not the factors at play within any single-domain genetics, behavior, social or economic circumstances, physical environment, health care—but the dynamics and synergies across domains. Medical and basic science research tend to examine these influences in isolation, which can distort interpretation of the results" (Bravewell Collaborative, 2010, p 27).

The integrative approach is not without its critics. Cassileth summed up the criticism by stating that "not all mainstream physicians are pleased with CAM, with current efforts to integrate CAM into mainstream medicine, or with a separate NIH research entity for 'alternative' medicine" (Cassileth, 1999, p 365).

The most effective treatment may involve using therapeutic applications from several different approaches. Successful primary health care providers benefit from moving between paradigms without prejudice, gleaning what is of value, and knowing when referral to a complementary medical practitioner is appropriate. Table 42-1 lists many of the complementary therapies in use. (Specific applications to pediatric or adolescent diagnoses are discussed at the end of the chapter in Table 42-5.)

THE ROLE OF PRIMARY HEALTH CARE PROVIDERS IN AN INTEGRATED HEALTH CARE SYSTEM

Medicine needs to return to an "art of healing," for "dependence on the 'quick fix' has made us less self-reliant regarding matters of health. The focus in medicine should be on creating an environment in which the body needs as few of these fixes as possible, and people become less dependent on the medical system, not more" (Rakel, 2003, p 8). The Bravewell Collaborative offers a Patient's Bill of Rights for delineating what individuals should expect from their health care system and providers (Box 42-1). The updated "role" of the clinician who uses the integrative medicine model focuses on the patient as a unique individual, looks at the complex phenomenon of health and disease, appreciates the concept of inherent healing capacity, and uses scientific research (Stumpf et al, 2008). Patients are seen as the primary agents influencing the status of their own health; the practitioner helps mobilize the interplay between biology, behavior, psychosocial factors, and environment. One practitioner describes the effort as one of augmenting host resistance (enhancing the overall immune response or constitutional state) rather than one of attacking the disease (treating, controlling, and suppressing symptoms) (Schoch, 1999).

Kreitzer and colleagues describe a future health care system that increases access to an integrative medical home and "teamlet" (comprised of primary care providers and "health coaches" in a 1:2 to 5 ratio). The focus would be on whole-person care, emphasizing lifestyle choices, behaviors, outcomes, health promotion, and disease prevention using conventional and CAM approaches. The health coach would spend more time with the patient; costs are predicted to decrease (unnecessary hospitalizations and emergency visits) because the health coaches would be intensively managing high-risk and high-use clinic patrons (Gawande, 2011; Kreitzer et al, 2009).

Health care providers who do not choose to integrate CAM therapies into their own practices can be effective by having sufficient knowledge, sensitivity, and willingness to support and help patients make informed decisions about their use. Sixty-three percent of adults believed that their own medical care would improve if communication between their medical doctor and their alternative care provider increased (Landmark Healthcare, 1998).

Complementary Practices of Health Care Providers in the U.

Eighty-one percent of surveyed health care providers i porate vitamins, minerals, or other nonherbal dietary s ments in their personal health regimens (Gardiner et al. Those that do not personally use herbs and dietary ments demonstrate a lower degree of general kn confidence, and communication skills about these (Kemper et al, 2006a).

The last periodic survey of pediatric fellows done by the American Academy of Pediatrics (A that 87% of them had at least one inquiry ab mentary medicine therapy from patients or prior 3 months; however, few proactively ask if they were using any type of CAM therap often were about the use of herbs, dietary ropractic therapies, or special diets. When thetical patient who had a recurrent uppe it was rare for the pediatricians to recor therapy (other than chicken soup or a v out eucalyptus oil). Yet, 72.8% of the they should be providing more infor

TABLE 42-1	Complementary Therapies and Their Applications	
Nonconventional Therapy	**Theory Behind Use**	**Treatment Applications***
Acupressure	Similar principle as acupuncture but uses fingertips instead of needles to apply pressure (see Acupuncture) Also incorporates breathing techniques to aid healing by balancing mind-body-spirit	Muscle tension, targeting a specific organ or glandular systems Usually more acceptable to children than acupuncture
Acupuncture	Hair-thin needles inserted at specific anatomical points to mobilize a limbic-paralimbic-neocortical network and its anticorrelated sensorimotor/paralimbic network at multiple levels of the brain The hemodynamic response is influenced by the psychophysical response (Hui et al, 2010) Blockages in energy flow patterns are altered along "meridians" and stimulate body to produce pain-relieving and mood-lifting chemicals or antiinflammatory substances (sterile, disposable needles should always be used) (University of California, Berkeley, 1998).	Morning sickness of pregnancy Postoperative dental pain Chronic pain (including headaches) Allergies Asthma Nausea and vomiting (including chemotherapy induced and postsurgical) Menstrual cramps Migraine headaches Low back pain Addictions (e.g., smoking) Musculoskeletal pain (e.g., arthritis, fibromyalgia, carpal tunnel syndrome, tendinitis)
Aromatherapy	Uses pure, essential, volatile oils containing oxygenated molecules to transport nutrients to cells of the body Believed to promote immunity and create a cellular environment in which disease-causing bacteria, fungi, and viruses cannot live Aromas of essential oils are either inhaled or absorbed through the skin. When inhaled, believed to activate the brain's amygdala (associated with memory and emotions). Taught in medical schools in France; used in Japanese in factories to increase productivity (Krebs, 2006).	Stress, anxiety, depression, agitation Fatigue Immune disorders Acute and chronic pain Insomnia Intrapartum: strengthens contractions
...vedic medicine	The traditional form of medicine practiced in Indian cultures Treats imbalances or "dosnas" within body that cause illness by using diet changes, herbal remedies, breath work, physical exercise, hatha yoga, meditation, and rejuvenation or detoxification programs Focuses on preventing disease by enhancing the mind-body connection.	For primary health care disorders involving GI systems, GYN, respiratory tract, bones and muscles, circulation (including cardiovascular), emotional, and psychological, addictions, ENT
	Therapy focuses on the beneficial effects of medicinal waters and involves bathing in water of various types (e.g., in reduced-sulfurous mineral water).	Low back pain, muscle spasm, stress, promotion of healing (Balogh et al, 2005)
	Empowers the mind to take control of conscious and autonomic ...processes (Frishberg, 1998); relaxation is focused on one muscle ...function rather than on the whole body.	Chronic pain, HTN Insomnia, circulation Tension and migraine headaches Incontinence (urine and fecal) Stroke rehabilitation PTSD and depression Chronic tinnitus Chronic facial nerve palsy Torticollis In children: chronic pain (e.g., sickle cell crises), JRA, RAP, functional voice disorders, improve sphincter control associated with urinary and fecal incontinence, postural training for scoliosis, ADHD (Allen, 2004)
	...of binding (chelating) agents that attach to toxic ...s in the body that are then excreted in the urine ...ation that uses diet or liquids to "cleanse" ...h as the liver, colon	Lead poisoning Arteriosclerosis Autism (experimental)
	...lumn as the center of body's well-being ...l massage of spinal vertebrae to restore ...impulses.	Musculoskeletal pain, including chronic low back pain, headaches Torticollis Whiplash following MVA

Text contin...

TABLE 42-1	Complementary Therapies and Their Applications—cont'd	
Nonconventional Therapy	**Theory Behind Use**	**Treatment Applications**[*]
Chromotherapy (color or light therapy)	Uses human sensitivity to color to identify energy pattern imbalances. Each of the seven colors used is regarded as having healing energies (e.g., blue is sedating).	Stress, depression Fatigue
Craniosacral mobilization	Manipulates craniosacral mechanisms to free the flow of cerebrospinal fluid pathways that surround brain and spinal cord; flow can be inhibited by injury to the brain, spinal cord, skull, sacrum, and related membranes	TMJ Headaches Skull injuries with resultant chronic pain Poorly fitting dentures Colic, vomiting, hypertonicity, tremor, irritability in infancy Obstetrically complicated delivery for infant ADHD
Deep breathing	Helps quiet the mind; involves taking slow, deep inhalations through the nose while counting to 10, then slowly and completely exhaling for another count of 10. This is repeated 5 to 10 times, a few times a day.	Stress and/or tension, anxiety Insomnia HTN, headaches
Diet (e.g., vegetarian, macrobiotic, Atkins, Ornish, Pritikin, Zone)	Desired effects achieved by eliminating calories, increasing fiber, decreasing fat, restricting fluids, or altering body's metabolism by manipulating production of key hormones	Weight loss Prevention of heart disease and arteriosclerosis, HTN, diabetes, to enhance athletic performance
Folk medicine (e.g., curanderismo, Native American healing, shamanism)	Form of healing embedded in many cultures; administered by folk healers who are often believed to have a gift passed down through generations Practices may involve prayer, healing touch, charms, herbal teas, tinctures, and magic rituals.	Maladies treated run the gamut of those seen in primary health care; many symptoms culturally based or have culturally based interpretation of disease
Guided imagery	Involves relaxation followed by visualization of calming images; technique practiced 20 to 30 minutes, several times a week	Chronic conditions including headaches, stress, HTN, anxiety; adjunct to cancer treatment
Herbalism (many phytomedicinals are not recommended for use in children (see Box 42-4)	Natural herbs are used over pharmaceutical derivatives; practitioners believe them to be as efficacious, gentler, and less toxic; used extensively by naturopathic, homeopathic, and holistic practitioners; appropriate preparation (tea, capsule, topical) of the herb important; the dried or extract form of the plant may be used.	Used in place of many pharmaceuticals to treat a myriad of primary health care entities, including PMS, cardiovascular, insomnia, stress, menopause, GI, respiratory, immunity, energy, and memory (see Table 42-5)
Hippotherapy	Uses the unique movements of a horse to achieve therapeutic benefits	Balance, fear, anxiety, lack of confidence, motor (may also improve energy expenditure during walking in those who have CP) and social delays in children Mental illness
Homeopathy	Stimulates a healing response by introducing a substance that is either the same as or similar to the patient's disease Infinitesimal doses of plants, minerals, and animal matter are used Medicinal products are prescribed on the basis of the "law of similars"—the medicine used is "homeopathic" to the symptoms presented.	Used by many for wide range of primary care illnesses (e.g., respiratory ailments, headaches, diarrhea, teething, toothaches, arthritis, dermatology problems, GI ailments, depression, and anxiety)
Hypnosis	Uses an altered state of consciousness to access various levels of the mind to effect changes Can be self-learned; usually practiced by a hypnotist or hypnotherapist	Weight loss, drug addictions, smoking cessation, insomnia, pain and stress reduction, phobias
Magnets, electromagnetic therapy (contraindications: pacemakers, defibrillators, acute injuries to bone and muscles, first-trimester pregnancy). Not to be confused with static magnetic therapy (sold as pads, shoe inserts, jewelry).	The use of magnetic field or biofields purport to produce vascular responses by releasing chemicals in response to injury and inflammation. The resulting vasodilation increases blood flow and directs it more quickly to stressed or injured areas, aiding the healing process; may interfere with electric impulses triggering pain or stimulate release of natural body painkillers (endorphins). Mechanism not clear (Miller, 2004).	Musculoskeletal pain Headaches Nausea Osteoarthritis of knee and cervical spine Neck pain Chronic pelvic pain Fracture therapy, soft tissue injury Parkinson disease (experimental)

Continued

TABLE 42-1 Complementary Therapies and Their Applications—cont'd

Nonconventional Therapy	Theory Behind Use	Treatment Applications*
Massage therapy (contraindications: clotting tendencies or communicable skin condition)	Hands-on bodywork techniques that knead and manipulate muscles, soft tissues, and connective tissues of the body Used to promote healing and relaxation, relieve sore and injured muscles, and improve one's overall sense of well-being and health	Premature infants, low birthweight Cocaine- and HIV-exposed infants Colic in infants Infants with disturbed sleep patterns Autistic children Diabetic children to help normalize glucose levels Asthma Arthritis HIV patients Chronic fatigue syndrome Stress-induced maladies Acute and chronic pain Digestive disorders Circulatory problems, lymphedema Musculoskeletal injuries Headaches
Meditation	A deep relaxation technique that can take many forms, from repeating a mantra to Sufi dancing	Stress-induced maladies Chronic illnesses
Megavitamin or high-dose vitamins	Use of vitamins beyond the RDA Can produce adverse and/or toxic effects	Prevention and treatment of a myriad of illnesses (e.g., cancer, heart disease, schizophrenia, viral infections)
Music therapy	Music used to provide rhythmic cues to stimulate brain's motor systems to help build and strengthen connections among nerve cells in the cerebral cortex Boosts immune function in children	Physical rehabilitation of stroke, cerebral palsy, Alzheimer, Parkinson, ADHD, learning disabilities, Down syndrome, depression and anxiety, hypertension Pain relief (surgical, during labor) Premature infants (increases weight gain in premature infants [Lubetzky et al, 2010])
Naturopathy	Natural remedies used to help restore health and balance in the body (e.g., diet, herbal medicine, hydrotherapy, acupuncture, homeopathy, and therapeutic massage) Practitioners often use similar diagnostic and testing procedures as Western medicine practitioners	Used by many for most primary health care issues (see Table 42-5)
Nutrition	Stresses wisdom of following healthy, balanced diet to affect diet-related health issues Advocates the food pyramid or FoodPlate guidelines	Weight loss Food allergies Vitamin and mineral deficiencies Nonpathological GI conditions (e.g., constipation) Chronic diseases
Osteopathy	Remobilization of joints and tissues to restore them to normal, structural positions and mobility, thus releasing tension in muscles and ligaments.	Musculoskeletal pain, including chronic back pain and headaches Torticollis Whiplash following MVA
Pet therapy	Therapy uses dogs, cats, and birds to help those with psychological issues.	Anxiety, social isolation, poor sense of well-being, antipathy
Pilates	Works on mind-body connection with exercise techniques Relies on exercising with firm support and stretching without straining to improve overall body flexibility and fitness	Restricted body flexibility
Prayer	Works on mind-body connection by using the strongly held belief of the connection between the self and a higher power. The most commonly relied on healing practice by people of all cultures and religious beliefs	All forms of health, illness, disease, and disability
Progressive relaxation	Successive tensing and relaxing each of the 15 major muscle groups, starting from the head; often used with deep breathing	Stress, tension, insomnia, anxiety, pain, HTN

TABLE 42-1	Complementary Therapies and Their Applications—cont'd	
Nonconventional Therapy	**Theory Behind Use**	**Treatment Applications***
Qi gong	Ancient Chinese practice combining gentle physical movements, mental focus, and deep breathing. Believed to integrate mind, body, spirit, and stimulate movement of vital life energy (qi). A learned series of movements—often organ specific—done 2+ times a week for 30 minutes.	Asthma, arthritis, stress, lower back pain, allergies, diabetes, headaches, CVD, HTN, chronic pain, autism (Silva et al, 2009)
Reflexology (use with caution in patients with deep vein thrombosis, leg ulcers, phlebitis in lower extremities, pregnancy, pacemakers; avoid renal reflexes in patients with suspected renal calculi; avoid kidney and gallbladder reflexes in patients with gallstones)	Massage technique based on the principle that proprioceptive nerve receptors in hands and feet correspond to all parts of the body, including organs and glands. Use thumb and fingers to massage reflex areas to detect diseases and to rebalance vital energy.	Stress and anxiety Promote circulation Colic, irritability and reflux in infants Headaches Low back pain Some allergic responses Some dermatology conditions GI tract disorders Menstrual problems Arthritis and sciatica
Reiki (aka energy healing therapy)	A bodywork technique to stimulate healing energy within body	Musculoskeletal maladies Low blood hemoglobin levels Pain control (including from cancer, fractured bones) Stress and grief
Tai chi	Stimulates and balances flow of chi or vital energy along acupuncture meridians	Restricted body flexibility, fitness, stamina and energy, stress
Traditional Oriental (Chinese) medicine	Combines practices and beliefs of acupuncture, acupressure, herbal remedies, massage, dietary changes, and bodywork, such as tai chi, breathing, and meditation, to stimulate vital body energy to rebalance life force	Used by one fourth of world's population for primary health care disorders involving GI systems, GYN, respiratory tract, ENT, bones and muscles, circulation (including cardiovascular), emotions and psychology addictions
Touch, therapeutic or healing	Based on autonomic nervous system effects using the subtle energy fields, vibration field, nonlinear electromagnetic energy, spirit or vital force Lowers heart rate; leads to relaxation, reduces anxiety, pain and enhances sense of well-being Similar to qi gong, Reiki	In children reduces anxiety, worry; insomnia, asthma, fatigue, isolation, pain (Kemper et al, 2009), abdominal, arthritis, backache, burn, bruises, cancer, fibromyalgia, headache, postoperative pain (Kemper and Kelly, 2004)
Yoga	Works on breathing, body alignment, and posture to improve health; preventive	Chronic musculoskeletal ailments Stress-related maladies Improving overall body flexibility, fitness, stamina, mental health Asthma Hypertension

*These applications may or may not be supported by scientific research; the listing of these therapies does not imply endorsement of proven efficacy.
Some data from Gasalberti D: Alternative therapies for children and youth with special health care needs, *J Pediatr Health Care* 20(2):133-136, 2006.
ADHD, Attention-deficit/hyperactivity disorder; *CP,* cerebral palsy; *CVD,* cardiovascular disease; *ENT,* ears, nose, and throat; *GI,* gastrointestinal; *GYN,* gynecology; *HIV,* human immunodeficiency virus; *HTN,* hypertension; *JRA,* juvenile rheumatoid arthritis; *MVA,* motor vehicle accident; *PMS,* premenstrual syndrome; *RAP,* recurrent abdominal pain; *RDA,* recommended dietary allowance (established by the National Academy of Science); *TMJ,* temporomandibular joint.

of treatment modalities to their patients (AAP, 2001). Physicians reported reluctance to respond to patients about CAM modalities because of their traditionally poor communication with CAM practitioners, doubts about CAM practitioner competence, their own inability to sort out efficacious complementary procedures, medical liability, and reluctance to participate in offering false hope of obtaining cures (Konefal, 2002).

Most national population-based surveys and studies are based on urban physician practices. In contrast, a study that surveyed 112 rural primary care providers (including NPs, physician assistants, and certified nurse-midwives) in Kentucky, found that of those returning the surveys, 94% of providers reported CAM use by their patients; most recommended CAM to patients, but few consistently asked about CAM use. The more providers were comfortable discussing

CAM use with patients, the more likely they were to view CAM in a positive light (Flannery et al, 2006).

Nurse Practitioners (NPs) recommend CAM therapies at a higher rate. One study reported that 9 out of every 10 NPs did so (Sohn and Loveland Cook, 2002). This interest in such therapies was also mirrored in another survey conducted of faculty and students employed or enrolled at the University of Minnesota schools of medicine, nursing, and pharmacology. Ninety percent of the combined groups believed that a model that integrated both CAM and allopathic medicine would be most efficacious for clinical care. Eighty-eight percent of the faculty members thought that CAM should be included in their school's curriculum; the nursing faculty reported the highest interest in practicing such therapies (Kreitzer et al, 2002).

■ Scientific Observation and Complementary Medicine

What might be conventional medical practice in one country—or even among allopathic medical providers (e.g., biofeedback is used in the discipline of physical medicine and rehabilitation but is regarded as alternative by other medical disciplines)—may be deemed complementary or alternative in another. Many mainstream medical providers still refute claims about the efficacy of CAM treatments and label them quackery or "not scientifically validated." Yet, allopathic medical procedures "...achieve widespread use without extensive clinical evaluation. Indeed, the extent of the variation in treatments may be

greatest when evidence about their relative effectiveness is lacking" (U.S. Congressional Budget Office, 2007, p 1, 4). Only 25% to 50% of all drugs marketed in the U.S. have been approved by the U.S. Food and Drug Administration (FDA) for use in some subset of children or have limited approval for use in children because of the lack of rigorous, scientific clinical trials regarding efficacy of the drugs (Murphy, 2009; Zito et al, 2008). Green notes that patient-centered medicine "challenges the supremacy of randomized controlled trials in evidence-based medicine. Research in integrative medicine can shift the spotlight from mediating variables that focus on the mechanisms of change to the moderating variables that focus on the characteristics of individual people and the context in which they live" (Green, 2010, p 28). Critics and advocates agree that whether or not the treatment is "mainstream" or "alternative," both need to be held to the standards of the scientific method.

CAM therapies can be effective and are increasingly being subjected to the rigorous scientific study that meets Western criteria. The most recent overall review of CAM randomized controlled trials (RCTs) in the pediatric population identified more than 1400 RCTs and 47 systematic reviews (Moher et al, 2002). The quality of the RCTs was judged as good as that in conventional medical studies (Klassen et al, 2005); the equality of systematic reviews of CAM exceeded that of conventional medicine (Lawson et al, 2005). Studies are readily available in the literature and from well-regarded Internet reference sites (PubMed, NCCAM, National Library of Medicine, Cochrane Collaboration to name of few). Kemper points out that when evaluating the efficacy of CAM treatments in children, the mere nature of CAM heterogeneity of products and practice methods can affect outcomes (Kemper, 2008a). This makes it difficult to measure treatment.

Homeopathy, based on the "like cures like" principle, continues to be one of the more controversial CAM treatments. According to critics it has failed to show efficacy in RCTs and systematic reviews (Baum and Ernst, 2009). Others refute this stance and cite outcomes research and numerous double-blind, placebo-controlled studies that show efficacy (Levatin, 2009a). *Homeopathic Family Medicine: Evidence Based Nanopharmcology* by Dana Ullman is regularly updated and can serve as a reference source. HP treatment for childhood upper and lower respiratory infections and ear complaints has been shown to stand up to scrutiny when compared to conventional medicine (Levatin, 2009a).

Advancements in such technologies as genomics, proteomics (study of proteins), metabolomics (study of chemical processes within living organisms), systems biology, and the analytic capacities of microprocessing and nanoprocessing will enable new scientifically based insight into an individual's expression of health and illness. This insight will lead to a greater appreciation about how "multiple variables interact in dynamic ways to further the understanding about how the connections can be harnessed to produce" personalized health and healing treatments (Green, 2010, p 27).

The NIH National Center for Complementary and Alternative Medicine (NCCAM) and more than 2500 research projects have been funded nationally and internationally to identify and study promising CAM practices using scientific methods to determine effectiveness. NCCAM does not include the pediatric population among its priority groups for federally funded research, and the AAP Section on Complementary, Holistic and Integrative Medicine (SOCHIM) has made a request that they do so. SOCHIM is also working with the Pediatric Research of Office Setting (PROS) Network and the NIH for more targeted CAM research. Examples of some current NCCAM-related research projects applicable to pediatrics involve supplements to support the immune system; use of yoga, massage, and meditation for anxiety and stress; the effect of nutrition on inflammation; and the use of qi gong massage therapy to calm autistic children (the results of these studies are incorporated into Table 42-5). Conventional institutions doing CAM research may not have adequate peer review resources or may face difficulties obtaining institutional review board approval for pediatric CAM studies (Kemper et al, 2008a).

Clinical evidence-based medicine research projects involving children have studied the use of echinacea, probiotics, and fish oil. The Pediatric Integrative Medicine Conference in the U.S. occurs annually each fall, and lectures are delivered by nationally recognized experts in their field. The conference focuses on ways to integrate CAM practices into clinical pediatric practice and how to evaluate current CAM research, and provides hands-on workshops. PedCAM (Pediatric Complementary and Alternative Medicine Research and Education Network) disseminates a wide range of CAM information and is building collaborative relationships among researchers, educators, clinicians, and policymakers, both nationally and internationally (www.care.ualberta.ca). It endeavors to develop a pediatric CAM research agenda through an international consensus-driven priority building process. The Center for Holistic Pediatric Education and Research (at Children's Hospital in Boston) is devoted to pediatric complementary therapies (acupuncture, therapeutic massage, bioenergetic therapies) especially as applicable to the management of pediatric pain.

A great body of research into complementary therapies has been generated outside the U.S. The number of studies using CAM are increasing; however, they may not include double-blind, placebo-controlled methodology that is the Western standard. European and Indian studies are most closely aligned with U.S. research designs; China is participating in some double-blind, placebo-controlled human studies. Many of the large, randomized, controlled studies have been done in Germany, where herbal extracts are regulated and used much the same way as pharmaceutical drugs to treat diseases. Negative studies regarding CAM are more likely to be published in well-known journals; positive ones are more likely to be found in foreign-language journals (Pham et al, 2005).

Do You Know If Your Patient Is Using Complementary/ Alternative Medicine?

In 1990 approximately 40% of patients told their conventional providers about using nonconventional treatments (Eisenberg et al, 1993). More recent studies continue to demonstrate that the rate of disclosure (including that by parents of pediatric patients) varies from 40% to 60% (Erlichman et al, 2010; Shorofi and Arbon, 2010). Caregivers may be combining both herbal preparations and prescription drugs without informing the pharmacist or care provider (Cala, 2003). Families may also seek treatment advice about childhood illness from commercial retailers that sell CAM (independent of a licensed clinician), and the advice may be contraindicated for age (Demattia et al, 2006).

TALKING WITH PATIENTS ABOUT THEIR USE OF CAM

The topic of CAM use must be broached nonjudgmentally to help the family clarify the safety issues and explore how these products or services might fit into their child's management plan. The provider-patient relationship and the trust that builds when they explore mutual goals form the foundation for ongoing dialogue (Wysocki, 1997). Furthermore, an open, sensitive attitude implies a commitment "to patients' welfare rather than to the particular system of medicine in which they trained" (Gordon, 1996, p 2209). The patient's health history should be expanded to include the following:

- Alternative products that the patient may be taking, including herbs, "natural products," and homeopathic and nutritional supplements from a health food store
- Other practitioners the patient may be seeing
- Other kinds of activities engaged in to address a particular problem
- The perception of any benefit gained from the complementary treatment
- The philosophy and self-care approaches to wellness and illness

An AAP policy statement and other health care providers offer guidance for clinicians counseling families about CAM to minimize legal risks of malpractice and/or professional discipline (AAP, 2005; Cohen and Kemper, 2005; Kemper et al, 2008a). Advice consists of the following:

- Determine whether the parents intend to abandon known effective, allopathic treatments if the child's illness is life threatening or serious.
- Maintain knowledge about popular complementary practices, being prepared to discuss them with patients, and provide information about different approaches to treatment; be respectful of the patient's values.
- Evaluate the scientific evidence for CAM therapies, including their safety and efficacy.
- Identify risks or possible deleterious effects, including diverting the child from an imminently necessary allopathic treatment.
- Educate families about evaluating information regarding CAM treatments.
- Avoid communication of a negative bias or defensiveness about CAM therapies.
- Offer to assist in monitoring and evaluating CAM therapies, if chosen by the family.
- Evaluate the risk-benefit ratio of the CAM therapy as if you were another equally qualified clinician considering the same therapy; base your judgment on support from medical literature.
- Understand the local and state statutes and regulations governing licensure of CAM providers and specific therapeutic modalities.
- Understand state abuse and neglect laws because knowledge of CAM that is used as a substitute for conventional medical treatment of children with life-threatening illnesses may be reportable.
- Be familiar with the diagnostic tests practitioners of CAM use (Table 42-2).

The American Society of Health-System Pharmacists offers a good patient handout, *Using Alternative Medicines Safely,* on their website.

TABLE 42-2	Laboratory Tests Used by Complementary Medicine Practitioners

TEST	EXPLANATION
Digestion/Nutrition	
Stool culture and analysis	Digestive stool analysis includes a number of stool markers to assess digestion, absorption, metabolism, pancreatic function, inflammation, and fecal flora
Intestinal permeability	Double-sugar test measuring the variable absorption of lactulose and mannitol after a challenge drink to measure permeability and absorption
Small bowel intestinal overgrowth	A lactulose challenge test that measures gas production (hydrogen and methane) over 2 hours to determine the level of bacterial fermentation in the distal small intestine
Lactose intolerance	A lactose challenge test that measures gas production to determine whether lactose is digested properly
Essential Fatty Acids	
Plasma fatty acids	Rapid turnover is an indication of current fatty acid intake; also allows assessment of triene-to-tetraene ratio
Red blood cell fatty acids	Measure of erythrocyte cell membrane fatty acids assesses fatty acid intake over past 2 to 4 months. Correlated with cardiovascular disease risk.
Heavy Metals	
Hair	Although of unknown value, hair tests for heavy metals have been used for the past 25 years by the U.S. Environmental Protection Agency to monitor environmental changes in toxic metals.
Urine	Random and timed urine tests can also provide another indication of exposure; used as a baseline evaluation before a chelating agent is given to determine total body burden.
Postprovocation urine	Chelating agent, including ethylenediaminetetraacetic acid (EDTA) (to bind lead) and dimercaptosuccinic acid (DMSA) or sodium dimercaptopropane sulfonate (DMPS) (to bind mercury) are given before a timed urine test to assess total body burden of a given heavy metal; useful to monitor treatment in an individual, but postprovocation reference ranges are not available.
Hormones	
Salivary/adrenal	Salivary hormone levels of dehydroepiandrosterone (DHEA) and cortisol measure free hormone availability and have been demonstrated to correspond with adrenal function.
Salivary/female	Salivary hormone levels of progesterone, testosterone, and estradiol have been normalized and correlate with free hormone availability. Data on changes in salivary levels with hormone therapy make its use as a tool for monitoring treatment levels unclear though.
Serum/hormone metabolites	2/16-hydroxyestrone ratio in blood has been demonstrated in Women's Health Initiative (WHI) cohort to be predictive of recurrence of breast cancer.
Urine/hormone metabolites	2/16-hydroxyestrone ratio in urine has been correlated with risk of breast cancer (low) and risk of osteoporosis (high)
Immunology	
Immune function	A flow cytometry evaluation of natural killer cell function, as well as presence/activity of immune cells and cytokines
Food allergies	Measures of immunoglobulin (Ig)E and IgG activation in the presence of various food antigens. IgE, true allergic reaction; IgG, delayed response
Nutrigenomics	Broad-based term to represent genomic testing that highlights individual biochemical needs for particular macro- and micronutrients. Purely experimental at this point; no outcome studies have demonstrated clinical validity.
Oxidative Stress Markers	
Lipid peroxides, isoprostane, 8-hydroxydeoxyguanosine	Markers of oxidative end tissue damage to fats, proteins, and deoxyribonucleic acid (DNA)
Glutathione, total antioxidant capacity (TAC)/total reactive antioxidant potential (TRAP) superoxide dismutase	Markers of capacity to deal with oxidative stress

From Rakel D: *Rakel's integrative medicine*, Philadelphia, 2007, Saunders.

Integrating Complementary and Alternative Medicine into a Primary Care Practice

For providers who are incorporating CAM therapies into their practices, it is recommended that informed consent be obtained and reference made to any conventional treatments that may be forgone. (A good patient intake form can be downloaded from www.integrativemedicine.arizona.edu/clinic/ptintakeform 118C3). One should not refer patients to a CAM practitioner without first having done a complete diagnostic evaluation that should also include (Kemper and Cohen, 2004; Adams et al, 2002):

- Determining the severity and acuteness of the illness and assessment of curability or effective treatment using conventional medicine
- Discussing treatment options, including the use and potential toxicity of CAM treatment
- Studying the literature about the degree of invasiveness, safety, and efficacy of the chosen CAM treatment for the particular malady
- Being aware of the licensure status of the recommended CAM practitioner
- Patient's knowledge of and willingness to accept the risk and benefits of therapy
- Reviewing any prescribed medications

After the diagnostic evaluation of the patient's complaint, the following steps should be taken to assist a patient who wishes to try CAM therapy:

- Assist the patient in identifying a suitable licensed practitioner.
- Provide the patient with questions to ask the alternative provider during the first consultative visit, including issues of safety, efficacy of any treatment, and reasonable expectations of measurable improvement.
- Monitor the patient to review the recommended treatment plan; encourage the patient to keep a symptom diary.
- Concurrent use of any prescribed medications
- Monitor the patient's response to treatment at monthly intervals.
- Document all interactions with the patient.

Many states have licensing boards and professional organizations that set standards for nonconventional practitioners, including a requirement to carry malpractice insurance. The Federation of State Medical Boards has established policy and model guidelines for the use of CAM therapies when recommending the therapy or when co-managing the patient with a CAM provider. Licensing requirements are subject to change, and patients should be encouraged to review the credentials of any practitioner whom they are considering using. Currently there is no national licensure for acupuncture, acupressure, homeopathy (except for those with conventional and osteopathic medical licenses), Ayurvedics, herbology, hypnotherapy, or naturopathy. State licensure requirements vary (University of California, San Diego, 2010).

NPs are advised to check the advanced nurse practice act of their state, the policies of their employer, and the relevant standards of practice before expanding their practice. NPs may have to pursue a broader interpretation and additional training or certification to ensure compliance with the terms of the nurse practice act.

Costs of Complementary Treatments and Health Care Insurance Coverage

Adults who were included in the 2007 NHIS spent approximately $22 billion on CAM products, classes, and materials and $11.9 billion on visits to CAM providers—all expenditures were out of pocket (NCCAM, 2008). Insurance companies are continuing to study the issue of offering premium coverage for "alternative medical treatments" in response to pressure from policy holders, including employers. State Medicaid programs may also offer CAM coverage. White and Ernst (2000) reported that there was a reduction in referrals and treatment costs when primary care providers included an array of CAM therapies in their treatment recommendations. Insurance companies mandated to cover CAM providers in Washington State noted a similar decrease in health care expenditures when comparing costs of treatment generated by CAM providers versus non-CAM providers that involved adults treated for back pain, fibromyalgia, or menopause symptoms (Lind et al, 2010).

Integrating Complementary and Alternative Medicine into Traditional Medical and Nursing Education

Forty-four academic health centers or medical schools in the U.S. and Canada now belong to the Consortium of Academic Health Centers for Integrative Medicine (CAHCIM). They offer clinical programs for medical students, residents, and other allied health professionals in integrative health care, clinical services, research, and/or education (CAHCIM, 2010). Outside the U.S., 40% of responding European medical universities offered some form of CAM training, and no conventional medical schools offered courses in CAM in England (Kemper et al, 2008a). Nine leading clinical centers deliver integrative care in the U.S. (e.g., Duke University, University of Maryland School of Medicine, and University of California, San Francisco Medical Center). The White House Commission on Complementary and Alternative Medicine Policy (WHCCAMP) recommended across-the-board "integration" of CAM into government health agencies, medical education, and insurance systems (WHCCAMP, 2002).

Nursing literature documents numerous articles that discuss or encourage the incorporation of holistic nursing practices and complementary and alternative modalities into schools of nursing curricula at both the baccalaureate and graduate levels. Nursing academicians acknowledge that nursing has been practicing CAM for years as part of the holistic approach to health (Kreitzer et al, 2009). Richardson (2003) showed that 77% of the 105 baccalaureate nursing programs surveyed offered some content or experiential learning on CAM therapies. Fenton and Morris (2003) documented that of 125 schools of nursing sampled, 60% incorporated such educational framework. In every case, the researchers and academicians noted that this integration was largely in response to consumer demand and that it was imperative that "nursing education find room for CAM in its curriculum to meet the needs of 21st century patients, so that nurses can

| **BOX 42-2** | Foods, Factors, and Labels Implicated in Hypersensitivity or Intolerance |

Foods Accounting for Hypersensitivity Reactions

Eggs
Wheat
Citrus
Peanuts, walnuts, pecans, almonds
Shellfish and fish
Milk and dairy products
Other gluten-containing grains (oats, rye, barley)
Soy

Substances Implicated in Food Intolerance (these occur naturally in food or are additives)

Lactose
Biogenic amines (histamine, tyramine)
Other disaccharides
Preservatives (benzoates, BHA [butylated hydroxyanisole], BHT [butylated hydroxytoluene], sulfites)
Artificial colors, especially tartrazine
Salicylates
Monosodium glutamate and other artificial flavors
Nitrates

Other Factors Implicated With Hypersensitivity (increase the likelihood of hypersensitivities in those genetically predisposed)

Family history of allergic reactions
Frequency of exposure
Other allergic reactions (e.g., inhalant allergies)

Increased intestinal permeability to allergens ("leaky gut")
Vigorous exercise
Concurrent consumption of alcohol
Hormone levels
Stress

Food Label Ingredients That May Signal Hyperallergenic Foods
Dairy

Casein, caseinate
Lactalbumin
Milk solids
Whey

Wheat

Semolina
Durum
Modified food starch
Malt, malt syrup

Soy

Hydrolyzed vegetable protein
Textured vegetable protein
Miso
Lecithin

Adapted from Johnson K: The elimination diet and diagnosing food hypersensitivities. In Rakel D: *Integrative medicine,* Philadelphia, 2003, Saunders.

effectively practice CAM with skills useful for participation in CAM research and safe clinical practice" (Wyatt and Post-White, 2005, p 2). Kemper (2007) offers a conceptual model (yin-yang model) as a method for teaching conventional medical professionals (including students) about different approaches of health care in order to find common ground with less conventional practitioners.

The NCCAM, American Medical Association, American Academy of Family Practice, American Nurses Association, American Nurse's Holistic Association, and other institutions (including hospitals) are providing patient and professional education (including hospital staff) in nonconventional treatment options. Many courses about CAM and herbal products are available online, and certifications of completion are offered.

Role of Allergens in Complementary Medicine

Complementary practitioners may be more likely to identify allergies as being the etiology for many common childhood conditions. Childhood afflictions such as otitis media, upper respiratory infections, and other immunological conditions, atopic dermatitis, asthma, headaches, and ADHD are regarded as being caused by allergies to foods and food additives as a result of reactions between the "inner being" and external environmental stimuli (i.e., foods) (Boxes 42-2 and 42-3) (Micozzi, 1996). Genetics, the early introduction of solids, early weaning, genetic reengineering of food components, limited consumption of a variety of foods, hidden foods,

additives and colorings, and impaired digestion are offered as possible reasons for an increase in food sensitivities. Conventional medicine suggests that blood tests for allergies (enzyme-linked immunosorbent assay [ELISA], immunoglobulin E [IgE], and ALCAT) remain unproven and controversial (Chafen et al, 2010); nutritionally oriented practitioners, such as naturopaths, may regard these tests as useful. See Chapter 10 for a discussion of allergies and allergy testing.

See Table 42-2 for a listing and explanation of other laboratory tests that are more commonly ordered by CAM practitioners.

Safety and Regulatory Issues

There have been few reported serious adverse side effects in children using CAM therapies (Kemper et al, 2008a). It is particularly important to ascertain the safety of certain treatment modalities by learning about any alternative product that the patient may be using, including its side effects, possible interactions with other medications, and mechanism of action. Mind-body techniques (e.g., prayer, guided imagery, spiritual healing, relaxation) and acupuncture are not likely to interact with conventional medications. Providers should be aware of the possible harmful effect of products that are taken at high doses, such as herbal or phytomedicinal products, megadose combination nutritional supplements, colonics, or products taken in unconventional ways. Any treatment must be viewed as hazardous if its use delays the provision of proven conventional care for a serious medical condition. Homeopathic

BOX 42-3	Elimination and Challenge Diet Regimen*

Elimination Phase

The initial step of the elimination diet is to completely stop one suspected food, a few suspected foods, or many foods at once depending on the clinician's initial evaluation. The help of a dietitian or nutritionist may be needed in the case of many foods being eliminated to ensure adequate nutrition and calories. This elimination step should be followed for at least 10 days (some suggest 2 to 4 weeks), but for no more than for 4 weeks.

Symptoms caused by food allergens will usually disappear by the fifth or sixth day of the diet, when the body has thoroughly cleansed itself of the allergen-antibody complexes, and the intestines have completely eliminated the allergen-containing food. Should symptoms not disappear, it is recommended that the diet become further restricted. Generally the fewer known allergens included in the diet, the easier it is to establish a cause (see Box 42-2). If used for ADHD,* behavioral changes may be evidenced. *Eat only these foods before reintroduction of other foods*: lamb, chicken, rice, potatoes, bananas, and vegetables in the cabbage family (cabbage, Brussels sprouts, broccoli, cauliflower, mustard, radish, turnip, watercress). Do not eat foods that contain artificial colors or preservatives (see Box 42-2).

Reintroduction Phase

This phase adds foods back one at a time; a diary or log needs to be kept to track symptoms. One food is reintroduced every 3 days. The challenged food should be introduced in sequential incremental doses, starting in the morning with a small bite and increasing the amount during the challenge day. The food should be in its most identifiable state (e.g., eating a scrambled egg rather than incorporating it in pancakes). Symptoms may be seen within hours, or a delayed response may take up to 3 days. No other foods should be reintroduced during this 3-day period. After a food is reintroduced, it should again be eliminated until all of the eliminated foods have been reintroduced per directions. If there is a positive response, more pronounced or acute symptoms will recur on reintroduction of the eliminated food.

On reintroduction, the most common foods that produce symptoms are often found to be eggs, wheat, chocolate, nuts, cow's milk, citrus, and cheese. Corn, soy, beef, food colorings and additives, refined sugar, and caffeine have also been implicated. Avoidance means both eliminating the food and identifying it in hidden foods (e.g., breads prepared with eggs).

A diary should be kept and wrist pulse recorded because the pulse may change when an allergen is eaten (Murray and Pizzorno, 1998). Children with atopy are more likely to respond to this diet (Boris and Mandel, 1994).

Final Phase

This can be done in one of two ways. A final diet can be planned that totally eliminates all of the foods that produced symptoms, or the foods can be eliminated for 3 to 6 months and then reintroduced on a rotational basis. This rotation diet adds the suspected food on an infrequent but consistent basis from every 4 days to once a month. This is believed to allow the levels of non-IgE antibodies to fall since the body is exposed to reduced antigen. The IgE levels are not likely to rise with this approach (Johnson, 2003).

General Guidelines

Is it important to be diligent about avoiding any exposure to the eliminated foods. Failing to do so may result in unclear symptoms during the reintroduction phase. Closely reading ingredient labels is imperative. If the elimination phase fails to reduce symptoms, one of three things may be occurring. Either food hypersensitivity or intolerance is not causing the symptoms, the child is still eating the potentially offending food, or something—besides or in addition to the food—may be causative. The elimination diet is only a tool, not a treatment. If possible ensure that the patient understands that this is not a "diet" in the traditional sense. Foods should not be permanently eliminated if they did not cause symptoms (Johnson, 2003).

*The role that diet plays as a causative factor of some ADHD symptoms is controversial. However, some studies (see following references) have demonstrated that children with ADHD have shown significant improvement in symptoms with the elimination of certain foods or additives or with diet modifications.
ADHD, Attention-deficit/hyperactivity disorder; *IgE,* immunoglobulin E.
Bateman B, Warner JO, Hutchinson E et al: The effects of a double blind, placebo controlled artificial food colouring and benzoate preservative challenge on hyperactivity in a general population sample of preschool children, *Arch Dis Child* 89(6):506-511, 2004; Johnson K: The elimination diet and diagnosing food hypersensitivities. In Rakel D: *Integrative medicine,* Philadelphia, 2003, Saunders; Schnoll R, Burshteyn D, Cea-Aravena J: Nutrition in the treatment of attention deficit hyperactivity disorder: a neglected but important aspect, *Appl Psychophysiol Biol Feedback* 28(1):63-75, 2003.

remedies are highly diluted (the basis for most of the criticism) and are generally safe for infants, children, and pregnant and lactating women; side effects are rare (Levatin, 2009a).

An estimated 80% of active ingredients and 40% of compounded drugs are imported into the United States. China and India are increasingly supplying these products (the largest drug companies are in North America, Europe, and Japan). Malaysia and Vietnam are gearing up to be international export suppliers. Though unlabeled, many dietary supplements are imported (e.g., almost all vitamin C found in supplements comes from China). Even though the FDA is charged with monitoring manufacturing plants supplying drugs to the U.S., Congress has noted problems with adequate oversight. For this reason, the FDA has opened offices in China, as well as India, Costa Rica, and other nations. The U.S. Pharmacopeia and Chinese Pharmacopeia have agreed to cooperate to ensure similar standards are met (University of California, Berkeley, 2010).

Contamination and potency are of concern when patients use herbal (notably Ayurvedic herbal medicines) or folk remedies. Some traditional folk remedies or herbal preparations manufactured in third world countries (notably South Asia) contain heavy metals (lead, zinc, mercury, arsenic, aluminum, and tin). Additional problems include content substitutions, adulterations or incorrect preparations, misleading advertising, improper labeling of contents, and failure to provide adequate amounts of the substance noted on the label (Gardiner and Kemper, 2000; Mortimore and Fischer, 2001; Saper et al, 2004). Prior, nonproblematic use of a product by an individual may not be a predictor of a future drug reaction because of potency inconsistency; lack of standardization regarding which parts of a plant are used; variations in plant ripeness, storage, and regional growth conditions; and the unknown influence of fertilizers, pesticides, and herbicides used during cultivation.

Few reports of adverse reactions to herbal preparations have been documented. The FDA summary report for 2009 showed that there were 13 reports of adverse effects from nutritional supplements; most were from supplements used for sexual enhancement, bodybuilding, and weight control

---

BOX 42-4 Herbals, Botanicals, and Diet Supplements: Precautions About Use in Children

Do Not Use

- Aristolochic acid–containing products (e.g., "Liqiang Xiao Ke Ling Thirst Quenching Efficacious" (aka birthwort, snakeroot, snake weed, sangree root, sangrel, serpentary, wild ginger)
- Arrow Brand Medicated Oil and Embrocation (aka Aceite Medicinal La Flecha [Spanish])
- Glyburide-containing supplements ("Liqiang 4")
- Tiratricol-containing supplements (often marketed for weight loss)
- Fenfluramine-containing products (often marketed for weight loss)
- "Better Than Formula Ultra Infant Immune Booster 17"
- Flu or avian flu preventive or treatment-promoting dietary supplements
- Body-building diet supplements (gamma hydroxybutyrate [GHB], gamma butyrolactone [GBL], 1,4-butanediol [BD] and may contain other harmful ingredients
- Dieter's teas containing senna, aloe, cascara, castor oil, rhubarb root, buckthorn, or other plant-derived stimulant laxative
- Dietary weight loss supplements (and see Tiratricol above)
- Ephedra (ma huang)
- Comfrey *(Symphytum officinale)*
- Crotalaria species (rattle pods) in herbal teas
- Borage *(Borago officinalis)*
- Coltsfoot *(Tussilago farfara)* in herbal teas

- Chaparral *(Larrea divaricata)*
- Foxglove *(Digitalis purpurea)*
- Germander *(Teucrium chamaedrys)*
- Ginkgo seeds (are toxic)
- Heliotropes
- Jin bu huan *(Lycopodium serratum)*
- Kava-kava *(Piper methysticum)*
- Monkshood/wolfsbane/aconite *(Aconitum napellus, A. columbianum)*
- Rattlebox *(Crotalaria* spp.)
- Sassafras
- Senecio (ragwort, groundsel, golden ragwort) in herbal teas
- St. Ignatius bean (contains strychnine and brucine)
- Strychnos Nux Vomica tree seeds (contain strychnine)
- Pennyroyal oil *(Mentha pulegium, Hedeoma* spp.)
- *Prunus* spp. (amygdalin, laetrile)
- Lobelia
- Organ or glandular extracts

Use With Restrictions

- Goldenseal/roots—not for use in infants younger than 1 month old
- Tea tree oil—do not prescribe for internal use
- Echinacea—do not use in children younger than 2 years old
- Pennyroyal—do not prescribe for internal use

Data from Clinical Advisor, editorial staff: Warn patients away from these supplements, *Clin Advisor* 7(5):12, 2004; Eisenberg DM: Advising patients who seek alternative therapies, *Ann Intern Med* 127:61-69, 1997; Fugh-Berman A: *Alternative medicine: what works,* Baltimore, 1997, Williams & Wilkins; Gardiner P, Kemper K: Herbs in pediatric and adolescent medicine, *Pediatr Rev* 21(2):44-57, 2000; Loo M: *Integrative medicine for children,* St Louis, 2009, Elsevier, Chapter 7; Mack R: "Something wicked this way comes"—herbs even witches should avoid, *Contemp Pediatr* 15(6):49-64, 1998; U.S. Food and Drug Administration: Medical product safety information. Available at www.fda.gov/medwatch/safety.htm (accessed Aug. 29, 2010).

(FDA, 2010). In children 5 years of age or younger, 2 of 47 deaths in 2009 were attributed to dietary supplements, herbals, or homeopathic substances as compared to 18 fatalities from pharmaceuticals (Bronstein et al, 2010). Deaths in prior years were attributable to preparations that had ma huang as an ingredient. Ingestion of toxic ornamental plants rather than herbs accounted for most reports of plant poisonings. In children, the most dangerous elements are the pyrrolizidine alkaloids, which can cause liver complications or death. These compounds occur in comfrey, borage, coltsfoot, and species of *Crotalaria* and *Senecio*. These plants are often found in herbal teas, particularly from Jamaica, Africa, and South and Central America. Chaparral, germander, and a Chinese medicine called jin bu huan can also cause liver toxicity. See Box 42-4 for a summary list of these herbs.

Even though 25% of pharmaceutical drugs are made from herbs, Western medical providers often regard herbal, natural health products (NHPs) as dangerous or ineffective. Since 1993 the FDA has had a voluntary system in place, called MedWatch, for reporting adverse reactions to nutritionals and botanicals. Access to MedWatch is available from the FDA's website.

With 250,000 flowering plant species, the burden of knowing what is safe to use or not use becomes cumbersome. Although many herbs are harmless even in large amounts, others should be prescribed only by a knowledgeable herbalist or botanical professional. More than 80 herbs or botanicals (e.g., plants, fungi, algae, and common constituents) can interact significantly with prescription and over-the counter medications (Ulbricht et al, 2008). The appropriate herb in

the appropriate quantity—like pharmaceutical medicines—is necessary to obtain the intended benefits. The medicinal effect of any one herb is thought to be the result of dozens of pharmacologically distinct actions. The herb may be causing physiological changes in numerous subtle ways, none of which alone would produce the desired response. This mechanism contrasts with conventional medicines, which generally act by one of a few mechanisms of action and use "physiologically more significant pharmacological" dosing.

Standardized extracts are more likely to ensure that a specific amount of an active compound is present. Western herbalists often use *simples* (the compound is made from one herb), whereas Chinese and Indian (Ayurvedic) medicines often blend together more than one herb. A general rule is that all herbs need to be respected; they are neither completely safe nor poisonous. See Table 42-3 for a list of drug categories and herbal product interactions and Table 42-4 for herbs contraindicated in pregnancy and lactation.

There are, however, some useful guidelines that clinicians can use when either advocating or advising about herbal and dietary supplements for their patients. These include (Gardiner et al, 2004; *The Oregonian,* 2006; Sego, 2006; Woolf et al, 2009a):

- Use only single-herb supplements instead of combinations to prevent side effect confusion.
- Stop herbal supplements at least 1 week before any scheduled surgical procedure to prevent any alterations in coagulation or interactions with anesthesia.
- Research the herb or NHP as thoroughly as possible:
  - USP Dietary Supplement Verified seal means the product has met certain manufacturing standards.

TABLE 42-3	Interactions Between Some Pharmaceuticals and Herbal Products	
Drug Category	**Herbs**	**Effect of Herb on the Drug's Action**
Acetaminophen	Ginkgo	May cause intracranial bleeding
Anesthetics	Kava, valerian	Prolonged sedation—an additive effect
Antibiotics (ampicillin, ciprofloxacin)	Dandelion, fennel, khat	Decrease drug availability
Anticonvulsants, general	Cis-gamma-linolenic acid–rich herbs (evening primrose oil) Thujone-containing herbs (cedar, tansy, sage) Ginkgo Salicylate-rich herbs (e.g., cramp bark, willow, wintergreen)	Decreased therapeutic effect—may decrease seizure threshold; mechanism of action unknown Prevents conversion of vitamin B_6 into a form that promotes GABA Increased therapeutic effect with transient effects, per case reports; mechanism of action unknown
Anticonvulsants (ethosuximide, fosphenytoin sodium, phenytoin, carbamazepine)	Shankhpushpi (an Ayurvedic product with many herbs) Gingko St. John's wort	Decreases effectiveness of phenytoin; reduced blood levels; lowered anticonvulsant action
Antidepressants—general Bupropion hydrochloride	Evening primrose oil, ginkgo, kava ginseng Cis-gamma-linolenic acid–rich herbs (evening primrose oil)	May interfere with seizure control May cause mania Lowers seizure threshold and may cause epileptic seizures
Tricyclics	Ma huang, St. John's wort, ginkgo, yohimbe	May enhance drug effects, causing restlessness May cause high blood pressure
SSRIs	St. John's wort, ma huang	Increased serotonergic effects and increased likelihood of adverse reactions (e.g., serotonin syndrome), restlessness
Barbiturates	Valerian, St. John's wort, kava	Potentiate side effects of drug, causing sleepiness, lethargy
Benzodiazepines	St. John's wort Kava, valerian	Decreased drug effect; may increase side effects and sedation; herb binds to GABA receptor sites, per animal and pharmacology studies Enhance drug effects of sleepiness, lethargy
Mood stabilizers	Psyllium, ginseng	Psyllium, decreases drug concentration; ginseng may cause mania
Monoamine oxidase inhibitors (MAOIs)	St. John's wort Yohimbe Ma huang Panax ginseng, bioactive amines, licorice	May decrease effect of MAOIs Increases toxic effect of MAOIs Potentiates action of MAOIs, possibly causing life-threatening high blood pressure, high fever, coma Increased side effects that may lead to toxicity; licorice is reported to be a very strong MAOI, per case reports
Corticosteroids	Laxative herbs (e.g., aloe, cascara, senna, yellow dock), diuretic herbs (e.g., celery seed, corn silk, horsetail, juniper) Licorice Panax ginseng	Increases side effects; increased potassium loss per theoretical evidence Increased plasma levels as a result of increase in bioavailability, per case reports and some pharmacological evidence CNS stimulation and insomnia, per case reports
Cyclosporine, tacrolimus	St. John's wort	Reduced blood levels; risk of transplant rejection
Diabetes medications, type 2 diabetes	Fenugreek, ginseng, karela or bitter melon Echinacea	May decrease blood sugar Can alter metabolic control
General medications	High-fiber herbs (e.g., flax, psyllium, acacia, slippery elm, marshmallow) "Hot" remedies (e.g., ginger, garlic, black pepper, red pepper)	Decreased absorption of drugs, per pharmacological studies Increased absorption by causing vasodilation of intestinal wall, per traditional use
Iron	Tannin-rich herbs (e.g., caffeine-containing herbs, cat's claw, tea, uva ursi)	Decreased drug effect because tannin binds with iron to decrease absorption, per theoretical and pharmacological evidence

Continued

TABLE 42-3 Interactions Between Some Pharmaceuticals and Herbal Products—cont'd

Drug Category	Herbs	Effect of Herb on the Drug's Action
Laxative, stimulant (e.g., bisacodyl)	Aloe, cascara sagrada, senna, yellow dock	May increase laxative effect
Minerals	Fiber-containing herbs (flax, psyllium, acacia, slippery elm, marshmallow)	Decreased bioavailability, especially of Ca, Mg, Cu, Zn with psyllium, per case reports
NSAIDs	Gastric irritant herbs (e.g., caffeine, rue, uva ursi) Nettles	Increased side effects and may increase gastric erosion and bleeding, per theoretical evidence Increased therapeutic effect—increases effect of antiinflammatory activity, per controlled trials
Oral contraceptives, combination	Licorice, St. John's wort	Both may increase blood pressure; St. John's wort may also cause breakthrough bleeding
Salicylates (e.g., aspirin)	Herbs that alkalinize urine (e.g., uva ursi) Tamarind Ginkgo, garlic	Decreased plasma levels caused by increased urine secretion, per pharmacology studies Increases blood level of aspirin May cause prolonged bleeding by decreasing platelet aggregation; eye hemorrhage
Theophylline	St. John's wort	May inhibit drug's effectiveness
Thyroid hormone	Horseradish Kelp	Decreased therapeutic effect by decreasing thyroid function Increased therapeutic effect because kelp contains iodine, which may lead to hyperthyroidism per theoretical evidence

Ca, Calcium; *CNS,* central nervous system; *Cu,* copper; *GABA,* gamma-aminobutyric acid; *Mg,* magnesium; *SSRIs,* selective serotonin reuptake inhibitors; *NSAIDs,* nonsteroidal antiinflammatory drugs; *Zn,* zinc.
Data from Golub C: Herb-medication interactions: what you don't know can hurt you, *Environ Nutr* 24(10):1-5, 2001; Graedon J, Graedon T: *The people's pharmacy: guide to home and herbal remedies,* New York, 1999, Graedon Enterprises; Hardy M: Herb-drug interactions: an evidence-based table, *Int Med Alert* Jan 29, 2001, pp 1-8; Rey JM, Walter G, Soh N: Complementary and alternative medicine (CAM) treatments and pediatric psychopharmacology, *J Am Acad Child Adolesc Psychiatry* 47(4):364-368, 2008; Simkins A, Thurston D, Colyar M et al: Nature's wrath? A closer look at complication with five popular herbs, *Adv Nurs Pract* 13(6):55-58, 2005.

TABLE 42-4 Herbs in Pregnancy and Lactation: Precautions About Use

Avoid in Pregnancy	Avoid During Lactation	May Be Used in Small, Limited Quantities During Lactation
Aloe	Aloe	Commercial herbal teas (available from Celestial Seasonings) such as orange, cinnamon, lemon lift, raspberry, rose hips
Autumn crocus	Black cohosh	Fennel (NOT in oil form)
Black cohosh root	Blue cohosh	Blessed thistle
Blue cohosh	Bladderwrack	Echinacea
Buckthorn bark and berry	Borage	
Cascara sagrada bark	Buckthorn bark	
Chaste tree fruit (limited data; Dugoua et al, 2008a)	Buckthorn berry	
Cinchona bark	Bugleweed	
Cinnamon bark	Caraway oil	
Coltsfoot leaf	Cascara sagrada bark	
Comfrey herb, leaf, and root	Chaste tree	
Dong quai	Comfrey	
Echinacea purpurea herb, injectable form	Coltsfoot leaf	
Ephedra	Elecampane	
Fennel oil and seed	Ephedra	
Gingerroot	Fenugreek (causes notable maple syrup smell in mother and infant) (*Note: Fenugeek is used widely in some communities to increase production of milk in lactating mothers*).	
Ginkgo biloba	Garlic	
Ginseng (use with caution, especially in first trimester) (Seely et al, 2008).	Ginkgo biloba	
Indian snakeroot	Ginseng	
Juniper root	Indian snakeroot	
Kava kava		

TABLE 42-4 Herbs in Pregnancy and Lactation: Precautions About Use—cont'd

Avoid in Pregnancy	Avoid During Lactation	May Be Used in Small, Limited Quantities During Lactation
Licorice root (>100 mg glycyrrhizin)	Joe-pye	
Mayapple root and resin	Kava kava	
Parsley herb and root	Licorice	
Pennyroyal	Male fern	
Petasites root	Peppermint oil	
Red raspberry leaf	Petasites root	
Rhubarb root	Rhubarb root	
Rosemary	Senna leaf	
Thuga	Stillinga	
Sage leaf	St. John's wort	
Senna leaf	Uva ursi	
St. John's wort	Valerian	
Uva ursi leaf	Wormwood	

Herbal Combinations

Angelica root with gentian root and fennel seed
Anise oil with fennel oil and caraway oil
Anise oil with fennel oil, licorice root, and thyme
Anise oil with fennel seed and caraway seed
Anise seed with ivy leaf, fennel seed, and licorice root
Anise seed with marshmallow root, eucalyptus oil, and licorice root >100 mg glycyrrhizin
Caraway oil and fennel oil
Caraway oil, fennel oil, chamomile flower
Caraway seed and fennel seed
Caraway seed, fennel seed, chamomile flower
Ivy leaf, licorice root (>100 mg glycyrrhizin), and thyme
Licorice root, peppermint leaf, German chamomile flower
Licorice root, primrose root, marshmallow root, and anise seed
Marshmallow root, fennel seed, Iceland moss, and thyme
Marshmallow root, primrose root, licorice root (>100 mg glycyrrhizin), and thyme oil
Peppermint leaf and fennel seed
Peppermint leaf, caraway seed, and fennel seed
Peppermint oil and fennel oil
Peppermint oil, caraway oil, fennel oil
Peppermint oil, caraway oil, fennel oil, chamomile flower
Peppermint oil, fennel oil, chamomile flower
Senna leaf, peppermint oil, caraway oil

Note: Botanical product elixirs and liquid preparations might be mixed with alcohol; such preparations should be avoided.
Adapted from Mattison D: *Herbal supplements: their safety, a concern for health care providers.* Available at www.marchofdimes.com/professionals/681_1815.asp (accessed Sept 2, 2010). Additional data from Conover E, Buehler BA: Use of herbal agents by breastfeeding women may affect infants, *Pediatr Ann* 33(4):235-240, 2004; Dugoua JJ, Seely D, Perri D et al: Safety and efficacy of chastetree *(Vitex agnus-castus)* during pregnancy and lactation, *Can J Clin Pharmacol* 15(1):e74-e79, 2008a; Dugoua JJ, Perri D, Seely D et al: Safety and efficacy of blue cohosh *(Caulophyllum thalictroides)* during pregnancy and lactation, *Can J Clin Pharmacol* 15(1):e66-e73, 2008b; Lawrence RA: *Herbs and breastfeeding.* Available at www.breastfeeding.com/reading_room/herbs.html (accessed Sept 2, 2010); McGuffin M, Goldberg A, editors: *American Herbal Products Association's botanical safety handbook,* New York, 1998, CRC Press, p 188; Seely D, Dugoua JJ, Perri D et al: Safety and efficacy of panax ginseng during pregnancy and lactation, *Can J Clin Pharmacol* 15(1):e87-e94, 2008.

○ Determine that the manufacturer complies with Good Manufacturing Practices (GMPs) that set standards for cleanliness, maintenance, and documented quality checks. Other quality standards are set by the National Nutritional Food Association TruLabel program, National Sanitation Foundation International certification program, and the U.S. Pharmacopeia (USP) Dietary Supplement Verification Program (USP noted on the product label).

○ Check the American Herbal Products Association safety rating system (discussion to follow).

○ Herbal and NHPs manufactured and imported from Europe are generally regarded as safe because they have to comply with standards set forth by Commission E (Europe's equivalent of the FDA) (e.g., a label noting "original German formula" would be a good choice).

○ Consumers in England can be relatively assured that an herbal product is licensed and meets standards of safety and quality if it has a PL (product license) or THR (Traditional Herbal Registration Scheme) number on the label. Consumers are cautioned about purchasing their herbal products over the Internet. The Medicines and Health Care Products Regulatory Agency (MHRA) evaluates, licenses, and prohibits and/or restricts the use of all herbal medicines sold in that country; a list of such products is available on their website.

○ Alternative medicine products in New Zealand are classified as food products and there are no regulations or safety standards. Toxic contaminants are monitored in herbal substances and noted in pharmacopoeial monographs in that country (Kemper et al, 2008a).

○ Avoid the use of herbs starting with the letter "G"—ginkgo, ginseng, garlic, ginger, or green tea if the patient is taking a drug that that is metabolized using the hepatic cytochrome P450 enzyme system (e.g., warfarin). The "G" herbs can either potentiate or inhibit the system, therefore altering the therapeutic effect or causing adverse effects.

Use websites, such as the American Botanical Council Herb-Clip Database, to determine if the product has been tested or reviewed. Also Natural Medicines Comprehensive Database (subscription fee) discusses clinically tested products and their interactions with pharmacological drugs. A list of herbal products that have been studied for specific conditions by NCCAM is available at www.nlm.nih.gov/medlineplus/herbalmedicine.html.

The Dietary Supplement Health and Education Act of 1994 requires cautionary labeling for all dietary supplements containing herbs. The American Herbal Products Association has evaluated herbal safety for all botanical ingredients sold in North America. Each herb has been placed in one of the following classes:

Class 1: Herb can be safely consumed when used appropriately
Class 2: The following use restrictions apply:
  2a: For external use only
  2b: Not to be used during pregnancy
  2c: Not to be used while nursing
  2d: Other specific use restrictions as noted
Class 3: Data exist to recommend the following labeling: "To be used only under the supervision of an expert qualified in the appropriate use of this substance"
Class 4: Insufficient data available for classification

■ Specific Complementary Treatments for Children and Adolescents

Table 42-5 lists some complementary treatments used to address health conditions present in the pediatric population. The complementary therapeutics in this table are also referenced based on evidence-based research as judged by the reference authors as being clinically reasonable or holding clues to promising areas needing further research. Physician authors from both Western medicine and naturopathic professions were used to compile this table. *Inclusion of a complementary treatment in Table 42-5 does not imply endorsement by this textbook's authors.* Clinicians are strongly encouraged to seek out further formal education regarding all aspects of CAM and to have a number of sound references on the subject that cite research and safety precautions. Loo (2009a,b,c) and Rakel (2007) are well researched and referenced. Knowledge of the following terms is useful when referencing Table 42-5:

• *Standardized:* An herbal product that contains a *specified concentration of one ingredient* of the plant; it may contain other nonstandardized ingredients from the same plant.

• *Essential oils:* Also known as volatile or aromatic oils that are found in many plants. These oils are highly concentrated and potent and are not to be taken internally.

• *Infusion:* Preparation similar to tea. The dried herb is steeped in boiling water for 5 to 10 minutes and strained; the preparation can be sweetened to make it more palatable; drink warm or cold.

• *Tincture:* A concentrated extract of an herb made with a mixture of cold water and alcohol (typically 25%, 40%, 60%, or 90% alcohol). The tincture usually is diluted four or five times with water or juice for children; tinctures should not be given internally to children younger than 2 years old.

TABLE 42-5 Complementary Treatments* for Some Common Conditions in Children and Adolescents

Diagnosis	Treatment Approach	Dosage	Benefit	Possible Side Effects†	Research/Citations
Abdominal pain, recurrent	Mind-body therapies (bio-feedback, touch, hypnosis, deep breathing)	Depends on practitioner	Causes relaxation of the proximal stomach	None	Kemper and Kelly (2004); Allen (2004) several studies cited; Culbert and Richtsmeier Cyr (2009a) (cite studies)
	Herbal Peppermint oil, enteric-coated Chinese herbal	1 capsule for children (that can swallow capsule) up to tid Depends on cause and practitioner	↓ Pain by relaxing stomach muscles and supporting peristalsis	None	Ditchek and Greenfield (2002); Scharff and Kemper (2003); Fitzgerald (2009a)—**only use enteric-coated peppermint oil stated explicitly for enteric use**
	Homeopathy	Depends on cause and practitioner		None	Levatin (2009b)
	Nutrition Use sucrose only; eliminate lactose, fructose, sorbitol				Weydert (2009a) cites study showing 40%-60% improvement
	Aromatherapy	Lavender, frankincense, mandarin, rosemary, sweet fennel, black pepper, roman chamomile, ginger		None	Fitzgerald (2009a)
Acne	*Herbal* Goldenseal, extract or tincture	Adolescents: used to wash face or apply on acne lesions	Antibacterial properties	Nontoxic at recommended dose *Class 2b*	University of Maryland Medical Center (2010) (few studies)
	Tea tree oil	Adolescents: 5% topically, diluted with water bid (use 15% concentration for severe acne)	Effective against *Propionibacterium acnes*—antiseptic and antifungal properties	Contact dermatitis	Studies show 5% tea tree oil as effective as 5% benzoyl peroxide and with less skin intolerance (Pizzorno, 2008; Woolf et al, 2009b)
	Salicylic acid	Adolescents: topically bid (start with 0.5% until tolerated and ↑ to 2% concentration)	Breaks apart sebum plugs	Redness and irritation	Kemper (2002a)
	Azelaic acid (20%)	Apply bid for 1-6 mo	Antibiotic for *P. acnes*	Redness, irritation	Pizzorno (2008)
	Diet	Omit refined and/or concentrated CHO, milk, and foods with trans fats, iodine	High concentrated CHOs decrease immunosuppression; milk may contain hormones; in acne-prone skin, glucose tolerance is impaired	None	Pizzorno (2008)
	Nutritional Vitamin A Vitamin E Vitamin C	100,000 IU daily for 3 mo 400 IU daily 1000 mg daily	For premenstrual aggravation of acne		Kemper (2002a) cites uncertain benefit; Pizzorno (2008)

Continued

TABLE 42-5 Complementary Treatments* for Some Common Conditions in Children and Adolescents—cont'd

Diagnosis	Treatment Approach	Dosage	Benefit	Possible Side Effects†	Research/Citations
	Selenium	200 mcg daily			
	Zinc	50 mg daily (picolinate, acetate, or monomethionine)			
	Brewer's yeast	1 Tbsp bid			Pizzorno (2008)
	Calendula soap	Twice daily	For cleansing	None	Pizzorno (2008)
	Homeopathy	Various compounds used		None	Levatin (2009c) (no controlled clinical trials)
Anxiety	Yoga		↓ Need for medication; ↑ self-esteem and ability to cope	Limit some yoga postures in pregnancy; after recent surgery; with HTN, glaucoma, acute sciatica, herniated disk, or joint replacement	Ott (2002) (cites studies)
	Aromatherapy				
	Chamomile	Infants/children: put in vaporizer using 2 or 3 gtt of the essential oil	↓ Irritability from illnesses (GI upset, varicella, fevers)	Rare allergic reactions if sensitive to ragweed, aster, chrysanthemums (daisy family of plants) (dermatitis, asthma, dyspnea, anaphylaxis) Class 2b	Kemper (2002a)
	Lavender, rosemary	Can be inhaled from vaporizer or added to massage oil	↑ In beta waves with lavender; ↓ in alpha and beta waves with rosemary	None	Krebs (2006)
	Belly breathing	Place child's hand over his or her belly button and picture it as a balloon. Have child breathe in through nose slowly, counting to 3-4, and blowing up "belly balloon"; breathe out through mouth slowly to a count of 6-8, deflating "balloon." Do for 1-2 min, working up to 10-20 min.	↓ Stress, anxiety, pain, panic, and heart rate	None	Ditchek and Greenfield (2002)

Music therapy		Listening to music directly influences pulse, BP, electrical activity of muscles; may help nerve cell connections within the cerebral cortex; leads to relaxation	None	Lin et al (2011); Kemper and Jennings (2005); Kemper et al (2008b)
Massage		Improved behavior, ↓ cortisol levels, BP	Rare reactions to too much pressure; allergy to oil	Reilly (2005); Sherman et al (2010)
Meditation		Calms via psycho-neuroendocrine-immune pathways		Culbert and Richtsmeier Cyr (2009b)
Therapeutic touch		↑ Relaxation, ↓ pain and anxiety	None	Kemper and Kelly (2004)
Aphthous stomatitis *Herbal* Deglycyrrhizinated licorice (DGL)	Lozenges: 1-2 (380 mg) chewable tablets melted in mouth in proximity of lesions; Mouthwash of DGL (200 mg powdered DGL dissolved in 200 mL warm water) swished in mouth qid	Accelerates healing; under investigation as antiviral and immunomodulator	Rare allergic reactions if taken internally; rare skin eruptions with topical use *Class 1*	Pizzorno (2008) (cites studies showing majority heal by 3rd day)
Tea tree oil	Apply topically bid	Antifungal, antibacterial	Rare allergic reaction **DO NOT INGEST**	LaValle et al (2000)
Lactobacillus acidophilus	<12 yr: 2 tabs daily up to 3 times daily >12 yr: 4 tabs up to tid	Antifungal, antibacterial	None	Graedon and Graedon (1999)
Nutritional Vitamins B, B$_2$, B$_6$, Zinc gluconate	Multivitamin with minerals for age	Deficiencies in B vitamins occur more frequently in those with canker sores	None	Graedon and Graedon (1999); Rini and Bloom (2002)
Black tea bag	Hold a tepid tea bag over ulcerated area for 3-5 min	Tannins ↓ pain and coat the sore to speed healing	None	Graedon and Graedon (2010a)
Sauerkraut juice	1 Tbsp swished in mouth, then swallowed			Graedon and Graedon (2010a)

Continued

TABLE 42-5 Complementary Treatments* for Some Common Conditions in Children and Adolescents—cont'd

Diagnosis	Treatment Approach	Dosage	Benefit	Possible Side Effects†	Research/Citations
Asthma	*Nutritional*				
	Diet exclusions (see in footnotes at end of table)		In severe asthma, combined treatment with pharmaceuticals is recommended—nutritionals reduce allergic threshold and can help prevent acute attacks. Diet should include foods high in antioxidants and supplement with antioxidant vitamins and minerals.	Requires diet compliance	Many studies cited in Pizzorno (2008) for nutritional recommendation Kemper (2002a); Weydert (2009b) (cites studies)
	Vegan diet	Vegan diet with exception of cold-water fish for their omega-3 fatty acids—try for 4 mo; use onions and garlic liberally *plus* Omega-3 fatty acids (supplement with fish oil)	Alters prostaglandin metabolism, increases intake of antioxidant nutrients and magnesium, eliminates food allergens; onions and garlic inhibit release of inflammatory chemicals; omega-3 fatty acids improve airway responsiveness to allergens; asthmatics that regularly eat fresh, fatty fish have significantly better lung function and decrease risk of asthma		Kemper (2002a) (flaxseed oil or fresh fish several times a wk rather than fish oil supplements); Pizzorno (2008); Weydert (2009b) (cites studies showing supplementation with omega-3 fatty acids is beneficial)
	Green tea extract *or*	Give as watered-down tea, prn	Inhibits histamine release from mast cells by ↑ absorption of flavonoids		Pizzorno (2008)
	Ginkgo biloba extract	<50 lb: 25 mg tid 50-100 lb: 40 mg tid >100 lb: 80 mg tid	Improves respiratory function; ↓ bronchial reactivity	Rare side effects (headaches, GI upset) *Class 2d*—may potentiate effect of MAOIs	McGuffin and Goldberg (1998); Pizzorno (2008)
	Astragalus	2-6 yr: 2 g in tea 6-12 yr: 5 g in tea	May boost the immune system	Can interfere with anesthesia and warfarin	Ditchek and Greenfield (2002); Graedon and Graedon (1999)
	Vitamin B₆ (effects seen after 1 mo)	<50 lb: 8-15 mg/bid 50-100 lb: 12-25 mg/bid >100 lb: 25-50 mg/bid	Reduces side effects in asthmatics being treated with theophylline and reduces number and severity of attacks and other medication use		Kemper (2002a); Pizzorno (2008); Weydert (2009b) (combination of several nutrients vs. a single nutrient produces the benefit)

Magnesium	<50 lb: 60-125 mg/tid 50-100 lb: 100-200 mg/tid >100 lb: 200-400 mg/tid	Adequate levels necessary for lung function; affects asthma severity		Fogarty et al (2003); Kemper (2002a); Patel et al (2006); Pizzorno (2008)
Vitamin B$_{12}$	<50 lb: 300 mcg/day 50-100 lb: 500 mcg/day >100 lb: 1000 mcg/day	Possibly ↓ reactions to sulfites		Pizzorno (2008)
Vitamin C	10-30 mg/kg/day in divided doses	A major antioxidant in lung lining; asthmatics have higher need for vitamin C; inhibits histamine release		Fogarty et al (2003); Kemper (2002a); Patel et al (2006); Pizzorno (2008); mixed results
Vitamin E	>100 lb: 200-400 international units daily			Pizzorno (2008)
Quercetin	>100 lb: 400 mg 20 min before meals			Pizzorno (2008)
Zinc (tablets or liquid)	1-10 yr of age: 15 mg daily >10 yr: 30-60 mg daily	Levels found to be lower in asthmatics	Take with food to avoid upset stomach	Baral (2009a)
Selenium	1 yr to adolescence: 50-100 mcg daily Teens: 200 mcg daily	Levels found to be lower in asthmatics		Baral (2009a)
Omega-3 fatty acids	Cold-water fish (wild salmon, sardines), fish or flax oil, walnuts			Weydert (2009b) (cites studies)
Probiotics *Lactobacillus GG,* *L. plantarum, L. paracasei,* *L. reuteri, or L. acidophilus*	<12 kg: 10 billion CFUs daily >12 kg: 20 billion CFUs Capsules may be opened and mixed into drinks or soft foods. If deemed to help, use indefinitely	↑ Interferon levels; ↓ inflammatory response	Well tolerated. Use as trial for 2-3 mo to see if helps. **Do not use in those immunosuppressed, with a central venous catheter, or in premature infants.**	Greenfield (2009a) (cites studies)
Acupuncture		Study results mixed; some show modest, temporary effect; ineffective for long-term control		Fugh-Berman (1997); Micozzi (1996); Loo (2009a) (better designed clinical studies needed; a popular treatment in China and Russia)
Hypnosis	Children can be good candidates	Reduced symptoms and medication use		Kemper (2002a) (controlled studies cited)
Biofeedback	Age-appropriate	Improved breathing, fewer and less severe asthma attacks		Kemper (2002a) (studies cited)
Massage		Improves peak airflow, ↓ asthma attacks, relieves anxiety, depression	None reported	Kemper (2002a) (studies cited); McLellan (2009a)

Continued

TABLE 42-5 Complementary Treatments* for Some Common Conditions in Children and Adolescents—cont'd

Diagnosis	Treatment Approach	Dosage	Benefit	Possible Side Effects†	Research/Citations
	Yoga		↓ Symptoms and Rx use; ↑ lung capacity	None	Kemper (2002a); Ott (2002) (cites studies)
	Qi gong	Regular, self-conducted exercises practiced up to bid for <30 min (depending on response)	↑ Peak air flow, ↓ asthma-related symptoms; ↓ costs, hospitalizations/ED visits, antibiotic use	None	Chow and Choy (2009) (cites study)
Attention-Deficit Disorder (ADD) or Attention-Deficit/ Hyperactivity Disorder (ADHD)	*Music therapy*	Have children listen to calm, low-pitched, slow-tempo music	↑ Work performance, ↓ tension and activity, calming effect on autonomic nervous system	High-pitched music creates tension; low pitch stimulates relaxation; slow tempo is soothing; fast or stimulating music increases anxiety and activity	Kemper (1996, 2002a) (cited one study done in Israel showing hyperactive boys doing as well as normal boys when listening to calming music vs no music vs fast-paced music); Rickson (2006) (cites study)
	Biofeedback (two types: electromyogram and electroencephalogram)	Takes 6-8 wk (35-50 sessions) to learn techniques; age dependent	More relaxed behavior, ↑ attention and language skills; technique focuses on reducing muscle tension in the forehead and ways to exercise different neurological pathways to control impulses, ↑ attention, and process information better		Kemper (2002a) (cites studies showing behavioral improvement equal to methylphenidate; technique works best if also used with structured scheduling and behavioral rewards)
	Homeopathy	Depends on characteristics of individual and practitioner		Considered safe alone or when combined with CAM or conventional medicine	Chan (2002); Levatin (2009d). No RCT for use in ADHD done; homeopathic literature contains evidence for use.
	Evening primrose oil (EPO)	Children: 500-1000 g/daily standardized to contain 8% gamma linolenic acid (GLA)	Improvement on parent and teacher behavioral scales	Safe; headache, diarrhea, nausea with high dose or chronic use; flatus, halitosis; ↑ bleeding time	Chan et al (2000) (2 studies cited); Ditcheck and Greenfield (2002)
	Nutritional Elimination diet (see footnote at end of table)		Decrease in irritability, insomnia, fidgetiness; improvement seen in up to 73% (Boris and Mandel, 1994) Vitamin deficiencies can result in impaired brain and nervous system function. Diet recommendations address principle that children are fast oxidizers (Ghuman et al, 2008).	Elimination diet can put strain on family; dietary management less likely to produce results with discordant marital relationships present (Carter et al, 1993); may need consultation with nutritionist. None reported with suggested foods	Pizzorno (2008); Kemper (2002a) (try elimination diet only after other measures have failed to help; does not recommend Feingold diet) Ghuman et al (2008) (cites some significant difference on ADHD outcome variables in at least one RCT supportive of an additive-free elimination diet)

Magnesium	<12 yr: 400 mg daily >12 yr: 400-600 mg daily. These doses are greater than RDA.	Regulates muscles and nerve function, helps with restlessness, irritability, anxiety	Diarrhea, drowsiness, weakness, lethargy if overdose	Starobrat-Hermelin and Kozielec (1997) (cite study)
Fish oil supplements (omega-3[EPA] and omega-6 [DHA]) plus diet changes noted in elimination diet	500-1000 mg/daily or more. Ration of omega-6 to omega-3 should be 4:1. Dietary omega-3: cold-water fish, walnuts, flaxseed/oil, hemp seeds/oil. Dietary omega-6: seeds, soy, canola oil, safflower oil, borage, red meats.	Improves visual processing and motor coordination in children with dyslexia and dyspraxia—may help with ADHD	Safe to try	Ditcheck and Greenfield (2002); Weydert (2009c) (cites studies) McDonough-Means and Cohen (2009)
Yoga, tai chi, qi gong	Twice weekly	↑ Relaxation; ↓ anxiety, hyperactivity, inappropriate emotions and improves conduct	None reported	Kemper (2002a); Culbert et al (2009) (cites study)
Meditation	Adolescents	Decrease in self-reported ADHD symptoms; ↑ attention and cognition when tested	None	Zylowska et al (2008) (cites one study showing efficacy of "mindfulness meditation")
Guided therapy Exercise Martial arts	Any sport that involves close interaction between child and coach		None	Kemper (2002a)
Aromatherapy	Lavender or rosemary essential oil	Improved behavior, calming effect	None	Fitzgerald (2009b) (cites studies)
Autism *Qi gong sensory training (QST)*	Ten hours (20 sessions) over 5 mo by QST trainers with 15-min massage protocol by parents	Opens sensory pathways so child can receive coherent data from senses that improve sensory impairment, digestion, and sleep	None	Silva et al (2009) (RCT study showed significant classroom improvement of social/language skills, reduction in autistic behaviors)
Nutritional Targeted amino acid therapy (TAAT) (uses dietary supplements)		Balances inhibiting neurotransmitters and the excitatory transmitters; urinary excretion of these neurotransmitters is monitored		Weydert (2009d) (cites studies, though they all have limitations)
Gluten-free/casein-free diet		Addresses abnormal intestinal permeability; peptidase deficiency leading to buildup of opioid-like peptides; food allergies		Same as above
Omega-3 fatty acids (EFAs)	1000 mg EFA daily (combo of EPA, DHA, GLA)			Same as above

Continued

TABLE 42-5 Complementary Treatments* for Some Common Conditions in Children and Adolescents—cont'd

Diagnosis	Treatment Approach	Dosage	Benefit	Possible Side Effects†	Research/Citations
Breastfeeding (mothers)	*Fish oil* (salmon oil is better than cod liver oil)	750 mg, bid or tid	Important for hormone, nervous tissue, cellular membrane production	Use with caution in those with diabetes, hypoglycemia, if taking aspirin, NSAIDs, anticoagulants **Do NOT use in those with bleeding disorders; stop before surgery or dental procedures.**	LaValle et al (2000)
Burns—first or second degree	*Herbal* Aloe vera	OTC gel (70% aloe vera) or squeezed from leaves: apply topically several times daily	Antiinflammatory, antibacterial, promotes wound healing	Contact dermatitis *Class 1*	Kemper (2002a) (recommends using fresh leaves)
	Calendula (no other homeopathic remedies recommended)	Popular skin soother, available in skin creams	Some antiinflammatory properties	Rare rash *Class 1*	Kemper (2002a); Levatin (2009e) (offers other homeopathic medicines)
	Nutritional Vitamin A	10,000 IU daily			Kemper (2002a)
	Vitamin C	60-250 mg tid or qid	Aids skin healing	Diarrhea with vitamin C; decrease dose if occurs	Kemper (2002a)
	Vitamin E	<100 lb: 100-200 IU PO daily >100 lb: 200-400 IU PO daily or as a salve	Improves resistance to infection		Kemper (2002a) (vitamin E is experimental)
	Hypnosis		↓ Pain and anxiety; improves sleep and appetite	None	Kemper (2002a) (cites studies)
	Therapeutic touch		Increased healing	None reported	Kemper (2002a) (double-blind study showed statistically significant results)
	Massage (of nonburned areas during healing; of burned areas after healing)		For comfort, relaxation, ↓ pain and stress hormones; ↓ itching, tightness, pain; ↑ circulation/flexibility	None	Kemper (2002a)
Cerebral palsy	*Therapeutic (subthreshold) electrical stimulation* (aka neuromuscular electrical stimulation [NES])		Pulses electricity into motor nerves, stimulating contraction in selective muscle groups		NINDS (2010) (Studies show increased range of motion and muscular strength. NES differs from threshold electrical stimulation [TENS] which has not shown to be effective (intensity of stimulation is too low)

	Hyperbaric oxygen therapy	40 treatments over 8 weeks	Forces high concentrations of oxygen to brain tissue surrounding the damaged brain areas to "wake it up"		NINDS (2010) (Study showed no added benefit to treatment)
	Nutritional 12% *sucrose solution*	Infants: 5½ tsp sugar in 8 oz water: give 2 mL over 30-60 sec for 1-2 days during inconsolable crying	Sucrose analgesia—works by stimulating secretion of endogenous endorphins	None	Markestad (1997) (small double-blind crossover study); Duygu et al (2008) (cites RCT)
	Probiotics Lactobacillus reuteri	10⁸ CFUs/day	Immature immune system may be struggling with bacterial imbalances in GI tract (i.e., high levels of *Escherichia coli*); probiotics improve gut motility and function that ↓ gas, abdominal pain, and cramping	None	Savino et al (2010) (cites blind, placebo-controlled study)
Colic	*Herbal* Tea with German chamomile, mint, fennel, licorice, or vervain. Other herbs used by different cultures (anise, catnip, peppermint leaf, fennel, caraway seed, gingerroot, dill)	Infants: Give in weak tea form (mix ½ to 1 tsp of herb in boiling water; steep 5 min): give ½ to 4 oz tid. German chamomile tea: ½ cup or 150 mL; no more than tid at times of colic episode	Calming, sedating effects (antispasmodic on smooth muscles of digestive tract)	Rare allergic reaction (dermatitis, asthma, dyspnea, anaphylaxis) in people with hypersensitivity to daisy family (see Anxiety section, chamomile) *Class 2b*	Kemper (2002a) (cites study. Discourages using any pharmacological drugs. Gardiner (2007) (cites RCT studies: colic eliminated over 1 week in 57% of infants)
	Chiropractic	Average of 3 treatments	Corrects rotational and/or distractive forces of spinal/neural injury due to abnormality in in utero positioning or from difficult labor or delivery	None reported	Spicer (2009a) (cites studies showing up to 94% resolution)
	Nutritional Eliminate certain foods in mother's diet if breastfed	For 1 wk no cow's milk, chocolate, coffee, tea, cola, soy, corn, wheat, eggs, cabbage, onion, broccoli, peppers, beans, garlic	Colic symptoms improved	None—counsel mother on other appropriate foods of equal nutritional value	Kemper (2002a) (studies equivocal—elimination diet helps in some infants
	Therapeutic touch		Calming	None reported	Kemper (2002a) (no studies cited)
	Massage	Can be taught to parents; used prn: massage tummy lightly with baby on side, head somewhat down and bottom elevated; give 20-30 min after a meal; can extend massage to include entire body. Use lavender oil as massage vehicle.	Calming, relaxes	None if done gently	Ditchek and Greenfield (2002); Kemper (2002a); McLellan (2009b) (study involved massage 3 times daily)

Continued

TABLE 42-5 Complementary Treatments* for Some Common Conditions in Children and Adolescents—cont'd

Diagnosis	Treatment Approach	Dosage	Benefit	Possible Side Effects†	Research/Citations
	Motion	Gentle rocking or rolling in rhythmic and relaxed manner	Calming, relaxes	None	Ditchek and Greenfield (2002); McLellan (2009b). Use front or backpack.
	Music therapy	When colicky baby is quiet, calm, not crying, play a recording of some music baby likes; pay extra attention at this time to infant. When infant starts crying, turn off the music and withdraw attention. Also, white noise in background may sooth (e.g., turn on the dryer).	Conditioning response	None; requires fair amount of discipline and dedication for parents to comply	Kemper (2002a) (cites study showing significant results). If procedure followed throughout day, within days colic should decrease significantly.
	Aromatherapy Essential oils of bergamot, Roman chamomile, ginger, mandarin	Place oil in a vaporizer/diffuser in infant's room.			Fitzgerald (2009c)
Common cold/flu	*Herbal* Echinacea purpurea	Adults: 2000-3000 mg crude extract once daily	May boost immunity	Allergy to aster family.	Nahas and Balla (2011) (moderate evidence to support use for the common cold; dose and formulation prevent it being recommended at this time)
	Astragalus root	2-6 yr: 4-8 gtt liquid standardized extract or tincture every 12 hr 6-12 yr: 8-15 gtt every 12 hr (capsules: 250-500 mg every 12 hr)	Stimulates immune system by boosting macrophages' ability to destroy germs, increases T-cell production, and may have interferon-like effects	None **Do NOT use in patients with progressive infections (e.g., tuberculosis, HIV) or autoimmune diseases; can interfere with immunosuppressive therapy.**	Kemper (2002a); Ditchek and Greenfield (2002). Astragalus root may be used as a daily tonic to prevent URIs.
	Maitake mushroom liquid extract or tincture (can also use shiitake or reishi)	1-5 yr: 5 gtt in chocolate syrup, 1-3 times daily 6+ yr: 10 gtt	May boost immunity	None	Ditchek and Greenfield (2002)
	Tea made from ginger, cinnamon, cloves, allspice, cardamom	Put ½ tsp of each into 2 cups of water to make a tea. Sip slowly. Or cut up 1-2 inches of gingerroot, boil pieces in a quart of water for 10-20 min; strain, let cool; sweeten if desired.	Helps fight chills and fatigue. Ginger combats one of the common cold viruses.	None	Kemper (2002a) (cites study)

Elderberry extract	Sambucol preparations	Antiviral properties, especially against influenza and herpes simplex; ↑ inflammatory cytokine production and activates immune system; shortens severity of headaches, nasal congestion, muscle aches, fever	None reported	Barak et al (2001); Zakay-Rones et al (2004) (cite studies showing ↓ in length of flu symptoms; studies done in 18+-yr-olds) Kong (2009): cites mid-level evidence of efficacy
Nutritional *Vitamin C*	Children: 250 mg qid or 4-5 glasses of OJ daily at onset of cold. ↑ Other citrus fruit, kiwi, berries, melon, bell pepper, broccoli. Adults: 1000 g daily for prevention; up to 10 g daily for treatment	↓ Symptoms and length of illness by activating neutrophils to oxidize inflammatory mediators and ↑ extracellular vitamin C	Regarded as safe; GI upset, diarrhea in high doses **(Do not exceed 10 g daily).**	Kemper (2002a); Ditchek and Greenfield (2002); Nabas and Balla (2011) (recommendation for use based upon review of clinical trials)
Chicken soup; peppers (including cayenne), mustard, horseradish, salsa, other spicy foods	Sip soup slowly throughout the day	Thins nasal secretions, increases nasal and sinus mucous mobility	None reported; use cautiously in children with diarrhea-associated illnesses because of chance of causing dehydration	Kemper (2002a) (proven efficacy incomplete in children but worthwhile to try)
Garlic	Raw clove minced in mashed potatoes (1 medium clove = 100,000 units penicillin); do not exceed 2 cloves in 1 day Kyolic liquid garlic: 1-5 yr: ½ tsp; 6+ yr: 1 tsp in grape juice bid	Kills cold viruses; supports immune function	Safe, occasional GI upset Class 2c	Ditcheck and Greenfield (2002a); Kemper (2002a)
Zinc lozenges (adolescents or older only)	Adults: 15-25 mg lozenge sucked every 2 hr for 7 days only; administer within 24 hours of onset of symptoms	May ↓ severity and length of illness by binding rhinoviral docking sites with somatic cells, inhibiting infectivity; works on the upper oropharynx and nasal passageways	Mouth irritation, nausea, vomiting, diarrhea, abdominal pain; can suppress immune system if taken longer than 7 days; smell and/or taste disturbances with nasal or lozenges (can be permanent with intranasal products) **DO NOT USE intranasal zinc** (Sego, 2009).	Singh and Das (2011) (studies show ↓ in duration and severity of URI symptoms; when taken for 5 months, ↓ in URI incidence, school absenteeism, and antibiotic use in children; optimum dose, formulation, length of treatment not established); Sego (2009)
Biochemical Saline nose drops or spray	Recipe: ½ tsp salt in 1 cup warm water; give as drops nasally prn	Helps thin nasal secretions	None reported at recommended dilution	Kemper (2002a)

Continued

TABLE 42-5 Complementary Treatments* for Some Common Conditions in Children and Adolescents—cont'd

Diagnosis	Treatment Approach	Dosage	Benefit	Possible Side Effects†	Research/Citations
	Aromatherapy Oils of camphor, eucalyptus, menthol, pine, rosemary, wintergreen, tea tree	Inhaled by vaporizer or steam	Helps relieve congestion; heats nasal passages to a degree that inhibits viral replication	*Class 1*	Kemper (2002a)
	Massage May use oil of menthol	Cradle infant/child on one's shoulder or chest. Massage face, head, back, shoulders, anterior chest wall, lymph glands with emphasis on intercostals, scalenes, serratus, pectorals, trapezius; downward motion. Mentholated ointment rubbed on soles of feet then covered with socks can decrease coughing and improve breathing.	Relieves musculoskeletal pain from coughing; calms; oil may cool the nose, causing perception of decreased nasal congestion	Safe, but do not apply directly under nose in order to avoid aspiration *Class 1*	Graedon and Graedon (2010b); Kemper (2002a); McLellan (2009c)
	Acupuncture		Aids blocked sinuses; ↑ speed of mucociliary transport; ↑ immune function	Included in 1979 WHO list of recognized therapies	Loo (2009b) (cites studies)
Crohn disease/IBD	*Nutritional* Coconut	Eat 2 coconut macaroon cookies daily or add flaked coconut to cereal (1-2 tsp) or as much as needed for control.	Possible antibacterial effect from lauric acid in coconut fat that decreases inflammation	None	Graedon and Graedon (1999) (anecdotal information of efficacy)
	↓ Undigested or unabsorbed CHO_3; ↑ complex CHO_3 and fiber; use fresh fruits and vegetables (steamed, not raw); vegetable protein, fish; ↓ animal proteins high in saturated fat; ↑ omega-3 foods (wild salmon, mackerel, herring, sardines, flaxseeds, hemp seeds, walnuts)	Diet available (see reference for Gottschalk under research/ citations column)	Avoids carbohydrate overload and excessive fermentation in the intestines	Diet very restrictive	Ditchek and Greenfield (2002) (patients have been able to avoid immunosuppressive therapy when on the diet) Gottschalk (1994); Weydert (2009e)
	Supplements: take all these daily	Omega-3 (fish oil): 1000 mg Folic acid: 1 mg Calcium: 1000-1500 mg Vitamin D: 2000 IU daily Vitamin B_{12}: 400 mcg Zinc: 15-20 mg Iron: 30 mg (take with source of vitamin C) Magnesium: 500-1000 mg (in form of gluconate, glycinate, or aspartate for better absorption)	Reduces clinical symptoms and disease activity; replaces lost nutrients from inflammation and malabsorption; helps avoid other clinical symptoms (e.g., osteopenia, growth delay, skin disorders)		Weydert (2009e) (studies cited)

Condition	Supplement	Dosage	Effects/Comments	Safety	References
	Probiotics	*Lactobacillus GG, L. reuteri,* bifidobacteria: <26 lb: 10 billion CFUs daily >26 lb: 20 billion CFUs daily Use on trial basis for 2-3 mo. Capsules can be opened and placed in liquids/soft foods.		Well tolerated. Do not use in immuno-compromised children, in those with central venous catheters, or premature infants.	Greenfield (2009) (cites studies)
Dental caries	*Xylitol*	6-10 g daily; 1 piece of gum chewed for 5 min qid (or 2 mints sucked).	Encourages remineralization; inhibits plaque; bacteria cannot colonize	None; diarrhea if recommended dose exceeded	Ly et al (2006) (cites well-documented, scientific studies); (See also Chapter 33)
Diabetes type 1	*Herbal/nutritionals* Cinnamon, zinc, nicotinamide, folate, pyridoxamine, vitamins D and E		No evidence to date of benefit	Safe	Shapiro and Rapaport (2009) (cites studies using these herbs that showed no improved glycemic control, no effect on HbA$_{1c}$ or c-peptide levels or on residual beta-cell function; *vitamin E:* transient reductions seen)
Diabetes, type 2	*Nutritional* Whey protein supplementation for those eating high-glycemic index meals		Whey proteins have insulinotropic effects and ↓ postprandial glycemia in healthy people; ↑ insulin release	None	Frid et al (2005) (study cited)
	Herbal cinnamon	½ tsp daily	Lowers blood-sugar levels; also lowers HDL cholesterol	None	Pratt and Matthews (2004) (cites study by USDA)
Diarrhea	*Herbal* Berberine-containing plants (goldenseal, barberry, or Chinese remedy "huanglian coptis chinonsis")	*Goldenseal:* Toddlers and older children: ¼-½ tsp tincture or ⅛ tsp fluid extract tid-qid can be mixed with water or juice *Berberine:* Children: 5-10 mg/kg; adults: 25-50 mg tid or daily dosage up to 150 mg *Giardia:* Children, 5 mg/kg/day for 6 days	Demonstrated benefits of ↑ antimicrobial activity against bacteria (includes *E. coli, Shigella, Salmonella, Klebsiella, E. aerogenes*), fungi, protozoa, including *Giardia.* When used with any indicated antibiotics, ↓ length of illness.	Hypotension or hypertension, nausea, vomiting, diarrhea. **NOT recommended for infants younger than 1 mo old.** *Class 2b* More effective than metronidazole in treating symptoms but not in clearing from GI tract; use with standard antibiotic therapy	Kemper (2002a) (also, stop vitamin C); Pizzorno (2008) (cites studies). Only use Chinese herbal preparations prepared by a licensed herbalist. Avoid herbal diarrhea remedies that contain agrimony or cocklebur, alder, and leaves and tops of betony because they contain high levels of cancer-causing tannins.
	Potentilla tormentilla	Children: 3 drops tormentil root extract per year of life tid until diarrhea ends (maximum 5 days and 60 drops/day) Adults: 60 drops of tincture bid	Shortens duration of diarrhea caused by rotavirus		Pizzorno (2008)
	Lactobacillus acidophilus or *Bifidobacterium bifidum*	5-7 billion organisms/day (check bottle ingredients). If using yogurt, make sure it contains these bacteria.	Can also be used to ↓ incidence of rotavirus diarrhea in infants 5-24 mo old; reinforces mucosal wall barrier	Flatulence, constipation **Do NOT use in those with impaired immune systems.**	Kemper (2002a) (study cited); Pizzorno (2008); Pettit (2002)

Continued

TABLE 42-5 Complementary Treatments* for Some Common Conditions in Children and Adolescents—cont'd

Diagnosis	Treatment Approach	Dosage	Benefit	Possible Side Effects†	Research/Citations
	5% carob pod powder (ceratonia siliqua)	Infants to 1 yr: 1.5 g/kg/day in formula or in oral rehydration solution (ORS) Children >1 yr: 1-15 g/kg/day in ORS or milk; stop 24 hr after appearance of formed stools	Acute diarrhea in infants and children; tannins inhibit growth of bacteria and bind bacterial toxins; controlled studies of hospitalized infants showed efficacy of treatment	None Used for centuries in Mediterranean regions *Class 1*	Kemper (2002a) (recommends not relying solely on this remedy until more studies prove its efficacy)
	Garlic Best formulations are enteric-coated tabs/caps, dried or powdered garlic, standardized for allicin content	>1 yr: ½-1 clove (or 2-4 g) chewed, chopped, bruised, or crushed; do not use more than 2 cloves of raw garlic daily	Treats *Entamoeba histolytica*; is antimicrobial; organosulfur compounds are believed to interfere with microbial structures and functions	Garlic breath (try chewing fennel, parsley, fenugreek to counter garlic breath); has anticlotting effect; GI upset, rash, burning mouth, sweating, lightheadedness; raw garlic is toxic in high doses	Baral (2009b); Castleman (1995); Pizzorno (2008)
	ORS for short-term use in an emergency: 5 cups potable water, 1 tsp table salt, 8 tsp sugar (may use instant Jell-O powder for flavor). Not to be used for more than 2 days before seeing a health care provider.	Offer 1 Tbsp to 1 oz every 15-30 min; increase as tolerated		**Best to use pack-aged ORS solution or specially formu-lated rehydration formulas to balance electrolytes**	Mother and Child Health and Education Rehydration Project (2010)
	Homeopathy	For acute diarrhea may include *Arsenic album, Podophyllum peltatum, Chamomilla vulgaris, sulphur, Veratrum album, Cal-carea carbonica*	↓ Number of stools and duration of symptoms	None; used with ORS in developing countries.	Kemper and Jacobs (2003) (2 studies cited that showed efficacy of homeopa-thy); Levatin (2009f) (cites studies)
Eczema/atopic dermatitis	*Herbal* Evening primrose oil, borage oil, black currant oil	3 g PO daily Requires 4-12 wk for benefit Borage oil: 40 gtt bid	↓ Scaling, itching, and general severity; con-tains high amounts of a fatty acid (GLA) that those with eczema are thought to have a defect in metabolizing	Very safe; rare, mild GI effects; headache *Class 1*	Kemper (2002a); Gardiner et al (2001) (studies cited); Weydert (2009f) (cites study about efficacy of borage oil)
	Echinacea	Apply topically	Promotes healing by stimulating formation of new tissue	Contact dermatitis; use with caution in patients allergic to ragweed and daisy family of plants *Class 1*	Kemper (2002a) (remains untested)

Oolong tea	3 cups daily	Improvement in skin symptoms	None	Kemper (2002a) (cites study showing 63% of patients with moderate or marked improvement; more than 50% benefited for up to 6 mo)
Licorice (Glycyrrhiza glabra)	Apply topically as pure glycyrrhetinic acid or as a compress, using licorice tea.	Exerts effect similar to hydrocortisone cream	None Class 2b	Kemper (2002a)
Chamomile extracts, witch hazel, calendula, aloe vera, St. John's wort oil	Apply topically	May help ↓ itching and inflammation; promotes healing	Contact dermatitis; use with caution in patients with allergy to ragweed or daisy family of plants	Gardiner and Kemper (2000); Kemper (2002a)
Nutritional and Naturopathic				
Rotation diet	See Boxes 42-2, 42-3. Also consider eliminating artificial colors, benzoates, berries, citrus, currants, fish, legumes, sulfites, tomatoes, and occasionally beef, chicken, pork.	Improvement in symptoms	Ensure adequate calcium, nutrients	Kemper (2002a) (does not recommend elimination diet unless eczema affects >20% of body); Pizzorno (2008); Rindfleisch (2007)
Vitamin C (after diet exclusion and rechallenge)	Infants/children: one 8-oz glass of orange juice daily		None at recommended doses	Kemper (2002a) (cites double-blind, controlled crossover trial of vitamin C with significant improvement of eczema. Do not give added vitamin A, vitamin E, or zinc to eczema-prone children)
Yogurt	Daily	Helps keep the immune system balanced		Kemper (2002a) (mothers who consume yogurt or probiotics 2wk before delivery and 6 mo after delivery had infants who developed eczema at half the rate of control group)
Increase foods high in omega-3 fatty acids: wild salmon, herring, mackerel, flaxseeds and oil, walnuts, algae or fish supplement	Fish oil supplement 1000 mg daily	Correct deficiencies in omega-3 fatty acids and prostaglandin metabolism; decreases inflammatory state		Weydert (2009f)
Mind-body techniques (all modalities)		Affects oversensitive immune system by ↓ stress		Kemper (2002a)
Massage	Add 1-2 gtt of chamomile or yarrow oil to 1 tsp vegetable oil	Enhances healing, ↓ stress		Kemper (2002a)
Elevated lead level	*Herbal* Garlic	Add liberally to foods; see under Common Cold/Flu for dosing information	Helps eliminate lead and heavy metals	*Use with caution in patients with clotting disorders*	Castleman (1995) (based on some European studies)

Continued

TABLE 42-5 Complementary Treatments* for Some Common Conditions in Children and Adolescents—cont'd

Diagnosis	Treatment Approach	Dosage	Benefit	Possible Side Effects†	Research/Citations
	Teas from red clover, lemongrass, milk thistle	Tea drinks	Herbalists believe these help detoxify heavy metals	Do not give red clover to children <2 yr old (Castleman, 1995)	Kemper (1996) (no scientific studies done to date)
	Nutritional	Ensure adequate intake of calcium and iron	May speed elimination of lead	None	Ditchek and Greenfield (2002)
Enuresis	*Biofeedback*	Children >4 yr: program—child voids in front of a uroflow device while being coached; pelvic floor relaxation techniques in front of electromyogram	80%-100% resolution; decreases postresidual void and improves voiding curves	None	Schulman et al (2001) (cites study)
	Acupuncture	Several weeks of acupuncture treatments		None	Kemper (2002a) (cites study showing comparable results to desmopressin acetate)
Headaches	*Herbal* Feverfew (*Tanacetum parthenium*)	Children >2 yr: 0.25-0.5 mg parthenolide bid (start with lower dose and increase as necessary) or Chew 1-3 leaves daily Change brands if no results seen after a few wks; try for several months	Prevention of migraines: inhibits release of blood vessel–dilating substances from platelets to ↓ production of inflammatory substances and reestablish proper blood vessel tone; benefits are similar to aspirin and NSAIDs; but if NSAIDs do not work, neither will feverfew because properties are similar.	Mouth sores, abdominal pain, allergic reactions usually within first wk of use; not to be used during pregnancy or in patients with clotting disorders; sudden cessation may result in rebound headaches Class 2b	Holroyd and Mauskop (2003) (study showed reduction in number of attacks but not duration; reduced nausea and vomiting); Pizzorno (2008) (reduces number and severity of migraines, not for acute attacks); Kemper (2002a)
	Ginger	Fresh: 6-mm slice daily Dried: 500 mg qid	Antiinflammatory	None	Pizzorno (2008) (needs further study; best results from fresh ginger or ginger oil)
	Thermal biofeedback	6 yr and up: as needed to master techniques (4-12 sessions over 6-10 wk); daily home practice results in greater improvement in pain	For tension and migraine headaches: patients learn to dilate blood vessels to affect blood flow to the head and relax muscles; ↓ pain frequency/intensity	None. Technique very popular with children familiar with computer age technology.	Allen, (2004) (for prophylaxis); Grazzi et al (2001); Kemper (2002a) (50% decrease in headaches); Pizzorno (2008)
	Massage	Face, head, neck, or shoulder: massage using 1-2 gtt lavender, peppermint, or eucalyptus oil to 1 tsp vegetable oil as massage lotion. Foot massage is an alternative, using reflexology points. *Tension headaches:* rosemary or sweet marjoram to back of neck and shoulders	Muscle relaxation; oil may help decrease pain sensitivity	None reported	Kemper (2002a) (cites studies showing proven effectiveness); Fitzgerald (2009d)

Modality	Usage/Dosing	Effect	Adverse effects	References
Self-hypnosis		Evidence of suppression in mast cell activation	None	Culbert and Richtsmeier Cyr (2009c) (cite RCT studies showing 60% reduction in migraine frequency)
Therapeutic touch				Kemper (2002a); Holroyd and Mauskop (2003)
Progressive relaxation				Culbert and Richtsmeier Cyr (2009c)
Acupuncture	Age: When tolerant to needles; non-needle techniques or Japanese-style acupuncture also available	Use in conjunction with massage and relaxation	None reported	Holroyd and Mauskop (2003); Kemper (2002a) (cites many studies showing effectiveness for migraine prevention and tension headaches).
Chiropractic	Chiropractors "adjust" all ages: manipulation of cervical and thoracic vertebrae	Pain reduction, acute and chronic	Few complications with cervical manipulation	Kemper (2002a) (cites studies showing no better relief of headaches than with massage alone); Spicer (2009b) (cites numerous studies showing efficacy and ↓ use of pharmaceuticals)
Naturopathy and nutritional				
Elimination diet (see footnotes at end of table)		Benefits children with other allergy symptoms and frequent headaches; vitamin A excess increases intracranial pressure; vitamin D and zinc can cause headaches	None reported	Kemper (2002a); Pizzorno (2008) (30% to 93% reduction in headaches); Rindfleisch (2007); Scharff and Kemper (2003)
Riboflavin (B_2)	400 mg daily for 3 mo	↑ Mitochondrial energy efficiency	None reported	Pizzorno (2008) (68% patients improved in studies)
Increase magnesium-rich foods (nuts, legumes, dark leafy green vegetables, whole grain cereals and breads, seafood) and include ginger and hot peppers, garlic, onion, vegetable oils, fish oils	Adolescents: Magnesium 250-800 mg daily in divided doses plus vitamin B_6 25 mg tid plus vitamin B_2 (see above dosing) Ginger: Daily ¼-inch slice fresh or 500 mg qid dried or 100-200 mg tid extract (20% gingerol and shogaol) (for prevention) and 200 mg every 2 hr acute migraine	Low magnesium levels often found in patients with all types of headaches; magnesium maintains blood vessel tone and prevents overexcitability of nerve cells; vitamin B_6 increases intracellular Mg; ginger (contains aspirin-like compounds) exerts antiinflammatory effects and ↓ platelet aggregation	Diarrhea, gastric irritation	Holroyd and Mauskop (2003) (double-blind study in children showed significantly decreased frequency and severity of headaches); Kemper (2002a); Pizzorno (2008)
Homeopathy	Individualized homeopathic remedies (belladonna, *Bryonia*, *Gelsemium*, *Nux vomica*)	Reduction in intensity and frequency of attacks	Not recommended for children (Kemper, 2002b)	Fugh-Berman (1997) (cites a double-blind, placebo-controlled study)
Aromatherapy	Peppermint oil in diffuser or vaporizer	Analgesic effect for tension headaches	None	Holroyd and Mauskop (2003); Fitzgerald (2009d)

Continued

TABLE 42-5 Complementary Treatments* for Some Common Conditions in Children and Adolescents—cont'd

Diagnosis	Treatment Approach	Dosage	Benefit	Possible Side Effects†	Research/Citations
Head lice	**Bug Buster kit** (contains 4 combs for use on wet conditioned hair)	Sequential combing regimen	Elimination of lice	None More advantageous than using pediculicides	Hill et al (2005); (significant efficacy over permethrin and malathion treatments; results may not be applicable outside UK, due to varying resistance patterns)
	Margarine; mayonnaise; petroleum jelly; Dr. Weil's mixture‡	Apply heavy coating to hair and scalp; cover with shower cap overnight; wash out; comb repeatedly with nit comb		None; messy	Ditchek and Greenfield (2002)
Herpes simplex labialis	**Herbal** 70:1 lemon balm extract cream	Apply fairly thickly (1 mm) to herpetic outbreak bid to qid	Antiviral compounds; may prevent recurrences if used for initial infection; speeds healing	Safe; use with caution if taking thyroid medication; ↑ effects of barbiturates	Gardiner et al (2001); Rakel (2007)
	Aloe vera	0.5% aloe extract cream applied topically several times daily at symptom onset	Speeds healing; antiinflammatory	Contact dermatitis Class 1	Gardiner et al (2001)
	Nutritional Vitamin C	Vitamin C, 1000 mg, with the addition of 1000 mg of bioflavonoids taken 5 times a day for 3 days at symptom onset	Speeds healing	None	Rakel (2007)
	L-Lycine	1 g daily to prevent recurrence	Better for preventing outbreak; has antiviral activity that blocks activity of arginine (arginine promotes HSV replication)	Diarrhea and abdominal pain if product used in excess (>10 g/day); may ↑ LDLs slightly	Same as above
	Vitamin E (D-alpha-tocopherol)	1 cap: break open and apply directly to lesion	Speeds healing; ↓ pain	Rare skin reactions	Same as above
Insomnia, onset	**Herbal** Melatonin	<40 kg: 3 mg >40 kg: 6 mg	Advances circadian rhythms of sleep-wake and endogenous melatonin; enhances total sleep time	No serious side effects or comorbidities	Hoebert et al (2009) (cite studies of use in children with ADHD); Van der Heijden et al (2007)
	Valerian root, crude herb or standardized extract	2-3 g before bed	Mild anxiolytic effects; promotes sleep		Rakel (2007)
Jaundice	**Prayer therapy**		Shown to prevent RBCs from breaking down in test tubes; ↑ hgb		Kemper (1996) (studies done in adults only)

Condition	Therapy	Dose/Ages	Mechanism	Side effects/Cautions	References
Jock itch (fungal infection)	Listerine mouthwash	Apply to groin area	Antifungal activity from herbal oils in product	Stings if placed in more delicate areas	Graedon and Graedon (2010c)
Mood disorders (depression, bipolar disorder)	*Herbal* St. John's wort (standardized to minimum of 2%-5% hyperforin or 0.3% hypericin): for treatment of mild to moderate depression	Adult: 300 mg tid	Inhibits reuptake of serotonin, dopamine, norepinephrine, and binds to GABA receptors; other unknown mechanisms that may result in an additional indirect antidepressant effect.	Usually well tolerated. Side effects: insomnia, vivid dreams, restlessness, anxiety, agitation, irritability, GI discomfort, fatigue, dry mouth, dizziness, headache. A potent inducer of cytochrome P450 and P-glycoprotein. Lower incidence of adverse side effects than with paroxetine and other SSRIs (Kasper et al, 2010). See Table 42-3.	Freeman et al (2010): herb better or equivalent to placebo and standard antidepressants (studies cited; some applied to major depressive disorder); Kemper and Gardiner (2007); Rakel (2007)
	Nutritional Omega-3 fatty acids, vitamin B		Omega-3 and fatty acid intake boosts mood and vagal tone, dampens nuclear factor-kappa B activation and responses to endotoxin, and modulates magnitude of inflammatory responses to stressors.	Omega-3: Rare interaction with anticoagulants in adult studies	Kiecolt-Glaser (2010); Rey et al (2008) (cites studies—few in children)
	Exercise (regimens more likely to be followed in those with mild or moderate depression)	All ages	Improves energy, mood, appetite, sleep, self-esteem	Not indicated if patient has anorexia nervosa that is already causing compulsive overexercising	Schneider and Levenson (2008)
	Mind-body techniques (yoga, meditation, hypnosis, imagery, tai chi)	Appropriate ages	Enhance efficacy of other treatments	None	Rakel (2007)
	Acupuncture	Depends on age	Certain acupuncture points can alter neurotransmitter levels.	Rare	Rakel (2007) (cites studies)

Continued

TABLE 42-5 Complementary Treatments* for Some Common Conditions in Children and Adolescents—cont'd

Diagnosis	Treatment Approach	Dosage	Benefit	Possible Side Effects†	Research/Citations
Nausea and vomiting	*Herbal*				
	Combination tea with chamomile, lemon balm, peppermint	Small, frequent sips	Soothing to stomach upsets	Safe unless existing allergy to ragweed or daisy family of plants *Class 1*	Kemper (2002a)
	Goldenseal or barberry	Tincture: 2-3 gtt in 4 oz water, sipped slowly over 1 hr	Especially helpful if child has vomiting and diarrhea	None reported at therapeutic levels; excessive levels: GI upset, CNS stimulation *Class 2b*	Kemper (2002a)
	Basil tea	Make with ½ oz dry basil and 1 cup boiling water, steeped 5 min and strained		Not recommended for infants or toddlers *Class 2b*	Kemper (2002a); McGuffin and Goldberg (1998)
	Gingerroot	<3 yr: 25 mg qid / 3-6 yr: 50-75 mg qid / 6-12 yr: 125 mg qid / >13 yr: 250 mg qid / or / Ginger tea: 1 cup water to 2 slices gingerroot (simmer 5 min) or ¼ tsp fresh grated ginger in juice, applesauce, or cereal / or / Ginger soda (with real ginger)	Helps to reduce nausea by promoting elimination of intestinal gas and reducing GI spasms	Not for long-term use; use only in recommended doses. Large doses can cause cardiac dysrhythmias, depress CNS, compromise platelet aggregation. **Do NOT use in pregnancy.** *Class 2b*	Kemper (2002a); King and Murphy (2009) (cite RCTs)
	Poultice	Soak cotton flannel cloth in castor oil, lay cloth over abdomen, and cover with towel for 1 hr; remove cloth and rinse abdomen with baking soda/water solution	Old folk remedy for nausea		Kemper (2002a)
	Nutritional Vitamin B_6	Motion sickness and nausea of radiation therapy: 10 mg 1 hr before traveling / Pregnancy: 10-25 mg every 8 hr	May help minimize nausea	None reported	Kemper (2002a)
	Hypnosis	Age dependent	Helpful in reducing recurrent vomiting and nausea associated with chemotherapy or motion sickness	None reported	Kemper (2002a)
	Therapeutic touch/Reiki				Kemper (2002a) (has found it useful in her practice)

	Treatment	Description	Effects	Notes	Reference
	Acupressure	Apply pressure 1 inch up from wrist crease, between the two tendons leading to the palm; repeat every 2 hr as needed to control nausea (can use travelers Nei-Kuan Point elastic wrist bands sold widely to control motion sickness)	Delays onset of motion sickness	None reported	Rakel (2007)
	Acupuncture		Controls postoperative and chemotherapy-induced nausea and vomiting in adults and children	None	Loo (2009c); Rakel (2007) (cite studies of efficacy; acupuncture found to be as effective as antiemetics in preventing vomiting and better than emetics for preventing nausea)
Onychomycosis					
Herbal	Tea tree oil Vicks VapoRub	Apply topically to affected nails bid for 3 mo	Antifungal, antibacterial	Allergic dermatitis in sensitive patients	Gardiner et al (2001); Graedon and Graedon (1999)
	Vinegar	Soak affected nails in 50-50 solution white vinegar/water 30 min daily for several mo			
	Vitamin E	Puncture one vitamin E capsule; apply oil to affected nail at bedtime (cover with cotton sock) until growth of new nail			
	Cornmeal soaks	Place 1 inch of cornmeal in dishpan; add hot water; dissolve cornmeal; when just cooled enough to tolerate, soak feet for 1 hr. Repeat regularly.			Graedon and Graedon (2010d)
Otitis media					
Nutritional	Elimination diet (see footnotes at end of table)		Boosts immune system by eliminating allergens known to impede it; decreases congestion of nasal mucous membranes that affect drainage of the eustachian tubes or insults to the integrity of the middle ear	None reported	Nsouli et al (1994) (After elimination diet 86% of food-sensitive patients [71% of subjects] showed significant improvement in serous otitis media recurrence] Baral (2009c)
Pain *Acute*	*Combination of acupuncture and hypnosis*	10-15 min tid	Significant ↓ in pain, per studies	None	Zeltzer et al (2002) (cites study)

Continued

TABLE 42-5 Complementary Treatments* for Some Common Conditions in Children and Adolescents—cont'd

Diagnosis	Treatment Approach	Dosage	Benefit	Possible Side Effects†	Research/Citations
Postsurgical or procedural	*Music therapy* *Deep breathing* *Guided imagery* *Distraction (videos, video games, stories, blowing bubbles)* *Relaxation* *Aromatherapy* *Massage* *Therapeutic touch* *Transcutaneous electrical nerve stimulation* *Hypnosis* (works especially well in pediatrics (Kemper et al, 2006b) Infants: Breastfeeding, bottle feeding with sucrose water, pacifiers		↓ Anxiety and pain by stimulating endogenous opioid and nonopioid systems. Significant decrease in pain scores (heart rate, crying, facial action) vs when infants swaddled or held for painful procedures		Cited studies showing efficacy: Good et al (2001); He et al (2006); Kankkunen et al (2003); Shah et al (2007); Voss et al (2004); Walach et al (2003); Kemper et al (2006b) (cites many studies)
Chronic	*Mind-body techniques* *Music therapy*		See Hyperactivity/ADHD section		Good et al (2001); Voss et al (2004)
	Yoga		↓ Functional disability and pain; ↓ use of pain Rx in those with chronic lower back pain (Iyengar yoga)		Boyle et al (2004) (cites study; consider for preseason training); Williams et al (2009) (cites study)
	Acupuncture		Acute and chronic pain analgesia	None reported	Kemper et al (2000); Kemper (2002a)
	Therapeutic touch			None reported	Kemper (2002a)
	Relaxation: Deep breathing, biofeedback, meditation, autogenics, diaphragmatic breathing		Alter states of arousal; facilitate sense of control; ↓ anticipatory anxiety	None reported	Culbert and Richtsmeier Cyr, (2009d); He et al (2006); Kemper (2002a); Koh et al (2005)
	Massage		↑ Plasma beta-endorphin levels	None	McLellen, 2009d (cites RCTs)
	Magnet therapy	Electromagnetic, not static	Mechanism not understood; suspected neuronal effect		Miller (2004) (cites efficacy with various pain syndromes, including soft tissue, musculoskeletal, OA)
	Nutritional Infants: *breastfeeding or breast milk supplementation*		Significant ↓ in pain scores vs when infants swaddled or held for painful procedures		Shah et al (2007); Walach et al (2003)

	Dose	Mechanism/Effects	Side effects	References
Omega-3 fatty acids	Fish oil omega-3 fatty acids (3 g/daily) plus 9.6 mL of olive oil daily	Inhibits proinflammatory eicosanoid and cytokine production by peripheral tissues and glial cells; blocks voltage-gated sodium channels	Mild GI distress	Berbert et al (2005) (adult study showed significant improvement in joint mobility, fatigue, pain over 12 wk; better than when taking omega-3 fatty acids alone)
Glucosamine, chondroitin, SAM-e	Adult doses: Glucosamine: 1600-2000 mg daily; Chondroitin: 400-500 mg bid-tid; SAM-e: 200-1600 mg daily	Reduces cartilage destruction, enhances chondrocyte anabolism, ↓ inflammation by inhibiting prostaglandins	Do not take if diabetic or have seafood allergies; None; None; very expensive	Soeken (2004) (adult studies show these help with mild knee pain caused by OA)
Natural proteases	Adults: 2 tabs qid (containing 325 mg pancreatic enzymes, 75 mg trypsin, 50 mg papain, 50 mg bromelain, 10 mg amylase, 10 mg lipase, 10 mg lysozyme, 2 mg chymotrypsin)	Promotes production of cartilage proteoglycans	None	Miller et al (2004) (study of men running downhill showed superior recovery of contractile function and decreased soreness)
Herbal				
Boswellia	>120 lb: 500 mg bid	Attenuates soft tissue injury after intense exercise	None to mild GI upset	Kimmatkar et al (2003) (adult studies show significant decrease in knee pain, swelling, mobility with OA and RA)
Bromelain	Individually tailored program	Antiinflammatory, antiarthritic, analgesic properties	Rare, including allergic reactions	Walker et al (2002) (adult studies show effective for ankle sprain, muscular trauma, OA and RA, mild knee pain)
Willow bark, rosa canina		Antiinflammatory, analgesic properties		Under study
Premature infants	*Massage* (moderate pressure; especially effective for weight gain when done with coconut or safflower oil)	Facilitates weight gain, bone density, and development; ↓ medical complications; ↑ vagal activity, GI motility, insulin, IGF-1 levels; shorter hospital stays and costs	None reported; shorter duration of massage produces less positive results	Fugh-Berman (1997) (cites several studies supporting massage or stroking); Field et al (2010a,b)
	Music therapy (slow, soothing music [e.g., harp])	↓ Stress; ↑ weight gain; ↓ activity	None	Kemper and Hamilton (2008)
Presurgery precautions	*STOP THE FOLLOWING:* Vitamin E, Ginkgo biloba, Ginseng, Garlic, Ginger, Green tea, Flax, NSAIDs, ASA, Fish oil	Interfere with platelet function, causing prolonged bleeding		Graedon and Graedon (1999); Sego (2006)

Continued

TABLE 42-5 Complementary Treatments* for Some Common Conditions in Children and Adolescents—cont'd

Diagnosis	Treatment Approach	Dosage	Benefit	Possible Side Effects†	Research/Citations
PMS	**Herbal** Black currant seed oil or Flaxseed oil or Evening primrose oil	As directed on label tid or 1000 mg tid	Important fatty acids help relieve PMS symptoms and aid glandular function	None Flaxseed needs to be taken with at least 6 oz of water; contra-indicated with bowel obstruction *Class 1*	Balch and Balch (1997) (other helpful suggestions offered in this reference); Gardiner and Kemper (2000); McGuffin and Goldberg (1998)
	Angelica or dong quai (*Angelica sinensis*)	Powered root or tea: 1-2 g tid Tincture (1:5): 4 mL tid Fluid extract: 1 mL tid	Roots contain phytoestro-gens, which nourish and tone female glandular and organ system	**Do NOT use if patient is pregnant, is nurs-ing, or has a history of cancer, cardiac disease, or photosen-sitivity;** occasional light laxative effect. *Class 2b*	Gardiner and Kemper (2000); Pizzorno (2008) (other helpful preparations offered in this reference)
	Licorice root (*Glycyrrhiza glabra*)	Powered root or tea: 1-2 g tid Fluid extract (1:1): 4 mL tid Dry powdered extract (1:4): 250-500 mg tid	↓ Water retention of PMS; believed to ↓ estrogen levels and ↑ progesterone levels	**Do NOT use if preg-nant, breastfeeding, has glaucoma, diabe-tes, HTN, or cardiac disease.**	McGuffin and Goldberg (1998); Pizzorno (2008)
	Black cohosh (*Cimicifuga racemosa*)	20 to 40 mg of the standardized extract bid (generally standard-ized to triterpene glycosides as a marker compound)	Useful for relieving cramps; may help with depres-sion, anxiety, tension, mood swings, breast pain, headaches	GI disturbance, weight gain, headaches, heavy feeling to legs Overdose symptoms: nausea, diarrhea, abdominal pain, vomiting, dizziness, headache, tremors, arthralgias **Use only if nonpreg-nant, nonnursing; not to be used in those with cardiac disease or estrogen-depen-dent cancers.** *Class 2b*	Rakel (2007)
	Chasteberry (*Vitex agnus-castus*)	250 to 1000 mg/day of dried fruit or liquid extract: 20-40 mg/day	Useful with breast tender-ness symptoms of PMS; appears to alter GnRH and FSH-RH to normalize secretion of prolactin and estrogen: progesterone ratio; dopaminergic effect	**Do NOT use if pregnant, lactating;** occasional minor skin irritations *Class 2b*	Mancho and Edwards (2005) (cite study showing 50% symptom relief); McGuffin and Goldberg (1998); Pizzorno (2008); Rakel (2007)

Nutritional and Naturopathic

	Dosage	Effect/Mechanism	Notes/Side Effects	Reference
Calcium	1200-1600 mg/day	Improves a number of mood and somatic symptoms (relieves cramping, backache, nervousness)	Should not be taken at the same time as tetracycline, iron supplements, thyroid hormones, or corticosteroids (can ↓ iron absorption up to 50%). Some calcium may contain lead—in U.S. ensure products bear USP on label.	Pizzorno (2008); Rakel (2007) (cites RCTs)
Magnesium	200 to 400 mg/day	Relieves dysmenorrhea, likely through inhibition of prostaglandin $F_{2\alpha}$		Rakel (2007)
Vitamin B complex plus extra vitamin B_6	100 mg tid (vitamin B_6 component: 50-100 mg/day)	B vitamins complement each other. ↓ Water and increases circulation to female organs; helps restore estrogen levels.	Reports of nerve damage occurring with prolonged ingestion of 150 mg/day	Pizzorno (2008); Rakel (2007)
Vitamin E	400 IU daily	Helps with breast tenderness, depression, irritability; improves oxygen profusion to body		Pizzorno (2008)
Zinc	30-40 mg/day piconilinic form	Promotes hormone balance; controls high prolactin secretion that results from low zinc levels		Pizzorno (2008)
Diet	Eat plenty of fresh fruits, vegetables, whole grain cereals and breads, beans, peas, lentil, nuts and seeds, broiled fowl, fish, high-protein foods as snacks, and soy products. Avoid salt, red meats, processed foods, junk and fast foods, caffeine, refined sugar, and dairy products 1 wk before menses; increase water intake to 1 qt distilled water/day both 1 wk before and after menses onset.	Red meats and dairy products believed to contribute to hormonal fluctuations; other recommended foods aid in metabolism, glucose, and absorption of nutrients, and decrease free estrogen in blood; excluding salt decreases bloating and water retention; dairy products and refined sugars also believed to increase excretion of magnesium with resulting impaired estrogen metabolism and moodiness		Micozzi (1996); Rakel (2007)
Isolated soy protein (ISP) containing soy isoflavones (IF)	ISP containing 68 mg (aglycone equivalents) of IF daily	Influence endogenous estrogen effects on specific tissues	None reported	Bryant et al (2005) (study showed some improvement in headaches and breast tenderness; significant improvement in swelling and cramps)

Continued

TABLE 42-5 Complementary Treatments* for Some Common Conditions in Children and Adolescents—cont'd

Diagnosis	Treatment Approach	Dosage	Benefit	Possible Side Effects†	Research/Citations
	Chiropractic		For cramps: Possibly alters prostaglandin levels		Fugh-Berman (1997) (cites studies)
	Acupuncture		For cramps		Fugh-Berman (1997) (cites studies); NIH (1998)
Skin irritation/ diaper rashes	*Herbal* Aloe vera	All ages: Pure gel form, applied topically several times daily	Antibacterial effects; accelerates healing	Contact dermatitis *Class 1*	Gardiner et al (2001); Kemper (2002a); Murray and Pizzorno (1998)
	Chamomile	Add essential oil to bath or make as tea and rub on affected area	Soothes diaper rash, varicella, contact dermatitis	Contact dermatitis; caution if allergic to ragweed or daisy family of plants *Class 1*	Kemper (2002a)
	Nutritional Live *Lactobacillus acidophilus* bacteria or *Bifidobacterium bifidum*	Infants ≥6 mo: Give as yogurt; ½ to 1 cup daily PO <6 mo: Apply directly to diaper area (may use yogurt or suspensions containing these probiotics)	Thought to help replace the yeast on the skin	None noted	Kemper (2002a)
Sleep/sedation	*Music therapy* (before sleep deprived EEG)	1-5 yr: Soothing music of voice, guitar, and/or soft percussion; culturally appropriate	Produces sleep for procedures	None	Loewy et al (2005) (study compared music therapy vs. chloral hydrate for successful completion of EEG: 97% of music therapy vs. 50% drug subjects successful)
Teething	*Herbal* Tea tree oil	Dilute with water and apply topically to gums with cotton-tipped swab	Antifungal, antibacterial; mouthwash for oral health	Allergic dermatitis in sensitive patients. **NOT FOR INGESTION.**	LaValle et al (2000)
	Clove oil	Apply topically; do not use >48 hr	Antiseptic: Good for toothaches, teething; analgesic on mucous membranes; antiviral and antibacterial		
Toothache, temporary relief	Acupressure	Rub ice cube in the V-shaped area where bones of your thumb and forefinger meet ("anatomical saltbox"; "Hoku" point) for 5-7 min.	Dulls pain	None	Shedletsky et al (1984) (repeated in later studies; 60%-90% effective)

	Herbal			
UTI prevention	Cranberry juice, juice extract capsules, or pure cranberry liquid extract mixed with orange juice to decrease tangy taste	Juice: 150-600 mL/day children and adolescents; 400 mg caps caps once or bid for adolescents	Reduces adhesion of gram-negative and gram-positive bacteria to bladder wall cells	Safe: can ↑ urinary oxalate levels; use cautiously in those with sugar sensitivity	Gardiner et al (2000) (cites studies); Pettit (2002)
Warts, common	Duct tape occlusive therapy	Cover wart(s) with piece of duct tape for 6 days (if falls off, replace); remove tape: soak wart in warm water and file with emery board; replace tape the next day and repeat regimen for 2 mo or until wart disappears (most resolve in 1 mo)		None unless develops allergic reaction to tape	Focht et al (2002)

*Inclusion of a complementary treatment in this table does not imply endorsement by this textbook's authors; for reference only.

†Food supplements and herbal labeling classifications. *Class 1*, Herb can be safely consumed when used appropriately; *Class 2*, the following use restrictions apply: *2a*, for external use only; *2b*, not to be used during pregnancy; *2c*, not to be used while nursing; *2d*, other specific use restrictions as noted; *Class 3*, requires label stating to be used only under supervision of an expert; *Class 4*, insufficient data for classification.

‡**DR. ANDREW WEIL'S MIXTURE FOR HEAD LICE.** Mix together: 2 oz olive or coconut oil; 20 gtt tea tree oil; 10 gtt either rosemary, lavender, or lemon essential oil. Rub into scalp and hair; cover with towel or shower cap for 1 hr only; wash thoroughly and comb repeatedly with nit comb (Ditcheck and Greenfield, 2002, pp 350-351).

SPECIFIC DIET EXCLUSIONS:

Asthma: Eliminate milk, chocolate, wheat, eggs, nuts, corn, soy, citrus, food colorings (tartrazine, sunset yellow, amaranth), food additives (sodium benzoate, 4-hydroxybenzoate esters, sulfites) and tryptophan (amino acid in milk, cheese, turkey, bananas). Ensure adequate vitamin C, magnesium, extra onions and garlic, fatty fish in diet.

Attention-Deficit Disorder (ADD) or *Attention-Deficit/Hyperactivity Disorder (ADHD):* See Box 42-3. Also recommended eliminations: apples, artificial colors, aspartame, butylated hydroxytoluene (BHT, often in packaged cereals), benzoates (chewing gum, margarine, pickles, prunes, tea, raspberries, cinnamon, anise, nutmeg), caffeine, corn, dairy, nitrates and nitrites (preserved meats), oranges, propyl gallate, sulfites (dried fruits, mushrooms, potatoes, baked goods, canned fish, relishes), peanuts, tomatoes (Rindfleisch, 2007). Supplement with a multivitamin that includes thiamin, niacin, vitamin B₆, magnesium, manganese, potassium, and zinc; fish oil supplement. Encourage diet high in protein, (good) fat, fruits and vegetables.

Headaches: Avoid nitrites (processed meats), aspartame, MSG (mushrooms, kelp, scallops, Chinese food), chocolate, aged cheeses, caffeine, wheat, oranges, eggs, milk, beef, corn, sugar, yeast, shellfish; avoid added vitamins A and D, zinc. Limit caffeine.

Otitis Media: Eliminate milk and dairy products, eggs, wheat, corn, citrus, peanut products, fish, tomatoes, concentrated simple carbohydrates (sugar, honey, dried fruit, concentrated fruit juices, etc.). Most subjects allergic to 2 to 4 foods, most to milk, wheat, egg, peanuts, soy, and corn (Nsouli et al, 1994).

ADHD, Attention-deficit/hyperactivity disorder; *ASA,* acetylsalicylic acid (aspirin); *bid,* twice daily; *BP,* blood pressure; *CAM,* complementary and alternative medicine; *cap,* capsule; *CFUs,* colony-forming units; *CHO,* carbohydrate; *CNS,* central nervous system; *DHA,* docosahexaenoic acid; *EEG,* electroencephalogram; *EPA,* eicosapentaenoic acid; *FDA,* U.S. Food and Drug Administration; *FSH-RH,* follicle-stimulating hormone releasing hormone; *g,* grams; *GABA,* gamma-aminobutyric acid; *GI,* gastrointestinal; *GLA,* gamma-linolenic acid; *GnRH,* gonadotropin-releasing hormone; *gtt,* drops; *HDL,* high-density lipoprotein; *HbgA₁c,* hemoglobin A concentration; *Hgb,* hemoglobin; *HIV,* human immunodeficiency virus; *HTN,* hypertension; *IGF,* insulin-like growth factor; *IU,* international units; *lbs,* pounds; *LDL,* low-density lipoprotein; *MAOIs,* monoamine oxidase inhibitors; *MSG,* monosodium glutamate; *NIH,* National Institutes of Health; *NSAID,* nonsteroidal antiinflammatory drug; *OA,* osteoarthritis; *OJ,* orange juice; *ORS,* oral rehydration solution; *OTC,* over-the-counter; *PMS,* premenstrual syndrome; *PO,* by mouth; *prn,* as needed; *qid,* 4 times daily; *RA,* rheumatoid arthritis; *RBC,* red blood cell; *RCT,* randomized-controlled trial; *Rx,* pharmaceutical medication; *SSRIs,* selective serotonin reuptake inhibitors; *tabs,* tablets; *Tbsp,* tablespoon; *tid,* 3 times daily; *tsp,* teaspoon; *UK,* United Kingdom; *URI,* upper respiratory infection; *USDA,* U.S. Department of Agriculture; *UTI,* urinary tract infection; *WHO,* World Health Organization.

43

Strategies for Managing a Health Care Practice

DENISE A. HALL

A successful health care practice requires the provision of excellent clinical care, a commitment to good customer service, sound business planning, efficient day-to-day operations, and ongoing attention to administrative and risk management operations. If the practice has excellent clinical providers but does not pay attention to or does not devote equal resources to its business operation, its future ability to operate will be compromised. This chapter is a primer for setting up and managing a health care practice and provides brief overviews of key administrative and clinical management strategies necessary for successful practice operations.

Paying attention to business operations in a medical practice can seem like a daunting task at times. Staying current with state and federal regulations, employment laws, and risk management issues requires constant vigilance and attention. Compliance with these legal requirements is only the beginning of ensuring good business operations. Strategic planning; financial management; staff recruiting, training, and retention; efficient administrative and clinical operations; ongoing practice benchmarking; risk management awareness; marketing; customer service and patient education are areas that can make a practice either mediocre or outstanding and are basic and necessary elements of successful medical practice management.

Developing a business plan and creating an operations plan are two practice management strategies that can provide the structure for many of the administrative and clinical recommendations that make the practice successful.

The Business Plan

Creating a business plan is a requisite first step for a new practice and is also recommended for established practices when considering a new project or change in business operations (e.g., adding a new provider, opening a new office, or offering new services). The business plan clearly declares the philosophy and goals of the practice on which an overall strategic plan will be based and how these goals will be reached. Even a simple one- or two-page plan can help provide a formal structure for present and future planning. A *vision statement, market analysis, strategic plan,* and *organizational chart* make up a simple business plan for

the practice and provide the necessary framework for clinical and administrative operations. If the practice is seeking funds from a financial institution or granting organization, a business plan will most certainly be requested as part of the application process.

VISION STATEMENT

This vision statement is the foundation for all clinical and administrative operations of the practice. It may be one or two simple sentences or one or two paragraphs, but it should summarize the practice's reason for being and the philosophy of the organization. It is a good idea to revisit the vision statement annually to ensure that it continues to reflect the mission and values of the practice.

MARKET ANALYSIS

A market analysis is a primary and critical key task that should be done to better understand the specific demographic makeup of the targeted patient population. This analysis looks at the current and future demand or need for (pediatric) health care services in a particular area and the current capacity or options for providing these services. Factors such as population data, growth projections, primary care competition, and the current economic and business climate, are important areas to review. Gathering this information requires time and effort but is important for good decision-making for new business operations as well as for short- and long-range planning.

STRATEGIC PLAN

The vision statement and market analysis are used together to formulate the strategic plan for the practice. A strategic plan is useful for starting a new practice, planning practice growth, or simply developing new projects. It provides both framework and direction for the task at hand and sets the business plan in motion. The strategic plan normally includes the following:
- Goals and objectives identified by the practice
- Budget or financial plan
- Physical and human resource requirements of the project
- Operations plan for development and implementation, including a timeline

ORGANIZATIONAL CHART

An organizational chart is a helpful administrative resource for the strategic plan and ongoing practice operations. The organizational chart normally shows names, titles, and reporting responsibilities of the people involved in implementing the business and operations plans of the practice. It not only provides a visual snapshot of the management structure of the practice but also connects its business plan with the practice's personnel resources.

■ The Operations Plan

Successfully moving the business plan from paper to reality requires additional planning and implementation. The operations plan provides structure during this process and helps ensure that key elements for successful practice management are not overlooked. It uses the formal business plan for its initial direction, but has a different purpose. Its goal is to take more of a micromanagement view of the business and strategic plan and make them fully functional. Developing an annual operations plan and corresponding budget is a valuable process and a tool for ensuring that the practice's clinical, administrative, and financial goals and operations are integrated. Although every practice is individual and distinct, and business plans differ by design and need, the operating plan establishes systems and processes to:

- Identify key practice management areas and practice resources.
- Develop policies and procedures to ensure administrative and clinical quality assurance.
- Monitor, report, and benchmark clinical and administrative results.
- Emphasize quality improvement and customer service.

Operational checklists are included in this chapter for the areas of legal, governance, financial, human resources, and clinical practice operations. The checklists include a basic list of elements and issues that are important in practice operations, regardless of size or strategy.

LEGAL AND GOVERNANCE OPERATIONS

Legal counsel and a certified public accountant (CPA) are necessary professionals to consult about legal, fiduciary, and financial issues that can affect a practice. Developing a strong business relationship with an attorney and accountant with experience in health care operations is valuable, not only during the start-up phase of a health care practice, but also for ongoing consultation. Box 43-1 includes a checklist of major items included in this category that need to be taken into consideration, especially for a new practice.

Organizational Structure and Tax Status

Choosing an organizational structure and a tax status are two initial decisions required when starting a practice or in subsequent years if the practice undergoes ownership changes or it is beneficial to take advantage of new tax laws relating to business structures. Because of the numerous legal and financial implications involved when choosing an organizational structure, it is imperative to have good legal advice during this process. Trusted financial and legal advice is also essential

---

BOX 43-1 Legal and Governance Checklist

- Legal counsel
- Accountant
- Organizational structure
  - Partnership, corporation
  - Tax status
  - Governance documents
- Federal tax employer identification number (EIN)
- National practice identification number (NPI)
- State and local tax identification numbers
- Business licenses
- Provider clinical license and Drug Enforcement Administration (DEA) number
- Insurance requirements
  - General liability
  - Professional liability
  - Workers' compensation
- Government regulations
  - Occupational Safety and Health Administration (OSHA)
  - Health Insurance Portability and Accountability Act (HIPAA)
  - Clinical Laboratory and Improvement Amendments of 1988 (CLIA)
- Legal guidelines
- Record retention

---

when drafting the practice's governance documents, such as bylaws, articles of incorporation, employment agreements, and buy-sell agreements, and when reviewing lease documents and contracts.

Federal Tax Identification, National Provider Identification and Required Licenses

In addition to appropriate legal documents, the practice will require a federal tax identification number, also called an employer identification number (EIN), and a national provider identification number (NPI). A state tax identification number is required for state tax reporting, and most cities require a local business license.

There are also identification and licensing requirements for health care providers. All providers should have an individual NPI. Most states require a state license and a Drug Enforcement Administration (DEA) number as minimum requirements.

Insurance Requirements

Basic insurance requirements for the practice include general liability, professional liability, and workers' compensation insurance.

General liability insurance protects the assets of the business from casualty damage, employee dishonesty, theft, business interruption, and personal injury. Pediatric practices are advised to add "spoilage" coverage to provide protection for their substantial vaccine inventories.

Professional liability insurance provides coverage for both individual providers and the practice in the event of a claim of medical malpractice. Professional liability insurance is written on either a claims-made or an occurrence basis. Because claims-made policies normally require the purchase of a "tail" or extended coverage in the event that the policy is terminated, it is important to understand the differences and which type of coverage is offered under the policy. When purchasing professional liability insurance, it is wise to insure the practice and the individual providers. Insuring the practice provides an added layer of protection in the event of a medical malpractice claim and includes coverage for clinical and administrative support staff. Limits of $1 million to $2 million for each occurrence with an aggregate limit of $3 million to $4 million are considered minimal standards of protection. Insurance payers will normally have coverage requirements in their provider contracts. Medical staff privileges also require a certain amount of coverage. The practice will need to review the pros and cons of individual policies for providers versus obtaining coverage on a group basis. This decision may vary based on practice preference, organizational structure, or legal or insurance company recommendations.

Workers' compensation insurance protects the practice and its employees against accidents or injuries on the job. Examples of accidents that most often happen in a health care practice are needlestick injuries; injuries caused by lifting or moving patients, equipment, or files; and repetitive motion types of injuries suffered by administrative staff. The practice's annual claims experience will impact its premiums for workers' compensation coverage; consequently an ongoing training program regarding safety in the workplace is important for good risk management and managing practice expenses.

Government Regulations

There are numerous and important regulations for health care practices. Special attention must be given to these regulations to ensure awareness, training, and compliance.

Health Insurance Portability and Accountability Act. Health care providers and managers should have a good understanding of the Health Insurance Portability and Accountability Act (HIPAA) and be aware of important and ongoing changes to this major piece of legislation. Although the section of this regulation dealing with the portability of health insurance (Consolidated Omnibus Budget Reconciliation Act [COBRA]) has been in effect since 1996, two more recent sections on privacy and security have important relevance for health care providers. The primary purpose of the privacy section of HIPAA is to protect the rights of patients. HIPAA regulations define how providers must treat protected health information (PHI). HIPAA regulations now require health care providers to provide all patients with a "Notice of Privacy Practices." This notice informs patients of their rights under HIPAA and how the practice will use and disclose their PHI for treatment, payment, or health care operations. Other parts of this regulation include requirements for the electronic transfer of PHI and for the development of business associate contracts with organizations with which the practice may share confidential information (outside billing or collection agencies, medical records couriers, transcription companies, answering services, etc.).

The security provisions of HIPAA require specific precautions for the safety and confidentiality of electronic health information. Being HIPAA compliant requires the practice to develop policies and procedures that ensure confidentiality of patient information within the practice and to orient and train staff in these areas.

The American Recovery and Reinvestment Act of 2009 (ARRA) includes the Health Information Technology for Economic and Clinical Health (HITECH) Act, which added new provisions to both the privacy and security sections of HIPAA. One of the more important additions to the privacy regulations is the fact that a patient who pays for medical services in full out of pocket can restrict a medical practice from disclosing PHI to a health plan (for payment and health care operations). Other important changes include guidelines for security breach notification and an expansion of HIPAA requirements for a practice's business associates.

The HITECH Act also includes stimulus funding to increase the use of electronic health records by health care providers. Financial incentives for providers as well as funding to support regional health information exchanges are significant pieces of this legislation.

Occupational Safety and Health Administration. The Occupational Safety and Health Administration (OSHA), a division of the Department of Labor, regulates health and safety in the workplace. Medical offices are required to meet safety standards regarding universal precautions, blood-borne pathogens, and tuberculosis and have written policies that enforce these standards. Practices must also provide education and annual training to staff and keep accurate records regarding any injuries and exposures that may have occurred. OSHA standards focus on infection control and contain guidelines for personal protective equipment, frequent handwashing, decontamination, and waste disposal.

Clinical Laboratory and Improvement Amendments of 1988. The Clinical Laboratory and Improvement Amendments of 1988 (CLIA) set performance standards and licensing requirements for hospital and physician-office laboratories based on the complexity of the tests being performed. CLIA standards focus on personnel qualifications of laboratory staff, quality control, quality assurance, and proficiency testing. A procedure manual that details how to perform every test conducted in the laboratory must be kept up-to-date. Based on the complexity of tests performed, the laboratory will have a CLIA designation of waived, physician-performed microscopy (PPM), moderate complexity, or high complexity. When determining what types of laboratory tests or services will be performed in the office, it is important to ensure that the practice has the necessary CLIA designation before providing those services. For example, a rapid strep test could be categorized as waived, PPM, or moderate based on the particular brand of the test. A cost-benefit analysis should be undertaken as part of any decision regarding laboratory services. The cost of CLIA compliance, proficiency testing, equipment, and staffing of the laboratory should be included along with the price of the individual tests when analyzing clinical needs, potential reimbursement, and customer service.

Retention of Records

There are specific guidelines for the retention of all records and business documents in the health care practice. Requirements vary depending on the type of records (medical records, financial records, claims and billing records, staff and employment records). Table 43-1 contains general recommendations for records retention. As the practice gets larger, the retention of records can become an expensive storage problem. Technologies such as optical scanners and "electronic file cabinets" can help practices meet these requirements efficiently.

TABLE 43-1	Guidelines for Record Retention

Document/Records	Months to Keep
Agenda or schedules	24
Bank statements	60
Budgets	60
Canceled checks	60
Committee meeting minutes	60
Contracts	60 (after expiration)
Employment applications	36
Financial reports	60
Financial statements	Life of organization
Insurance documents	36
Insurance policies	72 (after expiration)
Invoices	72
Policies	Life of organization
Accounts receivable	84
Account reconciliations	24
Reports	60
Tax returns	72
Medical records	Pediatric records should be kept a minimum of 7 years past age of majority

Developed from Recommendations of the American Society of Association Executives and the U.S. Code of Federal Regulations.

Financial Operations

Managing the revenues and expenses of a practice requires the establishment of good financial and accounting systems. This includes developing and implementing financial policies and processes to ensure necessary cash flow for the financial health of the practice and regular monitoring, review, and reporting of its revenues and expenses (Box 43-2). The following steps are recommended when establishing the financial operations of the practice.

- Establish a professional relationship with a bank or other financial institution for the purposes of opening a checking account, a payroll checking account, a savings account, and a line of credit.
- Work closely with an accountant to develop the bookkeeping and accounting systems to meet the needs of the practice. Depending on the size and sophistication of the practice this may mean that the accountant actively reviews financial operations on a monthly basis and prepares the financial reports or is used more as a business consultant. In either case, the accountant will probably be responsible for preparing annual tax returns.
- Choose computerized accounting software. A packaged accounting software, such as Quick Books or Quicken,

BOX 43-2	Financial Operations Checklist

- Accountant
- Bank accounts
- Accounting software
- Chart of accounts
- Budgets
  - Operations
  - Personnel
  - Capital expense
- Payroll
- Financial reports
- Revenue cycle

usually meets the needs of a small to medium-sized practice, whereas larger organizations with multiple locations and many cost centers may require a more powerful and sophisticated system. The accountant should be able to suggest a system that will best meet the needs of the practice. The system should not only be able to manage accounts payables and write checks but also be able to develop budgets, automate payroll, and provide a standard set of financial reports. The practice's accountant can also help decide whether to operate the accounting system on a cash basis, an accrual basis, or a modified cash basis. Most medical practices use a cash or modified cash basis of accounting.

- Establish a chart of accounts. The chart of accounts plays a key role in budgeting and financial reporting. Although any chart of accounts that can break out and report on revenue sources and track expenses by similar types will suffice, the practice may wish to adopt a chart of accounts similar to the one recommended by the Medical Group Management Association (MGMA). Setting up the chart of accounts so that financial reports are comparable with those of other similar medical groups can be helpful not only for the management of revenue and expenses in the practice, but also comparison or benchmarking purposes.
- Establish internal controls. Safeguarding the assets of the practice is an important part of responsible financial operations. Policies and procedures for handling and depositing cash and checks, reconciling bank statements, check signing, and petty cash management need attention in this area.
- Prepare an operations budget. The development of an operations budget is important as a tool for (1) synchronizing the clinical and administrative operations of the practice with the anticipated revenues and expenses, (2) monitoring the revenues and expenses throughout the year, and (3) reporting the status of actual financial operations compared with the budgeted plan.

OPERATIONS BUDGET

An annual operations budget should be developed in conjunction with the practice's operations plan and usually starts with a detailed look at the anticipated revenues of the practice (revenues from third-party payers or insurance payers, patient payments, and ancillary services). The fee schedule, insurance reimbursement data, average collection rates, and patient visit data are important elements that can be used to forecast practice revenues. Revenue projections should not only look back at historical data and current contracts but also take into account any anticipated changes that will affect the practice. Potential new sources of revenues, anticipated growth, and changes in contracts can affect practice revenue and should be included in the budget process.

Practice Expenses

Salaries and Benefits. In most instances the biggest expense for a health care practice is personnel. Personnel and supporting expenses are listed in the budget as salaries and benefits. Development of this part of the budget will also require projections based on past and anticipated patient visit data. The anticipated patient visit data are helpful in determining the number of providers and support staff required. A separate personnel budget developed using spreadsheet software, such as Excel, can help with planning this part of the expense budget. The personnel budget should identify titles, departments, full-time equivalent (FTE) status, hourly rate or salary, and projected annual compensation, including estimated salary increases and overtime. The chart of accounts normally specifies separate line items for budgeted salaries for physicians, nurse practitioners, physician assistants, management, and support staff. After the total salary expense is determined, the amount to budget for payroll taxes can be calculated (usually a percentage of the total salary expense). Benefit costs, such as health or dental insurance, can also be projected using a spreadsheet and then transferred to the operating budget. If practice policies or employment agreements provide additional benefits, such as continuing medical education or professional dues, these totals should also be added as a specific line item in the benefits budget category.

Other Expenses. Other operating expenses in the budget fall under the categories of physical resources, general and administrative expenses, or purchased services, and these should be included as separate sections in the budget and in financial reports. Examples of expenses budgeted as physical resources are occupancy costs (rent or mortgage payments), janitorial expense, medical supplies (including vaccines), printing of clinical forms, or any expense directly used in providing medical services. General and administrative expenses are those that pay for the administrative operations of the practice. Office supplies, administrative printing, telephone (including pagers), insurance, and depreciation expenses are examples of expenses that belong in this category. Expenses that fall under the classification of purchased services are fees paid to others for specific services provided. Accounting and legal services, answering service, telephone support, computer support, and marketing services are examples of purchased services.

Fixed Asset Expenses. If the practice is planning to purchase any furniture or equipment or make significant improvements to the facility that are considered "major" (usually more than $500), a capital expense budget and corresponding depreciation schedules should be developed. After the budget is finalized, the revenue and expense line items should be spread over a 12-month period so that they can be tracked, monitored, and reported by month. These expenses can either be spread equally over the 12 months of the year or adjusted based on known revenue or expense patterns.

FINANCIAL REPORTS

At a minimum, a basic set of monthly financial reports should include a profit and loss (income/expense), a year-to-date profit and loss compared with budget, and a balance sheet.

The practice's accounting software system should be able to produce these basic reports and other financial reports that are beneficial in tracking the financial performance of the practice. The practice may want to review additional reports on a quarterly or annual basis.

PAYROLL

In a small practice the accounting software can usually be used to prepare the payroll, calculate withholding taxes, and help ensure that tax deposits are made in a timely manner. Practices with more than 20 employees, or even small practices without the staff or the desire to manage this function, may want to explore using a payroll service for convenience and cost efficiencies. In any case, a method for hourly employees to record and report hours worked is necessary. There are a variety of ways for employees to track and report time—from manual time sheets to electronic systems that integrate with the payroll or accounting system. If the practice has exempt (salaried) and nonexempt (hourly) staff, it is usually advisable to have two separate payroll schedules. For example, hourly staff can be paid biweekly (every 2 weeks) and salaried staff semimonthly or monthly. This schedule assists with cash flow and balancing time management for payroll preparation.

REVENUE CYCLE

The revenue cycle of the practice is a critical concept to understand and manage. It is the all-inclusive system that starts with the development of a fee schedule and ends with appropriate reimbursement for services performed. Good policies and procedures and knowledgeable staff are important to ensure optimal revenue and cash flow for the practice.

Major elements of the revenue cycle include the following:
- Contracts with commercial insurance, Medicare, and Medicaid—Contracts may be for individual providers or for the practice with individual providers listed under the group contract. Providers will need to be "credentialed" with the insurance company before being added to a contract or receiving an individual contract. A standard universal credentialing is often used (e.g., Council for Affordable Quality Healthcare [CAQH]) for the initial and renewal credentialing process. Besides the reimbursement rate or fee schedule, important items to review in a contract include timely filing guidelines, methods for appeals, prompt payment guidelines, product lines, length of contract, specific requirements for patient access, and claims filing requirements.
- Fee schedule—The practice will need a fee schedule that lists its prices for the services it provides. A highly recommended process for development of the fee schedule is to use the Medicare Resource Based Relative Value Scales (RBRVS). The RBRVS is based on a formula of work values and practice and professional liability expenses and is adjusted by geographical region. The Medicare RBRVS table is adjusted annually and is the amount used for Medicare reimbursement. Many commercial payers also use the RBRVS formula in determining reimbursement rates. Similarly, the practice can use the RBRVS formula to develop its own fee schedule. It is important to coordinate the fee schedule with practice contracts (e.g., if the practice's highest reimbursement contract is negotiated at

130% of RBRVS, the practice's fee schedule will normally be set at a minimum of 135% to 140% of RBRVS). This ensures that the practice receives full reimbursement under its contracts and maintains a buffer for new contracts, contract changes, and those contracts that may not be based on RBRVS. At the same time, it is important to not set the RBRVS percentage of the fee schedule too high. A fee schedule that is too high will (1) falsely inflate the practice's accounts receivables and (2) place a higher burden on uninsured patients or patients with deductibles.

- Charge ticket—The charge ticket or "superbill" is the document the provider uses to communicate the services provided and the diagnosis for the visit. It should be as comprehensive as possible and easy for the provider to use to ensure that all services provided are identified and billed. It is also important to have a system that accounts for all charge tickets so that if one comes up missing it can be identified and re-created by the provider using the documentation in the medical record. Plan on reviewing and revising the charge ticket at least once a year to make annual current procedural terminology (CPT) and International Classification of Diseases and Related Health Problems (ICD-9) revisions (Box 43-3 lists coding concepts).

- Patient registration form—The patient registration form provides several important functions. Primarily, it is a record of the patient's current demographic and insurance information. It can also function as a consent-to-treat form and can often be a valuable resource for additional data if needed for collection purposes (employment, social security, additional family members, etc.). Patient demographic and insurance information should be reviewed at each visit to ensure the practice has accurate information on file and in the chart for both clinical and administrative operations.

- Verification of insurance eligibility—Verification of a patient's insurance eligibility or benefits should be done as early as possible in the revenue cycle. Ideally it should be done before the visit so that the correct copayment, coinsurance, or deductible can be collected at the time of service. Verifying eligibility or benefits prior to the patient visit or early in the revenue cycle is becoming easier with increasingly sophisticated claim submission software. Eligibility information is also normally available on insurance plan websites although checking those can be a manual and time-intensive process for the practice. Verifying insurance before the claim is submitted may add a day or two to the billing process, but is a proactive step that can prevent denials and save time and money for the practice.

- Accurate CPT and ICD-9 coding—Choosing the correct CPT code for services provided can be challenging for even the most experienced provider, and modifiers and special situations can add more uncertainty to the process. Continuing education and coding assistance for providers and billing staff are important not only for ensuring that the practice is getting adequate reimbursement, but also to guard against the potential for the submission of fraudulent claims.

- Charge entry (manual or electronic)—Entering the charges from the charge tickets into the practice management system by staff or by the providers into the electronic medical record should be done accurately and in a timely fashion. In most cases setting a guideline of having charges reviewed and ready for submission within 3 to 4 days after the date of service should give staff adequate time to ensure the correct insurance data and perform any necessary coding reviews. Having some type of audit process for charge tickets or charges is recommended to ensure that all charge tickets or charges are accounted for and all services have been captured and correctly coded before being submitted.

BOX 43-3 Coding Concepts

Current procedural terminology (CPT) codes are used by health care providers to report medical procedures and services to payers to provide them with clinical information and as a basis for reimbursement of services. CPT codes are designated as the national procedural coding standard under the Health Insurance Portability and Accountability Act (HIPAA). CPT codes are updated on an annual basis and revisions and new codes take effect each January.

International classification of disease (ICD-9) codes are the official code set based on the World Health Organization's classification of diseases and are used worldwide. Health care providers use ICD-9 codes to report symptoms and diagnoses to payers to provide them with clinical information. ICD codes are part of the standard code sets under HIPAA and are recognized and required by all payers. ICD codes are updated annually and revisions and new codes take effect each October. The current ICD-9 system is scheduled to be replaced by the ICD-10 system in 2013 and will require major changes for the entire industry.

Health care providers report services performed by use of CPT codes and ICD-9 codes. These two code sets provide information on what services were performed (e.g., evaluation and management, surgical, laboratory) and why they were performed (the diagnosis supporting the work). Centers for Medicare and Medicaid Services (CMS) documentation guidelines assist providers in choosing the correct CPT code.

A practice should determine whether to use CMS 1995 or 1997 documentation guidelines for coding. Many pediatric practices use 1995 guidelines because they are somewhat less complex.

Evaluation and management codes (CPT codes 99201-99499) are level 1 CPT codes used in office and outpatient settings. In addition, providers may use level II Healthcare Common Procedure Coding System (HCPCS) codes to report services and supplies not identified within CPT.

Good documentation and charting skills that incorporate CPT guidelines are important for the provider and the practice. The documentation of the patient visit should provide the structure for the codes chosen to report the visit. Analysis of a provider's charting skills is an important part of the practice's coding program and should share equal billing with regular coding audits and ongoing coding education.

A written compliance program, although not required, is highly recommended. The compliance program should communicate the practice's standards for documentation, coding, billing, fraud prevention, and retention of records. The following standards are widely recommended: (1) internal monitoring and auditing, (2) development and implementation of practice policies for documentation and coding, (3) identification of a compliance officer, (4) providing training and education for providers and practice staff, (5) method for responding to issues identified, (6) effective communication methods, and (7) enforcement of practice standards.

- Electronic claims submission—Most insurance companies require electronic claims submission for the majority of their claims. Exceptions are the few claims that require attachments or special handling. Sending claims electronically also allows better tracking and faster processing of the claims.
- Payment posting (manual or electronic)—Payment posting can be done several ways depending on the functions and sophistication of the practice management system. Insurance companies can still mail a check with a corresponding explanation of benefits (EOB), although more are requesting that offices be able to accept an electronic deposit with corresponding online EOB or even an automatic electronic posting to the practice management system. In any case it is important for the billing or payment staff to ensure that the correct reimbursement was received and that adjustments are posted correctly, that denials and adjustments are reviewed and appealed if necessary, and that there is a good system in place for quickly identifying claims that are overdue for payment.
- Patient statements—Patients should receive statements whenever there is activity on their account and, most importantly, should receive a statement as soon as there is a patient balance on the account. Statements should be "patient friendly" by being easy to read and understand.
- Accounts receivable management—The business office or billing staff should have processes in place to identify as early as possible any claims that have been billed but not paid. Most states have guidelines that require insurance companies to process and pay claims within 30 days.

Accounts receivable (AR) reports in the practice management system should be used to help this process. A process for monitoring, analyzing, and appealing denials is important. Accounts receivable management also includes development of collection policies and procedures, including collection letters and the potential use of a collection agency. This is often a good time for the practice to discuss what kind of charity care or discounts for payment at time of service the practice is prepared to offer.

- Practice management reports—In addition to financial reports, monthly practice management reports are important business tools. Individual and practice production reports, CPT distributions, average charge, average collection, and days in accounts receivable are all basic and important measurements for the practice to collect and monitor. A sample "dashboard" report is depicted in Figure 43-1.

FINANCIAL POLICIES

The development of policies and procedures for financial operations should include guidelines for internal cash controls, making bank deposits, collection of copayments at the time of service, insurance verification, methods of payment accepted (check, cash, credit card), timeliness of entry of charges into the practice management system, regular attention to accounts receivable, and collection policies, including potential discharge of patients from the practice. If the practice has decided to outsource any of its accounting, financial, or billing functions, similar policies should be developed and made part of any service contract.

ABC Pediatrics Key Indicator Report

	Prior Year	BUDGET	JAN	FEB	MAR	APR	MAY	JUNE	JULY	AUG	SEPT	OCT	NOV	DEC	*TOTAL*	*YTD%*
DOS Charges																
AR Charges																
Collections																
Average Charge																
Average Collection																
Total Visits																
Provider Visits																
MA Visits																
Hospital Visits																
Avg Patients/Day																
New Patients																
# Provider Days																
Provider RVUs / Avg Value RVU																
Well Care Visits																
Acute Care Visits																
Appointments Made																
Credit Balance																
Bad Debt Write-Off																
Vaccine Charges*																
Vaccine Revenue*																
Vaccine Costs*																
AR Insurance																
AR Responsible																
TOTAL AR																

FIGURE 43-1 A sample practice dashboard.

Human Resource Operations

The employees of a practice are instrumental in making a practice successful. They are either an asset to the practice or detrimental to its operations. The staff is not only the largest expense in the practice budget, but also functions as the day-to-day marketing and customer service team. Whether by providing clinical or administrative services, the staff represents the practice to current and potential patients every day. Managing staff and the human resource function of a practice is complex and requires a sound knowledge of employment law. Job descriptions are recommended for all employees and can be a valuable tool for use in the hiring, training, and evaluation of practice staff. Some practices have decided to outsource their personnel management and use a professional employee organization (PEO) to assist them with many human resource functions. A PEO employs the staff of a practice, provides benefits, and manages workers' compensation and unemployment insurance issues, while the practice manages and supervises the staff. Practices working with a PEO will still need to successfully manage employees and be knowledgeable about human resources functions. A basic human resources operations checklist is provided in Box 43-4.

LEGAL ISSUES FOR HUMAN RESOURCES

Knowledge of a state's wage and hour laws is necessary. These wage and hour laws help in the development of human resource policies and procedures for the practice. Some examples include:

- Identification of a "work week" for the practice (e.g., 12:01 AM Sunday to 12:00 PM Saturday). This standard is necessary for calculating overtime.
- Compliance with minimum hourly wage laws (federal and state).
- Identification of staff as "nonexempt" or "exempt" from overtime. Nonexempt staff members are normally paid hourly, whereas exempt staff members are paid by salary. The correct classification of staff is critical; misclassification and the failure to pay overtime when required can result in legal recourse, back pay, and fines.
- Development of policies for employee rest breaks during the workday.
- Payment of wages on involuntary or voluntary termination.
- Requirements of the practice for employee's civic obligations, such as jury duty or military leave.

The practice, depending on its size and its contracts, must be in compliance with the following federal employment laws:

- Americans with Disabilities Act (ADA)
- Family and Medical Leave Act (FMLA)
- Equal Employment Opportunity Commission (EEOC)
- Fair Labor Standards Act (FLSA)
- Consolidated Omnibus Budget Reconciliation Act (COBRA)

Other legal requirements that affect the human resource function include the completion by employees of I-9 (immigration) and W-4 (payroll withholding) forms. These two forms should be completed before the beginning of employment. It is generally recommended that the I-9 form be kept separately from the employee's personnel file for confidentiality purposes in the event of an audit. A separate medical file should be created if an employee has documents relating to medical treatments, such as workers' compensation or FMLA medical reports.

COMPENSATION AND BENEFITS

Compensation and the use of salary structures or salary ranges are an essential part of human resource management. The marketplace normally plays a large role in establishing these ranges by cities, states, or other specific regions of the country. In addition, the development of job descriptions and a method to evaluate employees' performance affect salary structure and consequently the personnel costs of the practice. Many human resource consultants suggest directly linking the performance evaluation to the job description. Various professional organizations and websites provide salary statistics that may be helpful in developing salary ranges or structures and at the very least can be used as a method of comparison with the local market.

Decisions about provider compensation can be more complex. The provider compensation model chosen should take into account the goals and philosophy of the practice. The most used compensation models are (1) straight salary, (2) base salary with a production component, (3) salary with bonus or incentives, and (4) pure production-based.

Benefits are an important part of the entire compensation package. By offering good benefits the practice can increase its competitiveness in the marketplace and provide security for employees. A basic benefit package usually includes health and dental insurance, life insurance, vision insurance, vacation, sick leave, or a combination of vacation and sick leave in a paid time off (PTO) account. Liability insurance may also be a benefit. More extensive benefits can include a 401(k) retirement plan, tuition allowance, uniform allowance, continuing education, bus passes, parking allowances, long- or short-term disability insurance, or employee assistance programs. A standard benefit package combined

---

BOX 43-4 Human Resources Checklist

- State wage and hour laws
- Federal employment laws
  - Americans with Disabilities Act (ADA)
  - Fair Labor Standards Act (FLSA)
  - Family and Medical Leave Act (FMLA)
  - Equal Employment Opportunity Commission (EEOC)
  - Consolidated Omnibus Budget Reconciliation Act (COBRA)
- Staffing
  - Exempt and nonexempt
  - Employment agreements
  - Personnel forms
- Salaries and benefits
- Employee handbook
- Job descriptions
- Performance evaluation process
- Orientation and training
- Important policies
  - Confidentiality
  - Harassment
  - Nonviolence

BOX 43-5 A Sample Table of Contents for an Employee Handbook

1. Welcome page
2. Important information about this handbook (an important section that provides the organization protection)
3. Equal employment opportunity (EEO) statement—includes policy on EEO, Americans with Disabilities Act (ADA), harassment, and complaint procedures
4. Employment—classification, outside employment, rehire, etc.
5. Working hours and attendance, standard work week, break periods, attendance, overtime
6. Compensation
7. Payroll, direct deposit, travel expense, garnishment
8. Benefits—holidays, insurance, 401(k), training, paid time off (PTO) guidelines, time off without pay, Family and Medical Leave Act (FMLA), bereavement leave, jury duty, parental leave, military leave, domestic abuse leave
9. Professional conduct, customer service, confidentiality, drugs and alcohol, antiviolence, smoking, dress code, personal phone calls, e-mail and Internet policies, company property, personal property, solicitation, parking, visitors, inclement weather
10. Communication—open door policy, patient communication standards
11. Safety, on the job injuries

BOX 43-6 Practice Operations Checklist

- Appointment scheduling and phones
  - Patient flow
  - Phone system
  - Patient communication
  - Telephone triage
  - Answering service
- Medical records
  - Electronic medical record
  - Charting and documentation
  - Quality assurance
  - Medical record forms
- Practice management information system
- Standardized procedures
- Emergency procedures
- Quality assurance
- Risk management

---

with required payroll taxes can add an additional 10% to 20% to the personnel costs of the practice.

EMPLOYEE HANDBOOK

An employee handbook is an excellent way to communicate personnel policies to staff members. The handbook should include the practice's mission statement, confidentiality requirements and agreements, and policies on benefits, vacation, sick leave, time off for bereavement or jury duty, calling in when ill, and leaves of absence. It also communicates the practice's compliance with state and federal regulations. In addition, the practice should develop and include policies on a professional code of conduct, harassment, and nonviolence for inclusion in the handbook. An employee handbook is a legal document and should always be reviewed by an attorney or a professional human resources organization to ensure that it does not contain or imply any language that could be construed as a contract of employment. A sample table of contents for an employee handbook is included in Box 43-5.

EMPLOYMENT AGREEMENTS

Health care practices often incorporate employment agreements or a contract of employment for their professional and senior management staff. An employment agreement is a legal contract that specifies the employees' and employers' duties to each other in detail. Counsel from the practice's attorney should be sought when deciding if employment agreements are right for the practice. In any event, an employment agreement should never be construed as a guarantee of employment and should always include a method for termination of the employment by either the employee or the employer during the contract term.

■ Practice Operations

An efficient and well-run health care practice often gives the impression that operating or managing a practice is an easy task. Nothing could be further from the truth! A health care practice is a complex business requiring multiple clinical and administrative systems that work well together. Successful day-to-day operations require that both systems operate in conjunction with good customer service. A basic practice operations checklist is provided in Box 43-6.

APPOINTMENT SCHEDULING

The practice's scheduling system provides the structure for the clinician's day and either helps to create an office that runs smoothly or contributes to one that is in constant chaos. Important issues in pediatric scheduling require decisions on how to handle well-child visits, sick-child visits, and newborns—how they should be arranged in the schedule and how much time should be allotted for each type of visit. In a multiprovider practice, a single scheduling philosophy and consistent scheduling rules for the entire practice are highly recommended. Close attention and ongoing monitoring of patient demand and access is critical for providing effective clinical care and customer satisfaction, and ensuring efficient use of provider and staff resources.

Most pediatric practices keep a substantial portion of the daily schedule open for same-day visits. Additionally the practice may want to consider keeping a few early morning slots open for patients who have been instructed to come to the office during that time by the provider or after-hours service taking night calls. Patients like the fact that they can be assured of being seen first thing in the morning without having to wait until the office opens to phone for an appointment. Some offices have reported success with open access types of schedules in which some well-care appointments are available on a same-day basis.

Other scheduling concerns that should be addressed in office policy statements and standard protocols include how the practice will confirm appointments and how it will deal with late patients, no-show patients, walk-in patients, and urgent or emergency patients. Practices serving pediatric patients also have found it beneficial to have seasonal schedules. For example, during the winter months it is optimal to reduce the number of well-care appointments and increase the number of acute-care appointments. Likewise, practices can implement a schedule in the summer months that contains more slots for well-child visits or physical examinations to help meet the demand for school and camp physicals. A pediatric practice may have a summer schedule for June, July, and August; a winter schedule for January, February, and March; and "transitional" schedules that cover the remaining 6 months of the year and are built based on a historical or ongoing analysis of demand for those months.

PATIENT COMMUNICATION

Communicating with patients is one of the most important responsibilities of a medical practice. Whether calling to schedule an appointment, for a prescription refill, for test results, to request a referral, or to ask for advice on home care suggestions during an illness, patients want their concerns handled efficiently and in a timely manner. Increasingly, patients are requesting and practices are implementing more online capabilities for some of these services. However, patient phone calls continue to be a significant factor in the day-to-day operations of most health care practices. The practice should have policies and procedures on how patient communications will be handled and by which staff members. Many of these responsibilities or requests can be handled by clinical support staff, such as registered nurses and medical assistants, or administrative staff. Registered nurses can take patient phone calls, assess the patient, and depending on the situation and following specific triage protocols, either give health care advice or recommend that an appointment be made. Medical assistants or nurses can process prescription refill requests per practice protocols. Medical assistants or administrative support staff can assist the patient in obtaining a referral or an appointment to instigate a referral. Safeguards should be in place to ensure that staff members functioning in these capacities are neither expected nor allowed to act outside of their clinical competency or scope of practice as designated by state laws.

The phone system itself plays a critical role in the scheduling process, practice operations, and good customer service. Does the practice want to have an automated greeting or a live person answer the phone? Both require backup systems to make them work successfully. If the practice uses an automated system, the greeting and subsequent choices for obtaining service should be simple, with only a few choices. If the practice opts for live operators, it should make sure that there are sufficient lines and staff members to handle anticipated volume at various times of the day and week.

MEDICAL RECORDS

Developing an effective medical records system to meet the needs of the practice has traditionally revolved around determining how to organize the paper medical chart, what type of filing system to use, and development of the policies and procedures required for the medical record functions. With numerous electronic systems available, a new practice should seriously consider an electronic medical records (EMR) system as a way to not only record the clinical information on

each patient but also improve coordination of care. Established practices should consider an EMR system for all of the aforementioned benefits, realizing, however, that additional planning for incorporating current paper records with the electronic system will be required. Large practices and practices with multiple locations often find that the many benefits of the EMR system outweigh the difficulties involved in moving to the electronic system, even if it is a time- and labor-intensive process. There are many types of EMR and electronic medical chart (EMC) systems. Adequately researching how a system works and knowledge of practice styles and outcomes are necessary when deciding on an EMR system. The federal government through the Certification Commission for Healthcare Information Technology (CCHIT) has developed standards for EMR systems and publishes these standards and lists the companies that have successfully met the CCHIT standards.

PRACTICE MANAGEMENT INFORMATION SYSTEM

A practice management computer system or practice management information system is essential to a health care practice. The basic system should integrate patient demographic information, the scheduling process, and billing functions. If the practice is interested in adopting an EMR or electronic health record (EHR) system immediately or in the future, the software should have an EMR component or be compatible with the desired EMR or EHR system. Many good systems have basic or entry-level systems for small offices that can be upgraded as the size and demands of the practice increase. When considering the purchase of a new system, it is a good idea to arrange to visit another practice of similar size that is using the system to see the functions demonstrated in a real-time environment. Scheduling functions, reporting capabilities, and billing functions—including the ability to send claims electronically—are key areas to research in a system. In addition, technical support, initial and ongoing training, and system upgrades are important aspects about which to become knowledgeable.

STANDARDIZATION IN THE PRACTICE

A medical practice can realize some important benefits by standardizing its practices and procedures. In addition to an appointment schedule, policies and procedures for chart organization and documentation, immunization and well-child schedules, and nursing procedures should be standardized. For example, if there are uniform policies and procedures for preparing patients before the clinician's entry into the examination room (vital signs, weighing, measuring, appropriate charting and graphing), support staff can more easily cover for each other and the provider can be confident that all necessary tasks are accomplished.

EMERGENCY PROCEDURES

Practices should develop and implement policies and procedures for handling emergencies in the office. Some topics to consider when developing these policies and procedures include:
- Identification of an emergency
- Calling 911—who and when?

- Definition of levels of emergency to be handled in the practice
- Leadership and communication during the emergency
- Provider and support staff responsibilities
- Stocking and monitoring of an "emergency cart"
- Initial and ongoing staff training in cardiopulmonary resuscitation (CPR), basic life support (BLS), or advanced life support (ALS) as appropriate
- Documentation and charting of emergencies
- Staff training for emergency situations
- Assessment or critique of emergencies or training sessions

QUALITY ASSURANCE

Developing clinical quality standards for the practice should be a major focus of any clinical checklist for risk management, in addition to improving clinical care. Organizations, such as the National Committee for Quality Assurance (NCQA), the American Health Information Management Association (AHIMA), and The Joint Commission (TJC), can provide valuable information and guidance for the development of clinical quality standards. The NCQA is a national organization that has long provided accreditation and certification to managed care plans. They provide certification for organizations that provide health care services. Certification by the NCQA requires health care organizations to meet basic standards along with a demonstrable commitment to quality improvement. NCQA standards are often used by health plans when setting quality assurance

guidelines for providers in their networks. Many professional liability insurers also use NCQA standards when developing risk management guidelines for their policyholders.

RISK MANAGEMENT

Risk management is an extremely important aspect of practice operations. Keeping up-to-date on legal requirements and developing and implementing policies and processes that encourage sound clinical and administrative practices can prevent many problems. Some areas that require special attention include medical record documentation, confidentiality and adolescent issues, informed consent, release of records, and clinical practices, such as communicating test results, and follow-up of recommended tests and treatment. Being proactive in the area of risk management will benefit the practice by ensuring optimal clinical care and follow-up, and will also prevent potential care oversights or patient compliance issues.

The Medical Record

A review of the medical chart is a primary focus of accreditation and impromptu site visits by insurance companies. This is because the record serves as legal documentation of all clinical activity. Consequently, the organization, content, and completeness of the medical record can be valuable to ensure quality assurance. Guidelines suggested by AHIMA and TJC are included in Box 43-7.

BOX 43-7 Medical Records Guidelines

- Only authorized individuals may make entries in the medical record, and individuals should be trained in documentation practices and documentation standards.
- Every page in the medical record must identify the patient by name and an identifying number.
- Entries made into the medical record should be made as soon as possible after the visit or communication with the patient.
- Every entry in the medical record must be signed or initialed and include a complete date (month, day, year) and time. Entries must be dated at the date and time they are made.
- A signature legend should be maintained by the practice that identifies all signatures and initials appearing in the medical record.
- The medical record should always use factual information. Documentation should clearly identify speculation versus factual information.
- A standard set of abbreviations to be used in the medical record should be developed by the practice.
- All entries in the medical record should be legible.
- If using forms or checklists, all fields should have some entry. If a field is not applicable, an entry, such as "N/A," should be made.
- Informed consent should be documented whenever applicable.
- All pertinent communication (and attempts at communication) with the patient or the patient's family should be documented. Messages left on answering machines or voice mail are not considered a valid form of notification.
- When an incident occurs, document the facts of the occurrence in the progress note. Do not chart that an incident report has been completed or refer to the report in charting.
- All entries in the medical record are considered permanent.
- All entries in the medical record should be in blue or black ink. Pencils should never be used.

- If an error is made in an entry, it should be corrected by (1) drawing a thin line through the incorrect entry, ensuring that the inaccurate information is still legible; (2) signing and dating the entry; (3) stating the reason for the error in the margin or above the note; and (4) documenting the correct information.
- If a late entry, addendum, or clarification is added to the medical record, identify it as such and enter the current date and time. The reason for the late entry should also be noted.
- The medical record should not be removed from the practice site. If it is necessary to transport the medical record, a tracking system and safeguards should be in place to protect confidentiality and protect against loss.
- Policies and procedures should be developed for the destruction of medical records.
  Other components of the medical record that ensure both good clinical processes and risk management include:
- A problem list that identifies the patient's chronic and significant illnesses. The problem list should appear in a prominent location in the medical record (usually at the front of the medical record).
- Allergy flags that indicate known allergies or no known allergies. Allergy flags should be documented on the outside of the medical record and on the problem list. Patients should be questioned about allergies at each visit.
- A medication list that contains the patient's acute and chronic medications. This list should be maintained in a prominent location in the medical record. The medication prescribed, the dosage, the date prescribed, and the prescriber should be entered on the medication list. The medication list should also include a record of prescription refills.

Note: Although this list was originally developed for a paper medical record system, most of the recommendations remain for electronic medical record systems.

Clinical Tracking Systems

Systems that focus on tracking necessary medical follow-up appointments, high-risk referrals, and clinical tests ordered are other risk management tools that benefit coordination of care and customer service. A newborn requiring a repeat bilirubin test is an example of a critical appointment that requires tracking to ensure that the patient complies with the provider's order for the repeat testing.

Appointment Tracking

An appointment tracking system helps ensure that patients return to the office as instructed (e.g., attention-deficit/hyperactivity disorder [ADHD] medication evaluations, annual well-care examinations).

Referral Tracking

If the provider refers the patient to a specialist for a high-risk problem, a tracking system will ensure that the visit was completed and the report from the specialist was received and reviewed.

Tests Ordered

A tracking and follow-up system should be implemented to ensure that diagnostic test results are completed and the results are received and reviewed in a timely manner. The system should also include verification that the patient was notified of the test results.

■ Summary

The topics reviewed in this chapter briefly touch on many important components of the successful medical practice, with most of the operational examples focused on pediatric or family medicine. In one chapter it is simply not possible to be completely thorough or to discuss many other interesting and important subjects pertaining to practice management. New technologies are bringing exciting possibilities along with new challenges to medical practices today as patients expect their health care providers to use modern technology for clinical and administrative operations and for communications. Practice websites, online communication between patient and provider, electronic prescribing, and EMR are just a few examples of ways technology is changing medical practices.

It is extremely important for the principals of a medical practice to be business savvy and to take advantage of business management knowledge and expertise that is available. There is a wealth of excellent information available through websites, books, journals, educational offerings, and networking that can help answer a specific question, explain a complicated subject, assist with solving a problem, or introduce a new concept. Good practice management is good business, and business resources offer new ideas and perspectives on technology, finance, operations, and personnel that can benefit the medical practice. Although medical practice management often seems complex and overwhelming, there are many resources to help manage the challenges and establish the practice as a leader in the community for children's health care.

Appendixes

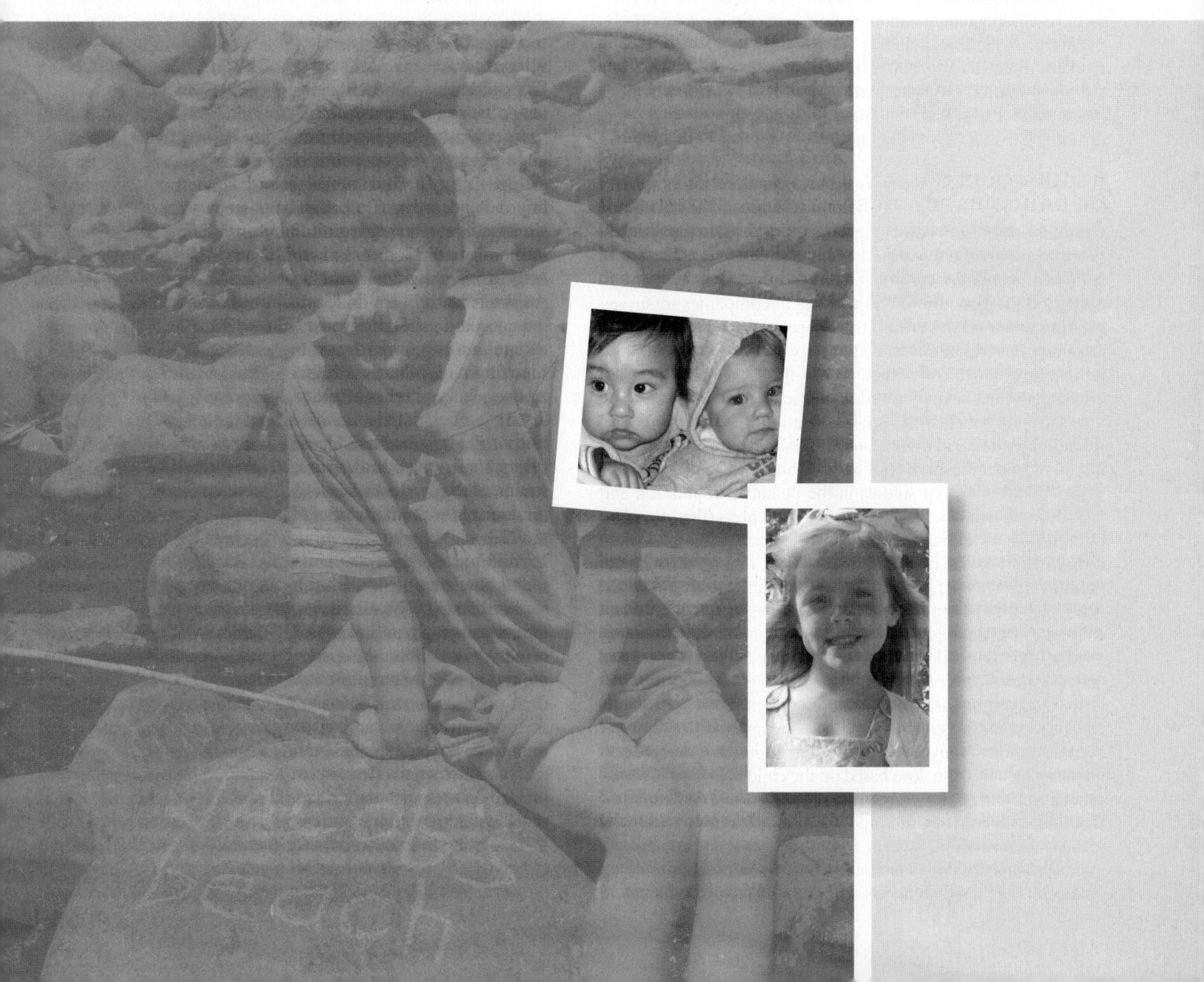

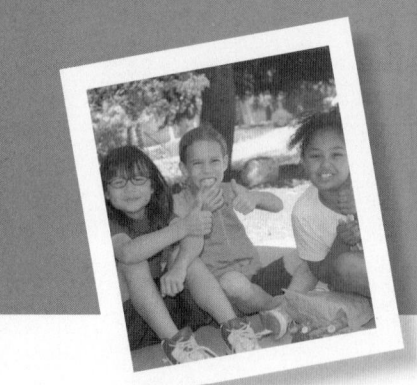

Appendix A

Prescribing Medications in Pediatrics

CATHERINE G. BLOSSER

■ Pediatric Prescription Medication Use

The following discussion will enable the healthcare provider to have a better understanding about prescribing drugs to the pediatric population, including ways to enhance adherence. The reader is directed to consult a drug reference, the Food and Drug Administration (FDA), or pharmaceutical manufacturer regarding specific drugs, their classification, preparation, indications, dosing, side effects, interactions and other considerations.

REGULATION, SAFETY, AND LABELING OF DRUGS USED IN PEDIATRICS

Only 25% to 50% of drugs approved by the FDA in the U.S. have been specifically tested for use in some subset of the pediatric population (Zito et al, 2008; Murphy, 2009). In 1994, the FDA required pharmaceutical companies to survey existing data and determine that there was sufficient support to use various drugs in the pediatric population with pediatric indications and dosages included in the labeling; controlled clinical studies that supported pediatric use did not need to be done. If there was insufficient information to support a pediatric indication, the labeling statement "safety and effectiveness in pediatric patients have not been established" was allowed.

Despite the lack of studies in the pediatric population and lack of pediatric labeling, many drugs are prescribed for children (i.e., used "off label"). "Off label" refers to prescribing the drug outside of the approved indications, dosing recommendations, or age groups according to the official FDA-approved drug's labeling. Using a drug off label does not imply unethical use. An estimated 6.7% to 33.2% of anticancer drugs are used off-label in children and adults, particularly for palliative care (*Medical News Today,* 2008) while the majority of pediatric psychotropic use is off label (Zito et al, 2008).

The dosage for pediatric patients using an off-label drug has been determined by extrapolating from the adult dose and proportionately reducing the dose based on the child's weight and drug side effect profiles. However, this does not take into account pediatric metabolism, the drug's pharmacokinetics, adverse effects (e.g., the connection between SSRIs and potential suicide risk in adolescents), and medication delivery form. Furthermore, the field of ethnopharmacology is adding to a better understanding

of how genetic variations of certain enzymes (e.g., CYP2D6) are influenced by ethnicity and race. These differences affect drug metabolism and an individual's response to dosage.

The historic lack of drug testing in the pediatric population stems from several factors: unprofitability of the pediatric pharmaceutical market (it is relatively small, except for vaccines and some cough/cold medications); difficulty setting up child-friendly environments within which to carry out testing; difficulty taking biologic samples from this population; and inability to obtain informed consent from either parents or children ages 7 or older (cancer research is the exception) (FDA, 2009; Murphy, 2009).

Drug safety and efficacy for pediatric use is currently addressed in the U.S. by two legislative acts: the Best Pharmaceuticals for Children Act (BPCA) and the Pediatric Research Equity Act (PREA); both have been renewed and amended since their inception in the FDA Amendment Act [FDAAA]). The BPCA grants a patent extension when drug companies voluntarily study an old or new drug in children. The PREA gives the FDA more leverage over the types of new drugs developed for children, and the pharmaceutical companies can be required to conduct pediatric studies if the FDA declares a drug possibly beneficial to ill children or one that might be used by a substantial number of children. Additionally, the FDA can require pediatric studies if a new drug application is for a new indication, contains a new active ingredient in an already marketed drug, proposes a change in dosage, or a new route of delivery. Under the BPCA, if companies refuse to conduct studies for children on off-patent drugs (i.e., generics), the National Institutes of Health can be requested to conduct the appropriate research. Forty drugs (referred to as the "List of Drugs for Which Additonal Pediatric Studies Are Needed") are on the off-patent priority list by the FDA for such study; seven have been studied (Sinha, 2008). An internal review committee (Pediatric Advisory Committee [PAC]) at the FDA evaluates the post-market safety of all drugs granted patent exclusivity by the FDA; the PAC can request labeling modifications, areas where further investigation is efficacious, or where further clinical trial data are necessary.

Under the FDAAA, 305 medications have been studied (FDA, 2010). Such studies have revealed underdosing, overdosing, ineffectiveness, and safety problems (FDA, 2009).

Eighty drugs have had label changes pertinent to their use in pediatrics, including ibuprofen (now lists dosing for those 6 months to 2 years); ranitidine (labeling now includes accurate dosing information for use in infants); loratadine; fluvoxamine maleate; gabapentin; and famotidine (FDA, 2009). However, more than one third of the published drug trials in pediatrics have been carried out, at least partly, in developing countries. This practice raises an ethical issue, since many of the drugs may not be made available or affordable to the participating countries despite their efficacy (Joelving, 2010).

Pharmaceutical labeling is required to make drug information easily accessible and understandable for providers. The most important prescribing information about the benefits and risk of a drug (in a section called Highlights), the date of initial product approval, and the phone number and web address to report adverse effects are now placed at the beginning of prescribing information and package inserts. Similar formatting must be included in electronic prescribing tools and other information resources. The American Academy of Pediatrics offers an online, subscription-based continuing education program (PediaLink) to providers that includes information about labeling changes. The PAC also recommends that pharmaceutial labels carry warnings about suicide, neonatal withdrawal/toxicity, and risks of off-label use for some drugs in pediatrics. However, many clinical adverse effects of drugs in this age group may go unreported, and the true nature of a drug's safety may not be fully understood. Providers are responsible for reporting adverse effects and for monitoring use of off-label drugs. All providers are encouraged to report adverse effects to the FDA Medwatch website at www.fda.gov/medwatch.

In the European Union, any company that applies to the European Medicines Agency (EMA) is mandated to include a pediatric investigation plan or obtain a waiver if a drug is not applicable for use in children. This regulation, the Pediatric Rule, also provides funding to study off-patent drugs in children, with the results made available to the public (Sinha, 2008).

PRESCRIBING MEDICATIONS FOR CHILDREN

Prescribing medications for pediatric patients presents a special challenge. Decisions about which drugs to use are not based simply on which will be most effective in treating the child's clinical condition nor which are most typically prescribed. Ethical considerations must be taken into account when prescribing, particularly where evidence of efficacy is weak or anecdotal and safety is a concern. The child's age and developmental level, and any family social and functional issues must be considered. Factors that influence adherence, such as taste, dosing regimen, and collaborative decision making, also need to be considered.

A child's developmental level and age influence the amount of control parents have over administration of medications and assist the provider to structure a successful teaching strategy. For *infants* it is important to take the following into consideration:

- The parent is in total control of administering the medication.
- The parent should be taught how to properly administer medications.
- Determine whether other caregivers will be administering the medication.
- Determine whether a simplified dosing schedule is necessary for a family with children in day care.

Toddlers and *preschoolers* are beginning to exert their independence, and administering medication to this age can be challenging. The keys to success with this age group are to:

- Discuss medication administration with the parent (see Table A-1).
- Choose a medication regimen with the fewest problems with administration.
- Take into account palatability and doses per day to increase compliance.

School-age children developmentally are industrious, and are often the most willing to take medications. Education should focus on:

- Both the parent *and* the child who will be taking the medication.
- Letting the child choose the formulation, if possible (liquid, chewable, or pills to swallow).
- Avoid dosing during school hours, if possible, to increase compliance.

Adolescent patients often administer their own medication, and compliance rates may vary. The provider needs to closely collaborate with adolescent patients regarding their medication regimen by:

- Allowing them to have input on dosing schedule and what will work best for them.
- Assisting the family with the transition from parent-controlled to teen-controlled administration.

MEDICATION ADHERENCE

Approximately 71% of visits to healthcare providers result in at least one prescription medication being written (USDHHS, 2009). However, Fischer and colleagues' study (2010) revealed that, overall, only 72% to 78% of prescriptions are actually filled. The highest rates of filled prescriptions (84%) are written by primary care physicians (notably pediatricians) and filled for individuals 18 years and younger (87% of the time). Lower rates are seen overall for newly prescribed medications that treat chronic conditions, such as hypertension, hyperlipidemia, and diabetes (Fischer et al, 2010).

Historically whether or not a patient was taking the recommended pharmaceutical or following a recommended treatment regimen was referred to as *compliance* or *noncompliance*. The term *adherence* is currently used more often in the medical literature. Nonadherence needs to be proactively managed in order to improve clinical and cost effectiveness. A myriad of research studies about adherence has led to the following conclusions:

- Providers obtain a better idea of the actual adherence rate if the question is framed in terms of nonadherence, such as "How many doses did you miss?" rather than "Did you take all of your medicine?"
- Adolescents are less likely to be adherent. Adherence rates can be increased with directly observed therapy for depressed youth (Gaur et al, 2010); greater maternal involvement in the treatment regimen (Reed-Knight et al, 2010); for those with a chronic illness, acknowledgement of the need for a future life on medication (Longhofer and Floersch, 2010); experiencing the rewards of treatment (improvement in symptoms, school performance, family relationships) (Hamrin et al, 2010); and improved understanding of their medication and how to manage it if it conflicts with other activities (Edgecombe et al, 2010).

TABLE A-1	Factors That Influence Adherence to Taking Prescribed Pediatric Medications
Factors that Influence Adherence	**Interventions that Improve Adherence**
Length of treatment: Longer treatment contributes to poorer adherence.	*Shorten length of treatment if possible.* An example would be to use 5 days of therapy for otitis media rather than 10; this can be accomplished with a number of antibiotics (azithromycin and cefpodoxime at all ages, amoxicillin in children >age 5 yr).
Chronic illness: Adherence rates vary with chronic illness.	*Develop creative solutions to encourage adherence* (e.g., sticker charts or calendars with a small reward for completing a set amount of therapy).
Doses per day: Adherence research in children indicates that the more doses of a medication that need to be administered per day, the poorer the adherence rate. This is particularly true with working parents and children in school, who often miss midday doses.	*Simplify dosing regimen.* Prescribing medications that require fewer doses per day will increase adherence. Rates range from 65%-93% for once-a-day dosing and 54%-84% for twice-daily regimens, compared with 49%-81% for three times a day and 31%-71% for a four times daily dosing regimen (Claxton et al, 2001). When the child needs to take the medication at day care or school, dispense two bottles: one for school and one for home. This will ensure fewer missed doses due to forgetting to transport the medication back and forth.
Palatability and ease of ingestion: Unpalatable medications are resisted by children, especially young children. Some children have difficulty swallowing some formulations (e.g., pills).	*Choose the best-tasting medication or mask the taste.* If a medication has the same efficacy profile, the best-tasting medication will be easier to administer to young children. There is also the option of using flavoring syrups or crushing tablets such as prednisone and mixing with sweet foods such as chocolate syrup, jam, applesauce, or pudding. Before crushing any tablet or mixing a medication with syrup, the provider should check with a pharmacist to determine if the flavoring is compatible with the medication. *Facilitate swallowing of pills and capsules.* Place pill in mouth and take a mouthful of water; turn head as far to the right as possible and swallow. Repeat on the left side and rotate sides, depending upon the number of pills in the treatment regimen. Pill(s) should be swallowed easily (Barron, 2010).
Expense: Out-of-pocket costs may be difficult for some families to meet.	*Choose the medication that has the lowest out-of-pocket expense for the family.* Ask families about insurance coverage and resources, and problem solve with them to increase the likelihood that they will fill the prescription (Daiichi Pharmaceutical Corporation, 2004).
Family issues: Family issues such as working parents, lack of social support, fatigue, family disruption, and dysfunction all affect the family's ability to adhere to the prescribed treatment regimen.	*Assess the family for issues that affect successful outcome.* If there is poor or less than expected outcome with a treatment regimen, the provider will need to determine if family issues are a factor in adherence and address interventions to assist the family in identifying strategies that will improve success.

- Adherence is not a steady state; individuals take into consideration the perceived risks and benefits for each medication separately (McHorney and Gadkari, 2010); therefore adherence needs to be assessed as part of each office visit. Seeing the same health care provider at clinical visits may improve adherence rates (Bell, 2005).
- A provider's credibility (trustworthiness and expertise) influences a patient's perceptions about the need for prescribed therapy. Switching between medicines to find the appropriate one can undermine this credibility. Better adherence results when the provider clearly outlines the treatment process at the beginning of treatment, the efficacy of treatment, and expectations for finding the appropriate drug (Ledford et al, 2010).
- The fewer regularly scheduled follow-up visits and the less time spent discussing the individual's/parents' perception about illness and medication, the lower the adherence rate; such constraints occur more frequently in primary care settings than speciality settings (Klok et al, 2010).
- Reinforcement techniques increase rates of adherence; have patients and/or parents identify and use reinforcement strategies (e.g., stickers, special treats [a day at the zoo, etc.]).
- Encourage the patient and/or parent to devise a plan for when they will take or administer the medicine, especially if they link the administration with a specific activity (e.g., toothbrushing, eating breakfast); focus on ways to eliminate barriers.

- Adherence rates decrease for more complex treatment regimens, longer time since diagnosis, and lower perceived level of disease severity (Reed-Knight et al, 2010).
- Past experience regarding the ease or difficulty in administering a drug will increase or decrease adherence (Daiichi Pharmaceutical Corporation, 2004).
- Written instructions increase adherence rates. However, consumer medication information (CMI) leaflets dispensed through retail pharmacies are unregulated and the content, format, reading level, and length can be problematic (Winterstein et al, 2010).
- Combining instructional methods (e.g., verbal and written) addresses different learning styles and can improve adherence rates (Bell, 2005).
- Establishing a provider/pharmacist collaborative management program for chronic treatment regimens increases adherence rates and ensures optimal medication regimens (Carter and Foppe van Mil, 2010; Chisholm-Burns et al, 2010).

Further research has shown that adherence rates increase with the following interventions: pictogram-based instruction sheets (language appropriate); teach-back demonstrations by parents after review of the pictogram; use of medication logs; use of a standardized dosing cup, spoon, or measuring dropper or dosing syringe (Yin et al, 2008); and telephone counseling (Cook et al, 2009). Use of a standardized dosing vehicle is important because spoon-dosing is one of the primary causes of administration errors and pediatric poisonings

(Wansink and van Ittersum, 2010). Educational video games show promise toward increasing knowledge, disease management adherence, and clinical outcomes (Deshazo et al, 2010). Technological applications, such as automated cell phone reminders and telephone alert systems are also available and can be product specific by manufacturer. Table A-1 discusses additional factors that predispose to lower adherence rates and suggests strategies to increase those rates.

DISPOSAL OF DRUGS

Most over-the-counter and prescription drugs should not be flushed down the drain or toilet. Trace amounts are showing up in rivers, streams, and treated water (University of California, Berkeley, 2006). Providers should know which pharmacies in their area will take back unused or expired products, or encourage patients to dispose of unused medications at hazardous recycling facilities or at a community-sponsored "take-back" program. The city or county Board of Health or household trash/recycling service companies can provide information about drug take-back programs. If these actions are not possible, proper disposal of unused drugs is offered as an Environmental Health Tip on the inside back cover of this textbook.

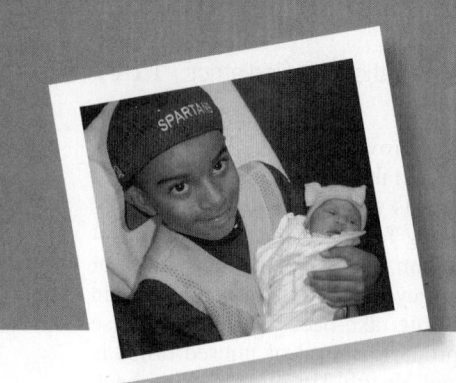

Appendix B

Growth Charts

CATHERINE E. BURNS

Growth in height, weight, and head circumference is an important indicator of health for children. Growth is modified by a variety of factors including, but not limited to, nutrition, general health, and genetics. It is also related to the environment in which the child lives. Sleep, exercise, nurturing, and psychosocial factors all influence a child's growth. Height, weight, and head circumference must be measured often enough to discern the rate and pattern of growth over time. Growth velocity is the most critical factor to identify. Measurements at 6 month intervals with plotting on the linear growth curve to the year and month of age is the easiest way to look at velocity over time (Rose et al, 2005). Assessing the child's absolute height and weight in comparison to children of similar sex and age is also important. Rose and colleagues (2005) propose that growth analysis should include 4 areas:

1. *Reliability of measurement*: Both careful measurement and careful plotting of measures are essential.
2. *Absolute height and weight*: The child who lies 2 standard deviations above or below the 3rd and 95th percentiles on the growth grids should receive additional consideration, though this may not be pathologic given other factors such as family stature genetics.
3. *Growth velocity*: At least three points in time over at least a 3- to 6-month period will give good information about velocity.
4. *Weight-for-height ratio*: Endocrine disorders are more commonly associated with normal weight but retarded height, while "systemic disorders" such as renal, respiratory, or cardiac conditions, more often result in poorer weight gain over time compared to height gain, resulting in a thin child. The Body Mass Index (BMI) is now used for assessing the height-weight proportions for all children older than 2 years. Using a BMI chart is the easiest way to assess the BMI for a given age.

To calculate BMI:

$$[\text{Weight (kg)} / \text{stature (cm)}] / \text{status (cm)} \times 10,000$$
or
$$[\text{Weight (lb)} / \text{stature (inches)} / \text{stature (inches)}] \times 703$$

For genetic potential, one can determine the target height using the formulas:

Boys: $\dfrac{(\text{Father's height in inches}) + (\text{Mother's height} + 5 \text{ inches})}{2}$

or

$$\dfrac{(\text{Father's height in cm}) + (\text{Mother's height} + 13 \text{ cm})}{2}$$

Girls: $\dfrac{(\text{Father's height} - 5 \text{ inches}) + (\text{Mother's height in inches})}{2}$

or

$$\dfrac{(\text{Father's height} - 13 \text{ cm}) + (\text{Mother's height in cm})}{2}$$

Most children achieve an adult height within 10 cm (4 inches) of their target height.

MEASUREMENT TECHNIQUES

The health care provider must remember that growth must be assessed accurately to be valid. Some of the following points may be helpful:

- Measure height of infants and children less than 2 years old in a recumbent position, holding the head stable against a headboard and using a footboard against both feet.
- Measure height of children greater than 2 years old using a stadiometer or against a wall using a right angle against the head rather than the height measure on a standing scale.
- Measure the head circumference for all infants less than 2 years old and older children who seem to have a small or large head. Measure the largest circumference 3 times and take the largest of the three measures.
- Arm span should approximate linear height by 8 years. For children with scoliosis or an inability to stand erect, an arm span measure may be a useful proxy for height.
- Head circumference is especially important to measure in children less than 2 years of age since it is the best indicator of brain growth, which is 90% complete by 2 years. Sometimes children older than 2 years may also need a head circumference measurement (e.g., for neurologic assessments).
- Measure height without shoes and infant weight without diapers.
- Chart the height, weight, and head circumference on grids for all visits, not just well-child visits.

The Centers for Disease Control and Prevention now recommends using the World Health Organization growth charts for children less than 2 years of age and the CDC charts for

Text continued on page 1157

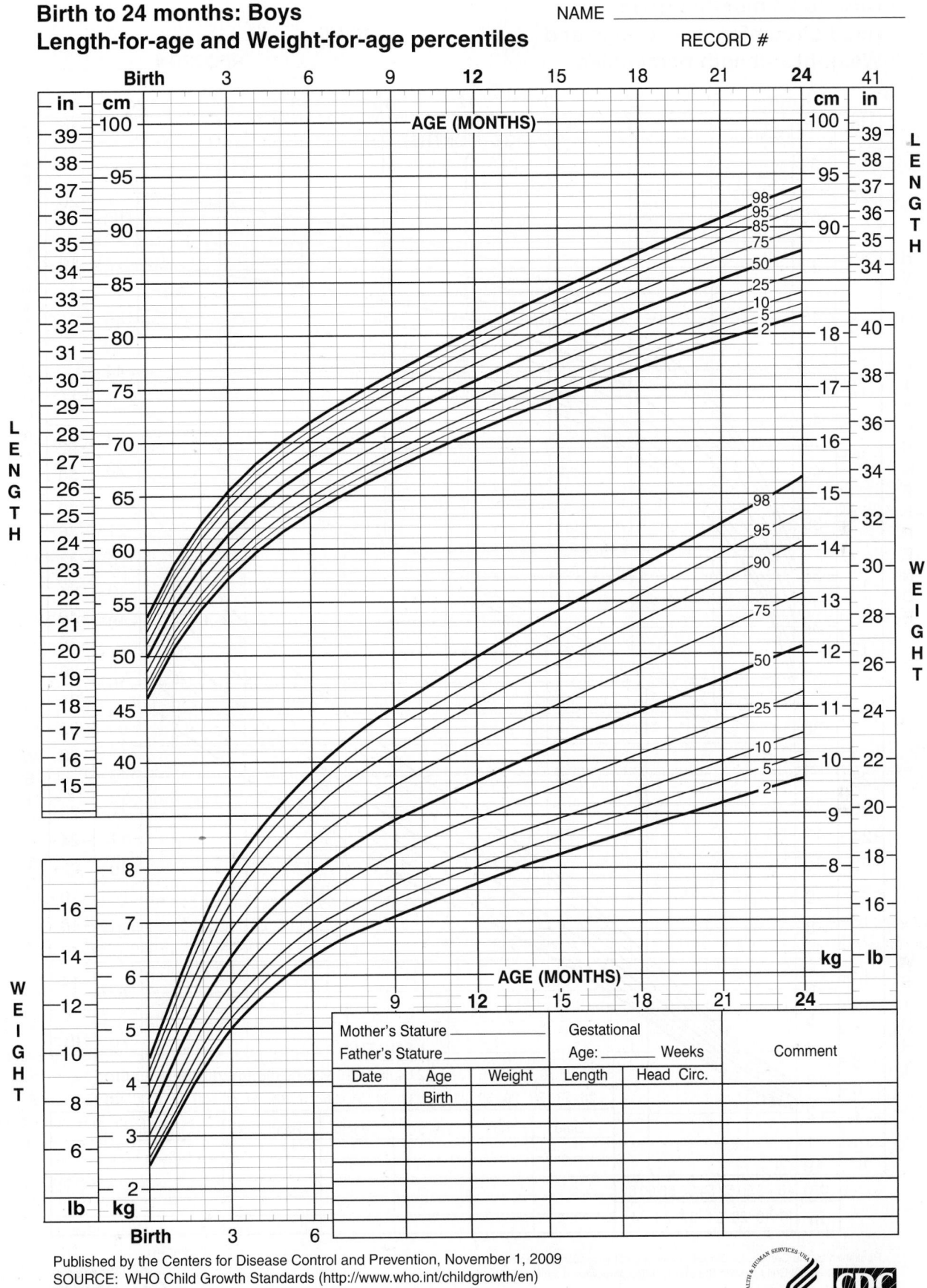

Birth to 24 months: Boys
Length-for-age and Weight-for-age percentiles

NAME _____

RECORD # _____

Published by the Centers for Disease Control and Prevention, November 1, 2009
SOURCE: WHO Child Growth Standards (http://www.who.int/childgrowth/en)

FIGURE B-1 Birth to 24 months: boys' length-for-age and weight-for-age percentiles. (Published by the Centers for Disease Control and Prevention, November 1, 2009. From WHO Child Growth Standards. Available at www.cdc.gov/growthcharts.)

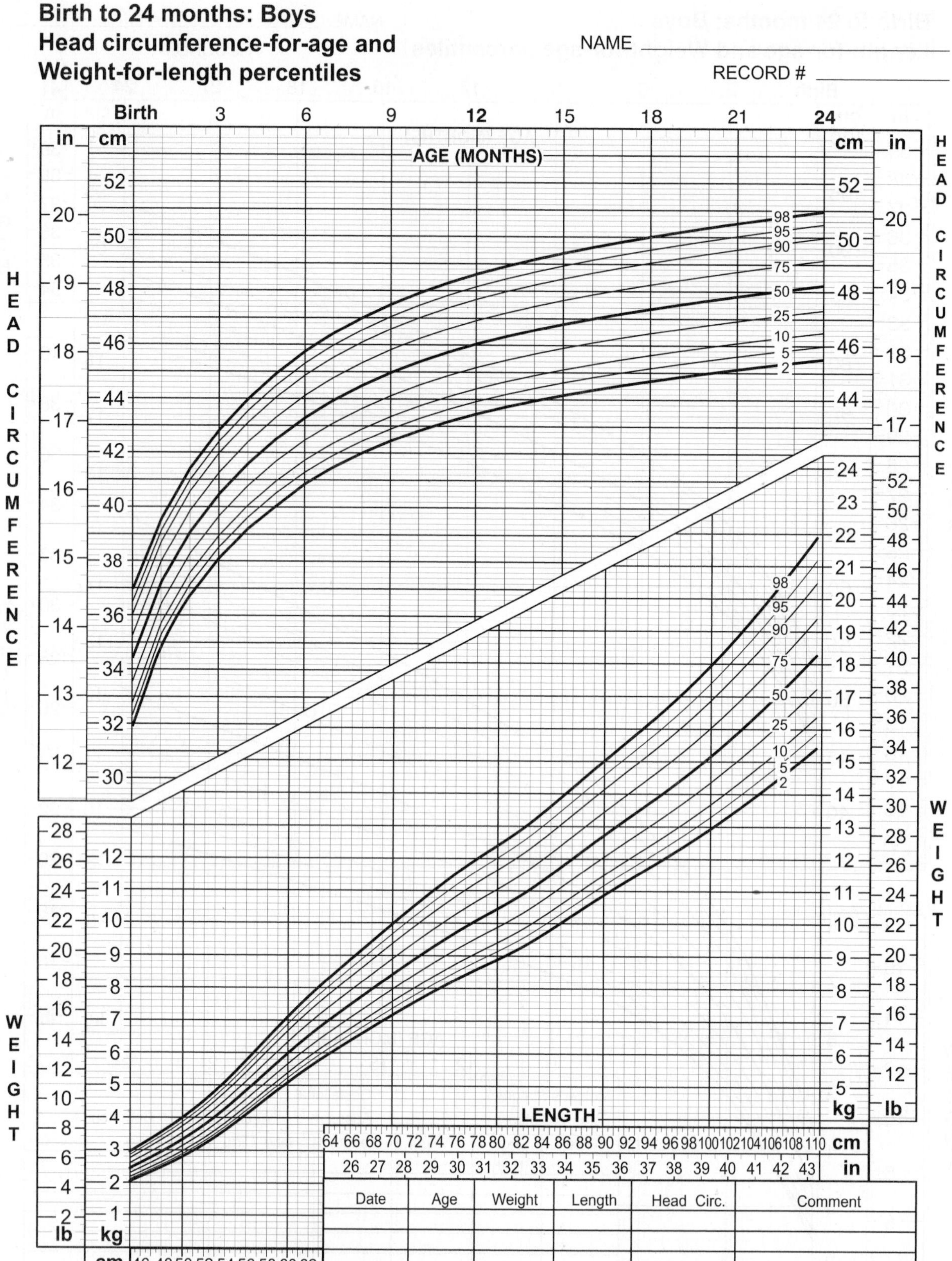

Birth to 24 months: Boys
Head circumference-for-age and
Weight-for-length percentiles

NAME _____

RECORD # _____

Published by the Centers for Disease Control and Prevention, November 1, 2009
SOURCE: WHO Child Growth Standards (http://www.who.int/childgrowth/en)

FIGURE B-2 Birth to 24 months: boys' head circumference-for-age and weight-for-length percentiles. (Published by the Centers for Disease Control and Prevention, November 1, 2009. From WHO Child Growth Standards. Available at www.cdc.gov/growthcharts.)

Birth to 24 months: Girls
Length-for-age and Weight-for-age percentiles

NAME _____

RECORD # _____

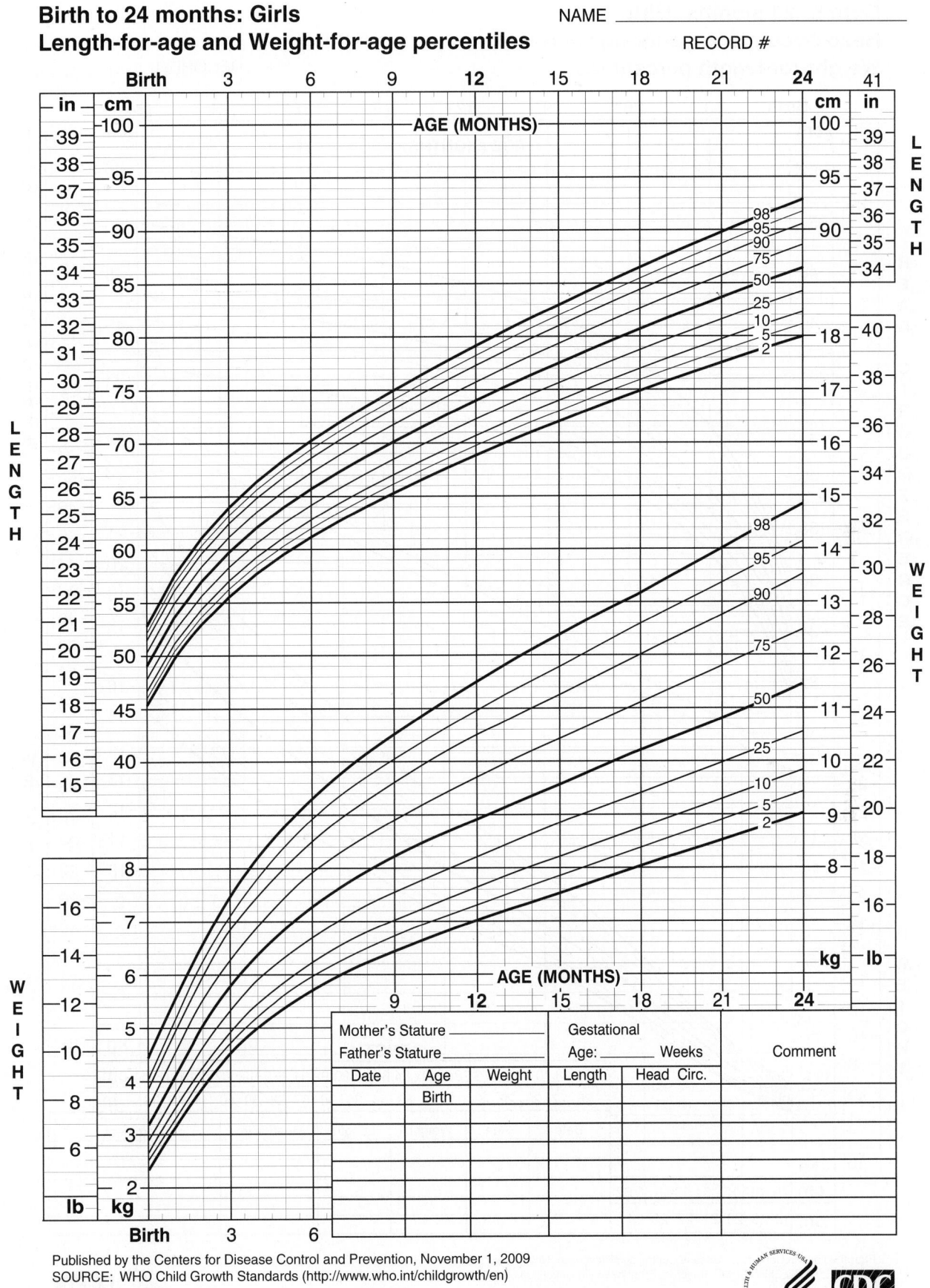

FIGURE B-3 Birth to 24 months: girls' length-for-age and weight-for-age percentiles. (Published by the Centers for Disease Control and Prevention, November 1, 2009. From WHO Child Growth Standards. Available at www.cdc.gov/growthcharts.)

Birth to 24 months: Girls
Head circumference-for-age and
Weight-for-length percentiles

NAME _____

RECORD # _____

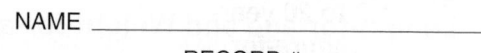

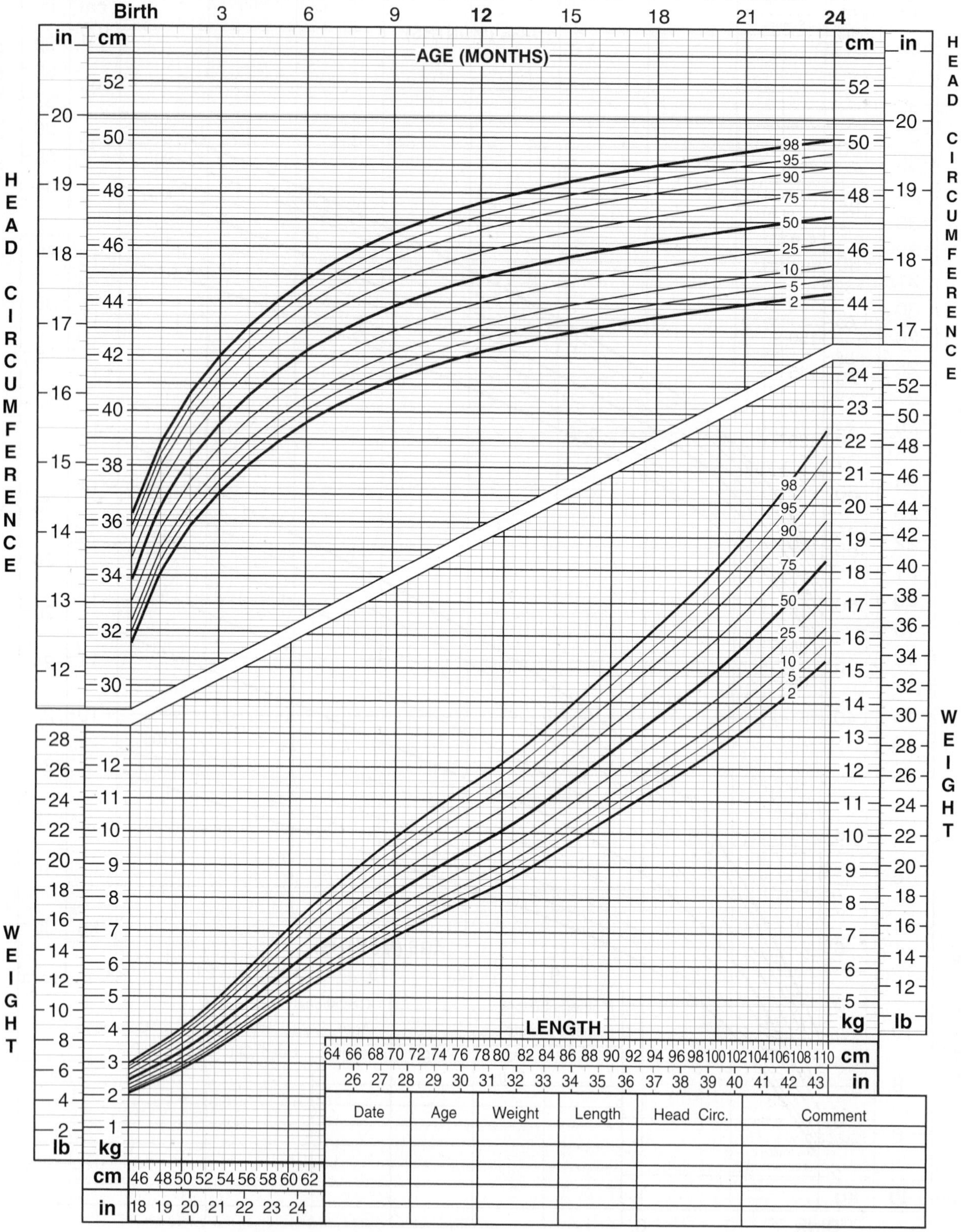

Published by the Centers for Disease Control and Prevention, November 1, 2009
SOURCE: WHO Child Growth Standards (http://www.who.int/childgrowth/en)

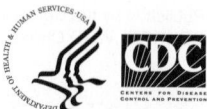

FIGURE B-4 Birth to 24 months: girls' head circumference-for-age and weight-for-length percentiles. (Published by the Centers for Disease Control and Prevention, November 1, 2009. From WHO Child Growth Standards. Available at www.cdc.gov/growthcharts.)

2 to 20 years: Boys
Stature-for-age and Weight-for-age percentiles

NAME _____

RECORD# _____

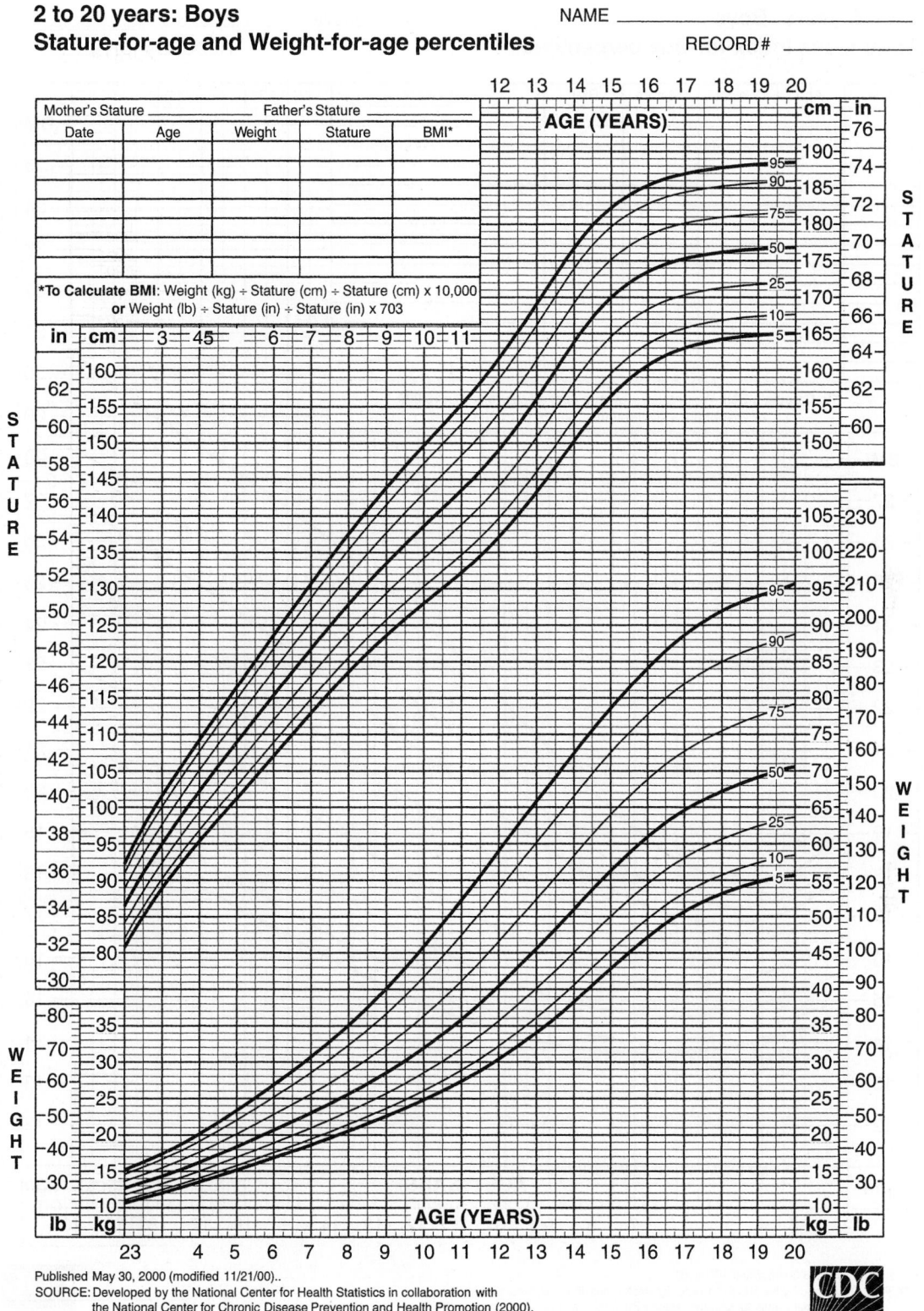

Published May 30, 2000 (modified 11/21/00)..
SOURCE: Developed by the National Center for Health Statistics in collaboration with
the National Center for Chronic Disease Prevention and Health Promotion (2000).
http://www.cdc.gov/growthcharts

FIGURE B-5 2 to 20 years old: boys' stature-for-age and weight-for-age percentiles. (From the National Center for Health Statistics in collaboration with the National Center for Chronic Disease Prevention and Health Promotion, 2000.)

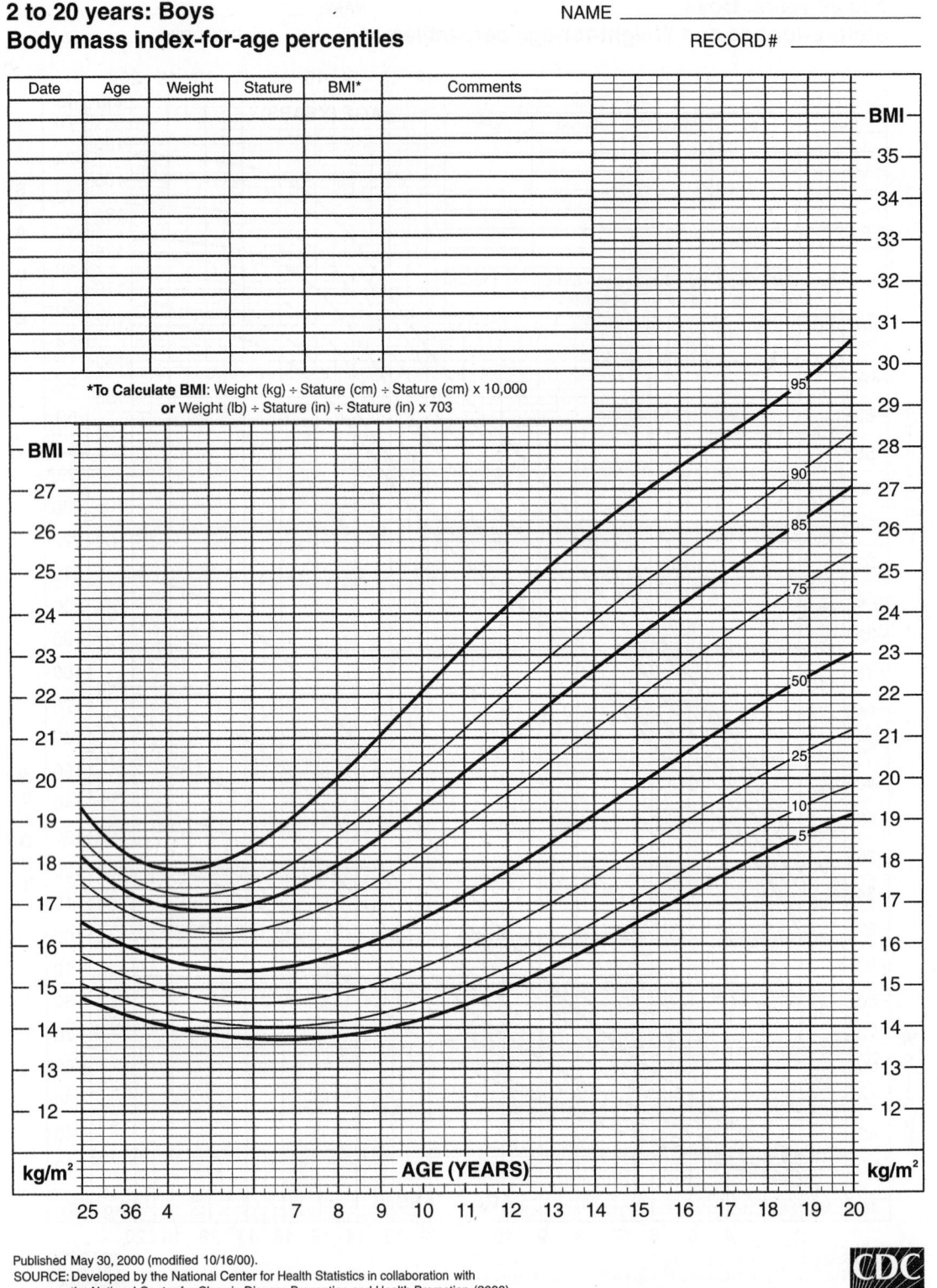

2 to 20 years: Boys
Body mass index-for-age percentiles

NAME _____

RECORD# _____

Date	Age	Weight	Stature	BMI*	Comments

*To Calculate BMI: Weight (kg) ÷ Stature (cm) ÷ Stature (cm) x 10,000
or Weight (lb) ÷ Stature (in) ÷ Stature (in) x 703

AGE (YEARS)

Published May 30, 2000 (modified 10/16/00).
SOURCE: Developed by the National Center for Health Statistics in collaboration with
the National Center for Chronic Disease Prevention and Health Promotion (2000).
http://www.cdc.gov/growthcharts

SAFER·HEALTHIER·PEOPLE™

FIGURE B-6 2 to 20 years old: boys' body mass index-for-age percentiles. (From the National Center for Health Statistics in collaboration with the National Center for Chronic Disease Prevention and Health Promotion, 2000.)

2 to 20 years: Girls
Stature-for-age and Weight-for-age percentiles

NAME _____

RECORD# _____

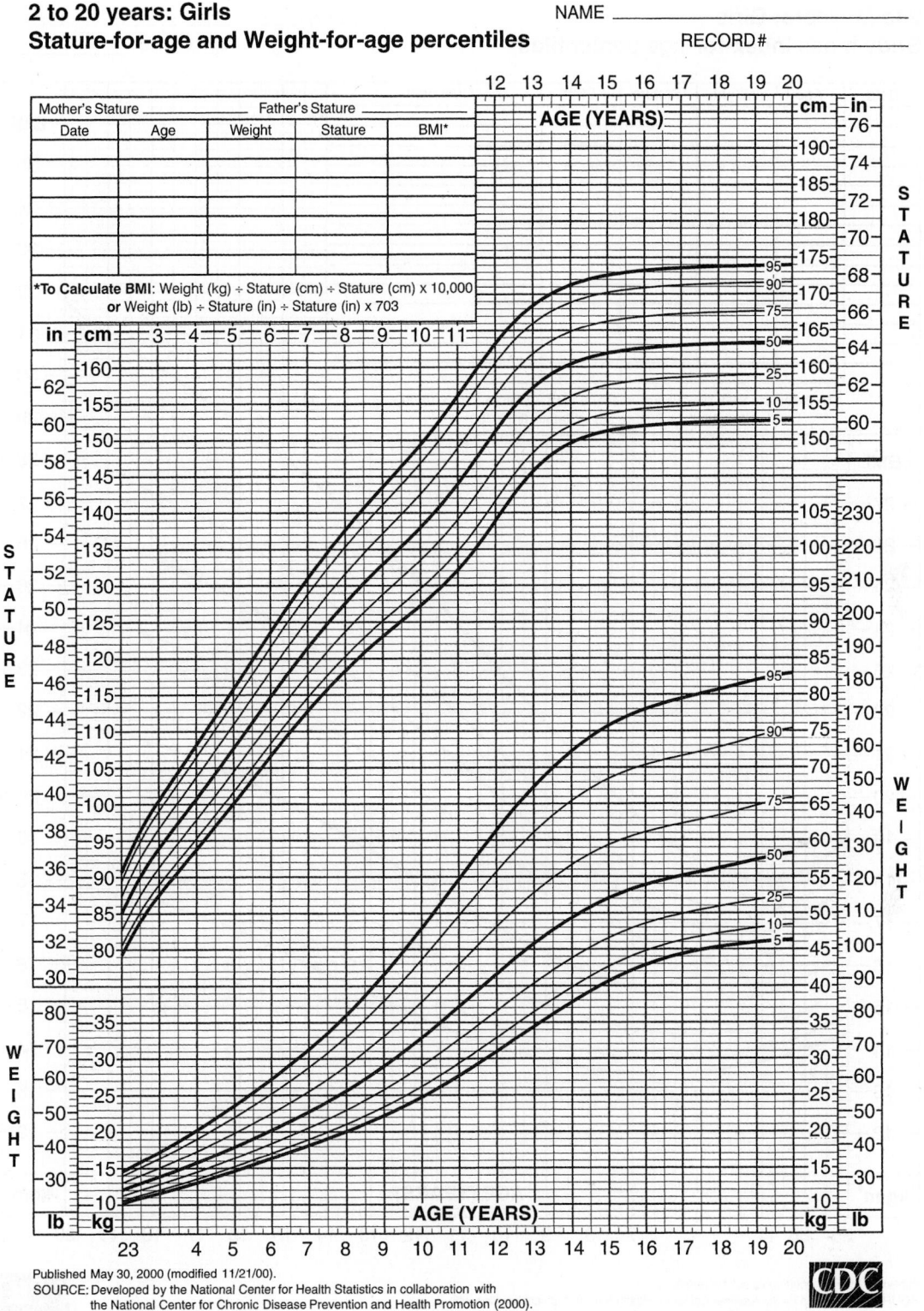

*To Calculate BMI: Weight (kg) ÷ Stature (cm) ÷ Stature (cm) x 10,000
or Weight (lb) ÷ Stature (in) ÷ Stature (in) x 703

Published May 30, 2000 (modified 11/21/00).
SOURCE: Developed by the National Center for Health Statistics in collaboration with
the National Center for Chronic Disease Prevention and Health Promotion (2000).
http://www.cdc.gov/growthcharts

FIGURE B-7 2 to 20 years old: girls' stature-for-age and weight-for-age percentiles. (From the National Center for Health Statistics in collaboration with the National Center for Chronic Disease Prevention and Health Promotion, 2000.)

2 to 20 years: Girls
Body mass index-for-age percentiles

NAME _____

RECORD# _____

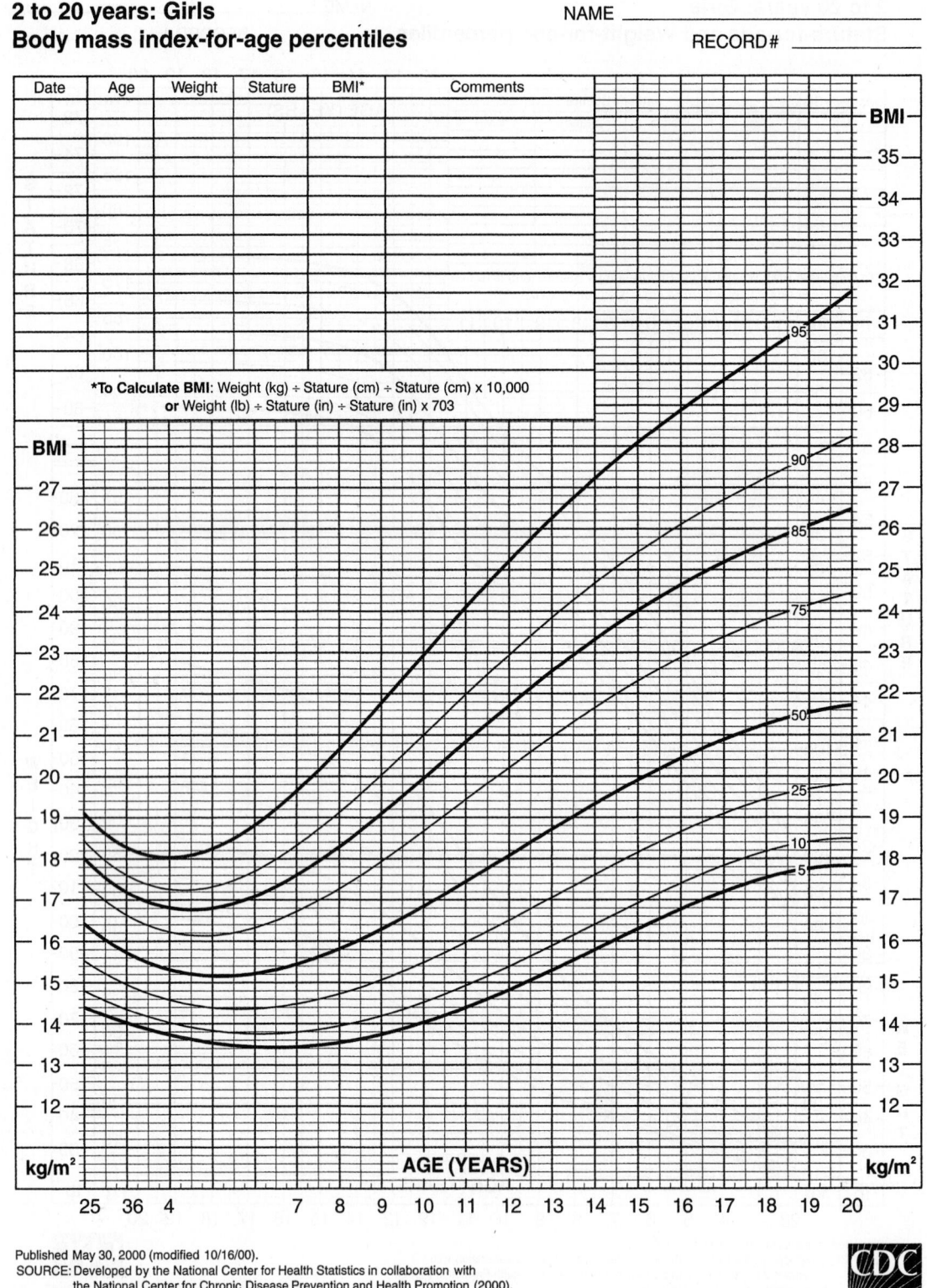

*To Calculate BMI: Weight (kg) ÷ Stature (cm) ÷ Stature (cm) x 10,000
or Weight (lb) ÷ Stature (in) ÷ Stature (in) x 703

Published May 30, 2000 (modified 10/16/00).
SOURCE: Developed by the National Center for Health Statistics in collaboration with
the National Center for Chronic Disease Prevention and Health Promotion (2000).
http://www.cdc.gov/growthcharts

CDC
SAFER·HEALTHIER·PEOPLE

FIGURE B-8 2 to 20 years old: girls' body mass index-for-age percentiles. (From the National Center for Health Statistics in collaboration with the National Center for Chronic Disease Prevention and Health Promotion, 2000.)

children older than 2 years. The combined charts are found at the CDC website and included among the figures to follow. When possible use growth charts that are specific for children with certain genetic conditions. Down syndrome, Turner syndrome, Williams syndrome, quadriplegic cerebral palsy, achondroplasia, and others have growth charts. A new set of growth charts have also been developed for preterm infants (Olsen et al, 2010).

BOYS

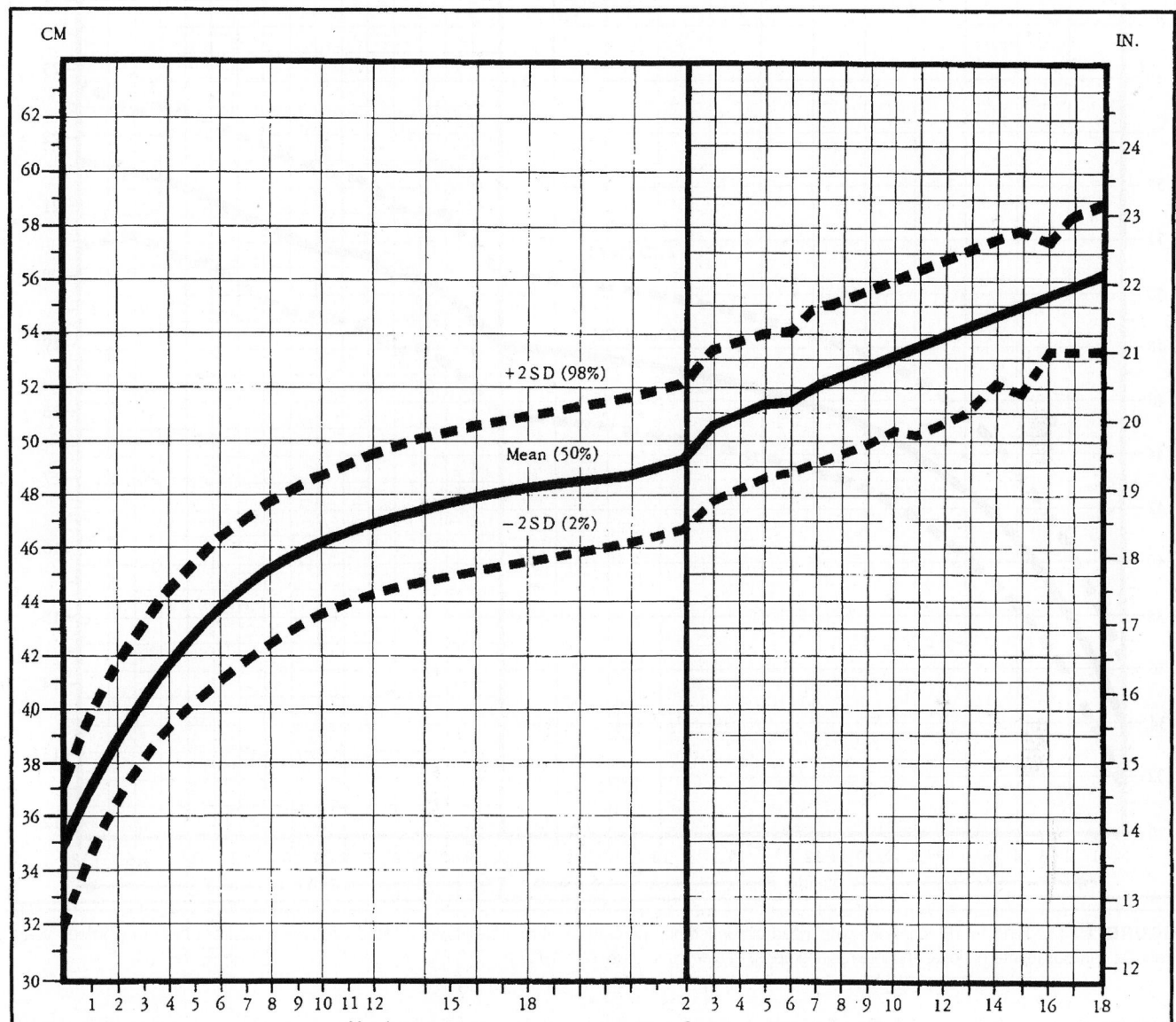

FIGURE B-9 Birth to 18 years old: boys' head circumference percentiles. (From Nellhaus G: Head circumference from birth to eighteen years. Practical composite international and interracial graphs, *Pediatrics* 41:106-114, 1968.)

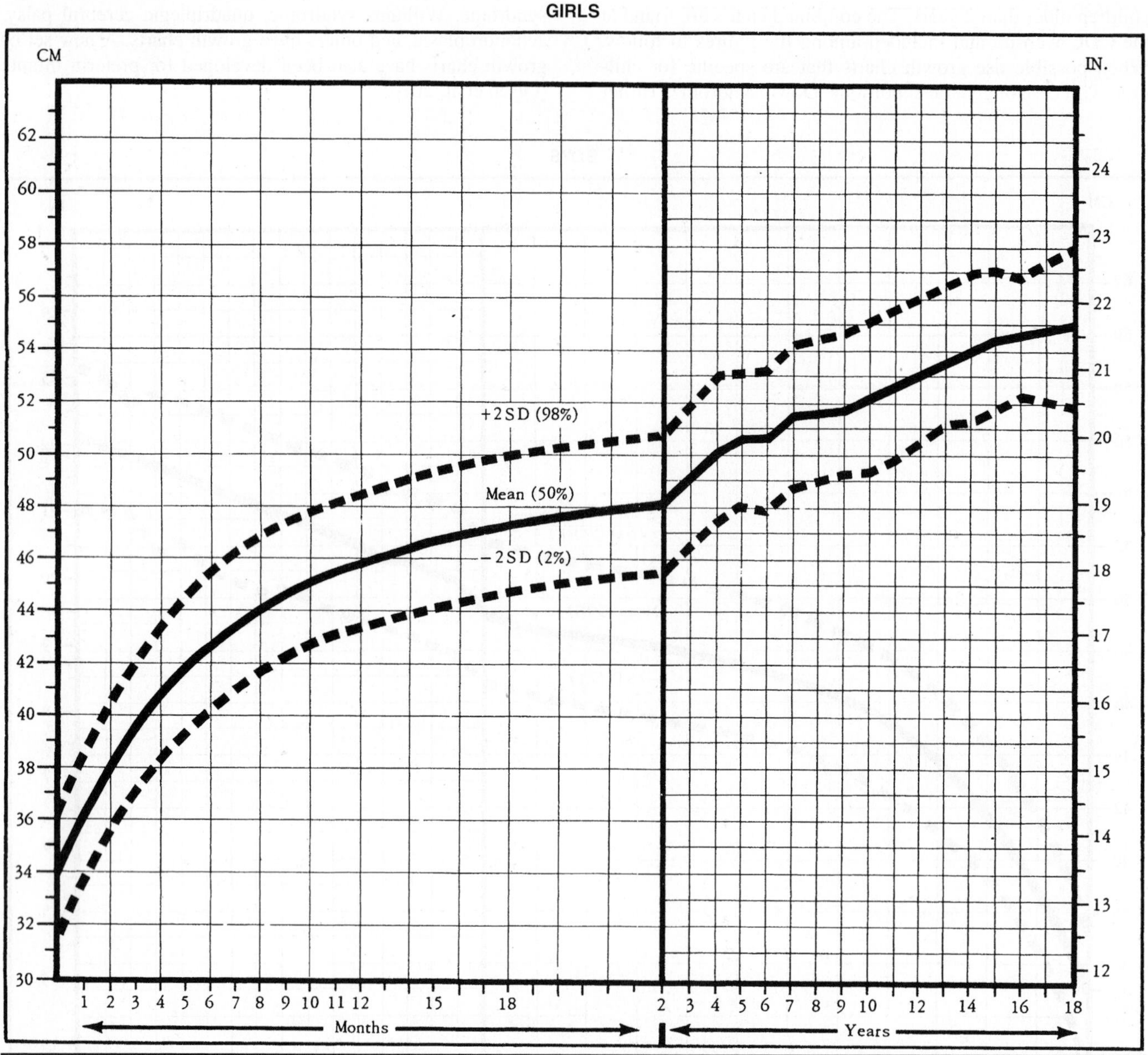

GIRLS

FIGURE B-10 Birth to 18 years old: girls' head circumference percentiles. (From Nellhaus G: Head circumference from birth to eighteen years. Practical composite international and interracial graphs, *Pediatrics* 41:106-114, 1968.)

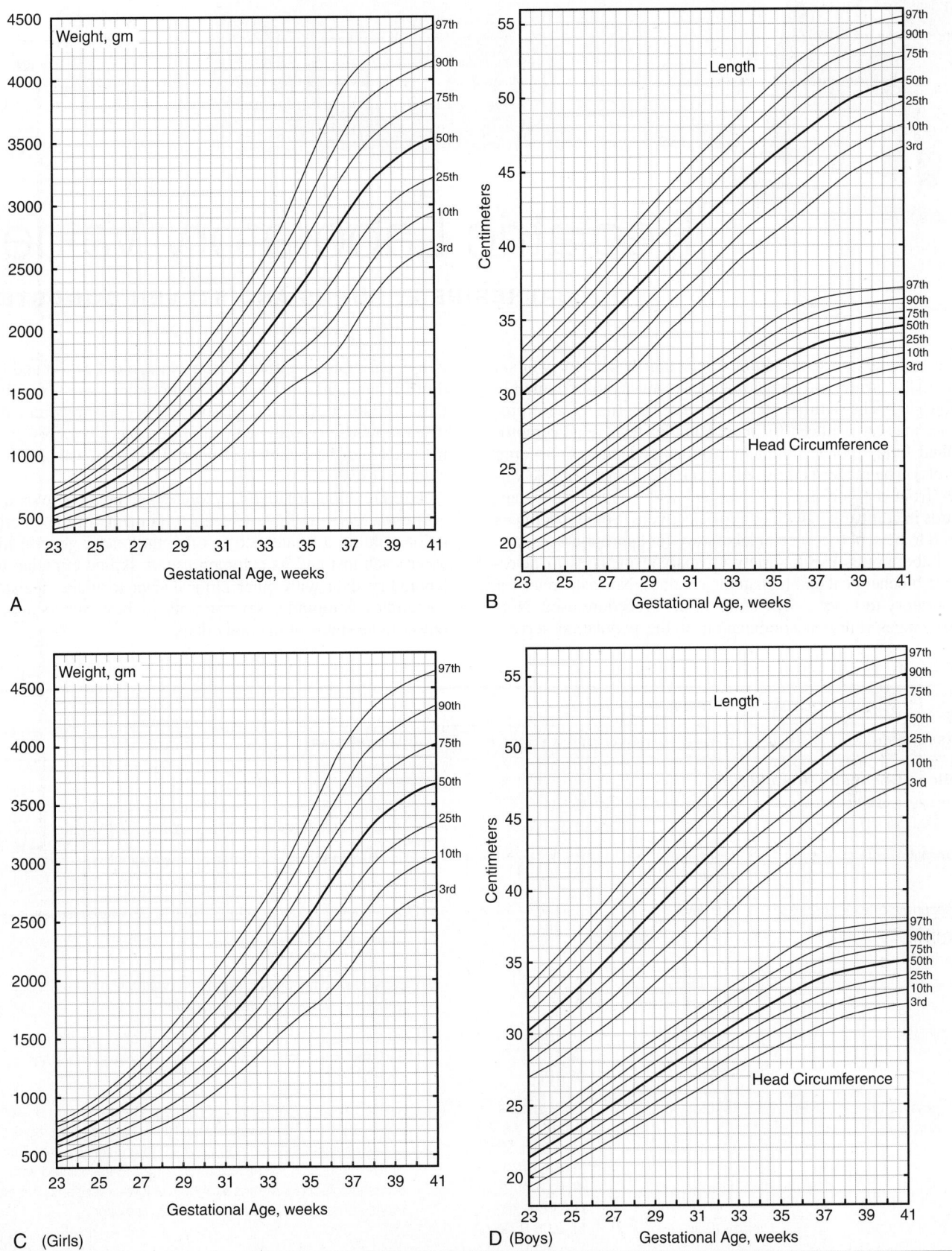

FIGURE B-11 New gender-specific intrauterine growth curves for girls' weight-for-age **(A)**, girls' length- and HC-for-age **(B)**, boys' weight-for-age **(C)**, and boys' length- and HC-for-age **(D)**. Of note, 3rd and 97th percentiles on all curves for 23 weeks should be interpreted cautiously given the small sample size; for boys' HC curve at 24 weeks, all percentiles should be interpreted cautiously because the distribution of data is skewed left. (From Olsen IE, Grovemen SA, Lawson ML et al: New intrauterine growth curves based on United States data, *Pediatrics* 125[2]:e214-224, 2010.)

Appendix C

Pediatric Laboratory Values

CATHERINE E. BURNS AND STEVEN GOODSTEIN

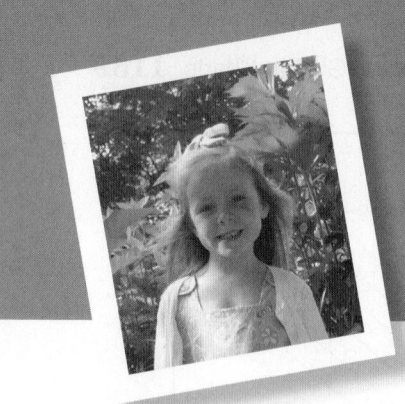

This appendix presents a limited selection of laboratory blood chemistry, urine, and hematologic test values most commonly requested. The authors recognize that the primary care provider may have a need for more complex tests (e.g., cerebrospinal fluid studies, immunoglobulins, and therapeutic drug levels). The reader is directed to seek the source of these values from the performing laboratory and its respective standards in comparison with control specimens. Some specimens need to be sent to a special laboratory for appropriate testing.

Laboratories use a variety of analytic methods to determine biochemical and hematologic values. Normal values for laboratory tests vary depending on the procedure used. Normal ranges reflect a combination of the population served,

individual biologic differences, specimen collection and handling techniques, and intrinsic laboratory variation. Given these variabilities, if any questions arise, it is recommended that the reader consult with the reference laboratory for its methods and the established normal range of values for the methods used.

Interpretation of laboratory values can be a complex diagnostic exercise. In Table C-1, the comments in the Interpretation column are intended to offer the reader general ideas about each test and its common use. A skilled clinician uses laboratory data with other clinical data to make decisions, sometimes combining several tests to best understand the physiologic status of the individual.

TABLE C-1 Pediatric Laboratory Values

Test Name	Reference Range (U.S.A.)		Interpretation
Blood Chemistry (from Serum)			
Alanine aminotransferase (ALT, SGPT) (units/L)	Newborn/infant	8-78	Liver, heart, and skeletal muscle have significant levels.
	>2 mo	8-36	High levels are associated with hepatic cell damage.
Amylase (units/L)	Newborn	0-60	Marked rise generally indicates acute pancreatitis.
	Adult	30-110	
Aspartate aminotransferase (AST, SGOT) (units/L)	0-5 days	35-140	Elevated levels occur with heart, liver, and muscle disease.
	1-9 yr	15-65	
	Adult	8-45	
Bilirubin, total (mg/dL)	0-3 days	2.0 -10.0	Elevated levels occur with increased destruction of RBCs or impairment of liver excretory function.
	1 mo to adult	0-1.5	
Chloride (mEq/L)	Cord blood	96-104	Values increase in metabolic acidosis and other conditions.
	0-30 days	98-113	Decreased values occur with diuresis, GI losses, and other conditions.
	>30 days	98-107	
C-reactive protein (CRP) (mg/dL)	0-90 days	M: 0.08-1.58	Increased in certain inflammatory states due to infection or tissue injury. Compared with ESR, CRP increases more rapidly, peaks earlier, and returns to normal more quickly on resolution of the stimulating agent. Values >10 mg/dL associated with bacterial infections versus viral (with a few exceptions). Serial measurements often used to monitor resolution.
		F: 0.09-1.58	
	91 days-12 mo	M: 0.08-1.12	
		F: 0.05-0.79	
	13 mo-3 yr	M: 0.08-1.12	
		F: 0.08-0.79	
	4-10 yr	M: 0.06-0.79	
		F: 0.5-1.0	
	11-14 yr	M: 0.08-0.76	
		F: 0.06-0.81	
	14-18 yr	M: 0.04-0.79	
		F: 0.06-0.79	

TABLE C-1 Pediatric Laboratory Values—cont'd

Test Name	Reference Range (U.S.A.)		Interpretation
Creatinine (mg/dL)	Cord blood	0.6-1.2	Elevated levels indicate impaired renal function, muscle disease, congestive heart failure, shock, dehydration, and other conditions.
	Newborn	0.3-1	
	Infant	0.2-0.4	
	Child	0.3-0.7	
	Adolescent	0.5-1	
	Adult		
	M	0.6-1.2	
	F	0.5-1.1	
Ferritin (ng/mL)	Newborn	25-200	Ferritin is a more sensitive indicator than iron or TIBC for diagnosing iron deficiency or overload.
	1 mo	200-600	
	2-5 mo	50-200	
	6 mo- 15 y	7-140	
	Adult		
	M	15-200	
	F	12-150	
Glucose (fasting) (mg/dL)	Cord blood	45-96	Fasting low levels may indicate a physiologic response or a disorder in glucose metabolism. Increased fasting levels may indicate diabetes mellitus, pancreatic disorders, endocrine diseases, drugs, and other conditions.
	Premature	20-60	
	Neonate	30-60	
	1 day	40-60	
	>1 day	50-80	
	Child	74-106	
	Adult	70-105	
Iron (mcg/dL)	Newborn	100-250	Decreased levels occur with iron deficiency, blood loss, and other conditions. Elevated levels occur with hemolytic anemias, iron intoxication, hepatitis, and other conditions.
	Infant	30-70	
	Child	50-120	
	Thereafter		
	M	65-175	
	F	50-170	
Lead (whole blood specimen) (mcg/dL)	Child	<10	Increased levels indicate lead toxicity. Any level indicates some degree of toxicity.
	Toxic	≥70	
Potassium (mmol/L)	Newborn	3-7	Decreased levels may indicate shifting of potassium into cells, GI loss, biliary loss, renal loss, and reduced uptake. Increased levels occur with shifts to intracellular fluid, decreased excretion, or increased uptake.
	2-12 mo	3.5-6.0	
	Thereafter	3.5-5.1	
Procalcitonin (Pro-CT; PCT) (ng/mL)	Children and adults	<0.1	Increased during onset and control of bacterial infections; values higher than seen with viral infections. Shows promise to be more specific than ESR and CRP; clinical usefulness as biomarker for bacterial infections in children is under study.
Sodium (mmol/L)	Newborn	133-146	Decreased levels indicate sodium loss or water excess (caused by numerous conditions). Increased levels may occur with an increase in sodium or an excessive loss of water (caused by numerous conditions).
	Child and adult	135-148	
Thyrotropin (thyroid-stimulating hormone [TSH]) (microunits/L)	Cord blood	3-22	Decreased levels are associated with hyperthyroidism. Increased levels are associated with hypothyroidism.
	Birth-3 days	<40	
	3-7 days	<25	
	>7 days	0-10	
Thyroxine, free (FT$_4$) (ng/dL)	Newborn	2.0-4.9	Decreased levels are associated with hypothyroidism or overproduction of T3. Increased levels are associated with Graves disease and thyrotoxicosis from overproduction of T$_4$.
	Infant	0.9-2.6	
	Prepubertal child	0.8-2.2	
	Pubertal child and adult	0.8-2.3	
Thyroxine, total (T$_4$) (mcg/dL)	1-3 days	8.2-19.9	T$_4$ serves as a good index of thyroid function only if binding globulin (TBG) is normal.
	1-2 wk	6.0-15.9	
	1-12 mo	6.1-14.9	
	1-5 yr	6.8-13.5	
	5-10 yr	6.4-12.8	
	Pubertal child and adult	4.2-13.0	

continued

TABLE C-1	Pediatric Laboratory Values—cont'd		
Test Name	**Reference Range (U.S.A.)**		**Interpretation**
Urea nitrogen (BUN) (mg/dL)	Premature (1 wk)	3-25	Measures glomerular function and production/excretion of urea. Decreased with liver failure, malnutrition, and other conditions. Increased with impaired renal function, congestive heart failure, salt/water depletion, shock, and other conditions.
	Newborn	4-12	
	Infant/child	5-18	
	Adult	7-18	
Hematology (Whole Blood Specimens)			
Erythrocyte count (RBC) (millions of cells/mm^3 [microliters])	1-3 days (capillary)	4-6.6	Measures total number of RBCs. Decreased with anemia, cell destruction, and decreased production. Elevated with increased RBC production, renal disease, tumors, altitude, pulmonary disease, cardiovascular diseases, and other conditions. A relative increase may occur with dehydration.
	1 wk	3.9-6.3	
	2 wk	3.6-6.2	
	1 mo	3-5.4	
	2 mo	2.7-4.9	
	3-6 mo	3.1-4.5	
	5 mo-2 yr	3.7-5.3	
	2-6 yr	3.9-5.3	
	6-12 yr	4-5.2	
	12-18 yr		
	M	4.5-5.3	
	F	4.1-5.1	
	18-49 yr		
	M	4.5-5.9	
	F	4-5.2	
Erythrocyte sedimentation rate (ESR, sed rate) (mm/hr)			Not diagnostic, but indicates a disease process. Increases occur with collagen diseases, infections, inflammatory conditions, neoplasms, heavy metal poisoning, tissue destruction, and other conditions.
Westergren, modified	Child	0-10	
	Adult		
	M <50 yr	0-15	
	F <50 yr	0-20	
Wintrobe	Child	0-13	
	Adult		
	M	0-9	
	F	0-20	
Hematocrit (HCT, Hct) (% packed erythrocyte volume [erythrocyte volume/ whole blood × 100])	1 day	48-69	Low values indicate blood loss or inadequate production or excess destruction of RBCs. High values indicate erythrocytosis, severe dehydration, shock, and other conditions.
	2 days	48-75	
	3 days	44-72	
	2 mo-6 yr	28-42	
	6-12 yr	35-45	
	12-18 yr		
	M	37-49	
	F	36-46	
	18-49 yr		
	M	41-53	
	F	36-46	
Hemoglobin, total (Hb) (g/dL)	1-3 days	14.5-22.5	Decreased levels are found with anemia, hyperthyroidism, cirrhosis, severe hemorrhage, hemolysis, and systemic diseases. Very low values may lead to heart failure and death.
	2 mo-6yr	9-14	
	6-12 yr	11.5-15.5	
	12-18 yr		
	M	13-16	
	F	12-16	
	18-49 yr		
	M	13.5-17.5	
	F	12-16	
Leukocyte count (white blood cell [WBC] count) (× 1000 cells/mm^3)	Birth	9-35	Indicates total WBC count circulating in the blood. With some infections, WBCs increase as cells are transported. A low count may occur in overwhelming bacterial infection (sepsis) or with the use of immunosuppressive agents. Elevated levels may occur in response to an underlying disease, a primary cellular disorder (leukemia), pregnancy, corticosteroid treatment, strenuous exercise, and other conditions.
	1-2 wk	5.0-20.0	
	1-6 mo	6-17.5	
	7 mo-2 yr	6-17.0	
	2-5 yr	5.5-15.5	
	5-8 yr	5.0-14.5	
	13-18 yr	4.5-13.0	
	Adult	4.5-11.0	

TABLE C-1 Pediatric Laboratory Values—cont'd

Test Name	Reference Range (U.S.A.)		Interpretation
Leukocyte differential (%)	Myelocytes	0-0	Describes the proportion of the types of WBCs. Used in conjunction with the total leukocyte count to determine absolute cell counts.
	Neutrophils ("bands")	3-5	Myelocytes: involved in the early maturation of neutrophils, eosinophils, basophils, and monocytes.
	Neutrophils ("segs")	54-62	Neutrophils: usually increased during bacterial infections. May be decreased in viral infections. Bands are immature; segmented are more mature forms.
	Lymphocytes	25-33	Lymphocytes: increased in viral infections. T-cell, B-cell, and natural killer cell types.
	Monocytes	3-7	Monocytes: increased in severe and recovery stages of infections (phagocytosis).
	Eosinophils	1-3	Eosinophils: increased during allergic responses and parasitic infections.
	Basophils	0-0.75	Basophils: increased in allergic reactions, hematologic disorders, and other conditions.
Platelet count (thrombocyte count)	Newborn	84-478 × 10³/mm³	Decreased platelet counts occur with anemias, some infections, congestive heart failure, bone marrow lesions, and other conditions. Increases occur with malignancies, splenectomy, collagen diseases, some anemias, and other conditions.
	1 wk-adult	150-400 × 10³/mm³	
Reticulocyte count (%)	Newborn	0-6	Provides an estimate of the rate of RBC production. The percentage may be used to calculate the absolute value. An elevated count with normal hemoglobin indicates RBC loss with bone marrow compensation. A normal reticulocyte count with a low hemoglobin level indicates an inadequate response to anemia. Reticulocyte turns to erythrocyte in 24 hr.
	1-6 mo	0-2.8	
	Adults	0.5-1.5	
Urine			
Urine, macroscopic	All ages		
Bilirubin		Negative	Increased in hepatocellular disease or intrahepatic/extrahepatic biliary obstruction.
Blood, occult		Negative	RBCs increased in acute glomerulonephritis, acute infections, renal calculi, trauma, and other conditions.
Glucose, qualitative		Negative	Increased when blood glucose level exceeds the reabsorption capacity of the renal tubes (pathologic or benign).
Hemoglobin		Negative	Hemoglobinuria may occur in intravascular hemolysis and other conditions.
Ketones		Negative	Increased with adequate carbohydrate intake or a defect in carbohydrate metabolism. Especially significant with diabetes mellitus.
Leukocyte esterase		Negative	Measures WBCs. Increase indicates inflammation or infection (or both). Associated with certain renal diseases and diseases of the urinary tract or vaginitis.
Nitrite		Negative	Positive associated with urinary tract infection.
pH		4.6-8	Indication of acid-base balance.
Protein, qualitative		Negative	Increased in pathologic or physiologic conditions (e.g., fever, stress, strenuous exercises).
Specific gravity		1.001-1.030	Measures the concentrating and diluting ability of the kidney. Associated with tubular damage.
Urobilinogen		0.2-1 mg/dL	Increased in liver disease. Decreased in obstruction of bile ducts and other conditions.

Continued

TABLE C-1	Pediatric Laboratory Values—cont'd		
Test Name	**Reference Range (U.S.A.)**		**Interpretation**
Urine, microscopic			
Casts	Hyaline	0-1/lpf	Hyaline casts: increased in pathologic or physiologic conditions. Implies damage to the glomerular capillary membrane permitting leakage of proteins through the glomerular filtrate.
	Other	None	Other casts: involved in a variety of conditions depending on the type of cast. Involved in tubular epithelial damage (epithelial cell cast), renal infection (WBC cast), vascular disorder (RBC cast), renal disease (granular cast), chronic renal condition (waxy cast), severe renal disease (broad cast), and degenerative tubular disease (fatty cast).
Red blood cells (RBCs)		0-2/hpf	RBCs: denote bleeding into the urinary system.
White blood cells (WBCs)	M	0-3/hpf	WBCs: associated with an inflammatory process.
	F and children	0-5/hpf	
Urine volume (mL/24 hr)	Newborn	50-300	Decreased in dehydration, renal ischemia, renal disease, obstruction, and other conditions. Increased in diabetes insipidus, diabetes mellitus, chronic progressive renal failure, and other conditions.
	Infant	350-550	
	Child	500-1000	
	Adolescent	700-1400	
	Thereafter		
	M	800-1800	
	F	600-1600	

F, Female; *GI*, gastrointestinal; *hpf*, high-power field; *hr*, hours; *lpf*, low-power field; *M*, male; *mo*, month(s); *T3*, triiodothyronine; *TBG*, thyroxine-binding globulin; *TIBC*, total iron-binding capacity; *wk*, week(s); *yr*, years.

TABLE C-2	Evaluation of Bleeding Disorders		
Test	**Mechanism**	**Normal Values***	**Examples of Disorders**
Prothrombin time	Extrinsic to common pathway	Neonate: 10.1-15.9 sec Postneonate: 11-12 sec	Defect in vitamin K–dependent factors, hemorrhagic disease of newborn, malabsorption; liver disease, DIC, oral anticoagulants
Activated partial thromboplastin time (APTT, PTT)	Intrinsic and common pathway	Neonate: 42.9 sec Postneonate: 25-37 sec	Hemophilia, von Willebrand, heparin, DIC, deficient factors
Thrombin time (TT)	Fibrinogen to fibrin	Neonate: 12-17 sec Postneonate: 10-15 sec	Fibrin split products, DIC, low fibrin level, heparin, uremia
Bleeding time (BT)	Hemostasis, capillary and platelet function	Postneonate: 3-7min	Platelet dysfunctions, low platelet count, von Willebrand, aspirin
Platelet count (see Table C-1)	—	—	—
Peripheral blood smear	Number and shape of blood cells	—	Platelets: peripheral destruction disorder RBCs: suggest microangiopathic process (e.g., HUS, hemangioma, DIC) WBCs: number and differential suggest infections, leukemias, etc.

*Values will vary from laboratory to laboratory based on the technology used. The values here are typical, but should not be considered as absolute normal values. Use the norms recorded on laboratory slips as another guide to decide whether a given value is abnormal or normal. And, of course, use clinical judgment because most disorders are defined by a variety of signs, symptoms, and test values.
DIC, Disseminated intravascular coagulation; *HUS*, hemolytic-uremic syndrome; *min*, minutes; *RBCs*, red blood cells; *sec*, seconds; *WBCs*, white blood cells.

TABLE C-3   Red Blood Cell Indices (May Be Used to Differentiate Anemias)

Index	Definition	Calculation (Usually Done Electronically)
Mean corpuscular volume (MCV)	Average volume of RBC expressed as femtoliters (fL)	Hct (%) × 10/RBC count (×10^{12}/L)
Mean corpuscular hemoglobin (MCH)	Average weight of hemoglobin in an RBC expressed in picograms (pg)	Hb (g/dL) × 10/RBC count (×10^{12}/L)
Mean corpuscular hemoglobin concentration (MCHC)	Average concentration of hemoglobin in the RBC expressed as grams per deciliter (g/dL)	Hb (g/dL) × 100/Hct (%)
Red cell distribution width (RDW)	A measure of anisocytosis; the coefficient of variation of the RBC size determined on automated blood cell counting instruments expressed as a percent	Standard deviation of RBC size/mean corpuscular volume. Normal range: 11.5%-14.5%.

NOTE: Normal values will vary depending on the technology used. Generally all of these values are calculated electronically.

Age	MCV (fL)	MCH (pg)	MCHC (g/dL)
0-1 day	95-125	31-37	30-34
2-4 days	98-118	31-37	29-37
5-7 days	100-120	28-40	28-38
8-14 days	95-115	28-40	30-34
15-30 days	93-113	28-40	30-34
1-2 months	83-107	28-40	29-37
3-5 months	83-107	25-35	30-36
6-11 months	78-102	23-31	30-36
1-3 years	76-92	23-30	31-37
4-7 years	78-94	25-33	31-37

Hb, Hemoglobin; *Hct,* hematocrit; *RBC,* red blood cell.
Data from Rodak B: *Hematology clinical principles and applications,* ed 2, Philadelphia, 2002, Saunders.

TABLE C-4   Serum Lipid Concentrations by Age and Gender

	MALES (mg/dL)			FEMALES (mg/dL)		
	5-9 yr	10-14 yr	15-19 yr	5-9 yr	10-14 yr	15-19 yr
Total Cholesterol						
50th percentile	153	161	152	164	159	157
75th percentile	168	173	168	177	171	176
90th percentile	183	191	183	189	191	198
95th percentile	186	201	191	197	205	208
Triglycerides						
50th percentile	48	58	68	57	68	64
75th percentile	58	74	88	74	85	85
90th percentile	70	94	125	103	104	112
95th percentile	85	111	143	120	120	126
LDL-C						
50th percentile	90	94	93	98	94	93
75th percentile	103	109	109	115	110	110
90th percentile	117	123	123	125	126	129
95th percentile	129	133	130	140	136	137

Continued

TABLE C-4	Serum Lipid Concentrations by Age and Gender—cont'd					
	MALES (mg/dL)			**FEMALES (mg/dL)**		
	5-9 yr	**10-14 yr**	**15-19 yr**	**5-9 yr**	**10-14 yr**	**15-19 yr**
HDL						
5th percentile	38	37	30	36	37	35
10th percentile	43	40	34	38	40	38
25th percentile	49	46	39	48	45	43
50th percentile	55	55	46	52	52	51

Adapted from American Academy of Pediatrics Committee on Nutrition: Lipid screening and cardiovascular health in childhood, *Pediatrics* 122(1):198-208, 2008.

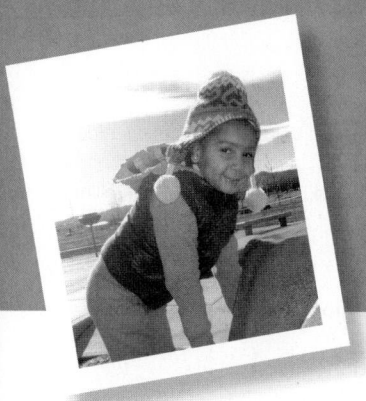

Appendix D

Additional Resources

CHAPTER 1: HEALTH STATUS OF CHILDREN: GLOBAL AND LOCAL PERSPECTIVES

Healthy People 2020
  http://healthypeople.gov/hp2020/default.asp
Millennium Development Goals
  www.un.org/millenniumgoals/bkgd.shtml
LiST: The Lives Saved Tool
  www.jhsph.edu/dept/ih/IIP/list/index.html
UNICEF Convention on the Rights of the Child
  www.unicef.org/rightsite/sowc

CHAPTER 3: CULTURAL PERSPECTIVES FOR PEDIATRIC PRIMARY CARE

American Refugee Committee International
  www.arcrelief.org
American Translators Association
  www.atanet.org
Centers for Medicare and Medicaid Services: American Indian/Alaska Native
  www.cms.gov/aian
Child Family Health International
  www.cfhi.org
Cross Cultural Health Care Program
  www.xculture.org
Diversity, Healing, and Health Care
  www.gasi-ves.org/diversity.htm
DiversityRX
  www.diversityrx.org
Ethnic American
  University of Buffalo, The State University of New York:
  http://ethnicamerican.smbs.buffalo.edu/eahome.shtml
EthnoMed
  www.ethnomed.org
Health Resources and Services Administration (HRSA) and Office of Minority Health Resource Center
  www.hrsa.gov/culturalcompetence
  www.omhrc.gov
  www.omhrc.gov/clas
National Center for Cultural Competence
  www.nccc.georgetown.edu
National Network of Libraries of Medicine: Cultural Competency Resources
  www.nnlm.gov/mcr/resources/community/competency.html
State University of New York Institute of Technology
  www.culturedmed.binghamton.edu
Think Cultural Health
  www.thinkculturalhealth.org

CHAPTER 4: DEVELOPMENTAL MANAGEMENT IN PEDIATRIC PRIMARY CARE

American Academy of Pediatrics, Section on Developmental and Behavioral Pediatrics (SODBP)
  www.dbpeds.org
Bright Futures **in Practice**
  www.brightfutures.org
Enhancing Developmentally Oriented Primary Care
  www.edopc.org
Facts for Families
  www.aacap.org
Growth Charts
  www.cdc.gov/nchs/about/major/nhanes/growthcharts/
    charts.htm
Growth Charts for Down Syndrome
  www.growthcharts.com
Hawaii Early Learning Program (HELP) at Home Manual
  www.vort.com
Healthy Steps
  www.healthysteps.org
Parents as Teachers
  www.parentsasteachers.org
NCAST
  www.ncast.org
The Commonwealth Fund
  www.thecommonwealthfund.org
Touchpoints
  www.touchpoints.org
Zero to Three
  www.zerotothree.org

CHAPTER 5: DEVELOPMENTAL MANAGEMENT OF INFANTS

Ages & Stages Questionnaire (ASQ)-3 and Ages & Stages Questionnaire: Social-Emotional (ASQ:SE)
  Birth through 5 years
  www.brookespublishing.com
Batelle Developmental Inventory Screening Test
  www.riversidepublishing.com
Brazelton TB, Sparrow JD: *Touchpoints—birth to three: your child's emotional and behavioral development,* Cambridge, MA, 2006, Perseus Publishing Services.
Bright Futures
  www.brightfutures.org
Bright Futures **Tool and Resource Kit**
  http://brightfutures.aap.org/tool_and_resource_kit.html

Child Development Inventories (CDI)

3 months through 6 years

www.dbpeds.org/screening/index.cfm

Communication and Symbolic Behavior Scales Developmental Profile (CSBSDP)

www.brookespublishing.com

Fields D, Brown A: *Baby 411: clear answers and smart advice for your baby's first year,* Boulder, CO, 2009, Windsor Peak Press.

Goldberg S: *Baby and toddler learning fun,* Cambridge, MA, 2001, DaCapo Press.

Gesell Developmental Screening Inventory (Revised)

Birth through school age

Order from Lorraine Coulson (e-mail: lrcoulson@ualr.edu)

Hagan JF, Shaw JS, Duncan PM, editors: Bright *Futures guidelines for health supervision of infants, children, and adolescents,* ed 3, Elk Grove Village, IL, 2008, American Academy of Pediatrics.

Healthy Steps for Young Children Program

A National Initiative to Foster Healthy Growth and Development

www.healthysteps.org

Home Observation for Measurement of the Environment (HOME) Scale

http://ualr.edu/case/index.php/home/home-inventory

Infant-Toddler and Family Instrument (ITFI)

Age 6 through 36 months

www.brookespublishing.com

Milani-Comparetti Motor Development

http://www.unl.edu/buros/bimm/index.html

National Capital Poison Center

1-800-222-1222

http://www.poison.org/actFast/1800.asp

Neonatal Behavioral Assessment Scale

www.brazelton-institute.com

Nursing Child Assessment Satellite Training (NCAST) Scales

Feeding and teaching scales (birth through 3 years)

Personal environmental assessments (manual only needed)

Sleep activity record (manual only needed)

www.ncast.org

Parents' Evaluation of Developmental Status (PEDS)

Birth through 8 years

www.pedstest.com

Prescreening Developmental Questionnaire, Inc. (PDQ-II)

www.denverii.com

Reach Out and Read National Center

www.reachoutandread.org

Receptive-Expressive Emergent Language (REEL) Scale, third edition

www.proedinc.com

Shelov SP, Altmann TR: *Caring for your baby and young child: birth to five years,* Elk Grove Village, IL, 2009, American Academy of Pediatrics.

Temperament and Atypical Behavior Scale (TABS)

www.brookespublishing.com

Zero to Three

www.zerotothree.org

CHAPTER 7: DEVELOPMENTAL MANAGEMENT OF SCHOOL-AGE CHILDREN

American Academy of Pediatrics

www.aap.org

Bright Futures

www.brightfutures.org

Guidelines for health supervision of infants, children, and adolescents (Hagan, Shaw, & Duncan, 2008)

Bright Futures in practice: mental health, Volume I, Practice Guide (Jellinek, Patel, & Froehle, 2002a)

Bright Futures in practice: mental health, Volume II, Tool Kit (Jellinek, Patel, & Froehle, 2002b)

Child Development Institute

www.childdevelopmentinfo.com

Institute for Multisensory Education

www.orton-gillingham.com

International Dyslexia Association

www.interdys.org

NAPNAP

Keep Your Child/Yourself Safe and Secure (KySS) Guide to Mental Health Screening, Intervention and Health Promotion

www.napnap.org

National Association for Child Development

www.nacd.org

School readiness

www.readyatfive.org

Search Institute

www.search-institute.org

CHAPTER 8: DEVELOPMENTAL MANAGEMENT OF ADOLESCENTS

Adolescent Health Transition Project

http://depts.washington.edu/healthtr

Alliance of Professional Tattooists, Inc. (APT)

www.safe-tattoos.com

American Academy of Family Physicians

www.aafp.org

American Academy of Pediatrics

www.aap.org

Centers for Disease Control and Prevention (CDC)

www.cdc.gov

Family Acceptance Project

http://familyproject.sfsu.edu

Ginsburg K: *A parent's guide to building resilience in children and teens: giving your child roots and wings,* Elk Grove Village, IL, 2006, American Academy of Pediatrics.

Kastner LS, Wyatt J: *Getting to calm: cool-headed strategies for parenting tweens + teens,* Seattle, 2009, Parent Map.

Kids Counsel: Center for Children's Advocacy

www.kidscounsel.org

National Runaway Switchboard

www.1800runaway.org

1-800-621-4000

1-800-RUNAWAY (786-2929)

National Sexual Assault Hotline

RAINN

www.rainn.org

1-800-HOPE (4673)

Resources for the prevention and victims of rape, abuse, and incest

Parenting Teens

www.parentingteens.com

Parents, Families, and Friends of Lesbians and Gays

www.pflag.org

Riera M: *Uncommon sense for parents with teenagers,* Berkeley, CA, 2004, Celestial Arts.

Search Institute

www.search-institute.org

Sex, etc.

www.sexetc.org

Sex education for teens by teens

Society for Adolescent Medicine

www.adolescenthealth.org

Wolfe AE: *Get out of my life, but first could you drive me & Cheryl to the mall: a parent's guide to the new teenager,* NY, 2002, Farrar, Straus, and Giroux.

CHAPTER 9: INTRODUCTION TO FUNCTIONAL HEALTH PATTERNS AND HEALTH PROMOTION

Partnership for Clear Health Communication

http://www.npsf.org/pchc

http://www.npsf.org/askme3/PCHC

CHAPTER 10: NUTRITION

2010 Dietary Guidelines for Americans

www.cnpp.usda.gov/dgas2010-dgacreport.htm

About Face

www.aboutface.ca

Allergy Information and Referral Hotline

800-822-2762

American Academy of Pediatrics

www.aap.org/obesity/index.html

American Diabetes Association

www.diabetes.org

American Dietetic Association

www.eatright.org

American School Food Service Association

www.asfsa.org

Association of Dieticians of Canada

www.dieticians.ca

Asthma and Allergy Foundation of America

www.aafa.org

BAM! Body and Mind

www.bam.gov

Best Bones Forever!

www.bestbonesforever.gov

Canadian Celiac Association

www.celiac.ca

Celiac Disease Foundation

www.celiac.org

Celiac Sprue Association/United States of America, Inc.

www.csaceliacs.org

Centers for Disease Control and Prevention (CDC)

www.cdc.gov/obesity/resources.html

School health guidelines to promote healthy eating and physical activity, *MMWR* 60 (RR-5): 1-76, 2011.

CDC's Community Strategies to Prevent Obesity

Centers for Disease Control and Prevention (CDC): Recommended community strategies and measurements to prevent obesity in the United States, *MMWR* 58(No. RR):1-29, 2009.

www.cdc.gov/search.do?queryText=Recommended+community+strategies+ and+measurements&searchButton.x=38&searchButton.y=10&action=search

Cleft Palate Association

www.cleftline.org

Crohn's and Colitis Foundation of America

www.ccfa.org

Cystic Fibrosis Foundation

www.cff.org

Division of Nutrition, Physical Activity, and Obesity

www.cdc.gov/nccdphp/dnpao/index.html

The Food Allergy and Anaphylaxis Network

www.foodallergy.org

Food Allergy and Anaphylaxis Alliance

www.foodallergyalliance.org

Gluten Intolerance Group

www.gluten.net

Growth Charts for Children With Special Conditions

In Hall JG, Allanson JE, Gripp KW, Slavotinek AM: *Handbook of physical measurements,* ed 2, Oxford, UK, 2007, Oxford University Press:

- Achondroplasia
- Correlia de Lange syndrome
- Cri du Chat syndrome
- Down syndrome
- Marfran syndrome
- Noonan syndrome
- Prader-Willi
- Pseudoachondroplasia
- Rubinstein-Taybi syndrome
- Russel-Silver syndrome
- Spondyloepiphyseal dysplasia congenital
- Trisomy 13
- Trisomy 18
- Turner syndrome
- Williams syndrome

From Child Development and Rehabilitation Center, Genetics Clinic (503)-494-8307:

- Myelomeningocele, male and female, 2 to 18 years old
- Asian children, 0 to 6 years old (also search Families With Children from China [www.fwcc.org] for "growth charts")

From Platt OS, Rosenstock W, Espeland MA: Influence of sickle hemoglobinopathies on growth and development, *N Engl J Med* 311(1):7-12, 1984: Sickle cell anemia growth chart.

International Pediatric Endosurgery Group (IPEG)

www.ipeg.org

www.ipeg.org/education/guidelines/morbidobesity.html

Juvenile Diabetes Research Foundation International

www.jdrf.org

Kids with Food Allergies

www.kidswithfoodallergies.org/index.html

KidsHealth

www.kidshealth.org

Healthy Eating and Activity Together (HEAT) Guidelines

www.guidelines.gov

Let's Move

www.letsmove.gov

MyPyramid

www.mypyramid.gov

www.mypyramidtracker.gov

www.mypyramid.gov/kids/index.html

National Agricultural Library/USDA

www.nutrition.gov

National Association of School Nurses

www.nasn.org

National Diabetes Education Program

www.ndep.nih.gov/diabetes/youth/youth.htm

National Digestive Diseases Information Clearinghouse

http://digestive.niddk.nih.gov/ddiseases/pubs/diarrhea

National Heart, Lung, and Blood Institute

www.nhlbi.nih.gov

National Institute for Health Care Management

www.nihcm.org

The North American Society for Pediatric Gastroenterology, Hepatology, and Nutrition

www.naspghan.org

Oregon Dairy Council
www.oregondairycouncil.org

Pediatric/Adolescent Gastroesophageal Reflux Association (PAGER)
www.reflux.org

School Nutrition Association
SNF Food Allergy Resources
www.schoolnutrition.org/Content.aspx?id=14376

Shapedown
www.shapedown.com
Child and adolescent obesity weight control program

U.S. Department of Agriculture
www.usda.gov

CHAPTER 11: BREASTFEEDING

Ameda
www.ameda.com

Human Milk Banking Association of North America
www.hmbana.org

International Board of Lactation Consultant Examiners (IBLCE)
www.iblce.org

International Lactation Consultant Association (ILCA)
www.ilca.org

Lactation Education Resources
www.leron-line.com

Lactation Institute
www.lactationinstitute.org

La Leche League International
www.lalecheleague.org

Medela, Inc.
www.medela.com

National Alliance for Breastfeeding Advocacy
www.naba-breastfeeding.org

National Conference of State Legislatures
www.ncsl.org

National Library of Medicine
www.toxnet.nlm.nih.gov

Nursing Mothers Counsel
www.nursingmothers.org

Wellstart
www.wellstart.org

WHO Global Data Bank on Breastfeeding and Complementary Feeding
www.who.int/nutrition/databases/infantfeeding/en/index.html

CHAPTER 12: ELIMINATION PATTERNS

American Gastroenterological Association
www.gastro.org

Bedwetting Store
www.bedwettingstore.com

Childhood Constipation
www.childhoodconstipation.com

Education and Resources for Improving Childhood Continence (ERIC)
www.eric.org.uk

Enuresis Alarms
www.wetbuster.com/alarms.htm

International Foundation for Functional Gastrointestinal Disorders
www.iffgd.org

Keep Kids Healthy
www.keepkidshealthy.com

Malem Ultimate Alarm
www.malem.co.uk

National Digestive Diseases Information Clearinghouse, National Institutes of Health
http://digestive.niddk.nih.gov/ddiseases/pubs/constipation/index.htm

National Kidney Foundation
www.kidney.org/patients/bw

National Kidney and Urologic Diseases Information Clearinghouse
www.kidney.niddk.nih.gov/kudiseases/pubs/uichildren

Nemours Foundation
www.kidshealth.org

Nite Train'r Alarm
www.nitetrain-r.com

North American Society of Pediatric Gastroenterology, Hepatology, and Nutrition
www.naspghan.org

Nytone Enuretic Alarm
www.nytone.com

PottyMD WET-STOP2 Alarm
www.pottymd.com

Potty Pager
www.pottypager.com

CHAPTER 13: PHYSICAL ACTIVITY AND SPORTS FOR CHILDREN AND ADOLESCENTS

2008 Physical Activity Guidelines for Americans
www.cdc.gov/Healthyyouth/physicalactivity/guidelines.htm#1

Adolescents Training and Learning to Avoid Steroids (ATLAS) Prevention Program
www.atlasprogram.com

American Academy of Family Physicians
www.aafp.org/online/en/home/clinical/publichealth/sportsmed/preparticipation-evaluation-forms0.html

American Academy of Pediatrics
www.aap.org

American College of Sports Medicine
www.acsm.org

American Dietetic Association: Sports, Cardiovascular, and Wellness Nutrition
www.scandp.org

American Orthopaedic Society for Sports Medicine (AOSSM)
www.sportsmed.org

Centers for Disease Control and Prevention
www.cdc.gov/concussion/headsup/physicians_tool_kit.html

Centers for Disease Control and Prevention, Kids Walk-to-School
www.cdc.gov/nccdphp/dnpa/KidsWalk.pdf

International Society of Sports Nutrition (ISSN)
www.sportsnutritionsociety.org

Los Angeles County Public Health Department
www.lapublichealth.org/acd/docs/MRSA/MRSAGuidelines.2007.pdf

Lids on Kids
www.lidsonkids.org

National Athletic Trainers' Association
www.nata.org/consensus-statement

National Safe Kids Campaign
www.safekids.org

National Highway Traffic Safety Administration
www.nhtsa.gov/people/injury/pedbimot/bike/kidsandbikesafetyweb

Santa Monica Orthopaedic and Sports Medicine Resource Foundation

www.sportsmedicine.about.com/cs/knee_injuries/a/aa22202a.htm

Special Olympics: Healthy Athletes

www.specialolympics.org/healthy_athletes.aspx

Standardized Concussion Assessment Tool 2 (SCAT2)

www.thinkfirst.ca/documents/Pocket_SCAT2_000.pdf

U.S. Youth Soccer Federation

www.usyouthsoccer.org/news/story.asp?story_id=4135

CHAPTER 14: SLEEP AND REST

National Sleep Foundation

www.sleepfoundation.org

Phone: (202) 347-3471

Fax: (202) 347-3472

E-mail: nsf@sleepfoundation.org

American Academy of Sleep Medicine

www.aasmnet.org

American Sleep Apnea Association

www.sleepapnea.org

Sleep for Kids website

www.Sleepforkids.org

CHAPTER 15: COGNITIVE-PERCEPTUAL DISORDERS: ATTENTION-DEFICIT/ HYPERACTIVITY DISORDER, LEARNING PROBLEMS, SENSORY PROCESSING DISORDER, AUTISM SPECTRUM DISORDER, BLINDNESS AND DEAFNESS

ADD WareHouse

www.addwarehouse.com

Alexander Graham Bell Association for the Deaf and Hard of Hearing (AGBAD)

www.agbell.org

American Academy of Pediatrics

Autism toolkit and patient handout, "Understanding Autism Spectrum Disorders (ASDs)"

www.aap.org

American Association of Deaf-Blind

www.aadb.org

American Council of the Blind (ACB)

www.acb.org

American Foundation for the Blind (AFB)

www.afb.org

American Society for Deaf Children (ASDC)

www.deafchildren.org

Autism Digest

www.autismdigest.com

Autism Research Institute

www.autism.com/ari

Autism Society of America

www.autism-society.org

Beginnings for Parents of Children Who are Deaf or Hard of Hearing

www.beginningsvcs.com

Blind Children's Fund (BCF)

www.blindchildrensfund.org

Centers for Disease Control and Prevention: Autism Information Center

www.cdc.gov/ncbddd/autism/index.html

Autism ALARM. Guidelines

http://www.cdc.gov/ncbddd/autism/hcp-recommendations.html

Children and Adults With Attention-Deficit/Hyperactivity Disorders (CHADD)

www.chadd.org

Cochlear Implant Association

www.listen-up.org/ci/ci-information.htm

Family Voices

www.familyvoices.org

First Steps

www.firstsigns.org

Imagery Language and Visual Communication

www.handspeak.com

Laurent Clerc National Deaf Education Center, Gallaudet University

www.clerccenter.gallaudet.edu

Learning Disabilities Association of America

www.ldanatl.org

LD Online

www.ldonline.org/index.php

My Baby's Hearing

www.babyhearing.org

National Association of the Deaf (NAD)

www.nad.org

National Association for Parents of Children with Visual Impairments (NAPVI)

www.spedex.com/napvi

National Attention Deficit Disorder Association

www.add.org

National Center for Learning Disabilities

www.ncld.org

National Disseminated Center for Children and Youth With Disabilities

www.nichcy.org

Source for age-appropriate books

National Family Association of the Deaf-Blind

www.nfadb.org

National Federation of the Blind—Division for Parents of Blind Children

www.nfb.org

National Institute on Deafness and Other Communication Disorders

www.nidcd.nih.gov

National Resource Center for ADHD

www.help4adhd.org

NIH NICHHD

www.nichd.nih.gov/health/topics/learning_disabilities.cfm

NINDS Learning Disabilities Information Page

www.ninds.nih.gov/disorders/learningdisabilities/learning disabilities.htm

Parents' Guide to ADHD Medication

www.parentsmedguide.org/pmg_adhd.html

Reach Out and Read

www.reachoutandread.org

S.E.E. (Signing Exact English) Center for Advancement of Deaf Children

www.seecenter.org

Sensory Processing Disorder Foundation

www.spdfoundation.net

Sensory Processing Disorder Resource Center

www.sensory-processing-disorder.com

Telecommunications for the Deaf and Hard of Hearing

www.tdi-online.org

Treatment and Education of Autistic and Communication related handicapped CHildren (TEACCH)

www.teacch.com

CHAPTER 16: SELF-PERCEPTION ISSUES

Arthur M. Blank Family Foundation

www.blankfoundation.org

Bright Futures

www.brightfutures.org

Campaign for Real Beauty

www.campaignforrealbeauty.com

Don't Buy It: Get Media Smart

http://pbskids.org/dontbuyit

Free Spirit Publishing, Inc.

www.freespirit.com

HEARTLIGHT GIRLS: Empowering Girls from the Inside Out

www.selfesteemforyounggirls.com

KidsHealth

www.kidshealth.org

Kid Source Online

www.kidsource.com

Marsh Media

www.marshmedia.com

Ms. Foundation for Women

www.ms.foundation.org

National Mental Health Information Center

http://mentalhealth.samhsa.gov

NYU Child Study Center

www.aboutourkids.org

National Association for Self-Esteem (NASE)

www.self-esteem-nase.org

Parent Further

www.parentfurther.com

Raising Resilient Children Foundation

www.raisingresilientkids.com

Redleaf Press

www.redleafpress.org

Resilience, Self-Esteem, Motivation, and Family Relationships

www.drrobertbrooks.com

Search Institute

www.search-institute.org

Soy Unica! Soy Latina!

www.sparkaction.org/node/1253

Sparks

www.ignitesparks.com/index.html

VERB: It's What You Do

www.cdc.gov/youthcampaign

Zero to Three

www.zerotothree.org

CHAPTER 17: ROLE RELATIONSHIPS

AARP Grandparent Information Center

www.aarp.org/families/grandparents

Adoption Information Clearinghouse

www.adoption.org/adopt/national-adoption-clearinghouse.php

Administration on Developmental Disabilities

www.acf.hhs.gov/programs/add

American Professional Society on the Abuse of Children

www.apsac.org

Big Brothers Big Sisters of America

www.bbbsa.org

Brady Campaign to Prevent Handgun Violence

www.handguncontrol.org

Brave Kids

www.bravekids.org

Casey Family Programs National Center for Resource Family Support

www.fostercaremonth.org

Child Care Aware

www.childcareaware.org

Child Welfare Information Gateway: U.S. Department of Health and Human Services, Children's Bureau, Administration for Children and Families

www.childwelfare.gov

Child Welfare League of America

www.cwla.org

Child Welfare League of America, Family Foster Care

www.cwla.org/programs/fostercare

Children's Bureau Express

www.cbexpress.acf.hhs.gov

Community Directory of International Adoption Medical Clinics

www.comeunity.com/adoption/health/clinics.html

Connect for Kids

www.connectforkids.org

Connected Kids: Safe, Strong, Secure

www.aap.org/ConnectedKids

The Dougy Center for Grieving Children and Families

www.dougy.org

Girls Health

www.girlshealth.gov/bullying

Grandparents **Magazine**

www.grandparentsmagazine.net

GrandsPlace

www.grandsplace.com

International Adoption Clinic

www.peds.umn.edu/iac

The Kempe Center for the Prevention and Treatment of Child Abuse and Neglect

www.kempe.org

KidsHealth

www.kidshealth.org

Medical Passports for Adopted Children

www.in.gov

Mothers of Twin Clubs, Inc.

www.momotc.org

National Adoption Center

www.adopt.org

National Center on Secondary Education and Transition

www.ncset.org

National Center for Victims of Crime

www.ncvc.org/ncvc/Main.aspx

National Children's Advocacy Center

www.nationalcac.org

National Child Care Information Center

www.nccic.org

National Coalition for the Homeless

www.nationalhomeless.org

The National Foster Parent Association

www.nfpainc.org

Online Resources for State Child Welfare Law and Policy

www.childwelfare.gov/systemwide/laws_policies/statutes/resources.cfm

Rowell Foster Children's Positive Plan
www.rowellfosterchildren.org
Stop Bullying Now
www.stopbullyingnow.hrsa.gov
Striving to Reduce Youth Violence Everywhere (STRYVE)
www.safeyouth.gov/Pages/Home.aspx

CHAPTER 18: SEXUALITY
American Academy of Pediatrics
www.aap.org
American Congress of Obstetricians and Gynecologists
www.acog.org
Association of Reproductive Health Professionals
www.arhp.org
ETR Associates
www.etr.org
Family Equality Council
www.familyequality.org
National Dissemination Center for Children and Youth with Disabilities
www.nichcy.org
Parents, Families, and Friends of Lesbians and Gays, Inc. (PFLAG)
www.pflag.org
Planned Parenthood Federation of America
www.plannedparenthood.org
Purdue University Cooperative Extension Service
www.ces.purdue.edu
ReproLine
www.reproline.jhu.edu
Sexual Assessment and History Taking
Davis CM, Yarber WL, Bauserman R et al: *Handbook of sexuality related measures,* Thousand Oaks, CA, 1998, Sage Publications.
Sexuality Information and Education Council of the United States (SIECUS)
www.SIECUS.org
The Society for Adolescent Medicine
www.adolescenthealth.org

CHAPTER 19: COPING AND STRESS TOLERANCE: MENTAL HEALTH AND ILLNESS
About Our Kids
www.aboutourkids.org
Achenbach Child Behavior Checklist
www.aseba.org/products/forms.html
Ages & Stages Questionnaire
www.agesandstages.com
American Academy of Child and Adolescent Psychiatry
www.aacap.org
American Academy of Pediatrics
www.aap.org
Bright Futures for Families
www.brightfuturesforfamilies.org
Bright Futures: Mental Health
www.brightfutures.org/mentalhealth
The Dougy Center: The National Center for Grieving Children
www.dougy.org
Family Voices
www.familyvoices.org

Infant & Toddler Social and Emotional Assessment (ITSEA) and Brief Infant & Toddler Social and Emotional Assessment (BITSEA)
www.pearsonassessments.com
Johns Hopkins Department of Mental Health Websites Related to Mental Health
www.jhsph.edu/dept/mh/related_links/index.html
KidsHealth
www.kidshealth.org
National Institute of Mental Health
www.nimh.nih.gov
Ounce of Prevention Fund
www.ounceofprevention.org
Pediatric Symptom Checklist
www.teenscreen.org
The Reach Institute: Guidelines for Adolescent Depression— Primary Care
www.glad-pc.org
Sensory Processing Disorder Foundation
www.spdfoundation.net
Substance Abuse and Mental Health Services Administration
www.family.samhsa.gov
Talking With Kids About Tough Issues
www.talkwithkids.org
Zero to Three
www.zerotothree.org

CHAPTER 20: VALUES AND BELIEFS
Beliefnet
www.beliefnet.com
Center for Compassion and Altruism Research and Education
http://ccare.stanford.edu/node
Native American Spirituality and Religion
www.academicinfo.net/nativeamrelig.html
Public Broadcasting System (PBS) Online Religion and Ethics
www.pbs.org/wnet/religionandethics/home.html
Puchalski CM, Ferrell B: *Making health care whole: integrating spirituality into patient care,* West Conshohocken, PA, 2010, Templeton Press.
OncoLink
www.oncolink.org
Search Institute
www.search-institute.org
Vanderbilt Kennedy Center
www.kc.vanderbilt.edu/site/services/disabilityservices/page.aspx?id=20

CHAPTER 21: INTRODUCTION TO DISEASE MANAGEMENT
DXplain
http://dxplain.org/dxp/dxp.pl
e-BUG
www.e-bug.eu
Gunning Fog Index
www.readabilityformulas.com/gunning-fog-readability-formula.php
To calculate the Gunning Fog Index, take the total number of words and divide it by the total number of sentences. This will give the average number of words in a sentence. The total number of words with more than three syllables is divided by the total

number of words to obtain the percentage of difficult words. When you total these two calculations (average number of words in a sentence plus the percentage of difficult words) and multiply it by 0.4, you will get the Fog Index in years of education. An index of 8 is considered necessary for general understanding.

Handwashing Guidelines
www.cdc.gov/Features/HandWashing

Healthy and Ready to Work National Center
www.hrtw.org

Helping Patient Make Choices
http://effectivehealthcare.ahrq.gov

Information About Medical Home Model
www.medhomeportal.org
www.medicalhomeinfo.org

The Institute for Child Health Policy
www.ichp.ufl.edu.ichp

Institute for Safe Medication Practices
www.ismp.org/Tools/errorproneabbreviations.pdf

Isabel
www.isabelhealthcare.com/home/default

GIDEON Informatics
www.gideononline.com

Gunning Fog Index
http.gunning-fog-index.com

Lifecom
www.lifecomhealth.com

Medication Administration
www.kidsmeds.com/admin.ccml
www.ces.purdue.edu/providerparent/Health-Safety/Tips.htm

The National Dissemination Centers for Children and Youths with Disabilities (NICHCY)
www.nichcy.org

National Organization for Rare Disorders (NORD)
www.rarediseases.org

Ounce of Prevention Campaign
www.cdc.gov/ounceofprevention

SMOG (Simple Measure of Gobbledygook)
www.harrymclaughlin.com/SMOG.htm

Support Groups for Families and Patients
www.imedix.com
www.dailystrength.org
www.organizedwisdom.com/home

Transitioning Resource Guide
www.hrtw.org/index.html

Utilities for Online Operating Systems (Reading Levels)
www.online-utility.org/english/readability_test_and_improve.jsp

VisualDx
www.visualdx.com

Youth Workbooks
http://hctransitions.ichp.edu/resources.html

CHAPTER 22: PEDIATRIC PAIN MANAGEMENT

American Academy of Pain Management
www.aapainmanage.org/links/Links.php

American Pain Society: Pediatric Chronic Pain
www.ampainsoc.org/library/bulletin/jan01.posi1.htm

American Society for Pain Management Nursing
www.aspmn.org

Doses of Tylenol for Children
http://www.tylenol.com/page.jhtml?id=tylenol/children/subchild.inc

Medication Adminsitration
www.kidsmeds.com/admin.ccml

National Organization for Rare Disorders (NORD)
www.rarediseases.org

Pediatric Pain—Science Helping Children
www.pediatric-pain.ca/links.html

Pediatric Pain Sourcebook of Protocols, Policies, and Pamphlets
http://psychology-of-pain.blogspot.com/2007/08/pediatric-pain-sourcebook-of-protocols.html

Tips for Providers
www.ces.purdue.edu/providerparent/Health-Safety/Tips.htm

UCLA Pain Assessment Tools
www.anes.ucla.edu/pdf/assessment_tool-cheops.pdf

U.S. Food and Drug Administration: How to Give Medicine to Children
www.fda.gov/ForConsumers/ConsumerUpdates/ucm164427.htm

Yale Anesthesiology, Yale University School of Medicine—pediatric pain management
http://medicine.yale.edu/anesthesiology/divisions/pediatrics/ped-pain.aspx

CHAPTER 23: INFECTIOUS DISEASES AND IMMUNIZATIONS

Advisory Committee on Immunization Practices
www.cdc.gov/vaccines/recs/acip

AIDS information (U.S. Department of Health and Human Services)
www.aidsinfo.nih.gov

American Academy of Pediatrics
www.aap.org

Association of State and Territorial Health Officials
www.astho.org

Centers for Disease Control and Prevention
www.cdc.gov

Childhood Immunization Support Program (CISP)
www.aap.org/immunization/pediatricians/pdf/RefusaltoVaccinate.pdf

Infectious Diseases Society of America (IDSA)
www.idsociety.org

International Lyme and Associated Diseases Society (ILADS)
www.ilads.org

Vaccines
www.cdc.gov/vaccines

Vaccine Adverse Event Reporting System (VAERS)
www.vaers.hhs.gov/professionals/index

Vaccine Shortages, Procurement, and Prioritization Information
www.cdc.gov/nip/news/shortages
www.cdc.gov/vaccines/vac-gen/shortages

World Health Organization
www.who.int

CHAPTER 24: ATOPIC AND RHEUMATIC DISORDERS

Allergy and Asthma Network—Mothers of Asthmatics, Inc.
www.aanma.org

American Academy of Allergy, Asthma, and Immunology
www.aaaai.org

American Arthritis Organization
www.arthritis.org

American Autoimmune Related Diseases Association
1-800-598-4668 (literature requests)
www.aarda.org

American College of Allergy, Asthma, and Immunology
www.acaai.org

American Lung Association
www.lungusa.org
Asthma and Allergy Foundation of America
www.aafa.org
Lupus Foundation of America, Inc.
www.lupus.org
National Asthma Education and Prevention Program
www.nhlbi.nih.gov/health/public/lung/asthma/resolut.htm
National Eczema Association for Science and Education
www.nationaleczema.org
National Heart, Lung, and Blood Institute
www.nhlbi.nih.gov
National Asthma Education and Prevention Program
www.nhlbi.nih.gov
National Institute of Allergy and Infectious Diseases
www.niaid.nih.gov
National Jewish Center Medical and Research Center
www.njc.org
U.S. Environmental Protection Agency (EPA)
www.epa.gov/asthma/programs.html
What you need to know about asthma
www.aboutasthma.com

CHAPTER 25: ENDOCRINE AND METABOLIC DISORDERS

American Association of Diabetes Educators (AADE)
www.diabeteseducator.org
American College of Medical Genetics
www.acmg.net
American Diabetes Association
www.diabetes.org
American Dietetic Association
www.eatright.org
American Heart Association
www.americanheart.org
American Thyroid Association
www.thyroid.org
Association for Glycogen Storage Disease UK
www.agsd.org.uk
Barbara Davis Center for Childhood Diabetes
University of Colorado Health Sciences Center
www.barbaradaviscenter.org
Children's Diabetes Foundation at Denver
www.childrensdiabetesfdn.com
Child Growth Foundation
United Kingdom
www.childgrowthfoundation.org
Children With Diabetes
www.childrenwithdiabetes.com
Dwarfism/Short Stature Resources
University of Kansas Medical Center
www.kumc.edu/gec/support/dwarfism.html
The Endocrine Society
www.endo-society.org
Gene Tests
http://genetests.org
www.ncbi.nlm.nih.gov/sites/GeneTests/?db=GeneTests
Genetics Home Reference
http://ghr.nlm.nih.gov
Human Growth Foundation
www.hgfound.org

Juvenile Diabetes Research Foundation International (JDRF)
www.jdrf.org
Little People of America
www.lpaonline.org
Magic Foundation
www.magicfoundation.org
MedicAlert
www.medicalert.org
The Online Metabolic and Molecular Bases of Inherited Disease
www.ommbid.com
National Diabetes Education Program
http://ndep.nih.gov
National Institutes of Health
www.nih.gov
National Newborn Screening and Genetics Resource Center
http://genes-r-us.uthscsa.edu
Online Mendelian Inheritance in Man (OMIM)
www.ncbi.nlm.nih.gov/omim
Pediatric Endocrinology Nursing Society (PENS)
www.pens.org
Pituitary Network Association
www.pituitary.org
Screening, Technology, and Research in Genetics (STAR-G)
www.newbornscreening.info
Treatment Options for Type 2 Diabetes in Adolescents & Youth (TODAY)
www.todaystudy.org/index.cgi

CHAPTER 26: HEMATOLOGIC DISORDERS

American Childhood Cancer Organization
www.candlelighters.org
Cooley's Anemia Foundation
www.cooleysanemia.org
CureSearch
National Childhood Cancer Foundation
www.curesearch.org
Leukemia and Lymphoma Society
www.leukemia.org
National Hemophilia Foundation
www.hemophilia.org
NIH: The Management of Sickle Cell Disease
www.nhlbi.nih.gov/health/prof/blood/sickle/sc_mngt.pdf
Sickle Cell Disease Association of America, Inc.
www.sicklecelldisease.org

CHAPTER 27: NEUROLOGIC DISORDERS

Brain Injury Association of America
www.biausa.org
International Rett Syndrome Association (IRSA)
www.rettsyndrome.org
National Headache Foundation
www.headaches.org
National Tourette Syndrome Association
www.tsa-usa.org
National Spinal Cord Injury Association
www.spinalcord.org
Spina Bifida Association
www.sbaa.org
United Cerebral Palsy
www.ucp.org

CHAPTER 28: EYE DISORDERS

American Academy of Ophthalmology
www.aao.org

American Association for Pediatric Ophthalmology and Strabismus
www.aapos.org

Blind Childrens Center
www.blindchildrenscenter.org

InfantSEE
www.infantsee.org

National Eye Institute
www.nei.nih.gov

National Federation of the Blind: National Organization of Parents of Blind Children
www.nfb.org/nfb/Parents_and_Teachers.asp

Prevent Blindness America
www.preventblindness.org

CHAPTER 29: EAR DISORDERS

AHQR National Guideline Clearinghouse
www.guideline.gov

American Academy of Audiology
www.audiology.org

American Academy of Family Physicians
www.aafp.org

American Academy of Pediatrics Virtual Classroom
www.aap.org/otitismedia
Online case studies and pneumatic otoscopy course

Centers for Disease Control and Prevention
www.cdc.gov

Intermountain Ear, Nose, and Throat Online Center
http://intermountainhealthcare.org/xp/public/managehealth/patiented/otitismedia

University of Michigan Health Topics Index
www.med.umich.edu/1libr/topics

University of Iowa Virtual Hospital Education Materials
www.uihealthcare.com/topics/medicaldepartments/otolaryngology/index.html

CHAPTER 30: CARDIOVASCULAR DISORDERS

American Heart Association
www.americanheart.org

Congenital Heart Information Network
www.tchin.org

Mended Hearts, Inc.
www.mendedhearts.org

National Center for Biotechnology Information
www.ncbi.nlm.nih.gov

Online Mendelian Inheritance in Man
www.ncbi.nlm.nih.gov/omim

PediHeart
www.pediheart.org

World Health Organization
www.WHO.int

CHAPTER 31: RESPIRATORY DISORDERS

Cincinnati Children's Hospital Medical Center
www.cincinnatichildrens.org
www.cincinnatichildrens.org/health/s/suction

Cystic Fibrosis Foundation
www.cff.org

Pertussis.com
www.pertussis.com

CHAPTER 32: GASTROINTESTINAL DISORDERS

Children's Digestive Health & Nutrition Foundation
www.cdhnf.org

Crohn's and Colitis Foundation of America (CCFA)
www.ccfa.org

Cyclic Vomiting Syndrome Association
www.cvsaonline.org

Gastroparesis and Dysmotilities Association
www.gpda.net

ImproveCareNow
www.improvecarenow.org

International Foundation for Functional Gastrointestinal Disorders (IFFGD)
www.iffgd.org

National Digestive Diseases Information Clearinghouse
www.digestive.niddk.nih.gov

National Institute of Diabetes and Digestive and Kidney Diseases
www.niddk.nih.gov

National Center on Shaken Baby Syndrome (NCSBS)
www.dontshake.com

North American Society for Pediatric Gastroenterology, Hepatology, and Nutrition
www.naspgn.org

National Organization for Rare Disorders
www.nord-rdb.com

The Period of PURPLE Crying (NCSBS)
www.purplecrying.info

Rehydrate Project
http://rehydrate.org/solutions/homemade.htm

Rome Foundation: Functional Gastrointestinal Disorders
www.romecriteria.org

CHAPTER 33: DENTAL AND ORAL DISORDERS

American Academy of Pediatric Dentistry
www.aapd.org

American Dental Association
www.ada.org

Colgate Duraphat Varnish
www.colgateprofessional.com

Duraflor Fluoride Varnish
www.medicom.com

Lift the Lip video and flipcharts (in multiple languages). Available at www.dental.washington.edu/conted/store/documents/lift%20the%20lip%20Brochure%202009.pdf (accessed Sept 29, 2010)

MEDLINE Plus (in Spanish and English)
www.medlineplus.gov

Milgrom P, Weinstein P: *Early childhood caries* and Weinstein P, Milgrom P: *Oral self care: strategies for preventive dentistry.* www.dentalbehavioralresources.com

MOUTH MIRRORS
www.practicewares.com
www.henryschein.com

MPL VarnishAmerica
www.medicalproductslaboratories.com/public-health/varnishamerica.html

National Maternal and Child Oral Health Resource Center
www.mchoralhealth.org

National Institutes of Dental and Cranial Research
Patient handout on temporomandibular joint disorder
www.nidcr.nih.gov/NR/rdonlyres/39C75C9B-1795-4A87-
8B46-8F77DDE639CA/0/TMJ_Disorders.pdf.

Premier Enamel Pro Varnish Clear
www.premusa.com/dental/hygiene.asp

Toothpaste and Toothbrushes
www.dentalcare.com
www.colgateprofessional.com

CHAPTER 34: GENITOURINARY DISORDERS

American Association of Kidney Patients
www.aakp.org

American Foundation for Urologic Disease
www.urologyhealth.org/auahome.asp

IgA Nephropathy Support Network
www.igansupport.org

National Cancer Institute: Wilms Tumor Information
www.cancer.gov/CancerInformation/CancerType/wilmstumor

National Institute of Diabetes and Digestive and Kidney Diseases
www2.niddk.nih.gov

National Kidney and Urologic Diseases Information Clearinghouse
www.kidney.niddk.nih.gov/index.htm

National Kidney Foundation
www.kidney.org

National Wilms Tumor Study
www.nwtsg.org

Testicular Cancer Awareness Week
www.tcaw.org

CHAPTER 35: GYNECOLOGIC DISORDERS

Abstinence Clearinghouse
www.abstinence.net

American Congress of Obstetricians and Gynecologists (ACOG) (pamphlets)
www.acog.com

American Social Health Association
www.ashastd.org

Association of Reproductive Health Professionals
www.arhp.org

Centers for Disease Control and Prevention (CDC) STD information
www.cdc.gov/std

Center for Young Women's Health, Children's Hospital Boston
www.youngwomenshealth.org

Education Training Resource Associates
www.etr.org

Medical Institute for Sexual Health
www.medinstitute.org

The National Campaign to Prevent Teen and Unplanned Pregnancy
www.thenationalcampaign.org

National Herpes Hotline
1-919-361-8488

National STD Hotline
1-800-227-8922

North American Society for Pediatric and Adolescent Gynecology (NASPAG)
www.naspag.org

Planned Parenthood Federation of America, Inc.
www.plannedparenthood.org

ReproLine
www.reproline.jhu.edu

Sexuality Information and Education Council of the United States (SIECUS)
www.siecus.org

Society for Adolescent Medicine
www.adolescenthealth.org

World Health Organization—Medical Eligibility Criteria for Contraceptive Use
www.who.int/reproductivehealth/publications/family_planning/
9789241563888/en/index.html

CHAPTER 36: DERMATOLOGIC DISORDERS

American Academy of Dermatology
www.aad.org

Association of Professional Piercers
www.safepiercing.org

Coppertone
www.coppertone.com

Dermatology Image Atlas
www.dermatlas.org

Dermatology Online Journal
http://dermatology.cdlib.org

Electronic Textbook of Dermatology
www.telemedicine.org/stamfor1.htm

FIRST: Foundation for Ichthyosis and Related Skin Types
www.firstskinfoundation.org

International OCD (Obsessive-Compulsive Disorder) Foundation
www.ocfoundation.org

Locks of Love
www.locksoflove.org

Loyola University Dermatology
www.meddean.luc.edu/lumen/meded/medicine/dermatology/
melton/atlas.htm

National Alopecia Areata Foundation
www.naaf.org

National Organization for Albinism and Hypopigmentation (NOAH)
www.albinism.org

National Pediculosis Association, Inc. (NPA)
www.headlice.org

National Psoriasis Foundation
www.psoriasis.org

National Vitiligo Foundation, Inc.
www.nvfi.org

Nevus Network
www.nevusnetwork.org

Prevent Cancer Foundation
www.preventcancer.org

Skin Cancer Foundation
www.skincancer.org

TLC Trichotillomania Learning Center, Inc.
www.trich.org

Trichotillomania: A Guide
www.miminc.org

CHAPTER 37: MUSCULOSKELETAL DISORDERS

American Academy of Family Practice
www.aafp.org

American Academy of Orthopaedic Surgeons (AAOS)

www.aaos.org

Backpack safety tips: http://orthoinfo.aaos.org/topic.cfm?topic=
A00043

Connecticut Children's Medical Center

www.ccmckids.org

Muscular Dystrophy Association

www.mdausa.org

Scoliosis Research Society

www.srs.org

The Spinal Connection

www.scoliosis.org/resources/spinalconnection.php

STEPS

National charity in the United Kingdom for those affected by a
lower limb condition

www.steps-charity.org.uk

**United Brachial Plexus Network, Inc.—Erb Palsy Support
and Information Network**

www.ubpn.org

CHAPTER 38: PERINATAL DISORDERS

Association for SIDS and Infant Mortality Programs

www.asip1.org

Birth Defect Research for Children, Inc.

www.birthdefects.org

Canada newborn screening

www.hc-sc.gc.ca/fniah-spnia/pubs/services/_nursing-infirm/
2001_ped_guide/chap_03-eng.php

**Centers for Disease Control and Prevention: Infectious
Disease Information**

www.cdc.gov/DiseasesConditions/Guidelines

Child Safety Seat Inspection Station Locator

www.seatcheck.org

Cleft Palate Foundation

www.cleftline.org

Compassionate Friends

www.compassionatefriends.org

**Family Empowerment Network: Families Affected by Fetal
Alcohol Syndrome/Fetal Alcohol Effects**

http://pregnancyandalcohol.org

Group B Strep Association

www.groupbstrep.org

March of Dimes (local chapters found online)

www.marchofdimes.com

National Highway Traffic Safety Administration

www.nhtsa.gov/cps/cpsfitting

National Newborn Screening and Genetics Resource Center

http://genes-r-us.uthscsa.edu

National Perinatal Association

www.nationalperinatal.org

National SIDS Resource Center

www.sidscenter.org

National Women's Health Information Center

www.4women.gov

**SIDS: Back to Sleep Campaign (National Institute of Child
Health and Human Development)**

www.nichd.nih.gov/sids

TEF/VATER International Support Network

www.tefvater.org

United Kingdom newborn screening

http://newbornbloodspot.
screening.nhs.uk

CHAPTER 39: COMMON INJURIES

American Burn Association

www.ameriburn.org

American Association of Poison Control Centers

www.aapcc.org/dnn/default.aspx

Car Seats for Larger Children with Special Needs

www.adaptivemall.com

**Centers for Disease Control and Prevention, National Center
for Injury Prevention and Control**

www.cdc.gov/ncipc

Child Restraint Systems

www.aap.org/healthtopics/carsafety.cfm

Child Passenger Safety: Fact Sheets

http://www.cdc.gov/Features/PassengerSafety/

**Council on Sports Medicine and Fitness Clinical Report on
Sport-Related Concussion in Children and Adolescents.**

http://aappolicy.aappublications.org/cgi/content/full/
pediatrics;126/3/597

Equipped to Survive

www.equipped.com

Healthy Children

http://www.healthychildren.org/

Kids Don't Leave Home Without It Equipment

www.equipped.com/kidequip.htm

**National Center for Injury Prevention and Control, Mild
Traumatic Brain Injury Resources for Health Professionals**

www.cdc.gov/concussion/HeadsUp/physicians_tool_kit.html

National Highway Traffic Safety Administration

www.nhtsa.dot.gov

Safe Kids USA

www.safekids.org

**Sage II Computerized Burn Diagramming: Free calculator to
estimate BSA and fluid resuscitation requirements**

www.SageDiagram.com

Snug Seat

www.snugseat.com

Traumatic Brain Injury Networking Team Resource Network

http://cokidswithbraininjury.com/mild-tbi-concussion-info

CHAPTER 40: GENETIC DISORDERS

**American Association for Klinefelter Syndrome Information
and Support (AAKSIS)**

www.aaksis.com

Birth Defect Research for Children, Inc.

www.birthdefects.org

**Centers for Disease Control and Prevention: Fetal Alcohol
Spectrum Disorders (FASDs)**

www.cdc.gov/ncbddd.fasd/index.html

**Family Empowerment Network: Families Affected by Fetal
Alcohol Syndrome/Fetal Alcohol Effects**

http://pregnancyandalcohol.org

Genetic Alliance

www.geneticalliance.org

Genetic and Rare Conditions

Medical Genetics, University of Kansas Medical Center

www.kumc.edu/gec/support

GeneTests

www.ncbi.nlm.nig.gov/sites/GeneTests/?db=GeneTests

Human Genome Project (U.S. Department of Energy)

genomics.energy.govwww.ornl.gov/hgmis

Klinefelter Syndrome and Associates

www.genetic.org

Little People of America
www.lpaonline.org

March of Dimes Foundation
www.marchofdimes.com/professionals/professionals.html

National Coalition for Health Professional Education in Genetics
www.nchpeg.org

National Coalition for Health Professionals Education in Genetics (NCHPEG): *Core competencies for all health professionals*. 2005. www.nhcpeg.org/index.php?option=com_content&;view=article&id=94&Itemid=84.

National Down Syndrome Congress
www.ndsccenter.org

National Down Syndrome Society
www.ndss.org

National Fragile X Foundation
www.fragilex.org

Newsletter, informational materials, networking, local chapters, advocacy, funds research

National Neurofibromatosis Foundation and Children's Tumor Foundation
www.ctf.org

National Organization on Fetal Alcohol Syndrome (NOFAS)
www.nofas.org

National Organization for Rare Disorders (NORD), Inc.
www.rarediseases.org

Neurofibromatosis Inc.
www.nfnetwork.org

Office of Public Health Genomics (Centers for Disease Control and Prevention)
www.cdc.gov/genetics

Office of Rare Diseases Research (National Institutes of Health)
www.rarediseases.info.nih.gov

Online Mendelian Inheritance in Man (OMIM)
www.ncbi.nlm.nih.gov/omim

Pregnancy Exposure InfoLine
www.thepeil.org

Support Organization for Trisomy 18, 13, and Related Disorders (SOFT)
www.trisomy.org

Turner Syndrome Society of the United States
www.turnersyndrome.org

Turner Syndrome Support Society
www.tss.org.uk

CHAPTER 41: ENVIRONMENTAL HEALTH ISSUES

Agency for Healthcare Research and Quality (AHRQ)
www.ahrq.gov

Agency for Toxic Substances and Disease Registry (ATSDR)
www.atsdr.cdc.gov

American Academy of Clinical Toxicology
clintox.org

Association of Occupational and Environmental Clinics (AOEC)
www.aoec.org

Children's Environmental Health Center
The Mount Sinai Medical Center
www.childenvironment.org

Centers for Disease Control and Prevention (CDC): National Center for Environmental Health
www.cdc.gov/nceh

Children's Environmental Health Network
www.cehn.org

Clean Water Action
www.cleanwateraction.org

Collaborative on Health and the Environment: CHE Toxicants and Disease Database
http://database.healthandenvironment.org

Consumer Product Safety Commission Office of Information
www.cpsc.gov

Environmental Health Perspectives
http://ehp.niehs.nih.gov/children

Environmental Working Group (EWG)
www.ewg.org

EnviRN (University of Maryland Environmental Health Site for Nurses)
www.enviRN.umaryland.edu

Health Care Without Harm
www.noharm.org

Green Guide for Health Care
http://www.gghc.org/

Pediatric Environmental Health Specialty Units (PEHSUs)
www.aoec.org/PEHSU.htm
www.ehp.niehs.nih.gov/children/resources.html

Material Safety Data Sheets
www.ilpi.com/msds

National Environmental Education Foundation (NEEF)
www.neefusa.org
www.neefusa.org/health/pesticides/index.htm
www.neefusa.org/health/PEHI/index.htm

National Environmental Health Association
www.neha.org

National Institute of Environmental Health Sciences
www.niehs.nih.gov

National Institute for Occupational Safety and Health
www.cdc.gov/niosh/topics/pesticides

National Pesticide Information Center (NPIC)
www.npic.orst.edu

National Safety Council
www.nsc.org

Rocky Mountain Poison & Drug Center
www.rmpdc.org

Scorecard: The pollution information site
www.scorecard.org

TOXNET: Hazardous Substances Data Bank
www.toxnet.nlm.nih.gov/cgi-bin/sis/htmlgen?HSDB

TOXMAP
www.toxmap.nlm.nih.gov/toxmap/main/index.jsp

U.S. Environmental Protection Agency (EPA)
www.epa.gov
The EPA has information on a wide range of environmental toxins.
For example:
Lead: www.epa.gov/lead/index.html
Fish: http://water.epa.gov/scitech/swguidance/fishshellfish/fish advisories/states.cfm
Molds: www.epa.gov/mold/index.html
Superfunds: www.epa.gov/superfund
Brownfields: www.epa.gov/brownfields
Worker Protection Standard: www.epa.gov/pesticides/safety/workers/PART170.htm
Radon and indoor air quality: www.epa.gov/iaq/whereyoulive.html

CHAPTER 42: COMPLEMENTARY MEDICINE

American Academy of Pediatrics Provisional Section on Complementary, Holistic, and Integrative Medicine
www.aap.org/sections/chim/p&r.htm

American Herbal Products Association
www.ahpa.org

Center for Studying Health System Change (HSC)
www.hschange.com

Cochrane Collaboration
www.cochrane.org

Consortium of Academic Health Centers for Integrative Medicine (CAHCIM)
www.imconsortium.org

Consumer Laboratory
www.consumerlab.com

Dietary Supplements Labels Database
www.dietarysupplements.nlm.nih.gov/dietary

Federation of State Medical Boards
www.fsmb.org

Harvard Medical School Osher Institute: Division for Research and Education in Complementary and Integrative Medicine
www.osher.hms.harvard.edu

Herbal Gram
www.herbalgram.org

HerbMed
www.herbmed

Kemper K: *The holistic pediatrician*, New York, 2002, HarperCollins.

Longwood Herbal Task Force
www.longwoodherbal.org

Loo M: *Integrative medicine for children,* St Louis, 2009, Saunders.

Mayo Clinic: *The Mayo Clinic Book of home remedies: what to do for the most common health problems,* N.Y., 2010, Time Home Entertainment, Inc.

National Center for Complementary and Alternative Medicine (NCCAM), National Institutes of Health
www.nccam.nih.gov

National Training Center and Clearinghouse
www.nnlm.gov/ntcc

Natural Medicines Comprehensive Database
www.naturaldatabase.com

NSF (National Sanitation Foundation) International
www.nsf.org

MedWatch (U.S. FDA)
www.fda.gov/medwatch

Rakel D: *Integrative medicine,* ed 2, Philadelphia, 2007, Saunders.

Ullman D: *Homeopathic family medicine: evidence based nanopharmacology,* an eBook. Available by subscription from Homeopathic Educational Services, www.homeopathic.com (regularly updated).

University of Arizona Program in Integrative Medicine
www.integrativemedicine.arizona.edu

Wake Forest University Baptist Medical Center: Program for Holistic and Integrative Medicine
www1.wfubmc.edu/phim

CHAPTER 43: STRATEGIES FOR MANAGING A HEALTH CARE PRACTICE

American Academy of Family Physicians (AAFP)
www.aafp.org

American Academy of Pediatrics (AAP)
www.aap.org

Centers for Medicare and Medicaid Services
www.cms.hhs.gov

Certification Commission for Healthcare Information Technology Standards
www.cchit.org

Council for Affordable Quality Healthcare (CAQH)
www.caqh.org

Health Insurance Portability and Accountability Act (HIPAA)
www.hipaa.org

Medical Group Management Association (MGMA)
www.mgma.com

National Committee for Quality Assurance (NCQA)
www.ncqa.org

Pediatric Coding Alert
www.codinginstitute.com

Resource Based Relative Value Scale (RBRVS)
aap.org/visit/rbrvsbrochure.pdf

Society of Human Resource Management (SHRM)
www.shrm.org

APPENDIX B: GROWTH CHARTS

Achondroplasia Growth Charts
Hoover-Fong JE, McGready J, Schulze KJ, et al: Weight for age charts for children with achondroplasia. *American Journal of Medical Genetics.* Part A 143A:2227-2235, 2007.

Asian Children
www.comeunity.com/adoption/health/growth.html

Cerebral Palsy, Quadriplegia
Kennedy Krieger Institute
http://www.kennedykrieger.org/

Down Syndrome Growth Charts
www.ndss.org/index.

Turner Syndrome Growth Charts
American Academy of Pediatrics: Health supervision guidelines for children with Turner syndrome, *Pediatrics* 111(3):692–702, 2003. aap.org/policy/0202.html

Williams Syndrome Growth Charts
American Academy of Pediatrics: Health supervision guidelines for children with Williams syndrome (RE0034), *Pediatrics* 107 (5):1192–1204, 2001. aap.org/policy/re0034.html

World Health Organization: Child Growth Standards
International growth charts, birth to 6 years old
www.who.int/childgrowth/standards/en/

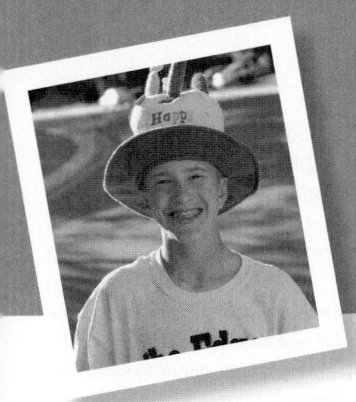

Appendix E

Discussion Questions

CHAPTER 1: HEALTH STATUS OF CHILDREN: GLOBAL AND LOCAL PERSPECTIVES

1. If you were to join a medical mission traveling to a country in Africa for 2 to 4 weeks, how would the Millennium Development Goals influence and inform your work objectives internationally?
2. How can organizations such as American Academy of Pediatrics and National Association of Pediatric Nurse Practitioners influence health policies related to promoting health equity among U.S. children?
3. Is evidence-based care (EBC) being implemented as policy in the United States? What else should be done to bring EBC into everyday clinical practice?
4. Discuss ways in which a patient- or family-centered health care home model could improve the pediatric health care infrastructure and improve child health outcomes.

CHAPTER 2: CHILD AND FAMILY HEALTH ASSESSMENT

1. How do the health effects of otitis media differ depending on whether the person uses the functional health, developmental, or disease problem orientation? Would there be a difference between a toddler and an adolescent? If so, discuss which frameworks would differ and provide examples of the differences.
2. How might a provider's personal definition of family and family roles affect the ability to assess a child and his or her family? List at least three strategies that the provider can use to assist families to make decisions that maximize health.
3. Compare and contrast history assessment techniques for a child from a blended family, a foster family, a single-parent family, and a grandparent-led family. How are these families similar? What unique issues are inherent in each of these family types?
4. Conduct a complete health history and physical examination on a child. Make sure you do a problem-oriented and a functional health history. What information is the same? What information is different?

CHAPTER 3: CULTURAL PERSPECTIVES FOR PEDIATRIC PRIMARY CARE

1. Your practice has begun to see clients from Somalia, Bhutan, and Eastern Europe (e.g., Khazakhstan and Georgia). Identify two reliable Internet sources for information about the cultural characteristics of each of these groups. Specifically look for health-related cultural characteristics. Identify resources in your community where you can find information and support for giving primary care to these clients. Where would you refer them for support services (e.g., nutrition, housing, safety)?

2. How do your cultural beliefs affect your ability to provide culturally competent care? List at least three strategies to overcome conflicts between your and your patient's cultural beliefs.
3. You see a child whose family believes in natural therapy for illnesses (e.g., diet therapy, massage, avoiding modern medical treatments). How can you incorporate the family's beliefs if the child has an upper respiratory infection? What if the child has a more serious condition, such as leukemia?
4. Compare how the two main cultural groups in your community view family, gender roles, childrearing, and health. Are there similarities? Differences?

CHAPTER 4: DEVELOPMENTAL MANAGEMENT IN PEDIATRIC PRIMARY CARE

1. List strategies that might be used by a pediatric primary care provider to incorporate developmental anticipatory guidance into the following sick visits: (1) an 18-month-old with an acute upper respiratory infection, (2) a 4-year-old with stool withholding and constipation, (3) a 9-year-old with chronic headaches, (4) a 15-year-old with dysmenorrhea.
2. Using the developmental theorists (where appropriate), explain the following child behaviors: a 3-year-old child has nighttime fears of the dark; an 8-year-old girl wants to be involved in a scouting group and is an avid collector of snow globes; a 13-year-old male wants to go to a camp sponsored by his religious denomination with a group of friends from school.
3. Conduct a developmental assessment on a child of your choice. Be sure to look at physical, developmental, social, and emotional growth. What changes to the assessment would you anticipate in 1 year? In 3 years?
4. You receive a phone call from a parent of a 4-year-old who fits the following temperament: high activity, high rhythmicity, low adaptability, low threshold of response, high intensity of reaction, outgoing and friendly mood, and high distractibility. His parent reports that the child is acting out against his younger sibling by kicking, hitting, and yelling. What anticipatory guidance related to discipline and parenting are appropriate for you to give the parents of this particular child and why?

CHAPTER 5: DEVELOPMENTAL MANAGEMENT OF INFANTS

1. Many providers are required to see 25 to 30 patients per day in their primary care practice. Discuss ways providers assess parents' sleep needs, expectations regarding crying and maternal depression while providing education about infant sleep-wake states, feeding patterns, and emotional development during a 15- to 20-minute newborn examination.

2. Identify developmental behaviors of a 6-month-old infant that would require an in-depth assessment and referral for developmental evaluation. How would your answer be different if the infant were 2 months old? Nine months old?

3. You get a phone call from a mother of a 10-day-old infant who tells you her son is crying "all the time." Further questioning reveals he wants to breastfeed every 3 hours (up from every 3½ to 4), and he has four or five loose bowel movements (BMs) daily that "look like they have birdseed in them." The mother denies any yellowing of the skin or sclera. Crying episodes last about 3 to 4 minutes at a time, and he quiets when the parent holds or swaddles him. What is the best response to this parent? What additional subjective or objective information do you need? What guidelines for management and follow-up will you use?

4. Create a caregiver education sheet that includes anticipatory guidance for one of the recommended infant well visits. Be sure to provide information regarding development, developmental red flags, nutrition, sleep, and safety. This handout should be written for caregivers and not health care professionals.

CHAPTER 6: DEVELOPMENTAL MANAGEMENT OF TODDLERS AND PRESCHOOLERS

1. A parent expresses concern that her 3-year-old is stuttering. Further questioning reveals the child repeats entire words, not syllables, and word repetitions are more common at the start of a sentence or thought. The physical examination is normal, and you detect no speech deficits. What management will you provide?

2. Create a plan for anticipatory guidance related to diet and discipline for a 15-month-old, a 24-month-old, a 3-year-old, and a 4-year-old. What developmental influences have the greatest effect on these areas during these ages?

3. A mother of an 18-month-old child tells you that she is very concerned about her son's lack of interest in playing with others. She says he plays side by side with other children without any problems, but becomes quite upset if other children use the toys he is playing with. The mother says she encourages him to share, but he does not always respond to her encouragement. Physical examination reveals a healthy child with no developmental deficits in fine motor, gross motor, or language. What techniques might be used to evaluate peer relationships for a child this age? How will you respond to the parent?

4. Compare and contrast the developmental assessment of a 13-month-old, a 30-month-old, a 3-year-old, and a 4-year-old. Which issues are unique to each of these ages?

5. Develop a management and educational plan for the management of toddler temper tantrums. How might these strategies differ for an older preschooler?

6. Identify resources in your community that can be used for the evaluation and management of toddlers and preschoolers with the developmental red flags identified in this chapter.

CHAPTER 7: DEVELOPMENTAL MANAGEMENT OF SCHOOL-AGE CHILDREN

1. A mother says she is concerned that her 7-year-old daughter "has no friends at school," seems "unhappy and very shy," and often "complains of a stomachache" before school begins. What assessment will you conduct to determine if there is a potential problem? What information can you share about development of children at this age? What guidance or suggestions will you give this mother?

2. While conducting an annual physical examination on a 12-year-old boy, you note that he is in the 85th percentile for weight, 50th percentile for height, has gynecomastia, and is at Tanner stage 1. What health issues are of greatest concern for you, and what will be your plan(s) for intervention?

3. The school nurse refers a 6-year-old boy for assessment of attention-deficit/hyperactivity disorder (ADHD). What might the long-term management plan for this child be? Consider assessment, anticipatory guidance for the child and family, consultation with the school nurse, arrangements for an individualized education plan, and treatments.

4. A 10-year-old girl's mother is killed in a motor vehicle accident; the family was very close, and the child is severely affected. Discuss the developmental characteristics and changes that guide the way this child might respond to her loss and examine how you will be able to help her most effectively.

CHAPTER 8: DEVELOPMENTAL MANAGEMENT OF ADOLESCENTS

1. A mother asks you if her daughter (13 years old) should get the "new sex shot" (human papillomavirus [HPV] vaccine). How do you solicit her concerns about the vaccine? What information and guidance do you give this mother? What other immunizations should this child receive? How would you answer her question if her child were a male?

2. You receive a phone call from a mother who tells you that her 15-year-old son is "angry all the time." She reports that when he was young they always got along but that they don't see eye to eye anymore and that he started "drifting away" when he entered high school. He is a good student, has friends, and no history of trouble at school or in the community. How would you respond to this mother? What additional questions are needed to determine if this behavior is developmentally normal?

3. Discuss the best approach to interviewing adolescent clients. What issues and challenges do adolescents present to the primary care provider's being able to gain their trust and confidence? How can you relate to adolescents to develop a healthy, interactive, and constructive patient-provider relationship?

4. Explain the importance of community involvement in an adolescent's development, using information from the Search Institute.

CHAPTER 9: INTRODUCTION TO FUNCTIONAL HEALTH PATTERNS AND HEALTH PROMOTION

1. How would you manage a health visit in which a child has an overweight problem using the principles found in Table 9-2 rather than in a more traditional visit?

2. Health literacy affects the information that clients have available to them to make decisions. What are some of the ways that providers could make use of technology and informatics to improve education of these families? What are some concepts that need to be considered in the development of these programs?

3. What strategies can busy practices use to help parents manage their children's growth and development needs until the next well-child visit?

4. What are some similarities and differences between anticipatory guidance and motivational interviewing? How can a provider use a motivational interview approach to make sure clients have the information they need to make healthy decisions?

CHAPTER 10: NUTRITION

1. What is the rationale regarding the use of infant formula with arachidonic acid (ARA) and docosahexaenoic acid (DHA)? What is the evidence regarding the benefits and risks of these formulas?

2. The mother of a toddler asks what she should be feeding her child. What advice will you give her? What resources will you use and why?

3. When taking a diet history from an immigrant family, you realize that you are unfamiliar with most of the foods they are feeding their child. What information do you need to ensure the child is

well nourished? How will you get that information? What is your approach to the family?

4. Select a school-aged client and analyze his or her 3-day diet (or analyze your own 3-day diet) using MyPyramid and Healthy Eating Index resources. What changes, if any, would you recommend?

5. As the primary care provider for a 10-year-old with cystic fibrosis, what goals will you set for the child's nutrition? What management plan and strategies will you use to achieve those goals? For a child with diabetes type 1?

6. Prepare a fact sheet for your local municipal government (e.g., city, county, township) presenting an argument for increased commitment to open, safe play spaces for children and youth. Incorporate national standards or recommendations regarding community action around issues of exercise and obesity. Present your data to your local elected officials.

CHAPTER 11: BREASTFEEDING

1. Only 50% of women in your community breastfeed beyond 1 month postpartum. Discuss measures you could initiate to improve rates of breastfeeding in your community.

2. A 25-year-old mother of a 2-month-old is upset because she has to stop breastfeeding for 2 weeks as a result of her medical problems. She is doing well with nursing her thriving infant. How can you help her? What conditions would allow her to resume breastfeeding in 2 weeks?

3. A mother of a 22-month-old states that she is still breastfeeding. She wants to stop but does not know how. What additional information do you need? What advice would you give her?

4. You see a couple for a prenatal visit at 8 months' gestation. You will be their primary pediatric provider. The woman states that she wants to breastfeed, but both members of the couple tell you that the father's family feels the baby should be fed formula. Discuss how you will approach this issue. What information and advice will you give to the couple?

CHAPTER 12: ELIMINATION PATTERNS

1. What are the dietary and medical options for treating constipation in a 1-year-old? Consider various causes. How would the treatment vary for a 5-year-old or a 15-year-old? Explain the pathophysiology of the relationship between constipation and urinary tract infections.

2. What are key points in the history and physical examination of a school-age child with dysfunctional voiding? Outline a plan to work with the family and child to treat this problem. When do you refer to a urologist?

3. A mother reports that despite following your advice about toilet training, her 4-year-old son insists on using diapers and has never urinated in the toilet. She states she is concerned. What will you review in the history and the physical examination? What suggestions do you have for this mother?

4. While conducting a sports physical for a 9-year-old boy, you discover he wets his bed at least three times a week. What information will you need to determine the cause of his enuresis and the best treatment for this child? You conclude that he has no organic disease for his enuresis. Outline a treatment plan you will develop with the child and his family. Explain your treatment choices.

CHAPTER 13: PHYSICAL ACTIVITY AND SPORTS FOR CHILDREN AND ADOLESCENTS

1. What physical assessment techniques should be done during a sport physical to screen for hypertrophic cardiomyopathy?

2. What role can the primary care provider play in ensuring that daily physical activities are part of the school curriculum?

3. How are preparticipation physical examinations done in your local community?

4. How can you affect the safety issues around organized and nonorganized sports in your community?

5. A 15-year-old is not wearing a bike helmet. The state law only mandates bike helmets until age 14. What can you do in the office to encourage bike helmet use? What effect can you have on a community and state level?

6. What are the signs and symptoms of steroid use in children and adolescents? How do you screen for them? What effect does screening athletes have on steroid use?

CHAPTER 14: SLEEP AND REST

1. How are the presentations of dyssomnias and medical reasons for awakening at night similar and different? How would you decide what sleep problem was presenting and thus how to manage it?

2. What expectations do you have for sleep patterns and sleep hygiene in children? How might your desires for a child to go to bed early, sleep late, sleep through the night, and sleep alone affect your ability to manage sleep problems in a family that didn't share those same expectations?

3. The mother of a healthy 9-month-old has a complaint that her child is awakening two or three times nightly. What are the likely causes at this age? What might the causes be if this child were school-age or an adolescent? How would your advice change?

4. Develop an intervention for a family with a 4-year-old child who awakens at 5 AM every day, is lively, and ready to get up for breakfast despite the fact that his parents usually work the swing shift and don't get to bed until midnight. Consider cultural, physiological, and psychological interventions.

CHAPTER 15: COGNITIVE-PERCEPTUAL DISORDERS: ATTENTION-DEFICIT/HYPERACTIVITY DISORDER, LEARNING PROBLEMS, SENSORY PROCESSING DISORDER, AUTISM SPECTRUM DISORDER, BLINDNESS AND DEAFNESS

1. Make a list of agencies in your community that provide services to help meet the educational, social, or physical needs of children with ADHD, visual deficits, auditory deficits, or pervasive developmental disorders.

2. You see a 7-year-old who was told by his teacher that "he needs treatment for ADHD." What assessment strategies will you use to establish this possible diagnosis? Create a plan of care to manage a child with ADHD that includes this child's physical, developmental, social, and family needs.

3. You see a 2-month-old for a well-child check. She has been blind since birth as a result of congenital cataracts. What anticipatory guidance related to this infant's visual deficit do you give this family? How will the anticipatory guidance change during the first and second years of life?

4. You are asked to speak to a group of mothers of preschoolers about how to distinguish behaviors that indicate ADHD and pervasive developmental disorder from normal preschool behavior. What information will you provide this group? What will you tell these parents about the comorbidities associated with these disorders?

5. The mother of a 4-year-old who was diagnosed with autism at 3 years old brings her younger, 2-yr-old, child in for a well-child examination. She is concerned that her younger child has autistic-like behaviors and wants the child evaluated for a pervasive developmental disorder (PDD). What screening is appropriate for a child this age? What pharmacologic and nonpharmacologic interventions would be

appropriate for a newly diagnosed 2-year-old with PDD? Make sure you include guidelines for referral and consultation and follow-up.

CHAPTER 16: SELF-PERCEPTION ISSUES

1. Compare and contrast the strategies used to assess the self-perception of a 5-year-old, an 11-year-old, and a 16-year-old. Identify at least four developmentally appropriate questions for each child.

2. Do a developmental asset evaluation on a child of your choosing. Pay special attention to identify family and environmental influences that affect the child's self-perception.

3. Create a plan of care to teach a parent parenting skills that promote a child's healthy self-perception. Focus on communication and discipline skills.

4. You identify altered self-perception and role performance problem in an adolescent female. Create a plan of care that addresses these issues and maximizes her developmental assets.

CHAPTER 17: ROLE RELATIONSHIPS

1. Conduct a family role assessment on the family of your choice. Be sure to identify each individual's roles, strengths, and weaknesses within the family. Which individual(s) is/are most critical to maintaining the family's dynamic?

2. After a careful assessment of family dynamics and strengths in question 1, what key anticipatory guidance issues should the pediatric provider address with the parent at this time related to the developmental needs of his or her children?

3. Parents of a 6-year-old child with terminal cancer seek counseling about how to best address this child's imminent death with her younger (3 years old) and older (14 years old) siblings. Discuss the areas of guidance you would provide and identify referrals to specific agencies in their community.

4. List three strategies that can be used by a pediatric provider to identify victims of child maltreatment. What biases and beliefs must the provider overcome to identify at-risk children? What are the local or regional resources available for abused or neglected children?

CHAPTER 18: SEXUALITY

1. How will you as a health care provider resolve any conflicts between your personal views and professional practice in discussing sexuality or birth control?

2. A mother of a 16-year-old refuses to leave the room during the well-child check. How are you going to handle a situation like this?

3. A father of a 17-year-old wants to know whether his child is sexually active. What will you tell him? What if the child is 14 years old? What if the child is 11 years old? What is your state law regarding parental notification?

4. A mother confides that she thinks her 8-year-old is going to be homosexual because he likes playing with dolls. What topics do you need to explore? How would you educate a mother who believes that homosexuality is a disease and can be changed?

5. Discuss what questions you could use to elicit parents' attitudes and ability to teach their children about sexuality as part of their child's life cycle?

6. How would you counsel the parents of a developmentally disabled 18-year-old who is going into a sheltered work and living environment about pregnancy prevention?

CHAPTER 19: COPING AND STRESS TOLERANCE: MENTAL HEALTH AND ILLNESS

1. Conduct a mental health assessment on a school-age child of your choice. Be sure to include stressors, parent-child interaction, and social, emotional, and behavioral development assessment.

How would your assessment be different if the child were an adolescent?

2. A concerned parent brings in her 3-year-old daughter because the child is "terrified of dogs." Further questioning reveals that the child cries and clings to the parent any time she sees a dog. There is no history of dog bite or attack, and the parents "can't figure where this came from" because they are both dog lovers. The child's growth and development are normal. The child's fears have become so intense that the family no longer visits the grandmother's home because she owns two dogs. What management will you provide? Would the management be different if the child were 8 years old, and her fear kept her from playing outside or taking the school bus? If so, how?

3. You see a 7-year-old child, MJ, in your office for a well visit. The parent reports that during the past 12 months MJ has become more "clingy." He will separate from his parents as long as he can see them nearby. For example, his mother reports that MJ will play soccer, but will turn around every 3 to 5 minutes to make eye contact with his mother and becomes quite agitated if he cannot find her in the crowd. Despite earlier excitement about the plans, MJ declined going to Boy Scout camp because his mother could not attend the overnight session. Also his mother reports that MJ has begun to have significant nightmares approximately four times a week, and MJ has moved from his bedroom to a pallet at the floor of the parents' bed because he is now afraid to go to sleep. What management do you suggest? Be sure to include pharmacologic and nonpharmacologic interventions if appropriate.

4. You are asked to speak to a Parent-Teacher Association at a local elementary school following a recent, well-publicized traumatic event in the community (weather-related, terrorism, child abduction, etc.). Specifically the group is interested in learning about how children between first and eighth grade respond to trauma and how parents can help their children cope. Create an educational plan for this meeting, making sure you identify normal and dysfunctional responses.

5. SH is a premenarchal 12-year-old female who has a 6-week complaint of difficulty concentrating, loss of appetite, and insomnia. Her mother notes that SH has stopped talking to her friends and seems "very withdrawn." There are no recent changes in the family and no history of trauma. What are the appropriate steps to evaluate this child for depression? What management will you recommend?

6. You receive a phone call from the parent of a 3-year-old child who was asked to leave his preschool because of fighting with the children and teachers, biting his classmates, and "dramatic" temper tantrums that often result in his throwing objects at others. His mother reports that he has "always been a difficult child" and does not respond to verbal redirection and timeouts "like his older brother does." In addition, he has always been a "physical child" and will often hit and push older children when angered. What disorder do you suspect, and what will be your management of this child?

CHAPTER 20: VALUES AND BELIEFS

1. How might a pediatric health care provider's own values, beliefs, and spirituality affect the ability to care for children and their families? Examine your own values, beliefs, and spirituality.

2. Discuss how health care providers can interact with children and their families to effectively include this component of health into their care.

3. What are unique issues related to values, beliefs, and spirituality of preschoolers? School-age children? Adolescents? How can

assessment of values and beliefs be incorporated into the preventive care of each of these age groups?

4. Conduct a values and beliefs assessment on a child. What anticipatory guidance strategies and family education strategies will you use in your wellness plan for this child that are based on your findings?

5. Conduct a spiritual screening on a child with a chronic or acute health condition. What interventions will you use in your plan of care based on your findings?

CHAPTER 21: INTRODUCTION TO DISEASE MANAGEMENT

1. Using each of the essential points of the shared decision model, create a comprehensive teaching plan for a 14-year-old teen newly diagnosed with type 1 diabetes mellitus and his family relative to his nutritional needs, monitoring of his blood glucose levels, and his insulin management.

2. Compare and contrast the primary care health needs of a child with normal growth and development with a child with a chronic physical or developmental condition.

3. List at least five strategies a pediatric provider can use to coordinate a multidisciplinary team to provide care for a chronically ill child. Develop at least one strategy that addresses advocacy for the parents, family, and siblings.

CHAPTER 22: PEDIATRIC PAIN MANAGEMENT

1. Explain how the pain assessment of a 9-month-old differs from that of a 7-year-old. How are they similar? Does pain assessment of a 15-year-old differ from that of a school-age child? If so, how?

2. Develop a pain management plan for the following children: an 18-month-old with an ear infection; a 3-year-old with toxic synovitis of the hip; a 9-year-old after a tonsillectomy, and a 12-year-old with juvenile arthritis. Include both pharmacological and nonpharmacologic interventions.

CHAPTER 23: INFECTIOUS DISEASES AND IMMUNIZATIONS

1. A new immigrant, who is a healthy 5-year-old, comes for his health care maintenance visit. The family does not have any documentation of prior vaccines. How do you proceed? Are there any vaccines that he no longer needs? What resources are available within your community for patients to get vaccines at no cost?

2. A healthy 43-day-old infant comes in for a health care maintenance visit. What is the minimum age for vaccines? Would you give vaccines today? Why or why not? If the family planned on traveling to Pakistan in 1 week, would that change your decision? How do you respond to a family's concerns about the variety of possible side effects/conditions that are attributed to vaccines?

3. Do all states require prenatal HIV screening? What are the issues about universal screening? How does HIV screening affect your practice?

4. What can be the role of the primary care provider in preventing infections in daycare centers?

5. Name at least four viruses and their different manifestations.

6. What is the local plan for emergency preparedness within your community? Within your state?

7. Identify the resources for health and safety services within your community that directly affect the quality of care children receive in out-of-home childcare facilities. Where are there gaps? Identify what you could do to improve the knowledge of childcare personnel in these facilities regarding health and safety of the children they serve.

CHAPTER 24: ATOPIC AND RHEUMATIC DISORDERS

1. A 12-year-old has recurrent spring time watery nasal discharge with nasal and eye itch. The common OTC medications have not worked. Discuss the following issues related to this child's presenting symptoms: (a) the probable diagnosis and its pathophysiology; (b) which if any diagnostic tests should be considered; (c) the likely offending allergens; and (d) key management issues.

2. A 15-month-old has a recurrent history of erythematous diffuse patches on both cheeks and is unable to sleep at night because of itching. How should this child be managed? Would the management change if a 7-year-old had a similar rash located in the antecubital fossa?

3. A 10-year-old has had a painful nonerythematous swelling in the right knee for 4 days. The pain is worse in the morning and with exercise. The family denies fever or flulike symptoms. The family history is remarkable for arthritis in the maternal side of the family, and it was noted that they went on a hiking trip in Massachusetts 2 months ago. The rest of history and physical examination is unremarkable. What diagnoses should be considered, and which laboratory studies should be ordered?

4. A 5-year-old is on albuterol MDI prn for rare episodes of wheezing. She recently moved to a apartment where the neighbor smokes and the fumes are coming into the apt. This has triggered wheezing every 2 to 3 weeks. Based on NIH guidelines, what medications would be used? What can be done to help her? What is the relationship between environmental pollutants and asthma?

CHAPTER 25: ENDOCRINE AND METABOLIC DISORDERS

1. The parent of a 3-week-old infant was just notified that the newborn screen on her infant was positive for hypothyroidism. She asks you, her primary care provider, why some of her baby's results were high (TSH) and some were low (T_3). How will you respond to her questions? What will be your management of this infant? Be sure to include pharmacologic and nonpharmacologic interventions.

2. Explain the workup and management for a 13-year-old female with growth failure over the last 3 years accompanied by pubertal-onset delay. What are your most likely differential diagnoses? How would your answer change if the child were an 8-year-old with growth failure?

3. You do a wellness examination on an 8-year-old female who has had a growth spurt of 4 inches in the last year and who is at Tanner 3 breast stage and Tanner 2 pubic hair. Her neurologic examination is normal. How will you manage this child? Be sure to include plans for pharmacologic management, consultation and/or referral, and anticipatory guidance.

4. You are asked by a local community group to talk about childhood diabetes. Prepare a discussion that includes the differences between type 1 and type 2 diabetes, specifically looking at pathologic conditions, epidemiology, risk factors, and clinical management.

5. You see a 2-month-old in your office for a wellness visit. Her weight gain was 7 ounces per week for the first 4 weeks, but it has decreased to 4 ounces per week. Her parents report she is increasingly irritable, and her suck is "not as strong as it used to be." Her bowel movements are less frequent and semiformed. Her abdominal girth has increased over her last visit. You note a high-pitched cry and generalized hypotonia and suspect galactosemia. What diagnostic testing is needed at this time? How will you manage this infant? Be sure to include anticipatory guidance, pharmacologic interventions, and guidelines for consultation and/or referral.

CHAPTER 26: HEMATOLOGIC DISORDERS

1. A 15-month-old has mild pallor. A spun Hgb is 9.5. What is your approach to this child? How might it be different if this child were an adolescent?

2. A 2-month-old is identified during newborn screening with sickle cell anemia. How would you manage this patient at 2 months, 2 years, 6 years, and at 13 years old? What are the issues for each stage in development? Where would you refer this child? How would you coordinate the care of this child?

3. An afebrile 10-year-old has new-onset petechiae. Her labs show a normal CBC except for a platelet count of 30,000/mm³, a normal PT, and PTT. What is your next step in the management of the patient? How might your management be different if her platelet count were 65,000/mm³?

4. How are you going to work with a hematologist in the co-management of a patient with chronic hematologic problems? What is the primary care provider's role in the management of children with chronic hematologic diseases?

CHAPTER 27: NEUROLOGIC DISORDERS

1. Are there different concerns about a new complaint of headache in a 3-year-old versus a 13-year-old? What are the similarities and differences in obtaining history, physical assessment, and differential diagnosis?

2. A 5-year-old has a tonic-clonic seizure and a temperature of 104° F (40° C). How would your management vary if this child were 3 months old? 8 years old?

3. A 10-year-old has a chief complaint of weakness. What are key physical assessment points? What are the differential diagnoses?

4. A 17-year-old football player received a severe head injury when in a motor vehicle accident in early May. He required hospitalization and was unconscious for 30 hours. He had one seizure the week following his injury. You see him 1 month after his discharge. What sort of examination (including all the elements) are you going to do? What do you tell him about his returning to play on the varsity football team in late August? What sort of prediction can you make about his recovery? What sort of follow-up do you recommend?

CHAPTER 28: EYE DISORDERS

1. You are vision screening a 4-year-old. The examination is 20/70 right eye and 20/30 left eye. Cover-uncover testing is normal, and the extraocular movements are intact. What is your next step? What is the risk of an untreated refractive error? If you get the same results in a 13-year-old, would it have the same significance?

2. A 13-year-old comes in during late April with bilateral red eyes without discharge and no history of trauma. What do you need to document on your note? What is the differential diagnoses? What would be included in your management plan?

3. How do resistance rates affect what drugs you prescribe for conjunctivitis? How are your prescribing practices affected by the pharmaceutical industries? Insurance companies?

CHAPTER 29: EAR DISORDERS

1. The treatments of relatively well children with otitis media have changed to a watch-and-see approach. How would you handle a resistant parent who wants to dictate how you prescribe?

2. The insurance company will not cover a fluoroquinolone-based otic preparation for an 8-year-old with an external otitis following swimming in his pool for a week. What is your next step and why?

3. A 3-year-old has a foreign body in the ear canal. It turns out the foreign object is a roach. How do you inform the parent? What factors need to be considered?

4. A mother reports that her febrile sick-appearing 18-month-old with acute otitis media is allergic to a variety of antibiotics. On careful questioning, the child gets diarrhea when these antibiotics are taken, but has no other side effects. Discuss this scenario.

CHAPTER 30: CARDIOVASCULAR DISORDERS

1. How does the assessment and evaluation of a 10-day-old infant with a new-onset systolic ejection murmur differ from that of a 2-year-old? How are they the same? Be sure to cover physical and developmental differences.

2. You see a 2-year-old with Down syndrome in your outpatient clinic. He has a large ventricular septal defect and is scheduled for surgical repair in 2 months. He is on digoxin at 7.5 mcg/kg/day for control of his congestive heart failure. Create a plan of care to coordinate this child's care through surgery, making sure you include interventions for this child's physical, developmental, and family needs.

3. How would you explain the need for subacute bacterial endocarditis prophylaxis to the mother of an infant with a patent ductus arteriosus? Would it be different if the child had a coarctation of the aorta or an atrioventricular canal?

4. You see a 3-year-old with hypertension (documented on three different visits) in your outpatient clinic. Describe the workup, differential diagnoses, assessment, and management. Be sure to include pharmacologic and nonpharmacologic interventions. How would your plan of care be different if the child were 10 years old?

CHAPTER 31: RESPIRATORY DISORDERS

1. A 3-year-old child has a 4-day history of temperature to 100.5° F (38.1° C) maximum, coughs mostly at night, and thick, yellow-green nasal discharge. Previous medical history is negative for allergies or any chronic disease. Mom reports that his appetite and activity levels are normal and states, "I'm sure he has a sinus infection because his drainage is yellow and green." Physical examination reveals a nontoxic-appearing child, lungs clear to auscultation, no cervical lymphadenitis, moderate nasal congestion, and copious clear postnasal drainage. What is your management plan for this child? What education regarding rhinosinusitis will you provide?

2. A mother calls because 10 days ago her 11-year-old daughter babysat an ill 4-month-old infant who has just been diagnosed with pertussis. Her daughter's last pertussis vaccine was at 4 years old (DTaP), and she is showing signs of upper respiratory infection (URI). What is your response to the parent?

3. A 10-month-old previously healthy child has a history of a URI with a fever of 101.5° F (38.7° C) for 2 days and now presents with acute-onset expiratory wheezing. On examination you note fine rales in the lung bases, and copious thick, clear rhinorrhea. The child's respiratory rate is 52, pulse is 134, and O₂ saturation in room air is 96%. The child is eating and drinking less than normal and had a wet diaper approximately 2 hours ago. Family history is positive for asthma in an older sibling. Social history is positive for daycare attendance. Do you need to do additional testing? Why or why not? What is your evidence-based plan of care for this child? Be sure to include physical, educational, and follow-up needs.

4. Compare and contrast the outpatient management of a 5-year-old and a 15-year-old with bacterial pneumonia. Be sure to consider the organism that causes pneumonia in these ages. How does that affect your management?

5. Develop a low-literacy handout to give parents who have a child with acute LTB that incorporates (1) essential management components, (2) signs that require further evaluation, (3) patient educational guidance, and (4) follow-up plan.

CHAPTER 32: GASTROINTESTINAL DISORDERS

1. A 2-month-old baby comes to clinic with his 19-year-old mother for persistent crying. There are no signs of infection. What specific history and physical findings will you be looking for? What plan of care will you recommend if you think the child has colic? What will you recommend if you think the child has reflux?

2. An 8-year-old walks into a clinic bent over holding her abdomen. She also has fever, nausea and vomiting that has become progressively worse over the last 12 hours. What physical exam findings will you look for? What labs will you order?

3. You are caring for a 6-year-old whose mother tells you she was just diagnosed with FAP. What clinical findings in the child would be associated with FAP? What is your role in caring for this child?

4. An 18-month-old who attends daycare and has been camping over the weekend presents with acute diarrhea. Outline the components of your assessment. Develop a management plan including both traditional and complementary modalities.

5. You suspect that a 9-year-old has Crohn disease. What tests do you order? What is your plan of care? What are some of the issues that can arise during adolescence? What techniques may be helpful in caring for a noncompliant adolescent?

CHAPTER 33: DENTAL AND ORAL DISORDERS

1. What is the level of fluoride in the water within the communities where you live? What information do you need before you prescribe fluoride? To what other sources of fluoride do children have access?

2. Why do children and adolescents with special health care needs have an increased risk for oral problems? What options are there for these children in your community and how can you help coordinate dental care for them?

3. Which groups of children need prophylactic antibiotics before dental care (refer also to Chapter 30 to more completely answer this question)?

4. Research your state's practice requirements for ordering, and learning how to apply, fluoride varnish as part of your practice. How would you incorporate its use in your practice?

CHAPTER 34: GENITOURINARY DISORDERS

1. How does your follow-up vary in a child 3 months of age with a urinary tract infection, a female 8 years of age, and a female 16 years of age? What things are you concerned about in each age group?

2. A 4-year-old male has a chief complaint of "his foreskin will not retract." The examination is otherwise normal. What do you want to advise the parent? How would this vary if the child were 13 years of age, Tanner 4?

3. What would you do if a 15-year-old adolescent refused a genitalia examination during a well visit? How would you manage this situation if it were a girl? A boy?

4. What are the recommendations for a screening urinalysis from the American Academy of Pediatrics, *Bright Futures,* and U.S. Preventive Services Task Force for a child who is 10 years of age? What are the recommendations for an adolescent? Why do the recommendations vary? Why do they vary by age?

CHAPTER 35: GYNECOLOGIC DISORDERS

1. As a provider you may have religious beliefs that are against abortion and birth control. In addition, you may work with providers with similar beliefs. How can you work with sexually active adolescents or adolescents who are pregnant and may want an abortion?

2. A sexually active 13-year-old is not using any contraceptive method. She does not want her parents to know that she is sexually active. How would you approach this adolescent? How would you counsel her about contraceptive use? What methods might be more suitable? What other things do you want to include in your discussion?

3. A 12-year-old female has had secondary amenorrhea for 3 months. She started her menses at 9 years old and has had a 28-day cycle for the past 2 years. What do you want to do and why? How would your approach vary if the patient were 10 years old and had her menses for only 6 months?

4. A 6-year-old has a yellow vaginal discharge. The examination is otherwise normal. What are key points in the history and physical examination? How would your approach differ if the patient were a sexually active 16-year-old? What are similarities and differences in the approach?

CHAPTER 36: DERMATOLOGIC DISORDERS

1. What factors do you need to consider when prescribing topical preparations for skin disorders?

2. You diagnose a 3-year-old to have eczema; the mother has a history of eczema and continues to suffer skin lesions as an adult. Describe your management of this child. What techniques will you use in counseling families about skin care for children with eczema?

3. There is an outbreak of lice in the community. What role can you play in helping to solve the problem?

4. A 13-year-old male comes for a well-child visit. He is doing well in school and is a star basketball player. Mom is very concerned about his acne and spends 5 minutes of the visit telling you how she had severe acne growing up. She does not want her son to get severe acne. On examination, there are several small whiteheads on his forehead and a few blackheads on his nose. There are no pustules, nodules, or cysts. How severe is his acne? What would be your treatment? What else do you need to discuss with this family?

5. A 5-year-old with impetigo was placed on Keflex 2 days ago. The family reports compliance with the medication, but the impetigo is spreading. What is the likely pathogen? How would you manage care for this child?

CHAPTER 37: MUSCULOSKELETAL DISORDERS

1. Compare and contrast the musculoskeletal assessment of a 2-month-old, a 4-year-old, and a 10-year-old. Include developmental variances and physiologic differences.

2. A brachial plexus injury is noted during the newborn examination of a postterm, large-for-gestational-age infant. The right shoulder, biceps, and forearm do not move, but the baby can flex the wrist. Create a plan of care for this child that includes diagnostic testing and management of the infant and family's physical, educational, and developmental needs.

3. An 11-year-old girl had a scoliosis screening done at school today. The school nurse told the mother that the child had a 9-degree lumbar curvature on the scoliometer. How do you respond to the mother? What treatment, diagnostic evaluation, and follow-up do you suggest?

4. What would be the differential for a 7-year-old male with a new-onset limp and complaint of anterior thigh pain? What physical examination, health history, and diagnostic testing findings would you expect for your top three diagnoses? How would your answers change if the boy were 13 years old?

5. A 12-month-old has marked in-toeing with a thigh-foot angle of −16 degrees. Other examination findings are normal, including the child's gait. What diagnostic testing and management do you prescribe?

6. A mother notes that her 18-month-old's foot is "curved," and the curving has worsened during the last 6 months since the toddler began walking. Physical examination reveals a normal right foot and a convex left foot. The defect can be straightened by applying lateral pressure to the anterior foot. Grandma told the mother that placing the child's shoes on the wrong foot would fix the problem. How do you respond? What management do you initiate?

CHAPTER 38: PERINATAL DISORDERS

1. Create a discharge plan for a healthy, term newborn. Make sure you include both newborn and family needs. Create a similar discharge plan for an infant with one of the high-risk conditions listed in Box 38-1. How do the plans differ? How are they the same?

2. You are called to the newborn nursery to evaluate a term, newborn with Apgar of 9/9 born via vaginal delivery to a 34-year-old primigravida. Pregnancy history was normal except for oligohydramnios. The nursery nurses inform you the infant has had one wet diaper in the last 8 hours and is now lethargic. Physical examination reveals a palpable abdominal mass. What diagnostic testing do you order, and what do you expect to find? What management do you prescribe?

3. Develop a plan of care for a 10-week-old with an acute life-threatening event. Be sure to list parameters for evaluation, referral, consultation, and follow-up.

4. You see a 36-week gestation newborn at 3 days old for follow-up following a discharge bilirubin of 9.4 mg/dL (obtained yesterday afternoon). The parents report an intake of 16 oz iron-fortified cow's milk formula over the last 24 hours. The newborn had three wet diapers and one bowel movement in the last 16 hours. Physical examination reveals marked jaundice of the face, trunk, and upper thighs with scleral yellowing. Prenatal history was negative, and the Coombs test was negative at birth. Total bilirubin today is 15.2. What management do you prescribe?

CHAPTER 39: COMMON INJURIES

1. You see an 11-year-old who received a mild traumatic brain injury 1 week ago during a football game. He did not lose consciousness at the time of injury and was managed during the game by a licensed athletic trainer. Today he still complains of headache but he has no other significant symptoms. He states he wants to return to play because the regional playoffs begin in 1 week. How do you respond? What additional management is needed at this time?

2. You are seeing a patient with a fractured wrist for the first time in an emergency department. What are key history points that may be helpful in trying to determine whether there is a pattern of injuries that may be suspicious of abuse?

3. You are seeing a 4-month-old in your office. What injury prevention anticipatory guidance should this patient receive? How would your answer be different if the patient were 30 months old? Five years old? Fourteen years old?

4. A family is planning a 1-week camping excursion. They ask you what they should bring on their trip in case of injuries. Develop a list for use in your practice based on recommendations from reliable resources.

5. A 15-year-old comes in following a fight at school. He has multiple abrasions and a few puncture wounds on the right knuckle. How do you treat these abrasions? The mother tells you that she put peroxide on them at home. What are key teaching points in this patient? What else about the presentation concerns you and why?

6. A 6-year-old complains of twisting his right ankle during a basketball game. He has point tenderness, edema, and mild ecchymosis of the right lateral malleolus. What is on your differential diagnosis? What are the physiologic differences between the skeleton of a 6-year-old versus the skeleton of a 15-year-old? What management do you recommend? Be sure to include diagnostic testing and pharmacologic and nonpharmacologic therapies.

CHAPTER 40: GENETIC DISORDERS

1. Conduct a family history on a child with asthma. Create a family pedigree, paying special attention to atopic diseases (i.e., asthma, allergies, and eczema). Look at the inheritance pattern. Does asthma appear to be a multifactorial problem or a single-gene disorder? Why?

2. The mother of a child with an autosomal recessive disorder wants to know the likelihood of her next child contracting the disease. What would you tell her? How would your answer be different if the disease were X-linked recessive?

3. How would you explain to the parent the role of spontaneous mutations in childhood genetic disease?

4. A 3-year-old child with fetal alcohol syndrome comes to your office for the first time. Create a care plan for this child that includes interventions for this child's physical, psychosocial, and emotional needs. Include interventions for the family's needs. Make sure you include referrals to agencies in your area.

CHAPTER 41: ENVIRONMENTAL HEALTH ISSUES

1. How can you integrate the use of the pediatric environmental health history into your well-child care visits? How can the use of survey tools like these improve your practice?

2. What are the principal environmental hazards in your local community? What community resources are there to assist families to clean up hazards?

3. What environmental hazards are more common in rural and urban settings? What do you need to think about in terms of environmental hazards in caring for children who travel or have extended families in other parts of the world?

4. What steps would you take if a parent brought a child in to you reporting that he had been playing with elemental mercury that he found? What information would you need to collect initially? What agencies would you call for help?

5. What steps would you take if your patient is the child of a migrant farm worker and the parent reports that pesticide spraying had drifted across the farm worker housing area several times in the past few weeks?

6. The majority of your client population is Medicaid-eligible and lives in housing built before 1960. Develop a protocol for your practice to manage exposure to lead, lead toxicity, and lead poisoning among your clients. Explain what you will do to prevent problems. Discuss your follow-up plan.

CHAPTER 42: COMPLEMENTARY MEDICINE

1. Are there medicolegal implications for the use of CAM therapy?

2. What principles govern the use of CAM therapies?

3. Discuss areas of your clinical practice you feel lend themselves to incorporating CAM practices.

4. You are asked about dosage of an herbal preparation. How do you answer? Where do you get your information? Are there risks in

giving information about herbal preparations? Does your malpractice cover you for using CAM?

5. Discuss how you would go about compiling a list of reliable complementary providers in your practice community. How would you go about setting up a collegial working relationship with them?

CHAPTER 43: STRATEGIES FOR MANAGING A HEALTH CARE PRACTICE

1. Create a vision statement that reflects your philosophy and role as a primary care provider.

2. Create a simple business plan for a one-provider practice. Be sure to cover organizational structure, insurance requirements, and financial operations.

3. Create an appointment scheduling process for a pediatric primary care provider.

References

CHAPTER 1

American Academy of Pediatrics (AAP): Recommendations for preventive pediatric health care: Committee on Practice and Ambulatory Medicine, *Pediatrics* 105(3):645–646, 2000.

Berwick D: What patient-centered should mean: confessions of an extremist, *Health Aff* 28(4):W555–W565, 2009.

Black RE, Cousens S, Johnson HL, et al: Global, regional, and national causes of child mortality in 2008: a systematic analysis, *Lancet* 375(9730):1969–1987, 2010.

Black RE, Allen LH, Bhutta ZA, et al: Maternal and child undernutrition: global and regional exposures and health consequences, *Lancet* 371(9608):243–260, 2008.

Centers for Disease Control and Prevention (CDC): National, state, and local area vaccination coverage among adolescents aged 13-17 years-United States, 2008, *MMWR* 58(36):997–1001, 2009.

Child Health Epidemiology Reference Group: *Objectives*. Available at http://cherg.org/about/objectives.html. Accessed Oct 20, 2010.

Crocker D, Brown C, Moolenaar R, et al: Racial and ethnic disparities in asthma medication usage and health-care utilization: data from the National Asthma Survey, *Chest* 136(3):1063–1071, 2009.

Duderstadt KG: Medical home: nurse practitioners' role in health care delivery to vulnerable populations, *J Pediatr Health Care* 22(6):390–393, 2008.

Fantuzzo JW, Mohr WK: Prevalence and effects of child exposure to domestic violence, *Fut Child* 9(3):21–32, 2003.

Forum on Child and Family Statistics: *America's children in brief: key national indicators of well-being 2010.* Available at www.childstats.gov/americaschildren/health.asp. Accessed Oct 20, 2010.

Foundation for Child Development: 2007 Special Focus Report on International Comparisons, *Child and Youth Well-Being Index (CWI) Project* 1–17, 2007.

Hagan JF, Shaw JS, Duncan PM: *Bright futures: guidelines for health supervision of infants, children, and adolescents*, ed 3, Elk Grove, IL, 2008, American Academy of Pediatrics.

Halfon N, DuPlessis H, Inkelas M: Transforming the U.S. child health system, *Health Aff* 26(2):315–330, 2007.

MacDorman MF, Mathews TJ: Behind international rankings of infant mortality: how the United States compares with Europe, *Int J Health Serv* 40(4):577–588, 2010.

National Association of Pediatric Nurse Practitioners: NAPNAP position statement on pediatric health care/medical home: key issues on delivery, reimbursement, and leadership, *J Pediatr Health Care* 23(3):A23–A24, 2009.

Naylor MD, Kurtzman ET: The role of nurse practitioners in reinventing primary care, *Health Aff* 29(5):893–899, 2010.

Ogden CL, Carroll MD, Curin LR, et al: Prevalence of high body mass index in US children and adolescents, 2007-2008, *JAMA* 303(3):242–249, 2010.

Schor EL: Rethinking well-child care, *Pediatrics* 114(1):210–216, 2004.

Tanner JL, Stein LM, Olson MP: Reflections on well-child care practice: a national study of pediatric clinicians, *Pediatrics* 124(3):849–857, 2009.

United Nations International Children's Fund: *The state of the world's children special edition, 2009.* Available at www.unicef.org/rightsite/sowc. Accessed Oct 20, 2010.

United Nations: *Millennium Development Goals, 2000.* Available at www.un.org/millenniumgoals/bkgd. Accessed Oct 20, 2010.

UN Millennium Project: *Halving hunger: it can be done, 2006.* Available at www.unmillenniumproject.org/reports/tf_hunger.htm. Accessed Oct 20, 2010.

U.S. Department of Health and Human Services (USDHHS): *National healthcare disparities report*, Rockville, MD, 2009, Agency for Healthcare Research and Quality.

United States Department of Health and Human Services (USDHHS): *Healthy People: Developing Healthy People 2020.* Available at http://healthypeople.gov/hp2020/Objectives/TopicAreas.aspx. Accessed Jan 6, 2011.

United States Department of Health and Human Services (USDHHS): *Healthy People 2010.* Available at www.healthypeople.gov/2020/topicsobjectives. Accessed Jan 6, 2012.

CHAPTER 2

Amer A, Fischer H: "Don't call me mom"—how parents want to be greeted by their pediatrician, *Clin Pediatr* 48:720–722, 2009.

American Academy of Pediatrics (AAP): Family pediatrics: report of the task force on the family, *Pediatrics* 111:1541–1571, 2003.

American Academy of Pediatrics (AAP): Council on Children With Disabilities, Section on Developmental Behavioral Pediatrics, *Bright Futures* Steering Committee, and Medical Home Initiatives for Children With Special Needs Project Advisory Committee: Identifying infants and young children with developmental disorders in the medical home: an algorithm for developmental surveillance and screening, *Pediatrics* 118:405–420, 2006.

American Academy of Sleep Medicine: *International classification of sleep disorders revised, diagnostic and coding manual*, Westchester, IL, 1997, American Academy of Sleep Medicine.

Benzies K, Mychasiuk R: Fostering family resiliency: a review of the key protective factors, *Child Fam Social Work* 14:103–114, 2009.

Brown JD, Wissow LS: Discussion of maternal stress during pediatric primary care visits, *Ambul Pediatr* 8:368–374, 2008.

Burns C: Development and content validity testing of a comprehensive classification of diagnoses for use by pediatric nurse practitioners, *Nurs Diagn* 2:93–104, 1991.

Burns C: A new assessment model and tool for nurse practitioners, *J Pediatr Health Care* 6:73–81, 1992a.

Burns C: Using a comprehensive taxonomy of diagnoses to describe the practice of pediatric nurse practitioners: findings of a field study, *J Pediatr Health Care* 7:115–121, 1992b.

Child and Adolescent Health Measurement Initiative: *2007 National Survey of Children's Health (2009). Data Resource Center for Child and Adolescent Health website.* Available at www.nschdata.org. Accessed August 29, 2010.

Cox ED, Raaum S: Discussion of alternatives, risks, and benefits in pediatric acute care, *Patient Educ Counsel* 72:122–129, 2008.

Cox ED, Smith M, Brown R: Evaluating deliberation in pediatric primary care, *Pediatrics* 120:e68–e77, 2007.

Curran D: *Traits of a healthy family*, New York, 1983, Ballantine.

deChesnay M: Promoting healthy family functioning in acute care units, *J Pediatr Nurs* 1:96–101, 1986.

Duffy ME: Health promotion in the family: current findings and directives for nursing research, *J Adv Nurs* 13:109–117, 1988.

Feetham SL, Humerick SS: The Feetham Family Functioning Survey. In Humerick SS, editor: *Analysis of current assessment strategies in the health care of young children and childbearing families*, East Norwalk, CT, 1982, Appleton-Century-Crofts.

Friedman MM: *Family nursing: theory and assessment*, ed 2, East Norwalk, CT, 1986, Appleton-Century-Crofts.

Garg A, Nelson CS, Burrell L, et al: Association of substance use discussion by pediatric providers with the parent-provider relationship and maternal behavior, *Clin Pediatr (Phila)* 49:240–248, 2010.

Glader B: Iron deficiency anemia. In Kliegman RM, Behrman RE, Jenson HB, et al: *Nelson textbook of pediatrics*, ed 18, Philadelphia, 2007, Saunders, pp 2015–2017.

Goldenring J, Rosen D: Getting into adolescent heads: an essential update, *Contemp Pediatr* 21:64–90, 2004.

Gordon M: *Manual of nursing diagnoses*, ed 12, Sudbury, MA, 2010, Jones and Bartlett.

Gordon M: *Nursing diagnosis: process and application*, New York, 1987, McGraw-Hill.

Halfon N, Regalado M, Sareen H: Assessing development in the pediatric office, *Pediatrics* 113:1926–1933, 2004.

Kazak A, Hoagwood K, Weisz JR, et al: A meta-systems approach to evidence-based practice for children and adolescents, *Am Psychol* 65:85–97, 2010.

Levetown M, Committee of Bioethics of AAP: Communicating with children and families: from everyday interactions to skill in conveying distressing information, *Pediatrics* 121:1441–1460, 2008.

Lehna C: Interpreter services in pediatric nursing, *Pediatr Nurs* 31:292–296, 2005.

Maradiegue A, Edwards QT: An overview of ethnicity and assessment of family history in primary care settings, *J Am Acad Nurs Pract* 18:447–456, 2006.

Margolis P, McLearn KT, Earls MF, et al: Assisting primary care practices in using office systems to promote early childhood development, *Ambul Pediatr* 8:383–387, 2008.

Mather M: *Children in immigrant families chart new path*, Washington DC, 2009, Population Reference Bureau. Available at www.prb.org. Accessed Aug 28, 2010.

McCubbin HI, Thompson AI, McCubbin MA: *Family assessment: resiliency, coping, and adaptation: inventories for research and practice*, Madison, WI, 1996, University of Wisconsin Publishers.

McGoldrick M, Gerson R, Shellenberger S: *Genograms: assessment and intervention*, New York, 2007, Norton.

McGuiness T, Noonan P, Dyer J: Family history as a tool for psychiatric nurses, *Arch Psychiatr Nurs* 19:116–124, 2005.

McKay K: Evaluation model programs to support dissemination: an evaluation of strengthening the developmental surveillance and referral practices of child health providers, *Dev Behav Pediatr* 27:S26–S29, 2006.

Minkovitz C, Strobino D, Scharfstein D, et al: Maternal depressive symptoms and children's receipt of health care in the first 3 years of life, *Pediatrics* 115:306–314, 2005.

Moos R, Moos B: *Family environment scale manual*, ed 3, Palo Alto, CA, 1994, Consulting Psychologists Press.

NANDA International: *Nursing diagnoses: definitions & classification 2009-2011*, Philadelphia, 2009, NANDA International.

Olsen S, Dudley-Brown S, McMullen P: Case for blending pedigrees, genograms, and ecomaps: nursing's contribution to the "big picture," *Nurs Health Sci* 6:295–308, 2004.

Olson DH, Gorall D: *FACES IV*, Roseville, MN, 2006, Life Innovations.

Otsuki M, Eakin MN, Arceneaux LL, et al: Prospective relationship between maternal depressive symptoms and asthma morbidity among inner-city African American children, *J Pediatr Psychol* 35:758–767, 2010.

Phelan K, Khoury J, Atherton H, et al: Maternal depression, child behavior, and injury, *Inj Prev* 13:403–408, 2007.

Raphael JL, Zhang Y, Liu H, et al: Parenting stress in US families: implications for paediatric healthcare utilization, *Child Care Health Dev* 36:216–224, 2010.

Richmond M, Stocker CM: Associations between family cohesion and adolescent siblings' externalizing behavior, *J Fam Psychol* 20:663–669, 2006.

Schonwald A, Horan K, Huntington N: Developmental screening: is there enough time? *Clin Pediatr* 48:648–655, 2009.

Smilkstein G: The family APGAR: a proposal for a family function test and its use by physicians, *J Fam Pract* 6:1231–1239, 1978.

Stein L, Malmberg K, Sylva J, et al: The influence of maternal depression, caregiving, and socioeconomic status in the postnatal year on children's language development, *Child Care Health Dev* 34:603–612, 2008.

Terkelsen KG: Toward a theory of the family life cycle. In Carter EA, McGoldrick M, editors: *The family life cycle: a framework for family theory*, New York, 1980, Gardner.

U.S. Department of Health and Human Services (USDHHS): *National Center for Health Statistics: International classification of diseases, ninth revision, clinical modification*, ed 6, Hyattsville, MD, 2003, Centers for Medicare and Medicaid Services.

Wattendorf D, Hadley D: Family history: the three-generation pedigree, *Am Fam Physician* 72:441–448, 2005.

Whall AL: The family as the unit of care in nursing: a historical review, *Public Health Nurs* 3:240–249, 1986.

Wright LM, Leahey M: *Nurses and families: a guide to family assessment and intervention*, ed 4, Philadelphia, 2005, FA Davis.

Zero to Three: *Diagnostic classification of mental health and developmental disorders of infancy and early childhood (rev.)*, Washington DC, 2005, Author.

Zink T, Levin L, Wollan P, et al: Mothers' comfort with screening questions about sensitive issues, including domestic violence, *J Am Board Fam Med* 19:358–367, 2006.

CHAPTER 3

Airhihenbuwa CO, Liburd L: Eliminating health disparities in the African American population: the interface of culture, gender, and power, *Health Educ Behav* 33:488–501, 2006.

Berger P, Luckmann T: *The social construction of reality*, New York, 1966, Doubleday.

Betancourt TS, Khan KT: The mental health of children affected by armed conflict: protective processes and pathways to resilience, *Int Rev Psychiatry* 20:317–328, 2008.

Bhui K, Warfa N, Edonya P, et al: Cultural competence in mental health care: a review of model evaluations, *BMC Health Serv Res* 7:15, 2007.

Birman D, Beehler S, Harris EM, et al: International Family, Adult, and Child Enhancement Services (FACES): a community-based comprehensive services model for refugee children in resettlement, *Am J Orthopsychiatry* 78:121–132, 2008.

Caldwell-Harris CL, Ayçiçegi A: When personality and culture clash: the psychological distress of allocentrics in an individualist culture and idiocentrics in a collectivist culture, *Transcult Psychiatry* 43:331–361, 2006.

Calvillo E, Clark L, Ballantyne JE, et al: Cultural competency in baccalaureate nursing education, *J Transcult Nurs* 20:137–145, 2009.

Centers for Disease Control and Prevention (CDC): *VitalStats—perinatal mortality*. Available at www.cdc.gov/nchs/data_access/vitalstats/VitalStats_Perinatal_Mortality.htm. Accessed June 24, 2010a.

Centers for Disease Control and Prevention (CDC): *Medical examination of immigrants and refugees*. Available at www.cdc.gov/immigrantrefugeehealth/exams/medical-examination.html. Accessed January 27, 2011b.

Chen Y, Nettles ME, Chen SW: Rethinking dependent personality disorder: comparing different human relatedness in cultural contexts, *J Nerv Ment Dis* 197:793–800, 2009.

Crowley C: The mental health needs of refugee children: a review of literature and implications for nurse practitioners, *J Am Acad Nurse Pract* 21:322–331, 2009.

Culhane-Pera KA, Allen M, Pergament SL, et al: Improving health through community-based participatory action research. Giving immigrants and refugees a voice, *Minn Med* 93:54–57, 2010.

Department of Homeland Security: *Immigration statistics: data and statistics*. Available at www.dhs.gov/files/statistics/data. Accessed June 24, 2010.

Dicker S, Stauffer WM, Mamo B, et al: Initial refugee health assessments. New recommendations for Minnesota, *Minn Med* 93:45–48, 2010.

Dunn AM: Culture competence and the primary care provider, *J Pediatr Health Care* 16:105–111, 2002.

Fadiman A: *The spirit catches you and you fall down*, New York, 1997, Farrar, Straus and Giroux.

Hall ET: *Understanding cultural differences*, Yarmouth, ME, 1990, Intercultural Press.

Hsieh E: Provider-interpreter collaboration in bilingual health care: competitions of control over interpreter-mediated interactions, *Patient Educ Couns* 78:154–159, 2010.

Hsieh E: Interpreters as co-diagnosticians: overlapping roles and services between providers and interpreters, *Soc Sci Med* 64:924–937, 2007.

Hsieh E, Ju H, Kong H: Dimensions of trust: the tensions and challenges in provider–interpreter trust, *Qual Health Res* 20:170–181, 2010.

Hulme P: Cultural considerations in evidence-based practice, *J Transcult Nurs* 21:271–280, 2010.

Karliner LS, Jacob EA, Chen AH, et al: Do professional interpreters improve clinical care for patients with limited English proficiency? A systematic review of the literature, *Health Serv Res* 42:727–754, 2007.

Kleinman A, Eisenberg L, Good B: Culture, illness and care: clinical lessons from anthropologic and cross-cultural research, *Ann Intern Med* 88:251–258, 1978.

Kripalani S, Bussey-Jones J, Katz MG, et al: A prescription for cultural competence in medical education, *J Gen Intern Med* 21:1116–1120, 2006.

Kroeber AL: *The nature of culture*, Chicago, 1952, University of Chicago Press.

Ku L: Health insurance coverage and medical expenditures of immigrants and native-born citizens in the United States, *Am J Public Health* 99:1322–1328, 2009.

Kumagai AK, Lypson ML: Beyond cultural competence: critical consciousness, social justice, and multicultural education, *Acad Med* 84:782–787, 2009.

Lie DA, Boker J, Crandall S, et al: Revising the Tool for Assessing Cultural Competence Training (TACCT) for curriculum evaluation: findings derived from seven US schools and expert consensus, *Med Educ Online* 13:1–11, 2008.

Maloney SA, Ortega LS, Cetron MS: Overseas medical screening for immigrants and refugees. In Walker PF, Barnett ED, editors: *Immigrant medicine*, Philadelphia, 2007, Saunders.

Mohanty SA, Woolhandler S, Himmelstein DU, et al: Health care expenditures of immigrants in the United States: a nationally representative analysis, *Am J Public Health* 95:1431–1438, 2005.

Mostow C, Crosson J, Gordon S, et al: Treating and precepting with RESPECT: a relational model addressing race, ethnicity, and culture in medical training, *J Gen Intern Med* 25:S146–S154, 2010.

Oberg K: Culture shock: adjustment to new cultural environment, *Practical Anthropol* 7:177–182, 1960.

Passel JS, Cohn D: *A portrait of unauthorized immigrants in the United States*, Washington, DC, 2009, Pew Research Center. Available at www.pewhispanic.org/reports/report.php?ReportID=107 Accessed June 24, 2010.

Pavlish CL, Noor S, Brandt J: Somali immigrant women and the American health care system: discordant beliefs, divergent expectations, and silent worries, *Soc Sci Med* 71:353–361, 2010.

Sequist TD, et al: Cultural competency training and performance reports to improve diabetes care for black patients: a cluster randomized, controlled trial, *Ann Intern Med* 152:40–46, 2010.

Steffen PR, Smith TB, Larson M, et al: Acculturation to Western society as a risk factor for high blood pressure: a meta-analytic review, *Psychosom Med* 68:386–397, 2006.

Suurmond J, Seelman C, Rupp I, et al: Cultural competence among nurse practitioners working with asylum seekers, *Nurse Educ Today* 30(8):821–826, 2010.

Turiel E: Beyond individualism and collectivism: a problem, or progress? *New Dir Child Adolesc Dev* (104):91–100, 2004.

Underwood SM, Buseh AG, Canales MK, et al: Nursing contributions to the elimination of health disparities among African-Americans: review and critique of a decade of research—part II, *J Natl Black Nurses Assoc* 16:31–47, 2005.

U.S. Department of Health and Human Services (USD-HHS) Office of Minority Health: *National standards for culturally and linguistically appropriate services in health care: final report*, Rockville, MD, 2001, USDHHS.

Walker PF, Barnett ED, editors: *Immigrant medicine*, Philadelphia, 2007, Saunders.

Watson OM: *Proxemic behavior: a cross-cultural study*, The Hague, Netherlands, 1980, Mouton.

Yanni EA, Marano N, Stauffer WM, et al: Health status of visitors and temporary residents, United States, *Emerg Infect Dis* 15(11):1715–1720, 2009.

CHAPTER 4

Ainsworth M, Bell S, Stayton D: Individual differences in strange-situation behavior of one year olds. In Schaffer HR, editor: *The origins of human social relations*, London, 1971, Academic Press.

American Academy of Pediatrics (AAP): Committee on Children with Disabilities: Care coordination: integrating health and related systems of care for children with special health care needs, *Pediatrics* 104:978–981, 1999.

American Academy of Pediatrics (AAP): Committee on Children with Disabilities: Identifying infants and young children with developmental disorders in the medical home: an algorithm for developmental surveillance and screening, *Pediatrics* 118:405–420, 2006.

American Academy of Pediatrics (AAP): Committee on Children with Disabilities: Role of the pediatrician in family-centered early intervention services, *Pediatrics* 107:1155–1157, 2001.

American Academy of Pediatrics (AAP): Committee on Psychosocial Aspects of Child and Family Health: Guidance for effective discipline, *Pediatrics* 101:723–728, 1998.

Antonelli RC, Antonelli DM: Providing a medical home: the cost of care coordination services in a community-based, general pediatric practice, *Pediatrics* 113:1522–1528, 2004.

Aylward GP: *Bayley infant developmental inventory*, San Antonio, TX, 1995, Psychological Corp.

Barnard K: *NCAST II learners' resource manual*, Seattle, 1976, NCAST Publications, University of Washington.

Barnard K: *NCAST instructors' manual*, Seattle, 1979, NCAST Publications, University of Washington.

Bhasin TK, Brocksen S, Aychen RN, et al: Prevalence of four developmental disabilities among children aged 8 years—metropolitan Atlanta Developmental Disabilities Surveillance Program, 1996 and 2000, *MMWR Surveill Summ* 55:1–9, 2006.

Bijou S, Baer D: *Child development II: universal stages of infancy*, New York, 1965, Appleton-Century-Crofts.

Blumberg SJ, Halfon N, Olson LM: The national survey of early childhood health, *Pediatrics* 113:1899–1906, 2004.

Bowlby J: *Attachment and loss, (vol 1), attachment*, New York, 1969, Basic Books.

Brazelton B, Sparrow JD: *Touchpoints: birth to three: your child's emotional and behavioral development*, Cambridge, MA, 2006, DaCapo Press.

Bronfenbrenner U: *The ecology of human development: experiments by nature and design*, Cambridge, MA, 1979, Harvard University Press.

Bronson MB: *Self-regulation in early childhood—nature and nurture*, New York, 2000, The Guilford Press.

Buhler C, Allen M: *Introduction to humanistic psychology*, Monterey, CA, 1972, Brooks/Cole.

Cech DJ, Martin S: *Functional movement development across the life span*, Philadelphia, 2002, Saunders.

Chess T, Thomas A: *Temperament in clinical practice*, New York, 1995, Guilford Press.

Dixon S, Stein M: *Encounters with children: pediatric behavior and development*, St Louis, 2006, Mosby.

Dworkin PH: British and American recommendations for developmental monitoring: the role of surveillance, *Pediatrics* 84(6):1000–1010, 1989.

Dworkin PH: Detection of behavioral, developmental, and psychosocial problems in pediatric primary care practice, *Curr Opin Pediatr* 5:531–536, 1993.

Earls MF, Hay SS: Setting the stage for success: implementation of developmental and behavioral screening and surveillance in primary care practice: the North Carolina Assuring Better Child Health and Development (ABCD) project, *Pediatrics* 118:e183–e188, 2006.

Emde RN: Development terminable and interminable. I. Innate and motivational factors from infancy, *Int J Psychoanal* 69:23–42, 1988.

Emde RN, Buchsbaum H: "Didn't you hear my mommy?" Autonomy with connectedness in moral self emergence. In Cicchetti D, Beeghly M, editors: *The self in transition: infancy to childhood*, Chicago, 1990, University of Chicago Press.

Emde RN, Mann TL, Bertacchi J: Organizational environments that support mental health, *Zero to Three* 22:67–69, 2001.

Erikson E: *Insight and responsibility*, New York, 1964, Norton.

Fiese BH: Routines of daily living and rituals in family life: a glimpse at stability and change during the early child-raising years, *Zero to Three* 22:10–13, 2002.

Flavell J: *Cognitive development*, Englewood Cliffs, NJ, 1977, Prentice-Hall.

Fowler J: *Stages of faith: the psychology of human development and the quest for meaning*, New York, 1981, Harper & Row.

Freud A: *The writings of Anna Freud*, (vol V), New York, 1974, International Universities Press.

Freud S: *An outline of psychoanalysis*, London, 1938, Hogarth.

Garzon DL, Thrasher C, Tiernan K: Providing optimal care for children with developmental disorders, *Nurse Pract* 35(10):30–39, 2010.

Gesell A: *The first five years of life*, New York, 1940, Harper.

Gilligan C: *In a different voice: psychological theory and women's development*, Cambridge, MA, 1982, Harvard University Press.

Glascoe FP: Detecting and addressing developmental and behavioral problems in primary care, *Pediatr Nurs* 26:251–257, 2000.

Hack M, Taylor HG, Drotar D, et al: Poor predictive validity of the Bayley Scales of Infant Development for cognitive function of extremely low birth weight children at school age, *Pediatrics* 116:333–341, 2005.

Hagan JF, Shaw JS, Duncan P: *Bright Futures: guidelines for health supervision of infants, children, and adolescent*, ed 3, Elk Grove Village, IL, 2008, American Academy of Pediatrics.

Havighurst R: *Human development and education*, New York, 1953, Longmans, Green.

Ireton H: *Child development inventory manual*, Minneapolis, MN, 1992, Behavior Science Systems, Inc.

Jackson Allen P, Vessey J, Shapiro NA: *Primary care of the child with a chronic condition*, ed 4, St Louis, 2010, Mosby.

Kelly JL, Barnard KE: Assessment of parent-child interaction: implications for early intervention. In Shonkoff JP, Meisels SJ, editors: *Handbook of early childhood education*, New York, 2000, Cambridge University Press.

Klaus M, Kennel J: *Maternal-infant bonding*, St Louis, 1976, Mosby.

Kochanska G, Coy KC, Murray KT: The development of self-regulation in the first four years of life, *Child Devel* 72:1091–1111, 2001.

Kohlberg L: Stage and sequence: the cognitive-development approach to socialization. In Gastin D, editor: *Handbook of socialization: theory and research*, New York, 1969, Rand McNally.

Kubicek L: Fresh perspectives on young children and family routines, *Zero to Three* 22:4–9, 2002.

Lewin K: *Principles of topological psychology*, New York, 1936, McGraw-Hill.

Lord C, Rutter M, Le Couteur A: Autism Diagnostic Observation Interview—Revised: a revised version of a diagnostic interview for caregivers of individuals with possible pervasive developmental disorders, *J Autism Dev Disord* 24:659–685, 1994.

Mahler M, Pine F, Bergman A: *The psychological birth of the human infant*, New York, 1975, Basic Books.

Mahrer A: *Experiencing: a humanistic theory of psychology and psychiatry*, New York, 1978, Brunner/Mazel.

Maslow A: *The farther reaches of human nature*, New York, 1971, Viking.

McCrory E, De Brito SA, Viding E: Research review: the neurobiology and genetics of maltreatment and adversity, *J Child Psychol Psychiatry*, 51(10):1079–1095, 2010.

McPherson M, Arango P, Fox H, et al: A new definition of children with special health care needs, *Pediatrics* 102:137–140, 1998.

Minkovitz C, Strobino D, Hughart N, et al: Early effects of the Healthy Steps for Young Children program, *Arch Pediatr Adolesc Med* 155:470–479, 2001.

Minuchin S: *Families and family therapy*, Cambridge, MA, 1974, Harvard University Press.

Moorthy LN, Peterson MGE, Baratelli MJ, et al: Preliminary cross-cultural adaptation of a new pediatric health-related quality of life scale in children with systemic lupus erythematosus: an international effort, *Lupus* 19:83–88, 2010.

Mott S: Developmental theories: how the child grows. In Mott S, James SR, Sperhac A, editors: *Nursing care of children and families*, New York, 1990, Addison-Wesley.

Mullen E: *Mullen Scales of Early Learning*, Cranston, RI, 1989, T.O.T.O.L. Child.

National Association of Pediatric Nurse Practitioners (NAPNAP): Position statement: the pediatric health care/medical home: Key issues on delivery reimbursement, and leadership, *J Pediatr Healthcare* 23:A23–A24, 2009.

Olson LM, Inkelas M, Halfron N, et al: Overview of the content of health supervision for young children: reports from parents and pediatricians, *Pediatrics* 113:1907–1916, 2004.

Perrin E, Stancin T: A continuing dilemma: whether and how to screen for concerns about children's behavior, *Pediatr Rev* 23:264–275, 2002.

Piaget J: *The theory of stages in cognitive development*, New York, 1969, McGraw-Hill.

Regalado M, Sareen H, Inkelas M, et al: Parents' discipline of young children: results from the National Survey of Early Childhood Health, *Pediatrics* 113:1952–1958, 2004.

Rogoff B: *Apprenticeship in thinking: cognitive development in social context*, New York, 1990, Oxford University Press.

Ruperto N, Ravelli A, Pistorio A, et al: Cross-cultural adaptation and psychometric evaluation of the Childhood Health Assessment Questionnaire (CHAQ) and the Child Health Questionnaire (CHQ) in 32 countries. Review of the general methodology, *Clin Exp Rheumatol* 19:S1–S9, 2001.

Rydz D, Shevell MI, Majnemer A, et al: Developmental screening, *J Child Neurol* 20:4–21, 2005.

Schopler E, Reichler RJ, Renner BR: *The Childhood Autism Rating Scale*, Los Angeles, 1986, Western Psychological Services.

Shonkoff JP, Phillips DA: *From neurons to neighborhoods: the science of early childhood development*, Washington, DC, 2000, National Academy Press.

Siegler R, Liebert D, Liebert R: Inhelder and Piaget's pendulum problem, *Dev Psychol* 9:97–101, 1973.

Skinner BF: *Science and human behavior*, New York, 1953, The Macmillan Free Press.

Squires J, Potter L, Bricker D: *The ASQ users guide*, ed 3, Baltimore, 2009, Paul H Brooks Publishing Co.

Stein M: Preparing families for the toddler and preschool years, *Contemp Pediatr* 15:88–97, 1998.

Stern D: *The interpersonal world of the infant: a view from psychoanalysis and developmental psychology*, New York, 1985, Basic Books.

Sullivan H: *The fusion of psychiatry and social sciences*, New York, 1964, Norton.

Thomas RM: *Comparing theories of child development*, Belmont, CA, 1985, Wadsworth.

Trevarthen C, Aitken KJ: Infant intersubjectivity: research, theory, and clinical applications, *J Child Psychol Psychiat* 42:3–48, 2001.

Vygotsky LS: *Mind in society*, ed 4, Cambridge, MA, 1978, Harvard University Press.

Webster-Stratton C: *The incredible years: a trouble shooting guide for parents of children aged 2-8*, Seattle, WA, 2005, Incredible Years Press.

Wolraich ML, Felice ME, Drotar D, editors: *The classification of child and adolescent mental health diagnoses in primary care: diagnostic and statistical manual for primary care (DSM-PC), child and adolescent version*, Elk Grove Village, IL, 1996, American Academy of Pediatrics.

CHAPTER 5

American Academy of Pediatrics (AAP) Committee on Children with Disabilities, et al: Identifying infants and young children with developmental disorders in the medical home: an algorithm for developmental surveillance and screening, *Pediatrics* 118:405–420, 2006.

American Academy of Pediatrics (AAP) Section on Breastfeeding: Breast-feeding and the use of human milk, *Pediatrics* 115:496–506, 2005.

American Academy of Pediatrics (AAP) Task Force on Sudden Infant Death Syndrome: The changing concept of sudden infant death syndrome: diagnostic coding shifts, controversies regarding the sleeping environment, and new variables to consider in reducing risk, *Pediatrics* 116:1245–1255, 2005.

American Academy of Pediatrics (AAP): AAP publication retired and reaffirmed, *Pediatrics* 123:188, 2009.

American Heart Association, American Academy of Pediatrics, Gidding SS, et al: Dietary recommendations for children and adolescents: a guide for practitioners, *Pediatrics* 117(2):544–559, 2006.

Cox JL, Holden JM, Sagovsky R: Detection of postnatal depression: development of the 10-item Edinburgh Postnatal Depression Scale, *Br J Psychiatry* 150:782–786, 1987.

Dixon SD, Stein M, editors: *Encounters with children: pediatric behavior and development*, St Louis, 2006, Mosby.

Hagan JF, Shaw JS, Duncan PM, editors: *Bright Futures: guidelines for health supervision of infants, children, and adolescents*, ed 3, Elk Grove Village, IL, 2008, American Academy of Pediatrics.

Hamilton BE, Martin JA, Ventura SJ: Births: preliminary data for 2008, *Natl Vital Stat Rep* 58(16):1–18, 2010.

Hauck FR, Omojokun OO, Siadatay MR: Do pacifiers reduce the risk of sudden infant death syndrome? A meta-analysis, *Pediatrics* 116:e716–e723, 2005.

Johnson CP, Myers SM, Council on Children with Disabilities: Identification and evaluation of children with autism spectrum disorders, *Pediatrics* 120:1183–1215, 2007.

Ma D: Babies should sleep on their backs, play on stomachs, *AAP News* 30(9):30, 2009.

Spinelli MG: Postpartum psychosis: detection of risk and management, *Am J Psychiatry* 166:405–408, 2009.

Tejada-Vera B, Sutton PD: Births, marriages, divorces and deaths: provisional data for 2009, *Natl Vital Stat Rep* 58(25):1–6, 2010.

Wisner KL, Parry BL, Pointek CM: Postpartum depression, *N Engl J Med* 347(3):194–199, 2002.

Xu J, Kochanek KD, Murphy SL, et al: Deaths, final data for 2007, *Natl Vital Stat Rep* 58(19):1–73, 2010.

CHAPTER 6

American Academy of Pediatrics (AAP) Section on Pediatric Dentistry: Oral health risk assessment timing and establishment of the dental home, *Pediatrics* 111:1113–1116, 2003; (reaffirmed in: policy statement-AAP publications retired and reaffirmed, *Pediatrics* 124:845, 2009).

American Academy of Pediatrics (AAP) Council on Communications and Media: Policy statement: media violence, *Pediatrics* 124:1495–1503, 2009.

Brazelton TB, Sparrow JD: *Touchpoints three to six, your child's emotional and behavioral development*, Cambridge, MA, 2006, Perseus Publishing.

Bureau of Labor Statistics: *Employment of characteristics of families statistics*. U.S. Department of Labor USDL publication number USDL-10–0721. Available at http://www.bls.gov/news.release/famee.nr0.htm. Accessed July 11, 2010.

Dixon S, Stein M: *Encounters with children: pediatric behavior and development*, ed 4, St Louis, 2006, Mosby.

Feldman HM: Evaluation and management of language and speech disorder in preschool children, *Pediatr Rev* 26:131–140, 2005.

Ginsburg KR, American Academy of Pediatrics (AAP) Committee on Communications and Committee on Psychosocial Aspects of Child and Family Health: The importance of play in promoting healthy child development and maintaining strong parent-child bonds, *Pediatrics* 119:182–191, 2007.

Hagan JF, Shaw JS, Duncan PM, editors: *Bright Futures: guidelines for health supervision of infants, children, and adolescents*, ed 3, Elk Grove Village, IL, 2008, American Academy of Pediatrics.

Hammer CS, Farkas G, Maczuga S: The language and literacy development of Head Start children: a study using the family and child experiences survey database, *Lang Speech Hear Serv Sch* 41(1):70–83, 2010.

Maughan A, Cicchetti D, Toth SL, Rogosch FA: Early occurring maternal depression and maternal negativity in predicting young children's emotional regulation and socioemotional difficulties, *J Abnorm Child Psychol* 35:685–703, 2007.

McCurdy LE, Winterbottom KE, Mehta SS, et al: Using nature and outdoor activity to improve children's health, *Curr Prob Adolesc Health Care* 40(5):102–117, 2010.

National Association of Pediatric Nurse Practitioners (NAPNAP): NAPNAP position statement on the identification and prevention of overweight and obesity in the pediatric population, *J Pediatr Health Care* 23(6):A15–A16, 2009.

Pascoe JM, Stolfi A, Ormond MB: Correlates of mothers' persistent depressive symptoms: a national study, *J Pediatr Health Care* 20:261–269, 2006.

Trifiletti LB, Shields W, Bishai D, et al: Tipping the scales: obese children and child safety seats, *Pediatrics* 117:1197–1202, 2006.

U.S. Census Bureau: *Who's minding the kids? Child care arrangements: Summer*, 2006, U.S. Census Bureau. Available at http://www.census.gov/population/www/socdemo/child/tables-2006.html. Accessed July 11, 2010.

Veitch J, Salmon J, Ball K: Individual, social and physical environmental correlates of children's active free-play: a cross-sectional study, *Intl J Behav Nutr Phys Act* 7:11, 2010.

CHAPTER 7

Beesdo K, Knappe S, Pine DS: Anxiety and anxiety disorders in children and adolescents: developmental issues and implications for DSM-V, *Psychiatr Clin North Am* 32:483–524, 2009.

Bernstein B: *Anxiety disorder, separation anxiety and school refusal*, 2008. Available at www.medicine.medscape.com. Accessed April 5, 2010.

Bierman KL, Domitrovich CE, Nix RL, et al: Promoting academic and social-emotional school readiness: the head start REDI program, *Child Dev* 79(6):1802–1817, 2008.

Boyer E: Ready to learn: a mandate for the nation, *Young Child* 48:54–57, 1993.

Brooks SJ, Kutcher S: Diagnosis and measurement of adolescent depression: a review of the commonly utilized instruments, *J Child Adolesc Psychopharmacol* 11:341–376, 2001.

Byrd RS: School failure: assessment, intervention, and prevention in primary pediatric care, *Pediatr Rev* 26(7):233–243, 2005.

Campbell WN, Skarakis-Doyle E: School-aged children with SLI: the ICF framework for collaborative service delivery, *J Commun Disord* 40:513–535, 2007.

Cartland J, Ruch-Ross HS: Health behaviors of school-age children: evidence from one large city, *J Sch Health* 76:175–180, 2006.

Currie J: Health disparities and gaps in school readiness, *Future Child* 15(1):117–138, 2005.

Dube SR, Orpinas P: Understanding excessive school absenteeism as school refusal behavior, *Child Sch* 31:87–95, 2009.

Dubow EF, Boxer P, Huesmann LR: Long-term effects of parents' education on children's educational and occupational success: mediation by family interactions, child aggression, and teenage aspirations, *Merrill Palmer Q* 55(3):1–19, 2009.

Foy JM, Perrin J, American Academy of Pediatrics Task Force on Mental Health: Enhancing pediatric mental health care: strategies for preparing community, *Pediatrics* 125:S75–S86, 2010.

Gall G, Pagano ME, Desmond DM, et al: Utility of psychosocial screening at a school-based health center, *J Sch Health* 70:292–298, 2000.

Hagan JF, Shaw JS, Duncan P: *Bright Futures: guidelines for health supervision of infants, children, and adolescents*, ed 3 rev, Elk Grove, IL, 2008, American Academy of Pediatrics.

Jellinek MS, Murphy JM, Little M, et al: Use of the pediatric symptom checklist to screen for psychosocial problems in pediatric primary care, *Arch Pediatr Adolesc Med* 153:254–260, 1999.

Jellinek MS, Murphy JM, Robinson J, et al: Pediatric symptom checklist: screening school-age children for psychosocial dysfunction, *J Pediatr* 112:201–209, 1988.

Jellinek MS, Patel BP, Froehle MC, editors: *Bright Futures in practice: mental health, practice guide*, (vol I), Arlington, VA, 2002a, National Center for Education in Maternal and Child Health.

Jellinek MS, Patel BP, Froehle MC, editors: *Bright Futures in practice: mental health, tool kit*, (vol II), Arlington, VA, 2002b, National Center for Education in Maternal and Child Health.

Jensen PS, Watanabe HK, Richters JE, et al: Scales, diagnoses, and child psychopathology: II. Comparing the CBCL and the DISC against external validators, *J Abnorm Child Psychol* 24:151–168, 1996.

Kearney C: Form and functions of school refusal behavior in youth: an empirical analysis of school absenteeism severity, *J Child Psychol Psychiatry* 48:53–61, 2007.

Kelly DP: Patterns of development and function in the school-aged child. In Kliegman RM, Behrman RE, Jenson HB, et al: *Nelson textbook of pediatrics*, ed 18, Philadelphia, 2007, Saunders, pp 139–145.

Kohlberg L: *The philosophy of moral development*, San Francisco, 1981, Harper & Row.

Levine MD: *Pediatric examination of educational readiness at middle childhood [Revised] (PEERA-MID-2)*, Cambridge, MA, 1995-1996, Educators Publishing Services.

Mahoney JL, Levine MD, Hinga B: The development of after-school program educators through university-community partnerships, *Applied Develop Sci* 14:89–105, 2010.

McAllister CL, Wilson PC, Green BL, et al: "Come and talk a walk:" listening to Early Head Start parents on school-readiness as a matter of child, family, and community health, *Am J Public Health* 95(4):617–625, 2005.

Myers K, Winters NC: Ten-year review of rating scales. II. Scales for internalizing disorders, *J Am Acad Child Adolesc Psychiatry* 41:634–659, 2002.

Noll JG, Shenk CE, Barnes JE, et al: Childhood abuse, avatar choices, and other risk factors associated with internet-initiated victimization of adolescent girls, *Pediatrics* 123:e1078–e1083, 2009.

Ogden CL, Caroll MD, Curtin LR, et al: Prevalence of high body mass index in US children and adolescents, 2007-2008, *JAMA* 303(3):242–249, 2010.

Shapiro L, Hurry J, Masterson J, et al: Classroom implications of recent research into literacy development: from predictors to assessment, *Dyslexia* 15:1–22, 2009.

Sharif I, Sargent JD: Association between television, movie, and video game exposure and school performance, *Pediatrics* 118(4):e1061–e1070, 2006.

Smith DK, Johnson AB, Pears KC, et al: Child maltreatment and foster care: unpacking the effects of prenatal and postnatal parental substance abuse, *Child Maltreat* 12:150–160, 2007.

Stafford B, Boris NW, Dalton R: Anxiety disorders. In Kliegman RM, Behrman RE, Jenson HB, et al, editors: *Nelson textbook of pediatrics*, ed 18, Philadelphia, 2007, Saunders, pp 117–120.

Tucker CJ, Updegraff K: The relative contributions of parents and siblings to child and adolescent development. In Kramer L, Conger KJ, editors: *Siblings as agents of socialization: new directions for child and adolescent development*, San Francisco, 2009, Jossey-Bass.

Tzoumas AC, Tzoumas JL, Burlingame JM, et al: The Y-OQ-12: psychosocial screening of youth in primary care medicine using items from an outcome measure, *Clin Psychol Psychother* 14:488–503, 2007.

U.S. Department of Health and Human Services (USD-HHS): *Substance Abuse and Mental Health Services Administration (SAMHSA): Fetal alcohol spectrum disorders: the basics*, Rockville, MD, 2006, SAMHSA.

U.S. Department of Health and Human Services (USDHHS): Substance Abuse and Mental Health Services Administration (SAMHSA): *Results from the 2008 National survey on drug use and health: national findings*, Rockville, MD, 2008, SAMHSA.

Vanderbilt-Adriance E, Shaw DS: Conceptualizing and re-evaluating resilience across levels of risk, time and domains of competence, *Clin Child Fam Psychol Rev* 11:30–58, 2008.

Wierzbicki M: A parent form of the children's depression inventory: reliability and validity in nonclinical populations, *J Clin Psychol* 43:390–397, 1987.

CHAPTER 8

Al Sabbah H, Vereecken CA, Elgar FJ, et al: Body weight dissatisfaction and communication with parents among adolescents in 24 countries: international cross-sectional survey, *BMC Public Health* 9:52, 2009.

American Academy of Pediatrics: Committee on Adolescence: Homosexuality and adolescence, *Pediatrics* 92(6):631–634, 1993.

Angle S, Keskinin S, Lapinleimu H, et al: Weight gain since infancy and prepubertal body dissatisfaction, *Arch Pediatr Adolesc Med* 159(6):567–571, 2005.

Berlan ED, Bravender T: Confidentiality, consent, and caring for the adolescent patient, *Curr Opin Pediatr* 21(4):450–456, 2009.

Blakemore SJ, Choudhury S: Development of the adolescent brain: implications for executive function and social cognition, *J Child Psychol Psychiatry* 47(3-4):296–312, 2006.

Botvin GJ, Griffin KW: School-based programmes to prevent alcohol, tobacco and other drug use, *Int Rev Psychiatry* 19(6):607–615, 2007.

Butt AL, Anderson HA, Gates DJ: Parental influence and effects of pro-smoking media messages on adolescents in Oklahoma, *J Okla State Med Assoc* 102(5):147–151, 2009.

Cabral L: Twenty-first century skills for students: hands-on learning after school builds school and life success, *New Dir Youth Dev* (110):155–161, 2006.

Centers for Disease Control and Prevention (CDC): Cigarette use among high school students—United States, 1991-2007, *MMWR* 57(25):686–688, 2008.

Centers for Disease Control and Prevention (CDC): "Choking game" awareness and participation among 8th graders—Oregon, 2008, *MMWR* 59(1):1–5, 2010.

Council on Scientific Affairs: American Medical Association: Health care needs of gay men and lesbians in the United States, *JAMA* 275(17):1354–1359, 1996.

Crone EA: Executive functions in adolescence: inferences from brain and behavior, *Dev Sci* 12(6):825–830, 2009.

Dalton MA, Adachi-Mejia AM, Longacre MR, et al: Parental rules and monitoring of children's movie viewing associated with children's risk for smoking and drinking, *Pediatrics* 118(5):1932–1942, 2006.

Dowshen N, Garofalo R: Optimizing primary care for LGBTQ youth, *Contemp Pediatr* 26(10):58–66, 2009.

Eaton DK, Kann L, Kinchen S, et al: Youth risk behavior surveillance—United States, 2005, *MMWR Surveill Summ* 55(ss5):1–108, 2006.

Eaton DK, Kann L, Kinchen S, et al: Youth risk behavior surveillance—United States, 2009, *MMWR Surveill Summ* 59(SS-5):1–142, 2010.

Elkind D: *All grown up and no place to go: teenagers in crisis*, Reading, MA, 1984, Addison-Wesley.

Ellickson PL, Tucker JS, Klein DJ: Reducing early smokers' risk for future smoking and other problem behavior: insights from a five-year longitudinal study, *J Adolesc Health* 43(4):394–400, 2008.

Elster A, Kuznets N: *A MA guidelines for adolescent preventive services (GAPS)*, Baltimore, 1994, Williams & Wilkins.

Emans SJ, Brown RT, Davis A, et al: Society for Adolescent Medicine position paper on reproductive health care for adolescents, *J Adolesc Health* 12(8):644–661, 1991.

Euling SY, Herman-Giddens ME, Lee PA, et al: Examination of US puberty-timing data from 1940 to 1994 for secular trends: panel findings, *Pediatrics* 121(S3):S172–S191, 2008.

Fleming MF, Balousek SL, Grossberg PM, et al: Brief physician advice for heavy drinking college students: a randomized controlled trial in college health clinics, *J Stud Alcohol Drugs* 71(1):23–31, 2010.

Forhan SE, Gottlieb SL, Sternberg MR, et al: Prevalence of sexually transmitted infections among female adolescents aged 14 to 19 in the United States, *Pediatrics* 124(6):1505–1512, 2009.

Goldenring JM, Rosen DS: Getting into adolescent heads: an essential update, *Contemp Pediatr* 21(1):64–90, 2004.

Guerri C, Pascual M: Mechanisms involved in the neurotoxic, cognitive, and neurobehavioral effects of alcohol consumption during adolescence, *Alcohol* 44(1):15–26, 2010.

Hagan JF, Shaw JS, Duncan PM, editors: *Bright Futures: guidelines for health supervision of infants, children, and adolescents*, ed 3, Elk Grove Village, IL, 2008, American Academy of Pediatrics.

Hall GS: *Adolescence: its psychology and its relations to physiology, anthropology, sociology, sex, crime, religion and education*, Englewood Cliffs, NJ, 1904, Prentice-Hall.

Halpern CT, Kaestle CE, Hallfors DD: Perceived physical maturity, age of romantic partner, and adolescent risk behavior, *Prev Sci* 8(1):1–10, 2007.

Heatherton TF, Sargent JD: Does watching smoking in movies promote teenage smoking? *Curr Dir Psychol Sci* 18(2):63–67, 2009.

Hendrik RE, Helvie MA: United States Preventative Health Services Task Force screening mammography recommendations: science ignored, *Am J Roentgenol* 196(2):W112–W116, 2011.

Henriksen L, Dauphinee AL, Wang Y, et al: Industry sponsored anti-smoking ads and adolescent reactance: test of a boomerang effect, *Tob Control* 15(1):13–18, 2006.

Herman-Giddens ME: Recent data on pubertal milestones in United States children: the secular trend toward earlier development, *Int J Androl* 29(1):241–246, 2006.

Herrmann M, King K, Weitzman M: Prenatal tobacco smoke and postnatal secondhand smoke exposure and child neurodevelopment, *Curr Opin Pediatr* 20(2):184–190, 2008.

Hicks KM, Hinck SM: Concept analysis of self-mutilation, *J Adv Nurs* 64(4):408–413, 2008.

Jackson C, Dickinson D: Enabling parents who smoke to prevent their children from initiating smoking: results from a 3-year intervention evaluation, *Arch Pediatr Adolesc Med* 160(1):56–62, 2006.

Janssen J, Reig S, Parellada M, et al: Regional gray matter volume deficits in adolescents with first-episode psychosis, *J Am Acad Child Adolesc Psychiatry* 47(11):1311–1320, 2008.

Joffe A, Morris RE: Adolescent substance use and abuse. In Neinstein LS, Gordon CM, Katzman DK, et al: *Adolescent healthcare: a practical guide*, Philadelphia, 2008, Lippincott Williams & Wilkins.

Kandel DB, Hu MC, Griesler PC, et al: On the development of nicotine dependence in adolescence, *Drug Alcohol Depend* 91(1):26–39, 2007.

Karp I, O'Laughlin J, Hanley J, et al: Risk factors for tobacco dependence in adolescent smokers, *Tob Control* 15(3):199–204, 2006.

Klonsky ED, Olino TM: Identifying clinically distinct subgroups of selfinjurers among young adults: a latent class analysis, *J Consult Clin Psychol* 76(1):22–27, 2008.

Laumann AE, Derick AJ: Tattoos and body piercings in the United States: a national data set, *J Am Acad Dermatol* 55(3):413–421, 2006.

Lee R: Health care problems of lesbian, gay, bisexual, and transgender patients, *West J Med* 172(6):403–408, 2000.

Luna B, Padmanabhan A, O'Hearn K: What has fMRI told us about the development of cognitive control through adolescence? *Brain Cogn* 72(1):101–113, 2010.

Maldonado-Devincci AM, Badanich KA, Kirstein C: Alcohol during adolescence selectively alters immediate and long-term behavior and neurochemistry, *Alcohol* 44(1):57–66, 2010.

McLeod K, White V, Mullins R, et al: How do friends influence smoking uptake? Findings from qualitative interviews with identical twins, *J Genet Psychol* 169(2):117–131, 2008.

Meckler GD, Elliott MN, Kanouse DE, et al: Nondisclosure of sexual orientation to a physician among a sample of gay, lesbian, and bisexual youth, *Arch Pediatr Adolesc Med* 160:1248–1254, 2006.

Moreira MT, Smith LA, Foxcroft D: Social norms interventions to reduce alcohol misuse in university or college students, *Cochrane Database Syst Rev* 8(3):CD006748, 2009.

Needleman IG, Binnie VI, Ainamo A, et al: Improving the effectiveness of tobacco use cessation (TUC), *Int Dent J* 60(1):50–59, 2010.

O'Loughlin J, Karp I, Koulis T, et al: Determinants of first puff and daily cigarette smoking in adolescents, *Am J Epidemiol* 170(5):585–597, 2009.

Pagsberg AK, Barre FC, Raabjerg AM, et al: Structural brain abnormalities in early onset first-episode psychosis, *J Neural Transm* 114(4):489–498, 2007.

Reiff MI: Adolescent school failure: failure to thrive in adolescence, *Pediatr Rev* 19(6):199–207, 1998.

Robinson TN, Chang JY, Haydel KF, et al: Overweight concerns and body dissatisfaction among third-grade children: the impacts of ethnicity and socioeconomic status, *J Pediatr* 138:181–187, 2001.

Ryan C, Huebner D, Diaz RM, et al: Family rejection as a predictor of negative health outcomes in white and Latino lesbian, gay, and bisexual young adults, *Pediatrics* 123(1):346–352, 2009.

Saab H, Klinger D: School differences in adolescent health and wellbeing: findings from the Canadian Health Behaviour in School-aged Children Study, *Soc Sci Med* 70(6):850–858, 2010.

Sanders RA, Kuo DZ, Levy E, et al: Transitioning adolescents to adult care and adulthood: is it time yet? *Contemp Pediatr* 26(12):46–55, 2009.

Schaus JF, Sole ML, McCoy TP, et al: Alcohol screening and brief intervention in a college student health center: a randomized controlled trial, *J Stud Alcohol Drugs Suppl* 16:131–141, 2009.

Schwartz PD, Maynard AM, Uzelac SM: Adolescent egocentrism: a contemporary view, *Adolescence* 43(171):441–448, 2008.

Shaw P, Greenstein D, Lerch J, et al: Intellectual ability and cortical development in children and adolescents, *Nature* 440(7084):676–679, 2006.

Sherar LB, Mirwald RL, Baxter-Jones ADG, et al: Prediction of adult height using maturity-based cumulative height velocity curves, *J Pediatr* 147(4):508–514, 2005.

Tanner J: *Growth at adolescence*, Oxford, UK, 1962, Blackwell.

Terry-McElrath YM, Wakefield MA, Emery S, et al: State anti-tobacco advertising and smoking outcomes by gender and race/ethnicity, *Ethn Health* 12(4):339–362, 2007.

U.S. Preventive Services Task Force (USPSTF): *Screening for testicular cancer*, February 2004. Available at www.uspreventiveservicestaskforce.org/uspstf.htm. Accessed May 11, 2011.

U.S. Preventive Services Task Force (USPSTF): Screening for breast cancer, *Ann Intern Med* 151:716–726, 2009.

Warren CW, Jones NR, Peruga A, et al: Global youth tobacco surveillance, 2000-2007, *MMWR Surveill Summ* 57(1):1–28, 2008.

Waters S, Cross D, Shaw T: Does the nature of schools matter? An exploration of selected school ecology factors on adolescent perceptions of school connectedness, *Br J Educ Psychol*, 80 (pt 3):381-402, 2010.

Whitlock J, Knox KL: The relationship between self-injurious behavior and suicide in a young adult population, *Arch Pediatr Adolesc Med* 161(7):634–640, 2007.

Whitlock J, Eckenrode J, Silverman D: Self-injurious behaviors in a college population, *Pediatrics* 117(6):1939–1948, 2006.

Wilkinson AV, Shete S, Prokhorov AV: The moderating role of parental smoking on their children's attitudes toward smoking among a predominantly minority sample: a cross-sectional analysis, *Subst Abuse Treat Prev Policy* 3:18, 2008.

Wilkinson AV, Shete S, Vasudevan S, et al: Influence of subjective social status on the relationship between positive outcome expectations and experimentation with cigarettes, *J Adolesc Health* 44(4):342–348, 2009.

Williams EC, Daley AM, DeSanto Iennaco J: Assessing non-suicidal selfinjurious behavior in adolescents, *Am J Nurse Pract* 4(5):18–26, 2010.

CHAPTER 9

American Academy of Pediatrics (AAP): Recommendations for preventive pediatric health care. In Hagan JF, Shaw JS, Duncan PM, editors: *Bright futures: guidelines for health supervision of infants, children, and adolescents*, ed 3, Elk Grove Village, IL, 2008, AAP, p 591.

Bandura A: Self-efficacy: the exercise of control, New York, 1997, WH Freeman and Company.

Bennett IM, Robbins S, Al-Shamali N, et al: Screening for low literacy among adult caregivers of pediatric patients, *Fam Med* 35(8):585–590, 2003.

Betz CL: Health literacy: the missing link in the provision of health care for children and their families, *J Pediatr Nurs* 22(4):257–258, 2007.

Betz CL, Ruccione K, Meeske K, et al: Health literacy: a pediatric nursing concern, *Pediatr Nurs* 34(3):231–239, 2008.

Borzekowski D: Considering children and health literacy: a theoretical approach, *Pediatrics* 124 (Suppl 3):S282–S288, 2009.

Brazelton TB, O'Brien M, Brandt K: Combining relationships and development: applying touchpoints to individual and community practices, *Infant Young Child* 10:74–84, 1997.

Brazelton TB, Sparrow J: *The touchpoints model of development*, Boston, 2003, Brazelton Touchpoints Center.

Cooper S, Guthrie B: Ecological influences on health-promoting and health-compromising behaviors: a socially embedded approach to urban African American girls' health, *Fam Community Health* 30(1):29–41, 2007.

Davis TC, Wolf MS, Arnold CL, et al: Development and validation of the Rapid Estimate of Adolescent Literacy in Medicine (REALM-Teen): a tool to screen adolescents for below-grade reading in health care settings, *Pediatrics* 118(6):e1707–e1714, 2006.

DeWalt D, Hink A: Health literacy and child health outcomes: a systematic review of the literature, *Pediatrics* 124(Suppl 3):S265–S274, 2009.

Downey LA, Zun L: Assessing adult literacy in urban healthcare settings, *J Natl Med Assoc* 11(11):1304–1308, 2008.

Dworkin P: Coming full circle: reflections at the interface of developmental-behavioral and general pediatrics, *J Dev Behav Pediatr* 28(2):167–172, 2007.

Eichler K, Weiser S, Brugger U: The costs of limited health literacy: a systematic review, *Int J Public Health* 54(5):313–324, 2009.

Glasgow RE, Emont S, Miller DC: Assessing delivery of the five "As" for patient-centered counseling, *Health Promot Int* 21(3):245–255, 2006.

Gordon M: *Nursing diagnosis: process and application*, New York, 1987, McGraw-Hill.

Gordon M: *Manual of nursing diagnosis*, ed 12, Sudbury, MA, 2010, Jones and Bartlett.

Griffiths F, Lindenmeyer A, Powell J, et al: Why are health care interventions delivered over the internet? A systematic review of the published literature, *J Med Internet Res* 8(2):e10, 2006.

Hagan JF, Shaw JS, Duncan PM: *Bright Futures: guidelines for health supervision of infants, children, and adolescents*, ed 3, Elk Grove Village, IL, 2008, AAP.

Institute of Medicine (IOM): *Crossing the quality chasm: a new health system for the 21st century*, Washington, DC, 2001, National Academies Press.

Koopman H, Baars RA, Chaplin J, et al: Illness through the eyes of the child: the development of children's understanding of the causes of illness, *Patient Educ Counsel* 55(3):363–370, 2004.

Mahat G, Scoloveno M, De Leon T, et al: Preliminary evidence of an adolescent HIV/AIDS peer education program, *J Pediatr Nurs* 23(5):358–363, 2008.

Mancuso J: Assessment and measurement of health literacy: an integrative review of the literature, *Nurs Health Sci* 11(1):77–89, 2009.

Mangione-Smith R, DeCristofaro AH, Setodji CM, et al: The quality of ambulatory care delivered to children in the United States, *N Engl J Med* 357(15):1515–1523, 2007.

Masters K: For what purpose and reasons do doctors use the internet: a systematic review, *Int J Med Inform* 77(1):4–16, 2008.

McGinnis M, Foege W: Actual causes of death in the United States, *JAMA* 270(18):2207–2212, 1993.

Miller WR, Rollnick S: *Motivational interviewing: preparing people to change addictive behavior*, New York, 1991, The Guilford Press.

Mokdad AH, Marks JS, Stroup DF, et al: Actual causes of death in the United States, 2000, *JAMA* 291(10):1238–1245, 2004.

Moyer V, Butler M: Gaps in the evidence for well-child care: a challenge for our profession, *Pediatrics* 114(6):1511–1521, 2004.

Myant KA, Williams JM: Children's concepts of health and illness: understanding of contagious illnesses, non-contagious illnesses and injuries, *J Health Psychol* 10(6):805–819, 2005.

Nicolas DB, Picone G, Vigneaux A, et al: Evaluation of an online peer support network for adolescents with chronic kidney disease, *J Technol Hum Serv* 27(1):23–33, 2009.

Nielsen-Bohlman L, Panzer AM, Kindig DA: *Health literacy: a prescription to end confusion*, Washington, DC, 2004, The National Academies Press.

Nutbeam D: Health literacy as a public health goal: a challenge for contemporary health education and communication strategies into the 21st century, *Health Promot Int* 15:259–267, 2000.

Pender N, Murdaugh CL, Parsons MA: *Health promotion in nursing practice*, ed 6, Upper Saddle River, NJ, 2011, Prentice-Hall.

Prochaska J: Disease management needs new paradigms, *J Gen Intern Med* 10(8):472–473, 1995.

Prochaska J, DiClemente C, Norcross J: In search of how people change: applications to addictive behaviors, *Am Psychol* 47(9):1102–1114, 1992.

Prochaska J, Velicer WF, Rossi JS, et al: Stages of change and decisional balance for 12 problem behaviors, *Health Psychol* 13(1):39–46, 1994.

Radecki L, Olson LM, Frintner MP, et al: What do families want from well-child care: including parents in the rethinking discussion, *Pediatrics* 124(3): 858–865, 2009.

Redman B: *Patient education,* ed 7, St Louis, 1993, Mosby.

Reinhardt C, Lopker N, Noack M, et al: Peer tutoring pilot program for the improvement of oral health behavior in underprivileged and immigrant children, *Pediatr Dent* 31(7):481–485, 2009.

Rogers EM: *Diffusion of innovations,* New York, 1983, Free Press.

Roose GA, Yazdani AF, John AM: A focus group investigation into young children's understanding of mental health and their views on appropriate services for their age group, *Child Care Health Dev* 29(6): 545–550, 2003.

Rubak S, Sandbaek A, Lauritzen T, et al: Motivational interviewing: a systematic review and meta-analysis, *Br J Gen Pract* 55(513):305–312, 2005.

Sanders LM, Federico S, Klass P, et al: Literacy and child health: a systematic review, *Arch Ped Adolesc Med* 163(2):131–140, 2009.

Shaw SJ, Huebner C, Armin J, et al: The role of culture in health literacy and chronic disease screening and management, *J Immigr Minor Health* 11:460–467, 2009.

Shea K: Reframing: a fresh outlook helps patients envision positive outcomes. In *2006 Pathways Professional Development,* Falls Church, VA, 2006, Gannett Healthcare Group, pp 56–60.

Sindelar H, Abrantes A, Hart C, et al: Motivational interviewing in pediatric practice, *Curr Prob Pediatr Adolesc Health Care* 34(9):322–339, 2004.

Suarez M, Mullins S: Motivational interviewing and pediatric health behavior interventions, *J Dev Behav Pediatr* 29(5):417–428, 2008.

Trifiletti LB, Shields WC, McDonald EM, et al: Development of injury prevention materials for people with low literacy, *Patient Educ Counsel* 64(1): 119–127, 2006.

Tyler DO, Horner SD: Family-centered collaborative negotiation: a model for facilitating behavior change in primary care, *J Am Acad NP* 20(4):194–203, 2008.

U.S. Department of Health and Human Services (USDHHS): *Healthy people 2020 public meetings.* Available at www.healthypeople.gov/hp2020/Objectives/files/Draft2009Objectives.pdf. Accessed June 17, 2010.

Wahl OF: Children's views of mental illness: a review of the literature, *Am J Psychiatr Rehabil* 6:134–158, 2002.

Wallace L, Lennon ES: American Academy of Family Physicians patient education materials: can patients read them? *Fam Med* 36(8):571–574, 2004.

Walsh J: Children's understanding of mental ill health: implications for risk and resilience in relationships, *Child Fam Soc Work* 14:115–122, 2009.

Wang J, Simons-Morton B, Farhart T, et al: Sociodemographic variability in adolescent substance use: mediation by parents and peers, *Prev Sci* 10(4): 387–396, 2009.

Watson AC, Miller F, Lyons J: Adolescent attitudes toward serious mental illness, *J Nerv Ment Dis* 193(11):769–772, 2005.

White S, Park Y, Israel T, et al: Longitudinal evaluation of peer health education on a college campus: impact on health behaviors, *J Am Coll Health* 57(5): 497–505, 2009.

Whitehead D: Evaluating health promotion: a model for nursing practice, *J Adv Nurs* 41(5):490–498, 2003.

Whitlock E, Orleans CT, Pender N, et al: Evaluating primary care behavioral counseling interventions: an evidence based approach, *Am J Prev Med* 22(4):267–284, 2004.

Williams D, Costa M, Odunlami A, et al: Moving upstream: how interventions that address the social determinants of health can improve health and reduce disparities, *J Public Health Manag Pract* 14(Suppl 6):S8–S17, 2008.

Yin HS, Johnson M, Mendelsohn AL, et al: The health literacy of parents in the United States: a nationally representative study, *Pediatrics* 124(Suppl 3): S289–S298, 2009.

CHAPTER 10

Agency for Healthcare Research and Quality: *2009 National Healthcare Quality Report,* Publication No. 10–0003, Rockville MD, 2010, HHS.

American Academy of Pediatrics (AAP) Section on Breastfeeding: breastfeeding and the use of human milk, *Pediatrics* 115:496–506, 2005.

American Dental Association (ADA): *Fluoridation facts,* Chicago, 2005, ADA.

American Medical Association (AMA): *Recommendations for physician and community collaboration on the management of obesity (A-05),* 2005. Available at www.ama-assn.org/ama/pub/. Accessed Jan 9, 2012.

Anderson J, Malley K, Snell R: Is 6 months still best for exclusive breast-feeding and introduction of solids? A literature review with consideration to the risk of the development of allergies, *Breastfeed Rev* 17(2):23–31, 2009.

August GP, Caprio S, Fennoy I, et al: Prevention and treatment of pediatric obesity: an Endocrine Society clinical practice guideline based on expert opinion, *J Clin Endocrinol Metab* 93(12):4576–4599, 2008.

Avena NM, Rada P, Hoebel BG: Evidence for sugar addiction: behavioral and neurochemical effects of intermittent, excessive sugar intake, *Neurosci Biobehav Rev* 32(1):20–39, 2008.

Bahna SL: Food challenge procedure: optimal choices for clinical practice, *Allergy Asthma Proc* 28(6): 640–646, 2007.

Barlow SE: Expert Committee: Expert Committee recommendations regarding the prevention, assessment, and treatment of child and adolescent overweight and obesity, *Pediatrics* 120(Suppl 14):S164–S192, 2007.

Blissett J, Haycraft E, Farrow C: Inducing preschool children's emotional eating: relations with parental feeding practices, *Am J Clin Nutr* 92(2):359–365, 2010.

Bonuck KA, Huang V, Fletcher J: Inappropriate bottle use: an early risk for overweight? Literature review and pilot data for a bottle-weaning trial, *Matern Child Nutr* 6(1):38–52, 2010.

Bouchard C: Childhood obesity: are genetic differences involved? *Am J Clin Nutr* 89(5):S1494–S1501, 2009.

Brandt ML, Harmon CM, Helmrath MA, et al: Morbid obesity in pediatric diabetes mellitus: surgical options and outcomes, *Nat Rev Endocrinol* 6(11):637–645, 2010.

Branner CM, Koyama T, Jensen GL: Racial and ethnic differences in pediatric obesity-prevention counseling: national prevalence of clinician practices, *Obesity (Silver Spring)* 16(3):690–694, 2008.

Branum AM, Lukacs SL: Food allergy among children in the United States, *Pediatrics* 124(6):1549–5155, 2009.

Brazelton TB, Sparrow J: *Feeding your child the Brazelton way,* Cambridge, MA, 2004, Da Capo Press, Perseus Books Group.

Brener ND, McManus T, Foti K, et al: *School health profiles 2008: characteristics of health programs among secondary schools,* Atlanta, 2009, Centers for Disease Control and Prevention.

Briefel R, Ziegler P, Novak T, et al: Feeding Infants and Toddlers Study: Do vitamin and mineral supplements contribute to nutrient adequacy or excess among U.S. infants and toddlers? *J Am Diet Assoc* 106(Suppl 1):S52–S65, 2006.

Byrd-Williams CE, Belcher BR, Spruijt-Metz D, et al: Increased physical activity and reduced adiposity in overweight Hispanic adolescents, *Med Sci Sports Exerc* 42(3):478–484, 2010.

Carver A, Timperio A, Crawford D: Playing it safe: the influence of neighbourhood safety on children's physical activity. A review, *Health Place* 14(2): 217–227, 2008.

Carver A, Timperio A, Hesketh K, et al: Are children and adolescents less active if parents restrict their physical activity and active transport due to perceived risk? *Soc Sci Med* 70(11):1799–1805, 2010.

Casey CF, Slawson DC, Neal LR: Vitamin D supplementation in infants, children, and adolescents, *Am Fam Physician* 81(6):745–748, 2010.

Centers for Disease Control and Prevention (CDC): Recommended community strategies and measurements to prevent obesity in the United States, *MMWR* 58(RR7):1–29, 2009.

Chafen JJ, Newberry SJ, Riedl MA, et al: Diagnosing and managing common food allergies: a systematic review, *JAMA* 303(18):1848–1856, 2010.

Chan GM, McElligott K, McNaught T, et al: Effects of dietary calcium intervention on adolescent mothers and newborns: a randomized controlled trial, *Obstet Gynecol* 108(3 Pt 1):565–571, 2006.

Chinapaw MJ, Mokkink LB, van Poppel MN, et al: Physical activity questionnaires for youth: a systematic review of measurement properties, *Sports Med* 40(7):539–563, 2010.

Clark AT, Ewan PW: Food allergy in childhood, *Arch Dis Child* 88(1):79–81, 2003.

Committee on Nutrition Standards for National School Lunch and Breakfast Programs, Institute of Medicine, Stallings VA, et al: *School meals: building blocks for healthy children,* Washington, DC, 2010, National Academies Press.

Cook S, Weitzman M, Auinger P, et al: Screening and counseling associated with obesity diagnosis in a national survey of ambulatory pediatric visits, *Pediatrics* 116(1):112–116, 2005.

Corsica JA, Pelchat ML: Food addiction: true or false? *Curr Opin Gastroenterol* 26(2):165–169, 2010.

Corwin RL, Grigson PS: Symposium overview—food addiction: fact or fiction? *J Nutr* 139(3):617–619, 2009.

Craig WJ, Mangels AR: Position of the American Dietetic Association: vegetarian diets, *J Am Diet Assoc* 109:1266–1282, 2009.

Crane JM, White J, Murphy P, et al: The effect of gestational weight gain by body mass index on maternal and neonatal outcomes, *J Obstet Gynaecol Can* 31(1):28–35, 2009.

Croll JK, Neumark-Sztainer D, Story M, et al: Adolescents involved in weight-related and power team sports have better eating patterns and nutrient intakes than non-sport-involved adolescents, *J Am Diet Assoc* 106(5):717–718, 2006.

Cruz NV, Bahna SL: Do foods or additives cause behavior disorders? *Pediatr Ann* 35(10):744–745, 748–754, 2006.

Dagnelie PC, van Staveren WA: Macrobiotic nutrition and child health: results of a population-based, mixed-longitudinal cohort study in The Netherlands, *Am J Clin Nutr* 59(Suppl 5):S1187–S1196, 1994.

Dan D, Harnanan D, Seetahal S, et al: Bariatric surgery in the management of childhood obesity: should there be an age limit? *Obes Surg* 20(1):114–117, 2010.

Daniels SR, Greer FR: American Academy of Pediatrics Committee on Nutrition: Lipid screening and cardiovascular health in childhood, *Pediatrics* 122(1):198–208, 2008.

Data Resource Center for Child and Adolescent Health: *2005-2006 National survey of children with special health care needs*, Portland, OR, 2010, Child and Adolescent Health Measurement Initiative. Available at www.cshcndata.org. Accessed Sept 24, 2010.

Day AS, Whitten KE, Sidler M, et al: Systematic review: nutritional therapy in paediatric Crohn's disease, *Aliment Pharmacol Ther* 27(4):293–307, 2007.

De La O A, Jordan KC, Ortiz K, et al: Do parents accurately perceive their child's weight status? *J Pediatr Health Care* 23(4):216–221, 2009.

Demerath EW, Reed D, Choh AC, et al: Rapid postnatal weight gain and visceral adiposity in adulthood: the Fels Longitudinal Study, *Obesity (Silver Spring)* 17(11):2060–2066, 2009.

Dubois L, Farmer A, Girard M, et al: Social factors and television use during meals and snacks is associated with higher BMI among pre-school children, *Public Health Nutr* 11(12):1267–1279, 2008.

Dubois L, Girard M: Early determinants of overweight at 4.5 years in a population-based longitudinal study, *Int J Obes (Lond)* 30(4):610–617, 2006.

Dunham L, Kollar LM: Vegetarian eating for children and adolescents, *J Pediatr Health Care* 20(1):27–34, 2006.

Faith MS, Hittner JB: Infant temperament and eating style predict change in standardized weight status and obesity risk at 6 years of age, *Int J Obes (Lond)* 34(10):1515–1523, 2010.

Fiocchi A, Martelli A: Dietary management of food allergy, *Pediatr Ann* 35(10):755–763, 2006.

Fleith M, Clandinin MT: Dietary PUFA for preterm and term infants: review of clinical studies, *Crit Rev Food Sci Nutr* 45(3):205–229, 2005.

Food and Nutrition Board (FNB): Institute of Medicine (IOM): *Dietary reference intakes for energy, carbohydrate, fiber, fat, fatty acids, cholesterol, protein, and amino acids*, Washington, DC, 2005, National Academies Press.

Fortuna JL: Sweet preference, sugar addiction and the familial risk of alcohol dependence: shared neural pathways and genes, *J Psychoactive Drugs* 42(2):147–151, 2010.

Fox MK, Reidy K, Novak T, et al: Sources of energy and nutrients in the diets of infants and toddlers, *J Am Diet Assoc* 106(Suppl 1):S28–S42, 2006.

Freedman LS, Guenther PM, Krebs-Smith SM, et al: A population's distribution of Healthy Eating Index-2005 component scores can be estimated when more than one 24-hour recall is available, *J Nutr* 140(8):1529–1534, 2010.

Gogakos A, Tzotzas TC, Krassas GE: Recent concepts of pharmacotherapy and bariatric surgery for childhood obesity: an overview, *Pediatr Endocrinol Rev* 7(2):83–94, 2009.

Gorton D, Bullen CR, Mhurchu CN: Environmental influences on food security in high-income countries, *Nutr Rev* 68(1):1–29, 2010.

Goodell LS, Wakefield DB, Ferris AM: Rapid weight gain during the first year of life predicts obesity in 2-3 year olds from a low-income, minority population, *J Community Health* 34(5):370–375, 2009.

Guenther PM, Reedy J, Krebs-Smith SM: Development of the Healthy Eating Index-2005, *J Am Diet Assoc* 108(11):1896–1901, 2008a.

Guenther PM, Reedy J, Krebs-Smith SM, et al: Evaluation of the Healthy Eating Index-2005, *J Am Diet Assoc* 108:1854–1864, 2008b.

Hahn NI: When food becomes a cry for help: how dietitians can combat childhood eating disorders. Interview with Monika M. Woolsey, *J Am Diet Assoc* 98:395–398, 1998.

Harbaugh BL, Bounds W, Kolbo J, et al: Prevalence estimates of overweight in Head Start preschoolers, *J Pediatr Nurs* 24(5):350–359, 2009.

Hatch EE, Nelson JW, Stahlhut RW, et al: Association of endocrine disruptors and obesity: perspectives from epidemiological studies, *Int J Androl* 33(2):324–332, 2010.

Holt K, Wooldridge N: *Bright Futures in practice: nutrition*, ed 3, Elk Grove Village, IL, 2011, American Academy of Pediatrics.

Hourihane JO: Prevalence and severity of food allergy—need for control, *Allergy* 53(Suppl 46):84–88, 1998.

Huh SY, Rifas-Shiman SL, Taveras EM, et al: Timing of solid food introduction and risk of obesity in preschool-aged children, *Pediatrics* 127(3):e544–e551, 2011.

Inge TH, Xanthakos SA, Zeller MH: Bariatric surgery for pediatric extreme obesity: now or later? *Int J Obes* 31(1):1–14, 2007.

Institute of Medicine (IOM): National Research Council (NRC): *Weight gain during pregnancy: reexamining the guidelines*, Washington, DC, 2009, National Academies Press.

Jacobs DR Jr, Haddad EH, Lanou AJ, et al: Food, plant food, and vegetarian diets in the US dietary guidelines: conclusions of an expert panel, *Am J Clin Nutr* 89(5):S1549–S1552, 2009.

Jordan AB, Kramer-Golinkoff EK, Strasburger VC: Does adolescent media use cause obesity and eating disorders? *Adolesc Med State Art Rev* 19(3):431–449, 2008.

Jordan AB, Robinson TN: Children, television viewing, and weight status: summary and recommendations from an expert panel meeting, *Ann Am Acad Pol Soc Sci* 615(1):119–132, 2008.

Kim JS, Sicherer S: Should avoidance of foods be strict in prevention and treatment of food allergy? *Curr Opin Allergy Clin Immunol* 10(3):252–257, 2010.

Kirby M, Danner E: Nutritional deficiencies in children on restricted diets, *Pediatr Clin North Am* 56(5):1085–1103, 2009.

Knight AK, Bahna SL: Diagnosis of food allergy, *Pediatr Ann* 35(10):709–714, 2006.

Koletzko B, von Kries R, Closa R, et al: Can infant feeding choices modulate later obesity risk? *Am J Clin Nutr* 89(5):S1502–S1508, 2009.

Koplin JJ, Osborne NJ, Wake M, et al: Can early introduction of egg prevent egg allergy in infants? A population-based study, *J Allergy Clin Immunol* 126(4):807–813, 2010.

Krebs-Smith SM, Guenther PM, Subar AF, et al: Americans do not meet federal dietary recommendations, *J Nutr* 140(10):1832–1838, 2010.

Larson NI, Neumark-Sztainer D, Hannan PJ, et al: Trends in adolescent fruit and vegetable consumption, 1999-2004: Project EAT, *Am J Prev Med* 32(2):147–150, 2007.

Lieberman JA, Sicherer SH: Diagnosis of food allergy: epicutaneous skin tests, in vitro tests, and oral food challenge, *Curr Allergy Asthma Rep* 11(1):58–64, 2011.

Lien L, Lien N, Heyerdahl S, et al: Consumption of soft drinks and hyperactivity, mental distress, and conduct problems among adolescents in Oslo, Norway, *Am J Public Health* 96(10):1815–1820, 2006.

Liu AH, Jaramillo R, Sicherer SH, et al: National prevalence and risk factors for food allergy and relationship to asthma: results from the National Health and Nutrition Examination Survey 2005-2006, *J Allergy Clin Immunol* 126(4):798–806, 2010.

Lustig RH: The "skinny" on childhood obesity: how our Western environment starves kids' brains, *Pediatr Ann* 35(12):899–907, 2006.

Madsen KA, Gosliner W, Woodward-Lopez G, et al: Physical activity opportunities associated with fitness and weight status among adolescents in low-income communities, *Arch Pediatr Adolesc Med* 163(11):1014–1021, 2009.

Merten MJ, Williams AL, Shriver LH: Breakfast consumption in adolescence and young adulthood: parental presence, community context, and obesity, *J Am Diet Assoc* 109(8):1384–1391, 2009.

Moissidis I, Chaidaroon D, Vichyanond P, et al: Milk-induced pulmonary disease in infants (Heiner syndrome), *Pediatr Allergy Immunol* 16(6):545–552, 2005.

Moran VH: A systematic review of dietary assessments of pregnant adolescents in industrialised countries, *Br J Nutr* 97(3):411–425, 2007.

Moss BG, Yeaton WH: Young children's weight trajectories and associated risk factors: results from the Early Childhood Longitudinal Study-Birth Cohort, *Am J Health Promot* 25(3):190–198, 2011.

Nadler EP, Brotman LM, Miyoshi T, et al: Morbidity in obese adolescents who meet the adult National Institutes of Health criteria for bariatric surgery, *J Pediatr Surg* 44(10):1869–1876, 2009.

National Association of Pediatric Nurse Practitioners (NAPNAP): *Healthy eating and activity together (HEAT): clinical practice guideline, identifying and preventing overweight in childhood*, Cherry Hill, NJ, 2006, NAPNAP.

Newbold RR: Impact of environmental endocrine disrupting chemicals on the development of obesity, *Hormones (Athens)* 9(3):206–217, 2010.

Nicholls D, Bryant-Waugh R: Eating disorders of infancy and childhood: definition, symptomatology, epidemiology, and comorbidity, *Child Adolesc Psychiatr Clin N Am* 18(1):17–30, 2009.

Nielsen JN, Gittelsohn J, Anliker J, et al: Interventions to improve diet and weight gain among pregnant adolescents and recommendations for future research, *J Am Diet Assoc* 106(11):1825–1840, 2006.

Ogden CL, Carroll M: *Prevalence of obesity among children and adolescents: United States, trends 1963-1965 through 2007-2008*. Available at www.cdc.gov/nchs/data/hestat/obesity_child_07_08/obesity_child_07_08.htm#table1. Accessed Sept 27, 2010.

Orenstein S, Peters J, Khan S, et al: The esophagus. In Kliegman RM, Behrman R, Jenson HB, et al: *Nelson textbook of pediatrics*, ed 18, Philadelphia, 2007, Saunders.

Otten JJ, Pitzi Hellwig J, Meyers LD, editors: *Dietary reference intakes: the essential guide to nutrient requirements*, Washington, DC, 2006, Institute of Medicine.

Panzer BM: Enhancing childhood obesity treatment, *ICAN: Infant Child Adolesc Nutr* 2(2):96–98, 2010.

Park MH, Kinra S, Ward KJ, et al: Metformin for obesity in children and adolescents: a systematic review, *Diabetes Care* 32(9):1743–1745, 2009.

Park K, Kersey M, Geppert J, et al: Household food insecurity is a risk factor for iron-deficiency anaemia in a multi-ethnic, low-income sample of infants and toddlers, *Public Health Nutr* 12(11):2120–2128, 2009.

Pollan M: Unhappy meals: thirty years of nutritional science has made Americans sicker, fatter and less well nourished, A plea for a return to plain old food, *New York Times Magazine*, Jan 28, 2007.

Prescott SL, Bouygue GR, Videky D, et al: Avoidance or exposure to foods in prevention and treatment of food allergy? *Curr Opin Allergy Clin Immunol* 10(3):258–266, 2010.

Reedy J, Krebs-Smith SM: Dietary sources of energy, solid fats, and added sugars among children and adolescents in the United States, *J Am Diet Assoc* 110(10):1477–1484, 2010.

Rideout VJ, Foehr UG, Roberts DF: *Generation M2: media in the lives of 8- to 18-year olds*, Menlo Park, CA, 2010, Kaiser Family Foundation.

Robinson-O'Brien R, Burgess-Champoux T, Haines J, et al: Associations between school meals offered through the National School Lunch Program and the School Breakfast Program and fruit and vegetable intake among ethnically diverse, low-income children, *J Sch Health* 80(10):487–492, 2010.

Robinson-O'Brien R, Perry CL, Wall MM, et al: Adolescent and young adult vegetarianism: better dietary intake and weight outcomes but increased risk of disordered eating behaviors, *J Am Diet Assoc* 109(4):648–655, 2009.

Rogovik AL, Goldman RD: Should weight-loss supplements be used for pediatric obesity? *Can Fam Physician* 55(3):257–259, 2009.

Rogovik AL, Chanoine JP, Goldman RD: Pharmacotherapy and weight-loss supplements for treatment of paediatric obesity, *Drugs* 70(3):335–346, 2010.

Royo-Bordonada, Garcés C, Gorgojo L, et al: Saturated fat in the diet of Spanish children: relationship with anthropometric, alimentary, nutritional and lipid profiles, *Public Health Nutr* 9(4):429–435, 2006.

Rudders SA, Banerji A, Corel B, et al: Multicenter study of repeat epinephrine treatments for food-related anaphylaxis, *Pediatrics* 125(4):e711–e718, 2010.

Ruottinen S, Lagström HK, Niinikoski H, et al: Dietary fiber does not displace energy but is associated with decreased serum cholesterol concentrations in healthy children, *Am J Clin Nutr* 91(3):651–661, 2010.

Russell S, Monroe K, Losek JD: Anaphylaxis management in the pediatric emergency department: opportunities for improvement, *Pediatr Emerg Care* 26(2):71–76, 2010.

Sabaté J, Wien M: Vegetarian diets and childhood obesity prevention, *Am J Clin Nutr* 91(5):S1525–S1529, 2010.

Schulze A, Matern D, Hoffman GF: Newborn screening. In Sarafoglou K, Hoffmann GR, Roth KS, editors: *Pediatric endocrinology and inborn errors of metabolism*, New York, 2009, McGraw-Hill Medical.

Scurlock AM, Jones SM: An update on immunotherapy for food allergy, *Curr Opin Allergy Clin Immunol* 10(6):587–593, 2010.

Scurlock AM, Vickery BP, Hourihane JO, et al: Pediatric food allergy and mucosal tolerance, *Mucosal Immunol* 3(4):345–354, 2010.

Sharma GD: *Cystic fibrosis, eMedicine.* Available at http://emedicine.medscape.com/article/1001602-overview. Accessed Sept 24, 2010.

Sicherer SH, Muñoz-Furlong A, Godbold JH, et al: U.S. prevalence of self-reported peanut, tree nut, and sesame allergy: 11-year follow-up, *J Allergy Clin Immunol* 125(6):1322–1326, 2010.

Singhal A: Does weight gain in infancy influence the later risk of obesity? *J Pediatr Gastroenterol Nutr* 51(Suppl 3):S119–S120, 2010.

Small L, Anderson D, Sidora-Arcoleo K, et al: Pediatric nurse practitioners' assessment and management of childhood overweight/obesity: results from 1999 and 2005 cohort surveys, *J Pediatr Health Care* 23(4):231–241, 2009.

Spruijt-Metz D, Li C, Cohen E, et al: Longitudinal influence of mother's child-feeding practices on adiposity in children, *J Pediatr* 148(3):314–320, 2006.

Strasburger VC, Jordan AB, Donnerstein E: Health effects of media on children and adolescents, *Pediatrics* 125(4):756–767, 2010.

Sukalich S, Mingione MJ, Glantz JC: Obstetric outcomes in overweight and obese adolescents, *Am J Obstet Gynecol* 195(3):851–855, 2006.

Taveras EM, Rifas-Shiman SL, Belfort MB, et al: Weight status in the first 6 months of life and obesity at 3 years of age, *Pediatrics* 123(4):1177–1183, 2009.

U.S. Department of Agriculture (USDA): U.S. Department of Health and Human Services (USDHHS): *Dietary Guidelines for Americans, 2010,* ed 7, Washington, DC, 2010, U.S. Government Printing Office. Available at www.cnpp.usda.gov/DGAs2010-Policy Document.htm. Accessed Feb 10, 2011.

U.S. Department of Health and Human Services (USDHHS): *2008 Physical activity guidelines for Americans,* Washington, DC, 2009, USDHHS. Available at www.health.gov/pageguidelines. Accessed Nov 8, 2010.

U.S. Preventive Services Task Force (USPSTF): *Screening for obesity in children and adolescents: recommendation statement.* Available at www.uspreventiveservicestaskforce.org/uspstf/uspschobes.htm. Accessed Sept 11, 2010.

Vandenplas Y, Rudolph CD, Di Lorenzo C, et al: Pediatric gastroesophageal reflux clinical practice guidelines: joint recommendations of the North American Society for Pediatric Gastroenterology, Hepatology, and Nutrition (NASPGHAN) and the European Society for Pediatric Gastroenterology, Hepatology, and Nutrition (ESPGHAN), *J Pediatr Gastroenterol Nutr* 49(4):498–547, 2009.

Vandewater EA, Rideout VJ, Wartella EA, et al: Digital childhood: electronic media and technology use among infants, toddlers, and preschoolers, *Pediatrics* 119(5):e1006–e1015, 2007.

Van Horn L, Obarzanek E, Barton BA, et al: A summary of results of the Dietary Intervention Study in Children (DISC): lessons learned, *Prog Cardiovasc Nurs* 18(1):28–41, 2003.

Vereecken CA, Todd J, Roberts C, et al: Television viewing behaviour and associations with food habits in different countries, *Public Health Nutr* 9(2):244–250, 2006.

Vitolo MR, Rauber F, Campagnolo PD, et al: Maternal dietary counseling in the first year of life is associated with a higher healthy eating index in childhood, *J Nutr* 140(11):2002–2007, 2010.

Wagner CL, Greer FR, American Academy of Pediatrics Section on Breast-feeding, et al: Prevention of rickets and vitamin D deficiency in infants, children, and adolescents, *Pediatrics* 122(5):1142–1152, 2008.

Watanabe F: Vitamin B_{12} sources and bioavailability, *Exp Biol Med (Maywood)* 232(10):1266–1274, 2007.

Westerterp KR, Speakman JR: Physical activity energy expenditure has not declined since the 1980s and matches energy expenditures of wild mammals, *Int J Obes (Lond)* 32(8):1256–1263, 2008.

Wiles NJ, Northstone K, Emmett P, et al: 'Junk food' diet and childhood behavioural problems: results from the ALSPAC cohort, *Eur J Clin Nutr* 63(4):491–498, 2009.

Woolford SJ, Clark SJ, Gebremariam A, et al: To cut or not to cut: physicians' perspectives on referring adolescents for bariatric surgery, *Obes Surg* 20(7):937–942, 2010.

Wosje KS, Specker BL, Giddens J: No differences in growth or body composition from age 12 to 24 months between toddlers consuming 2% milk and toddlers consuming whole milk, *J Am Diet Assoc* 101(1):53–56, 2001.

Wynne AL, Woo TM, Olyaei AJ: *Pharmacotherapeutics for nurse practitioner prescribers,* ed 2, Philadelphia, 2007, FA Davis.

Young VR, Pellett PL: Plant proteins in relation to human protein and amino acid nutrition, *Am J Clin Nutr* 59(Suppl 5):S1203–S1212, 1994.

Zutavern A, Brockow I, Schaaf B, et al: Timing of solid food introduction in relation to eczema, asthma, allergic rhinitis, and food and inhalant sensitization at the age of 6 years: results from the prospective birth cohort study LISA, *Pediatrics* 121(1):e44–e52, 2008.

CHAPTER 11

Agostoni C: Role of long-chain polyunsaturated fatty acids in the first year of life, *J Pediatr Gastroenterol Nutr* 47(Suppl 2):S41–S44, 2008.

Akus M, Bartick M: Lactation safety recommendations and reliability compared in 10 medication resources, *Ann Pharmacother* 41(9):1352–1360, 2007.

American Academy of Family Physicians (AAFP): *Breastfeeding, family physicians supporting (position paper, 2008).* Available at www.aafp.org/online/en/home/policy/policies/b/breastfeedingpositionpaper.html. Accessed Sept 8, 2010.

American Academy of Pediatrics (AAP): Breastfeeding and the use of human milk, *Pediatrics* 115:496–506, 2005.

Arroyo R, Martin V, Maldonado A, et al: Treatment of infectious mastitis during lactation: antibiotics versus oral administration of lactobacilli isolated from breast milk, *Clin Infect Dis* 50(12):1551–1558, 2010.

Baby-Friendly Hospital Initiative (BFHI) USA: 125 Baby-friendly hospitals and birth centers as of Dec 22, 2011. Available at www.babyfriendlyusa.org/eng/03.html. Accessed Jan 9, 2012.

Ball TM, Bennett DM: The economic impact of breastfeeding, *Pediatr Clin North Am* 48(1):253–262, 2001.

Bar-Yam N: Workplace lactation support, part I: a return-to-work breastfeeding assessment tool, *J Hum Lact* 14:249–254, 1998.

Benyamini L, Merlob P, Stahl B, et al: The safety of amoxicillin/clavulanic acid and cefuroxime during lactation, *Ther Drug Monit* 27(4):499–502, 2005.

Centers for Disease Control and Prevention (CDC): Breastfeeding report card—United States, 2010. Available at www.cdc.gov/breastfeeding/data/report_card.htm. Accessed February 7, 2011.

Chantry CJ, Howard CR, Auinger P: Full breastfeeding duration and associated decrease in respiratory tract infection in U.S. children, *Pediatrics* 117(2):425–432, 2006.

Chertok IR: Reexamination of ultra-thin nipple shield use, infant growth and maternal satisfaction, *J Clin Nurs* 18(21):2949–2955, 2009.

Correa S, Palmeira P, Carneiro-Sampaio MM, et al: Human colostrum contains IgA antibodies reactive to colonization factors I and II of enterotoxigenic, *Escherichia coli, FEMS Immunol Med Microbiol* 47(2):199–206, 2006.

De Silva M, Senarath U, Gunatilake M, et al: Prolonged breastfeeding reduces risk of breast cancer in Sri Lankan women: a case-control study, *Cancer Epidemiol* 34(3):267–273, 2010.

Eglash A, Ziemer AL, Chevalier A: Health professionals' attitudes and use of nipple shields for breastfeeding women, *Breastfeed Med* 5(4):147–151, 2010.

Greer FR, Sicherer SH, Burks AW, et al: Effects of early nutritional interventions on the development of atopic disease in infants and children: the role of maternal dietary restriction, breastfeeding, timing of introduction of complementary foods, and hydrolyzed formulas, *Pediatrics* 121(1):183–191, 2008.

Grummer-Strawn LM, Reinold C, Krebs NF: Use of World Health Organization and CDC growth charts for children aged 0-59 months in the United States: recommendations and reports, *MMWR* 59(RR-9):1–15, 2010. Available at www.cdc.gov/mmwr/preview/mmwrhtml/rr5909a1.htm?s_cid=rr5909a1_e. Accessed Sept 9, 2010.

Gunderson EP, Jacobs DR Jr, Chiang V, et al: Duration of lactation and incidence of metabolic syndrome in women of reproductive age according to gestational diabetes status: a 20 year prospective study in CARDIA—the Coronary Artery Risk Development in Young Adults study, *Diabetes* 59(2):495–504, 2010.

Hart S, Boylan LM, Carroll SR, et al: Brief report: newborn behavior differs with docosahexaenoic acid levels in breast milk, *J Pediatr Psych* 31:221–226, 2006.

Heird WC, Lapillonne A: The role of essential fatty acids in development, *Ann Rev Nutr* 25:549–571, 2005.

Hill DJ, Roy N, Heine RG, et al: Effect of a low-allergen maternal diet on colic among breastfed infants: a randomized, controlled trial, *Pediatrics* 116(5):e709–e715, 2005.

Human Milk Banking Association of North America (HMBANA): *2006 Best practice for expressing, storing, and handling human milk in hospitals, homes, and child care settings*, Raleigh, NC, 2006, Author.

Institute of Medicine Subcommittee on Lactation: *Nutrition during lactation*, Washington, DC, 1991, National Academies Press.

Ip S, Chung M, Raman G, et al: A summary of the Agency for Healthcare Research and Quality's evidence report on breastfeeding in developed countries, *Breastfeed Med* 4(Suppl 1):S17–S30, 2009.

Jahanfar S, Ng CJ, Teng CL: Antibiotics for mastitis in breastfeeding women, *Cochrane Database Syst Rev* 21(1):CD005458, 2009.

James DC, Lessen R, American Dietetic Association: Position of the American Dietetic Association: promoting and supporting breastfeeding, *J Am Diet Assoc* 109(11):1926–1942, 2009.

Konek S, Mascarenhas MR: Vitamin deficiencies and excesses. In Burg FD, Ingelfinger JR, Polin RA, et al: *Current pediatric therapy*, ed 18, Philadelphia, 2006, Saunders.

Lawrence RA, Lawrence RM: *Breastfeeding: a guide for the medical profession*, ed 6, St Louis, 2005, Mosby.

Marcobal A, Barboza M, Froehlich JW, et al: Consumption of human milk oligosaccharides by gut-related microbes, *J Agric Food Chem* 58(9):5334–5340, 2010.

Mayer-Davis EJ, Dabelea D, Lamichhane AP, et al: Breast-feeding and type 2 diabetes in the youth of three ethnic groups: the SEARCH for diabetes in youth case-control study, *Diabetes Care* 31(3):470–475, 2008.

Mills SP: Workplace lactation programs: a critical element for breastfeeding mothers' success, *AAOHN J* 57(6):227–231, 2009.

National Association of Pediatric Nurse Practitioners: NAPNAP position statement on breast-feeding, *J Pediatr Health Care* 21(2):A39–A40, 2007.

National Conference of State Legislatures (NCSL): *Breastfeeding state laws*. Available at www.ncsl.org. Accessed June 8, 2010.

Owen CG, Whincup PH, Kaye SJ, et al: Does initial breastfeeding lead to lower blood cholesterol in adult life? A quantitative review of the evidence, *Am J Clin Nutr* 88(2):305–314, 2008.

Pesonen M, Kallio MJ, Ranki A, et al: Prolonged exclusive breastfeeding is associated with increased atopic dermatitis: a prospective follow-up study of unselected healthy newborns from birth to age 20 years, *Clin Exp Allergy* 36(8):1011–1018, 2006.

Pisacane A, Continisio P, Palma O, et al: Breastfeeding and risk for fever after immunization, *Pediatrics* 25(6):e1448–e1452, 2010.

Preer GL, Philipp BL: Understanding and managing breast milk jaundice, *Arch Dis Child Fetal Neonatal Ed*, Aug 5, 2010. [Epub ahead of print].

Singhal A: Does weight gain in infancy influence the later risk of obesity? *J Pediatr Gastroenterol Nutr* 51(Suppl 3):S119–S120, 2010.

Singhal A, Cole TJ, Fewtrell M, et al: Breast milk feeding and lipoprotein profile in adolescents born preterm: follow-up of a prospective randomized study, *Lancet* 363(9421):1571–1578, 2004.

Stuebe AM, Schwarz EB: The risks and benefits of infant feeding practices for women and their children, *J Perinatol* 30(3):155–162, 2010.

Titus-Ernstoff L, Rees JR, Terry KL, et al: Breast-feeding the last born child and risk of ovarian cancer, *Cancer Causes Control* 21(2):201–207, 2010.

U.S. Department of Health and Human Services (USDHHS): *Maternal, Infant and Child Health*. Available at www.healthypeople.gov/hp2020/Objectives/ViewObjective.aspx?Id=177&;TopicArea=Maternal%2c+Infant+and+Child+Health&Objective=MICH+HP2020%E2%80%9312&TopicAreaId=32. Accessed August 9, 2010.

U.S. Department of Health and Human Services (USDHHS): *The Surgeon General's Call to Action to Support Breastfeeding*, Washington, DC, 2011, U.S. Department of Health and Human Services, Office of the Surgeon General. Available at www.surgeongeneral.gov. Accessed February 18, 2011.

United Nations International Children's Emergency Fund (UNICEF): *Baby-friendly hospital initiative training materials*. Available at www.unicef.org/nutrition/index_24850.html?q=printme. Accessed June 7, 2010a.

United Nations International Children's Emergency Fund (UNICEF): *Baby-friendly hospital initiative*. Available at www.unicef.org/nutrition/index_24806.html. Accessed June 7, 2010b.

van Dijk CE, Innis SM: Growth-curve standards and the assessment of early excess weight gain in infancy, *Pediatrics* 123(1):102–108, 2009.

Wagner CL, Greer FR, Section on Breastfeeding and Committee on Nutrition: Prevention of rickets and vitamin D deficiency in infants, children, and adolescents, *Pediatrics* 122(5):1142–1152, 2008.

Wijndaele K, Lakshman R, Landsbaugh JR, et al: Determinants of early weaning and use of unmodified cow's milk in infants: a systematic review, *J Am Diet Assoc* 109(12):2017–2028, 2009.

World Health Organization/United Nations International Children's Emergency Fund (WHO/UNICEF): *Protecting, promoting and supporting breastfeeding: the special role of maternity services: a joint WHO/ UNICEF statement*, Geneva, 1989, World Health Organization. Available at www.who.int/nutrition/publications/infantfeeding/9241561300/en/. Accessed Feb 7, 2011.

Zivkovic AM, German JB, Lebrilla CB, et al: Microbes and health Sackler colloquium: human milk glycobiome and its impact on the infant gastrointestinal microbiota, *Proc Natl Acad Sci U S A*, Aug 4, 2010. [Epub ahead of print].

CHAPTER 12

Allen HA, Austin JC, Boyt MA, et al: Initial trial of timed voiding is warranted for all children with daytime incontinence, *Urology* 69(5):962–965, 2007.

American Academy of Pediatrics (AAP) Committee on Practice and Ambulatory Medicine: *Bright Futures* Steering Committee: Recommendations for preventive pediatric health care, *Pediatrics* 120(6):1376, 2007.

Austin PF, Ferguson G, Yan Y, et al: Combination therapy with desmopressin and an anticholinergic medication for nonresponders to desmopressin for monosymptomatic nocturnal enuresis: a randomized, double-blind, placebo-controlled trial, *Pediatrics* 122(5):1027–1032, 2008.

Azrin NH, Foxx RM: *Toilet training in less than a day*, New York, 1974, Simon & Schuster.

Barone JG, Hanson C, DaJusta DG, et al: Nocturnal enuresis and overweight are associated with obstructive sleep apnea, *Pediatrics* 124(1):e53–e59, 2009.

Bekkali NL, Hamers SL, Reitsma JB, et al: Infant stool form scale: development and results, *J Pediatr* 154(4):521–516, 2009a.

Bekkali NL, van den Berg MM, Dijkgraaf MG, et al: Rectal fecal impaction treatment in childhood constipation: enemas versus high doses oral PEG, *Pediatrics* 124(6):e1108–e1115, 2009b.

Bergmann M, Corigliano T, Ataia I, et al: Childhood extraordinary daytime urinary frequency—a case series and a systematic literature review, *Pediatr Nephrol* 24(4):789–795, 2009.

Berkowitz CD: *Pediatrics: a primary care approach*, ed 2, Philadelphia, 2000, Saunders.

Blum NJ, Taubman B, Nemeth N: During toilet training, constipation occurs before stool toileting refusal, *Pediatrics* 113(6):e520–e522, 2004.

Blum NJ, Taubman B, Osborne ML: Behavioral characteristics of children with stool toileting refusal, *Pediatrics* 99(1):50–53, 1997.

Bolduc S, Moore K, Lebel S, et al: Double anticholinergic therapy for refractory overactive bladder, *J Urol* 182(Suppl 4):2033–2038, 2009.

Bolduc S, Moore K, Nadeau G, et al: Prospective open label study of solifenacin for overactive bladder in children, *J Urol* 184(Suppl 4):1668–1673, 2010.

Boris NW, Dalton R: Encopresis. In Kliegman RM, Behrman RE, Jenson HB, et al, editors: *Nelson textbook of pediatrics*, ed 18, Philadelphia, 2007a, Saunders.

Boris NW, Dalton R: Enuresis (bed-wetting). In Kliegman RM, Behrman RE, Jenson HB, et al, editors: *Nelson textbook of pediatrics*, ed 18, Philadelphia, 2007b, Saunders.

Brazelton TB, Sparrow J: *Toilet training—the Brazelton way*, Cambridge, MA, 2004, DaCapo Press Perseus Book Group.

Brazzelli M, Griffiths P: Behavioral and cognitive interventions with or without other treatments for the management of faecal incontinence in children, *Cochrane Database Syst Rev* 2:CD002240, 2006.

Burgers R, Benninga MA: Functional nonretentive fecal incontinence in children: a frustrating and long-lasting clinical entity, *J Pediatr Gastroenterol Nutr* 48(Suppl 2):S98–S100, 2009.

Butler RJ, Robinson JC: Alarm treatment for childhood nocturnal enuresis: an investigation of within-treatment variables, *Scand J Urol Nephrol* 36:268–272, 2002.

Candy D, Belsey J: Macrogol (polyethylene glycol) laxatives in children with functional constipation and faecal impaction: a systematic review, *Arch Dis Child* 94(2):156–160, 2009.

Carotenuto M, Esposito M, Pascotto A: Facial patterns and primary nocturnal enuresis in children, *Sleep Breath*, Jul 6, 2010. [Epub ahead of print].

Chandra M, Saharia R, Hill V, et al: Prevalence of diurnal voiding symptoms and difficult arousal from sleep in children with nocturnal enuresis, *J Urol* 172(1):311–316, 2004.

Chase J, Austin P, Hoebeke P, et al: The management of dysfunctional voiding in children: a report from the Standardisation Committee of the International Children's Continence Society, *J Urol* 183(4):1296–1302, 2010.

Choby BA, George S: Toilet training, *Am Fam Physician* 78(9):1059–1064, 2008.

De Bruyne E, Van Hoecke E, Van Gompel K, et al: Problem behavior, parental stress and enuresis, *J Urol* 182(Suppl 4):2015–2020, 2009.

De Guchtenaere A, Van de Walle C, Van Sintjan P, et al: Nocturnal polyuria is related to absent circadian rhythm of glomerular filtration rate, *J Urol* 178(6):2626–2629, 2007.

Dhondt K, Raes A, Hoebeke P, et al: Abnormal sleep architecture and refractory nocturnal enuresis, *J Urol* 182(Suppl 4):1961–1965, 2009.

Duel B: Non-surgical management of urinary incontinence in children, *Sci World J* 9:1306–1307, 2009.

Elder JS: Voiding dysfunction. In Kliegman RM, Behrman RE, Jenson HB, et al, editors: *Nelson textbook of pediatrics*, ed 18, Philadelphia, 2007, Saunders.

Evans J, Malmsten B, Maddocks A, et al: Randomized comparison of longterm desmopressin and alarm treatment for bedwetting, *J Pediatr Urol* 7(1):21–29, 2011.

Feldman AS, Bauer SB: Diagnosis and management of dysfunctional voiding, *Curr Opin Pediatr* 18(2):139–147, 2006.

Gelotte CK, Prior MJ, Gu J: A randomized, placebo-controlled, exploratory trial of ibuprofen and pseudoephedrine in the treatment of primary nocturnal enuresis in children, *Clin Pediatr (Phila)* 48(4):410–419, 2009.

Glazener CM, Evans JH, Peto RE: Alarm interventions for nocturnal enuresis in children, *Cochrane Database Syst Rev* 2:CD002911, 2005.

Gold JI, Kant AJ, Belmont KA, et al: Practitioner review: clinical applications of pediatric hypnosis, *J Child Psychol Psychiatry* 48(8):744–754, 2007.

Horn IB, Brenner R, Rao M, et al: Beliefs about the appropriate age for initiating toilet training: are there racial and socioeconomic differences? *J Pediatr* 149(2):151–152, 2006.

Humphreys MR, Vandersteen DR, Slezak JM, et al: Preliminary results of sacral neuromodulation in 23 children, *J Urol* 176(5):2227–2231, 2006.

Jansson UB, Hanson M, Sillén U, et al: Voiding pattern and acquisition of bladder control from birth to age 6 years—a longitudinal study, *J Urol* 174(1):289–293, 2005.

Jindal V, Ge A, Mansky PJ: Safety and efficacy of acupuncture in children: a review of the evidence, *J Pediatr Hematol Oncol* 30(6):431–442, 2008.

Joinson C, Heron J, Butler U, et al: Psychological differences between children with and without soiling problems, *Pediatrics* 117(5):1575–1584, 2006.

Joinson C, Heron J, von Gontard A, et al: A prospective study of age at initiation of toilet training and subsequent daytime bladder control in schoolage children, *J Dev Behav Pediatr* 30(5):385–393, 2009.

Joinson C, Heron J, von Gontard A, et al: Early childhood risk factors associated with daytime wetting and soiling in school-age children, *J Pediatr Psychol* 33(7):739–750, 2008.

Kamperis K, Hagstroem S, Rittig S, et al: Combination of the enuresis alarm and desmopressin: second line treatment for nocturnal enuresis, *J Urol* 179(3):1128–1131, 2008.

Kaugars AS, Silverman A, Kinservik M, et al: Families' perspectives on the effect of constipation and fecal incontinence on quality of life, *J Pediatr Gastroenterol Nutr* 51(6):747–752, 2010.

Kibar Y, Piskin M, Irkilata HC, et al: Management of abnormal postvoid residual urine in children with dysfunctional voiding, *Urology* 75(6):1472–1475, 2010.

Kilic N, Balkan E, Akgoz S, et al: Comparison of the effectiveness and side effects of tolterodine and oxybutynin in children with detrusor instability, *Int J Urol* 13(2):105–108, 2006.

Kistner M: Dysfunctional elimination behaviors and associated complications in school-age children, *J Sch Nurs* 25(2):108–116, 2009.

Lee-Robichaud H, Thomas K, Morgan J, et al: Lactulose versus polyethylene glycol for chronic constipation, *Cochrane Database Syst Rev* 7:CD007570, 2010.

Libonate J, Evans S, Tsao JC: Efficacy of acupuncture for health conditions in children: a review, *Sci World J* 8:670–682, 2008.

Long PW: *Imipramine: drug monograph.* Available at www.mentalhealth.com/drug/p30-t03.html. Accessed July 19, 2010.

Lottmann HB, Alova I: Primary monosymptomatic nocturnal enuresis in children and adolescents, *Int J Clin Pract Suppl* 155:8–16, 2007.

Lottmann HB, Baydala L, Eggert P, et al: Long-term desmopressin response in primary nocturnal enuresis: open-label, multinational study, *Int J Clin Pract* 63(1):35–45, 2009.

Mota DM, Barros AJ: Toilet training: methods, parental expectations and associated dysfunctions, *J Pediatr (Rio J)* 84(1):9–17, 2008.

Mulders MM, Cobussen-Boekhorst H, de Gier RP, et al: Urotherapy in children: Quantitative measurements of daytime urinary incontinence before and after treatment According to the new definitions of the International Children's Continence Society, *J Pediatr Urol*, Jun 10, 2010. [Epub ahead of print].

Nevéus T: Diagnosis and management of nocturnal enuresis, *Curr Opin Pediatr* 21(2):199–202, 2009.

Nevéus T, Eggert P, Evans J, et al: Evaluation of and treatment for monosymptomatic enuresis: a standardization document from the International Children's Continence Society, *J Urol* 183(2):441–447, 2010.

Pakarinen MP, Koivusalo A, Rintala RJ: Functional fecal soiling without constipation, organic cause or neuropsychiatric disorders? *J Pediatr Gastroenterol Nutr* 43(2):206–208, 2006.

Philichi L: When the going gets tough: pediatric constipation and encopresis, *Gastroenterol Nurs* 31(2):121–130, 2008.

Pijpers MA, Tabbers MM, Benninga MA, et al: Currently recommended treatments of childhood constipation are not evidence based: a systematic literature review on the effect of laxative treatment and dietary measures, *Arch Dis Child* 94(2):117–131, 2009.

Pohl HG, Bauer SB, Borer JG, et al: The outcome of voiding dysfunction managed with clean intermittent catheterization in neurologically and anatomically normal children, *BJU Int* 89(9):923–927, 2002.

Robson WL: Clinical practice. Evaluation and management of enuresis, *N Engl J Med* 360(14):1429–1436, 2009.

Robson WL, Leung AK: An approach to daytime wetting in children, *Adv Pediatr* 53:323–365, 2006.

Robson WL, Leung AK, Norgaard JP: The comparative safety of oral versus intranasal desmopressin for the treatment of children with nocturnal enuresis, *J Urol* 178(1):24–30, 2007.

Rocha MM, Costa NJ, Silvares EF: Changes in parents' and self-reports of behavioral problems in Brazilian adolescents after behavioral treatment with urine alarm for nocturnal enuresis, *Int Braz J Urol* 34(6):749–757, 2008.

Roth TJ, Vandersteen DR, Hollatz P, et al: Sacral neuromodulation for the dysfunctional elimination syndrome: a single center experience with 20 children, *J Urol* 180(1):306–311, 2008.

Rugolotto S, Sun M, Boucke L, et al: Toilet training started during the first year of life: a report on elimination signals, stool toileting refusal and completion age, *Minerva Pediatr* 60(1):27–35, 2008.

Schaumburg HL, Kapilin U, Blåsvaer C, et al: Hereditary phenotypes in nocturnal enuresis, *BJU Int* 102(7):816–821, 2008.

Schum TR, Kolb TM, McAuliffe TL, et al: Sequential acquisition of toilet training skills: a descriptive study of gender and age differences in normal children, *Pediatrics* 109(3):e48–e55, 2002.

Shrago LC, Reifsnider E, Insel K: The Neonatal Bowel Output Study: indicators of adequate breast milk intake in neonates, *Pediatr Nurs* 32(3):195–201, 2006.

Shreeram S, He JP, Kalaydjian A, et al: Prevalence of enuresis and its association with attention-deficit/hyperactivity disorder among U.S. children: results from a nationally representative study, *J Am Acad Child Adolesc Psychiatry* 48(1):35–41, 2009.

Sun M, Rugolotto S: Assisted infant toilet training in a Western family setting, *J Dev Behav Pediatr* 25(2):99–101, 2004.

Taubman B: Toilet training and toileting refusal for stool only: a prospective study, *Pediatrics* 99:54–58, 1997.

Taubman B, Blum NJ, Nemeth N: Children who hide while defecating before they have completed toilet training: a prospective study, *Arch Pediatr Adolesc Med* 157(12):1190–1192, 2003a.

Taubman B, Blum NJ, Nemeth N: Stool toileting refusal: a prospective intervention targeting parental behavior, *Arch Pediatr Adolesc Med* 157(12):1193–1196, 2003b.

Tunc VT, Camurdan AD, Ilhan MN, et al: Factors associated with defecation patterns in 0-24-month-old children, *Eur J Pediatr* 167(12):1357–1362, 2008.

U.S. Preventive Services Task Force (USPSTF): *Guide to clinical preventive services*, ed 2, Baltimore, 1996, Williams & Wilkins.

Van de Walle J, Van Herzeele C, Raes A: Is there still a role for desmopressin in children with primary monosymptomatic nocturnal enuresis? A focus on safety issues, *Drug Saf* 33(4):261–271, 2010.

van Dijk M, Benninga MA, Grootenhuis MA, et al: Prevalence and associated clinical characteristics of behavior problems in constipated children, *Pediatrics* 125(2):e309–e317, 2010.

van Dijk M, Bongers ME, de Vries GJ, et al: Behavioral therapy for childhood constipation: a randomized, controlled trial, *Pediatrics* 121:e1334–e1341, 2008.

van Gool JD: Enuresis and incontinence in children, *Semin Pediatr Surg* 11:100–107, 2002.

Van Kampen M, Lemkens H, Deschamps A, et al: Influence of pelvic floor muscle exercises on full spectrum therapy for nocturnal enuresis, *J Urol* 182(Suppl 4):2067–2071, 2009.

Vermandel A, Van Kampen M, Van Gorp C, et al: How to toilet train healthy children? A review of the literature, *Neurourol Urodyn* 27(3):162–166, 2008.

Vogt M, Lehnert T, Till H, et al: Evaluation of different modes of combined therapy in children with monosymptomatic nocturnal enuresis, *BJU Int* 105(10):1456–1459, 2010.

von Gontard A, Freitag CM, Seifen S, et al: Neuromotor development in nocturnal enuresis, *Dev Med Child Neurol* 48(9):744–750, 2006.

Wolraich ML, Tippins S: *American Academy of Pediatrics guide to toilet training*, New York, 2003, Bantam Books.

Wu HY: Achieving urinary continence in children, *Nat Rev Urol* 7(7):371–377, 2010.

Yeung CK, Sreedhar B, Sihoe JD, et al: Differences in characteristics of nocturnal enuresis between children and adolescents: a critical appraisal from a large epidemiological study, *BJU Int* 97(5):1069–1073, 2006.

Yeung CK, Sit FK, To LK, et al: Reduction in nocturnal functional bladder capacity is a common factor in the pathogenesis of refractory nocturnal enuresis, *BJU Int* 90:302–307, 2002.

Yue Z, Wang M, Xu W, et al: Secretion of antidiuretic hormone in children with obstructive sleep apnea-hypopnea syndrome, *Acta Otolaryngol* 129(8):867–871, 2009.

Zink S, Freitag CM, von Gontard A: Behavioral comorbidity differs in subtypes of enuresis and urinary incontinence, *J Urol* 179(1):295–298, 2008.

CHAPTER 13

American Academy of Allergy: Asthma and Immunology (AAAAI): *Topic of the month-July-Keep exercise-induced asthma on the sidelines*, 2008. Available at www.aaaai.org/patients/topicof month/0708. Accessed Sept 16, 2010.

American Association of Clinical Endocrinologists (AACE) Diabetes Mellitus Clinical Practice Guidelines Task Force: Medical guidelines for clinical practice for the management of diabetes mellitus, *Endocr Pract* 13(Suppl 1):1–68, 2007.

American Academy of Family Physicians, American Academy of Pediatrics, American College of Sports Medicine, et al: *Preparticipation physical evaluation (PPE) monograph*, ed 4, Elk Grove Village, IL, 2010, American Academy of Pediatrics.

American Academy of Orthopaedic Surgeons: *Playground safety guide*, 2009a. Available at www.orthoinfo.aaos.org/topic.cfm?topic=A00313. Accessed Sept 21, 2010.

American Academy of Orthopaedic Surgeons: *Winter sports injury prevention*, 2009b. Available at www.orthoinfo.aaos.org/topic.cfm?topic=A00062. Accessed Sept 21, 2010.

American Academy of Pediatrics: Guidelines for pediatricians: exertional heat-related illness. In *Sports Shorts*, issue 2, 2000. Available at www.aap.org/sections/sportsmedicine/SportsShorts.cfm. Accessed Sept 3, 2010.

American Academy of Pediatrics, Committee on Sports Medicine and Fitness, Committee on School Health: Organized sports for children and adolescents, *Pediatrics* 107(6):1459–1462, 2001; reaffirmed 2007a.

American Academy of Pediatrics: Policy statement: health supervision for children with Down syndrome, *Pediatrics* 107(2):442–449, 2001; reaffirmed 2007b.

American Academy of Pediatrics (AAP): Committee on Sports Medicine and Fitness: Climatic heat stress and the exercising child and adolescent, *Pediatrics* 106(1):158–159, 2000; reaffirmed 2007c.

American Academy of Pediatrics: Policy statement: all-terrain vehicle injury prevention: two-, three-, and four-wheeled unlicensed motor vehicles, *Pediatrics* 105(6):1352–1354, 2000; reaffirmed 2007d.

American Academy of Pediatrics: Committee on Sports Medicine and Fitness: Policy statement: strength training by children and adolescents, *Pediatrics* 121(4):835–840, 2008a.

American Academy of Pediatrics: Committee on Sports Medicine and Fitness: Policy statement: use of performance-enhancing substances, *Pediatrics* 11(4):1103–1106, 2005; reaffirmed 2008b.

American Academy of Pediatrics: Committee on Injury and Poison Prevention: Policy statement: skateboard and scooter injuries, *Pediatrics* 109(3):542–543, 2002; reaffirmed 2009.

American Academy of Pediatrics: Policy statement: active healthy living: prevention of childhood obesity through increased physical activity, *Pediatrics* 117(5):1834–1842, 2006; reaffirmed 2010a.

American Academy of Pediatrics: Promoting physical activity. Available at www.aap.org/family/physicalactivity/physicalactivity.htm. Accessed Sept 12, 2010b.

American Academy of Pediatrics Committee on Sports Medicine and Fitness: Policy statement: athletic participation by children and adolescents who have systemic hypertension, *Pediatrics* 125(6):1287–1293, 1997; revised 2010c.

American Academy of Pediatrics: Committee on Sports Medicine and Fitness: Policy statement: intensive training and sports specialization in young athlete, *Pediatrics* 106(1):154–157, 2000; reaffirmed 2010d.

American Association of Neurological Surgeons: *Sports related head injury*, updated July 2010. Available at www.aans.org/Patient Information/Conditions%and% treatments/Sports-related%Head% Injury.aspx. Accessed Sept 8, 2010.

American College of Cardiology: 36th Annual Bethesda conference on eligibility requirements for competitive athletes with cardiovascular abnormalities, *J Am Coll Cardiol* 45(8):1373–1375, 2005.

American College of Sports Medicine: *Female athlete issues for the team physician: a consensus statement*, 2003. Available at www.acsm.org/AM/Template.cfm? Section=Home_Page&;SECTION=Team_Physician_ Consensus_Statements&TEMPLATE=/CM/ContentDisplay.cfm&CONTENTID=1617. Accessed Sept 22, 2010.

American College of Sports Medicine: Young "extreme" athletes underuse protective equipment: injuries, high-risk behaviors linked to infrequent usage, *News Release*, June 1, 2005. Available at www.acsm.org /AM/Template.cfm?Section=Search&;TEMPLAT E=/CM/HTMLDisplay.cfm&CONTENTID=4179. Accessed Feb 7, 2011.

American College of Sports Medicine: Selected issues for the adolescent athlete and the team physician: a consensus statement, *Med Sci Sports Exer* 40(11):1997–2012, 2008. Available at www.journals.lww.com/acsm-msse/Fulltext/2008/11000/Selected_Issues_for_the_ Adolescent_Athlete_and_the.18.aspx. Accessed Mar 27, 2010.

Baker RJ: Sports nutrition. In Patel DP, Greydanus DE, Baker RJ, editors: *Pediatric practice: sports medicine*, New York, 2009, McGraw-Hill. Chapter 6.

Brennan Ramirez LK, Baker EA, Metzler M: *Promoting health equity: a resource to help communities address social determinants of health*, 2008. Available at www.cdc.gov/NCCDPHP/DACH/chaps/libra ryhealth_disparities.htm. Accessed July 5, 2010.

Brenner JS for the American Academy of Pediatrics Council on Sports Medicine and Fitness: Overuse injuries, overtraining, and burnout in child and adolescent athletes, *Pediatrics* 119(6):1242–1245, 2007.

Brent RL, Weitzman M: The pediatrician's role and responsibility in educating parents about environmental risks, *Pediatrics* 113:1167–1172, 2004.

Brian R, Glazer G: Taming the little tigers: golf-related head injuries in children, *Adv Nurs Pract* 13(6):59–60, 2005.

Browne GJ, Lam LT: Concussive head injury in children and adolescents related to sports and other leisure physical activities, *Br J Sports Med* 40:163–168, 2006.

Calfee R, Fadale P: Popular ergogenic drugs and supplements in young athletes, *Pediatrics* 117:e577–e589, 2006.

Cantu RC, Cantu RV: Head injuries. In DeLee JC, Drez D Jr, Miller MD, editors: ed 3, *DeLee and Drez's orthopaedic sports medicine: principles and practice*, vol 1, ed 3, Philadelphia, 2009, Saunders. Chapter 15.

Casa DJ, Csillan D: Preseason heat-acclimatization guidelines for secondary school athletes, *J Athl Train* 44(3):332–333, 2009.

Centers for Disease Control and Prevention: Non-fatal traumatic brain injuries from sports and recreational activities—United States, 2001-2005, *MMWR Morbid Mortal Wkly Rep* 56(29):733–737, 2007.

Centers for Disease Control and Prevention: Can I get HIV while playing sports? Available at www.cdc. gov/hiv/resources/qa/transmission.htm. Accessed Sept 15, 2010a.

Centers for Disease Control and Prevention: Heat illness among high school athletes—United States, 2005-2009, *MMWR Morbid Mortal Wkly Rep* 59(32):1009–1013, 2010b.

Chaddock L, Erickson KI, Prakash RS, et al: Basal ganglia volume is associated with aerobic fitness in preadolescent children, *Dev Neurosci* 32(3):249–256, 2010.

Chelminski PR: Preparticipation sports physical, 2010. In *ACP PIER AHFS DI Essentials*. Online reference updated regularly.

Cincinnati Children's Hospital: *Dynamic Neuromuscular Analysis (DNA) training program*. Available at www.cincinnatichildrens.org/svc/alpha/s/sports-med/dna-training/dna.htm. Accessed Aug 23, 2010.

Clarke M: *Type 2 diabetes mellitus (T2DM). 2008.* Evidence-based nursing monographs. Available at www.nursingconsult.com/das/ebnm/view/220868 205-2?DOCID=191979&sid=1062199734&SE QNO=1. Accessed Sept 27, 2010.

DeBerardino TM, Owens BD: The team physician: preparticipation examination, on-field emergencies, and ethical and legal issues. In DeLee JC, Drez D Jr, Miller MD, editors: *DeLee and Drez's orthopaedic sports medicine*, ed 3, Philadelphia, 2009, Saunders. Chapter 12.

Eaton DK, Kann L, Kinchen S, et al: Youth risk behavior surveillance—US, 2009, *MMWR Morb Mortal Wkly Rep* 59(SS05):1–142, 2010.

Editorial Staff of Infectious Diseases in Children: Panel endorses pre-participation sports physicals for every child, *Infect Dis Child* 23(4):1, 2010. 10–11.

Eichner ER: Asthma in athletes: scope, risks, mimics, trends, *Curr Sports Med Rep* 7(3):118–119, 2008.

Enoch JS: *ATV deaths, injuries climbing after 20 years, feds no closer to a solution*, 2008. Available at www.consumeraffairs.com/news04/2008/02/cpsc-atvs.htm. Accessed Sept 18, 2010.

Faigenbaum AD, Micheli LJ, American College of Sports Medicine: Current comments, report on youth strength training, *Sports Med Bull* 32(2):28, 2007.

Fountain NB, May AC: Epilepsy and athletics, *Clin Sports Med* 22:605–616, 2003.

Giese EA, O'Connor FG, Depenbrock PJ, et al: The athletic preparticipation evaluation: cardiovascular assessment, *Am Fam Physician* 75(7):1008–1014, 2007.

Goldberg L, MacKinnon DP, Elliot DL, et al: The adolescents training and learning to avoid steroid (ATLAS) prevention program: background and results of a model intervention, *Arch Pediatr Adolesc Med* 150(7):713–721, 1996.

Greydanus DE, Feucht C: Performance-enhancing drugs and supplements. In Patel DR, Greydanus DE, Baker RJ, editors: *Pediatric practice: sports medicine*, New York, 2009, McGraw-Hill. Chapter 7.

Greydanus DE, Patel DR: Preparticipation evaluation. In Patel DR, Greydanus DE, Baker RJ, editors: *Pediatric practice: sports medicine*, New York, 2009, McGraw-Hill. Chapter 8.

Groeger M: Injury risks for the female athlete, *Am Coll Sports Med Health Fitness J* 14(4):14–21, 2010.

Healthy Children: *Water safety for children*, 2010. Available at www.healthychildren.org.english/ safety-prevention/at-play/water-safety-for-older-children.aspx? Accessed Sept 21, 2010.

Heneman K, Zidenberg-Cherr S: *Nutrition and health information sheet: some facts about energy drinks*, 2007. Available at www.nutrition.ucdavis.edu/content/ infosheets/EnergyDrinks.pdf. Accessed Sept 10, 2010.

Hergenroeder AC: The preparticipation sports examination in children and adolescents. *UpToDate*. Available at www.uptodateonline.com. (updated Sept 29, 2008). Accessed May 4, 2010.

Holland-Hall C: Performance-enhancing substances: is your adolescent patient using? *Pediatr Clin North Am* 54(4):651–662, 2007.

Homnick DN: Chest and pulmonary conditions. In Patel DR, Greydanus DE, Baker RJ, editors: *Pediatric practice: sports medicine*, New York, 2009, McGraw-Hill. Chapter 12.

Horn P, Badowski E, Von Stein D: A new zip in playground injuries, *Consult Pediatricians* 9(9):313–314, 2010.

Hosick MB: Protocol decided for sickle cell testing, *NCAA News*, April 13, 2010. Available at www.ncaa. org/wps/portal/ncaahome?WCM_GLOBAL_CON TEXT=/ncaa/NCAA/NCAA+News/NCAA+News+ Online/2010/Division+I/Protocol+decided+for+sick le+cell+testing_04_13_10_NCAA_News. Accessed July 5, 2010.

Housh TJ, Johnson GO: *Growth in young wrestlers*. posted 2007. Available at www.acsm.org/AM/Template. cfm?Section=Home_Page&CONTENTID=8682& SECTION=Updated_single_page&TEMPLATE=/ CM/ContentDisplay.cfm. Accessed Feb 7, 2011.

Howard GM, Radloff M, Sevier TL: Epilepsy and sports, *Curr Sports Med Rep* 3(1):15–19, 2004.

Howe M, Leidel A, Krishnan SM, et al: Patient-related diet and exercise counseling: do providers' own lifestyle habits matter? *Prev Cardiol* 13(4):180–185, 2010.

Insurance Institute for Highway Safety: *Fatality facts*, 2008. Available at www.bhsi.org/stats/htm. Accessed Aug 31, 2010.

Jenkins RR, Adger H: Substance abuse. In Kliegman RM, Behrman RE, Jenson HB, et al, editors: *Nelson textbook of pediatrics*, ed 18, Philadelphia, 2007, Saunders, pp 824–834.

Jimenez CC, Corcoran MH, Crawley T, et al: National Athletic Trainers' Association position statement: management of the athlete with type 1 diabetes mellitus, *J Athl Train* 42(4):536–545, 2007.

Kamboj MK, Draznin MB: Diabetes mellitus. In Patel DR, Greydanus DE, Baker RJ, editors: *Pediatric practice: sports medicine*, New York, 2009, McGraw-Hill. Chapter 15.

Kant AK, Miner P: Physician advice about being overweight: association with self-reported weight loss, dietary, and physical activity behaviours of US adolescents in the National Health and Nutrition Examination Survey, *Pediatrics* 119(1):3142–3147, 2007.

Kapner DA, the Higher Education Center for Alcohol and Other Drug Abuse and Violence Prevention, U.S. Department of Education: Ephedra and energy drinks on college campuses, *Info Facts Resources*, August 2008. Available at www.higheredcenter.org/Services/publications/ephedra-and-energy-drinks-college-campuses. Accessed Sept 10, 2010.

Klein JD, Postle CK, Kreipe RE, et al: Do physicians discuss needed diet and nutrition health topics with adolescents? *J Adolesc Health* 38(5):608.e1–e6, 2006.

Koutures CG, Simpson CD, Munyak J: *Atlantoaxial injury and dysfunction*, 2008. Available at www.emedicine.medscape.com/article/93546-overview. Accessed Aug 15, 2010.

Krajnik S, Fogarty KJ, Yard EE, et al: Shoulder injuries in U.S. high school baseball and softball athletes, 2005-2008, *Pediatrics* 125(3):497–501, 2010.

Landry GL: Heat injuries. In Kliegman RM, Behrman RD, Jenson HB, et al, editors: *Nelson textbook of pediatrics*, ed 18, Philadelphia, 2007, Saunders, p 2864.

Lovell MR, Fazio V: Concussion management in the child and adolescent athlete, *Curr Sports Med Rep* 17(1):12–15, 2008.

Magee LM: *Return to play: a common sense guide for coaches*, 2005. Available at www.ascm.org/AM/Template.cfm?Section=brochures2&;Template=/CM/ContentDisplay.cfm&ContentID=1532. Accessed Sept 9, 2010.

Malinauskas BM, Aeby VG, Overton RF, et al: A survey of energy drink consumption patterns among college students, *Nutrition J* 6:35, 2007.

Martin TJ, American Academy of Pediatrics (AAP) Committee on Sports Medicine and Fitness: Technical report: knee brace use in the young athlete, *Pediatrics* 108(2):503–507, 2001.

McCarthy VM: Getting to the big game: keys to performing an efficient sports physical, *Adv Nurs Pract* 14(6):67–69, 2006.

McCrory P, Meeuwisse W, Johnston K, et al: Consensus statement on concussion in sports: the 3rd International Conference on Concussion in Sports, 2008, *J Athl Train* 44(4):434–448, 2009.

McDevitt ER, Brown DE: Sports pharmacology: ergogenic drugs in sports. In DeLee JC, Drez D Jr, Miller MD, editors: *DeLee and Drez's orthopaedic sports medicine*, ed 3, Philadelphia, 2009, Saunders. Chapter 8.

Metzl JD: Overtraining in children and adolescents. In *American Academy of Sports Medicine: Fit Society: youth sports and health*. Spring 2003. Available at www.acsm.org/AM/Template.cfm?Section=Home_Page&;CONTENTID=1276&TEMPLATE=/CM/ContentDisplay.cfm. Accessed Sept 21, 2010.

Mitchell JH, Haskell W, Van Camp SP: 36th Bethesda Conference: Task Force 8: Classification of Sports, *J Am Coll Cardiol* 45(8):1364–1367, 2005.

Murphy NA, Carbone PS, American Academy of Pediatrics Council on Children with Disabilities: Promoting the participation of children with disabilities in sports, recreation and physical activities, *Pediatrics* 121(5):1057–1061, 2008.

National Athletic Trainers' Association: *Sickle cell trait and the athlete: consensus statement*, 2007. Available at www.nata.org/statements/consensus-statements. Accessed July 25, 2010.

National Collegiate Athletic Association (NCAA): *NCAA guideline 21: Blood borne pathogens, 2009-2010 NCAA sports medicine handbook*, 2009. National Collegiate Athlete Association. Available at www.ncaa.org/health-safety. Accessed August 15, 2010.

National Collegiate Athletic Association (NCAA): *2010-2011 NCAA sports medicine handbook*. Available at www.ncaapublicatiions.com/productdownloads/MD11.pdf. Accessed Sept 14, 2010.

Nattiv A, Loucks AB, Manore MM, et al: American College of Sports Medicine position stand: the female athlete triad, *Med Sci Sports Exerc* 39(10):1867–1882, 2007.

Nemet D, Eliakim A: Pediatric sports nutrition: an update, *Curr Opin Clin Nutr Metab Care* 12:304–309, 2009.

Neumark-Sztainer D, Goeden C, Story M, et al: Associations between body satisfaction and physical activity in adolescents: implications for programs aimed at preventing a broad spectrum of weight-related disorders, *Eat Disord* 12(2):125–137, 2004.

O'Brien MC, McCoy TP, Rhodes SD, et al: Caffeinated cocktails: energy drink consumption, high-risk drinking, and alcohol-related consequences among college students, *Acad Emerg Med* 15(5):453–460, 2008.

Olsen OE, Myklebust G, Engebretsen L, et al: Exercises to prevent lower limb injuries in youth sports: cluster randomized controlled trial, *BMJ* 330:449–452, 2005.

Pantano KJ: Coaching concerns in physically active girls and young women—Part 1: the female athlete triad, *Strength Cond J* 31(6):38–43, 2009.

Patel DR: Cardiovascular considerations. In Patel DR, Greydanus DE, Baker RJ, editors: *Pediatric practice: sports medicine*, New York, 2009a, McGraw-Hill. Chapter 14.

Patel DR: Hematologic conditions. In Patel DR, Greydanus DE, Baker RJ, editors: *Pediatric practice: sports medicine*, New York, 2009b, McGraw-Hill. Chapter 16.

Patel DR, Greydanus DE: Physically challenged athletes. In Patel DR, Greydanus DE, Baker RJ, editors: *Pediatric practice: sports medicine*, New York, 2009, McGraw-Hill. Chapter 35.

Pennington C: *The effects of energy drinks on adolescents*, 2010. Available at www.today.uconn.edu/?p=17083. Accessed Sept 10, 2010.

Physical Activity Collaborative: *Moving to the future: the critical need for public health leadership and capacity to improve health through physical activity: recommendations from the Physical Activity Collaborative*, 2008. Available at www.health.state.mn.us/divs/.../physicalactivity/.../paccalltoaction.pdf. Accessed June 6, 2010.

Pianosi PT, Davis HS: Determinants of physical fitness in children with asthma, *Pediatrics* 113:3225–e229, 2004.

Pitetti KH, Beets MW, Combs C: Physical activity in children with intellectual disabilities during school, *Med Sci Sports Exerc* 41(8):1580–1586, 2009.

Putukian M, O'Connor FG, Stricker P: Mononucleosis and athletic participation: an evidence-based subject review, *Clin J Sports Med* 18(4):309–315, 2008.

Quinn C: ACL injury prevention training program, 2008. Available at www.sportsmedicine.about.com/cs/knee_injuries/a/aa022202a.htm. Accessed Sept 16, 2010.

Rice SG, American Academy of Pediatrics Council on Sports Medicine and Fitness: Medical conditions affecting sports participation, *Pediatrics* 121(4):841–848, 2008.

Safe Kids USA: *Headed for injury: an observational study of helmet use among children ages 5 to 14 participating in wheeled sports*, 2004. Available at www.safekids.org/assets/docs/ourwork/research/research-report-bike-2004.pdx. Accessed Sept 8, 2010.

Safe Kids Worldwide: *Sports and recreation safety*, 2007. Available at www.safekids.org/assets/docs/ourwork/research/2007-fact-sheet-sport-rec.doc. Accessed Aug 26, 2010.

Saglimbeni AJ: *Exercise-induced asthma: treatment and medication*, 2009. Available at www.emedicine.medscape.com/article/88849-treatment. Accessed Nov 28, 2010.

Savage JS, Dinallo JM, Downs DS: Adolescent body satisfaction: the role of perceived parental encouragement for physical activity, *Int J Behav Nutr Phys Act* 6:90, 2009.

Sesselberg TS, Klein JD, O'Connor KG, et al: Screening and counseling for childhood obesity: results from a national survey, *J Am Board Fam Med* 23(3):334–342, 2010.

Shealy JE: *If you wear a helmet, ski or snowboard as if you're not wearing one*, 2010. Available at www.lidsonkids.org/ski-or-snowboard-as-if-youre-not-wearing-one.asp. Accessed Sept 21, 2010.

Sheerin KA: The link between asthma and obesity. In American Academy of Allergy, Asthma, and Immunology: Asthma and advocate, 2005. Available at www.aaaai.org. Accessed Aug 4, 2006.

Silverstein J, Klingensmith G, Copeland K, et al: Care of children and adolescents with type 1 diabetes: a statement of the American Diabetes Association, *Diabetes Care* 28(1):186–212, 2005.

Smith AM, Link AA: Sport psychology and the adolescent athlete, *Pediatr Ann* 39(5):310–316, 2010.

Special Olympics: *Healthy athletes program*. Available at www.specialolympics.org/Special+Olympics+Public+Website/English/Coach/Coaching_Guides/Basics+of+Special+Olympics/Down+Syndrome+and+Restrictions+Based+on+Atlantoaxial+Instability.htm. Accessed Aug 15, 2010.

Stanford KI, Mickleborough TD, Ray S, et al: Influence of menstrual cycle phase on pulmonary function in asthmatic athletes, *Eur J Appl Physiol* 96(6):703–710, 2006.

Strong WB, Malina RM, Blimkie CJ, et al: Evidence-based physical activity for school-age youth, *J Pediatr* 146(6):732–737, 2005.

Ternouth A, Collier D, Maughan B: Childhood emotional problems and self-perceptions predict weight gain in a longitudinal regression model, *BMC Med* 7:46, 2009.

Thompson PD, Buchner D, Piña IL, et al: American Heart Association scientific statement: exercise and physical activity in the prevention and treatment of atherosclerotic cardiovascular disease, *Circulation* 107:3109–3116, 2003.

U.S. Consumer Protection Safety Committee: *Skiing helmets; an evaluation of the potential to reduce head injury*, 1999. Available at www.cpsc.gov/library/skihelm.pdf. Accessed Sept 21, 2010.

U.S. Consumer Protection Safety Committee: *Trampolines*, 2000. Available at www.cpsc.gov/library/tramp00.pdf. Accessed Sept 21, 2010.

U.S. Consumer Product Safety Commission: *Gear up, strap it on—helmets can save lives and reduce injuries*, 2006. Available at www.cpsc.gov/cpscpub/prerel/prhtml06/06122.html. Accessed Sept 8, 2010.

U.S. Department of Health and Human Services (USDHHS): *Healthy People 2010 midcourse review: physical activity and fitness*, Washington, DC, 2006, US Government Printing Office.

U.S. Department of Health and Human Services National Heart, Lung, and Blood Institute: *Expert panel report 3: guidelines for the diagnosis and management of asthma*, 2007. Available at www.nhlbi.nih.gov/guidelines/asthma/index.htm. Accessed Mar 27, 2010.

U.S. Department of Health and Human Services: *2008 Physical activity guidelines for Americans*, 2008a. Available at www.health.gov/paguidelines. Accessed Aug 14, 2010.

U.S. Department of Health and Human Services: *Healthy People 2010: progress report focus area 22—physical activity and fitness*, 2008b. Available at www.healthypeople.gov/data/2010prog/focus22. Accessed July 13, 2010.

U.S. Department of Health and Human Services: *Developing Healthy People 2020: physical activity and fitness*, 2009. Available at www.healthypeople.gov/hy2020/objectives?TopicArea.aspx?id=39&TopicArea=Physical+Activity+and+Fitness. Accessed July 5, 2010.

U.S. Preventive Services Task Force: Behavioral counseling in primary care to promote physical activity: recommendations and rationale, *Guidelines from guide to clinical preventive service*, ed 3, (2000-2003), Washington, DC, 2002, U.S. Department of Health and Human Services.

Watson DS, Mehan TJ, Smith GA, et al: Golf-cart-related injuries in the USA, *J Prev Med* 35(1):55–59, 2008.

World Health Organization (WHO): *Global strategy on diet, physical activity and health: resolution WHA55.23*, 2004. Available at www.who.int/dietphysicalactivity/strategy/eb11344/strategy_english_web.pdf. Accessed Sept 12, 2010.

World Health Organization (WHO): *Interventions on diet and physical activity: what works: summary report*, 2009. Available at www.who.int/dietphysicalactivity/summary-report.pdf. Accessed July 5, 2010.

World Health Organization (WHO): *Physical activity: a global public health problem*. Available at www.who.int/dietphysicalactivity/factsheet_inactivity/en/index.html. Accessed July 5, 2010a.

World Health Organization (WHO): *Childhood overweight and obesity*. Available at www.who.int/dietphysicalactivity/childhood/en/index.html. Accessed July 5, 2010b.

World Health Organization (WHO): *Global infobase: chronic diseases, global comparable estimates, risk factors*. Available at www.apps.who/int/infobase. Accessed July 5, 2010c.

Young WK, Metzi JD: Strength training for the young athlete, *Pediatr Ann* 39(5):293–299, 2010.

CHAPTER 14

Alfano CM, Zakem AH, Costa NM, et al: Sleep problems and their relation to cognitive factors, anxiety, and depressive symptoms in children and adolescents, *Depress Anxiety* 26:503–512, 2009.

American Academy of Pediatrics (AAP) Task Force on Sudden Infant Death Syndrome: The changing concept of sudden infant death syndrome: diagnostic coding shifts, controversies regarding the sleeping environment, and new variables to consider in reducing risk, *Pediatrics* 116:1245–1255, 2005.

American Academy of Sleep Medicine: *International classification of sleep disorders, revised: diagnostic and coding manual (ICSD-R)*, Westchester, IL, 2001, The Academies.

American Academy of Sleep Medicine: *Restless legs syndrome*, 2006a. Available at www.aasmnet.org/Resources/FactSheets/RLS.pdf. Accessed Jan 17, 2010.

American Academy of Sleep Medicine: *Sleep walking and sleep talking*, 2006b. Available at www.aasmnet.org/Resources/FactSheets/SleepwalkingTalking.pdf. Accessed Jan 17, 2010.

American Academy of Sleep Medicine: *Nightmares & other disturbing parasomnias*, 2008. Available at www.aasmnet.org/Resources/FactSheets/NightmareParasom.pdf. Accessed Jan 17, 2010.

Anders T: Night waking in infants during the first year of life, *Pediatrics* 63:860–864, 1979.

Archbold K, Pituch KJ, Panahi C, et al: Symptoms of sleep disturbances among children at two general pediatric clinics, *J Pediatr* 140:97–102, 2002.

Barone J, Hanson C, DaJusta DG, et al: Nocturnal enuresis and overweight are associated with obstructive sleep apneas, *Pediatrics* 124:e53–e59, 2009.

Boergers J, Hart C, Owens JA, et al: Child sleep disorders: associations with parental sleep duration and daytime sleepiness, *J Fam Psychol* 121(1):88–94, 2007.

Burnham M, Goodlin-Jones B, Gaylor B, et al: Use of sleep aids during the first year of life, *Pediatrics* 109:594–601, 2002.

Carey W: Night waking and temperament in infancy, *J Pediatr* 84:756–758, 1974.

Chaput A-P, Brunet M, Tremblay A: Relationship between short sleeping hours and childhood overweight/obesity: results from the 'Quebec en Forme' project, *Int J Obes* 30:1080–1085, 2006.

Connelly K: *Sleep disorder, night terrors*, 2005. Available at www.emedicinehealth.com/night_terrors/article_em.htm.

Connor JR, Ponnuro P, Wang X-S, et al: Profile of altered brain iron acquisition in restless leg syndrome, *Brain* 134(4):959–968, 2011.

Cubero J, Chancion B, Sanchez S, et al: Improving the qualities of infant sleep through the inclusion at supper of cereals enriched with tryptophan, anenosine-5-phosphate, and uridine-5-phosphate, *Nutr Neurosci* 12(60):272–280, 2009.

Davis K, Parker K, Montgomery G: Sleep in infants and young children: part 1: normal sleep, *J Pediatr Health Care* 18:65–71, 2004.

Dewar G: *Baby sleep patterns: a guide for the science-minded parents*, 2008a. Available at www.parentingscience.com/baby-sleep-patterns. Accessed Jan 10, 2010.

Dewar G: *Baby sleep requirements: a guide for the science-minded parents*, 2008b. Available at www.parentingscience.com/baby-sleep-requirements.html. Accessed Jan 10, 2010.

Dewar G: *Newborn sleep patterns: a guide for the science-minded parents*, 2008c. Available at www.parentingscience.com/newborn-sleep.html. Accessed Jan 10, 2010.

Eidelman AI, Gartner LM: Bed sharing with unimpaired parents is not an important risk for sudden infant death syndrome: to the editor, *Pediatrics* 117:991–992, 2006.

Ferber R: *Solve your child's sleep problems: new, revised, and expanded edition*, New York, 2006, Simon & Schuster.

Gessner BD, Porter TJ: Bed sharing with unimpaired parents is not an important risk for sudden infant death syndrome, *Pediatrics* 117:990–991, 2006.

Goldberg W, Keller M: Co-sleeping during infancy and early childhood: key findings and future directions, *Infant Child Dev* 16:457–469, 2007.

Goodlin-Jones B, Waters S, Andrews T: Objective sleep measurement in typically and atypically developing preschool children with ADHD-like profiles, *Child Psychiatry Hum Dev* 40:257–268, 2009.

Howard B, Wong J: Sleep disorders, *Pediatr Rev* 22:327–341, 2001.

Jan JE, Owens JA, Weiss MD, et al: Sleep hygiene for children with neurodevelopmental disabilities, *Pediatrics* 122(6):1343–1350, 2008.

Jenni O, Deboer T, Achermann P: Development of the 24-h rest-activity pattern in human infants, *Infant Behav Dev* 29:143–152, 2006.

Jenni O, Molinari L, Caflisch J, et al: Sleep duration from ages 1 to 10 years: variability and stability in comparison with growth, *Pediatrics* 120:769–776, 2007.

Johnson EO, Roth T: An epidemiological study of sleep-disordered breathing symptoms among adolescents, *Sleep* 29(9):1135–1142, 2006.

Johnson KP: Malow BA: Sleep in children with autism spectrum disorders, *Curr Neurol Neurosci Rep* 8:155–161, 2008.

Kieckhefer G, Lentz M, Tsai S, et al: Parent-child agreement in report of nighttime respiratory symptoms and sleep disruptions and quality, *J Pediatr Health Care* 23(5):315–326, 2009.

Koren A, Reece S, Kahn-DeAngelo L, et al: Parental information and behaviors and provider practices related to tummy time and back to sleep, *J Pediatr Health Care* 24(4):222–230, 2010.

Krakowiak P, Goodlin-Jones B, Hertz-Picciotto I, et al: Sleep problems in children with autism spectrum disorders, developmental delays, and typical development: a population-based study, *J Sleep Res* 17:197–206, 2008.

Lee K, Ward T: Critical components of a sleep assessment for clinical practice settings, *Issues Ment Health Nurs* 26:739–750, 2005.

Liu X, Buysee D, Gentzler A, et al: Insomnia and hypersomnia associated with depressive phenomenology and comorbidity in childhood depression, *Sleep* 30:83–90, 2007.

Maheswaran M, Kushida C: Restless legs syndrome in children, *Medscape Gen Med* 8:79, 2006.

Meltzer L, Johnson C, Crosette J, et al: *Prevalence of diagnosed sleep disorders in pediatric primary care practices*. Available at www.pediatrics.aappublications.org. Accessed Jan 14, 2010.

Meltzer L, Mindell J: Nonpharmacologic treatments for pediatric sleeplessness, *Pediatr Clin North Am* 51:135–151, 2004.

Mindell J, Emslie G, Blumer J, et al: Pharmacologic management of insomnia in children and adolescents: consensus statement, *Pediatrics* 117:e1223–e1232, 2006.

National Sleep Foundation: *Children and sleeping*, 2009. Available at www.sleepfoundation.org/article/sleep-topics/children-and-sleep. Accessed Jan 10, 2010.

Noland H, Price JH, Dake J, et al: Adolescents' sleep behaviors and perception of sleep, *J Sch Health* 75(5):224–230, 2009.

Owens JA: Sleep medicine. In Kliegman R, Behrman R, Jenson H, et al, editors: *Nelson textbook of pediatrics*, ed 18, Philadelphia, 2007, Saunders, pp 91–99.

Owens JA: Sleep disorders and attention deficit/hyperactivity disorder, *Curr Psychiatry Rep* 10:439–444, 2008.

Owens JA, Mehlenbeck R, Lee J, et al: Effect of weight, sleep duration, and comorbid sleep disorders on behavioral outcomes in children with sleep disordered breathing, *Arch Pediatr Adolesc Med* 162(4):31–34, 2008.

Pelayo R, Owens J, Mindell J, et al: Bed sharing with unimpaired parents is not an important risk for sudden infant death syndrome: to the editor, *Pediatrics* 117:993–994, 2006.

Petit D, Touchette E, Tremblay RE, et al: Dyssomnias and parasomnias in early childhood, *Pediatrics* 119:e1016–e1025, 2007.

Picchietti D, Allen RP, Walters AS, et al: Restless leg syndrome: prevalence and impact in children and adolescents–the Peds REST study, *Pediatrics* 120:253–266, 2007.

Rodriguez A: Pediatric sleep and epilepsy, *Curr Neurol Neurosci Rep* 7:342–347, 2007.

Sadeh A: A brief screening questionnaire for infant sleep problems: validation and findings for an internet sample, *Pediatrics* 113:e570–e577, 2004.

Schredl M, et al: Longitudinal study of nightmares in children: stability and effect of emotional symptoms, *Child Psychiatry Hum Dev* 40:439–449, 2009.

Sheldon SH: Parasomnias in childhood, *Pediatr Clin North Am* 51:69–88, 2004.

Smaldone A, Honig JC, Byrne MW: Does assessing sleep inadequacy across its continuum inform associations with child and family health? *J Pediatr Health Care* 23(6):394–404, 2009.

Sobralske M, Gruber M: Risks and benefits of parent/child bed sharing, *Am Acad Nurse Pract* 21:474–479, 2009.

Souders MC, Mason TB, Valladares O, et al: Sleep behaviors and sleep quality in children with autism spectrum disorders, *Sleep* 32(12):1566–1578, 2009.

Stevens MS: *Normal sleep, sleep physiology, and sleep deprivation.* (updated Oct 29, 2008). Available at emedicine.medscape.com/article/118826. Accessed Apr 26, 2010.

Szuhay G, Rotenberg J: Sleep apnea in pediatric neurological condition, *Curr Neurol Neurosci Rep* 9:145–152, 2009.

Thompson DA, Christakis DA: The association between television viewing and irregular sleep schedules among children less than 3 years of age, *Pediatrics* 116:851–856, 2005.

Touchette E, Petit D, Paquet J, et al: Factors associated with fragmented sleep at night across early childhood, *Arch Pediatr Adolesc Med* 159:242–249, 2005.

Touchette E, Mongrain V, Petit V, et al: Development of sleep-wake schedules during childhood and relationship with sleep duration, *Arch Pediatr Adolesc Med* 162(4):343–349, 2008.

Ward T, Mason T: Sleep disorders in children, *Nurs Clin North Am* 37:693–706, 2002.

Wills L, Garcia J: Parasomnias: epidemiology and management, *CNS Drugs* 16:803–810, 2002.

CHAPTER 15

Adesman A: A diagnosis of ADHD? Don't overlook the possibility of a co-morbidity, *Contemp Pediatr* 20(12):91–106, 2003.

All Kinds of Minds: *Learning framework.* Available at http://allkindsofminds.org/learning-framework. Accessed Nov 28, 2010.

American Academy of Pediatrics (AAP): Newborn and infant hearing loss: detection and intervention, *Pediatrics* 103:527–530, 1999.

American Academy of Pediatrics (AAP) Committee on Quality Improvement, Subcommittee on Attention Deficit/Hyperactivity Disorder: Clinical practice guideline: diagnosis and evaluation of the child with attention-deficit/hyperactivity disorder, *Pediatrics* 105(5):1158–1170, 2000.

American Academy of Pediatrics (AAP) Committee on Quality Improvement, Subcommittee on Attention Deficit/Hyperactivity Disorder: Clinical practice guideline: treatment of the school-aged child with attention-deficit/hyperactivity disorder, *Pediatrics* 108(4):1033–1044, 2001.

American Academy of Pediatrics (AAP): *Children's health topics.* Available at www.aap.org/healthtopics/autism.cfm. Accessed Nov 3, 2010.

American Psychiatric Association (APA): *Diagnostic and statistical manual of mental disorders,* ed 4, text revision, Washington, DC, 2000, American Psychiatric Association.

Arnsten AFT: Toward a new understanding of attention-deficit hyperactivity disorder pathophysiology, *CNS Drugs* 23(Supp 1):33–41, 2009.

Asberg KK, Vogel J, Bowers CA: Exploring correlates and predictors of stress in parents of children who are deaf: implications of perceived social support and mode of communication, *J Child Family Studies* 17(4):486–499, 2008.

Barbaresi WJ, Katusic SK, Voight RG: Autism: a review of the state of the science for pediatric primary health care clinicians, *Arch Pediatr Adolesc Med* 160:1167–1175, 2006.

Barker DH, Quittner A, Fink N, et al: Predicting behavior problems in deaf and hearing children: the influence of language, attention and parent-child communication, *Dev Psychopathol* 21(2):373–392, 2009.

Barkley RA, Murphy KR: *Attention deficit hyperactivity disorder: a clinical workbook,* ed 3, New York, 2005, Guilford Press.

Buitelaar J, Barton J, Danckaerts M, et al: Comparison of North American versus non-North American ADHD study populations, *Eur Child Adolesc Psychiatry* 15:177–181, 2006.

Butter EM, Mulick JA: Autism. In McInerny TK, Adam HM, Campbell DE, et al, editors: *American Academy of Pediatrics textbook of pediatric care,* Elk Grove Village, IL, 2009, American Academy of Pediatrics, pp 1196–1200.

Case-Smith J, Ratliff-Schaub K: Other sensory problems. In Carey W, Crocker A, Coleman W, et al, editors: *Developmental-behavioral pediatrics,* ed 4, Philadelphia, 2009, Saunders, pp 730–736.

Centers for Disease Control and Prevention (CDC). Prevalence of autism spectrum disorders—autism and developmental disabilities monitoring network, six sites, United States, 2000, *MMWR* 56(SS01):1–11, 2007.

Centers for Disease Control and Prevention (CDC): ADHD: Increasing prevalence of parent-reported attention deficit/hyperactivity disorder among children—United States, 2003 and 2007, *MMWR* 59(44):1439–1443, November 12, 2010a.

Centers for Disease Control and Prevention (CDC): *ADHD in the United States: data and statistics.* Available at www.cdc.gov/ncbddd/ADHD/data.html. Accessed Nov 3, 2010b.

Chilosi AM, Comarini A, Scusa MF, et al: Neurodevelopmental disorders in children with severe to profound sensorineural hearing loss: a clinical study, *Dev Med Child Neurol* 52(9):856–862, 2010.

Dupaul GJ, Power TJ, Anastopoulos A, Reid R: *ADHD rating scale IV: checklists, norms, and clinical interpretation,* New York, 1998, Guilford Press.

Dworkin PH: School learning problems and developmental differences. In McInery T, Adam H, Campbel D, et al, editors: *Textbook of pediatric care,* Elk Grove Village, IL, 2009, American Academy of Pediatrics, pp 1149–1155.

DynaMed Database: *Attention-deficit hyperactivity disorder (ADHD) in children.* Available at www.ebscohost.com.liboff.ohsu.edu/dynamed/what.php. Accessed Nov 30, 2010.

Elisa F, Josée L, Oreste FG, et al: Gross motor development and reach on sound as critical tools for the development of the blind child, *Brain Dev* 24(5):269–275, 2002.

Evans SW, Schultz BK, Sadler JM: Safety and efficacy of psychosocial interventions used to treat children with attention-deficit/hyperactivity disorder, *Pediatr Ann* 37(1):52–59, 2008.

Faraone SV, Sergeant J, Gillberg C, et al: The worldwide prevalence of ADHD: is it an American condition? *World Psychiatry* 2(2):104–113, 2003.

Fazzi E, Azccagnino M, Gahagan S, et al: Sleep disturbances in visually impaired toddlers, *Brain Dev* 30(9):572–578, 2008.

Froehlich TE, Lanphear BP, Auinger P, et al: Association of tobacco and lead exposures with attention-deficit/hyperactivity disorder, *Pediatrics* 124(6):e1054–e1063, 2009. Available at http://pediatrics.aappublications.org. Accessed Oct 30, 2010.

Geraghty ME, Depasquale GM, Lane AE: Nutritional intake and therapies in autism: a spectrum of what we know, *Infant Child Adolesc Nutr* 2(1):62–69, 2010a.

Geraghty ME, Bates-Wall J, Ratliff-Schaub KR, et al: Nutritional interventions and therapies in autism, *Infant Child Adolesc Nutr* 2(2):120–133, 2010b.

Gilchrist RH, Arnold LE: Long-term efficacy of ADHD pharmacotherapy in children, *Pediatr Ann* 37(1):46–51, 2008.

Glascoe FP, Hamilton S: Making developmental behavioral screening work for school-aged kids, *Contemp Pediatr,* 2010. Available at www.modernmedicine.com/modernmedicine/Modern+Medicine+Now/Making-developmental-behavioral-screening-work-for/Article Standard/Article/detail/687355. Accessed Jan 7, 2011.

Gliga T, Volein A, Csibra G: Verbal labels modulate perceptual object process in 1-year-old children, *J Cog Neurosci* 22(12):2781–2789, 2010.

Gordon M: *Manual of nursing diagnosis,* ed 12, Sudbury, MA, 2010, Jones and Bartlett.

Gregory S, Mogford K: Early language development in deaf children. In Kyle WJ, Deucher M, editors: *Perspectives on British sign language and deafness,* London, 1981, Croon Helm.

Haddad J: Hearing loss. In Kliegman R, Behrman R, Jenson H, et al, editors: *Nelson textbook of pediatrics,* ed 18, Philadelphia, 2007, Saunders, pp 2620–2628.

Hagan JF, Shaw JS, Duncan PM, editors: *Bright futures: guidelines for health supervision of infants, children, and adolescents,* ed 3, Elk Grove Village, IL, 2008, American Academy of Pediatrics.

Hansen RL, Ulrey GL: The spectrum of social cognition. In Carey W, Crocker A, Coleman W, et al, editors: *Developmental-behavioral pediatrics,* ed 4, Philadelphia, 2009, Saunders, pp 373–380.

Institute for Clinical Systems Improvement (ICSI): *Health care guideline: diagnosis and management of attention deficit hyperactivity disorder in primary care for school-age children and adolescents,* March 2010. Available at www.icsi.org. Accessed Oct 30, 2010.

Jacobson L, Hard AL, Horemuzova E, et al: Visual impairment is common in children born before 25 gestational weeks—boys are more vulnerable than girls, *Acta Paediatr* 98(2):261–265, 2009.

Kelly D: Hearing impairment. In Carey WB, Crocker AC, Coleman WL, et al, editors: *Developmental-behavioral pediatrics,* ed 4, Philadelphia, 2009, Elsevier, pp 687–695.

Kendall J: Outlasting disruption: the process of reinvestment in families with ADHD children, *Qual Health Res* 8:839–857, 1998.

Knafl K, Breitmayer B, Gallo A, et al: Family response to childhood chronic illness: description of management styles, *J Pediatr Nurs* 11:315–326, 1996.

Knafl K, Dietrick J, Kirby A: Normalization promotion. In Craft-Rosenberg M, Denehy J, editors: *Nursing interventions for infants, children, and families,* Thousand Oaks, CA, 2001, Sage, pp 377–388.

Korver AM, Konings S, Dekker FW, et al: Newborn hearing screening vs later hearing screening and developmental outcomes in children with permanent childhood hearing impairment, *JAMA* 304(15):1701–1708, 2010.

Krull K: Attention deficit hyperactivity disorder in children and adolescents: *Epidemiology and pathogenesis.* UpToDate, May 2010. Available at www.uptodate.com. Accessed Oct 13, 2010a.

Krull K: Attention deficit hyperactivity disorder in children and adolescents: *Pharmacotherapy.* UpToDate, May 2010. Available at www.uptodate.com. Accessed Oct 13, 2010b.

Kushalnagar P, Mathur G, Moreland CJ, et al: Infants and children with hearing loss need early language access, *J Clin Ethics* 21(2):143–154, 2010.

Lambros KM, Leslie LK: Management of the child with a learning disorder, *Pediatr Ann* 34(4):259–261, 2005.

LD Online: *What is a learning disability?* Available at www.ldonline.org/ldbasics. Accessed Nov 23, 2010.

Lerner M, Wigal T: Long-term safety of stimulant medications used to treat children with ADHD, *Pediatr Ann* 37(1):37–45, 2008.

Levy S, Maadell D, Schultz R: Autism, *Lancet* 374:1627–1638, 2009.

Liptak GS, et al: Satisfaction with primary health care received by families of children with developmental disabilities, *J Pediatr Health Care* 20(4):245–252, 2006.

Marcason W: What is the current status of research concerning use of a gluten-free, casein-free diet for children diagnosed with autism? *J Am Diet Assoc* 109(3):572, 2009.

Meadow K: *Deafness and child development*, Berkeley, CA, 1980, University of California Press.

Meadow-Orlans KP: Research on developmental aspects of deafness. In Moores DE, Meadow-Orlans KE, editors: *Educational and developmental aspects of deafness*, Washington, DC, 1990, Gallaudet University Press.

Meinzen-Derr J, Lim LH, Choo DI, et al: Pediatric hearing impairment caregiver experience: impact of duration of hearing loss on parental stress, *Int J Pediatr Otolaryngol* 72(11):1693–1703, 2008.

Miller KJ: Executive functions, *Pediatr Ann* 34(4):310–317, 2005.

Miller LJ: *Sensational kids: hope and help for children with sensory processing disorder*, New York, 2006, GP Putnam's Sons.

Miller L, Nielson D, Schoen S, et al: Perspectives on sensory processing disorder: a call for translational research, *Front Integr Neurosci* 3(22):1–12, 2009.

Morton CC, Nance WE: Newborn hearing screening – a silent revolution, *N Engl J Med* 354:2151–2164, 2006.

Myers SM: Management of autism spectrum disorders in primary care, *Pediatr Ann* 38(1):42–49, 2009.

National Initiative for Children's Healthcare Quality (NICHQ): *Caring for children with ADHD: a resource toolkit for clinicians.* Available at www.nichq.org/resources/ADHD_toolkit.html. Accessed Nov 28, 2010.

National Resource Center on ADHD: *Online resource of children and adults with attention deficit hyperactivity disorder (CHADD)*, July 2009. Available at www.help4ADHD.org/faq.cfm?fid=40&;varLang =en. Accessed Oct 30, 2010.

Olaniyan O, dosReis S, Garriett V, et al: Community perspectives of childhood behavioral problems and ADHD among African-American parents, *Ambul Pediatr* 7(3):226–231, 2007.

Olitsky S, Hug D, Smith L: Disorders of vision. In Kliegman R, Behrman R, Jenson H, et al, editors: *Nelson's textbook of pediatrics*, ed 18, Philadelphia, 2007, Saunders, pp 2573–2576.

Pastor PN, Reuben CA: Diagnosed attention deficit hyperactivity disorder and learning disability: United States, 2004-2006, *Vital Health Stat* 10(237):1–14, 2008.

Perrin JM, Friedman RA, Knilans TK, et al: Cardiovascular monitoring and stimulant drugs for attention-deficit/hyperactivity disorder, *Pediatrics* 122(2):451–452, 2008.

Phillips S, Hartley JT: Developmental differences and interventions for blind children, *Pediatr Nurs* 14(3):201–204, 1988.

Pliszka S: American Academy of Child and Adolescent Psychiatry (AACAP) work group on quality issues: Practice parameter for the assessment and treatment of children and adolescents with attention-deficit/hyperactivity disorder, *J Am Acad Child Adolesc Psychiatry* 46(7):894–921, 2007.

Quigley S, Kretschmer R: *The education of deaf children: issues, theory, and practice*, Baltimore, 1982, University Park Press.

Rahi JS, Manaras I, Tuomainen H, et al: Meeting the needs of parents around the time of diagnosis of disability among their children: evaluation of a novel program for information, support, and liaison by key workers, *Pediatrics* 114:e477–e482, 2004.

Ryan R: Hearing and speech assessment. In Ballard R, editor: *Pediatric care of the ICN graduate*, Philadelphia, 1988, Saunders.

Schlumberger E, Narbona J, Manrique M: Non-verbal development of children with deafness with and without cochlear implants, *Dev Med Child Neurol* 46:599–606, 2004.

Sensory Processing Foundation: *Ten fundamental facts about SPD.* Available at www.spdfoundation.net. Accessed Nov 23, 2010.

Shelton K: *The family experience with school when an adolescent has ADHD*, Unpublished doctoral dissertation, Portland, 2001, Oregon Health & Science University.

Singh I: Beyond polemics: science and ethics of ADHD, *Nat Rev Neurosci* 9:957-964, 2008. Available at www.nature.com/reviews/neuro. Accessed Oct 30, 2010.

Sininger YS, Grimes A, Christensen E: Auditory development in early amplified children: factors influencing auditory-based communication outcomes in children with hearing loss, *Ear Hear* 31(2):166–185, 2010.

Smith MK: *Howard Gardner, multiple intelligences and education.* Available at www.infed.org/thinkers/gardner.htm#issues. Accessed Nov 29, 2010.

Spencer TJ, Biederman J, Mick E: Attention-deficit/hyperactivity disorder: diagnosis, lifespan, comorbidities and neurobiology, *Ambul Pediatr* 7(3):73–81, 2007.

Strine TW, Lesense CA, Okoro CA, et al: Emotional and behavioral difficulties and impairments in everyday functioning among children with a history of attention-deficit/hyperactivity disorder, *Prev Chron Dis* 3(2):1–10, 2006. Available at www.cdc.gov/pcd/issues/2006/apr/05_0171.htm. Accessed Oct 21, 2010.

Teplin SW, Greeley S: Anthony TL: Blindness and visual impairment. In Carey WB, Crocker AC, Coleman WL, et al, editors: *Developmental-behavioral pediatrics*, ed 4, Philadelphia, 2009, Elsevier, pp 698–716.

Tobin MJ: Conservation of substance in the blind and partially blind, *Br J Edu Psychol* 42(2):192–197, 1972.

Tornqvist K, Kallen B: Risk factors in term children for visual impairment without a known prenatal or postnatal cause, *Paediatr Perinat Epidemiol* 18(6):425–430, 2004.

U.S. Department of Health and Human Services (USD-HHS): *Healthy People 2020: health promotion and disease prevention objectives for the year 2020.* Available at www.healthypeople.gov/hp2020/objectives. Accessed Oct 21, 2010.

U.S. Food and Drug Administration (FDA): *FDA approves the first drug to treat irritability associated with autism, Risperdal*, 2006. Available at www.fda.gov/bbs/topics/NEWS/2006/NEW01485.html. Accessed Nov 11, 2006.

U.S. Preventive Services Task Force (USPSTF): *Child and adolescent recommendations.* Available at www.uspreventiveservicestaskforce.org/tfchildcat.htm#top. Accessed Nov 11, 2010.

Van Cleave J, Leslie K: Approaching ADHD as a chronic condition: implications for long-term adherence, *Pediatr Ann* 37(1):19–26, 2008.

Venali F, Vieu A, Artieres F, et al: Educational and employment achievements in prelingually deaf children who receive cochlear implants, *Arch Otolaryngol Head Neck Surg* 136(4):366–372, 2010.

Vogel I, Bruq J, van der Ploeg C, et al: Young people's exposure to loud music: a summary of the literature, *Am J Prev Med* 33(2):124–133, 2007.

Wake M, Hughes EK, Poulakis Z, et al: Outcomes of children with mild-profound hearing loss at 7 to 8 years: a population study, *Ear Hear* 25:1–8, 2004.

Wegner LM: School achievement and underachievement. In Carey WB, Crocker AC, Coleman WL, et al, editors: *Developmental-behavioral pediatrics*, ed 4, Philadelphia, 2009, Elsevier, pp 698–716.

Wilks T, Gerber R, Erdie-Lalena C: Developmental milestones: cognitive development, *Pediatr Rev* 31(9):364–367, 2010.

Wolraich M, et al: Attention deficit/hyperactivity disorder among adolescents: a review of the diagnosis, treatment, and clinical implications, *Pediatrics* 115(6):1734–1746, 2005.

Zaidman-Zait A: Everyday problems and stress faced by parents of children with cochlear implants, *Rehabil Psychol* 5(2):139–152, 2008.

Ziegler R, Holden L: Family therapy for learning disabled and attention deficit disordered children, *Am J Orthopsychiatry* 58:196–210, 1988.

CHAPTER 16

Allison SE, von Wahlde L, Shockley T, et al: The development of the self in the era of the Internet and role-playing fantasy games, *Am J Psychiatry* 163(3):381–385, 2006.

Altschul I, Oyserman D: Racial-ethnic identity in mid-adolescence: content and change as predictors of academic achievement, *Child Dev* 77(5):1155–1169, 2006.

American Academy of Pediatrics (AAP) Council on Communications and Media: Impact of music, music lyrics, and music videos on children and youth, *Pediatrics* 124:1488–1494, 2009.

*Benson PL: *Sparks: how parents can help ignite the hidden strengths of teenagers*, San Francisco, 2008, Jossey-Bass.

*Benson PL, Galbraith J, Espeland P: *What kids need to succeed*, Minneapolis, 1998a, Free Spirit Publisher.

*Benson PL, Galbraith J, Espeland P: *What teens need to succeed*, Minneapolis, 1998b, Free Spirit Publisher.

*Brooks R: *What is resilience?*. Available at www.raisingresilientkids.com. Accessed Nov 18, 2010.

Burton S, Mitchell P: Judging who knows best about yourself: developmental change in citing the self across middle childhood, *Child Dev* 74(2):426–443, 2003.

Costello EJ, Compton SN, Keeler G, et al: Relationships between poverty and psychopathology, *JAMA* 290(15):2023–2029, 2003.

Dahlbeck DT, Lightsey OW: Generalized self-efficacy, coping, and self-esteem as predictors of psychological adjustment among children with disabilities or chronic illness, *Child Health Care* 372:93–315, 2008.

Dalgas-Pelish P: Effects of self-esteem intervention program on school-age children, *Pediatr Nurs* 32(4):341–348, 2006.

Davis-Kean PE, Sandler HM: A meta-analysis of measures on self-esteem for young children: a framework for future measures, *Child Dev* 72(3):887–906, 2001.

DeBate RD, Gabriel KP, Zwald M, et al: Changes in psychosocial factors and physical activity frequency among third-to-eighth grade girls who participated in a developmentally focused youth sports program: a preliminary study, *J School Health* 79(10): 474–484, 2009.

Dixon SD, Stein MT: *Encounters with children: pediatric behavior and development*, ed 4, St Louis, 2006, Mosby.

*Dobson J: *The new hide or seek: building self-esteem in your child*, Grand Rapids, MI, 1999, FH Revell.

Donaldson SJ, Ronan KR: The effects of sports participation on young adolescents' emotional well-being, *Adolescence* 41(162):369–389, 2006.

Eisenberg ME, Newmark-Sztainer D, Story M: Associations of weight based teasing and emotional well-being among adolescents, *Arch Pediatr Adolesc Med* 157:733–738, 2003.

Finn R: Clues from social networks can be valuable, *Pediatr News* 44(1):33, 2010.

*Forbes HT, Post BB: *Beyond consequences, logic and control*, Orlando, FL, 2006, Beyond Logic Consequences Institute.

Glascoe FP, Leew S: Parenting behaviors, perceptions, and psychosocial risk: impacts on young children's development, *Pediatrics* 125(2):313–319, 2010.

Gray-Little B, Hafdahl AR: Factors influencing racial comparisons of self-esteem: a quantitative review, *Psychol Bull* 126(1):26–54, 2000.

Gurian A: *How to raise girls with healthy self-esteem*, NYU Child Study Center. Available at www.about ourkids.org/articles/how_raise_girls_healthy_selfes teem?print=1. Accessed Nov 15, 2010.

Hagan JF, Shaw JS, Duncan PM, editors: *Bright Futures: guidelines for health supervision of infants, children, and adolescents*, ed 3, Elk Grove Village, IL, 2008, American Academy of Pediatrics.

Hahn-Smith AM, Smith JE: The positive influence of maternal identification on body image, eating attitudes, and self-esteem of Hispanic and Anglo girls, *Int J Eat Disord* 29(4):429–440, 2001.

Hall H: *Ways to enhance your child's self-esteem*, Chicago, 1998, Presentation at the NAPNAP National Conference.

Hart L: *The winning family: increasing self-esteem in your children and yourself*, Oakland, CA, 1990, LifeSkills Press.

Hedden SL, Davidson S, Smith CB: Cause and effect: the relationship between acne and self-esteem in the adolescent years, *J Nurse Pract* 4(8):595–600, 2008.

Hitlin S, Brown JS, Elder GH: Racial self-categorization in adolescence: multiracial development and social pathways, *Child Dev* 77(5):1298–1308, 2006.

Jackson LA, Zhao Y, Witt ED, et al: Self-concept, self-esteem, gender, race, and information technology use, *Cyberpsychol Behav* 12(4):437–440, 2009.

Jellinek M, Patel BP, Froehle MC, editors: *Bright futures in practice: mental health,* vol. 1, Practice guide, vol 2, Tool kit, Arlington, VA, 2002, National Center for Education in Maternal and Child Health.

Kim J, Cicchetti D: Longitudinal trajectories of self-system processes and depressive symptoms among maltreated and nonmaltreated children, *Child Dev* 77(3):624–639, 2006.

*Kurcinka MS: *Raising your spirited child*, New York, 2006, Harper Perennial.

Lee A, Hankin BL: Insecure attachment, dysfunctional attitudes, and low self-esteem predicting prospective symptoms of depression and anxiety during adolescence, *J Clin Child Adolesc Psychol* 38(2):219–231, 2009.

Lemeshow AR, Fisher L, Goodman E, et al: Subjective social status in the school and change in adiposity in female adolescents, *Arch Pediatr Adolesc Med* 162(1):23–28, 2008.

Lewis M, Ramsay D: Development of self-recognition, personal pronoun use, and pretend play during the 2nd year, *Child Dev* 75(6):1821–1831, 2004.

McLean KC: Late adolescent identity development: narrative meaning making and memory telling, *Dev Psychol* 41(4):683–691, 2005.

Mendelson BK, Mendelson MJ, White DR: Body esteem scale for adolescents and adults, *J Pers Assess* 76(1):90–106, 2001.

Neifert MA: Self-esteem and emotional health, *A Dr Mom Presentation*, Denver, 2005.

Ozmen D, Ozmen E, Ergin D, et al: The association of self-esteem, depression and body satisfaction with obesity among Turkish adolescents, *BMC Public Health* 7(80):1–7, 2007.

Perry PD: Creating novelty, *Scholas Parent Child* 9:67–68, 2001.

Phillips D, Haga T, Dodfiels E, et al: Exploring the impact of group work and mentoring for multiple heritage children's self-esteem, well being and behaviors, *Health Soc Care Comm* 16(3):310–321, 2008.

*Post BB: *From fear to love*, Palmyra, VA, 2010, Post Institute & Associates.

Putnick D, Bornstein M, Hendricks C, et al: Parenting stress, perceived parenting behaviors, and adolescent self-concept in European American families, *J Fam Psychol* 22(5):752–762, 2008.

Quatman T, Watson CM: Gender differences in adolescent self-esteem: an exploration of domains, *J Genet Psychol* 162(1):92–117, 2001.

Quintana SM, Aboud FE, Chao RK, et al: Race, ethnicity, and culture in child development: contemporary research and future directions, *Child Dev* 77(5):1129–1141, 2006.

Ransdell LB, Dratt J, Kennedy C, et al: Daughters and mothers exercising together (DAMET): a 12-week pilot project designed to improve physical self-perception and increase recreational physical activity, *Womens Health* 33(3/4):101–116, 2001.

*Reasoner R: *The true meaning of self-esteem*, 2002. Available at www.self-esteem-nase.org/what.php. Accessed Nov 18, 2010.

Rees CA: Thinking about children's attachments, *Arch Dis Child* 90:1058–1065, 2005.

Riesch SK, Anderson LS, Krueger HA: Parent-child communication processes: preventing children's health-risk behavior, *J Special Pediatr Nurs* 11(1):41–56, 2006.

Rochat P, Striano T: Who's in the mirror? Self-other discrimination in specular images by four- and nine-month-old infants, *Child Dev* 73(1):35–46, 2002.

Salmivalli C, Ojanen T, Haanpaa J: "I'm OK but you're not" and other peer-relational schemas: explaining individual differences in children's social goals, *Dev Psychol* 41(2):363–375, 2005.

Sanders-Phillips K, Settles-Reaves B, Walker D, et al: Social inequality and racial discrimination: risk factors for health disparities in children of color, *Pediatrics* 124:S176–S186, 2009.

Scharf M, Mayseless O: Socioemotional characteristics of elementary school children identified as exhibiting social leadership qualities, *J Genet Psychol* 170(1):73–94, 2009.

Schmalz DL, Deane GD, Birch LL, et al: A longitudinal assessment of the links between physical activity and self-esteem in early adolescent non-Hispanic females, *J Adolesc Health* 41:559–565, 2007.

Schmidt LA, Miskovic V, Boyle MH, et al: Shyness and timidity in young adults who were born at extremely low birth weight, *Pediatrics* 122:e181–e187, 2008.

Schore AN: Attachment, affect regulation, and the developing right brain: linking developmental neuroscience to pediatrics, *Pediatr Rev* 26(6):204–211, 2005.

Schott ER, Bellin W: The relational self-concept scale: a context specific self-report measure for adolescents, *Adolescence* 36(141):85–103, 2001.

*Search Institute: *About developmental assets*. Available at www.search-institute.org. Accessed Oct 19, 2010a.

*Search Institute: *Developmental assets research*. Available at www.search-institute.org/research/assets. Accessed Oct 19, 2010b.

*Search Institute: *Sparks*. Available at www.search-institute.org/what-kids-need-sparks. Accessed Oct 19, 2010c.

*Search Institute: *Thriving*. Available at www.search-institute.org/thriving. Accessed Oct 19, 2010d.

*Search Institute: *What are developmental assets*. Available at www.search-institute.org/content.what-are-developmental-assets. Accessed Oct 19, 2010e.

Sharaf AY, Thompson EA, Walsh E: Protective effects of self-esteem and family support on suicide risk behaviors among at-risk adolescents, *J Child Adolescent Psych Nurs* 22(3):160–168, 2009.

Shebloski B, Conger KJ, Widaman KF: Reciprocal links among differential parenting, perceived partiality, and self-worth: a three-wave longitudinal study, *J Fam Psych* 19(4):633–642, 2005.

Slattery J, Self-esteem: *Tween years, focus on your child, CD*, Summer 2008.

Slattery J, Self-esteem: *Discovery years, focus on your child, CD*, Dec 2005.

Solomon CR, Serres F: Effects of parental verbal aggression on children's self-esteem and school marks, *Child Abuse Negl* 23(4):339–351, 1999.

Spencer JM, Zimet GD, Aalsma MC, et al: Self-esteem as a predictor of initiation of coitus in early adolescents, *Pediatrics* 109(4):581–584, 2002.

Spratt E: Assessing and reinforcing your child's self-esteem. In Jellinek M, Patel BP, Froehler MC, editors: *Bright futures in practice: mental health*, vol. 2, Arlington, VA, 2002, National Center for Education in Maternal and Child Health.

Strasburger VC: Risky business: what primary care practitioners need to know about the influence of the media on adolescents, *Prim Care Clin Office Pract* 33:317–348, 2006.

Supple AJ, Ghazarian SR, Frabutt JM, et al: Contextual influences on Latino adolescent ethnic identity and academic outcomes, *Child Dev* 77(5):1427–1433, 2006.

Ternouth A, Collier D, Maughan B: Childhood emotional problems and self-perceptions predict weight gain in a longitudinal regression model, *BMC Med* 46(7), 2009. Available at www.biomedcentral.com/1741-7015/7/46. Accessed Feb 19, 2010.

Troop-Gordon W, Ladd GW: Trajectories of peer victimization and perceptions of the self and schoolmates: precursors to internalizing and externalizing problems, *Child Dev* 76(5):1072–1091, 2005.

Trzesniewski KH, Donnelan MB, Robins RW: Stability of self-esteem across the life span, *J Pers Soc Psych* 84(1):205–220, 2003.

U.S. Department of Health and Human Services (USDHHS) Substance Abuse and Mental Health Services Administration (SAMHSA): *Your child's mental health: building self-esteem in children*. Available at http://mentalhealth.samhsa.gov/allpubs/Ca-0048/default.asp. Accessed Feb 18, 2010a.

U.S. Department of Health and Human Services (USDHHS): *Healthy People 2020*. Available at www.healthypeople.gov/hp2020/objectives. Accessed Oct 21, 2010b.

U.S. Preventive Services Task Force (USPSTF): *The guide to clinical preventive services*. Available at www.uspreventiveservicestaskforce.org/tfchildcat. htm#top. Accessed Nov 10, 2010.

Valkenburg PM, Peter J, Schouten AP: Friend networking sites and their relationship to adolescents' well-being and social self-esteem, *Cyberpsychol Behav* 9(5):584–590, 2006.

Verschueren K, Buyck P, Marcoen A: Self-representations and socioemotional competence in young children: a 3-year longitudinal study, *Dev Psychol* 37(1):126–134, 2001.

Wang F, Veugelers PJ: Self-esteem and cognitive development in the era of the childhood obesity epidemic, *Obes Rev* 9:615–623, 2008.

Wang F, Wild TC, Kipp W, et al: The influence of childhood obesity on the development of self-esteem, *Stat Canada Health Rep* 20(2):21–27, 2009.

*Webster-Stratton C: *The incredible years: a troubleshooting guide for parents of children aged 3-8*, Toronto, 1997, Umbrella Press.

Zuckerman B, Zuckerman PM, Siegel DJ: Promoting self-understanding in parents—for the great good of your patients, *Contemp Pediatr* 22(4):77–90, 2005.

Designates parent-friendly resources.

CHAPTER 17

Adoption History Project: *Adoption Statistics*. Available at http://darkwing.uoregon.edu/~adoption/topics/ adoptionstatistics.htm. Accessed Dec 27, 2010.

Ahrons C: Family ties after divorce: long-term implications for children, *Family Process* 46:53–65, 2007.

American Academy of Pediatrics (AAP): Family pediatrics: report of the task force on the family, *Pediatrics* 111:1541–1571, 2003.

American Academy of Pediatrics (AAP): Medical evaluation of internationally adopted children for infectious diseases. In Pickering LK, Baker CJ, Kimberlin DW, et al, editors: *Redbook: 2009 report of the Committee on Infectious Diseases*, ed 28, Elk Grove Village, IL, 2009, AAP, p 183.

American Academy of Pediatrics Committee on Injury, Violence, and Poison Prevention: Policy statement—role of the pediatrician in youth violence prevention, *Pediatrics* 124(1):393–402, 2009.

Anderson JE: Sibling rivalry: when the family circle becomes a boxing ring, *Contemp Pediatr* 23(2):72–90, 2006.

Annie E. Casey Foundation: *2010 Kids count data book*. Available at www.datacenter.kidscount.org. Accessed Oct 11, 2010.

Barrett AE, Turner RJ: Family structure and mental health: the mediating effects of socioeconomic status, family process, and social stress, *J Health Soc Behav* 46:156–169, 2005.

Bauman LJ, Silver EJ, Stein RE: Cumulative social disadvantage and child health, *Pediatrics* 117:1321–1328, 2006.

Black CM, Driebe EM, Howard LA, et al: Multicenter study of nucleic acid amplification tests for detection of *Chlamydia trachomatis* and *Neisseria gonorrhoeae* in children being evaluated for sexual abuse, *J Pediatr Infect Dis* 28(7):608–613, 2009.

Bloom B, Cohen RA, Freeman G: Summary of health statistics for US children: National Health Interview Survey, 2008, *Vital Health Stat* 10(244):1–149, 2009.

Bureau of Labor Statistics: *Employment of characteristics of families statistics*, U.S. Department of Labor USDL Publication Number USDL-10–0721. Available at www.bls.gov/news.release/famee.nr0.htm. Accessed July 11, 2010.

Carter B: Becoming parents: the family with young children. In Carter C, McGoldrick M, editors: *The expanded family life cycle: individual, family, and social perspectives*, ed 3, Boston, 1999, Allyn & Bacon.

Centers for Disease Control and Prevention (CDC): *National vital statistics reports: births, marriages, divorces, and deaths: provisional data for 2009*. Available at www.cdc.gov/nchs/data/nvsr/nvsr58/ nvsr58_25.pdf. Accessed Dec 27, 2010.

Chadwick DL, Bertocc G, Castillo E, et al: Annual risk of death resulting from short falls among young children: less than 1 in 1 million, *Pediatrics* 121:1213–1224, 2008.

Chandra A, Sandraluz LC, Jaycox L, et al: Children on the homefront: the experience of children from military families, *Pediatrics* 125:16–25, 2010.

Child Care Aware: *High-quality child care*. Available at www.childcareaware.org. Accessed Dec 28, 2010.

Child Welfare Information Gateway: *Foster care statistics*, 2010. Available at www.childwelfare.gov/pubs/ factsheets/foster.cfm. Accessed Oct 9, 2010.

Children's Defense Fund: *The State of American's Children 2010 Report*. Available at http://ww w.childrensdefense.org/child-research-data-publications/data/state-of-americas-children-2010-report.html. Accessed March 18, 2011.

Christian CW, Blum NJ: Psychosocial issues. In Kliegman RM, Marcdante K, Jenson HB, et al, editors: *Nelson essentials of pediatrics*, ed 5, Philadelphia, 2006, Saunders.

Coffey J: Parenting a child with a chronic illness: a metasynthesis, *Pediatr Nurs* 32(1):51–59, 2006.

Coley R: : Fathers; and mothers' parenting predicting and responding to adolescent sexual risk behaviors, *Child Dev* May/June(80)808–827, 2009, May/June.

Cowell K, Horstman S, Linebarber J, et al: A "vaccine" against violence: coping power, *Pediatr Rev* 29(10):362–363, 2009.

Dziak E, Janzen B, Muhajarine N: Inequalities in the psychological well-being of employed, single and partnered mothers: the role of psychosocial work quality and work-family conflict, *Int J Equity Health* 9:6, 2010.

Ellerman C: Influences on the mental health of children placed in foster care, *Fam Comm Health Care* 30(Suppl 2S):S23–S32, 2007.

Forum on Child and Family Statistics: *America's Children: Key National Indicators of Well-Being*, 2009. Available at www.childstats.gov/americaschildren09/ famsoc1.asp. Accessed March 18, 2011.

Garfield C: Variations in family composition. In Carey WB, Crocker AC, Coleman WL, et al: *Developmental-behavioral pediatrics*, ed 4, Philadelphia, 2009, Elsevier, pp 94–102.

Ge X, Natsuaki MN, Conger RD: Trajectories of depressive symptoms and stressful life events among male and female adolescents in divorced and nondivorced families, *Dev Psychopathol* 18:253–273, 2006.

Gibbs D, Siebenaler K, Barth RP: *Assessing the field of post-adoption services: family issues, program models and evaluation issues*. Available at aspe.hhs.gov/hsp/post-adoption01/summary/ chapt1–2. Accessed Nov 16, 2010.

Ginsburg K, Durbin D, Garcia-Espana JF, et al: Associations between parenting styles and teen driving, safety-related behaviors and attitudes, *Pediatrics* 124:1040–1051, 2009.

Girardet RG, Lahoti S, Howard LA, et al: Epidemiology of sexually transmitted infections in suspected child victims of sexual assault, *Pediatrics* 124:79–86, 2009.

Glew GM, Frey KS, Walker WO: Bullying update: are we making any progress? *Pediatr Rev* 31(9):e68–e74, 2010.

Goodman C, Potts M, Pasztor M, et al: Grandmothers as kinship caregivers: private arrangements compared to public child welfare oversight, *Child Youth Serv Rev* 26(3):287–305, 2004.

Greeff AP, Ritman IN: Individual characteristics associated with resilience in single-parent families, *Psychol Rep* 96:36–42, 2005.

Halpern D: Psychology at the intersection of work and family, *Am Psychologist* 60:397–409, 2005.

Harris TS: Bruises in children: normal or child abuse? *J Pediatr Health Care* 24(4):216–221, 2010.

Hayslip B, Kaminski P: Grandparents raising their grandchildren: a review of the literature and suggestions for practice, *Gerontologist* 45:262–269, 2005.

Heaton J, Noyes J, Sloper P, et al: Families' experiences of caring for technology-dependent children: a temporal perspective, *Health Soc Care Community* 13(5):441–450, 2005.

Hildebrandt E, Stevens P: Impoverished women with children and no welfare benefits: the urgency of researching failures of the Temporary Assistance for Needy Families Program, *Am J Pediatr Health* 99(5):793–801, 2009.

Hoffman SD: *Kids having kids: economic costs and social consequences of teen pregnancy*, New York, 2008, Urban Institute Press.

Hymel KP, Hall CA: Diagnostic pediatric head trauma, *Pediatr Ann* 34(5):358–370, 2005.

Jellinek MS: Children living in a violent world, *Pediatr News* 41(1):30, 2007.

Johnson SJ, Sherman MD, Hoffman JS, et al, for the Presidential Task Force on Military Deployment Services for Youth, Families and Service Members: *The psychological needs of US military service members and their families: a preliminary report (Presidential Task Force on Military Deployment Services for Youth, Families and Service Members)*, Washington, DC, 2007, American Psychological Association.

Kepreotes E, Keatinge D, Stone T: The experience of parenting children with chronic health conditions: a new reality, *J Nurs Health Chron Illness* 2(1):51–62, 2010.

Knafl KA, Deatrick JA, Kirby A: Normalization promotion. In Craft-Rosenberg M, Denehy J, editors: *Nursing interventions for infants, children, and families*, Thousand Oaks, CA, 2001, Sage.

Kneipp SM: The relationships among employment, paid sick leave, and difficulty obtaining health care for single mothers with young children, *Policy Polit Nurs Pract* 3(1):20–30, 2002.

Kratz L, Uding N, Trahms C, et al: Managing childhood chronic illness: parent perspectives and implications for parent-provider relationships, *Fam Syst Health* 27(4):303–313, 2009.

Lauver L: Parenting foster children with chronic illness and complex medical needs, *J Fam Nurs* 14(1):74–96, 2008.

Lemmon KM, Chartrand MM: Caring for America's children: military youth in time of war, *Pediatr Rev* 30:e42–e48, 2009. Available at pedsinreview.aap-publications.org/cgi/contentfull/30/6/e42. Accessed Dec 27, 2010.

Lincoln A, Swift E, Shorteno-Fraser M: Psychological adjustment and treatment of children and families with parents deployed in military combat, *J Clin Psychol* 64:984–992, 2008.

Liptak G, Orlando M, Yingling JT, et al: Satisfaction with primary health care by families of children with developmental disabilities, *J Pediatr Health Care* 20(4):245–252, 2006.

McPherson M, Arango P, Fox H, et al: A new definition of children with special health care needs, *Pediatrics* 102(1):137–140, 1998.

Montgomery C, Fisk J, Craig L: The effects of perceived parenting style on the propensity for illicit drug use: the importance of parental warmth and control, *Drug Alcohol Rev* 27:640–649, 2008.

National Center for Health Statistics: *NCHS data on teenage pregnancy*. Available at www.cdc.gov/nchs/data/factsheets/factsheet_teen_pregnancy.htm. Accessed Dec 27, 2010.

National Center on Family Homelessness: *Report card: America's youngest outcasts*. Available at www.homelesschildrenamerica.org. Accessed Sept 4, 2010.

National Center for Injury Prevention and Control: *Understanding youth violence: fact sheet 2010*. Available at www.cdc.gov/violenceprevention/pdf/YV-FactSheet-a.pdf. Accessed Dec 27, 2010a.

National Coalition for the Homeless: *Homeless families with children NCH fact sheet. July 2009*. Available at www.nationalhomeless.org/factsheets/families.html. Accessed Dec 27, 2010.

Pasztor E, Hollinger D, Inkelas M, et al: Health and mental health services for children in foster care: the central role of foster parents, *Child Welfare* 85(1):33–57, 2006.

Perou R: *Impact of deployment on the health of service members and their families—why clinicians should ask: family and child issues*. Available at http://emergency.cdc.gov/coca/calls/2010/callinfo_092110.asp.

Raina P, O'Donnell M, Rosenbaum P, et al: The health and well-being of caregivers of children with cerebral palsy, *Pediatrics* 115(6):e626–e636, 2005.

Resch JA, Mireles G, Benz MR, et al: Giving parents a voice: a qualitative study of the challenges experienced by parents of children with disabilities, *Rehab Psychol* 55(2):39–50, 2010.

Simmons R: *Odd girl out: hidden culture of aggression in girls*, New York, 2002, Harvest Book Harcourt Brace.

Stirling J: Child maltreatment. In Burg FD, Polin RA, Gershon AA, et al, editors: *Current pediatric therapy*, ed 18, Philadelphia, 2006, Elsevier.

Tanner JL: Separation, divorce, and remarriage. In Carey WB, Crocker AC, Coleman WL, et al, editors: *Developmental-behavioral pediatrics*, ed 4, Philadelphia, 2009, Elsevier, pp 125–133.

Tasker F: Lesbian mothers, gay fathers, and their children: a review, *J Dev Behav Pediatr* 26(3):224–240, 2005.

Thorne SE, Robinson CA: Health care relationships: the chronic illness perspective, *Res Nurs Health* 11:293–300, 1988.

U.S. Census Bureau: *Who's minding the kids? Child care arrangements: summer*, 2006. Available at www.census.gov/population/www/socdemo/child/tables-2006.html. Accessed July 11, 2010.

U.S. Census Bureau: *2007 American Community Survey*. Available at www.census.gov/acs/www/products/users_guide/2007*. Accessed Sept 3, 2010.

U.S. Conference of Mayors: *A status report on hunger and homelessness in America's cities*, 2007. Available from US Conference of Mayors, 1620 Eye St., NW, 4th floor, Washington, DC, 20006-4005.

U.S. Department of Health and Human Services (USD-HHS): *Healthy People 2020: understanding and improving health*. Washington, DC, 2010a. Available at www.healthypeople.gov/hp2020.objectives. Accessed Dec 27, 2010.

U.S. Department of Health and Human Services, Administration for Children and Families, Children's Bureau: *The AFCARS report*, 2010. Available from www.acf.hhs.gov/programs/cb/stats_research/afcars/tar/report. Accessed Dec 28, 2010b.

U.S. Department of Health and Human Services: Administration for Children and Families, Children's Bureau: *Child maltreatment 2008*, 2010. Available at www.acf.hhs.gov/programs/cb/stats_research/index.htm#can. Accessed Dec 28, 2010c.

Ventura A, Burch L: Does parenting affect children's eating and weight status, *Int J Behav Nutr Phys Act* 5:5–15, 2008.

Wallerstein JS: Children of divorce: the psychological tasks of the child, *Am J Orthopsychiatry* 53:230–243, 1983.

Warrington SA, Wright CM, Team AS: Accidents and resulting injuries in premobile infants: data from the ALSPAC study, *Arch Dis Child* 85:104–107, 2001.

Weber S: Parenting, family life, and well-being among sexual minorities: nursing policy and practice implications, *Issues Ment Health Nurs* 29(6):601–618, 2008.

Wekerle C, Miller AL, Wolfe DA, et al: *Childhood maltreatment*, Cambridge, MA, 2006, Hogrefe & Huber Publishers.

Wise P: Chronic illness in childhood. In Kliegman R, Behrman RE, Jenson HB, et al, editors: *Nelson textbook of pediatrics*, ed 18, Philadelphia, 2007, Saunders.

CHAPTER 18

Ahmed SF, Morrison S, Hughes IA: Intersex and gender assignment; the third way? *Arch Dis Child* 89:847–850, 2004.

Ailey SH, Marks BA, Crisp C, et al: Promoting sexuality across the life span for individuals with intellectual and developmental disabilities, *Nurs Clin North Am* 38:229–252, 2003.

American Academy of Family Physicians (AAFP), *Policy & advocacy, adolescent health care, confidentiality*, 2008. Available at www.aafp.org/online/en/home/policy/policies/a/adol2.html. Accessed Sept 3, 2010.

American Academy of Family Physicians (AAFP): *Policy & advocacy, adolescent health care, sexuality and contraception*, 2010. Available at www.aafp.org/online/en/home/policy/policies/a/adol3.html. Accessed Sept 3, 2010.

American Academy of Pediatrics (AAP): Committee on Adolescence: Contraception and adolescents, *Pediatrics* 120(5):1135–1148, 2007.

American Academy of Pediatrics (AAP), Tanski S, Garfunkel LC, et al, editors: *The Bright Futures clinical guide to performing preventive services*, Elk Grove Village, IL, 2010, American Academy of Pediatrics.

American Congress of Obstetricians and Gynecologists (ACOG), Committee on Adolescent Healthcare: *Resource guide, adolescent sexuality and sex education*, 2005. Available at www.acog.org/departments/dept_notice.cfm?recno=7&;bulletin=3271. Accessed Sept 2, 2010.

American Medical Association (AMA): *Guidelines for adolescent preventive services (GAPS): recommendations monograph*, Chicago, 1997, American Medical Association.

American Nurses Association (ANA): *Position statement, HIV infection and U.S. teenagers*, 1991. Available at www.nursingworld.org/BloodborneandAirborneDiseases. Accessed Sept 3, 2010.

Association of Women's Health, Obstetric and Neonatal Nurses: *Confidentiality in adolescent health care: policy position statement revised and reaffirmed*, 2009. Available at www.awhonn.org. health policy and legislation. Accessed Sept 2, 2010.

American Psychological Association: *Answers to your questions: for a better understanding of sexual orientation and homosexuality*. Washington, DC, 2008. Available at www.apa.org/topics/sorientation.pdf. Accessed July 25, 2012.

Bell AP, Weinberg MS, Hammersmith SK: *Sexual preference*, Bloomington, IN, 1981, University Press.

Bidwell RJ: Gay, lesbian, and bisexual youth. In McInerny TK, Adam HM, Campbell DE, et al: *American Academy of Pediatrics Textbook of Pediatric Care*, Elk Grove Village, IL, 2009, American Academy of Pediatrics, pp 1358–1365.

Brown RT, Brown JD: Adolescent sexuality, *Prim Care* 33:373–390, 2006.

Busseri MA, Willoughby T, Chalmers H, et al: On the association between sexual attraction and adolescent risk behavior involvement: examining mediation and moderation, *Dev Psychol* 44(1):69–80, 2008.

Centers for Disease Control and Prevention: *Update on HPV vaccine recommendations for pre-teens*. Available at www.cdc.gov/podcasts/media/pdf/Wharton/HPV.pdf. Accessed Sept 23, 2010.

Friedrich WN, Fisher J, Broughton D, et al: Normative sexual behavior in children: a contemporary sample, *Pediatrics* 101(4), 1998. Available at www.pediatrics.org/cgi/content/full/101/4/e9. Accessed Sept 25, 2010.

Garofalo R, Wolf RC, Wissow LS, et al: Sexual orientation and risk of suicide attempts among a representative sample of youth, *Arch Pediatr Adolesc Med* 153(5):487–493, 1999.

Garofalo R, Harper G: Not all adolescents are the same: addressing the unique needs of gay and bisexual male youth, *Adolesc Med* 14:595–611, 2003.

Ginsburg KR, Winn RJ, Rudy BJ, et al: How to reach sexual minority youth in the health care setting: the teens offer guidance, *J Adolesc Health* 31:407–416, 2002.

Glasier A, Gülmezoglu AM, Schmid GP, et al: Sexual and reproductive health: a matter of life and death, *Lancet* 368(9547):1595–1607, 2006.

Gooren L: The biology of human psychosexual differentiation, *Horm Behav* 50(4):559–501, 2006.

Guttmacher Institute: *Facts on American teens' sexual and reproductive health*, 2011. Available at www.guttmacher.org/pubs/FB-ATSRH.html. Accessed Feb 21, 2011.

Hines M: Sex hormones and human destiny, *J Neuroendocrinol* 21(4):437–438, 2009.

Kellogg ND, American Academy of Pediatrics, Committee on Child Abuse and Neglect, 2008-2009: Clinical report—the evaluation of sexual behaviors in children, *Pediatrics* 124(3):994–998, 2009.

Kirby D: *Emerging answers: research findings on programs to reduce teen pregnancy and sexually transmitted diseases*, Washington, DC, 2007, National Campaign to Prevent Teen Pregnancy. Available at www.thenationalcampaign.org/EA2007/EA2007_full.pdf. Accessed Sept 2, 2010.

Lehrer JA, Pantell R, Tebb K, et al: Forgone health care among U.S. adolescents: associations between risk characteristics and confidentiality concern, *J Adolesc Health* 40(3):218–226, 2007.

Meininger E, Remafedi G: Gay, lesbian, bisexual and transgender adolescents. In Neinstein L, editor: *Adolescent health care: a practical guide*, ed 5, Philadelphia, 2008, Lippincott Williams & Wilkins.

Möller B, Schreier H, Li A, et al: Gender identity disorder in children and adolescents, *Curr Probl Pediatr Adolesc Health Care* 39(5):117–143, 2009.

Monasterio E, Hwang LY, Shafer MA: Adolescent sexual health, *Curr Probl Pediatr Adolesc Health Care* 37:302–325, 2007.

Murphy NA, Elias ER: Sexuality of children and adolescents with developmental disabilities, *Pediatrics* 118:398–403, 2006.

Mustanski B, Garofalo R, Herrick A, Donenberg G: Psychosocial health problems increase risk for HIV among urban young men who have sex with men: preliminary evidence of a syndemic in need of attention, *Ann Behav Med* 34(1):37–45, 2007.

National Association of Pediatric Nurse Practitioners (NAPNAP) Executive Board: Position statement on health risks and needs of gay, lesbian, bisexual, and transgender (GLT) adolescents, *J Pediatr Health Care* 20:29A–30A, 2006.

National Campaign to Prevent Teen and Unplanned Pregnancy: *State personal responsibility education program*. Washington, DC, 2010. Available at www.thenationalcampaign.org/federalfunding/prep.aspx. Accessed Sept 1, 2010.

Rakel RE, Rakel DP: *Textbook of family medicine,* ed 8, Philadelphia, 2011, Elsevier/Saunders. pp 1008–1011.

Remafedi G: Adolescent homosexuality. In Kliegman RM, Behrman RE, Jenson HB, et al: *Nelson textbook of pediatrics,* ed 19, Philadelphia, 2011, Elsevier/Saunders, pp 658–659.

Remafedi G, Resnick M, Blum R, et al: Demography of sexual orientation in adolescents, *Pediatrics* 89:714–721, 1992.

Russell ST, Toomey RB: Men's sexual orientation and suicide: evidence for adolescent-specific risk, *Soc Sci Med,* 2010. [Epub ahead of print].

Santelli J, Ott MA, Lyon M, et al: Abstinence-only education policies and programs: a position paper of the Society of Adolescent Medicine, *J Adolesc Health* 38(1):83–87, 2006.

Sexuality Information and Education Council of the United States (SIECUS) National Guidelines Task Force: *Guidelines for comprehensive sexuality education: kindergarten-12th grade,* ed 3, New York, 2004, Sexuality Information and Education Council of the United States. Available at www.siecus.org/pubs/pubs0004.html. Accessed Mar 9, 2010.

Sexuality Information and Education Council of the United States (SIECUS): *Position statements: human sexuality,* 2010. Available at www.siecus.org/index.cfm?fuseaction=Page.viewPage&;pageId=494&parentID=472. Accessed Aug 9, 2010.

Sison AC, Greydanus DE: Deconstructing adolescent same-sex attraction and sexual behavior in the twenty-first century, *Prim Care* 34(2):293–304, 2007.

Society for Adolescent Medicine (SAM): Protecting adolescents: ensuring access to care and reporting sexual activity and abuse, *J Adolesc Health* 35:420–423, 2004.

Society of Pediatric Nurses Position Statement: *The role of the pediatric nurse working with sexually active teens, pregnant adolescents, and young parents, prepared by Herrman JW,* 2004. Available at www.pedsnurses.org/all.php?l=positions. Accessed Sept 3, 2010.

Suellentrop K: *What works 2010: curriculum-based programs that help prevent teen pregnancy,* Washington, DC, 2010, The National Campaign to Prevent Teen and Unplanned Pregnancy.

Thornton AC, Collins JD: Teaching parents to talk to their children about sexual topics, *Clin Fam Pract* 6:801–819, 2004.

Troiden RR: Homosexual identity development, *J Adolesc Health Care* 9:105–113, 1988.

Tu W, Batteiger BE, Wiehe S, et al: Time from first intercourse to first sexually transmitted infection diagnosis among adolescent women, *Arch Pediatr Adolesc Med* 163:1106–1111, 2009.

Workowski KA, Berman S: Sexually transmitted disease treatment guidelines, *MMWR Morb Mort Wkly Rep* 59(RR12):1–110, 2010.

World Health Organization, United Nations Population Fund: *Promoting sexual and reproductive health for persons with disabilities: WHO/UNPF guidance note,* 2010. Available at www.wholibdoc.who.int/publications/2009/9789241598682_eng.pdf. Accessed Sept 23, 2010.

CHAPTER 19

American Academy of Child and Adolescent Psychiatry (AACAP): Practice parameter for the assessment and treatment of children and adolescents with substance use disorders, *J Am Acad Child Adolesc Psychiatry* 44:609–621, 2005.

American Academy of Child and Adolescent Psychiatry (AACAP): Practice parameter for the assessment and treatment of children and adolescents with anxiety disorders, *J Am Acad Child Adolesc Psychiatry* 46:267–283, 2007.

American Academy of Child and Adolescent Psychiatry (AACAP): Practice parameter for the assessment and treatment of children and adolescents with bipolar disorders, *J Am Acad Child Adolesc Psychiatry* 46:107–125, 2007a.

American Academy of Child and Adolescent Psychiatry (AACAP): Practice parameter for the assessment and treatment of children and adolescents with depressive disorders, *J Am Acad Child Adolesc Psychiatry* 46:1503–1526, 2007b.

American Academy of Child and Adolescent Psychiatry (AACAP): Practice parameter for the assessment and treatment of children and adolescents with oppositional defiant disorder, *J Am Acad Child Adolesc Psychiatry* 46:126–141, 2007c.

American Academy of Child and Adolescent Psychiatry (AACAP): Practice parameter on the use of psychotropic medication in children and adolescents, *J Am Acad Child Adolesc Psychiatry* 48:961–973, 2009a.

American Academy of Child and Adolescent Psychiatry (AACAP): *Workforce Fact Sheet,* 2009b. Available at www.aacap.org/cs/root/legislative_action/aacap_workforce_fact_sheet. Accessed Sept 17, 2010.

American Academy of Pediatrics (AAP), Committee on Psychosocial Aspects of Child and Family Health: The pediatrician and childhood bereavement, *Pediatrics* 105:445–447, 2000.

American Academy of Pediatrics (AAP), Committee on Psychosocial Aspects of Child and Family Health and Task Force on Mental Health: Policy statement- The future of pediatrics: Mental health competencies for pediatric primary care, *Pediatrics* 124:410–421, 2009.

American Dietetic Association: Position of the American Dietetic Association: nutrition intervention in the treatment of anorexia nervosa, bulimia nervosa, and other eating disorders, *J Am Diet Assoc* 106(12):2073–2082, 2006.

American Psychiatric Association (APA): *Diagnostic and statistical manual of mental disorders (DSM IV-TR),* ed 4, text revision, Washington, DC, 2000, American Psychiatric Association.

American Psychiatric Association: *Practice Guideline for the treatment of patients with eating disorders,* ed 3, Washington, DC, 2006, American Psychiatric Association.

Barbaresi WJ: Oppositional behavior/noncompliance. In Carey WB, Crocker AC, Coleman WL, et al, editors: *Developmental-behavioral pediatrics,* Philadelphia, 2009, Saunders, pp 381–388.

Bernstein GA, Victor AM, Pipal AJ, et al: Comparison of pediatric autoimmune neuropsychiatric disorders associated with streptococcal infections and childhood obsessive-compulsive disorder, *J Child Adolesc Psychopharmacol* 20:333–340, 2010.

Beydoun H, Saftlas AF: Physical and mental health outcomes of prenatal maternal stress in human and animal studies: a review of recent evidence, *Paediatr Perinat Epidemiol* 22:438–456, 2008.

Blum NJ: Repetitive behaviors and tics. In Carey WB, Crocker AC, Coelman WL, et al: *Developmental-behavioral pediatrics,* Philadelphia, 2009, Saunders, pp 629–641.

Boris N, Dalton R, Forman M: Mood disorders. In Kliegman R, Behrman RE, Jenson H, et al: *Nelson textbook of pediatrics,* ed 18, Philadelphia, 2007a, Saunders, pp 121–124.

Boris N, Dalton R, Forman M: Disruptive behavioral disorders. In Kliegman R, Behrman RE, Jenson H, et al, editors: *Nelson textbook of pediatrics,* ed 18, Philadelphia, 2007b, Saunders, pp 131–133.

Burt SA: Rethinking environmental contributions to child and adolescent psychopathology: a meta-analysis of shared environmental influences, *Psychol Bull* 135:608–637, 2009.

Carmody DP, Bendersky M: Early risk, attention, and brain activation in adolescents born preterm, *Child Dev* 77:384–394, 2006.

Centers for Disease Control and Prevention (CDC): *Web-based Injury Statistics Query and Reporting System (WISQARS),* Atlanta, 2007, Department of Health and Human Services, Centers for Disease Control. Available at www.cdc.gov/ncipc/wisqars/default.htm. Accessed Feb 19, 2010.

Chang K: Challenges in the diagnosis and treatment of pediatric bipolar depression, *Dialog Clin Neurosci* 111:73–80, 2009.

Choi J, Jeong B, Rohan ML, et al: Preliminary evidence for white matter tract abnormalities in young adults exposed to parental verbal abuse, *Biol Psychiatry* 65:227–234, 2009.

Cheung A, Jensen P: Major disturbances of emotion and mood. In Carey WB, Crocker AC, Coleman WL, et al: *Developmental-behavioral pediatrics,* Philadelphia, 2009, Saunders, pp 461–473.

Committee on Psychosocial Aspects of Child and Family Health and Task Force on Mental Health: Policy statement: The future of pediatrics: mental health competencies for pediatric primary care, *Pediatrics* 124:410–421, 2009.

Copelan R: Assessing the potential for violent behavior in children and adolescents, *Pediatr Rev* 27:e36–e41, 2006.

Council on Community Pediatrics: The role of preschool home visiting programs in improving children's developmental and health outcomes, *Pediatrics* 123:598–603, 2009.

Delahanty DL, Ostrowski SA: Recent advances in the pharmacological treatment/prevention of PTSD. In Delahanty DL, editor: *The psychobiology of trauma and resilience across the lifespan,* Plymouth, UK, 2008, Rowman & Littlefield Publishing Group, Inc, pp. 233–254.

DelBello MP, Adler CM, Strawski SM: The neurophysiology of child and adolescent bipolar disorder, *CNS Spectr* 11:298–311, 2006.

Demeter CA, Townsend LD, Wilson M, et al: Current research in child and adolescent bipolar disorder, *Dialogues Clin Neurosci* 10:215–228, 2008.

Eaton DK, Kann L, Kinchen S, et al: Youth risk behavior surveillance—United States, 2009, *MMWR Surveill Summ* 59(SS-5):1–142, 2010.

Forum on Child and Family Statistics: *America's children report,* 2009. Available at www.childstats.gov/americaschildren. Accessed Feb 19, 2010.

Foy JM, Perrin J, and the American Academy of Pediatrics Task Force on Mental Health: Enhancing pediatric mental health care: strategies for preparing a community, *Pediatrics* 125:S75–S86, 2010.

Foy JM, Kelleher KJ, Laraque D, et al: Enhancing pediatric mental health care: strategies for preparing a pediatric primary care practice, *Pediatrics* 125:S87–S108, 2010.

Garzon DL: Childhood depression: diagnosis and management in an era of black-box warnings, *Adv Nurs Pract* 15(2):35–48, 2007.

Garzon DL, Nelson J, Figgemeier M: A primary care provider's guide to the diagnosis and management of childhood depression, *Clin Adv* 10:24–32, 2009.

Gilbert AR, Maalouf FT: Pediatric obsessive-compulsive disorder: management in primary care, *Curr Opin Pediatr* 20:544–550, 2008.

Gleason M, Boris NW, Dalton R: Habit and tic disorders. In Kliegman R, Behrman RE, Jenson H, et al, editors: *Nelson textbook of pediatrics,* ed 18, Philadelphia, 2007, Saunders, pp 15–116.

Gowers SG: Management of eating disorders in children and adolescents, *Arch Dis Child* 93:331–334, 2008.

Hagan JF, Shaw JS, Duncan PM, editors: *Bright Futures: guidelines for health supervision of infants, children and adolescents,* Elk Grove Village, IL, 2008, American Academy of Pediatrics.

Hankin B: Adolescent depression: description, causes, and interventions, *Epilepsy Behav* 8:102–114, 2006.

Hanna GL, Fischer DJ, Fluent TE: Separation anxiety disorder and school refusal in children and adolescents, *Pediatr Rev* 27:56–62, 2006.

In-Albon T, Schneider S: Psychotherapy of childhood anxiety disorders: a meta-analysis, *Psychother Psychosom* 76(1):15–24, 2007.

Isper JC, Stein DJ, Hawkridge S, et al: Pharmacotherapy for anxiety disorders in children and adolescents, *Cochrane Database Syst Rev* 3:CD005170, 2009.

Jellinek MS, Murphy JM, White GW: Using the PSC in the pediatrician's office, *Contemp Pediatr* 26:48–52, 2009.

Kelleher KJ, Stevens J: Evolution of child mental health services in primary care, *Academic Pediatr* 9:7–14, 2009.

Kirkby R, Brown C: Stat consult: a quick review of common conditions, using the best global evidence. Anorexia nervosa, *Clin Advisor Nurs Pract* 10:84–85, 2007.

Knight JR, Harris SK, Sherritt L, et al: Prevalence of positive substance abuse screen results among adolescent primary care patients, *Arch Pediatr Adolesc Med* 161:1035–1041, 2007.

Kowatch RA, Youngstrom EA, Danielyan A, et al: Review and meta-analysis of the phenomenology and clinical characteristics of mania in children and adolescents, *Bipolar Disord* 7:483–496, 2005.

Leckman JF, Bloch MH, King RA: Symptoms dimensions and subtypes of obsessive-compulsive disorder: a developmental perspective, *Dialog Clin Neurosci* 11:21-33.

Leff SS, Tulleners C, Posner JC: Aggression, violence, and delinquency. In Carey WB, Crocker AC, Coleman WL, et al: *Developmental-behavioral pediatrics*, Philadelphia, 2009, Saunders, pp 389–396.

Lewin AB, Storch EA, Adkins J, et al: Current directions in pediatric obsessive-compulsive disorder, *Pediatr Ann* 34:129–134, 2005.

Lieberman A, Van Horn P: Giving voice to the unsayable: repairing the effects of trauma in infancy and childhood, *Child Adolesc Psychiatr Clin N Am* 18:707–720, 2009.

Mancuso E, Faro A, Joshi G, et al: Treatment of pediatric obsessive-compulsive disorder: a review, *J Child Adolesc Psychiatry* 20:299–308, 2010.

McDonough SC: Interaction guidance: promoting and nurturing the caregiving relationship. In Sameroff AJ, McDonough SC, Rosenblum KL, editors: *Treating parent-infant relationship problems*, New York, 2005, Guilford Press.

Meiser-Stedman R, Smith P, Glucksman E, et al: The post-traumatic stress disorder diagnosis in preschool- and elementary school-ages children exposed to motor vehicle accidents, *Am J Psychiatry* 165:1326–1337, 2008.

Merikangas KR, He JP, Brody D, et al: Prevalence and treatment of mental disorders among U.S. children in the 2001-2004 NHANES, *Pediatrics* 125:75–81, 2010.

Meyer RE, Salzman C, Youngstrom EA, et al: Suicidality and risk of suicide—definition, drug safety concerns, and a necessary target for drug development: a brief report, *J Clin Psychiatry* 71:1040–1046, 2010.

Miklowitz DJ, George EL, Axelson DA, et al: Family-focused treatment for adolescents with bipolar disorder: results of a 2-year randomized trial, *Arch Gen Psychiatry* 65:1053–1061, 2008.

Miller CA, Golden NH: An introduction to eating disorders: clinical presentation, epidemiology, and prognosis, *Nutr Clin Pract* 25:110–115, 2010.

National Association of Pediatric Nurse Practitioners: NAPNAP position statement on integration of mental health care in pediatric primary care settings, *J Pediatr Health Care* 21:29A–30A, 2007.

National Institute for Health and Clinical Excellence: *Clinical guideline 31—Obsessive-compulsive disorder: core interventions in the treatment of obsessive-compulsive disorder and body dysmorphic disorder*, London, 2005, NICE.

Olantunji BO, Cisler JM, Tomlin DF: Quality of life in the anxiety disorders: a meta-analytic review, *Clin Psychol Rep* 27:572–581, 2007.

Parraga HC, Harris KM, Parraga KL, et al: An overview of treatment of Tourette's disorder and tics, *Child Adolesc Psychopharmacol* 20:249–262, 2010.

Pfefferle SG, Spitznagel EL: Children's mental health service use and maternal mental health: a path analytic model, *Child Youth Serv Rev* 31:378–382, 2009.

Reinblatt SP, Riddle MA: The pharmacological management of childhood anxiety disorders: a review, *J Psychopharmacol* 191:67–86, 2007.

Report of Healthy Development: *A Summit on Young Children's Mental Health. Partnering with communication scientists, collaborating across disciplines and leveraging impact to promote children's mental health*, Washington, DC, 2009, Society for Research in Child Development.

Rubin KH, Root AK, Bowker J: Parents, peers and social withdrawal in childhood: a relationship perspective, *New Dir Child Adolesc Dev* 127:79–84, 2010.

Serwint JR: Separation, loss and bereavement. In Kliegman R, Behrman RE, Jenson H, editors: *Nelson textbook of pediatrics*, Philadelphia, 2007, Saunders, pp 86–91.

Sigel E: Disordered eating behaviors: Anorexia nervosa and bulimia nervosa. In Carey WB, Crocker AC, Coleman WL, editors: *Developmental-behavioral pediatrics*, Philadelphia, 2009, Saunders Elsevier, pp 569–581.

Stafford B, Boris N, Dalton R, et al: Anxiety disorders. In Kliegman R, Behrman RE, Jenson H, editors: *Nelson textbook of pediatrics*, ed 18, Philadelphia, 2007, Saunders, pp 117–120.

Sturm R: Obsessive-compulsive disorder in children: the role of nurse practitioners, *J Am Acad Nurs Pract* 21:393–401, 2009.

Stufferin-Roberts S, Joyce PR, Kennedy MA: Role of epigenetics in mental disorders, *Aust N Z J Psychiatry* 42:97–107, 2008.

Szyf M, Weaver ICG, Champagne FA, et al: Maternal programming of steroid receptor expression and phenotype through DNA methylation in the rat, *Front Neuroendocrinol* 26:139–162, 2005.

Taketomo CK, Hodding JH, Kraus DM: *Pediatric dosage handbook*, ed 17, Hudson, OH, 2010, Lexi-Comp.

Thomas CR, Holzer CE: The continuing shortage of child and adolescent psychiatrists, *J Am Acad Child Adolesc Psychiatry* 45:1023–1031, 2006.

Tottenham N, Hare TA, Quinn BT, et al: Prolonged institutional rearing is associated with atypically large amygdala volume and difficulty in emotional regulation, *Dev Sci* 13:46–61, 2010.

U.S. Preventive Services Task Force (USPSTF): *The guide to clinical preventive services*, ed 2, Rockville, MD, 2006, Agency for Healthcare Research and Quality. Available at www.ahrq.gov/clinic/pocketgd .htm. Accessed Feb 19, 2010.

Zepf FD: Attention deficit-hyperactivity disorder and early-onset bipolar disorder: two faces of one entity? *Dialog Clin Neurosci* 11:63–72, 2009.

Zero to Three: *Diagnostic classification of mental health and developmental disorders of infancy and early childhood: revised edition (DC: 0-3R)*, Washington, DC, 2005, Zero to Three Press.

CHAPTER 20

Anandarajah G, Craigie F Jr, Hatch R, et al: Toward competency-based curricula in patient-centered spiritual care: recommended competencies for family medicine resident education, *Acad Med* 85(12):1897–1904, 2010.

Anandarajah G, Hight E: Spirituality and medical practice: using the HOPE questions as a practical tool for spiritual assessment, *Am Fam Physician* 63:81–89, 2001.

Barnes LL, Plotnikoff GA, Fox K, et al: Spirituality, religion, and pediatrics: intersecting worlds of healing, *Pediatrics* 106(Suppl 4):899–908, 2000.

Barriga AQ, Sullivan-Cosetti M, Gibbs JC: Moral cognitive correlates of empathy in juvenile delinquents, *Crim Behav Ment Health* 19(4):253–264, 2009.

Bennett L: Narrative methods and children: theoretical explanations and practice issues, *J Child Adolesc Psychiatr Nurs* 21(1):13–23, 2008.

Eisenberg N, Eggum ND: Empathic responding: sympathy and personal distress. In Sullivan B, Snyder M, Sullivan J, editors: *Cooperation: the political psychology of effective human interaction*, Malden, MA, 2008, Blackwell Publishing.

Erikson EH: *Childhood and society*, ed 2, New York 1963, Norton.

Fanti KA, Henrich CC: Trajectories of pure and co-occurring internalizing and externalizing problems from age 2 to age 12: findings from the National Institute of Child Health and Human Development Study of Early Child Care, *Dev Psychol* 46(5):1159–1175, 2010.

Fontaine RG, Ming Yang C, Dodge KA, et al: Development of response evaluation and decision (RED) and antisocial behavior in childhood and adolescence, *Dev Psychol* 45(2):447–459, 2009.

Fowler JW: *Stages of faith: the psychology of human development and the quest for meaning*, New York, 1981, HarperSanFrancisco.

Fowler JW, Dell ML: Stages of faith and identity: birth to teens, *Child Adolesc Psychiatr Clin North Am* 13(1):17–33, 2004.

Fumagalli M, Vergari M, Pasqualetti P, et al: Brain switches utilitarian behavior: does gender make the difference? *PLoS One* 5(1):e8865, 2010.

Gibbs JC, Basinger KS, Fuller RL: *Moral maturity: measuring the development of sociomoral reflection*, Hillsdale, NJ, 1992, Erlbaum.

Gilligan C: *Mapping the moral domain*, Cambridge, MA, 1990, Harvard University Press.

Grossoehme DH: Development of a spiritual screening tool for children and adolescents, *J Pastoral Care Counsel* 62(1):71–85, 2008.

Gutzwiller-Helfenfinger E, Gasser L, Malti T: Moral emotions and moral judgments in children's narratives: comparing real-life and hypothetical transgressions, *New Dir Child Adolesc Dev* 129:11–31, 2010.

Highfield MEF: Providing spiritual care to patients with cancer, *Clin J Oncol Nurs* 4(3):115–120, 2000.

Johansson E: Morality in children's worlds—rationality of thought or values emanating from relations? *Stud Philos Educ* 20:345–358, 2001.

Kochanska G, Aksan N: Children's conscience and self-regulation, *J Pers* 74(6):1587–1617, 2006.

Kochanska G, Aksan N, Knaack A, et al: Maternal parenting and children's conscience: early security as moderator, *Child Dev* 75(4):1229–1242, 2004.

Kochanska G, Philibert RA, Barry RA: Interplay of genes and early mother-child relationship in the development of self-regulation from toddler to preschool age, *J Child Psychol Psychiatry* 50(11):1331–1338, 2009.

Kochanska G, Koenig JL, Barry RA, et al: Children's conscience during toddler and preschool years, moral self, and a competent, adaptive developmental trajectory, *Dev Psychol* 46(5):1320–1332, 2010a.

Kochanska G, Woodward J, Kim S, et al: Positive socialization mechanisms in secure and insecure parent-child dyads: two longitudinal studies, *J Child Psychol Psychiatry* 51(9):998–1009, 2010b.

Kohlberg L: Stage and sequence: the cognitive-development approach to socialization. In Gastin D, editor: *Handbook of socialization: theory and research*, New York, 1969, Rand McNally.

Leman PJ: Argument structure, argument content, and cognitive change in children's peer interaction, *J Genet Psychol* 163:40–58, 2002.

Malti T, Buchmann MJ: Socialization and individual antecedents of adolescents' and young adults' moral motivation, *Youth Adolesc* 39(2):138–149, 2010.

McEvoy M: An added dimension to the pediatric health maintenance visit: the spiritual history, *J Pediatr Health Care* 14(5):216–220, 2000.

McGowan PO, Sasaki A, D'Alessio AC, et al: Epigenetic regulation of the glucocorticoid receptor in human brain associates with childhood abuse, *Nat Neurosci* 12(3):342–348, 2009.

McGowan PO, Szyf M: The epigenetics of social adversity in early life: implications for mental health, *Neurobiol Dis* 39(1):66–72, 2010.

McLeod DL, Wright LM: Living the as-yet unanswered: spiritual care practices in family systems nursing, *J Fam Nurs* 14(1):118–141, 2008.

McPherson K: Pastoral crisis intervention with children: recognizing and responding to the spiritual reaction of children, *Int J Emerg Ment Health* 6(4):223–233, 2004.

Mueller CR: Spirituality in children: understanding and developing interventions, *Pediatr Nurs* 36(4):197–203, 208, 2010.

Narvaez D: The emotional foundations of high moral intelligence, *New Dir Child Adolesc Dev* 129:77–94, 2010.

National Consensus Project for Quality Palliative Care (NCPQPC): *Clinical guidelines for quality palliative care*, ed 2, Pittsburgh, 2009, NCPQPC.

North American Nursing Diagnosis Association (NANDA) International: *NANDA-I nursing diagnoses: definitions and classification, 2009-2011*, Philadelphia, 2009, NANDA.

Pearson J: Teaching the art of healing, *Minn Med* 92(4):38–39, 2009.

Puchalski CM, Romer AL: Taking a spiritual history allows clinicians to understand patients more fully, *J Palliat Med* 3(1):129–137, 2000.

Quinn J: Perspectives on spiritual development as part of youth development, *New Dir Youth Dev* 118:73–77, 2008.

Robinson MR, Thiel MM, Backus MM, et al: Matters of spirituality at the end of life in the pediatric intensive care unit, *Pediatrics* 118(3):e719–e729, 2006.

Shirtcliff EA, Vitacco MJ, Graf AR, et al: Neurobiology of empathy and callousness: implications for the development of antisocial behavior, *Behav Sci Law* 27(2):137–171, 2009.

Stilwell BM, Galvin MR, Kopta SM, et al: Moral volition: the fifth and final domain leading to an integrated theory of conscience understanding, *J Am Acad Child Adolesc Psychiatry* 37(2):202–210, 1998.

The Joint Commission (TJC): *Advancing effective communication, cultural competence, and patient- and family-centered care: a roadmap for hospitals*, Oakbrook Terrace, IL, 2010, The Joint Commission.

U.S. Preventive Services Task Force: *Screening and treatment for major depressive disorder in children and adolescents, recommendation statement*, 2009. Available at www.uspreventiveservicestaskforce.org/uspstf09/depression/chdeprrs.htm. Accessed Nov 18, 2010.

Walker LJ, Hennig KH, Krettenauer T: Parent and peer contexts for children's moral reasoning development, *Child Dev* 71(4):1033–1048, 2000.

Wolf AD: How to nurture the spirit in nonsectarian environments, *Young Child* 55:34–36, 2000.

Wong YJ, Rew L, Slaikeu KD: A systematic review of recent research on adolescent religiosity/spirituality and mental health, *Issues Ment Health Nurs* 27(2):161–183, 2006.

CHAPTER 21

Abrams MA, Klass P, Dreyer BP: Health literacy and children: recommendations for action, *Pediatrics* 124(Suppl 3):S327–S331, 2009.

Allen PJ: The primary care provider and children with chronic conditions. In Allen PJ, Vessey JA, Schapiro NA, editors: *Primary care of the child with a chronic condition*, ed 5, St Louis, 2010, Mosby.

Al-Mukhaizeem F, Allen U, Komar L, et al: Comparison of temporal artery, rectal and esophageal core temperatures in children: results of a pilot study, *Paediatr Child Health* 9(7):461–465, 2004.

American Academy of Pediatrics, Committee on Drugs and Committee on Hospital Care: Prevention of medication errors in the pediatric inpatient setting, *Pediatrics* 112(2):431–439, 2003. Reaffirmed 2007.

American Academy of Pediatrics: Committee on Genetics: Health supervision for children with Down syndrome, *Pediatrics* 107(2):442–449, 2001. reaffirmed 2007.

American Public Health Association (APHA), American Academy of Pediatrics (AAP): *Caring for our children. National health and safety standards: guidelines for out-of-home child care programs*, ed 2, Elk Grove Village, IL, 2002, American Academy of Pediatrics.

Avner J: Acute fever, *Pediatr Rev* 30(1):5–13, 2009.

Berner E, Graber M: Overconfidence as a cause of diagnostic error in medicine, *Am J Med* 121(5A):S2–S23, 2008.

Black KL: Standardization of telephone triage in pediatric oncology, *J Pediatr Oncol Nurs* 24(4):190–199, 2007.

Brenner D, Elliston C, Hall E, et al: Estimated risks of radiation-induced fatal cancer from pediatric CT, *AJR Am J Roentgenol* 176(2):289–296, 2001.

Brenner DJ, Hall EJ: Computed tomography—an increasing source of radiation exposure, *N Engl J Med* 357(22):2277–2284, 2007.

Briggs J: *Telephone triage for nurses*, Philadelphia, 2006, Lippincott Williams & Wilkins.

Butz A, Walker JM, Pulsifer M, et al: Shared decision making in school age children with asthma, *Pediatr Nurs* 33(2):111–116, 2007.

Carstairs KL, Tanen DA, Johnson AS, et al: Pneumococcal bacteremia in febrile infants presenting to the emergency department before and after the introduction of heptavalent pneumococcal vaccine, *Ann Emerg Med* 49(6):772–777, 2007.

Cohen MD: Pediatric CT radiation dose: how low can you go? *AJR Am J Roentgenol* 192(5):1292–1303, 2009.

Cox ED, Smith MA, Brown RL: Evaluating deliberation in pediatric primary care, *Pediatrics* 120(1):e68–e77, 2007.

El-Radhi AS, Barry W: Thermometry in paediatric practice, *Arch Dis Child* 91(4):351–356, 2006.

Elstein AS: Thinking about diagnostic thinking: a 30-year perspective, *Adv Health Sci Educ Theory Pract* 14(Suppl 1):7–18, 2009.

Erlewyn-Lajeunesse MD, Coppens K, Hunt LP, et al: A randomized controlled trial of combined paracetamol and ibuprofen for fever, *Arch Dis Child* 91(5):414–416, 2006.

Fielding D, Duff AJ: Adherence to treatment in children and adolescents living with chronic illness. In Burg FD, Ingelfinger JR, Polin RA, et al, editors: *Gellis and Kagan's current pediatric therapy*, ed 18, Philadelphia, 2006, Saunders.

Fiks AG, Localio AR, Alessandrini EA, et al: Shared decision-making in pediatrics: a national perspective, *Pediatrics* 126(2):306–314, 2010.

Gavin L, Wysocki TJ: Associations of paternal involvement in disease management with maternal and family outcomes in families with children with chronic illness, *J Pediatr Psychol* 31(5):481–489, 2006.

Haddadin RB, Shamo'on HI: Study between axillary and rectal temperature measurements in children, *East Mediterr Health J* 13(5):1060–1066, 2007.

Hay AD, Costelloe C, Redmond NM, et al: Paracetamol plus ibuprofen for the treatment of fever in children (PITCH): randomized controlled trial, *BMJ* 337:a1302, 2008.

Herz AM, Greenhow TL, Alcantara J, et al: Changing epidemiology of outpatient bacteremia in 3- to 36-month-old children after the introduction of the heptavalent-conjugated pneumococcal vaccine, *Pediatr Infect Dis J* 25(4):293–300, 2006.

Hing E, Hall MJ, Ashman JJ, et al: National Hospital Ambulatory Medical Care Survey: 2007 outpatient department summary, *Natl Health Stat Report* (28)1–32, 2010.

Hirsch O, Keller H, Albohn-Kühne C, et al: Satisfaction of patients and primary care physicians with shared decision making, *Eval Health Prof* 33(3):321–342, 2010.

Hobdell E: Chronic sorrow and depression in parents with children with neural tube defects, *J Neurosci Nurs* 36(2):82–88, 94, 2004.

Holzhauer JK, Reith V, Sawin KJ, et al: Evaluation of temporal artery thermometry in children 3-36 months old, *J Spect Pediatr Nurs* 14(4):239–244, 2009.

Ishimine P: The evolving approach to young child who has fever and no obvious source, *Emerg Med Clin North Am* 251087–251115, 2007.

Jackson C, Cheater FM, Reid I: A systematic review of decision support needs of parents making child health decisions, *Health Expect* 11:232–251, 2008.

John R: Beneficence, prescriptions, and the nurse practitioner. An ethics case study, *Adv Nurse Pract* 15(9):55–56, 2007.

Kempe A, Bunik M, Ellis J, et al: How safe is triage by an after-hours telephone call center? *Pediatrics* 118(2):457–463, 2006.

Kon AA: The shared decision-making continuum, *JAMA* 304(8):903–904, 2010.

Kramer LC, Richards PA, Thompson AM, et al: Alternating antipyretics: antipyretic efficacy of acetaminophen versus acetaminophen alternated with ibuprofen in children, *Clin Pediatr* 47(9):907–911, 2008.

Leape LL, Brennan TA, Laird N, et al: The nature of adverse events in hospitalized patients. Results of the Harvard Medical Practice Study II, *N Engl J Med* 324(6):377–384, 1991.

Ledford CJ, Villagan MM, Kreps GL, et al: "Practicing medicine": patient perceptions of physician communication and the process of prescription, *Patient Educ Couns* 80(3):384–392, 2010.

Légaré F, Ratté S, Stacey D, et al: Interventions for improving the adoption of shared decision making by healthcare professionals, *Cochrane Database Syst Rev* (5):CD006732, 2010.

Levine DA: Growth and development. In Marcdante KJ, Kliegman RM, Jenson HB, et al, editors: *Nelson essentials of pediatrics*, ed 6, Philadelphia, 2011, Saunders.

Major P, Thiele EA: Seizures in children: determining the variation, *Pediatr Rev* 28(10):363–371, 2007.

Mayo AM, Chang BL, Omery A: Use of protocols and guidelines by telephone nurses, *Clin Nurs Res* 11(2):204–219, 2002.

McAllister JW, Presler E, Turchi RM, et al: Achieving effective care coordination in the medical home, *Pediatr Ann* 38(9):491–497, 2009.

McPherson M, Arango P, Fox H, et al: A new definition of children with special health care needs, *Pediatrics* 102(1):137–140, 1998.

McCarthy PL: Evaluation of the sick child in the office and clinic. In Kliegman RM, Behrman RE, Jenson HB, et al, editors: *Nelson textbook of pediatrics*, ed 18, Philadelphia, 2007, Saunders.

Medical Home Initiatives for Children with Special Needs Project Advisory Committee, American Academy of Pediatrics: The medical home, *Pediatrics* 110(1):184–186, 2002. reaffirmed 2008.

Merenstein D, Diener-West M, Krist A, et al: An assessment of the shared decision model in parents of children with acute otitis media, *Pediatrics* 116(6):1267–1275, 2005.

Miller JE: How to write low literacy materials, *J Extension* 39(1), 2001. Available at www.joe.org/joe/2001february/tt2.php. Accessed Nov 3, 2010.

Nabulsi MM, Tamim H, Mahfoud Z, et al: Alternating ibuprofen and acetaminophen in the treatment of febrile children: a pilot study [ISRCTN30487061], *BMC Med* 4:4, 2006.

National Institute for Health and Clinical Excellence (NICE): *Feverish illness in children*, 2007. Available at http://publications.nice.org/uk/feverish.illness-in-children-cg47. Accessed Jan 7, 2012.

Niska R, Bhuiya F, Xu J: National Hospital Ambulatory Medical Care Survey: 2007 emergency department summary, *Natl Health Stat Report* 26:1–31, 2010.

Partnership for Clear Health Communication: *Ask me three*. Available at http://www.pfizerhealthliteracy.com/public-poliy-researchers/PcheAskme 3.aspx. Accessed Jan 6, 2012.

Poole SR: *Developing a telephone triage and advice system for a pediatric office practice*, Elk Grove Village, IL, 2003, American Academy of Pediatrics.

Roos S: *Chronic sorrow: a living loss*, New York and London, 2002, Brunner-Routledge.

Sadof MD, Nazarian BL: Caring for children who have special health-care needs: a practical guide for the primary care practitioner, *Pediatr Rev* 28(7):e36–e42, 2007.

Sarrell EM, Wielunsky E, Cohen HA: Antipyretic treatment in young children with fever: acetaminophen, ibuprofen, or both alternating in a randomized, double-blind study, *Arch Pediatr Adolesc Med* 160(2):197–202, 2006.

Schmitt BD: *Pediatric telephone protocols: office version*, ed 13, Elk Grove Village, IL, 2010, American Academy of Pediatrics.

Schmitt BD: *Your child's health: the parents' one-stop reference guide to symptoms, emergencies, common illnesses, behavior problems and healthy development*, New York, 2005, Bantam Dell Publishing Group.

Schwartz RP: Motivational interviewing (patient-centered counseling) to address childhood obesity, *Pediatr Ann* 39(3):154–158, 2010.

Shepard MP, Mahon MM: Family considerations. In Hayman LL, Mahon MM, Turner JR, editors: *Chronic illness in children*, New York, 2002, Springer.

Smith S: Infectious diseases. In Marcdante KJ, Kliegman RM, Jenson HB, et al, editors: *Nelson essentials of pediatrics*, ed 6, Philadelphia, 2011, Saunders.

Stille CJ: Communication, comanagement, and collaborative care for children and youth with special healthcare needs, *Pediatr Ann* 38(9):498–504, 2009.

Suarez M, Mullins S: Motivational interviewing and pediatric health behavior interventions, *J Dev Behav Pediatr* 29(5):417–428, 2008.

Taketomo CK, Hodding JH, Kraus DM: *Pediatric dosage handbook*, ed 18, Hudson, OH, 2011, Lexi-Comp.

The Joint Commission: *"What did the doctor say?" Improving health literacy to protect patient safety*, 2007. Available at www.jointcommission.org/1/18/improving-health-literacy.pdf. Accessed Jan 7, 2012.

Titus MO, Hulsey T, Heckman J, et al: Temporal artery thermometry utilization in pediatric emergency care, *Clin Pediatr* 48(2):190–193, 2009.

Wilson M: Readability and patient education materials used for low-income populations, *Clin Nurse Spec* 23(1):33–40, 2009.

Wise PH: Chronic illness in childhood. In Kliegman RM, Behrman RE, Jenson HB, et al, editors: *Nelson handbook of pediatrics*, ed 18, Philadelphia, 2007, Saunders.

World Health Organization: *WHO guidelines on hand hygiene in healthcare*. 2009. Available at www.whqlibdoc.who.int/publications/2009/9789241597906_eng.pdf. Accessed Sept 1, 2010.

Yin HS, Johnson M, Mendelsohn AL, et al: The health literacy of parents in the United States: a nationally representative study, *Pediatrics* 124(Suppl 3):S289–S298, 2009.

CHAPTER 22

American Academy of Pediatrics (AAP), Committee on Psychosocial Aspects of Child and Family Health, American Pain Society, Task Force on Pain in Infants, Children, and Adolescents: The assessment and management of acute pain in infants, children, and adolescents, *Pediatrics* 108(3):793–797, 2001.

Bear LA, Ward-Smith P: Interrater reliability of the Comfort Scale, *Pediatr Nurs* 32(5):427–434, 2006.

Betz CL, Sowden LA: *Mosby's pediatric nursing reference*, ed 6, Philadelphia, 2007, Mosby.

Beyer JE: *The oucher: a user's manual and technical report*, Denver, 1989, University of Colorado.

Buie VC, Owings MF, DeFrances CJ, Golosinskiy A: National hospital discharge survey: 2006 summary, *National Center for Health Statistics Vital Health Stat* 13(168), 2010.

Cline ME, Herman J, Shaw ER, et al: Standardization of the visual analogue scale, *Nurs Res* 41:378–380, 1992.

Craig KD, Korol CT: Developmental issues in understanding, assessing and managing pediatric pain. In Walco GA, Goldschneider KR, editors: *Pain in children: a practical guide for primary care*, Totowa, NJ, 2008, Humana Press, pp 9–20.

Eland J: Children with pain. In Jackson OB, Saunders RB, editors: *Child health nursing*, Philadelphia, 1993, JB Lippincott.

Golianu B, Krane EJ, Galloway KS, et al: Pediatric acute pain management, *Pediatr Clin North Am* 47:559–587, 2000.

Greco C, Berde C: Pain management for the hospitalized pediatric patient, *Pediatr Clin North Am* 52:995–1027, 2005.

Guite JW, Logan DE, McCue R, et al: Parental beliefs and worries regarding adolescent chronic pain, *Clin J Pain* 25(5):223–232, 2009.

Hester NO, Foster RL, Kristensen K, et al: Measurement of children's pain by children, parents, and nurses: psychometric and clinical issues related to the poker chip tool and pain ladder. Generalizability of procedures assessing pain in children: final report. Research funded by NIH, National Center for Nursing Research under grant no. R23NR01382, 1989.

Hicks CL, von Baeyer CL, Spafford PA, et al: The Faces Pain Scale, revised: toward a common metric in pediatric pain, *Pain* 93(2):173–183, 2001.

Jordan-Marsh M, Yoder L, Hall D, et al: Alternate Oucher form testing gender, ethnicity, and age variations, *Res Nurs Health* 17:111–118, 1994.

Kraemer FW, Rose JB: Pharmacologic management of acute pediatric pain, *Anesthesiol Clin* 27:241–268, 2009.

Malviya S, Vopel-Lewis T, Burke C, et al: The revised FLACC observational pain tool: improved reliability and validity for pain assessment in children with cognitive impairment, *Paediatr Anaesth* 16:258–265, 2006.

Marie B, editor: *Core curriculum for pain management in nursing*, ed 2, Dubuque, Iowa, 2009, Kendall-Hunt.

Melzack R, Wall PD: Pain mechanisms: a new theory, *Science* 150(699):971–979, 1965.

National Institutes of Health, National Heart, Lung, and Blood Institute: *The management of sickle cell disease*, ed 4, Bethesda, MD, 2002, NIH Publication No. 02–2117.

Overlander TF, O'Donell ME, Montgomery CJ: Pain in children with significant neurological impairment, *J Dev Behav Pediatr* 20(4):235–243, 1999.

Palermo TM, Zeltzer LK: Recurrent and chronic pain. In Carey WB, Crocker AC, Coleman WL, et al, editors: *Developmental-behavioral pediatrics*, ed 4, Philadelphia, 2009, Saunders.

Phillips DM: JCAHO pain management standards are unveiled: Joint Commission on Accreditation of Healthcare Organizations, *JAMA* 284:428–429, 2000.

Schechter WS: Pediatric pain management. In Burg FD, Ingelfinger JR, Polin RA, et al, editors: *Gellis and Kagan's current pediatric therapy*, ed 18, Philadelphia, 2006, Saunders.

Schechter NL, Zempsky WT, Cohen LL, et al: Pain reduction during pediatric immunizations: evidence-based review and recommendations, *Pediatrics* 119:1184–1198, 2007.

Scheffer R: Psychiatric disorders. In Marcdante KJ, Kliegman RM, Jenson HB, et al, editors: *Nelson essentials of pediatrics*, ed 6, Philadelphia, 2011, Saunders.

Sihna M, Christopher NC, Fenn R, et al: Evaluation of non-pharmacologic methods of pain and anxiety management for laceration repair in the pediatric emergency room, *Pediatrics* 117:1162–1168, 2006.

Taketomo CK, Hodding JH, Kraus DM: *Pediatric dosage handbook*, ed 17, Hudson, OH, 2011, Lexi-Comp.

Tesler MD, Savedra MC, Holzemer WL, et al: The word-graphic rating scale as a measure of children's and adolescent's pain intensity, *Res Nurs Health* 14:361–371, 1991.

Thompson LA, Knapp CA, Feeg V, et al: Pediatrician's management practices for chronic pain, *J Palliat Med* 13(2):171–178, 2010.

Tsao JC, Evans S, Meldrum M, et al: Part I. Sucrose and non-nutritive sucking, *Evid Based Complement Altern Med (eCAM)* 5(4):371–381, 2008.

Villarruel AM, Denyes MJ: Pain assessment in children: theoretical and empirical validity, *ANS Adv Nurs Sci* 14:32–41, 1991.

Weisman SJ, Bernstein B, Schecter NL: Consequences of inadequate analgesia during painful procedures in children, *Arch Pediatr Adolesc Med* 152:147–149, 1998.

Wendell VI: Analgesia and pain management. In Winterton-Edmunds M, Mayhew MS, editors: *Pharmacology for the primary care provider*, St Louis, 2009, Mosby.

Wolraich ML, Drotar DD, Dworkin PH, et al: *Developmental-behavioral pediatrics*, St Louis, 2008, Mosby.

Wong DL: The Wong-Baker FACES pain rating scale, *Home Health Focus* 2(8):62, 1996.

Wong D, Baker C: Pain in children: comparison of assessment scales, *Pediatr Nurs* 14:9–14, 1988.

Zeltzer LK, Krell H: Pediatric pain management. In Kliegman RM, Behrman RE, Jenson HB, et al, editors: *Nelson textbook of pediatrics*, ed 18, Philadelphia, 2007, Saunders.

Zempsky WT, Cravero JP: Committee on Pediatric Emergency Medicine and Section on Anesthesiology and Pain Medicine: Relief of pain and anxiety in pediatric patients in emergency medical systems, *Pediatrics* 114:1348–1354, 2004.

CHAPTER 23

Abzug MJ: Nonpolio enteroviruses. In Kliegman RM, Behrman RE, Jenson HB, et al, editors: *Nelson textbook of pediatrics*, ed 18, Philadelphia, 2007, Saunders, pp 1350–1356.

Advisory Committee on Immunization Practices (ACIP): *ACIP provisional recommendations for measles-mumps-rubella (MMR) evidence of immunity requirements for healthcare personnel*, 2009. Available at www.cdc.gov/vaccines/recs/provisional/downloads/mmr-evidence-immunity-Aug2009-508.pdf. Accessed Dec 12, 2010.

Amer A: *Point-counterpoint: responding to common reasons for vaccine refusal*, 2009. Available at www.pediatricsconsultantlive.com/display/article/1803329/1466497. Accessed May 6, 2011.

American Academy of Pediatrics: Committee on Pediatric AIDS: Prophylaxis to prevent mother-to-child transmission in the United States, *Pediatrics* 122(5):1127–1134, 2008.

American Academy of Pediatrics: *Vaccine studies: examine the evidence*, 2010. Available at www.aap.org/immunization/families/faq/VaccineStudies.pdf. Accessed Dec 4, 2010a.

American Academy of Pediatrics: *Summer safety tips—part 1, 2010b*. Available at www.aap.org/advocacy/releases/summertips.cfm. Accessed Nov 12, 2010.

American Veterinary Medical Association: *US pet ownership and demographics sourcebook*, Schaumburg, IL, 2007.

Beasley RP: Nature usually favors females, *J Infect Dis* 192:1865–1866, 2005.

Bhutta ZA: Acute gastroenteritis in children. In Kliegman RM, Behrman RE, Jenson HB, et al, editors: *Nelson textbook of pediatrics*, ed 18, Philadelphia, 2007, Saunders, p 1608. Table 337–2.

Bitnum A, Read S: Coronaviruses. In Kliegman RM, Behrman RE, Jenson HB, editors: *Nelson textbook of pediatrics*, ed 18, Philadelphia, 2007, Saunders, pp 1396–1398.

Blumberg HM, Leonard MK: Tuberculosis. In Dale DC, editor: *WebMD infectious diseases: the clinician's guide to diagnosis, treatment, and prevention*, 2010, WebMD Corporation.

Burrascano JJ: *Advanced topics in Lyme disease; diagnostic hints and treatment guidelines for Lyme and other tick borne illnesses*, 2008. Available at www.ilads.org/lyme_disease/B_guidelines_12_17_08.pdf. Accessed Nov 15, 2010.

Butler KH: Incision and drainage. In Roberts JR, Hedges JR, editors: *Clinical procedures in emergency medicine*, ed 5, Philadelphia, 2009, Saunders.

Centers for Disease Control and Prevention: Notice to Readers: Revised ACIP Recommendation for Avoiding Pregnancy After Receiving a Rubella-Containing Vaccine, *MMWR Morb Mort Wkly Rep* 50(49):1117, 2001.

Centers for Disease Control and Prevention: Interim guidelines for the evaluation of infants born to mothers infected with West Nile virus during pregnancy, *MMWR Morb Mortal Wkly Rep* 53(07):154–157, 2004.

Centers for Disease Control and Prevention: Antiretroviral postexposure prophylaxis after sexual, injection-drug use, or other nonoccupational exposure to HIV in the United States, *MMWR Morb Mortal Wkly Rep* 54(RR2):1–20, 2005.

Centers for Disease Control and Prevention: Enterovirus surveillance—United States, 1970-2005, *MMWR Morb Mortal Wkly Rep* 55(SS08):1–20, 2006a.

Centers for Disease Control and Prevention: Epidemiology of HIV/AIDS—United States, 1981-2005, *MMWR Morb Mortal Wkly Rep* 55(21):589–592, 2006b.

Centers for Disease Control and Prevention: Increased detections and severe neonatal disease associated with coxsackievirus B1 infection—United States, 2007, *MMWR Morb Mortal Wkly Rep* 57(20):553–556, 2008a.

Centers for Disease Control and Prevention: *Avian influenza: current situation*, 2008b. Available at www.cdc.gov/flu/avian/outbreaks/current.htm. Accessed Nov 19, 2010.

Centers for Disease Control and Prevention: Updated recommendation from the Advisory Committee on Immunization Practices (ACIP) for revaccination of persons at prolonged increased risk for meningococcal disease, *MMWR Morb Mortal Wkly Rep* 58(37):1042–1043, 2009a.

Centers for Disease Control and Prevention: Surveillance for acute viral hepatitis—United States, 2007, *MMWR Morb Mortal Wkly Rep* 58(SS-3):1–27, 2009b.

Centers for Disease Control and Prevention: *Hepatitis E FAQs for health professionals*, Updated 2009c. Available at www.cdc.gov/hepatitis/HEV/HEVfaq.htm#section2. Accessed Nov 30, 2010.

Centers for Disease Control and Prevention: *Varicella disease*, 2009d. Available at www.cdc.gov/vaccines/vpd-vac/varicella/dis-faqs-clinic.htm. Accessed Jan 6, 2011.

Centers for Disease Control and Prevention: *What you should know about a smallpox outbreak*, 2004, Reviewed 2009e. Available at www.bt.cdc.gov/agent/smallpox/basics/outbreak.asp. Accessed Dec 12, 2010.

Centers for Disease Control and Prevention: *Clostridium difficile— information for healthcare providers*, 2004, Updated 2010a. Available at www.cdc.gov/ncidod/dhqp/id_CdiffFAQ_HCP.html. Accessed Nov 28, 2010.

Centers for Disease Control and Prevention: FDA licensure of bivalent human papillomavirus vaccine (HPV2, Cervarix) for use in females and updated HPV vaccination recommendations from the Advisory Committee on Immunization Practices (ACIP), *MMWR Morb Mortal Wkly Rep* 59(20):626–629, 2010b.

Centers for Disease Control and Prevention: FDA licensure of quadrivalent human papillomavirus vaccine (HPV4, Gardasil) for use in males and guidance from the Advisory Committee on Immunization Practices (ACIP), *MMWR Morb Mortal Wkly Rep* 59(20):630–632, 2010c.

Centers for Disease Control and Prevention: Licensure of a meningococcal conjugate vaccine (Menveo) and guidance for use—Advisory Committee on Immunization Practices (ACIP), *MMWR Morb Mortal Wkly Rep* 59(09):273, 2010d.

Centers for Disease Control and Prevention: Licensure of a 13-valent pneumococcal conjugate vaccine (PCV13) and recommendations for use among children—Advisory Committee on Immunization Practices (ACIP), *MMWR Morb Mortal Wkly Rep* 59(09):258–261, 2010e.

Centers for Disease Control and Prevention: Outbreak following wild polio importations—Europe, Africa, and Asia, *MMWR Morb Mort Wkly Rep* 59(43):1393–1399, 2010f.

Centers for Disease Control and Prevention: *The ABCs of hepatitis*, publication no. 21-2076, 2010g. Available at www.cdc.gov/hepatitis. Accessed Nov 30, 2010.

Centers for Disease Control and Prevention: *Guidance for clinicians on the use of rapid influenza diagnostic tests for the 2010-2011 influenza season*, 2010h. Available at www.cdc.gov/flu/professionals/diagnosis/clinician_guidance_ridt.htm. Accessed Jan 6, 2011.

Centers for Disease Control and Prevention: *HIV/AIDS today*, 2010i. Available at www.cdcnpin.org/scripts/hiv/hiv.asp. Accessed Nov 12, 2010.

Centers for Disease Control and Prevention, National Center for Emerging and Zoonotic Infectious Diseases (NCEZID): *Toxocara infection*. Available at www.cdc.gov/ncidod/dpd/parasites/toxocara/default.htm. Accessed Oct 20, 2010j.

Centers for Disease Control and Prevention: *HIV surveillance report: diagnosis of HIV infection and AIDS in the United States*, 2009, Vol 21, 2011. Available at www.cdc.gov/hiv/surveillance/resources/reports/2009report/pdf/cover.pdf. Accessed May 9, 2011.

Chatterjee A, O'Keefe C: Current controversies in the USA regarding vaccine safety, *Expert Rev Vaccines* 9(5):497–502, 2010.

Clinician Reviews editorial staff: The mandate debate: how can we increase clinicians' flu vaccination rates? *Clin Rev* 20(10):1, 29-30.

Cohen JI: Human herpesvirus types 6 and 7. In Mandell GL, Bennett JE, Dolin R, editors: *Mandell, Douglas, and Bennett's principles and practice of infectious diseases*, ed 7, Philadelphia, 2009, Churchill Livingstone.

Cushing K, Cohn A: Meningococcal disease. In Centers for Disease Control and Prevention: *Manual for the surveillance of vaccine-preventable diseases*, ed 4, Atlanta, 2008, Centers for Disease Control and Prevention.

Davis C: *MRSA infection*, 2008. Available at www.emedicinehealth.com/mrsa_infection/article_em.htm. Accessed Nov 18, 2010.

Demas P, Webber MP, Schoenbaum EE, et al: Maternal adherence to the zidovudine regimen for HIV-exposed infants to prevent HIV infection: a preliminary study, *Pediatrics* 110(3):e35, 2002.

Dent AE, Kazura JW: Toxocariasis (visceral and ocular larva migrans). In Kliegman RM, Behrman RE, Jenson HB et al, editors: *Nelson textbook of pediatrics*, ed 18, Philadelphia, 2007, Saunders, pp 1506–1507.

Diekema DS: American Academy of Pediatrics Committee on bioethics: responding to parental refusals of immunization of children, *Pediatrics* 115(5):1428–1431, 2005.

Eaton DK, Kann L, Kinchen S, et al: Youth risk behavior surveillance—United States 2009, *MMWR Morb Mortal Wkly Rep* 59(SS05):1–142, 2010.

Fan JH, Zhu YM, Zhang XP: Correlation of hypoproteinuria with C-reactive protein and procalcitonin in children with sepsis, *Zhongguo Dang Dei Er Ke Za Zhi* 12(11):870–873, 2010. (available in translation).

Ferri FF: West Nile virus infection. In Ferri FF, editor: *Ferri's clinical advisor*, ed 1, Philadelphia, 2010, Mosby, p 1188.

Fiore AE, Wasley A, Bell BP: Prevention of hepatitis A through active or passive immunization: recommendations from the Advisory Committee on Immunization Practices (ACIP), *MMWR Morb Mortal Wkly Rep* 55(RR07):1–23, 2006.

Fitzgerald DW, Sterling TR, Haas DW: Mycobacterium tuberculosis. In Mandell GL, Bennett JE, Dolin R, editors: *Mandel, Douglas, and Bennett's principles and practice of infectious diseases*, ed 7, Philadelphia, 2009, Churchill Livingstone.

Galetto-Lacour A, Gervaix A: Identifying severe bacterial infection in children with fever without source, *Expert Rev Anti Infect Ther* 8(11):1231–1237, 2010.

1214 References

Gerber MA: Group A streptococcus. In Kliegman RM, Behrman RE, Jenson HB, et al, editors: *Nelson textbook of pediatrics*, ed 18, Philadelphia, 2007, Saunders, pp 1135–1140.

Hasty MB, Klasner A, Kness S, et al: Cutaneous community-associated methicillin-resistant *Staphylococcus aureus* among all skin and soft-tissue infections in two geographically distant pediatric emergency departments, *Acad Emerg Med* 14(1):35–40, 2007.

Hatzistilianou M: Diagnostic and prognostic role of procalcitonin in infections, *Sci World J* 10:1941–1946, 2010.

Havens PL, Committee on Pediatric AIDS: Postexposure prophylaxis in children and adolescents for non-occupational exposure to human immunodeficiency virus, *Pediatrics* 111(6):1475–1489, 2003.

Hayden GF: The newly licensed pneumococcal conjugate vaccine: questions—and answers, *Consult Pediatricians* 9(6):203–206, 2010.

Heilmann C, Grandjean P, Weihe P, et al: Reduced antibody responses to vaccinations in children exposed to polychlorinated biphenyls, *PLoS Med* 3(8):e11, 2006.

Helb D, Jones M, Story E, et al: Rapid detection of *Mycobacterium tuberculosis* and rifampin resistance by use of on-demand, near-patient technology, *J Clin Microbiol* 48(1):229–237, 2010.

Hermos CR, Vargas SO, McAdam AJ: Human metapneumovirus, *Clin Lab Med* 30(1):131–148, 2010.

Hsiao AL, Baker MD: Fever in the new millennium: a review of recent studies of markers of serious bacterial infection in febrile children, *Curr Opin Pediatr* 17(1):56–61, 2005.

Illinois Department of Public Health: *Methicillin-resistant Staphylococcus aureus in Illinois: guidelines for the primary care provider*, 2008. Available at www .idph.state.il.us/health/infect/MRSA_Provider.htm. Accessed Dec 14, 2010.

Infectious Disease Society of America: *Final report of the Lyme disease review panel of the Infectious Diseases Society of America (IDSA)*, 2010. Available at www.idsociety.org/uploadedFiles/IDSA/Resources/ Lyme_Disease/Final_Report/IDSA-Lyme-Disease-Final-Report.pdf. Accessed Dec 14, 2010.

Institute of Medicine (IOM): *Immunization safety review: vaccines and autism*, Washington, DC, 2004, National Academies Press.

Jenson HB: Epstein-Barr virus. In Kliegman RM, Behrman RE, Jenson HB, et al, editors: *Nelson textbook of pediatrics*, ed 18, Philadelphia, 2007, Saunders, pp 1372–1377.

Johannsen EC, Kaye KM: Epstein-Barr virus (infectious mononucleosis, Epstein-Barr virus-associated malignant diseases, and other diseases). In Mandell GL, Bennett JE, Dolin R, editors: *Mandell, Douglas, and Bennett's principles and practice of infectious diseases*, ed 7, Philadelphia, 2009, Churchill Livingstone.

Jusko TA, De Roos AJ, Schwartz SM, et al: A cohort study of developmental polychlorinated biphenyl (PCB) exposure in relation to post-vaccination antibody response at 6-months of age, *Environ Res* 110(4):388–395, 2010.

Kaye D, Levison M, Yuill T: *ID physicians speculate on potential emerging disease in the next decade*, February 2010. Available at www.pediatricsupersite. com/view.aspx?rid=60899. Accessed Nov 15, 2010.

Koch WC: Parvovirus B19. In Kliegman RM, Behrman RE, Jenson HB, et al, editors: *Nelson textbook of pediatrics*, ed 18, Philadelphia, 2007, Saunders, pp 1357–1360.

Kwong JC, Maaten S, Upshur RE, et al: The effect of universal influenza immunization on antibiotic prescriptions: an ecological study, *Clin Infect Dis* 49(5):750–756, 2009.

Lampe MA, Nesheim S, Shouse RL, et al: Racial/ethnic disparities among children with diagnosis of prenatal HIV infection—34 states 2004-2007, *MMWR Morb Mortal Wkly Rep* 59(04):97–101, 2010.

Lee E, Worsley DF: Role of radionuclide imaging in the orthopedic patient, *Orthop Clin North Am* 37(3):485–501, 2006.

Leroy S, Mosca A, Landre-Peigne C, et al: Ibuprofen in childhood: evidence-based review of efficacy and safety, *Arch Pediatr* 14(5):477–484, 2007.

Levine AM: Hematologic manifestations of AIDS. In Hoffman R, Benz EJ Jr, Shattil SJ, et al, editors: *Hematology: basic principles and practice*, ed 5, Philadelphia, 2008, Churchill Livingstone.

Lewis P: *MRSA and kids*. Lecture presented at the 2nd Annual Pediatric Review and Update series, Portland, December 1, 2006, Oregon Health and Science University.

Litman N, Baum SG: Mumps. In Mandell GL, Bennett JE, Dolin R, editors: *Mandel, Douglas, and Bennett's principles and practice of infectious diseases*, ed 7, Philadelphia, 2009, Churchill Livingstone.

Liu C, Bayer A, Cosgrove SE, et al: *Clinical practice guidelines by the Infectious Diseases Society of America for the treatment of methicillin-resistant Staphylococcus aureus infections in adults and children*, 2011. Available at www.cid.oxfordjournals.org /content/early/2011/01/04/cid.ciq146.full.pdf+html. Accessed Jan 8, 2011.

Long SS, Nyquist AC: Laboratory manifestations of infectious diseases: acute-phase response. In Long SS, Pickering LK, Prober CG, editors: *Principles and practice of pediatric infectious diseases*, ed 3, Philadelphia, 2008, Churchill Livingstone.

Long SS, Edwards KM: Prolonged, recurrent, and periodic fever syndromes. In Long SS, Pickering LK, Prober CG, editors: *Principles and practice of pediatric infectious diseases*, ed 3, Philadelphia, 2008, Churchill Livingstone.

Luzuriaga K, Sullivan JL: Immunopathogenesis of HIV-1 infection. In Long SS, Pickering LK, Prober CG, editors: *Principles and practice of pediatric infectious diseases*, ed 3, Philadelphia, 2008, Churchill Livingstone.

Maheshwari N: How useful is C-reactive protein in detecting occult bacterial infection in young children with fever without apparent focus? *Arch Dis Child* 91(6):533–535, 2006.

Maldonado YA: Measles virus. In Long SS, Pickering LK, Prober CG, editors: *Principles and practice of pediatric infectious diseases*, ed 3, Philadelphia, 2008, Churchill Livingstone.

Marin M, Güris D, Chaves SS, et al: Prevention of varicella: recommendations of the Advisory Committee on Immunization Practices (ACIP), *MMWR Morb Mortal Wkly Rep* 56(RR04):1–40, 2007.

Marin M, Broder KR, Temte JL, et al: Use of combination measles, mumps, rubella, and varicella vaccine recommendations of the Advisory Committee on Immunization Practices (ACIP), *MMWR Morb Mortal Wkly Rep* 59(RR03):1–12, 2010.

Marrazzo JM, Hofman J: Infections due to *Neisseria*. In Dale DC, editor: *Infectious diseases: the clinician's guide to diagnosis, treatment, and prevention*, New York, 2010, WebMD Professional Publishing.

Mason WH: Measles. In Kliegman RM, Behrman RE, Jenson HB, et al, editors: *Nelson textbook of pediatrics*, ed 18, Philadelphia, 2007a, Saunders, pp 1331–1337.

Mason WH: Mumps. In Kliegman RM, Behrman RE, Jenson HB, et al, editors: *Nelson textbook of pediatrics*, ed 18, Philadelphia, 2007b, Saunders, pp 1341–1344.

Mason WH: Rubella. In Kliegman RM, Behrman RE, Jenson HB, et al, editors: *Nelson textbook of pediatrics*, ed 18, Philadelphia, 2007c, Saunders, pp 1337–1341.

Miller LG, Kaplan SL: *Staphylococcus aureus:* a community pathogen, *Inf Dis Clin North Am* 23(1):35–52, 2009.

Myers MG, Seward JF, LaRussa PS: Varicella-zoster virus. In Kliegman RM, Behrman RE, Jenson HB, et al, editors: *Nelson textbook of pediatrics*, ed 18, Philadelphia, 2007, Saunders, pp 1366–1372.

Nash TE: Visceral larva migrans and other unusual helminth infection. In Mandell GL, Bennett JE, Dolin R, et al, editors: *Mandell, Douglas, and Bennett's principles and practice of infectious diseases*, ed 7, Philadelphia, 2009, Elsevier.

National Network for Immunization Information: *Vaccines and autism*, 2009. Available at www.immuni zationinfo.org/issues/thimerosal-mercury/vaccines-and-autism-2009. Accessed Dec 3, 2010.

Norrby-Teglund A, Low DE: Myositis, pyomyositis, and necrotizing fasciitis. In Long SS, Pickering LK, Prober CG, editors: *Principles and practice of pediatric infectious diseases*, ed 3, Philadelphia, 2008, Churchill Livingstone.

Pickering LK, Baker CJ, Kimberlin DW, et al, editors: *Red book: 2009 report of the committee on infectious diseases*, ed 28, Elk Grove Village, IL, 2009, American Academy of Pediatrics.

Phillips U: Should patients be discharged because parents refuse to have their child vaccinated, *Consult Pediatricians* 9(10):S16, 2010.

Pollack A: Rising threat of infection unfazed by antibiotics, *New York Times*, February 26, 2010. Available at www.nytmes.com/2010/02/27/business/ 27germ.html. Accessed Nov 18, 2010.

Poutanen SM: Human coronaviruses. In Long SS, Pickering LK, Prober CG, editors: *Principles and practice of pediatric infectious diseases*, ed 3, Philadelphia, 2008, Churchill Livingstone.

Powell KR: Fever without a focus. In Kliegman RM, Behrman RE, Jenson HB, et al, editors: *Nelson textbook of pediatrics*, ed 18, Philadelphia, 2007, Saunders, pp 1087–1093.

Price CS, Thompson WW, Goodson B, et al: Prenatal and infant exposure to thimerosal from vaccines and immunoglobulins and risk of autism, *Pediatrics* 126(4):656–664, 2010.

Prymula R, Siegrist CA, Chlibek R, et al: Effect of prophylactic paracetamol administration at time of vaccination on febrile reactions and antibody responses in children: two open-label, randomized controlled trials, *Lancet* 374(9698):1339–1350, 2009.

Puder JJ, Schindler C, Zahner L, et al: Adiposity, fitness and metabolic risk in children: a cross-sectional and longitudinal study, *Int J Pediatr Obes*, 2010, Nov 22.

Read JS, Committee on Pediatric AIDS: Human milk, breastfeeding, and transmission of human immunodeficiency virus type 1 in the United States, *Pediatrics* 112(5):1196–1205, 2003, reaffirmed 2007.

Review Panel of the Infectious Diseases Society of America (IDSA): *Final report of the Lyme disease review panel of the Infectious Diseases Society of America, April 2010*. Available at www.idsociety.org/uploadedFiles/IDSA/Resources- /Lyme_Disease/Final_Report/IDSA-Lyme-Disease-Final-Report.pdf. Accessed Nov 15, 2010. (This was a review and endorsement of Wormser et al, 2006 guidelines listed below.)

Reynolds SA, Levy F, Walker ES: *Hand sanitizer alert (letter)*, 2006. Available at www.cdc.gov/NCIDOD/EID/vol12no03/05-0955.htm. Accessed Dec 3, 2010.

Riley L: Barriers to best-practice vaccination in rural areas can be modified, *Infect Dis Child* 19(6):26, 2006.

Rodewald L, Orenstein W: Vaccines for Children Program entitling children to protection, *Infect Dis Child* 19(10):4–5, 2006.

Rongkavilit C: Importance of immunization: a serious disease is just a plane ride away, *Consult Pediatricians* 9(10):S17–S21, 2010.

Rosenthal M: CA-MRSA becoming fact of life for some athletes involved in contact sports, *Infect Dis Child* 18(11):52–53, 2005.

Rosenthal M: Treatment of skin and soft tissue infections changing in an age of MRSA, *Infect Dis Child* 19(4):52, 2006.

Rusk J: More work needed to increase adolescent vaccination coverage levels, research says, *Infect Dis Child* 19(6):37–38, 2006.

Savely GR: Update on Lyme disease, *Clin Rev* 16(4):45–50, 2006.

Schwartz A: Budget crisis shrinks vital program for child care providers, *Sci Caring* 22(2):16, 2010.

Shapiro ED: Lyme disease *(Borrelia burgdorferi)*. In Kliegman RM, Behrman RE, Jenson HB, et al, editors: *Nelson textbook of pediatrics*, ed 18, Philadelphia, 2007, Saunders, pp 1274–1278.

Shapiro ED: Fever without localizing signs. In Long SS, Pickering LK, Prober CG, editors: *Principles and practice of pediatric infectious diseases*, ed 3, Philadelphia, 2008, Churchill Livingstone.

Shapiro ED: *Chronic Lyme disease presents challenges for physicians, patients*, 2010. Available at www.pediatricsupersite.com/view.aspx?rid=68456. Accessed Nov 14, 2010.

Sherman C: Treating HIV infection in primary care, *Clin Adv* 13(10):67–69, 2010.

Shetty AK, Maldonado YA: Epidemiology and prevention of HIV infection in children and adolescents. In Long SS, Pickering LK, Prober CG, editors: *Principles and practice of pediatric infectious diseases*, ed 3, Philadelphia, 2008, Churchill Livingstone.

Simoes EAF: Polioviruses. In Kliegman RM, Behrman RE, Jenson HB, et al, editors: *Nelson textbook of pediatrics*, ed 18, Philadelphia, 2007, Saunders, pp 1344–1350.

Smith JC: *The structure, role, and procedures of the U.S. Advisory Committee on Immunization Practices*, 2010. Available at www.cdc.gov/vaccines/recs/acip/downloads/article-2010-role-procedures-ACIP-508.pdf. Accessed Dec 7, 2010.

Sosinsky LS, Giliam WS: Child care. In Kliegman RM, Behrman RE, Jenson HB, et al, editors: *Nelson textbook of pediatrics*, ed 18, Philadelphia, 2007, Saunders, pp 81–86.

Stanberry LR: Herpes simplex virus. In Kliegman RM, Behrman RE, Jenson HB, et al, editors: *Nelson textbook of pediatrics*, ed 18, Philadelphia, 2007, Saunders, pp 1360–1366.

Starke RJ, Jacobs RF: Mycobacterium tuberculosis. In Long SS, Pickering LK, Prober CG, editors: *Principles and practice of pediatric infectious disease*, ed 3, Philadelphia, 2008, Churchill Livingstone.

Starke JR, Munoz FM: Tuberculosis *(Mycobacterium tuberculosis)*. In Kliegman RM, Behrman RE, Jenson HB, et al, editors: *Nelson textbook of pediatrics*, ed 18, Philadelphia, 2007, Saunders, pp 1240–1254.

Stechenberg BW: Bartonella. In Kliegman RM, Behrman RE, Jenson HB, et al, editors: *Nelson textbook of pediatrics*, ed 18, Philadelphia, 2007, Saunders, pp 1219–1222.

Stevens DL: Infections due to Gram-positive cocci. In Dale DC, editor: *Infectious diseases: the clinician's guide to diagnosis, treatment, and prevention*, New York, 2010, WebMD Professional Publishing.

Stevenson AM: Factors influencing immunization rates, *Clin Adv* 12(11):19–26, 2009.

Stratton K, Alamario DA, Wizemann T, et al, editors: *Immunization safety review: influenza vaccines and neurological complications*, Appendix A. Written for Institute of Medicine. Washington DC, 2004, National Academies Press.

Sykes DL, Truax SR: *The window period re-examined: an update for HIV counselors*, 2010. UCSC AIDS Health Project: online resources for the basic 1. Available at www.ucsf-ahp.org/HTML2/Online_Resources/WindowPeriodExamined.pdf. Accessed Nov 12, 2010.

Tasabehji WR, Al-Quobaili FA, Al-Daher NA: Usefulness of procalcitonin and some inflammatory parameters in septic patients, *Saudi Med* 29(4):520–525, 2008.

Tufts G, Connor Hardman ME: Community-acquired methicillin-resistant *Staphylococcus aureus*, *Clin Rev* 16(1):52–58, 2006.

Van Voorhis WC, Weller PF: Intestinal nematoid infections. In Dale DC, editor: *Infectious diseases: the clinicians guide to diagnosis, treatment, and prevention*, New York, 2010, WebMD.

Waggoner-Fountain LA: Child care and communicable diseases. In Kliegman RM, Behrman RE, Jenson HB, et al, editors: *Nelson textbook of pediatrics*, ed 18, Philadelphia, 2007, Saunders, pp 1074–1077.

Won K, Kruszon-Moran D, Schantz PM, et al: *National seroprevalence and risk factors for zoonotic Toxocara spp. infection*. Philadelphia, 2007, Abstracts of the 56th American Society of Tropical Medicine and Hygiene. Nov 4–8.

World Health Organization: BCG vaccine, *Wkly Epid Record* 4(79):25–40, 2004.

World Health Organization: *Hepatitis B, fact sheet No. 204*, 2008. Available at www.who.int/mediacentre/factsheets/fs204/en. Accessed Nov 30, 2010.

World Health Organization: *Meeting report: WHO informal consultation on standardization and evaluation of BCG vaccines*, 2009. Available at www.who.int/biologicals/publications/meetings/areas/vaccines/bcg/BCG_meeting_report2009v7_FOR_WEB_10JUNE.pdf. Accessed Dec 10, 2010.

World Health Organization: *BCG vaccine, 2010*. In the WHO essential medicines library. Available at www.apps.who.int/emlib/MedicineDisplay.aspx?Language=EN&MedIDName=36%40BCG vaccine. Accessed Dec 10, 2010.

World Health Organization: *Polio Global Eradication Initiative: polio this week*, 2011. Available at www.polioeradication.org/Dataandmonitoring/Poliothisweek.aspx. Accessed May 11, 2011.

Woods CR: *Neisseria meningitidis* (meningococcus). In Kliegman RM, Behrman RE, Jenson HB, et al, editors: *Nelson textbook of pediatrics*, ed 18, Philadelphia, 2007, Saunders, pp 1164–1168.

Wormser GP, Dattwyler RJ, Shapiro ED, et al: The clinical assessment, treatment, and prevention of Lyme disease, human granulocytic anaplasmosis, and babesiosis: clinical practice guidelines by the Infectious Diseases Society of America. *Clin Infect Dis* 43:1089–1134, 2006. These recommendations were reviewed and endorsed by a Review Panel of the Infectious Diseases Society of America (IDSA) in April, 2010. Available at www.idsociety.org/uploadedFiles/IDSA/Resources/Lyme_Disease/Final_Report/IDSA-Lyme-Disease-Final-Report.pdf. Accessed November 15, 2010.

Wright P: Parainfluenza viruses. In Kliegman RM, Behrman RE, Jenson HB, et al, editors: *Nelson textbook of pediatrics*, ed 18, Philadelphia, 2007, Saunders, pp 1387–1388.

Wrubel J, Moskowitz JT, Richards TA, et al: Pediatric adherence perspective of mothers of children with HIV, *Soc Sci Med* 61(11):2423–2433, 2005.

Yalçin SS, Gümüş A, Yurdakök K: Prophylactic use of acetaminophen in children vaccinated with diphtheria-tetanus-pertussis, *World J Pediatr* 4(2):127–129, 2008.

Yogev R, Chadwick E: Acquired immunodeficiency syndrome (human immunodeficiency virus). In Kliegman RM, Behrman RE, Jenson HB, et al, editors: *Nelson textbook of pediatrics*, ed 18, Philadelphia, 2007, Saunders, pp 1427–1443.

Zou S, Foster GA, Dodd RY, et al: West Nile fever characteristics among viremic persons identified through blood donor screening, *J Infect Dis* 202(9):1354–1361, 2010.

CHAPTER 24

American Lung Association: *Trends in asthma morbidity and mortality*, 2010. Available at www.lungusa.org/finding-cures/our-research/trend-reports/asthma-trend-report.pdf. Accessed Nov 16, 2010.

Becker JM: *Allergic rhinitis*, 2009. Available at http://emedicine.medscape.com/article/889259-overview. Accessed Oct 23, 2010.

Buskila D: Pediatric fibromyalgia, *Rheum Dis Clin North Am* 35:253–261, 2009.

Centers for Disease Control and Prevention (CDC): *Chronic fatigue syndrome*. Available at www.cdc.gov/cfs. Accessed Oct 30, 2010.

Dedeoglu F, Kim S, Sundel R: *Clinical manifestations and diagnosis of Henoch-Schonlein purpura*. Available at www.uptodate.com. Accessed Nov 10, 2010.

Gaffin JM, Sheehan WJ, Morrill J, et al: Tree nut allergy, egg allergy, and asthma in children, *Clin Pediatr* 50(2):133–139, 2011.

Gamboa DG, Sugarman JL: An update on selected connective tissue diseases in adolescents, *Curr Opin Pediatr* 20:413–418, 2008.

Grüber C, van Stuijvenberg M, Mosca R, et al: Reduced occurrence of early atopic dermatitis because of immunoactive prebiotics among low-atopy-risk infants, *J Allergy Clin Immunol* 126(4):791–797, 2010.

Haftel HM: Rheumatic diseases of childhood. In Marcdante KJ, Kliegman RM, Jenson HB, et al, editors: *Nelson essentials of pediatrics*, ed 6, Philadelphia, 2011, Saunders.

Heim C, Nater UM, Maloney E, et al: Childhood trauma and the risk for chronic fatigue syndrome: association with neuroendocrine dysfunction, *Arch Gen Psychiatry* 66(1):72–80, 2009.

Huang JT, Abrams M, Tlougan B, et al: Treatment of *Staphylococcus aureus* colonization in atopic dermatitis decreases disease severity, *Pediatrics* 123:e808–e814, 2009.

Jenson HB, Jones JF: Chronic fatigue syndrome. In Kliegman RM, Jenson HB, Behrman RE, Jenson HB, et al, editors: *Nelson textbook of pediatrics*, ed 18, Philadelphia, 2007, Saunders.

Kelly WF, Oppenheimer JJ: *Allergic and environmental asthma: treatment and medication*, 2010. Available at http://emedicine.medscape.com/article/137501-treatment. Accessed Dec 22, 2010.

Klein-Gitelman MS, Miller ML: Systemic lupus erythematosus. In Kliegman RM, Berhrman RE, Jenson HB, et al, editors: *Nelson textbook of pediatrics*, ed 18, Philadelphia, 2007, Saunders, pp 1015–1019.

Klein-Gitelman MS: *Systemic lupus erythematosus*, 2010. Available at http://emedicine, medscape.com/article/1008066-overview. Accessed Sept 10, 2010.

Krafchik BR: *Atopic dermatitis*, 2010. Available at http://emedicine.medscape.com/article/1049085-overview. Accessed Dec 20, 2010.

Lasley MV: Allergy. In Kliegman RM, Marcdante KJ, Jenson HB, et al, editors: *Nelson essentials of pediatrics*, ed 5, Philadelphia, 2006, Saunders.

Lasley MV, Hetherington K: Allergy. In Marcdante KJ, Kliegman RM, Jenson HB, et al, editors: *Nelson essentials of pediatrics*, ed 6, Philadelphia, 2011, Saunders.

Lee JL: Acute rheumatic fever, *Autoimmune Rev* 1:117–123, 2009.

Liu AH, Covar RA, Spahn JD, et al: Childhood asthma. In Kliegman RM, Behrman RE, Jenson HB, et al, editors: *Nelson textbook of pediatrics*, ed 18, Philadelphia, 2007, Saunders.

Liu AH, Spahn JD, Leung DYM: Childhood asthma. In Behrman RE, Kliegman RM, Jenson HB, et al, editors: *Nelson textbook of pediatrics*, ed 17, Philadelphia, 2004, Saunders.

McBride JT: The association of acetaminophen and asthma prevalence and severity, *Pediatrics* 128(6):1181–1185, 2011.

Miller ML, Pachman LM: Vasculitis syndromes. In Kliegman RM, Behrman RE, Jenson HB, et al, editors: *Nelson textbook of pediatrics*, ed 18, Philadelphia, 2007, Saunders.

National Heart, Lung, and Blood Institute (NHLBI): *Full report of the expert panel: guidelines for the diagnosis and management of asthma*. Available at www.nhlbi.nih.gov/guidelines/asthma/epr-3/index.htm. Accessed Oct 27, 2007.

Paller AS, Mancini AJ: *Hurwitz clinical pediatric dermatology: a textbook of skin disorders of childhood and adolescence*, ed 3, Philadelphia, 2006, Saunders.

Pongmarutani T, Alpert P, Miller SK: Pediatric systemic lupus erythematosus: management issues in primary practice, *J Am Acad Nurse Pract* 18(6):258–267, 2006.

Rabinovich CE: *Juvenile rheumatoid arthritis*, 2010. Available at http://emedicine.medscape.com/article/1007276. Accessed Sept 10, 2010.

Scheffer R: Psychiatric disorders. In Marcdante KJ, Kliegman RM, Jenson HB, et al, editors: *Nelson essentials of pediatrics*, ed 6, Philadelphia, 2011, Saunders.

Schneider DS: The cardiovascular system. In Marcdante KJ, Kliegman RM, Jenson HB, et al, editors: *Nelson essentials of pediatrics*, ed 6, Philadelphia, 2011, Saunders.

Sharma GD, Gupta R: *Asthma*, 2010. Available at http://emedicine.medscape.com/article/1000997-overview. Accessed Oct 25, 2010.

Sheikh J, Najib U: *Rhinitis, allergic*, 2010. Available at http://emedicine.medscape.com/article/134825-overview. Accessed Oct 25, 2010.

Spergel J: Epidemiology of atopic dermatitis and atopic march in children, *Immunol Allergy Clin North Am* 30:269–280, 2010.

Stanley L, Ward-Smith P: The diagnosis and management of juvenile idiopathic arthritis. *J Pediatr Health Care* 25:191–194, 2011. doi.10.1016/j.pedhc.2010.12.003.

Steer AC, Carapetis JR: Acute rheumatic fever and rheumatic heart disease in indigenous populations, *Pediatr Clin North Am* 56:1401–1419, 2009.

Storms WW: *Asthma, exercise induced: treatment and medication*, 2010. Available at http://emedicine.medscape.com/article/1547626-treatment. Accessed Dec 22, 2010.

Taketomo CK, Hodding JH, Kraus DM: *Pediatric dosage handbook*, ed 17, Hudson, OH, 2010, Lexi-Comp.

Waits J: Rational use of laboratory testing in the initial evaluation of soft tissue and joint complaints, *Prim Care Clin Office Pract* 27:673–689, 2010. doi:10.1016/j.pop.2010.07.010.

Von Venrooij WJ, Pruijin GJ: Citrullination: a small change for a protein with great consequences for rheumatoid arthritis, *Arthritis Res* 2(4):249–251. doi:10.1186/ar95.

Wollenberg A, Schnopp C: Evaluation of conventional therapy in atopic dermatitis, *Immunol Allergy Clin North Am* 30:351–368, 2010.

Young TW, Strong WB: Acute rheumatic fever. In Burg FS, Ingelfinger JR, Polin RA, et al, editors: *Current pediatric diagnosis and treatment*, ed 18, Philadelphia, 2006, Saunders.

CHAPTER 25

Adams MA, Caparosa S, Thompson S, et al: Translating physical activity recommendations for overweight adolescents to steps per day, *Am J Prev Med* 37(2):137–140, 2009.

Aksglaede L, Juul A, Leffers H, et al: The sensitivity of the child to sex steroids: possible impact of exogenous estrogens, *Hum Reprod Update* 12(4):341–349, 2006.

Alemzadeh R, Wyatt DT: Diabetes mellitus in children. In Kliegman RM, Behrman RE, Jenson HB, et al, editors: *Nelson textbook of pediatrics*, ed 18, Philadelphia, 2007, Saunders.

American Diabetes Association (ADA): Type 2 diabetes in children and adolescents, *Diabetes Care* 23(3):381–389, 2000.

American Diabetes Association (ADA): Standards of medical care in diabetes-2010, *Diabetes Care* 33(Suppl 1):S11–S61, 2010.

Antal Z, Zhou P: Congenital adrenal hyperplasia: diagnosis, evaluation, and management, *Pediatr Rev* 30:e49–e57, 2009.

Butcher Z, Fairclough S, Stratton G, et al: The effect of feedback and information on children's pedometer step counts at school, *Pediatr Exerc Sci* 19(1):29–38, 2007.

Carroll TB, Findling JW: Cushing syndrome of nonpituitary causes, *Curr Opin Endocrinol Diabetes Obes* 16(4):308–315, 2009.

Carroll KN, Arbogast PG, Dudley JA, et al: Increase in incidence of medically treated thyroid disease in children with Down syndrome after rerelease of American Academy of Pediatrics health supervision guidelines, *Pediatrics* 122(2):493–498, 2008.

Cesario SK, Hughes LA: Precocious puberty: a comprehensive review of the literature, *J Obstet Gynecol Neonatal Nurs* 36(3):263–274, 2007.

Chia D, Boston B: Childhood obesity and the metabolic syndrome, *Adv Pediatr* 53:23–53, 2006.

Churchill JN, Ruppe RL, Smaldone A: Use of continuous insulin infusion pumps in young children with type 1 diabetes: a systematic review, *J Pediatr Health Care* 23:173–179, 2009.

Clar C, Waugh N, Thomas S: Routine hospital admission versus out-patient or home care in children at diagnosis of type 1 diabetes mellitus, *Cochrane Database Sys Rev* 2:CD004099, 2007.

Cooke DW, Plotnick L: Type 1 diabetes mellitus in pediatrics, *Pediatr Rev* 29(11):374–384, 2008.

Cope JU, Morrison AE, Samuels-Reid J: Adolescent use of insulin and patient-controlled analgesia pump technology: a 10-year Food and Drug Administration retrospective study of adverse events, *Pediatrics* 121(5):e1133–e1138, 2008.

Counts D, Varma SK: Hypothyroidism in children, *Pediatr Rev* 30(7):251–258, 2009.

Cowell KM: Type 2 diabetes mellitus, *Pediatr Rev* 29(8):289–292, 2008.

Daniels SR, Greer FR: Committee on Nutrition: Lipid screening and cardiovascular health in childhood, *Pediatrics* 122(1):198–208, 2008.

de Jager J, Kooy A, Lehert P, et al: Long term treatment with metformin in patients with type 2 diabetes and risk of vitamin B-12 deficiency: randomised placebo controlled trial, *BMJ* 340:c2181–c2188, 2010.

Diabetes Control and Complications Trial Research Group: The effect of intensive treatment of diabetes on the development and progression of long-term complications in insulin-dependent diabetes mellitus, *N Engl J Med* 329(14):977–986, 1993.

Diabetes Control and Complications Trial Research Group: Effect of intensive diabetes treatment on the development and progression of long-term complications in adolescents with insulin-dependent diabetes mellitus, *J Pediatr* 125(2):177–188, 1994.

Ehehalt S, Gauger N, Blumenstock G, et al: Hemoglobin A$_{1c}$ is a reliable criterion for diagnosing type 1 diabetes in childhood and adolescence, *Pediatr Diabetes* 11(7):446–449, 2010.

Ehtisham S, Hattersley AT, Dunger DB, et al: First UK survey of paediatric type 2 diabetes and MODY, *Arch Dis Child* 89(6):526–529, 2004.

Greiner MV, Kerrigan JR: Puberty: timing is everything, *Pediatr Ann* 35(12):916–922, 2006.

Guthrie R, Susi A: A simple phenylalanine method for detecting phenylketonuria in large populations of newborn infants, *Pediatrics* 32(3):338–343, 1963.

Hoffmann B, Mayatepek E: Neurological manifestations in lysosomal storage disorders—from pathology to first therapeutic possibilities, *Neuropediatrics* 36(5):285–289, 2005.

Hopkins RL, Leinung MC: Exogenous Cushing's syndrome and glucocorticoid withdrawal, *Endocrinol Metab Clin North Am* 34(2):371–384, 2005.

Ibáñez L, Díaz R, López-Bermejo A, et al: Clinical spectrum of premature pubarche: links to metabolic syndrome and ovarian hyperandrogenism, *Rev Endocr Metab Disord* 10(1):63–76, 2009.

Juvenile Diabetes Research Foundation Continuous Glucose Monitoring Study Group: Effectiveness of continuous glucose monitoring in a clinical care environment: evidence from the Juvenile Diabetes Research Foundation continuous glucose monitoring (JDRF-CGM) trial, *Diabetes Care* 33(1):17–22, 2010.

Kaplowitz P: Treatment of central precocious puberty, *Curr Opin Endocrinol Diabetes Obes* 16(1):31–36, 2009.

Keane V: Assessment of growth. In Kliegman RM, Behrman RE, Jenson HB, et al, editors: *Nelson textbook of pediatrics*, ed 18, Philadelphia, 2007, Saunders.

Kolon TF: Disorders of sexual development, *Curr Urol Rep* 9:172–177, 2008.

LaFranchi S: Hyperthyroidism. In Kliegman RM, Behrman RE, Jenson HB, et al, editors: *Nelson textbook of pediatrics*, ed 18, Philadelphia, 2007, Saunders.

Lanpher B, Brunetti-Pierri N, Lee B: Inborn errors of metabolism: the flux from Mendelian to complex diseases, *Nat Rev Genet* 7(6):449–460, 2006.

Liese AD, D'Agostino RB Jr, Hamman RF, et al: The burden of diabetes mellitus among US youth: prevalence estimates from the SEARCH for Diabetes in Youth Study, *Pediatrics* 118(4):1510–1518, 2006.

Loscalzo ML: Turner syndrome, *Pediatr Rev* 29(7):219–227, 2008.

Louis GMB, Gray LE Jr, Marcus M, et al: Environmental factors and puberty timing: expert panel research needs, *Pediatrics* 121(S3):S192–S207, 2008.

Ma RCW, Chan JCN: Incidence of childhood type 1 diabetes: a worrying trend, *Nat Rev Endocrinol* 5(10):529–530, 2009.

Mayer-Davis EJ, Bell RA, Dabelea D, et al: The many faces of diabetes in American youth: type 1 and type 2 diabetes in five race and ethnic populations: the SEARCH for Diabetes in Youth Study, *Diabetes Care* 32(Suppl 2):S99–S101, 2009.

Mohamadi A, Cooke DW: Type 2 diabetes mellitus in children and adolescents, *Adolesc Med State Art Rev* 21(1):103–119, 2010.

Muir A: Precocious puberty, *Pediatr Rev* 27(10):373–381, 2006.

Nathan BM, Palmert MR: Regulation and disorders of pubertal timing, *Endocrinol Metab Clin North Am* 34(3):617–641, 2005.

National Diabetes Information Clearinghouse: *National diabetes statistics*, 2007. National Institute of Health publication 08-3892. Available at http://diabetes.niddk.nih.gov/DM/PUBS/statistics/#i_young people. Accessed Feb 11, 2010.

National Newborn Screening & Genetics Resource Center: *Current newborn screening (NBS) conditions—US by state*, 2009. Available at http://genes-r-us.uthscsa.edu. Accessed Mar 10, 2010.

Nieman P, McKnight T: Medical management of pediatric obesity 2009, *Obes Weight Manage* 6(1):27–30, 2010.

Patterson CC, Dahlquist GG, Gyürüs E, et al: Incidence trends for childhood type 1 diabetes in Europe during 1989-2003 and predicted new cases 2005-20: a multicentre prospective registration study, *Lancet* 373(9680):2027–2033, 2009.

Prasad VK, Kurtzberg J: Cord blood and bone marrow transplantation in inherited metabolic diseases: scientific basis, current status and future directions, *Br J Haematol* 148(3):356–372, 2010.

Raghuveer TS, Garg U, Graf WD: Inborn errors of metabolism in infancy and early childhood: an update, *Am Fam Physician* 73(11):1981–1990, 2006.

Rezvani I: Urea cycle and hyperammonemia. In Kliegman RM, Behrman RE, Jenson HB, et al, editors: *Nelson textbook of pediatrics*, ed 18, Philadelphia, 2007, Saunders.

Roche EF, Menon A, Gill D, et al: Clinical presentation of type 1 diabetes, *Pediatr Diabetes* 6(2):75–78, 2005.

Rosenfield RL, Lipton RB, Drum ML: Thelarche, pubarche, and menarche attainment in children with normal and elevated body mass index, *Pediatrics* 123(1):84–88, 2009.

Schulze A, Matern D, Hoffman GF: Newborn screening. In Sarafoglou K, Hoffmann GR, Roth KS, editors: *Pediatric endocrinology and inborn errors of metabolism*, New York, 2009, McGraw-Hill Medical.

Schwenk WF: Growth hormone therapy–established uses in short children, *Acta Paediatr* 95(Suppl 452): 6–8, 2006.

SEARCH for Diabetes in Youth: *SEARCH study findings.* Available at www.searchfordiabetes.org. Accessed Aug 4, 2010.

Shankarappa RK, Moorthy N, Bhat SP, et al: The challenge produced by familial homozygous hypercholesterolemia when treating premature coronary arterial disease in the young, *Cardiol Young* 19(3):257–263, 2009.

Sondike SB, Jeffrey J: In defense of metabolic syndrome, *J Adolesc Health* 44(3):305–306, 2009.

Stanley CA, Bennett MJ: Disorders of mitochondrial fatty acid oxidation. In Kliegman RM, Behrman RE, Jenson HB, et al, editors: *Nelson textbook of pediatrics*, ed 18, Philadelphia, 2007, Saunders.

Stochholm K, Gravholt CH, Laursen T, et al: Incidence of GH deficiency—a nationwide study, *Eur J Endocrinol* 155(1):61–71, 2006.

Tan JM: Nephrology. In Custer JW, Rau RE, editors: *The Harriet Lane handbook: a manual for pediatric house officers*, ed 18, Philadelphia, 2009, Mosby.

Treatment Options for type 2 Diabetes in Adolescents and Youth (TODAY) Study Group: Design of a family-based lifestyle intervention for youth with type 2 diabetes: the TODAY study, *Int J Obes (Lond)* 34(2):217, 2010.

The Environmental Determinants of Diabetes in the Young [TEDDY] Study Group: The TEDDY study, *Ann N Y Acad Sci* 1150:1–13, 2008.

Thomas JA, Van Hove LK: Inborn errors of metabolism. In Hay WH, Levin M, Deterding R, et al: *Current pediatric diagnosis & treatment*, ed 19, New York, 2009, McGraw-Hill.

Walter JH: Tolerance to fast: rational and practical evaluation in children with hypoketonaemia, *J Inherit Metab Dis* 32(2):214–217, 2009.

CHAPTER 26

American Academy of Pediatrics (AAP), Committee on Genetics: Health supervision for children with sickle cell disease, *Pediatrics* 1009:526–535, 2002.

American Academy of Pediatrics (AAP), Committee on Practice and Ambulatory Medicine: Recommendations for preventative pediatric health care, *Pediatrics* 105:645, 2000.

Andrews NC, Ullrich CK, Fleming MD: Disorders of iron metabolism and sideroblastic anemia. In Orkin SH, Nathan DG, Ginsburg D, et al, editors: *Nathan and Oski's hematology of infancy and childhood*, ed 7, Philadelphia, 2008, Saunders.

Ashok BR, Bertolone S: *Sickle cell anemia*, 2010. Available at http://emedicine.medscape.com/article/958614-overview. Accessed Oct 5, 2010.

Baker RD, Greer FR: Committee on Nutrition: Clinical report—diagnosis and prevention of iron deficiency and iron-deficiency anemia in infants and young children (0-3 years of age), *Pediatrics* 126(5):1040–1050, 2010.

Berkow RL, Schwartz JH: Hemolytic anemias. In Burg F, Ingelfinger J, Polin R, et al, editors: *Current pediatric therapy*, ed 18, Philadelphia, 2006, Elsevier.

Briones M, Abshire T: Disorders of coagulation, platelet number and function. In Burg F, Ingelfinger J, Polin R, et al, editors: *Current pediatric therapy*, ed 18, Philadelphia, 2006, Elsevier.

Brotanek JM, Halterman JS, Auinger P, et al: Iron deficiency, prolonged bottle-feeding, and racial disparities in young children, *Arch Pediatr Adolesc Med* 159:1038–1042, 2005.

Burns K, Camitta BM: Polycythemia (erythrocytosis). In Kliegman R, Behrman R, Jenson HB, et al, editors: *Nelson textbook of pediatrics*, ed 18, Philadelphia, 2007, Saunders.

Cairo MS, Bradley MB: Lymphoma. In Kliegman R, Behrman R, Jenson HB, et al, editors: *Nelson textbook of pediatrics*, ed 18, Philadelphia, 2007, Saunders.

Cunningham MJ: Update on thalassemia: clinical care and complications, *Hematol Oncol Clin North Am* 24:215–227, 2010.

de Alarcon PA, Metzger M: *Hodgkin disease*, 2008. Available at http://emedicine.medscape.com/article/987101-overview. Updated Oct 2011. Accessed Jan 6, 2012.

DeBaun MR, Vichinsky E: Hemoglobinopathies. In Kliegman R, Behrman R, Jenson HB, et al, editors: *Nelson textbook of pediatrics*, ed 18, Philadelphia, 2007, Saunders.

Fuleihan R: Immunology. In Marcdante K, Kliegman R, Jenson HB, et al, editors: *Nelson essentials of pediatrics*, ed 6, Philadelphia, 2011, Saunders.

Gaziev J, Sodani P, Lucarelli G: Hematopoietic stem cell transplantation in thalassemia, *Bone Marrow Transpl* 42(Suppl 1):S41, 2008.

Glader B: Anemias of inadequate production. In Kliegman R, Behrman R, Jenson HB, et al, editors: *Nelson textbook of pediatrics*, ed 18, Philadelphia, 2007, Saunders.

Guyton A, Hall J: *Textbook of medical physiology*, ed 12, Philadelphia, 2010, Saunders.

Huang LH, Portwine C: *Transient erythroblastopenia of children*, 2009. Available at http://emedicine.medscape.com/article/959644. Accessed Sep 30, 2010.

Institute of Medicine: *Dietary reference intakes for vitamin A, vitamin K, arsenic, boron, chromium, copper, iodine, iron, manganese, molybdenum, nickel, silicon, vanadium, and zinc*, Washington, DC, 2003, National Academic Press.

Johnston JM: *Non-Hodgkin lymphoma*, 2010. Available at http://emedicine.medscape.com/article/987540-overview. Accessed Sep 30, 2010.

Kupfer GM: *Childhood cancer epidemiology*, 2009. Available at http://emedicine.medscape.com/article/989841-overview. Accessed Sep 30, 2010.

Levine DA: Disorders of development. In Marcdante R, Kliegman R, Jenson HB, et al, editors: *Nelson essentials of pediatrics*, ed 6, Philadelphia, 2011, Saunders.

Mahachoklertwattana P, Sirikulchayanonta V, Chuansumrit A, et al: Bone histomorphometry in children and adolescents with beta-thalassemia disease: iron-associated focal osteomalacia, *J Clin Endocrinol Metab* 88(8):3966–3972, 2003.

Markowitz M: Lead poisoning. In Kliegman R, Behrman R, Jenson HB, et al, editors: *Nelson textbook of pediatrics*, ed 18, Philadelphia, 2007, Saunders.

McPherson M, Tender J: Iron deficiency anemia. In Burg F, Ingelfinger J, Polin R, et al, editors: *Current pediatric therapy*, ed 18, Philadelphia, 2006, Elsevier.

Meck MM, Leary M, Sills RH: Late effects in survivors of childhood cancer, *Pediatr Rev* 27:257–262, 2006.

Mitchell BL: Sickle cell trait and sudden death—bringing it home, *J Natl Med Assoc* 99(3):300–305, 2007.

Modell B, Darlison M: Global epidemiology of haemoglobin disorders and derived service indicators, *Bull World Health Org* 86(6):480–487, 2008.

Monteleone PM, Meadows: *Late effects of childhood cancer and treatment*, 2009. Available at http://emedicine.medscape.com/article/990815-overview. Accessed Oct 5, 2010.

National Cancer Institute: *SEER Cancer Statistics Review 1975-2007*, 2010. Available at http://seer.cancer.gov/csr/1975_2007/index.html. Accessed Nov 2, 2010.

Ohls RK, Christensen RD: Diseases of the blood. In Kliegman R, Behrman R, Jenson HB, et al, editors: *Nelson textbook of pediatrics*, ed 18, Philadelphia, 2007, Saunders.

Orkin SH, Nathan DG, Ginsburg D, et al: *Nathan and Oski's hematology of infancy and childhood*, ed 7, Philadelphia, 2008, Saunders.

Panepinto JA, Scott JP: Hematology. In Marcdante K, Kliegman R, Jenson HB, et al, editors: *Nelson essentials of pediatrics*, ed 6, Philadelphia, 2011, Saunders.

Pitts RHB, Record E: Sickle cell disease. In Allen P, Vessey J, editors: *Primary care of the child with a chronic condition*, ed 5, St Louis, 2010, Mosby.

Recht M: Thrombocytopenia and anemia in infants and children, *Emerg Med Clin North Am* 27:505–523, 2009.

Satake N, Yoon JM: *Acute lymphoblastic leukemia*, 2010. Available at http://emedicine.medscape.com/article/990113-overview. Accessed Oct 5, 2010.

Schnitzer B: Hodgkin lymphoma, *Hematol Oncol Clin North Am* 23:4, 2009.

Scott JP, Montgomery RR: Hemorrhagic and thrombotic diseases. In Kliegman R, Behrman R, Jenson HB, et al, editors: *Nelson textbook of pediatrics*, ed 18, Philadelphia, 2007, Saunders.

Segel GB: Hereditary spherocytosis. In Kliegman R, Behrman R, Jenson HB, et al, editors: *Nelson textbook of pediatrics*, ed 18, Philadelphia, 2007, Saunders.

Segel G, Hirsh M, Feig S: Managing anemia in a pediatric office practice: part 1, *Pediatr Rev* 23:75–83, 2002a.

Segel G, Hirsh M, Feig S: Managing anemia in a pediatric office practice: part 2, *Pediatr Rev* 23:111–121, 2002b.

Silverman LB: Acute lymphoblastic leukemia. In Orkin SH, Nathan DG, Ginsburg D, et al, editors: *Orkin: oncology of infancy and childhood*, Philadelphia, 2009, Saunders.

Stoll BJ: Infections in the neonatal infant. In Kliegman R, Behrman R, Jenson HB, et al, editors: *Nelson textbook of pediatrics*, ed 18, Philadelphia, 2007, Saunders.

Sulis M, Morris E, Cairo M: Neonatal and childhood neutropenia. In Burg F, Ingelfinger J, Polin R, et al, editors: *Current pediatric therapy*, ed 18, Philadelphia, 2006, Saunders.

Takeshita K: *Beta-thalassemia*, 2010. Available at http://emedicine.medscape.com/article/206490-print. Accessed Oct 5, 2010.

Taketomo C, Hodding J, Kraus D: *Pediatric dosage handbook*, ed 17, Hudson, Ohio, 2010, Lexi-Comp.

Tubergen DG, Bleyer A: The leukemias. In Kliegman R, Behrman R, Jenson HB, et al, editors: *Nelson textbook of pediatrics*, ed 18, Philadelphia, 2007, Saunders.

Weinblatt ME: *Pediatric acute myelocytic leukemia*, 2010. Available at http://emedicine.medscape.com/article/987228-overview.

Woolf AD, Goldman R, Bellinger DC: Update on the clinical management of childhood lead poisoning, *Pediatr Clin North Am* 54:2, 2007.

Wu AHB: *Tietz clinical guide to laboratory tests*, ed 4, Philadelphia, 2006, Saunders.

Zitelli BJ, Davis HW: *Atlas of pediatric physical diagnosis*, ed 5, Philadelphia, 2007, Elsevier.

CHAPTER 27

American Academy of Pediatrics: Pertussis. In Pickering LK, Baker CJ, Kimberlin DW, et al, editors: *2009 Red book: report of the Committee on Infectious Diseases*, ed 28, Elk Grove Village, IL, 2009, American Academy of Pediatrics, pp 504–519.

Bale JF: Meningitis and encephalitis. In Maria BL, editor: *Current management in child neurology*, ed 4, Hamilton, Ontario, 2009, BC Decker, pp 618–623.

Banwell BL: Acquired demyelination of the central nervous system. In Maria BL, editor: *Current management in child neurology*, ed 4, Hamilton, Ontario, 2009, BC Decker, pp 580–590.

Baren JM: LP is not needed for young children with first simple febrile seizure, *J Watch Emerg Med*, 2009. Available at www.emergency-medicine. jwatch.org/cgi/cntent/fll/2009/227/1#. Accessed Oct 1, 2010.

Behrman AJ, Adler J: *Latex allergy*, 2008. Available at www.emedicine.medscape.com/article/756632-overview#a0199. Accessed June 9, 2011.

Beutler AI, Chestnut GT, Mattingly JC, et al: Aspirin use in children for fever or viral syndromes, *Am Fam Physician* 80(12):1472–1474, 2009.

Bigal ME, Lipton RB, Winner P: Epidemiology and classification of headache. In Winner P, Lewis DW, Rothner AD, editors: *Headache in children and adolescents*, ed 2, Hamilton, Ontario, 2008, BC Decker, Chapter 1.

Boes CJ, Capobianco DJ, Cutrer FM, et al: Headache and other craniofacial pain. In Bradley WG, Daroff RB, Fenichel GM, et al: *Neurology in clinical practice*, ed 5, Philadelphia, 2008, Butterworth Heinemann, pp 2011–2059.

Brunstrom J, Tilton A: Cerebral palsy. In Maria BL, editor: *Current management in child neurology*, ed 4, Hamilton, Ontario, 2009, BC Decker, pp 307–312.

Camfield P, Camfield C: What is epilepsy? In Maria BL, editor: *Current management in child neurology*, ed 4, Hamilton, Ontario, 2009, BC Decker, pp 95–98.

Centers for Disease Control and Prevention (CDC): Folate status in women of childbearing age, by race/ethnicity—United States, 1999-2000, 2001-2002, and 2003-2004, *MMWR Morb Mort Wkly Rep* 55(51):1377–1380, 2007.

Centers for Disease Control and Prevention (CDC): *Preventing neural tube birth defects: a prevention model and resource guide*, 2009. Available at www.cdc.gov/ncbddd/orders/pdfs/09_202063-A_Nash_Neural Tube BD Guide FINAL508.pdf. Accessed March 22, 2011.

Centers for Disease Control and Prevention (CDC): *Traumatic brain injury in the U.S.*, 2010a. Available at www.cdc.gov/Features/dsTBI_BrainInjury/. Accessed July 29, 2010.

Centers for Disease Control and Prevention (CDC): CDC Grand Rounds: additional opportunities to prevent neural tube defects with folic acid fortification, *MMWR Morb Mort Wkly Rep* 59(31):980–984, 2010b.

Daniel SJ: The upper airway: congenital malformations, *Paediatr Resp Rev* 7S:S260–S263, 2006.

Dawodu ST: *Traumatic brain injury (TBI)—definition, epidemiology, pathophysiology*. updated 2009. Available at www.emedicine.medscape.com/article/326510-overview. Accessed March 22, 2011.

Di Muzio B: *Benign enlargement of the subarachnoid space in infancy*, 2011. Available at www.radio paedia.org/articles/benign-enlargement-of-the-subarachnoid-space-in-infancy. Accessed March 22, 2011.

DeMyer W: Small, large and abnormally shaped head. In Maria BL, editor: *Current management in child neurology*, ed 4, Hamilton, Ontario, 2009, BC Decker, pp 413–420.

DiRocco F, Arnaud E, Renier D: Evolution in the frequency of nonsyndromic craniosynostosis, *J Neurosurgery* 4(1): online ed 1–4, 2009.

Djukic A: Folate-responsive neurologic diseases, *Pediatr Neurol* 37(6):387–397, 2007.

Dodson WE: Epilepsy, cerebral palsy and IQ. In Pellock JM, Bourgeois BFD, Dodson WE, editors: *Pediatric epilepsy diagnosis and therapy*, ed 3, New York, 2008, Demos. Chapter 67.

Duchowny M: Surgical evaluation. In Pellock JM, Bourgeois BFD, Dodson WE, editors: *Pediatric epilepsy diagnosis and therapy*, ed 3, New York, 2008, Demos. Chapter 60.

Fu PP, Xia Q, Guo L, et al: Toxicity of kava-kava, *J Environ Carcin Ectotoxicol Rev* 26(1):89–112, 2008.

Ghotbi F, Shiva F: An assessment of the necessity of lumbar puncture in children with seizure and fever, *J Pak Med Assoc* 59(5):292–296, 2009.

Haslam RHA: Headaches. In Kliegman RM, Behrman RE, Jenson HB, et al, editors: *Nelson textbook of pediatrics*, ed 18, Philadelphia, 2007, Saunders, pp 2479–2483.

Hawkes CH, Giovannoni G: The McDonald criteria for multiple sclerosis: time for clarification, *Mult Scler*, Mar 1, 2010. epub.

Hershey AD, Powers SW, Vockell AL, et al: Coenzyme Q10 deficiency and response to supplementation in pediatric and adolescent migraine, *Headache* 47(1):73–80, 2007.

Hill CM, Parker RC, Allen P, et al: Sleep quality and respiratory function in children with severe cerebral palsy using night-time postural equipment: a pilot study, *Acta Paediatr* 98:1809–1814, 2009.

Johnston MV: Encephalopathies: cerebral palsy. In Kliegman RM, Behrman RE, Jenson HB, et al, editors: *Nelson textbook of pediatrics*, ed 18, Philadelphia, 2007, Saunders, pp 2494–2499.

Katz RT: Life expectancy for children with cerebral palsy and mental retardation, *Neurorehabilitation* 18:261–270, 2003.

Kinsman SL, Johnston MV: Congenital anomalies of the central nervous system: myelomeningocele. In Kliegman RM, Behrman RE, Jenson HB, et al, editors: *Nelson textbook of pediatrics*, ed 18, Philadelphia, 2007, Saunders, pp 2444–2447.

Kinsman SL: Neural tube defects and spinal dysraphism. In Maria BL, editor: *Current management in child neurology*, ed 4, Hamilton, Ontario, 2009, BC Decker, pp 756–761.

Kossoff EH, Zupec-Kania BA, Rho JM: Ketogenic diets: an update for child neurologists, *Child Neurol* 24(8):979–988, 2009.

Kronenberger WG, Dunn DW: Conversion reaction. In Maria BL, editor: *Current management in child neurology*, ed 4, Hamilton, Ontario, 2009, BC Decker, pp 544–550.

Leszczyszyn DJ, Pellock JM: Status epilepticus and acute seizures. In Pellock JM, Bourgeois BFD, Dodson WE, editors: *Pediatric epilepsy diagnosis and therapy*, ed 3, New York, 2008, Demos.

Lewis D, Ashwal S, Hershey A, et al: Practice parameter: pharmacological treatment of migraine headache in children and adolescents, *Neurology* 63(12):2215–2224, 2004.

Lewis DW, Bigal ME, Winner P: Migraine and the childhood periodic syndromes. In Winner P, Lewis DW, Rothner AD, editors: *Headache in children and adolescents*, ed 2, Hamilton, Ontario, 2008a, BC Decker, Chapter 3.

Lewis DW, Rothner AD, Linder SL: Evaluation of headache. In Winner P, Lewis DW, Rothner AD, editors: *Headache in children and adolescents*, ed 2, Hamilton, Ontario, 2008b, BC Decker, Chapter 2.

Lewis DW: Pediatric migraine, *Neurol clin* 27(2):481–501, 2009.

Mahajan PV: Status epilepticus: evaluation and management, *Consult Pediatricians* 8(12):421–424, 2009.

Martin Sanz E, Barona de Guzman R: Benign paroxysmal vertigo of childhood: categorization and comparison with benign positional paroxysmal vertigo in adults, *Acta Otorhinolaringol* 58(7):296–301, 2007.

Menkes JH, Ellenbogen RG: Traumatic brain and spinal cord injuries in children. In Maria BL, editor: *Current management in child neurology*, ed 4, Hamilton, Ontario, 2009, BC Decker, pp 624–637.

Menkes J, Moser R: *Child neurology*, ed 7, Philadelphia, 2006, Lippincott Williams & Wilkins.

Morrison LA: Guillain-Barre syndrome. In Maria BL, editor: *Current management in child neurology*, ed 4, Hamilton, Ontario, 2009, BC Decker, pp 752–755.

Msall ME: Children at risk: social disadvantage and neurodevelopmental functioning. In Maria BL, editor: *Current management in child neurology*, ed 4, Hamilton, Ontario, 2009, BC Decker, pp 300–306.

National Institute of Neurology Disorders and Stroke (NINDS): *NINDS Rett syndrome information page*, 2010a. Available at www.ninds.nih.gov/disorders/disorder_index.htm. Accessed July 29, 2010.

National Institute of Neurology Disorders and Stroke (NINDS): *Cerebral palsy: hope through research.* NIH publication no. 10-159, Bethesda, MD, 2010b. National Institutes of Health. Available at www.ninds. nih.gov/disorders/cerebral_palsy/detail_cerebral_palsy.htm?css=print#154513104. Accessed Aug 12, 2010.

National Institute of Neurology Disorders and Stroke (NINDS): *NINDS tethered cord syndrome information page*, 2010c. Available at www.ninds.nih.gov/disorders/thertherd_cord/tethered_cord.htm. Accessed Apr 29, 2010.

National MS Society: *Epidemiology of MS*, 2010. Available at www.nationalmssociety.org/about-multiple-sclerosis/what-we-know-about-ms/who-gets-ms/epidemiology-of-ms/index.aspx. Accessed Aug. 20, 2010.

Nelson MR: Birth brachial plexus palsy. In Maria BL, editor: *Current management in child neurology*, ed 4, Hamilton, Ontario, 2009, BC Decker, pp 663–668.

Nordli DR, DeVivo DC: The ketogenic diet. In Pellock JM, Bourgeois BFD, Dodson WE, editors: *Pediatric epilepsy diagnosis and therapy*, ed 3, New York, 2008, Demos. Chapter 57.

Percy AK, Lane JB: Rett syndrome. In Maria BL, editor: *Current management in child neurology*, ed 4, Hamilton, Ontario, 2009, BC Decker, pp 375–382.

Prasad AN: Status epilepticus in the PICU: state of the art, *Can J Neurol Sci* 36(Suppl 2):S92–S98, 2009.

Proud VK, Elias ER: Genetic syndromes and dysmorphology. In Carey WB, Crocker AC, Coleman WL, et al: *Developmental-behavioral pediatrics*, ed 4, Philadelphia, 2009, Saunders, p 253.

Quality Standards Subcommittee of the American Academy of Neurology and the Practice Committee of the Child Neurology Society, Delgado MR, Hirtz D, Aisen M, et al: Practice parameter: pharmacologic treatment of spasticity in children and adolescents with cerebral palsy (an evidence based review): report of the Quality Standards Subcommittee of the American Academy of Neurology and the Practice Committee of the Child Neurology Society, *Neurology* 74(4):336–343, 2010.

Raieli V: Headache: what do children and mothers expect from pediatricians? *Headache* 50(2):290–300, 2010.

Richardson I, Palmer LS: Clinical and urodynamic spectrum of bladder function in cerebral palsy, *J Urol* 182(Suppl 4):1945–1948, 2009.

Robinson S, Proctor M: Diagnosis and management of deformational plagiocephaly a review, *J Neurosurg* 3(4), 2009. online, and 1–9.

Rosman NP: Head injury. In Burg FD, Ingelfinger JR, Polin RA, et al, editors: *Current pediatric therapy*, ed 18, Philadelphia, 2006, Saunders.

Rubin DH, Kornblau DH, Conway EE, et al, editors: Neurologic disorders: headache in children. In Marx JA, Hockberger RS, Walls RM, et al, editors: *Rosen's emergency medicine: concepts and clinical practice*, ed 7, Philadelphia, 2010, Mosby, pp 2234–2238.

Ryan MM: Neonatal hypotonia. In Maria BL, editor: *Current management in child neurology*, ed 4, Hamilton, Ontario, 2009, BC Decker, pp 638–644.

Salman MS, Maria BL: Brainstem and cerebellar malformations. In Maria BL, editor: *Current management in child neurology*, ed 4, Hamilton, Ontario, 2009, BC Decker, pp 573–579.

Sarnat HB: Neuromuscular disorders. In Kliegman RM, Behrman RE, Jenson HB, et al: *Nelson textbook of pediatrics*, ed 18, Philadelphia, 2007, Saunders, pp 2531–2567.

Shevell MI: Diagnostic approach to developmental delay. In Maria BL, editor: *Current management in child neurology*, ed 4, Hamilton, Ontario, 2009, BC Decker, pp 292–299.

Shih JJ, Ochoa JG: A systematic review of antiepileptic drug initiation and withdrawal, *Neurologist* 15(3):122–131, 2009.

Shinnar S, O'Dell C: Treatment decisions in childhood seizures. In Pellock JM, Bourgeois BFD, Dodson WE, editors: *Pediatric epilepsy diagnosis and therapy*, ed 3, New York, 2008, Demos. Chapter 29.

Singer HS: Treatment of tic disorders. In Maria BL, editor: *Current management in child neurology*, ed 4, Hamilton, Ontario, 2009, BC Decker, pp 516–521.

Steinfeld R, Grapp M, Kraetzner R, et al: Folate receptor alpha defect causes cerebral folate transport deficiency: a treatable neurodegenerative disorder associated with disturbed myelin metabolism, *Am J Hum Genet* 85:354–363, 2009.

Taub E, Ramey SL, DeLuca S, et al: Efficacy of constraint-induced movement therapy for children with cerebral palsy with asymmetric motor impairment, *Pediatrics* 113(2):305–312, 2004.

Taub PJ, Pierce P: Positional plagiocephaly, part 2: prevention and treatment, *Consultant Pediatricians* 10(1):13–15, 2011.

Terzis JK, Kokkalis ZT: pediatric brachial plexus reconstruction, *Plast Reconstr Surg* 124(Suppl 6):e370–e385, 2009.

Tiamkao S, Sawanyawisuth K, Towanabut S, et al: Epilepsy investigators: seizure attacks while driving: quality of life in the persons with epilepsy, *Can J Neurol Sci* 36(4):475–479, 2009.

Vajsar J: Neuromuscular junction disorders. In Maria BL, editor: *Current management in child neurology*, ed 4, Hamilton, Ontario, 2009, BC Decker, pp 488–493.

Waknine Y: *FDA approves glycopyrrolate oral solution for chronic severe drooling*, 2010. Available at www.medscape.com/viewarticle/726048. Accessed March 23, 2011.

Wilkinson IA: Migraine variants and mimics. In Maria BL, editor: *Current management in child neurology*, ed 4, Hamilton, Ontario, 2009, BC Decker, pp 55–61.

Williams VC, Maria BL: Bell's palsy. In Maria BL, editor: *Current management in child neurology*, ed 4, Hamilton, Ontario, 2009, BC Decker, pp 451–454.

Wilson-Costello D, Friedman H, Minich N, et al: Improved neurodevelopmental outcomes for extremely low-birth weight infants in 2000-2002, *Pediatrics* 119(1):37–45, 2007.

Wolf P, Shinnar S: Febrile seizures. In Maria BL, editor: *Current management in child neurology*, ed 4, Hamilton, Ontario, 2009, BC Decker, pp 99–104.

Worster A, Keim SM, Sahsi R, et al: Do either corticosteroids or antiviral acyclovir reduce the risk of long-term facial paresis in patients with new-onset Bell's palsy? *J Emerg Med* 38(4), 518–312, 2010.

CHAPTER 28

Ajudua S, Mello M: Shedding some light on laser pointer eye injuries, *Pediatr Emerg Care* 23(9):669–672, 2007.

American Academy of Ophthalmology (AAO): *Protective eyewear for young athletes: joint policy statement*, revised 2003. Available at www.aao.org/about/policy/upload/Protective-Eyewear-for-young-athletes.pdf. Accessed Oct 24, 2010.

American Academy of Ophthalmology (AAO): *Academy applauds second study on unregulated plano contact lenses confirming need for legislation*, 2005. Available at www.ophthalmologyweb.com/News.aspx?spid=23&newsid=99081&headerid=23. Accessed Nov 8, 2010.

American Academy of Ophthalmology (AAO), Refractive Management/Intervention Panel: *Preferred practice pattern guidelines: refractive errors and refractive surgery*, 2007a. Available at www.one.aao.org/ce/practiceguidelines/ppp_content.aspx?cid=e6930284-2c41-48d5-afd2-631dec586286. Accessed Oct 25, 2010.

American Academy of Ophthalmology (AAO), Pediatric Ophthalmology/Strabismus Panel: *Preferred practice pattern guidelines: esotropia and exotropia*, 2007b. Available at www.one.aao.org/ce/practiceguidelines/ppp_content.aspx?cid=89921a42-f4b1-47e4-a5ef-6cbbce4d0197. Accessed Oct 25, 2010.

American Academy of Ophthalmology (AAO), Pediatric Ophthalmology/Strabismus Panel: *Amblyopia*, 2007c. Available at www.one.aao.org/CE/Practice Guidelines/PPP_Content.aspx?cid=930d01f2-740b-433e-a973-cf68565bd27b. Accessed Oct 23, 2010.

American Academy of Ophthalmology (AAO): *Summary recommendations for LASIK*, 2002, revised 2008a. Available at www.aao.org/ce/practiceguidelines/clinicalstatements_content.aspx?cid=Id8a8b79-4952-4140-9680-50bd53da3f55. Accessed Oct 24, 2010.

American Academy of Ophthalmology (AAO): *Eye injuries: recent data and trends in the United States*, 2008b. Available at www.aao.org/newsroom/guide/upload/eye-injuries-bkgrndlongversfinal-1.pdf. Accessed Nov 6, 2010.

American Academy of Ophthalmology (AAO), Pediatric Ophthalmology Panel: *Policy statement: frequency of ocular examinations*, 2009. Available at www.one.aao.org/CE/PracticeGuidelines/ClinicalStatements_Content.aspx?cid+810eaf61-181e-41c8-a0e8-e1d122efe5a4. Accessed Oct 25, 2010.

American Academy of Pediatrics (AAP) Committee on Practice and Ambulatory Medicine and Section on Ophthalmology, American Association of Certified Orthoptists, American Association of Pediatric Ophthalmology and Strabismus, American Academy of Ophthalmology (AAO): Eye examination in infants, children, and young adults by pediatricians: policy statement, *Pediatrics* 111(4):902–907, 2003, reaffirmed 2007.

American Academy of Pediatrics (AAP) (Section on Ophthalmology), the American Association of Pediatric Ophthalmology and Strabismus, the American Academy of Ophthalmology, and the American Association of Certified Orthoptists: *Red reflex examination in neonates, infants and children (a joint statement)*, 2008. Available at www.one.aao.org/CE/PracticeGuidelines/ClinicalStatements_Content.aspx?cid=b2d084bd-00e7-4a33-aa18-b186d1d8714d. Accessed Oct 25, 2010.

American Academy of Pediatrics (AAP): Use of photo screening for children's vision screening, *Pediatrics* 109(3):524–525, 2002, reaffirmed 2008a.

American Academy of Pediatrics (AAP): Policy statement: red reflex examination in infants, *Pediatrics* 109(5):980–981, 2002, reaffirmed 2008b.

American Academy of Pediatrics (AAP): Learning disabilities, dyslexia, and vision: a subject review, *Pediatrics* 102:1217–1219, 1998, reaffirmed 2008c.

American Academy of Pediatrics (Section on Ophthalmology, Council on Children with Disabilities), the American Academy of Ophthalmology, the American Association for Pediatric Ophthalmology and Strabismus, and the American Association of Certified Orthoptists: *Learning disabilities, dyslexia and vision (a joint statement)*, 2009. Available at www.one.aao.org/CE/PracticeGuidelines/Clinical Statements_Content.aspx?cid=8aa39ca4-039a-4329-beec-42e5a3007329. Accessed Oct 31, 2010.

American Academy of Pediatrics (AAP): Prevention of neonatal ophthalmia. In Pickering LK, editor: *Red book: 2009 report of the Committee on Infectious Diseases*, ed 28, Elk Grove Village, IL, 2009a, AAP, pp 827–829.

American Academy of Pediatrics (AAP): Nongonococcal, nonchlamydial ophthalmia. In Pickering LK, editor: *Red book: 2009 report of the Committee on Infectious Diseases*, ed 28, Elk Grove Village, IL, 2009b, AAP, pp 828–829.

American Academy of Pediatrics (AAP): Chlamydia trachomatis. In Pickering LK, editor: *Red book: 2009 report of the Committee on Infectious Diseases*, ed 28, Elk Grove Village, IL, 2009c, AAP, pp 255–259.

American Academy of Pediatrics (AAP): Pneumococcal infections. In Pickering LK, editor: *Red book: 2009 report of the Committee on Infectious Diseases*, ed 28, Elk Grove Village, IL, 2009d, AAP, pp 524–535.

American Association for Pediatric Ophthalmology and Strabismus (AAPOS), American Academy of Ophthalmology (AAO): *Vision screening for infants and children (a joint statement)*, 2007. Available at www.one.aao.org/CE/PracticeGuidelines/ClinicalStatements_Content.aspx?cid=0ad11e02-6a8b-437e-8d01-f45eb18bc0b6. Accessed Oct 25, 3010.

American Optometric Association (AOA), Consensus Panel on Pediatric Eye and Vision Examinations: *Optometric clinic practice guideline: pediatric eye and vision examination, reference guide for clinicians*, 2002. Available at www.aoa.org/documents/CPG-2.pdf. Accessed Nov 8, 2010.

American Optometric Association (AOA): *Shopping guide for sunglasses*, 2008. Available at www.aoa.org/documents/SunglassShopppingGuide0810.pdf. Accessed Nov 6, 2010.

Augsburger JJ, Bornfeld N, Giblin M: Retinoblastoma. In Yankoff M, Duker JS, editors: *Ophthalmology*, ed 3, Maryland Heights, MO, 2008, Mosby, pp 887–894.

Bashour M, Menassa J, Gerontis C: *Cataract, congenital*, 2009. Available at www.emedicine.medscape.com/article/1210837-overview. Accessed Nov 8, 2010.

Bielory L, Friedlaender MH: Allergic conjunctivitis, *Immunol Allergy Clin North Am* 28(1):43–58, 2008.

Bishop R, National Eye Institute, National Institutes of Health: *What kind of eyewear can I use to protect my eyes?* 2009. Available at www.nei.nih.gov/eyeonnei/askthedoctor/archive/1009.asp. Accessed Nov 7, 2010.

Brandt JD: Congenital glaucoma. In Yankoff M, Duker JS, editors: *Ophthalmology*, ed 3, Maryland Heights, MO, 2008, Mosby. Chapter 10.21.

Braverman RS: Eye. In Hay WW, Levin MJ, Sondheimer JM, et al, editors: *Current pediatrics: diagnosis and treatment*, ed 19, New York, 2009, McGraw-Hill, Chapter 15.

Centers for Disease Control and Prevention (CDC): *Dear colleague letter, August 31*, 2009a. Available at www.cdc.gov/std/treatment/DCL-ErythromycinOintmentShortage-8-31-2009.pdf. Accessed Nov 6, 2010.

Centers for Disease Control and Prevention (CDC): *CDC guidance on shortage of erythromycin (0.5%) ophthalmic ointment*, 2009b. Available at www.cdc.gov/std/treatment/2006/erythromycinOintmentShortage.htm. Accessed Nov 6, 2010.

Crouch ER Jr, Crouch ER, Grant T: Ophthalmology. In Rakel RE, editor: *Textbook of family medicine*, Philadelphia, 2007, Saunders, p 1262.

Custer PL: Blepharoptosis. In Yankoff M, Duker JS, editors: *Ophthalmology*, ed 3, Maryland Heights, MO, 2008, Mosby, pp 1397–1403.

Dahan E: Pediatric cataract surgery. In Yankoff M, Duker JS, editors: *Ophthalmology*, ed 3, Maryland Heights, MO, 2008, Mosby, pp 479–483.

Daoud YJ, Hutchinson A, Wallace DK, et al: Refractive surgery in children: treatment options, outcomes, and controversies, *Am J Ophthalmol* 147(4):573–582, 2009.

Diamond GR: Sensory status in strabismus. In Yanoff M, Duker JS, editors: *Ophthalmology*, ed 3, Maryland Heights, MO, 2008, Mosby, pp 1323–1327.

Drenser KA, Capone A: Retinopathy of prematurity. In Yankoff M, Duker JS, editors: *Ophthalmology*, ed 3, Maryland Heights, MO, 2008, Mosby, pp 606–612.

Fecarotta CM, Kim M, Wasserman BN: Refractive surgery in children, *Curr Opin Ophthalmol* 21(5):350–355, 2010.

Frederick DR: Special subjects of pediatric interest. In Riordan-Eva P, Whitcher JP, editors: *Vaughan and Asbury's general ophthalmology*, ed 17, NY, 2008, Lange Medical Books/McGraw-Hill, Chapter 17.

Ganatra JB, Goldstein MH: Blepharitis. In Yankoff M, Duker JS, editors: *Ophthalmology*, ed 3, Maryland Heights, MO, 2008, Mosby, pp 219–221.

Grabowski E: Intraocular and extraocular retinoblastoma. In Burg FD, Ingelfinger JR, Polin RA, et al, editors: *Current pediatric therapy*, ed 18, Philadelphia, 2006, Saunders.

Hammerschlag M: Chlamydia trachomatis. In Kliegman RM, Behrman RE, Jenson HB, et al, editors: *Nelson textbook of pediatrics*, ed 18, Philadelphia, 2007, Saunders, pp 1285–1287.

Harper RA, Shock JP: Lens. In Riordan-Eva P, Whitcher JP, editors: *Vaughan and Asbury's general ophthalmology*, ed 17, New York, 2008, Lange Medical Books/McGraw-Hill, Chapter 8.

Haslam RHA: Neurologic evaluation. In Kliegman RM, Behrman RE, Jenson HB, et al, editors: *Nelson textbook of pediatrics*, ed 18, Philadelphia, 2007, Saunders, pp 2433–2443.

Hautala N, Koskela M, Hautala T: Major age group-specific differences in conjunctival bacteria and evolution of antimicrobial resistance revealed by laboratory data surveillance, *Curr Eye Res* 33(11):907–911, 2008.

Jacobs DS: *Conjunctivitis, UpToDate Online*, 2009. Available at www.uptodate.com/online/content/topic.do?topicKey=priophth/6879&selectedTitle=1~23&source=search_result#H22. Accessed Nov 2, 2010.

Jones L, Sinnott L, Chitkara M, et al: *Ohio State study: kids with contact lenses like their looks better than kids with glasses, The Ohio State University News Room*, 2009. Available at www.osu.edu/news/newsitem2365. Accessed Nov 6, 2010.

Jones-Jordan LA, Walline JJ, Mutti DO, et al: Gas permeable and soft contact lens wear in children, *Optom Vis Sci* 87(6):414–420, 2010.

Jun J, Bielory L, Raizman MB: Vernal conjunctivitis, *Immunol Allergy Clin North Am* 28(1):59–82, 2008.

Lanier AP, Holck P, Ehrsam Day G, et al: Childhood cancer among Alaska Natives, *Pediatrics* 112(5):e396–e403, 2003.

Li T, Shotton K: Conventional occlusion versus pharmacologic penalization for amblyopia, *Cochrane Database Syst Rev*(4):CD006460, 2009.

Listman DA: Paintball injuries in children: more than meets the eye, *Pediatrics* 113(1Pt1):e15–e18, 2004.

Meltzer JA, Kunkov S, Crain EF: Identifying children at low risk for bacterial conjunctivitis, *Arch Pediatr Adolesc Med* 164(3):263–267, 2010.

Mills M, Khazaeni L: Red eye. In Burg FD, Ingelfinger JR, Polin RA, et al, editors: *Current pediatric therapy*, ed 18, Philadelphia, 2006, Saunders.

Mills TJ: *Corneal ulceration and ulcerative keratitis*, 2009. Available at www.emedicine.medscape.com/article/798100. Accessed Nov 8, 2010.

Murphee AL, Christensen LE: Retinoblastoma and other malignant intraocular tumors. In Wright LB, Spiegel SE, editors: *Pediatric ophthalmology and strabismus*, New York, 2003, Springer.

Nageswaran S, Woods CR, Benjamin DK, et al: Orbital cellulitis in children, *Pediatr Infect Dis J* 25(8):695–699, 2006.

National Eye Institute: *Vision in preschool study (VIP study)*. Available at www.clinicaltrials.gov. Accessed Oct 25, 2010.

Neal CR, Engmann C: Retinopathy of prematurity. In Donn SM, editor: *The Michigan manual of neonatal intensive care*, ed 3, Philadelphia, 2003, Hanley & Belfus.

Neff AG, Carter KD: Benign eyelid lesions. In Yankoff M, Duker JS, editors: *Ophthalmology*, ed 3, Maryland Heights, MO, 2008, Mosby, pp 1422–1433.

Olitsky SE, Hug D, Smith LP: Disorders of the eye. In Kliegman RM, Behrman RE, Jenson HB, et al, editors: *Nelson textbook of pediatrics*, ed 18, Philadelphia, 2007, Saunders, pp 2569–2615.

Palay DA, Krachmer JH: *Primary care ophthalmology*, Philadelphia, 2005, Mosby.

Patel PB, Diaz MCG, Bennett J, et al: Clinical features of bacterial conjunctivitis in children, *Acad Emerg Med* 14(1):1–5, 2007.

Phelps DL: Retinopathy of prematurity. In Martin F, Fanaroff A, Walsh MC, editors: *Fanaroff and Martin's neonatal-perinatal medicine*, ed 9, Philadelphia, 2010, Mosby, pp 1764–1768.

Prevent Blindness America: *Our vision for children's vision: a national call to action for the advancement of children's vision and eye health*, 2008. Available at www.preventblindness.net/site/DocServer/08-045_OVFCV_small.pdf?docID=1601. Accessed Nov 8, 2010.

Quiros PA, Yee RD: Nystagmus, saccadic intrusions, and oscillations. In Yankoff M, Duker JS, editors: *Ophthalmology*, ed 3, Maryland Heights, MO, 2008, Mosby, pp 1040–1048.

Reynolds JD: Retinopathy of prematurity. In Nelson LB, Olitsky SE, editors: *Harley's pediatric ophthalmology*, ed 5, Philadelphia, 2005, Lippincott Williams & Wilkins.

Rodriguez-Galindo C, Wilson MW, Chantada G, et al: Retinoblastoma: one world, one vision, *Pediatrics* 122(3):e763–e770, 2008.

Rubenstein JB, Virasch V: Conjunctivitis: infectious and noninfectious. In Yankoff M, Duker JS, editors: *Ophthalmology*, ed 3, Maryland Heights, MO, 2008, Mosby, pp 227–236.

Scheiman MM, Hertle RW, Beck RW, et al: Randomized trial of treatment of amblyopia in children aged 7 to 17 years, *Arch Ophthalmol* 123(4):437–447, 2005.

Sharma R, Brunette DD: Ophthalmology. In Marx JA, Hockberger RS, Walls RM, et al, editors: *Rosen's emergency medicine: concepts and clinical practice*, Philadelphia, 2010, Mosby, p 860.

Shields JA, Shields CL: Ocular tumors of childhood. In Nelson LB, Olitsky SE, editors: *Harley's pediatric ophthalmology*, ed 5, Philadelphia, 2005, Lippincott Williams & Wilkins.

Smith AF, Waycaster C: Estimate of the direct and indirect annual cost of bacterial conjunctivitis in the United States, *BMC Ophthalmol* 9:13, 2009.

Teplin SW, Greeley J, Anthony TL: Blindness and visual impairment. In Carey WB, Crocker AC, Coleman WL, et al, editors: *Developmental-behavioral pediatrics*, ed 4, Philadelphia, 2009, Saunders, pp 698–716.

Tesser RA, Hess DB, Buckley EG: Pediatric cataracts and lens anomalies. In Nelson LB, Olitsky SE, editors: *Harley's pediatric ophthalmology*, ed 5, Philadelphia, 2005, Lippincott Williams & Wilkins.

Tomsak RL: Neuro-ophthalmology: afferent visual system. In Barkley WG, Daroff RB, Fenichel GM, et al, editors: *Neurology in clinical practice*, ed 5, Philadelphia, 2008, Butterworth-Heinemann, pp 730–737.

U.S. Department of Health and Human Services (USDHHS): *Healthy People 2020: Proposed HP2020 objectives: vision*, 2009. Available at www.healthypeople.gov/hp2020/Objectives/TopicArea.aspx?id=48&TopicArea=Vision. Accessed Oct 26, 2010.

U.S. Food and Drug Administration (FDA): *Focusing on contact lens safety*, 2008. Available at www.fda.gov/forconsumers/consumerupdates/ucm048893.htm#DecorativeContactLenses. Accessed Oct 30, 2010.

U.S. Food and Drug Administration (FDA): *Important information for laser pointer manufacturers*, 2009. Available at www.fda.gov/Radiation-EmittingProducts/RadiationEmittingProductsandProcedures/HomeBusinessandEntertainment/LaserProductsandInstruments/ucm116373.htm. Accessed Oct 30, 2010.

U.S. Preventive Services Task Force (USPSTF): Screening for visual impairment in children younger than age 5 years: recommendation statement. In *Guide to clinical preventive services*, ed 3, Rockville, MD, 2004, Agency for Healthcare Research and Quality. Available at www.ahrq.gov/clinic/3rduspstf/vision scr/vischrs.htm. Accessed Oct 25, 2010.

Wagner RS, D'Arienzo PA, Dorfman MS: Conjunctivitis in children: challenges and choices. *Healthcare solutions: Monthly prescribing reference monograph*, August 2010, Alcon Laboratories.

Wald ER: Periorbital and orbital infections, *Infect Dis Clin North Am* 21(2):393–408, 2007.

Wald ER: Periorbital and orbital infection. In Long SS, Pickering LK, Prober CG, editors: *Principles and practice of pediatric infectious diseases*, Philadelphia, 2008, Churchill Livingstone, pp 511–516.

Walton RC: *Uveitis, anterior, childhood*, 2010. Available at www.emedicine.medscape.com/article/1209403-overview. Accessed Nov 8, 2010.

Weaver CNM, Rosen CL: *Burns, ocular*, 2010. Available at www.emedicine.medscape.com/article/798696-overview. Accessed Nov 8, 2010.

Weichel ED, Vander JF, Tasman W, et al: Diseases of the retina and vitreous. In Nelson LB, Olitsky SE, editors: *Harley's pediatric ophthalmology*, ed 5, Philadelphia, 2005, Lippincott Williams & Wilkins.

Weiss AH: Uveitis, retinitis, and chorioretinitis. In Long SS, editor: *Principles and practice of pediatric infectious diseases*, ed 3, Philadelphia, 2008, Elsevier, pp 504–508.

Wilson MW, Haik BG, Karcioglu ZA, et al: Pediatric conjunctival tumors. In Wright KW, Spiegel PH, editors: *Pediatric ophthalmology and strabismus*, Philadelphia, 2003, Springer.

Wright KW: Pediatric ocular trauma. In Wright KW, Spiegel PH, editors: *Pediatric ophthalmology and strabismus*, New York, 2003, Springer.

Wyrsch S, Baenninger PB, Schmid MK: Retinal injuries from a handheld laser pointer, *N Engl J Med* 363(11):1089–1091, 2010.

Zhou Y, Huang C, Xu P, et al: Perceptual learning improves contrast sensitivity and visual acuity in adults with anisometropic amblyopia, *Vision Res* 46(5):739–750, 2006.

CHAPTER 29

American Academy of Pediatrics (AAP): American Academy of Family Physicians: Clinical practice guideline: diagnosis and management of acute otitis media, *Pediatrics* 113(5):1451–1465, 2004a.

American Academy of Pediatrics (AAP): Clinical practice guideline: otitis media with effusion, *Pediatrics* 113(5):1413–1429, 2004b.

Bakaletz LO: Bacterial biofilms in otitis media: evidence and relevance, *Pediatr Infect Dis J* 26(10):S17–S19, 2007.

Browning GG, Rovers MM, Williamson I, et al: Grommets (ventilation tubes) for hearing loss associated with otitis media with effusion in children, *Cochrane Database Syst Rev*(10): CD001801, 2010.

Casey JR, Aldowitz DG, Pichichero ME: New patterns in the otopathogens causing acute otitis media six to eight years after introduction of pneumococcal conjugate vaccine, *Pediatr Infect Dis J* 29(4):304–309, 2010.

Casey JR, Pichichero ME: Changes in frequency and pathogens causing acute otitis media in 1995-2003, *Pediatric Infect Dis J* 23(9):824–828, 2004.

Centers for Disease Control and Prevention (CDC): Announcement: better hearing and speech month, *MMWR Morb Mort Wkly Rep* 59(18):561, 2010.

Clegg AJ, Loveman E, Gospodarevskaya E, et al: The safety and effectiveness of different methods of ear wax removal: a systematic review and economic evaluation, *Health Technol Assess* 14(28):1–192, 2010.

Coco A, Vernacchio L, Horst M, et al: Management of acute otitis media after publication of the 2004 AAP and AAFP Clinical Practice Guideline, *Pediatrics* 125(2):214–220, 2010.

Coker TR, Chan LS, Newberry SJ, et al: Diagnosis, microbial epidemiology, and antibiotic treatment of acute otitis media in children: a systematic review, *JAMA* 304(19):2161–2169, 2010.

Daly KA, Hoffman HJ, Kvaerner KJ, et al: Epidemiology, natural history, and risk factors: panel report from the Ninth International Conference on Otitis Media, *Int J Pediatr Otorhinolaryngol* 74(3):231–240, 2010.

Dowell SF, Marcy SM, Phillips WR, et al: Otitis media—principles of judicious use of antimicrobial agents, *Pediatrics* 101(Suppl 1):165–171, 1998.

Dwivedi RC, Dwivedi RC, Bhatia N, et al: Low cost dual-action aural foreign-body extractor, *Laryngoscope* 119(2):351–354, 2009.

Gifford KA, Holmes MG, Bernstein HH: Hearing loss in children, *Pediatrics in Review* 30(6):207–216, 2009.

Goodrich T, Rubio F, Cutler JL: Otitis media and antihistamines, *Curr Allergy Asthma Rep* 9(6):456–459, 2009.

Gould JM, Matz PS: Otitis media, *Pediatr Rev* 31(3):102–116, 2010.

Granath A, Rynnel-Dagöö B, Backheden M, et al: Tube associated otorrhea in children with recurrent acute otitis media: results of a prospective randomized study on bacteriology and topical treatment with or without systematic antibiotics, *Int J Pediatr Otorhinolaryngol* 72(8):1225–1233, 2008.

Gregg R, Au DL, Wiorek M, et al: Pediatric audiology: a review, *Pediatr Rev* 25(7):224–233, 2004.

Haddad J: Ear. In Kliegman RM, Behrman RE, Jenson HB, et al, editors: *Nelson textbook of pediatrics*, ed 18, Philadelphia, 2007, Saunders, pp 2617–2649.

Hagan JF, Shaw JS, Duncan PS, editors: *Bright futures: guidelines for health supervision for infants, children, and adolescents*, ed 3, Elk Grove, IL, 2008, American Academy of Pediatrics.

Hall-Stoodley L, Hu FZ, Gieseke A, et al: Direct detection of bacterial biofilms on the middle-ear mucosa of children with chronic otitis media, *JAMA* 296(2):202–211, 2006.

Harlor AD, Bower C: Committee on Practice and Ambulatory Medicine and the Section on Otolaryngology Head and Neck Surgery: Hearing assessment in infants and children: recommendations beyond neonatal screening, *Pediatrics* 124(4):1252–1263, 2009.

Heim SW, Maughan KL: Foreign bodies in the ear, nose, and throat, *Am Fam Physician* 76(8):1185–1189, 2007.

Ho D, Rotenberg BW, Berkowitz RG: The relationship between acute mastoiditis and antibiotic use for acute otitis media in children, *Arch Otolaryngol Head Neck Surg* 134(1):45–48, 2008.

Joint Committee on Infant Hearing: Year 2007 position statement: principles and guidelines for early hearing detection and intervention programs, *Pediatrics* 120(4):898–921, 2007.

Kaushik V, Malik T, Saeed S: Interventions for otitis externa, *Cochrane Database Syst Rev*(1):CD004740, 2010.

Kershner JE: Otitis media. In Kliegman RM, Behrman RE, Jenson HB, et al, editors: *Nelson textbook of pediatrics*, ed 18, Philadelphia, 2007, Saunders, pp 2617–2649.

Laury AM, Casey S, McKay S, et al: Etiology of unilateral neural hearing loss in children, *Int J Pediatr Otorhinolaryngol* 73:417–427, 2009.

Lieu JEC, Tye-Murray N, Karzon RK, et al: Unilateral hearing loss is associated with worse speech-language scores in children, *Pediatrics* 125(6):e1348–e1355, 2010.

Marchisio P, Bellussi L, DiMauro G, et al: Acute otits media: from diagnosis to prevention: summary of the Italian guideline, *Int J Pediatr Otolaryngol* 74:1209–1216, 2010.

Marchisio P, Esposito S, Bianchini S, et al: Efficacy of injectable trivalent virosomal-adjuvanted inactive influenza vaccine in preventing acute otitis media in children with recurrent or noncomplicated acute otitis media, *Pediatr Infect Dis J* 28(10):855–859, 2009.

McCormick DP, Chandler SM, Chonmaitree T: Laterality of acute otitis media: different clinical and microbiologic characteristics, *Pediatr Infect Dis J* 26:583–588, 2007.

Mehra S, Eavey RD, Keamy DG Jr: The epidemiology of hearing impairment in the United States: newborns, children, and adolescents, *Otolaryngol Head Neck Surg* 140(4):461–472, 2009.

Moody SA, Strasnick B: *Inner ear, genetic sensorineural hearing loss*, 2010. Available at http://emedicine.medscape.com/article1855875. Accessed Oct 23, 2010.

National Institute on Deafness and other Communication Disorders: *Healthy People 2010 hearing health programs review*, 2004. Available at www.nidcd.nih.gov/health/heatlhyhearing. Accessed Oct 11, 2010.

Nelson HD, Bougatsos C, Nygren P: Universal newborn hearing screening: systematic review to update the 2001 US Preventive Services Task Force recommendation, *Pediatrics* 122:e266–e276, 2008.

O'Brien MA, Prosser LA, Paradise JL, et al: New vaccines against otitis media: projected benefits and cost-effectiveness, *Pediatrics* 123(6):1452–1463, 2009.

Ologe FE, Dunmade AD, Afolabi OA: Aural foreign bodies in children, *Indian J Pediatr* 74(8):755–758, 2007.

Paradise JL, Feldman HM, Campbell TF, et al: Tympanostomy tubes and developmental outcomes at 9 to 11 years of age, *N Engl J Med* 356(3):248–261, 2007.

Pelton SI, Leibovitz E: Recent advances in otitis media, *Pediatr Infect Dis J* 28(10):S133–S137, 2009.

Roland PS, Smith TL, Schwartz SR, et al: Clinical practice guideline: cerumen impaction, *Otolaryngol Head Neck Surg* 139(3 Suppl 2):S1–S21, 2008.

Sabirov A, Casey JR, Murphy TF, et al: Breastfeeding is associated with a reduced frequency of acute otitis media and high serum antibody levels against NTHi and outer membrane protein vaccine antigen candidate P6, *Pediatr Res* 66(5):565–570, 2009.

Schmelzle J, Birtwhistle R, Andre K: Acute otitis media with tympanostomy tubes, *Can Fam Physician* 54:1123–1127, 2008.

Shafi M, Yousufani AH, Hussain SI: Foreign bodies in external auditory canals: experience of 653 cases over 8 years, *JLUMHS* 9(2):70–75, 2010.

Shaikh N, Havey K, Paradise JL, et al: The Cochrane library and acute otitis media in children: an overview of reviews, *Evidence-Based Child Health: A Cochrane Review Journal* 4(2):390–399, 2009.

Shaikh N, Hoberman A, Kaleida PH, et al: Diagnosing otitis media: otoscopy and cerumen removal, *N Engl J Med* 362(20):e62–e64, 2010.

Siegel RM: Acute otitis media guidelines, antibiotic use, and shared decision-making, *Pediatrics* 125(2):384–386, 2010.

Spektor Z: AOE: predisposing factors and pathogens, *Infect Dis Child*, June 2010. Monograph, 3–6.

Spielmann PM, McKee H, Adamson RM, et al: Follow up after middle-ear ventilation tube insertion: what is needed and when? *J Laryngol Otol* 122(6):580–583, 2008.

Spilsbury K, Miller I, Semmens JB, et al: Factors associated with developing cholesteatoma: a study of 45,980 children with middle ear disease, *Laryngoscope* 120(3):625–630, 2010.

Tonnaer ELGM, Graamans K, Sanders EAM, et al: Advances in understanding the pathogenesis of pneumococcal otitis media, *Pediatr Infect Dis J* 25(6):546–552, 2006.

U.S. Preventive Services Task Force (USPSTF): Universal screening for hearing loss in newborns: US Preventive Task Force recommendation statement, *Pediatrics* 122(1):143, 2008.

Vergison A, Dagan R, Arguedas A, et al: Otitis media and its consequences: beyond the earache, *Lancet* 10:195–203, 2010.

Vernacchio L, Vezina R, Mitchell A: Tolerability of oral xylitol solution in young children: Implications for otitis media prophylaxis, *Int J Pediatr Otolaryngol* 71(1):89–94, 2006.

Vernacchio L, Vezina R, Mitchell A: Management of acute otitis media by primary care physicians: trends since the release of the 2004 American Academy of Pediatrics/American Academy of Family Physicians Clinical Practice Guideline, *Pediatrics* 120(2):281–287, 2007.

Wall GM, Stroman DW, Roland PS, et al: Ciprofloxacin 0.3%/dexamethasone 0.1% sterile otic suspension for the topical treatment of ear infections, *Pediatr Infect Dis J* 28(2):141–144, 2009.

Wang MC, Liu CY, Shiao AS: Water penetration into the middle ear through ventilation tubes in children while surface diving, *J Chinese Med Assoc* 72(2):72–75, 2009.

Williamson I, Benge S, Barton S, et al: Topical intranasal corticosteroids in 4-11 year old children with persistent bilateral otitis media with effusion in primary care: double blind randomized placebo controlled trial, *BMJ* 339:b4984, 2009.

Younis RT: Proper diagnosis essential for treatment of AOE, *Infect Dis Child Monograph*, 7–9, June 2010.

CHAPTER 30

Aboulhosn J, Child J: Congenital heart disease in adults. In Fuster V, O'Rourke RA, Walsh RA, et al, editors: *Hurst's the heart*, ed 12, New York, 2008, McGraw-Hill.

Allen H, Phillips JR, Chan DP: History and physical examination. In Allen HD, Driscoll DJ, Shaddy RE, et al, editors: *Moss and Adams' heart disease in infants, children, and adolescents, including the fetus and young adult*, ed 7, Philadelphia, 2008, Lippincott Williams & Wilkins.

Alexander ME: Syncope. In Burg FD, Polin RA, Gershon AA, et al, editors: *Current pediatric therapy*, ed 18, Philadelphia, 2006, Saunders.

American Academy of Pediatrics (AAP): *2009 Red Book: report of the Committee on Infectious Diseases*, ed 28, Elk Grove Village, IL, 2009, American Academy of Pediatrics.

Beekman R: Coarctation of the aorta. In Allen HD, Driscoll DJ, Shaddy RE, et al, editors: *Moss and Adams' heart disease in infants, children, and adolescents, including the fetus and young adult*, ed 7, Philadelphia, 2008, Lippincott Williams & Wilkins.

Botto LD, Goldmuntz E, Lin AE: Epidemiology and prevention of congenital heart defects. In Allen HD, Driscoll DJ, Shaddy RE, et al, editors: *Moss and Adams' heart disease in infants, children, and adolescents, including the fetus and young adult*, ed 7, Philadelphia, 2008, Lippincott Williams & Wilkins.

Cetta F, Minich L, Edwards WD, et al: Atrioventricular septal defects. In Allen HD, Driscoll DJ, Shaddy RE, et al, editors: *Moss and Adams' heart disease in infants, children, and adolescents, including the fetus and young adult*, ed 7, Philadelphia, 2008, Lippincott Williams & Wilkins.

Doniger SJ, Sharieff GO: Pediatric dysrhythmias, *Pediatr Clin North Am* 53(1):85–105, 2006.

Driscoll DJ: Chest pain in children and adolescents. In Allen HD, Driscoll DJ, Shaddy RE, et al, editors: *Moss and Adams' heart disease in infants, children, and adolescents, including the fetus and young adult*, ed 7, Philadelphia, 2008, Lippincott Williams & Wilkins.

Enright P, Goodwin J, Sherrill D, et al: Blood pressure elevation associated with sleep-related breathing disorder in a community sample of white and Hispanic children, *Arch Pediatr Adolesc Med* 157:901–904, 2003.

Epstein ML: Tricuspid atresia, stenosis and regurgitation. In Allen HD, Driscoll DJ, Shaddy RE, et al, editors: *Moss and Adams' heart disease in infants, children, and adolescents, including the fetus and young adult*, ed 7, Philadelphia, 2008, Lippincott Williams & Wilkins.

Fukazawa R, Ogawa S: Long-term prognosis of patients with Kawasaki disease: at risk for future atherosclerosis? *J Nippon Med Sch* 76:124–133, 2009.

Flynn J: Pediatric hypertension: Recent trends and accomplishments, future challenges, *Am J Hypertens* 21:605–612, 2008.

Goldmuntz E, Lin A: The genetics of congenital heart defects. In Allen HD, Driscoll DJ, Shaddy RE, et al, editors: *Moss and Adams' heart disease in infants, children, and adolescents, including the fetus and young adult*, ed 7, Philadelphia, 2008, Lippincott Williams & Wilkins.

Grinsell M, Norwood V: At the bottom of the differential diagnosis list: unusual causes of pediatric hypertension, *Pediatr Nephrol* 24:2137–2146, 2009.

Hansen M, Gunn P, Kaelber D: Underdiagnosis of hypertension in children and adolescents, *JAMA* 298:874–879, 2007.

Harmon WG, Sleeper LA, Cuniberti L, et al: Treating children with idiopathic dilated cardiomyopathy (from the Pediatric Cardiomyopathy Registry), *Am J Cardiol* 104(2):281–286, 2009.

Hsu D, Pearson G: Heart failure in children part I: history, etiology and pathophysiology, *Circ Heart Failure* 2:63–70, 2009a.

Hsu D, Pearson G: Heart failure in children part II: diagnosis, treatment and future directions, *Circ Heart Failure* 2:490–498, 2009b.

Johnston MV: Conditions that mimic seizures. In Kliegman RM, Behrman RE, Jenson HB, et al, editors: *Nelson textbook of pediatrics*, ed 18, Philadelphia, 2007, Saunders.

Kleinman CS, Glickstein JS, Shaw R: Fetal echocardiography and fetal cardiology. In Allen HD, Driscoll DJ, Shaddy RE, et al, editors: *Moss and Adams' heart disease in infants, children, and adolescents, including the fetus and young adult*, ed 7, Philadelphia, 2008, Lippincott Williams & Wilkins.

Latal B, Helfricht S, Fischer JE, et al: Psychological adjustment and quality of life in children and adolescents following open-heart surgery for congenital heart disease: a systematic review, *BMC Pediatrics* 9:6, 2009.

Mahle WT, Newberger JW, Matherne GP, et al: Role of pulse oximetry in examining newborns for congenital heart disease: a scientific statement from the AHA and AAP, *Pediatrics* 124(2):823–834, 2009.

Majnemer A, Limeropoulos C, Shevell M, et al: Developmental and functional outcomes at school entry in children with congenital heart defects, *J Pediatr* 153:55–60, 2008.

Maron B, Zipes D, Ackerman M, et al: 36th Bethesda Conference: eligibility recommendations for competitive athletes with cardiovascular abnormalities, *J Am Coll Cardiol* 45(8):1313–1377, 2005.

Maron B, Doerer J, Haas T, et al: Sudden deaths in young competitive athletes. Analysis of 1866 deaths in the United States, 1980-2006, *Circulation* 119:1085–1092, 2009.

McCormack J: The role of genetic testing in paediatric syndromes of sudden death: state of the art and future considerations, *Cardiol Young* 19(Suppl 2):54–65, 2009.

McDaniel NL, Gutgesell HP: Ventricular septal defects. In Allen HD, Driscoll DJ, Shaddy RE, et al, editors: *Moss and Adams' heart disease in infants, children, and adolescents, including the fetus and young adult*, ed 7, Philadelphia, 2008, Lippincott Williams & Wilkins.

Miller S, McQuillen P, Hamrick S, et al: Abnormal brain development in newborns with congenital heart disease, *N Engl J Med* 357:1928–1938, 2007.

Moore P, Brook MM, Heymann MA: Patent ductus arteriosus and aortopulmonary window. In Allen HD, Driscoll DJ, Shaddy RE, et al, editors: *Moss and Adams' heart disease in infants, children, and adolescents, including the fetus and young adult*, ed 7, Philadelphia, 2008, Lippincott Williams & Wilkins.

National Institutes of Health, National High Blood Pressure Education Program Working Group on High Blood Pressure in Children and Adolescents (NIH-NHBPEP): The fourth report on the diagnosis, evaluation, and treatment of high blood pressure in children and adolescents, *Pediatrics* 114:555–576, 2004.

Newburger J, Takahashi M, Gerber M, et al: Diagnosis, treatment and long-term management of Kawasaki diseases: a statement for health professionals from the committee on rheumatic fever, endocarditis, and Kawasaki disease, council on cardiovascular disease in the young, American Heart Association, *Pediatrics* 114:1708–1733, 2004.

Newburger JW, Alexander ME, Fulton DR: Innocent murmurs, syncope, and chest pain. In Keane JF, Lock JE, Fyler DC, editors: *Nadas' pediatric cardiology*, ed 2, Philadelphia, 2006, Saunders.

Nishimura RA, Carabello BA, Faxon DP, et al: ACC/AHA 2008 guideline update on valvular heart disease: focused update on infective endocarditis. A report of the American College of Cardiology/American Heart Association task force on practice guidelines: endorsed by the Society of Cardiovascular Anesthesiologists, Society for Cardiovascular Angiography and Interventions, and Society of Thoracic Surgeons, *Circulation* 118:887–896, 2008.

Park MK: *Pediatric cardiology for practitioners*, ed 5, Philadelphia, 2008, Mosby.

Pereira BA, da Silva NA, Andrade LE, et al: Jones criteria and underdiagnosis of rheumatic fever, *Indian J Pediatr* 74:117–121, 2007.

Pierpont ME, Basson CT, Benson DW, et al: Genetic basis for congenital heart defects: current knowledge, *Circulation* 115:3015–3038, 2007.

Porter CJ, Edwards WD: Atrial septal defects. In Allen HD, Driscoll DJ, Shaddy RE, et al, editors: *Moss and Adams' heart disease in infants, children, and adolescents, including the fetus and young adult*, ed 7, Philadelphia, 2008, Lippincott Williams & Wilkins.

Prieto LR, Latson LA: Pulmonary stenosis. In Allen HD, Driscoll DJ, Shaddy RE, et al, editors: *Moss and Adams' heart disease in infants, children, and adolescents, including the fetus and young adult*, ed 7, Philadelphia, 2008, Lippincott Williams & Wilkins.

Rheuban KS: Pericardial diseases. In Allen HD, Driscoll DJ, Shaddy RE, et al, editors: *Moss and Adams' heart disease in infants, children, and adolescents, including the fetus and young adult*, ed 7, Philadelphia, 2008, Lippincott Williams & Wilkins.

Schneider DJ, Moore JW: Aortic stenosis. In Allen HD, Driscoll DJ, Shaddy RE, et al, editors: *Moss and Adams' heart disease in infants, children, and adolescents, including the fetus and young adult*, ed 7, Philadelphia, 2008, Lippincott Williams & Wilkins.

Siwek ES, Erenberg FG, Zahka KG: Tetralogy of Fallot. In Allen HD, Driscoll DJ, Shaddy RE, et al, editors: *Moss and Adams' heart disease in infants, children, and adolescents, including the fetus and young adult*, ed 7, Philadelphia, 2008, Lippincott Williams & Wilkins.

Sondheimer HM, Darst JR, Shaffer EM, et al: Cardiovascular diseases: syncope. In Hay W, Levin M, Deterding R, et al, editors: *Current diagnosis and treatment pediatrics*, ed 19, Chicago, 2009, McGraw-Hill.

Steelman R, Rosen DA, Nelson ER, et al: Gingival colonization with selective HACEK microbes in children with congenital heart disease, *Clin Oral Invest* 7(1):38–40, 2003.

Taubert KA, Gewetz M: Infective endocarditis. In Allen HD, Driscoll DJ, Shaddy RE, et al, editors: *Moss and Adams' heart disease in infants, children, and adolescents, including the fetus and young adult*, ed 7, Philadelphia, 2008, Lippincott Williams & Wilkins.

Tierney E, Newberger J: Are patients with KD at increased risk for premature atherosclerosis? *J Pediatr* 151:225–228, 2007.

Towbin JA: Myocarditis. In Allen HD, Driscoll DJ, Shaddy RE, et al: *Moss and Adams' heart disease in infants, children, and adolescents, including the fetus and young adult*, ed 7, Philadelphia, 2008, Lippincott Williams & Wilkins.

Tweddell JS, Hoffman GM, Ghanayem NS, et al: Hypoplastic left heart syndrome. In Allen HD, Driscoll DJ, Shaddy RE, et al, editors: *Moss and Adams' heart disease in infants, children, and adolescents, including the fetus and young adult*, ed 7, Philadelphia, 2008, Lippincott Williams & Wilkins.

Wiesen J, Adkins M, Fortune S, et al: Evaluation of pediatric patients with mild-to-moderate hypertension: yield of diagnostic testing, *Pediatrics* 122:e988–e993, 2008.

Wernovsky G: Transposition of the great arteries. In Allen HD, Driscoll DJ, Shaddy RE, et al, editors: *Moss and Adams' heart disease in infants, children, and adolescents, including the fetus and young adult*, ed 7, Philadelphia, 2008, Lippincott Williams & Wilkins.

Wood LE, Tulloh RM: Kawasaki disease in children, *Heart* 95:787–792, 2009.

World Health Organization: *Rheumatic Fever and Rheumatic Heart Disease: Report of a WHO Expert Consultation, 2001*. Technical Report Series 923, 2004. Available at www.who.int/cardiovascular_diseases/resources/trs923/en/. Accessed July 22, 2010.

Yani L: Rheumatic fever and rheumatic heart disease. In Allen HD, Driscoll DJ, Shaddy RE, et al, editors: *Moss and Adams' heart disease in infants, children, and adolescents, including the fetus and young adult*, ed 7, Philadelphia, 2008, Lippincott Williams & Wilkins.

CHAPTER 31

Alberta Clinical Practice Guidelines Working Group: *Guidelines for diagnosis and management of croup, 2003*. Alberta, ON, Canada. Available at www.albertadoctors.org/bcm/ama/ama-website.nsf/. Accessed Dec 20, 2011.

American Academy of Pediatrics (AAP): Summaries of infectious diseases. In Pickering LK, Baker CJ, Kimberlin DW, et al, editors: *Red Book: 2009 report of the committee on infectious diseases*, ed 28, Elk Grove Village, IL, 2009, American Academy of Pediatrics.

American Academy of Pediatrics Subcommittee on Diagnosis and Management of Bronchitis (AAPB): Diagnosis and management of bronchiolitis, *Pediatrics* 118:1774–1793, 2006.

American Academy of Pediatrics Subcommittee on Management of Sinusitis and the Committee on Quality Improvement: Clinical practice guidelines: management of sinusitis, *Pediatrics* 108:798–808, 2001.

Bell AT, Fortune B: What test is the best for diagnosing infectious mononucleosis? *J Fam Pract* 55(9):799–802, 2006.

Bjornson C, Johnson D: Croup, *Lancet* 371:329–339, 2008.

Boyer K: Nonbacterial pneumonia. In Cherry J, Kaplan S, Demmler-Harrison G, et al, editors: *Feigin & Cherry's textbook of pediatric infectious diseases*, ed 6, Philadelphia, 2010, Saunders, pp 288–302.

Braman S: Chronic cough due to acute bronchitis, *Chest* 129:S95–S103, 2006.

British Thoracic Society Standards of Care Committee: British Thoracic Society guidelines for the management of community acquired pneumonia in childhood, *Thorax* 57(Suppl 1):i1–i24, 2002.

Brook I: Chronic sinusitis in children, *Pediatr Ann* 39(1):41–47, 2010.

Bukutu C, Le C, Vohra S: Complementary, holistic, and integrative medicine: the common cold, *Pediatr Rev* 29:e66–e71, 2008.

Burton MJ, Glasziou PP: Tonsillectomy or adeno-tonsillectomy versus non-surgical treatment for chronic/recurrent acute tonsillitis, *Cochrane Database Syst Rev*(1):CD001802, 2009.

Bush A: Recurrent respiratory infections, *Pediatr Clin North Am* 56:67–100, 2009.

Carter ER, Marshall SG: The respiratory system. In Marcdante KJ, Kliegman RM, Jenson HB, et al, editors: *Nelson essentials of pediatrics*, ed 6, Philadelphia, 2011, Saunders.

Centers for Disease Control and Prevention (CDC): Revised product labels for pediatric over-the-counter cough and cold medicines, *MMWR Morb Mort Wkly Rep* 57(43):1180, 2008.

Chang AB: Cough, *Pediatr Clin N Am* 56:19–31, 2009.

Cherry JD: Croup, *New England J of Med* 358(4):384–391, 2008.

Cherry JD: Pharyngitis (pharyngitis, tonsillitis, tonsillopharyngitis, and nasopharyngitis). In Cherry J, Kaplan S, Demmler-Harrison G, et al, editors: *Feigin & Cherry's textbook of pediatric infectious diseases*, ed 6, Philadelphia, 2010a, Saunders, pp 160–168.

Cherry JD: Croup (laryngitis, laryngotracheitis, spasmodic croup, laryngotracheobronchitis, bacterial tracheitis, and laryngotracheobronchopneumonitis). In Cherry J, Kaplan S, Demmler-Harrison G, et al, editors: *Feigin & Cherry's textbook of pediatric infectious diseases*, ed 6, Philadelphia, 2010b, Saunders, pp 254–268.

Cherry JD: Epiglottitis. In Cherry J, Kaplan S, Demmler-Harrison G, et al, editors: *Feigin & Cherry's textbook of pediatric infectious diseases*, ed 6, Philadelphia, 2010c, Saunders, pp 244–254.

Cherry JD: Acute bronchitis. In Cherry J, Kaplan S, Demmler-Harrison G, et al, editors: *Feigin & Cherry's textbook of pediatric infectious diseases*, ed 6, Philadelphia, 2010d, Saunders, pp 269–277.

Cherry JD, Heininger U: Pertussis and other *Bordetella* infections. In Cherry J, Kaplan S, Demmler-Harrison G, et al, editors: *Feigin & Cherry's textbook of pediatric infectious diseases*, ed 6, Philadelphia, 2010, Saunders, pp 1683–1706.

Cherry JD, Nieves D: The common cold. In Cherry J, Kaplan S, Demmler-Harrison G, et al, editors: *Feigin & Cherry's textbook of pediatric infectious diseases*, ed 6, Philadelphia, 2010, Saunders.

Cherry JD, Shapiro NL: Rhinosinusitis. In Cherry J, Kaplan S, Demmler-Harrison G, et al, editors: *Feigin & Cherry's textbook of pediatric infectious diseases*, ed 6, Philadelphia, 2010, Saunders.

Chin ES: Pediatric reactive airway disease: treatment & medication, *eMedicine*, 2010. Available at http://emedicine.medscape.com/article/800119-overview. Accessed Sep 7, 2010.

Christ-Crain M, Opal SM: Clinical review: the role of biomarkers in the diagnosis and management of community acquired pneumonia, *Crit Care* 14:203, 2010.

Congeni B: Antibiotic susceptibility, *Pediatr Rev* 30:499–501, 2009.

DeMuri G, Wald ER: Sinusitis: clinical manifestations and treatment approaches, *Pediatr Ann* 39(1):34–40, 2010.

Everard M: Acute bronchiolitis and croup, *Pediatr Clin North Am* 56:119–133, 2009.

Garavello W, Romagnoli M, Gaini RM: Effectiveness of adenotonsillectomy in PFAPA syndrome: a randomized study, *J Pediatr* 155(2):250–253, 2009.

Gerber M, Baltimore R, Eaton C, et al: Prevention of rheumatic fever and diagnosis and treatment of acute streptococcal pharyngitis: a scientific statement from the American Heart Association Rheumatic Fever, Endocarditis, and Kawasaki Disease Committee of the Council on Cardiovascular Disease in the Young, the Interdisciplinary Council on Functional Genomics and Translational Biology, and the Interdisciplinary Council on Quality of Care and Outcomes Research, *Circulation* 119:1541–1551, 2009.

Gifford TO, Orlandi RR: Epistaxis, *Otolaryngol Clin North Am* 41(3):525–536, 2009.

Gokhale J, Selbst S: Chest pain and chest wall deformity, *Pediatr Clin North Am* 56:49–65, 2009.

Guinto-Ocampo H, McNeil BK: Pertussis, *eMedicine*, 2010. Available at http://emedicine.medscape.com/article/967268-overview. Accessed Sep 24, 2010.

Haddad J: Acquired disorders of the nose. In Kliegman RM, Behrman RE, Jenson HB, et al, editors: *Nelson textbook of pediatrics*, ed 18, Philadelphia, 2007, Saunders.

Hanson IC, Shearer W: Chronic bronchitis. In Cherry J, Kaplan S, Demmler-Harrison G, et al, editors: *Feigin & Cherry's textbook of pediatric infectious diseases*, ed 6, Philadelphia, 2010, Saunders, pp 272–277.

Hwang P: A 51 year old woman with acute onset of facial pressure, rhinorrhea, and tooth pain: Review of acute rhinosinusitis, *JAMA* 301(17):1798–1807, 2009.

Klein J: Bacterial pneumonias. In Cherry J, Demmler-Harrison G, Kaplan S, editors: *Feigin & Cherry's textbook of pediatric infectious diseases*, ed 6, Philadelphia, 2010, Saunders, pp 302–314.

Kubba H: Childhood epistaxis, *Clin Otolaryngol* 31:212–213, 2006.

Kumar P, McKean MS: Evidence based paediatrics: review of BTS guidelines for the management of community acquired pneumonia in children, *J Infect* 48(2):134–138, 2004.

Licameli G, Jeffrey J, Luz J: Effect of adenotonsillectomy in PFAPA syndrome, *Arch Otolaryngol Head Neck Surg* 134(2):136–140, 2008.

Linde K, Barrett B, Bauer R, et al: Echinacea for preventing and treating the common cold, *Cochrane Database Syst Rev*(1):CD000530, 2006.

Loughran S, Spinou E, Clement W, et al: A prospective, single-blind, randomized controlled trial of petroleum jelly (Vaseline) for recurrent paediatric epistaxis, *Clin Otolaryngol* 29:266–269, 2004.

Manes RP: Evaluating and managing the patient with nosebleeds, *Med Clin North Am* 94:903–912, 2010.

Martin JM: Pharyngitis and streptococcal throat infections, *Pediatr Ann* 39(1):22–27, 2010.

Mellis C: Respiratory noises: how useful are they clinically? *Pediatr Clin North Am* 56:1–17, 2009.

Moore M, Little P: Humidified air inhalation for treating croup, *Cochrane Database Syst Rev* 3:CD002870, 2006.

Morer A, Viñas O, Lázaro L, et al: Antineuronal antibodies in a group of children with obsessive-compulsive disorder and Tourette syndrome, *J Psychiatr Res* 42(1):64–68, 2006.

Morris P: Upper respiratory tract infections (including otitis media), *Pediatr Clin North Am* 56:101–117, 2009.

O'Sullivan B, Freedman SD: Cystic fibrosis, *Lancet* 373:1891–1904, 2009.

Paul IM, Beiler J, McMonagle A, et al: Effect of honey, dextromethorphan, and no treatment on nocturnal cough and sleep quality for coughing children and their parents, *Arch Pediatr Adolesc Med* 161:1140–1145, 2007.

Pearlman A, Conley D: Review of current guidelines related to the diagnosis and treatment of rhinosinusitis, *Curr Opin Otolaryngol Head Neck Surg* 16:226–230, 2008.

Powell KR: *Pediatric infectious diseases: volume 1*, Elk Grove Village, IL, 2007, American Academy of Pediatrics.

Ranganathan S, Sonnappa S: Pneumonia and other respiratory infection, *Pediatr Clin North Am* 56:135–156, 2009.

Ratjen F: Cystic fibrosis: pathogenesis and future treatments, *Respir Care* 54(5):595–605, 2009.

Robinson PD, Van Asperen P: Asthma in childhood, *Pediatr Clin North Am* 56(1):191–226, 2009.

Russell K, Wiebe N, Saenz A, et al: Glucocorticosteroids for croup, *Cochrane Database Syst Rev* 4:CD001955, 2004.

Saiman L, Hiatt P: Cystic fibrosis. In Cherry J, Kaplan S, Demmler-Harrison G, et al, editors: *Feigin & Cherry's textbook of pediatric infectious diseases*, ed 6, Philadelphia, 2010, Saunders, pp 342–364.

Sarnaik AP, Heidemann SM: Respiratory system. In Kliegman RE, Behrman RE, Jenson HB, et al, editors: *Nelson textbook of pediatrics*, ed 18, Philadelphia, 2007, Saunders.

Schechter MS, Section on Pediatric Pulmonology Subcommittee on Obstructive Sleep Apnea Syndrome: Technical report: diagnosis and management of childhood obstructive sleep apnea syndrome, *Pediatrics* 109(4):e69, 2002.

Schlosser R: Epistaxis, *N Engl J Med* 360(8):784–789, 2009.

Scottish Intercollegiate Guidelines Network (SIGN): *Bronchiolitis in children*. Available at www.sign.ac.uk. Accessed Jan 17, 2010.

See K, Evans A: Sinusitis and its management, *BMJ* 334:348–361, 2007.

Smellie WS, Forth J, Smart S, et al: Best practice in primary care pathology: review 7, *J Clin Pathol* 60:458–465, 2007.

Smith S: Infectious diseases. In Marcdante KJ, Kliegman RM, Jenson HB, et al, editors: *Nelson essentials of pediatrics*, ed 6, Philadelphia, 2011, Saunders.

Taketomo CK, Hodding JH, Kraus DM: *Pediatric dosage handbook*, ed 17, Hudson, OH, 2010, Lexi-Comp.

Tom LW, Shah UK: Foreign bodies in the ears, nose, and pharynx. In Burg FD, Ingelfinger JR, Polin RA, et al, editors: *Current pediatric therapy*, ed 18, Philadelphia, 2006, Saunders.

Wald E: Croup: common syndromes and therapy, *Pediatr Ann* 39(1):15–21, 2010.

Welliver R: Bronchiolitis and infectious asthma. In Cherry J, Kaplan S, Demmler-Harrison G, et al, editors: *Feigin & Cherry's textbook of pediatric infectious diseases*, ed 6, Philadelphia, 2010, Saunders, pp 277–288.

Winther B, Bronfeldt S, Gronborg H, et al: Study of bacteria in the nasal cavity and the nasopharynx during naturally acquired common colds, *Acta Otolaryngol* 98:315, 1984.

Zaimanovici A, Yaphe J: Steroids for acute sinusitis, *Cochrane Database Syst Rev* 2:CD005149, 2007.

CHAPTER 32

Ables AZ, Simon MD, Melton ER: Update on Helicobacter pylori treatment, *Am Fam Physician* 75(3):351–358, 2007.

Akobeng AK, Zachos M: *Tumor necrosis factor-alpha antibody for induction of remission in Crohn's diseases (Review)*, The Cochrane Collaboration, 2009, John Wiley & Sons, Ltd.

Alkhouri N, Franciosi JP, Mamula P: Familial adenomatous polyposis in children and adolescents, *J Pediatr Gastroenterol Nutr* 51(6):727–732, 2010.

Allen C, Etzwiler L, Miller M, et al: Recombinant human hyaluronidase-enabled subcutaneous pediatric rehydration, *Pediatrics* 124(5):e585–e867, 2009.

Allen SJ, Martinez EG, Gregorio GV, et al: Probiotics for treating acute infectious diarrhea, *Cochrane Database Syst Rev* 10(11):CD003048, 2010.

American Academy of Otolaryngology-Head and Neck Surgery (AAO-HNS): *Fact sheet: pediatric GERD (gastroesophageal reflux disease)*. Available at www.entnet.org/HealthInformation/pediatricGERD.cfm. Accessed Jan 12, 2011.

Amir L: Ondansetron for the management of vomiting in children with gastroenteritis: a critical review of the literature, *Israeli J Emerg Med* 7:26–30, 2007.

Ammoury RF, Pfefferkorn MD: Significance of esophageal Crohn disease in children, *J Pediatr Gastroenterol Nutr* 52(3):291–294, 2011.

Apley J, Naish N: Recurrent abdominal pains: a field survey of 1000 school children, *Arch Dis Child* 168:165–170, 1958.

Ardizzone S, Cassinotti A, Manes G, et al: Immunomodulators for all patients with inflammatory bowel disease? *Ther Adv Gastroenterol* 3(1):31–42, 2010.

Aviner S, Berkovitch M, Dalkian H, et al: Use of a homeopathic preparation for "infantile colic" and an apparent life-threatening event, *Pediatrics* 125(2):e318–e323, 2010.

Barnard J: Screening and surveillance recommendations for pediatric gastrointestinal polyposis syndromes, *J Pediatr Gastroenterol Nutr* 48(Suppl 2):S75–S78, 2009.

Bauchner H: Failure to thrive. In Kliegman RM, Behrman RE, Jenson HB, et al: *Nelson textbook of pediatrics*, ed 18, Philadelphia, 2007, Saunders, pp 184–187.

Bell EA: Pharmacology consult: ORS for dehydration: are you using it? *Inf Dis Childr* 23(12), 2010. Available at www.pediatricsupersite.com/print.aspx?rid=78398. Accessed Jan 17, 2011.

Benavente L, Morís G: Neurologic disorders associated with inflammatory bowel disease, *Eur J Neurol* 18(1):138–143, 2011.

Benchimol EI, Fortinsky KJ, Gozdyra P, et al: Epidemiology of pediatric inflammatory bowel disease: a systematic review of international trends, *Inflamm Bowel Dis* 17(1):423–439, 2011.

Benchimol EI, Guttmann A, Griffiths AM, et al: Increasing incidence of paediatric inflammatory bowel disease in Ontario, Canada: evidence from health administration data, *Gut* 58(11):1490–1497, 2009.

Bhutta ZA: Acute gastroenteritis in children. In Kliegman RM, Behrman RE, Jenson HB, et al: *Nelson textbook of pediatrics*, ed 18, Philadelphia, 2007, Saunders, pp 1605–1618.

Bhutta ZA, Nelson EA, Lee WS, et al: Recent advances and evidence gaps in persistent diarrhea, *J Pediatr Gastroenter Nutr* 47(2):260–265, 2008.

Bishop WP: The digestive system. In Marcdante KJ, Kliegman RM, Jenson HB, Behrman RE, et al: *Nelson essentials of pediatrics*, ed 6, Philadelphia, 2011, Saunders, pp 463–498.

Blanchard S, Czinn S: Peptic ulcer disease in children. In Kliegman RM, Behrman RE, Jenson HB, editors: *Nelson textbook of pediatrics*, ed 18, Philadelphia, 2007, Saunders, pp 1572–1574.

Blanco FC, Chahine AA: *Intussusception*, 2010. Available at www.emedicine.medscape.com/article/930844. Accessed Jan. 11, 2011.

Boles R, Adams K, Li B: Maternal inheritance in cyclic vomiting syndrome, *Am J Med Genet* 133:71–77, 2005.

Bourreille A, Ignjatovic A, Aabakken L, et al: Role of small-bowel endoscopy in the management of patients with inflammatory bowel disease: an international OMED-ECCO consensus, *Endoscopy* 41(7):618–637, 2009.

Bryant RV, van Langenberg DR, Holtmann GJ, et al: Functional gastrointestinal disorders in inflammatory bowel disease: impact on quality of life and psychological status, *Gastroenterol Hepatol* 26(5):916–923, 2011.

Campo JV, Perel J, Lucas A, et al: Citalopram treatment of pediatric recurrent abdominal pain and co-morbid internalizing disorders: an exploratory study, *J Am Acad Child Adolesc Psychiatry* 43(10):1234–1242, 2004.

Carey WB: Clinical applications of infant temperament measurements, *J Pediatr* 81:823–828, 1972.

Casey PH: Failure-to-thrive. In Carey WB, Crocker AC, Coleman WL, et al, editors: *Developmental-behavioral pediatrics*, ed 4, Philadelphia, 2009, Saunders, pp 583–591.

Centers for Disease Control and Prevention Disaster Safety: Information for Health Care Providers: *Guidelines for the Management of Acute Diarrhea*, 2008. Available at www.emergency.cdc.gov/disasters/hurricanes/pdf/dguidelines.pdf. Accessed Jan 21, 2011.

Centers for Disease Control and Prevention (CDC): *Inflammatory bowel disease*, 2010. Available at www.cdc.gov/ibd/. Accessed Jan 20, 2011.

Chandran L, Chitkara M: Vomiting in children: reassurance, red flag, or referral? *Pediatr Rev* 29(6):183–192, 2008.

Chang HY, Kelly EC, Lembo AJ: Current gut-directed therapies for irritable bowel syndrome, *Curr Treat Options Gastroenterol* 9(4):314–423, 2006.

Chiappini E, de Martino M, Mangiantini F, et al: Crohn disease and mycobacterial infection in children: an intriguing relationship, *J Pediatr Gastroenterol Nutr* 49(5):550–558, 2009.

Cirgin-Ellett M, Perkind S: Examination of the effect of Dr. Brown's Natural Flow Baby Bottles on infant colic, *Gastroenterol Nurs* 29(3):226–231, 2006.

Clayton K: Focus on diagnosis: pediatric abdominal imaging, *Pediatr Rev* 31(12):506–510, 2010.

Conners GP: *Pediatrics, foreign body ingestion*, updated 2010. Available at www.emedicine.medscape.com/article/80182-overview. Accessed Jan 16, 2011.

Dafer RM: *Migraine variants*, 2010. Available at www.emedicine.medscape.com/article/1142731. Accessed Jan 11, 2011.

Damen GM, van Krieken JH, Hoppenreijs E, et al: Overlap, common features, and essential differences in pediatric granulomatous inflammatory bowel disease, *J Pediatr Gastroenterol Nutr* 51(6):690–697, 2010.

Daniel M, Kleis L, Ayse PC: Etiology of failure to thrive in infants and toddlers referred to a pediatric endocrinology outpatient clinic, *Clin Pediatr* 47(8):762–765, 2008.

Day AS, Whitten KE, Sidler M, et al: Systematic review: nutritional therapy in paediatric Crohn's disease, *Aliment Pharmacol Ther* 27(4):293–307, 2007.

Decker E, Engelmann G, Findeisen A, et al: Cesarean delivery is associated with celiac disease but not inflammatory bowel disease in children, *Pediatrics* 125(6):1433–1440, 2010.

de Zoeten E, Mamula P: What are the guidelines for using biologics in pediatric patients? *Inflamm Bowel Dis* 14(Suppl 2):S259–S261, 2008.

Diamante A, Panetta F, Basso MS, et al: Diagnostic work-up of inflammatory bowel disease in children: the role of calprotectin assay, *Inflamm Bowel Dis* 16(11):1926–1930, 2010.

Dranove JE: New technologies for the diagnosis of gastroesophageal reflux disease, *Pediatr Rev* 29(9):317-320.

El-Baba MF: *Irritable bowel syndrome*, 2010. Available at www. emedicine.medscape.com/article/930708-overview. Accessed Jan 11, 2011.

Evanoo G: Infant crying: a clinical conundrum, *J Pediatric Health Care* 21(5):333–338, 2007.

Fasano A, Araya M, Bhatnagar S, et al: Federation of International Societies of Pediatric Gastroenterology, Hepatology, and Nutrition Consensus Report on Celiac Disease, *J Pediatr Gastroenterol Nutr* 47(2):214–219, 2008.

Ficicioglu C, an Haack K: Failure to thrive; when to suspect inborn errors of metabolism, *Pediatrics* 124(3):972–979, 2009.

Fiocchi A, Brozek J, Schünemann H, et al: World Allergy Organization (WAO) diagnosis and rationale for action against cow's milk allergy (DRACMA) guidelines, *WAO J*, April 2010.

Fireman L: Colic, *Pediatr Rev* 27(9):357–358, 2006.

Freedman S, Adler M, Seshadri R, et al: Oral ondansetron for gastroenteritis in a pediatric emergency department, *N Engl J Med* 354:1698–1705, 2006.

Freedman S, Al-Harthy N, Thull-Freeman J: The crying infant: diagnostic testing and frequency of serious underling disease, *Pediatrics* 123(3):841–848, 2009.

Freedman S, Cho D, Boutis K, et al: Palatability of oral rehydration solutions varies but does not impact quantity consumed, *Arch Pediatr Adolesc Med* 164:L696–L702, 2010.

Gelfond D, Fasano A: Celiac disease in the pediatric population, *Pediatr Ann* 35(4):275–279, 2006.

Glickman JN, Odze RD: Does rectal sparing ever occur in ulcerative colitis? *Inflamm Bowel Dis* 14(Supp 2):S166–S167, 2008.

Goerg K, Spilker T: Effect of peppermint oil and caraway oil on gastrointestinal motility in healthy volunteers: a pharmacodynamic study using simultaneous determination of gastric and gallbladder emptying and oral ceocal transit time, *Ailment Pharmacol Ther* 17(2):445–451, 2003.

Goldman R, Friedman J, Parkin P: Validation of the clinical dehydration scale for children with acute gastroenteritis, *Pediatrics* 122:545–549, 2008.

Gottsegen D: Complementary, holistic, and integrative medicine: recurrent abdominal pain, *Pediatr Rev* 31:e36–e39, 2010.

Gower-Rousseau C, Dauchet L, Vernier-Massouille G, et al: The natural history of pediatric ulcerative colitis: a population-based cohort study, *Am J Gastroenterol* 104(8):2080–2088, 2009.

Grimwood K, Forbes DA: Acute and persistent diarrhea, *Pediatr Clin North Am* 56(6):1343–1361, 2009.

Grishan FK: Chronic diarrhea. In Kliegman RM, Behrman RE, Jenson HB, et al, editors: *Nelson textbook of pediatrics*, ed 18, Philadelphia, 2007, Saunders, pp 1621–1627.

Guandalini S, Frye R, Tamer MA: *Diarrhea*, updated 2010. Available at www.emedicine.medscape.com/article/928598. Accessed Jan 17, 2011.

Guariso G, Gasparetto M, Visonà Dalla Pozza L, et al: Inflammatory bowel disease developing in paediatric and adult age, *J Pediatr Gastroenterol Nutr* 51(6):698–707, 2010.

Hadjivassiliou M, Rao DG, Wharton SB, et al: Sensory ganglionopathy due to gluten sensitivity, *Neurology* 75(11):1003–1008, 2010.

Haque R: Human intestinal parasites, *J Health Popul Nutr* 25(4):387–391, 2007.

Harrison D, Bueno M, Yamada J, et al: Analgesic effects of sweet-tasting solutions for infants: current state of equipoise, *Pediatrics* 126(5):894–902, 2010.

Hegar B, Dewanti N, Kadim M, et al: Natural evolution of regurgitation in healthy infants, *Acta Paediatr* 98(7):1189–1193, 2009.

Henderson P, van Limbergen JE, Schwarze J, et al: Function of the intestinal epithelium and its dysregulation in inflammatory bowel disease, *Inflamm Bowel Dis* 17(1):382–395, 2011.

Heyman MB, Garnett EA, Wojcicki J, et al: Growth hormone treatment of growth failure in pediatric patients with Crohn's disease, *J Pediatr* 153(5):651–658, 2008.

Hill D, Toy N, Heine R, et al: Effect of low-allergen maternal diet on colic among breastfed infants: a randomized controlled trial, *Pediatrics* 116(5):709–715, 2006.

Huertas-Ceballos AA, Logan S, Bennett C, Macarthur C: Dietary interventions for recurrent abdominal pain (RAP) and irritable bowel syndrome (IBS) in childhood, *Cochrane Database Syst Rev* 21(1):CD003019, 2009.

Hughes LE: Clinical classification of perianal Crohn's disease, *Dis Colon Rectum* 35(10):928–932, 1992.

Humphreys EH, Smith NA, Azman H, et al: Prevention of diarrhea in children with HIV infection or exposure to maternal HIV infection, *Cochrane Database Syst Rev* 16(6):CD008563, 2010.

Illingsworth S: Infantile colic revisited, *Arch Dis Child* 60:981–985, 1985.

Johnston BC, Supina AL, Ospina M, et al: Probiotics for the prevention of pediatric antibiotic-associated diarrhea, *Cochrane Database System Rev* 11:CD004827, 2011.

Jones K: Probiotics: preventing antibiotic-associated diarrhea, *J Special Pediatr Nurs* 15(2):160–162, 2010.

Kappelman MD, Grand RJ: Does inflammatory bowel disease develop in infants? *Inflamm Bowel Dis* 14(Supp2):S6–S8, 2008.

Karp H: Safe swaddling and healthy hips: don't toss the baby out with the bathwater, *Pediatrics* 121(5):1075–1076, 2008.

Katz MS, Freitas MS, Tucker JR, et al: *Appendicitis*, 2009. Available at www. emedicine.medscape.com/article/926795. Accessed Jan 11, 2011.

Keating J: Chronic diarrhea, *Pediatr Rev* 26(1):5–13, 2005.

Keefe M: Irritable infant syndrome: theoretical perspective and practice implications, *Adv Nurs Sci* 10(3):70–78, 1988.

Keefe M, Karlson K, Dudley W, et al: Reducing parenting stress in families with irritable infants, *Nurs Res* 55(3):198–205, 2006a.

Keefe M, Lobo M, Froese-Fretz A, et al: Effectiveness of an intervention for colic, *Clin Pediatr* 45:123–13, 2006b.

Kelsen J, Baldassano RN: Inflammatory bowel disease: the difference between children and adults, *Inflamm Bowel Dis* 14(Supp 2):S9–S11, 2008.

Kharbanda A, Taylor G, Fishman S, et al: A clinical decision rule to identify children at low risk for appendicitis, *Pediatrics* 116(3):709–716, 2005.

Kimball SJ, Park AH, Rollins MD, et al: A review of esophageal disk battery ingestion and a protocol for management, *Arch Otolaryngol Head Neck Surg* 136(9):866–871, 2010.

Kohli R, Li B: Differential diagnosis of recurrent abdominal pain: new considerations, *Pediatr Ann* 33(2):113–122, 2004.

Koskinen O, Villanen M, Korponay-Szabo I, et al: Oats do not induce systemic or mucosal autoantibody response in children with celiac disease, *J Pediatr Gastroenterol Nutr* 48(5):559–565, 2009.

Krebs NF, Primak LE: Normal childhood nutrition and its disorders: pediatric under- and over nutrition. In Hay WW, Levin MJ, Sondheimer JM, et al, editors: *Current diagnosis and treatment pediatrics*, ed 19, New York, 2009, McGraw-Hill.

Kunz JH, Hommel KA, Greenley RN: Health-related quality of life of youth with inflammatory bowel disease: a comparison with published data using the PedsQL 4.0 generic core scales, *Inflamm Bowel Dis* 16(6):939–946, 2010.

Lee HJ, Lee JH, Lee JS, et al: Is colonoscopy necessary in children suspected of having colonic polyps? *Gut Liver* 4(3):326–331, 2010.

Levine A, Griffiths A, Markowitz J, et al: Pediatric modification of the Montreal classification for inflammatory bowel disease: the Paris classification, *Inflamm Bowel Dis* 17(6):1314–1321, 2010.

Li B, Lefevre F, Chelimsky GG, et al: North American Society for Pediatric Gastroenterology, Hepatology, and Nutrition consensus statement on the diagnosis, and management of cyclic vomiting syndrome, *J Pediatr Gastroenterol Nutr* 47:379–393, 2008.

Li ST, Grossman DC, Cummings P: Loperamide therapy for acute diarrhea in children: systematic review and meta-analysis, *PLoS Med* 4(3):e98, 2007.

Litovitz T, Whitaker N, Clark L, et al: Emerging battery-ingestion hazard: clinical implications, *Pediatrics* 125(6):1168–1677, 2010.

Lochs H, Dejong C, Hammarqvist F, et al: ESPEN guidelines on enteral nutrition: gastroenterology, *Clin Nutr* 25(2):260–274, 2006.

Logan I, Bowlus CL: The geoepidemiology of autoimmune intestinal diseases, *Autoimmun Rev* 9(5):A372–A378, 2010.

Loo M: *Integrative medicine for children*, Philadelphia, 2009, Saunders, p 134.

Lu Y, Jacobson D, Bousvaros A: Immunizations in patients with inflammatory bowel disease, *Inflamm Bowel Dis* 15(9):1417–1423, 2009.

Mahajan P: Dehydration. In McInerny T, Adam H, Campbell D, et al, editors: *American Academy of Pediatrics textbook of pediatric care*, Elk Grove, IL, 2009, American Academy of Pediatrics.

Malik S, Wong SC, Bishop J, et al: Improvement in growth of children with Crohn disease following anti-TNF-a therapy can be independent of pubertal progress and glucocorticoid reduction, *J Pediatr Gastroenterol Nutr* 52(1):31–37, 2011.

Mallon DP, Suskind DL: Nutrition in pediatric inflammatory bowel disease, *Nutr Clin Pract* 25(4):335–339, 2010.

Mamula P, Markowitz JE, Baldassano RN, editors: *Pediatric inflammatory bowel disease*, New York, 2008, Springer.

Manfredi M: Hereditary hamartomatous polyposis syndromes: understanding the disease risks as children reach adulthood, *Gastroenterol Hepatol* 6(3):185–196, 2010.

Markowitz J, Hyams J, Mack D, et al: Corticosteroid therapy in the age of infliximab: acute and 1-year outcomes in newly diagnosed children with Crohn's disease, *Clin Gastroenterol Hepatol* 4:1124–1129, 2006.

Matricardi PM, Bockelbrink A, Beyer K, et al: Primary versus secondary immunoglobulin E sensitization to soy and wheat in the Multi-Centre Allergy Study cohort, *Clin Exp Allergy* 38(3):493–500, 2008.

Mazumder S, Taneja S, Bhandari N, et al: Effectiveness of zinc supplementation plus oral rehydration salts for diarrhea in infants aged less than 6 months in Haryana state, India, *Bull World Health Org* 88(10):754–760, 2010.

Megel M, Wilson M, Bravo K, et al: Baby lost and found: mothers' experiences of infants who cry persistently, *J Pediatr Health Care* 25(3):144–152, 2011.

Mitchell WG: *Childhood migraine variants*, 2009. Available at www. emedicine.medscape.com/article /1178141. Accessed Jan 11, 2011.

Mones RL, Atienza KV, Youssef NN, et al: Celiac crisis in the modern era, *J Pediatr Gastroenterol Nutr* 45(4):480–483, 2007.

Moon A, Solomon A, Beneck D, et al: Positive association between *Helicobacter pylori* and gastroesophageal reflux disease in children, *J Pediatr Gastroenterol Nutr* 49(3):238–288, 2009.

Moore D: Inflamming the debate on infant colic, *J Pediatr* 155:772–773, 2009.

Moore JC, Thompson K, LaFleur B, et al: Clinical variables as prognostic tools in pediatric-onset ulcerative colitis: a retrospective cohort study, *Inflamm Bowel Dis* 17(1):15–21, 2011.

Mubarak A, Wolters VM, Gerritsen SA, et al: A biopsy is not always necessary to diagnose celiac disease, *J Pediatr Gastroenterol Nutr* 52(5):554–557, 2011.

Mustalahti K, Catassi C, Reunanen A, et al: The prevalence of celiac disease in Europe: results of a centralized, international mass screening project, *Ann Med* 42(8):587–595, 2010.

National Institute for Health and Clinical Excellence (NICE): *Coeliac disease: recognition and assessment of coeliac disease*, London, 2009, National Institute for Health and Clinical Excellence. Available at www.nice.org.uk/CG86. Accessed Jan 9, 2011.

Navaneethan U, Shen B: Hepatopancreatobiliary manifestations and complications associated with inflammatory bowel disease, *Inflamm Bowel Dis* 16(9):1598–1619, 2010.

Newby EA, Croft NM, Green M, et al: Natural history of paediatric inflammatory bowel diseases over a 5-year follow-up: a retrospective review of data from the register of paediatric inflammatory bowel diseases, *J Pediatr Gastroenterol Nutr* 46(5):539–545, 2008.

Ng SC, Kamm MA: Therapeutic strategies for the management of ulcerative colitis, *Inflamm Bowel Dis* 15(6):935–950, 2009.

Noble A, Turner D: Clinical indices for pediatric inflammatory bowel disease research. In Mamula P, Markowitz JE, Baldassano RN, editors: *Pediatric inflammatory bowel disease*, New York, 2008, Springer, pp 507–530.

Norman G, Pedley S, Takkouche B: Effects of sewerage on diarrhea and enteric infections: a systematic review and meta-analysis, *Lancet* 10(8):536–544, 2010.

North American Society for Pediatric Gastroenterology: Hepatology, and Nutrition (NASPGHAN): Guideline for the diagnosis and treatment of celiac disease in children, *JPGN* 40:1–19, 2005.

Olsen EM, Petersen J, Skovgaard AM, et al: Failure to thrive: the prevalence and concurrence of anthropometric criteria in a general infant population, *Arch Dis Child* 92:109–114, 2007.

Olsen EM, Skovgaard AM, Weile AM, et al: Risk factors for weight faltering in infancy according to age at onset, *Paediatr Perinat Epidemiol* 24(4):370–382, 2010.

Orenstein S: Foreign bodies in the esophagus. In Kliegman RM, Behrman RE, Jenson HB, et al: *Nelson textbook of pediatrics*, ed 18, Philadelphia, 2007, Saunders, pp 1552–1553.

Orenstein S, Peters J, Khan S, et al: Gastroesophageal reflux disease. In Kliegman RM, Behrman RE, Jenson HB, et al: *Nelson textbook of pediatrics*, ed 18, Philadelphia, 2007, Saunders, pp 1547–1550.

Pacilli M, Eaton S, Fell JM, et al: Surgery in children with Crohn disease refractory to medical therapy, *J Pediatr Gastroenterol Nutr* 52(3):286–290, 2011.

Pakarinen MP, Natunen J, Ashom M, et al: Long-term outcomes of restorative proctocolectomy in children with ulcerative colitis, *Pediatrics* 123(5):1377–1382, 2009.

Panetta F, Magazzu D, Sferlazzas C, et al: Diagnosis on a positive fashion of nonorganic failure to thrive, *Acta Paediatr* 97(9):1281–1284, 2008.

Pashankar DS, Corbin Z, Shah S, et al: Increased prevalence of gastroesophageal reflux symptoms in obese children evaluated in an academic medical center, *J Clin Gastroenterol* 43(5):410–413, 2009.

Passariello A, Terrin G, De Marco G, et al: Efficacy of a new hypotonic oral rehydration solution containing zinc and prebiotics in the treatment of childhood acute diarrhea: a randomized controlled trial, *J Pediatr* 158(2):288–292, 2011.

Patel AB, Dibley MJ, Mamtani M, et al: Influence of zinc supplementation in acute diarrhea differs by the isolated organism, *Int J Pediatr* 2010:671587, 2010. Epub 2010 May 31.

Patro B, Szymanski H, Szajewska H: Oral zinc for the treatment of acute gastroenteritis in Polish children: a randomized, double-blind, placebo-controlled trial, *J Pediatr* 157(6):984–988, 2010.

Peyrin-Biroulet L, Loftus EV Jr, Colombel JF, et al: Long-term complications, extraintestinal manifestations, and mortality in adult Crohn's disease in population-based cohorts, *Inflamm Bowel Dis* 17(1):471–478, 2011.

Pigneur B, Seksik P, Viola S, et al: Natural history of Crohn's disease: comparison between childhood- and adult-onset disease, *Inflamm Bowel Dis* 16:953–961, 2010.

Pirotta M: Irritable bowel syndrome—the role of complementary medicines in treatment, *Aust Fam Physician* 38(12):966–968, 2009.

Portela F, Magro F, Lago P, et al: Ulcerative colitis in a southern European country: a national perspective, *Inflamm Bowel Dis* 16(5):822–829, 2010.

Pulido OM, Gillespie Z, Zarkadas M, et al: Introduction of oats in the diet of individuals with celiac disease: a systematic review, *Adv Food Nutr Res* 57:235–285, 2009.

Pulling M, Surawicz CM: Loperamide use for acute infectious diarrhea in children: safe and sound? *Gastroenterology* 134(4):1260–1262, 2008.

Rabinowitz SS, Katturupalli M, Rogers G: *Failure to thrive*, updated 2010. Available at www.emedicine. medscape.com/article/985007-overview. Accessed Jan 12, 2011.

Rao M, Brenner R, Schisterman T, et al: Long term cognitive development in children with prolonged crying, *Arch Dis Child* 89:989–992, 2004.

Rasquin A, DiLorenzo C, Forbes D, et al: Childhood functional gastrointestinal disorders: child/adolescent, *Gastroenterology* 130:1527–1537, 2006.

Reynolds SA, Levy F, Walker ES: *Emerging infectious diseases, letter: hand sanitizer alert*, 2006. Available at www.cdc.gov/NCIDOD/EID/vol12no03/05-0955.htm. Accessed Jan 17, 2011.

Rhoads J, Fatheree N, Norori J, et al: Altered fecal microflora and increased calprotectin in infants with colic, *J Pediatr* 155(6):823–828, 2009.

Roberts D, Ostapchuk M, O'Brien J: Infantile colic, *Am Fam Physician* 70(4):735–740, 2004.

Rosen L, Bukutu C, Le C, et al: Complementary, holistic, and integrative medicine: colic, *Pediatr Rev* 28(10):381–385, 2007.

Roslund G, Hepps T, McQuillen K: The ED role of ondansetron in oral rehydration of children in with gastroenteritis related vomiting, *Acad Emerg Med* 13(5):5147–5153, 2006.

Ross A, LeLeiko NS: Acute abdominal pain, *Pediatr Rev* 31:135–144, 2010.

Satsangi J, Silverberg MS, Vermeire S, et al: The Montreal classification of inflammatory bowel diseases: controversies, consensus, and implications, *Gut* 55(6):749–753, 2006.

Savage MO: Growth-promoting hormone therapy in inflammatory bowel disease, *J Pediatr Gastroenterol Nutr* 51(Suppl 3):S135–S136, 2010.

Savino F, Cordisco L, Tarasco V, et al: Molecular identification of coliform bacteria from colicky breastfed infants, *Acta Paediatr* 98(10):1582–1588, 2009.

Savino F, Cordisco L, Tarasco V, et al: *Lactobacillus reuteri* DSM 17938 in infantile colic: a randomized, double-blind, placebo-controlled trial, *Pediatrics* 126(3):e526–e533, 2010.

Scheffer R: Psychiatric disorders. In Marcdante KJ, Kliegman RM, Jenson HB, et al, editors: *Nelson essentials of pediatrics*, ed 6, Philadelphia, 2011, Saunders, pp 63–80.

Schuppan D, Junker Y, Barisani D: Celiac disease: from pathogenesis to novel therapies, *Gastroenterology* 137(6):1912–1933, 2009.

Segal K, Otley A, Issenman R, et al: Low prevalence of *Helicobacter pylori* infection in Canadian children: a cross-sectional analysis, *Can J Gastroenterol* 22(5):485–489, 2008.

Setty M, Hormaza L, Guandalini S: Celiac disease: risk assessment, diagnosis, and monitoring, *Mol Diagn Ther* 12(5):289–298, 2008.

Shamir R: Nutrition and growth in inflammatory bowel disease, *J Pediatr Gastroenterol Nutr* 51(Suppl 3):S131–S132, 2010.

Shane AL: *Choosing right drug, probiotic supplementation effective in prevention of antibiotic-associated diarrhea*, 2010. Available at www.pediatricsupersite. com/print.aspx?rid=78253. Accessed Jan 12, 2011.

Sondheimer JM: Gastrointestinal tract. In Hay WW, Hayward A, Levin M, et al, editors: *Current pediatric diagnosis and treatment*, ed 17, New York, 2005, Lange Medical Books.

Steiner M, DeWalt D, Byerly J: Is this child dehydrated? *JAMA* 291(22):2746–2754, 2004.

Stene L, Honeyman M, Hoffenber E, et al: Rotavirus infection frequency and risk of celiac disease autoimmunity in early childhood: a longitudinal study, *Am J Gastroenterol* 101:2333–2340, 2006.

Stephens MB, Gentry BC, Michener MD, et al: What is the clinical workup for failure to thrive? *J Fam Pract* 57(4):264–266, 2008.

Suchy FJ, Brannon PM, Carpenter TO, et al: National Institutes of Health Consensus Development Conference: lactose intolerance and health, *Ann Intern Med* 152(12):792–796, 2010.

Sultan MI, Li BUK, Shah A: *Peptic ulcer disease*, 2009. Available at www. emedicine.medscape.com/ article/932308. Accessed Jan 15, 2011.

Suwandhi E, Ton M, Schwarz S: GER in infancy and childhood, *Pediatr Ann* 35(4):259–266, 2006.

Szajewska H, Setty M, Mrukowic J, et al: Probiotics in gastrointestinal disease in children: hard and not so hard evidence of efficacy, *J Pediatr Gastroenterol Nutr* 42:454–475, 2006.

Tam YH, Lee KH, To KF: *Helicobacter pylori*-positive versus *Helicobacter pylori*-negative idiopathic peptic ulcers in children, *J Pediatr Gastroenterol Nutr* 48:299–305, 2009.

Thomas DW, Greer FR: Committee on Nutrition: Section on gastroenterology, hepatology, and nutrition: probiotics and prebiotics in pediatrics, *Pediatrics* 126(6):1217–1231, 2010.

Turner D, Griffiths AM: Acute severe ulcerative colitis in children: a systematic review, *Inflamm Bowel Dis* 17(1):440–449, 2011.

Turner D, Otley AR, Mack D, et al: Development, validation, and evaluation of a pediatric ulcerative colitis activity index (PUCAI): a prospective multicenter study, *Gastroenterology* 133(2):423–432, 2007.

Turner D, Shah PS, Steinhart AH, et al: Maintenance of remission in inflammatory bowel disease using omega-3 fatty acids (fish oil): a systematic review and meta-analyses, *Inflamm Bowel Dis* 17(1):336–345, 2011.

Ulshen MH: Vomiting. In McInery TK, Adam HM, Campbell DE, et al: *American Academy of Pediatrics textbook of pediatric care*, Elk Grove, IL, 2009, American Academy of Pediatrics, pp 1783–1785.

Vandenplas Y, Rudolph C, Di Lorenzo C, et al: Pediatric gastroesophageal reflux clinical practice guidelines: joint recommendations of the North American Society for Pediatric Gastroenterology, Hepatology, and Nutrition (NASPGHAN) and the European Society for Pediatric Gastroenterology, Hepatology, and Nutrition (ESPGHAN), *J Pediatr Gastroenterol Nutr* 49(4):498–547, 2009.

van Sleuwen B, Engelberts A, Boere-Boonekamp M, et al: Swaddling: a systematic review, *Pediatrics* 120(4):e1097–e1106, 2007.

von Roon AC, Reese G, Teare J, et al: The risk of cancer in patients with Crohn's disease, *Dis Colon Rectum* 50(6):839–855, 2007.

Walker LS, Dengler-Crish CM, Rippel S, et al: Functional abdominal pain in childhood and adolescence increases risk for chronic pain in adulthood, *Pain* 150(3):568–572, 2010.

Welander A, Tjernberg AR, Montgomery SM, et al: Infectious disease and risk of later celiac disease in childhood, *Pediatrics* 125(3):530–536, 2010.

Weng M, Walker WA: Bacterial colonization, probiotics, and clinical disease, *J Pediatr* 149(5):S107–S114, 2006.

Wessel M, Cobb J, Jackson E, et al: Paroxysmal fussing in infancy, sometimes called "colic," *Pediatrics* 14:421–433, 1954.

World Health Organization: *News release: global use of rotavirus vaccines recommended*, 2009. Available at www.who.int/mediacentre/news/releases/2009/rotavirus_vaccines_20090605/en. Accessed Jan 17, 2011.

Wyllie R: Foreign bodies and bezoars. In Kliegman RM, Behrman RE, Jenson HB, et al: *Nelson textbook of pediatrics*, ed 18, Philadelphia, 2007, Saunders, p 1571.

Xavier RJ, Podolsky DK: Unraveling the pathogenesis of inflammatory bowel disease, *Nature* 448(7152):427–434, 2007.

CHAPTER 33

Al Agili DE, Pass MA, Bronstein JM, et al: Medicaid participation by private dentists in Alabama, *Pediatr Dent* 29:293–302, 2007.

Alexander RE: Readability of published dental educational materials, *J Am Dent Assoc* 131(7):937–942, 2000.

Altarum Institute: *Topical fluoride recommendations for high-risk children: development of decision support matrix—recommendations from MCHB expert panel*, 2009. Available at www.mchoralhealth.org/PDFs/TopicalFluorideRpt.pdf. Accessed Dec 22, 2009.

American Academy of Pediatric Dentistry (AAPD): Reference manual 2009-2010: policy on use of a caries-risk assessment tool (CAT) for infants, children, and adolescents, *Pediatr Dent* 31(special issue):29–33, 2009a.

American Academy of Pediatric Dentistry (AAPD): Reference manual 2009-2010: periodontal diseases of children and adolescents, *Pediatr Dent* 31(special issue):255–262, 2009b.

American Academy of Pediatric Dentistry (AAPD): Reference manual 2009-2010: policy on prevention of sports-related orofacial injuries, *Pediatr Dent* 31(special issue):56–58, 2009c.

American Academy of Pediatric Dentistry (AAPD): Reference manual 2009-2010: policy on the use of dental bleaching for child and adolescent patients, *Pediatr Dent* 31(special issue):59–61, 2009d.

American Academy of Pediatric Dentistry (AAPD): Council on Clinical Affairs: *Policy on the use of xylitol in caries prevention*, 2006, revised 2010a. Available at www.aapd.org/media/policies_guidelines/p_xylitol.pdf. Accessed Sept 26, 2010.

American Academy of Pediatric Dentistry (AAPD), Clinical Affairs Committee, Temporomandibular Joint Problems in Children Subcommittee: *Guidelines on acquired temporomandibular disorders in infants, children, and adolescents*, 1990, revised 2010b. Available at www.aapd.org/media/Policies_Guidelines/G-TMD.pdf. Accessed Sept 8, 2010.

Azevedo TD, Bezerra AC, de Toledo OA: Feeding habits and severe early childhood caries in Brazilian preschool children, *Pediatr Dent* 27(1):28–33, 2005.

Bailey DL, Adams GG, Tsao CE, et al: Regression of post-orthodontic lesions by a remineralizing cream, *J Dent Res* 88(12):1148–1153, 2009.

Beil HA, Rozier RG: Primary health care providers' advice for a dental checkup and dental use in children, *Pediatrics* 126(2):e435–e441, 2010.

Beltrán-Aguilar ED, Barker LK, Canto MT, et al: Surveillance for dental caries, dental sealants, tooth retention, edentulism, and enamel fluorosis—United States, 1988-1991 and 1999-2002, *MMWR Morb Mort Wkly Rep* 54(03):1–44, 2005.

Beltrán-Aguilar ED, Barker L, Dye BA: Prevalence and severity of dental fluorosis in the United States, 1999–2004, *NCHS Data Brief* 53:1–8, 2010.

Berkowitz RJ, Koo H, McDermott MP, et al: Adjunctive chemotherapeutic suppression of *Mutans streptococci* in the setting of severe early childhood caries: an exploratory study, *J Public Health Dent* 69(3):163–167, 2009.

Blackwell DL: Family structure and children's health in the United States: findings from the national Health Interview Survey 2001-2007, National Center for Health Statistics, *Vital Health Stat* 10(246), 2010. Available at www.cdc.gov/nchs/data/series/sr_10/sr10_246.pdf. Accessed March 30, 2011.

Bloom B, Cohen RA, Freeman G: Summary health statistics for U.S. children: National Health Interview Survey, 2008, National Center for Health Statistics, *Vital Health Stat* 10(244), 2009.

Bobetsis YA, Barros SP, Offenbacher S: Exploring the relationship between periodontal disease and pregnancy complications, *J Am Dent Assoc* 137(S2):7s–13s, 2006.

California Dental Association Foundation: *Oral health during pregnancy and early childhood: evidence-based guidelines for the health professional*, 2010. Available at www.cdafoundation.org/library/docs/poh_guidelines.pdf. Accessed Sep 25, 2010.

Centers for Disease Control and Prevention (CDC), Chronic Disease Prevention and Health Promotion: *Oral health: preventing cavities, gum disease, tooth loss, and oral cancers: at a glance*, 2010a. Available at www.cdc.gov/chronicdisease/resources/publications/AAG/doh.htm. Accessed Sep 25, 2010.

Centers for Disease Control and Prevention (CDC): *Recommendation for using fluoride to prevent and control dental caries in the United States*, 2001, reviewed 2010b. Available at www.cdc.gov/fluoridation/fact_sheets/fl_caries.htm. Accessed Aug 26, 2010.

Cheifetz AT, Osganian SK, Allred EN, et al: Prevalence of bruxism and associated correlates as reported by parents, *J Dent Child* 72:67–73, 2005.

Chi D, Kanellis M, Himadi E, et al: Lip biting in a pediatric dental patient after dental local anesthesia: a case report, *J Pediatr Nurs* 23(6):490–493, 2008.

Chi D, Milgrom P: Preventive dental service utilization for Medicaid-enrolled children in New Hampshire: a comparison of care provided by pediatric dentists and general dentists, *J Health Care Poor Underserved* 20(2):458–472, 2009.

Chung NY, Batra R, Itzkevitch M, et al: Severe methemoglobinemia linked to gel-type topical benzocaine use: a case report, *J Emerg Med* 38(5):601–606, 2010.

Crawford PJM, Aldred MF: Anomalies of tooth formation and eruption. In Welbury R, Duggal M, Department of Child Dental Care: *Paediatric dentistry*, ed 3, Oxford, 2005, Oxford University Press.

Danielson R, Dillenberg J, Bay C: Oral health competencies for physician assistants and nurse practitioners, *J Phys Assist Educ* 17(4):12–16, 2006.

Davies GM, Duxbury JT, Boothman NJ, et al: A staged intervention dental health programme to reduce early childhood caries, *Community Dent Health* 22(2):118–122, 2005.

Deery C, Wagner ML, Longbottom C, et al: The prevalence of dental erosion in a United States and a United Kingdom sample of adolescents, *Pediatr Dent* 22:505–510, 2000.

Do LG, Spencer AJ: Risk-benefit balance in the use of fluoride among young children, *J Dent Res* 86:723–728, 2007.

Donly KJ, Segura A, Henson T, et al: Randomized controlled trial of professional at-home tooth whitening in teenagers, *Gen Dent* 55(7):669–674, 2007.

Dworkin SF, Drangsholt M: Clinical trials in temporomandibular disorders. In Max MJ, Lynn J, editors: *Interactive textbook on clinical symptom research*, 2003. Available at www.symptomresearch.nih.gov/chapter_22. Accessed Sep 29, 2010.

Edelstein BL, Chinn CH: Update on disparities in oral health and access to dental care for America's children, *Acad Pediatr* 9(6):415–419, 2009.

Friedman JW: The prophylactic extraction of third molars: a public health hazard, *Am J Pub Health* 97(9):1554–1559, 2007.

Gould JM, Cies JJ: *Dental abscess: treatment and medication*. updated Feb 2010. Available at www.emedicine.medscape.com/article/909373-treatment. Accessed Aug 26, 2010.

Hasson H, Ismail AI, Neiva G: Home-based chemically-induced whitening of teeth in adults, *Cochrane Database Syst Rev* 4:CD006202, 2006.

Hayes C, Thornton K: Nutrition in the growth and development of oral structures. In Palmer CA, editor: *Diet and nutrition in oral health*, ed 2, Upper Saddle River, NJ, 2007, Prentice-Hall.

Herrera JA, Parra B, Herrera E, et al: Periodontal disease severity is related to high levels of C-reactive protein in pre-eclampsia, *J Hypertens* 25(7):1459–1464, 2007.

Holve S: An observational study of the association of fluoride varnish applied during well child visits and the prevention of early childhood caries in American Indian Children, *Matern Child Health J* 12(Suppl 1):64–67, 2008.

Hosey MT, Welbury RR: Medical disability. In Welbury R, Duggal M, editors: *Paediatric dentistry*, ed 3, Oxford, 2005, Oxford University Press.

Iben P, Kanellis MJ, Warren J: Appointment-keeping behavior of Medicaid-enrolled pediatric dental patients in eastern Iowa, *Pediatr Dent* 22:325–329, 2000.

Isokangas P, Söderling E, Pienihäkkinen K, et al: Occurrence of dental decay in children after maternal consumption of xylitol chewing gum: a follow-up from 0 to 5 years of age, *J Dent Res* 79(11):1885–1889, 2000.

Jasper J, Losh G, Endom E: *Evaluation and repair of tongue lacerations, UpToDate Online* 18.2. Available at www.uptodateonline.com. Accessed Oct 9, 2010.

Keels MA, Clements DA: *Herpetic gingivostomatitis in young children, UpToDate Online* 18.2. Available at www.uptodateonline.com. Accessed Aug 25, 2010.

Klasser GD, Epstein J: Methamphetamine and its impact on dental care, *J Can Dent Assoc* 71:759–762, 2005.

Klein U: Oral medicine and dentistry. In Hay W, Levin M, Deterding R, et al, editors: *Current diagnosis and treatment—pediatrics,* ed 19, New York, 2009, McGraw-Hill.

Kwan SY, Petersen PE, Pine CM, et al: Health-promoting schools: an opportunity for oral health promotion, *Bull World Health Organ* 83(9):677–685, 2005.

Lam A, Kiyak A, Gossett AM, et al: Assessment of the use of xerogenic medications for chronic medical and dental conditions among adult day health participants, *Consult Pharm* 24(10):755–764, 2009.

LeResche L, Mancl LA, Drangsholt MT, et al: Predictors of onset of facial pain and temporomandibular disorders in early adolescence, *Pain* 129(3):269–278, 2007.

Leung AK, Robson WL: Natal teeth: a review, *J Natl Med Assoc* 98(2):226–228, 2006.

Ly KA, Milgrom P, Rothen M: Xylitol, sweeteners and dental caries, *Pediatr Dent* 28(2):154–163, 2006.

McIntyre J, Lee JY, Trope M, et al: Permanent tooth replantation following avulsion: using a decision tree to achieve the best outcome, *Pediatr Dent* 31(2):137–144, 2009. An adaptation of this decision tree is available at www.aapd.org/media/policies_guidelines/rs_traumaflowsheet.pdf. Accessed Sep 8, 2010.

Milgrom P, Weinstein P: *Early childhood caries,* Seattle, 2001, Behavioral Dental Publications. Available from www.Dentalbehavioralresources.com. Accessed Sep 29, 2010.

Milgrom P, Weinstein P, Huebner C, et al: Empowering Head Start to improve access to good oral health for children from low-income families, *Matern Child Health J* 15(7):876–882, 2011.

Milgrom P, Ly KA, Tut OK, et al: Xylitol pediatric topical oral syrup to prevent dental caries: a double-blind randomized clinical trial of efficacy, *Arch Pediatr Adolesc Med* 163(7):601–607, 2009.

Mitchell L: *An introduction to orthodontics,* ed 3, Oxford, 2007, Oxford University Press.

Morgan R, Tsang J, Harrington N, et al: Survey of hospital doctors' attitudes and knowledge of oral conditions in older patients, *Postgrad Med J* 77(908):392–394, 2001.

Muscari ME: *A tough one to chew on: smokeless tobacco and teens,* 2010. Available at www.medscape.com/viewarticle/724317. Accessed Sep 27, 2010.

Nash DA: Expanding dental hygiene to include dental therapy: improving access to care for children, *J Dental Hyg* 83:39–44, 2009.

National Institutes of Dental and Craniofacial Research (NIDCR), National Institutes of Health: *TMJ disorders,* revised March 2010. Available at www.nidcr.nih.gov/oralhealth/Topics/TMJ/TMJDisorders.htm. Accessed Sep 8, 2010.

Nilsson IM, List T, Drangsholt M: Prevalence of temporomandibular pain and subsequent dental treatment in Swedish adolescents, *J Orofac Pain* 19(2):144–150, 2005.

Nilsson IM, List T, Drangsholt M: The reliability and validity of self-reported temporomandibular disorder pain in adolescents, *J Orofac Pain* 20(2):138–144, 2006.

Prober CG: Herpes simplex virus. In Long SS, Pickering LK, Prober CG, editors: *Principles and practice of pediatric infectious diseases,* ed 3, Philadelphia, 2008, Churchill Livingstone.

Proffit WR, Fields HW Jr, Moray LJ: Prevalence of malocclusion and orthodontic treatment need in the United States: estimates from the NHANES III survey, *Int J Adult Orthodon Orthognath Surg* 13:97–106, 1998.

Rizzolo D, Sedrak M: Oral pathology, *Clin Rev* 19(6):26–30, 2009.

Singh SM, Chopra S, Thomas AM: Efficacy of 10% povidone iodine in children affected with early childhood caries: an in vivo study, *J Am Dent Assoc* 141(3):307–318, 2010.

Smith TA, Heaton LJ: Fear of dental care: are we making any progress? *J Am Dent Assoc* 134(8):1101–1108, 2003.

Smitherman LC, Janisse J, Mathur A: The use of folk remedies among children in an urban black community: remedies for fever, colic, and teething, *Pediatrics* 3:e297–e304, 2005.

Stanberry LR: Herpes Simplex virus. In Kliegman RM, Behrman RE, Jenson HB, et al, editors: *Nelson textbook of pediatrics,* ed 18, Philadelphia, 2007, Saunders, pp 1360–1366.

Tinanoff N, Reisine S: Update on early childhood caries since the Surgeon General's report, *Acad Pediatr* 9(6):396–403, 2009.

Truelove E, Huggins KH, Mancl L, et al: The efficacy of traditional, low-cost and nonsplint therapies for temporomandibular disorder: a randomized controlled trial, *J Am Dent Assoc* 8:1099–1107, 2006.

Tut OK, Milgrom PM: Topical iodine and fluoride varnish combined is more effective than fluoride varnish alone for protecting erupting first permanent molars: a retrospective cohort study, *J Public Health Dent* 70(3):249–252, 2010.

University of California, Berkeley, School of Public Health: Chew this over, *UC Berkeley Wellness Letter* 35(10):2–3, 2009.

U.S. Department of Health and Human Services (USD-HHS): *National call to action to promote oral health,* Rockville, MD, 2003, Spring, U.S. Department of Health and Human Services, National Institutes of Health, National Institute of Dental and Craniofacial Research. NIH Publication No. 03-5303.

U.S. Department of Health and Human Services (USDHHS): Summary health statistics for U.S. children: National Health Interview Survey, 2009, National Center for Health Statistics, *Vital Health Stat* 10(247), 2010. Available at www.cdc.gov/nchs/data/series/sr_10/sr10_247.pdf. Accessed Sep 29, 2010.

U.S. Department of Health and Human Services (USD-HHS): *Proposed HHS Recommendation for Fluoride Concentration in Drinking Water for Prevention of Dental Caries,* 2011. Available at www.hhs.gov/news/press/2011pres/01/pre_pub_frn_fluoride.html. Accessed April 4, 2011.

U.S. Food and Drug Administration (FDA): *About dental amalgam fillings,* 2009. Available at www.fda.gov/medicaldevices/productsandmedicalprocedures/dentalproducts/dentalamalgam/ucm171094.htm. Accessed Sep 9, 2010.

van Palenstein Helderman WH, Soe W, van't Hof MA: Risk factors of early childhood caries in a Southeast Asian population, *J Dent Res* 85(1):85–88, 2006.

Warren JJ, Slayton RL, Bishara SE, et al: Effects of nonnutritive sucking habits on occlusal characteristics in the mixed dentition, *Pediatr Dent* 27(6):445–450, 2005.

Weinstein P, Harrison R, Benton T: Motivating parents to prevent caries in their young children: one-year findings, *J Am Dent Assoc* 135(6):731–738, 2004.

Weinstein P, Milgrom P: *Oral self care: strategies for preventive dentistry,* ed 4, Seattle, 2006, Behavioral Dental Publications. Available from www.Dentalbehavioralresources.com. Accessed Sept 29, 2010.

Weiss A, Nelson P, Dym H: Oral pathology for the primary-care clinician, *Clin Adv* 13(4):17–22, 2010.

Zhan L, Featherstone JD, Gansky SA, et al: Antibacterial treatment needed for severe early childhood caries, *J Public Health Dent* 3:174–179, 2006.

CHAPTER 34

Aiken JJ, Oldham KT: Inguinal hernias. In Kliegman RM, Behrman RE, Jenson HB, et al: *Nelson textbook of pediatrics,* ed 18, Philadelphia, 2007, Saunders.

American Academy of Family Physicians (AAFP), American Academy of Pediatrics (AAP), American College of Sports Medicine (ACSM), et al: Preparticipation physical evaluation. In Bernhardt DT, Roberts WO, editors: *Preparticipation physical evaluation,* ed 4, Elk Grove Village, IL, 2010, AAP.

American Academy of Pediatrics (AAP): The diagnosis, treatment, and evaluation of the initial urinary tract infection in febrile infants and young children. In *Pediatric clinical practice guidelines and policies: a compendium of evidence-based research for pediatric practice,* ed 7, Elk Grove Village, IL, 2007, AAP.

American Academy of Pediatrics (AAP): Committee on Practice and Ambulatory Care: Recommendations for preventive pediatric health care, *Pediatrics* 105(3):645–646, 2000. reaffirmed 2007. Available at http://aappolicy.aappublications.org/cgi/content/full/pediatrics;105/3/645. Accessed May 30, 2010.

American Academy of Pediatrics (AAP): Antimicrobial therapy. In Pickering LK, Baker CJ, Kimberlin DW, et al, editors: *The Red Book: 2009 report of the committee on infectious disease,* ed 28, Elk Grove Village, IL, 2009, AAP.

American Academy of Pediatrics (AAP), Subcommittee on Urinary Tract Infection, Steering Committee on Quality Improvement and Management: Urinary tract infection: clinical practice guideline for the diagnosis and management of the initial UTI in febrile infants and children 2 to 24 months. Pediatrics 128(9):595–610, 2011. doi:10.1542/peds. 2011–1330.

Bloom TL, Kolon TF: Gross hematuria in a healthy adolescent, *Clin Adv* 8:99–100, 2005.

Bressan S, Andreola B, Zucchetta P, et al: Procalcitonin as a predictor of renal scarring in infants and young children, *Pediatr Nephrol* 24(6):1199–1204, 2009.

Cataldi L, Zaffanello M, Gnarra M, et al: Urinary tract infection in the newborn and the infant: state of the art, *J Matern Fetal Neonat Med* 23(Suppl 3):90–93, 2010.

Chang SL, Shortliffe LD: Pediatric urinary tract infections, *Pediatr Clin North Am* 53(3):379–400, 2006.

Custer JW, Rau RE: *The Harriet Lane handbook,* ed 18, Philadelphia, 2009, Elsevier.

Dai B, Liu Y, Jia J, et al: Long-term antibiotics for the prevention of recurrent urinary tract infection in children: a systematic review and meta-analysis, *Arch Dis Child* 95(7):499–508, 2009.

Davis ID, Avner ED: Conditions particularly associated with hematuria. In Kliegman RM, Behrman RE, Jenson HB, et al, editors: *Nelson textbook of pediatrics,* ed 18, Philadelphia, 2007, Saunders.

Dell KM, Avner ED: Tubular disorders. In Kliegman RM, Behrman RE, Jenson HB, et al, editors: *Nelson textbook of pediatrics,* ed 18, Philadelphia, 2007, Saunders.

Edmunds MW, Mayhew MS: *Pharmacology for the primary care provider,* St Louis, 2009, Mosby.

Elder JS: Anomalies of the penis and urethra. In Kliegman RM, Behrman RE, Jenson HB, et al, editors: *Nelson textbook of pediatrics*, ed 18, Philadelphia, 2007a, Saunders.

Elder JS: Disorders and anomalies of the scrotal contents. In Kliegman RM, Behrman RE, Jenson HB, et al, editors: *Nelson textbook of pediatrics*, ed 18, Philadelphia, 2007b, Saunders.

Elder JS: Urinary lithiasis. In Kliegman RM, Behrman RE, Jenson HB, et al: *Nelson textbook of pediatrics*, ed 18, Philadelphia, 2007c, Saunders.

Elder JS: Urinary tract infections. In Kliegman RM, Behrman RE, Jenson HB, et al, editors: *Nelson textbook of pediatrics*, ed 18, Philadelphia, 2007d, Saunders.

Elder JS: Vesicoureteral reflux. In Kliegman RM, Behrman RE, Jenson HB, et al, editors: *Nelson textbook of pediatrics*, ed 18, Philadelphia, 2007e, Saunders.

Feld LG, Mattoo TK: Urinary tract infections and vesicoureteral reflux in infants and children, *Pediatr Rev* 31(11):451–463, 2010.

Fitzgerald A, Lee CW, Mori R: Antibiotics for treating uncomplicated urinary tract infections in children (Protocol), *Cochrane Database Syst Rev* 3:CD006857, 2009.

Fouzas S, Krikelli E, Vassilakos P, et al: DSMA scan for revealing vesicoureteral reflux in young children with urinary tract infection, *Pediatrics* 126(3):e513–e519, 2010.

Garin EH, Olavarria F, Garcia Nieto V, et al: Clinical significance of primary vesicoureteral reflux and urinary antibiotic prophylaxis after acute pyelonephritis: a multicenter, randomized, controlled study, *Pediatrics* 117(3):626–632, 2006.

Gatti JM, Murphy JP: Acute testicular disorders, *Pediatr Rev* 29(7):235–241, 2008.

Gholoum S, Baird R, Laberge JM, et al: Incarceration rates in pediatric inguinal hernia: do not trust the coding, *J Pediatr Surg* 45(5):1007–1011, 2010.

Gordillo R, Spitzer A: The nephrotic syndrome, *Pediatr Rev* 30(3):94–105, 2009.

Greenbaum LA, Mesrobian HG: Vesicoureteral reflux, *Pediatr Clin North Am* 53(3):413–427, 2006.

Hagan JF, Shaw JS, Duncan PM, editors: *Bright Futures: guidelines for health supervision of infants, children and adolescents*, ed 3, Elk Grove Village, IL, 2008, American Academy of Pediatrics.

Halverson L, Alper BS: Hematuria, *Clin Adv* 9(3):93–94, 2006.

Hannula A, Venhola M, Renko M, et al: Vesicoureteral reflux in children with suspected and proven urinary tract infection, *Pediatr Nephrol* 25(8):1463–1469, 2010.

Hodson EM, Willis NS, Craig JC: Corticosteroid therapy for nephrotic syndrome in children, *Cochrane Database Syst Rev* 4:CD001533, 2008a.

Hodson EM, Willis NS, Craig JC: Non-corticosteroid therapy for nephrotic syndrome in children, *Cochrane Database Syst Rev* 1:CD002290, 2008b.

Hutchings F, Jadresic L: GPs should evaluate all children following a UTI, *Practitioner* 254(1731):17–19, 21, 22, 2010.

Jaffe N, Huff V: Neoplasms of the kidney. In Kliegman RM, Behrman RE, Jenson HB, et al: *Nelson textbook of pediatrics*, ed 18, Philadelphia, 2007, Saunders.

Kallen RJ: Renal tubular acidosis. In McInerny TK, Adam HM, Campbell DE, et al, editors: *AAP textbook of pediatric care*, Elk Grove Village, IL, 2009, American Academy of Pediatrics.

Kis E, Nyitrai A, Várkonyi I, et al: Voiding urosonography with second-generation contrast agent versus voiding cystourethrography, *Pediatr Nephrol* 25(11):2289–2293, 2010.

Koski ME, Makari JH, Adams MC, et al: Infant communicating hydroceles—do they need immediate repair of might some clinically resolve? *J Pediatr Surg* 45(3):590–593, 2010.

Lee MD, Lin CC, Huang FY, et al: Screening young children with first febrile urinary tract infection for high–grade vesicoureteral reflux with renal ultrasound scanning and technetium-99m-labeled dimercaptosuccinic acid scanning, *J Pediatr* 154(6):797–802, 2009.

Lennon R, Watson L, Webb JA: Nephrotic syndrome in children, *Paediatr Child Health* 20(1):36–42, 2010.

Long E, Vince J: Evidence behind the WHO guidelines: hospital care for children: what are appropriate methods of urine collection in UTI? *J Trop Pediatr* 53(4):221–224, 2007.

Lum GM: Kidney and urinary tract. In Hay WW, Levin MJ, Sondheimer JM, et al, editors: *Current pediatric diagnosis and treatment*, ed 19, New York, 2009, McGraw-Hill.

Mahesh S, Woroniecki: Proteinuria. In McInerny TK, Adam HM, Campbell DE, et al, editors: *AAP textbook of pediatric care*, Elk Grove Village, IL, 2009, American Academy of Pediatrics.

Massengill SF: Hematuria, *Pediatr Rev* 29(10):342–348, 2008.

Menezes M, Puri P: Familial vesicoureteral reflux: is screening beneficial? *J Urol* 182(4 Suppl):1673–1677, 2009.

Michael M, Hodson EM, Craig JC, et al: Short versus standard duration oral antibiotic therapy for acute urinary tract infection in children, *Cochrane Database Syst Rev* 1:CD003966, 2003.

National Collaborating Center for Women's and Children's Health: *Urinary tract infection in children: diagnosis, treatment, and long-term management*. NICE clinical guideline 54, London, 2007, National Institute for Health and Clinical Excellence (NICE).

North AC, Gearhart JP: Hypospadias, epispadias and cryptorchidism. In McInerny TK, Adam HM, Campbell DE, et al, editors: *AAP textbook of pediatric care*, Elk Grove Village, IL, 2009, American Academy of Pediatrics.

Nguyen HT: Obstructive uropathy and vesicoureteral reflux. In McInerny TK, Adam HM, Campbell DE, et al, editors: *AAP textbook of pediatric care*, Elk Grove Village, IL, 2009, American Academy of Pediatrics.

Palmer LS: Scrotal swelling and pain. In McInerny TK, Adam HM, Campbell DE, et al, editors: *AAP textbook of pediatric care*, Elk Grove Village, IL, 2009, American Academy of Pediatrics.

Peters CA, Skooj SJ, Arant BS Jr, et al: Summary of the American Urological Association guideline on management of primary vesicoureteral reflux in children, *J Urol* 184(3):1134–1144, 2010.

Pileggi F, de O, Vincente YA: Phimotic ring topical corticoid cream (0.1% mometasone furoate) treatment in children, *J Pediatr Surg* 42(10):1749–1752, 2007.

Pohl A: Modes of administration of antibiotics for symptomatic severe urinary tract infections, *Cochrane Database Syst Rev* 4:CD003237, 2007.

Quigley R: Diagnosis of urinary tract infections in children, *Curr Opin Pediatr* 21(2):194–198, 2009.

Schnitzer JJ: Hernias and hydroceles. In Burg FD, Polin RA, Gershon AA, et al, editors: *Current pediatric therapy*, ed 18, Philadelphia, 2006, Saunders.

Sekhar DL, Wang L, Hollenbeak CS, et al: A cost-effectiveness analysis of screening urine dipsticks in well-child care, *Pediatrics* 125(4):660–663, 2010.

Shaikh N, Morone NE, Bost JE: Prevalence of urinary tract infection in childhood: a meta-analysis, *Pediatr Infect Dis J* 27(4):302–308, 2008.

Sobel JD, Kaye D: Urinary tract infection. In Mandell GL, Bennett JE, Dolin R, editors: *Mandell, Douglas, and Bennett's principles and practice of infectious diseases*, ed 7, Philadelphia, 2009, Churchill Livingstone.

Tan JM: Nephrology. In Custer JW, Rau RE, editors: *The Harriet Lane handbook*, ed 18, Philadelphia, 2009, Elsevier.

U.S. Preventive Services Task Force (USPSTF): *Healthcare guideline: preventive services for children and adolescents*, 2009, National Guideline Clearinghouse at Agency for Healthcare Research and Quality (AHRQ). Available at www.ahrq.gov/clinic/tfchfocus.htm. Accessed April 24, 2010.

VanDeVoorde RG, Bissler JJ: Hematuria and proteinuria. In Burg FD, Polin RA, Gershon AA, et al, editors: *Current pediatric therapy*, ed 18, Philadelphia, 2006, Elsevier.

Varade WS: Nephritis. In McInerny TK, Adam HM, Campbell DE, et al, editors: *AAP textbook of pediatric care*, Elk Grove Village, IL, 2009, American Academy of Pediatrics.

Vogt BA, Avner ED: Conditions particularly associated with proteinuria. In Kliegman RM, Behrman RE, Jenson HB, et al, editors: *Nelson textbook of pediatrics*, ed 18, Philadelphia, 2007, Saunders.

CHAPTER 35

Abma JC, Martinez GM, Mosher WP, et al: Teenagers in the U.S.: sexual activity, contraceptive use, and childbearing, 2002, National Center for Health Statistics, *Vital Health Stat* 23(24), 2004. Available at www.cdc.gov/nchs/data/series/sr_23/sr23_024.pdf. Accessed Sep 6, 2010.

American College of Obstetricians and Gynecologists (ACOG): Committee opinion, endometriosis in adolescents, *Obstet Gynecol* 105:921–927, 2005.

American College of Obstetricians and Gynecologists (ACOG): Committee opinion, cervical cancer in adolescents: Screening, evaluation, and management, *Obstet Gynecol* 116(2):469–472, 2010a.

American College of Obstetricians and Gynecologists (ACOG): Committee opinion, the initial reproductive health visit, *Obstet Gynecol* 116(1):240–243, 2010b.

Blythe MJ: Gonorrhea. In Neinstein L, editor: *Adolescent health care: a practical guide*, ed 5, Philadelphia, 2008, Lippincott Williams & Wilkins.

Braverman PK: Dysmenorrhea and premenstrual syndrome. In Neinstein L, editor: *Adolescent health care: a practical guide*, ed 5, Philadelphia, 2008, Lippincott Williams & Wilkins.

Centers for Disease Control and Prevention (CDC): Sexually transmitted diseases: treatment guidelines, *MMWR Morb Mortal Wkly Rep* 55(RR-11):i–100, 2006.

Centers for Disease Control and Prevention (CDC): *Sexually transmitted disease surveillance, 2008*, Atlanta, 2009, U.S. Department of Health and Human Services. Available at www.cdc.gov/std/stats08/surv2008-Complete.pdf. Accessed Sep 1, 2010.

Centers for Disease Control and Prevention (CDC): *Sexually transmitted diseases treatment guidelines*, 2010a, U.S. Department of Health and Human Services. Available at www.cdc.gov/std/treatment/2010/STD-Treatment-2010-RR5912.pdf. Accessed Apr 15, 2011.

Centers for Disease Control and Prevention (CDC): Youth risk behavior surveillance—United States, 2009, *MMWR Morb Mortal Wkly Rep* 59(SS-5):1–142, 2010b.

Centers for Disease Control and Prevention (CDC): *Adolescent pregnancy and childbirth-United States, 1991-2008*, Atlanta, 2011, U.S. Department of Health and Human Services. Available at http://www.cdc.gov/mmwr/preview/mmwrhtml/su6001a23.htm?s_cid=su6001a23_w#tab. Accessed Apr 15, 2011.

Chen C, Cho SI, Damokosh AI, et al: Prospective study of exposure to environmental tobacco smoke and dysmenorrhea, *Environ Health Perspect* 108:1019–1022, 2000.

Cox JE: Teenage pregnancy. In Neinstein LS, editor: *Adolescent health care, a practical guide*, ed 5, Philadelphia, 2008, Lippincott Williams & Wilkins.

Dryfoos JG: Thirty years in pursuit of the magic bullet, *J Adolesc Health* 23:338–343, 1998.

Durain D: Primary dysmenorrhea: assessment and management update, *J Midwifery Womens Health* 49:520–528, 2004.

Emans SJ: Amenorrhea in the adolescent. In Emans SJ, Laufer MR, Goldstein DP, editors: *Pediatric and adolescent gynecology*, ed 5, Philadelphia, 2005a, Lippincott Williams & Wilkins.

Emans SJ: Contraception. In Emans SJ, Laufer MR, Goldstein DP, editors: *Pediatric and adolescent gynecology*, ed 5, Philadelphia, 2005b, Lippincott Williams & Wilkins.

Emans SJ: Dysfunctional uterine bleeding. In Emans SJ, Laufer MR, Goldstein DP, editors: *Pediatric and adolescent gynecology*, ed 5, Philadelphia, 2005c, Lippincott Williams & Wilkins.

Emans SJ: Vulvovaginal problems in the prepubertal child. In Emans SJ, Laufer MR, Goldstein DP, editors: *Pediatric and adolescent gynecology*, ed 5, Philadelphia, 2005d, Lippincott Williams & Wilkins.

Gupta N, Corrados S, Goldstein M: Hormonal contraceptives for the adolescent, *Pediatr Rev* 29(11):386–397, 2008.

Hagan JF, Shaw JS, Duncan PM: *Bright futures: guidelines for health supervision of infants, children, and adolescents*, ed 3, Elk Grove Village, IL, 2008, American Academy of Pediatrics.

Hamel-Teillac D: Vulvo-vaginal disorders. Pediatric and adolescent gynecology. Evidence-based clinical practice, *Endocr Dev* 7:39–56, 2004.

Harel Z: In training, approach to the adolescent girl as she transits from irregular to regular menstrual cycles, *J Pediatr Adolesc Gynecol* 18:193–200, 2005.

Hatcher RA, Trussell J, Nelson AL, et al: *Contraceptive technology*, ed 19, New York, 2007, Ardent.

Holland-Hall C, Hewill G, Breech L: Tips for clinicians, the 'well girl' exam, *J Pediatr Adolesc Gynecol* 18:289–291, 2005.

Kahn JA, Lan D, Kahn RS: Sociodemographic factors associated with high-risk human papillomavirus infection, *Obstet Gynecol* 110(1):87–95, 2007.

Kaplowitz PB, Oberfield SE: Reexamination of the age limit for defining when puberty is precocious in girls in the United States: implications for evaluation and treatment, *Pediatrics* 104:936–941, 1999.

Klein JD: Adolescent pregnancy: current trends and issues, *Pediatrics* 116:281–286, 2005.

Laufer MR, Goldstein DP: Gynecologic pain: dysmenorrhea, acute and chronic pelvic pain, endometriosis, and premenstrual syndrome. In Emans SJ, Laufer MR, Goldstein DP, editors: *Pediatric and adolescent gynecology*, ed 5, Philadelphia, 2005, Lippincott Williams & Wilkins.

Levine SB: In training, dysfunctional uterine bleeding in adolescents, *J Pediatr Adolesc Gynecol* 19:49–51, 2006.

Lohr PA: Barrier contraceptives and spermicides. In Neinstein LS, editor: *Adolescent health care, a practical guide*, ed 5, Philadelphia, 2008, Lippincott Williams & Wilkins.

Mama ST: Dysmenorrhea and irregular uterine bleeding, *Pediatr News* 44(8):40, 2010.

Mansfield JM, Neinstein LS: Abnormal growth and development. In Neinstein L, editor: *Adolescent health care: a practical guide*, ed 5, Philadelphia, 2008, Lippincott Williams & Wilkins.

Matytsina LA, Zoloto EV, Sinenko LV, et al: Dysfunctional uterine bleeding in adolescents: concepts of pathophysiology and management, *Prim Care* 33:503–515, 2006.

Meininger E, Remafedi G: Gay, lesbian, bisexual and transgender adolescents. In Neinstein L, editor: *Adolescent health care: a practical guide*, ed 5, Philadelphia, 2008, Lippincott Williams & Wilkins.

Mitan LA, Slap GB: Dysfunctional uterine bleeding. In Neinstein LS, editor: *Adolescent health care, a practical guide*, ed 5, Philadelphia, 2008, Lippincott Williams & Wilkins.

The National Campaign to Prevent Teen and Unwanted Pregnancy: *Ten tips for parents to help their children avoid teen pregnancy*, 2008. Available at www.thenationalcampaign.org/resources/pdf/pubs/10Tips_final.pdf. Accessed Sep 6, 2010.

Nelson AL, Neinstein LS: Combination hormonal contraceptives. In Neinstein LS, editor: *Adolescent health care, a practical guide*, ed 5, Philadelphia, 2008, Lippincott Williams & Wilkins.

Nicoletti AM: Teen pregnancy. In Emans SJ, Laufer MR, Goldstein DP, editors: *Pediatric and adolescent gynecology*, ed 5, Philadelphia, 2005, Lippincott Williams & Wilkins.

Nield LS: Labial Adhesions. In McInery TK, editor: *Textbook of pediatric care*, Washington, DC, 2009, American Academy of Pediatrics.

Proctor ML, Farquhar CM: Dysmenorrhoea, *Clin Evid* 12:2524–2547, 2004.

Shrier LA: Bacterial sexually transmitted infections: gonorrhea, chlamydia, pelvic inflammatory disease, and syphilis. In Emans SJ, Laufer MR, Goldstein DP, editors: *Pediatric and adolescent gynecology*, ed 5, Philadelphia, 2005, Lippincott Williams & Wilkins.

Shrier LA: Pelvic inflammatory disease. In Neinstein LS, editor: *Adolescent health care, a practical guide*, ed 5, Philadelphia, 2008, Lippincott Williams & Wilkins.

Speroff L, Darney PD: *A clinical guide for contraception*, ed 4, Philadelphia, 2005, Lippincott Williams & Wilkins.

Speroff L, Fritz MA: *Clinical gynecologic endocrinology and infertility*, ed 7, Philadelphia, 2005, Lippincott Williams & Wilkins.

Speroff L, Glass RH, Kase NG: *Clinical gynecologic endocrinology and infertility*, Baltimore, 1973, Williams & Wilkins.

Sugar NF, Graham EA: Common gynecologic problems in prepubertal girls, *Pediatr Rev* 27:213–222, 2006.

Syed TS, Braverman PK: Vaginitis in adolescents, *Adolesc Med Clin* 15:235–251, 2004.

U.S. Department of Health and Human Services: *Healthy people 2010: understanding and improving health,* ed 2, 2000. Available at www.healthypeople.gov/Document/tableofcontents.htm#topofpage. Accessed Sep 6, 2010.

U.S. Department of Health and Human Services: *Healthy people 2010: 2009 draft objectives,* 2009. Available at www.healthypeople.gov/hp2020/Objectives/TopicAreas.aspx. Accessed Mar 8, 2010.

U.S. Preventive Services Task Force: *Guide to clinical preventive services,* 2009. Available at www.ahrq.gov/clinic/pocketgd09/pocketgd09.pdf. Accessed Sep 4, 2010.

Wilson GR, Haddad JE, Haddad CJ: Amenorrhea: common causes and evaluation, *Comp Ther* 31:270–278, 2005.

Wong CL, Farquhar C, Roberts H, Proctor M: Oral contraceptive pill for primary dysmenorrhoea, *Cochrane Database Syst Rev*, 2009. Available at www2.cochrane.org/reviews/en/ab002120.html. Accessed Sep 1, 2010.

World Health Organization, Reproductive Health and Research: *Medical eligibility criteria for contraceptive use,* ed 4, Geneva, 2009. Available at www.who.int/reproductivehealth/publications/family_planning/9789241563888/en/index.html. Accessed Feb 2, 2010.

CHAPTER 36

American Academy of Dermatology: *Sun protection for children,* 2010. Available at www.aad.org/public/publications/pamphlets/sun_sunprotection.html. Accessed Jan 12, 2011.

American Academy of Pediatrics (AAP): *Red Book: report of the committee on infectious diseases,* ed 27, Elk Grove Village, IL, 2009, American Academy of Pediatrics.

Aronson PL, Florin TA: Pediatric dermatologic emergencies: a case-based approach for the pediatrician, *Pediatr Ann* 38(2):109–116, 2009.

Baron J, Levine N: *Acanthosis nigricans,* updated Oct, 2006. Available at www.emedicine.com. Accessed Jan 12, 2011.

Berk DR, Bayliss SJ: MRSA, staphylococcal scalded skin syndrome, and other cutaneous bacterial emergencies, *Pediatr Ann* 39(10):627–633, 2010.

Bloch MH: Trichotillomania across the life span, *J Am Acad Child Adolesc Psychiatry* 48(9):879–883, 2009.

Cole C, Gazewood J: Diagnosis and treatment of impetigo, *Am Fam Physician* 75(6):859–864, 2007.

Connelly EA, Schachter L: Seborrheic dermatitis. In McInerny TK, Adam HM, Campbell DE, et al: *Textbook of pediatric care*, Elk Grove Village, IL, 2009, American Academy of Pediatrics.

Connelly EA, Friedlander SF: Fungal infections of the skin, hair, and nails. In Burg FD, Ingelfinger JR, Polin RA, et al, editors: *Current pediatric therapy,* ed 18, Philadelphia, 2006, Saunders.

Diamantis SA, Morrell DS, Burkhart CN: Pediatric infestations, *Pediatr Ann* 38(6):326–332, 2009.

Dyer JA: Childhood viral exanthems, *Pediatr Ann* 36(1):21–29, 2007.

Fisher RG, Chen C, Williams JV: Bacterial skin infections. In McInerny TK, Adam HM, Campbell DE, et al, editors: *Textbook of pediatric care*, Elk Grove Village, IL, 2009, American Academy of Pediatrics.

Frankowski BL, Bocchini JA Jr: AAP Council on School Health and Committee on Infectious Diseases: Head lice, *Pediatrics* 126(2):392–403, 2010.

Gerber MA: Group A streptococcus. In Kliegman RM, Behrman RE, Jenson HB, et al, editors: *Nelson textbook of pediatrics,* ed 18, Philadelphia, 2007, Saunders, pp 1135–1140.

Ghali FE: Allergic contact dermatitis. In Burg FD, Ingelfinger JR, Polin RA, et al, editors: *Current pediatric therapy,* ed 18, Philadelphia, 2006, Saunders.

Goates BM, Atkin JS, Wilding KG, et al: An effective nonchemical treatment for head lice: a lot of hot air, *Pediatrics* 118(5):1962–1970, 2006.

Koning S, van der Wouden JC, Chosidow O, et al: Efficacy and safety of retapamulin ointment as treatment of impetigo: randomized double-blind multicentre placebo-controlled trial, *Br J Dermatol* 158(5):1077–1082, 2008.

Leung AK, Eneli I, Davies HD: Necrotizing fasciitis in children, *Pediatr Ann* 37(10):704–710, 2008.

Liptak GS: Diaper rash. In McInerny TK, Adam HM, Campbell DE, et al, editors: *Textbook of pediatric care*, Elk Grove Village, IL, 2009, American Academy of Pediatrics.

Lyon VB: Dermatology. In Marcdante KJ, Kliegman RM, Jenson HB, et al, editors: *Nelson essentials of pediatrics,* ed 6, Philadelphia, 2011, Saunders.

Mayers LM, Chiffriller SH: Body art (piercing and tattooing) among undergraduate university students: "then and now," *J Adolesc Health* 42(2):201–203, 2008.

Mikula C: Balneo phototherapy for psoriasis: modern application of an age-old treatment, *Adv Nurse Pract* 11(1):53–56, 2003.

Morelli J: Disorders of the mucus membranes. In Kliegman RM, Behrman RE, Jenson HB, et al: *Nelson textbook of pediatrics*, ed 18, Philadelphia, 2007, Saunders, pp 2734–2736.

National Pediculosis Association: *Treatment*, 2009. Available at www.headlice.org. Accessed Dec 23, 2010.

Newell BD, Horii KA: Cutaneous drug reactions in children, *Pediatr Ann* 39(10):618–625, 2010.

Paller AS, Mancini AJ: *Hurwitz clinical pediatric dermatology: a textbook of skin disorders of children and adolescence*, ed 4, Philadelphia, 2011, Elsevier.

Parish LC, Parish JL: Retapamulin: a new topical antibiotic for the treatment of uncomplicated skin infections, *Drugs Today* 44(2):91–102, 2008.

Patel T, Ishiuji Y, Yosipovitch G: Menthol: a refreshing look at this ancient compound, *J Am Acad Dermatol* 57(5):873–878, 2007.

Poindexter GB, Burkhart CN, Morrell DS: Therapies for pediatric seborrheic dermatitis, *Pediatr Ann* 38(6):333–338, 2009.

Putgen C: Traction folliculitis and traction alopecia: recognition and treatment, *Contemp Pediatr* 25(10)(Suppl 2–3), 2008.

Taketomo CK, Hodding JH, Kraus DM: *Pediatric dosage handbook*, ed 17, Hudson, OH, 2011, Lexi-Comp.

Theos A: Diagnosis and management of superficial cutaneous fungal infections in children, *Pediatr Ann* 36(1):46–54, 2007.

Thielitz A, Gollnick H: Overview of new therapeutic developments for acne, *Expert Rev Dermatol* 4(1):55–65, 2009.

Treat J: Stevens-Johnson syndrome and toxic epidermal necrolysis, *Pediatr Ann* 39(10):667–669, 2010. 672–674.

Weinberg JM, Tyring SK: Retapamulin: an antibacterial with a novel mode of action in an age of emerging resistance to Staphylococcus aureus, *J Drugs Dermatol* 9(10):1198–1204, 2010.

Weston WL, Lane AT, Morelli JG: *Color textbook of pediatric dermatology*, ed 4, St Louis, 2007, Mosby.

Yang LP, Kearn SJ: Spotlight on retapamulin in impetigo and other uncomplicated superficial skin infections, *Am J Clin Dermatol* 9(6):411–413, 2008.

CHAPTER 37

Adler B: *Imaging slipped femoral capital epiphysis*, 2008. Updated May 2011. Available at http://emedicine.medscape.com/article/413810-print. Accessed Jan 7, 2012.

Atalar H, Sayli U, Yavuz Y, et al: Indicators of successful use of the Pavlik harness in infants with developmental hip dysplasia of the hip, *Int Orthop* 31:145–150, 2007.

Beaty J: Congenital and developmental anomalies of the hip and pelvis. In Canale ST, Beaty JH, editors: *Campbell's operative orthopaedics*, ed 11, Philadelphia, 2007, Elsevier.

Benjamin H, Hang B: Common acute upper extremity injuries in sports, *Clin Pediatr Emerg Med* 8(1):15–30, 2007.

Bernstein R, Cozen H: Evaluation of back pain in children and adolescent, *Am Fam Physician* 76(11):1669–1676, 2007.

Boyd A, Benjamin H, Asplund C: Principles of casting and splinting, *Am Fam Physician* 79(1):16–22, 2009a.

Boyd A, Benjamin H, Asplund C: Splints and casts: indications and methods, *Am Fam Physician* 80(5):491–499, 2009b.

Brenner J, the Council of Sports Medicine and Fitness: Overuse injuries, overtraining, and burnout in child and adolescent athletes, *Pediatrics* 119(6):1242–1246, 2007.

Bui-Mansfield L, Youngberg R: *Baker cyst*, 2009. Available at http://emedicine.medscape.com/article/387399-print. Accessed Jan 7, 2012.

Canale ST, Beaty J: Muscular dystrophy. In Canale ST, Beaty JH, editors: *Campbell's operative orthopaedics*, ed 11, Philadelphia, 2007, Elsevier.

Chang A: *Osgood-Schlatter disease in emergency medicine*, 2010. Available at http://emedicine.medscape.com/article/827380-print. Accessed Jan 7, 2012.

Dolan M, Waters P: Fractures and dislocation of the forearm, wrist and hand. In Green NE, Swiontkowski MF, editors: *Skeletal trauma in children*, ed 4, Philadelphia, 2008, Saunders.

Duderstadt KG, Schapiro NA: Musculoskeletal system. In Duderstadt KG, editor: *Pediatric physical examination: an illustrated handbook*, Philadelphia, 2006, Mosby.

Garry J: Pediatric costochondritis. eMedicine, *Pediatrics*, 2010. Available at http://emedicine.medscape.com/article/1006486. Accessed Oct. 22, 2010.

Gholve PA, Hosalkar HS, Wells L: Common fractures. In Kliegman RM, Behrman RE, Jenson HB, et al, editors: *Nelson textbook of pediatrics*, ed 18, Philadelphia, 2007, Saunders.

Green N, Swiontkowski M: Differences between pediatric and adult fracture healing. In Green N, editor: *Skeletal trauma in children*, ed 4, Philadelphia, 2008, Saunders.

Harris G: *Legg-Calve-Perthes disease*, 2009. Available at http://emedicine.medscape.com/article/1248267-print. Accessed Oct 22, 2010.

Hart E, Grottkau B, Albright M: Slipped capital femoral epiphysis: don't miss this pediatric hip disorder, *Nurse Pract* 32(3):14–21, 2007.

Hosalkar H, Gholve P, Wells L: Torsional and angular deformities. In Kliegman RM, Behrman RE, Jenson HB, et al, editors: *Nelson textbook of pediatrics*, ed 18, Philadelphia, 2007a, Saunders.

Hosalkar H, Horn D, Friedman JE, et al: The hip. In Kliegman RM, Behrman RE, Jenson HB, et al, editors: *Nelson textbook of pediatrics*, ed 18, Philadelphia, 2007b, Saunders.

Hosalkar H, Spiegel D, Davidson R: The foot and toes. In Kliegman RM, Behrman RE, Jenson HB, et al, editors: *Nelson textbook of pediatrics*, ed 18, Philadelphia, 2007c, Saunders.

Hosalkar H, Wells L: Growth and development. In Kliegman RM, Behrman RE, Jenson HB, et al, editors: *Nelson textbook of pediatrics*, ed 18, Philadelphia, 2007, Saunders.

Jandial S, Myers A, Wise E, et al: Doctors likely to encounter children with musculoskeletal complaints have low confidence in their clinical skills, *J Pediatr* 154(2):267–271, 2009.

Joshi A: *Osgood-Schlatter disease imaging*, 2010. Updated May 2011. Available at http://emedicine.medscape.com/article/411842-print. Accessed Jan 7, 2012.

Khan A, Seriki D, Hutchinson S, et al: *Legg-Calve-Perthes disease*, 2008. Updated May 2011. Available at http://emedicine.medscape.com/article/410482-print. Accessed Jan 7, 2012.

Koifman A, Nevo O, Toe A, et al: Diagnostic approach to prenatally diagnosed limb abnormalities, *Ultrasound Clin* 3(4):595–608, 2008.

Legano L, McHugh M, Palusci V: Child abuse and neglect, *Curr Prob Pediatr Adolesc Health Care* 39(2):1–26, 2009.

Moore W, Smith TH: *Salter-Harris fracture imaging*, 2009. Available at http://emedicine.medscape.com/article/412956-overview. Accessed Jan 7, 2012.

Owens J: Sleep medicine. In Kliegman RM, Behrman RE, Jenson HB, et al, editors: *Nelson textbook of pediatrics*, ed 18, Philadelphia, 2007, Saunders.

Sabharwal S, Bhrens F: Fractures with soft tissue injuries. In Green N, editor: *Skeletal trauma in children*, ed 4, Philadelphia, 2008, Saunders.

Sawyer J, Kapoor M: The limping child: a systemic approach to diagnosis, *Am Fam Physician* 79(3):215–224, 2009.

Sawyer JR, Drendel AL: Rotational orthopedic problems of the extremities. In Burg FD, Ingelfinger JR, Polin RA, et al: *Current pediatric therapy*, ed 18, Philadelphia, 2006, Saunders.

Shipman S, Helfand M, Moyer V, et al: Screening for developmental dysplasia of the hip: a systemic literature review for the US Preventive Services Task Force, *Pediatrics* 11:e557–e567, 2006.

Smith JR: The role of bracing, casting, and vertical expandable prosthetic titanium rib for the treatment of infantile idiopathic scoliosis: a single-institution experience with 31 consecutive patients, *J Neurosurg Spine* 11(1):3–8, 2009.

Soprano J, Fuchs S: Common overuse injuries in pediatric and adolescent athlete, *Clin Pediatr Emerg Med* 8(1):7–14, 2007.

Spiegel D, Hosalkar H, Dormans: The spine. In Kliegman RM, Behrman RE, Jenson HB, et al, editors: *Nelson textbook of pediatrics*, ed 18, Philadelphia, 2007, Saunders.

Stevens P: *Genu valgum, Pediatrics*, 2010. Available at http://emedicine.medscape.com/article/1259772-print. Accessed Oct. 22, 2010.

Torres M, DiPietro M: Developmental dysplasia of the hip, *Ultrasound Clin* 4:445–455, 2009.

Uziel Y, Hashkes PJ: Growing pains in children, *Pediatr Rheumatol Online J* 5:5, 2007. Available at http://www.ncbi.nlm.nih.gov/pmc/articles/PMC1869025/?tool=pubmed. Accessed April 6, 2011.

Wynshaw-Boris A, Biesecker L: Dysmorphology. In Kliegman RM, Behrman RE, Jenson HB, et al, editors: *Nelson textbook of pediatrics*, ed 18, Philadelphia, 2007, Saunders.

Zafeirious D, Psychogious K: Obstetrical brachial plexus palsy, *Pediatr Neurol* 38(4):235–242, 2008.

CHAPTER 38

Adams-Chapman I, Stoll BJ: Nervous system disorders. In Kliegman RM, Behrman RE, Jenson HB, et al, editors: *Nelson textbook of pediatrics*, ed 18, Philadelphia, 2007, Saunders.

American Academy of Pediatrics (AAP): Selecting and using the most appropriate car safety seats for growing children: guidelines for counseling parents, *Pediatrics* 109:550–553, 2002.

American Academy of Pediatrics (AAP): Clinical practice guideline: management of hyperbilirubinemia in the newborn infant 35 or more weeks of gestation, *Pediatrics* 114:297–316, 2004.

American Academy of Pediatrics (AAP): The changing concept of sudden infant death syndrome: diagnostic coding shifts, controversies regarding the sleeping environment, and new variables to consider in reducing risk, *Pediatrics* 116:1245–1255, 2005.

American Academy of Pediatrics (AAP): The Apgar score, *Pediatrics* 117:1444–1447, 2006.

American Academy of Pediatrics (AAP): Recommendations for preventive pediatric health care, *Pediatrics* 120:1376, 2007.

American Academy of Pediatrics (AAP): AAP publications retired and reaffirmed, *Pediatrics* 123(1):188, 2009a.

American Academy of Pediatrics (AAP): *Red book: 2009 report of the committee on infectious diseases*, ed 28, Elk Grove Village, IL, 2009b, American Academy of Pediatrics.

American Academy of Pediatrics (AAP): *Where we stand: folic acid*. Available at www.healthychildren.org/English/ages-stages/prenatal/pages/Where-We-Stand-Folic-Acid.aspx. Accessed Sep 9, 2010.

Ater JL: Neuroblastoma. In Kliegman RM, Behrman RE, Jenson HB, et al, editors: *Nelson textbook of pediatrics*, ed 18, Philadelphia, 2007, Saunders.

Bauer CR, Shankaran S, Bada H, et al: The maternal lifestyle study: drug exposure during pregnancy and short-term maternal outcomes, *Am J Obstet Gynecol* 186:487–495, 2002.

Brady-Fryer B, Wiebe N, Lander JA: Pain relief for neonatal circumcision, *Cochrane Database Syst Rev* 18:CD004217, 2004.

Brown RE, Neu J: Necrotizing enterocolitis. In Burg FD, Ingelfinger J, Polin R, et al, editors: *Current pediatric therapy*, ed 18, Philadelphia, 2006, Saunders.

Centers for Disease Control and Prevention (CDC): Effectiveness in disease and injury prevention use of folic acid for prevention of spina bifida and other neural tube defects—1983-1991, *MMWR Morbid Mortal Wkly Rep* 40(30):513–516, 1991.

Centers for Disease Control and Prevention (CDC): Prevention of perinatal group B streptococcal disease: revised guidelines from CDC, *MMWR Morbid Mortal Wkly Rep* 51(RR-11):1–22, 2002.

Centers for Disease Control and Prevention (CDC): Sexually transmitted diseases guidelines, 2006, *MMWR Morbid Mortal Wkly Rep* 55(R-11):1–94, 2006.

Centers for Disease Control and Prevention (CDC): *Folic acid: recommendations.* Available at www.cdc.gov/ncbddd/folicacid/recommendations.html. Accessed Sep 8, 2010a.

Centers for Disease Control and Prevention (CDC): Recommended adult immunization schedule—United States, 2010, *MMWR Morbid Mortal Wkly Rep* 59:1–4, 2010b.

Cornwall R: Upper limb. In Kliegman RM, Behrman RE, Jenson HB, et al, editors: *Nelson textbook of pediatrics*, ed 18, Philadelphia, 2007, Saunders.

Custer JW, Rau RE: *The Harriet Lane handbook*, ed 18, Philadelphia, 2009, Elsevier.

Davis ID, Avner ED: Anatomic abnormalities associated with hematuria. In Kliegman RM, Behrman RE, Jenson HB, et al, editors: *Nelson textbook of pediatrics*, ed 18, Philadelphia, 2007, Saunders.

Dudell GG, Stoll BJ: Respiratory tract disorders. In Kliegman RM, Behrman RE, Jenson HB, et al: *Nelson textbook of pediatrics*, ed 18, Philadelphia, 2007, Saunders.

Ehrlich PF, Coran AG: Diaphragmatic hernia. In Kliegman RM, Behrman RE, Jenson HB, et al: *Nelson textbook of pediatrics*, ed 18, Philadelphia, 2007, Saunders.

Elder JS: Congenital anomalies and dysgenesis of the kidneys. In Kliegman RM, Behrman RE, Jenson HB, et al, editors: *Nelson textbook of pediatrics*, ed 18, Philadelphia, 2007, Saunders.

Fanaroff AA, Martin RJ: *Fanaroff & Martin's neonatal-perinatal medicine: diseases of the fetus and infant*, ed 8, Philadelphia, 2006, Mosby Yearbook.

Feldstein NA, Anderson RCE: Diagnosis and management of hydrocephalus. In Burg FD, Ingelfinger J, Polin R, et al, editors: *Current pediatric therapy*, ed 18, Philadelphia, 2006, Saunders.

Frank DA, Augustyn M, Knight WG, et al: Growth, development, and behavior in early childhood following prenatal cocaine exposure: a systematic review, *JAMA* 285:1613–1625, 2001.

Hagan JF, Shaw JS, Duncan PM, editors: *Bright futures: guidelines for health supervision of infants, children, and adolescents*, ed 3, Elk Grove Village, IL, 2008, American Academy of Pediatrics.

Hendricks-Munoz: Infants of diabetic mothers. In Burg FD, Ingelfinger J, Polin R, et al, editors: *Current pediatric therapy*, ed 18, Philadelphia, 2006, Saunders.

Hosalkar HS, Spiegel DA, Davidson RS: The foot and toes. In Kliegman RM, Behrman RE, Jenson HB, et al, editors: *Nelson textbook of pediatrics*, ed 18, Philadelphia, 2007, Saunders.

Hunt CE, Hauck FR: Sudden infant death syndrome. In Kliegman RM, Behrman RE, Jenson HB, et al, editors: *Nelson textbook of pediatrics*, ed 18, Philadelphia, 2007, Saunders.

Kinsman S, Johnston MV: Congenital anomalies of the central nervous system. In Kliegman RM, Behrman RE, Jenson HB, et al, editors: *Nelson textbook of pediatrics*, ed 18, Philadelphia, 2007, Saunders.

Klein MD, Thomas RP: Surgical conditions of the anus, rectum, and colon. In Kliegman RM, Behrman RE, Jenson HB, et al, editors: *Nelson textbook of pediatrics*, ed 18, Philadelphia, 2007, Saunders.

Lemnos JA, Lockwood CJ, editors: *Guidelines for perinatal care*, ed 6, Elk Grove Village, IL, 2008, American Academy of Pediatrics and American College of Obstetricians and Gynecologists.

Lin RL, Tinkle LL, Janniger CK: Skin care of the healthy newborn, *Cutis* 75:25–30, 2005.

Madden JM, Soumerai SB, Lieu TA, et al: Length-of-stay policies and ascertainment of postdischarge problems in newborns, *Pediatrics* 113:442–449, 2004.

Mahon BE, Rosenman MB, Kleiman MB: Maternal and infant use of erythromycin and other macrolide antibiotics as risk factors for infantile hypertrophic pyloric stenosis, *J Pediatr* 139:380–384, 2001.

McLeod R, Remington JS: Toxoplasmosis *(Toxoplasma gondii)*. In Kliegman RM, Behrman RE, Jenson HB, et al: *Nelson textbook of pediatrics*, ed 18, Philadelphia, 2007, Saunders.

Middlesworth W, Kadenhe-Chiweshe A: Neonatal intestinal obstruction. In Burg FD, Ingelfinger J, Polin R, et al: *Current pediatric therapy*, ed 18, Philadelphia, 2006, Saunders.

Myers MG, Seward JF, LaRussa PS: Varicella-zoster virus. In Kliegman RM, Behrman RE, Jenson HB, et al, editors: *Nelson textbook of pediatrics*, ed 18, Philadelphia, 2007, Saunders.

Orenstein S, Peters J, Khan S, et al: Embryology, anatomy & function of the esophagus. In Kliegman RM, Behrman RE, Jenson HB, et al, editors: *Nelson textbook of pediatrics*, ed 18, Philadelphia, 2007, Saunders.

Perlman JM: Intracranial hemorrhage in the newborn. In Burg FD, Ingelfinger J, Polin R, et al, editors: *Current pediatric therapy*, ed 18, Philadelphia, 2006, Saunders.

Piazza AJ, Stoll BJ: Digestive system disorders. In Kliegman RM, Behrman RE, Jenson HB, et al, editors: *Nelson textbook of pediatrics*, ed 18, Philadelphia, 2007, Saunders.

Remington JS, Klein J: *Infectious diseases of the fetus and newborn infant*, ed 6, Philadelphia, 2005, Elsevier.

Roberts D, Dalziel S: Antenatal corticosteroids for accelerating fetal lung maturation for women at risk of preterm birth, *Cochrane Database Syst Rev* 19:CD004454, 2006.

Singer LT, Minnes S, Sort E, et al: C. Cognitive outcomes of preschool children with prenatal cocaine exposure, *JAMA* 291:2448–2456, 2004.

Stoll BJ: The fetus and the neonatal infant: overview of mortality and morbidity. In Kliegman RM, Behrman RE, Jenson HB, et al, editors: *Nelson textbook of pediatrics*, ed 18, Philadelphia, 2007a, Saunders.

Stoll BJ: The fetus and the neonatal infant: the umbilicus. In Kliegman RM, Behrman RE, Jenson HB, et al, editors: *Nelson textbook of pediatrics*, ed 18, Philadelphia, 2007b, Saunders.

Stoll BJ: The fetus and the neonatal infant: metabolic disturbances. In Kliegman RM, Behrman RE, Jenson HB, et al, editors: *Nelson textbook of pediatrics*, ed 18, Philadelphia, 2007c, Saunders.

Suchy FJ: Cystic diseases of the biliary tract and liver. In Kliegman RM, Behrman RE, Jenson HB, et al, editors: *Nelson textbook of pediatrics*, ed 18, Philadelphia, 2007, Saunders.

Tinanoff N: The oral cavity. In Kliegman RM, Behrman RE, Jenson HB, et al, editors: *Nelson textbook of pediatrics*, ed 18, Philadelphia, 2007, Saunders.

Ulshen MH: Intestinal malformations. In Burg FD, Ingelfinger J, Polin R, et al, editors: *Current pediatric therapy*, ed 18, Philadelphia, 2006, Saunders.

U.S. Department of Health and Human Services: *Healthy People 2020 objectives*, Washington, DC. 2010. Available from www.healthypeople.gov/hp2020/default.asp. Accessed Feb 2010.

U.S. Preventive Services Task Force: *Guide to clinical preventive services*, 2009. Available from www.ahrq.gov/clinicpocketgd.htm. Accessed Feb 2010.

Vain NE, Szyld EG, Prudent LM, et al: Oropharyngeal and nasopharyngeal suctioning of meconium-stained neonates before delivery of their shoulders: multicentre, randomised controlled trial, *Lancet* 364:597–602, 2004.

Wyllie R: Intestinal atresia, stenosis, and malrotation. In Kliegman RM, Behrman RE, Jenson HB, et al editors: *Nelson textbook of pediatrics*, ed 18, Philadelphia, 2007, Saunders.

Zupan J, Garner P, Omari AA: Topical umbilical cord care at birth, *Cochrane Database Syst Rev* 3:CD001057, 2004.

CHAPTER 39

American Academy of Pediatrics (AAP) Committee on Infectious Diseases: Bite wounds. In Pickering LK, Baker CJ, Kimberlin DW, et al, editors: *2009 Red Book: report of the committee on infectious diseases*, ed 29, Elk Grove Village, IL, 2009, American Academy of Pediatrics.

Anderson AC: Injury-ankle. In Fleisher GR, Ludwig S, Silverman BK, et al, editors: *Textbook of pediatric emergency medicine*, ed 6, Philadelphia, 2010, Lippincott Williams & Wilkins, pp 328–336.

Antoon AY, Donovan MK: Burn injuries. In Kliegman RM, Behrman RE, Jenson HB, et al, editors: *Nelson textbook of pediatrics*, ed 18, Philadelphia, 2007, Saunders, pp 450–458.

Baddour LM: Overview of puncture wounds. In Sexton DJ, Baron EL, editors: *Up to date*, 2009. Available at www.uptodate.com. Accessed Feb 2, 2010.

Borse NN, Gilchrist J, Dellinger A, et al: *CDC childhood injury report: patterns of unintentional injuries among 0-19 year-olds in the United States, 2000-2006*, Atlanta, 2008, Centers for Disease Control and Prevention, National Center for Injury Prevention and Control.

Brook I: Management of human and animal bite wound infection, *Curr Infect Dis Rep* 11:389–395, 2009.

Burge MD, ten Napel SJC: Upper extremity trauma. In Baren JM, Rothrock SG, Brennan J, et al, editors: *Pediatric emergency medicine*, Philadelphia, 2008, Saunders.

Buttaravoli P: *Minor emergencies: splinters to fractures*, St Louis, 2007, Mosby.

Canty G: Pediatric sports injuries in the ED. In Strange GR, Ahrens W, Schafermeyer R, et al, editors: *Pediatric emergency medicine*, ed 3, New York, 2009, McGraw-Hill.

Centers for Disease Control and Prevention: *Heads Up: Facts for Physicians about Mild Traumatic Brain Injury*. Available online at http://www.cdc.gov/concussion/headsup/pdf/Facts_for_Physicians_booklet-a.pdf. Accessed Nov 29, 2010.

Christian CW, Blum NJ: Abuse and neglect. In Marcdante KJ, Kliegman RM, Jenson HB, et al, editors: *Nelson essentials of pediatrics*, ed 6, Philadelphia, 2011, Elsevier/Saunders, pp 84–90.

Cornwall R: Upper limb. In Kliegman RM, Behrman RE, Jenson HB, et al, editors: *Nelson textbook of pediatrics*, ed 18, Philadelphia, 2007, Saunders, pp 2826–2828.

Covar RA, Fleischer DM, Boguniewicz M: Allergic disorders. In Hay WH, Levin MJ, Sondheimer JM, et al, editors: *Current diagnosis & treatment: pediatrics*, ed 20, New York, 2011, McGraw Hill, pp 1054–1088.

Diaz JH: Recognition, management and prevention of *Hymenoptera* stings and allergic reactions in travelers, *J Travel Med* 16:357–364, 2009.

Dowling S, Spooner CH, Liang Y, et al: Accuracy of Ottawa ankle rules to exclude fractures of the ankle and midfoot in children: a meta-analysis, *Acad Emerg Med* 16:277–287, 2009.

Elston DM: Tick bites and skin rashes, *Curr Opin Infect Dis* 23:132–138, 2010.

Ewald MB, Baum CR: Environmental emergencies. In Fleisher GR, Ludwig S, Silverman BK, editors: *Synopsis of pediatric emergency medicine*, ed 6, Philadelphia, 2010, Lippincott Williams & Wilkins, pp 783–804.

Faul M, Xu L, Wald MM, et al: *Traumatic brain injury in the United States: emergency department visits, hospitalizations and deaths, 2002-2006*, Atlanta, 2010, Centers for Disease Control and Prevention, National Center for Injury Prevention and Control.

Garcia-Gubern CF, Colon-Rolon L, Bond MC: Essential concepts of wound management, *Emerg Med Clin North Am* 28:951–967, 2010.

Ginsburg CM: Animal and human bites. In Kliegman RM, Behrman RE, Jenson HB, et al, editors: *Nelson textbook of pediatrics*, ed 18, Philadelphia, 2007, Saunders, pp 2928–2932.

Hagan JF, Shaw JS, Duncan PM, editors: *Bright Futures: guidelines for health supervision of infants, children, and adolescents*, ed 3, Elk Grove Village, IL, 2008, American Academy of Pediatrics.

Halstead ME, Walter KD, the Council on Sports Medicine and Fitness: Clinical report—sport-related concussion in children and adolescents, *Pediatrics* 126:597–615, 2010.

Harley JR: Pediatric sports injuries in the ED. In Strange GR, Ahrens W, Schafermeyer R, et al, editors: *Pediatric emergency medicine*, ed 3, New York, 2009, McGraw-Hill.

Hisea A, Sirotnak AP: Child abuse & neglect. In Hay WW, Levin M, Deterding R, et al, editors: *Current diagnosis & treatment in pediatrics*, ed 19, New York, 2009, McGraw-Hill, pp 212–239.

Hodge D: Bites and stings. In Fleisher GR, Ludwig S, Bachur RG, et al, editors: *Textbook of pediatric emergency medicine*, ed 6, Philadelphia, 2010, Lippincott Williams & Wilkins, pp 671–689.

Hosalkar HS, Spiegel DA, Davidson RS: The foot and toes. In Kliegman RM, Behrman RE, Jenson HB, et al, editors: *Nelson textbook of pediatrics*, ed 18, Philadelphia, 2007, Saunders, pp 2776–2784.

Jacome GCC, Waxler JL, Sweeney-McMahon P: Digital injuries and infections part 1 injuries. In Baren JM, Rothrock SG, Brennan J, et al, editors: *Pediatric emergency medicine*, Philadelphia, 2008, Saunders.

Jarjosa JL: Trauma, burns, and common critical care emergencies. In Custer JW, Rau RE, editors: *The Harriet Lane handbook*, ed 18, Philadelphia, 2009, Elsevier.

Landry GL: Management of musculoskeletal injury. In Kliegman RM, Behrman RE, Jenson HB, et al, editors: *Nelson textbook of pediatrics*, ed 18, Philadelphia, 2007, Saunders, pp 2851–2861.

Latterman C, Armfield D, Wukich DK: Lower leg, ankle, & foot injuries. In McMahon PJ, editor: *Current diagnosis & treatment sports medicine*, New York, 2007, McGraw-Hill.

Linzer JF: Pediatric anaphylaxis, *eMedicine*, 2011. Available at http://emedicine.medscape.com/article/799744-overview#a1. Accessed April 22, 2011.

McMahon PJ: *Current diagnosis & treatment sports medicine*, New York, 2007, McGraw-Hill.

National Center for Health Statistics: *Health, United States, 2009: with special feature on medical technology*. Hyattsville, MD, 2010. Available at www.cdc.gov/nchs/data/hus/hus09.pdf. Accessed Dec 4, 2010.

National Highway Traffic Safety Administration (NHTSA): *Traffic safety facts, 2009 data: children*, 2009a. Available at http://www-nrd.nhtsa.dot.gov/Pubs/811387.pdf. Accessed April 22, 2011.

National Highway Traffic Safety Administration (NHTSA): *Traffic safety facts, 2009 data: occupant protection*, 2009b. Available at http://www-nrd.nhtsa.dot.gov/Pubs/811390.pdf. Accessed April 22, 2011.

National Highway Traffic Safety Administration (NHTSA): *Traffic safety facts, research note: fatal crashes involving young drivers*, 2009c. Available at http://ddot-hso.com/ddot/hso/documents/Publications/Young_Drivers/2009/NHTSA%20Traffic%20Safety%20Facts%202009.pdf. Accessed April 22, 2011.

National Highway Traffic Safety Administration (NHTSA): *NHTSA releases new child seat guidelines*, 2011. Available at http://www.nhtsa.gov/PR/NHTSA-02-11. Accessed April 22, 2011.

Polousky JD, Eilert RE: Orthopedics. In Hay WW, Levin M, Deterding R, et al, editors: *Current diagnosis & treatment in pediatrics*, ed 19, New York, 2009, McGraw-Hill, pp 778–795.

Quinlan KP, O'Connor A, Robinson M, et al: Protecting children from fires and burns, *Pediatr Ann* 39:709–713, 2010.

Reddy K, Parke Maier L: Pediatric burns. In Strange GR, Ahrens W, Schafermeyer R, et al, editors: *Pediatric emergency medicine*, ed 3, New York, 2009, McGraw-Hill.

Russell S, Lozano D, Monroe K, et al: Anaphylaxis management in the pediatric emergency department: Opportunities for improvement, *Pediatr Emerg Care* 26:71–76, 2010.

Schutzman SA: Injury-head. In Fleisher GR, Ludwig S, Silverman BK, editors: *Synopsis of pediatric emergency medicine*, ed 6, Philadelphia, 2010, Lippincott Williams & Wilkins, pp 337–344.

Schwartz HS, Holt GE: Pathologic fractures in children. In Green NE, Swiontkowski MF, editors: *Skeletal trauma in children*, ed 4, Philadelphia, 2008, Elsevier.

Selbst SM, Attia M: Minor trauma—lacerations. In. Fleisher GR, Ludwig S, Henretig FM, editors: *Textbook of pediatric emergency medicine*, ed 6, Philadelphia, 2010, Lippincott Williams & Wilkins, pp 1256–1270.

Shea K, Edmonds E, Chambers H: Skeletal trauma in young athletes. In Green NE, Swiontowski MF, editors: *Skeletal trauma in children*, ed 4, Philadelphia, 2008, Elsevier.

Sheridan RL: Burns. In Wolff K, Goldsmith L, Katz S, et al: *Fitzpatrick's dermatology in general medicine*, ed 7, New York, 2008, McGraw-Hill.

Singer AJ, Dagum AB: Current management of acute cutaneous wounds, *N Engl J Med* 359:1037–1046, 2008.

Staheli LT: *Fundamentals of pediatric orthopedics*, ed 4, Philadelphia, 2008, Lippincott Williams & Wilkins.

Stiell IG, Wells G, Laupacis A, et al: Multicentre trial to introduce the Ottawa Rules for use of radiography in acute ankle injuries, *BMJ* 311:594–597, 1995.

Sullivan DM: Soft tissue injury and wound repair. In Strange GR, Ahrens W, Schafermeyer R, et al, editors: *Pediatric emergency medicine*, ed 3, New York, 2009, McGraw-Hill.

Taketomo CK, Hodding JH, Kraus DM: *Pediatric dosage handbook*, ed 17, Hudson, OH, 2011, Lexi-Comp.

Toy BJ: Conditions involving the foot, ankle, and leg. In Toy BJ, Healy PF, editors: *Primary care for sports and fitness: a lifespan approach*, Philadelphia, 2009, FA Davis, pp 179–226.

Tsarouhas N, Agosto P: Burns. In Baren JM, Rothrock S, Brennan J, et al, editors: *Pediatric emergency medicine*, Philadelphia, 2008, Saunders.

Vaillancourt C, Shrier I: Compartment syndrome. In Baren JM, Rothrock S, Brennan J, et al: *Pediatric emergency medicine*, Philadelphia, 2008, Saunders.

Vijayasankar D, Boyle AA, Atkinson P: Can the Ottawa knee rule be applied to children? A systematic review and meta-analysis of observational studies, *Emerg Med J* 26:250–253, 2009.

Zivna I, Ellison RT: Tick-borne illness. In Irwin RS, Rippe JM, editors: *Manual of intensive care medicine*, ed 5, Philadelphia, 2009, Lippincott Williams & Wilkins, pp 466–467.

CHAPTER 40

American Academy of Pediatrics (AAP), Committee on Bioethics: Ethical issues with genetic testing in pediatrics (RE9924), *Pediatrics* 107:1451–1455, 2001.

American Academy of Pediatrics (AAP), Committee on Genetics: Health supervision for children with fragile X syndrome, *Pediatrics* 98:297–300, 1996a.

American Academy of Pediatrics (AAP), Committee on Genetics: Health supervision of children with Marfan syndrome, *Pediatrics* 98:978–982, 1996b.

American Academy of Pediatrics (AAP), Committee on Genetics: Health supervision for children with Down syndrome, *Pediatrics* 107:442–449, 2001a, reaffirmed Sept 1, 2007.

American Academy of Pediatrics (AAP), Committee on Genetics: Health care supervision for children with Williams syndrome, *Pediatrics* 107:1192–1204, 2001b.

American Academy of Pediatrics (AAP), Committee on Genetics: Health supervision for children with sickle cell disease, *Pediatrics* 109:526–535, 2002.

American College of Obstetricians and Gynecologists Committee on Practice Bulletins: Practice Bulletin No. 77: screening for fetal chromosomal abnormalities, *Obstet Gynecol* 109(1):217–228, 2007.

Bagot RC, Meaney MJ: Epigenetics and the biological basis of gene x environment interactions, *Am Acad Child Adolesc Psychiatry* 49(8):752–771, 2010.

Boada R, Janusz J, Hutaff-Lee C, et al: The cognitive phenotype in Klinefelter syndrome: a review of the literature including genetic and hormonal factors, *Dev Disabil Res Rev* 15:284–294, 2009.

Bojesen A, Gravholt CH: Klinefelter syndrome in clinical practice, *Nat Clin Pract Urol* 4(4):192–204, 2007.

Bojesen A, Kristensen K, Birkebaek NH, et al: The metabolic syndrome is frequent in Klinefelter syndrome and is associated with abdominal obesity and hypogonadism, *Diabetes Care* 29(7):1591–1598, 2006a.

Bojesen A, Juul S, Birkebaek NH, et al: Morbidity in Klinefelter syndrome: a Danish register study based on hospital discharge diagnoses, *J Clin Endocrinol Metab* 91(4):1254–1260, 2006b.

Bondy C: Turner syndrome 2008, *Horm Res* 7(Suppl):52–56, 2009.

Borry P, Goffin T, Nys H, et al: Predictive genetic testing in minors for adult-onset genetic diseases, *Mt Sinai J Med* 75(3):287–296, 2008.

Carrel AL, Myers SE, Whitman BY, et al: Long term growth hormone therapy changes the natural history of body composition and motor function in children with Prader-Willi syndrome, *J Clin Endocrinol Metab* 95:1131–1136, 2010.

Carroll KN, Arbogast PG, Dudley JA, et al: Increase in incidence of medically treated thyroid disease in children with Down syndrome after rerelease of American Academy of Pediatrics health supervision guidelines, *Pediatrics* 122(2):e493–e498, 2008.

Centers for Disease Control and Prevention (CDC) key findings: updated national birth defects prevalence estimates for selected birth defects in the United States, 2004-2006, 2006. Available at www.cdc.gov/ncbddd/features/birthdefecs-keyfindings.html. Accessed Dec 27, 2010.

Cheng T, Cohn RD, Dover GJ: The genetics revolution and primary care pediatrics, *JAMA* 299(4):451–453, 2008.

Cohen W: Down syndrome: care of the child and family. In Carey W, Crocker AC, Coleman WL, et al, editors: *Developmental-behavioral pediatrics*, ed 4, Philadelphia, 2009, Saunders, pp 235–245.

Creavin AL, Brown RD: Ophthalmic abnormalities in children with Down syndrome, *J Pediatr Ophthalmol Strabismus* 46(2):76–82, 2009.

Defendi GL: Fetal alcohol spectrum disorder: how to recognize the various manifestations, *Consult Pediatricians* 343–351, 2010.

Denson LA: Growth hormone therapy in children and adolescents: pharmacokinetic/pharmacodynamic considerations and emerging indications, *Expert Opin Drug Metab Toxicol* 4(12):1569–1580, 2008.

Descartes M, Carroll D: Cytogenetics. In Kliegman RM, Behrman RE, Jenson HB, et al, editors: *Nelson textbook of pediatrics*, ed 18, Philadelphia, 2007, Saunders, pp 502–517.

Dolan SM, Moore C: Linking family history in obstetric and pediatric care: assessing risk for genetic disease and birth defects, *Pediatrics* 120(Suppl 2):s66–s70, 2007.

Epigenome Network of Excellence: *What is epigenetics?* 2009. Available at www.epigenesys.eu.aboutus/epigenetics.php. Accessed Jan 14, 2010.

Feinberg A: Review article: phenotypic plasticity and the epigenetics of human disease, *Nature* 447:433–440, 2007.

Ferguson MA, Mulvihill JJ, Schaefer GB, et al: Low adherence to national guidelines for thyroid screening in Down syndrome, *Genet Med* 11f(7):548–551, 2009.

Frias JL, Davenport ML: Committee on Genetics and Section on Endocrinology: Health supervision for children with Turner syndrome, *Pediatrics* 111(3):692–702, 2003.

Gallo AM, Angst DB, Knafl KA: Disclosure of genetic information within families, *Am J Nurs* 109(4):65–69, 2009.

Giedd JN, Clasen LS, Wallace GL, et al: XXY (Klinefelter syndrome): a pediatric quantitative brain magnetic resonance imaging case-control study, *Pediatrics* 119(1):232–240, 2007.

Grafodatskaya D, Chung B, Szatmari P, et al: Autism spectrum disorders and epigenetics, *J Am Acad Child Adolesc Psychiatry* 49(8):797–809, 2010.

Guerrero-Bosagna CM, Skinner MK: Epigenetic transgenerational effects of endocrine disruptors on male reproduction, *Semin Reprod Med* 27(5):403–408, 2009.

Hawli Y, Nasrallah M, El-Hajj Fuleihan G: Endocrine and musculoskeletal abnormalities in patients with Down syndrome, *Nat Rev Endocrinol* 5(6):327–334, 2009.

Hersh J: AAP Committee on Genetics: Health supervision guidelines for children with neurofibromatosis, *Pediatrics* 121(3):633–642, 2008.

Ishikawa T, Yamaguchi K, Kondo Y, et al: Metabolic syndrome in men with Klinefelter syndrome, *Urology* 7(6):1109–1113, 2008.

Issa J: *The ghost in your genes: epigenetic therapy, PBS—NOVA*. Available at www.pbs.org/wgbh/nova/body/epigenetic-therapy.html. Accessed Jan 14, 2010.

Itti E, Gonzalo IT, Pawlikowska-Haddal A, et al: The structural brain correlates of cognitive deficits in adults with Klinefelter syndrome, *J Clin Endocrinol Metab* 9(4):1423–1427, 2006.

Jablonka E, Raz G: Transgenerational epigenetic inheritance: prevalence, mechanisms, and implications for the study of heredity and evolution, *Q Rev Biol* 84(2):131–176, 2009.

Jones KL: *Smith's recognizable patterns of human malformation*, ed 6, Philadelphia, 2006, Saunders.

Jorde LB, Carey JC, Bamshad MJ, et al: *Medical genetics*, ed 3, St Louis, 2006, Mosby.

Kaye CI and the Committee on Genetics: Introduction to the newborn screening fact sheets, *Pediatrics* 118(3):1304–1312, 2006.

Korenberg JR: Down syndrome: the crucible for treating genomic imbalance, *Genet Med* 11(9):617–619, 2009.

Kupferman JC, Druschel CM, Kupchik GS: Increased prevalence of renal and urinary tract anomalies in children with Down syndrome, *Pediatrics* 124(4):e615–e621, 2009.

Loscalzo ML: Turner syndrome, *Pediatr Rev* 29(7):219–226, 2008.

Lose EJ: The emerging role of primary care in genetics, *Curr Opin Pediatr* 20:634–636, 2008.

McBride CM, Guttmacher AE: Commentary: trailblazing a research agenda at the interface of pediatrics and genomic discovery—a commentary on the psychological aspects of genomics and child health, *J Pediatr Psychol* 34(6):662–664, 2009.

McKusick-Nathans Institute of Genetic Medicine, Johns Hopkins University and National Center for Biotechnology Information, National Library of Medicine: *Online Mendelian Inheritance in Man (OMIM) (TM)*. Available at www.ncbi.nlm.nih.gov/omim/. Accessed Dec 7, 2010.

Morgan T: Turner syndrome: diagnosis and management, *Am Fam Physician* 76:405–410, 2007.

Morris JK, Alberman E: Trends in Down syndrome live births and antenatal diagnoses in England and Wales from 1989 to 2008: analysis of data from the National Down Syndrome Cytogenetic Register, *BMJ* 339:b3794, 2009.

Morris M, Jackson S, Hancock J: *The psychological and social impact of Klinefelter syndrome: report for the Klinefelter Syndrome Association*, Bristol, England, September, 2009, University of the West of England.

National Newborn Screening & Genetics Resource Center, 2006. Available at http://genes-r-us.uthscsa.edu. Accessed Dec 27, 2010.

Nelson K, Holmes LB: Malformations due to presumed spontaneous mutations in newborn infants, *N Engl J Med* 320(1):19–23, 1989.

Paduch DA, Bolyakov A, Cohen P, et al: Reproduction in men with Klinefelter syndrome: the past, the present, and the future, *Semin Reprod Med* 27(2):137–148, 2009.

Patterson D: Molecular genetic analysis of Down syndrome, *Hum Genet* 126(1):195–214, 2009.

Patwardhan AJ, Eliez S, Bender B, et al: Brain morphology in Klinefelter syndrome: extra X chromosome and testosterone supplementation, *Neurology* 54(12):2218–2223, 2000.

Proud VK, Elias ER: Genetic syndromes and dysmorphology. In Carey W, Crocker AC, Coleman WL, et al, editors: *Developmental-behavioral pediatrics*, ed 4, Philadelphia, 2009, Saunders, pp 246–257.

Robin N: Patterns of genetic transmission. In Kliegman RM, Behrman RE, Jenson HB, et al, editors: *Nelson textbook of pediatrics*, ed 18, Philadelphia, 2007, Saunders, pp 492–502.

Ross LF: Ethical and policy issues in pediatric genetics, *Am J Med Genet* 148C(1):1–7, 2008.

Simm PJ, Zacharin MR: The psychosocial impact of Klinefelter syndrome—a 10 year review, *J Pediatr Endocrinol* 19(4):499–505, 2006.

Skotko BG, Capone G, Priya SK: Postnatal diagnosis of Down syndrome: synthesis of the evidence about how best to deliver the news, *Pediatrics* 124(4):e751–e758, 2009.

Trott AA, Matalon R: When should children be tested for genetic diseases? *Pediatrics* 124(4):3807–3808, 2009.

Trotter TL, Hall JG, AAP Committee on Genetics: Health supervision for children with achondroplasia, *Pediatrics* 116(3):771–783, 2005.

Tsai AC, Pickler L, Tartaglia N, et al: Chromosomal disorders and fragile x syndrome. In Carey W, Crocker AC, Coleman WL, et al, editors: *Developmental-behavioral pediatrics*, ed 4, Philadelphia, 2009, Saunders, pp 224–234.

U.S. Department of Health and Human Services: *Surgeon General's Family History Initiative*, 2005. Available at www.hhs.gov/familyhistory. Accessed Dec 27, 2010.

U.S. Department of Health and Human Services (USD-HHS), Office for Civil Rights—HIPAA: *Medical privacy: national standards to protect the privacy of personal health information*. Available at www.hhs.gov/ocr/privacy/hipaa/administrative/index.html. Accessed Dec 27, 2010.

Weinhold B: Epigenetics: the science of change, *Environ Health Perspect* 114(3):A160–A167, 2006.

Wikstrom AM, Painter JN, Raivio T, et al: Genetic features of the X chromosome affect pubertal development and testicular degeneration in adolescent boys with Klinefelter syndrome, *Clin Endocrinol* 65(1):92–97, 2006.

Wilson L: *Preventive care for adults with Down syndrome*. Available at www.cme.medscape.com/viewarticle/715382. Accessed Feb 2, 2010.

Xavier AC, Ge Y, Taub JW: Down syndrome and malignancies: a unique clinical relationship: a paper from the 2008 William Beaumont hospital symposium on molecular pathology, *J Mol Diagn* 11(5):371–380, 2009.

CHAPTER 41

Agency for Toxic Substances and Disease Registry (ATSDR): *Case studies in environmental medicine: lead toxicity*, 2010. Available at www.atsdr.cdc.gov/csem/lead/docs/lead.pdf. Accessed Apr 2, 2011.

Akinbami LJ, Lynch CD, Parker JD: The association between childhood asthma and prevalence of monitored air pollutants in metropolitan areas, 2001-2004, *Environ Res* 110(3):294–301, 2010.

Alessandrini F, Schulz H, Takenaka S, et al: Effects of ultrafine carbon particle inhalation on allergic inflammation of the lung, *J Allergy Clin Immunol* 117(4):824–830, 2006.

American Academy of Pediatrics (AAP) Committee on Environmental Health: Lead exposure in children: prevention, detection, and management, *Pediatrics* 116(4):1036–1046, 2005.

American Academy of Pediatrics (AAP) Committee on Environmental Health: Policy statement: ambient air pollution: health hazards to children, *Pediatrics* 114(6):1699–1707, 2004.

American Academy of Pediatrics (AAP) Committee on Injury, Violence, and Poison Prevention: Policy statement: poison treatment in the home, *Pediatrics* 112:1182–1185, 2003.

Aschner M, Ceccatelli S: Are neuropathological conditions relevant to ethylmercury exposure? *Neurotox Res* 18(1):59–68, 2010.

Atkins D: Leung D: Principles of treatment of allergic disease. In Kliegman RM, Behrman RE, Jenson HB, et al, editors: *Nelson textbook of pediatrics*, ed 18, Philadelphia, 2007, Saunders, pp 942–948.

Beitz J, de Castro AB: Integrating environmental health into nurse practitioner training-childhood pesticide exposure risk assessment, prevention, and management, *AAOHN J* 58(8):349–355, 2010.

Benuck I: Tobacco, heart disease, and practical counseling, *Pediatr Ann* 35(11):802–807, 2006.

Berglund B, Lindvall T, Schwela DH: *Guidelines for community noise*, Geneva, 1999, WHO.

Bhattacharyya N, Shapiro N: Air quality improvement and the prevalence of frequent ear infections in children, *Otolaryngol Head Neck Surg* 142(2):242–246, 2010.

Bird S: Organophosphate and carbamate poisoning. *UpToDate*, 2009. Available at www.uptodate.com/patients/content/topic.do?topicKey=~p8NLmnyw.MEP&;selectedTitle=1~55&source=search_result. Accessed Nov 1, 2010.

Bouchard M, Bellinger D, Wright R, et al: Attention deficit/hyperactivity disorder and urinary metabolites of organophosphate pesticides, *Pediatrics* 125:e1270–e1277, 2010.

Brent RL: Environmental causes of human congenital malformations: the pediatrician's role in dealing with these complex clinical problems caused by a multiplicity of environmental and genetic factors, *Pediatrics* 113(4):957–968, 2004.

Briggs D: *Making a difference: indicators to improve children's environmental health*, Geneva, 2003, WHO.

Bronstein AC, Spyker D, Cantilena LR, et al: 2008 Annual report of the American Association of Poison Control Centers' National Poison Data System (NPDS): 26th Annual Report, *Clin Toxicol* 47:911–1084, 2009.

Bruchova H, Vasikova A, Merkorova M: Effect of maternal tobacco smoke on the placental transcriptome, *Placenta* 31(3):186–191, 2010.

Brunnberg E, Lindén-Boström M, Berglund M: Tinnitus and hearing loss in 15- to 16-year-old students: mental health symptoms, substance use, and exposure in school, *Int J Audiol* 47(11):688–694, 2008.

Canfield RL, Henderson CR Jr, Cory-Slechta DA, et al: Intellectual impairment in children with blood lead concentrations below 10 microg per deciliter, *N Engl J Med* 348(16):1517–1526, 2003.

Centers for Disease Control and Prevention (CDC): *Screening young children for lead poisoning: guidance for state and local public health officials*, 1997, updated 2009. Available at www.cdc.gov/nceh/lead/publications/screening.htm. Accessed Oct 29, 2010.

Chepesiuk R: Decibel hell: the effects of living in a noisy world, *Environ Health Perspect* 113(1):A34–A41, 2005.

Chervenak FA, McCullough LB, Brent RL: The perils of the imperfect expectation of the perfect baby, *Am J Obstet Gynecol* 203(2):101.e1–e5, 2010.

Clardy P, Manaker S, Perry H: Carbon monoxide poisoning, *UpToDate*, 2009. Available at www.uptodate.com/patients/content/topic.do?topicKey=~RqWRDMJl2tNq&;selectedTitle=1~36&source=search_result. Accessed Nov 1, 2010.

Clark C, Martin R, van Kempen E, et al: Exposure-effect relations between aircraft and road traffic noise exposure at school and reading comprehension: the RANCH project, *Am J Epidemiol* 163(1):27–37, 2006.

Cohen Hubal EA, Richard A, Aylward L, et al: Advancing exposure characterization for chemical evaluation and risk assessment, *J Toxicol Environ Health B Crit Rev* 13(2-4):299–313, 2010.

Colborn T, Dumanoski D, Myers JP: *Our stolen future: are we threatening our fertility, intelligence, and survival? A scientific detective story*, New York, 1996, Penguin Group.

Counter SA, Buchanan LH: Mercury exposure in children: a review, *Toxicol Appl Pharmacol* 198(2):209–230, 2004.

Crain DA, Janssen SJ, Edwards TM, et al: Female reproductive disorders: the roles of endocrine-disrupting compounds and developmental timing, *Fertil Steril* 90(4):911–940, 2008.

de Vendômois JS, Roullier F, Cellier D, et al: A comparison of the effects of three GM corn varieties on mammalian health, *Int J Biol Sci* 5(7):706–726, 2009.

Duderstadt KG: Chemical policy and the impact on child health, *J Pediatr Health Care* 23(6):421–424, 2009.

Eaton DK, Kann L, Kinchen S, et al: Youth risk behavior surveillance—United States, 2009, *MMWR Surveill Summ* 59(SS-5):1–142, 2010.

Edwards SC, Jedrychowski W, Butscher M, et al: Prenatal exposure to airborne polycyclic aromatic hydrocarbons and children's intelligence at 5 years of age in a prospective cohort study in Poland, *Environ Health Perspect* 118(9):1326–1331, 2010.

Engle S, Miodovnik A, Canfield R, et al: Prenatal phthalate exposures associated with childhood behavior and executive functioning, *Environ Health Perspect* 118(4):565–571, 2010.

Environmental Protection Agency (EPA): *About pesticides: 2000-2001 pesticide market estimates*, 2006. Available at www.epa.gov/pesticides/pestsales/01pestsales/introduction2001.htm. Accessed Nov 12, 2010.

Environmental Protection Agency (EPA): *What you need to know about mercury in fish and shellfish, 2004 EPA and FDA advice*, 2004. Available at http://water.epa.gov/scitech/swguidance/fishshellfish/outreach/advice_index.cfm. Accessed Nov 1, 2010.

Environmental Protection Agency (EPA) Office of Children's Health Protection: *1997 declaration of the environment leaders of the eight on children's environmental health*, 1997. Available at http://yosemite.epa.gov/ochp/ochpweb.nsf/content/declara.htm. Accessed Nov 1, 2010.

Etzel RA, Balk SJ: *Handbook of pediatric environmental health*, ed 2, Elk Grove Village, IL, 2003, American Academy of Pediatrics.

Etzel RA, Balk SJ, Bearer CF, et al: Noise: a hazard for the fetus and newborn, *Pediatrics* 100(4):724–727, 1997.

Fiore MC, Jaôn CR, Baker TB, et al: *Treating tobacco use and dependence: 2008 update, clinical practice guideline*, Rockville, MD, 2008, USDHHS, Public Health Service.

Franklin R, Rodgers G: Unintentional child poisoning treated in United States hospital emergency departments: national estimates of incident cases, population-based poisoning rates, and product involvement, *Pediatrics* 122:1244–1251, 2008.

Froehlich TE, Lanphear BP, Auinger P, et al: Association of tobacco and lead exposures with attention-deficit/hyperactivity disorder, *Pediatrics* 124(6):e1054–e1063, 2009.

Gilbert SG, Weiss B: A rationale for lowering the blood action level from 10 to 2 microg/dL, *Neurotoxicology* 27(5):693–701, 2006.

Gilmour M, Jaakkola M, London S, et al: How exposure to environmental tobacco smoke, outdoor air pollutants, and increased pollen burdens influences the incidence of asthma, *Environ Health Perspect* 114:627–633, 2006.

Goksor E, Amark M, Alm B, et al: The impact of pre- and post-natal smoke exposure on future asthma and bronchial hyperresponsiveness, *Acta Pediatr* 96(7):1030–1035, 2007.

Goldman RH: Occupational and environmental risks to reproduction in females, *UpToDate*, 2010. Available at www.uptodate.com/patients/content/topic.do?topicKey=~/hI_eWM9axg9MxX&;selectedTitle=3~150&source=search_result. Accessed Nov 1, 2010.

Grandjean P, Landrigan PJ: Developmental neurotoxicity of industrial chemicals, *Lancet* 368(9553):2167–2178, 2006.

Grigg J: Particulate matter exposure in children: relevance to chronic pulmonary obstructive disease, *Proc Am Thorac Soc* 6(7):564–569, 2009.

Groner J, Hoshaw-Woodard S, Koren G, et al: Screening for children's exposure to environmental tobacco smoke in a pediatric primary care setting, *Arch Pediatr Adolesc Med* 159(5):450–455, 2005.

Guillette EA: A broad-based evaluation of pesticide-exposed children, *Cent Eur J Public Health* 8(Suppl):58–59, 2000.

Hall AG: Nurses: taking precautionary action on a pediatric environmental exposure: DEHP, *Pediatr Nurs* 32(1):91–94, 2006.

Han YY, Lee YL, Guo YL: Indoor environmental risk factors and seasonal variation of childhood asthma, *Pediatr Allergy Immunol* 20(8):748–756, 2009.

Hauser R, Meeker JD, Duty S, et al: Altered semen quality in relation to urinary concentrations of phthalate monoester and oxidative metabolites, *Epidemiology* 17(6):682–691, 2006.

Herrick R, McClean MD, Meeker JD, et al: An unrecognized source of PCB contamination in schools and other buildings, *Environ Health Perspect* 12(10):1051–1053, 2004.

Herrmann M, King K, Weitzman M: Prenatal tobacco smoke and postnatal secondhand smoke exposure and child neurodevelopment, *Curr Opin Pediatr* 20(2):184–190, 2008.

Hightower JM, O'Hare A, Hernandez GT: Blood mercury reporting in NHANES: identifying Asian, Pacific Islander, Native American and multiracial groups, *Environ Health Perspect* 114(2):173–175, 2006.

Hill WG, Butterfield P, Larsson LS: Rural parents' perceptions of risks associated with their children's exposure to radon, *Public Health Nurs* 23(5):392–399, 2006.

Hornung RW, Lanphear BP, Dietrich KN: Age of greatest susceptibility to childhood lead exposure: a new statistical approach, *Environ Health Perspect* 117(8):1309–1312, 2009.

Iossifova YY, Reponen T, Ryan PH, et al: Mold exposure during infancy as a predictor of potential asthma development, *Ann Allergy Asthma Immunol* 102(2):131–137, 2009.

Jacobs DE, Clickner RP, Zhou JY, et al: The prevalence of lead-based paint hazards in US housing, *Environ Health Perspect* 110(10):A599–A606, 2002.

Jamil H, Campbell-Voytal K, Arnetz JE: Perceptions of training in occupational and environmental medicine among family medicine residents, *J Occup Environ Med* 52(2):202–206, 2010.

Jan J, Sovcikova E, Kocan A, et al: Developmental dental defects in children exposed to PCBs in eastern Slovakia, *Chemosphere* 67(9):S350–S354, 2007.

Jedrychowski W, Galas A, Pac A, et al: Prenatal ambient air exposure to polycyclic aromatic hydrocarbons and the occurrence of respiratory symptoms over the first year of life, *Eur J Epidemiol* 20(9):775–782, 2005.

Jedrychowski W, Perera F, Jankowski J, et al: Gender specific differences in neurodevelopmental effects of prenatal exposure to very low-lead levels: the prospective cohort study in three-year olds, *Early Hum Dev* 85(8):503–510, 2009.

Judson R, Richard A, Dix DJ, et al: The toxicity data landscape for environmental chemicals, *Environ Health Perspect* 117(5):685–695, 2009.

Jusko TA, Henderson CR, Lanphear BP, et al: Blood lead concentrations < 10 microg/dL and child intelligence at 6 years of age, *Environ Health Perspect* 116(2):243–248, 2008.

Karvonen AM, Hyvarinen A, Roponen M, et al: Confirmed moisture damage at home, respiratory symptoms and atopy in early life: a birth-cohort study, *Pediatrics* 124(2):e329–e338, 2009.

Kavlock R, Dix D: Computational toxicology as implemented by the U.S. EPA: providing high throughput decision support tools for screening and assessing chemical exposure, hazard and risk, *J Toxicol Environ Health B Crit Rev* 13(2-4):197–217, 2010.

Kemper AR, Cohn LM, Fant KE, et al: Follow-up testing among children with elevated screening blood lead tests, *JAMA* 293(18):2232–2237, 2005.

Kosnett MJ: Chelation for heavy metals (arsenic, lead, and mercury): protective or perilous? *Clin Pharmacol Ther* 88(3):412–415, 2010.

Kum-Nji P, Meloy L, Herrod H: Environmental tobacco smoke exposure prevalence and mechanisms of causation of infections in children, *Pediatrics* 117(5):1745–1754, 2006.

Laks DR: Assessment of chronic mercury exposure within the U.S. population, National Health and Nutrition Examination Survey, 1999-2006, *Biometals*, 22(6):1103–1104, 2009.

Landrigan PJ, Schechter CB, Lipton JM, et al: Environmental pollutants and disease in American children: estimates of morbidity, mortality, and costs of lead poisoning, asthma, cancer, and developmental disabilities, *Environ Health Perspect* 110(7):721–728, 2002.

Landrigan PJ, Forman JA: Chemical pollutants. In Kliegman RM, Behrman RE, Jenson HB, et al, editors: *Nelson textbook of pediatrics*, ed 18, Philadelphia, 2007, Saunders, pp 2906–2908.

Lang IA, Galloway TS, Scarlett A: Association of urinary bisphenol A concentration with medical disorders and laboratory abnormalities in adults, *JAMA* 300(1):1303–1310, 2008.

Lanphear B, Hornung R, Khoury J, et al: Low-level environmental lead exposure and children's intellectual function: an international pooled analysis, *Environ Health Perspect* 113(7):894–899, 2005.

Latini G, Vecchio A, Massaro M, et al: In utero exposure to phthalates and fetal development, *Curr Med Chem* 13(21):2527–2534, 2006.

Lee R, Middleton D, Caldwell K, et al: A review of events that expose children to elemental mercury in the United States, *Environ Health Perspect* 117(6):871–878, 2009.

le Moal J, Reis J: Do we need a specialization in environmental medicine? *J Neurol Sci* 302(1-2):106–107, 2011.

Lu C, Toepel K, Irish R, et al: Organic diets significantly lower children's dietary exposure to organophosphorus pesticides, *Environ Health Perspect* 114(2):260–263, 2006.

Mahajan PV: Heavy metal intoxication. In Kliegman RM, Behrman RE, Jenson HB, et al, editors: *Nelson textbook of pediatrics*, ed 18, Philadelphia, 2007, Saunders, pp 2909–2913.

Mahler BJ, Metre PC, Musgrove JT, et al: Coal-tar-based parking lot sealcoat: an unrecognized source of PAH to settled house dust, *Environ Sci Technol* 44(3):894–900, 2010.

Mar TF, Koenig JQ: Relationship between visits to emergency departments for asthma and ozone exposure in greater Seattle, Washington, *Ann Allergy Asthma Immunol* 103(6):474–479, 2009.

Markowitz M: Lead poisoning. In Kliegman RM, Behrman RE, Jenson HB, et al, editors: *Nelson textbook of pediatrics*, ed 18, Philadelphia, 2007, Saunders, pp 2913–2918.

Marsee K, Woodruff TJ, Axelrad DA, et al: Estimated daily phthalate exposures in a population of mothers of male infants exhibiting reduced anogenital distance, *Environ Health Perspect* 114(6):805–809, 2006.

Mattison DR: Environmental exposures and development, *Curr Opin Pediatr* 22(2):208–218, 2010.

Mazur LJ, Kim J, Committee on Environmental Health: Technical report: spectrum of noninfectious health effects from molds, *Pediatrics* 118(6):e1909–e1926, 2006.

Mazurek B, Olze H, Haupt H, et al: The more the worse: the grade of noise-induced hearing loss associates with the severity of tinnitus, *Int J Environ Res Public Health* 7(8):3071–3079, 2010.

McConnell R, Islam T, Shankardass K, et al: Childhood incident asthma and traffic-related air pollution at home and school, *Environ Health Perspect* 118(7):1021–1026, 2010.

Ng DK, Chan CH, Soo MT, et al: Low-level chronic mercury exposure in children and adolescents: meta-analysis, *Pediatr Int* 49(1):80–87, 2007.

Occupational Safety and Health Administration (OSHA): *Asbestos, Federal regulation 755889*, 2008, U.S. Department of Labor. Available at www.osha.gov/pls/oshaweb/owadisp.show_document?p_id=10862&;p_table=STANDARDS. Accessed Apr 3, 2011.

Opler MGA, Buka SL, Groeger J: Prenatal exposure to lead, delta-aminolevulinic acid, and schizophrenia: further evidence, *Environ Health Perspect* 116(11):1586–1590, 2008.

Perera FP, Rauh V, Whyatt RM, et al: A summary of recent findings on birth outcomes and developmental effects of prenatal ETS, PAH, and pesticide exposures, *Neurotoxicity* 26(4):573–587, 2005.

Perera FP, Li Z, Whyatt R, et al: Prenatal airborne polycyclic aromatic hydrocarbon exposure and child IQ at age 5 years, *Pediatrics* 124(2):e195–e202, 2009.

Prabhu N, Smith N, Campbell D, et al: First trimester maternal tobacco smoking habits and fetal growth, *Thorax* 65(3):235–240, 2010.

Prüss-Ustün A, Bonjour S, Corvalán C: The impact of the environment on health by country: a meta-synthesis, *Environ Health* 25(7):7, 2008.

Rahman A, Persson LÅ, Nermell B, et al: Arsenic exposure and risk of spontaneous abortion, stillbirth, and infant mortality, *Epidemiology* 21(6):797–804, 2010.

Ritz B, Wilhelm M, Hoggart K, et al: Ambient air pollution and preterm birth in the environment and pregnancy outcomes study at the University of California, Los Angeles, *Am J Epidemiol* 166(9):1045–1052, 2007.

Rodgers GC, Condurache T, Reed MD, et al: Poisonings. In Kliegman RM, Behrman RE, Jenson HB, et al, editors: *Nelson textbook of pediatrics*, ed 18, Philadelphia, 2007, Saunders, pp 329–357.

Samet JM, Sockrider M: Secondhand smoke exposure: effects in children, *UpToDate*, 2010. Available at: www.uptodate.com/contents/secondhand-smoke-exposure-effects-in-children?source=search_result&;selectedTitle=1~150. Accessed Apr 3 10, 2011.

Savitz DA, Ness R: Saving the National Children's Study, *Epidemiology* 21(5):598–601, 2010.

Schapiro M: *Exposed: the toxic chemistry of everyday products and what's at stake for American power*, White River Junction, VT, 2007, Chelsea Green Publishing Company.

Schildcrout JS, Sheppard C, Lumley T, et al: Ambient air pollution and asthma exacerbations in children: an eight-city analysis, *Am J Epidemiol* 164(6):505–517, 2006.

Shargorodsky J, Curhan SG, Curhan GC, et al: Change in prevalence of hearing loss in U.S. adolescents, *JAMA* 304(7):772–778, 2010.

Shrader-Frechette K: *Taking action, saving lives: our duties to protect environmental and public health*, New York, 2007, Oxford University Press.

Singh GK, Siahpush M, Kogan MD: Disparities in children's exposure to environmental tobacco smoke in the United States, 2007, *Pediatrics* 126(1):4–13, 2010.

Sleiman M, Gundel LA, Pankow JF, et al: Formation of carcinogens indoors by surface-mediated reactions of nicotine with nitrous acid, leading to potential thirdhand smoke hazards, *Proc Natl Acad Sci USA* 107(15):6576–6581, 2010.

Söderlund GB, Sikström S, Loftesnes JM, et al: The effects of background white noise on memory performance in inattentive school children, *Behav Brain Funct* 29(6):55, 2010.

TEDX: *The endocrine disruption exchange*, 2010. Available at www.endocrinedisruption.com. Accessed Oct 16, 2010.

Tercyak KP, Britto MT, Hanna KM, et al: Prevention of tobacco use among medically at-risk children and adolescents: clinical and research opportunities in the interest of public health, *J Pediatr Psychol* 33(2):119–132, 2008.

Trasande L, Landrigan PJ, Schechter C: Public health and economic consequences of methylmercury toxicity to the developing brain, *Environ Health Perspect* 113(5):590–596, 2005.

Trasande L, Newman N, Long L, et al: Translating knowledge about environmental health to practitioners: are we doing enough? *Mt Sinai J Med* 77(1):114–123, 2010.

U.S. Department of Health and Human Services (USDHHS): *Bisphenol A information for parents*. Available at www.dhhs.gov/safety/bpa. Accessed June 27, 2010.

U.S. Department of Health and Human Services (USDHHS): *Nurse practitioner primary care competencies in specialty areas: adult, family, gerontological, pediatric, and women's health*, Rockville, MD, 2002, USDHHS.

U.S. Department of Health and Human Services (USDHHS): *The health consequences of involuntary exposure to tobacco smoke: a report of the Surgeon General*, 2006, USDHHS, CDC, Coordinating Center for Health Promotion, National Center for Chronic Disease Prevention and Health Promotion, Office on Smoking and Health. Available at www.surgeongeneral.gov/library/secondhandsmoke. Accessed Apr 2, 2011.

U.S. Department of Health and Human Services (USDHHS), Centers for Disease Control and Prevention (CDC): *Fourth national report on human exposure to environmental chemicals*, Atlanta, GA, 2009, National Center for Environmental Health. Available at www.cdc.gov/exposurereport. Accessed Nov 1, 2010.

U.S. Food and Drug Administration (FDA): *Rapid lead screening test*, 2009a. Available at www.fda.gov/MedicalDevices/ProductsandMedicalProcedures/InVitroDiagnostics/LabTest/ucm126101.htm. Accessed Oct 29, 2010.

U.S. Food and Drug Administration (FDA): Dental devices: classification of dental amalgam, reclassification of dental mercury, designation of special controls for dental amalgam, mercury, and amalgam alloy. Final rule, *Fed Regist* 74(148):38685–38714, 2009b.

van Kempen E, van Kamp I, Lebret E, et al: Neurobehavioral effects of transportation noise in primary schoolchildren: a cross-sectional study, *Environ Health* 1(9):25, 2010.

Van Metre PC, Mahler BJ, Wilson JT: PAHs underfoot: contaminated dust from coal-tar sealcoat pavement is widespread in the United States, *Environ Sci Technol* 43(1):20–25, 2009.

Vivier PM, Hauptman M, Weitzen SH, et al: The important health impact of where a child lives: neighborhood characteristics and the burden of lead poisoning, *Matern Child Health J*, 2010 Oct 23. [Epub ahead of print].

Vogel S: *Battles over bisphenol A*, April 16, 2008. Available at www.defendingscience.org/case_studies/battles-over-bisphenol-a. Accessed Oct 16, 2010.

Wang S, Chonock S, Tang D, et al: Effect of gene-environment interaction on mental development in African American, Dominican, and Caucasian mothers and newborns, *Ann Hum Genet* 74(1):46–56, 2010.

Warniment C, Tsang K, Galazka SS: Lead poisoning in children, *Am Fam Physician* 81(6):751–757, 2010.

Weinhold B: Mystery in a bottle: will the EPA require disclosure of inert pesticide ingredients? *Environ Health Perspect* 118(4):a168–a171, 2010.

Whyatt RM, Adibi JJ, Calafat AM, et al: Prenatal di(2-ethylhexyl)phthalate exposure and length of gestation among an inner city cohort, *Pediatrics* 124(6):e1213–e1220, 2009.

Wigle DT, Arbuckle TE, Turner MC, et al: Epidemiologic evidence of relationships between reproductive and child health outcomes and environmental chemical contaminants, *J Toxicol Environ Health B Crit Rev* 11(5-6):373–517, 2008.

Wright JP, Dietrich KN, Ris MD, et al: Association of prenatal and childhood blood lead concentrations with criminal arrests in early adulthood, *PLoS Med* 5(5):e101, 2008.

World Health Organization (WHO): *The global burden of disease, 2004 update*, Geneva, 2008, WHO.

Yiin LM, Rhoads GG, Rich DQ, et al: Comparison of techniques to reduce residential lead dust on carpet and upholstery: the New Jersey assessment of cleaning techniques trial, *Environ Health Perspect* 110(12):1233–1237, 2002.

Zeft AS, Prahalad S, Lefevre S: Juvenile idiopathic arthritis and exposure to fine particulate air pollution, *Clin Exp Rheumatol* 27(5):877–884, 2009.

CHAPTER 42

Adams KE, Cohen MH, Eisenberg D, et al: Ethical considerations of complementary and alternative medical therapies in conventional medical settings, *Ann Intern Med* 137(8):660–664, 2002.

Allen K: Using biofeedback to make childhood headaches less of a pain, *Pediatr Ann* 33(4):241–245, 2004.

American Academy of Pediatrics (AAP): Policy statement: counseling families who choose complementary and alternative medicine for their child with chronic illness or disability (RE0049), *Pediatrics* 107(3):598–601, 2001, reaffirmed 2005.

American Academy of Pediatrics (AAP): *Periodic survey #49: complementary and alternative medicine (CAM) therapies in pediatric practices*, 2001. Available at www.aap.org/research/periodicsurvey/ps49b exs.htm. Accessed Sept 3, 2010.

Balch J, Balch P: *Prescription for nutritional healing*, ed 2, Garden City, NY, 1997, Avery.

Balogh Z, Ordough J, Gasz A, et al: Effectiveness of balneotherapy in chronic low back pain—a randomized single-blind controlled follow-up study, *Forsch Komplementarmed Klass Naturheilkd* 12(4):196–201, 2005.

Barak V, Halperin T, Kalickman I: The effect of Sambucol, a black elderberry-based, natural product, on the production of human cytokines: I. inflammatory cytokines, *Eur Cytokine Netw* 12(2):290–296, 2001.

Baral MI: Asthma: naturopathy. In Loo M, editor: *Integrative medicine for children*, St. Louis, 2009a, Saunders, pp 169–170.

Baral MI: Diarrhea: naturopathy. In Loo M, editor: *Integrative medicine for children*, St. Louis, 2009b, Saunders, pp 302–303.

Baral MI: Otitis externa and otitis media: naturopathy. In Loo M, editor: *Integrative medicine for children*, St. Louis, 2009c, Saunders, p 417.

Barnes PM, Bloom B, Nahin R: *CDC National health statistics report #12, complementary and alternative medicine use among adults and children: United States, 2007*, December 2008. Available at www.nccam. nih.gov/news/camstats.htm. Accessed July 17, 2010.

Baum M, Ernst E: Should we maintain an open mind about homeopathy? *Am J Med* 122(11):973–974, 2009.

Berbert AA, Kondo CR, Almendra CL, et al: Supplementation of fish oil and olive oil in patients with rheumatoid arthritis, *Nutrition* 21(2):131–136, 2005.

Birdee GS, Phillips RS, Davis RB, et al: Factors associated with pediatric use of complementary and alternative medicine, *Pediatrics* 125(2):249–256, 2010.

Boris M, Mandel F: Foods and additives are common causes of the attention deficit hyperactive disorder in children, *Ann Allergy* 72:462–468, 1994.

Boyle CA, Sayers SP, Jensen BE, et al: The effects of yoga training and a single bout of yoga on delayed onset muscle soreness in the lower extremity, *J Strength Cond Res* 18(4):723–729, 2004.

Bravewell Collaborative: *Bravewell Collaborative Report: improving health care for patients and health care delivery for providers and payors.* Presented at the Institute of Medicine's Summit on Integrative Medicine and the Health of the Public, 2010. Available at www.bravewell.org/ integrative_medicine/integrativemedicine_report. Accessed July 12, 2010.

Bronstein AC, Spyker DA, Cantilena LR, et al: 2009 Annual report of the American Association of Poison Control Centers' National Poison Data System (NPDS): 27th annual report, *Clin Toxicol* 48:979–1178, 2010. Available at www.aapcc.org/dnn/ Portals/0/correctedannualreport.pdf. Accessed on Feb 28, 2011.

Bryant M, Cassidy A, Hill C, et al: Effect of consumption of soy isoflavones on behavioral, somatic and affective symptoms in women with premenstrual syndrome, *Br J Nutr* 93(5):731–739, 2005.

Cala S: A survey of herbal use in children with attention-deficient-hyperactivity disorder or depression, *Pharmacotherapy* 23(2):222–230, 2003.

Carter CM, Urbanowicz M, Hemsley R, et al: Effects of a few food diet in attention deficit disorder, *Arch Dis Child* 69:564–568, 1993.

Cassileth BR: Evaluating complementary and alternative therapies for cancer patients, *CA Cancer J Clin* 49(6):362–375, 1999.

Castleman M: *The healing herbs: the ultimate guide to the curative power of nature's medicines*, New York, 1995, Bantam.

Chafen JJ, Newberry SJ, Riedl MA, et al: Diagnosing and managing common food allergies: a systematic review, *JAMA* 303(18):1848–1856, 2010.

Chan E: The role of complementary and alternative medicine in attention-deficit hyperactivity disorder, *J Dev Behav Pediatr* 23(1S):S37–S44, 2002.

Chan E, Gardiner P, Kemper KJ: "At least it's natural..." herbs and dietary supplements in ADHD, *Contemp Pediatr* 17(9):116–130, 2000.

Chow EPY, Choy M: Asthma: qigong. In Loo M, editor: *Integrative medicine for children*, St. Louis, 2009, Saunders.

Cohen MH, Kemper KJ: Complementary therapies in pediatrics: a legal perspective, *Pediatrics* 115(3):774–780, 2005.

Consortium of Academic Health Centers for Integrative Medicine (CAHCIM): *About us.* Available at www. ahc.umn.edu/cahcim/about/home.html. Accessed July 26, 2010.

Culbert T, Richtsmeier Cyr L: Abdominal pain: mind/body. In Loo M, editor: *Integrative medicine for children*, St. Louis, 2009a, Saunders, pp 136–137.

Culbert T, Richtsmeier Cyr L: Mind-body approaches: biofeedback, hypnosis, spirituality. In Loo M, editor: *Integrative medicine for children*, St. Louis, 2009b, Saunders, pp 5–14.

Culbert T, Richtsmeier Cyr L: Headache: mind/body. In Loo M, editor: *Integrative medicine for children*, St. Louis, 2009c, Saunders, pp 355–356.

Culbert T, Richtsmeier Cyr L: Chronic pain: mind/body. In Loo M, editor: *Integrative medicine for children*, St. Louis, 2009d, Saunders, p 240.

Culbert T, Richtsmeier Cyr L, Olness K: Attention-deficit hyperactivity disorder. In Loo M, editor: *Integrative medicine for children*, St. Louis, 2009, Saunders, p 184.

Demattia A, Moskowitz H, Kemper KJ, et al: Disparities in complementary and alternative medical therapy recommendations for children in two different socioeconomic communities, *Ambul Pediatr* 6(6):312–317, 2006.

Ditchek SH, Greenfield RH: *Healthy child, whole child: integrating the best of conventional and alternative medicine to keep your kids healthy*, New York, 2002, Quill.

Duygu A, Handan A, Gözüm S, et al: Effectiveness of massage, sucrose solution, herbal tea or hydrolysed formula in the treatment of infantile colic, *J Clin Nurs* 17(13):1754–1761, 2008.

Eisenberg DM, Kessler KC, Foster C, et al: Unconventional medicine in the United States: prevalence, costs and patterns of use, *N Engl J Med* 328:246–252, 1993.

Erlichman J, Salam A, Haber BA: Use of complementary and alternative medicine in pediatric chronic viral hepatitis, *J Pediatr Gastroenterol Nutr* 50(4):417–421, 2010.

Fenton MV, Morris DL: The integration of holistic nursing practices and complementary and alternative modalities into curricula of schools of nursing, *Altern Ther Health Med* 9(4):62–67, 2003.

Field T, Diego M, Hernandez-Reif M: Moderate pressure is essential for massage therapy effects, *Int J Neurosci* 120(5):381–385, 2010a.

Field T, Diego M, Hernandez-Reif M: Preterm infant massage therapy research: a review, *Infant Behav Dev* 33(2):115–124, 2010b.

Fitzgerald MA: Abdominal pain: aromatherapy. In Loo M, editor: *Integrative medicine for children*, St. Louis, 2009a, Saunders, p 134.

Fitzgerald MA: Attention-deficit hyperactivity disorder: aromatherapy. In Loo M, editor: *Integrative medicine for children*, St. Louis, 2009b, Saunders, p 181.

Fitzgerald MA: Colic: aromatherapy. In Loo M, editor: *Integrative medicine for children*, St. Louis, 2009c, Saunders, p 250.

Fitzgerald MA: Headache: aromatherapy. In Loo M, editor: *Integrative medicine for children*, St. Louis, 2009d, Saunders, pp 352–353.

Flannery MA, Love MM, Pearce KA, et al: Communication about complementary and alternative medicine: perspectives of primary care clinicians, *Altern Ther Health Med* 12(1):56–63, 2006.

Focht D, Spicer C, Fairchok M: The efficacy of duct tape vs cryotherapy in the treatment of *verruca vulgaris* (the common wart), *Arch Pediatr Adolesc Med* 156(10):971–977, 2002.

Fogarty A, Lewis SA, Scrivener SL, et al: Oral magnesium and vitamin C supplements in asthma: a parallel group randomized placebo-controlled trial, *Clin Exp Allergy* 33(10):1355–1359, 2003.

Freeman MP, Mischoulon D, Tedeschini E, et al: Complementary and alternative medicine for major depressive disorder: a meta-analysis of patient characteristics, placebo-response rates, and treatment outcomes relative to standard antidepressants, *J Clin Psychiatry* 71(6):667–668, 2010.

Frid AH, Nilsson M, Holst JJ, et al: Effect of whey on blood glucose and insulin responses to composite breakfast and lunch meals in type 2 diabetic subjects, *Am J Clin Nutr* 82(1):69–75, 2005.

Frishberg M: Alternative medicine gaining wider acceptance, *Common Ground Reflections* 8–24, Jan 1998.

Fugh-Berman A: *Alternative medicine: what works*, Baltimore, 1997, Williams & Wilkins.

Gardiner P: Complementary, holistic, and integrative medicine: chamomile, *Ped Rev* 28(4):e16–e18, 2007.

Gardiner P, Buettner C, Davis RB, et al: Factors and common conditions associated with adolescent dietary supplement use: an analysis of the National Health and Nutrition Examination Survey (NHANES), *BMC Complement Altern Med* 8:9, 2008.

Gardiner P, Coles P, Kemper KJ: The skinny on herbal remedies for dermatologic disorders, *Contemp Pediatr* 18(7):103–113, 2001.

Gardiner P, Dvorkin L, Kemper KJ: Supplement use growing among children and adolescents, *Pediatr Ann* 33(4):227–232, 2004.

Gardiner P, Kemper K: Herbs in pediatric and adolescent medicine, *Pediatr Rev* 21(2):44–57, 2000.

Gardiner P, Wood C, Kemper KJ: Dietary supplement use among healthcare professionals enrolled in an online curriculum on herbs and dietary supplements, *Complement Altern Med* 6:21, 2006.

Gaudet T quoted in *The Bravewell Collaborative report*, Bravewell Collaborative, 2010, p 29. Available at www.bravewell.org/integrative_medicine/integrativemedicine_report. Accessed July 12, 2010.

Gawande A: Medical report; the hot spotters: can we lower medical costs by giving the neediest patients better care? *The New Yorker* 40–51, 2011(Jan 24).

Ghuman JK, Arnold LE, Anthony BJ: Psychopharmacological and other treatments in preschool children with attention-deficit/hyperactivity disorder: current evidence and practice, *J Child Adolesc Psychopharmacol* 18(5):413–447, 2008.

Good M, Stanton-Hicks M, Grass JA, et al: Relaxation and music to reduce postsurgical pain, *J Adv Nurs* 33(2):208–215, 2001.

Gordon J: Alternative medicine and the family physician, *Am Fam Physician* 54:2205–2212, 1996.

Gottschalk E: *Breaking the vicious cycle: intestinal health through diet*, Baltimore, 1994, Kirkton Press.

Graedon J, Graedon T: *The people's pharmacy: guide to home and herbal remedies*, New York, 1999, Graedon Enterprises.

Graedon J, Graedon T: *Home remedy may ease misery of canker sores*. Available at www.peoplespharmacy.com/2003/09/22/home-remedy-may-ease-misery-of. Accessed Sept 3, 2010a.

Graedon J, Graedon T: *Vicks helps relieve persistent cough*. Available at www.peoplespharmacy.com/2005/05/09/vicks-helps-releive-persistant. Accessed Sept 3 2010b.

Graedon J, Graedon T: *Listerine works against jock itch and dandruff*. Available at www.peoplespharmacy.com/2006/01/09/listerine-works/. Accessed Sept 3, 2010c.

Graedon J, Graedon T: *Cornmeal fights fungus on rose and toes*. Available at www.peoplespharmacy.com/2005/04/18/cornmeal-fights-Fungus-on-rose/. Accessed Sept 3, 2010d.

Green L: quoted in *The Bravewell Collaborative report*, Bravewell Collaborative, 2010, p 27–28. Available at www.bravewell.org/integrative_medicine/integrativemedicine_report. Accessed July 12, 2010.

Greenfield RH: Asthma: probiotics. In Loo M, editor: *Integrative medicine for children*, St. Louis, 2009a, Saunders, p 171.

Greenfield RH: Inflammatory bowel disease: probiotics. In Loo M, editor: *Integrative medicine for children*, St. Louis, 2009b, Saunders, p 386.

Grazzi L, Andrasik F, D'Amico D, et al: Electromyographic biofeedback-assisted relaxation training in juvenile episodic tension-type headache: clinical outcome at three-year follow-up, *Cephalalgia* 21(8):798–803, 2001.

He HG, Polkki T, Pietila AM, et al: Chinese parent's use of nonpharmacological methods in children's postoperative pain relief, *Scand J Caring Sci* 20(1):2–9, 2006.

Hill N, Moor G, Cameron MM, et al: Single blind, randomized, comparative study of the Bug Buster kit and over the counter pediculocide treatments against head lice in the United Kingdom, *BMJ* 331(7513):326–333, 2005.

Hoebert M, van der Heijden KB, van Geijlswijk IM, et al: Long-term follow-up of melatonin treatment in children with ADHD and chronic sleep onset insomnia, *J Pineal Res* 47(1):1–7, 2009.

Holroyd KA, Mauskop A: Complementary and alternative treatments, *Neurology* 60(7):S58, 2003.

Hui KK, Napadow V, Liu J, et al: Monitoring acupuncture effects on human brain by FMRI, *J Vis Exp* 38, 2010. Available at www.jove.com/details.stp?id=1190. Accessed July 12, 2010.

Janiger O, Goldberg P: *A different kind of healing*, New York, 1993, Putnam's.

Johnson K: The elimination diet and diagnosing food hypersensitivities. In Rakel D, editor: *Integrative medicine*, Philadelphia, 2003, Saunders.

Kankkunen P, Vehviläinen-Julkkunen K, Pietilä AM, et al: Parents' use of nonpharmacological methods to alleviate children's postoperative pain at home, *J Adv Nurs* 41(4):367–375, 2003.

Kasper S, Gastpar M, Möller JH, et al: Better tolerability of St. John's wort extract WS 5570 compared to treatment with SSRIs: a reanalysis of data from controlled clinical trials in acute major depression, *Int Clin Psychopharmacol* 25(4):204–213, 2010.

Kemper KJ: *The holistic pediatrician*, New York, 1996, HarperCollins.

Kemper KJ: *The holistic pediatrician*, ed 2, New York, 2002a, HarperCollins.

Kemper KJ: Otitis media: when parents don't want antibiotics or tubes, *Contemp Pediatr* 4:47, 2002b.

Kemper KJ: The yin and yang of integrative clinical care, education, and research, *Explore (NY)* 3(1):37–41, 2007.

Kemper KJ, Cohen M: Ethics meet complementary and alternative medicine: new light on old principles, *Contemp Pediatr* 21:61, 2004.

Kemper KJ, Gardiner P: Herbal medicines. In Kliegman RM, Behrman RE, Jenson HB, et al, editors: *Nelson textbook of pediatrics*, ed 18, Philadelphia, 2007, Saunders.

Kemper KJ, Hamilton C: Live harp music reduces activity and increases weight gain in stable premature infants, *J Altern Complement Med* 14(10):1185–1186, 2008.

Kemper KJ, Jacobs J: Homeopathy in pediatrics—no harm likely, but how much good? *Contemp Pediatr* 20(5):97, 2003.

Kemper KJ, Jennings D: Consider the benefits of music therapy for your patients, *Contemp Pediatr* 22(2):59, 2005.

Kemper KJ, Kelly EA: Treating children with therapeutic and healing touch, *Pediatr Ann* 33(4):249–252, 2004.

Kemper KJ, Sarah R, Silver-Highfield E, et al: On pins and needles? Pediatric pain patients' experience with acupuncture, *Pediatrics* 105(4 pt 2):941–947, 2000.

Kemper KJ, Gardiner P, Gobble J, et al: Expertise about herbs and dietary supplements among diverse health professionals, *BMC Complement Altern Med* 28(6):15, 2006a.

Kemper KJ, Butler LD, Culbert T, et al: Letter: pediatric guidelines, *EXPLORE: J Sci Healing* 2(5):386–387, 2006b.

Kemper KJ, Vohra S, Walls R: The use of complementary and alternative medicine in pediatrics, *Pediatrics* 122(6):1374–1386, 2008a.

Kemper KJ, Hamilton CA, McLean TW, et al: Impact of music on pediatric oncology outpatients, *Pediatr Res* 4(1):105–109, 2008b.

Kemper KJ, Fletcher NB, Hamilton CA, et al: Impact of healing touch on pediatric oncology outpatients: pilot study, *J Soc Integr Oncol* 7(1):12–18, 2009.

Kiecolt-Glaser JK: Stress, food, and inflammation: psychoneuroimmunology and nutrition at the cutting edge, *Psychosom Med* 72(4):365–369, 2010.

Kimmatkar J, Thawani V, Hingorani L, et al: Efficacy and tolerability of *Boswellia serrata* extract in treatment of osteoarthritis of the knee—a randomized double blind placebo controlled trial, *Phytomedicine* 10(1):3–7, 2003.

King T, Murphy PA: Evidence-based approaches to managing nausea and vomiting in early pregnancy, *J Midwifery Women's Hlth* 54(6):430–444, 2009.

Klassen TP, Pham B, Lawson ML, et al: For randomized controlled trials, the quality of reports of complementary and alternative medicine was as good as reports of conventional medicine, *J Clin Epidemiol* 58(8):763–768, 2005.

Koh JL, Harrison D, Palermo TM, et al: Assessment of acute and chronic pain symptoms in children with cystic fibrosis, *Pediatr Pulmonol* 40(4):330–335, 2005.

Konefal J: The challenge of educating physicians about complementary and alternative medicine, *Acad Med* 77(9):847–850, 2002.

Kong F: Pilot clinical study on a proprietary elderberry extract: efficacy in addressing influenza symptoms, *Online J Pharmacol Pharmacokin* 5:32–43, 2009.

Krebs M: The sweet smell of healing: promote wellness with aromatherapy, *Adv Nurs Pract* 14(5):41–44, 2006.

Kreitzer MJ, Kligler B, Meeker WC: Health professions education and integrative healthcare, *J Sci Healing* 5(4):212–227, 2009.

Kreitzer MJ, Mitten D, Harris I, et al: Attitudes toward CAM among medical, nursing, and pharmacy faculty and students: a comparative analysis, *Altern Ther Health Med* 8(6):50–53, 2002.

Landmark Healthcare: *Landmark report on public perceptions of alternative care*, Sacramento, CA, 1998, Landmark Healthcare.

LaValle J, Krinsky DL, Hawkins EB, et al: *Natural therapeutics pocket guide 2000-2001*, Hudson, OH, 2000, Lexi-Comp.

Lawson ML, Pham B, Classen TP, et al: Systematic reviews involving complementary and alternative medicine interventions had higher quality of reporting than conventional medicine reviews, *J Clin Epidemiol* 58(8):777–784, 2005.

Lazar K: Parents turn to alternative cures, *The Oregonian*, Thursday, Dec 11, 2008, pp A1, A4.

Levatin JL: Alternative systems: homeopathy. In Loo M, editor: *Integrative medicine for children*, St. Louis, 2009a, Saunders, pp 58–65.

Levatin JL: Abdominal pain: homeopathy. In Loo M, editor: *Integrative medicine for children*, St. Louis, 2009b, Saunders, p 136.

Levatin JL: Acne: homeopathy. In Loo M, editor: *Integrative medicine for children*, St. Louis, 2009c, Saunders, pp 143–144.

Levatin JL: Attention-deficit hyperactivity disorder. In Loo M, editor: *Integrative medicine for children*, St. Louis, 2009d, Saunders, pp 183–184.

Levatin JL: Burns: homeopathy. In Loo M, editor: *Integrative medicine for children*, St. Louis, 2009e, Saunders, pp 218–219.

Levatin JL: Diarrhea: homeopathy. In Loo M, editor: *Integrative medicine for children*, St. Louis, 2009f, Saunders, pp 301–302.

Lin ST, Yang P, Lai CY, et al: Mental health implications of music: insight from neuroscientific and clinical studies, *Harv Rev Psychiatry* 19(1):34–46, 2011.

Lind BK, Lafferty WE, Tyree PT, et al: Comparison of health care expenditures among insured users and nonusers of complementary and alternative medicine in Washington State: a cost minimization analysis, *J Altern Complement Med* 16(4):7, 2010.

Loewy J, Hallan C, Friedman E, et al: Sleep-sedation in children undergoing EEG testing: a comparison of chloral hydrate and music therapy, *J Perianaesth Nurs* 20(5):323–332, 2005.

Loo M: Asthma: acupuncture. In Loo M, editor: *Integrative medicine for children*, St. Louis, 2009a, Saunders, pp 163–164.

Loo M: Upper respiratory tract infection. In Loo M, editor: *Integrative medicine for children*, St. Louis, 2009b, Saunders, pp 451–452.

Loo M: Vomiting: acupuncture. In Loo M, editor: *Integrative medicine for children*, St. Louis, 2009c, Saunders, pp 463–464.

Lubetzky R, Mimouni FB, Dollberg S, et al: Effect of music by Mozart on energy expenditure in growing preterm infants, *Pediatrics* 125(1):e24–e28, 2010.

Ly KA: Xylitol, sweeteners, and dental caries, *Pediatr Dent* 28(2):154–163, 2006.

Mancho P, Edwards QT: Chaste tree for premenstrual syndrome, *Adv Nurs Pract* 13(5):43–46, 2005.

Markestad T: Use of sucrose as a treatment for infant colic, *Arch Dis Child* 76:356–358, 1997.

McDonough-Means SI, Cohen MW: Attention deficit disorder. In Rakel D, editor: *Rakel's integrative medicine*, Philadelphia, 2003, Saunders.

McGuffin M, Goldberg A, editors: *American Herbal Products Association's botanical safety handbook*, New York, 1998, CRC Press.

McLellan MC: Asthma: massage therapy. In Loo M, editor: *Integrative medicine for children*, St. Louis, 2009a, Saunders, p 168.

McLellan MC: Colic: massage therapy. In Loo M, editor: *Integrative medicine for children*, St. Louis, 2009b, Saunders, p 253.

McLellan MC: Cough: massage therapy. In Loo M, editor: *Integrative medicine for children*, St. Louis, 2009c, Saunders, p 284.

McLellan MC: Chronic pain: massage therapy. In Loo M, editor: *Integrative medicine for children*, St. Louis, 2009d, Saunders, pp 239–240.

Micozzi M: *Fundamentals of complementary and alternative medicine*, New York, 1996, Churchill Livingstone.

Micozzi M: The common principles of complementary health care systems: enduring concepts with current clinical relevance, *Complement Med Physician* 2(8):1, 1997.

Miller SK: Magnet therapy for pain control, *Adv Nurs Pract* 12(5):49–52, 2004.

Miller PC, Bailey SP, Barnes ME, et al: The effects of protease supplementation on skeletal muscle function and DOMS following downhill running, *J Sports Sci* 22(4):365–372, 2004.

Moher D, Soeken K, Sampson M, et al: Assessing the quality of reports of randomized trials in pediatric complementary and alternative medicine, *BMC Pediatr* 2:3, 2002.

Mortimore J, Fischer S: Are we ready to give herbal remedies to children? Health Care Agency, County of Orange, California, *Nutrition Times* 3(1):1–3, 2001.

Mother and Child, Health and Education Trust, Rehydration Project: *Oral rehydration salts*, updated April 2010. Available at www.rehydrate.org/ors/made-at-home.htm. Accessed Sep 6, 2010.

Murphy D: *Science and research*: October 19, 2009 presentation for the American Academy of Pediatrics meeting: section on clinical pharmacology and therapeutics program. Available at www.fda.gov/ScienceResearch/SpecialTopics/Pediatric TherapeuticsResearch/ucm189451.htm. Accessed Oct 2, 2010.

Murray M, Pizzorno J: *Encyclopedia of natural medicine*, ed 2, Rocklin, CA, 1998, Prima Health.

Nabas R, Balla A: Complementary and alternative medicines for prevention and treatment of the common cold, *Can Fam Physician* 57(1):31–36, 2011.

National Center for Complementary and Alternative Medicine (NCCAM): *National Institutes for Health, National Center for Health Statistics National Health Interview Survey—2007*, 2008. Available at www.NCCAM.nih.gov/health/financial. Accessed July 8, 2010.

National Institutes of Health (NIH): Consensus conference: acupuncture, *JAMA* 280:1518–1524, 1998.

National Institute of Neurology Disorders and Stroke (NINDS): *Cerebral palsy: hope through research*. NIH publication no. 10-159, Bethesda, 2010, National Institutes of Health. Available at www.ninds.nih.gov/disorders/cerebral_palsy/detail_cerebral_palsy.htm?css=print#154513104. Accessed Aug 12, 2010.

Nsouli TM, Nsouli SM, Linde RE, et al: Role of food allergy in serous otitis media, *Ann Allergy* 73:215–219, 1994.

Ott M: Yoga as a clinical intervention: pain control and stress reduction may be just a breath away, *Adv Nurse Pract* 10(1):81–90, 2002.

Patel BD, Welch AA, Bingham SA, et al: Dietary antioxidants and asthma in adults, *Thorax* 61(5):388–393, 2006.

Pettit J: Alternative medicine: cranberry, *Clin Rev* 12(1):43–44, 2002.

Pham B, Klassen TP, Lawson ML, et al: Language of publication restrictions in systematic reviews gave different results depending on whether the intervention was conventional or complementary, *J Clin Epidemiol* 58(8):769–776, 2005.

Pizzorno J: *The clinician's handbook of natural medicine*, ed 2, Philadelphia, 2008, Churchill Livingstone.

Pratt SG, Matthews K: *SuperFoods Rx: fourteen foods that will change your life*, New York, 2004, HarperCollins.

Rakel D: *Rakel's integrative medicine*, Philadelphia, 2003, Saunders.

Rakel D: *Integrative medicine*, ed 2, Philadelphia, 2007, Saunders.

Reilly AM: Massage therapy: integration with traditional medicine, *Adv Nurs Pract* 13(5):37–42, 2005.

Rey JM, Walter G, Soh N, et al: Complementary and alternative medicine (CAM) treatments and pediatric psychopharmacology, *J Am Acad Child Adolesc Psychiatry* 47(4):364–368, 2008.

Reznik M, Ozuah PO, Franco K, et al: Use of complementary therapy by adolescents with asthma, *Arch Pediatr Adolesc Med* 156(10):1042–1044, 2002.

Richardson SF: Complementary health and healing in nursing education, *J Holistic Nurs* 21(1):20–23, 2003.

Rickson DJ: Instructional and improvisational models of music therapy with adolescents who have attention deficit disorder (ADHD): a comparison of the effects on motor impulsivity, *J Music Ther* 43(1):39–62, 2006.

Rindfleisch JA: Adverse food reactions and the elimination diet. In Rakel D, editor: *Integrative medicine*, ed 2, Philadelphia, 2007, Saunders.

Rini A, Bloom K: Down in the mouth: update on treatment of oral aphthous ulcers, *Clin Adv* 5(2):67–72, 2002.

Sanders H, Davis MF, Duncan B, et al: Use of complementary and alternative medical therapies among children with special health care needs in southeastern Arizona, *Pediatrics* 111(3):584–587, 2003.

Saper RB, Kales SN, Paquin J, et al: Heavy metal content of ayurvedic herbal medicine products, *JAMA* 292(23):2868–2873, 2004.

Savino F, Cordisco L, Tarasco V, et al: *Lactobacillus reuteri* DSM 17938 in infantile colic; a randomized, double-blind, placebo-controlled trial, *Pediatrics* 126(3):e526–e533, 2010.

Scharff C, Kemper KJ: For chronic pain, complementary and alternative medical approaches, *Contemp Pediatr* 20:117, 2003.

Schneider RK, Levenson JL: *Psychiatry essentials for primary care*, Philadelphia, 2008, American College of Physicians.

Schoch R: A conversation with Dana Ullman, *Calif Monthly* 27–30, Feb 1999.

Schulman SL, Von Zuben FC, Plachter N, et al: Biofeedback methodology: does it matter how we teach children how to relax the pelvic floor during voiding? *J Urol* 166(6):2423–2426, 2001.

Sego S: What clinicians should know about herbals, *Clin Adv* 10(1):46–51, 2006.

Sego S: What you should know about the herbs and supplements patients use: zinc, *Clin Adv* 12(10):67–69, 2009.

Shah PS, Aliwalas L, Shah V: Breastfeeding or breast milk to alleviate procedural pain in neonates: a systematic review, *Breastfeed Med* 2(2):74–82, 2007.

Shapiro S, Rapaport R: The role of complementary and alternative therapies in pediatric diabetes, *Endocrinol Metab Clin North Am* 38(4):791–810, 2009.

Shedletsky P, Gale EN, Levine MS: The effects of ice massage applied over the "Hoku" acupuncture point in reducing spontaneous pain of endodontic origin, *J Can Dent Assoc* 50(8):635–638, 1984.

Sherman KJ, Ludman EJ, Cook AJ, et al: Effectiveness of therapeutic massage for generalized anxiety disorder: a randomized controlled trial, *Depress Anxiety* 27(5):441–450, 2010.

Shorofi SA, Arbon P: Complementary and alternative medicine (CAM) among hospitalized patients: an Australian study, *Complement Ther Clin Pract* 16(2):86–91, 2010.

Silva L, Schalock M, Ayers R, et al: Qigong massage treatment for sensory and self-regulation problems in young children with autism: a randomized controlled trial, *Am J Occup Ther* 63(4):423–432, 2009.

Singh M, Das RR: Zinc for the common cold, *Cochrane Database Syst Rev* 2:CD001364, 2011 Feb.

Snyderman R, website quote introducing Snyderman radio interview— *Bravewell Collaborative*. Available at www.bravewell.org/integrative_medicine/national_summit/Snyderman_Radio. Accessed Sept 3, 2010.

Snyderman R, Weil A: *Integrative medicine: bringing medicine back to its roots*. Available at www.bravewell.org/content/pdf/14_Snyderman_Weil_Article.pdf. Accessed Sept 3, 2010.

Soeken KL: Selected CAM therapies for arthritis-related pain: the evidence from systematic reviews, *Clin J Pain* 20(1):13–18, 2004.

Sohn PM, Loveland Cook CA: Nurse practitioner knowledge of complementary alternative healthcare, *J Adv Nurs* 39(1):9–16, 2002.

Spicer A: Colic: chiropractic. In Loo M, editor: *Integrative medicine for children*, St. Louis, 2009a, Saunders, pp 250–251.

Spicer A: Headache: chiropractic. In Loo M, editor: *Integrative medicine for children*, St. Louis, 2009b, Saunders, pp 353–354.

Starobrat-Hermelin B, Kozielec T: The effects of magnesium physiological supplementation on hyperactivity in children with ADHD. Positive response to magnesium oral loading test, *Magnet Res* 10(2):149–156, 1997.

Stumpf SH, Shapiro SJ, Hardy ML: Divining integrative medicine, *Evid Based Complement Altern Med* 5:409–413, 2008.

The Oregonian: *Want to know if natural remedies work?* April 5, 2006, p F3.

Thompson EA, Bishop JL, Northstone K: The use of homeopathic products in childhood: data generated over 8.5 years from the Avon longitudinal study of parents and children (ALSPAC), *J Altern Complement Med* 16(1):69–79, 2010.

Ulbricht C, Chao W, Costa D, et al: Clinical evidence of herb-drug interactions: a systematic review by the natural standard research collaboration, *Curr Drug Metab* 9(10):1063–1120, 2008.

University of California Berkeley: *Wellness letter: acupuncture scores points* 14(8):2, 1998.

University of California, Berkeley: *Wellness letter: the newsletter of nutrition, fitness, and self-care* 26(6):1–2, 2010.

University of California, San Diego Medical Center: *Complementary and alternative therapies for cancer patients: Appendix C: Education, training, licensing and accreditation of health care practitioners.* Available at www.cancer.ucsd.edu/outreach/PublicEducation/CAMs/appendixc.asp. Accessed Aug 3, 2010.

University of Maryland Medical Center: *Goldenseal.* Available at www.umm.edu/altmed/articles/goldenseal-000252. Accessed Oct 30, 2010.

U.S. Congressional Budget Office: *Research on the comparative effectiveness of medical treatment,* 2007, Congressional Budget Office. Available at http://www.cbo.gov/ftpdocs/88xx/doc8891/12-18-comparativeeffectiveness.pdf. Accessed Dec 21, 2011.

U.S. Food and Drug Administration: *Medical product safety information.* Available at www.fda.gov/medwatch/safety.htm. Accessed July 7, 2010.

Van der Heijden KB, Smits MG, van Someren EJ, et al: Effect of melatonin on sleep, behavior, and cognition in ADHD and chronic sleep-onset insomnia, *J Am Acad Child Adolesc Psychiatry* 46(2):233–241, 2007.

Voss JA, Good M, Yates B, et al: Sedative music reduces anxiety and pain during chair rest after open-heart surgery, *Pain* 112(1-2):197–203, 2004.

Walach J, Guthlin C, Konig M: Efficacy of massage therapy in chronic pain: a pragmatic randomized trial, *J Altern Complement Med* 9(6):837–846, 2003.

Walker AF, Bundy R, Hicks SM, et al: Bromelain reduces mild acute knee pain and improves well-being in a dose-dependent fashion in an open study of otherwise healthy adults, *Phytomedicine* 9(8):681–686, 2002.

Weydert JA: Abdominal pain: nutrition. In Loo M, editor: *Integrative medicine for children,* St. Louis, 2009a, Saunders, pp 137–138.

Weydert JA: Asthma: nutrition. In Loo M, editor: *Integrative medicine for children,* St. Louis, 2009b, Saunders, pp 170–171.

Weydert JA: Attention-deficit hyperactivity disorder: nutrition. In Loo M, editor: *Integrative medicine for children,* St. Louis, 2009c, Saunders, pp 184–185.

Weydert JA: Autism: nutrition. In Loo M, editor: *Integrative medicine for children,* St. Louis, 2009d, Saunders, p 202.

Weydert JA: Inflammatory bowel disease: nutrition. In Loo M, editor: *Integrative medicine for children,* St. Louis, 2009e, Saunders, pp 385–386.

Weydert JA: Eczema: nutrition. In Loo M, editor: *Integrative medicine for children,* St. Louis, 2009f, Saunders, pp 314–315.

White AR, Ernst E: Economic analysis of complementary medicine: a systematic review, *Complement Ther Med* 8(2):111–118, 2000.

White House Commission on Complementary and Alternative Medicine Policy (WHCCAMP): *Final report,* March 2002. Available at www.whccamp.hhs.gov. Accessed Sept 4, 2010.

Williams K, Abildso C, Steinberg L: Evaluation of the effectiveness and efficacy of Iyengar yoga therapy on chronic low back pain, *Spine* 34(19):2066–2076, 2009.

Wilson KM, Klein JD, Sesselberg TS, et al: Use of complementary medicine and dietary supplements among U.S. adolescents, *J Adolesc Health* 38(4):385–394, 2006.

Woolf AD, Gardiner PM, Dvorkin-Camiel L, et al: Herbs and biological agents—Western. In Loo M, editor: *Integrative medicine for children,* St. Louis, 2009a, Saunders, p 3.

Woolf AD, Gardiner PM, Dvorkin-Camiel L, et al: Acne: herbs—Western. In Loo M, editor: *Integrative medicine for children,* St. Louis, 2009b, Saunders, p 143.

World Health Organization: *Traditional medicine, fact sheet* 134, 2008. Available at www.who.int/mediacentre/factsheets/fs134/en/. Accessed July 26, 2010.

Wyatt G, Post-White J: Future direction of complementary and alternative medicine (CAM) education and research, *Semin Oncol Nurs* 21(3):215–224, 2005.

Wysocki S: Unconventional and conventional medicine: searching for common ground, *Contemp Nurse Pract* 3–15, Winter 1997.

Zakay-Rones A, Thom E, Wollan T, et al: Randomized study of the efficacy and safety of oral elderberry extract in the treatment of influenza A and B virus infections, *J Int Med Res* 32(2):132–140, 2004.

Zeltzer LK, Tsao JC, Sterling C, et al: A phase I study on the feasibility and acceptability of an acupuncture/hypnosis intervention for chronic pediatric pain, *J Pain Symptom Manage* 24(4):437–446, 2002.

Zito JM, Derivan AT, Kratochvil CJ, et al: Off-label psychopharmacologic prescribing for children: history supports close clinical monitoring, *Child Adolesc Psychiatry Mental Health* 2(24), 2008. Available at www.capmh.com/content/2/1/24. Accessed October 12, 2010.

Zylowska L, Ackerman DL, Yang MH, et al: Mindfulness meditation training in adults and adolescents with ADHD: a feasibility study, *J Atten Disord* 11(6):737–746, 2008.

APPENDIX A

Barron JR: Advisor Forum: helping the medicine go down, *Clin Adv* 13(10):78, 2010.

Bell E: Are your patients taking their medication? *Infect Dis Child* 18(9):12–13, 2005.

Carter BL, Foppe van Mil JW: Comparative effectiveness research: evaluating pharmacist interventions and strategies to improve medication adherence, *Am J Hypertens* 23(9):949–955, 2010.

Chisholm-Burns MA, Kim Lee J, Spivey CA, et al: U.S. pharmacists' effect as team members on patient care: systematic review and meta-analyses, *Med Care* 48(10):923–933, 2010.

Claxton AJ, Cramer J, Pierce C: A systematic review of the associations between dose regimens and medication compliance, *Clin Ther* 23(8):1296–1310, 2001.

Cook PF, McCabe MM, Emiliozzi S: Telephone nurse counseling improves HIV medication adherence: an effectiveness study, *J Assn Nurs in AIDS Care* 20(4):316–325, 2009.

Daiichi Pharmaceutical Corporation: Adherence and dosing, *Sound Advice* 1(12):1–8, 2004.

Deshazo J, Harris L, Pratt W: Effective intervention or child's play? A review of video games for diabetes education, *Diabetes Technol Ther* 12(10):815–822, 2010.

Edgecombe K, Latter S, Peters S, et al: Health experiences of adolescents with uncontrolled severe asthma, *Arch Dis Child* 95(12): 985–991, 2010.

Fischer MA, Stedman MR, Lii J, et al: Primary medication non-adherence: analysis of 195,930 electronic prescriptions, *J Gen Intern Med* 25(4):284–290, 2010.

Gaur AH, Belzer M, Britto P, et al: Directly observed therapy (DOT) for nonadherent HIV-infected youth: lessons learned, challenges ahead, *AIDS Res Hum Retroviruses* 26(9):947–953, 2010.

Hamrin V, McCarthy EM, Tyson V: Pediatric psychotropic medication initiation and adherence: a literature review based on social exchange theory, *J Child Adolesc Psychiatr Nurs* 23(3):151–172, 2010.

Joelving F: *Many drugs for U.S. kids tested in poor countries,* August 23, 2010. Available at www.uk.reuters.com/article/idUKTRE67M1VO20100823. Accessed Sept 27, 2010.

Klok T, Brand PL, Bomhof-Roordink H, et al: Parental illness perceptions and medication perceptions in childhood asthma, a focus group study, *Acta Paediatr,* 2010 Sept 22. [Epub ahead of print].

Ledford CJ, Villagran MM, Kreps GL, et al: "Practicing medicine": patient perceptions of physician communication and the process of prescription, *Patient Educ Couns* 80(3):384–392, 2010.

Longhofer J, Floersch J: Desire and disappointment: adolescent psychotropic treatment and adherence, *Anthropol Med* 17(2):159–172, 2010.

McHorney CA, Gadkari AS: Individual patients hold different beliefs to prescription medications to which they persist vs nonpersist and persist vs nonfulfill, *Patient Pref Adherence* 4:187–195, 2010.

Medical News Today, the Lancet Oncology: *Anticancer drugs are often used off-label in children and adults, particularly for palliative care,* 2008. Available at www.medicalnewstoday.com/articles/126929.php. Accessed October 12, 2010.

Murphy D: *Science and research.* October 19, 2009 presentation for the American Academy of Pediatrics meeting: section on clinical pharmacology and therapeutics program, 2009. Available at www.fda.gov/ScienceResearch/SpecialTopics/PediatricTherapeuticsResearch/ucm189451.htm. Accessed October 2, 2010.

Reed-Knight B, Lewis JD, Blount RL: Association of disease, adolescent, and family factors with medication adherence in pediatric inflammatory bowel disease, *J Pediatr Psychol,* 2010, Aug 26. [Epub ahead of print].

Sinha G: EU law mandates drug testing in children, *J Natl Cancer Inst* 100(2):84–85, 2008.

University of California, Berkeley: *Wellness letter* 23(2):8, 2006.

U.S. Department of Health and Human Services (USDHHS): *Health, United States, 2009, with special feature on medical technology.* Available at www.cdc.gov/nchs/data/hus/hus09.pdf#095. Accessed Oct 14, 2010.

U.S. Food and Drug Administration (FDA): *Drugs: Drug research and children, updated 2009.* Available at www.fda.gov/Drugs/ResourcesForYou/Consumers/ucm143565.htm. Accessed Oct 13, 2010.

U.S. Food and Drug Administration (FDA): *Breakdown of FDAA completed pediatric studies,* 2010. Available at www.fda.gov/Drugs/DevelopmentApprovalProcess/DevelopmentResources/ucm190622.htm. Accessed Oct 13, 2010.

Wansink B, van Ittersum K: Spoons systematically bias dosing of liquid medicine, *Annal Int Med* 152(1):66–67, 2010.

Winterstein AG, Linden S, Lee AE, et al: Evaluation of consumer medication information dispensed in retail pharmacies, *Arch Intern Med* 170(15):1317–1324, 2010.

Yin HS, Mendelsohn AL, Wolf MS, et al: Parents' medication administration errors: role of dosing instruments and health literacy, *Arch Pediatr Adolesc Med* 164(2):181–186, 2010.

Zito JM, Derivan AT, Kratochvil CJ, et al: Off-label psychopharmacologic prescribing for children: history supports close clinical monitoring, *Child Adol Psychiatry Mental Hlth* 2:24, 2008. Available at www.capmh.com/content/2/1/24. Accessed Oct 12, 2010.

APPENDIX B

Olsen I, Groveman MS, Lawson ML: New intrauterine growth curves based on United States data, *Pediatrics* 125(2):e214–e224, 2010.

Rose SR, Vogiatzi MG, Copeland KC: A general pediatric approach to evaluating a short child, *Pediatrics in Review* 26(11):410–419, 2005.

APPENDIX C

American Academy of Pediatrics: *Normal laboratory values for children.* Available at www.pediatriccareonline.org/pco/ub/view/Pediatric-Drug-Lookup/153930/0/normal-laboratory-values-for-children. Accessed Nov 30, 2010.

Burtis C, Ashwood E: *Tietz textbook of clinical chemistry*, ed 3, Philadelphia, 1999, Saunders.

Fishbach F: *A manual of laboratory and diagnostic tests*, ed 6, Philadelphia, 2000, Lippincott.

Free HM, editor: *Modern urine chemistry*, Tarrytown, NY, 1996, Bayer.

Long SS, Nyquist A-C: Laboratory manifestations of infectious diseases. In Long SS, Pickering LK, Prober CG, editors: *Principles and practice of infectious diseases*, ed 3, Philadelphia, 2008, Churchill Livingstone/Elsevier. Chapter 288.

Pesce MA: Laboratory medicine. In Kliegman RM, Behrman RE, Jenson HB, et al, editors: *Nelson textbook of pediatrics*, ed 18, Philadelphia, 2007, Saunders, pp 2949–2954.

Index

Page numbers followed by *f* indicate figures; *t,* tables; *b,* boxes.

■ Current Procedural Terminology (CPT) Codes

PREVENTIVE SERVICES CODES

- Codes are not time based.
- Illnesses identified during preventive care are coded separately. Insignificant illnesses or abnormalities not requiring additional work are not reported.
- Immunizations are coded separately.
- Includes age-appropriate pelvic examination.

New Patient CPT Codes	Established Patient CPT Codes	ICD-9-CM Codes
99381 <1 yr 99382 1-4 yrs 99383 5-11 yrs 99384 12-17 yrs 99385 18 yrs or older	99391 <1 yr 99392 1-4 yrs 99393 5-11 yrs 99394 12-17 yrs 99395 18 yrs or older	V20.2 Routine infant or child health check V70.0 Routine general medical examination at a health care facility

HEALTH RISK ASSESSMENT CODE

CPT Code	ICD-9-CM Code
99420 Administration and interpretation of health risk assessment instrument (e.g., health hazard appraisal)	V79.8 Special screening for other specified mental disorders and developmental handicaps. Use for administration of instruments such as the AMA Guidelines for Adolescent Preventive Services (GAPS).

COUNSELING, RISK FACTOR REDUCTION, AND BEHAVIOR CHANGE INTERVENTION CODES

- Codes are used to report activities to prevent illness and/or promote health; not used for specific disease management. Family dynamics, nutrition, sexual practices, injury prevention are examples.
- Counseling must be recorded specifically.
- Codes are time based.
- Not used for group counseling.

CPT Codes	ICD-9-CM Code Examples
99401 Preventive medicine counseling or risk reduction intervention provided to an individual; approximately 15 min 99402 Approximately 30 min 99403 Approximately 45 min 99404 Approximately 60 min	V15.89 Other specific personal history presenting as hazards to health (e.g., tobacco use) V25.09 Encounter for contraceptive management; general counseling and advice V65.3 Dietary surveillance and counseling V65.40 Counseling not otherwise specified V65.41 Exercise counseling V65.42 Counseling on substance use and abuse V65.43 Counseling on injury prevention V65.49 Other specified counseling

CPT Codes	ICD-9-CM Code Examples
99406 Smoking and tobacco use cessation counseling visit; intermediate, greater than 3 minutes, up to 10 minutes 99407 Smoking and tobacco use cessation counseling visit; intensive, greater than 10 minutes 99408 Alcohol or substance (other than tobacco) abuse "structured screening" (e.g., Alcohol Use Disorder Identification Test [AUDIT], Drug Abuse Screening Test [DAST]) and brief intervention (SBI) services; 15 to 30 minutes 99409 Alcohol or substance (other than tobacco) abuse structured screening (e.g., AUDIT, DAST) and brief intervention (SBI) services; greater than 30 minutes	V65.49 (Other specified counseling) primary and V61.49 (Health problems within family; other) (secondary) when tobacco cessation counseling is administered to the parent because the child benefits from a reduction in environmental tobacco smoke exposure

CASE MANAGEMENT AND CARE OVERSIGHT CODES

Telephone Care Management

- Cannot be related to evaluation and management (E/M) service or procedure from past 7 days or code to be used in next 24 hours or soonest available appointment.

99441	Telephone E/M service provided by a physician to an established patient, parent, or guardian; 5 to 10 minutes of medical discussion
99442	11 to 20 minutes of medical discussion
99443	21 to 30 minutes of medical discussion

Online Management

99444	Online E/M service provided by a physician to an established patient, guardian, or health care provider using the Internet or similar electronic communications network

Care Plan Oversight

- Reported once per calendar month
- Use telephone service codes for each call made or received from patient or parent excluding those occurring 7 days after or 24 hours before a face-to-face visit.
- If the online medical evaluation refers to an E/M service previously performed and reported by a physician within the previous 7 days (either physician requested or unsolicited patient follow-up) or within the postoperative period of the previously completed procedure, the service is considered covered by the previous E/M service or procedure.
- For the online medical evaluation codes, a reportable service encompasses the sum of communication (e.g., related telephone calls, prescription provision, laboratory orders) pertaining to the online patient encounter.